MW00845749

Textbook of Natural Medicine

Dedication

This book is dedicated to Dr John Bastyr and all the natural healers of the past and future who bring the virtues of the "healing powers of nature" to all the people of the world. Dr Bastyr, the namesake for Bastyr University, exemplified the ideal physician/healer/teacher we endeavour to become in our professional lives.

We pass on a few of his words to all who strive to provide the best of health care and healing: "Always touch your patients – let them know you care", and "Always read at least one research article or learn a new remedy before you retire at night".

For Churchill Livingstone

Commissioning Editor: Inta Ozols
Head of Project Management: Ewan Halley
Project Development Manager: Dinah Thom
Design Direction: Judith Wright

Textbook of Natural Medicine

VOLUME 1

Edited by

Joseph E. Pizzorno Jr ND

President and Faculty, Bastyr University, Kenmore, Washington, USA

Michael T. Murray ND

Faculty, Bastyr University, Kenmore, Washington, USA

SECOND EDITION

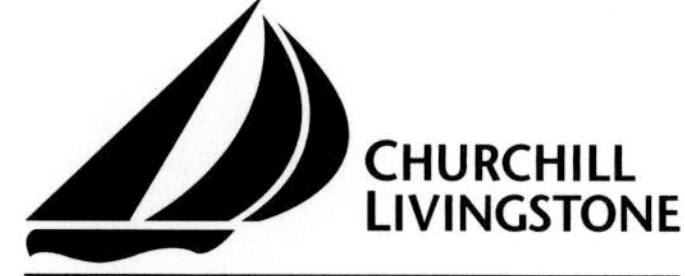

CHURCHILL LIVINGSTONE

EDINBURGH LONDON NEW YORK PHILADELPHIA SYDNEY TORONTO 1999

CHURCHILL LIVINGSTONE
An imprint of Harcourt Publishers Limited

First edition 1993
Second edition 1999
Reprinted 1999
Reprinted 2000

ISBN 0 443 05945 4

British Library Cataloguing in Publication Data
A catalogue record for this book is available from the British Library

Library of Congress Cataloging in Publication Data
A catalog record for this book is available from the Library of Congress

Notice
This is a textbook and reference for students and practitioners of natural medicine and other professionals interested in learning about this healing art.
For several important reasons, this work should not be viewed as providing a single answer applicable to all individuals.
First, the practice of natural medicine is constantly evolving. New research and ongoing clinical experience continue to give us a better understanding of the human body, its interaction with the physical environment, its reaction to the stresses of modern life, and its response to various forms of therapy and treatment.
Second, diagnosis and therapy are so personalized and individualized that the same problem for the same person may call for different treatment at different ages or in different settings.
Third, all readers need to be aware of the times at which more invasive interventions are more appropriate.
The Publisher, the Editors, and the Contributors do not assume any responsibility for any injury and/or damage to persons or property arising out of or related to any use of the material contained in this textbook. The reader is advised to check the appropriate literature and the product information currently provided by the manufacturer of each therapeutic substance to verify dosages, the method and duration of administration, or contraindications. It is the responsibility of the treating practitioner, relying on independent experience and knowledge of the patient, to determine dosages and the best treatment for the patient. There is no substitute for individualized diagnosis and treatment.
This personalized approach is at the heart of naturopathic medicine.
These recommendations are particularly important for new forms of treatment and for rare or serious health problems.

Most of the laboratory procedures presented in Section 2 are on the cutting edge of our understanding of the assessment of the physiological function of metabolically unique individuals. As an emerging field, few experts exist and most are employed by the commercial laboratories providing the procedures. The following is a list of the Textbook authors employed by laboratories providing these tests:

Stephen Barrie, ND
J. Alexander Bralley, PhD
Richard S. Lord, PhD
Carl P Verdon, MS, PhD
Aristo Vojdani, PhD, MT

Printed in China
CTPS/02

The publisher's policy is to use **paper manufactured from sustainable forests**

Contents

VOLUME 2

Contributors

Steve Austin ND
Chief Science Officer, HealthNotes Inc, Portland, Oregon, USA

Stephen Barrie ND
President, Great Smokies Diagnostic Laboratory, Asheville, North Carolina, USA

Robert Barry ND
Private Practitioner, Seattle, Washington, USA

Peter Bennett ND
Chief Medical Officer, Helios Clinic, Saanichton, British Columbia, Canada

Jeffrey S. Bland PhD
Chief Executive Officer of HealthComm International Inc., Tacoma, Washington, USA

Jennifer Booker ND
Private Practitioner, Olympia, Washington, USA

Randall S. Bradley ND DHNAP
Private Practitioner, Omaha, Nebraska, USA

J. Alexander Bralley PhD
Chief Executive Officer, MetaMetrix Clinical Laboratory, Norcross, Georgia, USA

Donald J. Brown ND
Editor, Quarterly Review of Natural Medicine, Seattle, Washington, USA

Qiang Cao MD(China) ND LAc
Professor, Acupuncture and Oriental Medicine, Bastyr University, Kenmore, Washington, USA

Leon Chaitow ND DO
Practitioner and Senior Lecturer, Centre for Community Care and Primary Health, University of Westminster, London, UK

Anthony J. Cichoke MA DC
Director, Wellness Institute, Portland, Oregon, USA

George Wm Cody JD
Instructor, Jurisprudence, Bastyr University, Kenmore, Washington, USA

Walter J. Crinnion ND
Director, Healing Naturally Inc, Kirkland, Washington, USA; Instructor, Department of Environmental Medicine, Bastyr University, Kenmore, Washington, USA

Beth DiDomenico ND
Federal Way Naturopathy, Federal Way, Washington, USA

Patrick M. Donovan ND
Naturopathic Staff Physician, Seattle Cancer Treatment and Wellness Center; Private Practitioner, University Health Clinic, Seattle, Washington, USA

Cathryn M. Flanagan ND
Private Practitioner, Old Saybrook, Connecticut, USA

Alan R. Gaby MD
Professor, Nutrition, Bastyr University, Kenmore, Washington, USA

Kjersten Gmeiner MD
Research Assistant, Bastyr University, Kenmore, Washington, USA

Mark D. Groven ND
Faculty, Physical Medicine, Bastyr University Natural Health Clinic, Kenmore, Washington, USA

Kathi Head ND
Senior Editor, Alternative Medicine Review; Technical Advisor, Thorne Research, Dover, Idaho, USA

Gregory S. Kelly ND
Private Practitioner, Stamford, Connecticut, USA

Richard Kitaeff MA ND DAc
Naturopathic Physician, Acupuncturist and Director, New Health Medical Center, Edmonds, Washington, USA

Allen M. Kratz PharmD
Chief Executive Officer, HVS Laboratories Inc, Naples, Florida, USA

Elizabeth Kutter PhD
Faculty, Evergreen State College, Olympia, Washington, USA

Andrew Lange ND
Private Practice, Boulder, Colorado, USA

Martin J. Lee PhD
Lee Research Laboratory, Asheville, North Carolina, USA

Buck Levin PhD RD
Professor, Nutrition, Bastyr University, Kenmore, Washington, USA

Douglas C. Lewis ND
Instructor, Physical Medicine, Bastyr University, Kenmore, Washington, USA

Richard S. Lord PhD
Chief Information Officer, MetaMetrix Inc, Norcross, Georgia, USA

Dan Lukaczer ND
Director of Clinical Research, Functional Medicine Research Center, HealthComm International, Gig Harbor, Washington, USA

Bobbi Lutack MS ND
Private Practitioner, Evergreen Natural Health Clinic, Seattle, Washington, USA

Stephen P. Markus MD
Private Practitioner, Moss Bay Center for Integrative Medicine, Bellevue, Washington, USA

Robert M. Martinez DC ND
Private Practitioner, Kirkland, Washington, USA

Alan L. Miller ND
Senior Editor, Alternative Medicine Review; Senior Technical Advisor, Thorne Research, Dover, Idaho, USA

Gaetano Morello ND
Lecturer, Consultant and Private Practitioner, West Coast Clinic of Integrative Medicine, Vancouver, British Columbia, Canada

M. Harrison Nolting ND LAc
Associate Professor, Acupuncture and Oriental Medicine, Bastyr University, Kenmore, Washington, USA

Lara E. Pizzorno MA (Divinity)
Medical Writer and Editor, Seattle, Washington, USA

Terry A. Pollock MS
Clinical Services Director, MetaMetrix Clinical Laboratory, Norcross, Georgia, USA

Dirk Wm Powell ND
Private Practitioner, Kent, Washington, USA; Faculty, Bastyr University, Kenmore, Washington, USA

Peter T. Pugliese MD
President, Peter T. Pugliese and Associates, Reading, Pennsylvania, USA

Paul Reilly ND
Private Practitioner, Tacoma; Clinical Staff, Seattle Cancer Treatment and Wellness Center, Seattle, Washington, USA

Corey Resnick ND
Chief Technology Officer, Tyler Encapsulations, Gresham, Oregon, USA

Nancy Roberts ND
Private Practitioner, Seattle, Washington, USA

Sally J. Rockwell PhD CCN
Nutritionist, Seattle, Washington, USA

Robert A. Ronzio PhD
Laboratory Director, Biotics Research, Houston, Texas, USA

John F. Ruhland ND
Research Assistant, Bastyr University, Kenmore, Washington, USA

Trevor K. Salloum ND
Private Practitioner, Kelowna, British Columbia, Canada

Alexander G. Schauss PhD
Director, Natural and Medicinal Products Research, Life Sciences Division, American Institute for Biosocial and Medical Research, Tacoma, Washington, USA

Michael A. Schmidt PhD CNS
Visiting Professor, Applied Biochemistry and Clinical Nutrition, Bellingham, Washington, USA

David K. Shefrin ND
Private Practitioner, Beaverton, Oregon; Chair, Board of Trustees, Southwest College of Naturopathic Medicine and Health Sciences, Tempe, Arizona, USA

Virender Sodhi MS(Ayurveda) ND
Medical Director, Ayurvedic, Naturopathic Medical Clinic, Bellevue, Washington, USA

Nick Soloway LMT DC LAc
Private Practitioner, Helena, Massachusetts, USA

Leanna J. Standish ND PhD
Principal Investigator, Bastyr University AIDS Research Center, Bastyr University, Kenmore, Washington, USA

Carl P. Verdon PhD
Vice President, Science and Development, MetaMetrix Inc, Norcross, Georgia, USA

Aristo Vojdani PhD MT
Director of Immunosciences Laboratory Inc, Beverly Hills; Associate Professor, Department of Medicine, Charles Drew University, Compton, California, USA

Terry Willard PhD
President of Canadian Association of Herbal Practitioners; Director, Wild Rose College of Natural Healing, Calgary, Alberta, Canada

Preface

The scientific support for the philosophical and therapeutic foundation of natural medicine has evolved remarkably over the past 25 years. Concepts that were once considered "quaint" at best, are now recognized as fundamental to good health and the prevention and treatment of disease. This textbook, with its some 10 000 citations to the peer-review research literature, provides well-documented standards of practice for natural medicine. Based on a sound combination of philosophy and clinical studies, this work provides the astute practitioner with a reliable informational resource to provide health care that identifies and controls the underlying causes of disease, is supportive of the body's own healing processes, and considerate of each patient's unique biochemistry.

The Textbook is composed of six Sections, each focused on a fundamental aspect of the practice of natural medicine. "Philosophy of natural medicine" covers the history and conceptual basis of natural medicine. "Supplementary diagnostic procedures" provides a primer on diagnostic procedures not commonly taught in conventional medical schools. Diet analysis, food allergy testing, immune function assessment, fatty acid profiling, and hair mineral analysis are examples of these analytical procedures. The next section, "Therapeutic modalities", provides a descriptive, practical, scientific, and historical review of the common modalities of natural medicine, including botanical medicine, nutritional therapy, therapeutic fasting, exercise therapy, hydrotherapy, counselling, acupuncture, homeopathy, and soft tissue manipulation. "Syndromes and special topics" considers underlying issues relevant to many diseases. "Pharmacology of natural medicines" covers the pharmacognosy, pharmacology and clinical indications for the most commonly prescribed botanical medicines, special nutrients, and other natural agents. Finally, "Specific health problems" provides an in-depth natural medicine approach to over 70 specific diseases and conditions. The comprehensive therapeutic rationales are well documented and based on the pathophysiology and causes of each condition.

Kenmore, 1999

Joe Pizzorno
Michael Murray

SECTION 1

Philosophy of natural medicine

SECTION CONTENTS

Nature is doing her best each moment to make us well. She exists for no other end. Do not resist. With the least inclination to be well, we should not be sick.

(Henry David Thoreau)

One of the differentiating features of naturopathic medicine compared with conventional (allopathic) medicine is its strong philosophical foundation. The basic philosophical premise of naturopathic medicine is that there is an inherent healing power in nature and in every human being. It is the physician's role to bring out or enhance this innate healing power within their patients.

In many ways, this was the most difficult section of the textbook to write, as no comprehensive history of the social, political and philosophical development of naturopathic medicine had ever been written, and, even in the halcyon years of the 1920s and 1930s, the profession was never able to agree upon a concise philosophy. This has now changed.

We provide here a well-documented chapter detailing the roots of American naturopathy. After a century of maturation, the profession has now widely agreed to a comprehensive definition, a set of principles and system of case analysis that provide a systematic guide for the application of these concepts in a clinical setting.

There are seven fundamental principles of naturopathic medicine:

1. The healing power of nature (*vis medicatrix naturae*)
2. First do no harm (*primum non nocere*)
3. Find the cause (*tolle causam*)
4. Treat the whole person
5. Preventive medicine
6. Wellness
7. Doctor as teacher.

These principles translate into the following questions the practitioner applies when analyzing a case:

- What is the first cause; what is contributing now?
- How is the body trying to heal itself?
- What is the minimum level of intervention needed to facilitate the self-healing process?
- What are the patient's underlying functional weaknesses?
- What education does the patient need to understand why they are sick and how to become healthier?
- How does the patient's physical disease relate to their psychological and spiritual health?

We have further expanded on the philosophical basis of naturopathic medicine by having these concepts addressed by several authors, whose backgrounds allow each of them a unique and, we feel, complementary insight into some of the fundamental questions of the goals of health care. Although the dominant school of medicine has essentially ignored these issues, we believe that the true physician cannot function without a sound philosophical basis to guide his or her actions. Without a more than superficial understanding of health and disease, the physician can only function as a technician, temporarily alleviating symptoms while allowing the real disease to progress past the point of recovery.

CHAPTER CONTENTS

1

Functional medicine in natural medicine

Buck Levin, PhD RD

Michael A. Schmidt, PhD CNS

Jeffrey S. Bland, PhD

PART I: THE PHILOSOPHY OF FUNCTIONAL MEDICINE

INTRODUCTION

This textbook bears witness to the remarkable evolution of naturopathic medicine in the USA since Benedict Lust first opened his American School of Naturopathy at the end of the 19th century. During the intervening century, naturopathic physicians have become recognized as primary health care providers in about one-fourth of all states; naturopathic practice has become part of publicly funded clinics, and accredited training has become available in all regions of the country. In addition, naturopathic philosophy has influenced medical philosophy as a whole, including the functional approach which we have espoused in our own work. Naturopathic recognition of key medical principles, including *tolle causam* (identify and treat the causes), *primum non nocere* (first do no harm) and *docere* (doctor as teacher), has helped us clarify our vision of a functional approach to health which derives from a patient-centered, self-care, outcomes-based model.

Through functional medicine, we have worked to develop an approach to health care which can be incorporated into the everyday practice of all health care practitioners regardless of training or specialty. Moreover, we have tried to carve out an approach which capitalizes not only upon the foremost accomplishments of basic and applied science, but also upon the strengths of specialty fields and specialized approaches to clinical practice. It is our hope that naturopaths, osteopaths, chiropractors, medical doctors, nutritionists, dietitians, herbalists, homeopaths, acupuncturists, Ayurvedic physicians, and other diversely trained practitioners will be able to find in functional medicine an approach which naturally extends and enhances their current practice. Functional medicine is not an "alternative" approach which requires a change in basic clinical orientation or political allegiance. It requires only a willingness to take seriously one's basic medical philosophy, and to engage the science of our time with the spirit of true discovery, open-mindedness, and due diligence. In this chapter, we specifically address the consequences of such an approach for naturopathy and its clinical practice.

THEORETICAL ASPECTS

The philosophy of function in a medical context

Most dictionary definitions of "function" indicate that the word is derived from the Greek term *ergon*, which means "the kind of action or activity proper to a person or thing; the purpose for which something is designed or exists".[1] This definition tells us the concept of function must be viewed in the same category as the concepts of "purpose" and "design". It tells us we cannot understand the function of a person or thing without also understanding the purpose for which that person or thing is designed.

In early Greek philosophy, the term *ergon* was frequently contrasted with the term *pathemata* – things that happened to a person or thing.[2] This comparison focused on the difference between things with the capacity to act (*poiein*) and things that were, in contrast, "passive activations" (*pathe*).[2] *En-ergia* – being in activity, or functioning – was considered to be the *telos* (end purpose) of being alive. Today, when we refer to disease as "pathology-based", we are actually linking disease, etymologically, to this realm of *pathemata* and *pathe*. We are defining disease as something that "happens to" a person, something that is not a part of that person's purposeful activity. Etymologically, the term "functional medicine" moves us away from this pathological model and aligns us with a medicine that views disease as part of something that is purposeful and is proceeding actively in accordance with some design.

The history of philosophy – at least as far back as the writings of Aristotle in the third century BC – has witnessed an ongoing debate between "vitalistic" and "mechanistic" approaches to life and health. Naturopathic medicine has consistently aligned itself with the vitalistic side of this argument. Naturopathy recognizes a vital force – *vis medicatrix naturae,* or healing power of nature – that is present in all living things, including the human body. For naturopaths, it is this vital force which is ultimately responsible for healing.

The functional medicine emphasis on purpose and design is closely related to this recognition of vital force in naturopathy. When functional practitioners recognize purpose and design in physiological events (including "disease of unknown origin"), they are acknowledging that body function is guided by a universal, supra-individual set of principles. They are acknowledging that physiological function originates from an infinite, complex, patterned matrix of occurrences which both precede and transcend individual human experience. The purpose and design of functional medicine therefore echo the spirit of vitalism.

This spirit of vitalism does not mean, however, that the healing force is totally mysterious or unapproachable. While the universal, patterned matrix of events is infinite and cannot be fully understood, it is nevertheless a complex pattern which can be observed and analyzed within the limits of a human perspective. Pursuit of this possibility is essential to a functional approach. The more that can be learned about the patterned matrix of universal events, the better able is the practitioner to support healing.

The terms "form" and "function" are probably most familiar to us from the field of architecture. At the turn of the 20th century, US architect Louis Sullivan coined the phrase "form follows function", recognizing that purpose precedes the blueprint. But in our philosophy of the body's architecture, how do these terms apply? In the case of several body systems – the musculoskeletal system or the circulatory system, for example – shape and form give an initial hint about function, design, and purpose. It is difficult to observe the body's skeleton without concluding that it has been designed for structural support. With other physiological systems, these connections are not nearly so obvious.

Phrenology, described by English historian J. C. Flugel a century after its origin as "psychology's greatest *faux pas*", argued that the quality of a person's mental faculties was determined by the size of the brain area upon which those faculties depended, and this quality could be judged by the contours of the skull adjacent to the area.[3] This literal equating of brain function with brain form, proposed in 1810 in Paris by François Joseph Gall and his student J. C. Spurzheim, met with some immediate difficulty in application. After discovering that the skull of French philosopher René Descartes was particularly small in the anterior and superior regions of the forehead, understood to be the seat of a person's rational faculties, Spurzheim reportedly commented:[3] "Descartes was not so great a thinker as he was held to be."

The inability of phrenologists to make sense of function by reference to form alone is one example of a difficulty that continues to permeate 20th century medicine. Naturopathy has made great strides in linking form with function, by accommodating into its practice long-standing medical traditions which treat function by working with form. Naturopathy's embrace of physical medicine – from craniosacral therapy and osseous manipulation to hydrotherapy and physiotherapy – has made the connection between form and function more accessible.

A final common ground between functional and

naturopathic medicine involves the very idea of a "medical *philosophy*". The need for practical solutions in everyday medical practice is great (so great that most practitioners will not see themselves as having the time – or inclination – to "philosophize"). Yet from a functional and naturopathic perspective, it is impossible to approach health without paying continual attention to one's *philosophy* of medicine. In the remainder of this section, we look at several examples of philosophical thinking that we believe continue to represent stumbling blocks for an integrated 21st century medicine. Each of these examples thinks "dualistically" about medical concepts and in so doing, we believe, loses sight of function.

Function as a mediator for opposition thinking in the sciences

Part/whole

The traditional philosophical dualism of "part/whole" has been directly addressed in the field of holistic health. Two national organizations – the American Holistic Health Association (AHHA), with headquarters in Anaheim, California, and the American Holistic Medical Association (AHMA), located in Raleigh, North Carolina – have each referred to this dualism in defining their field of study.

According to the American Holistic Health Association:[4]

> Rather than focusing on illness or specific parts of the body, holistic health considers the *whole person* and how it interacts with its environment. It emphasizes the connection of body, mind, and spirit. Holistic Health is based on the law of nature that *a whole is made up of interdependent parts.* The earth is made up of systems, such as air, land, water, plants, and animals. If life is to be sustained, they cannot be separated, for what is happening to one is also felt by all of the other systems. In the same way, an individual is a whole made up of interdependent parts, which are the physical, mental, emotional, and spiritual. When one part is not working at its best, it will impact all the other parts of that person. Further, this whole person, including all of the parts, is constantly interacting with everything in the surrounding environment.

And according to the American Holistic Medical Association:[5]

> Wellness is defined as a state of well-being in which an individual's body, mind, emotions, and spirit are in harmony with and guided by an awareness of society, nature, and the universe. ... [It] encompasses all safe modalities of diagnosis and treatment, including the use of medications and surgery, emphasizing the necessity of looking at the whole person.

On its Internet website, the AHMA states:[6] "Optimal health is much more than the absence of sickness. It is the conscious pursuit of the highest qualities of the spiritual, mental, emotional, physical, environmental, and social aspects of the human experience."

With respect to their characterization of "part" and "whole", these definitions of holistic medicine are largely compatible with a functional approach. Because the concept of function asks us to consider why a thing is here, i.e., what it is "doing" in the universe, it asks us to be holistic and take into account the *holon* – which in early Greek philosophy meant both "universe" and "organism". Wholeness becomes a necessary concept for understanding function, and holistic medicine has done medical philosophy an important service by renewing its focus on the whole.

At the same time, we invite supporters of holistic medicine to consider an extension of their philosophy in two ways. First, we invite consideration of a multi-level understanding of wholeness that does not predetermine a frame of reference or specific context in which wholeness is to be evaluated. For example, if we do not presently know whether planetary indices of geomagnetic disturbance – such as sunspot relative number, area, and geomagnetic activity – are as valuable a "whole" or "universe" against which to evaluate and treat cardiovascular disease as homocysteine imbalances (the "whole" or "universe" of the cell) or "heartlessness" and "disheartenment" (a psychological or sociocultural "whole" or "context"), we might expect to benefit by keeping a radical open-mindedness about frames of reference, levels of wholeness, and their ultimate interrelationship in a holistic model. Instead of trying to simplify with three or four frames of reference based on early 20th century psychology (i.e., wholeness as the sum of physical, emotional, mental, and spiritual frames of reference) or a few contexts based on specialty (physical body, immediate external environment, global environment), we might simply postpone such conclusions until we learn more about levels of wholeness and their relationship. From a functional perspective, we suspect this relationship will closely resemble the one described by US engineer, designer, and architect, Buckminster Fuller, in his discussion of "functions" in his 1975 opus, *Synergetics*:[7] "Functions occur only as inherently cooperative and accommodatively varying subaspects of synergistically transforming wholes."

The relationship of part *to* whole is a second area in which a holistic perspective could be logically extended. We believe the concept of function necessitates a view of "part" and "whole" that is quite different from the image of a disassembled jigsaw puzzle or a shattered china teacup, which can be reassembled or glued back together to re-establish the "whole" from which it came. In both of these examples, the parts have a visible connection to the whole, but in and of themselves are a diverse array of pieces in all shapes and sizes, bearing no individual resemblance to the whole from which they came. From a functional perspective, we believe this image of part and whole should be changed. Instead of a shattered teacup or a disassembled puzzle, we propose a shattered *hologram*. When a hologram breaks, it does not shatter into discrete pieces with different sizes and shapes that individually bear no resemblance to the original hologram. It splits into separate pieces, each of which visibly contains the complete and original hologram.

From a medical perspective, this change means that we would stop assigning partial functions to anatomically distinct body parts or systems and begin treating all parts as visibly containing the original hologram, i.e., whole-body capability. For example, we have traditionally viewed the gastrointestinal (GI) tract, brain, and immune system as separate, identifiable parts unable to carry out each other's basic functions. In the case of the GI tract, these functions have traditionally been limited to digestion, absorption, secretion, and motility. We now know the GI tract has its own immune system (GALT) and its own brain (memory T-cells disseminated to the intestinal epithelium and lamina propria providing the functional basis for oral tolerance),[8] and that it can carry on functions traditionally reserved for other systems of the body. Similarly, we now recognize that the eye does not simply "see". We know it helps set the body's circadian rhythms through the production of melatonin,[9] and that it may therefore coordinate reproductive signaling as well.[10] These findings encourage recognition of the whole inside each part. Equally encouraging have been the many "reflexologies" that have dotted the landscape of alternative medicine, and which have been given open-minded consideration in naturopathy – foot reflexology, iridology, intestinal reflexology in colonics, contact reflex analysis – each pointing toward a "shattered hologram" model in which the unbroken whole is visible in its seemingly separate parts.

Inside/outside

The classic debate over nature vs. nurture, heredity/environment, and genetics/experience has had troublesome consequences for a patient-centered approach to well-being. We have seen what can happen when the "insides", in their purest form, are equated with the chromosomal material inside the nucleus of the cell. What can happen is a philosophy of development that treats the three billion base pairs in the human genome as a largely unalterable blueprint working from the inside to define a person's potential with respect to the "great taskmaster outside", i.e., the environment. This extremist view of inside/outside, equating inside – the true "inner sanctum" – with the gene, has given us a national eugenics movement based on misinterpretation of ethnic differences in IQ, a national backlash against elementary school "mainstreaming" based on misinterpretation of learning disorders, and a popular anthropology of racial difference based on misinterpretation of the anthropological facts.

Two examples from the history of biology can help place the dualism of "inside/outside" in a more functional context. The first example involves a chapter of a book written by Swiss zoologist Adolph Portmann in 1967. In his chapter, titled "The Outside and the Inside", Portmann writes:[11]

> Biologists ... have worked from the outside inwards, from what is visible and tangible to what is more and more deeply hidden. ... But such probing makes us strangers to the appearance of the living creatures around us. ... With a knowledge of the developmental conditions under which, for instance, a feather primordium develops and its pigment is formed, it is only the problem of shape that has been solved. But it still remains to be shown what brings about that special distribution of color in the pattern on the feather germ which is specifically directed towards the whole form in its final condition.

In his book, Portmann argues that outsides of animals are in fact expressions of their inwardness, i.e., their developmentally unfolding uniqueness and individuality. He also concludes that the ultimate purpose of this "insides-becoming-outsides" is to help living creatures find each other and "break the ban of isolation".[11]

What we hear in Portmann's writing is a desire to blur (or even erase) the line between inside and outside. What is innermost "feels a desire" to become outermost, and for the purpose of connecting up with the innermost sanctum of another.

As health care practitioners, we are all familiar with the notion of a *milieu interieur* – an interior, homeostatic, calm harbor maintained in the wake of outside, stormy seas. Pasteur's contemporary, Claude Bernard, first wrote about this concept in 1865 in his classic text *An Introduction to the Study of Experimental Medicine*,[12] and it still serves as a cornerstone of our understanding of cellular events. But what we are not familiar with, in this second example, is the extent to which Bernard was forced to dismiss the relevance of purpose and design in positing the *milieu interieur*:[12]

> Neither physiologists nor physicians need imagine it their task to seek the cause of life or the essence of disease. That would be entirely wasting one's time in pursuing a phantom. The words life, death, health, disease have no objective reality.
>
> Sickness and death are merely a dislocation or disturbance of the mechanism which regulates the contact of vital stimulants with organic units.

It is, of course, the interior milieu that regulates this contact. But by making such an absolute division between inside and outside, Bernard ends up placing all responsibility and focus on this "mechanism" that connects "in" with "out", and turning his back on the purpose and essence of life/death and health/disease.

Both of these examples caution us against drawing

absolute lines between inside and outside. So does the concept of function itself. When we recognize that function requires purpose – some goal or end-point toward which activity is directed – we are also recognizing that function requires *potential*, a goal or end-point that is capable of being reached but has not yet been attained in actuality. Without potentiality, there is no function.

In functional medicine, no question is more critical than the question of this potentiality and its "location". To what extent is potential "inside" of us, inside of our cells, our thought, our genes? How are "outside" events related to this potential? In immunology, at least since the end of World War II, we've developed a self/non-self model that is forcing us to relabel long lists of diseases as diseases of autoimmunity, diseases in which the distinction between self and non-self has become confused. But from a functional perspective, an absolute division between self and non-self is a too-literal separation of inside from out. Autoimmune diseases cannot be a set of inside, interior dynamics in which "self" mistakes "self" for "non-self" and self-destructs. If this were the case, we wouldn't be discovering all the risk factors for autoimmune disorders on the outside, removed from the self. Yet that is exactly where we are finding them. The 17-amino acid sequence in bovine serum albumin that travels from cow's milk formulas to pancreatic beta-cell surface proteins (protein 69) and increases risk for the autoimmune disease we call juvenile-onset diabetes,[13] the links between xenobiotic exposure and systemic lupus erythematosus,[14] and the newly designated "autoimmune polyendocrine syndromes" and their responsiveness to dietary modification are all examples that point to dangers *outside* the self and their key role in the development of autoimmune disease.

But it is not only negative potential that gets locked outside the self when we draw a line too absolutely between inside and out; it is positive potential as well. Function requires purpose. Purpose requires potential. To be "pluri-functioning" organisms, we must also be "pluri-potential". And because the unbroken whole is visible in the parts, this pluripotential must reside in the parts as well, even in that innermost part we call the human genome, locked away inside the nucleus of the cell.

Molecular medicine is teaching us that there is no untouchable inside. Our outside experience – including our dietary intake – continually modifies the expression of our genes. Control of gene expression is highly encrypted, i.e., genes have inducer binding sites and promoter sequences that modify their expression. Numerous nutritional components have been shown to modify that expression, including linoleic and alpha-linolenic acid, isoflavones, quercetin, ellagic acid, vitamin A, and vitamin B_6.[15] The potentiality is ever-present, even when IQ suggests otherwise. At our innermost, genetic selves, we are always also outside of ourselves, linked to wholes through our potential.

Cause/effect

In the fourth century BC, in a treatise entitled *Physica*, the Greek philosopher Aristotle described a doctrine of four causes: formal cause (*eidos*), producing in a thing its constitutive essence; material cause (*hyle*), providing a thing with its matter and embodiment; efficient cause (*kinoun*), initiating change in a thing; and final cause (*telos*), providing an ultimate purpose for the change. Since the word "cause" has several meanings, Aristotle wrote: "It follows that there are several causes of the same thing (not merely in virtue of a concomitant attribute), e.g., both the art of the sculptor and the bronze are causes of the statue."[16]

What appears treatable or preventable to us as practitioners depends entirely on our philosophy of medicine. Whether dysfunction is treatable or preventable depends on what caused the dysfunction in the first place, i.e., on our concept of causality. Keith Block, MD, medical director of the Cancer Institute at Edgewater Medical Center in Chicago, Illinois, has recently argued that the labeling of any cancer as "terminal" is both scientifically and spiritually unjustifiable.[17] His argument is based on a view of cancer causality that includes an active role for the self in deciphering and acting upon the cosmic event that cancer represents.

But the views of Aristotle and Block, welcoming a complex view of causality into our understanding of health, are far from our classic heritage in the sciences. As French Nobel Prize winner Jacques Monod wrote, in his classic 1970 work *Chance and Necessity*:

> The cornerstone of the scientific method is … *systematic* denial that "true" knowledge can be got at by interpreting phenomena in terms of final causes – that is to say of "purpose".[18]
>
> Against this notion, this powerful feeling of destiny, we must be constantly on guard.[18]

Monod's philosophy is our reigning medical philosophy – a philosophy steeped in the Darwinian legacy of a universe with minimal original essence, minimal momentary stability, and an indefinite horizon of possibilities.[19] It is a philosophy that tells us we must be careful when reading purpose into dysfunction, and that we should accept whole categories of disability and death as purposeless, chance events that are essentially not preventable.

Naturopathy, with its focus on prevention, has helped to transform this perspective. Most naturopaths would readily subscribe to the mission statement of the Foundation for Preventive Medicine, based in New York City, when it describes its mission as "enhancing the public's awareness of recent information indicating that most causes of death in our society … are now regarded as potentially preventable". Preventive, functional, and naturopathic medicine all seem to agree that lack of well-being, lack of vitality, depression, and deficiency in energy are also associated with largely preventable conditions,[20] and that each time we transfer a health condition from the category of "not preventable" to "preventable", we are honoring our medical philosophy.

Energy/matter

As scientists, most of us subscribe to an energy-based view of human function. We believe that healthy function rests on the shoulders of gated ion channels, electrolyte balance, membrane potential, redox, electrochemical gradients, and high-energy phosphate bonds. In our view, the release of heat energy from cells is what makes biological order actually possible in the first place.[21] Yet in spite of its acceptance at a biological and biochemical level, this energy-based paradigm has yet to become fully integrated into our *medicine*. While electrocardiographic, magnetic resonance, and single photon emission imaging have become standard parts of our diagnostic repertoire, electroacupuncture biofeedback devices, despite their research record and use in many countries,[22] remain unapproved for clinical use in the USA.

Once again, naturopathic medicine has provided leadership in this area. Energy-based medicine has been given open-minded consideration in naturopathy, and whole traditions based on principles of energy, including acupuncture and Oriental medicine, have been treated as essential areas for understanding and research. Similarly, acceptance of homeopathy, an energy-based medicine used by a quarter of a million practitioners worldwide,[23] has been nurtured in the USA by the supportive position adopted by naturopaths and naturopathic institutions.

From a functional perspective, the rightful place of "energy medicine" in health care approaches is woven into the term "function" itself, which derives from the Greek *en-ergia*, literally "functioning" or "being in activity". But clearly, as practitioners, we are just starting to explore this energy–matter relationship in our medical philosophy. In nutrition, for example, we are just beginning to shed our 19th century steam engine model, which perceives the body as a large furnace combusting matter (food) for the sake of extracting caloric energy. In this model, energy is not useful unless extracted out of matter, and matter, once depleted of its energy, is of little use as well. This food-as-fuel model has left us with an under-appreciation of food's matter and its energy. As raw material for caloric extraction, food becomes most important for its gross, undifferentiated macronutrient content – its 20 g of fat or 100 g of carbohydrate. Subtler distinctions involving omega 3:omega 6 or oligosaccharide:polysaccharide ratio have been slow to evolve. Likewise, food energetics – including the issues of raw food, live food, food enzymes, and active cultures – have been negligibly addressed. Interestingly, we are finding the role of light – in the form of food pigments, including the hemes, chlorophylls, carotenoids, and flavonoids – is slowly revolutionizing our approach to food in the same way that light (and the frame of reference it represented) revolutionized our approach to mass and energy in physics.

Body systems from a functional medicine perspective

Historical and philosophical perspective

Students of science and medicine in the USA and other Western countries learn anatomy and physiology from a systems approach. They learn to view organ systems, individual organs, tissues, cells, and subcellular spaces as separate entities that interact with one another to create form and function. The better one understands any one system or entity, by this model, the more skilled one will be at treating dysfunction of that entity. This model served well in developing a rational method of inquiry into the etiology of many diseases. Indeed, the advancement of medical science has long been measured by progress made in understanding the mechanisms of disease related to dysfunction in the body's distinct compartments.

Fundamental to the systems model has been the assumption that the more we know about individual organs or systems, the better our medicine will be. Until very recently, this assumption had been widely validated throughout medical history by remarkable progress in diagnosis and treatment of disease, surgical practice, and the development of medications for symptom reduction related to specific diseases.

The progress that resulted from this compartmentalizing approach can be compared to advances in biology that followed Linnaeus's development of a system of taxonomic classification of living organisms in the 18th century. The formalized system of learning allowed for significant advancement in the field of biology. By the 1970s, however, many biologists had become aware of the limitations of description and classification as an epistemology. Their science had outgrown the model. Through advancements in the disciplines of ecology and environmental science, they knew they could classify all the plants and animals in an ecosystem and yet understand nothing about the functioning of the ecosystem as an integrated whole. The need had arisen to address the larger issues of how compartments within the ecosystem interacted to give rise to its function and survival.

From the perspective of these advancements in biology, one could view medicine as a specialized discipline within the broader field of human ecology. To understand health and disease, one would be required to examine the functional interaction of organ systems with the human environment. Furthermore, one would have to observe the functional interaction between the total human environment and the energy processing and control systems within it.

Examining any discipline from a new point of view makes it possible to ask new questions and gain new insights. Looking at human health and medicine from the point of view of interactive function raises questions about the homeodynamic interplay between the external and internal environments of the individual. The functional viewpoint is the longer, larger view; it moves away from the narrow focus on pathology of various parts of the body. It removes the principal focus from diagnosis of pathology and places it on evaluation of genetic pluripotential and its translation into homeodynamic function. It views disease not as an enemy with which to grapple, but as a manifestation of the breakdown of mechanisms that establish control and resilience. To restore these processes, functional medicine uses a broader range of methods than the cut-and-paste tools of compartmentalized medicine. Among others, it employs nutrition, environmental adaptation, lifestyle changes, activity or stress pattern adjustment, or molecular pharmacology, and its selection of tools is based on the unique needs of the individual.

The traditional anatomy / physiology model of Western medicine still has great value in diagnosis and treatment, and it has wide application in responding to many specific disease states. This traditional model breaks down, however, when it is applied to chronic conditions that transcend individual organs or organ systems. Among these chronic health problems are inflammation, fatigue, pain, immune dysfunction, and problems of digestion. All of these conditions are characterized, not by end-stage pathologies, but by altered physiological function, and they require a more integrative model to design a therapeutic approach that can improve long-term outcome. This more integrative model is built upon the understanding that dysfunction is not compartment- or organ-specific, but is an alteration in integrated homeodynamic processes.

The functional medicine approach incorporates evaluation of antecedents to a health problem, its triggering factors, mediators of altered physiological function, and the relationship to signs and symptoms, to develop an integrated view of the patient's health status. It focuses less on defining the disease and more on understanding the functions that give rise to the expression of symptoms.

A woman may approach her physician complaining of chronic intestinal pain and symptoms of irritable bowel syndrome, for example. A medical history and initial evaluation might uncover other symptoms, including joint pain, headache, low energy, sleep disturbances, and eczema. Rather than coming up with a primary and secondary diagnosis and prescribing symptom-relieving medications, a functional medicine practitioner would delve further in evaluating the source of the inflammation. The practitioner might assess gastrointestinal function, hepatic detoxification ability, and immunological status, and assess their relationship to oxidative stress mediators. Based on this "second tier" of assessments, the practitioner would develop an integrated approach to modify triggers and mediators using specific biological response modifiers and lifestyle alterations of the individual.

Systems integration and functional medicine

The emerging science of today has blurred distinctions among organs, and separation of function into distinct compartments is less useful as a concept. We now know, for example, that identical signalling molecules are released and received by all organ systems, and each influences the function of the others. The view of the body as a collection of separate, interconnected parts is being replaced by an image of the body as a hologram. The endocrine system synthesizes a neurotransmitter that is released by the nervous system and has a receptor site on the white blood cell. A blood cell synthesizes cytokines that are released by the immune system and have receptor cites on the glial cell in the brain. The liver synthesizes steroid hormones that are released by the endocrine system and have immune and nervous system receptors, and vice versa. In other words, all the organs and organ systems of the body are constantly engaging in "cross-communication", which makes distinctions among them a matter of definition rather than function.

In the past 10 years, medicine has witnessed a revolution in molecular biology. We now know, for example, that modifiers of gene expression are produced not only by different organs but also by exposure to various agents in the diet and environment, including chemicals and electromagnetic radiation. We have learned that the processes that give rise to an individual's health or disease are not controlled by genes alone. Instead, modification of function comes about through alteration in gene expression, transmitting new physiological messages about individual regulation and control.

This new view of health focuses on maintaining metabolic and homeodynamic freedom based on interconnectedness, pluripotential, diversity, and redundancy of function. Loss or decline in any of these parameters can be seen as an altered state of health. Altered physiological diversity, for example, translates to a loss of metabolic freedom and a subsequent state of lower health reserve. Assessing health, therefore, depends on measuring this reserve rather than evaluating pathology. Functional challenge tests, an integral part of the practice of functional medicine, make it possible to measure specific reserves under conditions of stress. Examples of functional tests include the exercise treadmill test for cardiac function, oral glucose tolerance testing for blood sugar management, and food provocation challenges for food sensitivity.

Functional medicine practitioners use the patient as his or her own "universe", or point of reference in which his or her unique set of interconnections, potentials, diversities, and redundancies is realized. Whether changing conditions involving time, temperature, electromagnetic energy gradients, infective organisms, or trauma will lower degrees of metabolic freedom is a question that can be answered only in the context of the individual and his or her ability to maintain reserve and avoid reduced stability that comes from lost potential.

Functional medicine focuses on maintenance of stability and pluripotential across organ domains. From this perspective, all organ-specific symptoms the patient possesses at any one moment reflect homeodynamic alterations at a broad, "weblike" level and result in new metastable physiological states characterized by lowered stability and reduced degrees of metabolic freedom and efficiency. The more freedom is lost at this "weblike" level, the more symptoms will become manifest, and the more closely they will resemble classical pathology. It is the integrative, homeodynamic, regulatory role of the web that is being altered, however, not a circumscribed set of functions within a specific organ domain. As a diagnostician, a practitioner might look through a focused lens such as an X-ray, blood chemistry, or CAT scan at an isolated, compartmentalized organ system. As a functional medicine practitioner, however, he or she will view alteration in this seemingly distinct compartment as a reflection of change in the web, the whole of which is the individual and his or her unique life experience in the world.

PART II: THE CLINICAL APPLICATION OF FUNCTIONAL MEDICINE

BASIC CONCEPTS IN FUNCTIONAL MEDICINE PRACTICE

The practice of functional medicine is guided by three basic concepts: biochemical individuality, health as positive vitality, and life processes as homeodynamic.

Biochemical individuality

Each individual is unique. This uniqueness encompasses voluntary activities, such as decision-making, personality development, and emotional response, and involuntary activities like metabolism of nutrients, cellular processing of information, and communications among the body's organ systems. The concept of biochemical individuality is central to every aspect of the practice of functional medicine, from clinical assessment and diagnosis to the broad spectrum of treatment modalities.

As traditionally practiced, medicine and nutrition have given only token consideration to the concept of individuality. In conditions such as phenylketonuria (PKU) or maple sugar urine disease (MSUD), for example, although medicine has long recognized that specific metabolic aberrations alter the afflicted individual's nutrition and health needs, it has taken the view that these defects are so rare as to be inconsequential. A functional medicine practitioner, on the other hand, considers that all individuals have unique metabolic patterns that affect their nutrition and health needs. In comparing two individuals whose blood levels of B vitamins are nearly identical, for example, one might have five times as high a level of B vitamins in his or her cells as the other. Individuals also respond uniquely to environmental toxins, food additives, and prescription medications.

Health as a positive vitality

Functional medicine views health as more than the absence of disease. Health, in the functional medicine model, is the state of positive vitality unique to each individual within his or her life context. Functional medicine employs new assessment tools to help quantify individual well-being and evaluate his or her physiological, cognitive/emotional, and physical function.

Functional medicine practitioners cannot narrowly focus on a patient's symptoms, complaints, or history of illness. They must also evaluate the patient's history of wellness by asking when in life the individual has felt best and what circumstances would be necessary to make that patient feel truly well again. Although relief of symptoms might be one goal of the application of functional medicine, the broader goal would be to support vitality in the patient's life experience.

Life processes as homeodynamic

Homeodynamics as a principle of functional medicine contrasts with the concept of "homeostasis" in conventional medicine. Homeostasis describes the balance of interconnected components that keep a physical or chemical parameter of the body relatively constant. Homeodynamics posits a similar control system functioning to maintain biochemical individuality.

Applied to the body, the term "homeodynamic" describes a range of continuously occurring metabolic and physiologic activities that enable an individual to adapt to changing circumstances, stresses, and experiences. The homeodynamics of one's health are constantly at work to enable a person to function as a unique individual. Supporting health at a homeodynamic level may require one to focus attention on cellular processes or organ function at sites that seem to be far removed from the patient's area of discomfort, and at levels that may be unusual from a conventional point of view.

ASSESSMENT AND TREATMENT FROM A FUNCTIONAL PERSPECTIVE

Healing practices in any society evolve within a cultural context and draw upon the belief systems and resources of the healers within that culture. In traditional societies, the background and support of healing derive from the natural world. In industrialized societies, evolving in a framework erected by Newton and Descartes, medicine formed a different understanding of the body and its function.

The term "diagnosis" derives from the Greek word *dia-gnosis*, which means, literally, "through gnosis, through the knowledge gained through a perspective". In conventional Western medicine, diagnosis is defined as "the art of distinguishing one disease from another" or "the determination of the nature of a case of a disease". *Clinical diagnosis* is "diagnosis based on symptoms, irrespective of the morbid changes producing them". *Differential diagnosis* is "determining which of two or more diseases or conditions a patient suffers from, by systematically comparing and contrasting their symptoms".

Key concepts in these definitions are "disease", "symptoms", and "suffers from", and analysis of these concepts yields clues to the philosophical perspective underlying the Western medical approach to managing health. This underlying perspective is the key factor that differentiates one healing system from another. It is the basis by which we examine patients and develop our plan of action or treatment. A physician whose perspective is oriented toward pharmacology views patients in terms of what drugs are needed. A nutritionist might look for specific nutrients or dietary changes that would benefit patients. A psychotherapist might ask which form of counseling or behavioral intervention is warranted. In each case, the course of action is dictated by the practitioner's underlying perspective.

The underlying perspective of functional medicine is based on process, dynamics, and purpose. Functional medicine focuses on dynamic processes that underlie and precede the pathological state. Acknowledging the existence and necessity to understand pathology, functional medicine focuses on underlying processes and seeks solutions that address these processes.

The practice of functional medicine does not focus on diagnosis that compartmentalizes diseases into known entities. Such a system, although it might be useful, is apt to presume that if we can name a disorder we can understand how it came about. Functional medicine practitioners recognize diagnosit categories, but they also investigate underlying dietary, nutritional, lifestyle, environmental, and psychosocial factors that might alter the patient's state of health and investigate the "purpose" behind the expression of illness.

Illness as information

From the traditional medical viewpoint, illness "happens" to a human being; an outside force upsets a system of the body. The clinician then seeks to discover precisely what it was that caused the illness. Although this method remains a useful view in diagnosis (since a number of factors, including food, chemicals, and microorganisms, affect our homeodynamics), it places constraints on both patient and clinician. On the other hand, if we take the view that the human body is an energy-driven, energy-sensitive system that interacts constantly with its surroundings, we can begin to view illness as a form of communication from one level to a level of conscious awareness. Conscious awareness enables the individual to begin to understand the factors that collectively led to the illness.

Because it has a purpose, illness can be seen as a functional condition. It may function as an agent for change. It may itself be an epiphenomenon that requires treatment, but paying heed to the "message" that is being communicated by the illness may be what finally enables healing to take place. Both scientific and popular literature often describe cases of recovery from serious illness that occurred as a result of the individual's paying attention to the message contained in the symptoms.

In clinical practice, illness communicates its messages in many ways, including symptoms arising from exposure to chemicals, rashes or breathing difficulties from consuming food allergens, neck pain from repetitive workplace activity, and stress-induced chest pains. Patients who present with these complaints are all getting messages about their bodies' interactions with their surroundings. In neurology, occurrences of hysterical blindness or hemiplegia are examples of illness as information. In both conditions, physical symptoms arising from deep psychological problems mimic severe organic disease.[24]

In making a diagnosis, the functional medicine practitioner must be aware of the message being sent and approach the patient's illness not as an adversary to be overcome but as information that must be understood and acted upon.

Treatment decisions

The experienced practitioner of functional medicine knows that illness typically arises from multiple influences, and his or her assessment and treatment take this array of influences into account. In dealing with a problem like migraine headaches, for example, this approach contrasts with the traditional approach of Western medicine. The latter would identify the symptom pattern, rule out vascular and intracranial pathology, and test for the presence of hypertension or renal disease. Treatment would be with drugs like sumatriptan, propranolol, or ergotamine. Biofeedback might be employed as an adjunctive therapy. The functional medicine practitioner, in contrast, would ask the migraine sufferer about dietary, nutritional, genetic, environmental, lifestyle, psychosocial, or spiritual factors that might be interacting in his or her life. The practitioner would inquire into functional changes that might underlie the expression of migraine symptoms. The goal would be to develop a range of potential patient-centered solutions to migraine headache. Remediation of migraine, for example, has been reported with oral magnesium therapy (M. A. Schmidt, unpublished data), essential fatty acid supplementation (S. Baker, personal communication, 1996), removal of food, chemical, and inhalant triggers,[25] sublingual neutralization therapy,[26] spinal manipulation (P. Bolin, personal communication, 1996), acupuncture, homeopathy, and the botanical feverfew (*Tanacetum parthenium*).[27] The functional medicine practitioner might employ any one or a combination of these therapies, realizing that no single approach is effective with all migraine sufferers. Rea[25] found that the headache symptoms of 100% of a group of 30 migraine sufferers were triggered by chemicals under controlled challenge, but these were patients who reported chemical sensitivity. A patient-centered approach that recognizes statistical tendencies and diagnostic categories, but is not constrained by them, is desirable.

Another example of the value of the functional medicine approach is in assessing microbe-associated illness. The traditional approach to infectious disease regards the organism as an external threat that must be eradicated by intervention that targets that organism specifically. The microbe is the enemy, and drug therapy is the typical weapon. A broader, functional medicine approach would view the microbe as just one (albeit important) factor contributing to poor health. The functional medicine practitioner would consider the state of the host's defenses and evaluate factors that influence host defenses by examining nutritional, metabolic, environmental, lifestyle, and psychosocial factors that influence immune vigilance.

The philosophical basis of functional medicine leads to treatment decisions that are quite different from those typically encountered in an infectious disease model. For example, a patient with Down's syndrome who suffers from recurrent infection with *S. pneumoniae* or *H. influenzae* may experience an increase in IgG_2 and IgG_4 production and a reduction in infection susceptibility with selenium supplementation.[28] A child with otitis media with effusion might be treated not with antimicrobials, but with elimination of allergenic foods.[29] An endurance runner who suffers from upper respiratory tract infection associated with heavy training might be given antioxidants.[30]

Concept of total load

Total load refers to the sum of influences affecting an individual's life. Initially advanced by environmental medicine practitioners, the concept is now widely adopted. Included in the total load are chemicals, food, microbes, psychological stressors, and other factors, each of which alone might not give rise to the symptoms of illness. Together, however, the factors that comprise the total load may overwhelm the patient's metabolic management system. According to Rea[25], more than 20,000 patients at his Environmental Health Center in Dallas, Texas, experienced relief of symptoms of a range of clinical disorders through reduction of total load.

A person's biochemical individuality affects his or her susceptibility to toxins, and intervention aimed at improving function can help reduce susceptibility or sensitivity. A defective sulfur metabolism pathway, for example, might cause an individual who reacts to sulfur-rich foods to react to other substances in ways that lead to metabolic disturbance. Nutrient modulation might lessen his or her sensitivity to these environmental substances. Efforts to reduce total load should be balanced by efforts to restore function, with the long-term goal being reduced susceptibility.

Depth of action

The functional perspective requires the practitioner to examine the processes that give rise to symptoms. Arriving at a diagnosis does not guarantee that we understand what is happening or what the patient needs. For example, we might arrive at a diagnosis of "mood disorder" in a depressed patient and assume that he or she would benefit from a drug like fluoxetine. If the depression arose from a spiritual or relationship crisis, however, the drug therapy might actually interfere with the problem-solving processes that would lead to true healing. Mood and quality of life might appear to improve with drugs, but the patient's long-term healing would not have been facilitated.

A group of epileptic children who were videotaped as they interacted with their families illustrates the point. Emotionally fraught family encounters were, in many cases, followed by seizures. When the epileptic patients were later shown films of these episodes, and they saw the relationship between emotional events and seizures, they were able, in many instances, to become almost seizure-free.[31] Granted, drug therapy might have helped these patients to control seizures, but if drugs were the only means of intervention employed, the epileptic children would not have had the opportunity to experience healing at a deeper level.

Mechanism and outcome

Understanding biochemical mechanisms enables functional medicine practitioners to apply them in diagnosis and treatment. Understanding the mechanism of homocysteine accumulation, for example, allows them to recommend nutritional strategies like folic acid and vitamin B_{12} therapy. By understanding fatty acid synthesis and the arachidonic acid cascade, they can develop nutritional therapies that modify inflammation. Knowing that copper accumulation leads to Wilson's disease allows them to utilize zinc therapy.

Some treatment modalities bring positive outcomes for which the mechanism is not yet well understood. Spinal manipulation in asthmatics admitted to the emergency room, for example, can lessen anxiety and ease breathing. This treatment typically brings about a 25–70% improvement in measurement of peak blood flow.[32] Using pre- and post-manipulation tympanographs, Fallon showed that spinal manipulation in children with otitis media led to normalization of abnormal tympanograms (J. Fallon, personal communication, 1995). Similarly, Fryman (personal communication, 1996) has shown that cranial manipulation normalizes tympanographic measurements in some children.

The knowledge that viscerosomatic and somatovisceral reflexes influence the flow of information within the human body suggests the possible mechanism by which manipulation affects visceral function, although the mechanism is not yet clearly understood. Improved function, patient outcome, and quality of life are central to the success of any healing system, however, whether or not we understand the mechanisms of action.

Homeopathic medicine is a discipline that is not bound by mechanism, but is rooted in careful analysis and pattern recognition. Reilly[33] demonstrated that asthmatic patients who took homeopathic preparations showed significant improvement in only 1 week compared with those taking placebo. These dramatic results led him to conclude that either homeopathic medicine worked beyond a shadow of a doubt, or the double-blind, placebo-controlled trial, the gold standard of proof upon which modern pharmacology is built, was essentially invalid.

Throughout the range of healing arts and sciences, there are numerous examples of positive treatment outcomes that occur even though the mechanism cannot be explained. In functional medicine, the value of understanding mechanisms is in improving human function and patient outcome.

Prevention, early detection, and functional medicine

"Prevention" has become a welcome and popular concept in recent years in the practice of medicine. A distinction must be made, however, between true prevention and "early detection". Although periodic mammography has been heralded as a form of preventive medicine, for example, it is clearly in the realm of early detection. Prevention assumes an understanding of factors that give rise to breast cancer and recommendation/adoption of habits or patterns that prevent disease occurrence.

Both prevention and early detection are included in the practice of functional medicine, but the patient's individuality remains paramount. Functional medicine practitioners work to prevent a specific disorder by managing risk factors, but they also strive to raise the individual's functional capacity within his or her unique life circumstances.

Approach to the patient

Functional medicine is always patient-centered, but it is not the only discipline that fits this description. Naturopathic medicine has helped to pioneer a patient-centered medical approach, not only by making the whole person the center of its practice, but also by incorporating highly patient-centered traditions into its repertoire, including traditional Chinese medicine, Ayurvedic medicine, homeopathy, chiropractic, and physical therapy, including manipulation and massage. The focus on the patient is important, however, because as methods of data management become more sophisticated, the tendency is to think in terms of probability instead of thinking in terms of the individual patient. Probability is useful in understanding the broad context of health and disease, but clinical practice is filled with so many exceptions that relying on statistics is difficult.

Laboratory and instrumental diagnosis from a functional perspective

In assessing a patient's health, the functional medicine practitioner uses tools that help in understanding how the patient functioned before developing the pathology. These tools also help the practitioner to understand function in the existence of pathology and to assist in predicting preventive measures.

Serum glucose measurement is a traditional assessment

of a fixed analyte at a fixed point in time. Although this measurement yields useful information, it does not reveal how serum glucose will respond under varying dietary conditions. The glucose challenge test, on the other hand, is a functional test that assesses glucose status over time. Similarly, although a resting ECG provides useful information, it does not indicate how the heart would respond to a physical challenge. The stress ECG shows how the heart responds upon exertion.

Assessment of magnesium is a third example. Magnesium is an intracellular element, which means that most of the body's magnesium stores are contained within cells, and only a small amount circulates in blood. A measurement of serum magnesium levels, therefore, does not reflect total body magnesium or the functional status of magnesium. Red cell magnesium is a better indicator of status, although it is a measurement of a fixed analyte at a fixed point in time and has limitations as well. Magnesium loading and subsequently assessing retention by measuring urinary excretion provide a means to assess the functional magnesium status and the unique needs of a particular patient.

For functional medicine practitioners, tools that view the body under challenge conditions give a more accurate assessment of body function. This is especially true when one wishes to examine the body's response to exogenous substances. Some individuals will experience an adverse reaction to any given drug, and these reactions are regarded as atypical and unavoidable. From a different perspective, however, the reactions are not atypical and unavoidable; they are typical and avoidable for that person, and he or she would typically be expected to have an adverse reaction on ingestion of this drug.

This understanding comes from developments in understanding the body's detoxification mechanisms. When a drug or medication is ingested, it is metabolized by the body and prepared for excretion. The process of detoxification and preparation for excretion takes place in two distinct biochemical phases, known as phase I and phase II. In the biotransformation of a drug or chemical, the agent is progressively converted to a more water-soluble, excretable substance. In phase I, which generally occurs first, a family of isozymes known as cytochrome P450 (cP450) converts the drug or substance into a reactive intermediate, which, although it may be excreted in its present form, typically is further acted upon by phase II processes.

In phase II, conjugating substances are attached to the phase I product to facilitate its excretion. Phase II reactions typically take place through glucuronidation, amino acid conjugation, glutathione conjugation, acetylation, and methylation.[34] The phase II process, which depends strongly on adequacy of specific nutrients, must be capable of transforming all of the phase I-generated reactive molecules into excretable compounds. If this process is incomplete, toxic intermediates can build up.

Acetaminophen is a typical drug that undergoes conversion for excretion through these two pathways. A common OTC and prescription pain-relieving drug, acetaminophen is a useful model because more than 70,000 incidents of acetaminophen overdose were reported to US poison control centers in 1994.[35] Acetaminophen normally undergoes phase II transformation through the sulfation and glucuronidation pathways, with a small amount being metabolized through glutathione conjugation after conversion in phase I.[36] When the drug is not efficiently converted for excretion, the metabolites that build up can have negative metabolic consequences. Accumulations of one extremely toxic metabolite, NAPQI, may cause liver and nervous system damage. An individual with an adequately functioning detoxification ability that facilitates efficient phase II conversion of acetaminophen is much less likely to have a negative experience than one whose ineffective conversion pathways allow toxic intermediates to accumulate.

If one ingests acetaminophen on a regular basis, the sulfur-bearing nutrients glutathione, methionine, and cysteine can be rapidly depleted, with accompanying liver cell damage.[37]

Adverse acetaminophen reactions may therefore result from alterations in detoxification pathways. The acetaminophen challenge test effectively assesses the function of these pathways. After the individual has consumed a challenge substance, measurements of acetaminophen metabolites in urine can determine the efficiency of the various conversion processes and provide information about the individual's unique susceptibility.

It may be that alterations in the detoxification pathways of many individuals who have "atypical" drug reactions are making them predictably susceptible to certain kinds of substances. If we can gather this information about them, we may be able to predict their response to drugs, as well as chemicals, foods, and plants. We may be able to understand the functional derangement that underlies the pathology that can result from interaction with the environment; and we may be able to use diet and nutrition to help these individuals restore function in these pathways.

Pattern recognition

The next step in the evolution of functional assessment will be to consider human physiology as a dynamic process, involving the interrelationship of multiple systems. Functional assessment of only one pathway or one series of pathways may yield useful information, but it still provides a very limited view. Functional testing will no doubt soon evolve to assess multiple analytes and utilize sophisticated pattern recognition methods.

Pattern recognition is not new. For centuries, in fact, traditional Chinese medicine has dealt with "patterns of disharmony". The clinician trained in this discipline learns to recognize the pattern and assign it to a specific diagnostic category. In homeopathic medicine, it was pattern recognition that led to the extensive *materia medica*. In psychotherapy, an evaluation of the patient's life events and stories is conducted in an effort to understand the patterns that produce disharmony. In all of these examples, the mechanisms are unimportant; the pattern leads to treatment decisions.

SUMMARY

Pattern recognition, depth of action, total load, energetics, information, and patient-centered decisions all describe the early stages of development of the evolving functional approach to assessment and treatment. They also characterize a functional approach with a strong focus on the integrative use of treatment modalities based on recognition of underlying purpose in the transformations viewed by practitioners as they work with individual patients. This is also the integrative paradigm which unites naturopathy with functional medicine.

REFERENCES

1. Urdang L, Flexner SB. Random House dictionary of the English language. New York: Random House. 1968: p 535
2. Peters FE. Greek philosophical terms. New York: New York University Press. 1967
3. Young R. Mind, brain and adaptation in the nineteenth century. Oxford: Clarendon Press. 1970
4. Walter S. Encyclopedia of body mind disciplines. New York, NY: Rosen Publishing Group. 1998. Reprinted on the AHHA Internet website at http://www.healthy.net/ahha
5. Anderson R. Wellness medicine. Lynnwood, Wash., American Health Press. 1987: p 6
6. American Holistic Medical Association. Raleigh, NC: http://www.doubleclickd/com/about_ahma.html
7. Fuller RB. Synergetics: explorations in the geometry of thinking. New York, NY: Macmillan Publishing. 1975: p 58
8. Weiner LH, Mayer LF (eds). Oral tolerance: mechanisms and applications. Ann NY Acad Sci 1996; 778; xiii–xvii: 6–7
9. Raloff J. Eyes possess their own biological clocks. Sci News 1996; 149: 245
10. Tamarkin L, Bond CJ, Baird J et al. Melatonin: a coordinating signal for mammalian reproduction? Science 1985; 227: 714–720
11. Portmann A. Animal forms and patterns: a study of the appearance of animals. New York, NY: Schocken Books. 1967
12. Bernard C. An introduction to the study of experimental medicine (1865). Greene HC (Transl.). New York, NY: Dover Publications. 1957
13. Karjalainen J, Martin JM et al. A bovine albumin peptide as a possible trigger of insulin-dependent diabetes mellitus. NEJM 1992; 327(5): 302–307
14. National Academy of Sciences. Biologic markers in immunotoxicology. Washington, DC: National Academy Press. 1992: p 55
15. Berdanier CD, Hargrove JL. Nutrition and gene expression. Boca Raton, Fla: CRC Press. 1993
16. McKeon R. Introduction to Aristotle. New York, NY: Modern Library. 1947: p 123
17. Block KI. The role of self in healthy cancer survivorship: a view from the frontlines of treating cancer. Advances: J Mind-Body Health 1997; 13: 6–25
18. Monod J. Chance and necessity. New York, NY: Vintage. 1971
19. Jonas H. The phenomenon of life: toward a philosophical biology. New York, NY: Delta. 1971: p 46–47
20. Foundation for Preventive Medicine. New York, NY. Website information: http://www.preventivemed.org
21. Alberts B, Bray D, Lewis J et al. Molecular biology of the cell. New York, NY: Garland Publishing. 1983: p 62
22. Zong-xiang Z. Recent advances in the electrical specificity of meridians and acupuncture points. Am J Acupunct 1981; 9(3): 203–215
23. Cook TM. Homeopathic medicine today. New Canaan, Conn.: Keats Publishing. 1989: p 21–30
24. DeMeyer WE. Technique of the neurological examination. 4th edn. New York, NY: McGraw-Hill. 1994: p 512–513
25. Rea WJ. Chemical sensitivity. Vol. IV. Boca Raton, Fla: CRC Press. 1996
26. Hoover S. Ménière's migraine and allergy. In: Claussen CF, Kirtan MV, Schlitter K, eds. Vertigo, nausea, tinnitus, and hypoacusia in metabolic disorders. New York: Elsevier Science. 1988: p 293–300
27. Awang DVC. Feverfew. Can Pharm J 1989; 122: 266–270
28. Anneren G, Magnusson CGM, Nordvall SL. Increase in serum concentrations of IgG2 and IgG4 have been observed with selenium supplementation in children with Down syndrome. Arch Dis Child 1990; 65: 1353–1355
29. Nsouli TM. Role of food allergy in serous otitis media. Ann Allergy 1994; 73(3): 215–219
30. Peters EM. Vitamin C supplementation reduces the incidence of post-race symptoms of upper respiratory tract infection. Am J Clin Nutr 1993: 57: 170–174
31. Brown B. Supermind: the ultimate energy. New York: Harper and Row. 1980: p 275
32. Paul FA, Buser BR. Manipulative treatment applications for the emergency department patient. J Am Ost Assoc 1996; 96(7): 403–409
33. Reilly DT. Is evidence for homeopathy reproducible? Lancet 1994; 344: 1601–1606
34. Murray R, Granner D, Mayes P, Rodwell V. Harper's biochemistry. Norwalk, Conn.: Appleton & Lange. 1990
35. Anil D, Sorrell MD. Acetaminophen overdose: need to consider intravenous preparation of N-acetylcysteine in the United States. Am J Gastroenterol 1996; 91(7): 1476
36. Patel M, Tang B, Kalow W. Variability of acetaminophen metabolism in Caucasians and Orientals. Pharmacogenetic 1992; 2: 38–45
37. Willson RA, Hall T. The concentration and temporal relationships of acetaminophen-induced changes in intracellular and extracellular total glutathione freshly isolated hepatocytes from untreated and 3-methylcholanthrene pretreated Sprague-Dawley and Fischer rats. Pharmacol Toxicol 1991; 69: 205–212

2

History of naturopathic medicine

George Cody, JD

CHAPTER CONTENTS

INTRODUCTION

"Naturopathy", as a generally used term, began with the teachings and concepts of Benedict Lust. Naturopathy, or "nature cure", is both a way of life, and a concept of healing employing various natural means of treating human infirmities and disease states. The earliest mechanisms of healing associated with the term, as utilized by Lust, involved a combination of hygienics and hydropathy (hydrotherapy). The term itself was coined in 1895 by Dr John Scheel of New York City, to describe his method of health care. But earlier forerunners of these concepts had already existed in the history of natural healing, both in America and in the Austro-Germanic European core.

Lust came to this country from Germany in 1892 as a disciple of Father Kneipp and as a missionary dispatched by Kneipp to bring hydrotherapy to America. Lust purchased the term "naturopathy" from Scheel in 1902 to describe the eclectic compilation of doctrines of natural healing that he envisioned to be the future of natural medicine. In January of 1902, Lust, who had been publishing the *Kneipp Water Cure Monthly* and its German language counterpart in New York since 1896, changed the name of the journal to *The Naturopathic and Herald of Health* and evoked the dawn of a new health care era with the following editorial:

> Naturopathy is a hybrid word. It is purposely so. No single tongue could distinguish a system whose origin, scope and purpose is universal – broad as the world, deep as love, high as heaven. Naturopathy was not born of a sudden or a happen-so. Its progenitors have for eons been projecting thoughts and ideas and ideals whose culminations are crystallized in the new Therapy. Connaro, doling out his few fixed ounces of food and drink each day in his determined exemplification of Dietotherapy; Priessnitz, agonizing, despised and dejected through the long years of Hydropathy's travail; the Woerishofen priest, laboring lovingly in his little parish home for the thousands who journeyed Germany over for the Kneipp cure; Kuhne, living vicariously and dying a martyr for the sake of Serotherapy; A.T. Still, studying and struggling and enduring for his faith

in Osteopathy; Bernarr Macfadden, fired by the will to make Physical Culture popular; Helen Willmans, threading the mazes of Mental Science, and finally emerging triumphant; Orrison Sweet Maraden, throbbing in sympathy with human faults and failures, and longing to realize Success to all mankind – these and hosts of others have brought into being single systems whose focal features are perpetuated in Naturopathy.

Jesus Christ – I say it reverently – knew the possibility of physical immortality. He believed in bodily beauty; He founded Mental Healing; He perfected Spirit-power. And Naturopathy will include ultimately the supreme forces that made the Man of Galilee omnipotent.

The scope of Naturopathy is from the first kiss of the new-found lovers to the burying of the centenarian whose birth was the symbol of their perfected one-ness. It includes ideally every life-phase of the id, the embryo, the foetus, the birth, the babe, the child, the youth, the man, the lover, the husband, the father, the patriarch, the soul.

We believe in strong, pure, beautiful bodies thrilling perpetually with the glorious power of radiating health. We want every man, woman and child in this great land to know and embody and feel the truths of right living that mean conscious mastery. We plead for the renouncing of poisons from the coffee, white flour, glucose, lard, and like venom of the American table to patent medicines, tobacco, liquor and the other inevitable recourse of perverted appetite. We long for the time when an eight-hour day may enable every worker to stop existing long enough to live; when the spirit of universal brotherhood shall animate business and society and the church; when every American may have a little cottage of his own, and a bit of ground where he may combine Aerotherapy, Heliotherapy, Geotherapy, Aristophagy and nature's other forces with home and peace and happiness and things forbidden to flat-dwellers; when people may stop doing and thinking and being for others and be for themselves; when true love and divine marriage and pre-natal culture and controlled parenthood may fill this world with germ-gods instead of humanized animals.

In a word, Naturopathy stands for the reconciling, harmonizing and unifying of nature, humanity and God.

Fundamentally therapeutic because men need healing; elementally educational because men need teaching; ultimately inspirational because men need empowering, it encompasses the realm of human progress and destiny.

Perhaps a word of appreciation is due Mr. John H. Scheel, who first used the term "Naturopathic" in connection with his Sanitarium "Badekur," and who has courteously allowed us to share the name. It was chosen out of some 150 submitted, as most comprehensive and enduring. All our present plans are looking forward some five or ten or fifty years when Naturopathy shall be the greatest system in the world.

Actually the present development of Naturopathy is pitifully inadequate, and we shall from time to time present plans and ask suggestions for the surpassing achievement of our world-wide purpose. Dietetics, Physical Culture and Hydropathy are the measures upon which Naturopathy is to build; mental culture is the means, and soul-selfhood is the motive.

If the infinite immensity of plan, plea and purpose of this particular magazine and movement were told you, you would simply smile in your condescendingly superior way and straightway forget. Not having learned as yet what a brain and imagination and a will can do, you consider Naturopathy an ordinarily innocuous affair, with a lukewarm purpose back of it, and an ebbing future ahead of it. Such is the character of the average wishy-washy health movement and tumultuous wave of reform.

Your incredulous smile would not discomfit us – we do not importune your belief, or your help, or your money. Wherein we differ from the orthodox self-labeled reformer, who cries for sympathy and cringes for shekels.

We need money most persistently – a million dollars could be used to advantage in a single branch of the work already definitely planned and awaiting materialization; and we need co-operation in a hundred different ways. But these are not the things we expect or deem best.

Criticism, fair, full and unsparing is the one thing of value you can give this paper. Let me explain. Change is the keynote of this January issue – in form, title, make-up. If it please you, your subscription and a word to your still-benighted friends is ample appreciation. But if you don't like it, say so. Tell us wherein the paper is inefficient or redundant or ill-advised, how it will more nearly fit into your personal needs, what we can do to make it the broadest, deepest, truest, most inspiring of the mighty host of printed powers. The most salient letter of less than 300 words will be printed in full, and we shall ask to present the writer with a subscription-receipt for life.

By to-morrow you will probably have forgotten this request; by the day after you will have dropped back into your old ways of criminal eating and foolish drinking and sagged standing and congested sitting and narrow thinking and deadly fearing – until the next progress paper of New Thought or Mental Science or Dietetics or Physical Culture prods you into momentary activity.

Between now and December we shall tell you just how to preserve the right attitude, physical and mental, without a single external aid; and how, every moment of every day, to tingle and pulsate and leap with the boundless ecstasy of manhood consciously nearing perfection.

A BRIEF HISTORY OF EARLY AMERICAN MEDICINE WITH AN EMPHASIS ON NATURAL HEALING

To understand the evolutionary history of naturopathic medicine in this country, it is necessary to view the internal development of the profession against the historical, social, and cultural backdrop of American social history.

Medicine in America: 1800–1875

In the America of 1800, although a professional medical class existed, medicine was primarily domestically oriented. When an individual fell ill, he was commonly nursed by a friend or family member who relied upon William Buchan's *Domestic Medicine* (1769), John Wesley's *Primitive Physic* (1747), or John Gunn's *Domestic Medicine* (1830).[1]

Professional medicine

Professional medicine transferred from England and Scotland to America in pre-revolutionary days. However, 18th- and early 19th-century America considered the concept of creating a small, elite, learned profession in violation of the political and institutional concepts of early American democracy.[1]

The first medical school in the American colonies was opened in 1765 at what was then the College of Philadelphia (later the University of Pennsylvania) and the school came to be dominated by revolutionary leader and physician Benjamin Rush, a signatory to the Declaration of Independence. The proliferation of medical schools to train the new professional medical class began seriously after the war of 1812. Between 1810 and 1820, new schools were established in Baltimore, Lexington and Cincinnati, and even in rural communities in Vermont and Western New York. Between 1820 and 1850, a substantial number of schools were established in the western rural states. By 1850, there were 42 medical schools recognized in the United States, while there were only three in all of France.

Generally, these schools were started by a group of five to seven local physicians approaching a local college with the idea of establishing a medical school in conjunction with the college's educational facilities. The schools were largely apprenticeship-based, and the professors received their remuneration directly from fees paid by the students.

The requirements for an MD degree in late 18th- and early 19th-century America were roughly the following:

- knowledge of Latin, natural and experimental philosophy
- 3 years of serving an apprenticeship under practicing physicians
- attending of two terms of lectures and passing of attendant examinations
- a thesis.

Graduating students had to be at least 21 years of age.[1]

The rise of any professional class is gradual and marked by difficulties, and varying concepts existed as to what was the demarcation of a "professional" physician. There were the graduates of medical school versus non-graduates, medical society members versus non-members, and licensed physicians versus unlicensed "doctors". Licensing statutes came into existence between 1830 and 1850, but were soon repealed, as they were considered "undemocratic" during the apex of Jacksonian democracy.[1]

Thomsonianism

In 1822, the rise in popularity of Samuel Thomson and his publication of *New Guide to Health* helped to frustrate the creation of a professional medical class. Thomson's work was a compilation of his personal view of medical theory and American Indian herbal and medical botanical lore. Thomson espoused the belief that disease had one general cause – "cold" influences on the human body – and that disease had therefore one general remedy – "heat". Unlike the followers of Benjamin Rush and the American "heroic" medical tradition who advocated blood-letting, leeching, and the substantial use of mineral-based purgatives such as antimony and mercury, Thomson believed that minerals were sources of "cold" because they come from the ground and that vegetation, which grew toward the sun, represented "heat".[1]

As noted in Griggs' *Green Pharmacy* (the best history of herbal medicine to date), Thomson's theory developed as follows:[2]

> Instead, he elaborated a theory of his own, of the utmost simplicity: "All diseases ... are brought about by a decrease or derangement of the vital fluids by taking cold or the loss of animal warmth ... the name of the complaint depends upon what part of the body has become so weak as to be affected. If the lungs, it is consumption, or the pleura, pleurisy; if the limbs, it is rheumatism, or the bowels, colic or cholera morbus ... all these different diseases may be removed by a restoration of the vital energy, and removing the obstructions which the disease has generated ...
>
> Thus the great object of his treatment was always to raise and restore the body's vital heat: "All ... that medicine can do in the expulsion of disorder, is to kindle up the decaying spark, and restore its energy till it glows in all its wonted vigor.

Thomson's view was that individuals could be self-treating if they had a sincere understanding of his "new guide to health" philosophy *and* a copy of his book, *New Guide to Health*. The right to sell "family franchises" for utilization of the Thomsonian method of healing was the basis of a profound lay movement between 1822 and Thomson's death in 1843. Thomson adamantly believed that no professional medical class should exist and that democratic medicine was best practiced by lay persons within a Thomsonian "family" unit.

By 1839, Thomson claimed to have sold some 100,000 of these family franchises called "friendly botanic societies". While he professed to have solely the interests of the individual at heart, his system was sold at a profit under the protection of a patent he had obtained in 1813.

The eclectic school of medicine

Some of the botanics (professional Thomsonian doctors) wanted to separate themselves from the lay movement by creating requirements and standards for the practice of Thomsonian medicine. Thomson, however, was adamantly against a medical school founded on his views. Thus, it was not until the decade after Thomson's death that independent Thomsonians founded a medical college (in Cincinnati) and began to dominate the Thomsonian movement. These Thomsonian doctors, or "botanics", were later absorbed into the medical sectarian movement known as the "eclectic school", which originated with the New Yorker, Wooster Beach.

Wooster Beach was another of medical history's fascinating characters. From a well-established New England family, he started his medical studies at an early age, apprenticing under an old German herbal doctor, Jacob Tidd, until Tidd died. Beach then enrolled in the Barclay Street Medical University in New York. As noted by Griggs (p. 180):[2]

> Beach's burning ambition was to reform medical practice generally – not to alienate the entire profession by savage attacks from without – and he was convinced that he would be in a stronger position to do so if he were himself a diplomatized doctor. The faculty occasionally listened to criticism from within their own number: against onslaughts of "illiterate quacks" like Samuel Thomson, they simply closed ranks in complacent hostility.

After opening his own practice in New York, Beach set out to win over fellow members of the New York Medical Society (into which he had been warmly introduced by the screening committee) to his point of view that heroic medicine was inherently dangerous to mankind and should be reduced to the gentler theories of herbal medicine. He was summarily ostracized from the medical society.

To Beach this was a bitter blow, but he soon founded his own school in New York, calling the clinic and educational facility "The United States Infirmary". However, due to continued pressure from the medical society, he was unable to obtain charter authority to issue legitimate diplomas. He then located a financially ailing, but legally chartered, school, Worthington College, in Worthington, Ohio. He opened there a full-scale medical college; out of its classrooms was launched what became known as the eclectic school of medical theory. As Griggs relates (p. 183):[2]

> Beach had a new name for his practice: while explaining to a friend his notions of combining what was useful in the old practice with what was best in the new, the friend exclaimed, "You are an eclectic!" to which, according to legend, Beach replied, "You have given me the term which I have wanted: I am an eclectic!"

Cincinnati subsequently became the focal point of the eclectic movement and the medical school remained until 1938 (the last eclectic school to exist in America).[1] The philosophies of the sect helped to form the theoretical underpinnings of Benedict Lust's naturopathic school of medicine.

Despite his criticism of the early allopathic medical movement (although the followers of Benjamin Rush were not as yet known by this term, reputed to have been coined by Samuel Hahnemann) for their "heroic" tendencies, Thomson's medical theories were "heroic" in their own fashion. While he did not advocate bloodletting, heavy metal poisoning and leeching, botanic purgatives – particularly *Lobelia inflata* (Indian tobacco) – were a substantial part of the therapy.

The hygienic school of thought

One other forerunner of American naturopathy, also originating as a lay movement, grew into existence at this time. This was the "hygienic" school, which had its genesis in the popular teachings of Sylvester Graham and William Alcott.

Sylvester Graham began preaching the doctrines of temperance and hygiene in 1830, and published, in 1839, *Lectures on the Science of Human Life*, two hefty volumes that prescribed healthy dietary habits. He emphasized a moderate lifestyle, recommending an anti-flesh diet and bran bread as an alternative to bolted or white bread.

William Alcott dominated the scene in Boston during this same period, and together with Grahm, saw that the American hygienic movement – at least as a lay doctrine – was well-established.[3]

Homeopathy

By 1840, the profession of homeopathy had also been transplanted to America from Germany. Homeopathy, the creation of an early German physician, Samuel Hahnemann (1755–1843), had three central doctrines:

- the "law of similars" (that like cures like)
- that the effect of a medication could be heightened by its administration in minute doses (the more diluted the dose, the greater the "dynamic" effect)
- that nearly all diseases were the result of a suppressed itch, or "psora".

The view was that a patient's natural symptom-producing disease would be displaced after homeopathic medication by a similar, but much weaker, artificial disease that the body's immune system could easily overcome.

Originally, most homeopaths in this country were converted orthodox medical men, or "allopaths". The high rate of conversion made this particular medical sect the arch-enemy of the rising orthodox medical profession. (For a more detailed discussion of homeopathy, see Ch. 41.)

The first homeopathic medical school was founded in 1850 in Cleveland; the last purely homeopathic medical school, based in Philadelphia, survived into the early 1930s.[1]

The rise and fall of the sects

Although these two non-allopathic sects were popular, they never comprised more than one-fifth of the professional medical class in America. Homeopathy at its highest point reached roughly 15%, and the eclectic school roughly 5%. However, their very existence for many years kept the exclusive recognition desired by the orthodox profession from coming within its grasp. Homeopathy was distasteful to the more conventional medical men not only because it resulted in the conversion of a substantial number of their peers, but also because homeopaths generally also made a better income. The rejection of the eclectic school was more fundamental: it had its roots in a lay movement that challenged the validity of a privileged professional medical class.

The existence of three professional medical groups – the orthodox school, the homeopaths, and the eclectics – combined with the Jacksonian view of democracy that prevailed in mid-19th century America, resulted in the repeal of virtually all medical licensing statutes existing prior to 1850. But by the 1870s and 1880s, all three medical groups had begun to voice support for the restoration of medical licensing.

There are differing views as to what caused the homeopathic and eclectic schools to disappear from the medical scene in the 50 years following 1875. One view defines a sect as follows:[4]

> A sect consists of a number of physicians, together with their professional institutions, who utilize a distinctive set of medically invalid therapies which are rejected by other sects ...

By this definition, the orthodox or allopathic school was just as sectarian as the homeopathic and eclectics. Rothstein's view is that these two 19th century sects disappeared because, beginning in the 1870s, the orthodox school grasped the European idea of "scientific medicine". Based on the research of such men as Pasteur and Koch, and the "germ theory", this approach supposedly proved to be the medically proper view of valid therapy and gained public recognition because of its truth.

Another view is that the convergence of the needs of the three sects for professional medical recognition (which began in the 1870s and continued into the early 1900s), and the "progressive era", led to a political alliance in which the majority orthodox school ultimately came to be dominant by sheer weight of numbers and internal political authority. As Starr[1] notes (p. 107):

> Both the homeopaths and eclectics wanted to share in the legal privileges of the profession. Only afterward did they lose their popularity. When homeopathic and eclectic doctors were shunned and denounced by the regular profession, they thrived, but the more they gained an access to the privileges of regular physicians, the more their numbers declined. The turn of the century was both the point of acceptance and the moment of incipient disintegration ...

In any event, this development was an integral part of the drive toward professional authority and autonomy established during the progressive era (1900–1917). It was acceptable to the homeopaths and the eclectics because they controlled medical schools that continued to teach and maintain their own professional authority and autonomy. However, it was after these professional goals were attained that the lesser schools of medical thought went into rapid decline.[1]

The American influence

From 1850 through 1900, the medical counterculture continued to establish itself in America. From its lay roots in the teachings of the hygienic movement, there grew professional medical recognition, albeit a small minority and "irregular" view, that hygiene and hydropathy were the basis of sound medical thought (much like the Thomsonian transition to botanic and eclectic medicine).

Trall

The earliest physician who came to have a significant impact on the later growth of naturopathy as a philosophical movement was Russell Trall MD. As noted in Whorton's *Crusaders for Fitness*,[3] he "passed like a meteor through the American hydropathic and hygienic movement" (pp. 138–139):

> The exemplar of the physical educator-hydropath was Russell Thatcher Trall. Still another physician who had lost his faith in regular therapy, Trall opened the second water cure establishment in America, in New York City in 1844. Immediately he combined the full Preissnitzian armamentarium of baths with regulation of diet, air, exercise and sleep. He would eventually open and or direct any number of other hydropathic institutions around the country, as well as edit the *Water-Cure Journal*, the *Hydropathic Review*, and a temperance journal. He authored several books, including popular sex manuals which perpetuated Graham-like concepts into the 1890's, sold Graham crackers and physiology texts at his New York office, was a charter member (and officer) of the American Vegetarian Society, presided over a short-lived World Health Association, and so on. His crowning accomplishment was the Hygeian Home, a "model Health Institution [which] is beautifully situated on the Delaware River between Trenton and Philadelphia." A drawing presents it as a palatial establishment with expansive grounds for walking and riding, facilities for rowing, sailing, and swimming, and even a grove for open-air "dancing gymnastics." It was the grandest of water cures, and lived beyond the Civil War period, which saw the demise of most hydropathic hospitals. True, Trall had to struggle to keep his head above water during the 1860's, but by the 1870's he had a firm financial footing (being stabilized by tuition fees from the attached Hygeio-therapeutic College). With Trall's death in 1877, however, the hydropathic phase of health reform passed.

As will be seen later in this chapter, this plethora of activity is very similar to that engaged in by Benedict Lust between 1896 and his death in 1945, when he worked to establish naturopathic medicine. The Hygeian Home and later "Yungborn" establishments at Butler, New Jersey, and Tangerine, Florida, were very similar to European nature cure sanitariums, such as the original

Yungborn founded by Adolph Just and the spa/sanitarium facilities of Preissnitz, Kneipp and Just.

Trall gave a famous address to the Smithsonian Institution in Washington, DC, in 1862, under the sponsorship of the Washington Lecture Association. "The true healing art: or hygienic vs drug medication", a 2.5 hour lecture purported to have received rapt attention, was devoted to Trall's belief in the hygienic system and in hydropathy as the true healing art. The address was reprinted by Fowler and Wells (New York, 1880) with an introduction written by Trall, prior to his death in 1877.

Trall also founded the first school of natural healing arts in this country to have a 4-year curriculum and the authorization to confer the degree of MD. It was founded in 1852 as a "hydropathic and physiological school" and was chartered by the New York State Legislature in 1857 under the name "New York Hygio-Therapeutic College", with the legislature's authorization to confer the MD degree.

In 1862, Trall went to Europe to attend the International Temperance Convention. At this meeting of reformers, he took prominent part, specifically relating to the use of alcohol as a beverage and as a medicine. He eventually published more than 25 books on the subjects of physiology, hydropathy, hygiene, vegetarianism, and temperance, among many others.

The most valuable and enduring of these was his *Hydropathic Encyclopedia*, a volume of nearly 1,000 pages that covered the theory and practice of hydropathy and the philosophy and treatment of diseases advanced by older schools of medicine. At the time of his death, according to the December 1877 *Phrenological Journal* cover article featuring a lengthy obituary of Trall, this encyclopedia had sold more than 40,000 copies since its original publication in 1851.

For more than 15 years, Trall was editor of the *Water-Cure Journal* (also published by Fowler and Wells). During this period, the journal went through several name changes including the *Hygienic Teacher* and *The Herald of Health*. When Dr Lust originally opened the American School of Naturopathy, an English-language version of *Kneipp's Water-cure* (or in German *Meine Wasser-kurr*) being unavailable, he used only the works and writings of Russell Trall as his texts.

By 1871, Trall had moved from New York to the Hygeian Home on the Delaware River. His water-cure establishment in New York became The New Hygienic Institute. One of the co-proprietors there was Martin Luther Holbrook, who later replaced Trall as the editor of *The Herald of Health*. As noted by Professor Whorton (pp. 139–140):[3]

> But Holbrook's greatest service to the cause was as an editor. In 1866 he replaced Trall at the head of *The Herald of Health*, which had descended from the *Water-Cure Journal* and *Herald of Reforms* (1845–1861) by the way of the *Hygienic Teacher* and *Water-Cure Journal* (1862). Under Holbrook's direction the periodical would pass through two more name changes (*Journal of Hygiene Herald of Health*, 1893–1897, and *Omega*, 1898–1900) before merging with *Physical Culture*.

Trall and Holbrook both advanced the idea that physicians should teach the maintenance of health rather than simply provide a last resort in times of health crisis. Besides providing a strong editorial voice espousing vegetarianism, the evils of tobacco and drugs, and the value of bathing and exercise, dietetics and nutrition along with personal hygiene were strongly advanced by Holbrook and others of the hygienic movement during this era. As described, again by Whorton (pp. 143–144):[3]

> The orthodox hygienists of the progressive years were equally enthused by the recent progress of nutrition, of course, and exploited it for their own ends, but their utilization of science hardly stopped with dietetics. Medical bacteriology was another area of remarkable discovery, bacteriologists having provided, in the short space of the last quarter of the 19th century, an understanding, at long last, of the nature of infection. This new science's implications for hygienic ideology were profound – when Holbrook locked horns with female fashion, for example, he did not attack the bulky, ground-length skirts still in style with the crude Grahamite objection that the skirt was too heavy. Rather he forced a gasp from his readers with an account of watching a smartly dressed lady unwittingly drag her skirt "over some virulent, revolting looking sputum, which some unfortunate consumptive had expectorated."

Holbrook expanded on the work of Graham, Alcott and Trall and, working with an awareness of the European concepts developed by Preissnitz and Kneipp, laid further groundwork for the concepts later advanced by Lust, Lindlahr and others:[3]

> For disease to result, the latter had to provide a suitable culture medium, had to be susceptible. As yet, most physicians were still so excited at having discovered the causative agents of infection that they were paying less than adequate notice to the host. Radical hygienists, however, were bent just as far in the other direction. They were inclined to see bacteria as merely impotent organisms that throve only in individuals whose hygienic carelessness had made their body compost heaps. Tuberculosis is contagious, Holbrook acknowledged, but "the degree of vital resistance is the real element of protection. When there is no preparation of the soil by heredity, predisposition or lowered health standard, the individual is amply guarded against the attack." A theory favored by many others was that germs were the effect of disease rather than its cause; tissues corrupted by poor hygiene offered microbes, all harmless, an environment in which they could thrive. (p. 144)

In addition to introducing the works of Father Kneipp and his teachings to the American hygienic health care movement, Holbrook was a leader of the fight against vivisection and vaccination:[3]

> Vivisection and vaccination were but two of the practices of medicine criticized in the late 19th century. Therapy also continued to be an object of protest. Although the heroism of

standard treatment had declined markedly since mid-century, a prescription was still the reward of any visit to the doctor, and drugless alternatives to healing were appearing in protest. Holbrook published frequent favorable commentaries on the revised water cure system of Germany's Father Kneipp. A combination of baths, herbal teas, and hardening exercises, the system had some vogue in the 1890's before flowering into naturopathy. Holbrook's journal also gave positive notices to osteopathy and "chiropathy" [chiropractic] commending them for not going to the "drugstore or ransack[ing] creation for remedies nor load[ing] the blood with poison." But though bathing and musculoskeletal manipulation were natural and nonpoisonous, Holbrook preferred to give the body complete responsibility for healing itself. Rest and proper diet were the medicines of this doctor who billed himself as a "hygienic physician" and censured ordinary physicians for being engrossed with disease rather than health. (pp. 146–147)

The beginnings of "scientific medicine"

While the hygienic movement was making its impact, the orthodox medical profession, in alliance with the homeopaths and eclectics, was making significant advances. The orthodox profession, through the political efforts of the AMA, had first tried to remove sectarian and irregular practitioners by segregating them from the medical profession altogether. It did so by formulating and publishing its first national medical code of ethics in 1847. (In 1846, the orthodox profession formed the American Medical Association to represent their professional views.) The code condemned proprietary patents (even carrying over into a physician's development of surgical or other medical implements, which led to its greatest criticism); encouraged the adoption of uniform rules for payment in geographical areas; condemned the practice of contract work, prohibited advertising and fee-sharing even among specialists and general practitioners; eliminated blacks and women; and, most significantly, prohibited any consultation or contact with irregulars or sectarian practitioners. As the code stated:[5]

> ... no one can be considered as a regular practitioner, or a fit associate in consultation, whose practice is based on an exclusive dogma, to the rejection of the accumulated experience of the profession, and of the aids actually furnished by anatomy, physiology, pathology, and organic chemistry. (pp. 234–279)

In the late 1870s and into the 1880s, the major sects – the orthodox, or allopathic school, the homeopaths and the eclectics – began to find more reason to cooperate to obtain common professional goals. These included the enactment of new licensing laws and the creation of a "respectable" medical educational system. Also at this time, the concept of "scientific medicine" was brought to America. (Although Starr differs with Rothstein about the cause of the death of the homeopathic and eclectic sectarian schools, he notes that Rothstein clearly documents the transition, during the 19th century, of medicine to a recognized professional class composed of both the minority sects and the orthodox school.)

This transition from conflict between the major sects resulted in the erosion of the implementation of the code of ethics, the cooperation among the sects to revive medical licensing standards, the admission of sectarian physicians to regular medical societies and, ultimately, a structural reorganization of the American Medical Association, which took place between 1875 and 1903.[1,4]

Once the cooperation between the three medical views had begun, the medical class as dominated by the regular school came fully into power. And the homeopathic and eclectic schools of thought met their demise, which was finally brought about by two significant events: the rapid creation of new medical educational standards between 1900 and 1910, culminating in the publication of the famous "Flexner Report" (1910); and the effective infusion of millions of dollars into selected allopathic medical schools by the newly created capitalistic philanthropic foundations, principally the Carnegie and Rockefeller foundations.

The foundations

The impact of the monies from the Carnegie and Rockefeller foundations has been clearly documented[6] and is described in detail, albeit for the advancement of a particular political point of view, in Brown's *Rockefeller Medicine Men*. The impact of the monies from these foundations, as contributed to medical schools that met the AMA's view of medical education and philosophy, cannot be underestimated.

This process has been well documented.[1,6–8] As discussed by Burrows,[8] this educational reform allowed the AMA to form a new alliance with legislators, and push quickly for medical licensing designed to reward the educational and medical expertise of the new orthodox "scientific medicine", and the exclusion of all others.[8]

Medical education in transition

Based upon the rising example of scientific medicine and its necessary connection to research, the educational laboratory, and a more thorough scientific education as a preamble to medical practice, Harvard University (under the presidency of Charles Elliott) created a 4-year medical educational program in 1871. The primal modern medical educational curriculum was devised and set in motion over 20 years later at Johns Hopkins University under the leadership of William Osler and William Welch, using the resources from the original endowment of the hospital and university from the estate of Johns Hopkins.[1]

Other schools followed suit. By the time the American Medical Association set up its Council on Medical

Education in 1904, it was made up of five members from the faculties of schools modeled on the Johns Hopkins prototype. This committee set out to visit and rate each of the (160) medical schools then in operation in the country. The ratings used were class "A" (acceptable), class "B" (doubtful), and class "C" (unacceptable).

Eighty-two schools received a class "A" rating, led by Harvard, Rush (Chicago), Western Reserve, the University of California and, notably, Johns Hopkins. Forty-six received a class "B" rating, and thirty-two a class "C" rating. The class "C" schools were mostly in rural areas and many of them proprietary in nature.

Flexner report

Subsequently to the AMA ratings, the Council on Medical Education applied to the Carnegie Foundation to commission an independent report to verify its work. Abraham Flexner, a young, energetic and noted educator was chosen for this task by the Carnegie Foundation and accompanied by the secretary (Nathan Colwell MD) of the Council on Medical Education, who had participated in all of the committee site visits.

Flexner visited each of the 162 United States medical schools then operating. The publication of the "Flexner Report", which was widely publicized, put the nails in the coffins of all schools with class "C" ratings and many with class "B" ratings. Significantly, the educational programs of all but one eclectic school (in Cincinnati) and one homeopathic school (in Philadelphia) were eliminated by 1918.

The eclectic medical schools, in particular, were severely affected by the report. According to Griggs (p. 251):[2]

> Of the eight Eclectic schools, the Report declared that none had "anything remotely resembling the laboratory equipment which is claimed in their catalogs." Three of them were under-equipped; the rest "are without exception filthy and almost bare. They have at best grimy little laboratories ... a few microscopes, some bottles containing discolored and unlabeled pathological material, in an incubator out of commission, and a horrid dissecting room." The Report found them more culpable than a regular school for these inadequacies: "... the Eclectics are drug-mad; yet, with the exception of the Cincinnati and New York schools, they are not equipped to teach the drugs or drug therapy which constitutes their sole reason for existence."

The other regular schools that had conducted homeopathic or eclectic programs had by that time phased them out in the name of "scientific medicine".

Pharmaceutical industry

During this same period of time, the American Medical Association, through several of its efforts, began a significant alliance with the organized pharmaceutical industry of the United States, shaping that industry in a manner acceptable to the allopathic profession.[1,7,9]

The new "sects"

The period from 1890 through 1905 saw the rise of three new medical sects and several other smaller "irregular" schools which replaced those soon to pass away. In Missouri, Andrew Taylor Still, originally trained as an orthodox practitioner, founded the school of medical thought known as "osteopathy", and in 1892 opened the American School of Osteopathy in Kirksville, Missouri. In 1895, Daniel David Palmer, originally a magnetic healer from Davenport, Iowa, performed the first spinal manipulation, which gave rise to the school he termed "chiropractic". He formally published his findings in 1910, after having founded a chiropractic school in Davenport, Iowa. And, in 1902, Benedict Lust founded the American School of Naturopathy in New York.

Although some of the following discussion will be devoted to the schools of healing called osteopathy and chiropractic, only that portion of their histories related to the history of naturopathy will be mentioned.[10] (A full study of osteopathic medicine in America may be found in *The D.O.'s* by Gevitz[11], and a reasonable sketch of chiropractic medicine may be found in Ronald Lee Kapling's chapter in Salmon.[10])

As noted by Starr,[1] these new sects, including Christian Science, formulated by Mary Baker Eddy (see Silberger[12] for further discussion), either rose or fell on their own without ever completely allying with orthodox medicine. Starr theorized that these sects arose late enough that the orthodox profession and its political action arm, the AMA, had no need to ally with them and would rather battle with them publicly. This made these sectarian views separate and distinct from the homeopathic and eclectic schools.

THE FOUNDING OF NATUROPATHIC MEDICINE

Benedict Lust

Benedict Lust came to the United States in 1892 at the age of 23. He had suffered from a debilitating condition in his late teens while growing up in Michelbach, Baden, Germany, and had been sent by his father to undergo the Kneipp cure at Woerishofen. He stayed there from mid-1890 to early 1892; not only was he "cured" of his condition, but he also became a protégé of Father Kneipp. Dispatched by Kneipp to bring the principles of the Kneipp water cure to America, he emigrated to New York City.

By making contact in New York with other German Americans who were also becoming aware of the Kneipp principles, Lust participated in the founding of the first "Kneipp Society", which was organized in Jersey City, New Jersey, on 3 October 1896.

Lust was also present at the first organizational

meeting (in the middle of October 1896) of the Kneipp Society of Brooklyn, and subsequently, through Lust's organization and contacts, Kneipp Societies were founded in Boston, Chicago, Cleveland, Denver, Cincinnati, Philadelphia, Columbus, Buffalo, Rochester, New Haven, San Francisco, the state of New Mexico, and Mineola on Long Island.

The members of these organizations were provided with copies of the *Kneipp Blatter*, and a companion English publication Lust began to put out called *The Kneipp Water-Cure Monthly*.

The first "sanatorium" using Kneipp's principles was organized in this country shortly before Lust's arrival. Charles Lauterwasser, an earlier student of Kneipp's who called himself a hydrophic physician and natural scientist, opened the Kneipp and Nature Cure Sanatorium in Newark, New Jersey, in 1891.

In 1895, the Brooklyn Light and Water-Cure Institute was established in Brooklyn, New York, by L. Staden and his wife Carola, both graduates of Lindlahr's Hygienic College in Dresden, Germany. According to their advertising, they specialized in natural healing, Kneipp water treatment, Kuhne's and Preissnitz's principles (including diet cure and electric light baths – both white and blue – electric vibration massage, Swedish massage and movements, and Thure-brandt massage).

In 1895, Lust opened the Kneipp Water-Cure Institute in New York City, listing himself as the owner and a Dr William Steffens as the residing physician. At the same address (on 59th Street) in October of that year, Lust opened the first "Kneipp store". In the originating November 1896 edition of *The Kneipp Water-Cure Monthly* and *Kneipp Blatter*, he advertised his store and sanitarium as personally authorized by Father Kneipp.

Father Kneipp died in Germany, at Woerishofen, on 17 June 1897. With his passing, Lust was no longer bound strictly to the principles of the Kneipp water cure. He had begun to associate earlier with other German American physicians, principally Dr Hugo R. Wendel (a German-trained *Naturarzt*) who began, in 1897, to practice in New York and New Jersey, as a licensed osteopathic physician. In 1896, Lust entered the Universal Osteopathic College of New York, graduated in 1898, and became licensed as an osteopathic physician. In 1897, Lust became an American citizen.

Once he was licensed to practice as a health care physician in his own right, Lust began the transition toward the concept of "naturopathy". Between 1898 and 1902, when he adopted the term "naturopath", Lust acquired a chiropractic education and changed the name of his Kneipp store to "health food store" (the original facility to utilize that name and concept in this country), specializing in providing organic foods and the materials necessary for drugless cures. He also began the New York School of Massage (listed as established in 1896) and the American School of Chiropractic, all within the same facility – Lust's Kneipp Institute.

Photographs of this facility taken between 1902 and 1907, when the facility moved to another location, show a five-story building listing "Benedict Lust – Naturopath, Publisher, Importer".

In the first part of 1896, just prior to his organizing of various Kneipp Societies around the New York area, Lust returned to Woerishofen to study further with Father Kneipp. He returned again in 1907 to visit with Dr Baumgarten, Kneipp's medical successor at the Woerishofen facility, which was then run, in cooperation with Baumgarten, by the Reverend Prior Reily, the former secretary to Father Kneipp and his lay successor at Woerishofen. As directed by Kneipp, Reily had completed, after Kneipp's death, Kneipp's master work *Das grosse Kneipp – Buch*. Lust was to maintain contact with the partnership of Reily and Baumgarten throughout the early part of the 20th century.

In 1902, when he purchased and began using the term naturopathy and calling himself a "naturopath", Lust, in addition to his New York School of Massage and American School of Chiropractic, his various publications and his operation of the Health Food Store, began to operate the American School of Naturopathy, all at the same 59th Street address.

By 1907, Lust's enterprises had grown sufficiently large that he moved them to a 55 room building. It housed the Naturopathic Institute, Clinic and Hospital; the American Schools of Naturopathy and Chiropractic; the now entitled "Original Health Food Store"; Lust's publishing enterprises; and New York School of Massage. The operation remained in this four-story building, roughly twice the size of the original facility, from 1907 to 1915.

In the period of 1912 through 1914, Lust took a "sabbatical" from his operations to further his education. By this time he had founded his large estate-like sanitarium at Butler, New Jersey, known as "Yungborn" after the German sanitarium operation of Adolph Just.

In 1912, he attended the Homeopathic Medical College in New York, which, in 1913, granted him a degree in homeopathic medicine and, in 1914, a degree in eclectic medicine. In early 1914, Lust traveled to Florida and obtained an MD's license on the basis of his graduation from the Homeopathic Medical College.

Thereafter, he founded another "Yungborn" sanitarium facility in Tangerine, Florida, and for the rest of his life, while continuing his publications, engaged in active lecturing. He also continued to maintain a practice in New York City, and operated the sanitariums at Tangerine, Florida, and Butler, New Jersey. His schools were operated by Hugo R. Wendel.

From 1902, when he began to utilize the term naturopathy, until 1918, Lust replaced the Kneipp Societies with the Naturopathic Society of America. Then, in December 1919, the Naturopathic Society of America was formally dissolved due to its insolvency and Lust founded the "American Naturopathic Association". Thereafter, the association was incorporated in some additional 18 states.

In 1918, as part of his effort to replace the Naturopathic Society of America (an operation into which he invested a great deal of his funds and resources in an attempt to organize a naturopathic profession) and replace it with the American Naturopathic Association, Lust published the first *Universal Naturopathic Directory and Buyer's Guide* (a "yearbook of drugless therapy").

Although a completely new version was never actually published, in spite of Lust's announced intention to make this volume an annual publication, annual supplements were published in either *The Naturopath and Herald of Health* or its companion publication, with which *The Naturopath* at one time merged, *Nature's Path* (which commenced publication in 1925). The *Naturopath and Herald of Health*, sometimes printed with the two phrases reversed, was published from 1902 through 1927, and from 1934 until after Lust's death in 1945.

This volume documents the merging of the German and American influences which influenced Lust in his development of the practice of naturopathy. The voluminous tome, which ran to 1,416 pages, is dedicated to:

> … the memory of all those noble pioneers and discoverers who have died in the faith of Naturopathy, and to their courageous successors in the art of drugless healing, all of whom have suffered persecution for saving human lives that medical autocracy could not save, this work is respectfully dedicated by its editor Benedict Lust, N.D., M.D., "The Yungborn", Butler, New Jersey, U.S.A., April 1, 1918.

Lust's introduction is reprinted here in its entirety to show the purpose of the directory and the status of the profession in the early 1900s:

Introduction

To the Naturopathic Profession, the Professors of Natural Healing in all its branches, the Professors of Scientific Diet, Hydrotherapy, Heliotherapy, Electrotherapy, Neuropathy, Osteopathy, Chiropractic, Naprapathy, Magnetopathy, Phytotherapy, Exercise, Swedish Movements, Curative Gymnastics, Physical and Mental Culture, Balneopathy, and all forms of Drugless Healing, the Faculties of all Drugless Colleges, Institutions, Schools, and all Professors of Hygiene and Sanitation; Manufacturers of Naturopathic Supplies; Publishers of Health Literature, and Natural Healing Societies, GREETINGS:

I have the honor to present to your consideration and goodwill, this Volume, No. 1, Year 1918–1919, of the Universal Naturopathic Directory, Year Book of Drugless Healing, and Buyers' Guide.

For twenty-two years past, the need of a directory for Drugless Therapy has been felt. The medical world is in a condition of intense evolution at the present time. It is evolving from the Drugging School of Therapy to the Drugless School. People by the million have lost confidence in the virtues of Allopathy and are turning with joyful confidence to the Professions of Natural Healing until it has been estimated that there are at least forty thousand practitioners of Naturopathic healing in the United States.

The motto that IN UNITY THERE IS STRENGTH is the foundation of the present enterprise.

Hitherto, the drugless profession has lacked that prestige in the eyes of the public, which comes from the continuous existence of a big institution, duly organized and wielding the immense authority which is derived no less from organization and history than from the virtues of the principles that are held and practiced by such institutions. The public at large instantaneously respects an institution that is thoroughly organized and has its root earthed in history.

The time has fully arrived when the drugless profession should no longer exist in the form of isolated units, not knowing one another and caring but little for such knowledge. Our profession has been, as it were, as sheep without a shepherd, but the various individuals that constitute this movement so pregnant with benefits to humanity, are now collected for the first time into a Directory and Year-Book of Drugless Healing, which alone will give immense weight and dignity to the standing of the individuals mentioned therein.

Not only will the book add to the prestige of the practitioner in the eyes of his patients, but when the scattered members of our profession in every State desire to obtain legislative action on behalf of their profession and themselves, the appeal of such a work as our directory will, in the eyes of legislators, gain for them a much more respectful hearing than could otherwise be obtained.

Now, for the first time, the drugless practitioner finds himself one of a vast army of professional men and women who are employing the most healthful forces of nature to rejuvenate and regenerate the world. But the book itself throws a powerful light upon every phase of drugless healing and annihilates time and distance in investigating WHO IS WHO in the realm of Drugless Therapy.

A most sincere effort has been made to obtain the name and address of every adherent of the Rational School of Medicine who practices his profession within the United States, Canada and the British Isles. It is impossible at this stage of Naturopathic history, which is still largely in the making, to obtain the name and address of every such practitioner. There were some who, even when appealed to, refused to respond to our invitation, not understanding the object of our work. Many of even the most intelligent members have refused to advertise their professional cards in our pages. But we can only attribute these drawbacks to the fact that every new institution that has suddenly dawned upon human intelligence will find that a certain proportion of people who do not understand the nature of the enterprise because the brain cells that would appreciate the benefits that are sought to be conferred upon them, are undeveloped, but a goodly proportion of our Naturopaths have gladly responded to the invitation to advertise their specialty in our columns. These, of course, constitute the brightest and most successful of our practitioners and their examples in this respect should be followed by every practitioner whose card does not appear in this book.

We take it for granted that every one of the forty thousand practitioners of Naturopathy is in favor of the enterprise represented by this Directory. This work is a tool of his trade and not to possess this book is a serious handicap in the race for success.

Here will be found an Index of by far the larger number of Naturopaths in the country arranged in Alphabetic, Geographic and Naturopathic sections. Besides this, there is a classified Buyers' Guide that gives immediate information regarding where you can find special supplies, or a certain apparatus, or a certain book or magazine, its name, and where it is published. The list of Institutions with the curriculum of each will be found exceedingly useful.

Natural healing, that has drifted so long, and, by reason of a lack of organization, has been made for so many years the football of official medicine, to be kicked by any one who thought fit to do so, has now arrived at such a pitch of power that it has shaken the old system of bureaucratic medicine to its foundations. The professors of the irrational theories of life, health and disease, that are looking for victims to be inoculated with dangerous drugs and animalized vaccines and serums, have begun to fear the growth of this young giant of medical healing that demands medical freedom, social justice and equal rights for the new healing system that exists alone for the betterment and uplifting of humanity.

I want every Professor of Drugless Therapy to become my friend and co-worker in the great cause to which we are committed, and those whose names are not recorded in this book should send them to me without delay. It will be of far greater interest and value to themselves to have their professional card included amongst those who advertise with us than the few dollars that such advertisement costs.

It will be noted that there are quite a number of Drugless Healers belonging to foreign countries (particularly those of the Western Hemisphere) represented in this Directory. The profession of medicine is not confined to any race, country, clime or religion. It is a universal profession and demands universal recognition. It will be a great honor to the Directory, as well as to the Naturopathic profession at large to have every Naturopathic practitioner, from the Arctic Circle to the furthest limits of Patagonia, represented in the pages of this immense and most helpful work.

I expect that the Directory for the year 1920 will be larger and even more important than the present Directory and that it will contain the names of thousands of practitioners that are not included in the present work.

The publication of this Directory will aid in abolishing whatever evils of sectarianism, narrow-mindedness and lack of loyalty to the cause to which we are devoted, that may exist. That it will promote a fraternal spirit among all exponents of natural healing, and create an increase of their prestige and power to resist the encroachments of official medicine on their constitutional rights of liberty and the pursuit of happiness, by favorably influencing Legislators, Law courts, City Councils and Boards of Health everywhere, is the sincere belief of the editor and publisher.

Having introduced the volume, Lust leads off with his article entitled "The principles, aim and program of the nature cure system". Again, this relatively brief article is reproduced here in its entirety, so that one can see the merging of influences:

The principles, aim and program of the nature cure system

Since the earliest ages, Medical Science has been of all sciences the most unscientific. Its professors, with few exceptions, have sought to cure disease by the magic of pills and potions and poisons that attacked the ailment with the idea of suppressing the symptoms instead of attacking the real cause of the ailment.

Medical science has always believed in the superstition that the use of chemical substances which are harmful and destructive to human life will prove an efficient substitute for the violation of laws, and in this way encourages the belief that a man may go the limit in self indulgences that weaken and destroy his physical system, and then hope to be absolved from his physical ailments by swallowing a few pills, or submitting to an injection of a serum or vaccine, that are supposed to act as vicarious redeemers of the physical organism and counteract life-long practices that are poisonous and wholly destructive to the patient's well-being.

From the earliest ages to the present time, the priests of medicine have discovered that it is ten times easier to obtain ten dollars from a man by acting upon his superstition, than it is to extract one dollar from him, by appealing to reason and common sense. Having this key to a gold mine within their grasp, we find official medicine indulging at all times in the most blatant, outrageous, freakish and unscientific methods of curing disease, because the methods were in harmony with the medical prestige of the physician.

Away back in pre-historic times, disease was regarded as a demon to be exorcized from its victim, and the medicine man of his tribe belabored the body of his patient with a bag in which rattled bones and feathers, and no doubt in extreme cases the tremendous faith in this process of cure that was engendered in the mind of the patient really cured some ailments for which mental science and not the bag of bones and feathers should be given credit.

Coming down to the middle ages, the Witches' Broth – one ingredient of which was the blood of a child murderer drawn in the dark of the moon – was sworn to, by official medicine, as a remedy for every disease.

In a later period, the "docteur a la mode", between his taking pinches of snuff from a gold snuff box, would order the patient bled as a remedy for what he denominated spirits, vapors, megrims, or miasms.

Following this pseudo-scientific diagnosis and method of cure, came the drugging phase in which symptoms of disease were unmercifully attacked by all kinds of drugs, alkalis, acids and poisons which were supposed, that by suffocating the symptoms of disease, by smothering their destructive energy, to thus enhance the vitality of the individual. All these cures have had their inception, their period of extensive application, and their certain desuetude. The contemporary fashion of healing disease is that of serums, inoculations and vaccines, which, instead of being an improvement on the fake medicines of former ages are of no value in the cure of disease, but on the contrary introduce lesions into the human body of the most distressing and deadly import.

The policy of expediency is at the basis of medical drug healing. It is along the lines of self-indulgence, indifference, ignorance and lack of self-control that drug medicine lives, moves and has its being. The sleeping swineries of mankind are wholly exploited by a system of medical treatment, founded on poisonous and revolting products, whose chemical composition and whose mode of attacking disease, are equally unknown to their originators, and this is called "Scientific medicine."

Like the alchemist of old who circulated the false belief that he could transmute the baser metals into gold, in like manner the vivisector claims that he can coin the agony of animals into cures for human disease. He insists on cursing animals that he may bless mankind with such curses.

To understand how revolting these products are, let us just refer to the vaccine matter which is supposed to be an efficient preventive of smallpox. Who would be fool enough to swallow the putrid pus and corruption scraped from the foulest sores of smallpox that has been implanted in the body of a calf? Even if any one would be fool enough to drink so atrocious a substance, its danger might be neutralized by the digestive juices of the intestinal tract. But it is a far greater danger to the organism when inoculated into the blood and tissues direct, where no digestive substances can possibly neutralize its poison.

The natural system for curing disease is based on a return to nature in regulating the diet, breathing, exercising, bathing and the employment of various forces to eliminate the poisonous products in the system, and so raise the vitality of the patient to a proper standard of health.

Official medicine has in all ages simply attacked the symptoms of disease without paying any attention to the causes thereof, but natural healing is concerned far more with removing the causes of disease, than merely curing its symptoms. This is the glory of this new school of medicine that it cures by removing the causes of the ailment, and is the only rational method of practicing medicine. It begins its cures by avoiding the uses of drugs and hence is styled the system of drugless healing. It came first into vogue in Germany and its most famous exponents in that country were Priessnitz, Schroth, Kuhne, Kneipp, Rickli, Lahmann, Just, Ehret, Engelhardt, and others.

In Sweden, Ling and others developed various systems of mechano-therapy and curative gymnastics.

In America, Palmer invented Chiropractic; McCormick, Ophthalmology. Still originated Osteopathy; Weltmer, suggestive Therapeutics. Lindlahr combined the essentials of various natural methods, while Kellogg, Tilden, Schultz, Trall, Lust, Lahn, Arnold, Struch, Havard, Davis, Jackson, Walters, Deininger, Tyrell, Collins and others, have each of them spent a lifetime in studying and putting into practice the best ideas of drugless healing and have greatly enlarged and enriched the new school of medicine.

Life Maltreated by Allopathy

The prime object of natural healing is to give the principle of life the line of least resistance, that it may enable man to possess the most abundant health.

What is life?

The finite mind of man fails to comprehend the nature of this mysterious principle. The philosopher says "Life is the sum of the forces that resist death," but that definition only increases its obscurity. Life is a most precious endowment of protoplasm, of the various combinations of oxygen, hydrogen, carbon and nitrogen, and other purely mineral substances in forming organic tissues. As Othello says, referring to Desdemona's life, which he compares to the light of a candle –

"If I quench thee thou flaming minister,
I can thy former light restore
Should I repent me; but once put out THY light,
I know not whence is that Promethean heat
That can thy light relume."

The spark of life flickers in the sockets of millions and is about to go out. What system of medicine will most surely restore that flickering spark to a steady, burning flame?

Will [it be] the system that employs poisonous vaccines, serums and inoculations, whose medical value has to be supported by the most mendacious statements, and whose practitioners are far more intent on their emoluments and fame, than they are in the practice of humanity?

The Allopathic system, which includes nine-tenths of all medical practitioners, is known by its fruits, but it is an appalling fact that infant mortality, insanity, heart disease, arteriosclerosis, cancer, debility, impoverished constitutions, degeneracy, idiocy and inefficiency have enormously increased, particularly during the last twenty-five years, that is, during the regime of inoculations, serums and vaccines.

Naturopathy, on the other hand, so far as it has been developed, and so far as official medicine will allow it to act, leaves no such trail of disease, disaster and death behind it. Natural healing is emancipation from medical superstition, ignorance and tyranny. It is the true Elixir of Life.

The Allopaths have endeavored to cure sick humanity on the basis of the highly erroneous idea that man can change the laws of nature that govern our being, and cure the cause of disease by simply ignoring it. To cure disease by poisoning its symptoms is medical manslaughter.

Dr. Schwenninger of Germany says: "We are suffering under the curse of the past mistakes of our profession. For thousands of years medical doctors have been educating the public into the false belief that poisonous drugs can give health. This belief has become in the public mind such a deep-seated superstition, that those of us who know better and who would like to adopt more sensible, natural methods of cure, can do so only at the peril of losing practice and reputation.

"The average medical man is at his best but a devoted bigot to this vain school-craft, which we call the Medical Art and which alone in this age of science has made no perceptible progress since the days of its earliest teachers. They call it recognized science! Recognized ignorance! The science of to-day is the ignorance of to-morrow. Every year some bold guess lights up as truth to which but the year before the schoolmen of science were as blind as moles."

And Dr. O.W. Holmes, Professor of Anatomy in Harvard University, states: "The disgrace of medicine has been that colossal system of self-deception, in obedience to which mines have been emptied of their cankering minerals, entrails of animals taxed for their impurities, the poison bags of reptiles drained of their venom, and all the inconceivable abominations thus obtained thrust down the throats of human beings, suffering from some fault of organization, nourishment, or vital stimulation."

And these misguided drug doctors are not only not ashamed of their work, but they have induced subservient legislators to pass laws that perpetuate the age-long scandal of allopathic importance, and the degenerative influence of the poisons, and to actually make it a crime on the part of nature doctors to cure a man of his ailment. The brazen effrontery of these medical despots has no limits. They boast of making the State legislators their catspaw in arresting, fining and imprisoning the professors of natural healing for saving human life.

Legislators have no right to sit in judgment over the claims of rival schools of healing. They see tens of thousands of sick people go down to their graves by being denied the cures that the employers of nature's forces alone can give them. It is their business to provide for the various schools of medicine a fair field and no favor.

A citizen has an inalienable right to liberty in the pursuit of happiness. Yet the real saviors of mankind are persecuted by the medical oligarchy which is responsible for compulsory vaccination, compulsory medical inspection of public school children, and the demands for State and Federal departments of health, all for the ostensible good of the people, but in reality for the gain of the Medical Trust.

The Naturopaths

The Naturopaths are desirous of freedom for all schools of medicine. They are responsible practitioners who are willing to be examined by an impartial council, appointed by and acting for the State, who will testify to the life and character of every drugless physician before he is entitled to practice medicine. Not one invidious discrimination should be made between the different schools of medicine. The state should see to it that each school should have a full opportunity to do its best for the up-lifting of its citizens.

The Program of Naturopathic Cure

1. ELIMINATION OF EVIL HABITS, or the weeds of life, such as over-eating, alcoholic drinks, drugs, the use of tea, coffee and cocoa that contain poisons, meat eating, improper hours of living, waste of vital forces, lowered vitality, sexual and social aberrations, worry, etc.

2. CORRECTIVE HABITS. Correct breathing, correct exercise, right mental attitude. Moderation in the pursuit of health and wealth.

3. NEW PRINCIPLES OF LIVING. Proper fasting, selection of food, hydropathy, light and air baths, mud baths, osteopathy, chiropractic and other forms of mechano-therapy, mineral salts obtained in organic form, electropathy, heliopathy, steam or Turkish baths, sitz baths, etc.

Natural healing is the most desirable factor in the regeneration of the race. It is a return to nature in methods of living and treatment. It makes use of the elementary forces of nature, of chemical selection of foods that will constitute a correct medical dietary. The diet of civilized man is devitalized, is poor in essential organic salts. The fact that foods are cooked in so many ways and are salted, spiced, sweetened and otherwise made attractive to the palate, induces people to over-eat, and over eating does more harm than under feeding. High protein food and lazy habits are the cause of cancer, Bright's disease, rheumatism and the poisons of auto-intoxication.

There is really but one healing force in existence and that is Nature herself, which means the inherent restorative power of the organism to overcome disease. Now the question is, can this power be appropriated and guided more readily by extrinsic or intrinsic methods? That is to say, is it more amenable to combat disease by irritating drugs, vaccines and serums employed by superstitious moderns, or by the bland intrinsic congenial forces of Natural Therapeutics, that are employed by this new school of medicine, that is Naturopathy, which is the only orthodox school of medicine? Are not these natural forces much more orthodox than the artificial resources of the druggist? The practical application of these natural agencies, duly suited to the individual case, are true signs that the art of healing has been elaborated by the aid of absolutely harmless, congenial treatments, under whose ministration the death rate is but five per cent of persons treated as compared with fifty per cent under the present allopathic methods.

The Germanic influence

The philosophical origins of naturopathy were clearly Germanic. The most significant influences, except those of Russell Trall and the Osteopathic concepts of A. T. Still (at this time strictly the correction of spinal lesions by adjustment), and the chiropractic principles of D. D. Palmer, were all Germanic. (This is well documented in the January 1902 editorial of *Water Cure Monthly*.)

The specific influences drawn upon by Lust for his work, in order of their chronological contributions to the system of naturopathy, are the following:

1. Vincent Preissnitz (1799–1851)
2. Johann Schroth (1798–1856)
3. Father Sebastian Kneipp (1821–1897)
4. Arnold Rickli (1823–1926)
5 Louis Kuhne (c. 1823–1907)
6. Henry Lahman (no dates known)
7. F. E. Bilz (1823–1903)
8. Adolph Just (?–1939).

Also of note were Theodor Hahn and Meltzer, who, in the 1860s, were well-known for their work in the movement called, in German, *Naturatz* or "naturism".

In photographs accompanying his article "The principles, aim and program of the nature cure system", Lust described each of these thinkers as follows:

1. VINCENT PREISSNITZ, of Graefenberg, Silesia. Founder of Hydropathy. Born October 4, 1799. A pioneer Naturopath, prosecuted by the medical authorities of his day, and convicted of using witchcraft, because he cured his patients by the use of water, air, diet and exercise. He took his patients back to Nature – to the woods, the streams, the open fields – treated them with Nature's own forces and fed them on natural foods. His fame spread over the whole of Europe, and even to America. His cured patients were numbered by the thousands. The Preissnitz compress or bandage is in the medical literature. Preissnitz is no more, but his spirit lives in every true Naturopath.

2. JOHANN SCHROTH, a layman, not described in Lust's directory, but often talked of in later works and prominently mentioned for his curative theories in Bilz's master work *The Natural Method of Healing*. Schroth smashed his right knee in an accident with a horse and it remained stiff in spite of repeated medical treatment. At last, a priest told Schroth that Preissnitz's methods might help, and Schroth decided to give them a try. In order to avoid frequent changing of the packs that were directed by Preissnitz, he placed several packs on top of one another, wrapping the whole portion with a woolen cloth. He left this pack on the injured knee for several hours and produced a moist heat which he theorized to cause the poisonous toxins to dissolve and be swept away. These packs are still used as part of the "Schroth cure" and have reportedly become famous for their blood-cleansing effect. (From an article in the March 1937 *Naturopath and Herald of Health* by Dr. T.M. Schippel.) As noted by Bilz, the Schroth cure, called by Bilz "the regenerative treatment," was developed for treatment of chronic diseases through the use of an extreme diet following total fasting by withdrawing of all food and drink and then the use of totally dry grain products and the eventual reintroduction of fluids.

3. FATHER SEBASTIAN KNEIPP, of course, is much described and the photos include one of Kneipp lecturing to the multitudes at Wandelhale at Woerishofen, attending Pope Leo XIII in 1893, noting this is the only consultation on health care matters that Kneipp ever consented to outside of Woerishofen, though many famous and aristocratic individuals desired his counsel, and a picture of Kneipp with

the Archdukes Joseph and Francis Ferdinand of Austria walking barefoot in new-fallen snow for purposes of hardening the constitution. It was noted that the older Archduke was cured by Father Kneipp of Bright's disease in 1892, and it noted that the Archduke Joseph, in appreciation of this cure, donated a public park in the town of Woerishofen at a cost of $150,000 florens. The Archduke Francis Ferdinand, the son of Archduke Joseph, was the individual whose murder precipitated World War I. There is a further picture of Father Kneipp surrounded by "Doctors" from different parts of the world while he gave consultation to numerous patients.

4. ARNOLD RICKLI, founder of the light and light and air cures (atmospheric cure). Dr. Rickli was one of the foremost exponents of natural living and healing. In 1848, he established at Veldes, Krain, Austria, the first institution of light and air cure or as it was called in Europe the "atmospheric cure". In a limited way (rather very late) his ideas have been adopted by the medical profession in America for the cure of consumption. He was an ardent disciple of the vegetarian diet and exemplified the principles of natural living in his own life. The enclosed photo shows him at the age of 97, when he was still active and healthy. He has since passed on, but his work still lives as a testimonial of his untiring efforts. He was the founder and for over 50 years the President of the National Austrian Vegetarian Association.

5. LOUIS KUHNE wrote, in 1891, *The New Science of Healing,* the greatest work of basic principles in natural healing. In the tradition of Natural Healing and prevention, Kuhne has been described as one who "... advocated sun, steam baths, a vegetarian diet, and whole-wheat bread ..." in these relatively early days". His renowned work constitutes the only true scientific philosophy for the application of all Drugless Methods. He was the first to give to the world the comprehensible idea of pathology and the first to proclaim the doctrine of the "unity of cure." His book *Facial Expression* gives the means of diagnosing a patient's pathological condition and determining the amount and location of the systemic encumbrance. He is the founder and first Master of Naturopathy.

6. DR. H. LAHMAN. When the University of Leipzig expelled H. Lahman for his spreading medical sedition among the students, it added a staunch advocate to natural healing. Dr. Lahman finished his medical education in Switzerland and returned to Germany to refute in practice the false ideas of medical science. He later founded the largest Nature Cure institution in the world at Weisser Hirsch, near Dresden, Saxony. He was a strong believer in the "Light and Air" cure and constructed the first appliances for the administration of electric light treatment and baths. He was the author of several books on Diet, Nature Cure and Heliotherapy. As noted in *Other Healers, Other Cures*: "Heinrich Lahmann came along to stress no salt on foods and no water with meals ..."* His works on diet are authoritative and his "nutritive salts theory" forms the basis of rational dietetic treatment. This work has but recently come to light in America, and progressive dietitians are forsaking their old, worn-out, high protein, chemical and caloric theories for the "organic salts theory." Carque, Lindlahr, McCann, and other wide awake food scientists have adopted it as a basis for their work. Dr. Lahman was a medical nihilist. He denounced medicine as unscientific and entirely experimental in its practice and lived to prove the saneness of his ideas as evidenced by his thousands of cured patients.

7. PROFESSOR F.E. BILZ. That real physicians are born, not made, is well illustrated in the case of Dr. Bilz, who achieved his first success in healing as a lay practitioner. As a mark of gratitude, a wealthy patient presented him with land and a castle in which to found a Nature Cure sanitarium... The Bilz institution at Dresden-Rdebeul, Germany, became world renowned and was long considered the center of the Nature Cure movement. Professor Bilz is the author of the first Naturopathic encyclopedia, *The Natural Method of Healing,* which has been translated into a dozen languages, and in German alone has run into 150 editions. He has written many works on Nature Cure and Natural Life, among them being *The Future State,* in which he predicted the present World War, and advocated a federation of nations as the only logical solution of international problems.

8. ADOLPH JUST, famous author of Return to Nature and founder of original 'Yungborn' in Germany.

Both Adolph Just's *Return to Nature* and Louis Kuhne's *The Natural Science of Healing* were translated into English by Lust and released through his publication house.

The convergence with American influences

The Universal Naturopathic Directory was truly eclectic in its compilation and composition. Besides the Lust article noted previously, the volume included: "How I became acquainted with nature cure" by Henry Lindlahr MD ND (which has been reproduced in large part in the introduction to volume 1 of Lindlahr[13]); "The nature cure" by Carl Strueh MD ND; "Naturopathy" by Harry E. Brook ND; "The present position of naturopathy and allied therapeutic measures in the British Isles" by J. Allen Pattreiouex ND; "Why all drugless methods?" by Per Nelson; and "Efficiency in drugless healing" by Edward Earle Purinton (a reprint of the 1917 publication, referred to earlier, which was composed of a series of articles published in *The Herald of Health and Naturopath* between August 14 and February 1916).

The volume also contained Louis Kuhne's "Neo-naturopathy (the new science of healing)" in the first publication of the translation by Lust, and articles on electrotherapy, neuropathy, dietology, chiropractic, mechanotherapy, osteopathy, phytotherapy, apyrtropher, physical culture, optometry, hydrotherapy, orthopedics, pathology, natural healing and living, astroscopy, phrenology, and physiology – all of which were specially commissioned for the directory from practitioners and authors considered expert in these subjects.

The volume also included the directory of drugless physicians in alphabetical order, geographically arranged, and itemized by profession; biographical notes on American contributors of note; the naturopathic book catalog; a guide to natural healing and natural life books and periodicals; a classified list of medical works, a series of book reviews; a buyer's guide for naturopathic supplies; and, in addition to extensive indexes, a "parting word" by Lust.

*See Kruger.[16]

In addition, the volume contained numerous advertisements for naturopathic schools, sanitariums and individual practices, and closed with the following note:

> This, then, completes Volume 1 of the Naturopathic Directory, Drugless Yearbook and Buyer's Guide for the years 1918 and 1919.
>
> Into it, has been placed the conscientious labor of many willing hearts, hands and minds. It is their contribution to the noble cause of natural healing. It will stand as a monument to their endeavors, as well as a memorial to the great souls, the fathers of natural healing, who have passed on.
>
> Let this, then, herald a new era – the era wherein man shall recognize the omniscience of Nature, and shall profit through conforming to her laws.

In the biographical section, it becomes apparent that Lust owed a great deal of the feeling of camaraderie in the nature cure movement to some varied American practitioners. The most prominent of these have had their biographical sections as contained in the 1918 directory. Two of them deserve specific note and attention: Palmer and Still.

Lust met *A. T. Still* in 1915 in Kirksville, Missouri, shortly before Still's death. From their meetings, Lust noted later in the *Naturopath and Herald of Health* (June 1937) that Still believed that osteopathy by "... compromising with medicine ... is doomed as the school that could have incorporated all the natural and biological healing arts ...". Lust wanted naturopathy to fill this void.

Lust also had lengthy acquaintance with B. J. Palmer (the son of D. D. Palmer, the founder of chiropractic), who, following in his father's footsteps, put Davenport, Iowa, and the Palmer Chiropractic College on the map.

Lust also became connected with Henry Lindlahr MD ND of Chicago, Illinois (as noted in the autobiographical sketch contained in the directory[14] and reprinted in the volume 1 of Lindlahr[13]). Lindlahr was a rising businessman in Chicago with all the bad habits of the "gay nineties" era. Only in his 30s, he had begun to be chronically ill. He had gone to the orthodox practitioners of his day and received no relief.

Then he was exposed to Schroth's works, and in following them began to feel somewhat better. Subsequently, he liquidated all his assets and went to Germany to stay in a German sanitarium to be cured and to learn nature cure. He then came back to Chicago and enrolled in the Homeopathic/Eclectic College of Illinois. In 1903, he opened a sanitarium, which included a residential sanitarium, located in Elmhurst, Illinois, a "transient" clinic (office) on State Street in Chicago, and "Lindlahr's Health Food Store".

Shortly thereafter he founded the Lindlahr College of Natural Therapeutics, which included hospital internships at the sanitarium. The institution became one of the leading naturopathic colleges of the day. In 1908, he began to publish *Nature Cure Magazine* and began publishing his series of *Philosophy of Natural Therapeutics*, with volume 1 ("Philosophy") in 1918. This was followed by volume 2 ("Practice") in 1919, volume 3 ("Dietetics"; republished with revisions as it had originally been published in 1914), and, in 1923, volume 6 ("Iridiagnosis"). The intended volumes 4 and 5 were in production at the time of Lindlahr's death in 1927. As described in *Other Healers, Other Cures*:

> Henry Lindlahr, another American, is remembered for his conviction that disease did not represent an invasion of molecules, but the body's way of healing something. In other words, he viewed symptoms as a positive physiological response-proof that the body is fighting whatever's wrong. Accordingly, a fever is a "healthy" sign and one should be let alone, unless it is dangerously high, of course.

The impact of all of these gentlemen on the development of naturopathy in America, under Lust's guidance, was profound.

From these beginnings, the naturopathic movement gathered strength and continued to grow through the 1920s and 1930s, having a major impact on natural healing and natural lifestyle in the United States.

Along the way, Lust was greatly influenced by the writings of *John H. Tilden* MD (largely published between 1915 and 1925). Tilden was originally a practicing physician in Denver, Colorado, who became disenchanted with orthodox medicine and began to rely heavily on dietetics and nutrition, formulating his theories of "autointoxication" (the effect of fecal matter remaining too long in the digestive process) and "toxemia".

Lust was also greatly influenced by *Elmer Lee* MD, who became a practicing naturopath in about 1910, and whose movement was called the "hygienic system", following the earlier works of Russell Trall. Lee published *Health Culture* for many years.

In addition to John Tilden MD and Elmer Lee MD, another medical doctor, *John Harvey Kellogg* MD, who turned to more nutritionally based natural healing concepts, was greatly respected by Lust. Kellogg was renowned through his connection with the Battle Creek Sanitarium. The sanitarium itself was originally founded in the 1860s as a Seventh Day Adventist institution designed to perpetuate the Grahamite philosophies of Sylvester Graham and William Alcott. The sanitarium was on the verge of being closed, however, due to economic failure, when in 1876 Kellogg, a new and more dynamic physician-in-chief, was appointed.

Kellogg, born in 1852, was a "sickly child" who, at the age of 14, ran across the works of Graham and converted to vegetarianism. At the age of 20 he studied for a term at Trall's Hygio-Therapeutic College and then earned a medical degree at New York's Bellevue Medical School. He maintained an affiliation with the regular schools of medicine during his lifetime, due more to his practice of surgery, than his beliefs in the area of health care.[3]

Kellogg designated his concepts, which were basically the hygienic system of healthful living, "biologic living". Principally, Kellogg defended vegetarianism, attacked sexual misconduct and the evils of alcohol, and was a prolific writer through the late 19th century and early 20th century. He produced a popular periodical, *Good Health*, which continued in existence until 1955. When Kellogg died in 1943 at the age of 91, he had had more than 300,000 patients through the Battle Creek Sanitarium (which he had renamed from Western Health Reform Institute shortly after his appointment in 1876), including many celebrities, and the "San" became nationally well known.

Kellogg, along with Tilden and Elie Metchnikoff (director of the prestigious Pasteur Institute and winner of the 1908 Nobel Prize for a contribution to immunology), wrote prolifically on the theory of "auto-intoxication". Kellogg, in particular, felt that humans, in the process of digesting meat, produced a variety of intestinal self-poisons that contributed to "auto-intoxication".

As a result, Kellogg became a near fanatic on the subject of helping humans to return to a more healthy natural state by returning to the naturally designed usage of the colon. He felt that the average modern colon was devitalized by the combination of sedentary living, the custom of sitting rather than squatting to defecate, and the modern civilized habit of ignoring "nature's call" out of an undue concern for politeness. Further, Kellogg concentrated on the fact that the modern diet had insufficient bulk and roughage to stimulate the bowels to proper action.

Kellogg was also extremely interested in hydrotherapy. In the 1890s, he established a laboratory at the San to study the clinical applications of hydrotherapy. This led, in 1902, to his writing *Rational Hydrotherapy*. The preface espoused a philosophy of drugless healing that came to be one of the bases of the hydrotherapy school of medical thought in America.

Tilden, as mentioned, was of a similar mind. Indeed, he had to have been to have provided natural health care literature with his 200-plus page dissertation entitled "constipation", with a whole chapter devoted to the evils of not responding when nature called.

This belief in the "evils" drawing away from the natural condition of the colon was extremely important to Kellogg's work.[3] Because of Lust's interest, Kellogg's *The New Dietetics* (1921) became one of the bibles of naturopathic literature.[15]

Lust was also influenced by the works of *Sidney Weltmer*, the father of "suggestive therapeutics". The theory behind Professor Weltmer's work was that whether it was the mind or the body that first lost its grip on health, the two were inseparably related. When the problem originated in the body, the mind nonetheless lost its ability and desire to overcome the disease because the patient "felt sick", and consequently slid further into the diseased state. Alternatively, if the mind first lost its ability and desire to "be healthy" and some physical infirmity followed, the patient was susceptible to being overcome by disease.

Weltmer's work dealt specifically with the psychological process of desiring to be healthy. Lust enthusiastically backed Weltmer's work and had him on the program at various of the annual conventions of the American Naturopathic Association (which commenced after its founding in 1919).

Lust was also personal friends with and a deep admirer of *Bernarr MacFadden*. MacFadden was the founder of the "physical culture" school of health and healing, also known as "physcultopathy". This school of healing gave birth across the country to gymnasiums at which exercise programs, designed to allow the individual man or woman to maintain the most perfect state of health and human condition possible, were developed and taught.[3] As described in *Other Healers, Other Cures* (p. 182):[16]

> The next Naturopathic star, after Kellogg, was Bernarr MacFadden, the physical culturist who built a magazine-publishing empire (his first magazine was *Physical Culture* founded in 1898.) MacFadden proselytizes for exercise and fresh vegetables, hardly eccentric notions. But his flamboyant efforts to publicize them and his occasional crack-pot ideas (like freezing the unemployed, then thawing them out when the Depression was over) alienated many people. Still, he was his own best advertisement. He fathered nine children by four wives and was parachuting from planes in his 80s. One of MacFadden's admirers was that arch-foe of the medical profession, George Bernard Shaw, the longevous eccentric in his own right …

Lust was also very interested in, and helped to publicize "zone therapy", originated by *Joe Shelby Riley* DC, a chiropractor based in Washington, DC, and one of the early practitioners of "broad chiropractic". Zone therapy was an early forerunner of acupressure as it related "… pressures and manipulations of the fingers and tongue, and percussion on the spinal column, according to the relation of the fingers to certain zones of the body …".[14]

Several other American drugless healers contributed to a broad range of "-opathies" that Lust merged into his growing view of naturopathy as the eclectic compilation of methods of natural healing. The *Universal Directory* also contained a complete list of osteopaths and chiropractors as drugless healers within the realm of Lust's view of naturopathic theory. His other significant compatriots at the time of the publication of the directory were Carl Stueh, described by Lust as "… one of the first medical men in this country who gave up medicine and operation for natural healing", F. W. Collings MD DO DC, an early graduate of the American School of Naturopathy (1907) who went on to graduate from the

New Jersey College of Osteopathy (1909) and the Palmer School of Chiropractic (1912), another "broad chiropractor", Anthony Matijaca MD ND DO, the naturopathic resident expert in electrotherapy and an associate editor of the *Herald and Health Naturopath* (the inverted name of the Lust journal at the time of the directory), and Carl Schultz ND DO MD, president and general manager of the Naturopathic Institute and Sanitorium of California, essentially the second school in the country to pursue the education of physicians under the name of "naturopathy."

EARLY 20th-CENTURY MEDICINE

The metamorphosis of orthodox medicine

In many ways, the progressive health era of 1900–1917 not only marked the formative years of naturopathy, but were also its halcyon days. In many jurisdictions, modern licensing laws, crafted during this time, were not yet in effect, so varied views of health care could be openly practiced. By 1920, however, the American world of medicine had undergone a sharp transition, culminating four decades of change.

A look at the structure of early medical care in the United States, even as practiced and dominated by the orthodox school, is instructive, when one notes the changes occurring between 1875 and 1920.

In 1875 the following was generally true of American medical practice:

- The practice, even in urban areas, sent the doctor to the patient; the "house call" was the norm.
- There was little modern licensing regulation.
- Hospitals were charitable institutions where persons too poor to otherwise receive health care were usually sent when ill.
- The AMA, although formed in 1846, and generally representative of the professional goals of the regular or orthodox school of medicine, had scarcely begun to make any political inroads at all.
- Medical schools required little or no college education for entrance, and were largely apprenticeship-based and proprietary in nature, having changed little throughout the century.
- Although some doctors had begun to specialize, to do so was far from the norm. The major recognized specialties were surgery, obstetrics and gynecology.
- There were many different types of doctors and society's recognition of the profession neither recognized specific expertise nor necessarily rewarded professionals in medical practice well.
- Although the orthodox school made up roughly 80% of the professional medical practitioners, the homeopaths and the eclectics were visible and respected in their own communities for their abilities and expertise, and much of the public relied on other "irregular" practitioners.

By comparison, in 1920, total metamorphosis of medicine as a profession had occurred:

- By 1920, practices had become office- and clinic-oriented.
- Modern licensing principles had become fully developed, and physicians and surgeons were licensed in all jurisdictions. Most other health care providers had some licensing restrictions placed upon them if they were recognized at all.
- Due largely to the introduction into surgery of the practice of antiseptic techniques and aseptic procedures, and a correspondent decline in operative mortality, institutional care in the hospital became increasingly accepted. Also, clinical pathology and diagnostic laboratory procedures had become well developed, the hospital had become a major training and clinical research facility, and generally more acceptable to the patient.
- The AMA was approaching the peak of its political power, having exercised, through its Council on Medical Education and its Council of Pharmacy and Chemistry, major effects on medical schools and the pharmaceutical industry.
- The transition to research and education-based medical schools, instead of practitioner apprenticeships and proprietary education, had become complete. All recognized medical schools had a 4-year curriculum, with an undergraduate degree or substantial undergraduate study required as a prerequisite. In addition, most schools, in conjunction with most licensing statutes, required a year's internship.
- Specialization was becoming well developed, and the number of specialty groups had increased considerably. This would continue through the 1930s and into the early 1940s.
- Professional authority and autonomy had undergone a substantial transition; and the allopathic physician was now recognized as the medical expert.
- By 1922, the last eclectic school was on the verge of closure, and in the early 1930s the last of the homeopathic schools in the United States was also on the verge of closure. The influence of these sects on orthodox medicine had dwindled to almost nothing. Naturopaths and other alternative health care practitioners had adopted the areas of expertise previously considered the territory of homeopaths and eclectics.

The halcyon years of naturopathy

In 1924, Morris Fishbein succeeded George Simmons as editor of the *Journal of the American Medical Association* (*JAMA*). Fishbein had joined the editorial staff of *JAMA* under Simmons immediately following his graduation from Chicago's Rush Medical School in 1913. As Campion points out:[7]

Over the years Fishbein not only established himself as the gifted editor of the most widely read medical journal in the United States; he also learned how to extend his editorial position, how to project his opinions nationwide. He became, as the saying went in those years, a "personality." TIME referred to him as "the nation's most ubiquitous, the most widely maligned, and perhaps most influential medico."

In addition to his development of *JAMA* as an editorial and personal voice, Fishbein also continually railed against "quackery". Lust, among others, including MacFadden, became Fishbein's epitome of quackery. When MacFadden became a wealthy man, after his publishing company included popular magazines like *True Confessions* and *True Detective,* he began campaigning for the 1936 Republican presidential nomination. In response, a physician submitted, under the initials "K.G.", a tongue-in-cheek listing of the cabinet that would exist under MacFadden, including the newly created "Secretary of Aviation" for Benedict Lust. Lust was a popular figure by this time who conducted such a busy lecture schedule and practice, alternating between the "Yungborns" in Butler, New Jersey, and Tangerine, Florida, that he had become almost as well known as an airline traveler. Lust devoted a complete editorial in *Nature's Path* to a response.

If Fishbein had *JAMA* as a personal editorial outlet, Lust had his own publications. Commencing with the *Naturopath and Herald of Health* in 1902 (which changed its name to *Herald of Health and Naturopath* in 1918), Lust continually published this and other monthly journals. In 1919, it became the official journal of the American Naturopathic Association, mailed to all members. Each edition contained the editorial column "Dr Lust speaking".

In the early 1920s, the "health fad" movement was reaching its peak in terms of public awareness and interest. As described, somewhat wistfully, in his June 1937 column, Lust announced the approach of the 41st Congress of Natural Healing under his guidance:

The progress of our movement could be observed in our wonderful congresses, in 1914 Butler, N.J., 1915 Atlantic City, 1916 in Chicago, 1917 Cleveland, 1918 New York, 1919 Philadelphia, 1920 and 1921 again New York, and 1922 in Washington, D.C., where we had the full support and backing of the Congress of the United States. President Harding received the president and the delegates of our convention and we were the guests of the City of Washington. Through the strenuous efforts of Dr. T.M. Schippel, Hon. Congresswoman Catherine Langley of Kentucky, and eight years of hard work financed and sustained by Dr. Schippel and her powerful friends in Congress, Naturopathy was fully legalized as a healing art in the District of Columbia and the definition was placed on record and the law affirmed and amended by another act which has been fully published over and over again in the official journal of the A.N.A., *Naturopath.*

In 1923 in Chicago, with the help and financing of the great and never-to-be forgotten Dr. Henry Lindlahr, we had a great convention. Not only were all the Naturopaths there but even to an extent our congress was recognized and acknowledged as official and of great importance by the medical people, particularly by the Health Commissioner of Chicago. We held a banquet, and there were discussions covering all platforms of the healing art. It was the first congress in the United States where medicine and Naturopathy in all its branches such as the general old-time Nature Cure, Hydrotherapy and Diet, Osteopathy, Naprapathy, Chiropractic, Neuropathy and Physiotherapy were represented on the same platform. The speakers represented every modern school of healing and the movement at that time was in the direction of an entirely recognized and independent school of healing. There were two camps, official medicine and official Naturopathy, the medical camp having all that is good and bad in medicine and surgery and all the other schools of healing that had sold their birthright and trusted to the allurement of organized medicine, such as Homeopaths, Eclectics, Physio-medics, and the Osteopaths to a large extent. The Osteopaths were always in the wrong camp when they went on mixed boards and Dr. Andrew Taylor Still, the father of Osteopathy, told me in 1915 that by compromising with medicine Osteopathy is doomed as the school that could have incorporated all of the natural and biological healing arts.

The year following we had the great congress in Los Angeles which has never been duplicated. We had to meet in two hotels because the crowds ran over 10,000. The glorious banquet will never be forgotten and the congress celebrated and demonstrated that the initial and first intent of the A.N.A. to teach the public Natural Living and Nature Cure was realized. We will never forget the glorious week in Los Angeles where the authorities and the whole city joined us. The success of that congress was largely due to the talent of Dr. Fred Hirsch, the successor to Prof. Arnold Ehret and the noble and generous Naturopaths of the A.N.A. of Cal. There was never a second congress like that.

Then we had the great congresses of New York in 1925, Indianapolis 1926, Philadelphia 1927, Minneapolis 1928, Portland, Oregon 1929, New York 1930, Milwaukee 1931, Washington, D.C., 1932, Chicago 1933, Denver 1934, San Diego 1935, and Omaha 1936.

In 1925, Lust began to try to reach more of the general populace through the lay publication *Nature's Path. The Naturopath* and *Nature's Path* were later merged because the self-supporting advertising and subscription monies were more available by publication to the general populace than to the members of the association (*The Naturopath,* 1902–1927; *Nature's Path,* 1925–1927; merged 1927–1933; separated 1934–1938; *Nature's Path,* 1939–?).

In January of 1934, Lust commenced republication under the title *Naturopath and Herald of Health* in addition to *Nature's Path.* Each of the volumes opened with his column, which was different for each publication. Both publications were issued continuing through 1938, when the *Nature's Path* again became the sole publication until Lust's death in 1945.

Although, after the *Universal Directory,* Lust continued to write volumes on naturopathic principles, he was more of a synthesizer, organizer, lecturer, and essayist than a lasting scientific author of naturopathic articles.

His most enduring contributions remain his early translations of Kuhne's and Just's works.

During the 1920s and up until 1937, Lust's brand of "quackery", as labeled by Fishbein, was in its most popular phase. Although the institutional markings of the orthodox school had gained ascendancy, prior to 1937 it had no real solutions to the problems of human disease.

Instructive in this regard is Louis Thomas' interesting work *The Youngest Science*. Thomas compares his education and internship as a physician to his father's life as a physician. His father believed that bedside manner was more important than any actual medication offered by the physician. Indeed, his father went into general surgery so that he could offer some service to his patients that actually made some change in their condition. Thomas points out that the major growth of "scientific medicine" up until 1937 advanced diagnosis rather than offering any hope of cure.

During this period of time, Lust's naturopathic medicine, and both chiropractic and osteopathic medicine, continued to be on the outside looking in. Practitioners of all three groups were continually prosecuted for practicing medicine without a license, although they often won their cases by establishing before juries that their practices were, even according to the testimony of medical men, not the same at all. Additionally, because the orthodox practitioners could offer little or no actual hope of cure for many diseases, the "health food and natural health" movement was generally popular.

During the 1920s, *Gaylord Hauser*, later to become the health food guru of the Hollywood set, came to Lust as a seriously ill young man. Lust, through application of the nature cure, removed Hauser's afflictions and was rewarded by Hauser's lifelong devotion. His regular columns in *Nature's Path* became widely read among the Hollywood set.

As noted in *Other Healers, Other Cures* (p. 183):[16]

> The last big name in Naturopathy was Gaylord Hauser, a Viennese-Born food scientist (as one of his early books identified him) turned to Naturopathy in his later years. He is best remembered for advising the eating of living foods, not dead foods, and for escorting Greta Garbo around. In addition to fresh fruits and vegetables, Hauser's "Wonder Foods" were skinned milk, brewers yeast, wheat germ, yogurt, and black strap molasses.

In 1937, however, all this began to change. The change came, as both Thomas and Campion note in their works, with the era of "miracle medicine". Lust recognized this and his editorializing became, if anything, even more strident. From the introduction of sulfa drugs in 1937 to the Salk vaccine's release in 1955, the American public became used to annual developments of miracle vaccines and antibiotics.

Benedict Lust died in September of 1945 in residence at the Yungborn facility in Butler, New Jersey, preparing to attend the 49th Annual Congress of his American Naturopathic Association. On 30 August 1945, for the official program of that congress which was held in October 1945 just after his death, he dictated the following remarks:

> What is the present condition of Naturopathy? What is its future? I can give my opinion in a very few words. For fifty years I have been in the thick of the fight to bring to the American people the Nature Cure. During that period I have had an opportunity to judge what Naturopathy has done, and can accomplish and the type of men and women, past and present, who make up the Naturopathic ranks.
>
> Let us take the present situation first. What is Naturopathy accomplishing? The answer to that is: "Everything." Naturopathy holds the key for the prevention, alleviation and cure of every ailment, to man and beast alike. It has never failed in the hands of a competent Naturopath. Whatever the body can "catch" – that same body, with proper handling, can eliminate. And that takes in cancer, tumors, arthritis, cataract and the whole gamut of "incurable medical" disease and ailments. During my years of practice I, personally, have seen every type of human ailment and so-called serious "disease" give way to the simple, proven Naturopathic methods. I make no exception to that statement.
>
> Now let us see the type of men and women who are the Naturopaths of today. Many of them are fine, upstanding individuals, believing fully in the effectiveness of their chosen profession – willing to give their all for the sake of alleviating human suffering and ready to fight for their rights to the last ditch. More power to them! But there are others who claim to be Naturopaths who are woeful misfits. Yes, and there are outright fakers and cheats masking as Naturopaths. That is the fate of any science – any profession – which the unjust laws have placed beyond the pale. Where there is no official recognition and regulation, you will find the plotters, the thieves, the charlatans operating on the same basis as the conscientious practitioners. And these riff-raff opportunists bring the whole art into disrepute. Frankly such conditions cannot be remedied until suitable safeguards are erected by law, or by the profession itself, around the practice of Naturopathy. That will come in time.
>
> Now let us look at the future. What do we see? The gradual recognition of this true healing art – not only because of the efforts of the present conscientious practitioners but because of the bungling, asinine mistakes of orthodox medicine – Naturopathy's greatest enemy. The fiasco of the sulpha drugs as emphasized disastrously in our armed forces is just one straw in the wind. The murderous Schick test – that deadly "prevention" of diphtheria – is another. All these medical crimes are steadily piling up. They are slowly, but inevitably, creating a public distrust in all things medical. This increasing lack of confidence in the infallibility of Modern Medicine will eventually make itself felt to such an extent that the man on the street will turn upon these self-constituted oppressors and not only demand but force a change. I may not be here to witness this revolution but I believe with all my soul that it is coming. Yes, the future of Naturopathy is indeed bright. It merely requires that each and every true Naturopath carry on – carry on – to the best of his and her abilities. May God bless you all.

The naturopathic journals of the 1920s and 1930s are instructive. Much of the dietary advice focused on poor eating habits, including the lack of fiber in the diet and an overreliance upon red meat as a protein source. Over half a century later in the 1980s, the pronouncements of the orthodox profession, the National Institute of Health and the National Cancer Institute finally became aware of the validity of the early assertions of the naturopaths that such dietary habits would lead to degenerative diseases, including cancers associated with the digestive tract and the colon.

The December 1928 volume of *Nature's Path* was the first American publication of the works of Herman J. DeWolff, a Dutch epidemiologist who was one of the first individuals to assert, based on studies of the incidence of cancer in the Netherlands, that there was a correlation between exposure to petrochemicals and various types of cancerous conditions. He saw a connection between chemical fertilizers and their usage in some soils (principally clay) that led to their remaining in vegetables after they had arrived at the market and were purchased for consumption. Again, it was 50 years later before orthodox medicine began to see the wisdom of such assertions.

The emerging dominance of AMA medicine

The introduction of "miracle medicine", the impact of World War II on health care, and the death of Benedict Lust in 1945, all combined to cause the decline of naturopathic medicine and natural healing in the United States. (During the war, the necessity for crisis surgical intervention techniques for battlefront wounds encouraged use of morphine and sulfa drugs, and penicillin for diseases not previously encountered by American citizens. This resulted in rapid development of high-technology approaches to medicine and highly visible successes.)

The effects of these events on osteopathy and chiropractic, however, were completely different. In the early days of osteopathy, there was a significant split between the strict drugless systems advocated by A. T. Still, and the beliefs of many MDs who were converted to osteopathy because of its therapeutic value. The latter group did not want to abandon all of the techniques they had previously learned and all of the drugs they had previously used when those therapy techniques were sometimes effective. Ultimately, most schools of osteopathy, commencing with the school based in Los Angeles, California, converted to more of an imitation of modern orthodox medicine. These developments led to more of an accommodation between the California osteopaths and the members of the California Medical Association. (This developing cooperation between the California Osteopathic and Medical Association was one of the major issues leading to the downfall, in 1949, of Fishbein's editorial voice in *JAMA*.) Thus, osteopathy found a place in professional medicine, at the cost of its drugless healing roots and therapies.[7]

The effect on chiropractic of the post-war years was somewhat different. Because of educational recognition under the G.I. Bill, the number of chiropractors in the country grew substantially, and their impact on the populace grew accordingly. The sect eventually grew powerful enough in terms of numbers and economic clout that it could pose a legal challenge to the orthodox monopoly of the AMA. However, in the immediate post-war years, the American Medical Association gained tremendous political clout. Combined with the American Legion and the National Board of Realtors,[17] these three groups posed a powerful political triumvirate before the United States Congress.

These years, called the years of the "great fear" in Caute's book by that name,[18] were the years during which to be unorthodox was to be "un-American".

Across the country, courts began to take the view that naturopaths were not truly doctors, as they espoused doctrines from "the dark ages of medicine" (something American medicine had apparently come out of in 1937) and that drugless healers were intended by law to operate without "drugs" (which became defined as anything a person would ingest or apply externally for any remedial medical purpose). In this regard, the Washington State Supreme Court case of *Kelly vs. Carroll* (the defendant being Otis G. Carroll of Spokane, Washington, a long-time follower, with his brother Robert V. Carrol, Sr, of Lust), and the Arizona State Supreme Court case of *Kuts-Cheraux vs. Wilson* document how significant limitations were placed on naturopaths under the guise of calling them "drugless healers".

In the state of Tennessee, as a reaction to the 1939 publication of the book *Back to Eden* by herbalist Jethro Kloss, court action initiated by the Tennessee State Medical Association led first to the publishers being forbidden to advertise the book for any therapeutic purpose. They were allowed only to acknowledge that it was in stock. The Tennessee State Legislature then declared that the practice of naturopathy in the state of Tennessee would be considered a gross misdemeanor, punishable by up to 1 year in jail.

Although it was under considerable public pressure in those years, the American Naturopathic Association undertook some of its most scholarly work, coordinating all the systems of naturopathy under commission. This resulted in the publication of a basic textbook on naturopathy (*Basic Naturopathy* published in 1948 by the ANA[19]) and a significant work compiling all the known theories of botanical medicine (as commissioned by the ANA's successor after its 1950 name change to the American Naturopathic Physicians and Surgeons Association), the *Naturae Medicina* published in 1953.[20] Naturopathic medicine began splintering when Lust's ANA was succeeded by six different organizations in the mid 1950s.

The primary organizations among these were the successor to the ANA, which underwent a name change in 1950 to the American Naturopathic Physician and Surgeon's Association, and subsequently changed to the American Association of Naturopathic Physicians in 1956, and the International Society of Naturopathic Physicians formed under the leadership of M. T. Campenella of Florida shortly after Lust's death, with its American offshoot, the National Association of Naturopathic Physicians.

By 1955, the AANP, as it ultimately became known, had recognized only two schools of naturopathic medicine, the Central States College of Physiatrics in Eaton, Ohio, under the leadership of H. Riley Spitler, and Western States College of Chiropractic and Naturopathy located outside Portland, Oregon, under the leadership of R. A. Budden. Budden was a Lindlahr graduate and among the group which took over control of the Lindlahr College after Lindlahr's death in the 1920s. He moved west after World War II when the north-west States, including Oregon, became the last bastion of naturopathic medicine in this country.

THE MODERN REJUVENATION

After the counter-culture years of the late 1960s and America's disenchantment with organized institutional medicine, which began after the miracle era faded and it became apparent that orthodox medicine had its limitations, alternative medicine began to gain new respect. Naturopathic medicine underwent an era of rejuvenation.

As succinctly described in Cassedy's *Medicine in America: A Short History*,[21] this phenomenon, which is not limited to naturopathic medicine, is consistent with the modern, and continuing, "search for health beyond orthodox medicine" (pp. 147–148):

> It should not have been surprising to anyone that certain organized therapeutic sects continue to exist in mid-twentieth century America as successful and conspicuous alternatives to regular medicine. This is not to say that they offer the same threats to the medical establishment or play the same roles as their nineteenth-century counterparts had, as complete therapeutic systems. But they do continue to hold a strong collective appeal for individuals who mistrust or are somehow disenchanted with main line medicine. They have appealed also to anti-authoritarian sentiments that flourish throughout society. Moreover, as earlier, they satisfy a variety of needs that regular medicine continues to neglect or ignore.

The same author, in describing the post-World War II decades and the changing fortunes of such healing theories as naturopathic medicine, observed as follows:

> The period also brought about the renewal or updating of certain previously widely used therapies and considerable experimentation with others, some of them exotic. To an extent this trend represented the rediscovery by trained physicians, nurses, and other regular health professionals of certain values and older styles of therapy. The participation of such professionals proved to be an essential ingredient in the rebirth of several such therapies. However, the major reason for the new successes was the wide-spread active interest and involvement of America's literate lay people in the search for more personal or humane forms of treatment.

As another author, John Duffy, has observed in *From Humors to Medical Science* (p. 350):[22]

> Since health is too closely related to cultural, social, and economic factors to be left exclusively to doctors, American lay people have always engaged in do-it-yourself medicine, resorted to "irregulars and quacks", and supported health movements. As a result of the current fad for physical fitness, our streets are beset by sweat-suited individuals of all ages doggedly jogging their way to health and long life. In addition, stores selling "natural" foods are flourishing, physical fitness salons have become a major business, and anti-smoking and weight-loss clinics and workshops are attracting thousands of individuals bent on leading cleaner and leaner lives. And those for whom physical activity in itself is not enough are seeking physical and mental well-being through faith healing, yoga, and a host of major and minor gurus.
>
> When neither mental effort nor physical exercise can solve medical problems, the sceptics of modern medicine can always turn to the irregulars. A recent estimate places a number of Americans who have relied on an irregular practitioner at some time in their lives at 60 million, and, aided by the high cost of orthodox medicine, irregular medical practice appears to be on the rise ...

At the beginning of this period of rejuvenation, the profession's educational institutions had dwindled to one, the National College of Naturopathic Medicine (which had branches in Seattle, Washington, and Portland, Oregon) which was created after the death of R. A. Budden and the conversion of Western States College to a straight school of chiropractic. As described in *Other Healers, Other Cures*, c. 1970 (p. 183):[16]

> Today, Naturopaths in seventeen states are licensed to diagnose, treat, and prescribe for any human disease through the use of air, light, heat, herbs, nutrition, electrotherapy, physiotherapy, manipulations, and minor surgery. At present, one can earn an D.N. [a misnomomer, actually – N.D.] degree at the National College of Naturopathic Medicine in Seattle and Emporia, Kansas, [where, by contract, the first two years of the four year medical education were then taught], or the new North American Naturopathic Institute in North Arlington New Jersey [there is also a school in Montreal]. The four-year curriculum covers many standard medical courses – anatomy, bacteriology, urology, pathology, physiology, X-ray reading etc. – but also includes botanical medicine, hydrotherapy, electrotherapy, and manipulative technique ...

The public, by the late 1970s, was particularly ripe for another rejuvenation of naturopathy's brand of "alternative" health care. As described in Murphy's *Enter The Physician: The Transformation of Domestic Medicine, 1760–1860*, when discussing this cyclical rejuvenation in the mid-20th century (pp. 226–227):[23]

> Contemporary crusaders still stress prevention as the lay

person's primary duty, but a growing chorus is calling for every person to assume the newly proactive role in his or her own health care. This is essential, say the analysts, because both lay people and doctors have placed far too much faith in the power of medicine and technology to work miracles. For a host of different reasons and from a variety of different perspectives, health advocates are calling on each person to "accept a certain measure of responsibility for his or her own recovery from disease or disability."

What would this entail? There are probably as many answers to this question as there are respondents, but it is striking to note how many of the solutions would have been familiar to our ancestors who lived between 1760 and 1860. One recurring idea, for instance, is that each person knows his or her own constitution history the best, and therefore has a duty to communicate that knowledge to medical personnel. Another is a refurbished concept of *vis, medicatrix, naturae,* the belief that many diseases are self-limiting and therefore do not require much medical intervention – and certainly not the amount or the sort to which contemporary Americans are accustomed. Most significantly, today's analysts are calling on professionals and non professionals to build and nurture a health-care partnership very much like that envisioned by nineteenth-century health publicists: a partnership based on mutual respect, clear understanding and faithful execution. In that scenario, both as it originally evolved and in its updated version, it is the doctor who directs treatment, but crucial to a successful outcome are the informed and responsible actions of the patients, other care givers, and the patient's family and friends.

In 1978, the John Bastyr College of Naturopathic Medicine was formed in Seattle, Washington, by Joseph E. Pizzorno, Jr, ND (founding president), Lester E. Griffith ND, and William Mitchell ND (all graduates of the National College of Naturopathic Medicine), who felt that it was necessary to have more institutions devoted to naturopathic care and the teaching of naturopathic therapeutics. During the late 1970s, other naturopathic doctors also recognized this need and naturopathic colleges were established in Arizona (the Arizona College of Naturopathic Medicine), Oregon (the American College of Naturopathic Medicine) and California (the Pacific College of Naturopathic Medicine). Unfortunately, none of these three survived. However, the current status of naturopathic medicine, as represented by Bastyr University and National College of Naturopathic Medicine, and now joined by the Southwest College of Naturopathic Medicine and Health Sciences in Arizona and a program in naturopathic medicine at the University of Bridgeport in Connecticut, is that of growth and presumably a solid future. There are currently favorable commentaries on the state of naturopathic medicine, and its continuing efforts to reinvest various diverse theories of "natural healing" with modern vigor.

In *Other Healers, Unorthodox Medicine In America* (edited by Norman Gevitz, the author of *The D.O.'s*),[24] a volume which was written to provide "a scholarly perspective on unorthodox movements and practices that have arisen in the United States" (from the editor's preface), part of this effort is described by Author Martin Kauffman, (from the Department of History at Westfield State College,) a modern expert on homeopathy (pp. 116–117):

In addition to the revival of classical homeopathy, a major development in recent times has been the teaching of homeopathy at naturopathic colleges on the West coast. In Seattle, John Bastyr, a Naturopath and Homeopath who had been practicing for fifty years, readied the move in 1956 to establish the national college of Naturopathic Medicine, which was later moved to Portland, Oregon. The College's four-year curriculum includes a required third-year course in homeopathy, with homeopathic electives being available to third and fourth year students.

In 1978, three naturopathic practitioners in Seattle founded the John Bastyr College of Naturopathic Medicine. During the sixth quarter all students at that school are required to take 44 hours of course work in homeopathy, after which they may elect another 66 hours and up to 238 hours of clinical homeopathic instruction. The significance of the naturopathic schools to the resurgence of homeopathy is demonstrated by the fact that "about one third of the graduating class specialized in homeopathic practice, a total of about 50 each year in all" (citing the American Homeopath in italics).

And, as described in the *Encyclopedia of Alternative Health Care* by Olsen (pp. 209–210):[25]

Today in Germany, the nature care movement in herbal remedies tradition has matured into a well-established health care practice, with about 5,000 professionals throughout the country. ...

One Kneipp practitioner, Benedict Lust, emigrated to America to begin teaching and practicing naturopathy here. By 1902, he had founded the American School of Naturopathy in New York City.

The practice quickly spread across the United States (California was the first State to pass a law regulating natural medicine, in 1919.)

Numerous schools offering a variety of training cropped up and disappeared. The movement peaked in America around 1950 and nearly died out by the early 1960's. The legal climate for naturopathy turned cold in many States, in the face of the powerful modern medical establishment. While naturopathy medicine is now legal (in several states) many naturopaths practicing in other states are old-timers, practicing under their original "drugless therapy" licenses, issued before laws prohibiting new naturopathic practices went into effect. Today, there are only two schools in naturopathic medicine in the United States: the National College in Portland Oregon, and John Bastyr College in Seattle, Washington. The American Association of Naturopathic Physicians is beginning to organize and unify the profession, with its own definition and philosophy of modern naturopathic medicine.

Alaska, Arizona, Connecticut, Oregon, Washington, and Hawaii recognize naturopathy as a primary medicine with specific licensing laws, as do the Canadian provinces of British Columbia, Manitoba, Ontario, and Saskatchewan. In other states, efforts are under way to gain licensure for naturopaths (this description was cerca in 1989).

And the movement continues to grow. And so, the impact of natural healing has come full circle. In an era where the statistical number of persons born who are expected to contract cancer, now recognized as a degenerative disease, has increased rather than declined, and the incidence of other degenerative diseases (arthritis, arteriosclerosis, atherosclerosis, etc.) has increased in direct relation to the lengthening of life expectancies produced by improved sanitation and nutrition (although speciously claimed by AMA medicine to be the result of their therapies), the early teachings of Lust, Lindlahr, et al appear to have more validity than ever.

REFERENCES

1. Starr P. Social transformation of American medicine. New York: Basic Books. 1983
2. Griggs B. Green pharmacy. London: Jill, Norman, & Hobhouse. 1981
3. Whorton J. Crusaders for fitness. Princeton, NJ: Princeton Press. 1982
4. Rothstein W. American physicians in the 19th century. Baltimore, MD: Johns Hopkins Press. 1972
5. Haller J. American medicine in transition, 1850–1910. Urbana, IL: University of Illinois Press. 1981: p 234–279
6. Rosen G. The structure of American medical practice. Philadelphia: University of Pennsylvania. 1983
7. Campion F. AMA & US Health Policy Since 1940. Chicago, IL: AMA Publishers. 1984
8. Burrows J. Original medicine in the progressive era. Baltimore, MD: Johns Hopkins Press. 1977: p 31–51
9. Coulter H. Divided legacy, vol II. Washington, DC: Wehawken Books. 1973: p 402–423
10. Salmon JW. Alternative medicines. NY: Tavistock. 1984: p 80–113
11. Gevitz N. The D.O.'s. Baltimore, MD: Johns Hopkins Press. 1982
12. Silberger J. Mary Baker Eddy. Boston, MA: Little Brown. 1980
13. Lindlahr H. Philosophy of natural therapeutics, vol. I. Maidstone, England: Maidstone Osteopathic. 1918. (Vol II – Practice: 1919; Vol III – Dietetics: 1914; Reprints: CW Daniel Co, Essex, England, 1975, 1981, 1983)
14. Lust B. Universal directory of naturopathy. Butler, NJ: Lust. 1918
15. Kellogg JH. New dietetics. Battle Creek, MC: Modern Medical Publications. 1923
16. Kruger, H. Other healers, other cures. A guide to alternative medicine. New York: Bobbs-Merrill. 1974
17. Goulden J. The best years. New York, NY: Athenium. 1976
18. Caute D. The great fear. New York, NY: Simon & Schuster. 1978
19. Spitler HR. Basic naturopathy. Des Moines, IA: ANA. 1948
20. Kuts-Cheraux AW. Naturae medicina. Des Moines, IA: ANPSA. 1953
21. Cassedy JH. Medicine in America: a short history. Baltimore: Johns Hopkins University Press. 1991
22. Duffy J. From humors to medical science: a history of American medicine, 2nd edn. Urbana, IL: University of Illinois Press. 1993
23. Murphy LR. Enter the physician: the transformation of domestic medicine, 1760–1860. University of Alabama Press. 1991
24. Gevitz, N. Other healers: unorthodox medicine in America. Baltimore: Johns Hopkins University Press. 1988
25. Olsen KG. The encyclopedia of alternative health care. NY: Pocket Books. 1989

FURTHER READING

General

Barrett S, Herbert V. The vitamin pushers: how the health food industry is selling America a bill of goods. NY: Prometheus Books. 1994

Barrett S, Jarvis W. The health robbers: a close look at quackery in America. NY: Prometheus Books. 1993

Berlinger H. A system of medicine: philanthropic foundations in the Flexner era. NY: Tavistock Publishers. 1985

Breiger G. Medical America in the 19th century. Baltimore, MD: Johns Hopkins Press. 1972

Brown ER. Rockefeller medicine men. CA: University of California Press. 1978

Burrows J. Organized medicine in the progressive era. Baltimore, MD: Johns Hopkins Press. 1977

Campion F. AMA & U.S. health policy since 1940. Chicago, IL: AMA Publishers. 1984

Cassedy JH. Medicine in America: a short history. Baltimore: Johns Hopkins University Press. 1991

Coulter H. Divided legacy, vol. III. Washington, DC: Wehawken Books. 1973

Coward R. The whole truth: the myth of alternative health. London: Faber and Faber. 1989

Duffy J. The healers. Urbana, IL: University of Illinois Press. 1976

Duffy J. From humors to medical science: a history of American medicine, 2nd edn. Urbana, IL: University of Illinois Press. 1993

Gevitz N. The D.O.'s. Baltimore, MD: Johns Hopkins University Press. 1982

Gevitz, N. Other healers: unorthodox medicine in America. Baltimore: Johns Hopkins University Press. 1988

Dr Goodenough's Home Cures & Herbal Remedies. Crown. 1982

Green H. Fit for America: health, fitness, sport & American society. NY: Pantheon Books. 1986

Griggs B. Green pharmacy. London, UK: Jill, Norman & Hobhouse. 1981

Haller J. American medicine in transition, 1850–1910. Urbana, IL: University of Illinois Press. 1981

Inglis B, West R. Alternative health guide. New York, NY: Knopf. 1983

Kruger H. Other healers, other cures: a guide to alternative medicine. NY: Bobbs-Merrill. 1974.

Ludmerer K. Learning to heal. NY: Basic Books. 1985

Manger LN. A history of medicine. NY: Marcel Dekker. 1992

McKeown T. The role of medicine: dream, mirage, or nemesis? London, UK: Nuffield Provincial Hospitals Trust. 1976

Murphy LR. Enter the physician: the transformation of domestic medicine, 1760–1860. Tuscaloosa, AL: University of Alabama Press. 1991

Rosen G. The structure of American medical practice: 1875–1941. Philadelphia: University of Pennsylvania. 1983

Rosenberg C. The care of strangers: the rise of America's hospital system. NY: Basic Books. 1987

Rothstein W. American physicians in the 19th century. Baltimore, MD: Johns Hopkins Press. 1972

Salmon JW. Alternative medicines. New York: Tavistock. 1984

Serrentino J. How natural remedies work. B.C.: Hartley & Marks. 1991

Silberger J. Mary Baker Eddy. Boston, MA: Little Brown. 1980

Starr P. Social transformation of American medicine. New York: Basic Books. 1983

Thomas L. The youngest science. Boston, MA: Viking. 1983

Whorton J. Crusaders for fitness. Princeton, NJ: Princeton Press. 1982

Wirt A. Health & healing. New York, NY: Houghton Mifflin. 1983

Wohl S. Medical industrial complex. New York, NY: Harmony. 1983

A naturopathic bibliography

Abbot JK (MD). Essentials of medical electricity. Philadelphia, PA: WB Saunders. 1915

Altman N. The chiropractic alternative: how the chiropractic health care system can help keep you well. Los Angeles, CA: J.P. Tarcher. 1948

Barber ED (DO). Osteopathy complete. Kansas City, MO: Private 1896

Baruch S (MD). An epitome of hydro-therapy. Philadelphia, PA: WB Saunders. 1920

Benjamin H (ND). Everybody's guide to nature cure, 7th edn. England: Thorsons. 1981
Bennet HC (MD). The electro-therapeutic guide. Lima, OH: National College of Electro-therapeutics. 1912
Bilz FE. The natural method of healing (2 vols). (English translation) New York, NY: Bilz, International News Co. 1898
Dejarnette MB (DC). Technic & practice of bloodless surgery. Nebraska City, NB: Private. 1939
Downing CH (DO). Principles & practice of osteopathy. Kansas City, MO: Williams. 1923
Filden JH (MD). Impaired health (its cause & cure), 2nd edn. Denver, CO: Private. 1921
Finkel H (DC, ND). Health via nature. New York, NY: Barness Printing & Society for Public Health Education. 1925
Foster AL (DC, ND). Foster's system of non-medicinal therapy. Chicago, IL: National Publishing Association. 1919
Fuller RC. Alternative medicine and American religious life. NY: Oxford University Press. 1989
Goetz EW (DO). Manual of osteopathy. Cincinnati, OH: Nature's Cure. 1909
Gottsschalk FB (MD). Practical electro-therapeutics. Hammond, IN: Frank Betz. 1904
Olsen KG. The encyclopedia of alternative health care. NY: Pocket Books. 1989
Graham RL (MD). Hydro-hygiene. New York, NY: Thompson – Barlow Co. 1923
Inglis B. Natural medicine. Great Britain: William Collins. 1979
Johnson AC (DC, ND, DWT). Principles & practice of drugless therapeutics. Los Angeles, CA: Chiropractic Education Extension Bureau. 1946
Kellogg JH (MD). New dietetics. Battle Creek, MI: Modern Medical Publications. 1923
Kellogg JF. Rational hydrotherapy. Battle Creek, MI: Modern Medical Publications. 1901, 1902
King FX. Rudolf Steiner and holistic medicine. York Beach, MA: Nicolas-Hays. 1987
Kuhne L. Neo-naturopathy (new science of healing). (Translated by B Lust), Butler, NJ: Lust Publ. 1918
Kuts-Cheraux AW (MD, ND). Naturae medicina. Des Moines, IA: ANPSA. 1953
Just A. Return to nature. (Translated by B Lust), Butler, NJ. Lust Publ. 1922
Lust B (ND). Universal directory of naturopathy. Butler, NJ: Lust Publ. 1918
Lindlahr H (MD). Philosophy of natural therapeutics, vol. I. Maidstone, England: Maidstone Osteopathic. 1918. (Vol II – Practice: 1919; Vol III – Dietetics: 1914; Reprints: CW Daniel Co, Essex, England, 1975, 1981, 1983)
MacFadden B (ND). Building of vital power. NJ: Physical Culture Publications. 1904
MacFadden B (ND). Power & beauty of superb womanhood. NJ: Physical Culture Publications. 1901
Murray CH (DO). Practice of osteopathy. Elgin, IL: Private. 1909
Murray MT (ND), Pizzorno JE (ND). Encyclopedia of natural medicine. Rocklin, CA: Prima. 1998
Pizzorno JE (ND). Total wellness. Rocklin, CA: Prima. 1996
Richter JT (DC, ND). Nature – the healer. Los Angeles, CA: Private. 1949
Spitler HR (MD, ND, PhD). Basic naturopathy. Des Moines, IA: ANA. 1948
Trall RT (ND). Hydropathic encyclopedia (3 vols). New York, NY: SR Wells. 1880
Turner RN (ND, DO, Bac, MBNOA). Naturopathic medicine: treating the whole person. Great Britain: Thorsons. 1984
Weltmer E. Practice of suggestive therapeutics. Nevada, MO: Weltmer Institute. 1913

CHAPTER CONTENTS

3

Philosophy of naturopathic medicine

Randall S. Bradley, ND DHANP

INTRODUCTION

This chapter examines the philosophical foundation of naturopathic medicine and its modern applications. Unlike most other health care systems, naturopathy is not identified by any particular therapy or modalities. In fact, there is a wide variety of therapeutic styles and modalities found within the naturopathic community (see Table 3.1). For example, there are still practitioners who adhere to the strict "nature cure" tradition and focus only on diet, "detoxification", lifestyle modification, and hydrotherapy. There are also those who specialize in homeopathy, acupuncture or natural childbirth. At the other end of the spectrum are found naturopathic physicians who extensively use natural medicinal substances to manipulate the body's biochemistry and physiology. Finally, there is the majority who practice an eclectic naturopathic practice that includes a little of everything.

From its inception 100 years ago, naturopathic medicine has been an eclectic system of health care. This has allowed it to adopt many of this century's more effective elements of natural and alternative medicine, as well as to adopt conventional medicine's basic and clinical sciences and diagnostics (see Ch. 2 for further discussion). Through all of this eclecticism, it has always identified the Latin expression *vis medicatrix naturae* (the healing power of nature) as its philosophical linchpin.

Table 3.1 Naturopathic modalities

Naturopathic physicians are trained to use a number of diagnostic and treatment techniques. These modalities include:

- *Diagnosis* – all of the conventional clinical laboratory, physical diagnosis, and imaging (i.e. X-ray, etc.) techniques, as well as holistic evaluation techniques
- *Counseling* – lifestyle, nutritional and psychological
- *Natural medicines* – nutritional supplements (i.e. all food constituents), botanical medicine, and homeopathy
- *Physical medicine* – hydrotherapy, naturopathic manipulative therapy, physiotherapy modalities, exercise therapy and acupuncture
- *Family practice* – natural childbirth, minor surgery, natural hormones, biologicals, and natural antibiotics

However, the expression *vis medicatrix naturae*, by itself, does not provide a clear picture of naturopathic medical philosophy, or an understanding of the practice of naturopathic medicine in all of its varied forms. With the profession's history of eclecticism, no two practitioners will treat any individual patient exactly alike. While this has its advantages (i.e. individualization of each patient's care, more therapeutic options, etc.), it also makes it difficult to perceive the profession's philosophic cohesiveness. Another major disadvantage of this eclecticism is the difficulty in developing consistent practice standards.

To attempt to solve this problem, the modern profession has articulated a general statement of naturopathic principles expanding on *vis medicatrix naturae* (see Table 3.2). However, this statement of principles is probably still not adequate to address the issues that concern modern students of naturopathic medicine or other professionals. Therefore, in order to gain a more in-depth understanding of naturopathic medicine, it is necessary to discuss medical philosophy in general.

MEDICAL PHILOSOPHY

The issues fundamental to medical philosophy have changed little since naturopathy first appeared as a distinct profession at the end of the 19th century. What has changed is the level of understanding of the biological process and the language of science. Most people who study the early writers on naturopathic medical philosophy quickly get lost in the archaic language and arguments used to justify the theories. This chapter translates these concepts and issues into modern terms.

Vitalism vs. mechanism

Historically, there have been two main medical philosophies, those of *vitalism* and *mechanism*. Their origins can be traced to the Hippocratic writings of ancient Greece. Throughout history, the line separating these two schools of thought has not always been clear, but their philosophical perspectives have generally been in opposition. The conflicting goals and philosophical foundations of these two concepts remain relevant as the modern practices of conventional and alternative physicians come into conflict. As will be seen, the foundations of naturopathic medical philosophy are found in vitalism. However, naturopathy also recognizes the practical value of the mechanistic approach to health care.

Mechanism

Up to the early part of the 20th century, there was considerable debate over the issue of vitalism vs. mechanism in the field of biology. The mechanists, or materialists, maintained that the phenomenon of life could be explained exclusively as the product of a complex series of chemical and physical reactions. They denied the possibility that the animate had any special quality that distinguished it from the inanimate. It was their contention that the only difference between life and non-life is the degree of complexity of the system.

Mechanism has several other distinctive characteristics. Its most obvious is that it is reductionistic. In fact, "reductionism" is often used as a synonym of mechanism. Mechanistic science is also characterized by an emphasis

Table 3.2 The principles of naturopathic medicine

- **The healing power of nature: *vis medicatrix naturae***
Nature acts powerfully through healing mechanisms in the body and mind to maintain and restore health. Naturopathic physicians work to restore and support these inherent healing systems when they have broken down, by using methods, medicines, and techniques that are in harmony with natural processes.
- **First do no harm: *primum non nocere***
Naturopathic physicians prefer non-invasive treatments that minimize the risks of harmful side-effects. They are trained to know which patients they can treat safely, and which ones they need to refer to other health care practitioners.
- **Find the cause: *tolle causam***
Every illness has an underlying cause, often in aspects of the lifestyle, diet or habits of the individual. A naturopathic physician is trained to find and remove the underlying cause of a disease.
- **Doctor as teacher: docere**
A principal objective of naturopathic medicine is to educate the patient and emphasize self-responsibility for health. Naturopathic physicians also recognize and employ the therapeutic potential of the doctor–patient relationship.
- **Treat the whole person**
Health or disease comes from a complex interaction of physical, emotional, dietary, genetic, environmental, lifestyle, and other factors. Naturopathic physicians treat the whole person, taking these factors into account.
- **Preventive medicine**
The naturopathic approach to health care can prevent minor illnesses from developing into more serious or chronic degenerative diseases. Patients are taught the principles with which to live a healthy life; by following these principles they can prevent major illnesses.

on linear causality. Without its emphasis on reductionism and linear causality, Western science and medicine would probably have not been so successful. As the 20th century advanced, each new discovery in biological and medical science reinforced the arguments for mechanism, until by the middle of the 20th century, the biology community had almost exclusively embraced the philosophy of mechanism.

Mechanism is the philosophical foundation of biomedical science and conventional medicine. Mechanistic medicine identifies disease and its accompanying signs and symptoms as simply the result of a disruption of normal chemical reactions and physical activities. Such disruptions are caused by the direct interference in these reactions and activities of a "pathogenic agent". (For the purposes of this discussion, the general expression "pathogenic agent" refers to any known or unknown etiological agent or condition. Examples include microbial agents, autotoxins, genetic defects, environmental toxins, non-end-product metabolites, and physical and emotional stress and trauma.) A living organism, then, is simply a very complex machine which, due to external agents and "wear and tear", breaks down. Because the signs and symptoms of disease are thought to be due only to these mechanical disruptions and interference with reactions, they are considered to be completely destructive phenomena and are therefore to be eliminated. Disappearance of the signs and symptoms indicates that the pathogenic agent and its resulting disease have been eradicated, or at least controlled. The goals of mechanistic medicine tend to be the quick removal of the signs, symptoms, and the pathogenic agent.

Mechanistic medicine is being practiced in cases where the intention of the therapy is to intervene in the perceived mechanism of the disease and/or relieve the symptoms. Examples would be the use of antihistamines to relieve rhinitis, vitamin B_6 to help PMS, surgery and emergency care for traumatic injuries, coronary bypass surgery, anti-inflammatory agents in systemic lupus erythematosus (SLE), or insulin in juvenile onset diabetes. Mechanism is also being used when an identified pathogenic agent is directly attacked or eliminated. Instances of this would be the use of antibiotics or the isolation of a patient from a particular allergen. Clearly, mechanistic medicine can be very effective in achieving its goals. In the face of modern medical technology, it is easy to see how this philosophy came to dominate biology, medicine, and the attention of the public.

However, the unsolved problems of mechanistic medicine – particularly those of chronic degenerative disease, authoritarianism which alienates patients from responsibility for their own health, and the increasing cost of health care – suggest that there are limits to the mechanistic perspective and explain why vitalism has not disappeared and is, in fact, in resurgence.

Vitalism

The philosophy of vitalism is based on the concept that life is too well organized to be explained simply as a complex assemblage of chemical and physical reactions (i.e. a living system is more than just the sum of its parts). This is in contrast to the mechanist's contention that "the only difference between life and non-life is the degree of complexity". Throughout the 19th century, the debate between vitalism and mechanism was mostly carried on by biologists whose interests were mainly in the study of the organism's specific cellular activities, such as morphological development. These activities were argued to be "vital" and, therefore, not explainable by mechanistic science. The tendency was to infer a metaphysical quality to this concept. As can be imagined, these earlier debates lurched from one specific argument to the next as modern biology unraveled the secrets of cellular metabolism. Fortunately, the debate has now shifted back to the relevant and holistic general concepts.

While modern vitalism is inherently holistic in its view and has an emphasis on circularity as its causality (i.e. feedback loops), there is no conflict with the findings of biomedical science. Eventually, all of the individual chemical and physical reactions that are found in the processes of life will probably be identified. What is significant is not the individual reaction, but the fact that they are all coordinated to such a degree as to produce the special activities of a living organism. An organism's unique complexity – as demonstrated by its ability to grow and develop, respond to stimuli, reproduce, and repair itself – requires a level of organization and co-ordination that suggests a distinct quality that is not readily explained by mechanism. This organization and coordination has been identified as "homeostasis" by physiology. All organisms, up to the point of death, are attempting to return to this ideal state when injured or ill. As there is no inanimate counterpart to this level of complexity and organization, this is the most dramatic general argument in favor of vitalism.

A less dramatic argument used to support the vitalistic perspective is the "problem of entropy". Entropy is the tendency of any closed system to find equilibrium, i.e. the state of least organization. In other words, systems tend to run down and become less complex over time. In defiance of this universal rule, life, up until the point of death, consistently creates more complex systems out of simple ones. To do this, life actively pursues external matter and energy to incorporate into itself, while at the same time selectively eliminating by-products from its utilization of this matter and energy.

When the problem of entropy is examined on the molecular level, the same individual chemical processes and elements may be found in both animate and inanimate systems. In the inanimate system, however, there is a constant move toward a state of chemical equilibrium. This type of system cannot maintain an unstable chemical state and always seeks stabilization. Even after the addition of external exciting energy, the system will return to the simplest, least reactive state possible. The animate system is virtually the opposite. It is continuously in a state of dynamic chemical instability, actively seeking energy to maintain this instability, and consistently moving to more complex and organized states (and back again). It is only at the onset of death that an animate system begins to move towards equilibrium.

The third general argument in favor of a vitalistic view of life is evolution. For evolution to exist as a force in nature, generations of living organisms have to survive long enough to grow, reproduce and then evolve. In order for this survival to take place, the organisms' homeostatic and repair processes must be consistently directed towards maintaining a state of balance with the external environment (i.e. health). Any organisms that did not behave biochemically and physiologically in this manner would have died and not evolved. Thus the phenomenon of evolution, as the action of countless living organisms over eons, multiplies life's anti-entropic quality and is incompatible with a mechanistic view of living systems.

These easily observable examples of life's "special quality" suggest an "organizing force" that goes beyond what is possible from mere chemistry. This quality that makes life unique should not be mistaken as a metaphysical concept, although is not intended to argue here for or against such concepts. The point is only that vitalism is a medical philosophy based on observable scientific phenomena. Unfortunately, a definitive definition of this quality (in the old literature called the "vital force", defense mechanism, or simply "Nature") will have to wait for more research.

At this point in the discussion, not many mechanistic practitioners would have reason to be uncomfortable, as the ideas proposed are relatively non-controversial and just follow generally accepted physiological principles. Interestingly, many of these practitioners probably have personal belief systems that are quite compatible with this stage of the vitalistic argument. However, the conflict becomes evident upon examination of the premises upon which the practice of vitalistic medicine is based. What truly separates vitalism from mechanism, and makes it useful as a medical philosophy, is its perspective on disease and the associated symptoms.

Meaning of disease

Vitalism maintains that the pathogenic agent does not directly cause the symptoms accompanying disease; rather, they are the result of the organism's intrinsic response or reaction to the agent and the organism's attempt to defend and heal itself. Symptoms, then, are part of a constructive phenomenon that is the best "choice" the organism can make, given the circumstances at any particular point in time.

These symptoms can be further described as arising from two situations. The first and most common situation is when they are from a "healing reaction", which is the organism's concerted and organized attempt to defend and heal itself. These healing reactions produce what can be called "benign symptoms". Examples include fever and inflammation in infections, almost any reaction of the immune system, and many of the symptoms of chronic disease.

This interpretation of symptoms is generally ignored by mechanism. Instead, it views them as the result of a destructive process and focuses on intervening by relieving the symptom or manipulating the pathological mechanism. Mechanistic medicine is therefore most often working contrary to homeostasis and the organism's healing attempt (in fact, this is usually its intent). When this therapeutic approach is effective, vitalists call the result a "suppression" (see Table 3.3). This approach to health care is so pervasive that most people, lay and professional alike, today routinely suppress mild fevers with antipyretics.

In contrast, vitalism considers these symptoms to be the product of a constructive phenomenon and therapeutically stimulates and encourages this directed healing process. Rather than simply trying to eliminate a pathogenic agent, as mechanistic therapy might, vitalism focuses more on augmenting the organism's resistance to that agent. That is not to say that vitalists object to removing the agent, only that it should be done in the context of simultaneously increasing resistance (in other words, decreasing susceptibility). The importance of this approach becomes evident when one recognizes that disease is only possible when both a pathogenic agent and a susceptibility to that agent are present.

Healing reactions can take several forms, as shown in Table 3.4. In the first type, an organism's response to a

Table 3.3 Cure, suppression and palliation

When symptoms improve following treatment (regardless of the therapeutic system), it is for one of three reasons:

- *Cure*. The symptoms go away and the patient's overall health improves. In this case the treatment can be discontinued and the patient continues to do well.
- *Suppression*. The symptoms go away but overall the patient becomes less healthy. The treatment can be discontinued and the symptoms will stay away, but the patient feels worse generally (i.e. deceased sense of well-being, energy or moods), or new, often more limiting, symptoms eventually develop (e.g. suppressed eczema leading to asthma).
- *Palliation*. The symptoms are improved but only as long as the treatment is continued. At best, palliation is something that is done while a curative treatment is given time to work. In and of itself, palliation will never lead to a cure, but unfortunately, continued palliation may eventually lead to suppression.

Table 3.4 The four types of healing reactions

Reaction	Description
Acute, asymptomatic	Organism easily defends itself
"Healing crisis"	Relative strength of pathogenic agent and organism similar; symptoms of body defending itself apparent
Vigorous but unsuccessful	Pathogenic agent stronger than organism; death if no intervention
Chronic, mildly symptomatic	Healing reaction feeble, but adequate to maintain life; progressive degeneration

pathogenic agent does not produce symptoms. When it is capable of easily defending itself from the agent, no symptoms will be perceivable. This is a common homeostatic process and is demonstrated when a potential pathogen, such as beta-hemolytic streptococcus, is cultured from a healthy person's throat. However, when the organism is more susceptible or the relative strength of the pathogenic agent is greater, a threshold is reached and symptoms become perceivable. Successful healing reactions of this type would include vigorous acute diseases that quickly resolve. The early naturopaths would have called these acute reactions "healing crises". As the susceptibility of the organism increases relative to the strength of the pathogenic agent, there is a greater likelihood that the healing attempt will not be successful. When such a reaction is unsuccessful but vigorous, death may result, unless there is timely application of vitalistic or mechanistic therapy. Examples of this situation might be acute bacterial meningitis or cholera.

When the healing attempt is feeble and therefore ineffective, it usually goes into the "chronic disease" stage of the reaction. Vitalists observe that suppression seems to increase the likelihood that the reaction will be forced to go into such a chronic stage. In this situation the reaction is "smoldering", and most often the organism cannot overcome the pathogenic agent unassisted. It just "holds its own", and if the organism's general health decreases over the years, the reaction gradually degenerates, producing symptoms that become less benign as it moves to an end-stage pathology. If the organism can be therapeutically stimulated to produce a more vigorous healing reaction, it can often successfully complete the original healing attempt. This augmented reaction is another example of a naturopathic healing crisis and would also be called an "aggravation" by the vitalists who practice homeopathic medicine.

Intervening in the mechanism of disease by relieving symptoms does little to stimulate or encourage the healing response; in fact it usually actually inhibits the healing response. In contrast, vitalistic therapies can be very effective in helping these healing reactions, because their goals are precisely the same as those of the organism. Thus, it is thought that vitalistic medicine works because, by honoring this process and thereby strengthening the whole organism, it encourages a more effective healing effort. Ideally, the organism is then able to accelerate and complete its reaction against the pathogenic agent, leading to the permanent disappearance of the symptoms as it returns to a state of health.

It would be naive to say that every stage of the healing reaction is positive and in the best interest of the organism, or that no symptoms should be palliated. The modern vitalist acknowledges that intervention is sometimes necessary. On the other hand, it is important to note that routine intervention can encourage its own worst-case scenarios. When mechanistic therapies successfully suppress an organism's chosen healing reaction, a less effective and less desirable response is often produced. Therefore, when suppression occurs, it can lead to a more complicated medical situation. Consequently, the very practice of mechanistic medicine tends to reinforce its practitioner's conviction that intervention is usually necessary. It should be noted, however, that not all intervention leads to suppression. It happens less often when the pathogenic agent can be readily eliminated, such as in non-recurring acute bacterial infections, or when relatively non-invasive therapies are used, such as natural medicines.

The second type of symptom-producing situation occurs when the organism produces symptoms in response to an organic lesion that arises from the direct pathological influence of a pathogenic agent. These can be called "morbid symptoms" and examples would include symptoms from the mass of an invasive tumor, shortness of breath from emphysema, and pain of an injury or MI. It should be mentioned that even these symptoms are the result of the organism's overall effort to maintain homeostasis; benign symptoms are also often present. In addition, a morbid symptom is not necessarily produced for a negative reason. For instance, pain is valuable as an indication of tissue damage. As can be seen, many, if not most, of these situations involve "end-stage" pathology. Here mechanistic therapies can be very positive when the goals of the therapy do not conflict with those of the organism.

There are instances when invasive intervention will probably be required to save "life and limb". These include such conditions as birth and genetic defects, serious traumatic injuries, crisis situations, overwhelming infections, and many malignancies. Unfortunately, conventional intervention does not guarantee a successful outcome either. Even in these situations, however, the effectiveness of vitalistic and natural therapy should not be underestimated, and their concurrent use will certainly augment any mechanistic intervention.

Although the concept of benign and morbid symptoms can be a useful tool to help understand the healing and disease process, in many situations it may not be possible to categorize the type of symptoms produced. A rough rule of thumb, however, would be that virtually all symptoms accompanying "reversible" or functional pathology are benign. On the other hand, many of the symptoms associated with traumatic injury and end-stage pathology would be morbid symptoms.

Changing society

After this discussion of vitalism's perspective on disease, the question that comes to mind is: "If most health problems are likely to respond to vitalistic medicine, then why is mechanism dominant?" The best answer is probably found in examination of the general attitudes held by society during the Industrial Age just ending. Mechanism came into dominance during this period because it neatly fit into the Industrial Age's world-view. This is the "man conquers nature" view that holds humanity as above and separate from the world in which it lives. It follows that nature is simply a resource that technology will eventually subdue or subjugate and put into order. Although this perspective is still very strong in Western society, there has been a dramatic change within the last 30 years.

Attitudes are now shifting in favor of the ecological integration of humanity into the environment. This "new" world-view holds that humanity is part of an orderly nature and that to ignore this creates situations that eventually become problems. Most ecological disasters are excellent examples of the results of the old view. In addition, the new view contends that if an effort is made to understand how nature functions and an attempt is made to work within that understanding, humanity's needs can be more efficiently met.

Mechanistic medicine, as part of the "old" world-view, generally sees disease as something to conquer and put into order. Vitalistic medicine, on the other hand, looks at the order that is already present and attempts to integrate its therapy into that orderly process. As a result, vitalism is becoming increasingly popular as society shifts from the old to the new world-view.

The belief systems of many mechanistic practitioners recognize this order. However, due to education and peer pressure, these personal beliefs are rarely translated into clinical practice. The mechanistic view is still relatively pervasive in society, and because mechanism is convenient (e.g. taking aspirin for a headache), vitalistic practitioners can generally shift their perspective and successfully use mechanistic therapy (although their therapeutic goals may be different). On the other hand, since mechanists dispute the premises upon which vitalistic medicine is based, they generally have great difficulty when attempting to practice or research a vitalistic therapy and frequently cannot demonstrate its efficacy.

Scientific medicine

While mechanism and vitalism represent opposing perspectives, the systems of medicine that represent these philosophies can be successfully tested and examined with the scientific method.* That is not to say that the philosophy of vitalism has been unquestionably proven – only that the validity of vitalistic interventions can be scientifically demonstrated. If a therapy can be proven effective, then that implies the accuracy of the philosophy upon which it is based. Unfortunately, very few of the vast resources of the 20th century biomedical community have been directed toward investigating vitalistic medicine.

Conventional medicine, as the dominant health care system and a representative of mechanism, has claimed for itself the title of "scientific medicine". However, it is inherently no more or less scientific than vitalistic medicine. A system is scientific only when it has met the criteria of the scientific method. This method requires the collection of data through observation and experimentation, and the formulation and testing of hypotheses. Non-prejudicial science can effectively study any system, but the researcher must understand the system's particular paradigm. Experiments on a vitalistic therapy based on a reductionistic and mechanistic model are going to be less than satisfactory.

The criteria of the scientific method can be met by vitalistic medicine, but only when the researchers recognize that it cannot be studied as though it is reductionistic or based on a simplistic model of linear causality. When the experimental model acknowledges the complexity of a living system in a social context (i.e. holism and circularity), vitalistic medicine proves to be both verifiable and reproducible, and thus scientific. Unfortunately, due to conventional medicine's current political and economic dominance, it is in the position to dictate (through economic and publication control) that research, and therefore the scientific method, will primarily be applied to itself. The result is that most conventional practitioners dismiss vitalistic medicine, along with all alternatives, as unscientific.

This is unfortunate because most vitalistic physicians also have extensive training in mechanistic and/or conventional medicine. Generally, they are capable of practicing mechanistically, and do so to greater or lesser

*A thorough review of all health care modalities in use today reveals a category that could be called "esotericia". While this category is not historically relevant to this discussion of medical philosophy, and its brief mention is not intended as an argument for or against "legitimacy", esotericia would include such things as prayer, faith healing, psychic healing, Healing Touch, Touch for Health and medical dowsing. Generally speaking, the actual operator of the therapy must call on God or have some special endogenous skill or "power" that goes beyond intellectual knowledge. These modalities are all "operator-dependent" and cannot be examined separate from the practitioner – thus greatly increasing the difficulty of their scientific verification.

degrees. The conflict between the practitioners of these different systems is very often due to a lack of constructive dialog. This can be attributed to two general causes: the first is simply that each system defines the world of "correct" medicine in terms of its own principles; the second is the issue of who controls the economic and political power.

NATUROPATHIC PHILOSOPHY

Historically, naturopathy is a vitalistic system of medicine. However, over the last 100 years it has also incorporated a number of therapies that can function mechanistically. What makes them acceptable, given naturopathic medicine's vitalistic foundation, is that they are natural therapies. Natural medicines and therapies, when properly used, generally have low invasiveness and there is little evidence that they cause suppression or side-effects. When used mechanistically, they allow some intervention while still allowing the organism's healing abilities the opportunity to continue unopposed, especially when used to support the body's own healing processes.

Vis medicatrix naturae

Naturopathic physicians assert that all true healing is a result of *vis medicatrix naturae* (the healing power of nature). Unfortunately, some people in the field of alternative medicine (including some naturopathic physicians and students) have mistakenly translocated this concept to the therapy. These practitioners tend to operate as though this "healing power" is an intrinsic property of the natural therapy or medicinal substance itself. In contrast, vitalism and naturopathic medicine have always understood that the "healing power of nature" is an inherent property of the living organism. *Vis medicatrix naturae* is the living organism's "desire" and ability to heal itself.

The application of this principle in practice is, of course, dependent upon the patient's needs. Ideally, it involves only the use of therapies that support the organism and encourage its intrinsic healing process to work more effectively. It also avoids the use of medicines and procedures that interfere with natural functions or have harmful side-effects. Natural medicines and therapies are therefore preferred, since, when used properly and in appropriate circumstances, they are the least harmful, least invasive, and best able to work in harmony with the natural healing process.

Since the total organism is involved in the healing attempt, the most effective approach to diagnosis and treatment is to consider the whole person. In addition to physical and laboratory findings, important consideration is given to the patient's attitude, psychological and spiritual state, social circumstances, lifestyle, diet, heredity, and environment. Careful attention to each person's unique individuality and susceptibility to disease is critical to the proper evaluation and treatment of any health problem.

Naturopathic physicians contend that most disease is the direct result of the ignorance and violation of what would be traditionally called "natural living laws". These general lifestyle (including diet) rules are based on the concept that there is an environment (both internal and external) that optimizes the health of an organism. Analysis of the lifestyles of Paleolithic and healthy primitive and modern cultures gave naturopathic physicians and their progenitors many clues as to what a healthy lifestyle should include.

Throughout most of modern history, biomedical science has focused primarily on researching the sick. Recently it has finally begun to evaluate what makes for a healthy lifestyle. To no-one's surprise, this lifestyle looks like the same one advocated by naturopaths for the last 100 years. A healthy lifestyle could be generalized to include: the consumption of natural unrefined foods; getting adequate amounts of exercise and rest; living a moderately paced lifestyle; having constructive and creative attitudes; avoiding toxins and polluted environments; and the maintaining of proper elimination. During illness, it is also important to control these areas in order to remove as many unnecessary stresses as possible and to optimize the chances that the organism's healing attempt will be successful. Therefore, patient education and responsibility, lifestyle modification and preventive medicine are fundamental to naturopathic practice.

While the practice of naturopathic medicine is grounded in *vis medicatrix naturae*, it also recognizes that intervention in the disease process is sometimes efficacious and, at times, absolutely necessary. Naturopathic physicians treat patients using a wide variety of therapeutic modalities. Some of these are vitalistic and some mechanistic. It is the goal of the therapy that ultimately determines which approach is utilized. Naturopathic physicians have a long-standing tradition of integrating the best aspects of traditional, alternative, and conventional medicine in the interest of the patient. As appropriate, patients are referred to other health care practitioners. Whenever possible, every effort is made to use all treatment techniques in a manner that is harmonious with the naturopathic philosophy.

Natural medicines and therapies

The medicines administered and prescribed by naturopathic physicians are primarily natural and relatively unprocessed. Although it is recognized that some situations may require the use of synthesized medicines, their use is considered less desirable. Some of the arguments in favor of natural medicinal substances have already been discussed. In addition to the reasons noted above, natural agents are preferred because their constituents have been encountered in nature for millions of years. This long period of exposure has enabled the body to develop metabolic pathways capable of effectively utilizing, processing, and detoxifying these medicines.

Four categories of natural medicines can be defined. The first includes substances found in nature that have been only minimally processed. Examples would include, but are not limited to, foods, clean air and water, and whole herbs. The early "nature cure" practitioners used this category primarily. The second category includes agents extracted or made from naturally occurring products. Although these have undergone pharmacological processing, the constituents of the medicines are still in the form found in the original natural substance. These first two types of natural medicinal substances have synergistic constituents that allow their use at lower doses with a resultant broader and safer therapeutic index. Examples of this category include tinctures and other botanical extracts, homeopathic medicines, glandulars and other substances of animal origin.

The third type of natural medicines are those highly processed medicinal substances that are derived from a natural source. These often have everything removed but the identified active ingredient and no longer have any synergistic constituents. Examples include many new phytotherapeutic agents, constituents of biochemical pathways, enzymes, amino acids, minerals, vitamins, and other food extracts.

The fourth category that may be considered "natural" are those manufactured medicines which are presumed to be identical to naturally occurring substances. These have the advantage of being less expensive and are typically available in higher concentrations. However, their use is less desirable due to:

- the difficulty of determining whether they are indeed the equivalent of the natural product
- their lack of natural synergistic components
- the inclusion of contaminates from the manufacturing process. These contaminates are often chemically and structurally similar to the desired medicine, but generally interfere with the normal pathways rather than enhance them.

Examples of these manufactured "natural" medicines include hormones, synthetic vitamins and analogs of plant and animal constituents.

Increasingly, medicines of the types identified in categories three and four are being grown "synthetically" by microorganisms specially engineered to produce the desired medicinal substance. It is difficult to say which of these categories best describes this situation. There are also potential problems with this kind of manufacturing process as evidenced by the tryptophan disaster of several years ago.

Naturopathic physicians also use many natural therapies. What makes a therapy "natural" is that it is derived from a phenomenon of nature and is used to stimulate the body to heal itself. Examples of these phenomena are air, light, heat, electricity, sound and mechanical force. Some of these natural therapies include mechanical and manual manipulation of the bony and soft tissues (naturopathic manipulative therapy), physiotherapy modalities (e.g. electrotherapy and ultrasound), hydrotherapy, and exercise therapy. Naturopathic physicians also use lifestyle modification, counseling and suggestive therapeutics. These therapies are all discussed in more detail in other chapters.

Family and specialty practice

Naturopathic physicians, like other types of primary care providers, develop practices that meet their personal interests and skills. While most are engaged in general and family practice, many have also specialized in particular therapeutic modalities and/or types of health problems. However, in all situations the emphasis is still on treating the whole person. The practice of family medicine requires the use of some techniques and devices that are not, in the strict sense of the word, natural therapies, but belong among the comprehensive family practice services offered by the naturopathic profession.

Included in family practice are such services as the prescription and fitting of birth control devices, first aid, and minor surgery. Minor surgery includes the repair of minor wounds and lesions and the removal of growths and foreign bodies from superficial tissues. When necessary, it includes the use of local anesthetics and appropriate first aid procedures. First aid includes the treatment of ambulatory acute injuries and conditions that are routinely seen and handled in general practice.

Many naturopaths have also developed advanced expertise in different natural therapeutic modalities. These practitioners have usually invested in postgraduate training, such as that available through residencies. Three therapeutic specialties that merit mention are natural childbirth, acupuncture, and homeopathy.

THE PHILOSOPHICAL CONTINUUM

When the various healing systems are examined and placed on a philosophical continuum, mechanism and vitalism are on different ends of the same health care spectrum. Both ends of this health care continuum have their strengths and weaknesses. Mechanistic medicine is effective for trauma, crisis care, end-stage pathology and many acute diseases. It is essentially a failure with chronic disease. In fact, conventional medicine considers most chronic diseases incurable. Vitalistic medicine, on the other hand, has its most dramatic successes with chronic disease and is effective with many kinds of acute disease. It is not very effective with trauma and crisis care and end-stage pathology, although it can be a very useful complement to conventional medicine. As can be seen, both ends of the health care spectrum are necessary if every patient's health care needs are going to be met.

Although aspects of naturopathic (e.g. constitutional hydrotherapy) and conventional medicine (e.g. chemotherapy) represent the archetypes of vitalism and mechanism, the area between the ends of this spectrum is a gray area within which both naturopathic and conventional physicians operate on a continual basis. While naturopathic physicians integrate vitalistic therapies with some mechanistic therapies, it is not possible for everyone to be experts in everything. The vast majority of naturopathic or conventional physicians are not going to be able to learn and competently practice all types of health care. Consequently, to effectively meet society's health care needs, it is necessary to create an integrated health care system. Such an integrated system would have both vitalistic and mechanistic practitioners working together in the same clinical settings.

The trends of popular culture and a biomedical science that is finally beginning to study alternative medicine suggest that the creation of an integrated health care system is now underway. However, it takes no great skill for a mechanistic medical doctor to switch from giving a synthetic drug for a disease to giving a natural medicinal substance. If naturopathic medicine becomes just another mechanistic system using natural medical substances to treat disease (instead of a system identified with treating the whole person vitalistically), it will lose its unique niche in an integrated health care system. For naturopathic medicine to survive and thrive in this new environment, it will need to keep its vitalistic roots. With a thorough grounding in *vis medicatrix naturae*, modern naturopathic medicine will flourish and achieve a leadership position as the dominant health care paradigm shifts to the integrated medicine of the future.

CONCLUSION

The practice of naturopathic medicine can be summarized most simply as helping the body/mind heal itself in the least invasive, most fundamentally curative manner possible. This approach is not tied to any particular therapy or modality, but rather is oriented to a rational blend of vitalistic and mechanistic principles working with the whole person, and educating the patient in the ways of health.

As naturopathic knowledge of health and disease grows, new therapies and approaches to health care will be added as they satisfy the principle of *vis medicatrix naturae*. As the larger health care system becomes more integrated, naturopathic medicine's place is assured as the profession that truly understands each unique human being's power to heal.

FURTHER READING

Baer HA. The potential rejuvenation of American naturopathy as a consequence of the holistic health movement. Medical Anthropology 1992; 13:369–383

Coulter HL. Divided legacy. Richmond, CA: North Atlantic Books. 1975 (vol. 1), 1977 (vol. 2), 1982 (vol. 3), 1994 (vol. 4)

Coulter HL. Homeopathic science and modern medicine. Richmond, CA: North Atlantic Books. 1980

Dubos R. Mirage of health: utopias, progress, and biological change. New York: Harper & Row. 1959: p 131

Kirchfeld F, Boyle W. Nature doctors: pioneers in naturopathic medicine. Portland, OR: Medicina Biologica. 1994

Lindlahr H. Philosophy of natural therapeutics. Reprinted by the Maidstone Osteopathic Clinic. 1975

McKee J. Holistic health and the critique of western medicine. Soc Sci Med 1988; 26(8): 775–784

McKeown T. The role of medicine: dream, mirage or nemesis? Oxford: Basil Blackwell. 1979

Payer L. Medicine and culture. New York: Henry Holt. 1988

Schubert-Soldern R. Mechanism and vitalism. University of Notre Dame Press. 1962

Selys H. The stress of life. McGraw-Hill. 1956

Sinnott E. The bridge of life. Simon and Schuster. 1966

Spitler HR. Basic naturopathy. American Naturopathic Association. 1948

Zeff JL. The process of healing: a unifying theory of naturopathic medicine. J Nat Med 1997; 7(1)

CHAPTER CONTENTS

4

Placebo and healing

Peter Bennett, ND

INTRODUCTION

The thoughts of a patient's mind and the physician's therapeutic intention on the patient have a profound effect on the health of the patient. The ability of the patient's mind to affect the process of virtually every disease has been well documented,[1,2] and the internal mechanisms and pathways by which the mind can positively or negatively affect the immune and healing processes has been investigated in the scientific literature of psychoneuroimmunology.[3,4] As the body of knowledge documenting the critical importance of the patient's psyche on the therapeutic environment has grown, it has become increasingly important for all schools of medicine to teach the healing potential of the human mind.

The potential of the mind to influence human healing has been explored to the greatest depth in medical literature discussing the placebo effect. The "power of placebo" draws upon the innate ability of the body to spontaneously heal itself, a fundamental principle of naturopathic medicine. This point separates the care delivered by naturopathic physicians from the pharmaceutical and surgical approaches of current medical "standard of care" procedures. If common medical texts on internal medicine or ambulatory care are examined, the word "healing" is not found in the index. Except for the diagnositic evaluation of "self-limiting diseases" and "spontaneous regression", the ability of the human organism to self-right and repair from a state of acute or chronic disease does not get explored in modern medicine except under the designation of "placebo response". The placebo response therefore represents all the "unknown" variables which conspire to heal a patient, in spite of pharmaceutical and surgical intervention.

Placebo response

Placebo response is the power of the mind through intention, to effect:

- a change in oneself

- a change in those around us
- a change in the environment we live in.

Intention has been seen to affect machines[5] and remote biological systems.[6] Distantly influenced systems include another person's electrodermal activity, blood pressure, and muscular activity; the spatial orientation of fish; the locomotor activity of small mammals and the rate of hemolysis of human red blood cells. Prayer, an example of intention, has been extensively studied as a therapeutic healing modality.[7] One study showed a dramatic result in cardiac ICU recovery when patients were prayed for by someone at a distant location.[8] Patients in this study were five times less likely to require antibiotics, three times less likely to develop pulmonary edema, 12 times less likely to require endotracheal intubation and less likely to suffer cardiac mortality.

Our biological systems must conform to the laws of physics. Modern physics has investigated the effect of an observer on the system observed. It has been shown that an electron will acquire a definite axis of measurement in the process of measurement. Bell's theorem supports the idea that our universe consists of particles unified instantly as an indivisible whole; our biological homeostatic systems cannot be analyzed in terms of independent parts. The interconnected nature of our biological systems has been known for thousands of years; the ancient Buddhist concept of "interdependent phenomena" accurately describes this paradigm.

Our current medical system has not shifted with the developments in modern physics. These modern ideas of biological systems are diametrically opposed to Cartesian paradigms that our internal and external environments consist of separate parts joined by local connections. Medicine must take a "quantum leap" to catch up with the knowledge we possess about our environment through quantum physics. We can see clearly that it is impossible for a doctor to observe a patient and not have that observation affect the health of the patient.

Pierre Teilhard de Chardin postulated, and Rupert Sheldrake proved, that the possibility of a "morphogenetic field" for the subliminal communication to all members of our species is possible.[9] The effect of human thought on other members of society has been described in human society since the beginning of our earliest cultures.

Naturopathic physicians believe that the body has a powerful ability to maintain health and repair to a healthy state after disease by virtue of its inherent power of vitality. This homeostatic healing mechanism has been selected by Nature in the same way that other organs which we consider to be vital to our survival have been selected. Healing occurs unaided by simply maintaining an environment that does not obstruct the path of cure.

Because placebo literature documents the philosophical foundations of the naturopathic health care model, it is important to review the full scope of this subject. Integrating known placebo initiators in clinical practice is essential for good patient care.

Why study the placebo effect?

For hundreds of years, physicians have watched their patients respond to therapies with a wide range of results. Some patients recover fully, while others, with apparently identical diseases and therapies, wither and die. Today, a skilled physician can correctly diagnose the condition of a patient by applying the sophisticated techniques of modern medicine. Then, an appropriate therapy, the efficacy of which has been thoroughly proven in research and clinical trials, can be prescribed. Through this process the patient will have received the best care available through current medical technology. But if the diagnosis, therapy, and therapeutic interaction do not stimulate the hope, faith, and belief of the patient, the chances of success are measurably diminished. It has been repeatedly demonstrated in the literature on the placebo effect,[10] psychoneuroimmunology,[3] and psychosomatic,[11] behavioral,[12,13] and psychiatric[14] medicine that the beliefs of both the patient and the doctor, and their trust in each other and the process, generate a significant portion of the therapeutic results.[15]

The placebo and its effect are not separate from any aspect of the therapeutic interaction, nor are they "nuisance variables" muddying a clear clinical picture. Rather, they send the physician a strong message: it is a patient's own belief systems that mobilize the inherent healing powers of the mind. By studying the placebo effect, a physician is better able to fully harness this power to trigger internal healing mechanisms. Yet, despite the amount of documentation, the placebo effect remains one of the most misunderstood areas in modern medicine.

The physician should always strive to stimulate self-healing, or the placebo effect, as fully as possible to maximize its potential for healing. Someday the physician will be able to explore the deepest recesses of the unconscious to directly access therapies that assist the body in the restoration of internal homeostasis. The optimal model for health care is the marriage of appropriate medical technology with the factors that have been shown to generate the placebo effect. This exciting scenario shines on the horizon as the health care of the future.

Since the doctor/patient relationship is such fertile ground for stimulating the healing response,[16–18] it serves a physician well to comprehend the nature of the placebo phenomena in order to fully realize this potential for healing.

HISTORY OF PLACEBO

The modern physician and the primitive medicine men and shamans of the past have both used ineffective therapies to stimulate healing in their patients. As Shapiro notes: "... the true importance of placebo emerges with a review of the history of medical treatment".[19] It has been noted that the historic therapies of the medical profession and traditional healers, "... purging, puking, poisoning, puncturing, cutting, cupping, blistering, bleeding, leeching, heating, freezing, sweating, and shocking",[20] worked because of the placebo effect. Although in retrospect these practices might seem ludicrous, all of these therapies were once considered effective. As an embarrassing epilogue, placebo literature has shown that ineffective procedures are just as pervasive in modern medicine as in the jungle hut of the shaman. We must therefore ask ourselves the following question: how can unfounded medical therapies survive peer review literature and centuries of cultural acceptance?

The power of the patient's belief in the potential for cure has been consistently observed throughout history. Both Galen and Hippocrates recognized the strong effect of the mind on disease and recommended that faith, treatment ritual, and a sound doctor/patient relationship could provide important therapeutic results.[21] Recognition of the power of positive expectation was recorded frequently in the medical literature of the 17th and 18th centuries. It was in the 18th century that placebo was first defined as a "... commonplace method of medicine".[22] As the importance of drug therapy grew in the 19th century, the term placebo became identified with medicines involving substances that resembled drugs. But in the 1940s, because of the increase in double-blind research, it became associated with inert substances that were used to replace active medication.

Origin of the term placebo

The original Latin meaning of placebo is "I shall please".[23] Although the term had a purely medical application in the first half of the 20th century, its meaning has been subject to various interpretations throughout the last several hundred years.

Before the 1940s, placebos were pharmacologically inactive substances, such as saline or lactose pills, used to satisfy patients that something was being done for them, i.e. the doctor was "pleasing" the patient. In the 1940s and 1950s, there was an explosion of the use of double-blind experimental procedures to evaluate the growing number of new drugs and medical procedures. Suspicion arose that all medical therapies contained an element of placebo phenomena.[24] This new understanding pressed the scientific community to offer new, far broader definitions.

Shapiro offered the classic definition of a placebo:[25]

> Any therapeutic procedure (or that component of any therapeutic procedure) which is given deliberately to have an effect, or unknowingly has an effect on a patient, symptom, syndrome, or disease, but which is objectively without specific activity for the condition being treated. The therapeutic procedure may be given with or without the conscious knowledge that the procedure is a placebo, may be an active (non-inert) or inactive (inert) procedure, and includes, therefore, all medical procedures no matter how specific – oral and parenteral medications, topical preparations, inhalants, and mechanical, surgical, and psychotherapeutic procedures. The placebo must be differentiated from the placebo effect which may or may not occur and which may be favorable or unfavorable. The placebo effect is defined as the changes produced by placebos. The placebo is also used to describe an adequate control in research.

A more accurate definition of placebo would be:

> Placebo effect is the process of a physician working with the self-healing processes of a patient. Placebo response means healing that results from the patient's own natural survival and homeostatic defense mechanisms.

Modern placebo definitions extend to its nature, properties, and effects. Placebo can be known or unknown, active or inactive, and positive or negative in results (placebo effect vs. nocebo effect), and can extend to all forms of diagnostic or therapeutic modalities, which are further defined in Table 4.1.

CLINICAL OBSERVATIONS OF "KNOWN" PLACEBO THERAPY

One of the more dramatic examples of the placebo effect reported in the medical literature involved a patient with advanced lymphosarcoma, which Klopfer[27] reported was

Table 4.1 Types of placebo

Placebo type	Definition
Known placebo	Placebo used in a single-blind experiment. The doctor knows it is a placebo but the patient does not
Unknown placebo	Double-blind placebo use. Neither the doctor nor the patient knows that the medication is a placebo
Active placebo	Any substance that has an intrinsic physiological effect that is irrelevant to the ensuing placebo effect. The vasodilating effect of niacin would make it a good active placebo
Inactive placebo	Any substance that is used with medicinal intent but which has no inherent physiological effect. Except for the glucose effect in a sugar pill (or, to complicate things, an allergic reaction to some component of the supposedly inert substance), it has no physiological effect
Placebo effect	Any changes that occur in a patient as the result of placebo therapy
Nocebo effect	Any changes that occur as a result of placebo therapy that are perceived as negative or counterproductive to the path of cure

highly susceptible to the patient's faith in an experimental drug called Krebozion. When the patient was placed on the drug, his enthusiasm was so intense that "the tumor masses had melted like snowballs on a hot stove, and in only a few days, they were half their original size!".

The injections were continued until the patient was discharged from the hospital and had regained a full and normal life, a complete reversal of his disease and its grim prognosis. Within 2 months of this recovery, reports that the drug Krebozion was ineffectual were leaked to the press.

Learning of this, the patient quickly began to revert to his former condition. Suspicious of the patient's relapse, his doctors decided to take advantage of the opportunity to test the dramatic regenerative capabilities of the mind; a single-blind study was done on the patient using pure placebo. He was told that a new version of Krebozion had been developed which overcame the difficulties described in the press, and some was promised to him as soon as it could be procured:[27]

> With much pomp and ceremony saline water placebo was injected, increasing the patient's expectations to a fevered pitch.
>
> Recovery from his second near terminal state was even more dramatic than the first. Tumor masses melted, chest fluid vanished, he became ambulatory, and even went back to flying again. At this time he was certainly the picture of health. The water injections were continued, since they worked such wonders. He then remained symptom-free for over two months. At this time the final AMA announcement appeared in the press – "nationwide tests show Krebiozen to be a worthless drug in the treatment of cancer".
>
> Within a few days of this report, Mr. Wright was readmitted to the hospital in extremis. His faith now gone, his last hope vanished, and he succumbed in less than 2 days.

Other famous placebo case studies include one reported by Cannon on belief causing "voodoo death",[28] and one reported by Kirkpatrick,[29] who documented the spontaneous regression of lupus erythematosus resulting, in part, from the patient's belief in the removal of a curse.

Other clinical observations

Belief sickens, belief kills, belief heals[30]

Evans[31] and Beecher[32] reviewed, between them, 26 double-blind studies on the efficacy of active analgesic drugs in the treatment of pain. Independently, they concluded that 35% of patients suffering from pain experienced a 50% reduction in their symptoms following placebo medication. These are particularly remarkable results when viewed in the context of Evans' observation that with a standard dose of morphine only 75% of the patients will get a 50% reduction in pain. In calculating the efficiency index of placebo analgesia, a method often used to determine the relative efficiency of drugs, placebo efficacy compared with a standard dose of morphine was 0.56 as effective. This prompted Evans to remark: "Thus, on average, placebo is not a third as effective as a standard injection of morphine in reducing severe clinical pain of various kinds but is in fact 56% as effective."[31]

Table 4.2 Symptoms and side-effects of placebo response

- Anger[33]
- Anorexia[34]
- Behavioral changes[35]
- Depression[33]
- Dermatitis medicamentosa[34]
- Diarrhea[34]
- Drowsiness[36]
- Epigastric pain[34]
- Hallucinations[37]
- Headache[38]
- Lightheadedness[34]
- Palpitation[34]
- Pupillary dilation[32]
- Rash[39]
- Weakness[34]

As discussed above, placebo has been evaluated in a wide variety of clinical settings besides pain management (see Table 4.2). When a phenomenon such as placebo has been observed to be active in diverse clinical situations, such as surgery, drug therapy, psychotherapy, and biofeedback, and over a range of physical and mental symptoms, the conclusion that it must be a factor in all aspects of medicine is inescapable.

In addition to the variety of positive effects that placebo produces are the nocebo effects, perceived as counterproductive to the therapeutic goals. These side-effects frequently are consistent with the medication that patients think they are getting. For example, the studies that measure the effects of a supposed aspirin usually show nocebo effects of ulcer-like pain.[40]

In homeopathy, aggravations and ameliorations are commonly seen when a placebo is given to fend off a patient's need to take a medication while the homeopathic physician is waiting to see if a high-potency remedy will effect a cure. Homeopathic doctors report that placebos can cause anxiety and loneliness, as well as calmness and immediate relief from insomnia.[41]

PLACEBO MYTHS

Investigation of the understanding of placebo found in the current medical literature reveals the misconceptions that prevail about the nature of placebo therapy and its effectiveness.[42] A study undertaken to examine doctors' and nurses' attitudes about placebo efficacy and use revealed that both groups underestimated the number of patients who could be helped by placebo.[42] Physicians showed a consistent pattern of placebo use:

- Placebos were used to prove the patient wrong by diagnosing psychogenic symptoms in patients who were thought to be exaggerating, imagining, or faking their symptoms.

• Placebos were used in the treatment of alcoholic, psychotic, and demanding patients who were disliked by the staff of the hospital.

• In situations where standard treatments had failed or the patient was getting worse, placebos were used as treatment.

These misconceptions regarding the nature of the placebo have accounted for its widespread misuse for patients who are perceived as uncooperative or who are suspected of malingering.

Myths about placebos continue to hinder a full understanding about the power inherent in this aspect of health care. The most common are discussed below.[43]

Myth 1

Since placebos tend to be physiologically inert, it is not possible for them to have an effect on physiological homeostasis.

Fact. Research shows that placebos have a wide range of effects (see Table 4.3) that are found throughout all aspects of human physiology.

Myth 2

Placebos are only useful with symptoms that are associated with psychological or psychosomatic complaints. Patients who need a placebo are hypochondriacs with vivid imaginations and need to be palliated with something "to please them".

Fact. Placebos have been shown to be effective in the care of all types of patients, with a consistent level of positive results for a wide variety of accurately diagnosed diseases.

Table 4.3 Physiologic changes induced by placebo

- Heart
  —improved exercise tolerance[44,45]
  —decreased serum lipoproteins[46]
  —improved T-waves[47]
  —decreased pulse rate and arterial pressure[48]
- Sympathetic stimulation
  —decreased tremulousness, sweating, and tachycardia[34]
- Claudication
  —increased walking distance[49]
  —addictive drug withdrawal[50]
- Post-surgical trauma
  —decreased facial swelling[51]
- Diabetic blood sugar dyscrasias (NIDDM)
  —lowered fasting blood sugar[52,53]
- Gastrointestinal secretion and motility
  —decreased gastric acid secretion[54]
  —changes in gastric motility[55,56]
  —healing of duodenal ulcers[57]
- Hypertension
  —lowered blood pressure[58–60]
  —reduced urinary catecholamines[61]
- Motor dysfunction
  —improved tremor magnitude[62]

Beecher was one of the first to compile a listing of the therapeutic effectiveness of placebo, thereby uncovering the wide range of therapeutic applications that were previously thought to be limited to only pain control.[15] He concluded:

> ... there is too little scientific as well as clinical appreciation of how important unawareness of these placebo effects can be and how devastating to experimental studies as well as to sound clinical judgement lack of attention to them can be.

The large and ever-growing number of studies on placebo and double-blind research (see Table 4.4) supports the assertion made by Beecher 30 years ago:[15]

> Many "effective" drugs have power only a little greater than that of placebo. To separate out even fairly great true effects above those of placebo is manifestly difficult to impossible on the basis of clinical impression. Many a drug has been extolled on the basis of clinical impression when the only power it had was that of a placebo.

Myth 3

The placebo effect is only found in substances that are inert.

Fact. Placebo phenomena have been observed across a wide spectrum of medical disciplines, including surgery,[103] drug therapy,[104] and biofeedback.[93]

Myth 4

The patient who responds to placebo can be characterized as someone who is of a typical neurotic disposition.[42]

Fact. Although many studies have tried to infer a

Table 4.4 Conditions that have been shown to respond to placebo

- Angina[44,63–66]
- Anxiety[67–69]
- Arthritis[40,70,71]
- Asthma[72–75]
- Behavioral problems[76]
- Claudication, intermittent[49]
- Common cold[77–80]
- Cough[81]
- Depression[82,83]
- Diabetes (NIDDM)[52,53]
- Drug dependence[55]
- Dysmenorrhea[84]
- Dyspepsia[85]
- Gastric ulcers[86]
- Hayfever[87,88]
- Temporal and vascular headaches[89–91]
- Hypertension[92,93]
- Labor and postpartum pain[94]
- PMS[95]
- Ménière's disease[96]
- Nausea of pregnancy[34]
- Pain[97,98]
- Psychoneuroses[99,100]
- Rhinitis[101]
- Sleep disturbances[102]
- Tremor[62]

personality type, disposition,[105,106] or certain epidemiological class of patient,[107] this has yet to be well demonstrated since, given the right circumstances, any person can become a placebo reactor.[108,109]

After reviewing the bulk of the research on this subject, Bush[110] and Wolf & Pinsky[34] concluded that the attempts to pigeonhole personalities into a clinical profile ignored the complexity of the human mind. Gliedman et al[99] similarly reported that age, sex, marital status, social class, and intelligence are unimportant factors in determining a patient's response to placebo. Wolf summarized that attempts to identify placebo reactors need to:[104]

> ... identify the nature of the symptom being treated, the motivation of the patient and physician, the nature of the test agent, its mode of administration and the life situation of the subject at the time he is tested. The significant point here is not the apparently conflicting findings of investigators with respect to placebo reactors, but rather that in any given situation, responses to a placebo may vary as compared to any other situation and the significance of situations to human subjects cannot be precisely duplicated.

PHARMACODYNAMICS

The physiological response of the "inert and inactive" placebo extends into the realm of drug pharmacodynamics. Dose–response time curves, cumulative effects (increasing therapeutic efficacy with repeated doses),[111] variable strengths of analgesia based on a patient's drug expectation,[63] drug interactions,[34,112] and carry-over effects[37,106] have all been demonstrated. The effects of placebo are so pronounced that some observers have suggested that they can exceed those attributable to potent pharmacological agents.[34]

Packaging and delivery

Several studies have found that the effectiveness of a placebo therapy is dependent on the mode of delivery.[47] For example, one study found that green tablets improved anxiety and yellow tablets improved depression,[113] while another study found that blue capsules were more sedative and pink capsules were more stimulating.[48] Placebo injections appear to be more effective than oral administration after oral placebo has failed to relieve the symptoms.[40]

Placebo interactions

Benson[114] writes that the patient's belief is also a powerful force in determining the degree of relief afforded by the placebo. An increase in patient expectation enhances the physician's ability to elicit a placebo response. Even if patients know that they are receiving placebos, the expectation and relief brought about by the therapeutic interaction provides positive results.[115] The importance of expectation is further demonstrated by the observation that the greater the stress level of the patient and the greater his or her need for assistance, the greater the effectiveness of placebo.[36] This is even seen in patient response to psychotropic drugs: LSD-25 can have no effect if the patient is told that the drug is a placebo.[105,116]

Patients, such as war heroes, who have severe injuries but do not have great mental suffering attached to their pain need less pain medication than similar injuries in persons who have pain that engenders anxiety and connotes disaster.[117]

PLACEBO HEALING MECHANISMS

Where animals or humans can react to their own deviations from homeostasis and where these deviations set off restorative processes, therapeutic intervention, including placebo, has an already existing substrate of recovery for exploitation.[12]

A human being has an intrinsic ability to "self-right" – *vis medicatrix naturae*. This is the keystone of a philosophy that has been held for thousands of years by naturally oriented physicians (see Ch. 3). The concept of a homeostatic, self-regulating mechanism is central to the understanding of basic concepts of physiology: negative feedback loops control virtually all systems of the body. According to Guyton:[118]

> ... the body is actually a social order of about 75 trillion cells organized into different functional structures ... each cell benefits from homeostasis and in turn each cell contributes its share towards the maintenance of homeostasis.

The body can maintain health and re-establish a healthy state after disease by virtue of its inherent vitality. This is part of the definition of a homeostatic mechanism; it has been selected by nature in the same way that organs vital to our survival have been selected. The surviving species are those most fitted and best able to cope with dysfunction. Those organisms that can tolerate the greatest stresses and still maintain a normal physiology are the hardiest survivors and ensure the species' ability to increase the limits of its adaptation. Therefore, given that an organism is self-maintaining when in an environment that it has been selected for, healing happens unaided by simply maintaining an environment that does not obstruct the path of cure. As Norman Cousins observed:[119]

> ... without any help, the human body is able to prescribe for itself. It does so because of a healing system that is no less real than the circulatory system, the digestive system, the nervous system, or any of the other systems that define human beings and enable them to function.

The role of emotions

Reviews of studies that explore how specific emotions can increase cancer susceptibility,[120,121] examine the effect of emotions and recovery from cancer,[122] examine the increased incidence of sudden and rapid death during psychological stress,[123] and monitor the changes in immune function during emotional stress[124,125] all confirm that emotions play a powerful role in the prognosis of a patient. Cannon and Tregear document dramatic case histories of pioneering anthropologists who witnessed the power of taboos and curses to kill strong healthy men and women in Third World cultures throughout Africa, South America, and the South Pacific: "I have seen a strong young man die the same day he was tauped; the victims die under it as though their strength ran out as water."[126]

The vis medicatrix naturae

The healing process described as *vis medicatrix naturae* demonstrates the significant power and potential of the self-generated healing capacity. For a physician, there is no more powerful stimulator of this healing mechanism, the placebo effect, than a strong doctor/patient interaction. Just by walking through the door of the physician's office, a patient's internal homeostatic mechanisms are nudged into seeking higher levels of health, healing, and adaptation. The placebo effect is a result or effect of the patient seeking the assistance of the doctor's ability to heal and cure. As Benson noted:[114]

> When we dissected the placebo effect a number of years ago, we found three basic components: one, the belief and expectation of the patient; two, the belief and expectation of the physician; and three, the interaction between the physician and the patient. When these are in concert, the placebo effect is operative. ... Perhaps nothing is being transmitted from the healer to the patient, but rather it's the belief the patient has in the healer that's helpful.

Conscious control over homeostasis

The body has two internal forces to maintain homeostasis: a lower and a higher drive. The lower drive is the inherent internal healing mechanism, the vital force, or primitive life support and repair mechanism that can operate even in a person who is asleep, unconscious, or comatose. The higher drive is the power of the mind and emotions to intervene and affect the course of health and disease by depressing or stimulating the internal healing capacities. This can be seen in the clinical observation of patients who move toward spontaneous remission of a life-threatening disease through positive emotional support[10,122] or in patients who fail to express emotions compatible with the body's attempts to survive.[122]

In any disease process, the consciousness of the patient decides the effectiveness of any therapy. Experiments in remote intention generated healing and prayer show that the intention of others is a factor in the homeostatic capabilities of the mind and body. The fact that the homeostatic mechanism can sense and respond to these remote intentions is a reflection of the power of the human mind. Some authors feel that there is a physiological basis for the unlimited possibility of human voluntary control.[127]

The ultimate control of psyche over soma demonstrates the priority of the conscious mind over physiologic processes such as immunity and pain control.[128] This puts an enormous responsibility on the physician. He or she must take full account of a patient's mental and emotional states when treating chronic or life-threatening disease.

Physiological mechanisms

Identification of a biochemical mechanism for placebo analgesia has done more to change the image of placebo than any amount of arguing about the importance of beliefs and the mind.[129]

The mechanisms of placebo response have been suggested to be a mixture of psychological interactions mediating physiological responses.[14] Psychological components of the patient's placebo effect have been shown to include the decreased anxiety and the increased relaxation,[63] conditioning,[13] expectation,[18] and well-being generated by the establishment of a sound doctor/patient relationship.[130,131]

The physiologic mechanisms of the placebo effect have been suggested to include chemicals, catalysts, and enzymes. It is believed that steroids, catecholamines,[10] the autonomic nervous system,[14,132] neuropeptides, and endorphins[133] are also involved. These physiologic mechanisms interrelate synergistically and are presently being researched under the rapidly developing field of psychoneuroimmunology,[4] through which the links between depression, affective disorders, emotions, and the immune and central nervous systems are being explored. Susceptibility to depression and sensitivity to pain have now been found to be mediated through neurotransmitters such as catecholamines, serotonin, and dopamine.

The current model for explaining the mechanism by which emotions, mood, and psychological stress suppress immune function involves cerebral-hypothalamic and pituitary interaction which translates stress and anxiety into an autonomic-endocrine response. This response adversely affects the immune function, particularly after chronic stimulation. Stressful stimulation is received in the sensory cortex of the brain and is then referred to the limbic system and the hypothalamus. This interface of the higher brain functions and homeostatic regulating centers provides the communication link between the psyche and soma. According to Rossi: "The hypothalamus is thus the major output pathway of the limbic system. It integrates the sensory-perceptual, emotional, and cognitive function of the mind with the biology of the body."[14]

In the hypothalamus are the nerve centers which

control both branches of the autonomic nervous system, parasympathetic and sympathetic, nerve cells that secrete endocrine-releasing factors, and neural pathways that release hormones directly into the posterior pituitary. The corticosteroids and catecholamines from sympathetic stimulation are key factors in altering disease susceptibility in response to stress. Corticosteroids inhibit the function of both macrophages and lymphocytes, as well as lymphocyte proliferation.[134] Corticosteroids also cause the thymic and lymphoid atrophy noted by Hans Selye in his experiments on stress-induced immune dysfunction.

The autonomic release of catecholamines stimulates receptors on the surface of lymphocytes, thereby increasing their maturation rate. When in a mature state, the lymphocytes' ability to kill bacteria and cancer cells and produce interferon seems to become paralyzed.[135] Thus a population of mature lymphocytes develops, ready to defend the body from infection and inflammation yet remaining paralyzed until the "red alert" signal of sympathetic fight or flight is turned off, signaling the appropriate time to rest and repair.

A number of other peptides, E-type prostaglandins, somatotropin, histamine, insulin, endorphins, ADH, and PTH, all have receptor sites on lymphocytes and can stimulate the same cAMP-mediated response resulting in lymphocyte maturation and inhibition.[134] A study of the effect of catecholamines on the human immune system showed that when a physiologic dose of epinephrine is injected into a healthy volunteer there is an increase in the number of circulating T-suppressor lymphocytes and a decrease in the number of circulating T-helper lymphocytes (changes similar to those found in AIDS).[134]

Placebo and stress physiology

Stress "let-down" of a patient in the therapeutic environment is one of the mechanisms producing the placebo effect. This results from the patient's perception that a transition from a stressful situation to a non-stressful situation has occurred. Mowrer[135] observed that with a decrease in anxiety there is a concomitant increase in hope, signifying that the period of suffering is over. Certain familiar images and signals, such as white coats, syringes, behavioral procedures, and clinical protocol, create a conditioned response – relief, now that help has arrived. Evans similarly observed that "... the reduction of fear through the shared expectations that the doctor's medicine will work – even if unknown to the patient it is placebo – mediates powerful therapeutic effects".[63]

The placebo effect in the clinical environment transforms the emotional and mental stress of the patient. These effects, also observed and described by Franz Alexander,[11] Hans Selye,[136] George Solomon,[137] and Walter Cannon,[138] allow the patient to escape the "fight and flight" response that can cause, and maintain, the state of illness.

Physiologic and psychologic stress

Selye[139] demonstrated that physiologic stress can have a dramatic effect on the immune and endocrine systems of the body. Laudenslager[140] went on to show that it is not just stress that creates these physiologic changes, but also the perception that stress is "inescapable" that is critical to the response. More recently, studies on the effects of psychological stress have demonstrated significant changes in immune capability. Maladjustment to "life-change stress" correlates with reduced activity of natural killer cells,[141] decreased T- and B-cell responsivity,[124] and decreased lymphocyte cytotoxicity.[142] For example, Riley[143] observed increased tumor activity in a controlled stress environment and concluded:

> Emotional, psychosocial, or anxiety-stimulated stress produces increased plasma concentrations of adrenaline, corticosteroids and other hormones through well-known neuroendocrine pathways. A direct consequence of these increased corticoid concentrations is the injury to elements of the immunological apparatus, which may leave the subject vulnerable to the action of the latent oncogenic viruses, newly transformed cancer cells, or other incipient pathological processes that are normally held in check by an intact immune system.

Current reviews of the literature relating psychological stress and immune dysfunction support the hypothesis that the homeostatic immune mechanisms, both humoral and cellular, are significantly impaired by both natural and experimental stress.[2,134,115,144] Hypertension,[145] common colds,[146] coronary artery disease,[147] and myocardial ischemia[148] have been linked to adverse stress physiology. Stress even has the ability to increase permeability of the blood–brain barrier.[149] The implication of stress altering the blood–brain barrier exposes important insights into enigmatic diseases like chronic fatigue syndrome and stress-induced neurological disorders.

Endorphins, hormones and neuropeptides

> ... one rapidly activated psychoneuroendocrine mechanism through which a placebo stimulus may reduce both depression and pain is produced by stimulating the endorphin system.[13]

Research on endorphins is a relatively new area of study in the field of psychoneuroimmunology. Original research by Levine et al[97] suggested that the pain relief noted in placebo studies could be explained by the simple mechanism of endorphin-mediated actions. The original emphasis on endorphins and enkephalins was plausible considering their known modulation of pain and mood functions. This position was further supported by later observations that depression increases chronic clinical pain[150] and that decreased activity in endogenous opioids may be part of the pathophysiology of depression.[151] With the information that placebo can stimulate endorphins,

Levine et al felt that an explanation for the action of placebos had finally been found. However, this hypothesis failed to account for the broad spectrum of placebo effects, nor did it account for the fact that the analgesia associated with hypnosis is not affected by an opioid antagonist.[152,153] It is important to note that recent literature suggests that Levine et al were not entirely wrong in implicating the role of endorphins with the placebo mechanism. Rather, they were right for the wrong reason.

Endorphins are mainly derived from three precursor proteins (by separate biochemical processes).[154] These opioid peptides are released from central and peripheral areas in response to pain, stress, and emotions and perform many physiological functions, of which analgesia is but one.[155] However, it is becoming evident that the boundaries between the central nervous system and the immune system are not as clear as once thought. The several known effects of endorphins on immune system function are listed in Table 4.5.[156]

When the functions of neurotransmitters such as endorphins are found to have such an intimate relationship with immune integrity, the paradigm of a body with functions performed independently by its parts – a Newtonian type of thinking – begins to lose credibility. To further blur the already hazy distinction between the central nervous system and the immune system, research has demonstrated that endorphins and peptide hormones such as ACTH, TSH, HCG, and LH are produced by lymphocytes.[156]

It is clear that the demarcation between the central nervous system and the immune system is impossible to distinguish. Both the brain and the immune system are the only tissues in the body which have a memory, and the level of communication between the two argues a taxonomy which identifies them as one. Evidence of the innervation of the thymus gland, bone marrow, spleen, and lymph nodes supports the finding that the immune system is subject to efferent CNS information.[156] In addition, studies demonstrating the atrophy of the thymus and lymphatic tissues in the absence of growth hormone,[157] corticotropin (ACTH), and increased steroid production by adrenal cells after interferon stimulation indicate that "... in the future it will be difficult to distinguish the receptors and signals that are used within and between the neuroendocrine and immune system".[156]

Table 4.5 Effects of endorphins on the immune system

Lymphocyte production	Increased and decreased
Chemotaxis	Increased
T-cell sensitivity to PGE_2	Increased
Antibody production	Increased and decreased
Complement	Binding of fractions C_{5B}–C_9
T-cell proliferation	Modulation of
NK-cell function	Modulation of
B-cell differentiation	Modulation of

CLINICAL APPLICATION

A physician with an interest in the psychopharmacologic treatment which also can be expensive, elaborate, detailed, time-consuming, esoteric, and dangerous will usually generate a strong placebo response. He or she will be interested in the symptoms of the patient, the differential response to various drugs and will be careful to observe side-effects which may be dangerous. The physician may encourage the patient to call at any time if side-effects develop.[21]

The application of placebo phenomena in clinical practice should not be a vague attempt to replace the skill of the medically trained physician with obscure "hand waving", incantations, and inert lactose pills. In primary care and specialty clinical practice, the physician's intent should be to optimize patient care through engaging restorative defense mechanisms. To effectively apply current placebo research, several principles (listed in Table 4.6 and discussed below) must be understood.

Prima non nocerum: prioritize a treatment program and establish a hierarchy of care

Prima non nocerum is the Hippocratic injunction dictating that a physician care for the patient so that self-healing mechanisms can engage. This ancient phrase means, "don't disturb the organism's ability to heal itself". The body must be given the full range of possibilities in allowing the power of homeostasis, *vis medicatrix naturae,* to have its optimum capability. Doing no harm means that a patient is supplied with the level of medical intervention that is appropriate to their ability to maintain life support. The job of the physician is to determine when homeostasis or defense mechanism has lost the ability to respond to disease.

Acute traumatic swelling and inflammation and shock are examples of the human defense mechanism responding in a way that threatens the health of the organism. It is most interesting that the organism would make choices, as in shock and inflammation, that could end up killing itself. To practice the principle of *prima non nocerum* a physician must learn when to act and when to let the body heal itself. This is the highest art of medicine; each case and situation will be different and it is up to the physician to interpret the needs of the moment.

Table 4.6 Six principles of optimizing placebo response in clinical practice

- *Prima non nocerum* – prioritize a heirarchy of therapeutic intervention
- *Tollum causum* – remove the obstacles
- Support the therapeutic relationship
- Enhance positive emotional states
- Implement therapeutic conditioning or learning
- Utilize altered states of consciousness

By implication, the physician who seeks to apply this principle understands the principles of physiology upon which human life depends for homeostasis.

Doing no harm means that a patient is supplied with the level of intervention that is appropriate to his or her own ability to maintain life support. *Prima non nocerum* does not necessarily mean that a physician withholds invasive therapy: it is the physician's responsibility to determine when the body is unable to re-establish homeostasis and therapy is indicated. If an arm must be severed to save the patient's life, there is no violation of *prima non nocerum*.

However, to enhance the principle of *prima non nocerum*, a physician sometimes must withhold therapies and be content to leave the patient to self-heal. Hippocrates understood the wisdom of letting the body heal on its own, implicit in the "do no harm" injunction. The treatment of Charles II is a case in point:[158]

> A pint of blood was extracted from his right arm and a half pint from his left shoulder, followed by an emetic, two physics, and an enema comprised of fifteen substances; the royal head was shaved and a blister raised; then sneezing powder, more emetics, and bleeding, soothing potions, a plaster of pitch and pigeon dung on his feet, poisons containing ten different substances, chiefly herbs, finally forty drops of extract of human skull and an application of bezoar stone; after which his majesty died.

When this treatment is compared with modern procedures such as mammary artery ligation for the relief of angina – a procedure which has no benefit when compared with sham artery ligation – it appears that throughout the centuries physicians have continued to rely on the placebo effect for the care and cure of their patients. Since it plays such an important role in health care, simple, non-invasive, and effective treatments should be the goal of all therapeutic approaches. Robert Burton wrote in 1628: "... an empiric oftentimes, and a silly chirurgeon, doth more strange cures than a rational physician ... because the patient puts confidence in him."[159]

The rational physician will also recognize that healing and curing are not necessarily the same. If a patient is helped in any way by the doctor, with or without the use of placebo, the path of cure has been assisted, although the specific pathology may not have responded. Not all patients can be cured but most patients can be helped.

Tollum causum: remove the cause of disease

Tollum causum is the principle that seeks to remove the obstacles to cure. The forces "inhibiting the floodgates of health from opening" must be removed for the full force of the patient's beliefs to effect the path of cure. This concept is fundamental to the philosophy of naturopathic medicine with its strong emphasis on diet, detoxification, and a pattern of living that is consistent and compatible with the context in which humans evolved. Obstacles to cure are defined as blocks to the self-healing capacity of the organism. Contamination with heavy metals and xenobiotics (see Ch. 37), focal infections, electromagnetic pollution, scar tissue, genetic metabolic abnormalities, and parenchymal organ damage defeat the best therapeutic intentions and must be addressed.

The patient's habitat is an important aspect of the therapeutic protocol, not only in the diagnosis and care of internal mental and physiological dysfunction, but also in determining which environmental factors may be contributing to dysfunction and disease. These factors might include diet, lifestyle, and living environment. It is of the utmost importance to remove a patient from surroundings that are associated with illness or to assist the patient in creating an environment more conducive to health.

Factors which provide conditioning that reinforce the disease process can be associated directly or indirectly with one's environment. For example, if animals are returned to situations where their experimental neuroses were induced, their pathological behavior reactivates.[160] When a patient leaves the offending environment to receive treatment from a physician, the prognosis is correspondingly more favorable.[12] The physician has the added advantage of a patient's heightened expectation during an office visit – a patient's positive associations with the "healing" environment increases their receptivity to treatment.[161] If the home or work environment is a source of "dis-ease", and an obstacle to cure, then providing an alternative environment may be a most helpful way to remove the obstacles to cure.

Support the therapeutic relationship

Confidence should surround all aspects of the therapeutic interaction. The patient must have confidence in the doctor's ability to assist a cure, the doctor must have confidence in the efficacy of his or her therapy,[162] and there must be an understanding or relationship between the doctor and the patient which is mutually conducive to respect, trust, and compassion.

The quality of the doctor/patient relationship is paramount. The therapeutic approach to a patient which optimizes the confidence of the patient in the skill of the doctor stimulates the inherent self-regulating healing mechanisms by relaxing the anxiety the patient has about their illness. Anxiety is a well-known immunosupressant and aggravates the body's defense mechanism. An optimum therapeutic relationship when combined with the clinical skill to remove the cause of homeostatic dysfunction is the height of therapeutic acumen. As Lewith so accurately states:[163]

> The general practitioner may therefore wish to employ all his knowledge, enthusiasm, consultation technique and

sympathy, to create the best possible atmosphere in which to elicit a placebo response from the patient.

Current research on factors contributing to the genesis of the placebo effect consistently documents the importance of the doctor/patient relationship.[164–166] The healing power of the therapeutic interaction has been demonstrated by the commencement of the placebo effect even before the actual administration of the pill.[167]

The physician facilitates the cultivation of a sound relationship through developing good communication skills. The art of bedside manner has been recognized throughout history as the primary skill a successful physician needs.[168] Indeed, the history of medicine is as much a history of the relationship between doctor and patient as it is the evolution of medical technology and techniques. Through centuries when doctors were doing more harm than good, little more than the esteem of their clientele sustained the medical profession. But however little real help the doctor had to offer, it was to him that people turned when illness struck.[169]

Bedside manner has been found in clinical studies to entirely alter the course of double-blind studies and the quality of a therapeutic encounter to facilitate or disrupt the efficacy of a treatment.[170] Listening to the patient,[170] verbal and non-verbal communication of the physician, amount of time spent with the patient,[171] patient education,[172] demeanor of the physician,[173] and interview skills[171] have been suggested as factors and components of effective physician communication skills.

Touch is an important form of communication and is sometimes forgotten as a key aspect of the doctor/patient relationship. Highly skilled clinicians with many years of experience, such as the late Dr John Bastyr (whose remarkable healing abilities inspired the founding of Bastyr University by those privileged to have been his students), frequently impressed upon clinicians the importance of always using diagnostic and therapeutic touch during a patient visit. The doctor's touch can be diagnostic, therapeutic, and, perhaps most important, a means of communicating that he or she is deeply attuned to the problems, needs, and fears of the patient.[174] Touch can heal by increasing tissue mobility and fluid exchange (as in massage), and by relieving pain, as demonstrated in research on healers who use their hands.[175] Touch has also been documented in well-designed double-blind research to extend an unusual healing power which can be transmitted through the hands to plants and animals.[176]

Regarding other methods of enhancing confidence between the doctor and patient, the setting in which a doctor provides therapy to a patient will also determine its effectiveness. The doctor's office setting is very important for optimum and effective treatment: tools and support systems are more accessible, and a heightened patient response results from seeking out the "healing" environment. In a clinical trial with hypertensive patients, placebo alone was not as effective as when it was administered in conjunction with hospitalization. The visit to the physician represents a search for changes that cannot be found through "self-care" or over-the-counter medicines. According to Frank:[177]

> In short, it appeared that the placebo situation relieved chiefly anxiety and depression, that the degree of relief was unrelated to personality and autonomic measures, and that the patients who responded strongly to a placebo at one time might not at another. In conjunction, these results suggest that the extent of responsiveness to a placebo depends on the interaction of the patient's state at a particular time with certain properties of the situation. The finding that administration of tests and questionnaires seemed to have at least as beneficial an effect as had the pill implies that any interaction between patient and situation that heightens expectations of help may lead to symptom reduction and improvement in mood. The aspects of the situation producing this effect include not only presentation of a symbol of the physician's healing powers (a pill), but any attention and interest shown by professional personal.

This phenomenon was also observed in industry and termed the "Hawthorne effect". As a direct result of the increased attention factory workers received during investigation, the quality of their work improved.[178] In conclusion, the importance of a doctor/patient relationship and the confidence that this engenders shows that all human beings need to share their feelings and experience the therapeutic benefits of touch: the doctor/patient relationship provides an ideal way to meet these fundamental needs.

Enhance positive emotional states

> Love in all its subtleties is nothing more and nothing less than … the psychical convergence of the universe upon itself. (*The Phenomenon of Man*, Pierre Teilhard de Chardin)

For optimum enhancement of the psychoneuroimmune system, the physician must assist the patient in developing practices that amplify positive emotional states and reduce negative emotional states. A negative mental state (anxiety, stress, panic, anger, depression, neurotic behavior, self-deprecation, self-destructive feelings and tendencies, and a weak will to live) hinders the ideal functioning of the psycho-neuro-immune-endocrine axis, disrupting homeostasis. Engle has termed this the giving-up/given-up complex:[179]

> Study of the life settings in which patients fall ill reveals that illness is commonly preceded by a period of psychological disturbance, during which the individual feels unable to cope. This has been designated the giving-up/given-up complex and has the following five characteristics: a feeling of giving up, experienced as helplessness or hopelessness; a depreciated image of the self; a sense of loss of gratification from relationships or roles in life; a feeling of disruption of the sense of continuity between past, present, and future; and a reactivation of earlier periods of giving-up. It is proposed that this state reflects the temporary failure of the mental coping

mechanisms with a consequent activation of neurally regulated biological emergency patterns. Changes in body economy so evoked may alter the organism's capability to deal with concurrent pathogenic processes, permitting disease to develop.

The importance of reducing negative mental states in acute and chronic conditions has been discussed extensively.[123] Acute psychological stress is documented to cause various forms of cardiopulmonary dysfunction, even death.[115]

Chronic mental and emotional strain causes immune system breakdown and disease. The homeostatic processes become overwhelmed by autoimmune, microbial, or neoplastic invasion. Major authors on the subject of acute and chronic stress emphasize the high priority of managing the physiologically and immunologically destructive effects of the human body's response to stress. Pelletier[180] lists hypertension, arteriosclerosis, migraine headache, cancer, chronic bronchitis, emphysema, asthma, and arthritis as disease processes which are caused or exacerbated by stress physiology. A study researching the relationship between resistance to streptococcal infections in families and stress load in the family found a positive correlation.[181] Another study on the psychosomatic susceptibility to infectious mononucleosis found that psychosocial factors of high motivation and poor academic performance significantly increased the risk of "dis-ease" infection.[182] In yet another study, anticipation of mood and menstrual discomfort were positively correlated and manipulated, thereby supporting the suspicion that expectations act as a determinant of mood.[183]

The conclusion that there is no acute, chronic, or degenerative disease that is not affected by a patient's mental and emotional state must be drawn from the pervasive immunoendocrine effects generated by the mind and emotions. Wolf[184] and Cousins[185] write of the power of panic as a factor in myocardial infarction, Marbach & Dworkin[150] describe depression as a component in myofascial pain dysfunction, and Shekelle[186] notes, in a 17-year follow-up study, a twofold increase in the incidence of cancer in depressed patients. The clinical scenarios these observers describe infer that the placebo effect can control the onset and advance of a disease by shutting down the destructive thoughts, images, and feelings that mediate stress.

Enhancing positive emotions is the corollary of controlling the damaging effects of negative mental and emotional states. Laughter,[187] hope,[188] acceptance,[117] and the reduction of suffering[189] have been shown to speed the course of healing and reduce the level of pain and distress reported by patients. Although pain is sometimes the only language nature can use to adequately communicate to the patient that something is in need of healing: "... the relief of suffering and the cure of disease must be seen as twin obligations of a medical profession that is truly dedicated to the sick".[189]

Acceptance has been observed to be a key factor that assists patients in greater understanding of their pain.[117] Acceptance does not mean complacency in the face of disease, but a rational understanding of the situation and the limitations that can sometimes accompany a disease process.

The importance of cultivating hope in a patient also cannot be underestimated.[190] The fact that a patient seeks the help of a physician or "care giver" already implies a substrate of hope and is a signal that the patient can visualize the potential for recovery. The treatment needs to merely stimulate this willingness to envision a future of health. Hope is an embodiment of the patient's and the doctor's ability to visualize an image of healing and recovery. This process is a recurrent theme in imagery therapy,[191] visualization therapy,[192] therapeutic touch,[193] and psychic healing.[194] Hope is both an active and a passive placebo. Passive hope placebo is that brought with the patient as the act of seeking help generates a level of unspoken faith in an image or potential for cure. Active hope placebo is generated by the physician, who consciously instills a vision or image of cure in the patient as an adjunct to therapy.

Frank performed a double-blind study where patients were divided into control and induction groups.[195] The induction group was led through a process whereby their hope was strengthened to conform with the expectations of the therapist:[177]

> It introduces some perceptual clarity into the process of treatment; and to the extent that all our therapists adhered roughly to the insight model of therapy, it helped to bring the patient's expectations in line with what actually occurred in treatment, and also helped him behave in accordance with the therapist's expectations of a good patient.

The induction group were actually being consciously strengthened to a level of optimal response, while not being led into false expectations.

This type of patient education or active placebo is a necessary and useful tool for framing and directing a positive outlook and prognosis. If a patient can conceive of a state of wellness, then that state of wellness can be achieved. It is the job and domain of the physician to discover those images, emotions, and perceptions which reside in the conscious and subconscious mind of the patient that block the image of a positive state of health. He or she must actively work to control these with the same level of intent as with any presenting gross complaint or physiological dysfunction. Finding these dysfunctional mental substrates and working with the patient to try and change them is fundamental to treating the true cause of disease (see *Tollum causum* on p. 60).

Research has demonstrated the importance of positive and negative thinking in heart disease and cancer, the two areas of disease which cause the highest death rate. Doctors' health care management protocols should reflect this research in the same way that attention to proper diet is a part of a management approach to high serum cholesterol. It is now clearly established, for instance, that even low levels of stress trigger the onset of myocardial ischemia.[196] We also know from the work of Steven Greer et al[197] and David Spiegel[198] that the attitude and emotional exploration are critical to breast cancer survival. Knowing these scientific facts, it is imperative that every doctor have strategies for helping their patients explore the areas of stress management, group therapy and support groups and skills in building positive attitude.

Implement therapeutic conditioning or learning

Those who remain at least dimly aware that everything they say or do to a patient conveys a major or minor, positive or negative, helpful or harmful psychological impact are likely to be more effective physicians.[199]

Conditioning of the mind has been suggested as a mechanism by which the placebo effect becomes a learned response.[12,14,177] The future of therapeutic application of placebo will probably hinge primarily on the use of conditioning. A doctor who can understand this will pay close attention to the stimuli of his patients and modify these stimuli in a scientific way to help treat immune and neurological related diseases.

Modern psychology acknowledges two models of conditioning or reinforcement of learning behavior: operant and classical conditioning. Operant conditioning is a behavior response that theoretically occurs in the presence of some stimulus that is a positive reinforcement, e.g. a rat will learn to press a conditioning bar if a food pellet is dispensed as a result. Classical conditioning is a behavior response created by the simultaneous pairing of unconditioned and conditioned stimuli prior to an evoked response. This is best illustrated by the experiments of Pavlov and his "salivating dog".

In Pavlov's experiment with the conditioning of a dog's salivary response to the ringing of a bell, the bell ring is the conditioned stimuli, the food the unconditioned stimuli. The salivation is the unconditioned response to the food that becomes the conditioned response. When the dog finally associates the bell ring with the food, the ringing alone causes salivation, the conditioned response.

The principle of classical conditioning has far-reaching implications for the diagnosis and treatment of disease because of the pervasive and permeating implications that conditioning has in all the sensory stimuli of daily existence, in sickness and in health:[200]

Pavlov's teachings, concepts and basic notions afford the real and ultimately scientific basis for the recognition of the potentialities of medical science attacking diseases from both the psychic and somatic sides.

For the purposes of this discussion, recognize that classical conditioning happens randomly in our environment and is closely linked to health and healing phenomena. Subconsciously, we note random events and associate them with previous events and observations, independent of an intended learning behavior. Operant conditioning happens in the context of reward, and classical conditioning happens in the context of associated stimuli. There is a much greater predominance and range of associated stimuli (classical conditioning) than operant conditioning for the genesis of the placebo effect. This is because the operant depends on reward, although operant conditioning can happen in the medical mode: "Pain killing drugs which I have taken in the past kills pain therefore this capsule which is a painkiller will kill my pain."

Gliedman et al[12] note that drugs that affect the CNS are readily conditioned, whereas drugs that affect the peripheral nervous system and are secretory stimulators (e.g. atropine and pilocarpine) do not result in the establishment of a conditioned response. The primary importance of psychological states to central nervous system excitation demonstrates that the pivotal loci of command for conditioning resides within the hypothalamus and the limbic system. Therefore, a doctor who can induce a state of central excitation in the patient can encourage and condition this patient to make those changes that are deemed necessary for the recovery of health.

The conditioning of a patient to a placebo response is modified by learning stimuli associated with the illness, the stimuli of the doctor and the therapeutic setting, the stimuli of the therapy, previous health, medical therapy, and authority-related experiences.[201] The way that all of these factors interact in the psyche of the patient determines the nature of the placebo response that is achieved.

Satiation obscures the conditioned response, while situations of increased stress seem to potentiate the responsiveness of the placebo effect.[117] Placebo, conditioning, and learning may therefore be subject to the nature of central excitatory states as well as to levels of stress and distress.

The physiological breadth of the placebo response in humans can now be understood in terms of the variety of interactions and effects that drugs, therapeutic procedures, and sensory phenomena of the medical environment have on the psychosomatic matrix of a patient's consciousness. Rossi[14] notes that this complicated web of sensory processing reveals how any facet of therapy:

... that alters any aspect of the body's sensory, perceptual or physiological responsiveness on any level can disrupt the more or less fragile state-dependent encoding of symptoms and thereby evoke a "nonspecific" but real healing effect that we call the placebo response.

In fact, the scientific basis of therapeutic applications of psychoneuroimmunology is based on classical conditioning. This research was done by Ader & Cohen[202] to show that the immune system could be conditioned for therapeutic purposes. Ader & Cohen conditioned immunosuppression in rats by injecting them with a conditioned stimulus of cyclophosphamide (a potent immunosuppressing agent) while feeding them a saccharine solution as an unconditioned stimulus. The idea of conditioning for immunomodulation in human patients is therefore a promising therapeutic modality. Applying conditioning techniques for the treatment of systemic lupus erythematosus resulted in a delay in the development of the disease using a dosage that normally had minimal results.[203]

To fully account for the extent of previous and future conditioning in a patient, the physician must take a complete and exhaustive history in order to explore the influences of family, work, accidents, emotional predispositions, past medical history, and neutral stimuli as contributing factors during the onset of an illness. Lifestyle and emotional, behavioral, or physiological factors might contribute to maintaining the state-dependent learning pattern of disease and dysfunction or give clues for a successful therapeutic intervention. A good example of this is Batterman & Lower's[204] demonstration of increased analgesic effectiveness based on similar previous therapy.

A physician who knows which therapies succeeded, and which failed, can take advantage of the patient's conditioning and encourage biochemical pathways that the body has learned. Drug or therapeutic interventions are not procedures that can be predicted in the same way as can in vivo experimental results. The variables involved in human responses to therapy are clearly underestimated in the current rush of research-oriented therapeutic evaluation.[55] Therefore, a patient who has been treated by a number of physicians or practitioners for a complaint and received no results or relief has been conditioned to believe that consultation and treatment by a physician will provide no positive changes. When the patient visits the next practitioner, even if this practitioner can offer a diagnosis and treatment that are correct answers to the long-sought cure, there are very real patient conditioning factors that must still be considered.

Consider the case of a young woman who was undergoing treatment for breast cancer and the clinical course of the ensuing metastases. Each time that she had a positive response to therapy, she experienced a subsequent remanifestation of the cancer. The result of this conditioning was that she came to equate each new course of chemotherapy as a herald of some new manifestation: "... she was torn between a desire to live and the fear that allowing hope to emerge again would merely expose her to misery if the treatment failed."[205]

The parameters of conditioning in a clinical setting extend to all aspects of the patient's sensory perceptions. Consciously, or unconsciously, the physician is providing an environment for patient learning. Lipkin[206] points out that every drug, every apparatus, every injection, and every piece of information or advice carries a suggestion of help and hope, regardless of the physiological effects that may accompany it. It is important to realize that the patients are taking in all the information about the surroundings, interactions, and therapy, and making associations that can potentially affect the course of their responsiveness to therapy.

Mower[135] observed that the "safety signals" of syringes, laboratory coats, and behavioral procedures are all retained in the patient's psyche for future association. A physician can skillfully take advantage of these by encouraging and cultivating response generalization or by associating previous therapeutic situations with subsequent treatments with unconditioned stimuli such as office music, odors, and images. Giving patients some sort of unconditioned stimulus that can be taken home allows them to associate with the conditioned response, eliciting the memory of the therapeutic interaction while away from the doctor's office. These unconditioned stimuli or placebos can be given in multiples at one time,[131] changed for more powerful stimuli,[70] and delivered at the end of an induction, suggestion, or imagery procedure. They should not be limited to pills or other apparent medicaments, but should extend to sounds, smells, visualizations, and feelings.

It should be remembered that therapeutic conditioning depends on a perceived physiological shift or change in the patient as described in the theory and research of biofeedback.[207] This shift can be experienced as a sense of relaxation, increased warmth or circulation, altered autonomic tone, or change in some sensory perception. Patients know immediately when there is no change in their disease or dysfunction after they have been given placebo.[208] Therefore some patients will need a more active form of therapeutic management that allows for some level of perceived change. Ideally this perception would be a sense of being free from pain, or a state of abnormal physiologic function altered to a state of improved physiologic function. Acupuncture, spinal manipulation, drug therapy, physiotherapy, hydrotherapy, and surgery are all therapies that can create an immediate biochemical impact perceived by the patient.

The optimum model to apply to the concept of conditioning therapy and the selection of an appropriate therapy or modality was proposed by Greene & Laskin[209] in their evaluation of myofascial pain dysfunction (MPD). During an 11-year follow-up study of MPD patients, they concluded that, when comparing the effectiveness of a wide variety of reversible and non-reversible (surgical) therapies, conservative and reversible therapies were the most important and appropriate treatment factors for the patient's health and well-being. Focusing on patient communication, educating patients regarding reversibility of the condition and the nature of muscle dysfunction as it relates to stress–pain–spasm, developing a therapeutic strategy based on increasing patient awareness and self-management skills, and selecting a flexible treatment strategy were all found to be essential for achieving a good initial response which could lead to long-term wellness. The specifics of which therapy was most indicated was not felt to be as important as the need to focus on the nature of presenting musculoskeletal problems and the factors and complexity of the treatment environment.

Routine use of active pharmacological substances reinforces the relationship between conditioned and unconditioned stimuli. However, routine use of unconditioned stimuli in the absence of a conditioned response weakens the therapeutic efficacy of the practitioner and has been described as "placebo sag".[13] Therefore, the learning of a conditioned response from unconditioned stimuli could diminish if the conditioned stimuli fail to produce an adequate or reliable conditioned response. Without the intermittent demonstration of active strength, the placebo effect will get weaker and weaker.

The implications of placebo sag for practitioners of alternative medicine, who try to work with the body's own defense mechanisms without overwhelming medical intervention, are that periodic use of perceptually active therapy is needed to support a patient who is not able to respond to, or responds too slowly to, a gentler therapeutic nudge. In this case, the physician must recondition the vital force to open a path to homeostasis.

In a sense, this may be a paradigm of the therapeutic situation where changes towards health are induced in the patient by a doctor who is able to cultivate a basic state of arousal, presumably central in nature. This state of arousal causes the patient to become accessible to the doctor's expectations of him.[12]

The typical placebo burst, where a therapy is initially effective after a short period, but then wanes, is now understood in terms of the placebo sagging from lack of effective unconditioned stimuli to maintain the conditioned framework.[70] Physicians who lack the ability to extract themselves from a series of unsuccessful therapies risk eventual placebo sag:[13]

> ... therapists who primarily use their active strengths (or unconditioned stimuli) paradoxically will get stronger placebo effects than quacks, will enjoy escalating credibility, and will seem as miracle men – when in fact perhaps only half their miracles can be traced to their active ingredients while the other half is a function of the anticipatory (or conditioned) response elicited by their conditioned features.

Since the visit to a physician is often initiated by the physical pain of the patient, it stands to reason that skillful pain management is a high priority in establishing a therapeutic conditioned response. Pain management by hypnosis, TENS, therapeutic touch, direct or indirect manipulation, imagery, acupuncture, meditation,[210] and an understanding that aims to elicit the nature of suffering[205] can all be valuable therapeutic adjuncts to establishing a therapeutic environment that conditions the patient for full potentiation of their healing capabilities (see Ch. 56 for a full discussion of these techniques.)

With the recent development of standardization, research, and concentration of the active components of plant medicines, vitamins, and biochemical precursors, naturopathic medicine (and other forms of alternative medicine) stands on a stronger therapeutic base because of an ever-growing verification of their pharmaceutical and therapeutic armamentarium. These therapeutic modalities are characterized by safe, yet physiologically active, substances and procedures; therefore they provide some defense against placebo sag.

Utilize altered states of consciousness

Since ancient times, aboriginal humans have recognized the tremendous therapeutic power that lies dormant in the subconscious mind. For thousands of years, shamans and medicine men have used trance states to engage the most subtle aspects of the patient's subconscious to effect factors in disease pathogenesis and prognosis.[211] In modern medicine, it has been documented that shamanistic healing involving altered states can offer dramatic "spontaneous remissions";[29] the mechanisms of this process have been explored in the theory and application of hypnosis.[1,128]

Most currently accepted techniques employed to trigger the subconscious to effect positive changes in somatic or psychic health involve hypnosis. Placebo effect has been linked with hypnosis, or "low arousal states", which are therefore believed to be critical factors in the evaluation of the mechanisms and perimeters of placebo.[200] A review of the literature documenting the potency of hypnosis and the observed results of placebo clearly demonstrates that these two areas yield remarkably similar clinical results. The inquiry into hypnosis grew out of the simple intent to validate the effectiveness of the mind in healing processes, whereas most placebo literature grew out of the intent to demonstrate a certain percentage of chance, fluke, spontaneous remission, or psychosomatic illness as a factor to be ruled out in the delivery of intelligent, scientific health care. Using these antiquated definitions of placebo and hypnosis, one is led to believe that hypnosis describes a process of healing based on the skillful guidance of a qualified practitioner, while placebo describes a process based on chance, regardless of the professional circumstances. On closer inspection, the distinction between the two blurs: they appear to be much the same process.

Illness, healing, and health states constantly shift in the homeostatic system, a system affected by stimuli received through the different levels of awareness, and can be accessed, investigated, and modified by a variety of techniques. These include placebo, hypnosis, and induced altered states of consciousness. Rossi[14] notes that since memory is dependent and limited to the level of awareness in which the memory was acquired, it is "state bound information":

> State dependent memory, learning, and behavior phenomena are the missing link in all previous theories of mind body relationships. ... The major thrust of these hypotheses is that mind-body information and state-dependent memory, learning and behavior mediated by the limbic-hypothalamic system, are the two fundamental processes of mind-body communication and healing. ... The new approach to mind-body healing and therapeutic hypnosis may be conceptualized as processes of accessing and utilizing state-dependent memory, learning and behavior systems that encode symptoms and problems and then reframing them for more integrated levels of adaptation and development.

Some psychosomatic phenomena are coded into the behavior of an individual through state-induced patterning. Until the patient can access the state in which somatic complaints are induced, possibly through hypnosis or other methods which break the sympathetic dominance of "encoded" shock,[212] the psyche cannot clear them from the soma:[14]

> A person in a traumatic car accident experiences an intense rush of the alarm reaction hormones. His detailed memories of the accident are intertwined with the complex psychophysiological state associated with these hormones. When he returns to his usual or "normal" psychophysiological states of awareness a few hours or days later, the memories of the accident become fuzzy or, in really severe cases ... the victim may be completely amnesic. The memories of the accident have become "state-bound" – that is, they are bound to the precise psychophysiological state evoked by the alarm reaction, together with its associated sensory-perceptual impressions.

In accessing these psychosomatic state-dependent areas of homeostatic dysfunction, the physician must use techniques that relax the conscious mind and allow access to subconscious content for reframing. The nature of the visit to a physician encourages a patient into more accessible unconscious states, as demonstrated by higher placebo effects when patients present to a hospital setting.[161] These labile states of consciousness are quite natural; humans constantly cycle in and out of different consciousness states.[161] These cycles, or ultradian rhythms, are described as alternating cycles of hemispherical dominance that change every 1.5 hours.

When these cycles are interrupted by behavioral stress, psychosomatic behavioral responses such as ulcers, gastritis, asthma attacks, and skin rashes develop.[213] A change in these rhythms manifests as a period of psychic repose. If an individual is in the midst of performing a task, day-dreaming or the felt need for a rest or coffee break may be the external manifestation of an internally sensed signal of a change in rhythm. This is also a period when one is highly susceptible to hypnotic suggestion. Because these rhythms are very flexible and labile, they can be invoked through hypnosis or, if the physician senses a natural lull indicating a hemispherical switch, a "natural" trance can be induced.

Centuries ago in India, practitioners of hatha yoga observed the effect of mental states on the breathing patterns of an individual. With anger, frustration, and mental instability, the breath reflected a short, arrhythmic pattern which mirrored the disturbed psyche of the person. Conversely, when a person is in a peaceful, relaxed, deep meditative state, the breath is long, rhythmic, and barely perceptible.

Their discovery formed the basis for the development of breathing exercises called *pranayama* (literally, regulation or restraint of the vital energy), which aimed to calm the breath so that deep states of meditation and focused concentration could be attained. Current research has affirmed the powerful effect these exercises have on asthma, diabetes, chronic gastrointestinal disorders, and psychosomatic and psychiatric dysfunction.[214]

Therapeutic exercises which use somatic stimuli to effect changes in the psyche create fertile environments for stimulating the placebo response. A breathing technique used to decrease sympathetic tone or alter nostril predominance for causing shifts in hemispherical activity,[215] an exercise to release fascial muscle tension and thereby effect mood-enhancing blood flow in the brain,[216,217] or a biofeedback treatment that aids in slowing the heart rate and decreasing negative emotional states[207] are all examples of how the psyche can be accessed by the soma. The whole process of eliciting the placebo response involves an attempt to marshal all the reserves and potential for healing through a doctor/patient interaction, engaging both the patient's mind and body to re-establish homeostatic equilibrium.

Health care professionals can use the wisdom of psychosomatic therapies as a central part of their therapeutic protocol. In addition to the specific therapeutic regimen, treatment of the whole patient can be achieved through these harmonious techniques. If physicians could persuade patients to care daily for their emotions, minds, and spirits the way they care for their hair or teeth, the effectiveness of any prescribed treatment would be greatly enhanced. As a primary therapeutic adjunct and important basis for preventive medicine, this line of treatment is all too often ignored.

ETHICS

It is important to remember that there are two forms of "conscious" placebo used by the physician. The use of placebo as a gentle therapeutic agent by a practitioner is very different from the use of placebo in a controlled trial where the possibility of a known therapy is withheld in a treatment group. Some authors feel that the use of placebo in clinical trial breeches the Declaration of Helsinki which states that every patient should be assured of the best proven diagnostic and therapeutic method.[218] The ethical problems of delivering health care in a research design where there is a possibility of favorable outcome and having half of the group be denied access to this possible favorable outcome is a troubling ethical issue.

The ethical use of placebo has also been questioned in an attempt to determine if a physician should be deceiving patients in the process of healing.[219] Although there are some authors who advocate a restricted use of pure and impure placebo because of its "deceptive" nature,[207] it becomes clear in a brief review of the current literature[4] that any argument for or against the use of placebo assumes that there are medical procedures that are free of potential placebo effect. Brody[24] concludes that placebo can be called the "lie that heals". However, on closer examination it can be seen that it is not the lie that does the healing, but rather the relationship between the patient and doctor which stimulates a natural self-healing mechanism via psychologic, symbolic, and biologic intervention:

> For some time, medical science has looked almost exclusively at technical means of diagnosis and treatment; the doctor/patient relationship that forms the setting for their application has been naively viewed as a non contributory background factor, relegated to the amorphous realm of the "art of medicine," or simply ignored. In this setting, the placebo effect has inevitably been viewed as a nuisance variable, interfering with our ability to elicit "clean data" from clinical trials; and deception in medicine has been seen either as an unimportant side issue or as a tolerated means toward an end. But as the doctor/patient relationship is rediscovered as a worthy focus for medical research and medical education, the placebo effect assumes center stage as one approach to a more sophisticated understanding of this relationship.[24]

While it has been observed that a physician's correct understanding of the nature of placebo therapy can coexist with its inaccurate use and abuse,[42] it has been recommended that:[219]

- Pure placebo should not be prescribed unless the physician has examined the exact indications even more carefully than when prescribing specific therapy.
- To avoid missing disease process that can be easily treated with an empirically proven protocol (e.g. vitamin B_{12}-deficient peripheral neuropathy), the physician should not relax a diagnostic protocol because a patient seems to be responding to placebo.

CONCLUSION

Health practitioners need to be equipped with a better understanding of placebo therapeutics.[6,220] For many years now, the study of placebo has been recommended to doctors and health care professionals. The ideal environment for the dissemination of the therapeutic implications of the doctor/patient relationship is in medical schools as a required part of the curriculum. After finding a pattern of misuse and misunderstanding about the nature and efficacy of placebo, Goodwin[42] recommended that better education might result in more effective placebo use.

In 1938, Houston[168] wrote of the need to reaffirm the art of medicine because he perceived a trend in medicine that invested in a concept of the therapeutic doctor/patient interaction as "undisciplined thought". Houston's remedy for the intellectual bias that viewed medicine as a "tight, fast-set science" was to emphasize the importance of psychobiology in medical schools:[168]

> One of the most hopeful moves in medical education is teaching to first-year students the elements of psychobiology. A system of belief is implanted best in the young. It would be my suggestion that psychobiology be taught in the premedical years, that the doctor/patient relationship be the beginning of medical studies. A deep insight into this fundamental philosophy is a chief concern of the internist.

REFERENCES

1. Hall H. Hypnosis and the immune system. Am J Clin Hyp 1982; 25: 92–103
2. Rogers M, Dubey D, Reich P. Influence of the psyche and brain on immunity and disease susceptibility. Psyche Som Med 1979; 41: 147–164
3. Ader R, ed. Psychoneuroimmunology. New York, NY: Academic Press. 1981
4. White LB, Tursky B, Schwartz G, eds. Placebos: theory, research and mechanisms. NY: Guilford. 1985
5. Thompson R. Numerical analysis and theoretical modeling of causal effects of conscious intention. Subtle Energies 1991; 2: 47–70
6. Braud W. Conscious interactions with remote biological systems. anomalous intentionality effects. Subtle Energies 1991; 2: 1–46
7. Dossey L. Healing Words. The power of prayer and the practice of medicine. New York: Harper Collins. 1993
8. Byrd R. Positive therapeutic effects of intercessory prayer in a coronary care unit population. Southern Med J 1988; 81: 826–829
9. Sheldrake R. The presence of the past: morphic resonance and the habits of nature. New York: New York Times Books. 1988
10. Benson H, Epstein MD. The placebo effect. JAMA 1975; 232: 1225–1227
11. Alexander F. Psychosomatic medicine. New York, NY: Norton. 1987
12. Gliedman LH, Gantt WH, Teitelbaum HA. Some implications of conditional reflex studies for placebo research. Am J Psych 1957; 113: 1103–1107
13. Wickramasekara I. The placebo as a conditioned response. Advances 1984; 1: 109–135
14 Rossi E. The psychobiology of mind-body healing. NY: Norton. 1986
15. Beecher HK. The powerful placebo. JAMA 1955; 159: 1602–1606
16. Everson TC, Cole WH. Spontaneous regression of cancer. Philadelphia: Saunders. 1966

17. Booth G. Psychological aspects of 'spontaneous' regressions of cancer. J Am Acad Psychoanalysis 1973; 1: 303–317
18. Cousins N. Anatomy of an illness. New Engl J Med 1976; 295: 1458–1463
19. Shapiro AK. A contribution to the history of the placebo effect. Behav Sci 1960; 5: 1109–1135
20. Shapiro AK. Factors contributing to the placebo effect: their implication for psychotherapy. Am J Psychother 1961; 18: 73–88
21. Shapiro AK. Placebogenics and iatroplacebogenics. Med Time 1964; 92: 1037–1043
22. Berg AO. The placebo effect reconsidered. J Fam Prac 1983; 17: 647–650
23. Webster's II, New Riverside University Dictionary. Boston, MA: Riverside Publ Co. 1984
24. Brody H. The lie that heals: the ethics of giving placebos. Ann Intern Med 1982; 97: 112–118
25. Shapiro AK. Factors contributing to the placebo effect: their implications for psychotherapy. Am J Psych 1961; 18: 73–88
27. Klopfer B. Psychological variables in human cancer. J Proj Tech 1957; 21: 331–340
28. Cannon WB. 'Voodoo' death. Psychosomatic Med 1957; 19: 182–190
29. Kirkpatrick RA. Witchcraft and lupus erythematosus. JAMA 1981; 245: 1937–1938
30. Hahn R. In: White L, Tursky B, Schwartz G, eds. Placebos: theory, research and mechanisms. New York, NY: Guilford Press. 1985
31. Evans FJ. Unraveling placebo effects. Advances 1984; 1: 11–19
32. Beecher HK. Measurement of subjective responses: quantitative effect of drugs. New York, NY: Oxford University Press. 1959
33. Linton HB, Langs RJ. Placebo reactions in a study of LSD-25. Arch Gen Psych 1962; 6: 53–67
34. Wolf S, Pinsky RH. Effects of placebo administration and occurrence of toxic reactions. JAMA 1954; 155: 339–341
35. Cytryn L, Gilbert A. The effectiveness of tranquilizing drugs plus supportive psychotherapy in treating behavior disorders of children: a double-blind study of eighty outpatients. Am J Orthopsychiatry 1960; 30: 113–129
36. Beecher HK. Evidence for increased effectiveness of placebos with increased stress. Am J Phys 1956; 187: 163–169
37. Lasagna L, von Felsinger JM, Beecher HK. Drug-induced changes in man. 1. Observations on healthy subjects, chronically ill patients, and 'postaddicts'. JAMA 1955; 157: 1006–1020
38. Keats AS, Beecher HK. Analgesic potency and side action liability in man of heptazone, WIN 1161–2, 6-methyl dihydromorphine, meptopon, levo-isomethadone and pentobarbitol sodium as a further effort to refine methods of evaluation of analgesic drugs. J Pharmacol Exp Ther 1952; 105: 109–129
39. Wolf S, Pinsky RH. Effects of placebo administration and occurrence of toxic reactions. JAMA 1954; 155: 339–341
40. Traut EF, Passarellu EW. Placebos in the treatment of rheumatoid arthritis and other rheumatic conditions. Ann Rheum Dis 1957; 16: 18–21
41. Elmore D. Personal communication, April 1988
42. Goodwin JS. Knowledge and use of placebos by house officers and nurses. Ann Int Med 1979; 91: 106–110
43. Vogel AV, Goodwin JS, Goodwin JM. The therapeutics of placebo, AFP 1980; 22: 107–109
44. Kostis JB, Krieger S, Cosgrove N et al. The mechanism of placebo effect on exercise tolerance in angina pectoris. Am J Card 1982; 49: 1001
45. Benson H, McCallie DP. Angina pectoris and the placebo effect. New Engl J Med 1979; 300: 1424–1429
46. Rinzler SH, Travell J. Effect of heparin in effort angina. Am J Med 1953; 14: 438–447
47. Shevchuk YM. A medical marvel. Can Pharm Rev 1987; Oct: 597–600
48. Blackwell B, Bloomfield SS, Buncher CR. Demonstration to medical students of placebo responses and non-drug factors. Lancet 1972; i: 1279–1282
49. Porter JM, Cutler BS, Lee BY et al. Pentoxifylline efficacy in the treatment of intermittent claudication. Multicenter controlled double-blind trial with objective assessment of chronic occlusive arterial disease patients. Am Heart J 1982; 104: 66–72
50. Viner O. Dependence on a placebo: a case report. Brit J Psychiat 1969; 115: 1189–1190
51. Hashish I, Harvey W. Anti-inflammatory effects of ultrasound therapy: evidence for a major placebo effect. Br J Rheumatol 1986; 25: 77–81
52. Katz HM, Bissel G. Blood sugar lowering effects of chlorpromamide and tolbutamide. Diabetes 1965; 14: 650–657
53. Singer DL, Hurwitz D. Long term experience with sulfonylureas and placebo. New Engl J Med 1967; 277: 450–456
54. Wolf S. Part iv. Placebo: problems and pitfalls. Clin Pharmacol Ther 1962; 3: 254–257
55. Wolf S. Effects of suggestion and conditioning on the action of chemical agents in human subjects – the pharmacology of placebos. J Clin Invest 1950; 29: 100–109
56. Abbot FK, Mack M, Wolf S. The action of banthine on the stomach and duodenum of man with observations on the effects of placebos. Gastroenterology 1952; 20: 249–261
57. Brogden RN, Carmine AA, Heel RC et al. Ranitidine: a review of its pharmacology and therapeutic use in peptic ulcer disease and other allied diseases. Drugs 1982; 24: 267–303
58. Grenfell RF, Briggs AH, Holland WC. Antihypertensive drugs evaluated in a controlled double study. South Med J 1963; 56: 1410–1416
59. Reader R. Therapeutic trials in mild hypertension. Med J Aust 1986; 144: 225–227
60. Gould BH, Davis AB, Altman ODG et al. Does placebo lower blood pressure? Lancet 1981; ii: 1377–1381
61. Hossman V, FitzGerald GA, Dollery CT. Influence of hospitalization and placebo therapy on blood pressure and sympathetic function in essential hypertension. Hypertension 1981; 3: 113–118
62. Calzetti S, Findley LJ, Gresty MA et al. Metoprolol and propranolol in essential tremor. A double blind, controlled study. J Neurol Neurosurg Psychiatry 1981; 44: 814–819
63. Evans W, Hoyle C. The comparative value of drugs used in the continuous treatment of angina pectoris. Q J Med 1933; 2: 311–338
64. Diamond EG, Kittle CF, Crockett JE. Comparison of internal mammary artery ligation and sham operation for angina pectoris. Am J Cardiology 1960; 5: 483–486
65. Benson H, McCallie DP. Angina pectoris and the placebo effect. New Engl J Med 1979; 300: 1424–1429
66. Cobb LA, Thomas GJ, Dillard DH et al. An evaluation of the internal mammary artery ligation by a double blind technique. New Engl J Med 1959; 269: 1115–1118
67. Wolf S, Pinsky RH. Effects of placebo administration and occurrence of toxic reactions. JAMA 1954; 155: 339–341
68. Uhlenhuth EH, Canter A, Neustadt JO, Payson HE. The symptomatic relief of anxiety with meprobamate, phenobarbital, and placebo. Am J Psychiatry 1959; 115: 905–910
69. Solomon K, Hart R. Pitfalls and prospects in clinical research on antianxiety drugs. Benzodiazepines and placebo – a research review. J Clin Psychiatry 1978; 39: 823–831
70. Morrison RAH, Woodsey A, Young AJ. Placebo responses in an arthritis trial. Ann Rheum Dis 1961; 20: 179–185
71. Cederlof S, Jonson G. Intraarticular prednisolone injection for osteoarthritis of the knee. Acta Chir Scand 1966; 132: 532–536
72. Wayne EJ. Placebos. Br Med J 1956; ii: 157
73. Godfrey S, Koing P. Suppression of exercise-induced asthma by salbutamol, theophylline, atropine, cromolyn, and placebo in a group of asthmatic children. Pediatrics 1975; 56: 930–934
74. Luparello T, Lyons HA, Bleecher ER, McFadden ER. Influences of suggestion on airway reactivity in asthmatic subjects. Psychosomatic Med 1968; 30: 819–825
75. Godfrey S, Silverman M. Demonstration by placebo response in asthma by means of exercise testing. J Psychosom Res 1973; 17: 293–297
76. Molling PA, Lockner AW, Sauls RJ et al. Committed delinquent boys. Arch Gen Psychiatry 1962; 7: 70–78
77. Green FHK, Andrews CH, Bain WA et al. Clinical trials of antihistamine drugs in the prevention and treatment of the common cold. Br Med J 1950; ii: 425–429

78. Diehl HS, Baker AB, Cowan DW. Cold vaccines: a further evaluation. JAMA 1940; 115: 593–594
79. Buck C. A clinical trial of a quaternary ammonium antiseptic lozenge in the treatment of the common cold. Can Med Assoc J 1962; 86: 489–491
80. Diehl HS. Medicinal treatment of the common cold. JAMA 1933; 101: 2042–2050
81. Hillis BR. The assessment of cough suppressing drugs. Lancet 1952; i: 1230–1235
82. Malitz S, Kanzler M. Are antidepressants better than placebos? Am J Psychiatry 1971; 127: 605–611
83. Morris JB, Beck AT. The efficacy of antidepressant drugs. Arch Gen Psych 1974; 30: 667–671
84. Budoff PW. Zomepirac sodium in the treatment of primary dysmenorrhea syndrome. New Engl J Med 1982; 307: 714–719
85. Nyren O, Adami HO, Bates S et al. Absence of therapeutic benefit from antacids or cimetidene in non-ulcer dyspepsia. New Engl J Med 1986; 314: 339–343
86. Sturdevant RAL, Isenberg JI, Secrist D, Ansfield J. Antacid and placebo produced similar pain relief in duodenal ulcer patients. Gastroenterology 1977; 77: 1–5
87. Wise PG, Rosenthal RR, Killian P et al. A controlled study of placebo treatment of hayfever (abstract). J Allergy Clin Immunol 1979; 63: 216
88. Baldwin H. Conference on therapy. Am J Med 1954; 17: 72
89. Frey GH. The role of placebo response in clinical headache evaluations. Headache 1961; July: 31–38
90. Jellinek EM. Clinical tests on comparative effectiveness of analgesic drugs. Biometrics Bull 1946; 2: 87–91
91. Sillaanpaa M. Clonidine prophylaxis of childhood migraine and other vascular headache. Headache 1977; 17: 28–31
92. Management Committee. Untreated mild hypertension. Lancet 1982; i: 185–191
93. Patel C, Marmot MG, Terry DJ. Controlled trial of biofeedback-aided behavioral methods in reducing mild hypertension. Br Med J 1981; 282: 2005–2008
94. Liberman R. An experimental study of the placebo response under three different situations of pain. J Psych Res 1964; 2: 233–246
95. Maddocks S, Hahn P, Moller F et al. A double-blind placebo-controlled trial of progesterone vaginal suppositories in the treatment of premenstrual syndrome. Am J Ob Gyn 1986; 154: 573–581
96. Thomsen J, Bretlau P, Tos M, Johnsen NJ. Placebo effect in surgery for Ménière's disease. Three-year follow-up. Otolaryngology 1983; 91: 183–186
97. Levine JD, Gordon NC, Fields HL. The mechanism of placebo analgesia. Lancet 1978; ii: 654–657
98. Posner J, Burke CA. The effects of nalaxone on opiate and placebo analgesia in healthy volunteers. Psychopharmacology 1985; 87: 468–472
99. Gliedman L, Nash EH, Imber SD et al. Reduction of symptoms by pharmacologically inert substances and by short-term psychotherapy. Am Med Assn Arch Neurol Psych 1958; 79: 345–351
100. Barron A, Beckering B, Rudy LH, Smith JA. A double blind study comparing RO4-0403, trifluoperazine and a placebo in chronically ill mental patients. Am J Psych 1961; 118: 347–348
101. Schultz JI, Johnson JD, Freedman SO. Double-blind trial comparing flunisolide and placebo for the treatment of perennial rhinitis. Clinical Allergy 1978; 8: 313–320
102. Straus B, Eisenberg J. Hypnotic effects of an antihistamine – methapyrilene hydrochloride. Ann Intern Med 1955; 42: 574–582
103. Beecher HK. Surgery as placebo. JAMA 1961; 176: 1102–1107
104. Wolf S. The pharmacology of placebos. Pharm Rev 1959; 11: 689–670
105. Linton HB, Langs RJ. Placebo reactions in a study of lysergic acid diethylamide. Arch Gen Psych 1962; 6: 368–383
106. Lasagna L. A study of the placebo response. Am J Med 1954; 16: 770–779
107. Moertel CG. Who responds to sugar pills? Mayo Clin Proc 1976; 51: 96–100
108. Parkhouse J. Placebo reactor. Nature 1963; 199: 308
109. Fisher S. The placebo reactor: thesis, anti-thesis, synthesis and hypothesis. Dis Nerv Syst 1967; 28: 510–515
110. Bush P. The placebo effect. J Am Pharm Assn 1974; 14: 671–674
111. Lasagna L, Laties VG, Dohan JL. Further studies on the 'pharmacology' of placebo administration. J Clin Invest 1958; 37: 533–537
112. Dinnerstein AJ, Halm J. Modification of placebo effects by means of drugs: effects of aspirin and placebo on self-rated moods. J Abn Psych 1970; 75: 308–314
113. Schapira K, McClelland HA, Griffiths NR, Newell DJ. Study on the effects of tablet color in the treatment of anxiety states. Brit Med J 1970; ii: 446–449
114. Benson H. Looking beyond the relaxation response. Revision 1984; 7: 50–55
115. Darko DF. A brief tour of psychoimmunology. Ann Allergy 1986; 57: 233–237
116. Reed CF, Witt PN. Factors contributing to unexpected reactions in two human drug-placebo experiments. Confin Psychiat 1963; 8: 57–68
117. Beecher HK. Relationship of significance of wound to pain experienced. JAMA 1956; 161: 1609–1613
118. Guyton AC. Textbook of medical physiology. Philadelphia, PA: WB Saunders. 1981
119. Cousins N. Foreword. In: Locke S, Colligen D, eds. The healer within. New York, NY: Dutton. 1986
120. Thomas CB, Duszynski KR, Shaffer JW. Family attitudes reported in youth as potential predictors of cancer. Psychosom Med 1979; 41: 287–301
121. Schekelle RB. Psychological depression and 17-year risk of death from cancer. Psychosom Med 1981; 43: 117–125
122. Dreher H. Cancer and the mind: current concepts in psycho-oncology. Advances 1987; 4: 27–43
123. Bartrop RW, Luckhurst E, Lazarus L et al. Depressed lymphocyte function after bereavement. Lancet 1977; i: 834–836
124. Schleifer SJ, Keller SE, Camerino M et al. Suppression of lymphocyte stimulation following bereavement. JAMA 1983; 250: 374–375
125. Engle GL. Sudden and rapid death during psychological stress. Ann Int Med 1971; 74: 771–782
126. Tregear E. J Anthr Inst 1890. 19: 100 [cited in Cannon[28]]
127. Gough WC, Shacklet. The science of connectiveness. Part 3: The human experience. Am J Clin Nutr 1980; 33: 71
128. Steggles S, Stam HJ, Fehr R, Aucoin P. Hypnosis and cancer: an annotated bibliography 1960–1985. Am J Clin Hyp, 1987; 29: 281–290
129. Weil A. Health and healing. Boston, MA: Houghton Mifflin. 1983
130. Freund J, Krupp G, Goodenough D, Preston LW. The doctor patient relationship and the drug effect. Clin Pharm Ther 1972; 13: 172–180
131. Greene CS, Laskin DM. Long-term evaluation of treatment for myofascial pain dysfunction syndrome. JADA 1983; 107: 235–236
132. Sternbach R. The effects of instructional sets on autonomic responsivity. Psychophys 1964; 1: 67–72
133. Levine JD, Gordon NC, Fields HL. The mechanism of placebo analgesia. Lancet 1978; ii: 654–657
134. Borysenko J. Psychoneuroimmunology: behavioral factors and the immune response. Revision 1984; 7: 56–65
135. Mower OH. Learning theory and behavior. New York, NY: Wiley. 1960
136. Selye H. The general adaptation syndrome and the diseases of adaptation. J Clin Endocrinology 1946; 6: 117–230
137. Solomon GF. The emerging field of psychoneuroimmunology, with a special note on AIDS. Advances 1985; 2: 6–19
138. Cannon W. Stresses and strains of homeostasis. Am J Med Sci 1935; 22: 1–18
139. Selye H. The general adaptation syndrome and the diseases of adaptation. J Clin Endocrinology 1940; 6: 117
140. Laudenslager ML. Coping and immunosuppression: inescapable but not escapable shock suppresses lymphocyte proliferation. Science 1983; 221: 568–570
141. Lloyd R. Possible mechanisms of psychoneuroimmunological interaction. Advances 1984; 1: 43–51
142. Monjan AA, Collector MI. Stress-induced modulation of the immune response. Science 1977; 196: 307–308

143. Riley V. Psychoneuroendocrine influences on immunocompetence and neoplasia. Science 1981; 212: 110, 1100–1109
144. Locke S, Colligen D. The healer within. New York, NY: Dutton. 1986
145. Schnall PL et al. The relationship between 'job strain' workplace diastolic blood pressure, and left ventricular mass index. Results of a case controlled study. JAMA 1990; 263: 1929–1935
146. Motional stress linked to common cold. Science News 1991; 140: 132
147. Stress puts squeeze on clogged vessels. Science News 1991; 140: 309
148. Editorial. Mittleman MA, Maclure M. Mental stress during daily life triggers myocardial ischemia. JAMA 1997; 277: 1558–1559
149. Stress may weaken the blood brain barrier. Science News 1996; 150: 375
150. Marbach JJ, Dworkin SF. Chronic MPD group therapy and psychodynamics. JADA 1975; 90: 827–833
151. Gold MS, Pottash AC, Sweeny D et al. Antimanic, antidepressant and antipanic effects of opiates: clinical, neuroanatomical and biochemical evidence. In: Verby K, ed. Opioids in mental illness. New York, NY: Academy of Sciences. 1982
152. Goldstein A, Grevert P. Placebo analgesia, endorphins and nalaxone. Lancet 1978; ii: 1385
153. Barber J, Mayer D. Evaluation of the efficacy and neural mechanism of a hypnotic analgesia procedure in experimental and clinical dental pain. Pain 1977; 4: 41–78
154. Krieger DT. Brain peptides. What, where and why. Science 1983; 222: 975–985
155. Heijnen CJ, Ballieux RE. Influence of opioid peptides on the immune system. Advances 1986; 3: 114–121
156. Blalock JE. The immune system as a sensory organ. J Immunol 1984; 132: 1067–1070
157. Pierpaoli W, Sorkin E. Hormones and immunologic capacity. J Immunol 1968; 101: 1036–1043
158. Haggard HW. Devils, drugs, and doctors. New York, NY: 1968. 1929
159. Burton R. The anatomy of melancholy. New York, NY: Empire State Book Company. 1929
160. Gantt WH. Principles of nervous breakdown – schizokinesis and autokinesis. Ann NY Acad Sci 1953; 56: 143–163
161. Klerman GL. Assessing the influence of the hospital milieu upon the effectiveness of psychiatric drug therapy. J Nerv Ment Dis 1963; 137: 143–154
162. Wheatly D. Influence of doctors' and patients' attitudes in the treatment of neurotic illness. Lancet 1967; ii: 1133–1135
163. Lewith GT. Every doctor a walking placebo. Comp Med Res 1987; 2: 10–18
164. Benson H, Epstein MD. The placebo effect. JAMA 1975; 232: 1225–1227
165. Brody HL. The lie that heals. Ann Int Med 1982; 97: 112–118
166. Jensen PS. The doctor-patient relationship. Headed for impasse or improvement? Ann Int Med 1981; 95: 769–771
167. Nash EH, Frank JD, Imber SD et al. Selected effects of inert medication on psychiatric patients. Am J Psychother 1964; 18: 33–48
168. Houston WR. The doctor himself as a therapeutic agent. Ann Int Med 1938; 11: 1416–1425
169. Freund J, Krupp G, Goodenough D et al. The doctor-patient relationship and the drug effect. Clin Pharm Ther 1972; 13: 172–180
170. Budd MA, Zimmerman ME. The potentiating clinician: combining scientific and linguistic competence. Advances 1986; 3: 40–45
171. Bogdonoff MD. The doctor-patient relationship. JAMA 1965; 192: 45–48
172. Egbert LD, Battit GE, Welch CE, Bartlett MK. Reduction of postoperative pain by encouragement and instruction of patients. New Engl J Med 1964; 270: 825–827
173. Shapiro AK. Placebo effects in psychotherpy and psychoanalysis. J Clin Pharm 1970; Mar–Apr: 73–77
174. Bruhn JG. The doctor's touch: tactile communication in the doctor-patient relationship. Southern Medical J 1978; 71: 1469–1473
175. Krieger D. The therapeutic touch. New York, NY: Prentice-Hall. 1979
176. Grad B. Some biological effects of the 'laying on of hands': a review of experiments with animals and plants. J Am Soc Psychical Res 1965; 59: 95
177. Frank J. The role of hope in psychotherapy. Int J Psych 1968; 5: 383–395
178. Roethlisberger FJ, Dickson WJ. Management and the worker. Cambridge, MA: Harvard University Press. 1961
179. Engle GL. A life setting conducive to illness: the giving-up–given-up complex. Ann Int Med 1968; 69: 293–300
180. Pelletier KR. Mind as healer, mind as slayer. New York, NY: Dell. 1977
181. Meyer RJ, Haggerty RJ. Streptococcal infections in families: factors altering individual susceptibility. Pediatrics 1962; April: 539–547
182. Kasl SV. Psychosocial risk factors in the development of infectious mononucleosis. Psychosom Med 1979; 41: 445–465
183. Olasov B, Jackson J. Effects of expectancies on women's reports of moods during the menstrual cycle. Psychosom Med 1987; 49: 55–78
184. Wolf S. The end of the rope: the role of the brain in cardiac death. Can Med Ass J 1967; 97: 1021–1025
185. Cousins N. The healing heart. New York, NY: Avon. 1983
186. Shekelle RB. Psychological depression and 17-year risk of death from cancer. Psychosom Med 1981; 43: 117–125
187. Cousins N. Anatomy of an illness. New Engl J Med 1976; 295: 1458–1463
188. Gottschalk LA. Hope and other deterents to illness. Am J Psychotherapy 1985; 39: 515–524
189. Cassel EJ. The nature of suffering and the goals of medicine. New Engl J Med 1982; 306: 639–645
190. Bruhn JG. Therapeutic value of hope. Southern Med J 1984; 77: 215–219
191. Achterberg J. Imagery in healing. Boston, MA: New Science Library. 1985
192. Simonton OC, Simonton S. Getting well again. Los Angeles, CA: Tarcher. 1978
193. Krieger D. The therapeutic touch. New York, NY: Prentice-Hall. 1979
194. Kunz D, ed. Spiritual aspects of healing. Wheaton, IL: Theosophical Publishing. 1985
195. Frank J. The role of hope in psychotherapy. Int J Psyc 1968; 5: 383–395
196. Editorial. Mittleman MA, Maclure M. Mental stress during daily life triggers myocardial ischemia. JAMA 1997; 277: 1558–1559
197. Greer S, Moorey S, Baruch JD et al. Adjuvant psychological therapy for patients with cancer: a prospective randomized trial. Br Med J 1992; 304: 675–680
198. Spiegel D. Psychological aspects of breast cancer treatment. Seminars in Oncology l24(suppl 1)S1-S47, 1997
199. Cornell Conference on Therapy. The use of placebos in therapy. NY State Med J 1946; 46: 1718–1726
200. Volgyesi A. 'School for patients,' hypnosis therapy and psychoprophylaxis. Br J Med Hyp 1954; 5: 8–17
201. Epstein JB. Understanding placebos in dentistry. JADA 1984; 109: 71–74
202. Ader R, Cohen N. Behaviorally conditioned immunosuppression. Psychosomatic Med 1975; 37: 333–340
203. Ader R. Behaviorally conditioned modulation of immunity. In: Guillemin R, Melnechuk T, eds. Neural modulation of immunity. New York, NY: Raven Press. 1985
204. Batterman RC, Lower WR. Placebo responsiveness – influence of previous therapy. Curr Ther Res 1968; 10: 136–143
205. Cassels EJ. The nature of suffering and the goals of medicine. New Engl J Med 1982; 306: 639–645
206. Lipkin M. Suggestion and healing. Perspectives Bio Med 1984; 28: 121–126
207. Schwartz GE. Biofeedback, self-regulation, and patterning of physiological processes. Am Scientist 1975; 63: 314–324
208. Modell W, Houde. Factors influencing clinical evaluation of drugs. JAMA 1958; 167: 2190–2199
209. Greene CS, Laskin DM. Long-term evaluation of treatment of myofascial pain dysfunction syndrome. Comparative analysis. JADA 1983; 107: 235–238

210. Kabat-zin J. An outpatient program in behavioral medicine for chronic pain patients based on the practice of mindfulness meditation: theoretical considerations and preliminary results. Gen Hosp Psychiatry 1982; 4: 33–47
211. Halifax J. Shamanic voices: a survey of visionary narratives. New York, NY: Dutton. 1979
212. Klinghardt DK. Neural therapy. J Neurol Orthop Med Surg 1993; 14: 109–114
213. Orr WC, Hoffman HJ, Hegge FW. Ultradian rhythms in extended performance. Aerospace Med 1974; 45: 995–1000
214. Goyeche J. Yoga as therapy in psychosomatic medicine. Psychother Psychosom 1977; 31: 373–381
215. Werntz D. Cerebral hemispheric activity and autonomic nervous function. Doctoral Dissertation, University of California, San Diego, CA
216. Zojonc RB. Emotion and fascial efference. A theory reclaimed. Science 1985; 228: 15–21
217. Critchly EMR. The human face. Br Med J 1985; 29: 1223–1224
218. Rothman KJ, Michaels KB. The continuing unethical use of placebo controls. New Engl J Med 1994; 331: 394–398
219. Bok S. The ethics of giving placebo. Sci Am 1974; 231: 17–23
220. Leslie A. Ethics and practice of placebo therapy. Am J Med 1954; 16: 854–862

CHAPTER CONTENTS

5

Women in the history of medicine

Jennifer Booker, ND

INTRODUCTION

Traditionally, women have been the healers, caring for their families and neighbors and helping each other through childbirth. Over centuries, women developed and utilized herbal remedies, poultices, diet therapies, water treatments, and techniques for bone setting and the suturing of wounds. Their methods were passed down to form not only the basis of naturopathic medicine, but also much of what is allopathic medicine.

Women have always been at the forefront in providing humane health care, from the venerated women healers of ancient Greece, to the persecuted medieval women lay healers, to the pioneering women of North America. The witch burnings of medieval Europe, the persecution of midwives in the 18th, 19th and 20th centuries, and the discrimination experienced by women in medicine today are all part of the history and development of medicine. To be unaware of women's role in medical history is to be ignorant of half the story of medicine.

Today, health care is primarily in the hands of men, with women playing helpmate roles. The history of women as primary health care givers has been almost completely obliterated. Information about women healers is not part of mainstream knowledge; the interested reader must seek out books specifically about women healers which, until recently, have been generally unavailable. Indeed, women are generally excluded from history books, not only those concerned with medicine (see Spender[1] for further discussion). This dearth of information is a reflection of the pervasive sexism of our civilization. It is the author's intent to reclaim here part of the history of women in medicine.

Today, 93% of allopathic physicians are male. Throughout the industrialized world there are still only few women physicians: England has 24%[2] and Canada 10%.[3] This phenomenon is the culmination of events that date back to early Greece. This chapter investigates the chronological events that have resulted in a medical system dominated by white, middle- and upper-class males.

FROM ANCIENT GREECE TO 13th-CENTURY ROME

Trotula lived in the 11th century and studied and taught in Salerno. Her gynecological work *De Mulerium Passionibus* (On the Suffering of Women), the earliest known compendium of women's health care, includes the treatments used by Greek, Roman and Arab physicians. During the following 300 years, this text was used across most of Europe. First typeset in 1544, it was reprinted many times in several languages.[4]

Unfortunately, in allowing women into medical schools and careers, Italy was an exception. The faculty of medicine at the University of Paris absolutely opposed female physicians. Since, in 1220, anyone who was not a faculty member was strictly prohibited by law from the practice of medicine, women were effectively eliminated. There was little need to enforce the law until 1322 when Jacoba Felicie, along with several other women, was charged with examining sick persons, prescribing remedies, curing patients and receiving fees without a license. Although many of Jacoba's patients testified in her favor, and she demonstrated her procedures were the same as those used by licensed physicians, she was still charged and fined. This discrimination continued in France, without remittance, until 1868 (600 years later), when the first woman was allowed entry into the Paris Medical School.

Generally, the tradition of women healers which had begun in the ancient world continued until around the 13th century. Surgery was commonly undertaken by nuns at the local convents or by the "lady of the manor" in wealthy homes as a charitable duty. Some women healers received payment for their skills. Cecelia of Oxford, designated wise woman of the village, was employed as court surgeon by Queen Phillippa, wife of Edward III (1327–1377).

In the 13th century, contact with Arabian scholars stimulated a revival of interest in learning which resulted in two major developments that directly led to excluding women from the healing professions: the appearance of medical schools in universities and the formation of barber-surgeon guilds.[4]

With the incorporation of medicine into universities, only licensed doctors were given the legal right to practice with the title of physician. With the exception of Italy, all European universities were closed to women. Official recognition of their medical skills was no longer available.

The development of universities and medicine was strictly controlled by church doctrine, and innovation suppressed. Medical students studied Plato, Aristotle, and Christian theology. Medical theory was restricted to Galen and the study of the "complexions" and "temperaments" of men. Students rarely, if ever, saw patients, and human dissection was outlawed by the church. Surgery was considered degrading and menial. Treatment consisted of bleeding, leeches and quasi-religious rituals. For example, the physician to Edward II, an Oxford graduate, prescribed writing "in the name of the Father, the Son and the Holy Ghost, Amen," on the patient's jaw for a toothache.[5]

In contrast, the women healers of this era, practicing illegally, followed the healing methods of Trotula and St Hildegarde of Bingen, Germany. Hildegarde (1098–1179) wrote a compendium of natural healing methods entitled *Liber Simplicis Medicine*. In it, at a time when male physicians had no use for such advice, she lists the healing properties of 213 plants and 55 trees and asserts the importance of cleanliness for proper treatment.[6] Although the natural healing methods of these women resulted in their being persecuted and burned at the stake as witches in the Middle Ages, many of these methods continue to be used in naturopathic medicine today.

Viewed from the perspective of the late 20th century, church doctrine was disturbingly misogynist. Pain in labor was perceived as the Lord's just punishment for Eve's original sin. In the 13th century, St Thomas Aquinas wrote:[2]

> As regards the individual nature, woman is defective and misbegotten, for the active power in the male seed tends to the production of a perfect likeness according to the male sex; while the production of women comes from defect in the active power, or some material indisposition. ... (*Summa Teleologica*)

This attitude towards women climaxed in the 15th century with the burning of witches or lay healers (discussed below).

The second development of the 13th century which served to exclude women from the healing professions was formation of barber-surgeon guilds. These guilds laid down regulations for apprenticeship and membership. In return for guaranteeing standards of practice, members were given exclusive rights to their home town's needs for surgical care and could prosecute non-guild members who dared to perform surgery. Those most affected were the midwives. Forceps, a surgeon's invention, could only be legally used by guild members; therefore, a midwife was required to call in a barber-surgeon during a difficult delivery. The surgeon would either remove the infant piecemeal by hooks and perforators or perform caesarian section once the mother was dead.[7] Occasionally women were allowed admittance into barber-surgeon guilds by patrimony or apprenticeship, but numbers were small.

By the end of the 14th century, organized medicine had effectively excluded women. The church joined in with witch-hunts in the 15th century, and the long tradition of women healers was almost completely eradicated.

THE 14th THROUGH 17th CENTURIES

By the 14th century, professional, university-trained physicians were in demand by the wealthy. Middle- and upper-class educated women healers were eliminated by excluding them from universities and licensing. This left only the women lay healers of the peasant class as competition. The medical profession appealed to the church for help, and the church responded by persecuting women in one of the most vicious rampages in history. There were two reasons for this victimization: the witch-healer was an empiricist in direct opposition to church doctrine, and women represented sexuality, a betrayal of faith through sensory awareness and alignment with the devil.

The church believed women to be the conduit of all evil. All pleasure was condemned, as the devil was considered the source. Women were associated with sex, and lust in either husband or wife was blamed on the woman. A newborn was immediately baptized by a male priest in order to ensure salvation of its soul, which had been exposed to the wickedness of the woman for 9 months while in the womb. Upon resurrection, it was believed that all humans would be reborn as men.[8]

Women healers had sins to atone for other than their sex. The so-called witches relied upon their senses and observation in treating their patients. The church believed that to trust one's senses was wrong – the senses were the devil's playground and used by the devil to lure men into the conceits of the intellect, delusions of carnality, and away from the faith.[8]

The methods of the witch-healer were based on years of experience. She maintained an attitude of active inquiry, learning through trial and error, cause and effect. Her repertoire included herbal remedies such as clary, hyssop, lily, ergot, belladonna and digitalis – many still used by naturopathic physicians today. Codified in the written works of Hildegarde of Bingen and Trotula of Italy, her approach was scientific according to today's standards. Even established medicine referred to these works for centuries.[8]

The approach of medical doctors, deeply anti-empirical with no concern for the material world and empirical observation, was more consistent with church doctrine. They did not search for the natural laws governing physical phenomena but instead abided by the belief that the Lord created the world anew each moment, and hence there was no point in questioning one's surroundings.

The witch-hunts

During the 14th through 17th centuries, witch-hunts spread across Europe. Thousands of executions, usually live burnings at the stake, were carried out, first in Germany and Italy and later in France and England.

In 1484, a witch-hunting manual, the *Malleus*, was written by reverends Kramer and Sprenger, beloved sons of Pope Innocent VIII. It contained specific instructions for conducting witch-hunts and methods of torture for extracting confessions and names of other witches. Witchcraft was defined as political subversion, religious heresy, lewdness, and blasphemy. Women were accused of every conceivable sex crime against men. They were accused of being organized, of having magical healing powers, and of harming with magic. According to the *Malleus*: "All witchcraft comes from carnal lust which in women is insatiable. … And blessed be the highest who so far has preserved the male sex from so great a crime. …"[8]

Women were often charged and burned at the stake simply for possessing medical knowledge and obstetrical skills. "If a woman dare to cure without having studied, she is a witch and must die" (*Malleus*).[8] Of course, women could not officially study as they were not allowed into medical schools.

English physicians complained to Parliament about the "worthless and presumptuous women who usurped the profession" and requested that fines and long imprisonment be the punishment for any woman "who dared to use the practice of Fisyk".[9] King Henry VIII heard their plea and secured nationwide regulation of medicine and surgery with the Act of 1512, which installed a system of licensing that approved practitioners and punished and suppressed all others.[7] In Europe, the church was given the responsibility of implementing the program to eliminate women healers and "witchcraft".

In several German cities, approximately 600 burnings occurred each year, two each day except Sundays. Over 900 "witches" were executed in 1 year in the Wertzberg area and over 1,000 in the area of Como. In Toulouse, 400 women were put to death in 1 day. In the Bishopric of Trier in 1585, so many woman were killed that two villages were left with only one woman each. It has been estimated that the total number of executed witches (85% of whom were women) was in the millions.[8]

The persecution of women healers greatly strengthened the relationship between the church and the medical profession. The doctor was considered the medical expert, providing an aura of authority to the witch-hunt as he decided whether the accused was a witch and what afflictions were the results of witchcraft. The dogma was that if a woman effected a cure, it was with the help of the devil, while if a male priest or doctor effected a cure, it was with the help of God – the Lord worked through male priests and doctors, not through women.[2]

The majority of witches were the general practitioners of the peasant population. The poor did not have access to hospitals or university-trained physicians and were bitterly afflicted with poverty and disease. The church upheld a double standard in terms of who should receive health care. For the upper classes and nobility, it was a given. For the poor, life experience in the world was fleeting and unimportant and so was their suffering. The peasants were offered little in the form of relief or even words of comfort from the church:[8]

> You have sinned and God is afflicting you. Thank him and you will suffer so much less the torment in the life to come. Endure, suffer, die. Has not the church its prayer for the dead?

The witch-hunts deprived the peasantry of the health care that was available to them and helped establish the dominance of a technological and rather violent male-dominated medical profession by eliminating the last of their competition. Not only during the medieval period in Europe, but also until about 1875, university-trained doctors depended on blood-letting and purgatives. Calomel, a mercury salt and the most popular purgative and cure-all medical remedy, was used in large doses for acute problems.[10] Through the 17th century, they derived their prognoses from astrology and the theory of "complexions and temperaments", partially treating their patients with incantations and quasi-religious rituals. A common treatment for leprosy was a soup made of black snake caught on dry land among stones.[5]

In contrast, the approach of the medieval woman healer emphasized the role played by the patient's innate power of healing – a view still held in naturopathic medicine today. Illness was regarded as part of the life process and an attempt on the part of the organism to regain homeostasis. Her methods included herbs, diet therapy, massage, water cures, poultices, and other gentle health-promoting approaches.[11] Women healers used their extensive knowledge of physiology, anatomy and herbs gained through experience and observation. Their superior healing abilities were acknowledged by Paracelsus who, in 1527, burned his texts on pharmaceuticals, confessing he "had learned from the Sorceress all he knew".[5]

The witch-hunts, however, branded women healers as superstitious and potentially malevolent and so thoroughly discredited women healers among the emerging middle class that, in the 17th and 18th centuries, devastating inroads were made into their last preserve, midwifery.

Discrediting the midwives

The English Act of 1512, which ultimately controlled the licensing of physicians, made no mention of midwives, probably on the basis that midwifery was considered part of surgery.[7] The system of licensing that did develop for midwives was concerned mainly with social and religious functions, for there was no way for a woman to become educated and therefore no possibility of achieving legitimate status through government licensing. Medical schools and universities were closed to women everywhere in Europe except Italy. The majority of midwives were peasants and could not afford to travel abroad to study. As a result, midwives lacked the knowledge of Latin and Greek necessary to read texts or communicate their knowledge of female anatomy and physiology. The few midwives who did manage to educate themselves, by witnessing dissections and reading medical works, still remained legally unqualified as they could not attain a university degree.[7]

Midwives in England organized in the mid-18th century to protest the Act of 1512 and the intrusion of male doctors into their realm. They charged doctors with commercialism, damaging infants' skulls with dangerous overuse of forceps, and causing undue harm to mothers. But as midwives did not know proper medical terminology and many of their members were being burned as witches even as they spoke, their protests were easily dismissed as "old wives' tales" based on ignorance and superstition.

So much was their skill and tradition discredited that they lost claim to their own techniques. For example, when Ambroise Pare (1510–1590), surgeon to the King of France, developed an interest in childbirth, he laid claim to discovery of podalic version, the method utilized and described by the woman physician Aspasia of second century Rome.[4] The male medical profession could now boast of their superior obstetrical methods.

By the early 1600s, male "midwives" began to establish themselves in earnest. They were called in for difficult cases, often with disastrous results. Nevertheless, by the end of the 18th century, throughout Europe childbirth had become the province of male physicians.[7]

Conclusion

The persecution of witches was a major exercise in medical and social control, eliminating women healers and removing the peasants' only source of health care. World-views that conflicted with church doctrine, i.e. that recognized the nature principle and the holistic quality of human life, were exorcised from the healing arts, not to be revived until the women's movement in North America in the 1700s and 1800s.

Perhaps most significant was the effect the witch-hunts had on society's perception of women, firmly establishing suspicion of evil, black magic and immoral sexuality of women in general, and women healers specifically.

THE BATTLE OF THE SECTS IN 19th-CENTURY AMERICA

Rise of the medical establishment

In early colonial America, the responsibility for healing was in the hands of women as was general family care. University-trained physicians, i.e. allopaths, did not emigrate to the colonies until the late 1700s, and then only a few came. In the New World, formal education, including medicine, was not available at the university level. In New Jersey, for example, medical practice, except in extraordinary cases, was mainly in the hands of women as late as 1818.[12] Colonial women brought centuries of healing lore with them handed down from the "witch" healers of medieval Europe. Knowledge of indigenous herbs learned from the American Indians was combined with the European traditions of massage, hydrotherapy, botanicals, and midwifery. Medical practice was open to anyone who could demonstrate healing skills, regardless of formal training, race, or sex.

Then, in the early 1800s, American university-trained doctors, modeled after the established European allopaths, began to become available. The four medical schools established by the turn of the century were far below European standards, and programs were only a few months in length. Most schools lacked clinical facilities and did not require even high school diplomas for entry. As the number of formally trained doctors grew, it became clear that much needed to be done before they could achieve the prestige and economic status of European medical doctors. One of their first tasks was to distinguish themselves from lay healers.

Allopaths were already easily identified as they were male, middle- and upper-class and almost always more costly. Their clientele consisted of middle- and upper-class citizens who could afford the prestige of being under their care. It was fashionable among upper-class women, for example, to employ male doctors for obstetrical care, much to the horror of the general populace who considered it immoral for a woman to expose herself in such a manner to a man.[12]

The allopaths, however, had little to offer in terms of theory or practice that was superior to what was available through folk medicine. Women healers used gentle botanical medications, offered dietary advice based on generations of experience, and, perhaps most importantly, did little or no harm. Allopathic doctors distinguished themselves by doing a great deal of harm in the form of "heroic medicine".

Benjamin Rush has been credited with playing a central role in establishing heroic medicine. Along with a small group of elite American medical doctors, he completed his medical education with a few years of study in Great Britain. Here they developed the style of the genteel, highly paid European physicians, and aspired to establish a similar medical model in the New World. To accomplish this, they had to convince the general public that the allopaths were able to offer medical care superior to the inexpensive and efficacious care provided by lay healers and midwives.

An all-encompassing theory and system of therapeutics was developed which resulted in immediate, although extremely dangerous, results. The purpose was to produce the strongest possible visible response in the patient. The stronger a drug or procedure, the greater its therapeutic value was purported to be. Blood-letting, purgatives, laxatives, enemas and blistering were among the most common treatments. A patient was bled until he either fainted or his pulse was no longer palpable. In 1847, one physician, after observing that extensive blistering of children often led to convulsions, gangrene or even death, concluded that blistering "ought to be held in high rank" in the treatment of childhood diseases.[10] Not all physicians were in agreement with these methods, however. Douglas observed that:[10]

> Frequently there is more danger from the physician than from the Distemper ... but sometimes not withstanding the Male Practice, Nature gets the better of the Doctor and the patient recovers.

Aside from the lack of effective therapeutic techniques, there was a total void where medical theory should have been. Air was considered the carrier of disease, and getting wet was thought to enhance susceptibility to disease. Those who listened lived in fear of bathing, sunlight, and breezes. Drinking water was kept from the ill, and windows were kept shut and covered with heavy drapes. Women were advised to keep themselves covered from the sun at all times with parasols and veils.

Heroic medicine gave regular doctors the appearance of being able to keep back disease, winning the "battle" against disease even if it killed the patient. Some of these doctors became very wealthy and gained much influence with statesmen and other influential members of the upper classes. Politically, this was essential to subsequent events in the development of allopathic dominance in North America.

Professions are the creation of the ruling class. To become sole providers of health care and succeed with the sham of heroic medicine, allopaths needed patronage from the ruling class. According to sociologist Elliot Friedson:[2]

> A profession attains and maintains its position by virtue of the protection and patronage of some elite segment of society which has been persuaded that there is some special value in it's work.

Between 1800 and 1820, allopaths used their newly acquired influence to pressure 17 states into passing licensing laws restricting the practice of medicine to their own kind. In 10 states, practicing without a license meant imprisonment.[13]

Two major unforeseen political problems, however, appeared to disrupt the allopaths' plans. First, the general populace and lower classes did not accept the hazards and pretensions of heroic medicine, preferring the more effective and much less painful and expensive health care provided by lay healers. The second problem was enforcement of licensing laws. The general populace was not prepared to persecute their own trusted healers, often the women of their own families or a well-known neighbor. The new laws incited public outrage. Fanned by the labor rebellion against upper class elitism and exploitation of burgeoning industrialization, the popular health movement emerged.

The popular health movement

In the early 1800s, the industrial revolution created a deep economic division between the upper and lower classes. Factory employees and unskilled laborers lived in abject poverty on the edge of starvation while working long hours for ridiculously low wages. Single family farmers and owners of small businesses were exploited by banks whose financial manipulations often pushed them into ruin. Upper class industrialists flaunted wealth gained at the expense of the lower classes. From this setting arose the labor movement with its membership of farmers, artisans and factory workers. At the same time, the women's movement began to take greater hold among working-class women.

In early industrialized society, many women were thrown together, free of the company of men. Women were either confined to home and church or worked in all-women factories such as those in the New England mill towns. Discovering their common aversion to heroic male medicine, women began to develop alternatives.[14] Among the hundreds of benevolent associations, charitable institutions and mutual support groups was the "Ladies Physiological Society", a feminist health care group. At society meetings, women learned about female anatomy, physiology and personal hygiene; old-time home remedies were recultivated and exchanged; and the lore of botanical healing and other techniques used by the pioneer women healers were recovered. In opposition to the dangerous therapies of allopathic doctors, they emphasized preventive care: frequent bathing, loose-fitting clothing, whole grains, and fresh air – all in direct opposition to the medical dogma of the day. The women's health movement was at the forefront of general social upheaval, a radical assault on medical elitism, and an affirmation of traditional "peoples'" medicine.

Women's outrage against allopathic medicine, shared by working-class men, resulted in a mass movement against medical professionalism and "expertism" of all forms. It was a class war, and the allopathic doctors were on the side of the aristocratic upper class. Regular doctors, with their claim to educational superiority, were denounced, along with the universities that trained them. It was popularly believed that students learned in the universities to look upon labor as "servile and demeaning".[11]

By the 1830s, the labor and feminist movements had converged into the popular health movement. According to historian Richard Shryock:[10]

> This crusade for women's health was related both in cause and effect to the demand for women's rights in general and the health and feminist movement became indistinguishable at this point.

The health movement was concerned with women's rights, and the women's movement was concerned with health care and access to medical training for women. However, it took a male voice to repeat what women had already said and done before any change took place.

Samuel Thomson is credited with laying the foundation of a theory (see Chs 2 and 35) and practice of folk medicine for the working class and feminists. A poor New Hampshire farmer, he had watched his wife and mother die at the hands of allopathic doctors. Outraged by their violent methods, he began to reconstruct the folk medicine he had learned from a woman healer and midwife named Mrs Benton. According to Thomson:[13]

> The whole of her practice was with roots and herbs applied to the patient, or given in hot drinks, to produce sweating which always answered the purpose. ... By her attention to the family, and the benefits they received from her skill, we became very much attached to her; and when she used to go out and collect roots and herbs, she would take me with her, and learn me their names, with what they were good for.

Thomson's methodology systemized Mrs Benton's methods, which she in turn had learned from native American Indians and the tradition of women healers before her. In 1822, he published *A New Guide to Health*, which described what was basically her entire healing system. His intention was to provide the public with self-sufficient health care and to remove healing as a commodity from the marketplace. (Although less toxic and more natural then the medical therapies of the day, Thomson's were not always particularly gentle. For example, lobelia was given as an emetic to cleanse the stomach and followed with capsicum to induce fever. He also used steam baths (his followers were often called "steamers") and sought to restore equilibrium through the use of *Myrica cerifera* (bayberry), *Nymphea odorata* (pond lilly), *Pinus canadensis* (spruce), and *Rhus glabrum* (sumac).)[15]

The Thomsonian Movement was in full swing by 1835, claiming just under one-quarter of the entire US population. There were five Thomsonian journals which included articles concerned with health, women's rights, and affronts to female health inflicted by "heroic" obstetrical practices. He felt that women were natural healers, and strongly believed that doctors, who graduated without ever having witnessed a delivery, should leave obstetrics to midwives. His son, John Thomson, wrote:[14]

> We cannot deny that women possess superior capacities for the science of medicine, and although men should reserve for themselves the exclusive right to mend broken limbs and fractured skulls, and to prescribe in all cares for their own sex, they should give up to women the office of attending upon women.

These ideas were in direct opposition to those of regular doctors, who felt that women had no place in medicine and continued to put much effort into keeping them out. Women were still not allowed into regular medical schools, and the new licensing laws forbade anyone who was not licensed and university educated from practicing the healing arts. Perhaps an extreme example of discrimination against women is that of Henrietta Faber who studied and practiced medicine in Havana, Cuba, disguised as a man. When, in 1820, she revealed her true sex in order to marry, she was sentenced to 10 years in prison.[16] It wasn't until 1849 that the first woman, Elizabeth Blackwell, entered a United States medical school. (When she was applying to the 42 all-male medical schools, a well-meaning professor at Jefferson Medical College recommended she attend classes disguised as a man.)

Healing systems similar to Thomson's grew in the radical climate of the 1830s. Sylvester Graham founded a movement of physiologically based healing called the Hygienic Movement. The Grahamites were so anti-medicine they rejected the use of botanicals as well as drugs. Instead, the system encouraged a vegetarian diet of raw fruits and vegetables and whole grains, while allopaths held that uncooked produce was injurious to your health and white bread was a status symbol.

Both the Thomsonians and the hygienists upheld that health care and healing skills belonged to the people and should not be a marketable commodity. Followers of Thomson and Graham fought the new licensing laws for physicians alongside the feminists and working-class activists:[17]

> Any system that teaches the sick that they can get well only through the exercise of the skill of someone else, and that they remain alive only through the tender mercies of the privileged class, has no place in nature's scheme of things, and the sooner it is abolished, the better off mankind will be.

(It should be noted, however, that while the Thomsonians and the hygienists actively recruited women and strongly believed in the importance of women improving their health and that of their families, they were not particularly supportive of feminism.)

By the mid-1830s, every state with restrictive licensing laws had either softened or repealed them. Some states, like Alabama and Delaware, exempted Thomsonians and Grahamites from any restrictions.[13] Regular doctors now became recognized as just another sect and were revealed as the sect that had attempted to monopolize health care at the expense of the working class. Unfortunately, however, the popular health movement began to decline shortly after its greatest victory.

By the late 1830s, some of the Thomsonian and Grahamian practitioners wanted professionalism and to establish schools and licensing for their graduates, seeking what they had fought so hard against and reversing some of the original tenets of the movement. In-fighting began over the loss of basic principles. Much competition developed between their schools for students, creating a larger rift. Along with these events occurred a loss of public support. Feminists turned away from health issues and refocused their efforts on women's rights in a world controlled by men. The radicalism of the working class trailed off toward Andrew Jackson's Democratic Party and away from socialist revolution. During the lull, allopaths began adopting enough of the principles of natural healing to appear credible.

The reputation of medical doctors was in a terrible state. Their professionalism had been significantly undermined, and uncontrollable growth of their ranks, from a few thousand in 1800 to over 40,000 in 1850, resulted in decreased medical fees and lowered economic status.[13] Many of the graduates, unable to make a living from their practice, chose to open schools of their own. Allopaths were also experiencing stiff competition from herbalists, hydropaths, midwives, homeopaths, and the eclectics who mixed natural healing with allopathy. Each healing art had its own schools, journals, and dedicated following. Homeopaths were particularly threatening as they appealed to the upper class, the patient population most coveted by allopathic physicians.

In 1847, a small group of allopathic doctors formed the American Medical Association (AMA). Upon surveying their affairs, they concluded:[13]

> No wonder the profession of medicine has measurably ceased to occupy the elevated position which once it did; one wonders that the merest pittance in the way of remuneration is scantily doled out even to the most industrious of our ranks.

One of the first acts of the newly formed AMA was to extend the length of required study from 4 to 6 months and to require 2 years of approved preceptorship. However, practically all hospitals barred women from internship programs. In 1857, Elizabeth Blackwell, after being barred from all New York hospitals (despite her degree), opened the first woman-dominated hospital in the world, the New York Infirmary for Women. Internships for women continued to be very limited (in the early 1940s, 607 of 712 hospitals would not accept women) until World War II when the shortage of male doctors opened the doors for women.

The problems for women were further aggravated by the AMA's Consultation Clause which barred women from membership in the AMA and prohibited members from providing consultations for irregular doctors.

Although the Consultation Clause was effective, it was not until the early 1900s that allopathic medicine was able to establish supremacy and essentially eliminate women allopaths and natural healers of both sexes from the field. This was accomplished through their adoption of the new religion of "science" and the infusion by the chemical and drug industry (primarily through the

Rockefeller and Carnegie foundations) of millions of dollars into their drug-oriented schools.

The threat of women doctors

From the 1850s through the turn of the century, allopathic doctors relentlessly attacked their competition: the sectarian or irregular and women practitioners. The natural healing-oriented groups were attacked for allowing women among the ranks, and women doctors were attacked for their sectarian methods. But the worst was yet to come.

By mid-century, middle- and upper-class women were aspiring to become regular doctors. They too were motivated by reform, as were the women of the popular health movement, but their spirit of reform was moral rather than social. Middle- and upper-class women were outraged by the implicit indecency of the male doctor treating a female patient. Catherine Beecher, a well-known doctor and journalist of her time, publicly raised charges of seduction and sexual abuse by male doctors.[18] A women's society in Philadelphia made it quite clear that "the Bible recognizes and approves only women in the sacred office of midwife".[19] A popular women's magazine, Godey's *Lady's Book*, argued strongly in favor of women physicians:[19]

> We would, in all deference, suggest that, first of all, there will be candor in the patient to the female physician, which would not be expected when a sense of native delicacy and modesty existed to the extent of preferring to suffer rather than divulge the symptoms.

Women began to force their way into allopathic medical schools. Elizabeth Blackwell gained admission into Geneva Medical College in upstate New York in 1849 after having been turned down by 16 other schools. After her graduation, Geneva College quickly passed a resolution barring entry of women.[19] In the same year, Harriet Hunt was admitted to Harvard Medical College, but the decision was reversed when the all-male student body threatened to riot. Instead, she attended and graduated from an irregular school.[19]

Emily Howard Jennings returned to Canada from the New York Medical College for Women in 1867 to become the first recognized Canadian woman doctor.[20] Ironically, the first woman doctor to practice in Canada was actually James Barry, who posed as a man right up to her death. Even in death her sex went unreported by the embalmer; only when her grave was exhumed did her sex become known. The truth had been too embarrassing for the male embalmer to reveal, since women were not believed to have the intellect required to become physicians let alone study (see Shyrock[10]), yet Barry had become chief military doctor for the country. Through the efforts of the sisters Augusta Jennings Kimball and Ella Jennings, the second and third Canadian women doctors, and those who followed, by 1900 there were approximately 5,000 women doctors in the US and Canada. Over 1,500 women were enrolled in medical colleges exclusively for women: seven in the United States[19] and two in Canada[20] (Toronto Women's Medical College and Queens Women's Medical College).

One of the strongest women physicians at the turn of the century, both as a feminist and leader of the natural health movement, was Dr Aloysia Stroebele. In the early 1890s, Stroebele, originally from Sigmaringen, Germany, opened the Bellevue Sanitarium in Butler, New Jersey, a nature cure retreat. As the personal aide to Lady Cooke, the famed suffragist leader, she became a strong advocate of "feminine independence and the emancipation of women".[21] During the several years she spent with Lady Cooke, she made three trips around the world, and in the process met with several natural healers, one of whom, Rikli, influenced her greatly. Her accomplishments were many: co-founding the first naturopathic college, co-founding the famed Yungborn sanitarium, funding the journal *Naturopath*, and authoring several articles and books. She married Benedict Lust, the founder of naturopathic medicine, in 1901 and changed her name to Louisa Lust. Her most telling contribution, besides her famous cures at "the Bellevue" through her integration of diet therapy, hydrotherapy, and the Rickli air cure, were the funds she contributed to fight 17 legal actions taken against practitioners of naturopathy.[22]

The male medical profession understood all too well the economic threat of these women physicians. Any middle- or upper-class woman who found the idea of revealing herself to a male doctor too repulsive could turn to a woman who was a regular, allopathic physician – still the preferred healers of the upper classes. She no longer had to quibble over going to see "irregular" women physicians. Male physicians fought back with all the misogynous slander they could muster.

They argued that women were too frail to practice medicine, incapable of operating while menstruating, and unable to survive the vulgarities of anatomy class or the shocking truths of reproduction.[19] The idea that women were too delicate and modest to survive medical training, let alone desire it, meant that women who insisted upon their rights were not really women at all. Alfred Stille, president of the AMA in 1871, explained the phenomenon of women in medicine in his presidential address:[10]

> Certain women seek to rival men in manly sports ... and the strange-minded ape them in all things, even in dress. In doing so they may command a sort of admiration such as all monstrous production inspires, especially when they tend towards a higher type of their own.

The editor of the *Buffalo Medical Journal* was more explicit:[17]

> If I were to plan with malicious hate the greatest curse I could conceive for women, if I could estrange them from the

protection of men, and make them as far as possible loathsome and disgusting to man, I would favor the so-called reform which proposes to make doctors of them.

In other words, women who became physicians, or even desired to become physicians, were not only less than women, they were less than human.

In addition to public slander, male MDs and medical students did all they could to make the lives of women aspiring to medical careers as miserable as possible. In class they were harassed with insolent and offensive language, and missiles of tobacco quid and garbage were thrown at them. Anatomy teachers often refused to lecture if women were present.[19] An 1848 obstetrics textbook explained how: "She (woman) has a head almost too small for intellect but just big enough for love."[10]

Once graduated, women doctors were allowed into few hospitals, and internships were almost non-existent. Nor were women doctors allowed to join medical societies or to publish in medical journals. Not until 1915 did the AMA admit its first female physician.

The entry of women into medicine was fiercely resisted by male doctors, not only because of their deeply rooted misogyny dating from the beginnings of Christianity and the economic threat they posed, but also because of their association with the popular health movement. The integrity of allopaths had been assaulted by the general public and the popular health movement in which women and feminism played a central role. The irregular schools of nature cure continued to welcome women students, and many of the irregular doctors were women providing a gentle and viable alternative to the dangers of regular health care. During the late 18th and early 19th centuries, women applying to medical school were considered guilty by association of being in opposition to regular medicine and of being feminists.[2]

Hydrotherapy: a haven for women

In terms of women's liberation and medical thought, the most revolutionary alternative system of healing was the hydrotherapy movement, or hydropathy as it was known in 19th century America. The original system consisted of using hot and cold water for bathing, wrapping, douching, and spritzing (spraying all or parts of the body). Allopathic medicines were excluded. Instead, a vegetarian diet, fresh air, exercise, regular bathing with cold water, and drinking numerous glasses of pure water were considered the pathways to health. Later, the principles of hydrotherapy were combined with those of the hygienic, Graham, and eclectic systems to form naturopathic medicine.

The formal practice of hydrotherapy began with Vincent Priessnitz who opened a water cure clinic in Graefenburg, Germany, in 1829.[23] A medical doctor, Joel Shew, and his wife, Mary Louise Shew, introduced hydrotherapy to the United States in 1843, where the cause was most visibly carried forward by Mary Gove Nichols and Russell Thatcher Trall.[23]

Women played a major role in hydrotherapy as practitioners, educators, and leaders in health reform and women's rights. Many women worked alongside husbands or male professionals, specializing in the care of obstetric and gynecological patients. Most prominent was Mary Gove Nichols who, in 1846, opened her own water cure establishment in New York.[23] In 1851, she and her physician husband Thomas Nichols opened a medical school based on water cure principles in New York. Other prominent water cure partners included Racheal Brooks Gleason and her physician husband Silas Gleason, James Jackson and Thodoria Gilbert (who opened the Glen Haven Water Cure), and Harriet Austin who later worked with Jackson.[23]

The concept of women as protectors of the family's health and morality was one of the major tenets guiding the hydrotherapist's insistence that women take control of their own health and personal power. They believed that by developing a healthy lifestyle and independence, women could work alongside men to improve society. These ideas were in direct opposition to the dominant social ethics and medical thought of the day.

Allopaths viewed puberty, menses, pregnancy, childbirth, and menopause as a series of potentially dangerous pathological events. Women were relegated to the domestic sphere due to their supposed weak physical and intellectual nature. In the home, they could be protected by the man.[24]

In contrast, the hydropaths viewed women's physiology and reproductive functions as normal, healthy processes. Water cure establishments provided a haven where women could receive sympathetic care, find relief from constant pregnancies, and receive psychological and emotional support.[24] Women were inspired to achieve beyond the domestic realm, and many went on to become hydropaths themselves.

Taking the cure at the hydrotherapy establishments became fashionable amongst the wealthy during the late 19th century. Between 1843 and 1900, 213 water cure sanitariums opened.[23] Numerous journals, books, and magazines devoted to the tenets of water cure and a natural lifestyle were published during this time. They became forums for disseminating hydropathic ideals of the perfect society where women no longer wore tight corsets, long dresses, or suffered the ill effects of the allopaths' over-medication with mercury (for postpartum hemorrhage), lead (for dyspepsia), opium, leeches, and blood-letting. Women were encouraged to avoid the meat-, salt- and stimulant-rich diet of the day. In the vision of the hydropaths, women were free to pursue any career they chose, with hydrotherapy and medicine being the most noble.[23–25]

Thomas Nichols' statement in the *Water Cure Journal* clearly states their intent: "Never has woman had such an opening for usefulness and influence as this. No water cure establishment is complete without a qualified woman physician."[26]

Mary Gove Nichols, in her inaugural address at the opening to the American Hydropathic Institute, professed: "Women are peculiarly fitted to the art of healing because of their tenderer love, the sublime devotion, the never to be wearied patience and kindness of woman."[27]

Women comprised between 30 and 50% of the graduates from the hydrotherapy schools. They worked diligently as the heads of the ladies' departments of the water cure establishments, attending to all facets of women's and children's health care. They provided prenatal care where allopaths had little to offer, recommending a diet of fruit, vegetables, whole grains, and milk. Loose clothing, daily exercise, and cold baths were recommended to tone the body in preparation for childbirth.[23] After the birth, women were encouraged to get out of bed within days, if not the same day, thus decreasing the risk of postpartum blood clots and pulmonary embolism. Women were taught to experience childbirth as an empowering, natural and holy function, rather than as an event to be dreaded as risking imminent death.

Hydrotherapy, more than any other 19th century medical sect, had the strongest connection with the women's movement.

Victory for a male profession

Until the early 20th century, allopaths had little to offer that was superior to the other types of health care practices. They had neither economic dominance nor elevated social status over the irregular or natural health care practitioners. In spite of the AMA's valiant attempts to establish allopathy as the only legitimate form of healing, only 8,000 out of 125,000 doctors in the United States were members of the AMA at the turn of the century.[28]

European allopaths had better success in establishing themselves among the upper class. With the introduction of the germ theory by French and German scientists came the first scientifically demonstrable basis for disease prevention and treatment. European medical men were the first to adopt scientific methodology into medical practice and education. This served to further enhance their already elevated status. Science had become the new religion of the general public and was held up as the answer to all social, economic and health problems. The new religion was received in North America with tremendous enthusiasm.

Science in North America became a national moral value; any discipline which wanted to justify its existence had to adopt scientific doctrine. Social work, philanthropy, housekeeping, child-rearing, business management, public administration, law, and medicine all began to search for a scientific basis. The adoption of scientific principles was synonymous with reform.[2]

In the late 19th century, a small group of American doctors traveled to German and French medical universities for further training and returned determined to install an elite medical educational system that would elevate their professional status. In 1893, they founded Johns Hopkins University, the first medical school in North America with laboratories and full-time professors. Eight years later, the Rockefeller Institute for Medical Research was opened. The institute was, and is still today, solely concerned with pure research and helped to exalt the mystery of European scientism. One of the founders of the institute and a close friend of the Rockefellers, described the place as "a theological seminary, presided over by the Reverend Simon Flexner, M.D.".[29]

Having finally created a credible academic and research model for medical education, the AMA began to effectively utilize economic and political pressure to ensure that all schools providing a medical education either ascribed to the model provided by the Rockefeller Institute and Johns Hopkins University or were closed.

This was accomplished through a cooperative effort between the AMA's Council on Medical Education (made up of faculty from the medical schools modeled on the Johns Hopkins prototype) and the Carnegie and Rockefeller Foundations. The Carnegie Foundation ostensibly agreed to conduct a study of the educational institutions found in the various healing professions. The results were then utilized to determine which schools and sects were to receive a portion of $150 million in endowments.

The study was conducted by Abraham Flexner, brother of the director of the Rockefeller Institute, Simon Flexner MD, a graduate of Johns Hopkins University. In the survey, schools such as Harvard were seen to be conforming to the new scientific model quite well, as they had the money (granted them by the foundations) to employ full-time professors and install expensive laboratories. These schools were given large endowments. The smaller, poorer schools, which provided medical education for women, blacks and those interested in natural healing, did poorly in meeting allopathic requirements and hence received no funds from the Rockefeller and Carnegie foundations. According to Flexner's report, these schools were not worth saving and their closure would be no loss.

Despite the 10 medical colleges in existence at the time that provided medical education solely for women, Flexner also decided that few women doctors were needed. He perceived a lack of "any strong demand for women physicians or any strong ungratified desire on the part of women to enter the profession"![30] Flexner did deduce that some black doctors were needed, but only enough to check the spread of disease from black to white neighborhoods for "ten millions of them live in close contact with sixty million whites".[30] Due to both economic and philosophical reasons, the irregular schools, which had been a haven for women, and women's medical colleges did not conform to the new allopathic model and were discredited by the Flexner report.

From 1904 to 1915, 92 medical schools closed or merged: five out of seven all-black medical schools closed, seven out of 10 medical schools for women shut their doors, and the majority of the alternative medical schools were eliminated. As a direct result, the number of women graduates from allopathic medical schools dropped from 4.3 to 3.2%. In the meantime, from 1910 to 1930, over $300 million was poured into the medical schools that ascribed to the Johns Hopkins model.[31] Not only women and blacks were affected by these events, for scientism became the domain of the upper classes.

The reforms which ruled the existence of medical schools included an entrance requirement of 2 years of university training. This effectively made a medical career impossible for all but the middle and upper classes due to the expense. Medical schools that had been economically accessible to the working class ceased to exist, and the entrance of blacks into medical schools was limited by racial discrimination. Women suffered sex discrimination in their attempts to enter the remaining medical colleges,[2] with percentages steadily shrinking until the 1970s and the resurgence of feminism.[32] The medical profession had become an institution composed almost entirely of white, middle- and upper-class males confirmed in their opposition to women and natural healing methods.

It is true that turn-of-the-century medicine needed some form of standardization of education and health care. However, in the fervor of scientism, sexism, racism, and the allopaths' rush for economic control, the alternatives to allopathic medicine were effectively eliminated. Despite the new reforms, the quality of medical care was not necessarily improved. The new system of lengthy scientific training did not guarantee that physicians were any more effective or humanely empathic than the irregular healers they replaced – in fact quite the opposite appears to have been the case (see Ivan Illich, *Limits to Medicine*[33] and other chapters of this textbook). While the scientific method has much to offer, it is arguable that, in the context of the stifling, one-dimensional philosophy and male elitism of the medical profession, the use of the banner of scientism to establish political and economic protection from competing ideas actually inhibited the development of health care in this country.

Midwives: the last of the women healers to fall

In 1900, approximately 50% of all births in North America were attended by midwives.[2] Middle- and upper-class women had their babies delivered by licensed MDs. Lower-class blacks and European immigrants could not afford MDs, nor did they want them. Midwifery was a respected tradition held in high esteem, particularly by Africans and Europeans. This meant fewer obstetrical cases for teaching medical students, as upper-class women certainly did not want a room full of men, medical students or not, witnessing their birthing efforts. Therefore, it was said that midwives, by providing affordable and readily available obstetrical care to the lower class, were depriving medical students of valuable learning experiences.

To remedy the situation, medical schools began to associate themselves with local charity hospitals, offering medical trainees as staff in return for patients they could learn on. In the meantime, the medical profession put considerable energy into making midwifery illegal. An editorial in the *Journal of the American Medical Association* by Charles Ziegler stated the situation:[11]

> It is at present impossible to secure cases sufficient for the proper training in obstetrics, since 75% of the material otherwise available for clinical purposes is utilized in providing a livelihood for midwives.

The "material," of course, was the bodies of pregnant women.

A campaign was launched to rally support among members of the profession to outlaw midwifery by appealing to their sense of what was best for medical education and by portraying midwives as "hopelessly dirty, ignorant and incompetent relics of a barbaric past" who could do only harm to mother and child:[34]

> They may wash their hands, but oh what myriads of dirt lurk under their fingernails. Numerous instances could be cited and we might well add to other causes of pyosalpinx "dirty midwives." She is the most virulent bacteria of them all and she is truly a micrococcus of the most poisonous kind.

An obvious solution to the problem of the "dirty and ignorant midwives" would have been to educate them in hygiene, in the use of an eyedropper to prevent gonococcal eye infections in the newborn, and in the use of forceps in difficult births. However, the medical profession wanted obstetrical "material", not to train midwives to further increase their effectiveness and legitimacy. Through cooperation with them, the MDs could have learned much about childbirth and improved their own reputations.

The medical doctors' version of childbirth was dangerous. If the labor was going too slowly for his schedule, he used forceps and caesarian section with considerable risk to mother and child.[7] In teaching hospitals, there was a definite bias in favor of surgery to provide experience for students in abnormal deliveries.[11] In fact, a 1912 study by Johns Hopkins University found the majority of American doctors less competent than the midwives they had replaced. According to the study, they were less experienced, less observant and less likely to be present at the critical moment.[35]

It appears that the MDs realized they could not fill the void of service left if midwives were eliminated. One obstetrician in 1915 admitted that of all births in New York State, 25% would be entirely deprived of assistance once midwifery was eliminated.[34] Yet between 1900 and 1930, midwives were almost totally eliminated from North America. With the demise of the midwife, American women lost their last independent role as healers.

More than one historian has referred to the years from 1900 to 1965 as the Dark Ages in terms of the progress of women in the healing arts.[36] Although there were women allopathic physicians, their numbers were small. In 1900, women comprised 5% of all physicians of all sects, and by 1926, they made up only 2%. Not until the 1970s, with the resurgence of feminism, did the number of women in allopathic medical schools approach even 6%.[32] The remaining irregular schools had continued accepting women students without discrimination, although the numbers were not as high as they are now. In the early 1970s, the naturopathic student body was approximately 33% female.

WOMEN IN MEDICINE TODAY

Today's dominant form of medicine is a refined form of the heroic techniques of turn-of-the-century allopaths, and women have only recently begun to make real progress in entering the ranks of male-dominated technological medicine. From 1968 to 1978, the number of women enrolled in regular medical schools has increased dramatically, from 7 to 25%. At McMaster Medical School in Hamilton, Ontario, more than 50% of the 1978 graduating class were women – the first time in North America that the number of women in an allopathic medical school was greater than that of men.[37] Discrimination against women in medicine persists, however.

According to a 1985–86 survey conducted by the AMA, women earn 62% of the salary of their male colleagues.[38] Women also fill less than 3% of administrative positions in medical schools, and, as of 1987, only two American medical colleges have a female dean. Academic ranking also shows discrimination as women make up 23.6% of assistant professors as compared with only 6% of full professors.[38,39]

Barriers to admitting women into medical schools have been lowered considerably for several reasons: the adoption of civil rights and affirmative action legislation, and resolutions on equal opportunity in the United States and Canada. The women's movement has encouraged women to seek non-traditional careers and to assert their rights to pursue them.[40] Although the number of women in medicine is increasing, sexist attitudes seem to have changed little since the turn of the century.

Ramey, referring to the scarcity of women in administrative positions, commented in 1980 that "women are prone to emotions, verbosity, pettiness and pregnancy".[41] In this author's opinion, the final proof of the continued existence of discrimination against women in allopathic medicine is this statistic: women comprise only 10% of practicing allopathic physicians. In contrast, they comprise 40% of practicing naturopathic physicians.

Continuing discrimination against women in medicine has manifested itself in many ways:[41–44]

- There is no school-supported recruitment of women such as there is for minority students.
- There is a reluctance to admit married women, as they may become pregnant and, if they have families, may not utilize their education.
- There is overt discrimination in the classroom, including baiting, hostility, and derogatory comments.

It has been documented that lecturers, in dealing with problems in medical practice, direct all of their questions and comments to male students.[43,45] The prevalence of stereotyping women as sex objects within the profession is exhibited by the number of female students who have been sexually embarrassed, harassed or abused by their male instructors. Reports of such incidents at a conference on women in medicine in Toronto in 1985 were too frequent to be considered extraordinary.[42] A 1988 study of the gender climate in medical school found that 80% of women students reported discrimination by faculty and other physicians, with faculty displaying subtle to blatant sexism.[43] Another recent study at a Midwest medical school indicated that gender discrimination increased in intensity as the women moved closer to graduation and licensing.[43] The types of discrimination reported included sexual remarks, jokes and innuendoes relegating women into stereotyped roles, sexual advances by married mentors, and blatant sexual manipulation.[44] The same study also found that two-thirds of practicing male physicians admitted they did not accept women as professional peers.

A prevalent argument used to justify reluctance in allowing women into allopathic medical school is that women MDs are less productive.[36] Evidence, however, suggests the opposite is true. The January 1976 *Bulletin of the Professional Corporation of Physicians of Quebec* indicated that although women doctors work only 66% of the hours that male doctors do, they provide 92% of the patient care that male doctors provide. While it is true that not all women physicians continue to practice throughout the entire span of their potential working years, it is also true that women doctors are still expected to carry on with traditional family roles – a continuing societal problem. A study of women doctors in Detroit indicated that only 59% had worked without interruption since graduation and that 76% of women physicians are still doing all of the cooking, shopping, housekeeping, and childcare.[44,46] Women's advancement within the profession is inversely related to marital status and family size.[36] As a direct result of carrying the lion's share of family responsibility, and the discrimination they experience in obtaining an education and competing for career opportunities, women allopathic physicians are severely underrepresented in private practice, surgical specialties, and administrative and policy-making positions.

Still, the future of women in allopathic medicine looks brighter since their numbers are increasing. It has been predicted that women will make up 35% of the medical profession within the next decade or two.[42] As to the types of medicine women will be practicing, it seems that women are returning to their traditional role of providing preventive health care. According to Spiro:[47]

> The long standing interest of women in preventive medicine, and the current public dissatisfaction with crisis-oriented care have led still others to predict that one contribution of women may be a more 'health-oriented' medical practice.

When one considers the percentage of women in naturopathic medicine, his statement is irrefutable.

The return of women to their role as primary providers of humane, holistic health care can be attributed to several events:

- the resurgence of irregular and naturopathic medicine in North America and Europe as indicated by the increasing number of colleges and institutions providing training in massage, herbal medicine, midwifery, acupuncture, homeopathy, and naturopathy
- the revival of the feminist movement since the late 1960s
- the increasing interest women are taking in self-health care as reflected by the growing number of women's organized health information groups
- the growing dissatisfaction of the general public with allopathic medicine, recognizing it as expensive and potentially dangerous to one's health.

(For further discussion, see Illich,[33] Mendelsohn,[48] and McKowen.[49])

These events and social conditions have created an atmosphere similar to the one in which the popular health movement became successful in the early 1800s. Now, as during that time, there is considerable public discontent with heroic medicine and a recultivation of folk medicine, with women at the forefront of the revolution in health care.

Today, women make up over 50% of the student bodies at Bastyr College and National College of Naturopathic Medicine. Much of the philosophy and therapeutic approach of naturopathic medicine has been derived from the work of women healers dating back to ancient Greece and the Roman empire. History seems to be repeating itself, with women once again playing a major role in providing preventive holistic health care.

CONCLUSION

The history of women in medicine is not well known outside of their traditional roles as helpmates and nurses to male physicians. It is not generally known that women have been primary health care providers from ancient Greece through the beginning of the 19th century. Many factors have created the low percentage of women in the medical profession today. Throughout the ages, women have been intensively persecuted for practicing medicine: Aspasia by Roman law, women folk healers of medieval times who were burned as witches, English midwives who were legislated out of practice in 1512, and women healers of all kinds in early America who were virtually barred from entering allopathic medical schools in North America until the end of the 19th century, and then allowed only in very limited numbers.

Today, women have made substantial progress in breaking into the allopathic medical profession despite continuing discrimination. The real changes for women in medicine may come with recent trends towards natural therapies and preventive health care, and the resurgence of midwifery and naturopathic medicine. Along with increasing public interest in irregular medicine and the resurgence of colleges providing credible training in alternative health care, an increasing number of primary health care givers are, once again, women.

REFERENCES

1. Spender D. Man made language. New York, NY: Routledge and Kegan. 1985
2. Ehrenreich B, English D. Witches, midwifes and nurses. Old Westbury, NY: The Feminist Press, SUNY/College. 1973: p 1–41
3. Avery ME. Women in medicine. J Am Med Wom Assoc 1981; 36: 279–281
4. Mead K, Hurd C. A history of women in medicine from the earliest times to the beginning of the 19th century. Haddam, CT: Haddam Press. 1938
5. Szasz TS. The manufacture of madness. New York, NY: Dell. 1970.
6. Thorndyke L. A history of magic and experimental science, Vol II. New York, NY: Columbia University Press. 1923
7. Donnison J. Midwifes and medical men. New York, NY: Schoken Books. 1977
8. Michelet J. Satanism and witchcraft. Secaucus, NY: Citadel Press. 1939
9. Hughes MJ. Women healers in medieval life and literature. Freeport, NY: Books for Libraries Press. 1943
10. Shryock RH. Medicine and society in America: 1660–1860. Ithaca, NY: Great Seal Books. 1960
11. Ehrenreich B, English D. For her own good, 150 years of the expert's advice to women. Garden City, NY: Anchor Books. 1979
12. Kett J. The foundation of the American medical profession: the role of institutions. New Haven, CN: Yale University Press. 1968

13. Rothstein WG. American physicians in the nineteenth century. Baltimore, MD: Johns Hopkins University Press. 1972
14. Ryan MP. Womanhood in America: from colonial times to the present. New York, NY: New Viewpoint. 1975
15. Kaufman M. Homeopathy in America. Baltimore, MD: Johns Hopkins Press. 1971: p 19
16. Faber. JAMA 1901; 37: 1403
17. Burns D, ed. The greatest health discovery: natural hygiene and its evolution past present and future. Chicago, IL: Natural Hygiene Press. 1972
18. Beecher C. On female health in America. In: Cott N, ed. Roots of bitterness: documents of the social history of American women. New York, NY: EP Dutton. 1972
19. Woody T. A history of women's education in the United States, Vol II. New York, NY: Octagon Books. 1974
20. Hacker C. The indomitable lady doctors. Toronto, Ontario: Irwin. 1974
21. Lust B. Autobiography. Bastyr University Press. 1998, in press
22. Kirchfield F, Boyle W. Pioneers in naturopathic medicine. Buckeye Naturopathic Press: Medicina Biologica. 1994
23. Donegan JB. Hydropathic highway to health: women and water-cure in antebellum America. Westport, CN: Greenwood Press. 1986
24. Cayleff SB. Wash and be healed. Philadelphia, PA: Temple University Press. 1987
25. Wevis HB, Kemble HR. The great American water cure craze, a history of hydrotherapy in the United States. Trenton, NJ: The Past Times Press. 1967
26. Nichols TL. Medical education. The American hydropathic institute. Water-Cure J 1851; 12: 66 (from Cayleff[43])
27. Gove Nichols MS. Woman the physician. Water-Cure J 1851; 12: 74 (from Cayleff[43])
28. Berliner HS. A larger perspective on the Flexner Report. Int J Health Serv 1975; 5: 573–592
29. Brown RE. Rockefeller medicine men: medicine and capitalism in the progressive era. Berkeley, CA: University of California Press. 1979
30. Flexner A. Medical education in the United States and Canada: a report to the Carnegie Foundation for the advancement of teaching. New York, NY: Arno Press. 1972 (c. 1910)
31. Markowitz G, Rosner DK. Doctors in crisis, a study of the use of medical education reform to establish modern professional elitism in medicine. Am Quart 1973; 25: 83
32. Walsh MR. Doctors wanted: no woman need apply. Boston, MA: Yale University Press. 1977
33. Illich I. Limits to medicine, medical nemesis: the expropriation of health. New York, NY: Harmondsworth Press. 1977
34. Barker-Benfield GJ. The horrors of the half-known life. New York, NY: Harper and Row. 1976
35. Kobrin FE. The American midwife controversy: a crisis of professionalization. Bull Hist Med 1966; 40: 350–363
36. Morantz RM, Pomerleau CS, Fenichel CH, eds. In her own words, oral histories of women physicians. Westport, CN: Greenwood Press. 1982
37. Carver C, Berlin S. Proposal for study on productivity of women doctors. Toronto, Ontario: Women's Research and Resource Center, The Ontario Institute for Studies in Education. 1978
38. Donahue GD. Eliminating salary inequities of women and minorities in medical academia. J Am Med Wom Assoc 1988; 43: 28–29
39. Bartlik BD, Smith CA. Women doctors meet to map working strategies. J Am Med Women's Assoc 1981; 36: 236–238
40. Braslow JB, Heins M. Women in medical education: a decade of change. New Engl J Med 1981; 304: 1129–1135
41. Levin BM. Women in medicine. Metuchen, NJ: Scarecrow Press. 1980
42. Proceedings of Symposium on murmurs of the heart: issues for women in medical training, February 9, 1985. Toronto, Ontario: Faculty of Medicine, Office of the Dean, University of Toronto Medical Sciences Building.
43. Grant L. The gender climate of medical school: perspectives of women and men students. J Am Med Wom Assoc 1988; 43: 109–119
44. Coombs RH, Hovanessian HC. Stress in the role constellation of women resident physicians. J Am Med Wom Assoc 1988; 43: 21–27
45. Campbell MA. Why would a girl go into medicine? Medical education in the United States. A Guide For Women. Westbury, NY: Feminist Press. 1974
46. Heins M, Smock S, Jacobs J et al. Productivity of women physicians. JAMA 1976; 236: 1961–1964
47. Spiro HM. Myths and mirths – women in medicine. New Engl J Med 1975; 292: 354–356
48. Mendelsohn RS. Confessions of a medical heretic. Lincolnwood, IL: Contemporary Publications. 1987
49. McKowen T. The role of medicine: dream, mirage, or nemesis. London: Nuffield Provincial Hospital Trust. 1976

SECTION 2

Supplementary diagnostic procedures

SECTION CONTENTS

Over the past 50 years, tremendous progress has been made in the development of laboratory procedures for the diagnosis of disease. However, this work has focused primarily on pathological processes – little has been done to aid the physician in recognizing physiological abnormalities before they progress to the pathological stage. The problem is further aggravated for doctors of preventive and natural medicine who need to evaluate in an objective manner the nutritional status, lifestyle, physiology and health of their patients. The few widely available tests that exist tend to be oriented to measuring absolute values rather than functional indices, and generally indicate abnormal values only after serious dysfunction develops.

We have compiled a number of useful procedures which we believe will greatly aid physicians who would like to utilize more objective tests in their evaluation of the pathophysiological status of their patients. These are not meant to replace the standard, pathologically oriented, diagnostic procedures, but rather to supplement them and aid in the early diagnosis of disease and the quantification of the processes that usually precede clinical disease. Where possible, preference is given to tests that measure function rather than abstract absolute values. In keeping with the metabolic and scientific orientation of the *Textbook*, heavy emphasis has been placed on those procedures which have good support in the scientific literature for the evaluation of nutritional status.

Most of these laboratory procedures are on the cutting edge of our understanding of the assessment of the physiological function of metabolically unique individuals. As an emerging field, few experts exist and most are employed by the commercial laboratories providing the procedures. Notification is made on the copyright page (p. iv) where such a potential conflict of interest exists.

Supplementary diagnostic procedures

CHAPTER CONTENTS

6

Apoptosis assessment

Aristo Vojdani, PhD MT

INTRODUCTION

Apoptosis is a distinct form of cell death controlled by an internally encoded suicide program. It is believed to take place in the majority of animal cells. It is a distinct event that triggers characteristic morphological and biological changes in the cellular life cycle. It is common during embryogenesis, normal tissue and organ involution, and cytotoxic immunological reactions and occurs naturally at the end of the life span of differentiated cells. Apoptosis can also be induced in cells by the application of a number of different agents, including physiological activators, heat shock, bacterial toxins, oncogenes, chemotherapeutic drugs, a variety of toxic chemicals, and ultraviolet and gamma radiation. When apoptosis occurs, the nucleus and cytoplasm of the cell often fragment into membrane-bound apoptotic bodies which are then phagocytized by neighboring cells. Alternatively, during necrosis, cell death occurs by direct injury to cells, resulting in cellular lysing and release of cytoplasmic components into the surrounding environment, often inducing an inflammatory response in the tissue. A landmark of cellular self-destruction by apoptosis is the activation of nucleases and proteases that degrade the higher-order chromatin structure of the DNA into fragments of 50–300 kilobases and subsequently into smaller DNA pieces of about 200 base-pairs in length. Using fluorescent-labeled reagents, it is possible to tag the DNA break and identify the percentage of apoptotic cells with a high degree of accuracy.[1–6]

Measurable features of apoptosis

One of the most easily measured features of apoptotic cells is the break-up of the genomic DNA by cellular nucleases. These DNA fragments can be extracted from apoptotic cells and result in the appearance of DNA laddering when the DNA is analyzed by agarose gel electrophoresis. The DNA of non-apoptotic cells, which remains largely intact, does not display this laddering on agarose gels during electrophoresis. The large number of DNA fragments appearing in apoptotic cells results in a multitude of 3′-hydroxyl termini of DNA ends. This property can also be used to identify apoptotic cells by labeling the DNA breaks with fluorescent-tagged deoxyuridine triphosphate nucleotides (F-dUTP). The enzyme terminal deoxynucleotidyl transferase (TdT) catalyzes a template-independent addition of deoxyribonucleotide triphosphates to the 3′-hydroxyl ends of double- or single-stranded DNA. A substantial number of these sites are available in apoptotic cells, providing the basis for the single-step fluorescent labeling and flow cytometric method. Non-apoptotic cells do not incorporate significant amounts of the F-dUTP owing to the lack of exposed 3′-hydroxyl DNA ends.

Apoptosis can also be characterized by changes in cell membrane structure. During apoptosis, the cell membrane's phospholipid asymmetry changes – phosphatidylserine (PS) is exposed on the outer membrane, while membrane integrity is maintained. Annexin V specifically binds phosphatidylserine (PS), whereas propidium iodide (PI) is a DNA-binding fluorochrome. When a cell population is exposed to both reagents, apoptotic cells will stain positive for annexin V and negative for PI; necrotic cells will stain positive for both and live cells will stain negative for both.[3]

This process of apoptosis and its analysis by flow cytometry are shown in Figures 6.1 and 6.2.

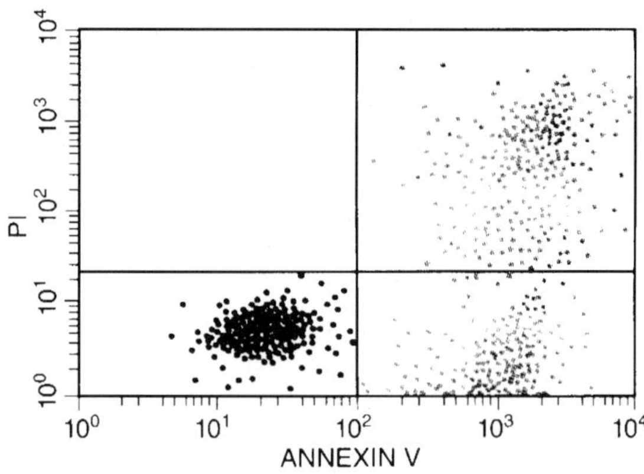

Figure 6.2 Separation of cells by flow cytometry and detection of apoptotic population.

Different stages of apoptosis

The process of apoptosis is divided into three different stages:

- induction
- sensing or triggering
- execution.

These stages of apoptosis are depicted in Figure 6.3. Induction represents the initial events that signal a cell so that apoptosis may begin. This induction phase may

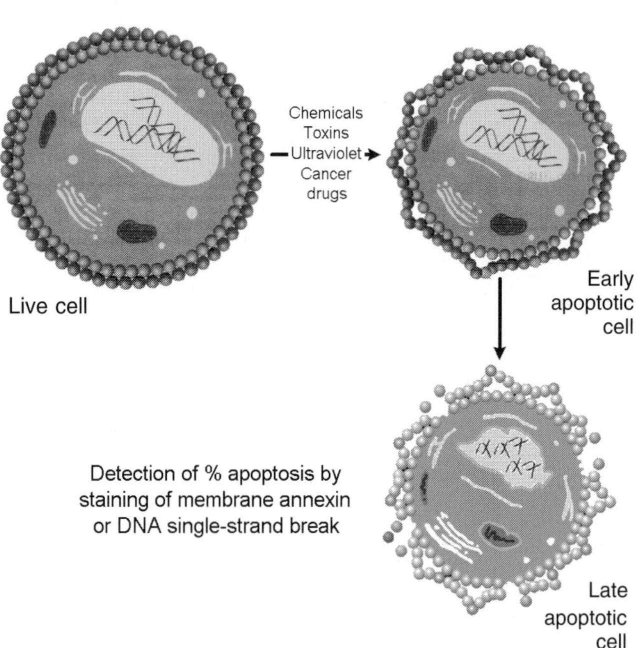

Figure 6.1 Detection of apoptosis using damaged membrane or DNA single-strand break and flow cytometry.

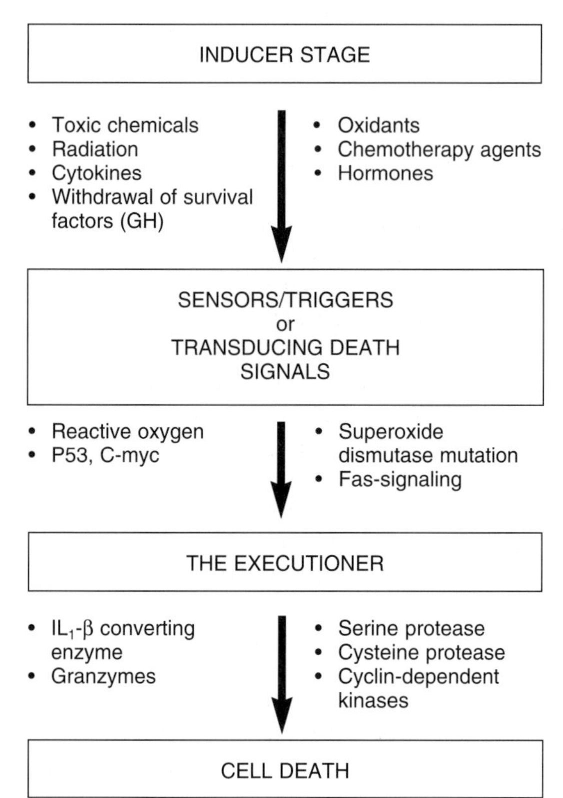

Figure 6.3 Various stages of "inside out" cell death or apoptosis.

be induced by a variety of physical agents such as toxic chemicals, radiation, chemotherapy agents, hormones and CD95 or Fas ligation. However, in a series of our recent experiments, we demonstrated that this induction stage of apoptosis is prevented by many antioxidants (vitamin C, beta-carotene and vitamin E) and also by a variety of biological response modifiers, including lentinan, thymic hormones, viral antigens and cytokines.

The induction stage is followed by a decision on whether or not the cell will undergo apoptosis. The decision to die is under the control of a number of different pathways or cellular sensors that induce the apoptosis signal which then triggers the central mechanisms. During this stage, several enzymes, such as IL_1-β* converting enzymes, serine protease, cysteine protease, granzymes and cyclin-dependent kinases, become activated. Once activated, these enzymes dismantle the cell and trigger the cell surface changes that cause direct cell recognition and engulfment of the dying cells by phagocytes. These central events are prevented by a variety of antioxidants and biological response modifiers.

Apoptosis is induced by chemicals to control malignancy

Many chemicals have the capacity to bind to DNA, form DNA adducts or cause DNA single-strand breaks, possibly leading to cancer. However, the body is equipped with many factors, enzymes, suppressor genes and cellular sensors, all with the capacity to prevent this action of chemicals on DNA by activating apoptosis-inducing signals.

The role of apoptosis in regulating tissue growth is readily apparent in the simple equation in which the rate of growth is equal to the difference between the rates of cell proliferation and cell death. Thus, tissues expand if the rate of proliferation exceeds the rate of cell death. This is one of the reasons for suggesting that defects in apoptosis may contribute to the transformed state.

An important prediction of the relevance of apoptosis to malignancy is that the rate of apoptosis versus mitosis should influence the behavior of a tumor. Recently, the relationship between the apoptotic and mitotic indices in a tumor was demonstrated predictive of outcome: higher ratios correlate with positive prognosis. Further, it was found that this is not simply a function of cell death per se. Tumors with a high incidence of necrosis rather than apoptosis were correlated with poor prognosis. It therefore follows that treatments or conditions that favor apoptosis should have desirable effects, and that defects in the pathway(s) leading to apoptosis are likely to play important roles in the process of oncogenesis.[4,5]

Many reactive chemicals and drugs, such as acetaminophen, diquat, carbon tetrachloride, quinones, cyanide, polyhydroxyl polyether, methyl mercury, organotin and others, have been implicated in apoptosis (programmed cell death) and necrosis (toxic cell death).[7–14]

Most of the research on chemical induction of apoptosis is carried out with primary cultures of cell lines (neurons, thymocytes, carcinoma cells, leukemia cells, neuroblastoma, breast cancer cells, lymphoma and others); little has been published on the in vivo effects of chemicals on apoptotic cells in animal models and none in humans. Therefore, it was of interest to examine the effects of exposure to low levels of benzene, as well as through drinking water concentrations of up to 14 ppb on the apoptotic cell population, and to examine possible changes in the cell-cycle progression.[7]

There is sufficient evidence for the carcinogenicity of benzene in humans; therefore, there is no safe level of exposure to this chemical or its metabolites. Published case reports, a case series, epidemiological studies, and both cohort and case–control studies have shown statistically significant associations between leukemia and occupational exposure to benzene and benzene-containing solvents.[15,16]

It is indicated that possibly 800,000 persons are exposed to benzene from coke oven emissions at levels greater than 0.1 ppm, and 5 million may be exposed to benzene from petroleum refinery emissions at levels of 0.1–1.0 ppm. Since then, numerous chemicals have been implicated in apoptosis (or programmed cell death) which arises from damage to DNA. We hypothesized that in individuals with a certain genetic make-up, benzene or its metabolites act as haptens, which may induce programmed cell death. The study involved a group of 60 male and female subjects who were exposed to benzene-contaminated water (at concentrations up to 14 ppm for a period of 3–5 years). For comparison, we recruited a control group consisting of 30 healthy males and females with a similar age distribution and without a history of exposure to benzene. Peripheral blood lymphocytes of both groups were tested for percentage of apoptotic cell population, using flow cytometry. When exposed individuals were compared with the control group, statistically significant differences between each mean group were detected (27.5 ± 2.4 and 10 ± 2.6, respectively), indicating an increased rate of apoptosis in 86.6% of exposed individuals ($P < 0.0001$, Mann–Whitney U-test). Flow cytometry analysis of apoptosis in a healthy control and a patient with CFS is shown in Figure 6.4.

We have already shown that benzene induction of apoptosis is caused by a discrete block of the cell cycle progression. Since it was shown that the ratio of apoptosis to mitosis is predictive of tumor growth, with increased apoptosis favoring positive prognosis, we analyzed our data and expressed them in terms of this ratio.[5]

As shown in Table 6.1, about 10% of the chemically exposed individuals demonstrated a rate of mitosis

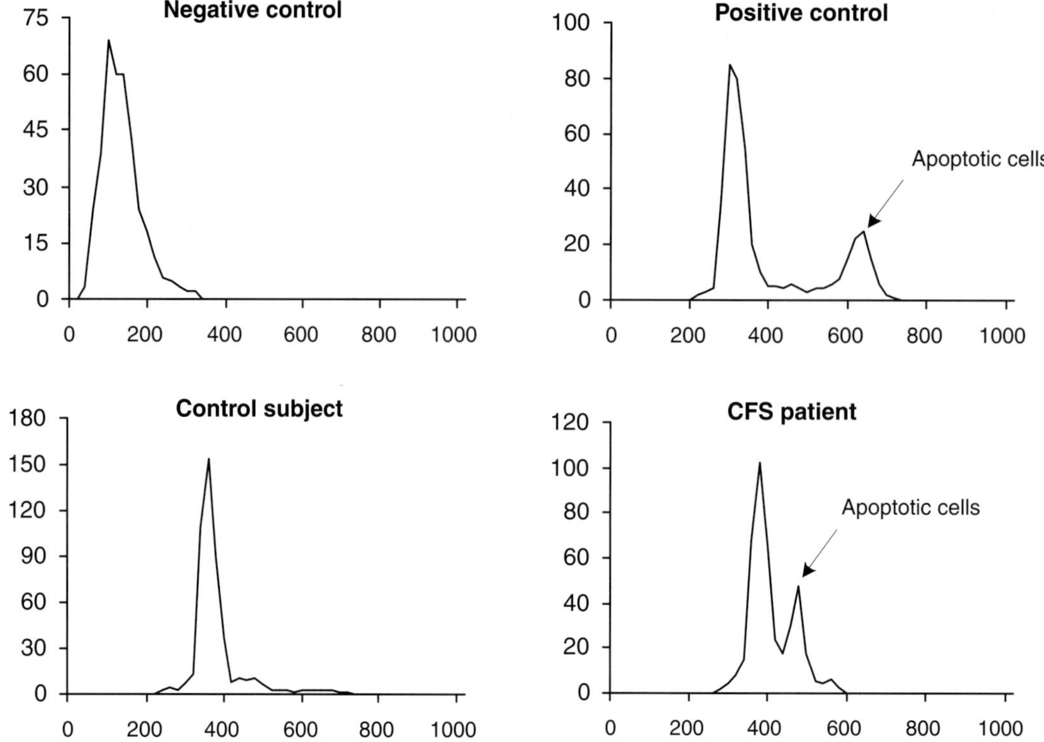

Figure 6.4 Enhanced apoptotic cell population in benzene-exposed CFS individuals. Flow cytometry analysis of apoptotic cell population in negative control cells (HL-60 leukemic cell line), positive control cells (HL-60 leukemic cells treated with the apogen camptothecin), control subjects and benzene-exposed individuals. PBL were isolated, cultured for 12 hours paraformaldehyde-fixed, F-dUTP-labeled and analyzed for apoptosis by flow cytometry.

greater than that of apoptosis, which is predictive of cancer development. Therefore, the tendency of normal cells to commit suicide when deprived of their usual growth factors, or of physical contact with their neighbors due to chemical exposure, is probably a built-in defense against metastasis. Prompt activation of apoptosis in tumor cells that leave their native tissue presumably eradicates many metastatic cells before they have a chance to proliferate. In cancer, it is tumor cells that neglect to sacrifice themselves or forget to die. Indeed, researchers increasingly describe cancer as a disease involving both excessive proliferation of cells and abandonment of their ability to die.

Cancer develops after a cell accumulates mutations in several genes that control cell growth and survival. When a mutation seems irreparable, the affected cell usually kills itself rather than risk becoming deranged and potentially dangerous. But if the cell does not die, it or its progeny may live long enough to accumulate mutations that enable it to divide uncontrollably and metastasize, to break away from the original tumor and establish masses at distant sites.

In many tumors, genetic damage apparently fails to induce apoptosis because the constituent cells have inactivated the gene that codes for the P53 protein. This protein, it will be recalled, can lead to activation of the cell's apoptotic machinery when DNA is injured by environmental agents such as benzene or its metabolites. Therefore, it is very important to study cell suicide in health and diseases.

CLINICAL APPLICATIONS

Apoptosis in autoimmune diseases

In cancer, it is the tumor cells that forget to die – in autoimmunity, immune cells fail to die when they are supposed to. Virtually all tissues harbor apoptotic cells at one time or another. Damaged cells usually commit suicide for the greater good of the body; when this does not occur, disease may develop. Autoimmunity occurs when the antigen receptors on immune cells recognize specific antigens on healthy cells and cause the cells bearing those particular substances to die. But true autoimmune diseases that involve apoptosis do exist. Under normal conditions, the body allows a certain number of self-reactive lymphocytes to circulate. These cells normally do little harm, but they can become overactive

Table 6.1 Ratio of apoptosis to mitosis in patients exposed to a carcinogenic chemical (benzene). In patients 11 and 14, the rate of mitosis is twice that of apoptosis, yielding a ratio of apoptosis to mitosis very close to 0.5. Others present ratios close to 1, which indicates normal homeostasis

Sample no.	Percentage apoptosis	Percentage mitosis	Ratio of apoptosis/mitosis
1	34	18.3	1.9
2	29	25	1.2
3	48	46	1.05
4	47	52	0.9
5	20	18	1.1
6	42	17	2.5
7	23	17	1.35
8	26	19	1.37
9	35	13	2.7
10	44	19	2.3
11	18	33	0.54
12	19	15	1.26
13	32	12	2.66
14	19	35	0.54
15	27	16	1.68
16	29	19	1.52
17	28	27	1.03
18	24	19	1.26
19	7	6	1.16
20	10	11	0.9

through several processes. For instance, if these reactive lymphocytes recognize some foreign antigen such as microbes on food and haptenic chemicals, then exposure to that antigen causes them to become excited. If, due to molecular mimicry, these antigens are similar to normal tissues, the activated cells may expand their numbers and attack the healthy tissue, thus causing an autoimmune disease.[1,17,18]

Autoimmune reactions usually are self-limited – they disappear when the antigens that originally set them off are cleared away. In some instances, however, the autoreactive lymphocytes survive longer than they should and continue to induce apoptosis in normal cells. Some evidence in animals and humans indicates that extended survival of autoreactive cells is implicated in at least two chronic autoimmune syndromes – systemic lupus erythematosus and rheumatoid arthritis. In other words, the lymphocytes undergo too little apoptosis, with the result that normal cells undergo too much.[19,20]

Apoptosis during viral infection

Disturbance in the regulation of apoptosis participates in a variety of diseases. Viral illnesses are among the diseases caused by apoptosis dysregulation. After entering a cell, viruses attempt to shut down the cell's ability to make any proteins except those needed to produce more virus. This act of stalling host protein synthesis is enough to induce many kinds of cells to commit suicide. If the host cell dies, the virus is also eliminated. Therefore, certain viruses have evolved ways to inhibit apoptosis in the cells they infect.

Epstein–Barr virus, which causes mononucleosis and has been linked to lymphomas in humans, uses a mechanism that has been seen in other viruses. It produces substances that inhibit apoptosis. Other viruses, such as P53, inactivate or degrade the induced apoptosis. Papillomavirus, a major cause of cervical cancer, is one example. Cowpox virus, a relative of which is used as the smallpox vaccine, is another. Both elaborate a protein that prevents proteases from carrying out the apoptotic program. Investigators interested in antiviral therapy are now exploring ways to block the activity of the anti-apoptotic molecules manufactured by viruses.[19]

Apoptosis in AIDS

Induction of apoptosis by viruses in healthy cells is believed to contribute to the immune deficiency found in AIDS patients. In these patients, infection with human immunodeficiency virus (HIV) causes T-helper cells to die. As T-helper cells gradually disappear, cytotoxic cells, such as NK cells, perish as well through apoptosis, since they cannot survive without the growth signals produced by T-helper cells. When the number of T-cells dwindles, so does the body's ability to fight infections, especially viral and parasitic. Researchers have shown that many more helper cells succumb than are infected with HIV. It is also highly probable that a large number of the cells probably die through apoptosis. Apparently, Fas plays a crucial role in this process.

Normally, T-cells make functional Fas only after they have been active for a few days and are ready to die. But helper cells from AIDS patients may display high amounts of functional Fas even before the cells have encountered an antigen. This display of Fas would be expected to cause the cells to undergo apoptosis prematurely whenever they encounter Fas ligand on other cells (such as on T-cells already activated against HIV or other microbes). In addition, if the primed cells encounter the antigen recognized by their receptors, they may trigger their own death.

It is also possible that oxygen free radicals trigger the suicide of virus-free T-cells. These highly reactive substances are produced by inflammatory cells drawn to infected lymph nodes in HIV patients. Free radicals can damage DNA and membranes in cells. They will cause necrosis if they do extensive damage, but they can induce apoptosis if the damage is more subtle. In support of the free-radical theory, researchers have found that molecules capable of neutralizing free radicals will prevent apoptosis in T-cells obtained from AIDS patients.[19,20]

Therapies with anti-apoptotic medication, such as Trolox, a water-soluble analog of vitamin E which prevents oxidative stress, and pyrrolidine dithiocarbamate, a potent inhibitor of nuclear factor kB (NF-kB), are now the focus of AIDS and autoimmune disease studies.[21,22]

Apoptosis in the heart and brain

In contrast to cancer, where cells forget to die and insufficient apoptosis occurs, excessive apoptosis accounts for much of the cell death that follows heart attacks and strokes. In the heart, vessel blockage decimates cells that were fully dependent on the vessel. Those cells die by necrosis, partly because they are catastrophically starved of the oxygen and glucose they need to maintain themselves and partly because calcium ions, which are normally pumped out of the cell, rise to toxic levels.

Over the course of a few days, cells surrounding the dead zone – which initially survive because they continue to receive nourishment from other blood vessels – can die as well. Later on, however, many cells die by necrosis after being overwhelmed by the destructive free radicals that are released when inflammatory cells swarm into the dead zone to remove necrotic tissue. The less injured cells commit suicide by apoptosis.

If the patient is treated by restoring blood flow, still more cells may die by necrosis or apoptosis, because reperfusion leads to a transient increase in the production of free radicals. Similarly, in strokes due to inflammation, release of such neurotransmitters as glutamate lead to necrosis and apoptosis. Understanding of the factors that lead to the tissue death accompanying heart attack, stroke, and reperfusion has led to new ideas for treatment. Notably, cell death might be limited by drugs and other agents that block free-radical production or inhibit proteases.

Apoptosis also accounts for much of the pathology seen in such diseases as Alzheimer's, Parkinson's, Huntington's and amyotrophic lateral sclerosis (Lou Gehrig's disease), which are marked by the loss of brain neurons. Elevated apoptosis in these neurological diseases seems to be related to lack of production of the nerve growth factor and to free radical damage. It seems likely that a combination of such factors could cause many cells to destroy themselves. Manipulation of this process of cell killing may help in treating these neurological diseases. In fact, studies in animal models imply that long-term delivery of nerve growth factors could protect against programmed cell death in these conditions. Therefore, a greater understanding of the mechanisms involved in cell death should greatly enhance those important steps.[17,21,23]

CONCLUSIONS

Apoptosis and cell proliferation play an important role in development, differentiation, homeostasis, and aging.[2–6] The balance established between these two processes depends on a variety of growth and death signals which are influenced by diet, nutrition, lifestyle and other environmental factors.

When the equilibrium between life and death is disrupted by aberrant signals (e.g. low levels of antioxidants in the blood or tissue cells), either tissue growth or atrophy occurs.

Under normal conditions with optimal nutritional factors, tissue homeostasis is sustained by balancing the effects of mitosis and apoptosis. The importance of this

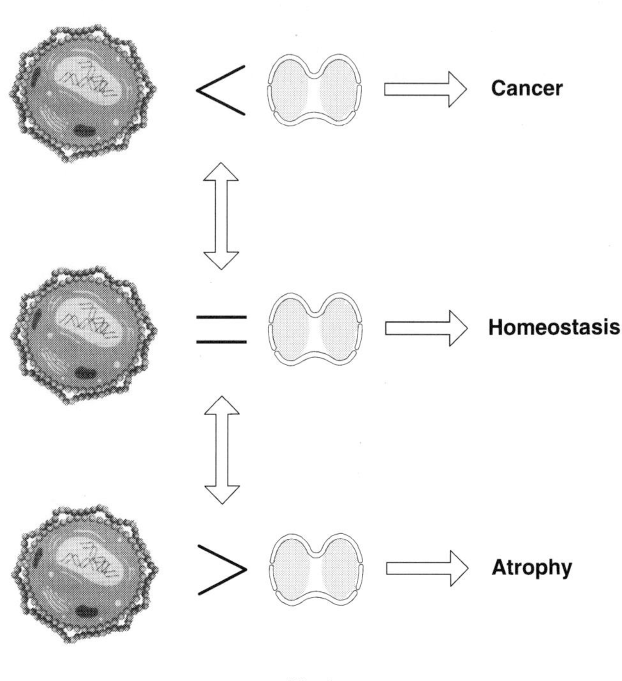

Figure 6.5 Balance or imbalance between the rate of apoptosis and mitosis determines tissue homeostasis, atrophy, cell proliferation, and development of cancer.

balance can clearly be seen when one of these processes becomes predominant (see Fig. 6.5).

During viral or chemical exposure and in pre-neoplastic tissue, the number of cells undergoing apoptosis increases, possibly to compensate for an increase in proliferation.

As the cell loses functional tumor-suppressor genes (the P53), the propensity to undergo apoptosis decreases and the population of tumor cells grows. Inefficient immune function such as low NK activity due to stress or antioxidant deficiencies may contribute further to this mitosis and apoptosis imbalance, which results in additional tumor cell growth.

REFERENCES

1. Wyllie AH, Kerr JF, Currie AR. Cell death. the significance of apoptosis. Int Rev Cytol 1980; 68: 251
2. White E. Life, death and the pursuit of apoptosis. Genes Dev 1996; 10: 1
3. Jarvis WD, Kolesnick RN, Fornari FA et al. Induction of apoptotic DNA damage and cell death by activation of the sphingomyelin pathway. Proc Natl Acad Sci USA 1994; 91: 73
4. Green DR, Martin SJ. The killer and the executioner: how apoptosis controls malignancy. Current Opinion Immunol 1995; 7: 694
5. Arends MJ, McGregor AH, Wyllie AH. Apoptosis is inversely related to necrosis and determines net growth in tumors bearing constitutively expressed myc, ras and HPV oncogenes. J Pathol 1994; 144: 1045
6. Marchetti P, Hirsch T, Zamzami M et al. Mitochondrial permeability triggers lymphocyte apoptosis. J Immunology 1996; 157: 4830
7. Vojdani A, Mordechai E, Brautbar N. Abnormal apoptosis and cell cycle progression in humans exposed to methyl tertiary-butyl ether and benzene contaminating water. Human Exp Toxicol 1997; 16: 485–494
8. Walker PR, Smith C, Youdale T et al. Topoisomerase II-reactive chemotherapeutic drugs induce apoptosis in thymocytes. Cancer Res 1991; 51: 1078–1085
9. Brown DB, Sun XM, Cohen GM. Dexamethasone-induced apoptosis involves cleavage of DNA to large fragments prior to internucleosomal fragmentation. J Biol Chem 1993; 268: 3037
10. Reynolds ES, Kanz MF, Chicco P, Moslen MT. 1.1-Dichloroethylene: an apoptotic hepatotoxin? Environ Health Perspect 1984; 57: 313
11. Aw TY, Nicotera P, Manzo L, Orrenius S. Tributyltin stimulates apoptosis in rat thymocytes. Arch Biochem Biophys 1990; 283: 46
12. Rossi AD, Larsson O, Manzo L et al. Modification of Ca^{2+} signaling by inorganic mercury in PC12 cells. FASEB 1993; 7: 1507
13. Kunimoto M. Methyl mercury induces apoptosis of rat cerebellar neurons in primary culture. Biochem Biophys Res Commun 1994; 204: 310
14. Vivian B, Rossi AD, Chow SC, Nicotera P. Organotin compounds induce calcium overload and apoptosis in PC12 cells. Neurotoxicology 1995; 16: 19
15. Ledda-Columbano GM, Coni P, Curto M et al. Induction of two different modes of cell death, apoptosis and necrosis in rat liver after a single dose of thioacetamide. Am J Pathol 1991; 139: 1099
16. ATSDR (Agency for Toxic Substances and Disease Registry) Toxicological profile for benzene, draft report. Atlanta, GA: Department of Health and Human Services, Agen. 1987
17. National Institute of Environmental Health Sciences. Sixth annual report on carcinogens. Benzene Case No. 71–43–2: 35. Research, 1991. Triangle Park, NC: National Institute of Environmental Health Sciences. 1991
18. Golstein P, Ojcius DM, Ding-E Young J. Cell death mechanisms and the immune system. Immunol Rev 1991; 121: 29
19. Cohen JJ, Duke RC, Fadok VA, Sellins KS. Apoptosis and programmed cell death in immunity. Ann Rev Immunol 1992; 10: 267
20. Duke RC, Ojcius DM, Ding-E Young J. Cell suicide in health and disease. Scientific American 1996; 275: 80
21. Martin SJ, Green DR. Protease activation during apoptosis: death by a thousand cuts. Cell 1995; 82: 349
22. Forrest VJ, Kang Y, McClain DE et al. Oxidative stress-induced apoptosis prevented by Trolox. Free-radical Biol Med 1994; 16: 675–684
23. Schreck R, Meier B, Mannel DN et al. Dithiocarbamates as potent inhibitors of nuclear factor kB activation in intact cells. J Exp Med 1992; 175: 1181

CHAPTER CONTENTS

7

Bacterial overgrowth of the small intestine breath test

Stephen Barrie, ND

INTRODUCTION

Bacterial overgrowth of the small intestine is a serious digestive disorder that is treatable after proper diagnosis. Although widespread, it is frequently unsuspected in cases of chronic bowel problems and carbohydrate intolerance because its symptoms often mimic other disorders.[1]

The incidence of bacterial overgrowth of the small intestine increases with age, particularly in people aged 80 years and more.[2] Elderly patients may develop malabsorption secondary to bacterial overgrowth. It has been suggested as the major cause of clinically significant malabsorption in the elderly and linked to the "failure to thrive syndrome" seen in older patients.[3]

Breath testing is a very useful procedure for distinguishing bacterial overgrowth of the small intestine from other problems with similar symptoms.

Symptoms of bacterial overgrowth

By inhibiting proper nutrient absorption, bacterial overgrowth of the small intestine can lead to systemic disorders such as altered permeability, anemia and weight loss, osteomalacia and vitamin K deficiency.[3] Bacterial overgrowth of the small intestine may also contribute to maldigestion and malabsorption. It frequently is a complication of parasitic infection. Patients with pancreatic insufficiency secondary to chronic pancreatitis are prone to developing bacterial overgrowth of the small intestine.[4]

As can be seen from Table 7.1, the signs and symptoms

Table 7.1 Symptoms of bacterial overgrowth

- Abdominal cramps
- Bloating
- Diarrhea
- Gas
- Steatorrhea
- Vitamin B_{12} malabsorption and deficiency
- Weight loss

of bacterial overgrowth are commonly seen in a clinical practice.

Causes of bacterial overgrowth

Normally, far fewer bacteria inhabit the small intestine than the ample growth found in the colon. Gastric acid secretion and intestinal motility keep the small intestine relatively free of bacteria. A wide range of abnormalities and malfunctions, however, can encourage bacteria to multiply in the small intestine.

The most common causes relate to a decrease in the production of hydrochloric acid or pancreatic enzymes, thereby creating an unsterile environment for the small intestine. Other causes of bacterial overgrowth of the small intestine include intestinal obstructions caused by Crohn's disease, adhesions, radiation damage and lymphoma (see Table 7.2). Many years may pass between the development of diverticula and symptoms of bacterial overgrowth.[5,6]

EFFECTS ON THE BODY

Bacterial flora function as small biochemical factories, which explains most of the effects of bacterial overgrowth of the small intestine.[7] The flora contain very high concentrations of different enzymes which act upon substrates presented through the diet. Some of these enzymes produce toxic fermentation products normally not found in the small intestine.

Gut flora metabolize biliary steroids, which contribute to the diarrhea common in bacterial overgrowth and which may contribute to colon cancer. As can be seen in Table 7.3, overgrowth of flora in the small intestine can have a wide variety of damaging effects to the intestines and health.

TESTING METHODS

While intubation and culture of intestinal aspirates are the standard for determining bacterial overgrowth of the small intestine, the less invasive breath trace-gas analysis is an attractive and effective alternative.[5,8–10]

Table 7.2 Causes of bacterial overgrowth of the small intestine

- Achlorhydria, hypochlorhydria or drug-induced hypoacidity
- Crohn's disease
- Diabetes mellitus
- Giardiasis and other parasitic infections
- Immunodeficiency syndromes (particularly sIgA)
- Intestinal adhesions
- Systemic lupus erythematosus
- Malnutrition
- Chronic pancreatitis
- Reduced motility in elderly patients
- Scleroderma
- Stasis due to structural changes – diverticulitis, blind loops, radiation damage

Table 7.3 Health effects of floral overgrowth in the small intestine

- Inactivate pancreatic and brush border digestive enzymes due to production of proteases
- Destroy dietary flavonoids, which serve as important natural antioxidants but are rapidly broken down and hydrolyzed by gut flora
- Hydrogenate polyunsaturated fatty acids
- Deconjugate bile salts
- Consume vitamin B_{12}
- Produce vitamin B_{12} antagonists
- Produce nitrosamines

Endoscopy and intestinal fluid culture have the advantages of providing a definitive diagnosis, but the method is expensive and requires invasive intubation. In addition, it assesses only one or a few sites and may miss flora elsewhere, leading to false-negative results.

On the other hand, hydrogen/methane breath tests are simple to administer and offer greater patient comfort and convenience. In addition, these breath tests have good sensitivity and specificity.

However, hydrogen/methane breath tests are not effective in patients who don't produce hydrogen or methane in response to carbohydrate challenge dose (less than 5%).

The bacterial overgrowth of the small intestine breath test uses a challenge dose of lactulose or glucose that the patient takes after an overnight fast. If bacteria exist in the small intestine, the bacteria will ferment the challenge substance and produce increases in breath hydrogen and methane. Each substance has advantages and disadvantages.

Lactulose challenge

Lactulose, a synthetic disaccharide not absorbed by the digestive system, produces hydrogen after contact with bacteria in the gut.[11] In the lactulose challenge test, patients collect a fasting breath sample, drink a 10 g lactulose solution, and collect breath samples every 15 minutes for 2 hours.[1]

Advantages

- Good sensitivity, because the challenge dose is carried farther toward the jejunum than glucose, so it checks for bacterial overgrowth farther down the intestinal tract
- Good specificity for bacterial overgrowth of the small intestine
- Suitable for patients with diabetes, hypoglycemia, and other blood sugar disorders because lactulose isn't absorbed.

Disadvantages

- Some difficulty in interpretation due to the possible late peak of colonic fermentation of lactulose
- Possible mild discomfort or diarrhea in some patients, although usually at higher doses than those used in the breath test.

Glucose challenge

Glucose is normally absorbed before it reaches the large intestine. If bacteria are present in the small intestine, the bacteria will metabolize glucose before it can be absorbed, producing breath gases. This test requires ingestion of a 75 g glucose solution.

Advantages

- Good sensitivity and specificity
- Easy to interpret because patients who don't have bacterial overgrowth of the small intestine absorb glucose and don't produce an increase in breath gases
- Can be performed at the same time as a glucose tolerance test (if both are medically indicated).

Disadvantages

- Test is not suitable for patients with diabetes, hypoglycemia, or other blood sugar disorders
- If the presence of yeast in the colon is regarded as a medical condition, ingestion of sugar may be inadvisable due to its potential for promoting yeast growth
- Sensitivity is reduced for distal ileum activity of bacterial overgrowth.[12]

Interpreting the results

Baseline responses

The typical fasting breath sample contains less than 10 ppm of breath hydrogen or methane. A high breath hydrogen or methane level greater than 20 ppm is likely in patients with bacterial overgrowth.

Because the fasting breath hydrogen level can be suppressed by methanogenic bacteria, testing for both hydrogen and methane is more sensitive than testing for hydrogen only.[1]

Lactulose response

The lactulose challenge typically causes a two-phase response. During the test, hydrogen increases early as lactulose comes into contact with bacteria in the small intestine. This rapid response distinguishes bacterial overgrowth from normal colonic flora, which produce a later, more prolonged increase in breath hydrogen.[1,12] The test monitors breath gas during the first 2 hours, so colonic fermentation either is not detected or is seen as a rise in the final breath specimens.

A breath hydrogen peak greater than 12 ppm above the fasting level within 30 minutes of ingesting lactulose and preceding the colonic excretion response by 15 minutes is considered indicative of bacterial overgrowth of the small intestine.[1,12,13]

Glucose response

With the glucose challenge, a rise of 12 ppm in breath hydrogen within 1 hour suggests bacterial overgrowth.[1] The 1 hour period avoids confusion between an increase in breath hydrogen due to bacterial fermentation and early colonic generation of breath hydrogen due to rapid transit.[14]

Combining the observation of elevated fasting breath hydrogen (greater than 20 ppm) and a positive hydrogen response (greater than 15 ppm) reduces the chance of false-positive responses.[1]

False-positives

The majority of false-positives reported in bacterial overgrowth of the small intestine breath test can be eliminated if patients follow proper instructions and preparation.[1] Typical problems include:

- Eating high-fiber foods within 24 hours of the test. This elevates the level of fiber in the colon at the beginning of the test and increases breath hydrogen production. No starches except rice should be eaten the night before the test. A protein and rice meal, such as beef, poultry, fish or tofu, should be eaten the night before. Fiber supplements should be discontinued 24 hours before the test.
- Smoking. Smoking in the area of the test produces high hydrogen levels and unstable baseline results. Breath samples should not be collected where patients are exposed to tobacco smoke.
- Sleeping. Sleeping during the test increases both hydrogen and methane levels due to the slow-down in removal of breath trace gases from blood.

False-negatives

False-negative results can be caused by severe diarrhea or recent use of an antibiotic, laxative, or enema. Any of these may inhibit bacterial fermentation of carbohydrates and thus production of breath trace gases.[15–19]

To reduce the possibility of false-negative results, patients should wait at least 1 week following completion of antibiotic treatment or after recovery from severe diarrhea to re-establish colonic flora. Hyperacidic colon contents do not affect the lactulose challenge because the test reports bacterial fermentation in the small intestine.[1]

CLINICAL APPLICATION

Once bacterial overgrowth of the small intestine has been diagnosed, two steps are necessary:

- treat the overgrowth symptoms
- investigate the underlying causes to keep bacterial overgrowth from recurring.

Antimicrobials

While tetracycline (250 mg four times daily) is the traditional antibiotic choice, research indicates that up to 60% of patients with bacterial overgrowth no longer respond to it.[5] Several broad-spectrum antibiotics have been used effectively. Augmentin (250–500 mg three times daily) is generally effective and well tolerated. Acceptable alternatives include the cephalosporin Keflex (250 mg four times daily) and Flagyl (250 mg three times daily).[5]

Antimicrobials such as penicillin, ampicillin, neomycin, kanamycin, and oral aminoglycosides are ineffective in treating bacterial overgrowth because of their poor activity against anaerobes. A non-absorbable rifamycin derivative, Rifaximin, has been used effectively against anaerobic intestinal bacteria in Italy.[20]

Several natural antimicrobials may be useful in the treatment of bacterial overgrowth syndromes. These include:

- bismuth, a broad-spectrum antimicrobial absorbed in the gut
- bentonite, which inhibits bacterial growth and activity, absorbing many by-products that bacteria produce
- berberine, an alkaloid from *Hydrastis canadensis*, with antimicrobial, antifungal and antiprotozoan activity
- herbal mixtures containing gentian and sanguinaria, which have very strong broad-spectrum antimicrobial activity.

Nutrition

A low-starch or low-sugar diet may be helpful in reducing diarrhea and steatorrhea. Whether starch or sugar needs to be restricted depends on the location of bacterial overgrowth. If bacteria are in the jejunum, patients tend to be more intolerant of sugars. If bacteria are in the ileum, starch may affect patients more.

Soluble fiber may exacerbate abnormal gut ecology. A diet free of cereal grains is generally helpful. Potential deficiencies of nutrients such as vitamin B_{12}, vitamin K, and calcium should be considered (see Ch. 19).[5]

Treatment of underlying causes

Bacterial overgrowth of the small intestine may recur if the root causes are not eradicated (Table 7.2). Hypochlorhydria and achlorhydria limit the body's ability to utilize nutrients from food and supplements. With low gastric acid, ingested food is not adequately sterilized, and normal colonic bacteria may move upstream into the small intestine, causing the return of bacterial overgrowth. Numerous studies have shown that acid secretion decreases with age, possibly due to atrophy of various digestive functions (see Ch. 19). Betaine hydrochloride may be useful in replacing hydrochloric acid in patients not producing sufficient amounts.

A sluggish digestive tract keeps food lingering in the intestinal system. Reduced motility may be caused by inadequate water intake, a low-fiber diet, or aging. Addition of insoluble fiber helps to create bulk and encourage motility.

SUMMARY

Bacterial Overgrowth of the Small Intestine Breath Test is a useful procedure for patients with chronic gastrointestinal problems. Table 7.4 lists the most appropriate clinical indications.

Table 7.4 Clinical conditions for the bacterial overgrowth of the small intestine breath test

- Patient has abdominal gas, bloating or diarrhea, usually within 1 hour of eating
- Patient cannot tolerate carbohydrates or starchy foods, fiber supplements and/or friendly flora supplements
- Evidence of hypochlorhydria and/or low transit time as indicated by patient history or the comprehensive digestive stool analysis
- When CDSA indicates maldigestion or malabsorption, patient is treated but symptoms persist. Also, when the CDSA suggests alkaline pH or dysbiosis
- Lactose intolerance is suspected but ruled out by lactose intolerance breath test
- Patient has abdominal symptoms coupled with unexplained symptoms such as vitamin B_{12} deficiency, chronic weight loss or chronic skin problems

REFERENCES

1. Hamilton LH. Breath testing and gastroenterology. QuinTron Division, The EF Brewer Company: Menomonee Falls, WI. 1992
2. Riordan SM, McIver CJ, Duncombe VM, Bolin TD. The association between small intestinal bacterial overgrowth and aging [abstract]. Gastroenterology 1994; 106: A266
3. Saltzman JR, Russell RM. Nutritional consequences of intestinal

bacterial overgrowth. Compr Ther 1994; 20: 523–530
4. Salemans JMJI, Nagengast FM, Jansen JBMJ. The 14C-xylose breath test in chronic pancreatitis: evidence for small intestinal bacterial overgrowth [abstract]. Gastroenterology 1994; 106: A320
5. Toskes PP. Bacterial overgrowth of the gastrointestinal tract. Adv Int Med 1993; 38: 387–407
6. Herlinger H. Enteroclysis in malabsorption: can it influence diagnosis and management? Radiologe 1993; 33: 335–342
7. Galland L. Clinical applications of breath testing. Great Smokies Diagnostic Laboratory Seminar, Greenwich, CT. 1994
8. Corazza GR, Menozzi MG, Strocchi A. The diagnosis of small bowel bacterial overgrowth. Reliability of jejunal culture and inadequacy of breath hydrogen testing. Gastroenterology 1990; 98: 302–309
9. King CE, Toskes PP. Comparison of the 1-gram [14C] xylose, 10-gram lactulose-H2, and 80-gram glucose-H2 breath tests in patients with small intestine bacterial overgrowth. Gastroenterology 1986; 91: 1447–1451
10. Kerlin P, Wong L. Breath hydrogen testing in bacterial overgrowth of the small intestine. Gastroenterology 1988; 95: 982–988
11. Davidson GP, Robb TA, Kirubakaran CP. Bacterial contamination of the small intestine as an important cause of chronic diarrhea and abdominal pain: diagnosis by breath hydrogen test. Pediatrics 1984; 74: 229–236
12. Rhodes JM, Middleton P, Jewell DP. The lactulose hydrogen breath test as a diagnostic test for small bowel bacterial overgrowth. Scand J Gastroenterol 1979; 14: 333–336
13. Rhodes JM. Lactulose hydrogen breath test in the diagnosis of bacterial overgrowth. Gastroenterology 1990; 98: 1547
14. Corazza G, Sorge M, Strocchi A. Glucose-H_2 breath test for small intestine bacterial overgrowth. Gastroenterology 1990; 98: 254
15. Lerch MM, Rieband HC, Feldberg W. Concordance of indirect methods for the detection of lactose malabsorption in diabetic and non-diabetic subjects. Digestion 1991; 48: 81–88
16. Gilat T, Ben Hur H, Gelman-Malachi E. Alterations of the colonic flora and the effect on the hydrogen breath test. Gut 1978; 19: 602
17. Solomons NW, Garcia R, Schneider R. H_2 breath tests during diarrhea. Acta Paediatr Scand 1979; 88: 171
18. Vogelsang H, Ferenci P, Frotz S. Acidic colonic microclimate – possible reason for false negative hydrogen breath test. Gut 1988; 29: 21–26
19. Perman JA, Modler S, Olson AC. Role of pH in production of hydrogen from carbohydrates by colonic bacterial flora. Studies in vivo and in vitro. J Clin Invest 1981; 67: 643
20. Corazza GR, Ventrucci M, Strocchi A. Treatment of small intestine bacterial overgrowth with rifaximin, a non-absorbable rifamycin. J Internat Med Res 1988; 16: 312–316

CHAPTER CONTENTS

8

Cell signaling analysis

Aristo Vojdani, PhD MT

INTRODUCTION

Signaling pathways in normal cells consist of growth and controlling messages from the outer surface deep into the nucleus. In the nucleus, the cell cycle clock collects different messages, which are used to determine when the cell should divide. Cancer cells often proliferate excessively because genetic mutations cause induction of stimulatory pathways and issue too many "go ahead" signals, or the inhibitory pathways can no longer control the stimulatory pathways.[1]

Over the past 5 years, impressive evidence has been gathered with regard to the destination of stimulatory and inhibitory pathways in the cell. These pathways converge on a molecular apparatus in the cell nucleus that is often referred to as the cell cycle clock. The clock is the executive decision-maker of the cell; apparently, it runs amok in virtually all types of human cancer. In a normal cell, the clock integrates the mixture of growth-regulating signals received by the cell and decides whether the cell should pass through its life cycle. If the answer is positive, the clock leads the process.

THE CELL CYCLE

A scheme of the classical cell cycle is shown in Figure 8.1. The cell cycle compartments are drawn such that their horizontal position reflects their respective DNA content. Cells that contain only one complement of DNA from each parent (2C) are referred to as diploid cells. Cells that have duplicated their genome, and thus have 4C amounts of DNA, are called tetraploid cells.

The cell cycle is classically divided into the following phases:

- G_0
- G_1
- S
- G_2
- M.

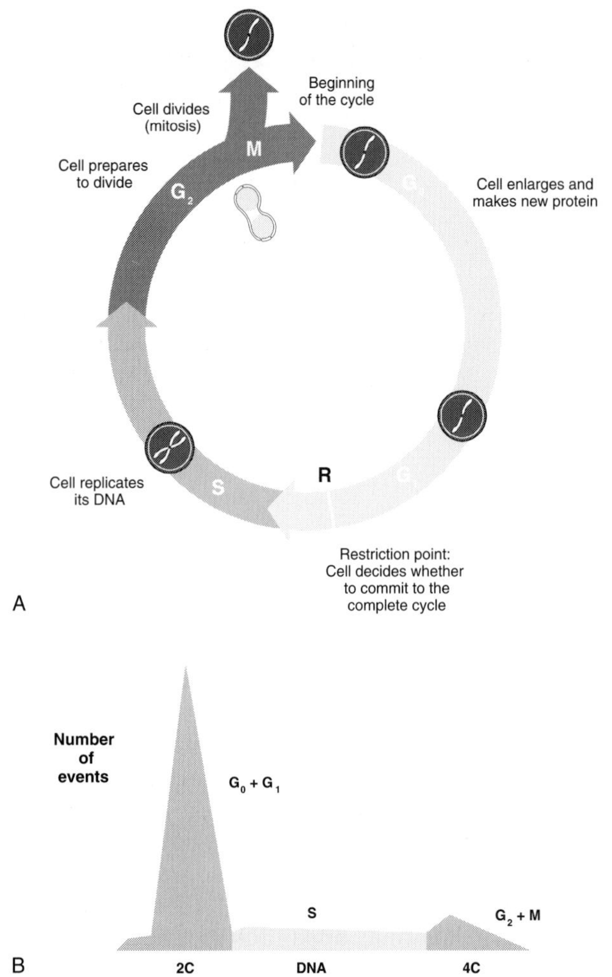

Figure 8.1 Stages of cell cycle (G_0, G_1, S, G_2, and M phases) (A) and DNA histogram (B) generated by flow cytometry.

The cell cycle phase of G_1 was historically considered to be a time when diploid (2C) cells had little observable activity. Since this time precedes DNA synthesis, the term Gap 1 (G_1) was coined. We now know that there is quite a bit of transcription and protein synthesis during this phase. At a certain point in the cell's life, the DNA synthetic machinery turns on. This phase of the cell's life is labeled "S" for synthesis. As the cell proceeds through this phase, its DNA content increases from 2C to 4C. At the end of S, the cell has duplicated its genome and now is in the tetraploid state. After the S phase, the cell again enters a phase that was historically thought to be quiescent. Since this phase is the second gap region, it is referred to as G_2. In the G_2 phase, the cell is producing the necessary proteins that will play a major role in cytokinesis. After a highly variable amount of time, the cell enters mitosis (M). DNA content remains constant at 4C until the cell actually divides at the end of telophase.

The enlarged parent cell finally reaches the point where it divides in half to produce its two daughters, each of which is endowed with a complete set of chromosomes. The new daughter cells immediately enter G_1 and may go through the full cycle again. Alternatively, they may stop cycling temporarily or permanently.[2–4]

FLOW CYTOMETRY TO ASSESS CELL CYCLE STATUS

Flow cytometry is a method of measuring cell properties as they "flow" through a detector while being illuminated with intense light. Tissues are generally disaggregated into single-cell suspensions and stained with one or more fluorescent dyes. The cells are forced to flow within a sheath of fluid, eventually being intersected and interrogated by an intense light source such as a laser beam. As the cell enters the laser beam, it scatters light in all directions. The measurement of light scattered in the forward direction yields information on the particle's size. Scattered light at right-angles to the incident light beam provides information on the internal granularity of the cell. If the cell has been stained with one or more fluorescent dyes, a correlated measurement of more than one cellular parameter can be achieved.

CLINICAL APPLICATION

Patients exposed to carcinogenic chemicals and patients with chronic fatigue syndrome

To determine whether peripheral blood lymphocytes (PBL) isolated from chronic fatigue syndrome (CFS) individuals and chemically exposed patients represent a discrete block in cell cycle progression, PBL isolated from CFS and control individuals were cultured, harvested, fixed, PI-stained, and analyzed by flow cytometry. The non-apoptotic cell population in PBL isolated from CFS individuals consisted of cells arrested in the late S and G_2/M boundaries, as compared with healthy controls. The arrest was characterized by increased S and G_2/M phases of the cell cycle (from 9 to 33% and from 4 to 21%, respectively) (Table 8.1, Fig. 8.2) at the expense of G_0/G_1. Such an abnormality in cell cycle progression is an indication of abnormal mitotic cell division in patients who have been exposed to chemicals and who suffer from chronic fatigue syndrome. From these results, we concluded that PBLs of patients with chemical exposure

Table 8.1 Percentage of different phases of cell cycle in healthy controls and patients exposed to chemicals

Phase	Healthy controls	Chemically exposed
G_0/G_1	88.6 ± 1.4	51.7 ± 2.4
S	8.6 ± 1.2	33.2 ± 4.3
G_2/M	3.6 ± 0.82	21.0 ± 2.6

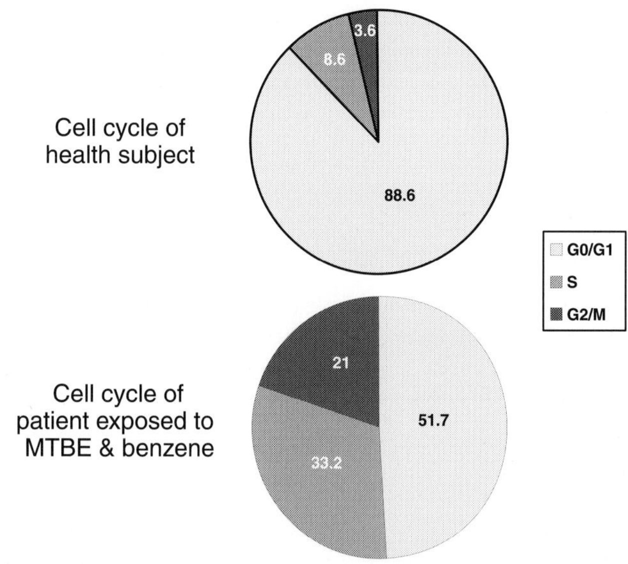

Figure 8.2 Cell cycle analysis of peripheral blood lymphocytes from healthy controls (A) and patients exposed to benzene (B). Note that in patients' samples, the majority of cells switched from G_0/G_1 to S and G_2/M phases.

and chronic fatigue syndrome grow inappropriately, not only because the signaling pathways in cells are perturbed, but also because the cell cycle clock becomes deranged and stimulatory messages become greater than the inhibitory pathways.[5,6]

However, in order to limit cell proliferation and avoid cancer, the human body equips cells with certain back-up systems that guard against runaway division. One such back-up system present in lymphocytes of CFS patients provokes the cell to undergo apoptosis. This programmed cell death occurs if some of the cell's essential components are deregulated or damaged. For example, injury to chromosomal DNA can trigger apoptosis.[1,5,6]

REFERENCES

1. Weinberg RA. How cancer arises. Scientific American 1996; 275: 62
2. Wheeless LL, Coon JS, Cox C et al. Precision of DNA flow cytometry in inter-institutional analyses. Cytometry 1991; 12: 405
3. Wersto RP, Liblit RL, Koss LG. Flow cytometric DNA analysis of human solid tumors: a review of the interpretation of DNA histograms. Hum Pathol 1991; 22: 1085
4. Shankey TV, Rabinovitch PS, Bagwell B et al. Guidelines for implementation of clinical DNA cytometry. Cytometry 1993; 14: 472
5. Vojdani A, Ghoneum M, Choppa PC et al. Elevated apoptotic cell population in patients with chronic fatigue syndrome: the pivotal role of protein kinase RNA. J Intern Med 1997; 242: 465–478
6. Vojdani A, Mordechai E, Brautbar N. Abnormal apoptosis and cell cycle progression in humans exposed to methyl tertiary-butyl ether and benzene contaminating water. Human Exp Toxicol 1997; 16: 485–494

CHAPTER CONTENTS

9

Comprehensive digestive stool analysis

Stephen Barrie, ND

INTRODUCTION

Nutrition and digestion are undeniably important to good health. We are, essentially, what we eat and then absorb. Over the long haul, excellent health is impossible without good nutrition. However, without adequate breakdown and assimilation, even the best diet offers little help. Additionally, incomplete or faulty digestive processes may lead to a variety of chronic disorders.

Gastrointestinal (GI) disorders have a major impact on health. One recent study found that, during a 3 month period, nearly 70% of American households experienced one or more gastrointestinal symptoms.[1] Maldigestion, malabsorption and abnormal gut flora and ecology, as well as many complex chronic illnesses and symptoms, lie at the root of most common GI complaints. Thus, nutrition and digestive processes are central to long-term health. The comprehensive digestive stool analysis (CDSA) provides clinicians with a critical tool for evaluating the status of the GI tract.

This assay helps to pinpoint imbalances, to provide clues about current symptoms and to warn of potential problems should the imbalances progress. With an accurate assessment, custom-tailored treatment can be easily applied, greatly increasing the chances for therapeutic success.

The CDSA is used in the evaluation of various gastrointestinal symptoms or systemic illnesses that may have started in the intestine. Because illnesses are often not discernible from symptoms, the CDSA is a valuable screen for all patients and frequently reveals critical imbalances previously unsuspected.

THE GASTROINTESTINAL TRACT

As most food molecules cannot be absorbed or utilized in their native state, a primary function of the gastrointestinal system is to break down complex molecules and absorb nutrients. This is a complex process, taking place primarily in the gastrointestinal mucosa, where the battle for health – to absorb nutrients and exclude toxins – is fought. The gastrointestinal mucosa does this through a combination of physical barriers to diffusion, mucosal fluids and active immune processes.[2]

The digestive process

Mouth

Teeth break up food and mix it with saliva. Saliva in turn helps to form a bolus and protects the pharyngeal and esophageal mucosa, primarily with secretory IgA antibodies. Saliva also helps to remineralize the teeth with calcium salts. The enzymes lingual lipase, salivary amylase and ptyalin initiate fat and starch digestion.[3]

Stomach

The stomach mechanically churns food, breaks up and emulsifies fats and exposes molecules to additional enzymes. In doing this, it produces 1–2 L of gastric juices per day.[4]

Gastric juice has several components:

- Hydrochloric acid is secreted by the parietal cells. It activates pepsinogens to convert to pepsin and renders some minerals (e.g. calcium and iron) more absorbable. Stomach acid all prevents bacterial overgrowth by creating an essentially sterile environment (a potential exception is *Helicobacter pylori*).
- Mucus forms an acid- and pepsin-resistant coating of the stomach lining.
- Gastric lipase begins the hydrolysis of fats.

Small intestine

Most digestion and absorption takes place in the small intestine and is mediated by pancreatic enzymes and bile.[4] The process involves several steps:

1. Secretion of pancreatic juices (about 2.5 L/day), which is controlled by the vagus nerve and the duodenal hormones secretin and cholecystokinin. Hormone production, in turn, is stimulated by the presence of fat, protein and acid chyme.
2. Secretion of bicarbonate which neutralizes stomach acid.
3. The proteases trypsinogen, chymotrypsinogen and procarboxypeptidase are activated to trypsin, chymotrypsin and carboxypeptidase. These enzymes digest proteins to oligopeptides and amino acids.
4. Amylase splits starch to maltose.
5. Lipase hydrolyzes diglycerides and triglycerides, producing long-chain fatty acids.
6. Bile secreted by the liver (about 700 ml daily) is stored in the gall bladder. Bile salts solubilize and emulsify fats, enabling enzymatic hydrolysis.

The crypts of Lieberkühn of the intestinal mucosa also produce immunoglobulins (which protect the gastric mucosa from microbes) and small amounts of digestive enzymes such as peptidase and disaccharidases.

Large intestine

A primary role of the large intestine is the absorption of water, about 1 L daily. The large intestine also provides an environment for microbial fermentation of soluble fiber, starch, and undigested carbohydrates.

Anaerobic colonic fermentation results in the production of short-chain fatty acids (SCFAs), the main energy source for colonic epithelial cells. It is these SCFAs, in combination with amines derived from protein degradation, that provide buffering and create the slightly acidic pH of fecal matter.

Absorption of specific nutrients[5]

Carbohydrate digestion

Salivary amylase initiates starch digestion in the mouth. However, this activity is short-lived as the enzyme is denatured by low gastric pH. In the duodenum, oligosaccharides and starch polymers undergo hydrolysis by pancreatic amylase. Specific disaccharides are hydrolyzed by brush border enzymes (lactase, maltase, sucrase) located on the enterocyte microvilli. Resulting monosaccharides are absorbed by specific sodium-dependent transport carrier mechanisms.

Protein digestion

Gastric acid and pepsin initiate the digestion of dietary protein. This is followed in the duodenum by hydrolysis into oligopeptides and amino acids by proteolytic pancreatic enzymes. Final protein digestion is accomplished by intestinal brush border peptidases. Dipeptides, tripeptides, free amino acids, and other short-chain peptides are then absorbed.

Fat digestion

Processing of dietary fat is the most complex of the digestive and absorptive processes. Fat is water-insoluble, so the GI tract must transform large water-insoluble particles into a soluble, absorbable form.

Digestion begins in the mouth with secretion of lingual lipases. The stomach disperses fat globules into an evenly divided phase, called chyme. Pancreatic enzymes then split triglycerides into fatty acids and monoglycerides, which then combine with bile acids and phospholipids to form micelles. This process transforms water-insoluble lipids into a water-soluble form absorbed in the proximal small intestine.

After absorption, fatty acids and other lipids are re-esterified in the intestinal cell to form chylomicrons, which are then secreted into the lymphatic system. Medium-chain triglycerides can be absorbed directly in the jejunum without forming chylomicrons.

DIGESTIVE ABNORMALITIES[6–8]

As discussed in Chapters 19 and 55, inadequate digestion and absorption of nutrients is a far more common problem than is generally recognized by clinicians. Not only does ingestion of even the best nutritional substances provide little benefit when breakdown and assimilation are inadequate, but also incompletely digested macromolecules can be inappropriately absorbed into the systemic circulation. This can lead to food allergy, immune complex deposition diseases, and toxic overload of the liver.

Maldigestion

Hypochlorhydria

Gastric acid secretion is a fundamental step in digestion and assimilation. Many clinical conditions originate with decreased gastric acidity (Tables 9.1 and 9.2). Acid secretion decreases with age, and low stomach acidity is found in more than 50% of patients over the age of 60.[22,23] Researchers speculate that malabsorption of nutrients in the elderly is due to atrophy of various digestive organs because of hypochlorhydria.[24]

Gastric acid has a fundamental role in activating pancreatic proenzymes and converting them from inactive precursors (chymotrypsinogen, trypsinogen, etc.) to their active forms (chymotrypsin, trypsin). Intestinal peristalsis and gastric acid secretion normally prevents excessive growth of bacteria in the small intestine. Bacterial overgrowth appears to interfere with fat digestion and irritate the intestinal mucosa.

Pancreatic exocrine insufficiency

Inadequate delivery of pancreatic lipases and proteases to the small intestine can lead to inadequate breakdown of fats and protein. The net effect is a failure to obtain nourishment from protein, carbohydrate and fiber foods and an unhealthy environment for the flora of the large colon. It has been argued that even small decreases in pancreatic output can contribute substantially to maldigestion and have far-reaching effects in chronically ill patients.

Table 9.1 Symptoms of low gastric acidity[9,10]

- Bloating, belching, burning, and flatulence immediately after meals
- Sense of fullness after eating
- Indigestion, diarrhea, or constipation
- Systemic reactions after eating
- Nausea after taking supplements
- Rectal itching
- Weak, peeling or cracked fingernails
- Dilated capillaries in cheeks and nose (in non-alcoholics)
- Post-adolescent acne
- Iron deficiency
- Chronic intestinal infections, parasites, yeast, bacteria
- Undigested food in stool

Table 9.2 Diseases linked to low gastric acidity[11–21]

- Addison's disease
- Asthma
- Celiac disease
- Chronic autoimmune disorders
- Dermatitis herpetiformis
- Diabetes mellitus
- Eczema
- Food allergies
- Gall bladder disease
- Gastric carcinoma
- Gastritis
- Graves' disease
- Hepatitis
- Lupus erythematosus
- Osteoporosis
- Pernicious anemia
- Psoriasis
- Rosacea
- Thyrotoxicosis
- Urticaria
- Vitiligo

Malabsorption

Malabsorption is characterized by abnormal fecal excretion of fat (steatorrhea) and variable malabsorption of fats, fat-soluble vitamins, other vitamins, proteins, carbohydrates, minerals and water. Common causes are listed in Table 9.3.

Important clinical diseases strongly associated with and possibly causal of mucosal malabsorption are listed in Table 9.4.

Table 9.3 Common causes of malabsorption

- Defective protein, fat, or carbohydrate breakdown
- Inadequate solubility of fatty acids (inadequate bile salts)
- Rapid transit (e.g. diarrhea), which doesn't allow sufficient time for absorption
- Mucosal cell abnormality and inadequate surface area
- Intestinal infection

Table 9.4 Diseases associated with mucosal malabsorption

- Sprue
- Whipple's disease
- Crohn's disease
- Giardiasis
- Cryptosporidiosis
- Lactose intolerance
- Eosinophilic gastroenteritis

Clinical considerations of malabsorption

The signs and symptoms of malabsorption, which increases with age, are varied.[25] Amino acids, carbohydrates, fats, vitamins, and trace elements may be absorbed by different processes, so an individual may suffer malabsorption of one nutrient but not of others. In fat malabsorption, essential fatty acid deficiency may result in addition to the loss of the highest dietary source of calories.

Table 9.5 Diseases associated with *Candida albicans* overgrowth[30–35]

- Food allergy
- Migraine headache
- Irritable bowel syndrome
- Asthma
- Indigestion and gas
- Depression related to PMS
- Vaginitis
- Chronic fatigue

MICROBIOLOGY

Bacteria

Because the oxygen content of the colon is low, the vast majority of bacteria are anaerobes. There are, however, hundreds of varieties of anaerobic flora in vastly different concentrations, all growing very slowly. The significance of most of these flora remains largely unknown. Most researchers, therefore, utilize the aerobic flora as an indication of bacterial health. Two frequently identified organisms, *Lactobacilli* sp. and *Escherichia coli*, are employed as indicators of eubiosis or healthy overall flora. Many researchers believe these two organisms have intrinsic benefit and aid digestion while helping to prevent overgrowth of abnormal flora.

Bacterial cultures also identify and show potential pathogens. The term "potential pathogens" is used because individuals may harbor traditional pathogens and appear healthy, while others harbor weak or questionable pathogens and have gastrointestinal complaints. While not necessarily causing acute GI tract disturbances, some intestinal bacteria may be involved in the etiology of various chronic or systemic problems. These include *Klebsiella, Proteus, Pseudomonas* and *Citrobacter*. These organisms may be involved, through molecular mimicry, in various autoimmune diseases. This has been reported in diabetes mellitus, meningitis, thyroid disease, ulcerative colitis, arthritis, ankylosing spondylitis and systemic lupus.[26,27] Some potential pathogens may cause clinical and subclinical malabsorption of nutrients and increase bowel permeability to large macromolecules. A number of clinicians speculate that this is directly related to the etiology of food and chemical sensitivity and intolerance.

Whipple's disease, although rare, presents an interesting model of the interaction of bacterial infection, absorptive processes and systemic health. This disease is known to be caused by an unusual bacteria which resists attempts to culture it in vitro. Symptoms include severe alterations in intestinal permeability and chronic fatigue.[28] There is strong scientific support for the profound relation between GI tract flora, malabsorption, permeability changes and overall health.

Yeast

In the last few years, colonic yeast infections have attracted attention and controversy as a possible cause of chronic complex illness.[29] Many investigators suggest that an intestinal overgrowth of *Candida albicans* (and other intestinal yeast) may be involved in several diseases, as listed in Table 9.5.

Although others have dismissed these claims as speculation, part of the problem is focusing on the terms "pathogen" and "commensal". It may be more accurate to use the terms "strong pathogen" and "weak pathogen". While it is obvious that yeasts are not strong pathogens, large amounts of weak pathogens are also a problem. A significant and surprising amount of peer-reviewed literature supports yeast as a weak pathogen.[36–38]

While the normal GI tract harbors small amounts of yeast, overgrowth may occur as a consequence of the wide use of antibiotics, corticosteroids, birth control pills and increased dietary carbohydrates.[39] Odds' text on *Candida* summarized more than 20 published studies which found that patients had a frequency of *C. albicans* in their feces more than twice as often as normal controls.[40] One study reported that chronic diarrhea and abdominal cramps may be caused by large numbers of dead or damaged yeast, as found in feces.[41] Other research indicates *Candida* as a cause of colitis in patients with AIDS, neoplastic disease and renal transplants.[42–44]

While the yeast pathogenicity debate continues, high-quality laboratory work is essential. Yeast may be observed directly via a microscope or indirectly through a culture. Both are necessary for proper analysis.

Dysbiosis

Dysbiosis is the state of disordered microbial ecology that causes disease. It may exist in the oral cavity, gastrointestinal tract or vaginal cavity. In dysbiosis, organisms of low intrinsic virulence, including bacteria, yeasts and protozoa, induce disease by altering the nutrition or immune responses of their host.[45] The major causes of intestinal dysbiosis are given in Table 9.6.

The concept of intestinal flora having a major impact on human health has increasingly gained support, particularly as the widespread use of antibiotics has been observed to disrupt the normal flora (Fig. 9.1 shows the microecology relationships). Published research has im-

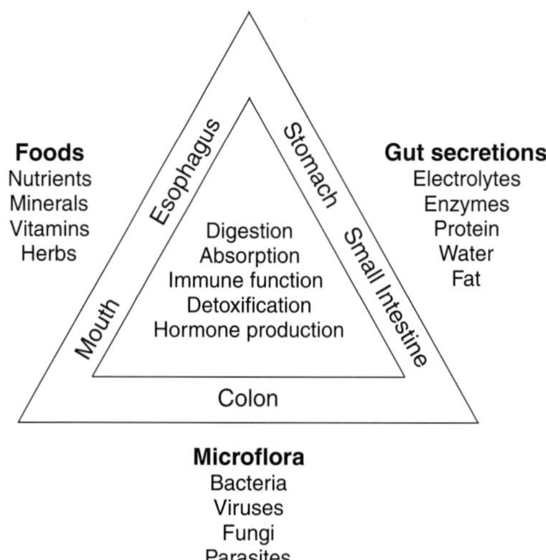

Figure 9.1 Microecology relationships.

Table 9.6 Major causes of intestinal dysbiosis[45–47]

- Poor diet/nutritional status (high fat, simple carbohydrates)
- Stress
- Antibiotic/drug therapy
- Decreased immune status
- Decreased gut motility
- Maldigestion
- Intestinal infection
- Presence of xenobiotics
- Increased intestinal pH

plicated intestinal dysbiosis as contributing to vitamin B_{12} deficiency, steatorrhea, irritable bowel syndrome, inflammatory bowel disease, autoimmune arthropathies, colon and breast cancer, psoriasis, eczema, cystic acne and chronic fatigue.[48–53]

GI tract and arthritis

Researchers increasingly acknowledge that there is a link between digestive processes and arthritis. In patients with altered bowel anatomy, chronic bacterial overgrowth can lead to the formation of circulating immune complexes and synovitis.[54] Changes in bowel permeability due to local gut inflammation may expose the host immune system to microbial or food antigens and even bacterial translocation.[55,56] In some cases, toxins derived from enteric organisms (e.g. *Clostridium difficile*) may play a direct role in the induction of arthritis.

Food allergy

Food allergy is a well-documented problem, although its prevalence, testing methods and treatment modalities are controversial. Some researchers have proposed that food allergy is not an immunological disease but a disorder of bacterial fermentation in the colon. The combined mechanisms of reduced gut enzyme concentrations, imbalanced bacterial flora and increased permeability may account for many cases of food intolerance.[57]

Four patterns of dysbiosis

Leo Galland MD has advanced the idea of four interlocking patterns of bacterial dysbiosis: putrefaction, fermentation excess, deficiency and sensitization.

Putrefaction

This is the Western degenerative disease pattern which results from diets high in fat and meat and low in insoluble fiber. This type of diet produces increased concentrations of *Bacteroides* sp. and induces bacterial urease and beta-glucuronidase activity. These enzymes may then metabolize bile acids to tumor promoters and deconjugate excreted estrogens, raising the plasma estrogen level. The fecal pH may increase as a result of increased ammonia production.

Epidemiologic data implicates this type of dysbiosis in the pathogenesis of colon cancer and breast cancer. It is usually corrected by decreasing dietary fat and animal flesh, increasing fiber consumption and consuming probiotic preparations.

Fermentation excess

This is a condition of carbohydrate intolerance induced by an excess of normal bacterial fermentation usually resulting from small bowel or fecal bacterial overgrowth. Abdominal distention, flatulence, diarrhea, constipation and feelings of malaise are commonly described. In small bowel bacterial overgrowth, degradation of intestinal brush-border and pancreatic enzymes by bacterial proteases may cause maldigestion.

Fecal short-chain fatty acids may be elevated. Patients with fermentation excess are usually intolerant of fiber supplements and often benefit from a reduction of carbohydrate consumption and antimicrobials.

Deficiency

Exposure to antibiotics or a diet depleted of soluble fiber may create a deficiency of normal fecal flora, including *Bifidobacteria*, *Lactobacillus* sp., and *E. coli*. Direct evidence of this condition is seen in stool cultures when concentrations of any of these organisms are reduced. This condition has been described in patients with irritable bowel syndrome and food intolerance.

Deficiency and putrefaction dysbiosis often occur together and respond to the same treatment. Probiotic supplementation as well as fructo-oligosaccharides are often helpful in re-establishing a normal flora.

Sensitization

Abnormal immune responses to components of the normal indigenous intestinal microflora may contribute to the pathogenesis of inflammatory bowel disease, spondyloarthropathies, and other connective tissue diseases or skin disorders such as psoriasis or acne. Endotoxins may activate the alternative complement pathway and sensitization may complement fermentation excess. Similar treatments may benefit both conditions.

THE CDSA MARKERS

The comprehensive digestive stool analysis provides diagnostic tools for analysis of digestion, colonic environment and absorption.

Digestion

The Great Smokies Diagnostic Laboratory (GSDL) has developed unique detergent extraction and enzymatic analysis procedures that allow quantitative, precise, and accurate measurements of digestion efficacy.[58,59] These methods give physicians the tools for differential diagnosis of digestive conditions as they relate to acute and chronic illness.

Triglycerides

Triglycerides are the major dietary fat component. Elevated fecal amounts reflect incomplete fat hydrolysis and suggest pancreatic insufficiency.

Chymotrypsin

Fecal chymotrypsin is a sensitive, specific measure of proteolytic enzyme activity.[60,61] Decreased values suggest diminished pancreatic output (pancreatic insufficiency), hypoacidity of the stomach, or cystic fibrosis. Elevated chymotrypsin values suggest rapid transit time, or, less likely, a large output of chymotrypsin from the pancreas.

Iso-butyrate, iso-valerate and n-valerate

New research suggests that these short-chain fatty acids (SCFAs) can be produced through bacterial fermentation of protein, thus reflecting the presence of undigested protein in the bowel. In a healthy colon, these SCFAs constitute less than 10% of the total concentrations of SCFAs due to the sparse amounts of polypeptides present in the large intestine compared with undigestible carbohydrates. However, an increase in the load of protein in the colon will alter these concentrations. Causes may include pancreatic insufficiency (insufficient proteases), malabsorption or gastrointestinal disease, leading to mucosal desquamation.[62]

Meat and vegetable fibers

These are microscopic, qualitative, indirect indicators of maldigestion from either gastric hypoacidity or diminished pancreatic output. Several studies report that fecal meat fibers were equal to other methods for non-specific maldigestion.[60,63,64] One study reported a correlation between excessive fecal meat fibers and hypochlorhydria or achlorhydria as measured by direct radiotelemetry.[65]

Absorption

Total fecal fat

This parameter is the sum of all the lipids except short-chain fatty acids. Elevation can be indicative of maldigestion or malabsorption. Elevated long-chain fatty acid levels may reflect malabsorption, and elevated triglyceride levels reflect maldigestion.

Long-chain fatty acids

These free fatty acids are readily absorbed by healthy mucosa. In cases of malabsorption, however, they accumulate and reach substantially elevated levels in the feces. Elevation can also indicate pancreatic insufficiency.

Cholesterol

Fecal cholesterol comes from both dietary sources and mucosal epithelial cell breakdown. Some of this cholesterol is absorbed, stored and used by the body, but some is excreted. The fecal cholesterol level remains surprisingly constant during fluctuating exogenous intake. An elevated cholesterol level in feces is abnormal and may reflect mucosal malabsorption.

Total short-chain fatty acids

A special property of colonic bacteria is their fermentation of soluble fibers to short-chain fatty acids (acetate, propionate, butyrate and valerate).[66] These molecules are normally readily absorbed so that fecal levels reflect a balance between production and absorption. SCFAs provide up to 70% of the energy for colonic epithelial cells.[67] SCFA production may be an important factor in establishing and maintaining a balanced ecosystem in the colon and may prevent establishment of pathogenic microbes such as *Salmonella* and *Shigella* spp. One interesting report suggests that diversion colitis might be successfully treated with rectal irrigations of SCFAs.[68] Elevated levels of the four main SCFAs may reflect colonic malabsorption or bacterial overgrowth. Elevated levels are also found in active colitis.[69] Decreased levels may reflect insufficient dietary fiber or disruption of the normal colonic flora.

Microbiology

Beneficial bacteria

Healthy amounts of *Lactobacilli*, *Bifidobacteria* and *E. coli* are essential to the maintenance of a healthy colon. *Lactobacilli* and *Bifidobacteria* spp., in particular, have long been noted for their contributions to intestinal health – from the inhibition of gut pathogens and carcinogens, control of intestinal pH and the reduction of cholesterol to the synthesis of vitamins and disaccharidase enzymes.

In a healthy gut, these organisms make up a substantial portion of the 400-plus species of bacteria; *Bifidobacteria* alone comprises up to one-quarter of the total flora in a healthy adult. Reduced numbers of these organisms, resulting from the use of broad-spectrum antibiotics, chronic maldigestion or bacterial overgrowth, leave the intestine susceptible to invasion by pathogens and production of carcinogens. Low levels may indicate the need to supplement with "friendly bacteria" to restore these important properties. While *E. coli* do not share some of these direct beneficial effects, clinical observation suggests that ample amounts of these organisms are present in healthy intestines.[70]

Additional bacteria

Bacteriology cultures quantitate normal flora (*Lactobacilli*, *Bifidobacteria*, *E. coli* and other frequently isolated organisms), imbalanced flora and potential pathogens. Serotyping for toxigenic *E. coli* and *Campylobacter* cultures is performed on diarrhetic specimens (see Tables 9.7 and 9.8).

Mycology

The CDSA includes a mycology culture that identifies and quantitates fecal yeast. Some of the more commonly identified species are *C. albicans*, *C. tropicalis*, *Rhodotorula* and *Geotrichum*. Broth dilution sensitivity analyses are performed on all yeast cultures of 2+ or greater, utilizing both pharmaceutical and natural substances. Quantitative MIC analysis determines the relative potency of differing antimycotic agents. This provides more information on the effective agents and dosages for each yeast.

Table 9.7 Common potential pathogens

- *Aeromonas*
- *Bacillus cereus*
- *Campylobacter*
- *Citrobacter*
- *Klebsiella*
- *Proteus*
- *Pseudomonas*
- *Salmonella*
- *Shigella*
- *Staphylococcus aureus*
- *Vibrio*

Table 9.8 Common imbalanced flora

- Beta-hemolytic streptococcus
- *Enterobacter*
- *Hafnia alvei*
- Hemolytic *E. coli*
- Mucoid *E. coli*

Metabolic markers

n-Butyrate

Butyric acid is a key SCFA because it is the main energy source for colonic epithelial cells. Adequate amounts are necessary for healthy metabolism of the colonic mucosa. A possible mechanism for the anticancer action of dietary fiber is the increased fermentation of fiber to butyrate. It has been suggested that failure to use butyric acid by colonic mucosal cells or inadequate amounts available in the colon could be a primary factor in the etiology of ulcerative colitis, inflammatory bowel disease and colon cancer.[66,71,72]

Beta-glucuronidase

Beta-glucuronidase is a bacterial enzyme, the activity of which serves as a valuable marker of cancer risk. This enzyme is elaborated by several microorganisms, including *E. coli*, *Bacteroides* and *Clostridium*. Via the uncoupling of glucuronides (compounds detoxified through the hepatic glucuronidation pathway), this enzyme catalyzes reactions which may result in the formation of carcinogens in the bowel as well as the persistence of certain hormones and drugs in the body. Thus, excess beta-glucuronidase activity correlates with increased cancer risk, including estrogen-related cancers through the enhanced enterohepatic recirculation of estrogen in the body. The activity of this enzyme is strongly influenced by diet, levels of *Lactobacilli* and *Bifidobacteria*, intestinal pH and nutrients such as calcium glucarate.[73–76]

pH

Fecal pH appears to be an indicator of the health or status of the colonic digestive processes. Abnormally acidic or alkaline pH usually reflects an abnormality in either acid production or absorption. There is increasing evidence that fecal pH is a useful indicator of risk for colon cancer.[77–79] There appears to be a correlation between alkaline pH and decreased short-chain fatty acids (particularly butyrate).[80] Elevated fecal pH and diminished SCFAs suggest inadequate digestion of fiber and/or inadequate intake of dietary fiber.

Short-chain fatty acid distribution

Adequate amounts and proportions of the different

SCFAs reflect the basic status of intestinal metabolism. The ratios of the individual SCFAs remain relatively constant in healthy colons, but become imbalanced in various disease states. Imbalanced ratios of the SCFAs reflect imbalanced metabolic processes due to disordered bowel flora. Researchers are beginning to identify unique SCFA "fingerprints" with specific bacterial infections.[71] The ratio among SCFAs has diagnostic value as a screening test for intestinal infections.[72] A significantly higher ratio of acetate/total SCFAs and a lower ratio of butyrate/total SCFAs have been found in the feces of patients with large bowel adenomas and cancer compared with control groups.[71]

Immunology

Fecal sIgA

Secretory IgA, derived from lymphoid tissue within the intestinal mucosa, acts as the first line of immunological defense against microbes and antigens in the GI tract. SIgA works by binding with pathogenic microorganisms, allergenic food proteins and carcinogens to form immune complexes which prevent them from binding to the surface of absorptive cells.

SIgA has been demonstrated to prevent the adhesion of *Vibrio cholerae* to mucosal epithelium, to neutralize cholera toxin and polio virus, and to reduce the absorption of ovalbumin and other allergenic food proteins. In patients with selective IgA deficiency, high titers of antibodies against food antigens can be detected. Depressed sIgA has also been observed in healthy, asymptomatic individuals, presumably from high antigenic exposure. Over time, this decreased resistance can lead to dysbiosis and increased risk for infection and allergy.[81–85]

Macroscopic observations

The color of feces provides important insight into various conditions, as listed in Table 9.9.

Table 9.9 Clinical interpretation of fecal color

Color	Probable significance
Light brown to brown	Normal
Yellow or green	Diarrhea or a bowel sterilized by antibiotics
Black	Upper GI tract bleeding
Tan or gray	Blockage of the common bile duct, pancreatic insufficiency (greasy stool) or steatorrhea
Red	Beets in diet; lower tract bleeding

The presence of mucus or pus can indicate irritable bowel syndrome, intestinal wall inflammation (caused by infection – typhoid, *Shigella* or amoebic), diverticulitis or other intestinal abscess. Absence of mucus and pus is normal.

The CDSA also includes an occult blood test. Although a positive result might be due to hemorrhoids or eating too much red meat, occult blood is a possible indicator of colon cancer. Follow-up is recommended, perhaps a second test using a meat-free diet or a sigmoidoscopic exam.

Dysbiosis index

Intestinal dysbiosis is marked by many indicators. Relevant results are weighed and an index is calculated to provide a quick assessment of the patient's GI tract. Factors used to determine the index include metabolic and microbiological markers.

SUMMARY

The CDSA's battery of integrated tests evaluates digestion, colonic environment, and absorption. It enables therapeutic intervention based not only on single test results, but also on patterns and relationships. The CDSA provides clinical insights not available with other diagnostic procedures, insights not limited to the gastrointestinal system. According to Mitch Kaminski MD: "More than 50% of the immune system takes its signals from the gut. Immune modulation, the cytokines, commonly produce oxidative stress. Free radicals cause aging and chromosomal damage associated with cancers."

REFERENCES

1. Drossman DA, Li Z, Andruzzi E, Temple RD, Talley NJ, Thompson WG et al. U.S. householder survey of functional GI disorders: prevalence, sociodemography and health impact. Dig Dis Sci 1993; 38: 1569–1580
2. Roberts S. Systems of life. Nursing Times 1991; 87: 45
3. Valdez IH, Fox PC. Interactions of the salivary and gastrointestinal systems. Dig Dis 1991; 9: 125–132
4. Davenport HW. A digest of digestion. 2nd edn. Chicago: Year Book Medical Publishers. 1978
5. Caspary WF. Physiology and pathophysiology of intestinal absorption. Am J Clin Nutr 1992; 55: 299S–308S
6. Heizer WD. Normal and abnormal intestinal absorption by humans. In: Schiller CM, ed. Intestinal toxicology. New York: Raven. 1984
7. Trier JS. Intestinal malabsorption: differentiation of cause. Hospital Practice 1988; May 15: 195–211
8. Cooke WT, Holmes GKT. Coelic disease. Edinburgh: Churchill Livingstone. 1984: p 130–143
9. Wright JV. Healing with nutrition. Emmaus, PA: Rodale Press. 1985
10. Rappaport, EM. Achlorhydria: associated symptoms and response to hydrochloric acid. New Eng J Med 1955; 25: 802–805
11. Howitz J, Schwartz M. Vitiligo, achlorhydria, and pernicious anaemia. Lancet 1971; June 26: 1331–1334
12. Bray GW. The hypochlorhydria of asthma in children. Br Med J 1930; 588–590

13. Hosking DJ, Moody F, Stewart IM, Atkinson M. Vagal impairment of gastric secretion in diabetic autonomic neuropathy. Br Med J 1975; June 14: 588–590
14. Rabinowitch IM. Achlorhydria and its clinical significance in diabetes mellitus. Am J Dig Dis 1949; 18: 322–333
15. Capper WM, Butler TJ, Kilby JO, Gibson MJ. Gallstones, gastric secretion, and flatulent dyspepsia. Lancet 1967; Feb 25: 413–415
16. Rawls WB, Ancona VC. Chronic urticaria associated with hypochlorhydria or achlorhydria. Rev Gastroenterol 1950; Oct: 267–271
17. Giannella RA, Broitman SA, Zamcheck N. Influence of gastric acidity on bacterial and parasitic enteric infections: a perspective. Ann Int Med 1973 78: 271–276
18. De Witt TJ, Geerdink PJ, Lamers CB, Boerbooms AM, van der Korst JK. Hypochlorhydria and hypergastrinaemia in rheumatoid arthritis. Ann Rheum Dis 1979; 38: 14–17
19. Ryle JA, Barber HW. Gastric analysis in acne rosacea. Lancet 1920; Dec 11: 1195–1196
20. Ayers S. Gastric secretion in psoriasis, eczemia and dermatitis herpetiformis. Arch Derm 1929; Jul: 854–859
21. Dotevall G, Walan A. Gastric secretion of acid and intrinsic factor in patients with hyper- and hypothyroidism. Acta Med Scand 1969; 186: 529–533
22. Vellas B, Bala D, Albarde JL. Effects of aging process on digestive functions. Comprehensive Therapy 1991; 17(8): 46–52
23. Rafsky HA, Weingarten M. The study of the gastric secretory response in the aged. Gastroenterol 1947; May: 348–352
24. Baker H, Frank O, Jaslow SP. Oral versus intramuscular vitamin supplementation for hypovitaminosis in the elderly. J Am Geriat Soc 1980; 48: 42–45
25. Russell RM. Changes in gastrointestinal function attributed to aging. Am J Clin Nutr 1992; 55: 1203S–1207S
26. Ebringer A, Khalafpour S, Wilson C. Rheumatoid arthritis and proteus: a possible aetiological association. Rheum Int 1989; 9: 223–228
27. Ebringer A, Cox NL, Abuljadayel I, Ghuloom M, Khalafpour S, Ptaszynska T et al. Klebsiella antibodies in ankylosing spondylitis and proteus antibodies in rheumatoid arthritis. Br J Rheum 1988; 27: 72–85
28. Robbins S, Cotran R. Pathologic basis of disease. 2nd edn. Philadelphia: WB Saunders. 1979
29. Crook WG. The yeast connection: a medical breakthrough. Jackson, TN: Professional Books. 1983
30. Romano TJ, Dobbins JW. Evaluation of the patient with suspected malabsorption. Gastroentero Clin N Am 1989; 18: 467–483
31. Palacios HJ. Hypersensitivity as a cause of dermatologic and vaginal moniliasis resistant to topical therapy. Ann Allergy 1976; 37: 110–113
32. Robinett RW. Asthma due to candida albicans. U Mi Med Ctr Bull 1968; 34: 12–15
33. Iwata K. A review of the literature on drunken symptoms due to yeasts in the gastrointestinal tract. In: Proceedings of the second international specialized symposium on yeasts. Tokyo: University of Tokyo Press. 1972: p 260–268
34. Truss CO. Tissue injury induced by candida albicans. Orthomol Psych 1977; 29: 17–37
35 Kudelko NM. Allergy in chronic monilial vaginitis. Ann Allergy 1971; 29: 266–267
36. Brabander JO, Blank F, Butas CA. Intestinal moniliasis in adults. Cand MAJ 1957; 77: 478–483
37. Bolivar R, Bodey GP. Candidiasis of the gastrointestinal tract. In: Bodey GP, Fainstein V, eds. Candidiasis. New York: Raven. 1985: p 181–201
38. Kane JG, Chretien JH, Garagusi VF. Diarrhea caused by candida. Lancet 1976; Feb 14: 335–336
39. Helstrom PB, Balish E. Effect of oral tetracycline, the microbial flora, and the athymic state on gastrointestinal colonization and infection of BALB/c mice with candida albicans. Infect and Immun 1979; 23: 764–774
40. Odds FC. Candida and candidosis: a review and bibliography. 2nd edn. London: Baillière Tindall. 1988
41. Caselli M, Trevisani L, Bighi S, Aleotti A, Balboni PG, Gaiani R et al. Dead fecal yeasts and chronic diarrhea. Digestion 1988; 41: 142–148
42. Eras P, Goldstein MJ, Sherlock P. Candida infection of the gastrointestinal tract. Medicine 1972; 51: 367–379
43. Stylianos S, Forde KA, Benvenisty AI, Hardy MA. Lower gastrointestinal hemorrhage in renal transplant recipients. Arch Surg 1988; 123: 739–744
44. Jayagopal S, Cervia JS. Colitis due to candida albicans in a patient with AIDS. Clin Inf Dis 1992; 15: 555
45. Haenl H, Bendig J. Intestinal flora in health and disease. Progress in Food and Nutr Sci 1975; 1: 21–64
46. Nord CE, Edlund C. Impact of antimicrobial agents on human intestinal microflora. J Chemotherapy 1990; 2: 218–237
47. Lizko NN. Stress and intestinal microflora. Die Nahrun 1987; 31: 443–447
48. Simon GL, Gorbach SL. The human intestinal flora. Dig Dis Sci 1986; 31: 147S–162S
49. Gorbach SL. Estrogens, breast cancer, and intestinal flora. Rev Infect Dis 1984; 6: S85–S90
50. Chung K-T, Fulk GE, Slein MW. Tryptophanase of fecal flora as a possible factor in the etiology of colon cancer. J Nat Cancer Inst 1975; 54: 1073–1078
51. Goldin BR. The metabolism of the intestinal microflora and its relationship to dietary fat, colon and breast cancer. Diet Fat and Cancer 1986; 655–685
52. Ionescu G, Kiehl R, Ona L, Schuler R. Abnormal fecal microflora and malabsorption phenomena in atopic eczema patients. J Advan Med 1990; 3: 71–89
53. Ionescu G, Kiehl R, Wichmann-Kunz F, Leimbeck R. Immunobiological significance of fungal and bacterial infections in atopic eczema. J Advan Med 1990; 3: 47–58
54. Inman RD. Antigens, the gastrointestinal tract, and arthritis. Rheum Dis Clin N Am (US) 1991; 17: 309–321
55. Wells CL, Jechorek RP, Gillingham KJ. Relative contributions of host and microbial factors in bacterial translocation. Arch Surg 1991; 126: 247–252
56. Husby S, Jensenius JC, Svehag SE. Passage of undegraded dietary antigen into the blood of healthy adults. Scand J Immunol 1985; 22: 83–92
57. Hunter JO. Food allergy or enterometabolic disorder? Lancet 1991; 338: 495–496
58. Crook T, Lee MJ, Noel C. Collection, extraction and enzyme assay methods for analysis of fecal fats [abstract]. American Association for Clinical Chemistry National Meeting; New Orleans, July 17–21, 1994
59. Lee MJ, Crook T, Noel C, Levinson U. Detergent extraction and enzymatic analysis for fecal long-chain fatty acids, triglycerides, and cholesterol. Clin Chem 1994; 40: 2230–2234
60. Lankisch PG. Exocrine pancreatic function tests. Gut 1982; 23: 777–798
61. Bode C, Bode JC. Usefulness of a simple photometric determination of chymotrypsin activity in stools: results of a multicentre study. Clin Biochem 1986; 19: 333–337
62. Rasmussen HS, Holtug K, Mortensen PB. Degradation of amino acids to short-chain fatty acids in humans: an in vitro study. Scand J Gastroenterol 1988; 23: 178–182
63. Arvanitakis C, Cooke AR. Diagnostic tests of exocrine pancreatic function and disease. Gastroenterol 1978; 74: 932–948
64. Moore JG, Englert E, Bigler AH, Clark RW. Simple fecal tests of absorption: a prospective study and critique. Am J Dig Dis 1971; 16: 97–105
65. Laird J, Barrie S. Presentation, American College for Advancement of Medicine. Fall. 1986
66. Royall D, Wolever TMS, Jeejeebhoy KN. Clinical significance of colonic fermentation. Am J Gastroenterol 1990; 85: 1307–1312
67. Araneo BA, Cebra JJ, Beuth J et al. Problems and priorities for controlling opportunistic pathogens with new antimicrobial strategies; an overview of current literature. Zentralbl Bakteriol 1996; 283: 431–465
68. Roediger WEW. The starved colon: diminished mucosal nutrition, diminished absorption, and colitis. Dis Col & Rect 1990; 33: 858–862
69. Roediger WEW, Heyworth M, Willoughby P, Piris J, Moore A, Truelove SC. Luminal ions and short chain fatty acids as markers of functional activity of the mucosa in ulcerative colitis. J Clin Pathol 1982; 35: 323–326

70. Modler HW, McKellar RC, Yaguchi M. Bifidobacteria and bifidogenic factors. J Inst Can Sci Technol Ailment 1990; 23: 29–41
71. Latella G, Caprilli R. Metabolism of large bowel mucosa in health and disease. Int J Colorect Dis 1991; 6: 127–132
72. Høverstad T. The normal microflora and short-chain fatty acids. In: Grubb R, Midtvedt T, Norin E, eds. The regulatory and protective role of the normal microflora. Proceedings of the fifth Bengt E. Gustafsson Symposium, Wenner-Gren Center, Stockholm, Sweden, 1–4 June 1988. Wenner-Gren International Symposium Series, Vol. 52. New York, NY: Stockton Press. 1989: p 89–108
73. Cummings JH, Macfarlane GT. Role of intestinal bacteria in nutrient metabolism. J Parenter Enteral Nutr 1997; 21: 357–365
74. Dwivedi C, Heck WJ, Downie AA, Larroya S, Webb TE. Effect of calcium glucarate on α-glucuronidase activity and glucarate content of certain vegetables and fruits. Biochem Med and Metabolic Bio 1990; 3: 83–92
75. Ling WH, Korpela R, Mykkanen H et al. Lactobacillus strain gg supplementation decreases colonic hydrolytic and reductive enzyme activities in healthy female adults. J Nutr 1994; 124: 18–23
76. Mallett AK, Bearne CA, Rowland IR. The influence of incubation pH on the activity of rat and human gut flora enzymes. J Appl Bacteriol 1988; 66: 433–437
77. Walker ARP, Walker BF, Walker AJ. Faecal pH, dietary fibre intake, and proneness to colon cancer in four South African populations. Br J Cancer 1986; 53: 489–495
78. Newmark HL, Lupton JR. Determinants and consequences of colonic luminal pH: implications for colon cancer. Nutr Cancer 1990; 14: 161–173
79. Malhotra SL. Faecal urobilinogen levels and pH of stools in population groups with different incidence of cancer of the colon, and their possible role in its aetiology. J Royal Soc of Med 1982; 75: 709–714
80. Lee MJ, Barrie S. Relationship between butyrate, pH, and microbial flora in stool samples. SOMED Sixteenth Internation Congress on Microbial Ecology and Disease; Mountain Lake, VA, September 1991
81. Buts JP, Bernasconi P, Vaerman J-P, Dive C. Stimulation of secretory IgA and secretory component of immunoglobulins in small intestine of rats treated with saccharomyces boulardii. Dig Dis and Sci 1990; 35: 251–256
82. Cash RA, Music SI, Libonati JP et al. Response of man to infection with Vibrio cholera. II. Protection from illness afforded by previous disease and vaccine. J Infect Dis 1974; 130: 325–333
83. Pierce NF, Cray WC, Jr, Engel PF. Antitoxic immunity to cholera in dogs immunized orally with cholera toxin. Infect and Immun 1980; 27: 632–637
84. Ogra PL, Karzon DT. Distribution of poliovirus antibody in serum, nasopharynx and alimentary tract following segmental immunization of lower alimentary tract with poliovaccine. J Immun 1969; 102: 1423–1430
85. Cunningham-Rundles C. Analysis of the gastrointestinal secretory immune barrier in IgA deficiency. Ann Allergy 1986; 57: 31–35

CHAPTER CONTENTS

10

ELISA/ACT test

Patrick M. Donovan, ND

INTRODUCTION

Antigens from the enteric environment are among the most common and constant challenges to our immune defense and repair systems, and hence to overall health and vitality.[1–5] Challenges can be from enteric organisms and seemingly innocuous, commonly encountered substances such as foods, chemicals, and microbial toxins (endo- and exotoxins). Maldigestion and increased intestinal permeability increase such exposure.[6–41]

The adaptive mechanisms for human immune defense and repair can be overwhelmed by these reactive substances. This enhances susceptibility to both infectious disease and hypersensitivity reactions. Clinically important immune overload dysfunction can then occur and present as recurrent infections, multisystem chronic inflammation, and/or autoimmune syndromes.[36–49]

Identifying the commonly encountered substances (foods, food additives, soaps, detergents, environmental chemicals, and pharmaceuticals) that cause delayed hypersensitivity reactions in an individual is often clinically challenging due to the time-delayed or late-phase reactions they elicit. The individual may slowly adapt to the impaired function and reduced performance caused by daily onslaught of reactive substances without being fully aware of the tax on his/her inner economy.[41] The identification of these reactive substances and their mitigation or elimination is the first step in preventing or correcting immune overload dysfunction and chronic inflammatory, degenerative or autoimmune diseases. A comprehensive, and clinically useful test for identifying such foreign reactants is the enzyme-linked immunosorbant assay.[50–52]

Reducing immunologic load allows an individual's physical economy to move from a state of "red alert" and hyperactivity to one of balance, regeneration, and repair. This shift is essential to the restoration of health.

REACTANTS AND THE IMMUNE RESPONSE

Chemical reactants are usually antigens, i.e. compounds that induce an immune response. The criteria are that the reactant be:[1–4]

- identified by the host organism as foreign
- of large enough molecular weight to be detected by the immune system
- of sufficient chemical complexity to induce a reaction.

Foreignness. Generally, the immune system does not respond to the body's own normal tissues (i.e. self-antigens), but it does respond to those antigenic compounds identified by the body as non-self or foreign. Autoimmune conditions are the exception where normally sequestered self-antigens are exposed to the immune system and treated as foreign. This is usually due to tissue damage significant enough to breach normal compartmentalization, decreased tissue repair, and increased tissue permeability which exposes antigens normally restricted from the circulation in states of health.

High molecular weight. A compound must have a certain molecular size to be antigenic. Low molecular weight compounds, such as many drugs and chemicals, can only be antigenic when they bind with a high molecular weight carrier such as a protein (haptenization).

Chemical complexity. There also must be a certain degree of structural and chemical complexity for a compound to be antigenic.

Classes of antigens

There are four major classes of antigens:

- polysaccharides
- lipids
- nucleic acids
- proteins.

These four are usually combined in reactive antigens, e.g. lipopolysaccharides, glycopeptides, nucleoproteins, etc.

Polysaccharides are part of more complex molecules found on the surface of most animal and human cells. They are also a major constituent in the cell walls of plants and microorganisms. Lipids are not antigenic of themselves. They are only antigenic when combined with other molecules such as polysaccharides, forming lipopolysaccharides (LPS). Lipopolysaccharides are products of many bacterial (endotoxins), fungal, and plant cell walls which can activate the immune system. Nucleic acids are also usually not themselves antigenic, but can become so when combined with protein carriers (histones). Proteins, especially glycopeptides, are the most antigenic of all compounds; virtually any protein can induce an immune response given the appropriate circumstances.

When an antigen enters the body, the healthy immune system is stimulated to respond. White blood cells such as macrophages, neutrophils, eosinophils, basophils, and lymphocytes, e.g. helper or natural killer (NK) cells, respond by phagocytosing and processing the antigen. Proinflammatory compounds and immunostimulating chemicals (interferons, interleukins, cytokines, and other growth factors and cellular modulators) play essential roles in modulating the immune response. Antibodies are produced from activated B-class lymphocytes which attack/bind to the antigen and stimulate complement amplification of the response. Immune complexes occur when humoral response exceeds cellular processing capacity. The reticuloendothelial system (RES), especially the Kuppfer cells of the liver, is responsible for removing immune complexes or cells with bound/absorbed immune complexes from the circulation.[1–4]

Hypersensitivity reactions

An amplified immune response to an antigen can occur, resulting in hypersensitivity reactions.[1–5,25,31,34,41,49] In a hypersensitive reaction or condition, the normally beneficial immune response becomes inappropriately over-responsive to normally innocuous, commonly encountered antigens, causing inflammation and tissue damage through the release of proinflammatory compounds. This can cause acute crises or lead to chronic allergies, asthma, autoimmune and inflammatory diseases, as well as other "environmentally sensitive" conditions. These reactions are increasingly common in the industrialized world where chemical dependence, environmental pollution, restructured diet patterns, and habitual distress are endemic.[5,28,34,37,39–41,48–49]

There are four basic types of hypersensitivity (allergic) responses (defined by Gel & Coombs in the 1960s). These responses are mediated by the release of proinflammatory compounds induced either by an antigen–antibody, cell-cytotoxic, or T-cell-mediated response. Delayed-type reactions (types II–IV) are not as easily identified clinically nor as closely linked to disease conditions due to their delayed nature and the variety and chronicity of the symptoms they cause. Type I reactions are typically readily identified as the reactions are immediate.

Type I: immediate hypersensitivity or immediate

This reaction is mediated by immunoglobulin E (IgE) which binds to the antigen and causes the release of pharmacologically active amines and cytokine compounds, most notably histamine. The classic allergic reaction of itchy eyes, runny nose, swelling and edema, hives, and bronchoconstriction, or more severe responses such as asthmatic attacks and anaphylaxis, can occur. It happens immediately (within minutes) on exposure to the antigen and can be life-threatening.

Type II: antibody-dependent cytotoxic hypersensitivity

This reaction occurs when antibodies (IgA, IgG, or IgM) are provoked against cellular antigens (this can be an antigen on an individual's own cells) leading to cell/tissue destruction via the activation of immune cells and proinflammatory compounds. This delayed reaction may take hours or days to develop. ABO and Rh incompatibility reactions, drug-induced reactions (via haptenization with cellular and/or circulating blood proteins), and many autoimmune conditions are examples.

Type III: immune complex-mediated hypersensitivity

This reaction occurs when immune complexes are formed when antibodies (IgG, IgM, or IgA) and antigens coalesce. These complexes deposit in the tissues causing the release of immunologically active cells and proinflammatory chemicals that damage those tissues. This delayed reaction may take hours or days to develop. The classic Arthus reaction, serum sickness, and autoimmune/infection-associated immune complex diseases (rheumatoid arthritis, rheumatic fever, glomerulonephritis, etc.) are examples of this type of reaction.

Type IV: T-cell-mediated hypersensitivity

This reaction is mediated by T-cells which have been previously sensitized to a specific antigen. The T-cells release lymphokines (interleukins) which induce an inflammatory reaction. This type of reaction is seen in the TB skin test, contact dermatitis, and tissue or organ rejection reactions. The classic delayed reaction can take days to develop.

Cross-reactive, cytotoxic antibodies, and disease

An antibody-dependent cytotoxic reaction directed against self-antigens can be initiated and propagated by environmental antigens (viruses, bacteria, food protein, chemical, etc.), similar enough to self-antigens to stimulate crosss-reactive antibodies to self. When this occurs, chronic exposure to the environmental antigen can potentiate this self-directed immune response by provoking continual production of cross-reactive antibodies – hence, the possible relationship between environmental antigens and autoimmune diseases.[1–4,41,53–55]

Immune complex-mediated diseases

High levels of circulating immune complexes can result in their deposition in susceptible tissues. This deposition can damage these tissues and organs and result in:

- metabolic dysfunction
- inflammation
- pain
- swelling
- fibrosis
- exposure of normally sequestered self-proteins to immunological recognition
- release of free radical and acidic oxidative products.

Chronic antigen exposure and systemic antigen load resulting in a delayed hypersensitivity response and immune complex deposition can often lead to autoimmune and chronic diseases, accelerated aging, and organ dysfunction and failure, if not corrected.[1–4,56–61]

These diseases/pathologies can be placed broadly into three groups (see Table 10.1) according to the source of the antigen and the organs most frequently affected.[3]

Persistent infection

When a low-grade persistent infection occurs with a weak antibody response, chronic immune complex formation can result. These complexes may then deposit in various tissues, producing such conditions as endocarditis, hepatitis, glomerulonephritis, and arthritis.

Autoimmunity

Immune complex-mediated inflammatory disease is a frequent complication of autoimmune disease. Such autoimmune diseases include rheumatoid arthritis and

Table 10.1 Immune complex-mediated diseases

Cause	Antigen	Sites of complex deposition
Persistent infection	Microbial antigen	Infected organ(s), kidneys, joints, heart
Autoimmunity	Self-antigen	Kidneys, joints, arteries, muscles, brain, lungs, liver, skin, bowel, connective tissue
Extrinsic or exogenous source	Environmental antigen (food, drugs, chemicals, etc.)	Generally the same as for autoimmunity

Modified from Roit et al[2] (p. 21).

other inflammatory joint diseases, systemic lupus, polyarteritis, vasculitis, polymyositis, glomerulonephritis, multiple sclerosis, colitis, Crohn's, and many of the mixed connective tissue diseases.

Extrinsic or exogenous antigens

Environmental antigens are generally contacted by the skin and mucosal surfaces (inhaled or ingested) and form immune complexes either at the body surfaces or in the tissues after absorption. Such antigens may include chemicals, drugs, endotoxins, food proteins, and antigenic material from moulds, plants, or animals. Prolonged immune complex formation and the production of cross-reactive autoantibodies may occur from chronic daily exposure to reactive environmental antigens leading to overload of the reticuloendothelial system and tissue deposition.

INTESTINAL ANTIGENS AND TOXICANTS

The most common portals of entry for foreign antigens are the skin and mucosal surfaces of the genitourinary, respiratory, and gastrointestinal tracts. Of primary clinical importance is the gastrointestinal tract because of its constant contact with a plethora of dietary materials, proteins, chemicals, and bacteria.[1–4,6–10,27,32,34,36–39]

Observations by clinicians since the time of Hippocrates and reports in the current scientific literature document the role of the colon and bowel in the etiology and propagation of many diseases and pathological conditions. This is due to the local and systemic effects of bowel antigens ("toxicants") in different tissues and organs, often mediated through a delayed hyperreactive mechanism.[6,26,28–29,32,41,49,56–61]

There is a significant release of toxicants from the bowel into systemic circulation when:

- colon health is compromised in any way (infection, irritation, inflammation, or ulceration)
- the microfloral homeostatic environment is disturbed (dysbiosis) resulting in overgrowth of pathogenic organisms
- there exists a hospitable environment for parasitic infection
- putrefaction occurs as a result of prolonged fecal transit time (constipation)
- prolonged distress has compromised normal protective mechanisms such as secretory IgA.

This release results in immune activation, delayed hypersensitivity, inflammation, and host disposition to chronic disease.

Antigenic bowel toxicants include dietary macromolecules (undigested or partially digested food proteins and other by-products of incomplete digestion), various food additives and chemicals, and microbial toxicants (bacterial lipopolysaccharides).[6–10,13,19,32,34,36–39,54–56,58,62] The bowel is partially permeable to these toxicants and many, particularly food, macromolecules can traverse the normal intestine in sufficient quantities to exceed the lymphatic system's surveillance capacity, resulting in their immunological recognition as foreign invaders.[6–10,32,56,58,62] This recognition causes activation of the body's immune mechanisms, particularly the activation of lymphocytes, resulting in the production of antibodies (IgA, IgG, IgE, IgM), the formation of immune complexes, and delayed hypersensitive reactions.

Food antigens

Normally, the digestive process completely breaks down foods into their component amino acids, tiny peptides, glycerides, and saccharides. All too often, however, digestion is not complete. In fact, appreciable quantities of these digestion remnants can penetrate the normal intestinal mucosal barrier and enter systemic circulation, where they provoke immune response.[6–10,32,56,58,62] Individuals with allergic conditions, gastrointestinal disease, poor digestive functions (especially low hydrochloric acid activity in the stomach and pancreatic insufficiency), constipation, and diets high in refined foods can absorb significant amounts of these food antigens, with resultant delayed hypersensitivity reactions.

These reactions are becoming more common.[28] Some researchers claim that they are the leading cause of many undiagnosed symptoms, and that at least 60% of the American population suffers some degree of disability from associated symptoms. Diet-induced hypersensitivity reactions are associated with:[25–34,18–20,62–80]

- migraine headache
- eczema
- arthritis
- systemic lupus erythematosus
- inflammatory bowel disease
- gall bladder disease
- asthma
- irritable bowel syndrome
- childhood hyperactivity
- disturbances of behavior
- sinus congestion
- indigestion
- intestinal gas
- diarrhea / constipation
- general fatigue.

Primary protective mechanisms against systemic antigen overload from the bowel

Secretory immunoglobulin A (sIgA)

Secretory IgA is found primarily in bodily secretions

(saliva, tears, breast milk, and gastrointestinal and respiratory mucus). Secretory IgA acts as a major protective mechanism in these areas by neutralizing biologically active antigens such as viruses, bacteria, enzymes, and toxins. It binds antigens crossing the mucosal barrier and mediates their transport from portal circulation through the liver into the bile for elimination, thus limiting the immunological response.[81–84]

Any deficiency of sIgA, transient or chronic, either from decreased production (immunodeficiency) or from overwhelming the sIgA system by repeated antigen exposure, can cause an influx of bowel antigens into the portal circulation. This influx, if prolonged and sufficient, can overwhelm the second line of defense: the liver's phagocytosis of these substances. When this occurs, the toxins enter systemic circulation and initiate both immediate and delayed reactions, immune complex deposition, complement activation, inflammation, tissue damage, and disease.[85–88] The increased levels of antibodies to dietary antigens found in patients with IgA deficiency (which occurs in one of 600 individuals of European origin)[53] further support the importance of this class of immunoglobulin in limiting the absorption of food macromolecules.[88] It is important to note that sIgA deficiency is the most common primary immunodeficiency.

Liver

The liver plays a crucial role by filtering the portal circulation and preventing antigen and immune complex entrance into systemic circulation. The Kuppfer cells of the liver, with the help of sIgA, phagocytize, process, and eliminate these toxins in the bile. However, if the liver is compromised in any way, either from (1) inflammation (e.g. hepatitis), (2) fatty infiltration and degeneration (e.g. cirrhosis), (3) excessive alcohol consumption, (4) drugs, and/or (5) chronic toxin overload, then these bowel antigens will more readily enter systemic circulation and generate disease.[81–84,89]

IDENTIFYING THE ANTIGENIC TOXICANTS OF DELAYED HYPERSENSITIVITY

The classic way of testing for delayed reactions to food and other environmental antigens is by the subjective method of provocative challenge.[5,25,31,34] Exposure to the reactive substance (food, chemical, etc.) will elicit various signs and symptoms. Often, as in the case of foods, it is necessary to eliminate the suspicious substance from the individual's immediate environment for 4 or more days, keeping all other variables constant, before reintroducing it (challenge). When multiple foods and other substances are suspected (as is usually the case), this process can be time-consuming and painfully frustrating to both patient and doctor. In such a case, an objective laboratory test may be the best method; however, no "gold standard" test has been developed which consistently recognizes all delayed reactions.

The tests currently available for delayed hypersensitivity reactions include:

- *the modified radioallergosorbent test (RAST)* – a solid-phase radioimmunoassay classically used to detect IgE (type 1) reactions modified for IgG
- *the radioallergosorbent procedure (RASP)* – a variant of the RAST, this is also a solid-phase radioimmunoassay classically used to detect IgE (type I) reactions but thought to be more sensitive to IgG reactions than the classic RAST
- *the food immune-complex assay (FICA)* – a solid-phase radioimmunoassay specific for IgG allergens and immune complexes
- *the IgG ELISA* – a solid-phase, monoclonal antibody test for an IgG subclass (IgG_4) reaction utilizing the ELISA technique (see below)
- *the ELISA/ACT* – a modification of the ELISA method which combines enzyme amplification with lymphocyte blastogenesis.

Of these tests, the ELISA/ACT appears to be the only one capable of testing for all (types II–IV) delayed hypersensitive reactions (see Fig. 10.1).[4–5,25,31,34,50–52]

The ELISA method

The ELISA method of immunologic testing is a solid-phase immunoassay (as are radioimmunoassays such as the RAST) which employs an enzyme-linked reactant (classically an anti-immunoglobulin). Positive results are obtained when the enzyme is activated in the presence of a substrate producing a measurable color change. The intensity of the color change can also be read to determine the strength of reaction. According to Benjamini & Leskowski:[4]

> The ELISA method is rapidly replacing many assays in which a radioactive label is used because it is less expensive. Also, it does not require the special precautions for the handling of radioactivity, and it is, in general, just as sensitive.

ELISA/ACT

The ELISA/ACT is a modification of the ELISA method. It combines enzyme amplification with lymphocyte blastogenesis (instead of monoclonal or anti-antibody binding) in an autologous environment (whole plasma, as opposed to serum, with all the immunologic constituents intact and inducible) to test for all phases (types II–IV) of delayed reactivity (see Fig. 10.1).[50,51] It is, in a sense, an ex vivo window on the immune system which can provide an "immunologic fingerprint" of an

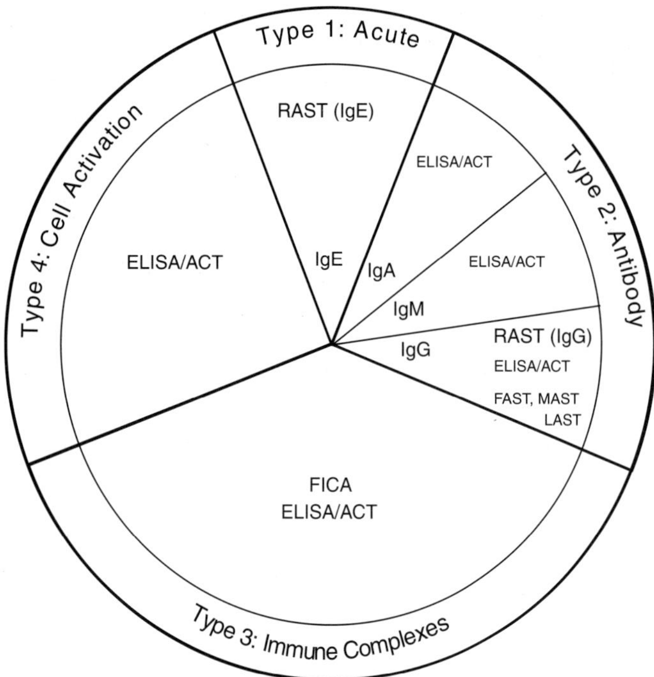

Figure 10.1 The immune response pie.

Table 10.2 ELISA/ACT categories tested

- Environmental chemicals
- Food preservatives
- Dairy products
- Fish/crustaceans/mollusks
- Fowl
- Fruit
- Grains
- Meat
- Oils
- Nuts/seeds
- Spices/seasoning
- Sugars
- Vegetables

individual's delayed reactivity via the pattern of reactivity to a large number of substances (see Tables 10.2 and 10.3). One of the key advantages of this procedure over other laboratory methods is its ability to measure IgG_4 antibodies. Although initially thought to act as a blocking antibody, thereby exerting protective effects against allergy, it now appears that IgG_4 antibodies are actually involved in producing allergic symptoms.[52]

As shown in Table 10.3, a positive result on the ELISA/ACT test (lymphocyte blastogenic reaction) can be due to one of four causes:

- immune recognition of a particular antigen specific to the compound tested
- immune recognition of a contaminant (such as a pesticide) not normally a constituent of the specific compound tested
- immune recognition contingent upon the presence of a specific hapten
- immune recognition of an identical epitope to another antigen.

While the common serum-based ELISA test, through several steps, builds up a molecular sandwich to improve the detection of small amounts of reactive substance, the ELISA/ACT is a one-step procedure taking unique advantage of the reactive cell surface on which enzymes become active when a substance is recognized as foreign. This reduction in steps contributes to greater precision.[50–52]

Table 10.3 Meaning of positive results

- Immune recognition
- Contaminant recognition
- Contingent recognition
- Cross-reaction to:
  —gut pathogen (identical epitope)
  —related food family (identical epitope)
  —patient's tissue (identical epitope)

Lymphocyte blastogenesis

Lymphocyte blastogenesis occurs during the early phase of all delayed hypersensitivity reactions. It represents lymphocyte activation from antigen/cytokine (see Table 10.4) stimulation where the lymphocytes are in a state of hyperactive metabolism resulting in a rapid increase in size and synthesis of DNA, RNA, and protein. By linking the enzyme reaction to lymphocyte blastogenesis (release of membrane-sequestered compound during the blastogenic reaction), the ELISA becomes an activated cell test (ACT) specific for all delayed responses.[52]

A blastogenic reaction can take place within hours as demonstrated by a change in the rate of protein formation. The measurement of such a reaction has traditionally taken up to 4–5 days using tests for thymidine and uptake of radiolabeled purine and pyrimidine. Because of a new technique, ELISA/ACT measures blastogenesis within hours, allowing for much quicker evaluation of sensitivity.[50–52]

Validity, reproducibility, sensitivity, and specificity

The classic way of determining the validity (the degree to which the results of a measurement correspond to

Table 10.4 Substances capable of eliciting a lymphocyte blastogenic response (positive result)

- Antigen
- Hapten
- Oxidant
- Lectin
- Other

the true state of the phenomenon being measured)[89] of a test is by comparing the observed measurement or results to some accepted, objective, physical standard (the "gold standard"). However, there is no such standard for determining delayed hypersensitivity reactions. Therefore, validity must be established by showing that the test results are predictive of or are directly related to clinically measurable or observable phenomena (signs and symptoms).[89]

To determine its validity (based on the predictive value of clinical phenomena), the ELISA/ACT was performed on a very refractory population: 81 patients suffering from an autoimmune or chronic viral syndrome for more than 5 years that had been progressive and had not responded more than briefly to any of several therapeutic interventions. Each patient filled out two symptom questionnaires (the Cornell Medical Index Questionnaire and a questionnaire prepared by Serammune Physicians' Laboratory) and rated the intensity of their primary symptoms on a scale of 1–100 prior to beginning the recommended ELISA/ACT program based on their test results. At 6–30 months after beginning the program, they again rated the intensity of their primary symptoms (these data are based on follow-up results regardless of how carefully the person followed the recommendations). The results showed a primary symptom intensity of 77.4 ± 14.5 before and 26.4 ± 18.2 after following the program ($P < 0.0001$), demonstrating a significant improvement (see Fig. 10.2).[90]

These results suggest a strong correlation between the reduction of symptom intensity and the elimination of the reactive foods and substances (as determined by the ELISA/ACT), and incorporation of the ELISA/ACT program, supporting the validity of the ELISA/ACT test and program.

During the 3 year development phase of the ELISA/ACT, two procedures were utilized to establish reliability (the extent to which repeated measurements of a relatively stable phenomenon fall closely to each other):[89]

1. In over 100 separate instances, multiple samples were taken at the same time, from the same subject, and analyzed with the technician blinded. Results replicated with $R > 0.999$ with only occasional differences where a strong reaction was read as an intermediate or a marginal intermediate was read as not reactive.
2. Many of the more than 3,000 different subjects tested were retested weekly, sometimes for months at a time. The results replicated with an $R = 0.998$.[91]

Determination of sensitivity (the proportion of positive reactions that are confirmed as truly positive – the greater the sensitivity, the fewer the false-positives)[89] and specificity (the proportion of negative reactions that are

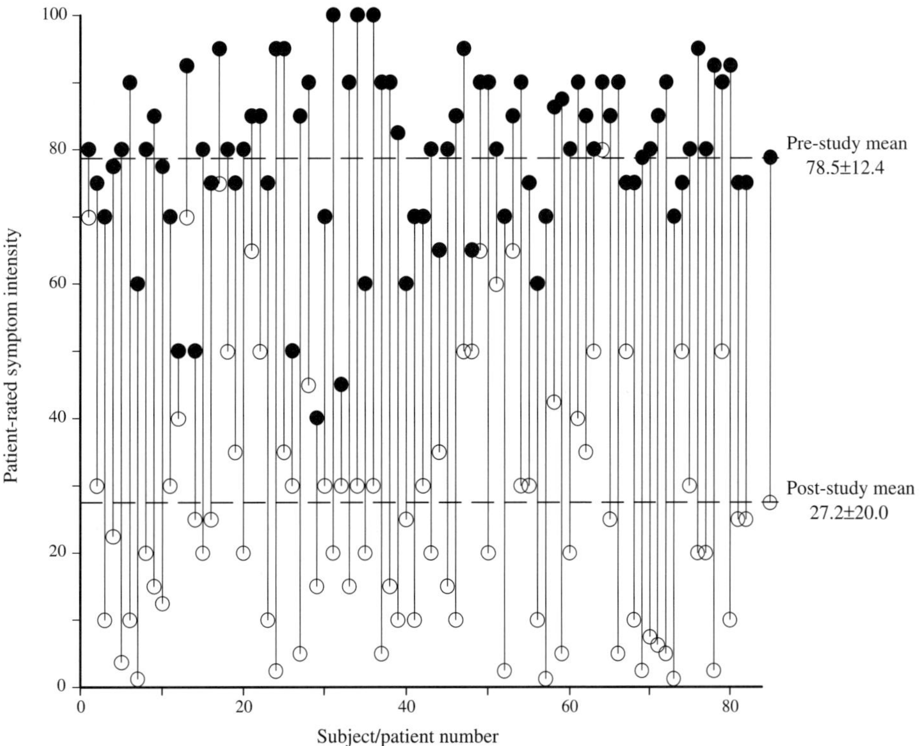

Figure 10.2 Response of autoimmune syndromes to ELISA/ACT – patient report (6–36 month follow-up)

Table 10.5 Measures to reduce error

Sources of error	Measures to reduce error
Glass contact	Sample drawn and shipped in plastic
Vacuum draw of sample	Sample drawn slowly using syringe
Tissue thromboplastin activated	Initial 3 ml of blood discarded
Heat	Sample refrigerated and shipped with ice pack
Leukopenia (<500 total WBC)	If suspected, must be checked for with CBC
Drugs (steroids, theophylline, anti-provided histamines, and all aspirin-containing compounds)	Detailed pre-test instructions

confirmed as truly negative – the greater the specificity, the fewer the false-negatives)[89] of a test like the ELISA/ACT is difficult. The physician is again faced with the lack of a "gold standard" to confirm a truly positive (induction of lymphocyte blastogenesis) or a truly negative (no induction of lymphocyte blastogenesis) result. At best, confirmation of such results can only be achieved by demonstrating the presence or absence of clinical signs and symptoms to the substances in question (provocative challenge test). However, reactivity to a substance does not always yield clinical signs and symptoms, so their elicitation may be due to a type 1 hypersensitivity reaction (not tested for with ELISA/ACT) or a psychologically programmed (dis-stress) response. Therefore, there are no clear-cut, confirming statistics available to determine the degree of sensitivity and specificity of the ELISA/ACT.

SUMMARY

The ELISA/ACT is a useful tool for the clinician in the treatment of autoimmune, chronic viral, and inflammatory conditions. It provides a comprehensive "immunologic fingerprint" of the substances to which a patient displays a delayed hypersensitivity reaction. After these substances are clearly identified, they can be eliminated from the patient's immediate environment, thereby reducing the immunologic stress and resultant pathology (immunologic disrepair, inflammation, and tissue destruction) induced by delayed hypersensitivity reactions.

Although the validity and sensitivity of the ELISA/ACT procedure must still be evaluated by other researchers, its theoretical premise and clinical relevancy for diagnosing late-phase hypersensitivities look very promising.

REFERENCES

1. Gel P, Coombs R, Lachman P, eds. Clinical aspects of immunology. Cambridge, MA: Blackwell. 1975
2. Barret J. Textbook of immunology. St Louis, MO: Mosby. 1983
3. Roit I, Brostoff J, Male D. Immunology. St Louis, MO: Mosby. 1986
4. Benjamini E, Leskowski S. Immunology: a short course. New York, NY: Alan Liss. 1988
5. Breneman J. Fundamentals of allergy. Springfield, IL: Thomas. 1984
6. Walker W. Transmucosal passage of antigens. In: Schmidt E, ed. Food allergy. New York, NY: Vevey/Raven Press. 1988
7. Mayron L. Portals of entry – a review. Ann Allergy 1978; 40: 399–405
8. Warshaw A, Bellini C, Walker W. The intestinal mucosal barrier to intact antigenic protein. Am J Surg 1977; 133: 55–58
9. Reinhardt M. Macromolecular absorption of food antigens in health and disease. Ann Allergy 1984; 53: 597
10. Editorial. Antigen absorption by the gut. Lancet 1978; ii: 715–717
11. Ecknaur R, Buck B, Breitig D. An experimental model for measuring intestinal permeability. Digestion 1983; 26: 24–32
12. Peled Y, Watz C, Gilat T. Measurement of intestinal permeability using 51Cr-EDTA. Am J Gastro 1985; 80: 770–773
13. Elia M, Behrens R, Northrop C et al. Evaluation of mannitol, lactulose, and 51Cr-EDTA as markers of intestinal permeability in man. Clin Sci 1987; 73: 197–204
14. Robinson G, Orrego H, Israel Y et al. Low-molecular weight polyethylene glycol as a probe of gastrointestinal permeability after alcohol ingestion. Dig Dis Sci 1981; 26: 971–977
15. Chadwick V, Phillips S, Hoffman A. Measurement of intestinal permeability using PEG 400. II Application to normal and abnormal permeability states in man and animals. Gastro 1977; 73: 247–251
16. Irving C, Lifschitz C, Marks L et al. Decreased intestinal permeability of Peg 400 polymers in children with mucosal damage. Gastro 1983; 84: 1195
17. Bjarnason I, Peters T. In vitro determination of small intestine permeability. Demonstration of a persistent defect in patients with coeliac disease. Gut 1984; 25: 145–150
18. Pearson A, Eastham L, Laker M et al. Intestinal permeability in children with Crohn's disease and coeliac disease. Br Med J 1982; 285: 20–21
19. Ukabam S, Clamp J, Cooper B. Abnormal small intestinal permeability to sugars in patients with Crohn's disease of the ileum and colon. Digestion 1983; 27: 70–74
20. Jachson P, Baker R, Lessof M et al. Intestinal permeability in patients with eczema and food allergy. Lancet 1981; i: 1285–1286
21. Kotler D, Gaetz H, Lange M et al. Enteropathy associated with the acquired immunodeficiency syndrome. Ann Int Med 1984; 101: 421–428
22. Chandra R, Jain VK. Intestinal infection and malnutrition initiate acquired immune deficiency syndrome (AIDS). Nutr Res 1984; 4: 537–543
23. Bjarnason I, Wise R, Peters T. The leaky gut of alcoholism: possible route of entry for toxic compounds. Lancet 1984; i: 179–182
24. Jenkins R, Rooney P, Jones D et al. Increased intestinal permeability in patients with rheumatoid arthritis: a side effect of oral nonsteroidal anti-inflammatory drug therapy? Br J Rheum 1987; 26: 103–107
25. Schmidt E, ed. Food allergy. New York: Vevey/Raven Press. 1988
26. Robertson D, Wright R. Food allergy and intolerance. Clin Gastro 1987; 1: 473–485
27. Buist R. The malfunctional "mucosal barrier" and food allergies. Int Clin Nutr Rev 1983; 3: 1–4

28. Buist R. Food intolerance – a growing phenomenon. Current concepts in development, manifestation and treatment. Int Clin Nutr Review 1986; 6: 1–10
29. Gerrard J. Food intolerance. Lancet 1984; ii: 413
30. Rinkel H. Food allergy. The role of food allergy in internal medicine. Ann Allergy 1944; 2: 504
31. Brostoff J, Challacombe S. Food allergy and intolerance. Philadelphia, PA: Baillière Tindall. 1987
32. Scadding G, Brostoff J. Immunological response to food. In: Hunter J, Jones V, eds. Food and the gut. England: Saunders. 1985
33. Trevino R. Food allergies and hypersensitivities. Ear Nose Throat 1988; 67: 42–49
34. Buist R. Food chemical sensitivity. New York, NY: Harper & Row. 1986
35. Mackaness G, Blanden R. Cellular immunity. Drug Allergy 1967; 11: 89
36. Lier H, Grune M. Progress in Liver Disease: endotoxins in liver disease. New York: Grune and Straten. 1979
37. Lappe M. When antibiotics fail: restoring the ecology of the body. Berkley, CA: North Atlantic Books. 1986
38. Lehner T. Candida infections. In: Gel P, Coombs R, Lachman P, eds. Clinical aspects of immunology. Cambridge, MA: Blackwell. 1975
39. Crook WG. The Yeast Connection. Jackson, TN: Professional Books. 1984
40. Buist R. Chronic fatigue syndrome and chemical overload. Int Clin Nutr Rev 1988; 8: 173–175
41. Jaffe R. Immune defense and repair system II. Clinical expression of impaired immune competence. In: Yanick P, Jaffe R, eds. Clinical chemistry and nutrition guidebook, vol. 1. Ariel, PA: T H Publishing. 1988
42. Cohen IR. The self, the world, and autoimmunity. Sci Amer 1988; 258: 52–60
43. Redfield R, Burke D. HIV infection: the clinical picture. Sci Amer 1988; 259: 90–99
44. Mazel S, Jaret P. In Self Defense. New York, NY: Harcourt, Brace & Jovanovich. 1985
45. Nilsson L. The body victorious: the illustrated story of our immune system and other defenses of the human body. New York, NY: Delcorte. 1987
46. O'Connor T, Gonzalez-Nunez A. Living with AIDS. San Francisco: Corwin. 1986
47. Sagan L. The health of the nations: the causes of sickness and well-being. New York, NY: Basic Books. 1987
48. Weissman J. Choose to live. New York, NY: Grove Press. 1988
49. Bell I. Clinical ecology. A new medical approach to environmental illness. Bolinas, CA: Common Knowledge Press. 1982
50. Jaffe R. Antigen detection (ELISA/ACT) immunology procedure. In: Yanick P, Jaffe R, eds. Clinical chemistry and nutrition guidebook, vol. 1. Ariel, PA: T H Publishing. 1988
51. Jaffe R. Health studies collegium information handbook. 10th edn. Reston, VA: Health Studies Collegium. 1989
52. AAAI Board of Directors. Measurement of specific and nonspecific IgG4 levels as diagnostic and prognostic tests for clinical allergy. J Allergy Clin Immunol 1995; 95: 652–654
53. Braunwald E, Isselbacher K, Petersdorf R et al, eds. Harrison's principles of internal medicine. 11th edn. New York, NY: McGraw-Hill. 1987: p 354, 364
54. Soderstrom T, Hansson G, Larson G. The Escherichia coli K1 capsule shares antigenic determinants with the human gangliosides GM3 and GD3. New Engl J Med 1984; 310: 726–727
55. Stephansson K, Dieperink M, Richman D et al. Sharing of antigenic determinants between the nicotinic acetylcholine receptor and proteins in *Escherichia coli*, *Proteus vulgaris*, and *Klebsiella pneumoniae*. New Engl J Med 1985; 312: 221–225
56. Paganelli R, Levinsky R, Atherton D. Detection of specific antigen within circulating immune complexes. Validation of the assay and its application to food antigen-antibody complexes formed in healthy and food-allergic subjects. Clin Exp Immunol 1981; 46: 44–53
57. Lawley T, Frank M. Immune-complex diseases. In: Braunwald E, Isselbacher K, Petersdorf R et al, eds. Harrison's principles of internal medicine. 11th edn. New York, NY: McGraw-Hill. 1987
58. Sancho J, Egido J, Rivera F, Hernando L. Immune complexes in IgA nephropathy: presence of antibodies against diet antigens and delayed clearance of specific polymeric IgA immune complexes. Clin Exp Immunol 1981; 45: 299–304
59. Hall R, Lawley T, Heck J, Katz S. IgA-containing circulating immune complexes in dermatitis herpetiformis, Henoch-Schonlein purpura, systemic lupus erythematosus and other diseases. Clin Exp Immunol 1980; 40: 431–437
60. Fiasse R, Lurhuma A, Cambiaso C et al. Circulating immune complexes and disease activity in Crohn's disease. Gut 1978; 19: 611–617
61. Levinsky R. The role of soluble immune complexes in disease. Arch Dis Child 1978; 53: 96–99
62. Egger J, Carter C, Wilson J et al. Is migraine food allergy? Lancet 1983; ii: 895–899
63. Monro J, Brostoff J, Carini C, Zilkha K. Food allergy in migraine. Lancet 1980; ii: 1–4
64. Buist R. Migraine and food intolerance. Int Clin Nutr Rev 1984; 4: 52–54
65. Price M. The role of diet in the management of atopic eczema. Human Nutr Applied Nutr 1984; 38A: 409–415
66. Finn RA. Serum IgG antibodies to gliadin and other dietary antigens in adults with atopic eczema. Clin Exp Dermatol 1985; 10: 222–228
67. Parke A, Hughes G. Rheumatoid arthritis and food. A case study. Br Med J 1981; 282: 2027–2029
68. Hicklin J, Mc Ewen L, Morgan J. The effect of diet in rheumatoid arthritis. Clin Allergy 1981; 47: 338–344
69. Panush RS, Stroud RM, Webster EM. Food-induced (allergic) arthritis. Inflammatory arthritis exacerbated by milk. Arth Rheum 1986; 29: 220–226
70. Reidenberg MM, Durant PJ, Harris RA et al. Systemic lupus erythematosus-like disease due to hydrazine. Am J Med 1983; 75: 365–370
71. Cooke H, Reading C. Dietary intervention in systemic lupus erythematosus. 4 cases of clinical remission and reversal of abnormal pathology. Int Clin Nutr Rev 1985; 5: 166–176
72. Workman E, Jones V, Wilson A et al. Diet in the management of Crohn's disease. Human Nutr Applied Nutr 1984; 38A: 469–473
73. Breneman JC. Allergy elimination diet as the most effective gallbladder diet. Ann Allergy 1968; 26: 83
74. Ficari A, De Muro P. Experimental studies on allergic cholecystitis. Gastroenterol 1946; 6: 302–314
75. Ogle K, Bullocks J. Children with allergic rhinitis and/or bronchial asthma treated with elimination diet: a five-year follow-up. Ann Allergy 1980; 44: 273–278
76. Jones V, McLaughlan P, Shuthouse M, Workman E. Food intolerance: a major factor in the pathogenesis of irritable bowel syndrome. Lancet 1982; ii: 1115–1117
77. Menzies IC. Disturbed children: the role of food and chemical sensitivities. Nutr Health 1984; 3: 39–54
78. Rapp DJ. Allergy and the hyperactive child. New York: Sovereign Books. 1979
79. O'Banion DR, Greenberg MR. Behavioral effects of food sensitivity. Int J Biosocial Res 1982; 3: 55–68
80. Speer F. The allergic-tension-fatigue syndrome in children. Int Arch Allergy Appl Immunol 1958; 12: 207–221
81. Brown TA, Russel MW, Mestecky J. Elimination of intestinally absorbed antigen into the bile by IgA. J Immunol 1984; 132: 780–782
82. Brown TA, Russel MW, Kulhavy R, Mestecky J. IgA-mediated elimination of antigens by the hepatobiliary route. Fed Proc 1983; 42: 3218–3221
83. Socken DJ, Simms ES, Smiley RE et al. Secretory component-dependent hepatic transport of IgA antibody-antigen complexes. J Immunol 1981; 127: 316
84. Russel MW, Brown TA, Claflin JL et al. Immunoglobulin A-mediated hepatobiliary transport constitutes a natural pathway for disposing of bacterial antigens. Infect Immunol 1983; 42: 1041–1048
85. Petty RE, Palmer NR, Cassidy JJ. The association of autoimmune disease and anti-IgA antibodies in patients with selective IgA deficiency. Clin Exp Immunol 1979; 37: 83–88

86. Ammann AJ, Hong R. Selective IgA deficiency: presentation of 30 cases and a review of the literature. Med 1971; 50: 223–236
87. Ammann AJ, Hong R. Selective IgA Deficiency and Autoimmunity. Clin Exp Immunol 1970; 7: 833–838
88. Rubenstein E, Federman DD. Scientific American medicine. New York, NY: Scientific American. 1991: p 6: II-6
89. Fletcher RH, Fletcher SW, Wagner EH. Clinical epidemiology. The essentials. 2nd edn. Baltimore: Williams & Wilkins. 1988
90. Jaffe R, Liers H. Improvement in immune performance: a 6–30 month follow-up of a cohort using the ELISA/ACT program. J Am Col Nutr 1989; 8: 424
91. Jaffe R. Accuracy and predictive value of ELISA/ACT test. Report from Serammune Physicians' Laboratory, Reston, VA. 1989

CHAPTER CONTENTS

11

Erythrocyte sedimentation rate

Michael T. Murray, ND

Joseph E. Pizzorno Jr, ND

INTRODUCTION

The erythrocyte sedimentation rate (ESR), the rate at which erythrocytes settle out of unclotted blood in one hour, has been one of the most widely performed laboratory tests for the past 50 years. Used primarily to detect occult processes and monitor inflammatory conditions, the ESR has undergone very little change since 1918, when Fahraeus discovered that erythrocytes of pregnant women sedimented in plasma more rapidly than they did in non-pregnant women. Since its incorporation into standard laboratory diagnosis, the ESR has been shrouded with medical myths and is often misinterpreted or misused. This chapter provides a rational guideline for its use as a non-specific measure of inflammatory, infectious, and neoplastic diseases.[1–3]

Normally, erythrocytes settle quite slowly, as the gravitational force of the erythrocyte's mass is counteracted by the buoyant force of the erythrocyte's volume. However, when erythrocytes aggregate, they sediment relatively rapidly because the proportional increase in their total mass exceeds the proportional increase in their volume.[1,2]

Therefore, the major determinant in the sedimentation rate of erythrocytes is erythrocyte aggregation, which usually occurs along a single axis (rouleaux formation). The aggregation of erythrocytes is largely determined by electrostatic forces. Under normal circumstances, the erythrocytes have a negative charge, and therefore repel each other. However, many plasma proteins are positively charged and neutralize the surface charge of erythrocytes, thereby reducing repulsive forces and promoting aggregation.[1–3]

The relative contribution of the various "acute-phase" reactant proteins to aggregation is shown in Table 11.1. One protein that has no direct effect on the ESR in physiological concentrations, but which is associated with certain inflammatory, degenerative, and neoplastic diseases, is the C-reactive protein. Its major function is

Table 11.1 Relative contribution of acute-phase reactant proteins to erythrocyte aggregation

Blood constituent	Relative contribution
Fibrinogen	10
Beta-globulin	5
Alpha-globulin	2
Albumin	1

facilitation of the complement system. Like the ESR, measurement of the C-reactive protein is used in the monitoring of patients with chronic inflammatory conditions.[1] An elevated C-reactive protein provides evidence of an inflammatory process despite a normal ESR. Therefore, when used in conjunction with the ESR, it greatly increases the sensitivity in detecting inflammatory/ infectious processes, especially when variables, such as anemia, confound the ESR.

The ESR will also be elevated in patients with proteinemias (myeloma, macroglobulinemia, cryoglobulinemia, and cold agglutinin disease).[1–3] Disorders of erythrocytes, such as anemias, alter the ESR and may interfere with accurate interpretation.[1–3] Since the ESR is directly proportional to the mass of the erythrocyte and inversely proportional to its surface area, large erythrocytes sediment more rapidly than smaller cells. Therefore, in macrocytic anemia there is an increased ESR, and in microcytic anemia there is a decreased ESR.

PROCEDURES

Various methods for determination of the ESR have been developed. Currently the Westegren method is recommended by the International Committee for Standardization in Hematology.

Westegren method

In the standard Westegren method, the following procedure is used:

1. Dilute venous blood 4:1 with anticoagulant sodium citrate.
2. Put in a 200 mm long, 2.5 mm internal diameter, glass tube (Westegren tube).
3. Allow to stand in a vertical position for 1 hour.
4. At the end of 1 hour, the distance from the meniscus to the top of the column of erythrocytes is recorded as the ESR.

The modified Westegren method uses edetic acid (EDTA) rather than sodium citrate as an anticoagulant and is more convenient, since the same tube of blood can be used for other hematological studies. The standard and modified methods give identical results.[1–3]

Wintrobe method

The second most commonly used method is the Wintrobe method. This method is performed with a 100 mm tube (Wintrobe tube) containing oxalate as the anticoagulant. It is more sensitive than the Westegren method in the "normal" to "mildly elevated" range; however, in the more highly elevated ESR, the short tube leads to relatively insensitive readings due to packing of cells.[2]

Results

- Westegren (normal results)
  —men: 0–10 mm/hour
  —women: 0–15 mm/hour
  —children: 0–10 mm/hour
- Wintrobe (normal results)
  —men: <6.5 mm/hour
  —women: <16 mm/hour.

INTERPRETATION

Several factors may result in false ESR values; the more significant of these are listed in Table 11.2. In addition, it is important to recognize that in acute disease, the change in rate may lag behind the temperature elevation and leukocytosis for 6–24 hours, and in *unruptured* acute appendicitis the rate may be normal. In convalescence, the increased rate tends to persist longer than the fever or leukocytosis. Table 11.3 lists the most common clinical implications of changes in the ESR.

Table 11.2 Factors interfering with the ESR[1,4]

False increase
- Elevated levels of fibrinogen, globulins, and cholesterol
- High room temperature
- Macrocytic anemia
- Menstruation
- Pregnancy
- Running a refrigerated blood sample before it has returned to room temperature
- Tilted ESR tube
- Certain drugs: dextran, methyldopa, methylsergide, OCA, penicillamine, procainamide, theophylline, trifluperidol, vitamin A

False decrease
- Cachexia
- Clotting of blood sample
- Elevated bile salts
- Elevated phospholipids
- Greater than 2 hour delay in running the test
- High doses of adrenal steroids
- Hypofibrinogenemia
- Hyperglycemia
- Hyperalbuminemia
- Leukocytosis
- Microcytic anemia
- Newborn
- Certain drugs: ACTH, cortisone, ethambutol, quinine, salicylates

Table 11.3 Clinical implications of changes in the ESR

Increased rate
- Acute heavy metal poisoning
- All collagen diseases
- Carcinoma
- Cell or tissue destruction
- Gouty arthritis
- Infections
- Inflammatory diseases
- Leukemia
- Myocardial infarction
- Multiple myeloma
- Nephritis
- Pneumonia
- Rheumatoid arthritis
- Syphilis
- Toxemia

Decreased rate
- Congestive heart failure
- Polycythemia
- Sickle cell disease

Elevated ESR

Asymptomatic patients

The presence of an elevated ESR as the only manifestation of a disease process is quite rare. However, when present, it can be highly significant. For example, in one study of 17 patients whose increased ESR was the sole initial clue to disease, two had tuberculosis and one had colon cancer (both of which are diseases whose outcome is improved by early detection), one had systemic lupus erythematosus and three had ankylosing spondylitis (diagnoses that become apparent only after several years of observation), and four men had a persistently elevated ESR several years before a myocardial infarction. The remaining patients developed myeloma, prostate cancer, psoriasis, benign monoclonal gammopathy, and pancreatic cancer.

Although, in general, the ESR makes a very small contribution to disease detection in asymptomatic persons, the presence of an elevated ESR as the only clue to illness in an asymptomatic indicates the need for a careful diagnostic work-up; it may be the first sign of an occult malignancy or a chronic inflammatory disease. Laboratory evaluation for an asymptomatic patient with an elevated sedimentation rate should include CBC with differential, BUN and creatinine, alkaline phosphatase measurement, serum protein electrophoresis, urinalysis, guaiac tests of stool, and chest X-ray.[1]

An ESR that exceeds 100 mm/hour is definitely associated (predictive value of greater than 95%) with infection, malignancy, or connective tissue disease. Rarely does disease remain undiagnosed when the ESR is greatly elevated.[1–3]

If, after further clinical evaluation, an elevated ESR cannot be explained, the ESR should be repeated in one month. In one study where 43 patients with an elevated ESR remained undiagnosed, the elevation was transitory in 32. The remaining 11 were followed for a period of 10 years: two developed cancer, one had a benign dysproteinemia, and no diagnosis was ever made for the remaining nine.[1]

Predictor of coronary artery disease. An elevated ESR in white men aged 45 to 64 years was found to be an independent risk factor for coronary heart disease in the National Health and Nutrition Examination Survey I. The risk was highest when the ESR was >22 mm/hr. It was hypothesized that an elevated ESR in these men reflected an elevated blood fibrinogen level (see Chapter 13 for further discussion of fibrinogen).[3]

Symptomatic patients

The ESR is sometimes used to provide confirmation of a disease process when the history and physical findings point toward a specific diagnosis. Although the ESR itself is not a specific test, when combined with information gathered in a history and physical, as well as in conjunction with other laboratory tests, it can be a great help in the formation of a specific diagnosis.

In patients with vague, unsubstantiated illness, the ESR offers limited benefit due to the lack of specificity and the presence of a normal ESR in a wide variety of illnesses. However, the ESR offers great diagnostic benefit when other signs, symptoms, and laboratory findings are present. This is particularly true in malignancies, temporal arteritis and polymyalgia rheumatica, inflammatory arthritis, and suspected infection.

ESR in cancer

Malignancy is quite common in symptomatic patients with an elevated ESR. In one study, 70 (or 8.8%) of 790 clinic patients with an elevated ESR had cancer.[1] However, of the 70 patients with malignancy and an increased ESR, 68 had local signs that led directly to the diagnosis. Thus, occult malignancy was present in only two of the 790 subjects. In addition, the ESR is often normal in patients with cancer, indicating that the ESR should not be relied upon as a test to exclude occult malignancy in patients with vague symptoms.

In a prospective follow-up of 300 patients with prostate cancer, an ESR greater than 37 mm/hr was associated with a higher incidence of disease progression and death. These findings paralleled other prognostic indicators such as M and T categories, grade, performance status, and age, but nonetheless indicate that ESR does provide additional value in the monitoring of these patients and presumably others with invasive cancer.[3]

Temporal arteritis and polymyalgia rheumatica

Temporal arteritis and polymyalgia rheumatica are

related syndromes that can occur together or alone. Both occur in older individuals and are associated with an increased ESR. Symptoms of temporal arteritis include unilateral throbbing headache, scalp sensitivity, visual symptoms, jaw claudication, and localized thickening or loss of pulsation of the temporal artery. Polymyalgia rheumatica is a fast-developing condition characterized by pain and stiffness of the pelvis and shoulder girdle, in association with fever, anemia, malaise, and weight loss. It is typically self-limited to 1–2 years.

Determination of the ESR is of critical importance in the diagnosis and management of patients with temporal arteritis, a condition that can result in blindness due to obstruction of the ophthalmic arteries. When the clinical evidence for temporal arteritis is limited, a normal ESR reduces the probability of the disease to less than 1%. When the clinical evidence is strong, it is extremely rare to have a normal ESR. Achievement of a normal ESR by the use of anti-inflammatory agents, such as cortisone or the natural medicines discussed in Section 5, greatly reduces the risk of developing blindness.[1,2]

Inflammatory arthritis

The ESR is sometimes used to distinguish inflammatory arthritis from other causes of joint symptoms. This is particularly true in the differentiation of rheumatoid arthritis, which has an elevated ESR, and osteoarthritis, which typically has a normal ESR. It is not appropriate to place much value on the ESR as an independent diagnostic predictor of rheumatoid arthritis. An elevated ESR in patients with joint symptoms simply indicates an active inflammatory process.[1,2]

Suspected infection

Leukocytosis and fever are better indicators than the ESR of an acute infectious process, as the ESR is typically normal during the first stages of infection. However, the ESR is of some value in the differentiation of an intact versus ruptured appendix. Researchers demonstrated that only two of 25 patients with non-ruptured appendicitis had an ESR of greater than 20 mm/hour. In contrast, 67% of patients with ruptured appendixes had an elevated ESR.[1]

Decreased ESR

The causes of a very low ESR (0–1 mm/hr) are listed in Tables 11.2 and 11.3. In one study of patients with a low ESR, 38% had no evidence of disease, and only 6% had one of the diseases commonly associated with a very low ESR. The remaining patients had a wide variety of diagnoses. A low ESR is generally of little significance and may actually indicate a healthy state.[1–3]

Monitoring of disease activity

The ESR is well recognized as an aid in monitoring the activity of such inflammatory diseases as temporal arteritis, polymyalgia rheumatica, and rheumatoid arthritis.[1,2]

Temporal arteritis and polymyalgia rheumatica

The ESR is the most widely used test for assessing disease activity in patients with temporal arteritis and polymyalgia rheumatica, because these conditions have few specific clinical indicators of disease activity. However, both the ESR and clinical status need to be monitored in these patients and appropriate therapy instituted if the ESR increases or if there is a worsening in the clinical picture.[1,2]

Rheumatoid arthritis

Although 5–10% of patients with rheumatoid arthritis have a normal ESR, the ESR generally parallels disease activity. Therefore, monitoring the patient's ESR provides invaluable feedback on therapeutic effect. An isolated elevated ESR is not useful for prognosis, but sustained extreme elevation of the ESR is associated with a very poor prognosis.[1,2]

Other inflammatory diseases

Other inflammatory diseases, particularly collagen diseases, such as systemic lupus erythematosus, can be monitored by the ESR in a fashion similar to that for rheumatoid arthritis.[1,2]

SUMMARY

The ESR is a simple, valuable, and useful laboratory procedure. Although it is a non-specific indicator, an elevated ESR (i.e. greater than 80 mm/hour) indicates the presence of significant disease in over 95% of individuals. The ESR should never be used as the sole diagnostic test. Clinical presentation, comprehensive history, laboratory investigation, and other diagnostic procedures should always be considered when interpreting ESR results. The ESR may be used as a non-specific gauge of therapeutic efficacy and as a monitoring tool in several inflammatory conditions, including temporal arteritis, polymyalgia rheumatica, rheumatoid arthritis, and certain malignancies.

REFERENCES

1. Sox HC, Liang MH. The erythrocyte sedimentation rate. Ann Int Med 1986; 104: 515–523
2. Bedell SE, Bush BT. Erythrocyte sedimentation rate, from folklore to facts. Am J Med 1985; 78: 1001–1009
3. Saadeh C. The erythrocyte sedimentation rate: old and new clinical applications. South Med J 1998; 91: 220–225
4. Fischbach FT. A manual of laboratory diagnostic tests. Philadelphia, PA: JB Lippincott. 1980: p 50–54

CHAPTER CONTENTS

12

Fantus test for urine chloride

Dirk Wm Powell, ND

INTRODUCTION

The Fantus test is a simple test for measuring urinary output of chlorides. It is generally used to estimate dietary sodium chloride intake. For this purpose, it has been shown to give accurate results if two factors are taken into consideration:[1–3]

- The concentration of urinary chloride is generally proportional to urinary sodium except when the patient is taking chloride salts without sodium, i.e. NH_4Cl or KCl.
- The urinary output of NaCl is indicative of intake, except when the patient is suffering from a salt-wasting disorder (see Table 12.1).

CLINICAL APPLICATION

This test was first described by J. B. Fantus in 1936.[4] Since then it has been used mainly in the diagnosis and treatment of salt and water depletion and edema.[5] However, one of the most useful applications of this procedure may be in the monitoring of patients with blood pressure disorders.

Since 1904 when Ambard & Beaujard[6] first implicated salt as a major factor in the pathogenesis of hypertension, conflicting opinions and data have confused this issue. In 1944, Kempner[7] published a classic article describing the effective treatment of essential hypertension using a very low-salt "rice diet". Since then, many studies have demonstrated the effectiveness of salt-restricted diets in hypertension.[8–12] There is now substantial evidence that sodium alone does not raise blood pressure as was commonly thought, but rather that chloride also

Table 12.1 Sodium-wasting conditions in which salt restriction can be deleterious

- Adrenal insufficiency
- Salt-wasting renal disease
- Heavy sweating or exercise
- Unusual losses via the GI tract

plays an important role in the elevation of blood pressure when consumed concomitantly as common table salt.[13,14] (See Ch. 178 for further discussion of the relative roles of dietary sodium and chloride.)

Since the Fantus test, which has been called an indirect test for sodium, actually measures chloride, it may therefore be preferable to direct tests of sodium in the management of hypertension.[13,14]

Two difficulties arise in the treatment of hypertensive patients with salt restriction:[15]

- salt must be carefully restricted to low levels, 3–6 g/day, as compared with the 6–18 g/day commonly consumed
- strict salt restriction is difficult to obtain and maintain because of the prevalence of salt in convenience and prepared foods, and the customary intake of large amounts of salt.

These problems make monitoring salt intake important and the Fantus test a valuable clinical tool.

The Fantus test may be used in other conditions where salt restriction is useful, i.e. congestive heart failure, premenstrual syndrome, edema, chronic kidney disorders, and where salt depletion may be contributing to the disorder, i.e. hypotension. It is important to recognize, however, that salt restriction is not always appropriate, as in the conditions listed in Table 12.1.

Another application is the identification of people who are ingesting excessive amounts of salt, but who are without overt disease. It has been observed that a high intake of sodium decreases longevity in animals,[16] and salt-induced angiotensin elevation may adversely affect the myocardium in humans, even though the blood pressure remains within normal limits.[17] The effects of excess salt may persist long after salt is withdrawn.[18,19]

Identifying those people at risk due to excessive salt consumption is a significant aspect of preventive medicine. People with risk factors for hypertension should restrict salt intake.[20] Included in this group are patients with chronic renal disease, those with one or both hypertensive parents, and most people over the age of 50.[20]

The potential benefits of identifying those people with excess salt intake suggest the usefulness of this non-invasive, low-cost test.

PROCEDURE

The Fantus reagent is prepared so that the number of drops of silver nitrate used in the titration step can be recorded as grams of NaCl per liter of urine (g NaCl/L urine).

Method

1. Collect a 24 hour urine sample
2. Measure and record volume (in L)
3. Add one drop of K_2CrO_4 solution to 10 drops of urine
4. Titrate (one drop at a time) with the $AgNO_3$ solution
5. Record the number of drops needed to turn color from yellow to brown.

(If chloride is present in too low a concentration, use 20 drops of urine. Each drop of $AgNO_3$ is then equal to 0.5 g NaCl/L.)

Reagents

- $AgNO_3$: 2.9% solution
- K_2CrO_4: 20% solution.

Results

- Typical Western diet: 12–27 g/24 hours
- Salt-restricted diet: 0.6–3.5 g/24 hours.

INTERPRETATION

Normally, urinary NaCl varies considerably, reflecting the salt content of the typical Western diet: 80–180 mEq/24 hours (12–27 g/24 hours).[21] On a salt-restricted diet, the goal is usually to reduce 24 hour urine NaCl to close to the minimum considered safe, i.e. 0.6–3.5 g/24 hours.[20] Water consumption is typically closely related to salt intake, and a salt intake of 3 g/day corresponds to an intake of 2,750 ml of water from both solids and fluids, which is the average water turnover for a 70 kg adult. After evaporation from the lungs and other losses, the urine volume is approximately 1500 ml/24 hours.[5] This would yield a urine NaCl of 2 g/L or 3 g/24 hours.

REFERENCES

1. Luft, Fineberg N, Sloan R. Overnight urine collections to estimate sodium intake. Hyperten 1982; 4: 494–498
2. DeGowin E, DeGowin R. Bedside diagnostic examination. New York, NY: Macmillan. 1969: p 37–38
3. Krupp M, Sweet N, Jawetz E et al. Physician's handbook. Los Altos, CA: Lange Medical. 1973: p 213
4. Fantus J. Fluids postoperatively. JAMA 1936; 107: 17
5. Marriott H. Water and salt depletion. Springfield, IL: CC Thomas. 1950: p 55–56
6. Ambard L, Beaujard F. Causes de l'hypertension arteriole. Arch Gen Med 1904; 1: 520–533
7. Kempner W. Treatment of kidney diseases and hypertensive diseases with rice diet. N C Med J 1944; 5: 125–133
8. Chapman C, Gibbons T, Henschel A. The effect of the rice-fruit diet on the composition of the body. New Engl J Med 1980; 243: 809–905
9. Grohman A, Harrison T, Masom M et al. Sodium restriction in the diet for hypertension. JAMA 1945; 129: 533

10. Dustan H, Bravo E, Tarazi R. Volume-dependent essential and steroid hypertension. Am J Card 1973; 31: 606–615
11. Dustan H, Tarazi R, Bravo E. Diuretic and diet treatment of hypertension. Arch Intern Med 1974; 133: 1007–1013
12. Partis J, Hoosens H, Linden L et al. Moderate sodium restriction and diuretics in the treatment of hypertension. Am Heart J 1973; 86: 22–34
13. Kotchen T, Luke R, Ott C et al. Effect of chloride on renin and blood pressure responses to sodium chloride. Ann Int Med 1983; 98: 817–822
14. Kurte T, Morris Jr R. Dietary chloride as a determinant of sodium-dependent hypertension. Science 1983; 222: 1139–1140
15. Hunt J, Margie J. The influence of diet on hypertension management. In: Hunt H, ed. Hypertension update. Bloomfield, NJ: Health Learn Sys Inc. 1981: p 197–207
16. Meneely G, Batterbee H. High sodium-low potassium environment and hypertension. A J Card 1976; 38: 775
17. Khairallah P, Sen S, Tarazi R. Angiotensin, protein biosynthesis and cardiovascular hypertrophy (abstr). Am J Card 1976; 37: 148
18. Tobian L, Ishii M, Duke M. Relationship of cytoplasmic granules in renal papillary interstitial cells to "post-salt" hypertension. J Lab Clin Med 1969; 73: 309–319
19. Dahl L. Effects of chronic excess salt feeding: induction of self-sustaining hypertension in rats. J Exp Med 1961; 114: 231–236
20. Scribner B. Salt and hypertension. JAMA 1983; 250: 388–389
21. Davidson I, Henry J, Todd-Sanford. Clinical diagnosis by laboratory methods. Philadelphia, PA: WB Saunders. 1974: p 1386

CHAPTER CONTENTS

13

Fatty acid profiling

Richard S. Lord, PhD

J. Alexander Bralley, PhD

INTRODUCTION

The analysis of fatty acids in blood provides useful information about fatty acid deficiencies and imbalances and can also reveal a functional need for certain vitamins and minerals. Clinical interventions involve changes in food selection or supplementation with selected nut or seed extract oils and required micronutrients. Laboratory reports of fatty acid profiles typically list the fatty acids by structural type in the following order: ω3-polyunsaturates, ω6-polyunsaturates, mono-unsaturates, even-numbered saturates, odd-numbered saturates, and, finally, *trans* mono-unsaturates. Several ratios may be calculated, and for plasma, the total fatty acid concentration may be calculated by summing the individual components and expressing the total in mg/dl, consistent with the units for serum triglycerides which are directly related to total fatty acid content.

METHODOLOGICAL ISSUES

A plasma fatty acid profile is an amplification of the standard serum triglyceride analysis. In both cases, the fatty acids are present in lipoprotein particles. Instead of measuring only the total of all fatty acids present, the profile test reports the individual concentrations of each fatty acid. An individual with high serum triglycerides will have higher levels of many individual fatty acids in plasma. Of course, any condition indicated by elevated serum triglycerides will likewise be revealed as elevated fatty acids. The pattern of the high and low levels will depend on recent dietary intake and, depending on the length of fasting state, the type of stored fatty acids.

Plasma vs. erythrocyte fatty acid profiles

Erythrocyte membrane fatty acid profiling is the most commonly used test to determine the presence of long-term insufficiencies and imbalances. The erythrocyte membrane is 45% fatty acids in the form of various phosphatides and glycolipids. The procedure used for profiling measures total concentrations of individual fatty acids. Erythrocyte data are generally preferred for assessing overall body status of fatty acids because the levels reflect those present in most tissues. For example, the fatty acid composition of brain has been found to be directly correlated with that in red blood cells in rat and primate studies.[1]

The triglyceride-lowering drug, gemfibrozil, causes a profound suppression of erythrocyte unsaturated fatty acids, even in the presence of high concentrations of the same compounds in plasma. The effect is apparently due to stimulation of the peroxisomal beta-oxidation system.[2]

Concentration vs. percentage

Prior to 1996, virtually all clinical laboratories reporting fatty acid fractionations had little choice but to express each fatty acid as a percentage of the total fatty acids present. Actual concentrations could not be reported due to the lack of pure standards necessary to build calibration curves. The reporting of "relative area" data has some utility but leaves important points obscured. The most abundant fatty acids are present at concentrations 50 times higher than those of the lesser components.[3] In percent area calculations, variations in the most abundant components have disproportionate impact. If linolenic acid is the same in two cases, for example, while palmitic acid is low in the first and high in the second, the percent linolenic can appear high in the first and normal in the second. This is due to the fact that palmitic acid makes up so much of the total, and the ratios of the minor components such as linolenic acid are calculated by dividing by the total.

With the availability of pure standards, it is now possible to measure the actual concentrations of each fatty acid. Since the molecular weights span a range of over 70-fold for these homologous compounds, molar units allow more meaningful comparisons. This unit also simplifies interpretation of plasma fatty acids where the total of all fatty acids is directly proportional (and closely equivalent) to the values for total triglycerides from a standard serum chemistry assay. For erythrocytes, the μM concentrations are based on packed cell volumes.

INTERPRETATION OF ABNORMAL FATTY ACID RESULTS

Table 13.1 provides a brief overview of the various fatty acid abnormalities. Table 85.4 (p. 729) lists the typical symptoms and diseases associated with various fatty acid abnormalities. The significance of abnormal levels and ratios of fatty acids is discussed below.

Individual fatty acids

Alpha-linolenic acid (ALA) (18:3ω3)

This polyunsaturated fatty acid is produced by many plants, but because of the small amounts of fresh vegetables consumed, it is one of the least abundant of the essential fatty acids in most diets. It is found in flax, hemp, rape (canola) seed, soybean, and walnut oils, and in dark green leaves and it must be supplied by such foods. Dietary insufficiencies and imbalances of this fatty acid and its counterpart, GLA, play a central role in many disease processes (see Tables 85.4 and 85.5, pp. 729 and 730). The wide range of symptoms and disease associations is due to the function of this fatty acid in critical cell processes of membrane integrity and eicosanoid local hormone production. The latter function utilizes the fatty acid eicosapentaenoic acid (EPA, see below), which can be produced from ALA by elongation and desaturation. This conversion is very efficient in most individuals. An inadequate conversion is indicated by low EPA and DHA in the presence of normal ALA.

Eicosapentaenoic acid (EPA) (20:5ω3)

Insufficiencies of EPA are likely the most prevalent fatty acid abnormality affecting the health of individuals in Western societies. Low levels in plasma or especially in erythrocytes are indicative of insufficiency. Arthritis and heart disease, as well as excessive aging, result from direct or indirect effects of unchecked inflammatory response. Supplementation with EPA-rich fish oils aids in the prevention of cardiac arrhythmias.[4] Significant reduction in total cholesterol and triglyceride has been achieved with a combination of garlic concentrate (900 mg/day) and fish oil supplementation.[5] EPA is the parent of the 3-series prostanoids and leukotrienes which moderate the proinflammatory effects of the 2-series derived from arachidonic acid (see below). Although EPA can be produced from the essential fatty acid, ALA, dietary intake of this fatty acid is generally poor. The conversion also requires the action of the Δ6 desaturase enzyme, which may be low due to inadequate Zn, Mg, or vitamins B_3, B_6, and C. Such an enzyme impairment would be indicated if EPA is low and ALA is normal or high. High levels of saturated, mono-unsaturated, and *trans* fatty acids, and cholesterol also slow the conversion of ALA to EPA (as well as GLA to DGLA). Fish oils are rich sources of EPA.

Docosapentaenoic acid (DPA) (22:5ω3), docosahexaenoic acid (DHA) (22:6ω3)

The growth and development of the central nervous system are particularly dependent upon the presence of an adequate amount of the very long-chain, highly

Table 13.1 Overview of fatty acid abnormalities

Name	Levels	Metabolic association	Potential responses*
Omega-3 polyunsaturated			
Alpha linolenic	L	Essential fatty acid	Add flax and/or fish oils
Eicosapentaenoic	L	Eicosanoid substrate	
Docosapentaenoic	L	Nerve membrane function	Add fish oils
Docosahexaenoic	L	Neurological development	
Omega-6 polyunsaturated			
Linoleic	L	Essential fatty acid	Add corn or borage oil
Gamma linolenic	L	Eicosanoid precursor	Add evening primrose oil
Eicosadienoic	H	Desaturase inhibition	Zn; 50 mg/day
DGLA	L	Eicosanoid substrate	Add borage oil
Arachidonic	H }	Eicosanoid substrate	Reduce red meats
Docosadienoic	H }		
Docosatetraenoic	H	Increase in adipose tissue	EFA and glycemic control
Mono-unsaturated			
Vaccenic	H	Biotin deficiency	Biotin; 50 mg BID
Myristoleic	H }		
Palmitoleic	H }	Membrane fluidity	See discussion
Oleic	H }		
11-Eicosenoic	H }		
Nervonic	L	Neurological development	Add fish or canola oils
Erucic	L	Nerve membrane function	Add peanut oil
Saturated			
Capric acid	H }	Multiple AcylCoA disorder (MAD)	Riboflavin; 50mg TID
Lauric	H }		
Myristic	H }		
Palmitic	H	Cholesterogenic	Reduce sat. fats; add niacin
Stearic	H	Elevated triglycerides	Reduce sat. fats; add niacin
	L	Cancer marker	
Arachidic	H }	Δ6 desaturase inhibition	Check eicosanoid ratios
Behenic	H }		
Lignoceric	H }	Nerve membrane function	Consider rape or mustard oils
Hexacosanoic	H }		
Odd-numbered			
Pentadecanoic	H }		
Heptadecanoic	H }		
Nonadecanoic	H }	Propionate accumulation	Vitamin B12; 1000 mcg, TID
Heneicosanoic	H }		
Tricosanoic	H }		
Trans fatty acids			
Palmitelaidic	H }	Eicosanoid interference	Eliminate hydrogenated oils
Elaidic	H }		
Ratios and indexes			
LA/DGLA	H }	Δ6 desaturase enzyme	Add blackcurrant oil
DGLA/EPA	L }		Add fish oils
	H	Eicosanoid imbalance	Add borage oil
AA/EPA	H		Add fish oils
P/S Ratio	H	Overall fatty acid status	Add dietary unsaturates
Stearic/oleic (rbc)	L	Cancer marker	See comments
Total fatty acids (pl)	H	Serum triglyceride (VLDL)	Evaluate hyperlipidemias

*Fatty acids are usually supplemented in the range of 1–3 g/day in the form of extracted nut and seed oils that may contain 30–60% of the fatty acid by weight.

unsaturated fatty acids, DPA and DHA.[6,7] Attention deficit hyperactivity disorder and failures in development of the visual system in essential fatty acid deficiencies are two examples of this dependency.[8] DHA is an important member of the very long-chain fatty acids (C22–C26) which characteristically occur in glycosphingolipids, particularly those in brain. Since this fatty acid is so important in early development, it is worth noting that the levels in breast milk are correlated with the mother's intake of fish oils, which are rich sources of DHA and DPA.[9]

Linoleic acid (LA) (18:2ω6)

LA is by far the most abundant polyunsaturated fatty acid in most human tissues. It is one of the essential fatty acids because it contains a double bond at the ω6 position which is beyond the reach of the human desaturase enzyme. Low levels indicate dietary insufficiency, which leads to a variety of symptoms (see Table 85.4, p. 729). Some of these symptoms result from a lack of linoleic acid in membranes, where it has a role in structural integrity. Most, however, are from failure to produce the 1-series and 3-series local hormones known as prostanoids. Linoleic acid is the starting point for this pathway. Normal neonatal status of this fatty acid is marginal, if not insufficient. Fetal linoleic and cervonic acid (DHA) are correlated with maternal RBC levels.[10] Since dietary sources (especially corn oil) are abundant, however, linoleic acid may be found to be above normal in some adults. Because of the need for balanced prostanoid and leukotriene synthesis, excessive linoleic acid can contribute to an overproduction of the proinflammatory 2-series local hormones. Compared with other fatty acids, linoleic acid caused growth inhibition of *Helicobacter pylori*, the bacterium thought to cause gastric ulcer.[11]

Gamma linolenic acid (GLA) (18:3ω6)

GLA is the precursor of DGLA, the parent of the 1-series prostanoids, as well as the precursor of arachidonic acid, the parent of the 2-series prostanoids. It is found in hemp, borage, blackcurrant, and evening primrose oils. It can be produced in human tissues by the action of desaturase enzymes on linoleic acid. Use of 1.4 g/day in the form of borage seed oil resulted in a clinically important reduction in the signs and symptoms of rheumatoid arthritis[12] (see Table 85.4, p. 729 for other clinical associations). In cases of cancer, it is especially important that low levels of GLA should not be supplemented without added ω3 fatty acids, because ω6 fatty acids enhance tumor formation and growth, while ω3 fatty acids inhibit tumors.[13] Gamma linolenic acid corrects most of the biological effects of zinc deficiency, indicating that the requirement of the Δ5 desaturase enzyme for zinc is a first-order essential function of zinc.[14]

Dihomogammalinolenic acid (DGLA) (18:3ω6)

Diets low in the essential fatty acid LA are almost universally also low in DGLA. The 1-series prostanoids and leukotrienes are derived from DGLA, so an insufficiency of this fatty acid impairs a wide range of cellular functions and tissue responses. The 1-series compounds act like the 3-series derived from ALA to moderate the proinflammatory 2-series. In tumor response, however, they are unique in being promoters of growth where the 3-series are inhibitors. When testing reveals low levels of DGLA, supplementation with borage or evening primrose oils should be considered, but if a history of tumor formation is known, always consider ALA sources (blackcurrant) as well. See EPA above (p. 136) for other factors affecting the desaturase enzyme required for conversion of GLA into DGLA.

Arachidonic acid (AA) (18:4ω6)

Because of the prevalence of corn and corn oil products in feed for cattle and hogs, diets high in these red meats are rich in AA. AA is a 20-carbon or eicosanoate fatty acid that serves as substrate for the cyclooxygenase and lipoxygenase enzymes, leading to the production of the 2-series prostanoids and leukotrienes. Several of these products have potent proinflammatory and thrombogenic activity. High AA also promotes gallstone formation by stimulating mucin production in the gall bladder mucosa.[15]

Docosadienoic acid (22:2ω6), docosatetraenoic acid (22:4ω6)

When ω6 dietary fatty acids are constantly supplied in overabundance, the intermediate products of further desaturation and elongation are not utilized as fast as they are produced. Under these conditions, the process of modification can continue through docosadienoic acid to the 22-carbon, four double bonded docosatetraenoic acid (DTA). These fatty acids can then accumulate in adipose tissue. Data from our own studies indicate a strong association of DTA acid in plasma with obesity. Apparently this fatty acid accumulates in adipose tissue from which it is mobilized in the fasting state. No such association has been seen in erythrocyte fatty acid profiles, indicating rapid utilization of these fatty acids once they are mobilized.

The level of DTA in plasma may be useful in monitoring the metabolic aspects of weight control and especially in avoiding the risk of essential fatty acid deficiencies while maintaining a very low-fat diet. A low level of DTA in an individual who is on a fat-restricted weight loss program may indicate a state of essential fatty acid deprivation.

Myristoleic acid (18:1ω7), palmitoleic acid (16:1ω9), vaccenic acid (14:1ω9)

The ratio of vaccenic acid to palmitoleic acid has been reported to be a valuable indicator of biotin deficiency.[16] Vaccenic acid also seems to have large effects on membrane fluidity, possibly due to the fact that the ω7 double bond does not align with the much more abundant ω9 positions of the majority of fatty acids present in the membrane. Inhibition of tumor growth in cell culture has been reported for vaccenic acid.[17]

Oleic acid (18:1ω9)

Oleic acid is present in all foods that contain fat and is

easily produced by the fatty acid synthetic pathways present in normal human hepatic cells. It constitutes 15% of the fatty acids in erythrocyte membranes. Because of the presence of the double bond in the center of the molecule, it helps to govern the critical nature of fluidity of the membrane matrix.

The pathogenesis of atherosclerosis involves accumulation of foam cells along the arterial wall. Lipids that transform macrophages into these foam cells are provided by oxidized low-density lipoproteins (LDLs). Oleic acid is the principal lipid of a class that makes LDLs resistant to oxidation, and thus a diet rich in this fatty acid reduces foam cell accumulation rates and thereby lowers the chances of atherosclerosis[18] (see Ch. 133 for a more complete discussion).

In tumors, the net result of modification in fatty acid enzymes is low stearic acid and high oleic acid, causing a profound shift in the ratio of stearic to oleic acids.[19] One likely outcome of this shift is an increased fluidity of the tumor cell membrane, resulting in more rapid movement of nutrients and waste products and allowing for faster metabolic rate. The stearic/oleic ratio is used as a monitor of the effectiveness of therapy.[20]

High oleic acid intake (usually as olive oil) can raise total oleic acid content of plasma above the reference range. This finding alone is not highly significant since oleic acid is a cholesterol neutral fatty acid and is produced in humans from stearic, so it is not an essential fatty acid.

Erucic acid (22:1ω12)

This fatty acid is apparently one of the components responsible for the favorable response of individuals with adrenal leukodystrophy to preparations containing rape and mustard seed oils.[21] Other studies using Lorenzo's oil containing glycerol trierucate revealed no appreciable changes in brain lipid content.[22] In Zellweger syndrome, where peroxisomes are absent, erucic and adrenic (docosatetraenoic) acids accumulate. It is speculated that either the anabolic enzymes are inhibited from producing sphingolipids or the catabolic enzymes are stimulated to faster clearance of the offending products.[23]

Capric acid (10:0), lauric acid (12:0), myristic acid (14:0)

These medium-chain fatty acids correspond to the dicarboxylic acids that accumulate in the fatty acid catabolic disorders known as multiple acyl-coenzyme A dehydrogenation disorders (MAD).[24] One type of this enzyme defect is responsive to riboflavin at levels far above normal intakes.[25] A pattern of low levels of the shorter chain fatty acids and high levels of longer chain fatty acids may indicate a fatty acid-restricted diet, in which case there is a stimulation of hepatic synthesis and elongation enzymes.

Palmitic acid (16:0)

The liver can convert fatty acids into cholesterol. Although any fatty acid can enter this pathway, palmitic acid is the most stimulatory one known and high levels lead to increased serum cholesterol levels and thus to increased risk of atherosclerosis, cardiovascular disease, and stroke. Most other fatty acids are either cholesterol neutral or have reverse effects, as in the case of EPA. Palm kernel and coconut oils are rich sources of palmitic acid. Palmitic is also the principal fatty acid product of human fatty acid synthesis, which is stimulated by dysinsulinemia and by diets high in simple carbohydrates.

Stearic acid (18:0)

Stearic acid is a saturated fatty acid that is two carbon atoms longer than palmitic and is similarly cholesterogenic. High levels in plasma are therefore a risk factor in atherosclerotic vascular disease (see 'Palmitic acid' above). Abnormal levels in erythrocyte membranes cause alteration in membrane fluidity with numerous consequences. Low levels give increased fluidity, which is associated with active tumor proliferation.

Arachidic acid (20:0)

Arachidic acid (20:0) can be utilized as an energy source or 1-position phospholipid, but it serves no other special function. Its accumulation is most likely to exacerbate essential fatty acid metabolism as it binds to the Δ6 desaturase enzyme and inhibits the insertion of double bonds needed to produce DGLA, EPA and AA.

Behenic acid (22:0), lignoceric acid (24:0), hexacosanoic acid (26:0)

Accumulation of certain very long-chain fatty acids is associated with degenerative diseases of the central nervous system such as adrenal leukodystrophy. There are a large number of known genetic disorders involving accumulation of sphingolipids, usually due to the lack of enzymes needed to maintain the turnover of membrane components. Behenic, lignoceric, and hexacosanoic acids, as well as the unsaturated members of the C22–24 classes, especially nervonic, are found elevated in such cases.

Pentadecanoic acid (15:0), heptadecanoic acid (17:0), nonadecanoic acid (19:0), heneicosanoic acid (21:0), tricosanoic acid (23:0)

Since the normal synthetic pathway for fatty acids leads to only even numbers of carbon atoms in the products, it may seem curious to find any odd-numbered chains present in human tissues. Fatty acids with odd numbers of carbon atoms are produced primarily by initiating the synthetic pathway with the three carbon compound, propionic acid. Vitamin B_{12} is required for the conversion of propionate into succinate for oxidation in the central energy pathways.[26] Deficiency of vitamin B_{12} results in accumulation of propionate and subsequent build-up of the odd-numbered fatty acids.

The bacteria in the gut of ruminants produce large amounts of propionate, which is absorbed and enters the metabolism. Consequently, the intake of animal and dairy products favors higher levels of odd-numbered fatty acids. Alternatively, it is possible that the bacteria in the human gut could produce sufficient amounts of propionate to lead to an elevation in the odd-carbon fatty acids. This would only occur under conditions of significant gut dysbiosis.

The association between vitamin B_{12} and abnormal fatty acid synthesis provides a rationale for the neuropathy of cobalamin deficiency. Odd-chain fatty acids would build up in membrane lipids of nervous tissue, resulting in altered myelin integrity and demyelination, leading eventually to impaired nervous system functioning.[27]

Palmitelaidic acid (16:1ω9t), elaidic acid (18:1ω9t)

The *trans* fatty acids, elaidic and palmitelaidic acid, are prevalent in most diets because of the widespread use of hydrogenated oils by manufacturers of margarine, bakery products, and peanut butters. These fatty acids contain one double bond and thus are included in the unsaturated category. Because of the geometry of the *trans* bond, however, they behave like saturated fats on the one hand, leading to higher cholesterol levels.[28] On the other hand, they mimic unsaturated fats in binding to desaturase enzymes and interfering with the normal production of critical products. The net effect is to raise plasma LDL and lower HDL.

The growing consensus among experts in lipid nutrition is that foods containing hydrogenated oils are to be avoided. These fatty acids are also produced by the bacteria in the gut of ruminant animals, which is the reason that beef and milk contain small amounts (1–3%) of elaidic acid. Moderate use of these foods is unlikely to provide *trans* fatty acids at levels that are of concern. If these synthetic fatty acids are elevated, foods containing hydrogenated oils may need to be avoided. Foods that generally contribute the greatest amounts of *trans* fatty acids include stick margarine, peanut butters, and bakery products such as breads, rolls, cookies, crackers, pies, and cakes. Products with labels that say simply "vegetable oil" should be substituted, avoiding those containing hydrogenated oils.

Fatty acid ratios

As with all ratios of reported laboratory values, the calculated value allows a comparison of the relative magnitudes of the two individual measurements. The added value lies in the use of the ratio as a quick guide to the balance between two parameters. Sometimes valuable insights into imbalances are found in ratio values, even though the individual components are normal.

The LA/DGLA ratio

The ratio of LA to DGLA increases when the Δ6 desaturase enzyme is inhibited by zinc deficiency or excesses of saturated, monoenoic, or *trans* fatty acids. Under these conditions, the enzyme cannot convert the substrate (LA) to the product (DGLA) fast enough. The production of all desaturation products is affected, including EPA and AA. These longer chain polyunsaturated fatty acids then must be supplied from the diet or supplemented forms.

The DGLA/EPA ratio

The balance of 20-carbon or eicosenoic fatty acids is critical for proper supply of the prostanoid and leukotriene 1-, 2-, and 3-series local hormones that control a host of cellular functions and responses. The DGLA/EPA ratio is typically high due to DGLA being elevated relative to EPA, indicating a need for EPA sources such as fish oils. When the ratio is low, sources of DGLA (borage or evening primrose oil) are indicated.

The AA/EPA ratio

This ratio allows a quick comparison of the relative amounts of these two eicosanoid precursors. An abundance of AA is quite common in Western diets high in meat and corn oil and can result in the elevation of the AA/EPA ratio. This is one of the indicators that extra ω3 fatty acids, including EPA of fish oils, would be beneficial.

Red cell stearic/oleic index

The ratio of stearic to oleic acids in red cell membranes has been found to be a strong indicator of the presence of malignant tissue, as it reflects the lowered ratio found in malignant tissue cell membranes.[29] Values below 1.1 are associated with the presence of malignancy. The ratio was found to respond to hormonal therapy for prostatic cancer and, in studies following surgical cures, individuals who maintained this ratio above 1.1 had no tumor recurrences.

The polyunsaturated to saturated fatty acid ratio (P/S)

Originating primarily as a measure of the quality of dietary fats, this ratio is sometimes used also as a general measure of physiological fatty acid balance. This ratio increases markedly during exercise, as the saturated fatty acids are preferentially utilized as energy sources, causing plasma levels to fall relative to the unsaturated fatty acids.[30] The availability of individual fatty acid data allows the inclusion of *trans* fatty acids in the saturated group since their physiological behaviour is the same. This has not normally been done in the food industry to date, giving misleadingly favorable ratios on labels. The overall effect of higher levels of the polyenoic fatty acids is suppression of hepatic lipogenesis.[31]

Total fatty acid concentration (calculated)

When the concentrations of total fatty acids present in plasma are summed and expressed in units of mg/100 dl, the result is closely equivalent to that of the routine serum triglyceride assay. In both cases, the fatty acids are normally present in the form of very low-density lipoprotein particles. The treatment of elevated levels by various actions involving dietary restriction of fats, the use of pharmacological doses of niacin and lipid-lowering drugs is in common practice, depending on the class of hyperlipidemia found by studies of lipoprotein subclasses and cholesterol levels.

When total fatty acids are low, there is the possibility of stimulation of peroxisomal oxidation of fatty acids. A number of structurally diverse chemicals have been found to cause proliferation of peroxisomes in liver and other tissues.[32] Paradoxically, high-fat diets also cause such proliferation. The increased oxidative activity leads to higher levels of hydrogen peroxide and development of liver tumors in laboratory animals.[33] In humans, the related disorder, hypobetalipoproteinemia, is associated with increased risk for a variety of cancers, pulmonary, and gastrointestinal diseases.[34]

SUMMARY

Recent advances in laboratory methodologies now allow measurement of absolute, as well as relative, levels of essential, non-essential and potentially damaging types of fatty acids in the blood. The research literature now provides guidance for interpretation of the clinical significance of various fatty acid patterns. Fatty acid manipulation through diet and supplementation is a very powerful therapeutic resource (see Ch. 85).

REFERENCES

1. Hoffman DR, Uauy R. Essentiality of dietary w-3 fatty acids for premature infants: plasma and red blood cell fatty acid composition. Lipids 1992; 27: 886
2. Hashimoto F, Ishikawa T, Hamada S et al. Effect of gemfibrozil on lipid biosynthesis from acetyl-CoA derived from peroxisomal beta-oxidation. Biochem Pharmacol 1995; 49: 1213–1221
3. Manku MS, Horrobin DF, Huang YS et al. Fatty acids in plasma and red cell membranes in normal humans. Lipids 1983; 18: 906
4. Nair SS, Leitch JW, Falconer J et al. Prevention of cardiac arrhythmia by dietary (n-3) polyunsaturated fatty acids and their mechanism of action. J Nutr 1997; 127: 383–393
5. Adler AJ, Holub BJ. Effect of garlic and fish-oil supplementation on serum lipid and lipoprotein concentrations in hypercholesterolemic men. Am J Clin Nutr 1997; 65: 445–450
6. Hoffman DR, Uauy R. Essentiality of dietary w-3 fatty acids for premature infants: plasma and red blood cell fatty acid composition. Lipids 1992; 27: 886
7. Innis S. n-3 Fatty acid requirements of the newborn. Lipids 1992; 27: 879–887
8. Stevens LJ, Zentall SS, Deck JL et al. Essential fatty acid metabolism in boys with attention-deficit hyperactivity disorder. Am J Clin Nutr 1995; 62: 761–768
9. Henderson RA, Jensen RG, Lammi-Keefe CJ et al. Effect of fish oil on the fatty acid composition of human milk and maternal and infant erythrocytes. Lipids 1992; 27: 863–869
10. Houwelingen AC, Puls J, Hornstra G. Essential fatty acid status during early human development. Early Human Dev 1992; 31: 97–111
11. Khulusi S, Ahmed HA, Patel P et al. The effects of unsaturated fatty acids on Helicobacter pylori in vitro. J Med Microbiol 1995; 42: 276–282
12. Leventhal LJ, Boyce EG, Zurier RB. Treatment of rheumatoid arthritis with gammalinolenic acid. Ann Int Med 1993; 119: 867–873
13. Noguchi M, Rose DP, Earashi M et al. The role of fatty acids and eicosanoid synthesis inhibitors in breast carcinoma. Oncology 1995; 52: 265–271
14. Huang YS, Cunnane SC, Horrobin DF et al. Most biological effects of zinc deficiency corrected by g-linolenic acid (18:3w6) but not by linoleic acid (18:2w6). Atherosclerosis 1982; 41: 193–207
15. Hayes KC, Livingston A, Trautwein EA. Dietary impact on biliary lipids and gallstones. Ann Rev Nutr 1992; 12: 299–326
16. Shigematsu YY, Bykov I, Nakai A et al. Abnormal fatty acid composition of lymphocytes of biotin-deficient rats. J Nutr Sci 1997; 40: 283–288
17. Awab AB, Herrmann T, Fink CS et al. 18:1 n7 fatty acids inhibit growth and decrease inositol phosphate release in HT-29 cells compared to n9 fatty acids. Cancer Lett 1995; 9: 55–61
18. Anonymous: How monounsaturates may save arteries. Science News 1990; 367, June 9
19. Wood CB, Habib NA, Thompson A et al. Increase of oleic acid in erythrocytes associated with malignancies. Br Med J 1985; 291: 163
20. Apostolov K, Barker W, Catousby D et al. Reduction in the stearic to oleic acid ratio in leukaemic cells – a possible chemical marker of malignancy. Blut 1985; 50: 349–354
21. Rizzo WB, Leshner RT, Odone A et al. Dietary erucic acid therapy for X-linked adrenoleukodystrophy. Neurology 1989; 39: 1415–1421
22. Poulos A, Gibson R, Sharp P et al. Very long chain fatty acids in X-linked. Ann Neurol 1994; 36: 741–746
23. Christensen E, Hagve TA, Christophersen BO. The Zellweger syndrome: deficient chain-shortening of erucic acid (22:1 (n-9)). Biochim Biophys Acta 1988; 959: 134–142
24. Saudubray JM, Mitchell G, Bonnefont JP et al. Approach to the patient with a fatty acid oxidation disorder. In: Coates PM, Tanaka K, eds. New developments in fatty acid oxidation. New York: Wiley-Liss. 1992: p 271–288
25. Roettger V, Marshall T, Amendt R. Multiple acyl-coenzyme A dehydrogenation disorders (MAD) responsive to riboflavin:

biochemical studies in fibroblasts. In: Coates PM, Tanaka K, eds. New developments in fatty acid oxidation. New York: Wiley-Liss. 1992: p 319–326

26. Metz J. Cobalamin deficiency and the pathogenesis of nervous system disease. In Olson RE, ed. Ann Rev Nutr 1992; 12: 59
27. Frenkel EP, Kitchens RL, Johnson JM. The effect of vitamin B_{12} deprivation on the enzymes of fatty acid synthesis. J Biol Chem 1973; 248: 7450
28. Abbey M, Nestel PJ. Plasma cholesterol ester transfer protein activity is increased when trans-elaidic acid is substituted for cis-oleic acid in the diet. Atherosclerosis 1994; 106: 99–107
29. Persad RA, Hillatt DA, Heinemann D et al: Erythrocyte stearic to oleic acid ratio in prostatic carcinoma. Brit J Urol 1990; 65: 268
30. Mougios V, Kotzamanidis C, Koutsari C et al. Exercise-induced changes in the concentration of individual fatty acids and triacylglycerols of human plasma. Metabolism 1995; 44: 681–688
31. Blake WL, Clarke SD. Suppression of hepatic fatty acid synthase and S14 gene transcription by dietary polyunsaturated fat. F Mutr 1990; 120: 1727–1729
32. Reddy JK, Lalwani ND. Carcinogenesis by hepatic peroxisome proliferators: evaluation of the risk of hypoilidemic drugs and industrial plasticizers to humans. CRC Crit Rev Toxicol 1983; 12: 1–58
33. Reddy JK, Lalwani ND. Peroxisome proliferation and hepatocarcinogenesis. In: Vainio H, Magee PN, McGregor DB, McMichael AJ, eds. Mechanism of carcinogenesis in risk identification. Lyon: International Agency for Research on Cancer. 1992: p 225–235

34 Schonfeld G. The hypobetalipoproteinemias. Ann Rev Nut 1995; 15: 23–34

CHAPTER CONTENTS

14

Folic acid status assessment

Michael T. Murray, ND

Joseph E. Pizzorno Jr, ND

INTRODUCTION

Folic acid is the nutritionally essential precursor of a large family of compounds collectively referred to as folates. It is a pteridine derivative linked through a methylene bridge to a molecule of para-amino-benzoyl-glutamic acid.

Folate coenzymes are widely distributed in the body and are involved in a diverse variety of metabolic processes: single carbon transfer reactions; biosynthesis of purines, the pyrimidine, thymidate (which is necessary for the formation of DNA), methionine, and choline; histidine degradation; methylation of biogenic amines, such as serotonin; the hydroxylation of proline for collagen formation; and the maturation of erythrocytes and leukocytes.[1]

Although widely distributed in nature, folic acid is thought to be the most common hypovitaminosis of humans, particularly of indigenous populations.[2] Deficiency is common during pregnancy (20% of women with otherwise normal pregnancies have been shown to have low folate levels),[3] lactation, early infancy, and adolescence;[4] and in those taking a wide range of anti-tumor, antimalarial, antibacterial, anticonvulsive, and contraceptive drugs.[1]

CLINICAL APPLICATION

Clinical conditions which can be caused by a folate deficiency include megaloblastic anemia, glossitis, diarrhea, affective disorders such as depression, and weight loss. Signs and symptoms may include ulcerative stomatitis, hyperpigmentation of the skin, cervical dysplasia (see Ch. 142), hepatomegaly, splenomegaly, ankle edema, and the typical non-specific signs of anemia, such as palpitations, angina, light-headedness, and faintness.[1,5] Folate deficiency has also been shown to impair the phagocytosis and bactericidal activity of neutrophils.[6]

A prolonged dietary folic acid deficiency, or the presence of folate antagonists, results in the progressive development of biochemical and hematological abnor-

Table 14.1 Progressive manifestations of folate deficiency[7,8]

Duration (weeks)	Abnormality
2–6	Decreased serum folate levels
6–11	Neutrophil hypersegmentation
13	High urinary formiminoglutamate
17	Low RBC folate
18	Macro-ovalocytosis
19	Megaloblastic marrow
20	Megaloblastic anemia

malities, as shown in Table 14.1. As can be seen, although an abnormal folate status is traditionally suspected by the presence of a megaloblastic anemia, this is a late-stage development. The measurement of neutrophil hypersegmentation is a far better indicator of incipient folate deficiency,[9] and is an inexpensive test that can be added to the repertoire of the nutritionally oriented doctor. Serum folate is somewhat unreliable since a vitamin B_{12} deficiency will result in invalidly high levels, and although RBC folate is more accurate, it is not widely available, expensive to run, and gives abnormally low values in patients with a vitamin B_{12} deficiency.[10]

Table 14.2 lists the typical causes of folic acid deficiency by mechanism.

Table 14.2 Causes of folic acid deficiency[11]

Mechanism	Cause
Inadequate intake	Alcoholism Dietary insufficiency
Increased requirements	Pregnancy Severe hemolysis Chronic hemodialysis
Inadequate absorption	Tropical sprue Gluten-sensitive enteropathy Crohn's disease Lymphoma of small bowel Amyloidosis of small bowel Diabetic enteropathy Intestinal resection or diversion Drugs that block absorption —cholestyramine —phenobarbital —biguanides
Impaired metabolism	Drugs blocking action of dihydrofolate reductase —methotrexate —trimethoprim —pyrimethamine —anticonvulsants Drugs interfering by other means —phenytoin —ethanol —antituberculous drugs —oral contraceptives —aspirin

PROCEDURE

The measurement of neutrophil hypersegmentation is a useful test that correlates well with serum folate levels ($R = -0.772$), and is easily performed in a clinical laboratory.[9]

Method

1. Take a standard peripheral blood smear on a 1 inch by 3 inches glass slide.
2. Stain with Leishman or other convenient stain.
3. Count the lobes on 100 neutrophils using an oil immersion objective.
4. Calculate the segmentation index (SI):

$$\text{SI} = \text{neutrophils with 5+ lobes} \times \frac{100}{\text{neutrophils with 4 lobes}}$$

Results

- Normal: SI = 2–30%
- Folate-deficient: SI = 31.5–116%

INTERPRETATION

Although abnormal folate levels are responsible for 90% of patients with neutrophil hypersegmentation in the absence of macrocytic anemia, other causes must be considered. It is seen in uremia, and 7% have a vitamin B_{12} deficiency.[12] It is also a congenital condition in as much as 1% of the population.[13]

REFERENCES

1. Roe DA. Drug-induced nutritional deficiencies. Westport, CN: AVI Publ. 1976: p 7–11
2. Worthington-Roberts BS. Contemporary developments in nutrition. St Louis: Mosby. 1981: p 225
3. Herbert V. Folic acid deficiency in the United States: folate assays in a prenatal clinic. Am J Obs Gyn 1975; 123: 175
4. Daniel WA, Gaines EG, Bennet DL. Dietary intakes and plasma folate in healthy adolescents. Am J Clin Nutr 1975; 28: 363–370
5. Shorvon SD, Carney MWP, Chanarin I et al. The neuropsychiatry of megaloblastic anemia. Br Med J 1980; 281: 1036
6. Youinou PY, Garre MA, Menez JF et al. Folic acid deficiency and neutrophil dysfunction. Am J Med 1982; 73: 652
7. Shamberger RJ. Implications of chronic vitamin undernutrition. In: Bland J, ed. Medical applications of clinical nutrition. New Canaan, CN: Keats. 1983: p 262–263
8. Herbert V. Biochemical and hematological lesions in folic acid deficiency. Am J Clin Nutr 1967; 20: 562–569

9. Bills T, Spatz L. Neutrophilic hypersegmentation as an indicator of incipient folic acid deficiency. AJCP 1977; 68: 263–267
10. Wagner C. Present knowledge in nutrition. 5th edn. Washington, DC: Nutrition Foundation. 1984: p 342–346
11. Schrier GM: SL: Anemia: Production defects. In Dale DC, Federman DD: Scientific American Medicine. 1997; 5: III: 1–19
12. Hattersley PG, Engels JL. Neutrophilic hypersegmentation without macrocytic anemia. West J Med 1974; 121: 179–184
13. Herbert V. Studies of folate deficiency in man. Proc R Soc Med 1964; 57: 377–384

CHAPTER CONTENTS

15

Food allergy testing

Stephen Barrie, ND

INTRODUCTION

The purpose of food allergy testing is to determine, in a reliable and reproducible manner, a patient's food sensitivities. When used in conjunction with a comprehensive history and food diary, the tests discussed here can help to determine what foods or chemicals an individual might be sensitive to.

Often, patients are unaware that they are sensitive to one or more foods because their reactions are either "masked" or "lost in the crowd". There are several well known immunological mediators of food sensitivity: IgE and IgG (immediate and delayed), and various immune complexes, as well as one or more unknown mechanisms of food allergy or food intolerance (see Ch. 51).[1,2]

There are two broad categories of applicable tests commonly used:

- laboratory methods that attempt to measure immune complex formation in a variety of ways (both in vitro and in vivo)
- experiential clinical tests which challenge the patient with suspected allergens while carefully monitoring for reactions.

LABORATORY METHODS

Enzyme linked immunosorbent assay (ELISA)

The ELISA is an in vitro test that requires serum from the patient (it is fully described in Ch. 10). This immunological procedure uses an enzyme bonding process to detect antibody levels and has been hailed as a "safe, economical, and highly sensitive test". It is currently the most popular method in use. The ELISA can measure IgE, IgG, IgG_4 and IgA antibodies, therefore identifying both immediate and delayed hypersensitivity reactions. In general, the ELISA method has replaced radioactive testing methods because it is less expensive and avoids the use and exposure to radioactive material, as used, for example, in RAST and RASP tests (discussed below).

In addition to the procedural advantages, one of the key advantages of the ELISA over other laboratory methods is its ability to measure IgG_4 antibodies. This subclass of antibody was initially thought to act as a blocking antibody, thereby exerting protective effects against allergy. However, it now appears that IgG_4 antibodies are actually involved in producing allergic symptoms.[3] For example, in a study in asthmatics it was demonstrated that asthma in these patients could be produced in response to inhaled antigens that did not bind to IgE antibodies, but did bind to IgG_4.[4] These results suggested that IgG_4 antibodies play a major role in atopic disease. In short, IgG_4 has been shown to act as an anaphylactic antibody, especially to food antigens.[5]

With regard to food allergy testing, it has been shown that the "combination of specific IgE and specific IgG_4 is a better correlate to positive food challenge than is skin testing alone".[6]

Radioallergosorbent test (RAST)

This is an in vitro test that requires serum from the patient. Suspected allergens are coupled to a solid matrix, followed by application of a sample of the patient's serum. If the patient's serum or plasma contains an antibody specific to the antigen, it will couple with the antigen, thus becoming attached to the solid matrix. A minute amount of radioactive-polyclonal antireaginic-antibody is then added. After incubation and subsequent washing, the residual radiation is measured to determine what percentage of the radioactive antibody became bound to the allergen-antibody solid matrix. The higher the radioactive bond, the greater the amount of reagenic antibody specific to the allergen tested is present in the patient's serum.[7]

The underlying assumption in this test is that a person without food sensitivity will have little or no food antigen specific antibodies in their blood. The RAST primarily measures immediate IgE-mediated sensitivities (i.e. type I reactions which occur in less than 1 hour). While traditional allergists believe that most food allergy is IgE-mediated, there is growing evidence that other immunological factors, especially IgG, may be considerably more important.[8–10] RAST seems to have better specificity and sensitivity for inhalants than for foods. Some studies have shown a poor correlation of RAST results with individual food challenge,[11] while others have demonstrated a positive correlation.[12]

RAST results are not influenced by B-receptor stimulants, ephedrine, antihistamines, or steroids, which can sometimes influence other tests (e.g. the skin scratch test). Results can be available within several days or up to several weeks, depending on where the laboratory is located (serum can be mailed without affecting the results). Many commercial laboratories offer the test, and it is availabile in kit form for in-office laboratories. Pharmacia was the first to market test kits for specific IgE (called Phadebas RAST). RAST results contain more false-negatives than false-positives.

A variant of this radioimmune assay (RIA) procedure is the enzyme immunoassay (EIA). In EIA, the same principles as in RIA are used. Using colorimetry or spectroscopy, EIA measures the enzyme broken off at the disulfide bridge on the anti-IgE to which the enzyme was tagged. Pharmacia offers EIA as Phadezym IgE (PRIST).

Radioallergosorbent procedure (RASP)

The RASP is a variant of the RAST, although it follows a slightly different protocol. It has been shown to have a higher degree of sensitivity and specificity for food allergens than the RAST.[9,11] In clinical practice, it appears to uncover a much higher degree of food allergy. Recent information suggests that the RASP may be measuring some IgG complexes in addition to IgE, which helps to explain the increased sensitivity.

Provocation-neutralization and serial dilution titration tests (P-N, S-D)

These controversial techniques are employed primarily by clinical ecologists. P-N testing is an in vivo technique which diagnoses a sensitivity by assessing the ability of a test dose to evoke symptoms and induce wheal growth. In the P-N method, 0.5 ml serial dilutions (in a 1:5 ratio) of each whole extract antigen dissolved in glycerin, phenol, or distilled water are administered intradermally.[13] The goals of this method are, first, to identify substances that provoke symptoms, and second, to discover which dilutions of those substances are appropriate for treatment (see Ch. 51).

Empirically, it has been found that certain dilutions of an offending substance will provoke, while other dilutions will relieve, various of the patient's characteristic symptoms during a 10 minute test period after each dilution.[14] The P-N method is applicable for a wide range of allergens – foods, pollens, dusts, molds, and chemicals.[15] In the P-N method, the neutralizing dose is a symptom-relieving dilution. Both stronger and weaker dilutions can provoke symptoms. Thus, the dose–response curve is often non-monotonic (i.e. biphasic). The P-N method may be used with wheal response alone, or in combination with symptom response.

A variant (especially useful in children) involves provocation through sublingual drops. With this approach, symptom provocation and neutralization are the only criteria for diagnosing sensitivities. Sublingual P-N is frequently used for testing food colorings and certain food chemicals, and is frequently effective for diagnosing sensitivities in hyperkinetic children.[16] While there have been both positive and negative studies, the P-N technique enjoys wide clinical use.[17–19] Due to its expense, patient time requirements (3 hours for four foods), and potential patient discomfort, the P-N is not a practical broad-screening technique for foods, except in special circumstances.

The serial dilution (S-D) technique is similar to the P-N technique. This titration method uses wheal changes alone to identify, and then neutralize, natural inhalants such as pollens, dusts, and molds.[20]

EAV acupuncture technique

The electroacupuncture diagnostic method utilizes a galvanometer designed to measure the skin's electrical activity at designated acupuncture points. Electroacupuncture, according to Voll (EAV), has been used in Europe for many years to determine the abnormalities or energy imbalances of the body. Proponents claim that allergy is a pathogenic and measurable entity. This controversial technique purports to measure both general allergic pathology and specific food sensitivity.[21] The patient holds a negative electrode in one hand, and the positive electrode probe is used to press selected acupuncture points. When a suspected food is placed on an aluminum tray which is connected into the circuit, certain galvanometer reading changes indicate sensitivity. If the appropriately diluted form of the extract is then placed on the tray, equilibrium of the reading should occur.

In order for this technique to gain wider acceptance, more research and clinical trials will have to be conducted, and a scientifically satisfactory explanation of its mode of operation will have to be developed.

Kinesiologic

Practitioners of applied kinesiology (AK) claim that kinesiologic muscle testing can diagnose food allergies. After either the patient has ingested a small amount of the antigen, or the antigen has been placed on the surface of the patient's body, certain of the muscles are tested kinesiologically for strength and weakness. This technique is widely used by AK practitioners (particularly chiropractors), and, if it is effective, does have the advantage of being inexpensive and fast.

More research needs to be done in order to confirm the limited clinical claims, and, as with the EVA technique, a satisfactory explanation of its mode of action must be developed.

EXPERIENTIAL CHALLENGE METHODS

Many physicians believe that oral food challenge is the definitive method ("gold standard") for diagnosing food sensitivities. Orthodox practitioners, clinical ecologists and naturopathic physicians agree that food challenge is an accurate and useful procedure when used with an appropriate patient. This is especially true considering research reports of food intolerance which is not detected by current immunological assessments.

For example, a recent study carefully evaluated antibody levels in four infants who had rice intolerance with symptoms which include shock, vomiting, diarrhea, and positive occult blood tests.[22] None of the immunologic tests was positive. All the symptoms disappeared during 6 weeks of a diet free of rice and flour. Histologic changes in the intestinal mucosa were noted after rice was reintroduced. This information is especially important since rice is commonly suggested as a component of an elimination diet in patients with food allergy.

When the relationship between ingestion of certain foods and resulting symptoms is unclear, the use of food challenge methods is warranted. There is, of course, a wide variety of protocols and indications among the physicians using these methods.

There are two broad categories of food provocation challenge testing:

- elimination or oligoantigenic diet, followed by food reintroduction
- pure water fast, followed by food challenge.

Food challenge may be performed in an open, single-blind, or double-blind manner.

Note. Food challenge testing should *not* be used in patients with symptoms that are potentially life threatening (such as airway constriction or other severe anaphylaxis).

Challenge/oligoantigenic diet method

The patient is placed on a limited diet; common foods are eliminated and replaced with either hypoallergenic and rarely eaten foods, or special hypoallergenic formulas (such as Vivonex).[23,24] The fewer the allergic foods, the greater the ease of establishing a diagnosis with an elimination diet. The patient stays on the limited diet for at least 1 week (up to 1 month). The first 4 days are considered the "cleansing period", with the GI tract being cleared of previously ingested foods, thus decreasing food sensitivity reactions. On the fifth or sixth day, symptoms due to food allergy usually disappear (if the food was eliminated), and the patient generally feels better. Care must be taken to ensure that suspected foods are not hidden in other foods and thus unknowingly consumed.

Beginning on day 7, individual foods are reintroduced according to some type of plan. Methods range from having the patient reintroduce only a single food every

2 days, to one every one or two meals. A careful record is made of any symptoms that may reappear.[25]

It can be useful to have patients track their wrist pulse during the trial, as it has been shown that pulse changes can occur in some people when a sensitive food is ingested.[26] During the cleansing period, the patient will typically develop an increased intolerance, or "hyper-reactivity", to sensitive foods. This explains why the reintroduction of foods may produce a more severe or recognizable symptom than before.

The challenge/elimination diet has proven clinically very useful in several studies. For example, one group of researchers studied 322 children under 1 year of age, 99% of whom had allergic rhinitis symptoms, while 85% had bronchial asthmatic symptoms.[27] The children, who were negative for inhalant skin tests, were placed on a 6 week hypoallergenic diet consisting of a meat-based formula: beef, carrots, broccoli, and apricots. Two hundred and ninety-two, or 91%, experienced improvement of respiratory symptom scores during the trial. Oral food challenge produced symptoms in 51% of the children. Milk, eggs, chocolate, soy, legumes, and cereals, in that order, were the most commonly offending foods. Only 6% of the children showed any evidence of food hypersensitivity 5 years later.

For patients with limited financial resources, as well as those with less severe health problems, elimination diets offer a viable means of detection. Because the patient can sometimes dramatically experience the effects of food reactions, motivation for therapy can be improved. The procedure is time-consuming and requires patient discipline and motivation.

Dietary fast with food challenge

A refinement which yields more results than the simple elimination diet is the 5 day water fast with subsequent challenge. Proponents of this approach believe that it is necessary for the patient to fast for at least 5 days in order to "clear" the body of all allergic responses.[28] This procedure can be performed on an outpatient basis, or in a hospital clinical ecology unit.[15] During the fast, patients are likely to experience "withdrawal" symptoms which will usually subside by the fourth day. As in the elimination diet, symptoms caused by food allergy will diminish or be eliminated after the fourth day.

After the 5 day fast, individual foods are singly reintroduced, with the patient monitoring symptoms and pulse. Due to the hyperreactive state, symptoms tend to be more acute and pronounced than before the fast. This method can produce dramatic results, greatly motivating the patient to follow whatever therapeutic procedures are appropriate.

This method is only advisable for people who are physically and mentally capable of a 5 day water fast. Close patient monitoring during the fast is a necessity.

Table 15.1 Advantages and disadvantages of the food allergy testing methodologies

Procedure	Advantages	Disadvantages
ELISA	Patient convenience Detects both IgE and IgG_4 Good sensitivity	Limited research substantiation
RAST	Patient convenience Good for inhalants Office kits available	Low sensitivity Expensive Detects IgE only
RASP	Patient convenience Good sensitivity	Expensive Not widely available Detects IgE and only some IgG
Skin prick	Widely available Good for inhalants	Poor sensitivity Inconvenient
Provocation	Good for chemicals Office procedure Aids therapy	Expensive Time-consuming
EAV acupuncture	Inexpensive Easily applied	No scientific basis Few clinical studies
Kinesiologic	Inexpensive Easily applied	No scientific basis Few clinical studies
Oligoantigenic	Sensitive to all types of food intolerance Inexpensive Improved patient motivation	Requires highly compliant patient Can be dangerous if severe reaction Susceptible to irrelevant events
Fast/challenge	Sensitive to all types of food intolerance Inexpensive Improved patient motivation	Requires highly compliant patient Can be dangerous if severe reaction Susceptible to irrelevant events

At times, careful interpretation of results is needed, due to the occurrence of delayed reactions.

SUMMARY

There is a wide variety of diagnostic food allergy test methods available. These procedures encompass a broad range of accuracy, sensitivity, specificity, patient economics, risk factors, suitability, and comfort, not to mention "medicophilosophical" paradigms. Table 15.1 summarizes the advantages and disadvantages of each methodology.

Each practitioner will have to develop his or her own operating plan, bearing in mind that different procedures are suitable in certain conditions and that new procedures are constantly being developed. No matter which methods are used, there is a wonderful cross-check for results: if the offending food is eliminated, the patient feels better; if it isn't, he/she doesn't!

REFERENCES

1. Galant SP, Bullock J, Frick OL. An immunological approach to the diagnosis of food sensitivity. Clin Allergy 1973; 3: 363–372
2. Todd S, Mackarness R. Allergy to food and chemicals. Investigation and treatment. Nurs Times 1978; 74: 506–510
3. AAAI Board of Directors. Measurement of specific and nonspecific IgG4 levels as diagnostic and prognostic tests for clinical allergy. J Allergy Clin Immunol 1995; 95: 652–654
4. Gwynn CM, Ingram J, Almousawi T et al. Bronchial provocation tests in atopic patients with allergen specific IgG4 antibodies. Lancet 1982; 1: 254–256
5. Shakib F, Brown HM, Phelps A et al. Study of IgG sub-class antibodies in patients with milk intolerance. Clin Allergy 1986; 16: 451–458
6. Rafei AE et al. Diagnostic value of IgG4 measurements in patients with food allergy. Annals Allergy 1989; 62: 94–99
7. Wide L. Clinical significance of measurement of reagenic (IgE) antibody by RAST. Clin All 1973; 3: 583–595
8. Perelmutter L. Non-IgE mediated atopic disease. Ann Allergy 1984; 52: 640–668
9. Hamburger R. Proceedings of the First International Symposium on Food Allergy, Vancouver, BC. 1982
10. Egger J, Carter CM, Wilson J et al. Are migraines food allergies? Lancet 1983; ii: 8355–8363
11. Wright JV, Moore R. Unpublished data.
12. Foucard T, Johansson S. Indications and Interpretations of RIST and RAST. Pediatrician 1976; 5: 228–236
13. Rinkel HJ. The diagnosis of food allergy. Arch Otolaryn 1964; 79: 71–79
14. Miller JB. Food allergy: provocative testing and injection therapy. IL: CC Thomas. 1972
15. Dickey LD, ed. Clinical ecology. IL: CC Thomas. 1976
16. Rapp DJ. Food allergy treatment for hyperkinesis. J Learning Dis 1979; 12: 608–616
17. Rapp DJ. Sublingual provocative food testing. Ann Allergy 1981; 46: 176
18. McGovern JJ, Rapp DJ et al. Reliability of provocative-neutralization procedure. (In press)
19. Breneman JC, Crook WC, Deamer W. Committee on provocative food testing. Ann Allergy 1973; 31: 375–383
20. Rinkel HJ. Inhalant allergy: the whealing response of the skin to serial dilution testing. Ann Allergy 1949; 7: 625–630
21. Tsuei JJ, Lehman CW et al. A food allergy study utilizing the EAV acupuncture technique. Am J Acupunc 1984; 12: 105–116
22. Cavataio F, Carroccio A, Montalto, Iacomo G. Isolated rice intolerance: clinical and immunologic characteristics in four infants. J Ped 1996; 128: 558–560
23. Dockhorn RJ, Smith TC. Use of a chemically defined hypoallergenic diet in the management of patients with suspected food allergy. Ann Allergy 1981; 47: 264–266
24. Rowe AH, Rowe A. Food allergy. Its manifestations and control and the elimination diets. IL: CC Thomas. 1972
25. Metcalfe D. Food hypersensitivity. J All Clin Imm 1984; 73: 749–761
26. Coca AF. Art of investigating pulse diet record in familial nonreagenic food allergy. Ann Allergy 1944; 2: 1
27. Ogle KA, Bullock JD. Children with allergic rhinitis and/or bronchial asthma treated with elimination diet: a five-year follow-up. Ann Allergy 1980; 44: 273–278
28. Rinkel HJ, Randolph T, Zeller M. Food allergy. IL: CC Thomas. 1951

CHAPTER CONTENTS

16

Functional assessment of liver phase I and II detoxification

Dan Lukaczer, ND

INTRODUCTION

The concept that toxins accumulate in the body and are the cause of various health problems has long been a fundamental tenet of traditional health care systems around the world. For centuries, societies have valued therapies which have promoted the idea of cleansing and detoxifying. From the simple water fast used since antiquity to the sometimes elaborate detoxifying regimens of spas, saunas, enemas, hydrotherapy treatments, and dietary modifications, detoxification as a therapeutic goal has long been pursued. In the late 20th century, as society has increasingly been exposed to toxic compounds in the air, water, and food, it has become apparent that an individual's ability to detoxify substances to which they are exposed is of critical importance in their overall health.

In any large population exposed to the same low levels of carcinogens, some individuals will develop cancer while others will not. The variability that one finds here and in other diseases appears to be associated, in part, with the individual's ability to detoxify various procarcinogens and other xenobiotics.[1] It is then not only the level of the toxin in the environment, but the individual's response that is significant. Until recently, science has had difficulty calculating and objectively analyzing the individual response to toxic compounds. New functional assessment tools have become available to the health professional which significantly enhance our understanding of interindividuality in detoxification. These tools allow clinicians to quantitatively analyze the body's ability adequately and properly to detoxify compounds to which it is exposed. In fact, new research suggests that the ability of the body to adequately transform toxic metabolites formed from both internal metabolism and external xenobiotic exposure may be related causally to various puzzling disease entities such as chronic fatigue syndrome, fibromyalgia, and multiple chemical sensitivities.[2] Research has also begun to validate the hypothesis that the dysfunction of the body's detoxification ability may underlie various chronic neurologic diseases such as Parkinson's and Alzheimer's.[3]

THE HEPATIC DETOXIFICATION SYSTEM

The process of conversion and excretion of toxic substances to non-toxic metabolites takes place at two major sites: the intestinal mucosal wall and, more significantly, the liver. There are two distinct phases in the biochemical processes related to detoxification. These two processes, traditionally known as phase I and phase II, chemically biotransform toxins into progressively more water-soluble, and hence excretable, substances, through a series of chemical reactions (see Fig. 16.1).

Phase I detoxification

The phase I reactions usually involve oxidation, reduction, or hydrolysis, the most important of which is performed by a family of enzymes commonly referred to as cytochrome P450 mixed function oxidases.[4] This system is actually a group of many isoenzymes which have specific affinity for differing substrates. They are responsible for beginning the process of detoxifying xenobiotics such as petrochemical hydrocarbons and medications, and endogenous substances such as steroid hormones and other end-products of metabolism, which would also be toxic if allowed to accumulate. In phase I, the biochemical reaction involves the adding or exposing of a functional group to the toxic molecule. In most cases, this biotransformation allows the phase I compound to undergo phase II conjugation reactions. In some cases, the compound may be eliminated directly after the phase I reaction.[5]

As is evident in Figure 16.1, a significant consequence of this biotransformation is the increase in oxidant stress and free radical generation.

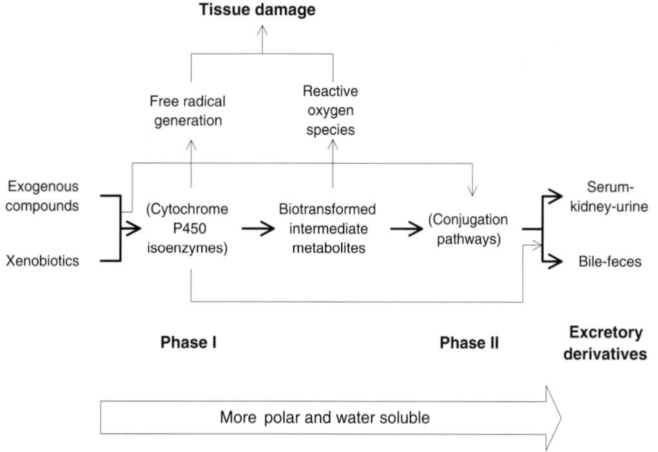

Figure 16.1 The major hepatic detoxification pathways.

Phase II

In the more common scenario, the phase I reaction produces an intermediate to be further transformed by phase II conjugation. This intermediate step in the process of transforming toxins to excretable harmless metabolites is referred to as "bioactivation". These biotransformed intermediates can be highly reactive and are, in fact, often more toxic than the original compound. Because of this, the more promptly and efficiently these metabolites are acted upon by the phase II reactions, the less tissue damage will occur. Therefore, of fundamental importance in detoxification is the balance of activities between the phase I and phase II processes. If phase II reactions are inhibited in some way, or if phase I has been up-regulated without a concomitant increase in phase II, that optimal balance is compromised.

Whereas the primary phase I reactions are a family of isoenzymes, phase II reactions, in which various biotransformed molecules are conjugated, are distinct reactions. The main conjugation reactions are glucuronidation, amino acid conjugation, sulfation, glutathione conjugation, acetylation, and methylation.[6] These conjugation reactions involve the addition of a molecule to the intermediate metabolite to further increase its hydrophilic qualities, allowing for final elimination in the urine or bile.[7]

PROCEDURE

In assessing the liver's detoxification ability, one is evaluating the functional capacity of this organ system. Measuring functional capacity and performance of an organ system is not new. Exercise EKG and the oral glucose tolerance tests are two examples in which the functional capacity, and therefore organ reserve, is appraised. Assessment of the activity of hepatic detoxifying systems is a new example of this challenge method. These tests differ substantially from the normal liver tests found in most panels, such as SGOT, GGPT, and SGPT. Those tests measure liver pathology, not liver metabolic function.[8] Elevation in the serum of these enzymes occurs as a consequence of necrosis of hepatic tissue. Functional liver testing, on the other hand, measures the detoxifying ability of the liver when challenged with a test substance. These tests allow assessment of the metabolic capacity of the liver, and thus provide a window to an individual's facility to adequately deal with his or her environment.

Laboratory assessment of the liver's detoxifying ability has been extensively studied.[9] To evaluate the various metabolic pathways of detoxification discussed above, probe substances, whose detoxification pathways are well established, are ingested, and their metabolites are measured in the urine, blood, or saliva.

Phase I assessment

Research over the past 20 years has shown that caffeine is a model substance for testing the phase I P-450 system.[10] A measured amount of caffeine is ingested, and then timed saliva samples are taken over the next 8 hours. Caffeine is almost completely absorbed by the intestine and is metabolized in the liver primarily by the isoenzyme P-4501A2. (To date, at least 20 different P450 isoenzymes have been identified.[11]) Its rate of clearance, as measured in saliva, has proven to be an ideal non-invasive way to assess activity of this P450 enzyme.[12,13] Genetics, nutrition,[14–16] medications,[17] and environmental factors[18,19] such as alcohol, heavy metals, and smoking can all influence the inducibility of this enzyme system.[20] Elevation or depression of the rate of caffeine clearance suggests up- or downregulation. Dietary elimination of caffeine-containing foods and medications is instituted 24 hours before the test.

Phase II assessment

As mentioned above, phase II reactions involve a number of distinct conjugating substances. The most important appear to be glycine conjugation, glutathione conjugation, glucuronidation, and sulfation. To accurately assess these pathways, two additional probe substances – acetaminophen and either aspirin or sodium benzoate – have been employed. Acetaminophen is metabolized through three phase II pathways: glutathione conjugation, sulfation, and glucuronidation to form urinary acetaminophen mercaptuates, acetaminophen sulfate, and acetaminophen glucuronide, respectively (see Fig. 16.2).[21]

Aspirin is readily degraded into salicylic acid, which is eventually conjugated and metabolized through glycine conjugation and glucuronidation to form salicyluric acid and salicyl glucuronide, respectively.[22] Alternatively, in individuals with salicylate sensitivities, the common food preservative, sodium benzoate, can be used to assess phase II glycine conjugation.[23] Either way, the metabolites are then measured in the urine.

These probe markers therefore serve as useful, well researched challenge substances for the functional evaluation of four important phase II detoxification pathways.[24] As with the caffeine challenge above, foods and medications containing aspirin, acetaminophen and sodium benzoate are eliminated 24 hours prior to the test.

Alternative pathways

Using these probe substances, one is provided with a tool for assessing the body's detoxification capacity which gives the clinician insight into the unique sensitivities the patient may have to his or her environment. For most toxins in need of detoxification, multiple pathways are utilized. Under optimal conditions, there is a particular affinity of a xenobiotic for a particular pathway.

When a pathway is underdeveloped, saturated, or bottlenecked, other pathways will be utilized in the metabolism of toxins. However, the alternative pathway may be less desirable because of incomplete detoxification or accumulation of toxic intermediates. A good example of this is the metabolism of acetaminophen. The usual pathways for this compound are primarily glucuronidation and sulfation. If these pathways are inhibited or depleted, an alternative pathway is through glutathione conjugation after acetaminophen is biotransformed by the phase I pathway. This biotransformed intermediate, *N*-acetyl-p-benzoquinoneimine (NAPQI), is a highly neurotoxic substance and, if not rapidly cleared by glutathione conjugation, can result in severe toxicity.[25] Not only are the sufficiencies of the various individual pathways of importance, but the relative balance of phase I and phase II detoxification is critical, as this determines the longevity of the biotransformed intermediates.

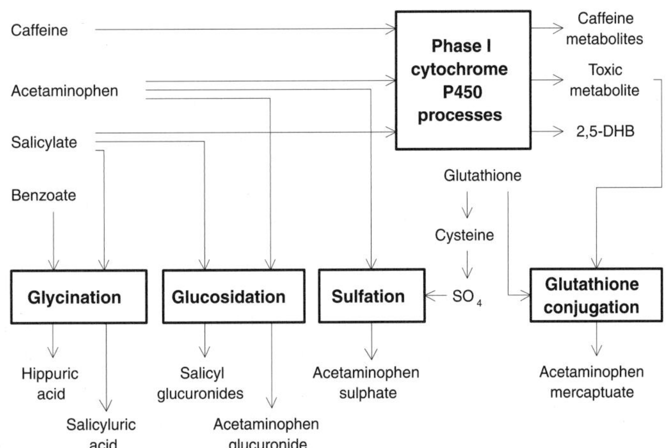

Figure 16.2 Degradation of acetaminophen and other probe substances.

Table 16.1 Interpretation of phase I and II marker excretion rates

Result	Interpretation	Possible causes	Possible consequences
Low caffeine clearance	Impaired phase I	Drugs (e.g. antihistamines, benzodiazapine antidepressants, amphetamines, H_2 blockers, isoniazid, oral contraceptives), deficiency (e.g. copper, magnesium, zinc or vitamin C), grapefruit juice, aging, spice curcumin	Increased susceptibility to toxins
High caffeine clearance	Overactive phase I	Drugs (alcohol, nicotine, phenobarbital, sulfonamides, steroids), heavy toxin exposure, charcoal broiled meats, herb sassafras	Excessive production of activated intermediates, increasing their potential for toxicity and carcinogenesis Depleted glutathione
Low salicyluric acid	Impaired phase II glycine congugation	Deficiency of glycine, low-protein diet	Increased susceptibility to toxins
Low acetaminophen mercaptuates	Impaired phase II glutathione conjugation	Deficiency (glutathione, vitamins B_2, B_6, selenium, zinc), excessive exposure to toxins, fasting	Poor detoxification of acetaminophen, nicotine from cigarette smoke, organophosphates, epoxides
Low acetaminophen sulfate	Impaired phase II sulfation	Deficiency (cysteine, methionine or molybdenum), drugs (NSAIDs), tartrazine, diet low in sulfur compounds (e.g. egg yolks, peppers, garlic, onions)	Increased susceptibility to neurotoxins, poor detoxification of neurotransmitters, estrogen, aniline dyes, coumarin, acetaminophen, methyl-dopa, increased risk of Parkinson's disease, Alzheimer's disease and rheumatoid arthritis
Low acetaminophen glucuronide	Impaired phase II glucuronidation	Deficiency (glucuronic acid), drugs (aspirin, probenecid), excessive oxidative stress	Poor detoxification of acetaminophen, morphine, diazepam, digitalis

INTERPRETATION

Table 16.1 lists the interpretation, possible causes, and possible consequences of the abnormal rates of phase I and II detoxification. As genetic variability affects all the detoxification pathways, it is not listed as a possible cause.

CLINICAL APPLICATIONS

Over the past 10 years, extensive research into the detoxification ability of the individual has resulted in the continuing evolution of our understanding.[26,27] Sluggish, imbalanced or impaired detoxification systems can result in the accumulation and deposition of metabolic toxins, increased free radical production and its ensuing pathology, and impairment of oxidative phosphorylation and consequent reduced energy production. Substances that upregulate phase I, such as alcohol, smoking, and certain medications, can have a deleterious effect upon this balance, because the phase II pathways may be unable to keep up with the demand. Conversely, various medications such as antidepressants (e.g. Prozac), oral birth control pills, and H_2 blockers (e.g. Tagamet) may inhibit phase I. This may also create problems, as endogenous and exogenous toxins may go unchanged and therefore lead to toxic reactions.

Cancer

The relative detoxification ability in an individual plays an important role in the toxicity or carcinogenicity of a specific substance. Upregulation of various P450 isoenzymes may be detrimental, as most chemical carcinogens are not capable of causing genetic damage by themselves, but require activation to electrophilic species.[28] For example, it has been shown that the risk for hepatic carcinoma is associated with the degree or activity of a particular isoenzyme of the cytochrome P450 system.[29] Elsewhere, it was shown that evaluations of detoxification rates were predictive of bladder cancer incidence when other factors were held constant.[30] Individuals with a high inducibility phenotype for P4501A1 appear to have a higher risk for cancer, regardless of exposure to smoking or other known carcinogens.[31] As the majority of all cancers can be related to environmental exposure or dietary intake, it is apparent that individual detoxification ability can be an important factor for their development.[32]

Gilbert's syndrome

Variability of detoxification may be involved in diseases previously thought to be benign. Gilbert's syndrome (GS), thought to be a condition with little morbidity, is a genetically induced, nutritionally exacerbated metabolic disorder determined to be caused by a deficit in the glucuronosyl transferase enzyme which catalyzes the phase II conjugation step of glucuronidation.[33] Recently, however, it has been seen that GS can predispose people to the bioactivation, and potentially the toxicity, of drugs for which glucuronidation constitutes a major, alternate pathway of elimination.[34] There is some evidence that nutritional support in GS patients improves a wide variety of symptomatology which previously had not been associated with this disorder.[35] Although further research is in order, this line of inquiry may open up a window to exploring how other detoxification "defects" may impinge upon health.

Chronic fatigue immunodeficiency syndrome

Current research on the etiology of chronic fatigue immunodeficiency syndrome (CFIDS) suggests that there may be a relationship between impairment in detoxifying pathways and symptomatology,[36] and that CFIDS may be a result of toxic exposure.[37] Correction of these imbalances and deficiencies has proven to be of significant benefit in alleviating some patients' symptoms.[38] A recent trial using nutritional modulation to support detoxifying pathways and a food elimination diet resulted in significant improvement in subjective symptom evaluation as well as objective improvement of phase I and II balance.[39]

Neurological diseases

Detoxification has clinical implications for chronic degenerative diseases as well. Research into the etiology of Parkinson's disease has discovered defects in patients' abilities to adequately metabolize sulfur-containing xenobiotics.[40] Altered detoxification, then, may render susceptible individuals at higher risk to neurotoxicity when exposed to sulfur-containing compounds.[41] A combination of genetic susceptibility, reduced detoxification capacity, and increased exposure to neurotoxins creates an increased risk of damage which, over the course of time, may lead to clinical disease. Connections with Alzheimer's and other motor neuron diseases have also been made.[42] Certainly genetic determination is but one factor and must be looked at in light of the strong support that has been found for the role of nutritional and environmental factors.[43]

Autoimmune disease

Emerging research is now showing a possible relationship role for altered hepatic detoxification ability in lupus erythematosus and rheumatoid arthritis.[44]

Endocrine disorders

As noted, various drugs or chemicals may have an inhibitory or stimulatory effect on the detoxification capacity. Because of this, other molecules detoxified through the same pathway may be slowed down or speeded up. For example, cigarette smoking upregulates certain phase I P450 isoenzymes. These same enzymes are involved in the detoxification of estrogen. As a consequence, it has been noted that serum estrogen levels are lower in women who smoke. This fact may in part explain the increased incidence of osteoporosis and menopausal symptoms in women smokers as compared with non-smokers.[45]

CONCLUSION

The consequences of defective drug metabolizing enzymes and pathways are varied. They may lead to:[46]

- functional overdose due to inefficient elimination of an active drug
- lack of efficacy due to inefficient activation of a drug
- idiosyncratic toxicity unrelated to the intended drug effect
- associations with apparently spontaneous diseases.

This opens up a huge field of inquiry to the identification and proper counseling of individuals, and dietary, environmental, or supplemental modification to take those biochemical individualities into account.

As we are increasingly exposed to higher levels of xenobiotics in the food we eat, the water we drink, and the air we breathe, as well as the increased endogenous load from faulty digestion, detoxification and our "detoxification personalities" will become increasingly important. Studies of detoxification function show that the enzymes that control the various phase I and phase II processes may vary significantly from person to person, with a wide variability in apparently healthy people.[47,48] There are numerous pharmacogenetic variants affecting drug disposition and which are manifested only upon drug or environmental challenge. This new understanding of detoxification brings us back full circle to a greater appreciation of Roger Williams' work some 40 years ago and his popularization of the term and concept of "biochemical individuality".[49] Differences among individual detoxification capacities based upon individual genetic disposition, environmental exposure and nutritional insufficiencies can have a profound effect upon susceptibility to a wide variety of diseases. Xenobiotics may act as immunotoxic agents, suggesting a biochemical connection between the immune, nervous, and hepatic detoxification systems.[50] The intriguing question is how many diseases we now consider idiopathic, or disorders of unknown origin, may be linked to atypical detoxification reactions? Disordered detoxification may have wide-ranging impact upon hepatic, renal, cardiovascular, neurological, endocrine, and immune system function. Certainly, the complicated interrelationship among exposure to various substances, genetically determined detoxification pathways, alteration of the pathways by foods, drugs, and chemicals, and sensitivity of tissues to secondary metabolites from toxins play an under-recognized role in contributing to the appearance of many health problems.

Identifying slow, fast, or otherwise imbalanced steps in the individuals' detoxification pathways can be extremely important to the clinician. Laboratory assessment of hepatic detoxification gives the health professional more precise and definitive assessment tools, an ability to define an individual's unique metabolic detoxification capacity, and then the opportunity to tailor nutritional support and environmental factors to reduce symptoms associated with metabolic toxicity.

REFERENCES

1. Hoffman D, Lavoie E, Hecht S. Nicotine: A precursor for carcinogens. Cancer Lett 1985; 26: 67–75
2. Bland J, Barrager E, Reedy R, Bland K. A medical food-supplemented detoxification program in the management of chronic health problems. Alt Therapies 1995; 1: 62–71
3. Steventon G, Healfield M, Waring R, Williams A. Xenobiotic metabolism in Parkinson's disease. Neurology 1989; 39: 883–887
4. Grant D. Detoxification pathways in the liver. J Inher Metab Dis 1991; 14: 421–430
5. Timbrell J. Principles of biochemical toxicology. 2nd edn. London: Taylor and Francis. 1991
6. Murray R, Granner D, Mayes P, Rodwell V. Harper's biochemistry. Norwalk, Conn.: Appleton & Lange. 1990
7. Grant D. Detoxification pathways in the liver. J Inher Metab Dis 1991; 14: 421–430
8. Neuschwnader-Tetri BA. Common blood tests for liver disease. Which ones are most useful? Postgrad Med 1995; 98: 49–63
9. Quick AJ. The synthesis of hippuric acid: a new test of liver function. Am J Med Sci 1933; 185: 630–637
10. Setchel K, Welsh M, Klooster M et al. Rapid high-performance liquid chromatography assay for salivary and serum caffeine following an oral load – an indicator of liver function. J Chromatography 1987; 385: 267–274
11. Nebert D, Nelson D, Coon J et al. The P450 superfamily: update on new sequences, gene mapping, and recommended nomenclature. DNA Cell Biol 1991; 10: 1
12. Brockmoller J, Roots I. Assessment of liver metabolic function. Clin Pharmacokinet Concepts 1994; 27: 216–247
13. Jost G, Wahllander A, Von Mandach R, Preisig R. Overnight salivary caffeine clearance: a liver function test suitable for routine use. Hepatology 1987; 7: 338–344
14. Guengerich F. Effects of nutritive factors on metabolic processes involving bioactivation and detoxication of chemicals. Ann Rev Nutr 1984; 4: 207–231
15. Kall M, Clausen J. Dietary effect on mixed function P450 1A2 activity assayed by estimation of caffeine metabolism in man. Human Exp Toxicol 1995; 14: 801–807
16. Anderson K. Dietary regulation of cytochrome P450. Ann Rev Nutr 1991; 11: 141–167
17. Jaw S, Jeffery E. Interaction of caffeine with acetaminophen. Biochem Pharmacol 1993; 46: 493–501
18. Fulton B, Jeffery E. The temporal relationship between hepatic GSH loss, hemeoxygenase induction, and cytochrome P450 loss following intraperitoneal aluminum administration to mice. Toxicol Appl Pharmacol 1994; 127: 291–297
19. Lieber C. Alcohol, liver, and nutrition. J Am Coll of Nut 1991; 10: 602–632
20. Parsons W, Neims AH. Effect of smoking on caffeine clearance. Clin Pharmacol Ther 1978; 24: 40–45
21. Patel M, Tang B, Kalow W. Variability of acetaminophen metabolism in Caucasians and Orientals. Pharmacogenetics 1992; 2: 38–45
22. Hutt A, Caldwell J, Smith R. The metabolism of aspirin in man: a population study. Xenobiotica 1986; 16: 239–249
23. Quick AJ. A new test for evaluating liver detoxification. Am J Med Sci 1993; 185: 630–637
24. Patel M, Tang B, Kalow W. Variability of acetaminophen metabolism in Caucasians and Orientals. Pharmacogenetics 1992; 2: 38–45
25. Whitcomb DC, Block G. Association of acetaminophen hepatotoxicity with fasting and ethanol use. JAMA 1994; 272: 845–509
26. Davies M. Sulphoxidation and sulphation capacity in patients with primary biliary cirrhosis. J Hepatol 1995; 22: 551–560
27. Bradley H. Sulfate metabolism is abnormal in patients with rheumatoid arthritis. Confirmation by in vivo biochemical findings. J Rheumatol 1994; 21: 1192–1196
28. Miller E, Miller J. Searches for ultimate chemical carcinogens and their reactions with cellular macromolecules. Cancer 1981; 47: 2327
29. Agundez JA, Ledisma MC, Benitiz J. CYP2D6 genes and risk of liver cancer. Lancet 1995; 345(8953): 830–831
30. Talaska G, Tannenbaum SR, Vineis P et al. Genetically based N-acetyltransferase metabolic polymorphism and low-level environmental exposure to carcinogens. Nature 1994; 369: 154–156
31. Kawajiri K, Nakaji K, Imai K et al. Identification of genetically high risk individuals to lung cancer by DNA polymorphisms of the cytochrome P4501A1 gene. FEBS Lett 1990; 263: 131
32. Ketterer B, Harris JM, Talaska G et al. The human glutathione S-transferase supergene family, its polymorphism, and low level environmental exposure to carcinogens. Nature 1994; 369: 154–156
33. Black M, Billings B. Hepatic bilirubin UDP-glucuronyl transferase activity in liver disease and Gilbert's syndrome. New Engl J Med 1969; 280: 1266–1271
34. De Morais S, Uetecht J, Wells P. Decreased glucuronidation and increased bioactivation of acetaminophen in Gilbert's syndrome. Gastroenterology 1992; 102: 577–586
35. Lonsdale D. Gilbert's disease: symptomatic response to nutritional supplementation in ten patients. J Nutr Med 1992; 3: 319–324
36. Rigden D, Brailey JA, Bland J. Nutritional upregulation of hepatic detoxification enzymes. J Appl Nutr 1992; 44: 2–15
37. Buist RA. Chronic fatigue syndrome and chemical overload. Int Clin Nutr Rev 1988; 8: 173–175
38. Rigden, S. Entero-hepatic resuscitation program for CFIDS. The CFIDS Chronicle 1995; Spring: 46–49
39. Bland J, Barrager E, Reedy RG, Bland K. A medical food supplemented detoxification program in the management of chronic health problems Alt Therapies 1995; Nov 1: 562–571
40. Steventon GB, Heafield MT, Waring RH, Williams AC. Xenobiotic metabolism in Parkinson's disease. Neurology 1989; 39: 883–887
41. Heafield MT, Fearn S, Steventon GB et al. Plasma cysteine and sulphate levels in patients with motor neurone, Parkinson's and Alzheimer's disease. Neurosci Lett 1990; 110: 216–220
42. Steventon GB, Heafield MTE, Waring RH et al. Xenobiotic metabolism in Alzheimer's disease. Neurology 1990; 40: 1095–1098
43. Wi JM. Carcinogen hemoglobin adducts, urinary mutagenicity, and metabolic phenotype in active and passive cigarette smokers. J Natl Cancer Inst 1991; 83: 963
44. McKinnon RA, Nebert DW. Possible role of cytochromes P450 in lupus erythematosus and related disorders. Lupus 1994; 3: 473–478
45. Michnovicz J. Environmental modulation of oestrogen metabolism in humans. Int Clin Nutr Rev 1987; 7: 169–173
46. Meyer U, Zanger U, Grant D et al. Genetic polymorphisms of drug metabolism. Adv Drug Res 1990; 19: 197–241
47. Temelli A, Mogavero S, Giulianotti PC et al. Conjugation of benzoic acid with glycine in human liver and kidney: a study on the interindividual variability. Xenobiotica 1993; 23: 1427–1433
48. Meyer U, Zanger U, Grant D et al. Genetic polymorphisms of drug metabolism. Adv Drug Res 1990; 19: 197–241
49. Williams RJ. Biochemical individuality: the basis of the genetrotropic concept. New York: John Wiley. 1956
50. Goldin F, Tatnayaka ID. Acetaminophen and macrophage activation. Int Hepato Comms 1995; 4: 16–18

CHAPTER CONTENTS

17

Hair mineral analysis

Steve Austin, ND

Nick Soloway, LMT DC LAc

INTRODUCTION

Despite several research studies since the original publication of this chapter in 1985, there has been little change in the *diagnostic* value of hair analysis (HA). Outside its accepted use for diagnosis of heavy metal toxicity (see Ch. 18), HA still has, at this time, only limited clinical application.

In recent years, several attempts have been made to standardize hair analysis testing techniques[1] and broaden the non-specific screening uses for which HA may be employed. However, its accepted use is still only in testing for heavy metal contamination.

Many conditions and diseases have been tested for abnormal HA patterns, and, indeed, a number have been shown to have patterns differing significantly from the norm, including, among others:

- learning disabilities[2,3]
- birth defects[4]
- hyperactivity[5,6]
- Down's syndrome[7,8]
- neurosis and psychosis[9]
- senile dementia[10]
- autism[11]
- alopecia areata[12]
- insulin-dependent diabetes mellitus[13,14]
- cystic fibrosis[15]
- beta-thalassemia.[16]

More recently, HA has been used successfully to test for drug abuse,[17,18] although the indices measured (drug metabolites) are not found on most commercial hair analyses.

In a few of the above-mentioned conditions, HA appears to offer real potential as a diagnostic tool. For example, the high hair sodium in infants with cystic fibrosis shows very little overlap with controls, and one study demonstrated that children with learning disabilities can be diagnosed with 98% accuracy due to a consistent pattern of high hair cadmium, manganese and chromium, in conjunction with low lithium and cobalt.[2] As a result of this progress, the non-invasive nature of the procedure, its low cost, and the philosophical relevance of mineral balance, HA has remained popular with nutritionally oriented practitioners.

Hair analysis' usefulness as a research tool can hardly be questioned. Significant controversy exists, however, over the use of HA for the clinical diagnosis of diseases, other than heavy metal toxicity, and as an indicator of nutritional status. The difference between research and clinical use is a significant one. Whereas it may be of interest in a research setting that patients with various skin conditions have lower mean levels of hair magnesium than controls, the two groups overlap so much that the procedure is useless diagnostically.[12] Moreover, even when an altered HA pattern has been associated with a disease, there is generally no investigation as to whether mineral supplementation would affect the clinical condition or even revert the hair mineral pattern to normal.

Wide overlap of disease and control groups is frequently the case with HA, resulting in excessive false-positives and -negatives. For example, mentally retarded patients have been found to have lead, sodium, and potassium hair levels approximately twice those of controls,[7] but when we consider the enormous standard deviations (for sodium, 1644.71 ± 1814.93 vs. 744.43 ± 1987;[12] and for potassium, 870.15 ± 1009.19 vs. 408.35 ± 689.99), we again see a pattern of overlap greatly reducing the clinical use of HA. In addition, many of the altered HA patterns associated with the diseases listed above are as yet unconfirmed.

SPECIFIC MINERALS

Calcium and magnesium

The literature on hair levels of calcium and magnesium is surprisingly sparse. Low magnesium levels have been found in autistic children[11] and in patients with various skin disorders,[12] while high levels have been reported with dyslexia,[19] and Prader–Willi syndrome.[20] The significance of these data is unknown. Elevations in both calcium and magnesium were correlated with a low dietary Ca/P ratio in one study whose author suggested that this may be indicative of an induced hyperparathyroidism.[21] Although there was little overlap between the groups, once again large standard deviations mar the clinical usefulness of these results. Passwater & Cranton[22] reviewed the limited literature on hair magnesium and calcium, but few if any conclusions can be drawn.

There is little evidence to support the use of hair calcium and magnesium in clinical diagnosis at this time.

Chromium

Hair chromium is low in insulin-dependent diabetics,[14] although there is much overlap with normals. Hair and tissue chromium levels vary greatly during pregnancy, being very high during the first few months of normal pregnancy and subsequently decreasing.[23,24] Late in pregnancy, hair chromium typically becomes low,[25] suggesting deficiency.[17] However, high hair chromium in pregnancy is associated with low-birth-weight infants[26] and gestational diabetes. Increasing dietary chromium has been linked to increasing hair chromium,[27] while supplemental chromium does not seem to alter hair levels.[23,28]

Although normal and deficiency ranges need to be more clearly defined, hair chromium appears to have potential future use in clinical settings.

Copper

Oral contraceptive use is associated with decreased hair copper and increased serum copper.[29] High hair copper is associated with being female, lactation,[30] idiopathic scoliosis,[31] and pregnancy in some,[30] but not all,[32] studies.

Unfortunately, conditions which affect systemic copper status have been shown not to affect hair levels. Copper deficiency,[33] Wilson's disease,[34] and cirrhosis[35] do not significantly alter hair copper. Copper levels also vary with geographical location.[36] However, fur and liver copper have been found to correlate in rats,[35] and one study has reported that supplemental copper raises hair levels.[37]

At this time, hair copper appears unreliable for clinical application.[30]

Manganese

Levels of hair manganese in mothers of infants with congenital malformations and their offspring were significantly decreased in one study,[4] which may allow maternal hair levels to be used as an indicator of the risk of malformations. Altered levels of manganese were also found in epileptics,[38] although the difference was not significant. Hair manganese levels were elevated in violent behavior with varying levels of significance.[39,40] Evidence that manganese supplementation will affect behavior does not appear to exist at present.

Hair manganese may serve as a useful research tool in the study of altered behavior, but the most promising value of hair manganese may lie in the prediction of congenital malformations.

Selenium

Well water and hair selenium levels show good correlation.[41] High hair levels are seen in toxicity,[42] and low levels are seen in deficiency.[43] Tissue values reflect short-term variations in intake[36] and hair levels increase significantly after supplementation.[44]

As with chromium, insufficient data are now available to establish reliable norms and the incidence of false-positives and -negatives remains unknown. When these problems are resolved, hair selenium shows promise for clinical use.

Sodium and potassium

It is generally accepted, even by HA proponents, that hair sodium and potassium do not reflect dietary status.[45] Very high elevations of hair sodium may be diagnostic in cystic fibrosis,[15] but require confirmation. A relatively low Na/K ratio has been reported in celiac disease.[46] Although many HA advocates site low hair sodium and potassium as indicative of "adrenal exhaustion", the only (preliminary) study on the subject reported that hair sodium and potassium do not correlate with adrenal function.[47]

Except for cystic fibrosis, hair sodium and potassium appear to hold little promise for clinical use.

Zinc

Hair zinc levels have received more research attention than any other mineral. Low hair zinc has been associated with zinc deficiency,[48] anorexia nervosa,[49] hyperactivity,[6] gender,[50] age,[51] atherosclerosis,[52] beta-thalassemia,[16] vegetarianism,[53] short stature in childhood,[54,55,50] poverty,[56–58] and insulin-dependent diabetes mellitus.[13]

Because a few of these conditions have been associated with potential zinc deficiencies and supplemental zinc has been shown to increase hair zinc levels,[48,49,55,59] practitioners who use HA often rely on hair zinc as an indicator of zinc status.

Unfortunately, shampooing and dying affect hair zinc levels,[60] as does the sex of the subject[60–63] and hair growth rate. Malnourished children have shown both low,[57,64,65] and high[66] hair zinc. Poor correlations between hair zinc and height, weight and zinc consumption have also been reported.[37,61] Although very low hair zinc levels have been reported in patients with insulin-dependent diabetes mellitus,[59] there is, in general, considerable overlap between cases and controls.

At this time there is no definitive explanation or correlations for hair zinc levels. The speculative interpretation is that high hair zinc levels reflect acute deficiency while low levels indicate chronic deficiency, an hypothesis which has yet to be proven.

Drug abuse

Recently, HA has been used to detect drugs of abuse and their metabolites when urine tests were negative.[17] Hair analysis has been used as evidence in a court of law concerning past drug abuse.[18] Although there are concerns about the role of HA in testing for drug abuse,[67] HA does seem to be a valuable tool in drug screening. As mentioned above, drug metabolites and not mineral levels are measured in these trials.

Ratios

The experimental documentation for the majority of the ideal ratios that have been published by several HA companies has not been found. The Zn/Cu ratio has been reported to be altered in violent patients.[40] This ratio was also elevated in survivors of myocardial infarcts,[68] but the clinical significance is not known.

DISCUSSION

Hair mineral analysis is conceptually very enticing and potentially a valuable clinical tool. However, problems abound. Many variables affect the results (see Austin[69] for a comprehensive review):

- gender
- hair color
- cold waving
- bleaching
- exogenous contamination
- variations in mineral content within a given sample, etc.

This is further aggravated by the reporting of different results on the same sample from different laboratories.[70] The distribution of elements within the lipid and non-lipid portions of hair and the treatment of the sample prior to testing may explain the variance.[71] As noted above, dietary intakes do not necessarily correlate with hair levels; and hair color, sex, age, and other variables appear important for some minerals. Separate norms are only now being established and reviews of the literature attempting to establish reference values show a large variance in mean values, standard deviations and ranges.[36,72]

As a result of the gulf between available information on the one hand, and the clinical interest by some practitioners on the other, several articles have appeared decrying the misuses of HA.[73–75] Hambidge[74] says:

> There is a wide gulf between the limited and mainly tentative justification for their use on an individual basis and the current exploitation of multielement chemical analysis of human hair.

Klevay et al[76] acknowledge the experimental usefulness of HA but go on to say that "... its use in clinical medicine for diagnosis, prognosis, and therapy will remain limited until validation by the standard methods of clinical investigation is achieved".

Widespread use of speculative diagnostic procedures

invites condemnation, especially when the burden of these speculations falls on the pocketbook and psyche of the patient. HA is a valid and useful screening tool for toxic metal exposure (lead, mercury, cadmium, arsenic, and selenium). It has the potential of becoming a clinical tool of considerable use in other areas. Current abuse is perhaps as likely to hinder this development as to help it.

REFERENCES

1. Passwater RA, Cranton EM. Trace elements, hair analysis and nutrition. New Canaan, CT: Heats Publ. 1983: p 291–303
2. Pihl RO, Parkes M. Hair element content in learning disabled children. Science 1977; 198: 204
3. Marlowe M, Moon C. Hair aluminum concentration and nonadaptive classroom behavior. J Adv Med 1988; 1: 135–142
4. Saner G, Dagoglu T, Ozden T. Hair manganese concentration in newborns and their mothers. Am J Clin Nutr 1985; 41: 1042–1044
5. Barlow PJ. A pilot study on the metal levels in the hair of hyperactive children. Med Hypoth 1983; 11: 309
6. Barlow PJ, Grancois PE, Goldberg IJL et al. Trace metal abnormalities in long-stay hyperactive mentally handicapped children and agitated senile dements. J Royal Soc Med 1986; 79: 581–583
7. Marlowe M, Moon C, Erra J, Stellern J. Hair mineral content as a predictor of mental retardation. J Orthomol Physchiatr 1983; 12: 26
8. Sherstha KP, Carrera AE. Hair trace elements and mental retardation among children. Arch Environ Health 1988; 43: 396–399
9. Kracke K. Biochemical bases for behavior disorders in children. J Orthomol Psychiatr 1982; 11: 289
10. Vobecky J, Hontela S, Shapcott D, Vicbecky K. Hair and urine content in 20 hospitalized female psychogeriatric patients and mentally healthy controls. Nutr Rep Int 1980; 22: 49
11. Marlowe M, Cossaairt A, Stellern J, Errera J. Decreased magnesium in the hair of autistic children. J Orthomol Psychiatr 1984; 13: 117
12. Cotton DWK, Porters JE and Spruit D. Magnesium content of the hair in alopecia areata atopica. Dermatologica 1976; 152: 60
13. Amador M, Hermelo M, Flores P, Gonzalez A. Hair zinc concentrations in diabetic children. Lancet 1975; ii: 1146
14. Hambidge KM, Rodgerson DO, O'Brien D. Concentration of chromium in the hair of normal children and children with juvenile diabetes mellitus. Diabetes 1968; 17: 517
15. Kopito L, Elian E, Shwachman H. Sodium, potassium, calcium, and magnesium in hair from neonates with cystic fibrosis and in amniotic fluid from mothers of such children. Pediatrics 1972; 49: 620
16. Dogru U, Arcasoy A, Cavdar AO. Zinc levels of plasma, erythrocyte, hair and urine in homozygote beta-thalassemia. Acta Haemat 1979; 62: 41
17. Graham K, Koren G, Kleen J et al. Determination of gestational cocaine exposure by hair analysis. JAMA 1989; 262: 2238–3330
18. Strang J, Marsh A, DeSouza N. Hair analysis for drugs of abuse. Lancet 1990; 335: 740
19. Capel ID, Pinnock M, Dorrell HM et al. Comparisons of concentrations of some trace, bulk, and toxic metals in the hair of normal and dyslexic children. Clin Chem 1981; 27: 879
20. Marlowe M, Medieros D, Errera J, Medeiros LC. Hair minerals and diet of Prader-Willi syndrome youth. J Autism Dev Disorders 1987; 17: 365–374
21. Bland J. Dietary calcium, phosphorus and their relationships to bone formation and parathyroid activity. J John Bastyr Col Nat Med 1979; 1: 3
22. See note, reference 1, p 306–310
23. Hambidge KM, Franklin ML, Jacobs MA. Changes in hair chromium concentrations with increasing distances from hair roots. Am J Clin Nutr 1972; 25: 380
24. Aharoni A, Tesler B, Palfieli Y et al. Hair chromium content of women with gestational diabetes compared with nondiabetic pregnant women. Am J Clin Nutr 1992; 55: 104–107
25. Jeejeebhoy KN, Chu RC, Marliss EB et al. Chromium deficiency, glucose intolerance, and neuropathy reversed by chromium supplementation, in a patient receiving long-term total parenteral nutrition. Am J Clin Nutr 1984; 30: 373
26. Rowland A. Trace metals leave more than trace effects. Sci News 1984; 125: 373
27. Hunt AE, Allen KGD, Smith BA. Effect of chromium supplementation on hair chromium concentration and diabetic status. Fed Proc 1983; 24: 925
28. Hambidge KM, Franklin ML, Jacobs MA. Hair chromium concentration. effects of sample washing and external environment. Am J Clin Nutr 1972; 25: 384
29. Deeming SB, Weber CW. Hair analysis of trace minerals in human subjects as influenced by age, sex, and contraceptive drugs. Am J Clin Nutr 1978; 31: 1175
30. Klevey LM. Hair as a biopsy material. II. Assessment of copper nutriture. Am J Clin Nutr 1970; 23: 1194
31. Pratt WB, Phippen WG. Elevated hair copper levels in idiopathic scoliosis. Preliminary observations. Spine 1980; 5: 230–233
32. Vir SC, Love AHG, Thompson W. Serum and hair concentrations of copper during pregnancy. Am J Clin Nutr 1981; 34: 2383
33. Bradfield RB, Cordano A, Baertl J, Graham GG. Hair copper in copper deficiency. Lancet 1980; ii: 343
34. Mediros D, Sturniolo GC, Martin A et al. Trace elements in human hair. Lancet 1982; ii: 608
35. Epstein O, Boss MB, Lyon DB, Sherlock S. Hair copper in primary biliary cirrhosis. Am J Clin Nutr 1980; 33: 965
36. Iyengar V, Woittiea JL. Trace elements in human clinical specimens: evaluation of literature data to identify reference values. Clin Chem 1988; 34: 474–481
37. Jacob RA, Klevay LM, Logan GM. Hair as a biopsy material. V. Hair metal as an index of hepatic metal in rats: copper and zinc. Am J Clin Nutr 1978; 31: 477
38. Papavasiliou PS, Kutt H, Miller ST et al. Seizure disorders and trace metals: manganese tissue levels in treated epileptics. Neurol 1979; 29: 1466–1473
39. Gottschal LA, Rebello T, Buchsbaum MS et al. Abnormalities in the hair trace elements as indicators of aberrant behavior. Comp Psych 1991; 32: 229–237
40. Cromwell PF, Abadie BR, Stephens JT, Kyler M. Hair mineral analysis: biochemical imbalances and violent criminal behavior. Psych Rep 1989; 64: 259–266
41. Valentine, JL, Kang HK, Spivey GH. Selenium levels in human blood, urine, and hair in response to exposure via drinking water. Env Res 1978; 17: 347
42. Yank G, Wang S, Zhou R, Sun S. Endemic selenium intoxication of humans in China. Am J Clin Nutr 1983; 37: 872
43. Keshan Disease Research Group of the Chinese Academy of Medical Sciences, Beijing. Epidemiological studies on the etiologic relationships of selenium and Keshan disease. Chin Med J 1979; 92: 477
44. Gallagher ML, Webb P, Crounse R et al. Selenium levels in new growth hair and in whole blood during injections of a selenium supplement for six weeks. Nutr Res 1984; 4: 577–582
45. See note, reference 31, p 85
46. Maugh TH. Hair: a diagnostic tool to complement blood serum and urine. Science 1978; 202: 1271
47. Wright JV, Severtson RB. Observations on the interpretations of hair mineral analysis in human medicine. J Intl Acad Prev Med 1982; April: 13
48. Pekarek RS, Sandstead HH, Jacob RA, Barcome DF. Abnormal cellular immune responses during acquired zinc deficiency. Am J Clin Nutr 1979; 32: 1466
49. Ward NI. Assessment of zinc status and oral supplementation in anorexia nervosa. J Nutr Med 1990; 1: 171–177
50. Gibson RS, Heywood A, Yaman C et al. Growth in children from

the Wosera subdistrict, Papua New Guinea, in relation to zinc status. Am J Clin Nutr 1991; 53: 782–789
51. Bales CW, Greeland-Graves JH, Askey S et al. Zinc, magnesium, copper and protein concentrations in human saliva: age- and sex-related differences. Am J Clin Nutr 1990; 51: 462–469
52. Strain WH, Pories WJ. Zinc levels of hair as tools in zinc metabolism. In: Prasad A, ed. Zinc metabolism. Springfield, IL: CC Thomas. 1966: p 363
53. Greeland-Graves JH, Bodzy PW, Epright MA. Zinc status of vegetarians. AJ Am Dietet Assoc 1980; 77: 655
54. Bradfield RB, Hambridge KM. Problems with hair zinc status as an indicator of zinc status. Lancet 1980; i: 363
55. Anonymous. Zinc supplementation in healthy short children. Int Clin Nutr Rev 1984; 4: 28 (citing Ann Nutr Metabol 1983; 27: 214)
56. Hambidge KM, Walravens PA, Brown RM et al. Zinc nutrition of preschool children in the Denver Head Start program. Am J Clin Nutr 1976; 29: 734
57. Weber W, Nelson G, de Vaquera MV, Pearson PR. Trace elements in the hair of healthy and malnourished children. J Trop Peds 1990; 36: 230–234
58. Gibson RS, Smit Vanderkooy PD, McDonald CA et al. A growth limiting, mild zinc deficiency syndrome in some southern Ontario boys with low height percentiles. Am J Clin Nutr 1989; 49: 1266–1273
59. Greger JL, Geissler AH. Effects of zinc supplementation on taste acuity of the aged. Am J Clin Nutr 1978; 31: 633
60. Clanet P, DeAntonio SM, Katz SA, Scheiner DM. Effects of some cosmetics on copper and zinc concentrations in human scalp hair. Clin Chem 1982; 28: 2450
61. McKenzie JM. Content of zinc in serum, hair, and toenails of New Zealand adults. Am J Clin Nutr 1979; 32: 570
62. Heinersdorff N, Taylor TG. Content of zinc in the hair of school children. Arch Dis Childhood 1979; 54: 958
63. Smit Vanderkooy PD, Gibson R. Food consumption patterns of Canadian preschool children in relation to zinc and growth status. Am J Clin Nutr 1987; 45: 609–616
64. Weber CW, Pearson PB, Nelson GW. Mineral levels in hair of malnourished children. Fed Proc 1980; 39: 551
65. Saner G. Hair trace element concentration in patients with protein-energy malnutrition. Nutr Rep Int 1985; 32: 263–268
66. Ertan J, Arcasoy A, Cavdar AO, Cin S. Hair zinc levels in healthy and malnourished children. AM J Clin Nutr 1978; 31: 1172
67. Bailey DN. Drug screening in an unconventional matrix: hair analysis. JAMA 1989; 262: 3331
68. Bialkowsa M, Hoser A, Szostak WB et al. Hair zinc and copper concentrations in survivors of myocardial infarction. Ann Nutr Metab 1987; 31: 327–332
69. Austin S. Hair analysis: a reappraisal. NCNM Review 1982; 3: 21
70. Spilker BA, Maugh TH. How useful is hair analysis? J Energy Med 1980; 1: 15
71. Attar K, Abdel-Aal MA, Debayle P. Distribution of trace elements in the lipid and non lipid matter of hair. Clin Chem 1990; 36: 477–480
72. Taylor A. Usefulness of measurements of trace elements in hair. Ann Clin Biochem 1986; 23: 364–378
73. Rivlin RS. Misuse of hair analysis for nutritional assessment. Am J Med 1983; 75: 489
74. Hambidge KM. Hair analysis: worthless for vitamins, limited for minerals. Am J Clin Nutr 1982; 36: 943
75. Barrett S. Commercial hair analysis. JAMA 1985; 254: 101–145
76. Klevay L, Bistrian BR, Fleming RC, Neumann CG. Hair analysis in clinical and experimental medicine. Am J Clin Nutr 1987; 46: 233–236

CHAPTER CONTENTS

18

Heavy metal assessment

Stephen Barrie, ND

INTRODUCTION

With the enormous amounts of toxic metals in the environment, assessing patients for heavy metal exposure is increasingly important. Consequently, elemental analysis is one of the most rapidly advancing fields in medicine. Rapid development of new technologies and the attendant possibility for new exposure patterns are a practical concern for the astute physician. In this chapter, the status of hair, urine and blood elemental analysis for providing a precise gauge of element exposure is examined.

Although measuring blood and urine are the traditional element assessment tools, the significance of measuring element concentrations in scalp hair has now been studied for more than 30 years. While blood and urine reflect the body's dynamic equilibrium, hair acts as a depot and indicates element storage over time. Numerous studies correlate elements in hair with environmental exposure (such as to smelters and mines) and with disease and physiologic or pathologic effects. Additionally, geographic variation and historical trends in hair element levels have been published, and hair analysis is used in forensic medicine. Consequently, hair analysis provides a long-term record that reflects normal and abnormal metabolism, assimilation, and exposure.[1–3]

ASSESSMENT METHODOLOGIES

Each of the three tissues regularly used to assess heavy metal load has its advantages and disadvantages. Hair is perhaps the best sample to screen patients for suspected heavy metal toxicities. It provides good long-term exposure assessment, is non-invasive, inexpensive and allows for investigation of nutrient/toxic interactions. Urine shows what elements the body is currently excreting. It provides good qualitative information if a person has been recently exposed to a toxic element (days–weeks), and gives quantitative information of excreted elements before, during and after provocative challenge. Blood provides information about what the body has recently (hours–days, in some cases weeks) absorbed. This is largely independent of tissue deposition. Blood levels vary according to the actual component analyzed (plasma, serum, RBCs). They can be transient in nature, and are subject to the body's homeostatic mechanisms.

Hair analysis

Numerous papers have been published evaluating the accuracy and efficacy of hair testing, particularly for toxic metals.[4,5] The EPA published a study in 1979 in which more than 400 reports on hair testing were reviewed. The authors concluded that hair is a "meaningful and representative tissue for biological monitoring of most of the toxic metals".[6] Hair element testing is best viewed as a screen and shouldn't be used to diagnose the presence or absence of disease, but rather to monitor element imbalances and environmental toxicity. Follow-up blood testing or provocative urine testing is useful to confirm hair element findings.

To understand how hair retains elements, it is important to know the structure of hair and how hair protein is synthesized and traps minerals. The hair shaft is a filament formed from the matrix of cells at the bottom of the hair follicle deep in the epidermal epithelium. Each follicle is a miniature organ that contains both muscular and glandular components. Human hair is composed of 80% protein, 15% water, and small amounts of lipids and inorganic materials. The mineral content of the hair is 0.25–0.95% of dry ash.[7] Of the approximately 100,000 hairs in the average human scalp, 10% are in the resting phase. During the growth phase, the scalp follicles produce hair at a rate of 0.2–0.5 mm/day or about 1 cm each month.

The growing hair follicle is richly supplied with blood vessels, and the blood that bathes the follicle is the transport medium for both essential and potentially toxic elements. These elements are then incorporated into the growing hair protein. Unlike other body tissues, hair is a metabolic end-product that incorporates elements into its structure while growing. As hair approaches the skin surface, it undergoes a hardening process, or keratinization, and the elements accumulated during its formation are sealed into the protein structure of the hair. Thus, element concentrations of the hair reflect concentrations in other body tissues.

Hair has a long history in human and animal studies of revealing chronic exposure to toxic metals. Because hair is biologically stable, accurate assays can be performed, even on hair that is hundreds of years old. For instance, hair samples taken from Napoleon were tested for arsenic poisoning.[8] In recent years, hair screening for toxic elements such as lead, mercury, cadmium, and arsenic has received substantial scientific validation.

Environmental exposure to toxic metals may be infrequent and highly variable, and hair element concentrations are most meaningful when cumulative intake and exposure over time are the case.[9–11] Research suggests that hair metal content provides a better estimate for long-term risk when compared with blood metal levels.[12] Hair is an excellent medium because concentrations often are up to 300 times higher than those of serum or urine. Because hair stores these elements, it is a barometer of early, chronic exposure and often reflects excess exposure before symptoms appear.

Urine analysis

Urine element testing is currently receiving a considerable amount of research attention.[13,14] The urine is an appropriate sample to assess the excretion of potentially toxic elements, providing a window on levels retained in the body and duration of exposure. As astutely stated by one researcher of heavy metal exposure in Denmark, a reasonable example of developed countries: "... high-dose environmental or occupational trace element exposure rarely occurs and health risk assessment is mainly pertained to the health effects of long-term low-dose exposure."[13] Under certain conditions, urine samples are optimal to gauge the effects of long-term, low-dose type deposition of toxic elements.

Provocative testing can help to determine toxic element deposition and provide the clinician with clear therapeutic direction and accurate monitoring of treatment response. In this technique, a strong excretory inducer is administered to the patient after a pretreatment urine sample is obtained. After a given time frame, dependent upon the agent used and the analytical technique applied, a second urine sample is collected and the post-treatment excretion of elements calculated. This method allows sampling of the stored deposits of toxic elements which have been sequestered from the blood.

Blood analysis

Minerals can be stored in various tissues where they may cause damage or metabolic interference in the depot structures (e.g. kidney, bone, nerve tissue) without causing particularly elevated blood levels. Cadmium, for example, accumulates in the renal tubules where it eventually reaches a threshold above which it causes damage and the potential for hypertension. The blood levels reflect only the last 2–3 months of absorption, whereas urine elemental analysis shows cadmium storage, mostly from the kidneys. Since cadmium has a biological half-life in humans of greater than 10 years, the cumulative deposition of this element can be of significant concern.[15]

The ability of the blood to counter changes in element concentration keeps many toxic levels within a narrow range, unless under heavy exposure. This homeostatic response illustrates the effective clearance mechanisms in the blood, and largely explains why blood analysis is best used only for short-term exposure. Exploring the depot storage of toxic metals is better met by urine and hair testing.

TOXIC METALS

Toxic metals used in industrial processes have increased human exposure dramatically during the last 50 years. These toxins can lead to a variety of symptoms (see Ch. 37).

Toxic elements have detrimental effects, even at minute levels, but the effects vary with the mode and degree of exposure and with individual metabolism and detoxification. Mechanisms of toxicity are multiple and include:

- enzyme or cofactor inhibition
- enzyme potentiation
- disruption of membrane and other transport processes
- decreases in neuronal functioning or nerve conduction processes.

Some of these effects are synergistic among elements or with toxic chemicals. Studies confirm that toxic elements can directly influence behavior by impairing brain function, influencing neurotransmitter production and utilization, and altering metabolic processes. The gastrointestinal, neurological, cardiovascular and urological systems are particularly sensitive to heavy metal-induced impairment and dysfunction.

The level of toxicity of these elements and corresponding adverse effects vary among individuals. Chronic, subacute exposure may lead to subtle or overt long-term problems in selected individuals and is of particular concern in children. Lead and mercury, in particular, show deleterious effects in children, in part due to their high growth rates and low body mass. The toxic elements may impair various enzymatic and neurologic processes gradually and progressively.

Below are some relationships that have been made between toxic elements and various types of dysfunction. Since hair analysis often serves as an easily available and inexpensive screening procedure, most of the following discussion focuses on this tissue for toxic element evaluation.

Aluminum

Aluminum is ubiquitous, being the most prevalent element in the Earth's crust. Sources of exposure may include drinking water (especially from areas exposed to acid rain), aluminum cookware, and aluminum-containing medications such as antacids. Urine levels of aluminum are observed to be elevated in people with a history of antacid intake.[16] The estimated half-life of aluminum found in the urine is 7.5 hours; however, the excretion kinetics vary according to the form of aluminum to which the patient was exposed.[17]

A disturbing pattern of aluminum accumulation and interference with normal neurological function appears to be supported in the literature. Dyslexic children have been shown to have higher levels of aluminum in their hair compared with controls, and other behavioral difficulties in school also correlated with elevated levels of this element.[18,19] There are geographical links with Alzheimer's disease and high aluminum in drinking water. Elevated hair aluminum has been observed in Alzheimer's patients, and some Alzheimer's patients experience stabilization of their symptoms upon treatment with the aluminum-chelating agent desferioxamine. Amyotrophic lateral sclerosis, another neurodegenerative disease, may also be linked with aluminum content of water supplies.[20,21] Aluminum also can interfere with phosphate absorption leading to hypophosphatemia.

Antimony

Antimony accumulates in the hair of exposed workers and their children, with higher levels accumulating in the children's hair.[22] Local environmental pollution (i.e. via airborne particles from phosphorus fertilizer production and smelting processes) leads to these elevated hair levels.[23] The smaller body mass of children combined with greater accumulations of antimony is perhaps cause for concern regarding potential toxicities in areas of high exposure. Antimony salts have in the past been used for the treatment of a wide range of parasitic infections, but, because of high toxicity, are now only used for the treatment of leishmaniasis. Chronic industrial exposure results in:

- itching skin pustules
- bleeding gums
- conjunctivitis
- laryngitis
- headache
- weight loss
- anemia.

Arsenic

Arsenic toxicity has been recognized for centuries. This toxicity manifests in a number of ways including muscular weakness and sensorimotor polyneuropathy, and in subacute exposure may lead to macrocytosis, anemia, jaundice, brown cutaneous pigmentation, hyperkeratosis of palms and soles, and white transverse banding of nails (Mee's lines). Continuing research is discovering new disease associations. One study which evaluated bladder cancer mortality over a 5-year period in 26 counties in the US, found that bladder cancer was significantly higher in counties with documented arsenic exposure. There was a dose–response relation between inorganic arsenic exposure from drinking water and bladder cancer.[24] Another study found a strong, dose-dependent relationship between ischemic heart disease and arsenic exposure.[25] Hair arsenic shows significant correlation with intake.[26]

Cereals are a major source of arsenic during infancy, and changes in hair arsenic levels during infancy correspond to the introduction of cereals in the diet.[27] Disturbing sources of arsenic, and other heavy metals, are a few contaminated, or adulterated, Chinese and Ayurvedic herbal remedies. In one study, imported traditional Chinese herbal balls used for fever, rheumatism, apoplexy and cataracts showed an arsenic level of 0.1–36.6 mg/ball. The recommended dose of two herbal balls daily could theoretically provide a daily dose of 73 mg of arsenic.[28]

Barium

The insoluble form of this element, barium sulphate, is used as an X-ray contrast medium and is non-problematic. Absorbable barium salts (hydroxide, chloride, or carbonate) may occur in some pesticides.[29] Few studies relate barium levels in the hair to pathologic processes; however, one retrospective study indicated that high levels in the hair along with an elevated calcium/magnesium ratio correlated with myocardial infarction.[30]

Cadmium

Cadmium is another toxic metal with a long history of detrimental effects. Industrialization has brought much higher levels of cadmium into the environment as a result of zinc and lead smelting, as well as industrial waste exposure, plastics production, paints, antiseptics and fungicides, and cigarette smoking. Cadmium exposure has been associated with hypertension, and studies show that hair levels of hypertensives are higher than controls.[31] Hair cadmium has also been shown to be significantly and inversely related to the activity of erythrocyte Na^+/K^+ ATPase among a group of male smokers. This enzymatic inhibition by cadmium was noted at levels far below toxic levels and may provide additional insight into the link between hypertension and cadmium exposure.[32] Cadmium appears to inhibit sulfhydryl-containing enzymes so that relatively low doses depress levels of norepinephrine, serotonin and acetylcholine.[33] Hair analysis is useful for evaluating cadmium in smoker and non-smoker populations of industrially non-exposed urban and rural areas.[34] Smoking itself causes significant elevation of toxic element levels in hair, particularly cadmium, lead, and nickel.[35] The urine level of cadmium is also a good measure of body stores, particularly relating to the kidney.[36] As it has been established that renal toxicity occurs once a threshold is exceeded, measurement of urine levels is a clinically useful technique.[37]

Lead

Lead is the best-known example of health problems associated with chronic low-level toxic element exposure. Studies show that lead toxicity is associated with deficits in central nervous system functioning that can persist into young adulthood.[38] Hair lead and cadmium are correlated with both reduced intelligence scores and lowered school achievement scores.[39] A recent study with 277 first-grade children gave some indication of the profound effects of lead on learning and behavior. There was a highly significant ($P < 0.0001$) relationship between hair lead and children with a high deficit rating in teacher questionnaires relating to concentration and task completion.[40] One study on lead noted a sevenfold increase in failure to graduate from high school.[41] The accepted level for lead-engendered neurotoxicity in children has declined steadily over the past decade as more sophisticated studies have been conducted. Sources are primarily from leaded solder joints, lead-based paint, and inner city urban environment.

Mercury

No metabolic functions are known for which mercury is required. Mercury is considered to be toxic at any level in the body, and at high concentrations causes liver and kidney damage and neurological symptoms.[42] Symptoms of mercury poisoning include:

- salivation
- stomatitis
- diarrhea
- neurologic signs (trembling, dysarthria, ataxia, irritability)
- changes in mood and affect.

Interest has grown in the possible ill health effects of mercury liberated from dental amalgam fillings as well as the increased consumption of fish contaminated with mercury.[43,44] Another potentially significant source may be contaminated or adulterated Chinese and Ayurvedic herbal medicines. One disturbing study of imported traditional Chinese herbal balls used for fever, rheumatism, apoplexy, and cataracts showed a mercury content ranging from 7.8 to 621.3 mg. The recommended dose of two herbal balls daily could theoretically provide more than 1,200 mg of mercury. Chronic mercury sulfide poisoning from ethnic Ayurvedic remedies has also been documented.[28]

There is intriguing evidence correlating increased hair mercury levels with certain disease conditions.[45,46] For instance, chronic mercury ingestion may be a risk factor for cardiovascular disease. Recent data suggest that a high intake of mercury from non-fatty freshwater fish and the consequent accumulation of mercury in the body is associated with an increased risk of acute myocardial infarction, as well as death from cardiovascular disease in general. This increased risk has been proposed to be due to the promotion of lipid peroxidation by mercury.[47]

Collaborative evidence for this finding comes from a Finnish case-controlled study in which higher numbers of dental fillings in individuals were associated with an increased risk of acute myocardial infarction.[48] There is other support that mercury from dental fillings results in increasing body burden: scalp hair mercury levels of British dentists and dental hygienists were two to three times higher than those of the support staff.[49] A study of dentists, dental nurses, and assistants showed that the average elevation of urine mercury levels were significantly related to the number of amalgam fillings the subjects had.[50]

Both hair and urinary mercury have been associated significantly with elevated titers of immune complexes containing oxidized LDL.[51] This supports other evidence which shows that mercury can induce autoimmune disease in both humans and experimental animals.[52] Mercury from dental fillings may also be a factor in multiple sclerosis, as hair mercury was found to be significantly higher in MS subjects than in the non-MS controls.[53] The above studies support the utility of hair and urine mercury measurement in situations of dietary, dental or environmental exposure.

Nickel

Nickel accumulates with age and smoking, perhaps explaining why tissue levels are highest in patients who died of cardiovascular disease.[54,55] Hair appears to be an accurate medium for evaluation of total tissue burden of nickel. Findings of elevated IgG, IgA, and IgM, and decreased levels of IgE have been observed in patients with high hair levels.[56] Most exposure leading to elevated hair levels is via dust from nearby industries including electrometallurgical emissions.[57,58]

Given nickel's ability to cause contact dermatitis, and its observed perturbation of immunoglobulin levels, elevated hair levels may serve as a warning sign for immune dysfunction along with its potential as a helpful marker of cardiovascular risk.

Uranium

Increased exposure to uranium dust has long been associated with increased incidence of lung cancer.[59] Although there are no strong studies linking hair uranium with either cancer risk or radon exposure, hair levels (measuring U238) do correlate with environmental exposure to this element. The accumulation of uranium in the hair may be related to blood group, with types AB and B having a higher apparent affinity for the element.[60] In animal studies, a condition of low iron nutriture led to greater retention of uranium as evidenced by hair levels.[61]

Vanadium

Correlations between hair vanadium levels and bipolar disorder indicate that the elevated vanadium found among patients with active symptoms tends to normalize during recovery.[62] Vanadate is reported to inhibit Na/K ATPase. This effect is decreased by a number of psychotropic drugs used to treat bipolar disorders and depression which catalyze the vanadate–vanadyl reaction. This results in a less inhibitory impact on the enzyme system and clinical improvement.[63] Here we see a correlation between changing hair levels of an element and movement toward clinical recovery, an affirmation of homeodynamic response mechanisms at work.

CONCLUSION

Research during the past three decades suggests that the relationship between hair, blood and urine element concentrations and human health is an important and complex process. Variables of key clinical relevance include exposure sources, absorption dynamics and tissue distribution of the various essential and toxic elements. As our understanding of the sophisticated relationships among nutrient and toxic elements grows, so will the utility of tissue elemental analysis for diagnosis and treatment applications.

REFERENCES

1. Chattopadhyay A, Roberts T, Jarvis RE et al. Scalp hair as a monitor of community exposure to lead. Arch Environ Health 1977; 32: 226–236
2. Suzuki T, Yamamoto R. Organic mercury levels in human hair with and without storage for eleven years. Bull Environ Contam Toxicol 1982; 28: 186–188

3. Airey D. Mercury in human hair due to environment and diet. A review. Env Health Perspectives 1983; 52: 303–316
4. Suzuki T, Yamamoto R. Organic mercury levels in human hair with and without storage for eleven years. Bull Environ Contam Toxicol 1982; 28: 186–188
5. Airey D. Mercury in human hair due to environment and diet. A review. Env Health Perspectives 1983; 52: 303–316
6. US EPA-600/4-79–049, August 1979
7. Katz S, Chatt A. Hair analysis: applications in the biomedical and environmental sciences. New York: VCH Publishers. 1988
8. Smith H, Forshufvud S. Distribution of arsenic in Napoleon's hair. Nature 1962; 194: 725
9. Foo S, Khoo N, Heng A et al. Metals in hair as biological indices for exposure. Int Arch Occup Environ Health 1993; 65: S83–86
10. Petering H, Yeager D, Witherup S et al. Trace element content of hair. cadmium and lead of human hair. Arch Environ Health 1973; 27: 327–333
11. Cigna-Rossi L, Clemente G, Santaroni G. Studies on the trace element distribution in the diets and population of Italy. Reviews on Environmental Health 1979; 3: 19–42
12. Bax M. Lead and impaired abilities. Develop Med Child Neurol 1981; 23: 565–566
13. Poulson O, Christensen J et al. Trace element reference values in tissues from inhabitants of the European community V: review of trace elements in blood, serum and urine and critical evaluation of reference values for the Danish population. Sci Total Environ 1994; 141: 197–215
14. Hamilton E, Sabbioni E, Van der Venne M. Element references values in tissues from inhabitants of the European community VI: review of elements in blood, plasma and urine and a critical evaluation of reference values for the United Kingdom population. Sci Total Environ 1994; 158: 165–190
15. Lauwerys R, Bernard A, Roels HA et al. Cadmium exposure markers as predictors of nephrotoxic effects. Clin Chem 1994; 40: 1391–1394
16. Bensryd I, Hagstedt B et al. Effect of acid precipitation on retention and excretion of elements in man. Sci Total Environ 1994; 145: 81–102
17. Pierre R, Diebold F et al. Effect of different exposure compounds on urinary kinetics of aluminum and flouride in industrially exposed workers. Occup Environ Med 1995; 52: 396–403
18. Capel I, Pinnock M, Dorrell HM et al. Comparison of concentrations of some trace, bulk and toxic metals in the hair of normal and dyslexic children. Clin Chem 1981; 6: 879–881
19. Moon C, Marlow M. Hair-aluminum concentrations and children's classroom behavior. Biol Trace Elem Res 1986; 11: 5–12
20. Savory J, Wills M. Trace minerals. Essential nutrients or toxins. Clin Chem 1992; 38: 1565–1573
21. Akanle O, Spyrou N et al. Investigation of elemental models in senile demential and depressives using neutron activation analysis. J Radioanal Nucl Chem 1987; 113: 405–416
22. Rafel Y, Popove Y, Zakusilova RM et al. Antimony accumulations in the hair of various population groups. Ad Ravorkhr Kirg 1985; 5: 13–14
23. Volokh A, Gorbunov A, Gundorina SF et al. Phosphorus fertilizer production as a source of rare-earth elements pollution of the environment. Sci Totl Environ 1990; 95: 141–148
24. Hopenhayn-Rich C, Biggs ML, Fuchs A et al. Bladder cancer mortality associated with arsenic in drinking water in Argentina. Epidemiology 1996; 7: 117–124
25. Chen CJ, Chiiou HY, Chiang MH et al. Dose-response relationship between ischemic heart disease mortality and long-term arsenic exposure. Arterioscler, Throm Vasc Biol 1996; 16: 504–510
26. Valentine J, Kang HK, Spivey G et al. Arsenic levels in human blood, urine, and hair in response to exposure via drinking water. Env Res 1979; 20: 24–32
27. Gibson R, Gage L. Changes in hair arsenic levels in breast and bottle fed infants during the first year of infancy. The Science of the Total Environment 1982; 26: 33–40
28. Espinosa EC. Arsenic and mercury in traditional Chinese herbal balls. New Eng J Med 1995; 333: 803–804
29. Dreisbach R. Handbook of poisoning. Prevention, diagnosis and treatment. 11th edn. Los Angeles. Lange Medical Publishers. 1983: p 245
30. Smith B. Cardiovascular risk as related to an element pattern in the hair. Trace Elements in Med 1987; 3: 130–133
31. Vivoli G, Bergomi M et al. Interaction between cadmium and some biochemical parameters involved with human hypertension. Heavy Met Environ Int Conf 4th 1983; 1: 545–548
32. Hajem S, Hannaert P, Moreau T et al. Cadmium and membrane ion transport in a French urban male population. Bull Environ Contam Toxicol 1991; 47: 850–857
33. Sutherland D, Robinson G. Role of cyclic AMP in control of carbohydrate metabolism. Diabetes 1973; 18: 797–800
34. Chattopadhyay P, Joshi H C, Samaddar KR et al. Hair cadmium level of smoker and nonsmoker human volunteers in and around Calcutta city. Bull Environ Contam Toxicol 1990; 45: 177–180
35. Wolfsperger M, Hauser G, Gossler W et al. Heavy metals in human hair samples from Austria and Italy: influence of sex and smoking habits. Sci Total Environ 1994; 156: 235–242
36. Lauwerys R, Bernard AM, Roels HA et al. Cadmium: exposure markers as predictors of nephrotoxic effects. Clin Chem 1994; 40: 1391–1394
37. Jonnalagadda S, Rao PV. Toxicity, bioavailability and metal speciation. Comp Biochem Physiol C 1993; 106: 585–595
38. Minder B, Das E et al. Exposure to lead and specific attentional problems in schoolchildren. J Learn Disabil 1994; 27: 393
39. Thatcher R, Lester M, McAlaster R et al. Effects of low levels of cadmium and lead on cognitive functioning in children. Arch Environ Health 1982; 37: 159–166
40. Tuthill R. Hair lead levels related to children's classroom attention-deficit behavior. Arch Environ Health 1996; 51: 214–220
41. Needleman H, Schell A, Bellinger D et al. The long-term effects of exposure to low doses of lead in childhood. New Engl J Med 1990; 322: 83–88
42. Clarkson T. Mercury. an element of mystery. N Engl J Med 1990; 323: 1137–1139
43. Lorscheider F, Vimy M, Summers AO et al. Mercury exposure from "silver" tooth fillings: emerging evidence questions a traditional dental paradigm. FASEB J 1995; 9: 504–508
44. Shahristani H, Shihab K, Al-Haddad IK et al. Mercury in hair as an indicator of total body burden. Bulletin of the World Health Organization 1976; 53: 105–112
45. Hac E, Krechniak J. Mercury concentrations in hair exposed in vitro to mercury vapor. Biol Trace Elem Res 1993; 39: 109–115
46. Chang Y, Yeh C, Wang JD et al. Subclinical neurotoxicity of mercury vapor revealed by a multimodality evoked potential study of chloralkali workers. Am J Ind Med 1995; 27: 271–279
47. Salonen J, Seppanen K, Nyyssonen K et al. Intake of mercury from fish, lipid peroxidation, and the risk of myocardial infarction and coronary, cardiovascular, and any death in eastern Finnish men. Circulation 1995; 91: 645–655
48. Mattila K, Nieminen M, Valtonen V et al. Association between dental health and acute myocardial infarction. Br Med J 1989; 298: 779–781
49. Lenihan J, Smith H, Harvey W et al. Mercury hazards in dental practice. Br Dent J 1973; 135: 365–396
50. Zander D, Ewers U, Freier I et al. Mercury exposure of the population V. Mercury exposure of male dentists and dental aides. Zentralbl Hyg Umweltmed 1992; 4(Dec): 318–328
51. Salonen J. Intake of mercury from fish, lipid peroxidation, and the risk of myocardial infarction and coronary, cardiovascular, and any death in Finnish men. Circulation 1995; 91: 645–655
52. Bigazzi P. Autoimmunity and heavy metals. Lupus 1994; 3: 449–453
53. Siblerus R, Kienholz E. Evidence that mercury from silver dental fillings may be an etiological factor in multiple sclerosis. Sci Total Environ 1994; 142: 191–205
54. Vienna A, Capucci E, Wolfsperger H, Hauser G et al. Exposure of the population to nickel. Cesk Hyg 1985; 30: 383–388
55. Vienna A, Capucci E, Wolfsperger M et al. Heavy metal concentration of hair of students in Rome. Anthropol Anz 1995; 53: 27–32
56. Bencko V, Wagner V, Wagnerova M et al. Human exposure to nickel and cobalt: biological monitoring and immunological response. Environ Res 1986; 40: 399–410
57. Creason J, Hinners T, Bumgarner JE et al. Trace elements in hair

as related to exposure in metropolitan NY. Clin Chem 1975; 21: 603–612
58. Wang J, Yang W, Li S et al. Effects of air pollution on health of residents in vicinity of an electrometallurgical factory in Chengdu. HuasHsi I Ko Ta Hseuh Hseuh Pao (China) 1993; 24: 198–201
59. Alexson O. Experiences and concerns on lung and radon daughter exposure in mines and dwellings in Sweden. Z Erke Atmungsorgane 1983; 161: 232–239
60. Zhuk L, Kist A. Mapping technique based on elemental hair composition and data. In: Shrauzer G, ed. Biological trace element research. Clifton, NJ: Havana Press. 1990
61. Sullivan M, Ruemmler P. Absorption of 233 U, 237 Np, 238 Np, 241 Am, and 244 Cm from the gastrointestinal tracts of rats fed on iron deficient diet. Health Phys 1988; 54: 311–316
62. Naylor G, Smith A, Bryce-Smith D et al. Tissue vanadium levels in manic-depressive psychosis. Psychol Med 1984; 14: 767–772
63. Naylor, G. Vanadium and manic-depressive psychosis. Nutr Health 1984; 3: 79–85

CHAPTER CONTENTS

19

Heidelberg pH capsule gastric analysis

Stephen Barrie, ND

INTRODUCTION

Proper digestion is a prerequisite for optimum health, and incomplete or disordered digestion can be a major contributor in the development of many diseases. The problem is not only that ingestion of the best nutritional substances may be of little benefit when breakdown and assimilation are inadequate, but also that incompletely digested macromolecules can be inappropriately absorbed into the systemic circulation. This can lead to various immune complex deposition diseases, and this process is now theorized to be an integral part in the etiology of food allergies.

Adequate gastric HCl is also necessary for protection of the gastrointestinal tract from ingested pathogens and for the maintenance of proper bowel flora. A healthy flora is known to be important for proper immune function, vitamin absorption, and the prevention of opportunistic infections, such as *Candida albicans*, in the gut.

The Heidelberg gastric analysis technique was developed to measure the pH of the digestive tract and determine the acid secretory ability of the parietal cells. Its use of radiotelemetry allows the gathering of this important information in a convenient and accurate manner.

The Heidelberg pH capsule system had its origin over 30 years ago at Heidelberg University in Germany. In research sponsored by Telefunken, a West German electronics firm, the inventor H. G. Noeller studied gastric acidity in 10,000 people. Since then, over 100 studies have utilized the Heidelberg system to investigate various aspects of digestion.[1–7] Physicians and researchers now utilize this technique for measuring the pH of the digestive system.

PHYSIOLOGY OF DIGESTION IN THE STOMACH

The epithelium of the stomach contains many gastric

glands. These tubular glands consist of parietal, chief, and mucous cells. The antral portion of the stomach produces the digestive hormone gastrin whose release is stimulated by

- vagal nerve stimulation
- the physical bulk of the ingested food distending the stomach
- partially digested proteins.

After gastrin is absorbed into the bloodstream, it is carried to the gastric glands where it stimulates the parietal cells to produce hydrochloric acid and, to a lesser extent, the chief cells to produce digestive enzymes (such as pepsin and intrinsic factor). With adequate stimulation, the parietal cells increase their production of HCl by as much as eightfold.

When the pH of the stomach reaches about 2.0, the gastrin mechanism becomes blocked, and feedback causes the parietal cells to decrease production of HCl. This concentration of hydrogen ions (by a factor of 100,000) is a very energy-dependent process.

Dietary protein is composed of amino acids held together by peptide linkages. Pepsin A, the major gastric protease, cleaves these in the stomach and is most active at pH values of between 2.0 and 3.0. It is inactive at a pH of 5.0 and above. Consequently, in order to have any significant digestive effect in the stomach, the gastric juices must be acidic.

Trypsin (a protein-splitting enzyme secreted by the pancreas) completes the process, yielding amino acids and dipeptides. The biochemical messenger which stimulates this pancreatic secretion is the acidic bolus of food moving from the stomach into the duodenum.

PROCEDURE

Equipment

The Heidelberg system consists of the following equipment:

- Radiotelemetry capsule – a hard plastic capsule (about 2 cm long × 0.8 cm in diameter) which contains a miniature radio transmitter, a pH sensing device and a saline activated battery.
- Waistband antenna – receives the signal from the capsule and relays it to the receiver.
- Receiver/recorder – receives and translates the signal. The pH reading is displayed on a meter and recorded by a continuous printer for a permanent record. The receiver also contains a calibration probe used to calibrate each capsule with known pH 1.0 and 7.0 solutions.
- Heater block – maintains the calibrating solutions at 37°C.

Methods

There are two ways in which to conduct the test: the tethered capsule repeat challenge and the flow-through method. Each gives different information and has its advantages and disadvantages. For both procedures, the test begins after the patient has fasted (food and liquid) for 8 hours.

The tethered capsule repeat challenge

In this procedure, the capsule is tethered so that it remains in the stomach while the stomach is challenged by the ingestion of a saturated sodium bicarbonate solution ($NaHCO_3$, i.e. baking soda).[8] The challenge solution triggers a rise in stomach pH and a subsequent attempt by the parietal cells to re-establish appropriate acidity. The majority of people have a normal initial pH of between 1.0 to 2.3. Abnormalities of stomach secretions are usually found only after the stomach is challenged. (A more involved protocol can be found in Wright.[8])

The procedure is as follows:

1. The waistband antenna is fastened around the patient's waist and the receiver/recorder is turned on and calibrated.
2. The patient swallows the capsule, which is attached to a 1 m long, thin cotton thread (a small amount of distilled water is allowed). The pH reading typically starts at 7.0 and falls towards 1.0. After about 5 minutes, the capsule reaches the bottom of the stomach (which normally displays a pH of between 1 and 2) and the remaining thread is taped to the cheek in order to prevent movement of the capsule out of the stomach and into the intestine.
3. If the fasting pH is normal, the patient swallows the first challenge of 5 ml of the alkaline solution. Within 30 seconds, the pH will normally rise to 7.0 and the patient is asked to lie down on his/her left side (to keep the stomach contents in as long as possible).
4. If stomach function is normal and acid is secreted sufficiently in response to the alkali challenge, the pH returns to normal (between 1.0 and 2.0) within 20 minutes.
5. The challenge is repeated up to four times, as long as the response time is within 20 minutes.

Flow-through capsule

In this procedure, the capsule is not tethered to a thread and is allowed to move freely from the stomach into the duodenum and the rest of the small intestine. The proponents of this method claim that this allows measurement of the gastric emptying time and intestinal pH, both of which are important parameters.

INTERPRETATION

Results may be classified as normal, hypochlorhydria, achlorhydria, and hyperchlorhydria.

Normal. The patient successfully reacidifies after four challenges (see Fig. 19.1). No. 1 shows the capsule entering digestive tract; no. 2 shows the capsule reaching bottom of stomach and alkaline challenge occurring; and no. 3 shows a pH rise after swallow and subsequent reacidification within 20 minutes.

Hypochlorhydria. The patient requires more than 20 minutes to reacidify (see Fig. 19.2). No. 4 shows a pH of 1.0 being reached after 30 minutes. Note that on the third challenge, the pH comes back only to about 5.0.

Achlorhydria. The patient's stomach shows little acid secretion and is not able to secrete enough acid to bring the pH below 4.0, even on the first challenge (see Fig. 19.3). The pH remains at about 4.2 for almost 2 hours.

Hyperchlorhydria. The gastrogram would show extremely rapid reacidification (within 5 minutes) after each challenge.

Depending on specific curve components, some investigators believe that mucous quantity, fresh or chronic ulcers, and acute gastritis conditions can at times be identified.

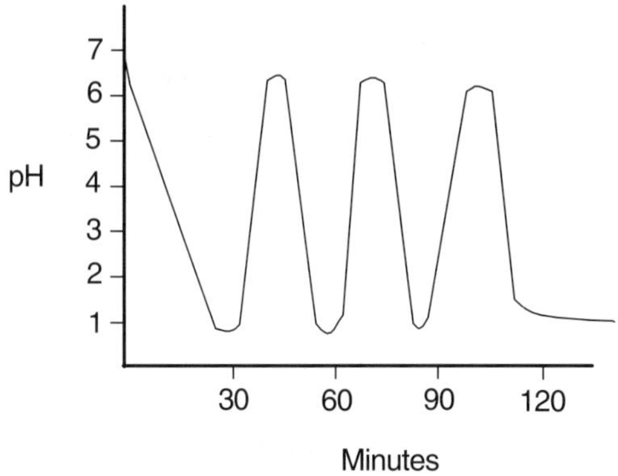

Figure 19.1 Normal Heidelberg gastrogram.

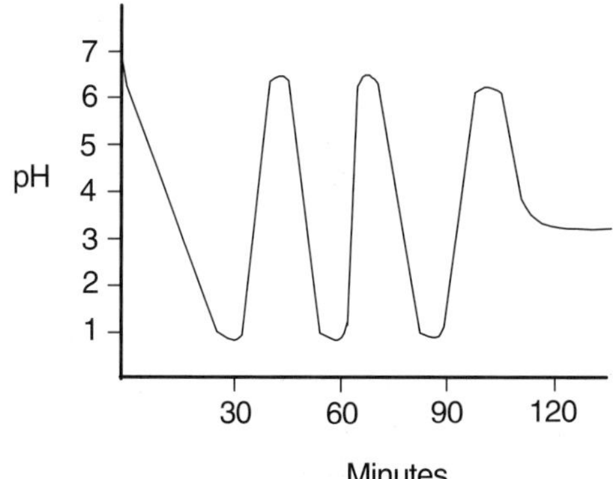

Figure 19.2 Hypochlorhydric gastrogram.

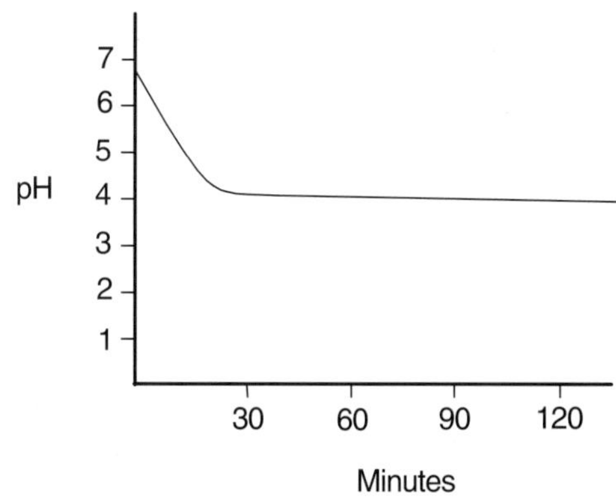

Figure 19.3 Achlorhydric gastrogram.

CLINICAL APPLICATION

Although much is said about hyperacidity conditions, probably more significant health problems are caused by hypochlorhydria and achlorhydria. Direct measurement of gastric acid secretion through intubation and aspiration is uncomfortable and unacceptable to many patients. The Heidelberg pH capsule system offers a convenient and accurate outpatient testing system to clinicians interested in evaluating gastric function.

Hydrochloric acid, pepsin and intrinsic factor are involved directly in digestion and contribute to the chemical changes in the intestines that assist in the absorption of many nutritional factors. For example, vitamin B_{12} absorption requires intrinsic factor, while zinc, calcium, and iron are poorly assimilated when gastric acidity is low.[9–11]

Indications

There are many symptoms and signs that suggest impaired acid secretory ability, and a number of specific diseases have been found to be associated with achlorhydria and hypochlorhydria (particularly HLA-B_8-related autoimmune diseases). These are listed in Tables 19.1, 19.2 and 19.3.

Aging

Numerous studies have shown that acid secretory ability decreases with age. Low stomach acidity has been found in over half of those over the age of 60.[24,25] One study of

Table 19.1 Common symptoms of low gastric acidity[12]

- Bloating, belching, burning, and flatulence immediately after meals
- A sense of "fullness" after eating
- Indigestion, diarrhea, or constipation
- Multiple food allergies
- Nausea after taking supplements
- Itching around the rectum

Table 19.2 Common signs of low gastric acidity[12]

- Weak, peeling and cracked fingernails
- Dilated capillaries in the cheeks and nose (in non-alcoholics)
- Post-adolescent acne
- Iron deficiency
- Chronic intestinal parasites or abnormal flora
- Undigested food in stool
- Chronic candidal infections
- Upper digestive tract gassiness

the elderly found that their tissue nutrient levels could be saturated only through the use of intramuscular supplementation; oral supplementation was ineffective. The authors speculated that this was due to atrophy of various digestive organs.[26]

CONCLUSION

The Heidelberg pH capsule system is an effective and convenient method to determine gastric acid secretory ability under conditions simulating ingestion of food. Results are extremely valuable in identifying the large number of people who have impaired secretion function. Ramifications of impaired acid secretion are widespread.

Table 19.3 Diseases associated with low gastric acidity[13–23]

- Addison's disease
- Asthma
- Celiac disease
- Dermatitis herpetiformis
- Diabetes mellitus
- Eczema
- Gall bladder disease
- Graves' disease
- Chronic autoimmune disorders
- Hepatitis
- Chronic hives
- Lupus erythematosus
- Myasthenia gravis
- Osteoporosis
- Pernicious anemia
- Psoriasis
- Rheumatoid arthritis
- Rosacea
- Sjögren's syndrome
- Thyrotoxicosis
- Hyper- and hypothyroidism
- Vitiligo

REFERENCES

1. Noeller HG. The use of a radiotransmitter capsule for the measurement of gastric pH. German Medical Monthly 1961; 6: 3
2. Noeller HG. Results of examinations of stomach functions with the endo-radio capsule - a new appliance for assisting stomach diagnosis. Fortschritte der Medizin 1962; 80: 351–363
3. Steinberg WJ, Mina FA, Pick PG. Heidelberg capsule. In vitro evaluation of a new instrument for measuring intragastric pH. J Pharm Sci 1965; 54: 772–778
4. Stavney LS, Hamilton T, Sircus W. Evaluation of the pH-sensitive telemetry capsule in the estimation of gastric secretory capacity. Am J Dig Dis 1966; 11: 10
5. Dabney R, Yarbrough I, McAlhany JC. Evaluation of the Heidelberg capsule method of tubeless gastric analysis. Am J Surgery 1969; 117: 185
6. Andres MR, Bingham JR. Tubeless gastric analysis with a radio-telemetry pill. CMA 1970; 102: 1087–1089
7. Mojaverian P, Ferguson RK, Vlasses PH et al. Estimation of gastric residence time of the Heidelberg capsule in humans. Gastroenterology 1985; 89: 392–397
8. Wright J. A proposal for standardized challenge testing of gastric acid secretory capacity using the Heidelberg capsule radiotelemetry system. J John Bastyr Col Nat Med 1979; 1(2): 3–11
9. Brewer GJ. Effect of intragastric ph on the absorption of oral zinc acetate and zinc oxide in young health volunteers. J Parent Ent Nutr 1995; 19: 393–397
10. Mahoney AW, Hendricks DG. Role of gastric acid in the utilization of dietary calcium by the rat. Nutr Metab 1974; 16: 375–382
11 Jacobs A, Rhodes J. Gastric factors influencing iron absorption in anaemic patients. Scan J Hemat 1967; 4: 105–110
12. Wright JV. Healing with nutrition. Emmaus, PA: Rodale Press. 1985
13. Howitz J, Schwartz M. Vitiligo, achlorhydria, and pernicious anemia. Lancet 1971; i: 1331–1334
14. Bray GW. The hypochlorhydria of asthma in childhood. Br Med J 1930; i: 181–197
15. Hosking DJ, Moody F, Stewart IM et al. Vagal impairment of gastric secretion in diabetic autonomic neuropathy. Br Med J 1975; i: 588–590
16. Rabinowitch IM. Achlorhydria and its clinical significance in diabetes mellitus. Am J Dig Dis 1949; 18: 322–333
17. Carper WM, Butler TJ, Kilby JO et al. Gallstones, gastric secretion and flatulent dyspepsia. Lancet 1967; i: 413–415
18. Rawls WB, Ancona VC. Chronic urticaria associated with hypochlorhydria or achlorhydria. Rev Gastroent 1950; Oct: 267–271
19. Gianella RA, Broitman SA, Zamcheck N. Influence of gastric acidity on bacterial and parasitic enteric infections. Ann Int Med 1973; 78: 271–276
20. De Witte TJ, Geerdink PJ, Lamers CB. Hypochlorhydria and hypergastrinaemia in rheumatoid arthritis. Ann Rheum Dis 1979; 38: 14–17
21. Ryle JA, Barber HW. Gastric analysis in acne rosacea. Lancet 1920; ii: 1195–1196
22. Ayres S. Gastric secretion in psoriasis, eczema and dermatitis herpetiformis. Arch Derm 1929; Jul: 854–859
23. Dotevall G, Walan A. Gastric secretion of acid and intrinsic factor in patients with hyper and hypothyroidism. Acta Med Scand 1969; 186: 529–533
24. Rafsky HA, Weingarten M. A study of the gastric secretory response in the aged. Gastroent 1946; May: 348–352
25. Davies D, James TG. An investigation into the gastric secretion of a hundred normal persons over the age of sixty. Brit J Med 1930; i: 1–14
26. Baker H, Frank O, Jaslow SP. Oral versus intramuscular vitamin supplementation for hypovitaminosis in the elderly. J Am Geriat Soc 1980; 48: 42–45

CHAPTER CONTENTS

20

Immune function assessment

Aristo Vojdani, PhD MT

INTRODUCTION

The human immune response is dependent on a diverse army of cells and molecules working in concert to protect the body against invaders. The ultimate target of all immune responses is an antigen, which is usually a foreign molecule from an invading microorganism or cancer cell. The immune system is composed of essentially two aspects: non-specific defenses, called cell-mediated immunity, and specific defenses, called humoral immunity.

Cell-mediated immunity, the first strike force, involves special white cells (typically T-cell lymphocytes and neutrophils) which immediately attack the invader and either prevent its entry into the body, or, if the invader manages to gain a foothold, quickly destroy it. Cell-mediated immunity is especially important in the body's ability to resist infection by yeasts (such as *Candida albicans*), fungi (such as athlete's foot), parasites (worms), and viruses (such as herpes simplex and Epstein–Barr). Cell-mediated immunity is also critical in protecting against the development of cancer and is commonly involved in allergic reactions.

Humoral immunity involves sensitized white cells and antibodies. Formed to uniquely match the surface of invaders, the humoral immunity team either damages them directly (sometimes by making them clump together) or alerts and activates other white cells to attack the pathogen. Although powerful, since these sensitized white cells and antibodies are tailored just to suit a specific invader, they take several days to develop.

Specialized antigen-presenting cells such as macrophages roam the body, ingesting the antigens they find and fragmenting them into antigenic peptides. This activates circulating T-cells that recognize the specific antigen. For a cell-mediated immune response to occur, antigen-specific T-cells must be stimulated. Interleukin-1, a product of activated macrophages, enhances this T-cell response. T-cell stimulation results in the clonal proliferation of helper T-cells, cytotoxic (killer) T-cells, suppressor T-cells and memory T-cells. When activated, T-cells produce and secrete a wide variety of immune chemicals, including interleukin-2, gamma-interferon and B-cell growth factors. These chemicals, known as cytokines, recruit and activate non-specific destructor cells such as natural killer (NK) cells, polymorphonuclear phagocytes (PMNs) and macrophages. Cytokines also stimulate the further growth and differentiation of T-cells and B-cells. In the presence of antigen and activated T-cells, B-cells will rapidly proliferate and differentiate into plasma cells. Plasma cells secrete antibody into the blood and lymph. The antibody binds to the antigen that stimulated its production. This response, also antigen-specific and known as humoral immunity, is shown in Figure 20.1.

Recent advances in immune function assessment

Unraveling the immune system's intricacies and finding better methods for diagnosing and treating its disorders are two of the most formidable challenges facing contemporary medicine. The best way to meet these challenges is through painstaking research that draws upon and combines the expertise of diverse disciplines. Only through leadership in research can a brighter future be anticipated by the estimated 65 million Americans with dysfunctional immune systems. Research into the immune system, how it functions and its relationship to health and disease, is therefore vital to identifying the cause and potential cure of the immunologically mediated diseases.

In the last several years, immunology as a section of the diagnostic clinical laboratory has increased in scope tremendously. New knowledge about cellular immunity, including lymphocyte subsets and advances in protein chemistry, bacteriology and cell biology has increased our understanding of human immunopathology and, at the same time, has made available clinically useful antigens and antibodies with great specificity and sensitivity. The developing technologies of monoclonal antibody production and genetic engineering have had tremendous impact on the quality of reagents available to the research and clinical laboratories.

Recognizing the need for research as well as the importance of education, the National Coalition on Immune System Disorders (NCISD) was established in 1987 to represent the millions of adults and children afflicted with immune system-related disorders and diseases. Since 1987, significant achievements in the field of immunology have been made which have contributed to the advancement of biomedical science. Based on these achievements, "our science is maturing, and the power of using the immune system for diagnosis and treatment of diseases is in place". Some of these developments of most interest are the ability to monitor T-helper 1, T-helper 2, T-suppressor 1, and T-suppressor 2 involvements in immune dysregulation, lymphokines and cytokines produced by these lymphocyte subsets, and the capability

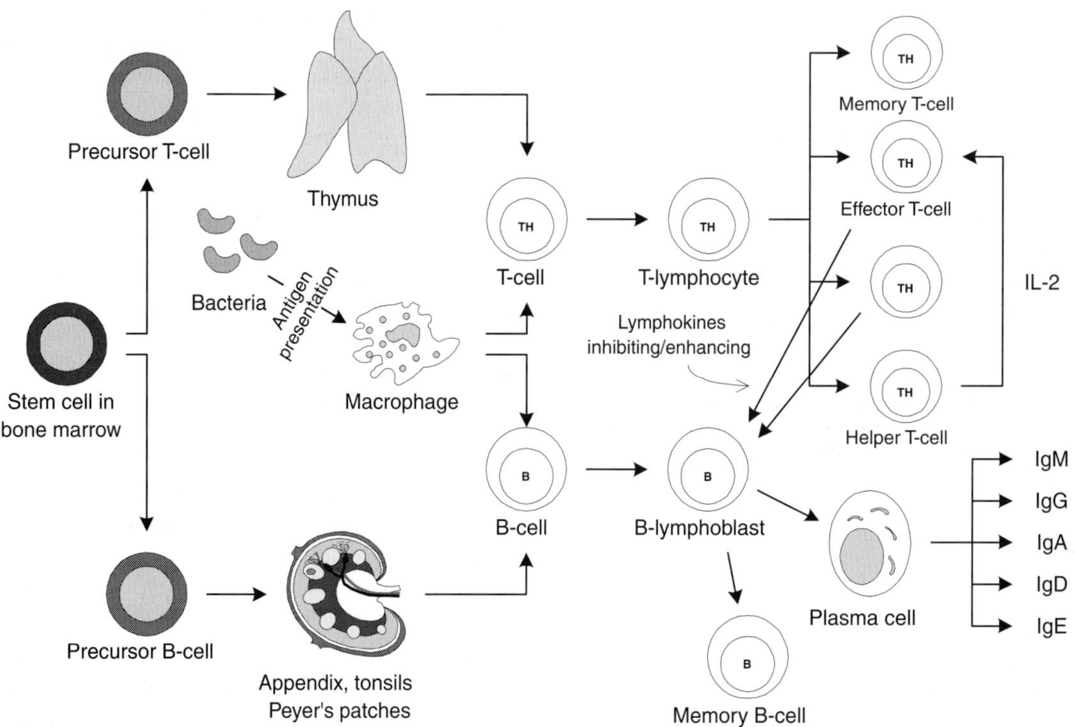

Figure 20.1 Humoral immunity.

of measuring these lymphocytes at the message as well as at the protein level.

All these are now possible, thanks to development of two major discoveries of the 1970s and 1980s in the field of molecular immunology: the monoclonal antibody and polymerase chain reaction.

Polymerase chain reaction (PCR) technology enables laboratories to detect genomes of many infectious agents at the level of femtograms. This makes PCR the most sensitive method of detection for viral and bacterial genomes in a clinical setting. Since many infectious agents have been implicated in immune dysregulation and immune dysfunction, early detection by PCR will help in the treatment of many immune disorders.

Disorders of the immune system underlie many diseases and disorders

Disorders and diseases of the immune system affect the health and quality of life of approximately one in four Americans. The data in Table 20.1 exemplify the magnitude of this problem.

Listing the incidence of these immune dysfunction diseases does not begin to estimate their costs in terms of number of work and school days lost, cost of medication, hospitalization, diminished quality of life and involvement of family and friends during illness. Although these diseases differ in terms of their severity, most have their roots in an immune system that has either failed to develop or gone awry.

The integrity of the immune system can be assessed in two different ways: by evaluation of cell number and by testing cell function.

MONOCYTE AND LYMPHOCYTE ENUMERATION

The number and functional capacity of circulating peripheral blood leukocytes reflects the overall state of immune competence of an individual. In a variety of clinical situations, tests for granulocyte, lymphocyte and monocyte number and function have become routine in the diagnosis of disease and in monitoring immunosuppressive and immunorestorative treatments. In recent years, flow cytometric tests for lymphocyte subsets have begun to take their place as useful diagnostic and prognostic indicators in several clinical situations, including bone marrow and organ transplantation, diagnosis of leukemias and lymphomas, and evaluation of immune deficiency disorders. Flow cytometric measurements allow the enumeration of different types of lymphocytes which are known to have distinctive functional activities.[1–3]

Table 20.1 Incidence of immune disorders in Americans

- 73 million have chronic respiratory problems
- 43 million have asthma or allergic disease
- 38 million, of which 250,000 are children, have arthritis
- 11 million have diabetes
- 2 million have ileitis and colitis
- 1 million are infected with the HIV virus
- 500,000 have systemic lupus erythematosus (8:1 are women)
- 250,000 have multiple sclerosis
- Over 200,000 have AIDS (the CDC has counted more than 500,000 AIDS cases since 1981 and 311,381 deaths; as of 1993, between 630,000 and 897,000 Americans were alive with HIV infection)
- 250,000 have a primary immune deficiency disorder

The techniques available to enumerate lymphocytes of various types have improved as a result of the development of monoclonal antibodies against cell surface differentiation antigens. These reagents are especially valuable when used in conjunction with flow cytometry to define lymphocyte cell surface phenotypes. T-lymphocytes, B-lymphocytes and natural killer (NK) cells, as well as subsets of these populations, can be discriminated. The close correlation of lymphocyte phenotype with function results in part from the fact that some of the molecules in the cell membrane of lymphocytes play a role in the specific functions that these cells perform. Such functions include recognition of antigen or other cells in the immune system, regulation of the immune response, cytotoxicity and a variety of other cellular interactions. Many of the monoclonal antibodies against lymphocytes react with molecules which play a role in one or more of these lymphocyte functions. Other monoclonal antibodies which are valuable in characterizing lymphocyte subpopulations react with receptors for soluble molecules which regulate the immune system. Overall, the cell surface phenotype of lymphocytes may reflect their lineage, differentiation state and immunological potential.[1–9] Enumeration of lymphocytes is done by the most reliable technique – flow cytometry.

Flow cytometry in clinical medicine

Flow cytometry in conjunction with monoclonal antibody staining has a number of advantages over alternative methods of lymphocyte enumeration. The technique is quick, precise, reproducible, and quantitative. Furthermore, it can be subjected to stringent quality control and standardization.

The lymphocyte population of human peripheral blood is composed of three cell types: T (thymus-derived), B (bone marrow-derived) and null cells. These cells are morphologically indistinguishable by microscopy but can be identified by characteristic antigenic differences in their cell membranes.[6,7]

Flow cytometry is a technique that enables rapid, multiparameter, correlated analysis of a large number of single cells. This method has been of particular importance in clinical immunology when used for the identification of human lymphocyte subsets based on the expression of cell surface antigens. This application has expanded over the past decade as a result of the development of specific monoclonal antibodies with specificity for lymphocyte surface antigens.

For preparation of flow cytometry samples, whole blood lysis is the most common technique used in the clinical laboratories. This method consists of mixing a fixed volume of whole blood with one or more directly conjugated monoclonal antibodies, then incubating the mixture at a designated temperature and time. Next, the red blood cells are lysed using Tris ammonium chloride or a hypotonic buffer. The sample is washed and then run into the flow cytometer, usually after being fixed in paraformaldehyde, which decreases the infectious risk of the sample and increases its stability.[7]

The LeucoGATE™ reagent is used to stain the first aliquot of whole blood from each subject with CD45 and CD14. The four parameters measured on this tube – two light scatter and two fluorescence – allow the SimulSET™ software to determine an optimal light scatter "gate", which identifies the lymphocyte cluster in all subsequent tubes from the same sample. This LeucoGATE™ analysis identifies lymphocytes, monocytes, and granulocytes by a combination of antigen expression and light scatter characteristics (shown in Fig. 20.2).

The use of this automated multiparameter procedure for setting the lymphocyte acquisition gate provides a significant advantage over operator-defined light scatter gating, because some overlap exists between the different cell lineages when light scatter is used as the sole criterion to identify lymphocytes.

Furthermore, with LeucoGATE™ analysis, uniform and reproducible acquisition gating is possible, and consistently more than 95% of the total lymphocytes can be located and evaluated with less than 10% contamination by either debris, granulocytes, or monocytes.

Macrophages play a central role in cell-mediated immunity because they are involved both in the initiation of responses as antigen-presenting cells and in the effector phase as inflammatory, tumoricidal and microbicidal cells. Using CD14 monoclonal antibodies, it is possible to define the percentage of monocytes in the blood.

Monoclonal antibodies for routine clinical enumeration of lymphocyte subpopulation

The nomenclature adopted by the International Leukocyte Differentiation Antigen Workshop is used in this chapter to designate the antigens with which various monoclonal antibodies react.[7–13] The following cluster designations (CDs) are used for determination of the lymphocyte subpopulation.

CD11 for identification of T-lymphocytes

The CD4 antigen is associated with the E-rosette receptor and has a molecular weight of 50 kDa. The T11 antigen normally is present on greater then 9% of thymocytes and 100% of E-rosetting positive lymphocytes, including T-lymphocytes and a fraction of null cells. It is also found on greater than 90% of tumor cells from patients with T-cell acute lymphoblastic leukemia (ALL) and Sezary syndrome, and in a rare leukemic population of myeloid lineage. The CD4 antigen is not present on non-T-cell acute lymphoblastic leukemia cells.

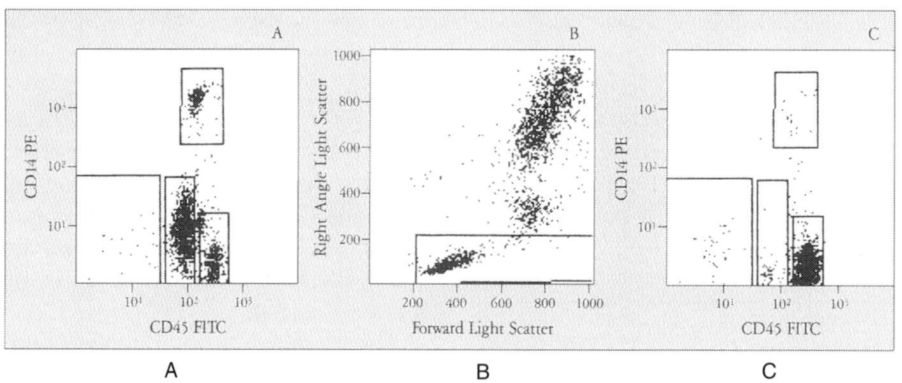

A B C

Figure 20.2 Lymphocyte gates set using LeucoGATE™. Lymphocyte gates for data acquisition were established using SimulSET™ software. Acquisition gates are defined by combining the fluorescence parameters from the LeucoGATE™ tube (A) with the forward- and right-angle light-scattering parameters (B). The light scatter gate (region 5, panel B) was set to include at least 95% of the lymphocytes. The cells of other lineages that also were included in this gate can be identified and enumerated by their characteristic immunofluorescence (C). Lymphocytes are confined to region 1, monocytes are found in region 2, while granulocyte and debris fall in regions 3 and 4, respectively. The analysis of subsequent tubes can be corrected by using the numbers of cells with each of the regions defined in (C), to obtain more precise values for enumeration of lymphocyte subsets.

Clinical relevance. The CD4 monoclonal antibody is used to quantitate total T-lymphocytes in circulating blood (both mature and immature) and to determine T-cell lineage of lymphoid tumor cells. Decreased numbers of T-lymphocytes are found in patients with autoimmune disorders including multiple sclerosis, systemic lupus erythematosus, and eczema. Thymic aplasia (DiGeorge syndrome) is associated with a decreased number of T-lymphocytes. Increased numbers of T-lymphocytes are noted in patients with acute infectious mononucleosis and some forms of acquired agammaglobulinemia due to the presence of activated suppressor cells.[14]

CD19 for identification of B-lymphocytes

The CD19 antigen defines a bimolecular structure of 40 and 80 kDa. The specificity of the CD19 monoclonal antibody for surface immunoglobulin of the B-lymphocyte was determined by removal of the CD19 positive population from peripheral blood by sorting the cell population that is induced to differentiate into Ig-secreting plasma cells in a pokeweed mitogen-driven system. The CD19 monoclonal antibody recognizes the CD19 antigen on human B-lymphocytes. The CD19 antigen is expressed on all normal B-lymphocytes, follows the Ia antigen in B-cell ontogeny and is only lost prior to the plasma cell. The CD19 antigen is present on all B-cells isolated from lymphoid organs and on approximately 5% of normal adult bone marrow cells. In addition, CD19 is expressed on greater than 95% of non-T-cell acute lymphoblastic leukemias (ALL), and on 90% of B-cell lymphomas and B-cell lymphocytic leukemias (CLL), but is not expressed on T-cell or myeloid tumors. The CD19 antigen appears to be the earliest B-cell-associated antigen demonstrated in fetal tissues.

Clinical relevance. The CD19 monoclonal antibody appears to be useful in defining the cellular lineage of non-T-cells. ALL cells and chronic myelogenous leukemia (CML) blast crisis cells and ALL non-T-cell and CML blast crisis cells are reactive with this antibody, suggesting a B-cell origin of these tumor cells. The CD19 monoclonal antibody may also be useful in defining early B-cells and in the study of immunodeficiency diseases.[15]

CD4 for identification of T-helper cell

Two main types of T-lymphocytes can be distinguished according to their function and surface proteins. These are the inducer/helper (CD4+) and suppressor/cytotoxic (CD8+) T-lymphocytes.

The CD4 antigen has a molecular weight of 62 kDa. It is normally present on a majority of thymocytes (approximately 80%) and approximately 60% of peripheral blood T-lymphocytes. The CD4+ lymphocytes play a central role in regulating the immune response. In peripheral blood, the CD4+ lymphocytes provide an inducer function for T-T, T-B and T-macrophage interaction. The CD4+ antigen reacts with the class II major histocompatibility complex (MHC) antigen on target cells.

Clinical relevance. Identification of abnormal levels of CD4+ lymphocytes may aid in the diagnosis and/or prognosis of immunodeficiency diseases such as agammaglobulinemia, thymic aplasia (DiGeorge syndrome), severe combined immunodeficiency and acquired immunodeficiency syndrome (AIDS). Measurement of CD4+ lymphocytes may also aid in phenotyping certain T-cell leukemias. Examples of these diseases include adult T-cell leukemia/lymphoma, T-cell acute lymphoblastic leukemia, and chronic T-cell leukemia.

Infection with human immunodeficiency virus (HIV), the etiologic agent of AIDS, results in profound immunosuppression due predominantly to a selective depletion of the CD4+ lymphocytes that express the receptor for the virus (the T4 antigen). Progressive clinical and immunologic deterioration generally correlates with a falling CD4+ lymphocyte count.[16]

CD8 for identification of T-suppressor cell

The CD8 antigen has a molecular weight of 76 kDa. It is normally present on a majority of thymocytes (approximately 80%) and approximately 30–35% of peripheral blood T-lymphocytes. The CD8+ lymphocytes play a central role in regulating the immune response through suppressor and cytotoxic action. The CD8 antigen reacts with the class I major histocompatibility complex (MHC) antigen on target cells.

Clinical relevance. Identification of abnormal levels of CD8+ lymphocytes may aid in the diagnosis and/or prognosis of immunodeficiency diseases such as agammaglobulinemia, thymic aplasia (DiGeorge syndrome) and severe combined immunodeficiency. Measurement of CD8+ lymphocytes may also aid in phenotyping certain T-cell leukemias. Examples of these diseases include adult T-cell acute lymphoblastic leukemia and chronic T-cell leukemia. The finding that increased levels of CD8+ cells are associated with viral infections such as hepatitis B, Epstein–Barr and cytomegalovirus may also be of diagnostic and/or prognostic significance.[17]

Ratio of CD4/CD8 for determination of T-helper/ T-suppressor ratio

Disease-related changes in CD4+ and/or CD8+ lymphocyte levels may alter the CD4/CD8 inducer to suppressor/ cytotoxic cell ratios. As a result, CD4 to CD8 ratios may also be useful as diagnostic and/or prognostic indicators of immune competence.

Clinical relevance. CD4/CD8 ratios in conjunction with CD4+ lymphocyte cell numbers have been the most widely used laboratory parameters for the evaluation of AIDS-related complex and AIDS. CD4/CD8 ratios fall toward zero in advanced AIDS patients with no detectable levels of CD4+ lymphocytes. In such cases, CD8+ lymphocyte levels may be normal, increased or decreased.

Modulations in CD4/CD8 ratios and CD4+ and T8+ lymphocyte levels may occur in autoimmune diseases such as multiple sclerosis (MS) and systemic lupus erythematosus (SLE). Increased CD4/CD8 ratios and decreased numbers of CD4+ and CD8+ lymphocytes have been observed in patients with progressive (active) MS. The lymphocyte response pattern in SLE, however, appears to reflect clinical disease activity and the level of organ involvement in the SLE disease process. For example, high T4/T8 ratios and elevated CD4+ lymphocyte percentages have been found in active/inactive SLE patients with multisystem disease including lymphadenopathy, but little or no renal disease. High T4/T8 ratios but decreased percentages of CD8+ lymphocytes have also been documented in similar active SLE patients. Further, high CD4+ and low CD8+ lymphocyte percentages have been measured in active SLE patients with central nervous system disease but no renal disease. In contrast, low CD4/CD8 ratios and decreased CD4+ lymphocyte percentages have been noted in active/inactive patients with SLE, manifested by severe renal disease and/or thrombocytopenia. In other active/inactive SLE patients, both low CD4+ and high CD8+ lymphocyte percentages have been recorded. Finally, normal CD4/CD8 ratios have been obtained in patients with widespread multisystem SLE, which often includes the renal and central nervous systems.

Increased CD4/CD8 ratios with high CD4+ and low CD8+ lymphocyte percentages have been reported in head and neck cancer patients with elevated circulating IgA and generalized hypergammaglobulinemia.

Decreased CD4+ and increased CD8+ lymphocyte percentages without significant changes in CD4/CD8 ratios have been observed in patients with stable renal allograft function after transplantation. Similar findings have been reported in patients with B-cell chronic lymphocytic leukemia, except that CD4/CD8 ratios were decreased.[16–19]

CD4+CD29 for determination of helper/inducer subpopulation of lymphocytes

The CD29 cell surface antigen has a molecular weight of 134 kDa and defines a common B1 subunit of the heterodimeric glycoprotein family called VLA. It appears on approximately 41% of unfractioned human T-lymphocytes, 41% of CD4+ inducer lymphocytes, 43% of CD8+ suppressor/cytotoxic lymphocytes, 5–30% of B-lymphocytes and over 30% of null cells, macrophages, and thymic lymphocytes. The CD29 antigen is not present on granulocytes. The monoclonal antibody identifies the helper/inducer (CD4+CD29) subpopulation of CD4 lymphocytes.

Research relevance. Disease-related changes in CD4+ lymphocyte levels may alter levels of the CD4+CD29 helper/inducer and suppressor/inducer subpopulations.

The presence of CD4+CD29+ cells in the joints of rheumatoid arthritis has been reported and may account for the inflammatory process. More recently, decreased numbers of these cells have been observed in HIV-positive patients in the early phases. Accumulation of CD4+CD29+ cells in tissues has also been reported in patients with tuberculoid leprosy and multiple sclerosis.[19]

CD16 and CD56 for determination of natural killer cells

NKH-1 (CD56 and CD16) defines a human natural killer cell antigen with a molecular weight of 200–220 kDa. It is expressed on a subpopulation of peripheral blood large granular lymphocytes (LGL) that demonstrate natural killer activity. More than 95% of cells capable of mediating spontaneous non-MHC restricted cytotoxicity in peripheral blood are contained within the 10–12% of peripheral blood mononuclear cells (PBMC) that express NKH-1. Seventy-five to 80% of NKH-1 cells co-express CD3 and T-cell receptor gene products. This latter population, which represents approximately 2% of PBMC in normal individuals, also mediates non-MHC restricted cytotoxic activity. NKH-1 is not expressed on other T- or B-lymphocyte, monocyte, granulocyte, or erythrocyte populations.

Research relevance. The NKH-1 antibody can aid in the detection and enumeration of natural killer cells in normal and disease states. For example, low numbers of NKH-1^+T3^- cells have recently been found in patients with chronic fatigue syndrome. When used with T3 antibodies, NKH-1 can be used to define distinct subsets of non-MHC restricted cytolytic cells within the NKH-1 population, i.e. NKH1^+CD3^- and NKH-1^+CD3^+. Also, this antibody can be used in the identification and enumeration of lymphoproliferative diseases involving NK cells and may be used in the purification of human NK cells and lymphokine-activated killer (LAK) cells.[20]

MEASUREMENT OF ACTIVATION MOLECULES AND LYMPHOCYTES

Many lymphocytes can be differentiated by measuring the level of activation markers on their surfaces.

CD25 antigen (Tac). Tac is a single-chain glycoprotein with a molecular weight of 55 kDa which is the low affinity receptor for IL-2. It is found on activated T- and B-cells, on activated macrophages and on T-cell clones. It is absent on thymocytes, resting T-cells, B-cells, and null cells.

CD26 (TA1). TA1 antigen has a molecular weight of 105 kDa and is a lymphocyte surface antigen. It is strongly expressed on activated human T-cells and IL-2-dependent human T-cell lines and clones. It is also weakly expressed on a small fraction of peripheral blood T-cells. This activation marker was found to be elevated in 80% of patients with chronic fatigue syndrome and in a high percentage of patients with a history of exposure to toxic chemicals.

CD69 antigen. CD69 antigen is a 60 kDa homodimer phosphorylated glycoprotein known as an activation inducer molecule (AIM). This structure contains two polypeptide chains of molecular weights 32 and 28 kDa. This activation antigen appears very early (before other activation antigens such as IL2-R) after T- or B-cell activation. It is also expressed by activated macrophages and by NK cells, but is absent in resting lymphocytes.

CD45RA epitope. The CD45RA epitope is present on all the CD45 restricted molecules in which the A axon is expressed. CD11 recognizes some peripheral T-cells, CD4+ T-lymphocytes and CD8+ T-lymphocytes, but specifically non-naive lymphocytes. The co-expression of CD4 and CD45RA antigens allows the identification of the suppressor/inducer subpopulation of CD4 lymphocytes. It also reacts with B-cells, monocytes, and granulocytes. This marker was found to be elevated in patients with rheumatoid arthritis.

CD45RO molecule. The CD45RO molecule is the 180 kDa isoform of the leukocyte common antigen. This isoform is the CD45 restricted form of the lowest molecular weight. CD45RO is a single-chain glycoprotein which is expressed by thymocytes, the CD4+ memory T-cell subset and activated T-cells. The CD45RO+, CD4+ T-cells which provide the helper-inducer function were found to be elevated in synovial tissue of patients with arthritis.

CD11a antigen. CD11a antigen (leukocyte function associated molecule-1 or LFA-1) is the 180/95 kDa integrin αL-chain, non-covalently associated with the 95 kDa CD19 (integrin β2). It promotes adhesion between lymphoid cells and the adhesion of lymphoid cells to the vascular endothelium. LFA-1 can interact with various ligands, the intercellular adhesion molecules: ICAM-1 (CD54), ICAM-2 (CD102) and ICAM-3 (CD50). CD11a antibodies have a strong reactivity with all leukocytes but do not recognize platelets. This antibody reacts with most peripheral blood T- and B- cells and with a portion of monocytes and granulocytes.

CD11b antigen (Mac1). Mac1 is the 165/95 kDa integrin αM chain, non-covalently associated with CD18 (integrin β2). It has been identified as the C3bi complement receptor (CR3). As a member of the β2 integrin family of adhesion molecules, Mac-1 mediates PMN and monocyte adherence to the endothelium. Additional CD11b ligands are ICAM-1 (CD54), factor X, fibrinogen, and endotoxin. CD11b antibodies mainly react with myeloid and natural killer cells. The Bear1 antibody recognizes some peripheral blood lymphocytes and a subset of T-cells (a portion of CD11b+ cells is also positive for CD8). It also reacts with granulocytes and monocytes. This population of CD8+CD11b lymphocytes is reported to be lower than normal in patients with chronic fatigue.[21–24]

I3 (HLA-DR antigen). The MHC class II HLA-DR antigen is expressed by human monocytes, macrophages, B-lymphocytes, and activated T-lymphocytes. Anti-I3 is used for classification and enumeration of Ia-positive B-cell lymphoproliferative malignancies (acute and chronic lymphocytic leukemias, non-Hodgkin lymphomas, etc.), acute myelogenous leukemias and identification of states of T-lymphocyte activation due to viral illnesses. Therefore, the number of HLA-DR+ positive cells is significantly increased in patients with chronic fatigue syndrome.

CD38. CD38 is a protein with a molecular weight of 45 kDa which is expressed on thymocytes, activated T-cells and plasma cells. Because of an increase in activated T-cells in chronic fatigue syndrome, the population of CD8 lymphocytes which carry the CD38 receptor are significantly elevated.[24]

Summary of lymphocyte enumeration

Immunophenotyping by flow cytometry is common in most larger clinical laboratories. The application of this technology has moved forward in response to significant improvements in instrumentation and an increase in the availability of reagents.

Properly performed, flow cytometry can identify lymphocyte subpopulations rapidly and accurately. The primary clinical uses of immunophenotyping are to quantitate CD4 T-cell counts in HIV infection and to assign lineage and/or monoclonality in leukemias and lymphomas. Additional uses include characterizing immune deficiency disorders, evaluating immune-mediated inflammatory diseases and assessing patients before and after organ transplantation.

Although certain surface antigens are associated with functional status, such as the isoforms of CD45 which appear to identify naive (CD45RA) or memory (CD45RO) T-cells, these classifications are not absolute and must not be considered determinants of cell function.

Immunophenotyping is a means of identifying cells, but it is not the equivalent of a functional evaluation. Therefore, for functional leukocyte capacity, macrophage function, NK cytotoxic activity, and T- and B-cell function should be measured.[21–26]

In many patients, lymphocyte subpopulation numbers are normal, but their functional capacity for killing bacteria or tumor cells and reaction to antigens are completely abnormal. Hence, the major emphasis of this chapter is on the functional capacity of lymphocytes.

ASSESSMENT OF MONOCYTE AND MACROPHAGE FUNCTION

The major function of monocytes and macrophages is host defense against the microorganisms, removal of necrotic and cellular debris, and interaction with lymphoid components in the generation and effector phase of immune responses. Patients suspected of having a deficiency of cell-mediated immunity are candidates for evaluation of monocyte functions, even if the number and function of T- and B-cells are normal. Various assays of monocyte competence are performed in the immunology laboratory, including mediating tumor cell-dependent cellular cytotoxicity, microbial killing, production of prostaglandins, generation of respiratory burst and the ability of monocytes' antigen-induced activation of T-cells and production of interleukin-1 (IL-1).

The test for IL-1 production, representing accessory function and antigen presentation, is the most useful in evaluating immunodeficiency. Other tests such as microbial killing, cytotoxicity, prostaglandin and generation of peroxide are more useful in the evaluation of patients suffering repeated infections by fungi, protozoans, saprophytic microorganisms and atypical mycobacteria.[27–30]

Production of IL-1 by monocytes

Measuring IL-1 production represents an important assay of monocyte function as it directly relates to accessory function and interaction with T-helper cells.

IL-1 is produced by monocyte-macrophages, endothelial cells and other non-leukocytic cell types. Monocytes can also release IL-1 in response to stimulation with the neuropeptide substance P, providing a potential link between the nervous system and immune system. The IL-1 family includes three peptides: IL-1α, IL-1β and IL-1 receptor antagonist (IL-1ra). IL-1 has numerous diverse effects including induction of fever, hypotension, sleep, and stimulation of T-cells and B-cells; IL-1ra binds the IL-1 receptor but does not activate it; and IL-1ra may diminish the disease-mediating effects of IL-1.[29,30]

IL-1 production can be measured by enzyme immunoassay and IL-1 messenger. RNA can also be measured by PCR with much higher sensitivity. In many clinical conditions, the message of cytokines may be abnormal but the protein level will be within the normal range. Therefore, a combination of both measurements (protein and message) is the logical step.

Procedure

Monocytes are isolated from peripheral blood mononuclear leukocytes by sequential buoyant density centrifugation over Ficoll-Hypaque, Percoll or similar gradients and adherence to glass or plastic surfaces. The buoyant density of monocytes is similar to that of other peripheral blood mononuclear leukocytes but is considerably less than that of polymorphonuclear leukocytes and erythrocytes. In separating monocytes from lymphocytes with similar density, advantage is taken of the greater adherent properties of the mononuclear phagocyte.

Heparinized venous blood is diluted with an equal volume of PBS or HBSS and carefully layered over 2 ml of Ficoll-Hypaque in sterile culture tubes. The diluted blood is added carefully so as to avoid turbulence which would disturb the interface. The tubes are centrifuged at approximately 500 × *g* at room temperature for 30 minutes. When the tubes are removed form the centrifuge, a distinct band can be seen between the plasma layer and the Ficoll-Hypaque layer. The top layer containing plasma is pipetted and discarded, and the bottom layer above the Ficoll-Hypaque is harvested with a sterile Pasteur pipette; the top one-third of the Ficoll-Hypaque layer is taken up in addition to the cells. The bands from several tubes are then combined in another tube and the cells are washed with either HBSS or PBS two or more times by centrifuging at $10^3 \times g$ for 8 minutes. This cell pellet should be relatively free of platelets and erythrocytes and should contain about 60–80% lymphocytes and 20–40% monocytes. The mixture of lymphocytes and monocytes is suspended in an RPMI medium with 10% human AB serum or fetal calf serum at a concentration of 2×10^6/ml in the presence or absence of endogenous activators such as bacterial lipopolysaccharide (LPS) with a concentration of 10 to 20 μg/ml. The cultures are kept in a CO_2 incubator for a period of 72 hours, and supernatant-containing cytokines are removed and measured for IL-1 concentration using ELISA methodology. Results are expressed as IL-1 picograms/million lymphocytes and used in a culture in the presence or absence of an endogenous activator (LPS).

Bacterial phagocytosis and killing by monocytes

The capacity of monocytes to ingest and digest bacteria is generally determined using a method in which the monocytes are allowed to ingest and subsequently kill a measured number of microorganisms. Once inside the monocyte, the microorganism is exposed to the microbicidal components of the cell. After an appropriate time, the monocytes are lysed and the intracellular organisms are released and assayed by a colony-counting method to determine the number of viable organisms remaining within the cell. Microbial killing is enhanced when resting monocytes undergo activation.

Procedure

The procedure for the microbial killing assay involves

preparation of a suspension of adherent monocytes in a glass Petri dish. Bacterial suspensions are prepared using either *Staphylococcus aureus* or *Streptomyces albus* and are cultured for 16–24 hours at 37°C in Trypticase soy broth. The bacterial culture is centrifuged, washed twice in PBS and adjusted to a concentration of approximately 10^8 bacteria/ml by measuring turbidity. The bacterial suspension is eventually diluted with HBSS to obtain a final working concentration of 10^7 bacteria/ml. Autologous or normal pooled AB serum can be used as a source of opsonin for the bacteria. In plastic culture tubes, 0.1 ml of medium, 0.2 ml of bacterial suspension at 10^7 bacteria/ml and 0.5 ml of monocyte suspension (10^6 monocytes/ml) are mixed. This mixture, along with proper controls, is then incubated for 1–2 hours at 37°C. Before culturing, a sample of the suspension is taken out for bacterial counts. After the 2 hour incubation, the cells are resuspended and colony counts are performed once more to determine the total amount of bacteria remaining. The tubes are then centrifuged and colony counts are performed on the supernatant using classical microbiology techniques. The colony-forming units are counted to quantitate the remaining viable bacteria.[31–33] The percentage of bacteria ingested and killed by the monocytes is calculated using the following formula:

$$\frac{(\text{CFU at zero time} - \text{CFU in 15 min sup.}) - (\text{CFU at 1 hour total} - \text{CFU in 1 hour sup.})}{\text{CFU at zero time} - \text{CFU in 15 min sup.}}$$

Measurement of bacterial phagocytes by flow cytometry

Similar measurements of bacterial engulfment and killing are possible using flow cytometry. For the assessment of phagocytosis by flow cytometry, 100 µl FITC-labeled yeast cells (5×10^6/ml) are mixed with 100 µl autologous plasma, 200 ml PBS and 100ml granulocytes (1×10^6/ml). After incubation at 37°C with continuous agitation for 1 hour, 1 ml of ice-cold PBS is added. After incubation at 20°C for 10 minutes, the cells are washed twice in ice-cold PBS. The cells are then taken up by the flow cytometer in 0.5 ml of PBS. The number of granulocytes showing green fluorescence (i.e. phagocytosing cells) is evaluated using the FACScan flow cytometer (Becton-Dickinson, USA). The gates are set around the granulocyte cluster in a cytogram, simultaneously evaluating forward-angle and right-angle light-scattering properties of the cell passing through the focused laser beam. The percentage of granulocytes with green fluorescence containing engulfed yeast cells in the histogram is determined on the FL1 channel (FITC filter transmission, 530 ± 30 nm) of the FACScan. Using this methodology, we found that the percentages of phagocytosing cells in healthy subjects were between 45 and 55%. Significant reduction in the percentage of phagocytosing cells was found in patients with chronic illnesses, including chronic fatigue immune dysfunction syndrome.[31–34]

In order to assess the percentage of yeast cells killed after phagocytosis, 100 µl of the yeast cell suspension (1×10^6/ml), are mixed with autologous plasma (100 µl), PBS (100 µl) and 100 µl of granulocyte (1×10^6/ml). A control consisted of 100 ml of yeast cells mixed with 100 ml of autologous plasma and 200 µl of PBS in the absence of cells. After incubation at 37°C with continuous agitation for 2 hours, 100 µl cold 0.5% Triton X-100 are added to lyse leukocytes. To remove DNA released from the lysed granulocytes, 1 ml of a warm (37°C) DNAse solution (40 µg deoxyribonuclease 1 from bovine pancrease = 2000 Kunitz units dissolved in PBS) is added and the mixture is incubated for 5 minutes with periodic agitation. The tubes are centrifuged (500 × *g* for 5 minutes) and the cell pellet is resuspended in 1 ml of PBS; 20 µl of propidium iodide (red fluorescence) 0.05 mg/ml is then added, and the tubes are incubated for 5 minutes at 4°C. The gate is set around the yeast cell cluster on the FL1 channel. The percentage of yeast cells showing red fluorescence (i.e. killed cells) is evaluated on the FL3 channel of the FACScan (red pass filter, transmission 650 ± 30 nm) within the gated region. The percentage of yeast cells killed is expressed as the percentage of cells killed in the test sample minus the percentage of cells killed in the control test tube.[35–37] In healthy controls examined in our laboratory, between 25 to 30% of yeasts were killed by this method, while in patients with chronic illnesses, these numbers may drop to below 10%.

Measurement of oxidative burst in monocytes

Phagocytosis and its associated oxidative burst are essential for certain monocyte functions. During the respiratory burst of hydrogen peroxide, hydroxyl radicals, nitric oxide and superoxide anion are produced as toxic oxygen metabolites.

Hydrogen peroxide released from monocytes can be measured as a function of oxidative burst activity in response to stimulation. Hydrogen peroxide can be assayed by a fluorescent scopoletin assay or by a photometer-based microassay requiring the horseradish peroxidase-dependent oxidation of phenol red. Hydrogen peroxide release is measured after in vitro stimulation by inducers of the oxidative burst such as phorbol myristate acetate (PMA) or serum-opsonized zymosan, which contains cell walls of *Saccharomyces cerevisiae.*

Recent studies have demonstrated that the production of nitric oxide (NO) by macrophages is important in the killing of intracellular parasites. Several different pathogens including *M. bovis* BCG and *Mycobacterium tuberculosis* are reported to be susceptible to NO. Furthermore, it is reported that activated macrophages contribute to the suppression of Ag-specific T-cell proliferation through their NO production during primary listerial infection. The suppressive effect of NO is also observed in Con A responsiveness and IFN-γ- and IL-2-induced production of T-cells. These findings suggest that NO is not only the molecule responsible for the tumoricidal and microbicidal effects, but also one of the crucial factors controlling immunologic responses.

In macrophages, NO is generated from oxidation of the terminal guanidino nitrogen atom of L-arginine by inducible NO-synthase (iNOS), an enzyme known to be induced by cytokines such as IFN-γ, TNF-α, IL-1 and LPS. Expression of iNOS is also inducible by infection with *L. moncytogenes, M. tuberculosis* and BCG in mice and by *M. avium* in humans. Therefore, measurement of NO is not only a measure of phagocytosis but also a measure of normal or abnormal immunologic responses. For measurement of nitric oxide generation, Ficoll-Hypaque-separated mononuclear cells (2×10^6/ml) are cultured in C-RPMI for 24 hours at 37°C. The non-adherent cells are removed by gentle washing with Hanks balanced salt solution (HBSS) and adherent cells are used as macrophages. Macrophages are stimulated with 10 μg/ml of LPS or 1×10^6 CFU/ml of BCG for 2 days at 37°C. After removal of the supernatant, the level of NO is measured by determining the amount of nitrite using Greiss reagent. Briefly, a 300 ml aliquot of each sample is mixed with an equal volume of Greiss reagent (0.5% sulfanilamide, 0.05% naphthylethylenediamin and 2.5% H_3PO_4) and absorbance at 550 nm is determined after 10–15 minutes' incubation at room temperature. Sodium nitrite is used as a standard. Results are expressed by nanogram of nitric oxide produced by 1 million monocytes.[38]

Defects in monocyte phagocytosis are reported in a variety of clinical conditions including systemic lupus erythematosus (SLE), monocytic leukemia and congenital deficiency of membrane-adherence glycoproteins (CD11-CD18 complex).

Impaired oxidative burst activity and defects in microbicidal activity characteristically involve the neutrophil and monocyte in chronic granulomatous disease (CGD). Generation of toxic oxygen intermediates may also be impaired by some malignancies and infectious diseases.

For the above reasons and for the general assessment of the immune function, monocyte phagocytosis should be recommended. Performance of this test will also be instrumental in evaluation of augmentative therapy using different biological response modifiers including antioxidants.

ASSESSMENT OF T- AND B-CELL FUNCTION

Assessment of T- and B-cell function is done by the standard lymphocyte proliferation assay or by the newly developed fast immune assay system of Becton-Dickinson using flow cytometry.

Lymphocyte proliferation or transformation is the process whereby new DNA synthesis and cell division takes place in lymphocytes after a stimulus of some type, resulting in a series of changes. The lymphocytes increase in size, the cytoplasm becomes more extensive, the nucleoli are visible in the nucleus and the lymphocytes resemble blast cells. The term "blast transformation" is also sometimes applied to this process. Lymphocytes from humans proliferate in response to antigens to which they are sensitized. This in vitro response correlates with the existence of delayed-type hypersensitivity in the host. Lymphocyte proliferation also occurs in response to different histocompatibility antigens when leukocytes from two donors are mixed in a mixed leukocyte culture. Mitogens, including pokeweed mitogen, phytohemagglutinin (PHA), LPS and concanavalin A, will induce proliferation of normal cells in culture.

Evaluation of lymphocyte proliferation can be quantitated by determination either of the percentage of lymphoblasts or of increased DNA synthesis. This evaluation may be achieved by the addition of a radiolabeled precursor of DNA (usually tritiated thymidine) to the culture medium and the subsequent detection of the amount of radioactivity incorporated into the cells. The assay involves the in vitro culture of a lymphocyte population in the presence or absence of a selected stimulus for various periods of time. The changes induced in the stimulated groups are compared with changes in the unstimulated cell populations. Radiolabeled amino acids are used most commonly for these comparisons, as they offer a means of quantitating the changes in a simple, reproducible manner. The use of automated harvesting procedures results in greater reproducibility and ease of performance of the assay.[39–41]

Lymphocyte proliferation assay procedure

After Ficoll-Hypaque separation, peripheral blood mononuclear cells are counted and adjusted to the concentration of 1×10^6/ml. Cells are cultured in quadruplicate in flat-bottom microtiter plate wells with 10 μg/ml of T-cell mitogens (PHA, CONA) or 5 μg/ml of B-cell mitogens (LPS or pokeweed). After 48 hours of incubation at 37°C in a water-saturated atmosphere of 95% air and 5% CO_2, cells are pulsed with 2 μci/well of tritiated thymidine for 16–18 hours. Incorporation of ^{3}H-thymidine into cellular DNA is determined by harvesting the cultures in a Mash II unit harvester. Radioactivity is measured by liquid scintillation counting.

The percentage of induction of ^{3}H-uptake is determined by the following formula:

$$\frac{\text{counts/minute in the presence of mitogen}}{\text{counts/minute in the absence of mitogen}}$$

Optimal DNA synthesis in response to mitogens is usually detected in 2–4 days, whereas 5–7 days are necessary to detect optimal responses to antigens and mixed allogenic leukocytes. Under suboptimal conditions (either low cell numbers or low concentrations of mitogen), the response to mitogens also peaks after 4 days, which suggests a relationship between the number of responding cells and the rate of DNA synthesis.

This method is not only lengthy, labor-intensive and involving radioactive material but also does not provide information about individual lymphocyte subsets responding to particular stimuli. In contrast, multiparameter flow cytometry offers the potential to analyze selected lymphocyte subset responses to a variety of stimuli (e.g. pathogens and bioresponse modifiers).

The graph in Figure 20.3 compares CD69 expression and ^{3}H-thymidine incorporation and suggests that T-cell activation, as measured by the expression of CD69 on CD3-positive cells, parallels the proliferative response determined by ^{3}H-thymidine incorporation.

In most cases, activation of T-cells requires the presence of accessory cells or antigen-presenting cells (APCs). Under appropriate conditions, in vitro, antigenic or mitogenic stimuli activate T-cells via the T-cell receptor complex. This results in a number of biochemical and morphological changes that culminate in T-cell differentiation and proliferation and expansion of memory cells.

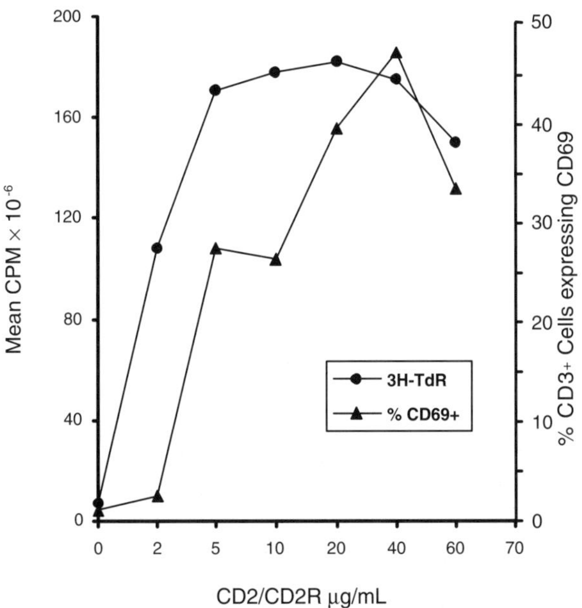

Figure 20.3 CD69 Expression vs. tritiated thymidine incorporation. Incorporation of ^{3}H-thymidine was compared with CD69 expression as a measure of T-cell response to varying concentrations of a co-mitogenic pair of antibodies, CD2 and CD2R. Tritiated thymidine incorporation was measured after 3 days of stimulation of PBMCs in media plus autologous plasma; the percentage of CD69 expression was measured by flow cytometry after 4 hours of stimulation under identical conditions.

One of the earliest changes noted is the expression of the activation antigen CD69, reaching peak expression within 8 hours of stimulation. Other activation markers, including CD25 (IL-2 receptor), CD71 (transferrin receptor) and HLA-DR, which are expressed later during this process, are shown in Figure 20.4.

Since expression of CD69 does not reflect some of the downstream events involved in signals for proliferation, such as IL-2 receptor expression, we use a combination of CD69+CD25 to cover the early and late signals involved in lymphocyte proliferation.

These properties suggest that the CD69+CD25 markers presented in Figure 20.3 are generic markers for lympho-

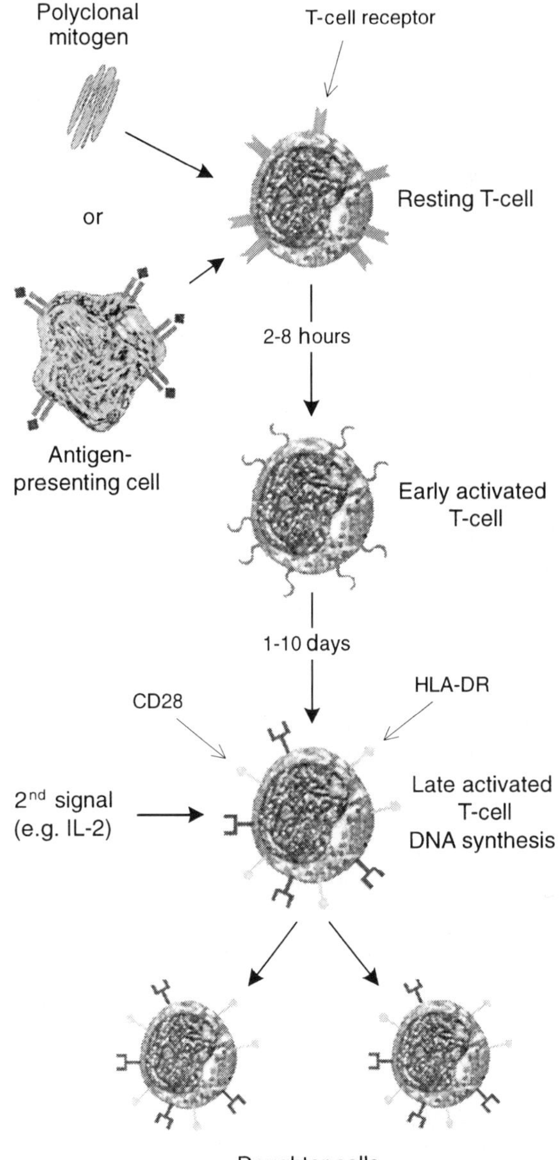

Figure 20.4 Expression of different activation markers on T-lymphocytes after polyclonal mitogenic stimulation.

cyte activation and are well suited to rapid analysis of functioning lymphocytes.

The assay utilizes fluorescence triggering on CD3-positive lymphocytes in the FL3 channel and subsequent two-color analysis of the activation marker (CD69 PE) versus the subpopulation marker (such as CD4 FITC or CD8 FITC). T-cell activation is measured as a function of the percentage of T-cell subsets (FL1) that express CD69 (FL2).

The FASTIMMUNE system includes a two-color reagent, CD69 PE/CD3 PerCP, that allows customized subset analyses. The functions of specific T-lymphocyte subpopulations may be studied by adding FITC-labeled T-cell subset markers to the two-color reagent. The open system utilizes isotype and activation controls.

Isotype control, γ1, FITC/γ1, PE/CD3 PerCP, is used to set the boundaries between positive and negative results for the FL1 and FL2 channels. The activation control, CD2/CD2R, is a combination of comitogenic monoclonal antibodies that assure that the activation system is working properly.[41,42]

Basic procedure

Sample preparation and mitogenic stimuli

1. Whole blood is collected using a sodium heparin anticoagulant.
2. Mitogenic or antigenic ligands and the FASTIMMUNE activation control are added to separate 200–500 μl aliquots of heparinized whole blood.
3. Stimulated samples and unstimulated control samples are incubated for 4 hours at 37°C in a water bath or an incubator.

Three-color immunofluorescent staining

1. FASTIMMUNE three-color antibody conjugate combinations, including fluorochrome-labeled isotype-matched staining controls, are added to 50 μl aliquots of stimulated and control samples.
2. Cells are stained for 15 minutes at room temperature.
3. Samples are lysed and fixed with 450 μl of FACS® lysing solution for 15–60 minutes at room temperature to analyze the percentage of activated lymphocytes by flow cytometry.

Clinical application

The lymphocyte transformation test has a broad range of applications, including:

- assessment and monitoring of congenital immunological defects
- assessment of either immunosuppressive or immunoenhancing therapies
- determination of histocompatibility matching in transplantation
- identification of serum or plasma factors which may suppress or enhance reactivity
- diagnostic testing for detection of previous exposure to a variety of antigens, allergens or pathogens
- determination of a variety of cytokines.

A wide variety of acquired conditions have been shown to have impaired lymphocyte transformation. These conditions include a variety of bacterial and viral infections as well as chemotherapy and autoimmune diseases such as Sjögren's syndrome and systemic lupus erythematosus. A variety of other clinical conditions have also been shown to affect lymphocyte transformation, including surgery and anesthesia, stress, aging, malnutrition, a variety of malignancies, uremia and major burns.

In patients with congenital immunological defects, lymphocyte transformation ranges from complete lack of function, as in severe combined immunodeficiency disease and DiGeorge syndrome, to a partial deficit, as in ataxia telangiectasia, Wiskott–Aldrich syndrome and chronic mucocutaneous candidiasis, to normal reactivity, as in X-linked hypogammaglobulinemia.

Lymphocyte transformation has also been used to monitor sequential samples from patients undergoing a variety of immunoenhancing or immunosuppressive therapies in the treatment of diseases states. This approach is especially sensitive when patients show nearly complete deficits before initiation of therapy, such as in immunodeficient subjects requiring bone marrow transplantation. Patients undergoing immunoenhancing therapy with lymphokines, such as recombinant interferon or the interleukins for cancer, can be monitored for increased reactivity after therapy.[39–43]

Therefore, enhancement of T- and B-cell function is the best screening method for selection of biological response modifiers, including botanicals.

T-HELPER 1 AND T-HELPER 2 FUNCTION

T-helper lymphocytes can be divided into at least two functionally distinct subpopulations, defined on the basis of clonal analysis as T-helper 1 (TH1) and T-helper 2 (TH2). However, at present, no phenotypic markers exist to distinguish between the TH1 and TH2 cells or between those that generate type 1 and type 2 responses. Thus, type 1 and type 2 responses are dependent on functional parameters that are more complex than the phenotypic markers based on cell surface analysis.[44–47]

TH1 lymphocyte clones are characterized by the production of type 1 cytokines or IL-2 and INF-δ. The TH2 lymphocyte clones produce type 2 cytokines, which are IL-4, IL-5, IL-6, IL-10 and IL-13. Therefore, measurements of these cytokines is an indirect way to assess T-helper 1 and T-helper 2 function.

The TH1–TH2 concept has been broadened to include the type 1 and type 2 responses, which reflect the functional profiles of interacting cell populations of the immune system and summarize the two modalities by which the immune system responds to antigenic stimuli. A type 1 response can be defined as a cytokine profile in which there is appreciable production of TH1 cytokines and/or expression of cytokine messenger RNA. This response is characterized by the activation of cell-mediated immunity and by certain isotypes of antibody. Type 2 responses can be defined as a cytokine profile characterized by a polarized production of TH2 cytokines, which induce strong humoral immunity and antibody production, including immunoglobulin, and switch from IgG to IgE production. Type 1 responses are negatively regulated by IL-4 and IL-10, and type 2 responses are down-modulated by INF-δ and IL-12. Increase in production of type 2 cytokines and decrease in production of type 1 cytokines have been described in a variety of immunological conditions, including immunodeficiencies and immune activations.

Clinical application

Evidence is accumulating that the pathogenesis of some human diseases may be conceptualized in terms of type 1 and type 2 helper cell cytokine profiles. Many of these diseases are due to infectious agents, including:

- viruses such as HIV-1 and the measles paramyxovirus
- mycobacteria such as *Mycobacterium leprae* (leprosy) and *M. tuberculosis*
- spirochetes such as *Treponema pallidum* (syphilis) and *Borrelia burgdorferi* (Lyme disease)
- parasitic diseases such as leishmaniasis and filariasis
- mycoplasma such as *M. fermentans* which have been described as a cofactor in AIDS and as one possible cause of chronic fatigue syndrome.

In this population of patients, a switch in the pattern of helper-1 to helper-2 population has been observed.

Stimulation of lymphocytes to produce INF-δ or other type 1 cytokines, but not IL-4, is the best method of screening biological response modifiers and botanical immunomodulators for treatment of immune diseases.[44–47]

NATURAL KILLER CELL CYTOTOXICITY

Natural killer (NK) cells are large granular lymphocytes which play an important role in a variety of human diseases. Compromised or absent natural immunity, as measured in vitro by decreased NK activity and/or depressed absolute numbers of circulating NK cells, has been linked to the development and progression of cancer, chronic and acute viral infections, including the acquired immunodeficiency syndrome (AIDS), chronic fatigue syndrome, psychological dysfunction, various immunodeficiencies, and certain autoimmune diseases.[1–4] Recent evidence indicates that NK cells are involved in multiple effector, regulatory, and developmental activities of the immune system and that deficiencies or abnormalities in NK cell function may contribute to, or be a biologic marker for, disease. For the above reasons, it is important to reliably detect abnormalities in NK cell function and monitor prognosis of chronic illnesses after therapy with biological response modifiers or other agents.[48–53]

T killer cell on the warpath

Although the main task of the immune system is to protect against the multitude of external microorganisms and other foreign perils, some of its weapons are reserved for combating abnormal cells. Their task is strongly reminiscent of the secret police in a dictatorship. Killer cells move constantly through the body's tissues, combing the tissues for deviant cells. T-lymphocytes originate in the bone marrow, enter the bloodstream, and settle in the thymus for a while. Here, they become immune-competent. Some of them are classed as helper T-cells, others as suppressors, and a third, exceedingly aggressive category as killer cells. The killer cells are equipped with special weapons which can kill the deviant cells.

While most white cells of the immune system react to foreign antigens on the surfaces of invading microorganisms, the killer cell reacts to both foreign antigens and the body's own antigens. Very often, for example, a virus conceals itself inside body cells, safe from antibodies, complement factors and scavenging cells. It is protected by the antigens of the infected cell, to which the body's defenses do not respond. The killer cell, however, detects the virus as the infected cell bears on its surface both the body's own antigens and foreign virus antigens.

Characteristics of NK cells

Morphologically, NK cells belong to a subset of large granular lymphocytes (LGLs). Using monoclonal antibodies, NK cells can be distinguished from other lymphocytes because they express a characteristic set of surface markers; they are $CD3^-$, $CD2^+$, $CD16^+$ and $CD56(NKH1)^+$. They do not productively rearrange T-cell receptor genes and do not express the CD3 complex. NK cells are cytotoxic effectors that are capable of spontaneously killing tumor or virus-infected cells.[18,19] Their cytolytic activity is not restricted by or dependent upon expression of the major histocompatibility complex (MHC) on target cells. Although the basis for target cell recognition by NK cells is not clear at this time, they are capable of distinguishing and sparing most normal tissue cells.[54,55]

Determination of NK activity

The number of NK cells in the blood or cellular suspensions is determined by staining mononuclear cell populations with monoclonal antibodies against surface antigens on NK cells such as CD56 or CD16.

NK activity is measured in a 4 hour cytotoxicity assay using cultured tumor cells as targets and mononuclear cells isolated from the blood or tissues as effectors. Tumor cells used as targets are sensitive to human NK cells and K562, a cell line derived from a patient with chronic myelogenous leukemia in blast crisis. The targets are first labeled with radioactive chromium (^{51}Cr) and extensively washed to remove any unbound radioisotope. The K562 line is maintained in culture in the presence of 10% (v/v) fetal calf serum (FCS) and is provided regularly with fresh medium to assure that cells used as targets are in the log phase of growth; this is important to ensure high viability and good uniform uptake of the radioisotope.

NK activity in the blood is measured by using unfractionated mononuclear cells. These are prepared fresh and maintained in medium supplemented with 5% (v/v) FCS prior to the assay. A constant number (usually 5×10^3) of ^{51}Cr-labeled K562 target cells is mixed with graded numbers of effector cells in triplicate wells of U-shaped microtiter plates. These plates are centrifuged briefly to bring effectors and targets into contact with each other, and then they are placed in a 37°C incubator for 4 hours. Killed targets are quantitated by measuring the amount of ^{51}Cr released into the supernatant following the 4 hour incubation of effectors and targets.

Each plate contains wells for determination of the spontaneous chromium release from target cells (i.e. target cells in medium only) and of the maximal chromium release from lysed tumor cells by adding acid or detergents. The harvested supernatants from control and experimental wells are counted in a gamma counter. The amount of ^{51}Cr released into the supernatant is directly related to the proportion of target cells killed by effector cells.[56–58]

Calculation of results in NK activity assay

Results of the NK cell assay for each effector/target (E:T) ratio can be expressed as a percentage of specific lysis, but more commonly NK activity is expressed in terms of "lytic-units" (LUs).

To calculate LUs of NK activity, we combine the percentage of specific lysis at all the measured E:T ratios. First, the E:T ratio yielding 20% lysis ($E{:}T_{20}$) is estimated from these measurements. The standard number of effectors (E_{std}) is typically chosen to be 10^7, and the standard number of target cells (T_{std}) is typically 5×10^3. Then the lytic activity is reported as:

$$\text{number of LUs} \times \frac{E_{std}/T_{std}}{E{:}T_{20}} = \frac{T{:}E_{20}}{T_{std}/E_{std}}$$

The size of a lytic batch, which is ($E{:}T_{20}$) (T_{std}) effector cells, represents 1 LU. Therefore, since lytic units (LUs) are a convenient way to quantitatively compare the relative cytotoxic activities of effector cell populations from different individuals or from the same individual over time, we use LUs to express NK activity of our clinical specimens. For this type of reproducibility, it is necessary to compare the percentage of specific lysis at all the measured E:T ratios.

First, the E:T ratio yielding 20% lysis ($E{:}T_{20}$) 20) is estimated from these measurements. The choice of 20% as a reference level of lysis is arbitrary; however, it is quite common and seems to be a good choice, since experimental E:T ratios can be chosen so that the calibration will rarely require extrapolation beyond the range of the experiment. The estimation of $E{:}T_{20}$ is usually accomplished by fitting a curve to the measured points on the graph of percentage of lysis versus E:T ratio and calibrating.

One feature of the LU, in contrast with using the percentage of lysis at a single E:T ratio, is that four values at four distinct ratios are used, implying greater amounts of information and, therefore, greater precision. For example, the mean of four measurements has half the standard deviation of a single measurement. Also, LUs provide a measure of potency and dosage, when effector cells are infused in a clinical trial or experiment. The total activity of a bolus of cells might be well represented as the size of the bolus divided by the size of a LU.[57]

These optimal conditions for NK cell cytotoxic assay and criteria for a reproducible assay were first established in Dr Herberman's laboratory at the Pittsburgh Cancer Institute in 1990.[57] Based on these criteria, we established conditions for obtaining a reproducible assay using 24-hour-old blood drawn in a yellow-top (ACD) tube and computer program; lytic units are calculated from 12 tubes used for each patient.

Examples of lytic units calculations for healthy subjects and patients are shown in Figures 20.5–20.7.

NK cell activity in human diseases

The biological roles of natural killer cells are shown in Table 20.2. As indicated in this table, NK cells are involved not only in defense against pathogens and elimination of metastases, but also in a variety of other biological interactions.

It has been well established that patients with a variety

Table 20.2 Role of NK cells in human health diseases

- Antitumor effects and elimination of cancer
- Antiviral and antibacterial activity
- Regulation of immune system
- Regulation of hematopoieses
- Interaction with the neuroendocrine system
- Effects on reproduction

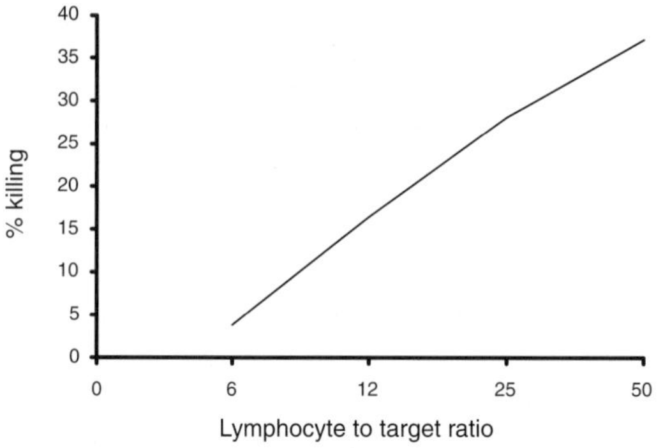

Figure 20.5 Normal natural killer cell activity of a healthy subject. Lymphocyte to target ratio giving 20% killing = 21.33. Results: lytic units = 1,000/21.33 = 46.89.

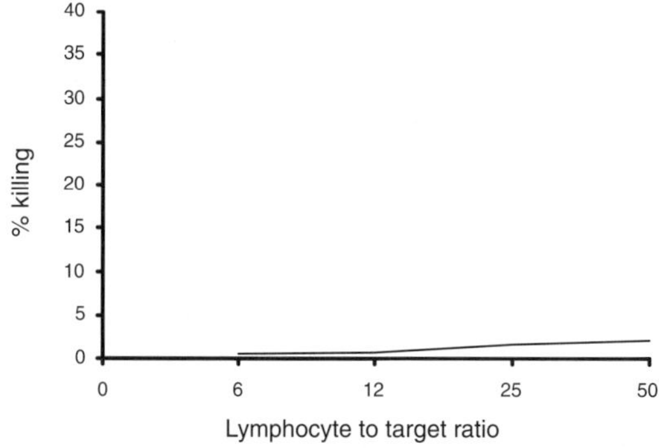

Figure 20.6 Very low natural killer cell activity of a cancer patient. Lymphocyte to target ratio giving 20% killing = 458.27. Results: lytic units = 1,000/458.27 = 2.18.

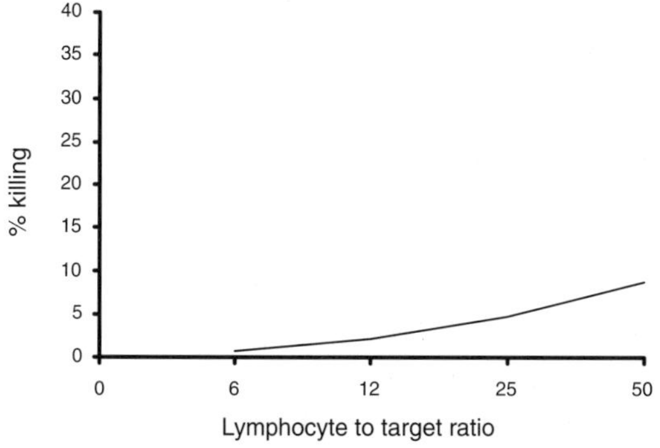

Figure 20.7 Low natural killer cell activity of a patient with chronic fatigue syndrome. Lymphocyte to target ratio giving 20% killing = 109.55. Results: lytic units = 1,000/109.55 = 9.13.

of solid malignancies and large tumor burdens have decreased NK activity in the circulation and that this low NK activity may be significantly associated with the development of distant metastases. Furthermore, in patients treated for metastatic disease, the survival time without metastases correlates directly with levels of NK activity.[59] In patients with hematologic malignancies, there appears to be a correlation between NK activity and the status of disease; the more advanced the disease, the lower the NK activity. Decreased NK activity may also be an important risk factor for the development of malignancy in humans. The prognostic significance of low NK activity in patients with cancer has been recently established; thus, low NK activity may have prognostic value in predicting relapses, poor responses to treatment and, especially, decreased survival time without metastases.[51–53]

NK cells are sensitive indicators of activation by biologic response modifiers and their monitoring has been used to document alterations in the activity of circulating immune cells during therapy with these agents. In cancer patients treated with radiation or chemotherapy, NK activity becomes depressed as a result of the therapy. Given a role for natural immunity in tumor control, it may be clinically important to monitor the extent and duration of suppression of NK activity in order to minimize it through adjustments to the extent and/or duration of cyto-reductive therapy. In human bone marrow transplantation, NK cells may influence the outcome by helping in engraftment and controlling viral infections and may mediate anti-leukemic effects important for the elimination of residual tumor cells. On the other hand, there is also evidence for the ability of NK cells to suppress hematopoietic development.[59] Furthermore, recent evidence indicates that there is a relationship between an individual's reaction to emotional stress and NK activity. Attempts are being made to define the mechanism responsible for low NK activity in individuals who have difficulties in handling stress and in those suffering from behavioral disorders.[60–62]

The role of NK cells in viral disease has been known for a long time. The correlation between low NK activity and serious viral infections in immunocompromised hosts, e.g. in AIDS, after transplantation and in certain congenital immunodeficiencies, has been well documented. Abnormalities in NK function have been described in a variety of autoimmune diseases, and since these diseases are frequently associated with serious viral infections and malignancy, low levels of NK activity may be biologically important in individuals with autoimmune disorders.[56] Finally, chronic fatigue immune dysfunction syndrome (CFIDS) is characterized by a number of immunologic abnormalities, the most consistent being a significant depression of NK activity.[61,62] A similar phenomenon (low NK cytotoxic activity) was recently reported by our laboratory in patients who have a history of toxic chemical exposure or silicone breast implants.[61–67]

Enhancement of NK cell activity by buffered vitamin C (ultra-potent C) in chronic fatigue syndrome patients exposed to toxic chemicals

After exposure to numerous toxic chemicals, NK function can be decreased significantly. Weeks or months later, NK function can rebound to normal levels in some persons and be suppressed for prolonged periods of time in others.

In view of these results, we decided to study the effect of buffered vitamin C on NK, T- and B-cell function in patients who had been exposed to toxic chemicals. After the first blood draw, 55 patients immediately ingested granulated buffered vitamin C in water at a dosage of 60 mg/kg body weight. Exactly 24 hours later, blood was again drawn for a follow-up study of NK, T- and B-cell function. In 78% of patients, vitamin C in a high oral dose enhanced NK activity up to 10-fold. Lymphocyte blastogenic responses to T- and B-cell mitogens were restored to the normal level after vitamin C usage. Signal transduction enzyme protein kinase C (PKC) appeared to be involved in the mechanism of induction of NK activity by vitamin C. We concluded that immune functional abnormalities after toxic chemical exposure can be restored by oral usage of vitamin C. The enhancement of NK activity in patients exposed to chemicals is shown in Figure 20.8.

We used a buffered preparation of vitamin C or ultra-potent C concentration of 60 mg/kg. This preparation was found to be very well tolerated at high doses. So far, a large number of patients have been followed by physical examination, hematology, and blood chemistry, including liver enzyme and complete urinalysis for a period of 3 years of post-ultra-potent C usage; no signs of tissue toxicity (liver or kidney) or other abnormalities were detected. While vitamin C was capable of enhancing the NK, T- and B-cell function, non-significant improvement in the described symptoms was observed. However, enhancement in functions of NK, T- and B-cells by vitamin C may prevent or delay infections or other health problems in patients who are at increased risk from toxic chemical exposure.

In our study, we proposed that immune function testing should become routine, not only in patients after toxic chemical exposure, but also in patients who suffer from malignant diseases and are undergoing chemotherapy and radiation therapy. These treatment modalities may further impair immune function; thus, the body's capacity to fight malignant cells will be reduced. In these patients, immune modulation or stimulation should be attempted. In our case, this was successfully accomplished with ultra-potent C in a majority (78%) of the patients studied. Other biological response modifiers, such as lentinan interleukin-2 and other cytokines, should be examined and then may be recommended for the other 22% of patients whose immune function did not respond to vitamin C.[68]

CONCLUSION

A collection of these tests not only reflects the function of the immune system but also represents the most important markers for detection of oxidative stress. Under normal conditions, T-cells, B-cells and natural killer cells maintain a suitable redox equilibrium by balancing cytoplasmic levels of oxidants and antioxidants.

Following activation by infectious agents, especially their superantigens and haptenic chemicals through different receptors, mitochondrial respiration increases, which results in higher levels of reactive oxygen intermediates.

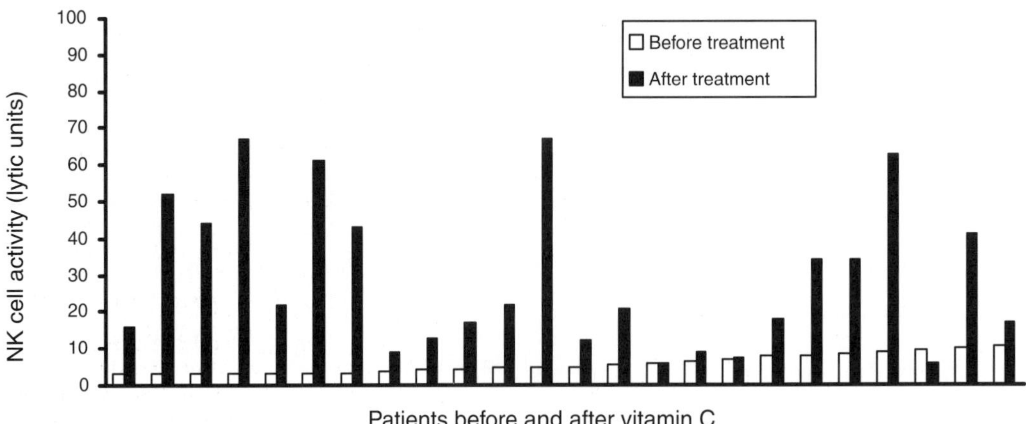

Figure 20.8 Effect of buffered vitamin C on NK cell activity in patients exposed to chemicals.

When cellular antioxidant levels are insufficient or cellular exposure to reactive oxygen intermediates occurs, oxidative stress may be invoked. This leads to activation of PKR, NF-kB, and finally, DNA damage.

Oxidative damage to DNA and activation of PKR and NF-kB first lead to malfunction of natural killer, T- and B-cells and then to the activation of death genes, which leads to a change in cell signaling (see Ch. 8) and programmed cell death (or apoptosis – see Ch. 6). Therefore, the measurement of NK cell activity along with cell cycle and apoptosis as shown in Figure 20.9 in patients with chronic illnesses will enable clinicians to simultaneously assess the function of the immune system and evaluate the cellular level of oxidative stress. Moreover, these tests are extremely important for the follow-up treatment and prognosis of diseases using biological response modifiers, antioxidants, growth hormone, cytokines, plant extracts and other modalities. In many chronic illnesses, the final goal of many clinicians is to reverse tissue abnormalities and sustain tissue homeostasis, and this could only be documented by laboratory examinations described in this chapter.

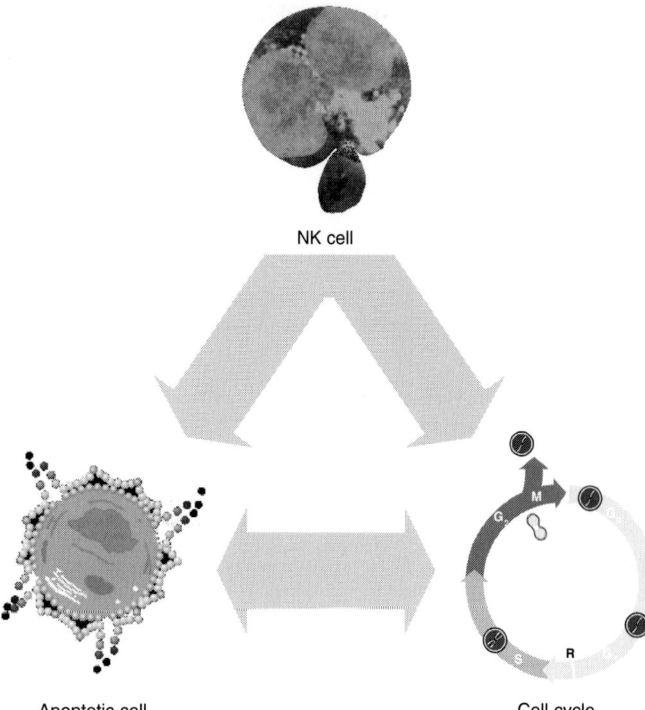

Figure 20.9 Natural killer cell activity, apoptosis and cell cycle in health and disease.

REFERENCES

1. Weiss A, Imboden J. Cell surface molecules and early events involved in human T lymphocyte activation. Adv Immunol 1987; 41: 1
2. Reinherz EL, Schlossman SF. Strategies for regulating the human immune response by selective T-cell subset manipulation. In: Feifer A, ed. The potential role of T-cell populations in cancer therapy. New York: Raven Press. 1982: p 253
3. Reinherz EL, Cooper MD, Schlossman SF. Abnormalities of T-cell maturation and regulation in human beings with immunodeficiency disorders. J Clin Invest 1981; 68: 699
4. Reinherz EL, Morimoto C, Fitzgerald KA et al. Heterogeneity of human T4+ inducer T-cells defined by a monoclonal antibody that delineates two functional subpopulations. J Immunol 1982; 128: 463
5. Reinherz EL, Meuer SC, Schlossman SF. The delineation of antigen receptors on human T-lymphocytes. Immunol Today 1983; 4: 5
6. Bass DA, Parse JW, DeChatelet LR et al. Flow cytometry studies of oxidative product formation by neutrophils: a graded response to membrane stimulation. J Immunol 1983; 130: 1910
7. Kammer GM. T-lymphocyte activation. In: Rose NR, DeMacario EC, Fahey JL et al, eds. Manual of clinical laboratory immunology. Washington, DC: American Society for Microbiology. 1992
8. Waggoner A, Ernst LA. Fluorescence reagents for flow cytometry. In: Bauer KD, Duque RE, Shankey TV, eds. Clinical flow cytometry, principles and application. Baltimore: Williams and Wilkins. 1993
9. Vowells SJ, Sekhsaria S, Malech HL et al. Flow cytometric analysis of the granulocyte respiratory burst: a comparison study of fluorescent probes. J Immunol Methods 1995; 178: 89
10. National Committee for Clinical Laboratory Standards. Clinical applications of flow cytometry: quality assurance and immunophenotyping of peripheral blood lymphocytes. NCCLS Document H42. Villanova, PA: NCCLS. 1992
11. Lewis DE, Rickman WJ. Methodology and quality control for flow cytometry. In: Rose NR, DeMacario EC, Fahey JL et al, eds. Manual of clinical laboratory immunology, 4th edn. Washington, DC: American Society of Microbiology. 1992
12. Renzi P, Ginns LC. Analysis of T-cell subsets in normal adults: comparison of whole blood lysis technique to Ficoll-Hypaque separation by flow cytometry. J Immunol Methods 1987; 98: 53
13. Yamada M, Tamura N, Shirai T et al. Flow cytometric analysis of lymphocyte subsets in the bronchoalveolar lavage fluid and peripheral blood of healthy volunteers. Scan J Immunol 1986; 24: 559
14. Campana D, Thompson JS, Amiot P et al. The cytoplasmic expression of CD3 antigens in normal and malignant cells of the T lymphoid lineage. J Immunol 1987; 138: 6481
15. Anker R, Conley ME, Pollock BA. Clonal diversity in the B-cell repertoire of patients with X-linked agammaglobulinemia. J Exp Med 1989; 169: 2109
16. Phillips AN, Lee CA, Elford J et al. Serial CD4 lymphocyte counts and development of AIDS. Lancet 1991; 337: 389
17. Morimoto C, Letvin NL, Distaso JA et al. The isolation and characterization of the human suppressor inducer T-cell subset. J Immunol 1985; 134: 1508
18. Ramos EL, Turka LA, Leggat JE et al. Decrease in phenotypically defined T-helper inducer cells (T4+4B4+) and increase in T-suppressor effector cells (T8+2H4+) in stable renal allograft recipients. Transplantation 1989; 47: 465
19. Raziuddin S, Nur MA, Alwabel AA. Selective loss of the CD4+ inducers of suppressor T-cell subsets (2H4+) in active systemic lupus erythematosus. J Rheumatol 1989; 16: 1315
20. Hercend T, Griffin JD, Bensussan S et al. Generation of monoclonal antibodies to a human natural killer clone: characterization of two natural killer-associated antigens (NKH-1A and NKH-2), expressed on subsets of large granular lymphocytes. J Clin Invest 1985; 75: 932

21. Jackson AL, Matsumoto H, Janszen M et al. Restricted expression of p55 interleukin 2 receptor (CD25) on normal T-cells. Clin Immunol Immunopathol 1990; 54: 126
22. Westermann J, Pabst R. Lymphocyte subsets in the blood. A diagnostic window on the lymphoid system? Immunol Today 1990; 11: 406
23. Sanders ME, Makgoba MW, Shaw S. Human naive and memory: reinterpretation of helper-inducer and suppressor-inducer subsets. Immunol Today 1988; 9: 195
24. Landay A, Jessop C, Lennette ET, Levy JA. Chronic fatigue syndrome. clinical condition associated with immune activation. Lancet 1991; 338: 707
25. Vojdani A, Ghoneum M, Brautbar N. Immune alteration associated with exposure to toxic chemicals. Toxicol Ind Health 1992; 8: 231
26. Vojdani A, Ghoneum M, Brautbar N. Immune functional abnormalities in patients with clinical abnormalities and silicone breast implants. Toxicol Ind Health 1993; 8: 415
27. Johnston RB. Monocytes and macrophages. N Engl J Med 1988; 318: 747
28. Smith PD, Ohura K, Masur H et al. Monocyte function in the acquired immune deficiency syndrome. J Clin Invest 1984; 74: 2121
29. Lotz M, Vaughan JH, Carson DA. Effect of neuropeptides on production of inflammatory cytokines by human monocytes. Science 1988; 241: 1218
30. Dinarello CA, Wolff SM. Mechanisms of diseases. The role of interleukin-1 in disease. N Engl J Med 1993; 328: 106
31. Gartner S, Markovits P, Markovits DM. The role of mononuclear phagocytes in HTLV-III/LAV infection. Science 1986; 233: 215
32. Lucey DR, Hensley RE, Ward WW et al. CD4+ monocyte counts in persons with HIV-1 infection: an early increase is followed by a progressive decline. J Acquir Immune Defic Syndr 1990; 4: 24
33. Weinberg JB, Hobbs MM, Misukonis MA. Phenotypic characterization of gamma-interferon-induced human monocyte polykaryons. Blood 1985; 66: 1241
34. Bandres JC, Trial J, Musher D. Increased phagocytosis and generation of reactive oxygen products by neutrophils and monocytes by men with stage 1 human immunodeficiency virus infection. J Infect Dis 1993; 168: 75
35. Gabrilovich D, Serebrovskaya L. Assessment of phagocytic activity in whole blood using laser flow cytometry. J Immunol Methods 1991; 140: 289
36. Malech HL, Gallin JI. Neutrophils in human diseases. N Engl J Med 1987; 317: 687
37. Buschman H, Winter M. Assessment of phagocytic activity of granulocytes using laser flow cytometry. J Immunol Methods 1989; 124: 231
38. Yang J, Kawamura I, Zhuh H, Mitsuyama M. Involvement of natural killer cells in nitric oxide production by spleen cells after stimulation with mycobacterium bovis BCG. J Immunol 1995; 155: 5728
39. Ling NR, Kay JE. Lymphocyte stimulation. Oxford: North Holland. 1975
40. Dean JH, Connor R, Herberman RB et al. The relative proliferation index as a more sensitive parameter for evaluating lymphoproliferative responses of cancer patients to mitogens and alloantigens. Int J Cancer 1977; 20: 359
41. Farrant J, Clark JC, Lee H et al. Conditions for measuring DNA synthesis in PHA stimulated human lymphocytes in 20 μl hanging drops with various cell concentrations and periods of culture. J Immunol Methods 1980; 33: 301
42. D'Ambrosio D, Trotta R, Vacca A et al. Transcriptional regulation of interleukin-2 gene expression by CD69-generated signals. Eur J Immunol 1993; 23: 2993
43. Oppenheim JJ, Dougherty S, Chen SC, Baker J. Utilization of lymphocyte transformation to assess clinical disorders. In: Vyas GN, ed. Laboratory diagnosis of immunological disorders. New York: Green and Stretton. 1975: p 87–109
44. Mossman TR, Coffman RL. TH1 and TH2 cells. Different patterns of lymphokine secretion lead to different functional properties. Ann Rev Immunol 1989; 7: 145
45. Romagnani S. Human TH1 and TH2 subsets: doubt no more. Immunol Today 1991; 12: 256
46. Shearer GM, Clerici M. Is HIV infection associated with a TH1®TH2 switch? Immunol Today 1993; 14: 107
47. Field EH, Noelle RJ, Rouse T et al. Evidence for excessive TH2 CD4+ subset activity *in vivo*. J Immunol 1993; 151: 48
48. Herberman RB, Ortaldo JR. Natural killer cells. Their role in defense against disease. Science 1981; 241: 24
49. Trunchieri G, Perussia B. Human natural killer cells: biologic and pathologic aspects. Lab Invest 1984; 50: 4489
50. Takayama H, Trenn G, Humphrey W et al. Antigen receptor-triggered secretion of a trypsin-type esterase from cytotoxic T lymphocyte. J Immunol 1987; 138: 566
51. Whiteside TL, Herberman RB. The role of natural killer cells in human disease. Clin Immunol Immunopathol 1988; 53: 1–23
52. Gorelik E, Wiltrout RH, Okumura K et al. Role of NK cells in the control of metastatic spread of tumor cells in mice. Int J Cancer 1982; 30: 107
53. Herberman RB, Holden HT. Natural cell-mediated immunity. Adv Cancer Res 1978; 27: 305
54. Abo T, Miller CA, Balch CM. Characterization of human granular lymphocyte subpopulations expressing NHK-1 (Leu-7 and Leu-11) antigens in the blood and lymphoid tissues from fetuses, neonates and adults. Eur J Immunol 1984; 1: 616
55. Timonen T, Ortaldo JR, Herberman RB. Characteristics of human large granular lymphocytes and their relationship to natural killer (NK) cells. J Exp Med 1981; 153: 569
56. Whiteside TL, Herberman RB. Role of human natural killer cells in health and disease. Clin Diag Lab Immunol 1994; 1: 125
57. Whiteside TL, Bryant J, Day R, Herberman RB. Natural killer cytotoxicity in the diagnosis of immune dysfunction: criteria for a reproducible assay. J Clin Lab Anal 1990; 2: 102
58. Whiteside TL, Herberman RB. The role of natural killer cells in immune surveillance of cancer. Curr Opinion Immunol 1995; 7: 704
59. Pross HR, Lotzova E. Role of natural killer cells in cancer. Nat Immunol 1993; 12: 279
60. Levy SM, Herberman RB, Simons A et al. Persistently low natural killer cell activity in normal adults: immunological, hormonal and mood correlates. Nat Immun Cell Growth Regul 1989; 8: 173
61. Aoki R, Usuda T, Miyakoshi H et al. Low NK syndrome (LNKS): clinical and immunologic features. Nat Immun Cell Growth Regul 1987; 6: 116
62. Eby N, Grufferman S, Huang M et al. Natural killer cell activity in the chronic fatigue-immune dysfunction syndrome. In:. Ades EW, Lopez C, eds. Natural killer cells and host defense. Karger: Basel. 1988: p 141
63. Biron C, Byron KS, Sullivan J. Severe herpes virus infections in an adolescent without natural killer cells. N Engl J Med 1989; 320: 1731
64. Purtilo DT, Strobach RS, Okano M et al. Epstein-Barr virus-associated lymphoproliferative disorders. Lab Invest 1992; 67: 5
65. Plaeger-Marshall S, Spina CA, Giorgi JV et al. Alterations in cytotoxic and phenotypic subsets of natural killer cells in acquired immunodeficiency syndrome (AIDS). J Clin Immunol 1987; 7: 16
66. Vojdani A, Campbell A, Brautbar N. Immune functional impairment in patients with clinical abnormalities and silicone breast implant. Toxicol Indus Health 1992; 8: 415
67. Campbell A, Brautbar N, Vojdani A. Suppressed NK cell activity in patients with silicone breast implant: reversal upon explanation. Toxicol Indus Health 1994; 10: 149
68. Heuser G, Vojdani A. Enhancement of natural killer cell activity and T and B cell function by buffered vitamin C in patients exposed to toxic chemicals: the role of protein kinase-C. Immunopharmacol Immunotoxicol 1997; 19: 291–312

CHAPTER CONTENTS

21

Intestinal permeability assessment

Martin J. Lee, PhD

INTRODUCTION

The small intestine has the paradoxical dual function of being a digestive/absorptive organ as well as a barrier to permeation of toxic compounds and macromolecules (Fig. 21.1).[1–3] Either one of these functions may be disrupted by various mechanisms, resulting in local as well as systemic problems.

In certain disease states of the small intestine, such as gluten-sensitive enteropathy, permeability to large molecules may increase while permeability to small molecules decreases. The explanation of this apparent paradox lies in the different routes of entry for readily absorbed, water-soluble molecules, such as mannitol, and normally excluded molecules like lactulose. Transcellular uptake of mannitol relies on properties of the luminal cell membrane, a relatively huge area compared to the minute intercellular junctional complexes or tight junctions. Increased porosity of tight junctions has little effect on mannitol uptake, but villous atrophy decreases mannitol diffusion into mucosal cells. Thus, decreased transcellular permeability to small, water-soluble molecules may lead to malnutrition. In contrast, increased porosity of junctional complexes may lead to increased uptake of food antigens and bacterial toxins, correlating with increased susceptibility to food allergies and autoimmune conditions such as rheumatoid arthritis.

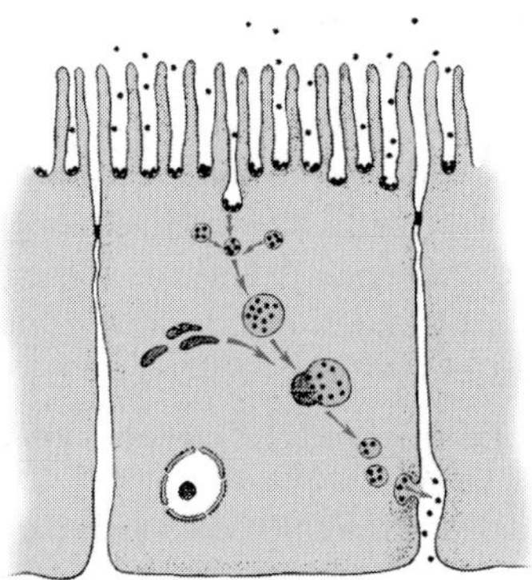

Figure 21.1 The intestinal barrier.

The large intestine contains numerous dietary and bacterial products with toxic properties. These include viable bacteria, bacterial cell wall polymers, chemotactic peptides, bacterial antigens capable of inducing antibodies which cross-react with host antibodies, and bacterial and dietary antigens which can form systemic immune complexes.[4] Abnormalities of the immune or mechanical barriers may lead to enhanced uptake of inflammatory luminal macromolecules and pathogenic bacteria. With intestinal injury, mucosal absorption of normally excluded substances increases dramatically. Intestinal inflammation enhances the uptake and systemic distribution of potentially injurious macromolecules.[4] Peters & Bjarnson[5] noted: "Measurement of intestinal permeability will play an increasing role in clinical investigation and monitoring of intestinal disease."

MEASURING INTESTINAL PERMEABILITY

Gut permeability has traditionally been measured by ingesting a non-metabolizable monomeric sugar and observing the degree to which it is adsorbed. The marker of absorption must be inert, so that it can be an indicator of the passive diffusion and uptake of nutrients. Xylose is an example of a molecule that fulfills this criteria.

Unfortunately, xylose absorption turns out to be a very insensitive test. There are two basic reasons for this. First, the amount of xylose absorbed is a function of the transit time and the contents of the gastrointestinal tract (osmotic strength, mucous flows, etc.). Thus, there is considerable within-individual biological variation. Secondly, and more importantly, it is incorrect and simplistic to view absorption with a model of a simple sieve.

Absorption can, in fact, be divided into transcellular (through the cell) and paracellular (between the cell) processes. A useful analogy to help understand this process is that of a train containing a number of boxcars, with each car representing a cell. Now, imagine that each boxcar was the length of a football field and each boxcar was held together with heavy-duty springs having an average distance between boxcars of perhaps 1 foot. Small molecules – monomers such as simple sugars, glycerol, amino acids, and many vitamins and nutrients – can go into the cells and be absorbed directly into the cells (boxcars). Large molecules, however, are excluded.

Interestingly, the spaces between the cells are not static. They vibrate with the springs that hold the cells together. These springs – called the tight junctions – are usually sufficient to keep out anything bigger than very small molecules. Some dipeptides and tripeptides can be absorbed, but larger peptides, disaccharides and larger carbohydrates cannot normally enter the body. However, when the cellular health is less than optimum, when nutrition is poor or digestive processes are compromised, in the presence of and possibly etiologically related to many gastrointestinal disorders, the tight junctions become less tight, the spaces between the cells become effectively larger, and bigger – even much bigger molecules can enter the body.

Thus, it can be seen that in many people there can be a paradoxical leakiness to gut antigens, proteins, food molecules and even bacteria, while at the same time there may be malabsorption of nutrients and vitamins when damage to the intestinal cells interferes with transcellular absorption of required nutrients.

An elegant method to evaluate this permeability and account for osmotic and biological variation has been developed in recent years. This system employs two non-metabolized molecules: mannitol, a monomeric sugar, and lactulose, a dimeric sugar. Mannitol, the monomer, is readily absorbed and serves as a marker of transcellular uptake. Lactulose is only slightly absorbed and serves as a marker for paracellular permeability. The ratio has been found in numerous clinical studies to be an exquisite marker of subtle changes in intestinal permeability. To perform the test, the patient ingests a pre-measured amount of lactulose and mannitol. Urine is then collected, usually for 6 hours, and the amount of each sugar recovered in the urine is then measured.

CLINICAL APPLICATIONS

Increased permeability of the intestinal mucosal barrier appears to correlate with a number of frequently seen clinical disorders, while decreased permeability appears to be a fundamental cause of malnutrition, malabsorption and failure to thrive. Increased permeability is seen in many disorders (Table 21.1).[6] Several of these disorders are discussed in detail below.

Inflammatory bowel disease

Increases in permeability have consistently been reported with small bowel inflammation.[7] In 1972, Shorter et al[8] proposed that a breach of the intestinal barrier is fundamental to the development of intestinal inflammation. Most current hypotheses about the pathogenesis of Crohn's disease posit the prime importance of mucosal

Table 21.1 Diseases associated with abnormal bowel permeability

- Inflammatory bowel disease
- Crohn's disease
- Inflammatory joint disease
- Food allergy
- Celiac disease
- Rheumatoid arthritis
- Ankylosing spondylitis
- Reiter's syndrome
- Chronic dermatological conditions
- Schizophrenia
- Allergic disorders

integrity in maintaining a healthy state, and suggest that increased mucosal permeability underlies the inflammatory process. Studies show Crohn's disease to be more extensive than is sometimes apparent using macroscopic approaches.[9] Pearson et al[10] showed a sixfold increase in permeability in people with Crohn's disease. When patients with Crohn's disease were placed on an elemental diet, their permeability improved significantly, coinciding with marked clinical improvement.[11] (See Ch. 163 for a full discussion.)

Inflammatory joint disease

The concept that the underlying etiology of inflammatory arthritides (including rheumatoid arthritis) is related to pathology in the gut has become accepted by many researchers.[12,13] All material that traverses the mucosa is inspected by the immune system and it is here that the immune system may have its greatest antigenic exposure. Increased gut permeability can permit exogenous antigens to enter the systemic circulation. If the antibodies generated against gut antigens cross-react with the body's own immunologically similar tissues, the resulting process may manifest itself as an autoimmune disease.[14]

Studies have demonstrated that patients with ankylosing spondylitis, rheumatoid arthritis and vasculitis have increased intestinal permeability; and suggest that this may be an important factor in the pathogenesis of these disorders.[13,15–17] There is a strong association between enteric infection and Reiter's syndrome or reactive arthritis. Intestinal infections of *Shigella, Salmonella, Yersinia,* and *Campylobacter* are known to cause this type of disorder. It has been suggested that the arthritis from these infections may be due to tissue deposition of circulating immune complexes arising from increased permeability of source antigens.[18,19] Darlington & Ramsey,[20] after studying the influence of diet on arthritis, concluded: "The mechanism by which fasting leads to improvement of rheumatoid arthritis may be a reduction in gut permeability". Mielants and co-workers[15,21] suggest that the joint disease in spondylarthropathies is triggered through the gut (see Ch. 185 for further discussion).

Food allergy

Development of food allergies depends on heredity, intestinal permeability, immune responsiveness, and exposure to food.[22] Food *sensitivity* is used to refer to all adverse reactions to the ingestion of food, including allergic, idiosyncratic, toxic, metabolic, and pharmacological. Food *allergies* are distinguished by being mediated by an immunologic mechanism, consistently reproduced by blinded food challenge and causing functional changes in target organs.[23]

In general, the intestinal tract provides an effective barrier against the excessive absorption of food antigens. When this mechanism is ineffective, antigens enter the system in excessive amounts, which leads to sensitization of the immune system in some individuals. Increased permeability is implicated in type I, type III and type IV allergies.[22] Andre et al,[24] in a study of food allergy, concluded that "evaluation of intestinal permeability... provides an objective means of diagnosing food allergy and assessing the effectiveness of anti-allergic agents". Their research has shown that people with food allergy have increased permeability during a fasting state; and that the permeability further increases after ingestion of an offending allergen. They concluded that using lactulose and mannitol to measure intestinal permeability allows objective diagnosis of food allergy. They also observed that permeability increases even after ingestion of an amount of food that is not large enough to cause a clinical reaction.[25]

Other researchers studied children with cow's milk allergy and found that the majority of children displayed changes in permeability after challenge, and that pretreatment with sodium cromoglycate diminished the changes.[26] Cromoglycate is believed to stabilize mast cells and IgE-producing plasma cells in the lamina propria of the gut, and thus to reduce the local inflammation which contributes to the increased intestinal permeability. Urticaria and atopic dermatitis can be caused by the ingestion of certain foods.[27] People with atopic dermatitis and those with urticaria demonstrated increased permeability when given an oral challenge of food that provoked symptoms[25] (see Chs 15 and 51 for further discussion).

Celiac disease

Intestinal permeability has been studied in patients with celiac disease.[10,28–30] Children with celiac disease suffer a significant alteration in permeability due to reduced absorption.[10] After exposure to a single oral dose of gluten, the intestinal permeability of people with celiac disease became transiently abnormal, returning to normal within 1 week.[28] Hamilton et al[28] concluded that the sugar ratio test is of value in assessing the response to gluten withdrawal and in monitoring patients who are already established on a gluten-free diet by detecting dietary lapses and "non-responders". In another study, a persistent functional and/or structural abnormality of the small intestine was found to be associated with celiac disease along with possible etiological implications.[29]

Non-steroidal anti-inflammatory drugs (NSAIDs)

Numerous studies have shown that NSAID usage disrupts the intestinal barrier function and causes increased permeability.[31–33] This is of particular importance in those people with arthritis who are being treated with NSAIDs, because the increased permeability may be a key factor in their disease process. The hypothesis that various bacterial and viral intestinal infections can cause altered permeability is well supported.[34,35] Studies show that host responses to infections are related to increased passage of microorganisms and endotoxins into the systemic circulation.[36] Several authors have claimed that this breach of the mucosal barrier is an important aspect in both acute and chronic systemic effects of intestinal infection. Deitch[37] reported that bacteria translocate across the mucosal barrier and cause systemic infections and various immunologic sequelae. Factors that promote translocation of bacteria include disruption of the ecologic balance of normal indigenous microflora (dysbiosis), bacterial overgrowth, impaired immune defense, trauma, and endotoxemia.

HIV infection and AIDS

Investigation has begun into intestinal permeability in patients testing positive for human immunodeficiency virus (HIV) and patients with acquired immunodeficiency syndrome (AIDS). One recent study evaluated intestinal permeability in HIV-positive patients and AIDS patients with and without diarrhea.[38] The researchers found that patients with AIDS and diarrhea have altered intestinal permeability and theorized that this alteration could allow increased transmucosal passage of opportunistic pathogens. Mannitol recovery decreased and lactulose/mannitol ratios increased incrementally as the disease progressed, suggesting that as HIV disease progresses, there is loss of functional absorptive capability, possibly contributing to the malnutrition that often characterizes AIDS.

Pancreatic insufficiency

Intestinal permeability was studied recently in patients with cystic fibrosis or pancreatic insufficiency.[39] Lactulose permeation increased with exocrine pancreatic insufficiency. The degree of increased intestinal permeability correlated with the level of duodenal trypsin and with the degree of undigested fat in the stool. The authors suggested that urinary lactulose might be useful in evaluating exocrine pancreatic function.

Malabsorption, malnutrition

Recent studies have shown that damage to the small intestine mucosa (resulting in decreased permeability) is linked to poor growth rates and failure to thrive in children. The intestinal damage is typically a result of infection and resulting diarrhea.[40,41]

Alcoholism

Studies of intestinal permeability in alcoholics have shown elevated intestinal permeability.[42] In many, the abnormality persisted for up to 2 weeks after cessation of drinking. This increased permeability may account for some of the extraintestinal tissue damage common in alcoholics. Gut-derived endotoxins may play a role in the initiation and aggravation of alcohol-induced liver disease.

Aging

In an intriguing study on aging, the authors concluded that "the intestinal barrier to the absorption of potentially harmful environmental substances may be less efficient in aging animals".[43] Various studies show that aging rats have diminishing capacity to prevent larger size molecules from penetrating the intestinal mucosa, possibly allowing antigenic or mutagenic compounds to reach the systemic circulation.[44]

Chemotherapy

Cytotoxic treatment has been shown to decrease permeability, a possible factor in malnutrition of cancer patients.[45]

CONCLUSION

Intestinal permeability is a widely applicable test. It measures the fundamental health of the mucosal epithelial membrane and its ability to carry out two of its primary functions: absorption of nutrients and the exclusion of toxic bowel constituents. Whenever digestive or nutritional dysfunction are suspected to impact systemic conditions, symptoms, or overall health, the measurement of intestinal permeability should be considered to provide information on this basic process.

REFERENCES

1. Antigen absorption by the gut [editorial]. Lancet 1978; 715–717
2. Crissinger KD, Kvietys PR, Granger DN. Pathophysiology of gastrointestinal mucosal permeability. J Int Med 1990; 732: 145–154
3. Madara JL. Pathobiology of the intestinal epithelial barrier. Am J Pathol 1990; 137: 1273–1281
4. Olaison G, Sjodahl R et al. Abnormal intestinal permeability in Crohn's disease. Scand J Gastroenterol 1990; 25: 321–328
5. Peters TJ, Bjarnason I. Uses and abuses of intestinal permeability measurements. Can J Gastroenterol 1988; 2: 127–132
6. Madara JL, Nash S, Moore R et al. Structure and function of the intestinal epithelial barrier in health and disease. Monogr Pathol 1990; 9: 306–324
7. Pironi L, Miglioli M et al. Relationship between intestinal permeability to [^{51}Cr]EDTA and inflammatory activity in

asymptomatic patients with Crohn's disease. Dig Dis Sci 1990; 35: 582–588
8. Shorter RG, Huizenga KA et al. A working hypothesis for the etiology and pathogenesis of nonspecific inflammatory bowel disease. Dig Dis 1972; 17: 1024–1032
9. Ukabam SO, Clamp JR, Cooper BT. Abnormal small intestinal permeability to sugars in patients with Crohn's disease of the terminal ileum and colon. Digestion 1983; 27: 70–74
10. Pearson AD, Eastham EJ, Laker MF et al. Intestinal permeability in children with Crohn's disease and coeliac disease. Br Med J 1982; 285(6334): 20–21
11. Sanderson IR, Boulton P, Menzies I et al. Improvement of abnormal lactulose/rhamnose permeability in active Crohn's disease of the small bowel by an elemental diet. Gut 1987; 28: 1073–1076
12. Bjarnason I. Experimental evidence of the benefit of misoprostol beyond the stomach in humans. J Rheumatol 1990; 17: 38–41
13. Rooney PJ, Jenkins RT, Buchanan WW. A short review of the relationship between intestinal permeability and inflammatory joint disease. Clin Exp Rheumatol 1990; 8: 75–83
14. Bjarnason I, Peters TJ. Intestinal permeability, non-steroidal anti-inflammatory drug enteropathy and inflammatory bowel disease: an overview. Gut 1989; (30 Spec No): 22–28
15. Mielants H, De Vos M, Goemaere S et al. Intestinal mucosal permeability in inflammatory rheumatic diseases. II. Role of disease. J Rheumatol 1991; 18: 394–400
16. Katz KD, Hollander D. Intestinal mucosal permeability and rheumatological diseases. Baillière's Clin Rheumatol 1989; 3: 271–284
17. Smith MD, Gibson RA, Brooks PM. Abnormal bowel permeability in ankylosing spondylitis and rheumatoid arthritis. J Rheumatol 1985; 12: 299–305
18. Lahesmaa-Rantala R, Magnusson KE et al. Intestinal permeability in patients with yersinia triggered reactive arthritis. Ann Rheum Dis 1991; 50: 91–94
19. Inman RD. Antigens, the gastrointestinal tract, and arthritis. Rheum Dis Clin N Am 1991; 17: 309–321
20. Darlington LG, Ramsey NW. Diets for rheumatoid arthritis [letter]. Lancet 1991; 338: 1209
21. Mielants H. Reflections on the link between intestinal permeability and inflammatory joint disease. Clin Exp Rheumatol 1990; 8: 523–524
22. Butkus SN, Mahan LK. Food allergies: immunological reactions to food. J Am Dietetic Assoc 1986; 86: 601–608
23. Schreiber RA, Walker WA. Food allergy: facts and fiction. Mayo Clin Proc 1989; 64: 1381–1391
24. Andre C, Andre F, Colin L et al. Measurement of intestinal permeability to mannitol and lactulose as a means of diagnosing food allergy and evaluating therapeutic effectiveness of disodium cromoglycate. Ann Allergy 1987; 59: 127–130
25. Andre C, Andre F, Colin L. Effect of allergen ingestion challenge with and without cromoglycate cover on intestinal permeability in atopic dermatitis, urticaria and other symptoms of food allergy. Allergy 1989; 44: 47–51
26. Falth-Magnusson K, Kjellman N-IM, Odelram H et al. Gastrointestinal permeability in children with cow's milk allergy: effect of milk challenge and sodium cromoglycate as assessed with polyethyleneglycols (PEG 400 and PEG 1000). Clin Allergy 1986; 16: 543–551
27. Paganelli R, Fagiolo U, Caucian et al. Intestinal permeability in patients with chronic urticaria-angioedema with and without arthralgia. Ann Allergy 1991; 66: 181–184
28. Hamilton I, Cobden I, Rothwell J et al. Intestinal permeability in coeliac disease: the response to gluten withdrawal and single-dose gluten challenge. Gut 1982; 23: 202–210
29. Bjarnason I, Peters TJ, Veall N. A persistent defect in intestinal permeability in coeliac disease demonstrated by a 51Cr-labelled EDTA absorption test. Lancet 1983; 1(8320): 323–325
30. Cobden I, Rothwell J, Axon ATR. Intestinal permeability and screening tests for coeliac disease. Gut 1980; 21: 512–518
31. Bjarnason I, Williams P, Smethhurst P et al. Effect of non-steroidal anti-inflammatory drugs and prostaglandins on the permeability of the human small intestine. Gut 1986; 27: 1292–1297
32. Bjarnason I, Zanelli G, Smith T et al. The pathogenesis and consequence of non steroidal anti-inflammatory drug induced small intestinal inflammation in man. Scand J Rheumatol 1987; 64: 55–62
33. Jenkins AP, Trew DR, Crump BJ et al. Do non-steroidal anti-inflammatory drugs increase colonic permeability? Gut 1991; 32: 66–69
34. Serrander R, Magnusson KE, Kihlstrome E et al. Acute yersinia infections in man increase intestinal permeability for low-molecular weight polyethylene glycols (PEG 400). Scand J Infec Dis 1986; 18: 409–413
35. Isolauri E, Juntunen M, Wiren S et al. Intestinal permeability changes in acute gastroenteritis: effects of clinical factors and nutritional management. J Ped Gastroenterol Nutr 1989; 8: 466–473
36. O'Dwyer ST, Michie HR, Ziegler TR et al. A single dose of endotoxin increases intestinal permeability in healthy humans. Arch Surg 1988; 123: 1459–1464
37. Deitch EA. Simple intestinal obstruction causes bacterial translocation in man. Arch Surg 1989; 124: 699–701
38. Tepper RE, Simon D et al. Intestinal permeability in patients infected with the human immunodeficiency virus. Am J Gastroenterol 1994; 89: 878–882
39. Mack DR, Flick JA, Durie PR et al. Correlation of intestinal lactulose permeability with exocrine pancreatic dysfunction. J Pediatrics 1992; 120: 696–701
40. Behrens RH, Lunn PG, Northrop CA et al. Factors affecting the integrity of the intestinal mucosa of Gambian children. Am J Clin Nutr 1987; 45: 1433–1441
41. Lunn PG, Northrop-Clewes CA, Downes RM. Intestinal permeability, mucosal injury, and growth faltering in Gambian infants. Lancet 1991; 338: 907–910
42. Bjarnason I, Peters TJ, Ward K. The leaky gut of alcoholism: possible route of entry for toxic compounds. Lancet 1984; 1(8370): 179–182
43. Hollander D, Tarnawski H. Aging-associated increase in intestinal absorption of macromolecules. Gerontology 1985; 31: 133–137
44. Katz D, Hollander D, Said HM et al. Aging-associated increase in intestinal permeability to polyethylene glycol 900. Dig Dis Sci 1987; 32: 285–288
45. Pledger JV, Pearson ADJ, Craft AW et al. Intestinal permeability during chemotherapy for childhood tumours. Eur J Pediatr 1988; 147: 123–127

CHAPTER CONTENTS

22

Laboratory tests for the determination of vitamin status

Michael T. Murray, ND

Joseph E. Pizzorno Jr, ND

INTRODUCTION

Laboratory assessment of vitamin status is a significant challenge for the clinician. Although measurement of blood and serum levels is easily available, their clinical value is limited to the detection of severe deficiencies. Detection of functional deficiencies requires far more sophistication.

ASSESSMENT OF VITAMIN STATUS (Table 22.1)

Ascorbic acid

Assessment of vitamin C is particularly difficult as ascorbate readily oxidizes in assay samples. In addition, serum levels reflect recent dietary uptake rather than actual tissues levels. Leukocyte levels are not as susceptible to dietary levels, but are also readily affected by infection, hypoglycemia and many common prescription and over-the-counter drugs. The popular lingual ascorbate test does not appear to be reliable as it does not correlate very well with leukocyte or serum levels. The loading test, if carefully controlled, is probably most accurate, although good standard ranges have yet to be determined.

Folate

Serum folate is also greatly affected by recent consumption. The neutrophil hypersegmentation test is a useful functional test. A deficiency of folate (as well as vitamin B_{12}) will cause an over-aging of white cells which results in increased lobulation of their nuclei. The test is not, however, reliable during pregnancy.

Niacin

While measurement of nicotinic acid in the blood is not very reliable, measurement of metabolites provides a clinically useful function assessment. Several metabolites tests are now available.

Table 22.1 Laboratory tests and optimal ranges for common vitamins[1–3]

Nutrient	Test	Acceptable level
Ascorbic acid	Serum	>0.3 mg/dl
	Leukocyte	30 ug/10^8 WBCs
	Load test	0.3–2.0 mg/h in control
		24–49 mg/h after 500 mg
Folate	RBC folacin	>160–650 ng/ml
	Neutrophil hypersegmentation	<30% with five or more lobes
Niacin	Urinary *N*-methylnicotinamide	>1.6 mg/gm creatinine
	RBC NAD/NADP	>1.0
Pyridoxine	Serum level	>50 ng/ml
	Tryptophan load	<35 mg/24 h xanthurenic acid
	Transaminase index	
	EGOT	<1.5 (ratio)
	EGPT	<1.25
	Plasma pyridoxal	>8 ng/ml
Riboflavin	RBC glutathione reductase	
	FAD-effect	<20% increase
Thiamine	RBC transketolase	<15% increase
Vitamin A	Plasma retinol	15–60 ug/dl
	0–5 months	>20
	6 months–17 years	>30
	Adult	>20
	Plasma carotene	80–400 ug/dl
	0–5 months	>10
	6–11 months	>30
	1–17 years	>40
	Adult	>40
	Pregnancy	>80
Vitamin B_{12}	Serum B_{12}	>150 pg/ml
	Urinary methylmalonic acid	<5 ug/mg creatinine
Vitamin D	Cholecalciferol (D_3)	10–80 ng/ml
	1,25 dihydroxycholecalciferol	21–45 pg/ml
Vitamin E	Serum tocopherol	>0.7 mg/100 dl
	RBC hemolysis in H_2O_2	<10%
	Serum tocopherol/triglyceride	35–120
Vitamin K	Abnormal prothrombin antigen assay	<20 ng/ml

Pyridoxine

Several procedures are available for assessing vitamin B_6 status. Unfortunately, substantial agreement on the best methodology has not been established as variations in phenotypes significantly alter the results of functional and loading tests.

Riboflavin

The most common measure of riboflavin is RBC glutathione reductase activity. The enzyme is stimulated in vitro by adding flavin adenine dinucleotide. Elevation of activity greater than 20% is suggestive of a functional deficiency.

Thiamine

The most common measure of thiamin is RBC transketolase activity. The enzyme is stimulated in vitro by adding thiamine pyrophosphate. Elevation in activity of greater than 15% indicates a functional deficiency. The test is not reliable in patients with diabetes mellitus, pernicious anemia or a significant negative nitrogen balance.

Vitamin A

While liver biopsy is the most accurate method of assessment, other less invasive and less expensive methodologies are more appropriate. As with most other nutrients, serum levels only fall significantly after tissue reserves have been depleted. Fortunately, the dark adaptation test will detect early deficiency (see Ch. 26 for a discussion of this useful, easily performed, office procedure).

Vitamin B_{12}

Serum levels are not very useful as they do not track cerebral spinal levels very well. Erythrocyte cell size is also not reliable, as neurological signs and symptoms can precede macrocytosis by 6–12 months. Measurement of urinary methylmalonic acid is sensitive and accurate, especially when expressed as a ration to urinary creatinine.

Vitamin D

Serum levels of vitamin D, especially its activated dihydroxy form, are clinically accurate and useful.

Vitamin E

Platelet vitamin E levels appear to be the most accurate measure of intake. However, a more clinically relevant measure appears to be the ratio of this important antioxidant to the one key molecule it protects: triglycerides.

Vitamin K

The various prothrombin and clotting time assays appear to be useful ways to assess vitamin K status.

CONCLUSION

As described above, many procedures are now available for the assessment of functional vitamin status. While research continues in this important area, the reader is advised to study carefully Chapter 29 on urinary organic acids profiling. Utilizing metabolic products excreted in the urine is now allowing the clinician far greater specificity in recognizing dysfunctional enzyme systems, whether due to genetic deviations or nutritional deficiencies.

REFERENCES

1. Tierney LM, McPhee SJ, Papdakis MA. Current diagnosis and treatment. Stamford, CT: Appleton Lange. 1997: p 1138–1142
2. Rubenstein E, Federman DD. Scientific American medicine. New York, NY: Scientific American. 1983: p 1–19
3. Werbach MR: Nutritional influences on illness, 2nd edn. Tarzana, CA: Third Line Press. 1993

CHAPTER CONTENTS

23

Lactose intolerance breath test

Stephen Barrie, ND

INTRODUCTION

More than 50 million Americans can't digest lactose (milk sugar) or other sugars because they lack the appropriate enzyme in their digestive systems. They may suffer from bloating, diarrhea, flatulence, abdominal cramps and discomfort and may never realize the cause of their symptoms.

The digestive system uses specific enzymes, such as dissaccharidases, to break down sugars into smaller components. Disaccharidases hydrolyze disaccharides into monosaccharides, smaller molecules that the body absorbs more easily.[1]

When an individual doesn't produce enough of a particular enzyme to break down a carbohydrate into simpler sugars, the carbohydrate passes into the colon. There, the bacteria ferment the carbohydrate, a side-effect of which is gas. Osmotic imbalances create diarrhea, and the gases cause the bloating seen in individuals with carbohydrate intolerances. Over time, the intestinal mucosal lining becomes irritated.

There are degrees of carbohydrate intolerance. Some individuals manufacture a small amount of the enzyme, while others lack the enzyme completely. Any degree of deficiency will result in malabsorption.[2]

Unfortunately, many people never relate their symptoms to their diet and continue to eat foods they cannot digest properly. Studies indicate that 70% of lactose-intolerant patients do not relate their symptoms to lactose ingestion. At times, individuals may even mislead their physicians by denying a connection to their symptoms and their diet.[3,4] Table 23.1 provides a list of lactase deficiency in various ethnic groups.

Ongoing carbohydrate malabsorption constantly damages the digestive system, leading to systemic disorders. The body cannot obtain needed nutrients when intestinal dysfunction disrupts absorption. The weakened digestive system is also more susceptible to attack by parasites, yeast and bacterial overgrowth, which further tip the scales of healthy intestinal balance.

Table 23.1 Incidence of lactase deficiency by ethnic group

Ethnic group	Incidence
African Blacks	97–100%
Asians	90–100%
N. American Blacks	70–75%
Mexicans	70–80%
Mediterraneans	60–90%
Jewish descent	60–80%
Middle Europeans	10–20%
North American Caucasians	7–15%
Northern Europeans	1–5%

Imbalanced gut flora, irritated mucosa, leaky gut, altered permeability, food allergies and chronic illness can result from these intestinal irritations. Therefore, suspected sugar malabsorption should be investigated and treated to ward off further damage to the body's digestive system.

TYPES OF SUGAR INTOLERANCE

Lactose

Lactose intolerance is the most common type of malabsorption because milk sugar is common in a typical diet. Without the lactase enzyme, the intestine cannot break down lactose into glucose and galactose (Fig. 23.1). Lactase retention is genetically determined as a dominant trait. Lactase reaches its maximum levels in the human intestine shortly after birth and declines after the age of 3½ years.[1]

Lactose malabsorption often is recognized for the first time in older patients, possibly because they are more sensitive to intestinal problems. They may have endured gas and other symptoms for years without connecting the symptoms to their diet.[5]

Conditions that damage the intestinal lining can create lactose malabsorption, such as infectious diarrhea, intestinal parasites or inflammatory bowel disease. Alcoholism, malnutrition, pelvic radiation therapy and drugs such as antibiotics can also trigger lactose malabsorption.[6]

Lactose intolerance is very different from milk allergy, and individuals who don't produce sufficient quantities of the lactase enzyme aren't necessarily allergic to milk proteins.

A reliable test for lactose intolerance can differentiate this disorder from other digestive problems such as milk allergy and irritable bowel syndrome. An accurate diagnosis is important because:

- Many patients don't relate intestinal troubles to what they eat. A lactose intolerance test can dramatically

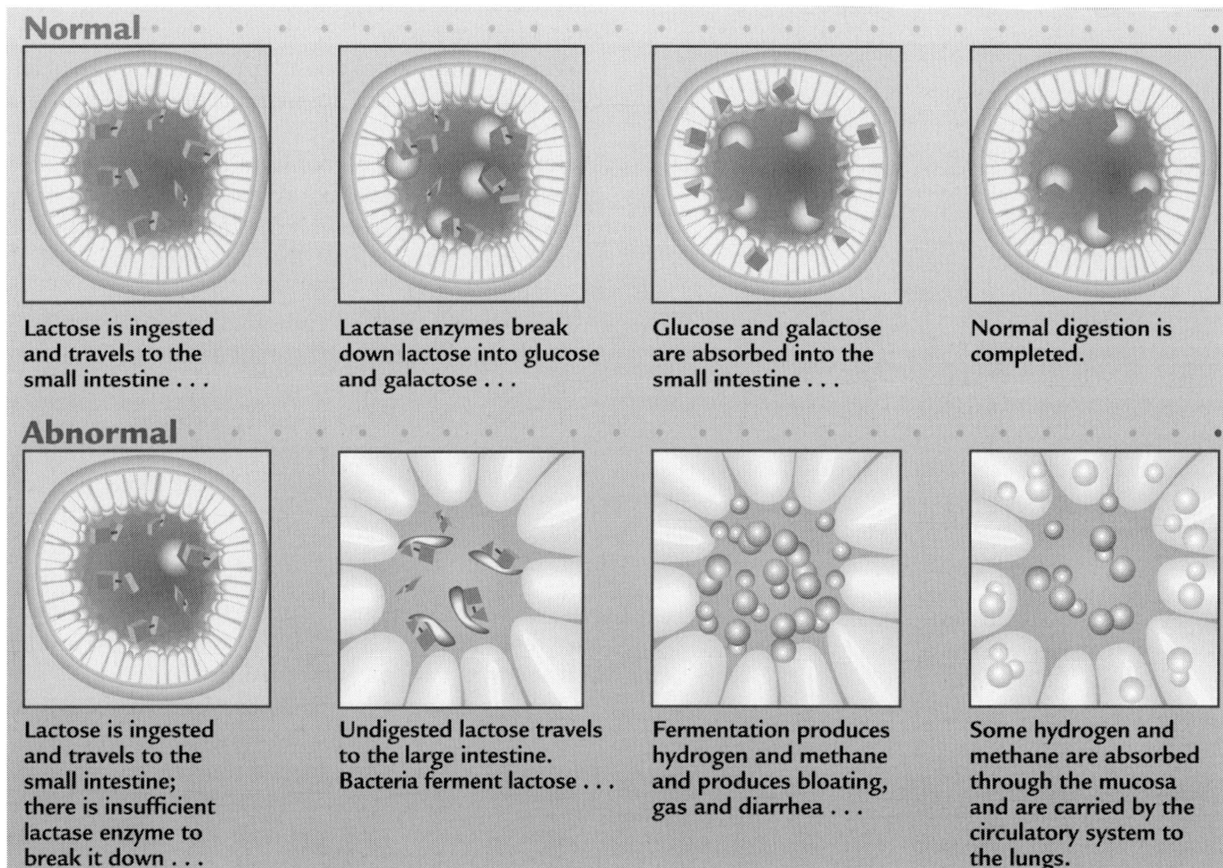

Normal
Lactose is ingested and travels to the small intestine . . .
Lactase enzymes break down lactose into glucose and galactose . . .
Glucose and galactose are absorbed into the small intestine . . .
Normal digestion is completed.
Abnormal
Lactose is ingested and travels to the small intestine; there is insufficient lactase enzyme to break it down . . .
Undigested lactose travels to the large intestine. Bacteria ferment lactose . . .
Fermentation produces hydrogen and methane and produces bloating, gas and diarrhea . . .
Some hydrogen and methane are absorbed through the mucosa and are carried by the circulatory system to the lungs.

Figure 23.1

demonstrate to patients the connection between symptoms and diet and the importance of following diet restrictions.[3] Studies show that some patients with lactose intolerance are not observant about food-related symptoms. In one study, 42% of lactose intolerant patients did not associate their symptoms with any food.[4]
- Patients may be unnecessarily avoiding dairy products. Since milk and dairy products can be important sources of nutrients for children, pregnant women, nursing mothers and older adults, they should not be eliminated from the diet without good reason.[7,8]

Treatment options, such as enzyme replacement therapy, can help individuals with lactose intolerance enjoy milk products. Lactase enzyme replacements will not benefit those people who are allergic to milk proteins or who cannot tolerate some other type of sugar.

Fructose

Fructose is used as a sweetener in many soft drinks and is present in a number of fruits. Individuals may be fructose malabsorbers and suffer symptoms similar to lactose intolerance.

Sucrose

Sucrose is common table sugar. The sucrase enzyme is needed to break down sucrose into glucose and fructose. If malabsorption symptoms exist but the lactose test is negative, sucrose intolerance should be considered.

Maltose

Maltose is also produced by some foods. The maltase enzyme is needed to break down maltose into two molecules of glucose. If malabsorption symptoms exist but the lactose test is negative, maltose intolerance should be considered.

LACTOSE INTOLERANCE TESTS

Eliminating milk from the diet

Excluding milk products from the diet is not a conclusive test because many patients don't follow the diet completely. Furthermore, many unsuspected foods and drugs use lactose as a filler, making it difficult to totally remove milk products from the diet (see Table 23.2). Patients who continue eating these foods may experience ongoing symptoms, leading to a false-negative diagnosis.[7]

Other common disaccharides and sweeteners can cause digestive disorders and symptoms, and removing milk from the diet does not resolve the underlying problem.

Table 23.2 Sources of lactose

Obvious sources
- All cheeses
- Butter
- Goat's milk
- Half-and-half cream
- Ice-cream and many sherbets
- Milk (whole, skim, dry powdered, evaporated)
- Yogurt

Hidden sources
- Artificial sweeteners containing lactose
- Breads, biscuits and crackers, doughnuts made with milk
- Breading on fried foods
- Breakfast and baby cereals containing milk solids
- Buttered or creamed foods (soups and vegetables)
- Cake and pudding mixes, many frostings
- Candies with milk chocolate
- Cookies made with milk
- Hot dogs, luncheon meats, sausage, hash, processed and canned meats
- Many margarines
- Mayonnaise and salad dressings made with milk
- Non-dairy creamers (except for Coffee Rich)
- Pancakes, waffles, toaster tarts
- Pizza
- Weight-reduction formulas
- Many prescription drugs
  - — birth control pills
  - — thyroid medication
  - — medications for gastrointestinal disorders (such as Reglan and Xanax)
- Many types of vitamins
- Foods containing whey, casein, caseinate, sodium caseinate and lactose

Histology

This test, while very accurate, is rarely used for disaccharide intolerance due to its expense and unpleasantness for patients. It requires an endoscopic biopsy of the small intestine, which is tested for its ability to generate glucose and galactose from lactose applied in vitro.

Blood and urine tests

After ingestion of large amounts of lactose (about 2 g/kg body weight), serial blood samples are drawn or serial urine samples collected to measure galactose change. If no change occurs over time, the test suggests lactose malabsorption. Because glucose is rapidly metabolized, a large dose of lactose is necessary, and this typically produces symptoms in lactase-deficient individuals.

The galactose serum and urine tests require prior oral ingestion of alcohol to suppress rapid galactose turnover by the liver, in addition to the large amount of lactose needed to produce measurable results. The alcohol can impair patients physically and mentally, making it impractical.[9]

Breath hydrogen/methane test

The breath hydrogen/methane test is the clinical standard

for testing lactose intolerance because of its many benefits:

- Breath sampling is simple, non-invasive, inexpensive and well tolerated by patients. It can be done at home by the patient or in the physician's office.[7,10]
- A breath test is highly sensitive and specific for lactose malabsorption. It is able to quantify incomplete absorption of even small amounts of lactose, leading to a more precise estimate as to the degree of malabsorption compared with other methods. This enables patients to moderate their diets and enjoy more foods.[4,5,11–14]
- The lower challenge dose of lactose causes significantly fewer side-effects than the dose used in blood tests and does not require blood samples.[15]
- False-positive results are rare and almost always due to improperly taking the test.[1,16]
- False-negative results are fewer than with the blood test, typically only 5%. These results can be reduced by testing suspected false-negative patients with another disaccharide carried to the colon.[4,11,12,17]
- The breath hydrogen/methane test is the standard in pediatric cases where other tests would be difficult to perform.[1,18–21]
- Testing for both breath hydrogen and methane provides a more comprehensive picture than testing for hydrogen alone because a minority of individuals do not produce hydrogen in response to some carbohydrate challenges.

PROCEDURE

In the breath hydrogen/methane test, a patient fasts overnight and then collects a breath sample. The patient then ingests a challenge dose of lactose (up to a maximum of 25 g) and collects breath samples at 1, 2 and 3 hour intervals.[16,22–24] Longer sample collection periods are optional.

INTERPRETATION

When lactose is not broken down by lactase enzyme in the small intestine, it travels to the colon and undergoes bacterial fermentation. Fermentation causes hydrogen and/or methane levels in breath to rise within 1–2 hours. As little as 2 g of carbohydrate reaching the colon will produce a detectable increase in breath hydrogen.[25] Using the total hydrogen and methane gas response increases the test's accuracy by reducing the number of false-negative responses.

Breath hydrogen

The normal breath hydrogen level in a healthy, fasting patient is less than 10 ppm.[26] Lactose malabsorbers will show an increase in breath hydrogen concentration of 20 ppm or more during the test period.[1,14,27] Lactose absorbers may show a small variation in breath hydrogen of a few ppm during the test period.

Breath methane

The normal breath methane level in a fasting patient is 0–7 ppm. An increase of at least 12 ppm of methane alone during test is considered positive for lactose malabsorption, regardless of the hydrogen response.[1,28,29]

Breath hydrogen plus methane

If both breath hydrogen and methane rise after a lactose challenge, the two responses are added to estimate the degree of malabsorption. An increase in methane will decrease the hydrogen response because methane is generated from the same substrate hydrolyzed by hydrogen-producing bacteria or produced by converting hydrogen to methane.

When breath hydrogen and methane are summed, the test interpretation requires a rise of 20 ppm or more to suggest lactose malabsorption:[1]

- rise of 20–40 ppm – mild malabsorption
- rise of 40–80 ppm – moderate malabsorption
- rise of 80+ ppm – severe malabsorption.

False-positive results

False-positive results are infrequent compared with other types of lactose intolerance testing. The majority of false positives reported in the breath hydrogen/methane test can be eliminated if patients follow proper procedures and preparation instructions.

Typical causes of interference include:

- taking fiber supplements or eating high-fiber foods prior to the test, as fiber increases hydrogen production
- smoking in the area of the test, which produces high hydrogen levels and unstable baseline results; breath samples should not be collected where patients are exposed to tobacco smoke
- sleeping during the test, which increases both hydrogen and methane levels.

False-negative results

Approximately 5% of patients tested for lactose intolerance with the breath hydrogen/methane test produce a false-negative result, compared with 8–12% if only hydrogen is measured. The majority of malabsorbers who do not produce hydrogen after ingesting lactose will generate methane instead. Therefore, the combined breath hydrogen/methane test identifies most malabsorbers.

Typical causes of interference include:

- the use of lactase enzyme supplements, which should be discontinued 24 hours prior to the test
- taking antibiotics prior to the test[9,30]
- the use of laxatives or enemas, which decrease hydrogen and methane response in malabsorbers and create reduced fermentation in the colon[31]
- severe diarrhea of hyperacidic colon contents. Hyperacidity inhibits the generation of hydrogen and causes generation of methane in addition to, or instead of, hydrogen by colonic bacteria.[32,33]

To reduce false-negative results, patients should wait at least 1 week after antibiotic treatment or recovery from severe diarrhea to reestablish colonic flora.

Suspected false-negative patients can also be tested with lactulose, another disaccharide carried to the colon and used to test for bacterial overgrowth. Lactulose determines whether patients produce hydrogen or do not react to lactose. A re-test on another day with a 10 g dose of lactulose as the challenge dose will produce positive breath hydrogen tests in patients capable of producing hydrogen.[34–36]

High baseline levels

A baseline level of hydrogen above 10 ppm indicates that the patient may have fasted improperly, eaten high fiber foods the day before the breath test, or performed the test immediately after awakening.[1] A baseline level above 20 ppm suggests patients have bacterial overgrowth of the small intestine. Levels typically rise during the first hour after lactose is ingested and fall to near-control levels during the test. Elevated methane levels are also seen with bacterial overgrowth.[1,37,38]

CONCLUSION

One advantage of the lactose intolerance breath test is its greater specificity compared to other tests. By determining a patient's degree of malabsorption, physicians can tailor therapeutic recommendations more accurately than simply removing all milk products from the diet.

Patients may be able to limit their avoidance of dairy products, depending upon the severity of their malabsorption. For a mild to moderate malabsorber, it may be enough to limit the intake of dairy products at any one time to avoid symptoms. Studies also indicate that milk is tolerated better if accompanied by food.[1] Decreasing the rate of gastric emptying by increasing the fat content and / or total caloric density of the lactose-containing meal may reduce symptoms, e.g. drinking whole rather than skim milk.[7]

For severe malabsorbers, lactase enzyme preparations that are added to milk and other products commercially available may provide relief from symptoms. These preparations can hydrolyze 70–99% of the lactose after 24 hours of refrigeration.[7,39,40]

REFERENCES

1. Hamilton LH. Breath tests and gastroenterology. Menomonee Falls, Wis.: QuinTron Division, The EF Brewer Company
2. Rosado JL, Allen LH, Solomons NW. Milk consumption, symptom response and lactose digestion in milk intolerance. Am J Clin Nutr 1987; 45: 1457–1460
3. Narvaez RM, Di Palma JA et al. Patient awareness of lactose associated symptoms. Gastroenterol 1986; 90: 1562
4. DiPalma JA, Narvaez RM. Prediction of lactose malabsorption in referral patients. Dig Dis Sci 1988; 33(3): 303–307
5. Solomons NW. Evaluation of carbohydrate absorption: the hydrogen breath test in clinical practice. Clin Nutr J 1984; 3: 71–78
6. Hoffman M et al. Disease free. Emmaus, PA: Rodale Press. 1993
7. Montes RG, Perman JA. Lactose intolerance. Postgraduate Med 1991; 89: 175–184
8. Newcomer AD, Hodgson SF, McGill DB, Thomas PJ. Lactase deficiency: prevalence in osteoporosis. Ann Intern Med 1978; 89: 218–220
9. Lerch M, Rieband HC et al. Concordance of indirect methods for the detection of lactose malabsorption in diabetic and nondiabetic subjects. Digestion 1991; 48: 81–88
10. Metz G, Jenkins DJA, Peters TJ et al. Breath testing as a diagnostic method for hypolactasia. Lancet 1975; 1(7917): 1155–1157
11. Davidson GP, Robb TA. Value of breath hydrogen analysis in management of diarrheal illness in childhood: comparison with duodenal biopsy. J Pediatr Gastroenterol Nutr 1985; 4: 381–387
12. Fernandes J, Vos CE, Douwes AC et al. Respiratory hydrogen excretion as a parameter for lactose malabsorption in children. Am J Clin Nutr 1978; 31: 597–602
13. Newcomer AD. Screening tests for carbohydrate malabsorption. J Pediatr Gastroenterol Nutr 1984; 3: 6–8
14. Douwes AC, Fernandes J et al. Improved accuracy of lactose tolerance test in children, using expired H_2 measurement. Arch Dis Child 1978; 53: 939–942
15. Jones DV, Latham MC, Kosikowski FV et al. Symptom response to lactose-reduced milk in lactose-intolerant adults. Am J Clin Nutr 1976; 29: 633–638
16. Solomons NW, Garcia-Ibanez R, Viteri FE. Hydrogen breath test of lactose absorption in adults: the application of physiological doses and whole cow's milk sources. Am J Clin Nutr 1980; 33: 545–554
17. Feibusch J, Holt PR. Impaired absorptive capacity for carbohydrate in the aging human. Dig Dis Sci 1982; 27: 1095–1100
18. Solomons NW, Garcia-Ibanez R, Viteri FE. Reduced rate of breath hydrogen excretion with lactose tolerance tests in young children using whole milk. Am J Clin Nutr 1979; 32: 783–786
19. Solomons NW, Barillas C. The cut-off criterion for a positive hydrogen breath test in children: a reappraisal. J Pediatr Gastroenterol Nutr 1986; 5: 920–925
20. Barillas-Mury C, Solomons NW. Test-retest reproducibility of hydrogen breath test for lactose maldigestion in preschool children. J Pediatr Gastroenterol Nutr 1987; 6: 281–285
21. Barillas-Mury C, Solomons NW. Variance in fasting breath hydrogen concentrations in Guatemalan preschool children. J Pediatr Gastroenterol Nutr 1987; 6: 109–113
22. Bond JH, Levitt MD. Quantitative measurement of lactose absorption. Gastroenterol 1976; 70: 1058–1062
23. Kolars JC, Levitt MD, Aouji M. Yogurt – an autodigesting source of lactose. N Eng J Med 1984; 310: 1–3

24. Robb TA, Davidson GP. Two-hour lactose breath hydrogen test. J Pediatr Gastroenterol Nutr 1987; 6: 481–482
25. Levitt MD. Production and excretion of hydrogen gas in man. N Eng J Med 1969; 281: 122–127
26. Jain NK, Patel VP et al. Geographical differences in fasting breath hydrogen levels. Gastroenterol 1985; 88: 1429
27. Caskey DA, Payne-Bose D, Welsh JD et al. Effects of age on lactose malabsorption in Oklahoma Native Americans as determined by breath H_2 analysis. J Digest Dis 1977; 22: 113–116
28. Cloarac D, Bornet F, Gouillond S et al. Breath hydrogen response to lactulose in healthy subjects: relationship to methane-producing status. Gut 1990; 31: 300–304
29. Fritz M, Siebert G, Kasper H et al. Dose dependence of breath hydrogen and methane in healthy volunteers after ingestion of a commercial disaccharide mixture, Palatinit. Br J Nutr 1985; 54: 389–400
30. Gilat T, Ben Hur H, Gelman-Malachi E et al. Alterations of the colonic flora and their effect on the hydrogen breath test. Gut 1978; 19: 602–605
31. Solomons NW, Garcia R, Schneider R et al. Breath tests during diarrhea. Acta Paediatr Scand 1979; 68: 171–172
32. Vogelsand H, Ferenci P, Frotz S et al. Acidic colonic microclimate – possible reason for false negative hydrogen breath tests. Gut 1988; 29: 21
33. Perman JA, Modler S, Olson AC et al. Role of pH in production of hydrogen from carbohydrates by colonic bacterial flora: studies in vivo and in vitro. J Clin Invest 1981; 67: 643–650
34. Douwes AC, Schapp C et al. Hydrogen breath test in school children. Arch Dis Child 1985; 60: 333–337
35. Roggero P, Offredi ML, Moscas F et al. Lactose absorption and malabsorption in healthy Italian children: do the quantity and malabsorbed sugar and the small bowel transit time play roles in symptom production? J Pediatr Gastroenterol Nutr 1985; 4: 82–86
36. Filali A, Ben Hassine L, Dhouib H et al. Detection of lactose malabsorption by hydrogen breath test in a population of 70 Tunisian adults. Gastroenterol Clin Biol 1987; 11: 554–557
37. Perman JA, Modler S, Barr RG et al. Fasting breath hydrogen concentration: normal values and clinical application. Gastroenterol 1984; 87: 1358–1363
38. Kerlin P, Wong L et al. An evaluation of breath hydrogen testing in the diagnosis of bacterial overgrowth of the small intestine. Gastroenterol 1986; 90: 1491
39. Solomons NW, Guerrero AM, Torun B et al. Dietary manipulation of postprandial colonic lactose fermentation: II. Addition of exogenous, microbial beta-galactosidases at mealtime. Am J Clin Nutr 1985; 41: 209–221
40. Goldberg DM. Enzymes as agents for the treatment of disease. Clin Chim Acta 1992; 206: 45–76

CHAPTER CONTENTS

24

Mineral status evaluation

Stephen Markus, MD

INTRODUCTION

The importance of trace mineral metabolism has only become appreciated in the past 30 years. Minerals play as important a role in the subtle biochemistry of the body as do vitamins. Virtually all reactions in the body require minerals as cofactors. With some trace elements, infinitesimally small amounts may be necessary, while others, such as calcium, make up a quarter of our body weight.

Assessment of body status for a particular trace element is extremely difficult (see Table 24.1 for recommended methods for the different elements).[1] For years there has been considerable controversy over hair mineral analysis. Although hair is the most convenient tissue for analyzing minerals, only a limited number of elements in the hair accurately reflect the true body content (see Ch. 17). Others are better measured intracellularly or extracellularly (depending on their state of equilibrium) or in specific cells, such as leukocytes. Many factors, such as specific protein carriers, the ionic charge of the element, or its capacity to be in equilibrium in the blood, affect the usefulness and reproducibility of a specific assay method and the appropriateness of a chosen tissue.

Table 24.1 Recommended methods for assessing essential mineral status

Mineral	Method	Normal range
Calcium	Hair analysis	340–850
Chromium	Hair analysis	0.5–1.5 ppm
Copper	Serum copper	0.8–1.5 ppm
	Hair analysis	8–22 ppm
Iron	Serum iron	0.65–1.75 ppm
	Serum ferritin	Male, 27–329 Female, 12–120
Magnesium	Mg retention test	<25%, normal
	Leukocyte Mg	0.98–2.82 ug/L
Manganese	Whole blood Mn	0.005–0.02 ppm
Potassium	Whole blood K	3741–4045 ppm
Selenium	Hair analysis	1.0–3.0 ppm
Zinc	Leukocyte zinc	0.082–0.57 ug/L

Over the last century, with increasing industrialization of our society, our exposure to toxic metals has increased enormously. Hair serves as an excellent source for measurement of continuous cumulative exposure more typical of environmental sources. Hair is also biologically stable and can be stored for analysis over a long period without degradation. Hair also concentrates toxic minerals several hundred times higher than blood, allowing for analytical determinations of ultra trace quantities. The fact that toxic minerals can have deleterious effects on multiple enzyme systems, neuronal structures, and organs, including the brain, heart, thyroid, liver, kidneys, and skin, at extraordinarily low levels suggests that hair mineral analysis should be an important screening test for many patients.[2–5]

ESSENTIAL MINERALS

Calcium

Despite detailed calcium balance studies measuring both intake and excretion with radiolabeled isotopes, determining calcium balance in an outpatient setting is extremely difficult.[6] Assessment of dietary intake of calcium is confounded by multiple factors which affect absorption, such as:

- the quantity of fiber and other natural chelators in the diet
- gastric acidity
- the ratio of dietary calcium to phosphorus (and dietary magnesium)
- gut transit time, etc.

When all of these are considered, multivariate analysis is currently very difficult with so many uncontrolled and difficult to measure variables.

Serum calcium, like other electrolytes, is so closely regulated (by the parathyroid gland) that its use as a measurement of calcium balance is rarely of value. Ionized calcium is currently being examined in more detail and may play a partial role in evaluation of calcium status in the future. Urinary calcium is of value in a patient with a known low total calcium intake and persistent calciuria.

At present, perhaps the most useful screening test for calcium balance is hair analysis. However, hair calcium levels are subject to considerable variability and should not be taken as a quantitative determination of calcium status. A few studies evaluating calcium content in hair have shown promising correlations. Two studies in particular were able to find a relationship between hair calcium and coronary disease.[7,8] Future studies need to be conducted for further verification. One team of researchers conducted careful studies of a group of patients and showed that calcium intake, and the ratio of calcium to phosphorus intake, significantly altered hair calcium. Those patients with high phosphorus/low calcium consistently showed hair calcium as much as three times higher than normal. Hair calcium returned to normal with proper supplementation and dietary changes.[9]

Chromium

Establishment of reliable laboratory assays for the assessment of chromium status has been a subject of considerable research. Only recently has analytical instrumentation of sufficient sensitivity been developed to allow accurate quantitative analysis of this ultra trace mineral. Plasma chromium is probably not a valid indicator of body status since it is not in equilibrium with tissue chromium, and plasma levels may be less than 1 ng/ml making measurement very difficult.

Since 80% of chromium is excreted in the urine, urinary chromium may be the most valid indicator of chromium status. Glucose consumption has been shown to increase plasma and, subsequently, urinary chromium. Pre- and post-glucose-load urinary chromium have been measured, but results have shown unacceptable variability.

Substantial GTF (glucose tolerance factor) activity has been found in hair follicles suggesting that hair chromium may be a useful indicator of body status.[10–12] This mineral is found in the hair at concentrations over 100 times that found in the blood, making measurement more technically feasible.

Copper

Under normal conditions, far more copper is absorbed than is needed by the body. Nearly all dietary copper is initially stored in the liver, leaving only a small percentage in the blood. Ninety-five per cent of plasma copper is bound to the protein ceruloplasmin, with almost no ionic copper; thus urinary output is nil. The principal homeostatic mechanism for controlling copper is by excretion through the biliary system.

As one might expect with such a large turnover of absorbed copper, assessing copper status is not easy. At present, serum copper may be the best indicator, if the clinical conditions which are known to cause abnormalities in copper metabolism (e.g. Wilsons's disease and cirrhosis of the liver) are first ruled out.[13]

Measurement of superoxide dismutase function has been used in the assessment of copper status, but since this enzyme also requires zinc and manganese, it is not adequately specific.

The usefulness of hair analysis as an indicator of chronic copper toxicity is well documented, although external contamination must be considered, and it is not reliable in Wilson's disease. Some studies have shown hair copper to be an acceptable method of assessment of copper status.[14,15] More studies are needed in this area.

Iron

Serum iron has a long history of use as an indicator of iron deficiency. It is not of much value by itself, however, since there is considerable variation in serum iron, even when samples are taken from the same person at the same time each day, and there is a considerable diurnal variation. The test is much more reliable when combined with measurement of serum transferrin or ferritin.

Ferritin is an iron storage protein accounting for 20% of the total body iron in normal adults. It is principally found in the cytoplasm of reticuloendothelial cells and liver cells, and, to some degree, in developing red cell precursors in bone marrow. It is involved in both iron absorption and recycling.

During the early stages of iron deficiency, a decreased serum ferritin level is the first sign that body stores are decreased. As iron deficiency progresses, anemia, decreased serum iron and elevated iron binding capacity become apparent.[16,17] The patient is done a disservice if the physician waits for hypochromia and microcytosis to appear before making a diagnosis of iron deficiency.[18] Table 24.2 compares the various methods of determining iron deficiency.

Serum ferritin levels are, however, not totally reliable since they are inappropriately elevated in several common medical conditions, including cancer, infections, inflammation, and acute and chronic liver disease. When iron overload is associated with hemochromatosis, hemosiderosis, or thalassemia, serum ferritin is also elevated. Overall serum ferritin is a convenient and usually reliable measurement of total body iron storage.

Magnesium

Measurement of magnesium status, like other minerals, has many problems. The magnesium retention test is probably the most accurate method of assessment currently available.[19] The test procedure is as follows:

1. The patient is injected with 2 ml of a 50% $MgSO_4$ solution.
2. 24 hour pre- and post-injection urine samples are collected and measured for magnesium and creatinine.
3. Retention of greater than 25% indicates magnesium deficiency.

Needless to say, this is a cumbersome procedure.

Serum magnesium is of little value since it is influenced by many factors. The degree of binding, complexing or chelating of magnesium to serum proteins and other fractions is subject to many uncontrollable variables. Values as low as 1.2 mEq/L have been measured in patients with normal total body magnesium.[19]

Although there has been interest in RBC magnesium, it has been shown that its value may vary by a factor of five depending on the age of the red blood cell, making this technique somewhat unreliable.[19] Early research is indicating that WBC magnesium is far easier to measure and may be nearly as accurate as the magnesium retention test. Its clinical usefulness awaits further studies.[20]

Manganese

Assessment of body status for manganese is difficult due to its low levels (1% of the level of copper or zinc in blood). Whole blood manganese is a valid indicator of body manganese and soft tissue levels.[21] Proper technique is essential in the collection procedure as well as the actual analysis. Hair manganese may be a rough indicator, especially in chronic toxicity, but is not as reliable as whole blood.

Potassium

Since potassium is primarily an intracellular ion, serum measurements do not accurately reflect body stores. A low serum potassium usually indicates an advanced intracellular deficit. However, an intracellular deficit may also occur with normal or high serum potassium. Several researchers have been studying red blood cell potassium which has been shown to reflect the potassium content of other tissue cells.[22,23] Although red blood cells do not have nuclei, the sodium–potassium membrane pump is intact, maintaining the proper influx and efflux of these ions. Whole blood potassium is almost as

Table 24.2 Comparison of various methods of determining iron status

	Normal	Iron deficiency		Severe iron deficiency
		With anemia	Without anemia	
Plasma iron level	75–150 ug/100 ml	Normal or reduced	Normal or reduced	<40 ug/100 ml
Iron-binding capacity	300–400 ug/100 ml	Normal or elevated	Normal or elevated	>400 ug/100 ml
Hemoglobin level	13–15 g/100 ml	13–15 g/100 ml	9–12 g/100 ml	6–7 g/100 ml
Hypochromia and microcytosis	Not present	Not present	Sl or not present	Profound
Ferritin level	12–300 ng/ml	<12 ng/ml	<12 ng/ml	<6 ng/ml
Free erythrocyte protoporphyrin	30–70 ug/100 ml	Normal or elevated	>100 ug/100ml	>100 ug/100 ml

accurate as RBC potassium since 98% of the potassium is intracellular.

An example of the validity of measuring intracellular potassium was demonstrated in a study which measured electrocardiographically the repolarization phase in the elderly. Alterations of repolarization correlated well with intracellular potassium levels but showed no correlation occurred with serum levels.[24]

Selenium

After absorption, selenium is distributed throughout the tissues but does not seem to be in equilibrium with the blood. Research currently indicates that blood selenium levels do not correlate with selenium intake, except at extremes.[25] Hair selenium does correlate well.[26–30] As with chromium and manganese, special analytical techniques must be used to ensure accuracy of measurements with this element.

Zinc

Since zinc is an intracellular ion, plasma and serum zinc are not sensitive indicators of depletion.[31] Erythrocyte zinc is an even less sensitive indicator of zinc status than plasma. Urine zinc is also not a good indicator. Low hair zinc levels indicate depletion, but normal values do not rule out low body stores.[15,32,33] Leukocyte zinc has been investigated and found to be an accurate index of body stores.[34]

CONCLUSION

No analysis is better than the laboratory performing it. Proper analytical procedures must be used and each step in the collection and preparation of a sample must be carefully monitored. For example, in hair analysis, proper washing of hair, and use of ultra-high pure digesting acid and distilled water are important. In blood analysis, collection tubes specially designed for the specific mineral being collected must be used.

Ultimately, it is the physician's responsibility to verify the validity of an analytical procedure. When in doubt, obtain a copy of the actual procedure for review and compare it with the limits of detection for the particular instrument being used.

Many of the reference articles listed here are reviews, and thus can serve as sources of additional information.

REFERENCES

1. Savory J, Wills M. Trace minerals. essential nutrients or toxins. Clin Chem 1992; 38: 1565–1573
2. Katz S, Chatt A. Hair analysis: applications in the biochemical and environmental sciences. New York: VCH Publishers. 1988
3. Vienna A, Capucci E, Wolfsperger M et al. Heavy metal concentration of hair of students in Rome. Anthropol Anz 1995; 53: 27–32
4. Foo S, Khoo N et al. Metals in hair as biological indices for exposure. Int Arch Occup Environ Health 1993; 65: 583–586
5. Jenkins D. Toxic metals in mammalian hair and nails. EPA report 600/4-79-049. Aug 1979. (Available through National Technical Information Service)
6. Albanese A. Bone loss. Causes, detection, and therapy. New York: Alan R Liss. 1977
7. Basco J. On determination of calcium in hair and its use for investigation of coronary heart disease and calcium metabolic rate. Atomki Kozl 1985; 26: 2324–2325
8. MacPherson A, Baklint J. Beard calcium concentration as a marker for coronary heart disease by supplementation with micro nutrients including selenium. Analyst 1995; 120: 871–875
9. Bland J. Dietary calcium, phosphorus and their relationships to bone formation and parathyroid activity. J John Bastyr Col Naturopathic Med 1979; 1: 1
10. Wallach S. Clinical and biochemical aspects of chromium deficiency. J Am Coll Nutr 1985; 4: 107–120
11. Hambidge K. Chromium nutrition in man. Am J Clin Nutr 1974; 27: 505–514
12. Aharomi A, Tesler B, Paltielei Y et al. Hair chromium content of women with gestational diabetes compared with non diabetic pregnant women. Am J Clin Nutr 1992; 55: 104–107
13. Solomons N. Biochemical, metabolic and clinical role of copper in human nutrition. J Am Coll Nutr 1985; 4: 83–105
14. Piccinni L, Borella P, Bargellini A et al. A case control study on selenium, zinc, and copper in plasma and hair of subjects affected by breast and lung cancer. Biol Trace Element Res 1990; 24: 105–109
15. Donma M, Donma O, Tas M et al. Hair zinc and copper concentrations and zinc/copper ratios in pediatric malignancies and healthy children from southeastern Turkey. Biol Trace Element Res 1993; 36: 51–58
16. Cook J. Serum ferritin as a measure of iron in normal subjects. Am J Clin Nutr 1974; 27: 9681–9687
17. Frank P, Wang S. Serum iron and total iron binding capacity compared with serum ferritin in assessment of iron deficiency. Clin Chem 1981; 27: 276–279
18. Rubenstein E, Federman DD. Scientific American medicine. New York: Scientific American Inc. 1985: p 5: II: 7–9
19. Seelig M. Magnesium deficiency in the pathogenesis of disease. New York: Plenum Medical Books. 1980
20. Hosseini JM, Johnson E, Elin RJ. Comparison of two separation techniques for the determination of blood mononuclear cell magnesium content. J Am Coll Nutr 1983; 2: 361–368
21. Keen C. Whole blood manganese as an indicator of body manganese. N Eng J Med 1983; 308: 1230
22. Bahemuka M, Hodkinson H. Red blood cell potassium as a practical index of potassium status in elderly patients. Age and Aging 1976; 5: 24–29
23. Lans K Stein IF, Meyer KA. The relationship of serum potassium to erythrocyte potassium in normal subjects and patients with potassium deficiency. Am J Med Sci 1952; 223: 65–74
24. Sangiorgi B, Barbagallo-Sangiorgi G, Costanga G et al. Serum potassium levels, red blood cell potassium and alternations of the repolarization phase of electrocardiography in old subjects. Age and Aging 1984; 13: 309–312
25. Lane HW, Warren DC, Taylor BJ, Stool E. Blood selenium and glutathione peroxidase levels and dietary selenium of free living and institutionalized elderly subjects. Proc Soc Exp Biol Med 1985; 173: 87–95
26. Schrauzer GN, Rhead WJ, Evans GA. Bioinorganic chemistry 1973; 2: 329–240
27. Shamberger R. Selenium in health and disease. Symposium on selenium and tellurium in the environment, University of Notre Dame, Ind. 1976: p 253–267

28. Observations on effect of sodium selenite in prevention of Keshan disease. Chinese Med J 1979; 92: 471–476
29. Spallholz JE, Martin JL, Gerbach ML, Heinzerling RH. Immunologic responses of mice feed diets supplemented with selenite selenium. Proceedings of the society of experimental biological medicine. 1973; 143: 685–698
30. Valentine JL, Kang HK, Spivey GH. Selenium levels in human blood, urine and hair in response to exposure via drinking water. Environ Res 1978; 17: 347–355
31. Davies S. Assessment of zinc status. Intl Clin Nutr Rev 1984; 4: 122–129
32. Hambidge KM, Hambidge C, Jacos M, Baum JD. Low levels of zinc in hair, anorexia, poor growth and hypogeusia in children. Ped Res 1972; 6: 868–874
33. Pekarek R, Sandstea HH Jacob RH, Barcome DF. Abnormal cellular immune response during acquired zinc deficiency. Am J Clin Nutr 1979; 32: 1466–1471
34. Jones R, Keeling P, Hilton P et al. The relationship between leukocyte and muscle zinc in health and disease. Science 1981; 60: 237–239

CHAPTER CONTENTS

25

Oral manifestations of nutritional status

Michael T. Murray, ND

Joseph E. Pizzorno Jr, ND

INTRODUCTION

The structures and lining of the oral cavity offer valuable, and easily accessible, information on the nutritional status of an individual. The lesions may indicate a nutrient deficiency or may be manifestations of gastrointestinal or other disease. Due to the very rapid cell turnover of the oral mucosa, these lesions often may precede other manifestations of nutrient deficiency or systemic disease. Some typical lesions are mucosal ulceration, cheilosis, gingivitis, and glossitis. Since between 5 and 10% of the people in the United States are deficient in one or more nutrients, signs of nutritional deficiency are common.

The healthy mouth

The ventral surface of the healthy tongue is covered with smooth, pink, mucous membrane and lymphoid follicles. On the dorsal surface, the filiform, fungiform, and circumvallate papillae (which contain the organs of taste) produce a rough, grayish-red appearance. The thick epithelial tufts of the filiform papillae give the tongue its characteristic grayish-white coating, whereas the globular, pale red fungiform papillae give it a speckled pink appearance. Furrows are not a characteristic of the healthy tongue.

The buccal mucosa has a grayish-red color and may be crossed by fine grayish ridges where it touches the closed teeth.

The healthy gums have a light reddish appearance and cover the roots of the teeth completely.[1]

ABNORMALITIES OF THE ORAL MEMBRANES

Table 25.1 summarizes the typical oral manifestations associated with a particular nutrient deficiency, while Table 25.2 summarizes common disorders associated with oral manifestations.

Table 25.1 Oral signs of nutrient deficiency[2–7]

Nutrient	Oral deficiency signs
Biotin	Geographic tongue, atrophy of lingual papillae
Folic acid	Gingivitis, glossitis with atrophy or hypertrophy of filiform papillae, cheilosis
Niacin	Intraoral burning, glossitis, tongue swollen with red tip and sides, swollen red fungiform papillae, filiform papillae become inflamed and lose their epithelial tufts (giving the characteristic slick red appearance)
Pyridoxine	Intraoral burning, glossitis, mucosal ulcerations and erosions, cheilosis
Vitamin B_{12}	Intraoral burning, mucosal ulcerations and erosions, painful glossitis with a beefy red or fiery appearance eventually resulting in an atrophic (smooth and shiny) tongue
Riboflavin	Soreness and intraoral burning, cheilosis, angular stomatitis, glossitis with a magenta tongue
Vitamin C	Sore and bleeding gums, gums deep blue-red color, loose teeth, follicular hyperkeratosis
Vitamin D	Intraoral burning
Vitamin E	Glossitis
Calcium	Periodontal disease, tooth decay
Iron	Cheilosis, atrophic glossitis, gingivitis, candidiasis, intraoral burning or pain, mucosal ulcerations and erosions, pallor
Zinc	Marked halitosis, cheilosis, stomatitis, discrete red, scaly plaques from short-lived vesicles, white coating on tongue and mucosa, intraoral burning

In general, *ulceration* should be considered a non-specific expression of a disease state. A search for the etiology will usually result in a specific therapy. Aphthous stomatitis is a common example of a mucosal ulceration and is discussed in detail in Chapter 130.

Similarly, *cheilosis* is a common expression for acquired nutrient deficiency. *Gingivitis* is associated with the classical signs of scurvy, but more recently other nutrients have been shown to play a role in gingival health. This subject is discussed in Chapter 181. *Glossitis* is associated with numerous vitamin deficiency states, each with a characteristic appearance.

Like glossitis, *intraoral burning* represents a non-specific expression of a possible nutrient deficiency or systemic disease. Besides those listed in Table 25.2, other possible causes include:

Table 25.2 Common disorders associated with oral manifestations[2–7]

Oral manifestation	Disorder
Cheilosis	Crohn's disease, acrodermatitis enteropathica, alcoholism, celiac disease, malabsorption syndrome
Gingivitis	Crohn's disease, anorexia nervosa, celiac disease, scurvy
Erythroplakia	Dysplasia or carconoma
Glossitis	Crohn's disease, diabetes, alcoholism, celiac disease, malabsorption syndrome, pernicious anemia, iron-deficiency anemia, amyloidosis, carcinoid syndrome, cigarette smoking, anemia
Intraoral burning	Menopause, diabetes mellitus, esophageal reflux, Sjögren's syndrome
Leukoplakia	Chronic irritation, dysplasia, early invasive squamous cell carcinoma
Ulcerations, erosions	Crohn's disease, ulcerative colitis, celiac disease, corticosteroid use, acrodermatitis enteropathica, anorexia nervosa, pernicious anemia, iron-deficient anemia, mercury poisoning, nicotine withdrawal

- xerostomia
- dentures
- deficiency states of iron, B_{12}, folic acid, B_6, and protein
- steatorrhea
- antibiotic use
- changes in mucosal innervation
- anxiety states.

In non-denture wearers, nutritional disorders are the most common causative factors.[8]

Leukoplakia is any white lesion of the oral cavity that cannot be removed by rubbing the mucosal surface. While they are usually only a sign of chronic irritation, 2–6% represent either dysplasia or early invasive squamous cell carcinoma.[4]

Erythroplakia is similar to leukoplakia, except that it has a definite erythematous component. This is a far more serious sign, with 90% representing dysplasia or carcinoma.

REFERENCES

1. Blackow RS: MacBryde's signs and symptoms. 6th ed. New York, NY: JB Lippincott. 1983: p 117–138
2. Beitman R, Frost S, Roth J. Oral manifestations of gastrointestinal disease. Dig Dis Sci 1981; 26: 741–747
3. Krause M, Mahan K. Food nutrition and diet therapy. Philadelphia, PA: WB Saunders. 1984: p 99–143
4. Tierney LM, McPhee SJ, Papdakis MA. Current diagnosis and treatment. Stamford, CT: Appleton Lange. 1997
5. Maragou P, Ibanyi L. Serum zinc levels in patients with burning mouth syndrome. Oral Surg Oral Med Oral Path 1991; 71: 447–450
6. Ship JA. Burning mouth syndrome: an update. J Am Dental Assoc 1995; 126: 843–853
7. Werbach MR. Nutritional influences on illness. 2nd edn. Tarzana, CA: Third Line Press. 1993
8. Basker R, Sturdee D, Davenport J. Patients with burning mouths. Brit Dent J 1978; 145: 9–16

CHAPTER CONTENTS

26

Rapid dark adaptation test

Dirk Wm Powell, ND

INTRODUCTION

The earliest sign of vitamin A deficiency is a decrease in dark adaptation, or night vision. Serum retinol levels are not predictive of subclinical deficiency states. However, classical dark adaptation testing is a cumbersome and time-consuming process (usually taking 45 minutes).

A rapid test (6 minutes) was described by Thornton[1] and evaluated by Vinton & Russell.[2] This rapid dark adaptation test (RDAT) has significant clinical utility. The basis for the test is the measurement of the time of the so-called Purkinje shift. This refers to the shifting of peak retinal wavelength sensitivity from the red toward the blue end of the visual spectrum during the transition from day (cone-mediated) vision to night (rod-mediated) vision. When color vision is non-functional, this shift causes the intensity, not the color, of blue to appear brighter than red under dim lighting.

CLINICAL APPLICATION

While the various dark adaptation tests have the advantage of being *in vivo* tests, and therefore directly relevant to function, they are also somewhat less specific. Table 26.1 lists conditions which may give abnormal dark adaptation results despite normal serum levels of vitamin A.

PROCEDURE

Method

1. The procedure is explained to the subject.

Table 26.1 Conditions causing abnormal DAT results with normal levels of vitamin A

- Zinc deficiency
- Cataract
- Retinitis pigmentosa
- Diabetic retinopathy
- Severe errors of refraction
- Miosis caused by pharmaceutical agents
- Tinted corrective lenses

2. The subject is light-adapted by fixation on a standard X-ray viewer for 1 minute at a distance of 0.5 m. The X-ray viewer is then turned off (the darkroom light is, of course, on).

3. The subject is given a pile containing all 18 discs mixed in random order and the stopwatch is started.

4. The subject separates the white and then the blue discs as fast as possible. Under these controlled lighting conditions, the subject will not be able to recognize the colors, since the cones cannot distinguish color with the limited light available. The ability to separate the discs by brightness is therefore dependent upon the rods. Any disc mistakenly separated by the subject is returned to the original pile until 100% accuracy of sorting is achieved.

5. The first test performed by a subject should be redone to allow for learning and standardization.

Equipment and supplies

- Light-proof room.
- A standard darkroom light fixture fitted with a 7.5 W bulb and a neutral density filter (allowing 1% transmittance). Alternately, an exposed X-ray film may serve as filter. The bottom of the fixture is suspended 1.2 m above the work surface, so that the target brightness on the work area is approximately 0.0068 candela/m^2.
- Munsell color discs with matte finish – five white discs (N9.5/-), six blue discs (5PB5/10), and seven red discs (5R5/10). Available from Munsell Color and Macbeth Division (Baltimore, MD).
- A non-reflective work surface.
- A stopwatch.
- A standard X-ray viewbox.

Results

- Normals
  —20–39 years old: 3.03 ± 1.00 min
  —40–60 years old: 4.41 ± 0.83 min
- Vitamin A-deficient
  —7.63 ± 1.79 min.

INTERPRETATION

The RDAT time will depend largely upon the individual setting. However, the difference in the RDAT time between normal and vitamin A-deficient individuals is significant, and therefore standardization is easily achieved. The normal values are dependent on the age of the subject, with older subjects having an increased RDAT time. Vinton & Russell's average RDAT time for normal subjects between the ages of 20 and 39 was 3.03 ± 1.00 minutes, while for the 40–60 years age group it was 4.41 ± 0.83 minutes. In vitamin A-deficient patients, the value was 7.63 ± 1.79 minutes. An increased RDAT time may also be indicative of a zinc deficiency.

REFERENCES

1. Thornton S. A rapid test for dark adaptation. Ann Ophthalmol 1977; 9: 731–734
2. Vinton N, Russell R. Evaluation of a rapid test of dark adaptation. Am J Clin Nutr 1981; 34: 1961–1966

CHAPTER CONTENTS

27

Serum bile acids assay

Michael T. Murray, ND

Joseph E. Pizzorno Jr, ND

INTRODUCTION

The standard serum enzyme studies (SGPT, GGTP, SGOT, LDH, alkaline phosphatase, etc.), which have traditionally been used for detecting hepatic damage, have been shown to be unreliable in identifying the early phases or progression of liver disease and the liver damage caused by a variety of toxic chemicals.[1–6] These enzyme studies are often of limited value because they measure acute disruption of cell membrane integrity (liver cell "leakage") rather than functional activity of the liver, i.e. uptake, metabolism, storage, and excretion. In subacute, chronic, and end-stage liver disease, the enzymes often return to normal levels after initial elevation and fail to reflect the decreased metabolic capacity of the remaining parenchyma.

Currently, measuring clearance rates of substances primarily removed from circulation by the liver provides the most sensitive and specific indicator of liver function. Such substances include exogenous anionic dyes (e.g. bromsulphalein (BSP) or indocyanine green) and endogenous metabolites (e.g. serum bile acids). The use of the anionic dyes does, however, carry with it significant risk of adverse reaction. In contrast, the measurement of serum bile acids represents a safe approach to measuring the functional capacity of the liver.

The usefulness of measuring serum bile acid concentrations for the detection of liver disease has been extensively studied in numerous clinical studies.[2–17] However, until recently, the use of this extremely sensitive liver function test has not been widely used in clinical practice, due to complex methodology and inadequate precision and standardization between laboratories. Now, several commercial assays are available.

The radioimmunoassay and bioluminescent enzymatic assay methodologies are sensitive, precise, and relatively inexpensive.[6,8] In contrast, enzymatic measurement based on bacterial dehydrogenases appears to be much less sensitive than the RIA and bioluminescent methods, especially when the elevation is only marginal. Accurate interpretation requires that the method being used by the laboratory be known.

There has been considerable disagreement as to whether fasting or postprandial serum bile acid measurement is the better determinant of abnormal liver function. As a postprandial rise is governed largely by non-hepatic factors, fasting levels are probably more reproducible. In addition, many studies have demonstrated fasting levels to be a more sensitive indicator than postprandial levels.[6–11]

DETERMINANTS OF SERUM BILE ACID LEVELS

In healthy subjects, the bile acid pool consists of primary, secondary, and tertiary bile acids. The two primary bile acids in humans, cholic acid and chenodeoxycholic acid (which are formed from cholesterol), are converted by intestinal bacteria (through deconjugation and 7-alpha-hydroxylation) to the secondary bile acids, deoxycholic acid and lithocholic acid. A fraction of chenodeoxycholic acid is transformed, via 7-ketolithocholic acid, into the tertiary bile acid, ursodeoxycholic acid.[6,8] All bile acids secreted by the liver are conjugated with either glycine or taurine, and about two-thirds of lithocholic acids are in addition sulphated. In health, only a small fraction of bile acids is glucuronidated.

The bile acid pool cycles five to 10 times daily through the enterohepatic circulation, where it is almost completely confined. The liver normally clears 20 g of bile salt from the blood each day.[12] Less than 1% of the total bile acid pool is present in the peripheral blood due to high efficiency of the hepatic transport mechanism for the bile acids.[8]

Serum bile acid levels at any moment are determined by the balance between intestinal absorption and hepatic elimination of bile acids. Input of bile acids from the intestine into the systemic circulation may occur via two pathways: portal-systemic shunts and the hepatic circulation.

Hepatic elimination of bile acids occurs as first-pass elimination from the portal blood and as systemic clearance from peripheral blood. Systemic clearance of bile acids depends on the intrinsic ability of the liver to remove bile acids and on hepatic blood flow. In patients with liver disease, diminished hepatic elimination of bile acids can be caused by reduced hepatic extraction, portosystemic shunting, or by a combination of both.

CLINICAL INDICATIONS FOR SERUM BILE ACID DETERMINATION

Fasting serum bile acid (SBA) determination can be used clinically in the diagnosis and prognosis of liver disease in conjunction with standard liver function tests. Because of the increased sensitivity of SBA determination as compared with standard liver function tests, SBA offers significant additional diagnostic information concerning liver function, especially in minor hepatic derangements. It is of particular benefit in the determination of hepatic dysfunction as a result of chemical and environmental injury.[2–17]

Liver injury as a result of occupational or environmental exposure to a wide variety of chemical substances can be determined to a much finer degree by SBA than by standard liver enzymes, especially when the liver has been only slightly damaged. In one study of individuals exposed to organic solvents, 73% of the exposed cases had elevated SBA levels, whereas increased levels of SGGT, alanine aminotransferase (ALT), aspartate aminotransferase (AST) and bilirubin were observed respectively in 8, 3, 2, and 1% of exposed workers.[2] These results and others support the hypothesis that standard liver function tests are not sensitive enough to determine hepatic dysfunction caused by such organic solvents as toluene, xylene, acetone, styrene, *n*-butlyacetate, *n*-butanol, ethylacetate, and other aromatic hydrocarbons and ketones.

Other indications for SBA determination include patients presenting with generalized pruritus[14] and pregnant women experiencing nausea and vomiting of pregnancy.[16] Both of these conditions can be a result of impaired hepatic function, yet standard liver function tests are usually not sensitive enough to be of value. In contrast, SBA determination has shown a significant correlation between hepatic dysfunction and both nausea and vomiting of pregnancy[16] and generalized pruritus.[14]

SBA determination also offers useful prognostic information in cases of cirrhosis. In one large study,[15] the SBA concentration correlated more closely with mortality than did the commonly used clinical and laboratory parameters such as the "number connection test", ascites, albumin, pseudocholinesterase, bilirubin, prothrombin time, and nutritional state. SBA levels below 20 μmol/L indicated a good prognosis, while those individuals with SBA levels exceeding 50 μmol/L had a very poor prognosis.

PROCEDURE

Method

1. Have the patient fast overnight.
2. Take 10 ml (in a red-top tube) from the antecubital vein.
3. Allow to clot, and separate within 20 minutes.
4. Freeze until delivered to laboratory.
5. Use only laboratories which use the radio-immunoassay and bioluminescent enzymatic assay methodologies.

Results

These values are for the radioimmunoassay technique:

- Normal: 1.3 ± 0.2 μmol/L
- Solvent exposure: 3.7 ± 2.8
- Mild liver dz: 5.5 ± .3
- Moderate liver dz: 12.5 ± 1.8
- Cirrhosis: 20.4 ± 3.2
- Cirrhosis (dying < 1 year): 79.6 ± 28.0.

INTERPRETATION

Bile sequestering agents, such as cholestyramine and cholestipol, will interfere with the test by decreasing reabsorption of bile acids from the intestine. Decreasing the total level of bile acids in the enterohepatic circulation may result in lower serum values, thus masking decreased liver function. The typical causes of elevated levels are listed in Table 27.1. Serum bile acid levels are normal in Gilbert's disease and are generally not useful in differentiating between the various types of liver disease.[6]

Table 27.1 Conditions with elevated fasting serum bile acids levels[18]

- Anicteric liver disease
- Alcoholic liver disease
- Biliary atresia
- Chemical-induced liver injury
- Cirrhosis
- Cholestasis
- Cystic fibrosis
- Drug-induced liver injury
- Generalized pruritus
- Hepatoma, primary
- Nausea and vomiting of pregnancy
- Neonatal hepatitis syndrome
- Protracted diarrhea of infancy
- Reye's syndrome
- Viral hepatitis

SUMMARY

Fasting serum bile acid determination by radioimmunoassay or bioluminescent enzymatic assay provides valuable information concerning the functional activity of the liver. SBA determination has a much greater specificity and sensitivity than standard liver function tests in the diagnosis of liver disease induced by chemical and environmental exposure and in diagnosing low levels of hepatic dysfunction.

REFERENCES

1. Lundberg I, Hakansson M. Normal serum activities of liver enzymes in Swedish paint industry workers with heavy exposure to organic solvents. Br J Industr Med 1985; 42: 596–600
2. Franco G, Fonte R, Tempinin G, Candura F. Serum bile acid concentrations as a liver function test in workers occupationally exposed to organic solvents. Int Arch Occup Environ Health 1986; 58: 157–164
3. Liss GM, Greenberg RA, Tamburro CH. Use of serum bile acids in the identification of vinyl chloride hepatotoxicity. Am J Med 1985; 78: 68–76
4. Edling C, Tagesson C. Raised serum bile acid concentration after occupational exposure to styrene: a possible sign of hepatotoxicity? Br J Industr Med 1984; 41: 257–259
5. Tobiasson P, Boerd B. Serum cholic and chenodeoxycholic acid conjugates and standard liver function tests in various morphological stages of alcoholic liver disease. Scand J Gastroent 1980; 15: 657–663
6. Editorial. Serum bile acids in hepatobiliary disease. Lancet 1982; ii: 1136–1138
7. Festi D, Labate AMM, Roda A et al. Diagnostic effectiveness of serum bile acids in liver diseases as evaluated by multivariate statistical methods. Hepatology 1983; 3: 707–713
8. Paumgartner G. Serum bile acids, physiological determinants and results in liver disease. J Hepatolo 1986; 2: 291–298
9. Einarsson K, Angelin B, Bjorkhem I, Glaumann H. The diagnostic value of fasting individual bile acids in anicteric alcoholic liver disease: relation to liver morphology. Hepatology 1985; 5: 108–111
10. Kishimoto Y, Hijiya S, Takeda I. Clinical significance of fasting serum bile acid in the long term observation of chronic liver disease. Am J Gastroenterol 1985; 80: 136–138
11. Simko V, Michael S. Bile acid levels in diagnosing mild liver disease. Arch Int Med 1986; 146: 695–697
12. Douglas JG, Beckett GJ, Nimmo IA et al. Clinical value of bile salt tests in anicteric liver disease. Gut 1981; 22: 141–148
13. Barnes S, Gallo GA, Trash DB, Morris JS. Diagnostic value of serum bile acid estimations in liver disease. J Clin Path 1975; 28: 506–509
14. Lawrence CM, Strange RC, Scriven AJ et al. Plasma bile salt levels in patients presenting with generalized pruritis: an improved indicator of occult liver disease. Ann Clin Biochem 1985; 22: 232–235
15. Mannes GA, Thieme C, Stellard F et al. Prognostic significance of serum bile acids in cirrhosis. Hepatology 1986; 6: 50–53
16. Jarnfelt-Samsioe A, Eriksson B, Wadenstrom J, Samsioe G. Serum bile acids, gamma-glutamyltransferase and routine liver function tests in emetic and nonemetic pregnancies. Gyn Obs Invest 1986; 21: 169–176
17. Sotaniemi EA, Sutinen S, Sutinen S, et al. Liver injury in subjects occupationally exposed to chemicals in low doses. Acta Med Scand 1982; 212: 207–215
18. Tietz NW. Clinical guide to laboratory tests. Philadelphia, PA: WB Saunders. 1983: p 78–81

CHAPTER CONTENTS

28

Tryptophan load test

Michael T. Murray, ND

Joseph E. Pizzorno Jr, ND

INTRODUCTION

The use of an oral loading dose of L-tryptophan to detect abnormalities in tryptophan and vitamin B_6 status is an under-utilized laboratory procedure. If used only to measure B_6 status, it may be less indicative than other indices, such as the methionine load test (urinary cystathionine), serum pyridoxal-5-phosphate, urinary vitamin B_6, or 4-pyridoxic acid. It may, however, be more accurate than erythrocyte aminotransaminases. The real value of the test is in the evaluation of tryptophan metabolism. Aberrations in tryptophan metabolism have been implicated in a wide range of diseases, including depression, autism, hypertension, and asthma. Correction of these aberrations is sometimes possible with supplementation of B_6 and magnesium, as these two nutrients play a major role in tryptophan metabolism. Even marginal B_6 or magnesium deficiencies cause significant alterations. A simplified schematic representation of tryptophan metabolism is shown in Figure 28.1.

PROCEDURE

The procedure is straightforward: tryptophan breakdown products are measured in the urine after a loading dose is orally administered.[2]

Method

1. Two grams of L-tryptophan are administered orally.
2. Urine is collected for the next 24 hours.
3. The urinary levels of 3-hydroxykynurenine, kynurenine, and xanthurenic acid are determined (xanthurenic acid is the easiest to measure and may be the only metabolite measured by some laboratories).

Results are interpreted as shown in Table 28.1.

INTERPRETATION

Kynurenine aminotransferase is apparently less sensitive

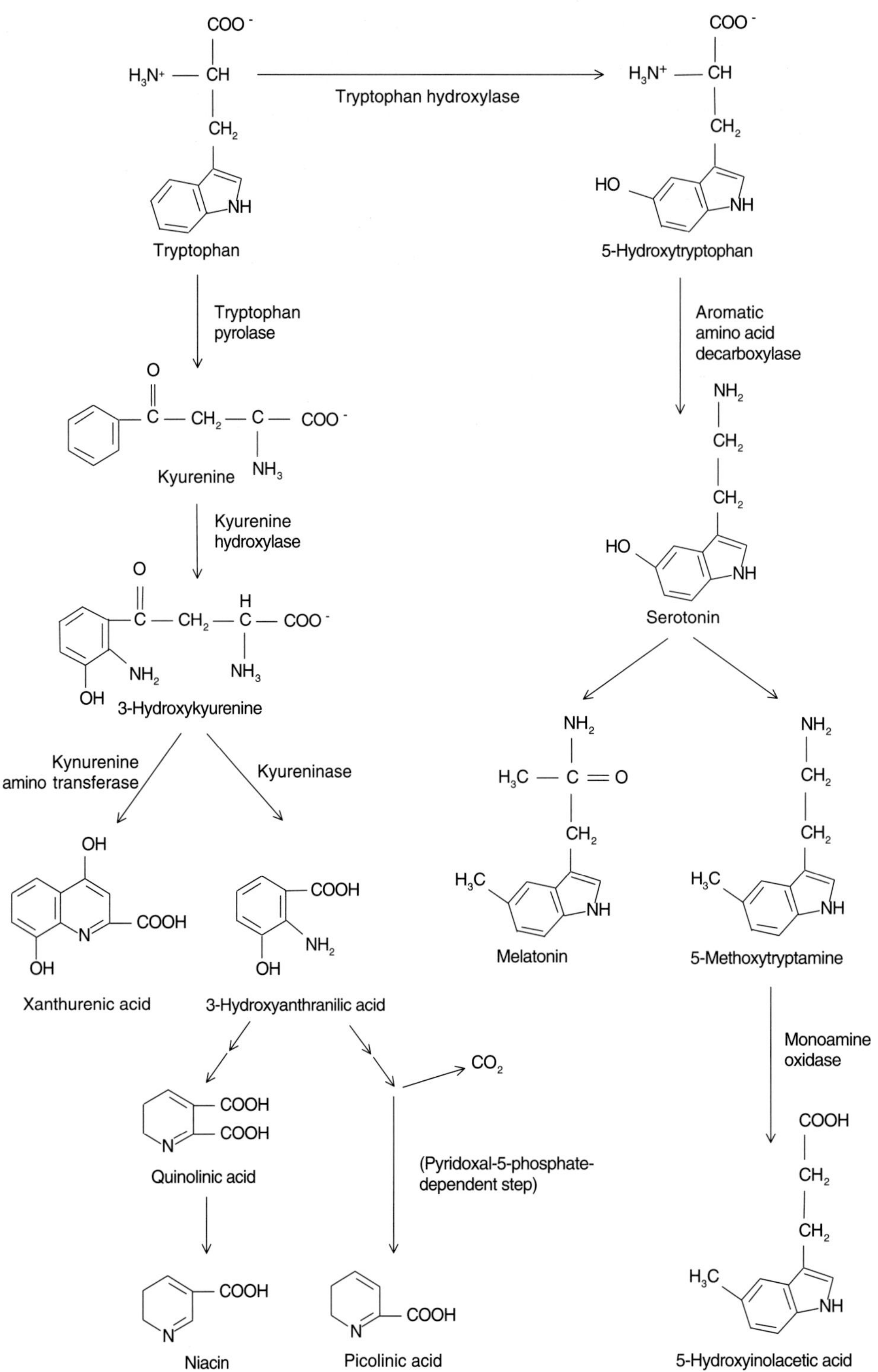

Figure 28.1 Tryptophan metabolism.[1]

Table 28.1 Vitamin B_6 and tryptophan metabolism status according to 24 hour urinary excretion of tryptophan metabolites

Metabolite	Abnormal (mg/24 h)	Normal (mg/24 h)
Xanthurenic acid	>50	<25
3-Hydroxykynurenine	>50	<25
Kynurenine	>50	<10

to a vitamin B_6 deficiency than kynureninase, resulting in a shunting to xanthurenic acid and, as the deficiency worsens, 3-hydroxykynurenic and kynurenine. The first two metabolites may also be increased in response to increased activity of tryptophan pyrrolase. This enzyme is stimulated by glucocorticoids, glucagon, and oral contraceptives, and inhibited by insulin. The tryptophan load test can be used to evaluate the therapeutic effect of vitamin B_6 supplementation.

REFERENCES

1. Brown R. Tryptophan metabolism in humans: perspectives and predictions. In: Hayaishi O, Ishimura Y, Kido R, eds. Biochemical and medical aspects of tryptophan metabolism. Amsterdam: Elsevier. 1980: p 227–235
2. Sauberlich H, Skala J, Dowdy R. Laboratory tests for the assessment of nutritional status. Cleveland, Oh: CRC Press. 1977: p 38–42

CHAPTER CONTENTS

29

Urinary organic acids profiling for assessment of functional nutrient deficiencies, gut dysbiosis, and toxicity

J. Alexander Bralley, PhD

Richard S. Lord, PhD

INTRODUCTION

Urinary organic acid analysis for metabolic profiling has traditionally only been used to assess and define inborn errors of metabolism that cause death within the first year of life or severe mental retardation. Profiling of organics in urine is a relatively recent addition to routine laboratory evaluation of chronic diseases. The identification of isovaleric acidemia in 1966 was soon followed by numerous additional acidurias as the severe enzyme impairments found in genetic diseases were found to result in greatly elevated amounts of organic compounds excreted in urine.[1]

The availability of instrumentation with improved reliability, sensitivity and reduced cost is now allowing greatly expanded clinical application. This valuable technique can be used for the detection of subtle functional nutritional deficiencies, identification of genetic variants and the source of toxicants from the environment and the gut.[2–4] For example, elevated methylmalonic acid in urine is a well-established and sensitive indicator of functional vitamin B_{12} deficiency.[5] This method of assessment of nutritional status is of far greater clinical applicability than serum levels of specific nutrients, as it allows a functional evaluation of nutritional status, thus incorporating the wide variability of biochemical individuality.

Organic acids

The term "organic acids" refers to a broad class of compounds used in fundamental metabolic processes of the body. Derived from dietary protein, fat and carbohydrate, they are used by the body to generate cellular energy and provide the building blocks necessary for cell function. Chemically they share the common features of water solubility, acidity, and ninhydrin-negativity which means that amino acids are usually excluded from this group. The term is generally considered to include all carboxylic acids, with or without keto, hydroxyl or other non-amino functional groups. Some nitrogen containing compounds are included such as pyroglutamate or amino conjugates like hippurate (benzoylglycine). Short chain fatty acids are also contained in this group. With the inclusion of neutral compounds of fungal origin such as arabinose and arabinitol in the metabolic profile, the name organic acid analysis is more correctly termed organics profiling.

URINARY ORGANICS PROFILING

The measurement of organic acids and neutrals in urine allows the simultaneous assessment of mitochondrial energy production efficiency, functional vitamin, mineral and certain amino acid deficiencies, neurotransmitter metabolism, clinically significant microflora imbalances in the gut, and metabolic toxicity problems.

The test is performed on an overnight urine sample from which the organic compounds are extracted and analyzed by gas chromatography with mass spectrometric detection. The basic methodologies are well known, but improvements are regularly reported.[6,7]

The information content of the profile is high, but the interpretation is simplified by keeping in mind that the data supply answers to four basic questions of clinical relevance:

- Is mitochondrial energy production adversely affected?
- Are functional nutrient deficiencies present?
- Are symptoms related to excessive growth of bacteria and fungi in the gut?
- Is there an undue toxic load and is this adversely affecting detoxification capacity?

Each of several compounds reported in the typical profiling of organics in urine is discussed briefly, with key references cited, to indicate why they are related to these clinical questions.

Figure 29.1 provides a graphic overview of the nutrient requirements for the citric acid cycle, while Table 29.1 shows various nutrient-related abnormalities that might appear on a typical quantitative report of organics in urine. The supplementary nutrient amounts are given as guides to starting points that might improve clinical outcomes for adults. For more information on how well the associations are established, see the discussions below.

Central energy pathway intermediates

Citrate, isocitrate, α-ketoglutarate (αKG), cis*-aconitate, succinate, fumarate*

These components are intermediates in the core metabolic pathway which generates cellular energy. The Krebs or citric acid cycle (CAC) is not only the final common pathway of food components, but also the source of basic structural or anabolic molecules that feed and support organ maintenance and neurological function. Therefore, the CAC serves both anabolic and catabolic functions of the body, representing the "crossroads" of food conversion and utilization.

Conversions of the CAC intermediates are under the control of enzymes that often require vitamin-derived cofactors and minerals for their function. Abnormal spilling of CAC intermediates indicates mitochondrial inefficiencies at specific steps in energy production. This fundamental pathway of energy flow is critical for all organ systems. The measurement of the intermediates listed above provides a unique perspective to energy metabolism, along with clues on how to improve energy production by supplying B complex vitamins to assure adequate coenzyme concentrations. In cytochrome C oxidase deficiency, for example, there is inefficient removal of the primary product of the CAC (NADH), and citrate, malate, fumarate, and αKG are all increased.[8] Coenzyme Q_{10} deficiency can also result in elevated CAC intermediates (see "Hydroxymethylglutarate" below).

Mild inborn errors of energy metabolism which may be compatible with survival at least into young adulthood, but not with normal development of mental and neurological functions, have been associated with the excretion of elevated αKG.[9] The clinical heterogeneity of neurometabolic disorders and the importance of organic acid analysis in the diagnosis of static encephalopathy were underscored by the finding of excretion of excess fumaric acid in a 5-year-old girl with a previous diagnosis of cerebral palsy.[10]

Intermediates of the cycle can also be derived from amino acids. This would explain the energy-boosting effect people often report when they take free form amino acid supplements. The effect is due to the conversion of specific amino acids directly into depleted CAC intermediates needed for the energy-producing cycle. The fatigue-reducing effect of supplementation of aspartate salts and α-ketoglutaric acid has been attributed to such a mechanism.[11,12] Supplementation of the precursors serves to drive the cycle and generate reducing equivalents used in the electron transport chain where ATP is produced via oxidative phosphorylation. Low levels of a specific metabolite may be indicative of suboptimal amino acid availability and need for supplemental amounts of these specific amino acids for improved function.

Lactate and pyruvate

These two compounds provide useful insight into basic metabolic factors due to their position in the energy production process. Pyruvate is the anaerobic breakdown product of glucose. Its further conversion to acetyl-CoA requires the pyruvate dehydrogenase enzyme complex.

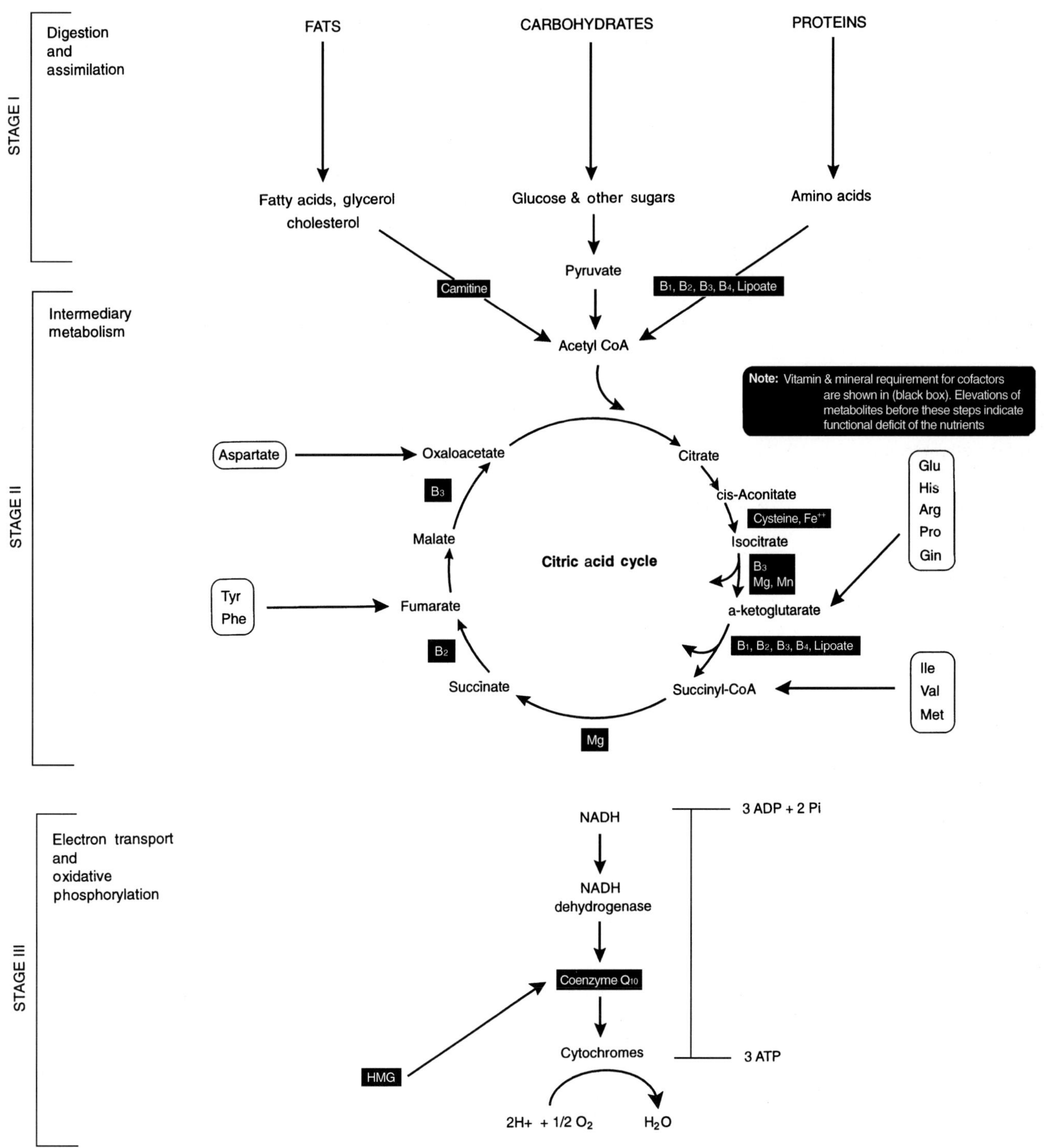

Figure 29.1 Vitamin and mineral cofactor requirements for the extraction of energy from food.

Pyruvate dehydrogenase requires cofactors derived from thiamin, riboflavin, niacin, lipoic acid, and pantothenic acid for optimal function. Elevated levels of pyruvate may reflect failure of the enzyme due to a functional need for increased B vitamins, particularly thiamin and pantothenic acid.

Levels of pyruvate in the tissues are further controlled by the biotin-containing protein, pyruvate carboxylase, which controls the first step in the reformation of glucose from pyruvate. Multiple forms of pyruvate carboxylase deficiency, some of which are biotin-responsive, have been reported.[13]

Lactate accumulates when there is a block in the final oxidative phosphorylation (ox/phos) stage of energy production. Such a block results in inactivation of the CAC. Coenzyme Q_{10} has been used in cases of lactic

Table 29.1 Quick reference to clinical significance of abnormal levels of organics in urine

Name	Abnormality	Potential intervention	Metabolic pathway
Energy production			
Citrate	L	Aspartic acid, 500 mg	
Cis-aconitate	H	Iron, 18 mg; cysteine, 1000 mg b.i.d.	
Isocitrate	H	αKG, 300mg t.i.d.; B_3, 100mg Magnesium, 400 mg; manganese, 20 mg	
α-Ketoglutarate	L	αKG, 300 mg; arginine, 1000 mg; glutamine, 1–5g	Citric acid cycle intermediates
	H	B-complex, 1 t.i.d.; lipoic acid 100 mg	
Succinate	L	Isoleucine, 1000 mg t.i.d.; valine, 1000 mg t.i.d.	
	H	Magnesium, 500 mg	
Fumarate	L	Tyrosine, 1000 mg b.i.d.; phenylalanine, 500 mg b.i.d.	
Malate	H	B_3, 100 mg t.i.d.	
Lactate	H	Coenzyme Q_{10}, 50 mg t.i.d.	
Pyruvate	H	B-complex, 1 capsule t.i.d.; B_1, 100 mg t.i.d.; lipoic acid, 100 mg t.i.d.	Aerobic/anaerobic energy production
Specific vitamin indicators			
α-Ketoisovalerate	H	B-complex, 1 capsule t.i.d.; B_1, 100 mg t.i.d.; lipoic acid, 100 mg t.i.d.	Amino acid catabolism utilizing B-complex vitamins
α-Ketoisocaproate	H		
α-Keto-β-methylvalerate	H		
Methylmalonate	H	B_{12}, 1000 mcg t.i.d.	BCAA input to Krebs cycle
β-Hydroxyisovalerate	H	Biotin, 5 mg b.i.d.; magnesium, 100 mg b.i.d.	Dicarboxylic acid metabolism requiring biotin
Hydroxymethylglutarate	H/L	Coenzyme Q_{10}, 50 mg t.i.d.	Co-Q_{10} synthesis
Carbohydrate metabolism			
β-Hydroxybutyrate	H	Chromium picolinate, 200 mcg b.i.d.	Balance of fat and CHO metabolism
α-Hydroxybutyrate	H		
Detoxication indicators			
Glucarate	H	Glycine, GSH, NAC, 500–5000 mg/day	Detox. liver enzyme induction
Orotate	H	αKG, 300 mg t.i.d.; arginine, 1–3 g/day; aspartic acid, 500 mg b.i.d.; magnesium, 300 mg	Ammonia clearance, pyrimidine synthesis
p-Hydroxyphenyllactate	H	Vitamin C up to 100 mg/kg	Prooxidant and carcinogen
2-Methylhippurate	H	Avoidance of xylene	Hepatic conjugation
Pyroglutamate	L/H	NAC, 1000 mg; glutathione, 300 mg	Renal amino acid recovery
Sulfate	L	Taurine, 500 mg b.i.d.; glutathione, 300 mg	Detox. and antioxidant functions
Fatty acid oxidation			
Adipate	H	L-carnitine, 250 mg t.i.d.; B_2, 100 mg b.i.d.;	
Suberate	H	B_5, 500 mg b.i.d.; choline, 100 mg t.i.d.;	Fatty acid oxidation
Ethylmalonate	H	vitamin C, 1000 mg t.i.d.: CoQ_{10}, 150 mg	
Neurotransmitter metabolism			
Vanilmandelate	L/H	Tyrosine, 1000 mg b.i.d.-t.i.d., between meals; contraindicated for patients taking MAO inhibitors	Catecholamine catabolism, neurotransmitter metabolites
Homovanillate	L/H		
5-Hydroxyindolacetate	L	5-Hydroxytryptophan, 100 mg t.i.d.	
Quinolinate	H	Magnesium, 300 mg	Serotonin catabolism
Dysbiosis markers (products of abnormal gut microflora)			
p-Hydroxybenzoate	H		
p-Hydroxyphenylacetate	H	If any of these compounds is high, the	
β-ketoglutarate	H	possibility of dysbiosis is reinforced.	Numerous interferences in pathways and
Hydrocaffeate	H	Glutamine, 10–30 g daily and free	cellular energy control mechanisms
Tartarate	H	form amino acids normalize gut permeability.	
Citramalate	H	Take appropriate steps to ensure favorable	
Arabinose	H	gut microflora population	
Arabinitol	H		
Tricarballylate	H		

acidosis associated with ox/phos impairments.[14,15] Increased lactate is a common acidotic condition that can be caused by a variety of metabolic problems. Decreased lactate is seen in people with very little physical activity. Highly trained athletes have such efficient conversion of lactate to glucose that they also demonstrate lower lactate levels.

Carbohydrate metabolism

α-Hydroxybutyrate, β-hydroxybutyrate

These two compounds are also called ketone bodies. Ketone body production occurs in conditions where glucose oxidation is impaired and free fatty acids are utilized as the predominant energy source. Ketone bodies can be thought of as a transportable form of acetate resulting from oxidation of fatty acids. β-Hydroxybutyrate is normally produced in much larger amounts than the α-isomer, but both compounds can serve the energy needs of most tissues. Elevations seen in an overnight urine collection may indicate inefficient utilization or mobilization of carbohydrate stores. Excessive fatigue on exertion is the most common symptom associated with ketosis. Chromium and vanadium supplementation may support the carbohydrate utilization by improving the action of insulin.

Indicators of a specific vitamin deficiency

β-Hydroxyisovalerate

This compound is elevated in multiple carboxylase insufficiency. This occurs due to genetic abnormalities and/or a biotin deficiency (biotin is the cofactor for three mitochondrial carboxylase enzymes). Symptoms of multiple carboxylase deficiencies include alopecia, skin rash, *Candida* dermatitis, unusual odor to the urine, immune deficiencies and muscle weakness. Biotin deficiencies of various degrees develop in a substantial minority of normal pregnancies and in patients on long-term therapy with anticonvulsants.[17,18] Other possible indications of biotin deficiency are elevations of lactate and alanine in urine, and accumulations of odd-chain fatty acids in plasma or red cell membranes.[19] Supplementation of biotin may improve these conditions.

Hydroxymethylglutarate (HMG)

HMG is the metabolic precursor of cholesterol and coenzyme Q_{10} (CoQ_{10}). Low levels may reflect inadequate synthesis and possible deficiency of the coenzyme Q_{10}. Cholesterol-lowering drugs that block utilization of HMG for cholesterol synthesis also lower coenzyme Q_{10} levels.[20] CoQ_{10} is utilized in the mitochondrial oxidative phosphorylation pathway for ATP synthesis and is a potent antioxidant. It has been used extensively as a cardiovascular protective agent.[21]

Coenzyme Q_{10} has been used successfully to improve mitochondrial function in clinical situations of cardiac and skeletal muscle weakness and cramping and, in the extreme, mitochondrial encephalomyopathy.[22,23] The coenzyme has been found useful in the treatment of fatigue, particularly when both lactate and pyruvate are elevated. Such responses reflect the inability of mitochondrial oxidative phosphorylation to proceed efficiently, possibly due to CoQ_{10} deficiency (see Ch. 76 for a full discussion of this useful nutrient).

α-Ketoisovalerate, α-ketoisocaproate, α-keto-β-methylvalerate

These compounds are the ketoacids of the branched chain amino acids, isoleucine, leucine and valine, respectively. They are formed by the removal of the amine group in the first step of their catabolism and are excreted in large amounts along with their amino acid precursors in the inherited disorder known as maple syrup urine disease. There are 10 known metabolic disorders in the pathways of catabolism of the ketoacids. The reactions require enzymes similar to pyruvate dehydrogenase that use the B-complex cofactors, B_1, B_2, B_3, B_5 and lipoic acid. Elevations of the branched chain ketoacids provide a functional assessment of the sufficiency of these vitamins, especially thiamin.[24]

Methylmalonate

This compound is converted into succinic acid using a vitamin B_{12}-dependent enzyme, methylmalonyl CoA mutase (see Fig. 29.2). The lack of vitamin B_{12} impairs this conversion, as well as the one in which methionine is recovered from homocysteine, leading to accumulation of homocysteine. As discussed above, high levels indicate a functional deficiency of vitamin B_{12}. A differential diagnosis can be made when considering both methylmalonate and the amino acid homocysteine. If homocysteine is also elevated, both B_{12} and folate functional deficiencies are indicated. If only homocysteine is high, folate and B_6 supplementation are suggested. If methylmalonate only is elevated, only B_{12} supplementation is needed.[25]

Fatty acid oxidation

Adipate and suberate, ethylmalonate

Adipate and suberate are short-chain dicarboxylic fatty acids. They are produced by an alternate oxidation pathway called omega-oxidation. Their production is normally very low because the predominant pathway is beta oxidation in the mitochondria. Transport of fatty acids into the mitochondria, however, requires carnitine as a carrier. Suboptimal levels of carnitine result in inadequate transfer of fatty acids into the mitochondria and subsequent compensation via omega oxidation, producing excess amounts of adipate and suberate. The same metabolic impairment leads to production of ethylmlalonate. All three of these compounds will be elevated in overt enzyme failure, but the patterns of elevations in milder carnitine deficiencies will vary.

Symptoms include periodic mild weakness, nausea, fatigue, hypoglycemia, "sweaty feet" odor, recurrent infections, and increased free fatty acids. Patients may also exhibit a Reye's-like syndrome with dicarboxylic aciduria, which has been associated with various metabolic toxins generated from viral infections that affect mitochondrial function. Mild, heterozygotic forms of dicarboxylic aciduria may be more commonly seen clinically and go unrecognized. The enzymes involved also respond to

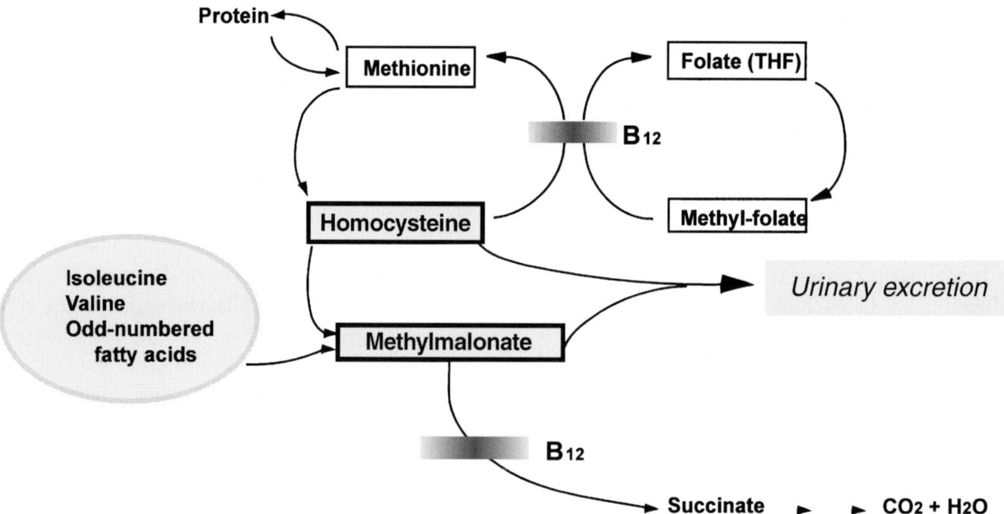

Figure 29.2 Methylmalonate is converted into succinic acid using a vitamin B_{12}-dependent enzyme, methylmalonyl CoA mutase.

environmental toxin exposure with altered lipid metabolism, which can lead to impaired immune responsiveness.[26,27] Supplementation of carnitine and other supportive nutrients is indicated when adipate, suberate or ethylmalonate are elevated.

Neurotransmitter metabolism

Vanilmandelate (VMA), homovanillate (HVA)

These two compounds are metabolites of the catecholamines, epinephrine and norepinephrine. Low urinary levels have been associated with low CNS levels of these neurotransmitters. Symptoms associated with this condition are depression, sleep disturbances, inability to deal with stress, and fatigue. Treatments aimed at improving protein digestion and supplementation of the amino acid precursors can normalize neurotransmitter levels in the CNS.[28] A further indication of need for these precursors is low fumarate, a metabolic intermediate that can also be derived from tyrosine and phenylalanine.

5-Hydroxyindolacetate (5-HIA)

Catabolic breakdown of serotonin leads to excretion of 5-hydroxyindoleacetate. Abnormal high levels of this metabolite result from increased release of serotonin from any of three primary sites: CNS, Argentiffin cells in the gut, or platelets. Carcinoid tumors composed of chromaffin tissue can also release large amounts of serotonin.

Serotonin is required for control of gut motility as it activates smooth muscle activity. Inadequate production of serotonin leads to constipation. Low levels have also been associated with depression, fatigue, insomnia, suicide, attention deficit and behavioral disorders. When HIA levels are low, dietary therapy should focus on improving protein digestion (see Ch. 19 for a discussion of hypochlorhydria and Ch. 101 for a discussion of pancreatic insufficiency) and increasing consumption of foods high in tryptophan, including turkey, bananas, low fat milk, lentils, and eggs. These actions minimize the need for oral tryptophan or 5-hydroxytryptophan use.

Products of gut microflora

Several studies have used the unique products of microbial metabolism as indicators of the abnormal overgrowth of unfavorable intestinal microflora, a condition sometimes referred to as "gut dysbiosis". Such a condition has been related to a wide variety of symptoms due to pathogenic toxins produced by these populations of microflora. No false-negative results and only 2% false-positive results for small bowel disease and bacterial overgrowth syndrome were found in a study of *p*-hydroxyphenylacetate in 360 acutely ill babies and children.[29] Some compounds are absorbed and enter the detoxification pathways of the liver to be excreted as products that can serve as sensitive indicators of changes in gastrointestinal flora.[30] One product of anaerobic bacteria, 3-phenylpropionic acid, is normally converted to common hippuric acid, but is excreted as 3-phenylpropionylglycine in individuals with a relatively common inborn error of fatty acid oxidation.[31] In people of north-western European origin, the incidence of this disorder may be 1 in 10,000.

p-Hydroxybenzoate, p-hydroxyphenylacetate, tricarballylate

For individuals with normal, healthy intestinal function, these compounds should not appear at more than background concentrations in urine, due to the efficient metabolic conservation or recycling of phenyl group compounds of which they are composed. They are produced by microbial action on tyrosine and phenylalanine and are markers of bacterial growth in the gut. *p*-Hydroxyphenylacetic aciduria has been found useful in detecting small bowel disease associated with *Giardia lamblia* infestation, ileal resection with blind loop, and other diseases of the small intestine associated with anaerobic bacterial overgrowth.[32] Use of antibiotics such as neomycin, which act primarily against aerobic bacteria, can encourage the growth of *Giardia* and anaerobic bacteria that then produce greater amounts of these compounds.[33]

Other GI disorders, including cystic fibrosis of the pancreas, celiac disease, and unclassified enteritis, have been associated with increased excretion of *p*-hydroxybenzoate, phenylacetate, and *p*-hydroxyphenylacetate. The patients with cystic fibrosis had elevated *p*-hydroxyphenylacetate even while on pancreatine therapy. Because of variations in the relative amounts of these compounds observed with this type of GI disturbance, the patterns of excretion are apparently determined by the microbial flora present in the patient's intestinal lumen.[34] Tricarballylate is produced by aerobic bacteria that quickly repopulate in the gut of germ-free animals.[35]

Arabinose, and arabinitol

Arabinose is a carbohydrate and arabinitol is the related sugar-alcohol which is a product specifically of anaerobic fungal growth in the gut. The D isomer of arabinitol is produced by fungal metabolism, and urinary excretion is elevated in patients with invasive candidiasis.[36,37]

Tartarate, citramalate, hydrocaffeate, β-ketoglutarate

The structures of these compounds are closely related to those of intermediates of normal human metabolism. They have accordingly been called anti-metabolites. The pathways that they impact upon are those of central energy production. They have been reported along with arabinose to be elevated in children who began to display autistic traits after repeated treatment with broad-spectrum antibiotics.[38] Patterns of elevations of any of the compounds in this category suggest treatments with bowel detoxification regimens to normalize the microbial flora of the gut.

Indicators of detoxification function

Glucarate

Glucaric acid (glucarate) is the oxidation product of glucuronic acid. It is a by-product of the predominant liver phase II detoxification reactions involving glucuronic acid conjugation. A great variety of drugs, environmental toxins, food components and products of gut microbial metabolism are prepared for excretion by glucuronidation. Decreased glucarate is an indicator of reduced overall hepatic function, while elevation is an indication of enzyme induction due to such potentially toxic exposures.[39,40]

The excretion of D-glucaric acid is considered a marker of the viability of hepatocytes and is a useful clinical prognostic predictor in biliary atresia.[41] Most exposures that result in stimulation of hepatic P-450 activity will result in increased excretion of glucarate. For example, urinary D-glucaric acid is elevated in pesticide-exposed groups.[42] Patients with clinically quiescent chronic pancreatitis also show elevated glucarate, indicating a relationship of toxic metabolite stress to heightened free radical activity and hence to the genesis of chronic pancreatitis.[43] The evidence of increased utilization of phase II conjugation pathways of xenobiotic disposal is in keeping with ongoing toxic metabolite stress from heightened phase I oxidative metabolism. Glucarate measurements have been advanced as useful biomarkers to xenobiotic exposure, being particularly useful as a screening tool in reproductive epidemiology.[44]

Orotate

Orotic acid accumulation is a sensitive marker of ammonia build-up. Ammonia (via glutamine) is normally disposed of by forming carbamoyl phosphate which enters the urea cycle. When there is insufficient capacity for detoxifying the load of ammonia, carbamoyl phosphate leaves the mitochondria and stimulates the synthesis of orotic acid.[45] Increased orotic acid production is a sensitive indicator of arginine availability. Most of the symptoms that develop following arginine deprivation can largely be accounted for by a decreased efficiency of ammonia detoxification. Increased orotic biosynthesis is observed with increasing ammonia concentrations in rat, mouse and human liver and is reduced by in vitro arginine supplementation.[46]

Medium-chain acyl coenzyme A dehydrogenase deficiency and other disorders of fatty acid oxidation may present long after infancy in patients such as those with a clinical diagnosis of Reye's syndrome. They may mimic the symptoms of defects in the urea cycle such as that reported for a 13-year-old girl with hyperammonemic encephalopathy and orotic aciduria due to ornithine transcarbamylase deficiency.[47] Responses should include steps to stimulate ureogenesis, including alpha-ketoglutarate, magnesium, aspartic and glutamic acids.

In addition, orotate requires magnesium for its metabolism. While a normal level in a urinary organic acid panel may not necessarily indicate magnesium sufficiency, high levels should alert one to a significant possibility of intracellular magnesium insufficiency. Red cell magnesium levels can confirm a deficiency condition. Symptoms of magnesium insufficiency include irritability, muscle cramping and twitching, irregular heart rhythm and fatigue.

p-Hydroxyphenyllactate (HPLA)

p-Hydroxyphenyllactate is a carcinogenic metabolite of tyrosine that increases lipid peroxidation in the liver.[48] Methyl *p*-hydroxyphenyllactate (MeHPLA) is an important cell growth-regulating agent, and tumor cells contain esterase enzymes that hydrolyse the compound to the free acid, HPLA.[49] HPLA is an important regulator of normal and malignant cell growth and it appears to mediate the cancer-promoting effects of estrogen. MeHPLA blocks uterine growth in vivo and inhibits MCF-7 human breast cancer cell growth in vitro.[50] High doses of ascorbic acid (100 mg/kg body weight daily) were shown to arrest or significantly inhibit the excretion of HPLA in patients with hemoblastoses and nephroblastoma.[51] HPLA is also produced by some microbes that could inhabit the gut, but the recently discovered cell proliferative and pro-oxidant functions are of far greater clinical relevance.[52]

2-Methylhippurate

This compound is a metabolite of the detoxification of the common solvent, xylene. Elevations indicate an exposure to this potentially toxic compound.[53,54] Methylhippurate, the product of hepatic oxidation and conjugation of xylene, is used to monitor xylene exposure.[55] A wide range of compounds which may be abused by inhalation can be detected by measuring the excretion of this compound or one of its metabolic products.[56] Spray-painting workers showed elevated methylhippurate, indicating recent exposure to zylene.[57] Patient counseling in avoidance of these compounds is indicated.

Pyroglutamate

Pyroglutamate is a cyclic form of glutamic acid. Small amounts are always present in overnight urine because it is produced as an intermediate in a cycle thought to be used in the active transport of amino acids.[58] This process utilizes glutathione as a carrier. With each molecule of amino acid resorbed, glutathione is split and then reformed by an ATP-requiring enzymatic step. When the energy-requiring step is impaired, the glutamic acid portion of glutathione is converted to pyroglutamate which is excreted. This shunt pathway conserves amino acids at the expense of glutathione. Glutamic acid, αKG, methionine and glutathione can replenish the intermediates in the amino acid recovery cycle and help rebuild total body glutathione.

Sulfate

Urinary sulfate is the only inorganic compound reported with the profiling of organics. It is measured in a separate assay and is included because of the added value in assessing the functioning of the detoxification pathways. Sulfation pathways are used in phase II liver detoxification for the important biotransformation of many drugs, steroid hormones, and phenolic compounds, among others. The ratio of sulfate to creatinine has been used to assess the body's reserve of sulfur-containing compounds (especially glutathione) used in phase II pathways. When the ratio of sulfate to creatinine is low, these stores need replenishment. Glutathione administration, in combination with oral cysteine and taurine and salts of sulfate, is used to replenish sulfur pathways and restore the hepatic supply of inorganic sulfate.[59,60] Glutathione levels in the liver can be increased 35% in normals by supplementation with *Silybum marianum* (see Ch. 111).

SUMMARY

Measurement of organics in the urine is rapidly becoming an indispensable tool for clinicians interested in deeply understanding the metabolic status of their patients. Through appropriate interpretation, energy production, carbohydrate metabolism, functional nutritional status, fatty acid metabolism, detoxification, gut biosis and neurotransmitter metabolism can all be assessed. Many of the detected abnormalities can then be corrected through the appropriate use of dietary changes, lifestyle improvements and nutritional and botanical supplements.

REFERENCES

1. Tanake K, Hine DG, West-Dull A, Lynn TB. Gas-chromatographic method of analysis for urinary organic acids. I. retention indices of 155 metabolically important compounds. Clin Chem 1980; 839–846
2. Scriver CR, Beaudet AL, Sly WS, Valle D. The metabolic and molecular bases of inherited disease, Vols 1–3. 7th edn. New York: McGraw-Hill. 1995
3. Ong CN, Lee BL, Shi CY, Ong HY, Lee HP. Elevated levels of benzene-related compounds in the urine of cigarette smokers. Int J Cancer 1994; 59: 177–180
4. Goodwin BL, Ruthven CR, Sandler M. Gut flora and the origin of some urinary aromatic phenolic compounds. Biochem Pharmacol 1994; 47: 2294–2297
5. Stabler SP et al. Assay of methylmalonic acid in the serum of patients with cobalamin deficiency using capillary gas chromatography-mass spectrometry. J Clin Invest 1986; 77: 1606–1612

6. Sweetman L. Qualitative and quantitative analysis of organic acids in physiologic fluids for diagnosis of the organic acidurias. In: Nyhan W, ed. Abnormalities in amino acid metabolism in clinical medicine. Norwalk: Appleton-Century-Crofts. 1984: p 419–453
7. Duez P, Kumps A, Mardens Y. GC-MS profiling of urinary organic acids evaluated as a quantitative method. Clin Chem 1996; 42: 1609–1615
8. Matsumoto I, Kuhara T, Matsumoto M, Yokota K. Urinary organic acid profile studies in a patient with cytochrome c oxidase deficiency. 39th ASMS Conf.
9. Hoffmann G, Mench-Hoinowski A, Knuppel H, Langenbeck U. Hyper-2-oxoglutaric aciduria in long-term mental handicap. J Ment Defic Res 1986; 30: 251–260
10. Elpeleg ON, Amir N, Christensen, E. Variability of clinical presentation in fumarate hydratase deficiency. J Pediatr 1992; 121: 752–754
11. Shaw DL et al. Management of fatigue. A physiological approach. Am J Med Sci 1962; 243: 758
12. Hicks JT. Treatment of fatigue in general practice. A double blind study. Clin Med 1964; Jan: 85
13. Robinson BH. Lactic acidemia (disorders of pyruvate carboxylase, pyruvate dehydrogenase). In: Nyhan W, ed. Abnormalities in amino acid metabolism in clinical medicine. Norwalk: Appleton-Century-Crofts. 1984: p 1478–1489
14. Wallace DC. Mitochondrial genetics. A paradigm for aging and degenerative diseases? Science 1992; 256: 628–632
15. Corral-Debrinksi M, Shoffener JM, Lott MT, Wallace DC. Association of mitochondrial DNA damage with aging and coronary atherosclerotic heart disease. Mutat Res 1992; 275: 169–180
16. Mock NI, et al. Increased urinary excretion of 3-hydroxyisovaleric acid and decreased urinary excretion of biotin are sensitive early indicators of decreased biotin status in experimental biotin deficiency, Am J Clin Nutr 1997; 65: 951–958
17. Dostalova L. Vitamin status during puerperium and lactation, Ann Nutr Metab 1984; 28: 385–408
18. Krause K-H, Berlit P, Bonjour J-P. Vitamin status in patients on chronic anticonvulsant therapy. Int J Vitam Nutr Res 1982; 52: 375–385
19. Nyhan WL. Inborn errors of biotin metabolism. Arch Dermatol 1987; 123(12): 1696–1698
20. Folkers K, Langsjoen P, Willis R et al. Lovastatin deceases coenzyme Q levels in humans. Proc Nat Acad Sci USA 1990; 87(22): 8931–8934
21. Mortensen SA, Vadhanavikit S, Muratsu K, Folkers K. Coenzyme Q_{10}. Clinical benefits with biochemical correleates suggesting a scientific breakthrough in the management of chronic heart failure. Int J Tissue React 1990; 12(3): 155–162
22. Nishikawa Y, Takahashi M, Yorifuji S et al. Long-term coenzyme Q_{10} therapy for a mitochondrial encephalomyopathy with cytochrome C oxidase deficiency. A ^{31}P NMR study. Neurology 1989; 39(3): 399–403
23. Ogasahara S, Engel AG, Frens D, Mack D. Muscle coenzyme Q deficiency in familial mitochondrial encephalomyopathy. Proc Natl Acad Sci USA 1989; 89(7): 2379–2382
24. Sweetman L and Williams JC. Branched chain organic acidurias. in Abnormalities in amino acid metabolism in clinical medicine, W Nyhan. Norwalk: Appleton-Century-Crofts. 1984: p 1387–1422
25. Lindenbaum J, Rosenberg I, Wilson P et al. Prevalence of cobalamin deficiency in the Framingham elderly population. Am J Clin Nutr 1994; 60: 2–11
26. Mullen PW. Immunopharmocological considerations in Reye's syndrome. a possible xenobiotic initiated disorder. Biochem Pharmacol 1978; 27: 145
27. Chalmers RA, Lawson AM. The dicarboxylic acidurias. In: Organic acids in man. London: Chapman & Hall. 1982: p 350–381
28. Braverman ER, Pfeiffer CC. Tyrosine. The antidepressant. In: The healing nutrients within. New Canaan, CT: Keats. 1987: p 44–58
29. Chalmers RA, Valman HB, Liberman MM. Measurement of 4-hydroxyphenylacetic aciduria as a screening test for small bowel disease. Clin Chem 1979; 25: 1791–1794
30. Lindblad BS, Alm J, Lundsjo A, Rafter JJ. Absorption of biological amines of bacterial origin in normal and sick infants. Ciba Found Symp 1979; 70: 281–291
31. Bennett MJ, Bhala A, Poirier SF et al. When do gut flora in the newborn produce 3-phenylpropionic acid? Implications for early diagnosis of medium-chain acyl-CoA dehydrogenase deficiency. Clin Chem 1992; 38(2): 278–281
32. Chalmers RA, Valman HB, Liberman NM. Measurement of 4-hydroxyphenylacetic aciduria as a screening test for small-bowel disease, Clin Chem 1979; 10: 1791–1794
33. Fellman JH, Buist NRM, Kennaway NG. Pitfalls in metabolic studies. The origin of urinary p-tyramine. Clin Biochem 1977; 10: 171
34. Van der Heiden C, Wauters EAK, Ketting D et al. Gas chromatographic analysis of urinary tyrosine and penylalanine metabolites in patients with gastrointestinal disorders. Clin Chim Acta 1971; 34: 289–296
35. McDevitt J, Goldman P. Effect of the intestinal flora on the urinary organic acid profile of rats ingesting a chemically simplified diet. Food Chem Toxicol 1991; 29(2): 107–113
36. Bernard EM, Wong B, Armstrong D. Sterioisomeric configuration of arabinitol in serum, urine, and tissues in invasive candidiasis. J Infect Dis 1985; 151(4): 711–715
37. Roboz J. Diagnosis and monitoring of disseminated candidaisis based on serum/urine D/L-arabinitol ratios. Chirality 1994; 6(2): 51–57
38. Shaw W, Kassen E, Chaves E. Increased urinary excretion of analogs of Krebs cycle metabolites and arabinose in two brothers with autistic features. Clin Chem 1995; 41(8): 1094–1104
39. Hunter J, Carrella M, Maxwell JD et al. Urinary D-glucaric acid excretion as a test for hepatic enzyme induction in man. Lancet 1971; i: 572–575
40. Sandle LN, Braganza JM. An evaluation of the low-pH enzymatic assay of urinary D-glucaric acid, and its use as a marker of enzyme induction in exocrine pancreatic disease. Clinica Chim Acta 1987; 162: 245–256
41. Fujimoto T, Ohya T, Miyano T. A new clinical prognostic predictor for patients with biliary atresia. J Pediatr Surg 1994; 29(6): 757–760
42. Edwards JW, Priestly BG. Effect of occupational exposure to aldrin on urinary D-glucaric acid, plasma dieldrin, and lymphocyte sister chromatid exchange. Int Arch Occup Environ Health 1994; 66(4): 229–234
43. Gut A, Chaloner C, Schofield D et al. Evidence of toxic metabolite stress in black South Africans with chronic pancreatitis. Clin Chim Acta 1995; 236: 145–153
44. Hogue CJ, Brewster MA. The potential of exposure biomarkers in epidemiologic studies of reproductive health. Environ Health Perspect 1991; 90: 261–269
45. Visek WJ. Nitrogen-stimulated orotic acid synthesis and nucleotide imbalance, Cancer Res 1992; 52: 2082–2084s
46. Milner JA. Metabolic aberrations associated with arginine deficiency. J Nutr 1985; 1154: 516–523
47. Marsden D, Sege-Petersen K, Nyhan WL et al. An unusual presentation of medium-chain acyl coenzyme A dehydrogenase deficiency. Am J Dis Child 1992; 146(12): 1459–1462
48. Levchuk AA, Pal'mina NP, Raushenbakh MO. Effect of the carcinogenic metabolites of aromatic amino acids on oxidative processes in lipids in vitro and in vivo. Biull Eksp Biol Med 1987; 104(7): 77–79
49. Markaverich BM, Gregory RR, Alejandro M et al. Methyl p-hydroxyphenyllactate and nuclear type II binding sites in malignant cells. metabolic fate and mammary tumor growth. Cancer Res 1990; 50(5): 1470–1478
50. Markaverich BM, Gregory RR, Alejandro MA et al. Estrogen regulation of methyl p-hydroxyphenyllactate hydrolysis. correlation with estrogen stimulation of rat uterine growth. J Steroid Biochem 1989; 33(5): 867–876
51. Baikova VN, Vares IM, Rybal'chenko VG et al. Congenital disorders of tyrosine metabolism and their correction in children with tumors. Vopr Onkol 1987; 33(11): 42–48
52. Montemartini M, Santome JA, Cazzulo JJ, Nowicki C. Production of aromatic alpha-hydroxyacids by epimastigotes of Trypanosoma cruzi, and its possible role in NADH reoxidation. FEMS Microbiol Lett 1994; 118(1–2): 89–92

53. Kira S. Measurement by gas chromatography of urinary hippuric acid and methylhippuric acid as indices of toluene and xylene exposure. Br J Ind Med 1977; 34(4): 305–309
54. Ogata M, Taguchi T. Quantitative analysis of urinary glycine conjugates by high performance liquid chromatography. excretion of hippuric acid and methylhippuric acids in the urine of subjects exposed to vapours of toluene and xylenes. Int Arch Occup Environ Health 1986; 58: 121–129
55. Inoue O, Seikji K, Watanabe T et al. Excretion of methylhippuric acids in urine of workers exposed to a xylene mixture. comparison among three xylene isomers and toluene. Int Arch Occup Environ Health 1993; 64: 533–539
56. Ramsey JD, Flanagan RJ. The role of the laboratory in the investigation of solvent abuse. Hum Toxicol 1982; 1: 299–311
57. Triebig G, Schaller KH, Weltle D. Neurotoxicity of solvent mixtures in spray painters. I. Study design, workplace exposure, and questionnaire. Int Arch Occup Environ Health 1992; 64: 353–391
58. Chalmers RA, Lawson AM. Organic acidurias due to disorders in other metabolic pathways. in Organic Acids in Man. London: Chapman & Hall. 1982: p 350–381
59. Levy, G. Sulfate conjugation in drug metabolism. role of inorganic sulfate. Fed Proc 1986; 45: 2235–2240
60. Gregus Z, White C, Howell S et al. Effect of glutathione depletion on sulfate activation and sulfate ester formation in rats. Biochem Pharmacol 1988; 37: 4307–4312

CHAPTER CONTENTS

30

Urinary porphyrins for the detection of heavy metal and toxic chemical exposure

Carl P. Verdon, PhD

Terry A. Pollock, MS

J. Alexander Bralley, PhD

INTRODUCTION

Toxic chemicals, at any level of chronic exposure, affect human biochemistry. Fortunately, the body has mechanisms for transforming, eliminating or compartmentalizing the many toxic chemicals encountered over a lifetime. Nonetheless, these "safety" mechanisms may be inadequate or even inappropriate in our modern industrialized society, especially for susceptible people such as the elderly, individuals with poor nutritional habits, and others who are physiologically stressed.[1,2]

Recognizing and identifying offending chemical(s) can present a difficult challenge for the clinician. Many chemicals exert their effect at such low concentrations that they escape detection except by very sophisticated laboratory methods. While measuring *effects* of toxicity by observing symptoms is a time-honored procedure, determination of the actual toxicant often requires the use of laboratory methods that measure *biomarkers*, which are specific indicators of the toxicant's action.

Porphyrins measured in urine serve as such a biomarker. The presence or elevation of various urinary porphyrin species can flag a potentially toxic condition. Metals and other toxic chemicals with pro-oxidant reactivity can inactivate porphyrinogenic enzymes, deplete glutathione and other antioxidants and increase oxidant stress, all of which lead to damaged membranes, enzymes and other proteins in cells.[3,4] In addition, porphyrinogens (precursors to porphyrins in the reduced state) themselves are easily non-enzymatically oxidized to porphyrins by toxic metals such as mercury (Fig. 30.1). Thus, the distribution pattern of porphyrins in the urine serves as a functional fingerprint of toxicity.[5]

The utility of urinary porphyrins as a diagnostic tool is not new – its use has been documented in the literature since 1934. Specific diseases collectively known as the *porphyrias*, which can be inherited or acquired (e.g. acute intermittent porphryia, porphyria cutanea tarda, variegate porphyria), are often diagnosed with the aid of

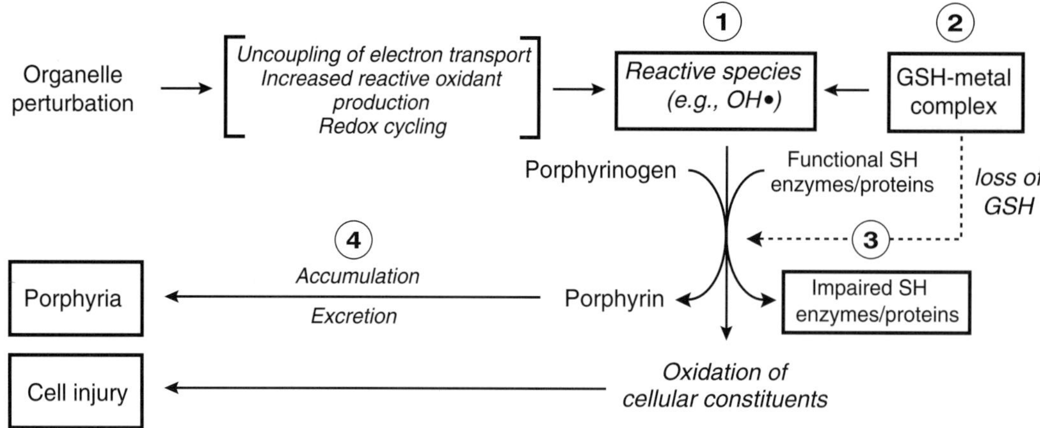

Figure 30.1 Toxic metal induction of porphyria and cell injury occurs as follows: (1) metals promote an increase in reactive prooxidants; (2) metals complex with glutathione compromising antioxidant and thiol status; (3) metals impair enzymes and other proteins via SH-complexation; (4) oxidant stress induced by metals causes cell injury and oxidation of porphyinogens to porphyrins which are excreted in the urine (porphyrinuria).[7]

information regarding the distribution profile of individual porphyrin species in human urine.

Definitions

Porphyrins are oxidized by-products that have escaped from the heme biosynthetic pathway, an essential pathway occurring in all nucleated mammalian cells. Heme is the all-important iron-binding molecule essential for the proper function of many proteins, including hemoglobin (oxygen transport), cytochrome c (energy production) and cytochrome P-450 (detoxification). Biosynthesis of heme involves eight enzymes (Fig. 30.2), five of which produce intermediate molecules that are collectively called *porphyrinogens*. Some porphyrinogens escape the intracellular pathway to become oxidized by other cellular processes to porphyrins. Some porphyrins, in turn, are excreted in urine and feces.

The different molecular species of porphyrins that occur in the urine of healthy individuals form a predictable, characteristic pattern. Elevated levels of one or more porphyrins is designated *porphyrinuria*. The term *porphyria* is reserved for primary conditions exhibiting specific clinical symptoms caused by an inherited defect in one or more of the heme biosynthetic enyzmes. *Porphyrinopathy* is an umbrella term for any disorder in porphyrin metabolism.

PORPHYRIAS

The porphyrias have been classified in the literature in several different ways. Most commonly, porphyrias are presented in textbooks with specific biochemical reference to the principal enzyme deficiency (e.g. ALA dehydratase deficiency, etc.) and the site of the deficiency (i.e. hepatic, erythropoietic, or both). Furthermore, the temporal pattern of appearance of overt clinical signs (acute vs. chronic) and the primary presentation of symptoms (neuropathic, dermatopathic, or mixed) are valid classifications that arrange porphyrias according to symptomatology. It is also useful to organize porphyrias according to etiology (hereditary vs. acquired or toxicant-induced).

PORPHYRINOPATHIES

Inhibition of an enzyme for heme biosynthesis can result in the inappropriate accumulation of that enzyme's substrate. The more severe the enzyme's inhibition, the greater the tissue accumulation of porphyrins, sometimes becoming severe enough to cause clinical porphyria.

One class of toxic chemicals capable of subtle yet insidious health effects that may mimic other disorders, especially in children, is the heavy metals. Lead, mercury, arsenic, aluminum, and cadmium are well-documented examples. Chronic exposure to these metals often results in organ-specific accumulation which compromises the physiology of that organ. Heavy metals damage many aspects of metabolism, as shown in Figure 30.1. Similarly, chronic exposure to organic chemicals such as herbicides, pesticides, and industrial and manufacturing by-products can have deleterious impact on the body's biochemistry which results in the decline of cellular function (Table 30.1).[3]

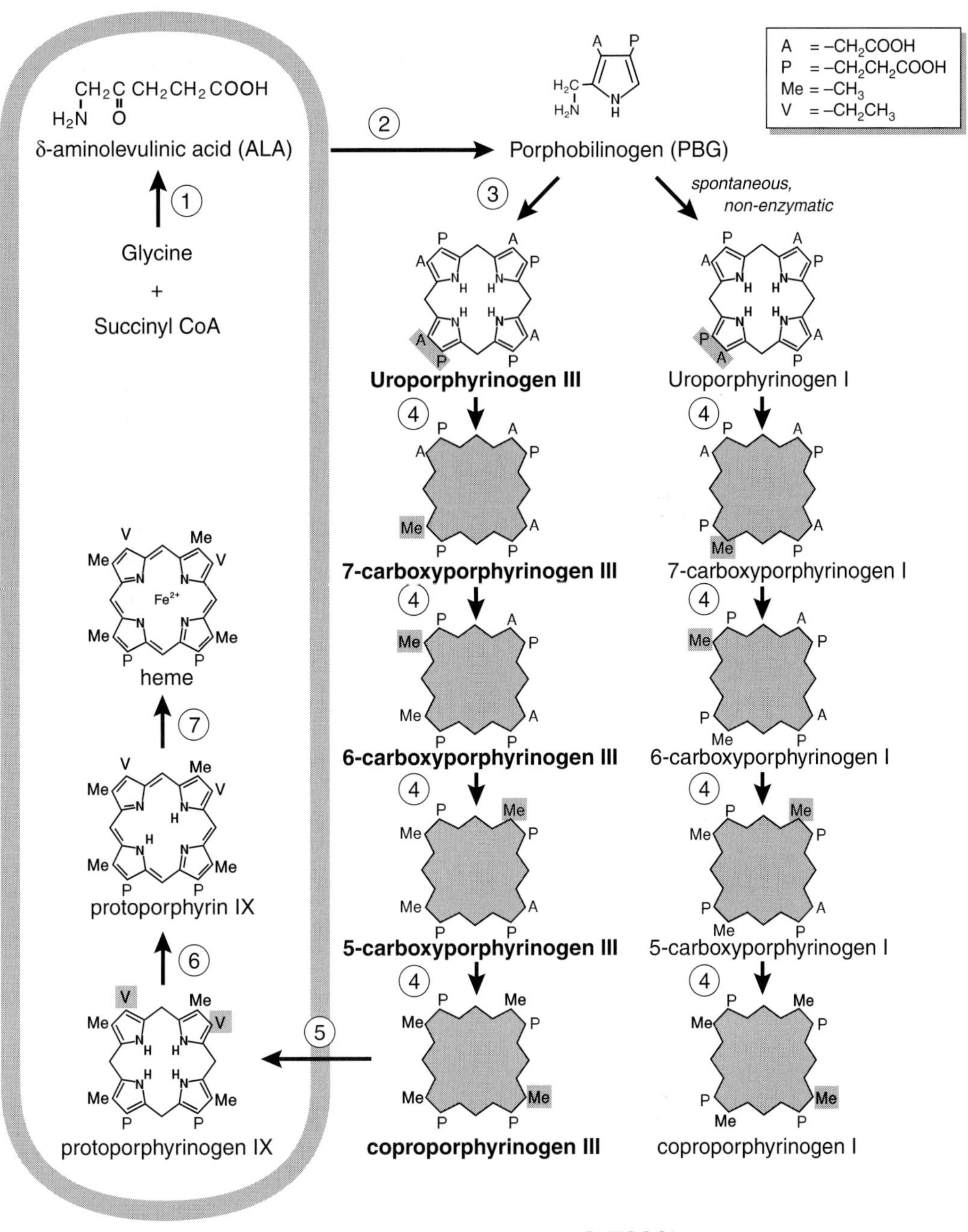

Figure 30.2 Biosynthesis of heme. The enzymes that drive the heme pathway are: (1) δ-aminolevulinate (ALA) synthetase, (2) ALA dehydratase, (3) uroporphyrinogen I synthetase (PBG deaminase) and uroporphyrinogen III cosynthetase, two enzymes that work in concert, (4) uroporphyrinogen decarboxylase, (5) coproporphyrinogen oxidase, (6) protoporphyrinogen oxidase, and (7) ferrochelatase (heme synthetase). Spilled porphyrins derived from porphyrinogens with 8-, 7-, 6-, 5-, and 4-carboxyl groups are largely excreted in the urine, while the less polar 2-carboxyporphyrin (protoporphyrin) is excreted exclusively in the feces. The physiologically relevant pathway leading to heme is via uroporphyrinogen III in which the propionyl and acetyl groups are "reversed" compared with the type I pathway, which "dead ends" with coproporphyrinogen I. The physiological significance of the type I pathway remains unclear; however, coproporphyrin I is elevated in hepatobiliary diseases.

Table 30.1 Symptomatology of the porphyrinopathies

Primary complaints	Associated symptoms	Condition exacerbated by
Neurologic presentations		
Abdominal pain; nausea; vomiting; constipation; seizures	Headaches; difficulty in concentration; personality changes; weakness; muscle and joint aches; unsteady gait, poor coordination; numbness, tingling of arms and legs; fluid retention; rapid heart rate; high blood pressure; increased sweating; intermittent fever	Low carbohydrate diets (skipped meals); intake of alcoholic beverages; medications, including sulfa-drug antibiotics, barbiturates, estrogen, birth control pills; exposure to toxic chemicals
Cutaneous presentations		
Changes in skin pigmentation; changes in facial hair; fragile skin; rashes; blistering	Dark-colored urine (especially after its exposure to sunlight), and above symptoms may be present	Above factors, and skin symptoms made worse by exposure to sunlight. Copper or brass jewelry exacerbates reaction

PROCEDURE

The clinical utility of urinary porphyrins is maximized when urine samples are taken when the patient is experiencing symptoms (see Table 30.4 below). Urine is best collected over a 24-hour period with 7 g of sodium carbonate added as a preservative. It may be useful with some patients to provoke their porphyria (e.g. a low carbohydrate diet for 2 days can be effective).

CLINICAL APPLICATIONS

Changes in the urinary porphyrins (i.e. porphyrinuria) coincident with provocation (e.g. fasting) or therapeutic intervention (e.g. medications, chelation therapy) are suggestive of some type of porphyrinopathy. If the patient's response upon provocation can be duplicated then the possibility of a diagnosis of porphyria should be investigated. Twenty-four hour output of any urinary porphyrin that is three or more times the upper limit of the reference range may indicate that organ accumulation of porphyrins is reaching pathological levels. In such cases, a comprehensive porphyria work-up is warranted. For out-of-range results that are lower than three times the upper limit, the rationale for further porphyria testing is predicated upon the availability of corroborating clinical and/or biochemical data such as complaints, family and patient medical history.

Elevations of the individual porphyrin species above the normal range have a number of causes, both inherited

Table 30.2 Enzymatic defects of the common porphyrias

Enzymatic defect	Porphyria
δ-Aminolevulinic acid (ALA) synthetase	
ALA dehydratase	Plumboporphyria
Porphobilinogen deaminase	Acute intermittent porphyria
Uroporphyrinogen cosynthetase	Congenital erythropoietic porphyria
Uroporphyrinogen decarboxylase	Porphyria cutanea tardia and hepatoerythropoeitic porphyria
Coproporphyrinogen	Hereditary coproporphyria
Prototporphyrinogen	Variegate porphyria
Ferrochelatase	Protoporphuria

Table 30.3 Various causes and conditions related to porphyria

- Intoxications
  —alcoholism
  —foreign and environmental chemicals, e.g. hexachlorobenzene, polyhalogenated biphenyls, dioxins (TCDD), vinyl chloride, carbon tetrachloride, benzene, chloroform
  —heavy metals such as lead, arsenic, mercury
  —drugs
- Liver diseases
  —cirrhosis
  —active chronic hepatitis
  —toxic and infectious hepatitis
  —fatty liver
  —alcoholic liver syndromes
  —drug injury
  —cholestasis
  —cholangitis
  —biliary cirrhosis
- Adverse effect of drugs
  —analgesics
  —sedatives
  —hypnotics
  —anesthetics
  —sex hormones
  —sulfa-drug antibiotics
- Infectious diseases
  —mononucleosis
  —acute poliomyelitis
- Diabetes mellitus
- Myocardial infarction
- Hematologic diseases
  —hemolytic, sideroachrestic, sideroblastic, aplastic anemias
  —ineffective erythropoiesis (intramedullary hemolysis)
  —pernicious anemia
  —thalassemia
  —leukemia
  —erythroblastosis
  —iron deficiency anemia
- Malignancies
  —hepatocellular tumors
  —hepatic metastases
  —pancreatic carcinoma
  —lymphomatosis
  —other systemic diseases
- Disturbance of iron metabolism
  —hemosiderosis
  —idiopathic and secondary hemochromatosis
- Hereditary hyperbilirubinemias
  —Dubin–Johnson syndrome
  —Rotor's syndrome
- Pregnancy
- Carbohydrate fasting
- Bronze baby syndrome
- Erythrohepatic protoporphyria
- Hereditary tyrosinemia

and environmental (see Tables 30.2 and 30.3).[6] The effect of chemicals on the porphyrin pathway has been the subject of many scientific reports. Lead, mercury or arsenic toxicity induces porphyrinuria,[7] as well as polychlorinated phenyls (e.g. dioxin, PCBs),[8] and many drugs (see Table 30.4).[9] A study of practicing dentists reported correlations between elevated urinary 5-carboxyporphyrin, precoproporphyrin, coproporphyrin and behavioral changes that were related to urinary excretion of mercury.[10,11] Together, elevations of these porphyrins served as biomarkers of mercury toxicity.

Upregulation of the heme biosynthetic pathway, with the concomitant increase in delta-aminolevulinic acid (ALA), is another mechanism by which porphyria can be precipitated. Increased ALA production is usually a normal physiological response to provide enough of this pre-porphyrin precursor to meet the body's demand for heme. However, overproduction of ALA can overwhelm even a normally functioning heme biosynthetic pathway, resulting in the inappropriate accumulation of ALA and/or the porphyrins.[6] Commonly, active porphyria occurs when ALA overproduction coincides with inhibition of one or more of the porphyrinogenic enzymes. Very often, porphyria is the result of a chemical insult to a porphyrinogenic enzyme combined with an external stressor that provokes dysregulation of the heme biosynthetic pathway. It is estimated that among cases of a porphyrinogenic enzyme deficiency, as many as 90% are healthy throughout adulthood until their porphyria is triggered mid-life by toxic chemicals or drugs, an acute illness or worsening chronic condition, or a major dietary change (Table 30.5).[12]

Table 30.4 Drugs known to cause or exacerbate porphyria[a]

- Antipyrine
- Amidopyrine
- Aminoglutethimide
- Barbiturates
- Carbamazepine
- Carbromal
- Chloropropramide
- Chloral hydrate
- Danazol
- Dapsone
- Diclofenac
- Diphenylhydrantoin
- Ergot preparations
- Ethanol (acute)
- Ethclorvynol
- Ethinamate
- Glutethimide
- Griseofulvin
- Isopropylmeprobamate
- Mephenyltoin
- Meprobamate
- Methylprylon
- *N*-butylscopolammaonium bromide
- Nitrous oxide
- Novobiocin
- Phenylbutazone
- Primadone
- Pyrazolone preparations
- Succinimides
- Sulfonamide antibiotics
- Sulfonthylmethane
- Sulfonmethane
- Synthetic estrogens, progestins
- Tolazamide
- Tolbutamide
- Trimethadone
- Valproic acid

[a]Although this list includes many of the better known drugs that can exacerbate porphyria, it should not be considered complete.

Table 30.5 Interpretation of abnormal urinary porphyrin test results: relationship to heme pathway defects and possible causes (with emphasis on toxic metals)

Abnormal test result[a]	Heme pathway defect[b]	Possible environmental cause[c]
Uroporphyrin and 7-carboxyporphyrin (sometimes)	Uroporphyrinogen decarboxylase	Arsenic[2] Certain organic chemicals
5-Carboxyporphyrin and coproporphyrin, 6-Carboxyporphyrin (sometimes)	Uroporphyrinogen decarboxylase Coproporphyrinogen oxidase	Mercury[5] Certain organic chemicals
Precoproporphyrin[d] (almost always accompanied by elevated coproporphyrin III)	Uroporphyrinogen decarboxylase (possibly)	Mercury[5]
Coproporphyrin III, coproporphyrin I (sometimes)	Coproporphyrinogen oxidase	Lead or mercury[2] Certain organic chemicals
Coproporphyrin I:coproporphyrin III ratio >1	Hepatobiliary dysfunction[3] PBG deaminase	Arsenic

[a]Reference ranges vary depending upon the laboratory doing the analysis. The following reference range (in units of nanomoles/24 h) was set to accentuate sensitivity (i.e. more patients with true porphyrinuria being detected at the risk of an increased false-positive rate). Multiplication factors to convert values to micrograms/24 h are shown in parentheses: uroporphyrin, 41 (0.830); 7-carboxyporphyrin, 14 (0.787); 6-carboxyporphyrin, 6 (0.743); 5-carboxyporphyrin, 5 (0.699); coproporphyrin I, 40 (0.654); coproporphyrin III, 79 (0.654). The reference range for the particular laboratory conducting the analysis should be used.
[b]Inherited disorders in the enzymes of heme biosynthesis are relatively rare, but such a possibility should be considered if urinary porphyrins are greatly elevated. Please consult a specialist in inherited disorders if such a disorder is suspected.
[c]When evaluating urinary porphyrin results to arrive at a diagnosis of metal or chemical toxicity, the following should be ruled out: use of ethanol, estrogens, oral contraceptives, antibiotics, sedatives, analgesics, dietary brewer's yeast; also rule out pregnancy, liver disease, malignancies, hematologic diseases such as pernicious or iron deficiency anemias. See Table 30.5 for a more complete list.
[d]The detection of precoproporphyrin is specifically diagnostic for mercury toxicity (see Woods et al[5]).

CONCLUSION

Use of porphyrin tests as biomarkers of chemical toxicity is reasonable in combination with other laboratory tests (e.g. hair analysis in cases of suspected metal toxicity). The clinician should realize that there are many conditions unrelated to primary or toxicant-induced porphyria that can cause porphyrinuria.[12] When considering a urinary porphyrin result, the clinician should be mindful that the distribution of normal urinary porphyrin values, representing healthy individuals, overlaps significantly with values representing those who have suffered from porphyria at one time or another.

Any patients testing positive on the urinary porphyrins test should be followed up with more specific testing for a differential diagnosis. Tests that assay toxic metals directly in biological samples (i.e. blood, urine and hair) are essential for confirming whether the toxicity symptoms are caused by a metal. Identification of toxic organic chemicals by laboratory methods is also possible. Ruling out porphyria as the primary cause of porphyria-like symptoms requires tests for porphyrinogenic enzyme activities (e.g. uroporphyrinogen decarboxylase), as well as tests for blood, fecal and urine porphobilinogen (PBG) and delta-aminolevulinic acid (ALA).

REFERENCES

1. Rowland I, ed. Nutrition, toxicity, and cancer. Boca Raton, FL: CRC Press. 1991
2. Baker S: Detoxification and healing. New Canaan, CT: Keats Publishing. 1997
3. Chang L, Magos L, Suzuki T, eds. Toxicology of metals. Boca Raton, FL: CRC Press. 1996
4. Fowler BA, Oskarsson A, Woods JS: Metal- and metalloid-induced porphyrinurias. Relationships to cell injury. Ann N Y Acad Sci 1987; 514: 172–182
5. Woods JS, Bowers MA, Davis HA. Urinary porphyrin profiles as biomarkers of trace metal exposure and toxicity: studies on urinary porphyrin excretion patterns in rats during prolonged exposure to methyl mercury. Toxicol Appl Pharmacol 1991; 110: 464–476
6. Kappas A, Sassa S, Galbraith RA, Nordmann Y. The porphyrias. In: Scriver CR, Beaudet AL, Sly WS, Valle D, eds. The metabolic and molecular bases of inherited disease. 7th edn. New York: McGraw-Hill. 1995: p 2103–2159
7. Woods JS. Porphyrin metabolism as indicator of metal exposure and toxicity. In: Goyer RA, Cherian MG, eds. Handbook of experimental pharmacology. Berlin: Springer-Verlag. 1995: p 19–52
8. Doss MO. Porphyrinurias and occupational disease. In: Silbergeld E, Fowler B, eds. Mechanisms of chemical-induced porphyrinopathies. 1987: p 204–218
9. Moore MR, Disler PB. Drug-induction of the acute porphyrias [Review]. Adv Drug React Ac Pois Rev 1983; 2: 149–189
10. Woods JS, Martin MD, Naleway CA, Echeverria D. Urinary porphyrin profiles as a biomarker of mercury exposure: Studies on dentists with occupational exposure to mercury vapor. J Toxicol Environ Health 1993; 40: 235–246
11. Woods JS. Altered porphyrin metabolism as a biomarker of mercury exposure and toxicity. Can J Physiol Pharmacol 1996; 74: 210–215
12. Donnay A, Ziem G. Porphyria protocol packet (on evaluating disorders of porphyrin metabolism in chemically-sensitive patients). Baltimore, MD: MCS Referral and Resources. 1995

CHAPTER CONTENTS

31

Urine indican test (Obermeyer test)

Dirk Wm Powell, ND

INTRODUCTION

The essential amino acid tryptophan is converted to indole by intestinal bacterial cleavage of the tryptophan side chain. Following absorption, indole is converted to 3-hydroxy indole (indoxyl or indican) in the liver, where it is then conjugated with potassium sulfate or glucoronic acid. It is then transported through the blood to the kidneys for excretion.

CLINICAL APPLICATION

As most of the endogenous indoles have a side chain which prevents cleavage and are instead metabolized to skatole, the production of indicans (indoxyl potassium sulfate and indoxyl glucoronate) reflects bacterial activity in the small and large intestines. Table 31.1 lists conditions in which increased levels are found. Elevated levels are considered by natural health care doctors as an indicator of intestinal toxemia and overgrowth of anaerobic bacteria.

PROCEDURE

Detection of indicans depends upon its decomposition to indoxyl and subsequent oxidation to indigo blue. It is then concentrated into a layer of chloroform for easier measurement.

Table 31.1 Conditions with elevated levels of urinary indican[1–4]

- Inflammatory bowel disease
- Celiac disease
- Hypochlorhydria
- Gastric ulcer
- Biliary and intestinal obstruction
- Jejunal diverticulosis
- Scleroderma
- Postgastrectomy
- Hartnup's disease
- Pancreatic insufficiency
- Diminished peristalsis
- Blue diaper syndrome

Method

1. Put 5 ml of fresh urine in a test tube.
2. Add 5 ml of Obermeyer reagent.
3. Mix.
4. Add 2 ml of chloroform and invert several times.
5. Allow the chloroform to settle and observe.
6. The results are then rated by the color present in the chloroform layer.

Reagents

- Obermeyer reagent – dissolve 0.8 g ferric chloride in 100 ml concentrated HCl (*caution*: caustic)
- Chloroform (*caution*: volatile, keep tightly capped).

Results

- Urine color: 0 (normal)
- Light blue: +1
- Blue: +2
- Violet: +3
- Jet black: +4

INTERPRETATION

A positive test may indicate one of the diseases listed in Table 31.1, hypochlorhydria, bacterial overgrowth in the small intestine, malabsorption of protein, or simply a high protein intake. The latter indication could be eliminated by the institution of a consistent dietary regime (moderate protein intake) for 2 days prior to testing.

False-negatives occur when formalin, methamine, or azulfidine are present.[2] Indigo red may form occasionally from slow oxidation. The presence of iodine, salcyluric acid, methylene blue or thymol will cause a violet color, which can be removed by the addition of a crystal of sodium thiosulfate. Bile pigments interfere with the reaction, but can be removed by shaking the urine with barium chloride and filtering.

REFERENCES

1. Todd J. Clinical diagnosis and management by laboratory methods. Philadelphia, PA: WB Saunders. 1979: p 592–593
2. Greenberger N, Saegh S, Ruppert R. Urine indican excretion in malabsorption disorders. Gastroenterol 1968; 55: 204–211
3. Curzon G, Walsh J. Value of measuring urinary indican excretion. Gut 1966; 7: 711
4. Asatoor A, London D, Craske J et al. Indole production in Hartnup's disease. Lancet 1963; i: 126–128

CHAPTER CONTENTS

32

Zinc status assessment

Michael T. Murray, ND

Joseph E. Pizzorno Jr, ND

INTRODUCTION

Zinc serves as the mineral cofactor in over 70 metalloenzymes. Severe zinc deficiency is manifested by bullous-pustular dermatitis, diarrhea, alopecia, mental disturbances, and recurrent infections as a result of cell-mediated disorders, while chronic zinc toxicity is characterized by copper deficiency.[1] Acute toxicity is quite rare, as the ingestion of amounts large enough to cause toxicity symptoms (2 g/kg body weight) will usually provoke vomiting. The area between severe deficiency and toxicity is termed the gray area of nutrition; somewhere between these two states lies a point of optimum zinc nutriture. In the USA, marginal zinc deficiency is widespread, particularly in the elderly.[2,3] Table 32.1 lists, alphabetically, clinical indications for zinc assessment, while Table 32.2 lists conditions predisposing to zinc deficiency.

ASSESSMENT OF ZINC STATUS

No "gold standard" yet exists for the assessment of zinc status. The following are functional and laboratory methodologies, each with strengths and weaknesses.

Functional tests of zinc status

Physical signs of zinc deficiency

Some physical findings that appear to correlate with low zinc status include poor wound healing, alopecia, skin disorders (e.g. acne, atopic dermatitis, and psoriasis), hypogeusia, hyposmia, poor dark adaptation, growth retardation, hypogonadism, stomatitis, a white coating on the tongue and buccal mucosa, and marked halitosis.[1,4]

It has also been reported that white spots on the fingernails reflect zinc status.[5] This may have some significance, as poor wound healing due to a zinc deficiency secondary to trauma to the nail bed may be responsible for the lesions in some subjects. Clinical judgment is

Table 32.1 Clinical indications for zinc assessment

- Acne
- Alcohol abuse
- Alopecia
- Amenorrhea
- Amnesia
- Anorexia
- Apathy
- Brittle nails
- Chronic fatigue
- Chronic and/or severe infections
- Connective tissue disease
- Dandruff and alopecia
- Delayed sexual maturation
- Delayed wound healing
- Depression
- Dermatological disorders (virtually all)
- Diuretic usage
- Eczema
- Growth retardation
- Hypercholesterolemia
- Hypogeusia, hyposmia
- Hypogonadism
- Impaired glucose tolerance
- Impotence, infertility
- Inflammatory bowel disease
- Irritability
- Malabsorption syndromes
- Memory impairment
- Night blindness
- Psychiatric illness
- Reduced appetite, anorexia
- Rheumatoid arthritis
- Sleep and behavioral disturbances
- White spots on nails
- Wound healing impairment

required to ascertain the significance of these lesions in a particular patient, i.e. do the lesions correspond to the level of trauma to the nail beds?

Two in-office tests that may indicate functional zinc deficiency are the zinc taste test (described below) and the dark adaptation response (described in Ch. 26).

Zinc taste test

Since loss of taste acuity is a well-documented sign of zinc deficiency, measurement of taste acuity is a useful functional test of zinc status. The taste solution is made by dissolving 1 g zinc sulfate heptahydrate ($ZnSO_4 \cdot 7H_2O$) in 1 L of distilled water. Responses to tasting 5 ml of this solution normally fall into one of the following four categories:

1. No specific taste or other sensation is noticed after the solution has been kept in the mouth for 10 seconds.
2. No immediate taste is noticed, but after a few seconds a slight taste variously described as "dry", "mineral", "furry", or "sweet" develops.
3. A definite, though not strongly unpleasant, taste is noted almost immediately and tends to intensify with time.
4. A strong and unpleasant taste is noted almost immediately.

Table 32.2 Conditions predisposing to zinc deficiency, decreased intake, and/or decreased utilization

Decreased intake
- Anorexia nervosa
- Fad diets
- Protein deficiency
- Vegetarianism
- Alcoholic cirrhosis
- Old age
- Acute infections/inflammation
- Low socioeconomic status
- Alcoholism

Increased body losses
- Starvation
- Burns
- Post-trauma

Decreased absorption
- Diabetes mellitus
- High phytate diet
- Alcoholism
- High dietary iron:zinc ratio
- Chelating agents
- Acrodermatitis enteropathica
- Dialysis
- Achlorhydria/hypochlorhydria
- Hepatic disease
- Celiac disease
- Inflammatory bowel disease
- Diarrhea
- Intestinal resection
- Chronic blood loss
- Short bowel syndrome
- Pancreatic insufficiency

Increased requirement
- Old age
- Pregnancy and lactation
- Oral contraceptive use
- Growth spurts and puberty

A reaction falling into categories 1 or 2 suggests a zinc deficiency and a favorable response to zinc supplementation.[6]

Laboratory determination of zinc status

A large number of laboratory analyses for determining zinc status have been developed, as listed in Table 32.3. Unfortunately, none has been determined to be the definitive methodology. A few of the procedures are discussed in detail below.

Plasma and serum zinc

Although these are perhaps the most widely used methods of zinc assessment, they are a poor measure of total body zinc status.[1,7] As zinc is bound primarily to albumin, changes in albumin concentrations will have a significant impact on zinc levels.[7] Total circulating zinc concentration reflects both serum albumin concentrations and the affinity of albumin for zinc, rather than zinc status.[7] Zinc's main functions are intracellular; therefore, like other minerals, serum and plasma levels do not reflect total body stores.

Table 32.3 Laboratory methods used in assessing zinc status

- Dark adaptation test
- Erythrocyte carbonic anhydrase
- Fingernail zinc content
- Hair zinc content
- Lymphoblast transformation
- Macrophage chemotaxis
- Neutrophil chemotaxis
- Plasma zinc concentration
- Radioisotope zinc turnover
- RBC zinc concentration
- Salivary zinc concentration
- Serum alkaline phosphatase
- Serum retinol binding protein concentration
- Serum ribonuclease activity
- Serum zinc concentration
- Sperm count
- Sweat zinc concentration and pool size
- WBC zinc concentration
- Zinc balance
- Zinc repletion test
- Zinc tolerance test

Plasma copper:zinc ratios have been used by some investigators as a clinical assessment aid in a variety of conditions.[1] This appears to be a more promising diagnostic aid, as it reflects the level of metallothionein uptake of zinc.[8] This protein is responsible for maintaining copper and zinc homeostasis. In inflammation or infection, macrophages release leukocyte endogenous mediator (LEM), which stimulates hepatic zinc uptake by metallothionein and ceruloplasmin.[9] Therefore, a high copper:zinc ratio – greater than 2 – is likely to be a result of an inflammatory process, either acute or chronic. Normal serum and plasma levels for zinc are 80–120 µg/dl. This ratio is commonly found in patients with psychiatric problems, which may suggest that a chronic inflammatory condition is taking place, rather than an overload of dietary copper or decreased intake of zinc.

Hair zinc

Hair mineral analysis has been a popular screening method for mineral deficiencies.[10] It has some procedural problems, and reference ranges are still being developed for all ages and hair colors (for further discussion, see Ch. 17). Low hair zinc content has been shown to be a good indicator of mild to moderate zinc deficiency.[1,7,10,11] However, in severe zinc deficiency, hair levels will be elevated as a result of concentration due to impaired hair growth.[7,10] A normal hair zinc level does not necessarily assure adequate tissue stores.[10] In addition, standard washing procedures are unable to remove exogenous zinc without removing endogenous zinc, making analysis unreliable where external contamination may have occurred. In summary, while low hair zinc levels may be indicative of low zinc status, further testing is required to confirm a clinical diagnosis.[7,10]

Serum alkaline phosphatase

The enzyme alkaline phosphatase (AP) is a zinc-dependent enzyme that is sensitive to dietary levels.[1] Although neutrophil AP is more reflective of zinc status, serum levels of AP are frequently assayed on routine chemistry screens.[1,12] Individuals with zinc deficiency will have low circulating levels of AP.[1,7,12] In one study, the ratio of maximal post-treatment to pretreatment serum activity (AP ratio) correlated inversely with pre-treatment serum zinc level in subjects who received a zinc-restricted diet initially, and who were later supplemented with zinc.[12] It was suggested that a serial determination of serum AP and calculation of the AP ratio during a trial of zinc therapy may provide biochemical confirmation of the adequacy of zinc replacement and may be useful in detection of mild zinc deficiency.[12] It should be kept in mind that AP levels will be increased in liver and bone disease and by many drugs, and decreased in hypothyroidism, pernicious anemia, and vitamin D excess.[13]

Zinc tolerance test (ZTT)

An oral loading dose of 220 mg zinc sulfate is used to determine zinc absorption. The normal patient usually shows a two- to threefold increase in plasma zinc concentrations 2 hours after supplementation.[7,14] This does not reflect zinc status as much as it determines the integrity of the small intestine mucosa and pancreatic sufficiency.[7,14,15] The zinc tolerance test has been used to assess intestinal absorption of zinc in patients treated for obesity by jejunal bypass, hepatic cirrhosis, Crohn's disease, pancreatic insufficiency, celiac disease, and dermatitis herpetiformis.[14] The procedure for the test is as follows:

1. A gelatin capsule containing 110 mg zinc sulfate heptahydrate (25 mg elemental zinc) is given to the subject following an overnight fast.
2. Samples are taken by venipuncture into trace metal-free heparinized tubes before administration of the zinc and at half-hour intervals for 3 hours.
3. The plasma is separated and stored until analysis.
4. Values are plotted as an increase above baseline, i.e. the initial reading is 0. The maximum reading is usually at 2 hours.

Normal readings for the test at various times are as follows:

- 0.5 hour – 40 ug/dl
- 1.0 hour – 65 ug/dl
- 1.5 hours – 80 ug/dl
- 2.0 hours – 90 ug/dl
- 2.5 hours – 70 ug/dl
- 3.0 hours – 65 ug/dl.

Patients with pancreatic insufficiency display an abnormal ZTT when zinc sulfate is used, but when zinc picolenate is used zinc absorption normalizes.[15] Picolinic acid is a metabolite of tryptophan and is believed to be the zinc-binding ligand secreted by the pancreas that facilitates transportation of zinc into the intestinal mucosa. If there is an abnormal ZTT using zinc sulfate, the test should be repeated using zinc picolenate to determine if pancreatic insufficiency contributes to the impaired ZTT.[15]

White and red cell zinc

The use of leukocytes, in particular the neutrophil, for assessing mineral status is gaining increasing support in the literature. The leukocyte zinc level appears to be the most reliable and reflective way of determining zinc status.[1,7] This test, however, is currently not widely available. Lymphocyte zinc also appears to be a more reliable assessment methodology than plasma, urine, or hair.[16]

Red cell zinc, while sometimes low in zinc deficiency, is unreliable, as RBC zinc levels are greatly altered by factors which affect zinc partitioning across cell membranes.[7] A more promising, newly defined erythrocyte ^{65}Zn uptake test will soon be clinically available. This methodology shows a much lower variance and is able to detect zinc deficiency more accurately in children suffering from such disorders as acrodermatitis enteropathica, diarrhea, chronic infections and growth retardation.[17] Reference standards for various population groups are now being established.

Another promising assessment is the alkaline phosphatase activity in erythrocyte membrane. In a nicely designed, controlled zinc depletion study, 15 normal men were fed a low-Zn diet with high phytates for 7 weeks, followed by a 2 week repletion period with 30 mg/day of supplemental zinc. While zinc concentrations in neutrophils, platelets, erythrocytes and erythrocyte membranes, and activity of alkaline phosphatase did not respond to the changes in zinc status, erythrocyte alkaline phosphatase showed significant and consistent changes.[18]

Sweat zinc

Sweat zinc appears to be a useful and sensitive index of zinc status. This simple, non-invasive test is more reliable than both hair and serum zinc, and may become clinically available.[7,19]

SUMMARY

Several methods of assessing zinc status have been presented. Each has some strong points and also some limitations. At this time the authors recommend the plasma copper:zinc ratio and neutrophil zinc test as the most accurate of those available. Serum zinc concentration is not considered useful, and hair zinc is useful only if the levels are low.

REFERENCES

1. Prasad A. Clinical, biochemical and nutritional spectrum of zinc deficiency in human subjects. Ann update. Nutr Rev 1983; 41: 197–208
2. Sandstead H. Zinc nutrition in the United States. Am J Clin Nutr 1973; 26: 1251–1260
3. Nordstrom J. Trace mineral nutrition in the elderly. Am J Clin Nutr 1982; 36: 788–795
4. Loeffel E, Koya D. Cutaneous manifestations of gastrointestinal disease. Cutis 1978; 21: 852–861
5. Pfeiffer C. Mental and elemental nutrients. New Canaan, Conn.: Keats Pub. 1975
6. Bryce-Smith D, Simpson R. Anorexia, depression and zinc deficiency. Lancet 1984; 2: 1163
7. Davies S. Assessment of zinc status. Int Clin Nutr Rev 1984; 4: 122–129
8. Webb M and Cain K. Functions of metallothionein. Biochem Pharmacol 1982; 31: 137–142
9. Powanda M, Beisel W. Hypothesis. leukocyte endogenous mediator/endogenous pyrogen/lymphocyte-activating factor modulates the development of nonspecific and specific immunity and affects nutritional status. Am J Clin Nutr 1982; 35: 762–768
10. Passwater R, Cranton E. Trace elements, hair analysis and nutrition. New Canaan, Conn.: Keats. 1983
11. Hambridge K. Hair analyses. worthless for vitamins, limited for minerals. Am J Clin Nutr 1982; 36: 943–949
12. Kasarskis E, Scuna A. Serum alkaline phosphatase after treatment of zinc deficiency in humans. Am J Clin Nutr 1980; 33: 2609–2612
13. Fishbach F. A manual of laboratory diagnostic tests. Philadelphia, PA: JB Lippincott. 1980
14. Crofton R, Glover S, Ewen S et al. Zinc absorption in celiac disease and dermatitis herpetiformis. A test of small intestinal function. Am J Clin Nutr 1983; 38: 706–712
15. Boosalis M, Evans G, McClain C. Impaired handling of orally administered zinc in pancreatic insufficiency. Am J Clin Nutr 1983; 37: 268–271
16. Terwolbeck K, Purmann J, Kuhn S et al. Zinc in lymphocytes--the assessment of zinc status in patients with Crohn's disease. J Trce Elem Electrol Health Dis 1992; 6: 117–121
17. Van Wouwe JP. Clinical and laboratory assessment of zinc deficiency in Dutch children. A review. Biol Trace Elem Res 1995; 49: 211–225
18. Ruz M, Cavan KR, Bettger WJ, Ginson RS. Erythrocytes, erythrocyte membranes, neutrophils and platelets as biopsy materials for the assessment of zinc status in humans. Br J Nutr 1992; 68: 515–527
19. Howard JMH. Serum, sweat and hair levels – a correlational study. J Nutr Med 1990; 1: 119–126

SECTION 3

Therapeutic modalities

SECTION CONTENTS

This section presents an historic, scientific, and functional review of the schools of thought and modalities of natural medicine. We have compiled the work of experts in their fields into what we hope the reader will find a concise, yet useful, description of these practices and modalities. Due to the clinically oriented and alternative nature of these disciplines, the scientific evaluation of their theories and efficacy has been limited. However, published research in natural medicine has increased dramatically since *A Textbook of Natural Medicine* was first published in 1985.

Although this textbook is strongly oriented to the scientific method and the use of the peer-review literature for documentation of the efficacy of a therapy, these modalities' widespread clinical use and long history of patient satisfaction demand they be given a place here even though the mechanism of action of several have yet to be elicited.

CHAPTER CONTENTS

33

Acupuncture

M. Harrison Nolting, ND LAc

INTRODUCTION

Around 210 AD, Zhang Ji, a highly revered Chinese doctor referred to as the "sage of medicine" in China's long history,[1] might have been found teaching students in the grottos of legendary Qing Chang Mountain outside of Chengdu, Sichuan Province, China. The philosophy was largely Taoist and Naturalist as well as quite practical, with roots probably linked to India. Out of these beginnings a distinctively Chinese system would arise that is referred to as traditional Chinese medicine and Oriental medicine. The science of classical China is an ancient science filled with myth, superstition, and unlimited wisdom – a wisdom that provided many medical "discoveries" such as the circulation of blood, circadian rhythms, thyroid hormone use, deficiency diseases, and a multitude of others long before their "rediscovery" in the West.[2] The basic question – How does acupuncture work? – awaits the scrutiny of the West. For thousands of Western-trained acupuncturists, acupuncture is a comprehensive system of medicine based in classical Chinese philosophy. Yin, Yang, Qi, Wu Hsing, Zang Fu – this is the language of traditional Chinese Medicine. While acupuncture is defined in many arenas as a comprehensive system of medicine, in others it is a modality, a treatment used alongside other practices. The needle defines acupuncture visually. For many acupuncturists, their practice is far more than needles, including moxibustion, cupping, shu sha (also called gua sha), herbs, tuina, and qigong. In order to properly respect and understand the field of acupuncture, a broad look is necessary.

HISTORY

The principles and theory underlying the techniques of acupuncture, so-called acuology, date to the ancient times of the great Yellow Emperor, Huangdi (~2698–2598 BC).[3,4] Huangdi has held a place of great legend and esteem in Chinese history. The question of whether this ruler actually authored the great medical work entitled *Huangdi Nei Jing* (*The Yellow Emperor's Inner Cannon*) will perhaps always remain a mystery.[5] Nevertheless it is attributed to the reign of Huangdi and is said to highlight questions and answers between the emperor and his ministers, chief among them a physician named Qi Bo. Huangdi discoursed on medicine, health, lifestyle, nutrition, and religious tenets of the times. He is ascribed such a high place in Chinese history that many Chinese consider themselves descendants. Huangdi is viewed as the "symbol of vital spirit of Chinese civilization".[6] Probably the most important text in the history of Chinese medicine, often "overshadowed" by the "reputation and authority of the original classic", the *Huangdi Nei Jing*, was the *Nan Jing* (*The Classic of Difficult Issues*), thought to have been compiled around the first or second century AD. According to Unschuld,[7] the *Nan Jing* was "a significant and innovative work that was the apex and conclusion of the developmental phase of the conceptual system unknown as the medicine of systematic correspondence". He goes on to describe the importance of the *Nan Jing* saying "the Nan-ching (jing in pinyin romanization) is comprehensive … discusses the origins and the nature of illness; outlines a system of therapeutic needling; and develops – in great detail – an innovative approach to diagnosis". The *Nei Jing* predates the historically available writings of ancient China, it delves strongly into "demonological medicine and religious healing", while the *Nan Jing* is homogeneous and highly systemized, basically intact and well focused.[7]

In terms of acupuncture specifically, Unshuld[8] cites no reliable references prior to 90 BC appearing in Chinese literature. Ancient works as a whole were written on bamboo strips and silk. These went through countless hands and copies, creating a body of written work that contained numerous errors and omissions. It was not until 26 BC that the Chinese government organized medical officials to collate and revise the royal collection of medical works preserved at the Mifu Natnal Royal Library.[9] The earliest recorded physician reputed to be versed in pulse-taking and acupuncture was Bian Que (~500 BC). Several medical works ascribed to him have all been lost.[4] Su Ma Qian, historian of the Han dynasty (206 BC–220 AD), writing in the Historical Note about 100 BC, wrote a chapter on the biography of Bian Que. This was the first reliable reference documenting acupuncture and moxibustion in Chinese.[10] He told many stories of Que's ability to treat with acupuncture.[11] Zhang Ji (AD 150–219) referred to as the sage of Chinese medicine authored the classic work *Shanghanlun*.[12] Statues of the legendary Zhong Ji are common on many of the TCM college campuses in mainland China today. Another of the famous ancient masters of Chinese medicine was Hua Tuo (?–208 AD), a surgeon and practitioner of an eclectic range of therapies including acupuncture and hydrotherapy, and originator of the therapeutice exercises called the "five animals".[4]

Huangfu Mi (214–282 AD), a famous acupuncturist, compiled *Zhen Jiu Jia Yi Jing* (*A Classic of Acupuncture and Moxibustion*), first monograph on acupuncture in history, around 282 AD. These 12 volumes covered all aspects of acupuncture practice and theory and are considered a monumental work.[13]

The first usage of the English term, acupuncture, meaning needle puncture, is attributed to a Dutch physician, Rhyne, who visited Japan sometime in early 17th century.[14] A Dr Berlioz in Paris, at the Paris Medical School, was attributed the first recorded use of acupuncture in the West. John Churchill, in 1821, was the first British acupuncturist publishing works highlighting treatment of tympany and rheumatism. Acupuncture is also mentioned in the *Lancet*'s first edition in 1823. Dr Elliotson published results of 42 cases of acupuncture treatment of rheumatism, concluding that acupuncture was effective as a treatment.[14]

In 1849, the Gold Rush in California brought about a large immigration of Chinese into the western America. Heading for "Gold Mountain", they brought all elements of their culture including their traditional medicine with its acupuncture and Chinese herbs. Writing in his book, *Chinese Medicine on the Golden Mountain*, Paul Buell states:[15]

> … [there] was an acute shortage of any form of medical care in Western America where most Chinese settled. … Well practiced Chinese medicine was often superior to contemporary Western practice. … Western medicine did not gain any real advantage over well practiced Chinese medicine until the coming of any 'wonder drugs' in the 1930s, and in some respects, as in many chronic ailments, (traditional) Chinese medicine is still superior.

In 1892, William Osler wrote, in his *Principles and Practice of Medicine*, about the use of acupuncture in the treatment of sciatica.[16]

FUNDAMENTALS OF ACUPUNCTURE

Acupuncture is a technique involving the insertion of fine needles into the skin at select points or points of tenderness. As discussed earlier, the theory, or acuology that surrounds the practice dates back as much as 4,000–5,000 years. For many contemporary practitioners, their practices are defined by the theory of the fundamental principles: five elements, Yin, Yang, Qi, and Zang Fu. For still others these ancient theories remain just that – ancient and removed from modern science – and they practice acupuncture based on recent theories of mechanism and anecdotal evidence.[17]

Yin and Yang, the base upon which all diagnosis and treatment in TCM arises

In perfect balance, in optimal health, Yin and Yang are

harmonious, the ebb and flow of the tides, day and night. The theory when translated can be set in quite poetic terms. A deficiency of liver and kidney Yin, for example, might result in clinical symptoms such as dizziness, vertigo, insomnia, dry throat, and lumbago, whereas a deficiency of spleen and kidney Yang may manifest clinically as cold limbs, lumbago, diarrhea, and scanty urine. Excess is usually seen as a relative state due to the deficiency of the other, as in deficient Yin resulting in an apparent excess of Yang.

Qi

Qi is the energy and potential energy that courses throughout the organism and defines what we call life. The lack of proper Qi flow in the system results in numerous maladies. Qi stagnation is often manifested as pain. Rebellious Qi manifests as belching, burping, and vomiting, a reversal of the normal downward movement of Qi digestively. There is also the potential energy, the Qi that occupies the rock, the board, this desk, that potential energy that lies in the way of being expressed. And then there is the Qi that waves through space connecting us to the web of the universe – a concept that begins to sound like theories in quantum physics.

Zang Fu

The Zang Fu are the Chinese organs, five solid Yin, and six hollow Yang. In the West, we use the English names for the organs – liver, heart, spleen, kidneys, and lungs – but depending solely on the Western name without a thorough understanding of the traditional Chinese meaning will lead to much confusion clinically. A complete and clinically sound synthesis of the Western biomedical understanding with the traditional Chinese understanding has not occurred to date. For example, the liver as we know it in the West is defined according to its anatomical structure and function, i.e. it is a large glandular organ that secretes bile and metabolizes blood-borne compounds. The Chinese gan stores blood and Qi and is responsible for the smooth transmission of Qi and blood throughout the body. Moreover, it has a chief role in emotions; an unbalanced gan (liver) results in anger, high blood pressure, and a general state of agitation. The liver in the Chinese sense is much more a functional system with many body-wide interactions. The hollow organs are the gall bladder, large and small intestines, triple burner, urinary bladder, and stomach. The triple burner is a good example of how different the Western and Chinese views are, since this has no meaning in the West. In the Zang Fu system, the triple burner corresponds to the thoracic and abdominal regions including all of the organs within. It has a specific function that distinguishes it as a fu organ, namely to transport water.

The five elements

The five elements (also called the five phases or in Chinese wu xing) are fire, metal, wood, earth, and water. The correspondences between these elements have become a method of diagnosing and treating patients. In the West, a school of thought following the teachings of Dr Worsley in England has evolved which has grown into a worldwide system of schools and practitioners associated with the so-called "law of five elements". There is a stark contrast between this system of acupuncture practice and the TCM systems.

Points and meridians

The other key aspect of the fundamentals of acupuncture is, of course, the theory of the channels. There are the basic 365 mapped acupuncture points along the 12 major and eight extra channels as well as over 1,000 extra points and special use points, including the microsystems such as the hand, ear, and scalp, all with very specialized functions. The so-called ashi points, or pain points, can literally be located anywhere on the body where there is a pain locus. Qi and blood flow throughout the channels and this is where the proper manipulation of the needle is critical in properly moving this flow.

RESEARCH

Western medical practice has grown within a system of great scrutiny and self-analysis. A massive research culture spins off studies by the thousands. The double-blinded, placebo-controlled trial has become the hallmark of the "appropriately conducted research trial". Acupuncture evolved in a completely different culture, that of China, where, ironically, as we were "discovering" the Chinese traditional system of acupuncture, not so many years previously the Chinese began a wholesale discovery of traditional Western medicine. Acupuncture, and indeed all that is traditional Chinese medicine, has been extensively researched in China.

Large research academies, the largest being the China Academy of Traditional Chinese Medicine in Beijing, and various universities and schools of TCM, have created a huge research culture in China. While there is considerable emphasis on herbal research, there is still quite a lot of research examining the other areas of TCM. But what does this Chinese research culture mean for Western medicine? This is a big question that is being sorted out in a number of ways today. The issues at hand are:

- poor translations
- a lack of studies utilizing "approved" Western research standards

- terminology problems
- major design problems
- cultural assumptions coloring the studies
- Western research arrogance.

To date, very few cross-cultural studies have been undertaken and we are really just making headway into reproducing studies with a Western perspective.

Acupuncture research is now occurring in many countries outside of China. Most notable since 1991 are the efforts by the Office of Alternative Medicine (OAM) at the National Institutes of Health (NIH) to generate research. Calls for research are increasing and a growing number of institutions are receiving grants. A positive sign of progress in this arena was the 1997 Consensus Conference on Acupuncture at the NIH.

China is the country where, since 1950, much of the research has been performed, from basic research to clinical trials, animal studies, and others, and this continues to be the case. In America, clinical research, outcome studies, are increasing but still are relatively few. Basic research is all but non-existent. An important step forward in documentation of the body of clinical outcomes-based research that exists in English can be found in a book titled *Acupuncture Efficacy*.[18]

The basic question posed in the West remains unanswered from a Western perspective: "How does acupuncture work?"

REFERENCES

1. Hoizey D, Hoizey M. A history of Chinese medicine. Vancouver: UBC Press. 1993: p 42
2. Unschuld P. Medicine and health. Berkeley: University of California Press. p 123–137
3. I-Yen Yang. Personal communication. 1997
4. Beijing Medical College. Dictionary of traditional Chinese medicine. Hong Kong: The Commercial Press. 1984: p 342
5. Veith I. The Yellow Emperor's classic of internal medicine. University of California Press. 1949
6. Maoshing Ni. The Yellow Emperor's classic of medicine. Boston, MA: Shambala. 1995
7. Unschuld PU. The classic of difficult issues. Berkeley, CA: University of California Press. 1986: p 3–4
8. Unschuld PU. Medicine in China, a history of ideas. Berkeley, CA: University of California Press. 1985
9. Unschuld P, ed. Approaches to traditional Chinese medical literature. Proceedings of an International Symposium on Translation Methodologies and Terminologies. Dordrecht: Kluwer. 1989
10. Porkert M, Hempen CH. Chinese Academy of TCM, classical acupuncture – the standard textbook. Dinkelscherben; Phainon Edititrus, and Media GmbH. 1995
11. Fu Wei Kang. The story of Chinese acupuncture and moxibustion. Beijing: Foreign Languages Press. 1975
12. Hoizey D, Hoizey M. A history of Chinese medicine. Vancouver, BC: Edinburgh University Press, UBC Press. 1993: p 42–43
13. Zhang Rui-fu, Wu Xiu-fen, Nissi Wang, Illustrated dictionary of Chinese acupuncture. Hong Kong: Sheep's Publication. 1985: p 403
14. Lewith GT. The history of acupuncture in China, acupuncture its place in Western medical science. Health World on-line. 1997
15. Buell P. Chinese medicine on the Golden Mountain, an interpretive guide. Idaho State Historical Society, ID. 1984
16. Osler W. Principles and practice of medicine. Common historic reference. 1892
17. Ross J, Zang Fu. The organ systems of traditional Chinese medicine. Edinburgh: Churchill Livingstone. 1985
18. Hammerschlag B. Acupuncture efficacy. Tarrytown, NY: National Academy of Acupuncture and Oriental Medicine. 1996

CHAPTER CONTENTS

34

Ayurveda: the science of life and mother of the healing arts

Virender Sodhi, MD(Ayurveda) ND

INTRODUCTION

Ayurveda is one of the most ancient systems of medicine known today. The origins of this science of life (*Ayu* – life, and *Veda* – knowledge), though difficult to pinpoint, have been placed by scholars of ancient Indian Ayurvedic literature at somewhere around 6000 BC.[1]

Ayurveda is a holistic science of balance and health. Disease is seen as an imbalance, and its treatment involves diverse strategies to restore optimal function and balance. Using dietary alterations, yoga, exercise, complex, integrated herbal formulas, and elaborate surgical techniques, the Ayurvedic physician treats the whole person, removing disease completely by ending the imbalance that created it.

HISTORY

In ancient India, it was the custom for a teacher's instruction to be recorded by his students, who would then repeat the information orally to their own disciples. Thus, according to the different interpretations given by the various disciples of Ayurveda, a number of treatises came to be written. Although specific instructions differed, the basic principles remained similar.

Ayurvedic teachings were orally transmitted for thousands of years, and then written down in melodious Sanskrit poetry. The contents of a number of Sanskrit verses, or *shlokas*, though written many centuries ago, still sound a note of familiarity in today's scientific environment. Ayurveda, in its first recorded form (in *vedas*, the world's oldest literature), is specifically called *Atharveda*.

The development of Ayurvedic medicine

Hindu legend holds that, seeing the suffering of human beings, Lord Brahma, the god of creation, elaborated ways to ease that suffering to Daksha, who, in turn, taught them to the Ashwin twins. Figure 34.1 presents the chronology of Ayurveda's development.

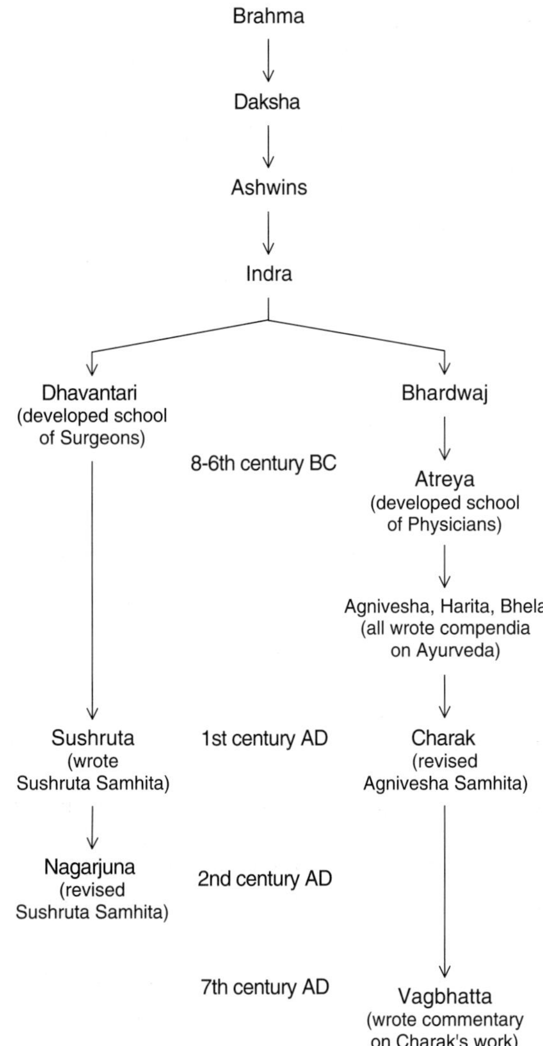

Figure 34.1 The chronology of Ayurveda.

Dhanvantari and Bhardwaj separately developed the surgical and medical aspects of Ayurveda around the 9th century BC. Their students recorded these principles in great detail in compendia which are called *Samhitas*.

The *Sushruta Samhita*, one of the most widely accepted Ayurvedic texts, emphasizes the surgical aspects of therapy. Its author, Sushruta, is considered the father of surgery (particularly of plastic and reconstructive surgery). The medical teachings of Charak were a synthesis of earlier work. His material has become a classic text of the non-surgical medical wisdom of Ayurveda. Successive generations have modified his work, the *Samhita*.

THE MAJOR SCHOOLS AND SPECIALTIES

School of physicians (Atreya sampradaya)

Charak wrote a complete text on Ayurvedic medicine in which he revised the work of Agnivesh. Charak's text described *Tridosh* physiology (*Vat*, *Pit*, and *Kaph*), seven *Dhatus* (tissues), and three *Malas* (excretions). Charak also presented in his text the pathophysiology and treatment of diseases, human constitution (*Pakriti*), classifications and preparations of drugs, diet, "right conduct", medical ethics, and many other aspects of medicine.

School of surgeons (Dhanvantri sampradaya)

Sushruta wrote the first comprehensive works on surgery. These were later revised by Nagarjuna in the 2nd century AD. Major subjects in his texts were:

- injections
- pre-operative care
- postoperative care
- suturing
- asepsis
- sterilization
- operation theaters
- hospitals.

He described 141 types of instruments and listed 40 types of surgeries, and surgical techniques for treating cataracts, hemorrhoids, hernias, and bone problems, for cosmetic and plastic purposes, and for the removal of renal and gallstones.

Branches of Ayurveda

There are eight specialties or branches in Ayurveda. They comprise a system developed to prevent and cure disease, as well as achieving and maintaining excellent health. The branches are listed in Table 34.1.

PHILOSOPHY

Ayurvedic philosophy is based on the *Samkhya* philosophy of creation. It has influenced major strains of philosophy in both the East and the West. The word *Samkhya* is derived from the Sanskrit *Sat* (truth) and *Khya* (to know). The Rishi Kapila (*Rishi* means realized beings or seers of truth) realized the *Samkhya* philosophy of creation. They perceived:

- the close relationship between humans and the universe (that humans are a microcosm, a universe

Table 34.1 Specialties in Ayurveda

Shalya Tantra	General surgery
Shalkya	Ophthalmology and otorhiolaryngology
Kaya Chikitsa	Medicine
Bhutvidya	Psychiatry
Kumar-Bhritya	Pediatrics, obstetrics, gynecology
Agada Tantra	Toxicology and jurisprudence
Rasayana	Geriatrics
Vajikaran	Fertility and sterility

within themselves, while the external environment is the macrocosm)
- that cosmic energy is manifest in all living and non-living things
- the 24 elements of the universe
- that the source of all existence is cosmic consciousness, manifest as male (*Shiva, Purusha*) and female (*Shakti, Prakriti*) energy.

Purusha is formless, colorless, and beyond attribute. It is choiceless, does not take an active part in the manifestation of the universe, and has passive awareness. *Prakriti* has form, color, awareness and choice. *Prakriti* creates all the forms of the universe and has three attributes (*Gunas*): *Satva* (essence), *Rajas* (movement), and *Tamas* (inertia). It is also represented by Brahma (the god of creation), Vishnu (god of protection), and Mahesh (god of destruction), which together comprise a cycle active in this universe.

In Pakriti, the three attributes are in balance. Whenever this balance is disturbed, they interact to bring about the evolution of the universe, yielding the cosmic vibration of *Aum*.

The cosmic intellect (the *Mahad*) manifests itself as ego (*Ahamkar*) which, through the help of Satva, manifests the five senses and five motor organs which together constitute the "organic universe". Ego further manifests into the five basic elements (space, air, fire, water, and earth) which, under the influence of *Tamas*, create the "inorganic universe".

Rajas is the active vital force which moves both the organic and inorganic universes to *Satva* and *Tamas*, respectively. *Satva* and *Tamas* are inactive, potential energies which need the active kinetic protective force of *Rajas*. *Satva* is a creative potential (*Brahma*), *Rajas* is a kinetic protective force (*Vishnu*), and *Tamas* is a potentially destructive force (*Mahesh*). These three – *Brahma, Vishnu*, and *Mahesh* – are constantly operating in the universe.

Five basic elements and the universe (Panchbhuta philosophy)

Ayurvedic knowledge is based on the concept of the five basic elements: ether (space), air, fire, water, and earth. The Rishis perceived that consciousness consists of these five basic elements or principles. At the beginning of the world, consciousness was without form, existing as the subtle vibration of the cosmic "soundless" sound *Aum*.

Within these vibrations appeared the element ether. Ether started to move, creating air. The movement of ether also produced friction and through friction, generated heat, then fire. From the heat of the fire, ethereal elements dissolved and liquified into water. Water then solidified to form molecules of earth. Thus was all matter born from the five elements. These five elements exist in subatomic forms.

Humans are a microcosm of nature and, as such, themselves comprise the five basic elements:

- Ether is represented in the hollow spaces of the mouth, nose, gastrointestinal tract, abdomen, thorax, respiratory apparatus, capillaries, lymphatics, tissues, and cells.
- Air exists as movement – as pulsation, expansion, or contraction of the various organs. Bodily movement is controlled by the central nervous system, itself governed by air.
- Fire is the source of heat and light somatically present as metabolism, gray matter, vision, temperature, digestion, and intelligence.
- Water exists as secretions of the salivary and digestive glands and the mucous membranes, and within plasma and cytoplasm.
- Earth is the solid structures, i.e. the bones, cartilage, nails, muscles, tendons, skin, and hair.

Five elements and the senses

The five elements also connect with the five senses – ether-hearing, air-touch, fire-vision, water-taste, and earth-smell – and they are present in certain physiological functions. Expressing the functions of the sensory organs are five actions (see Table 34.2). In this manner, the elements are directly related to humans' abilities both to perceive the external environment in which they live and to respond to it:

- Ether is the medium through which sound travels. The ear is the organ of hearing, expressing its action through the organ of speech, which creates meaningful sound.
- Air is related to skin and the sense of touch. Its organ of action is the hand, which is especially sensitive, and is the organ of the actions of holding, giving, and receiving.
- Fire produces light, heat, and color, and is thus related to vision and direction. Its organ is the eye.
- Water relates to the organ of taste. The tongue is also related to the action of the genitals, the penis, and clitoris. In Ayurveda, the penis and clitoris are called the lower tongues. By controlling the upper tongue, one naturally controls the lower tongue.
- The earth element relates to the sense of smell, and the nose is its organ.

Table 34.2 The five elements and the senses

Element	Sense	Organ	Action	Vehicle of action
Ether	Hearing	Ear	Speech	Mouth
Air	Touch	Skin	Holding, giving, receiving	Hand
Fire	Vision	Eye	Walking	Feet
Water	Taste	Tongue	Procreation	Genitals
Earth	Smell	Nose	Excretion	Anus

PHYSIOLOGY

The five elements manifest within the body as the *Tridosha* (*Dosha* means protective or, when out of balance, disease-producing). The *Tridosha* are the three humors, or basic principles, known as *Vat, Pit,* and *Kaph.*

From the bodily combination of ether and air comes the bodily air principle, *Vat Dosha.* Likewise, fire and water combine as *Pit Dosha,* or fire principle; and earth and water produce the *Kaph Dosha,* or water principle.

These three control all biological, psychological, and physiopathological functions of the body, mind, and consciousness. They produce natural urges and individual tastes in food, flavor, and temperature. They govern the maintenance and destruction of bodily tissue and the elimination of waste products. They also are responsible for psychological phenomena, including the emotions of fear, anger, and greed, as well as the highest order of emotions: understanding, compassion, and love.

Properties of *Dosha*

Vat, Pit and *Kaph* control all human biological, psychological and physiopathological functions, and have subtle properties, as shown in Table 34.3.

The *Doshas* increase by similar properties and are diminished by opposite properties. For example, *Vat* is dry, light and cold, so any food, medicine, lifestyle, or behavior which increases these qualities will increase *Vat* within the body. Conversely, oily, heavy, or hot factors will decrease *Vat.*

Functions of *Tridosha*

Each of the three humors has a specific action. *Vat* is the principle of movement, and may be called the bodily air principle, as opposed to the environmental air principle. *Vat* is a subtle energy governing all biological movement – breathing, blinking, muscle and joint movement, heartbeat, and all nerve and membrane contractions and expansions. In addition, it controls the psychological functions governing the emotions of fear and anxiety. *Vat* also controls pain, tremors, and spasms. Broadly speaking, the whole nervous system can be labeled as *Vat* function. The large intestine, pelvic cavity, bones, skin, ears, and thighs are the places of *Vat.* Any excess of *Vat* will accumulate in these areas.

Table 34.3 Properties of *Dosha*

Vat	*Pit*	*Kaph*
Dry	Oily	Oily
Light	Light	Heavy
Cold	Hot	Cold
Rough	Liquid	Slimy
Subtle	Penetrating	Soft
Mobile	Mobile	Static
Clear		Dense
Dispersing		Slow
	Smells sour	

Pit, or bodily fire, governs digestion, absorption, assimilation, nutrition, temperature, skin color, luster of the eye, intelligence, and understanding. It arouses anger, hate, and jealousy. The small intestine, stomach, blood, sweat glands, fat, eyes, and skin are the places of *Pit;* in fact all metabolism is governed by *Pit.*

Kaph, biological water, is the cement of the body, providing for physical structure. It is responsible for body resistance and biological strength. It lubricates the joints, provides moisture to skin, and promotes wound healing, strength, vigor, and stability. It supports memory, gives energy to the heart and lungs, and maintains immunity. *Kaph* is present within the throat, chest, head, sinuses, nose, mouth, stomach, joints, the cytoplasm, plasma, and liquid secretions. Psychologically, *Kaph* governs attachment, greed, long-standing envy, calmness, forgiveness, and love.

A balance of the *Dosha* is necessary for optimal health. Together, they govern all metabolic activities: anabolism (*Kaph*), catabolism (*Vat*), and metabolism (*Pit*). An excess of *Vat* results in an excess of catabolism, creating emaciation. When anabolism outstrips catabolism, there is an increase of growth and repair in the organs and tissues. Excessive *Pit* disturbs metabolism.

In childhood, *Kaph* elements, associated with growth, predominate. In adulthood, *Pit* is more apparent. As the body deteriorates in old age, *Vat* is most prominent.

Individual psychosomatic constitutions – *Prakriti*

Prakriti, a Sanskrit word composed of *pra* (before) and *akriti* (creativity), denotes the constitution of each individual as determined at conception. At the time of fertilization permutations of *Vat, Pit,* and *Kaph* determine the constitution of the new individual, with maleness or femaleness dominating other traits. These basic traits will also be shaped by other important factors, such as diet, lifestyle, behavior, emotions, seasons, etc.

As illustrated in Table 34.4, there can be up to seven different constitutions depending upon the permutation and combination of *Vat, Pit,* and *Kaph. Pakriti* is geneti-

Table 34.4 The seven types of constitution

- *Vat*
- *Pit*
- *Kaph*
- *Vat-Pit*
- *Pit-Kaph*
- *Kaph-Vat*
- *Vat-Pit-Kaph*

cally determined; the basic constitution, the combination of the three humors, remains unchanged throughout an individual's lifetime. The combination can, however, respond to environmental changes.

Life is considered a sacred path in Ayurveda, a ceaseless interaction between the internal (*Tridosha*) environment and the external environment, or the sum of cosmic forces. To counteract external change, an individual may create a balance in the internal forces by altering diet, lifestyle, and behavior. The characteristics of the corresponding pychosomatic constitutions are listed in Table 34.5.

Table 34.5 Psychosomatic constitutions (*Prakriti*)

Characteristic	*Vat*	*Pit*	*Kaph*
Body frame	Tall or small, thin, ill-nourished, hard, dry, cold	Medium, many moles, well nourished, pimples patches of pigment, tender appearance	Stout, well-nourished big, oily, greasy, cold, beautiful
Skin	Dry, cracked, tough, broken, brownish, black	Soft, thin, yellow, red, pink	Greasy, soft, yellow, white
Body hair	Scanty, coarse, dry, brown	Moderate, soft, pink	Plentiful, smooth, greasy, black
Hair on head	Brown, scanty, coarse, curved, wavy, wrinkled	Pinkish, yellow, moderate, soft, baldness, premature greyness	Black, plentiful, firm, wavy, curved
Head	Small size	Moderate in size	Big and steady
Forehead	Small	Moderate with many folds	Big, broad
Eyebrows	Small, thin, unsteady	Moderate	Thick, plentiful
Eyelashes	Small, dry, firm	Small, thin	Big, greasy, firm
Eyes	Small, dry, thin, muddy brown, unsteady gaze, not pleasant-looking	Thin, yellow, pink coppery, quickly become inflamed, pleasant-looking	Big, white, pink, pleasant-looking, thick, fixed, greasy
Nose	Small, dry, firm	Medium	Thick, big, greasy
Mustaches	Small, coarse, dry, blackish	Soft, pink, moderate	Heavy, thick, shining, black
Lips	Thin, small, blackish, brownish, dry, unsteady	Moderate, red, pink	Thick, big, smooth, firm, greasy
Teeth and gums	Dry, small, rough	Moderate	Thick, greasy, moist, soft, pink
Tongue	Thin, dry, fissured, unsteady	Moderate, pink, reddish	Thick, big, smooth, moist
Palate	Dry, blue, black	Pink	Moist, white
Lower jaw	Thin, small, dry	Moderate	Thick, big
Shoulders	Thin, small, unsteady, dry	Moderate	Thick, big, firm
Chest	Thin, small, not well-built	Moderate	Thick, big, well-developed
Arm	Thin, small, poorly built	Moderate	Thick, big, well-built
Hands	Thin, dry, small rough, fissured, unsteady	Moderate, pink	Thick, oily, big, hard
Calves	Small, hard	Loose soft	Shaped firmly, hard
Feet	Thin, small, coarse, dry, cracked, fissured, unsteady	Medium, soft, pink	Big, hard, steady
Joints	Thin, small, dry, unsteady, produce sound	Medium, soft, loose	Thick, big, well-built
Nails	Thin, small, dry, rough, black	Medium, soft, pink	Thick, big, greasy, smooth, white, firm
Body weight	Less	Moderate	Heavy
Action of body	Quick unsteady walk, quick actions and movements	Moderate, intelligent actions	Steady walk: slow and dignified
Eliminations	Less, constipated	Copious, watery	Moderate, solid
Strength	Less, tires quickly	Moderate	Strong, hard worker, can withstand strains
Body odor	No smell, less sweating	Heavy sweating, bad smell	Less sweating, pleasant smell
Voice	Feeble, broken, hidden, hoarse, unpleasant	High pitch	Pleasant, deep bass voice, good tone
Speech	Quick, very talkative	Moderate	Slow, definite

Table 34.5 (contd)

Characteristic	*Vat*	*Pit*	*Kaph*
Likes and dislikes	Poor quality things, irregular eating habits, likes roaming, journeys, dance, hunting, quarrels, stories, music, painting, artistic pursuits	Moderate, eats more, drinks more, likes sweet, bitter and astringent tastes, cold food, hates hot, eats very often, likes flowers, scents, music	Poor appetite, thirstless, likes sweet, pungent, hot, bitter, astringent and fat tastes, likes flowers and cosmetics
Mental and temperament	Poor memory, quick forgetting, quick mind; unsteady courage, quick passion and attachment, cowardice, sorrowful, steals, jealous, ungrateful; no control over senses, Atheist, impoverished, less resourceful, few friends	Loves opposite sex, intelligent, scholar, genius, quick to anger and cool off, brave, adventurous, active, alert, secretive, politician, cruel in punishing disobedience, speaks well of obedient subordinates, invincible in assemblies, moderate wealth, resourceful	Good insight and forethought; slow to grasp, scholar, courageous; firm belief in religion, science, faithful, intelligent, little anger or desire, calm, civilized, grateful, truthful, shy, obedient, wealthy, does not waste money, resourceful, many friends
Sleep	Less sleep, wakeful at night	Moderate	Sleeps a good deal
Dreams	Moving in sky, action	Cold, flowers, sun, fire, lightening, red, frightful dreams	Ponds, lakes, flowers, swans, beautiful sights
Sex	Less sex capacity, less semen/menses, few children	Less sex capacity, few children	Great sex capacity
Life expectancy	Short	Moderate	Long-lived
Reaction to disease	Quick to get diseases, usually nervous disorders	Moderate, usually inflammations	Good resistance, usually cold and phlegm type
Reaction to drugs	Minimum dosages required	Intolerance to drugs	Slow, tolerates at high dose

Mental constitutions

On the mental and astral planes, three *Gunas* (attributes of female energy or *Pakriti*) correspond to the three *humors* that make up the physical constitution. In the Ayurvedic system, the *Gunas* are *Satva*, *Rajas*, and *Tamas*. They provide the basis for the distinctions in human temperament and individual differences in psychological and moral dispositions. These attributes are further subdivided, but that is beyond the scope of this chapter.

Satva

This type of mind expresses essence, understanding, purity, clarity, compassion, and love. People of Satvic psyche (*Satva* temperament) have healthy bodies and very pure behavior and consciousness. They believe in the existence of God and are religious, often very holy, persons.

Rajas

This type of mind operates on the sensual level. Such persons are interested in business, prosperity, power, prestige, and position. They enjoy wealth, are generally extroverted, and are politically minded.

Tamas

This type is distinguished by its ignorance, inertia, heaviness, and dullness. Tamasic people are lazy, selfish, destructive by nature, and show very little respect to others. All their activities are egocentric.

The Satvic person attains self-realization without much effort, while those of Rajasic or Tamasic mind have difficulty. These three subtle mental energies are responsible for behavior patterns which may be altered and improved through practice and spiritual discipline, such as yoga and meditation.

HEALTH AND DISEASE

Health is defined in Ayurveda as soundness of body (*Shrira*), mind (*Manas*), and soul (*Atma*). Each part of this tripod of life should receive equal attention, to ensure that the individual achieves sound health. Ayurvedic medicine stresses that psychic influences strongly affect the body in health as well as disease, a fact which must also be taken into account in modern therapeutics.

Modern science takes pride in its understanding of physiology, but in so doing has emphasized fragmentation, isolation, and disunity. Instead of wholeness and interaction, this modern view accepts only physical objects as causes of disease, whereas these objects are merely the agents of disease, able to cause specific symptoms, but only in a susceptible host. Disease is the result of a disruption of the spontaneous flow of nature's intelligence within our physiology. When we violate nature's law and cannot adequately rid ourselves of the results of this action, then we have disease.

Ayurveda is based on certain fundamental doctrines (see Table 34.6) known as the *Darshnas*. It conceives of the body as being composed of three principal divisions: three *Dosha* (humors), seven *Dhatus* (tissues), and three *Malas* (excretions).

Table 34.6 *Doshas, Dhatus,* and *Malas*

Doshas (humors)
- Vat
- Pit
- Kaph

Dhatus (tissues)
- Ras (secretion)
- Rakata (blood)
- Mamsa (muscles)
- Meda (fat)
- Asthi (bone and cartilage)
- Majja (bone marrow)
- Shaukra (sex hormones and immunity)

Malas (excretions)
- Svet (sweat)
- Poorish (feces)
- Mutra (urine)

The three *Doshas* regulate cell functions. *Pit* gives energy and is responsible for cellular, enzymatic, and metabolic functions; *Kaph* helps in synthesizing blocks of cells; and *Vat* controls the other two. A balance of these *Doshas*, good quality tissues (the seven *Dhatus*), and a certain character of excretions are essential for maintaining health. All are, however, subject to qualitative and quantitative alterations.

As has been explained, an individual is born with a particular *Dosha* predominating in his or her constitution (*Pakriti*). This predominant *Dosha*, quite apart from genetic, age, environment, and dietary factors, may make an individual susceptible to a certain disease. For example, *Pit Pakriti* individuals are more prone to develop a disease syndrome with symptoms similar to a peptic ulcer. This is due to hyperactivity of the *Pit Dosha*, which regulates enzymatic activity. Now we know that hyperpepsinogenemic individuals are more susceptible to duodenal ulcer formation.[2]

Ayurveda teaches that the origin of most diseases is found either in an exogenous or endogenous *Dosha* imbalance, or in an inherent or acquired weakness of the tissues. Therefore, the successful treatment or prevention of disease will consist of normalizing cellular functions through correcting any *Dosha* imbalance or improving inherent tissue vitality. For example, in the treatment of cancer, the use of agents cytotoxic to the cancer cells is important. However, equally important is potentiation of the immune system and stimulation of the body's own healing mechanisms.

MODES OF THERAPY

Once a diagnosis is made, Ayurveda offers various modes of therapy. The treatment is chosen according to patient constitution as well as disease process. Modalities include dietary alterations, botanical medicines, minerals, animal products, exercise, yoga, meditation, counseling, and surgery.

Diet

Ayurveda places great emphasis on diet, for both its direct effect on the individual's physiological state and its influence upon the action of medicines. Proper assimilation of dietary constituents is essential for the maintenance of good health. Improper assimilation results in the formation of intermediary products of digestion which have toxic properties and are therefore treated as foreign by the body. Such toxic products are called *Ama* (this leads to the concepts of immune and autoimmune disorders).

Arthritic diseases, such as rheumatoid arthritis, are considered to originate due to an accumulation of *Ama*. Could these toxic intermediates – macromolecules absorbed transmucosally from the intestine (in nutritionally insignificant amounts) – provoke strong immune reactions? It is known that the human gut has a complex system to control the continuous onslaught of antigenic substances derived from food, microorganisms, and toxins.[3] It has been suggested that absorption of such compounds could underlie the pathogenesis of disease in the gut as well as in distant sites, such as the liver and spleen.[4]

Ayurveda stresses prevention of the formation and accumulation of *Ama* through appropriate diet and the use of therapies to improve digestion. It also considers various dietary factors which trigger or eliminate certain diseases.[5] That is why Ayurveda places emphasis on diet according to the patient's psychosomatic constitution (*Prakriti*), time of day (*Dincharya*), and season (*Ritucharya*). For example, a person with the *Pit* psychosomatic constitution should not eat foods which are very hot, pungent, or spicy at noon in the summer time, as this tends to increase diseases of inflammation.

Ayurveda prescribes specific diets for several psychiatric disorders. Recent research supports this approach. Brain levels of the neurotransmitters 5HT, catecholamine, and acetylcholine have been found to be influenced by dietary constituents. Consequently, it has been suggested that normal brain functions and mental disease can be altered by diet.[6] Recent exciting developments include the successful treatment of mental depression with neurotransmitter precursors.[7,8]

Ayurveda also prescribes certain diets (*Pathya*) during drug therapies, as dietary constituents are believed to influence drug action.

Individualization of medicinal therapy

Medicinal therapy is highly individualized in Ayurveda.[9] The choice and dose of medicine are influenced not only by disease, but by the individual's constitution and the environmental conditions likely to affect that individual's *Doshas*.

For example, *Piper rotudum* (black pepper) and *Zingiber officinale* (ginger), which increase *Pit* (increasing stomach acid and pepsin secretion), are used cautiously in individuals with a *Pit* constitution. Another example is in the treatment of the patient with hypertension. Ayurveda prescribes *Terminalia chebuli* for the treatment of hypertensive patients who have *Vat Pakriti*, while for the patient with *Pit Pakriti*, one uses *Terminalia arjuna*.

A parallel to this approach can be found in modern medicine. For example, it is well-known that hypertensive patients with normal renal status respond better to beta blockers or angiotensin-converting enzyme inhibitors than do those with a poor renal status.[10]

In the *Vimanastrana*, Charak presents a very interesting discussion of host- and drug-related factors which help in the determination of the drug and the dosage (see Table 34.7).

Ayurveda also emphasizes proper timing for the administration of medicines. Considering that chronopharmacology (the study of the timing of drug administration in relation to physiological function) has only recently been developed as a branch of modern therapeutics, it seems remarkable that such astute observations about the timing of medicaments were made so many centuries ago.

Pharmacy in Ayurveda

In Ayurveda, pharmacy is highly developed. There are almost 70 books containing more than 8,000 recipes for the preparation of different medicines, most of which are derived from minerals and plants. Many formulations, including simple distillates (*Arka*), decoctions (*Kwatha*), tinctures (*Avleha*), powders (*Churna*), pills (*Vati, Goti*, and *Modak*), fermented products (*Asva*), and medicated oils (*Taila* and *Ghrita*), are available. The oil preparations are particularly useful as they help to target the sites of actions.

There are also detailed descriptions of the methods recommended to ensure a medicine is suitable for human use.[11] One pharmaceutical technique, *Samskara* (refinement), is known as *Shudhi* (purification), a process which eliminates the toxicity of some minerals and plants. Another practice is the administration of drugs in combination (*Samyoga*) in order to reduce toxicity and increase efficacy.

At the beginning of the 20th century, Paul Ehrlich introduced the Western world to the concept of targeting drugs to the site of action, a concept that was used in the East since the teachings of Charak, who wrote, among other texts, the *Adhisthana* in the 1st century AD, in which he described using drugs that have an affinity for specific tissues.

Table 34.7 Host- and drug-related factors

Drug factors	
Pakiriti	Constitution of the drug
Guna	Properties
Prabhava	Activity (potency)
Desh	Place
Ritu	Season
Grahan	Storage
Nihit	Transport
Sanskar	Refinement
Matra	Dose
Sanyog	Combination
Adhishthan	Ability to reach site of action
Host factors	
Pakriti	Constitution of host
Vayam	Age
Vikriti	Pathological condition
Sar	System strength
Satamya	Tolerability
Satva	Psychological state
Ahar Shakti	Digestive capacity
Vyayam Shakti	Exercise tolerance
Balam	Strength of host

RESEARCH

Considerable modern research has proven the efficacy of Ayurvedic herbal preparations, and research has now moved to elucidating their mechanisms and sites of action.[12] Reserpine, an antihypertensive drug, was isolated from *Rauwolfia serpentina* (*Sarpgandha*, used for hypertension). *Curcumin*, the active principle of *Curcuma longa*, has been found to exert an anti-inflammatory effect by inhibiting prostaglandin synthesis. Further, it has been shown to selectively inhibit platelet prostaglandin production, while sparing vascular endothelial prostaglandin synthesis.

Many plant preparations have been used to strengthen general host resistance. These are called *Rasayna*, *Jeevaniya*, or *Balya* and they increase tissue resistance to disease, a concept similar to "prohost therapy" as put forward by Hadden.[13] Prohost therapy is claimed to augment cellular responses and, consequently, ameliorate disease states.[14]

Perhaps most exciting, however, is the current research demonstrating efficacy of Ayurvedic herbal preparations in conditions for which modern medicine has limited or no success. For example, animal studies have shown that *Winthania somnifera* (Ashwagandna) is able to reverse the immunosuppression cyclophosphamide, azathioprin, and prednisolone and a 50% alcoholic extract of *Phyllanthus emblica* protects the liver from paracetamol.[15,16] Recent human studies found that patients with acne vulgaris demonstrated substantial improvement, with no significant side-effects, of Sunder Vati when compared with placebo (interestingly, the study found three other Ayurvedic formulas ineffective) and patients with osteoarthritis experienced substantial, highly significant improvement in pain and disability with no significant side-effects (however, the radiological findings did not improve).[17]

AYURVEDIC AND MODERN MEDICINE

In evaluating Ayurvedic medicine by modern standards, one encounters a number of difficulties. First, there is in nature a wide variation in the quantity of pharmacologically active substances in plants. In addition, many findings are more subjective than objective. The modern scientist has difficulty recognizing subjective experiences because no reliable methodology has been developed to measure and reproduce such experiences. Yet we know that totally objective experience, which completely disregards the subjective, may be wrong and even dangerous.

In fact, there is no such thing as complete objectivity. What we claim as such is merely agreement among many minds. Subjective experience is limited. Our senses vary in ability, and reality for one is unreality for another. When using the tools of quantitative, technical science to describe biological and living systems phenomena, we soon encounter limits. We must impose artificial distinctions to reduce variables and interpret non-linear events intelligibly.

Science has often confused the map for the actual reality. Take the example of color vision in bees. The eye of a bee is more sensitive to blue, violet, and ultraviolet light, while receptors in the human eye more readily detect red, green, and blue wavelengths. Thus bees are nearly blind to red light, and humans are quite blind to ultraviolet light. These differing characteristics result in members of each species forming a completely different perception of the same object. Color, rather than being a part of the "reality" of a perceived object, is an expression of sensory apparatus, determined by each species' or individual's unique pattern of interneural connections. Even more interesting is the fact that, within the same species, perception may vary considerably.

Ayurvedic philosophy may strike the contemporary reader as unnecessarily complex for the conceptual territory it addresses. However, it is actually quite succinct and very relevant to modern life. Its precepts have influenced many systems of healing, including naturopathic medicine, through the several paths of its root traditions. It emerged alongside systems known to early Persians and Greeks, as well as the Chinese. Modern medicine is itself a distillation of these same rich traditions. Compare Ayurvedic concepts with those of pre-industrial Europe and much similarity becomes apparent.

SUMMARY

Only some glimpses of Ayurveda are presented here. This ancient system of medicine, developed over centuries, has a consistent and logical framework and gives detailed instructions for the preservation of health and the treatment of disease. Ayurveda faced a setback when modern medicine subjected all knowledge to experimental and statistical verification which, although useful, is limited by the tools available and the perceptions underlying the questions asked. Now that we have accumulated considerable knowledge of cellular physiology and have much more sensitive modern biomedical research tools, we may be able to evaluate the concepts of Ayurveda more effectively.

REFERENCES

1. Lee GB. In: Davis FA, ed. Medicine throughout antiquity. Philadelphia, PA: F.A. Davis Co. 1949: p 313–354
2. Rotter JI, Jones JQ, Samloff IN et al. Traditional medicine. New Engl J Med 1979; 300: 63–66
3. Walker WA. Antigen handling by the agent. Arch Dis 1978; Child 53: 527–531
4. Tagesson C, Sjodahl R, Thoren B. Passage of molecules through the wall of the gastrointestinal tract. Scand J Gastroent 1978; 13: 519–524
5. Gulablunverba S. Charak sutra 26, Charak samhita. Jamnagar: Ayurvedic Society. 1949: p 124–141
6. Ferstorm JD. Dietary precursors and brain neurotransmitter formation. Ann Rev Med 1981; 32: 413–425
7. Copen A, Shaw, DM, Farrell MB. Potentiation of the antidepressive effect of a monoamine oxidase inhibitor by tryptophan. Lancet 1963; 79–81
8. Gelenberg AJ, Wojcik JD, Growden JH et al. Tyrosine for the treatment of depression. Am J Psychiat 1980; 137: 622–623
9. Sasdri RD, Gulablunverba S. Charak sutra 8. Jamnagar: Ayurvedic Society. 1949: p 105
10. Laragh JH. In: Laragh JH, Buhler FR, Seldin, eds. Frontiers in hypertension research. Boston: Springer. 1981: p 183–194
11. Budar Peth YJB. Sharangdhar samhita, Part II. Pune: YJ Dixit. 1908
12. Satayavati GV, Raina MK, Sharma M. Medicinal plants of India, vols 1 and 2. New Delhi: Indian Council of Medical Research. 1976
13. Hadden JW. Immunomodulators in the immunotherapy of cancer and other diseases. Trends Pharm Sci 1982; 3: 191–194
14. Srivastva R, Puri V, Srimal RC, Dhwan BN. Drug Res 1986; 30
15. Ziauddin M, Phansalkar N, Patki P et al. Studies on the immunomodulatory effects of Ashwagandha. J Ethnopharmacol 1996; 50: 69–76
16. Agarwal S, Agrawal SS. Hepatoprotective studies on *Phyllanthus emblica* Linn. and quercetin. Indian J Exp Biol 1995; 33: 261–268
17. Paranjpe P, Kulkarni PH. Comparative efficacy of four Ayurvedic formulations in the treatment of acne vulgaris: a double-blind randomised placebo-controlled clinical evaluation. J Ethnopharmacol 1995; 49: 127–132

FURTHER READING

Budwar Peth YJB. Sharangdhai samhita, Part 1. Dixit: Pune. 1908: ch 2

Charak Samhita and Sushruta Shamita Shri Gulablunverba. Chaunkamba orientale, Varanasi. Jamnagar: Ayurvedic Society. 1980.

Dahanukar SA, Date SG, Karainchikar SM. Cytoprotective effect of Terminalia chebula and Asparagus racemosa on gastric mucosa. Indian Drugs 1983; 20: 442–495

Dahanukar SD, Karandikar SM. Evaluation of the antiallergic properties of Piper longum. Indian Drugs 1984; 21: 377–383

Kerup PVN. In: Bannerman RH, Burton J, Wrn-Chieh C, eds. Traditional medicine and health care coverage. Geneva: WHO. 1983: p 50–58

Kulkarni RR, Patki PS, Jog VP et al. Treatment of osteoarthritis with a herbomineral formulation. a double-blind, placebo-controlled, cross-over study. J Ethnopharmacol 1991; 33: 91–95

Lad V. Ayurveda, The Indian art and science of medicine. New York, NY: ASI. 1965

Lad V. Ayurveda, the science of self healing. Sante Fe, N Mexico: Lotus Press. 1984

Lad V. Ayurveda. A holistic medical approach. Probe 1987; XXVI: 293–297

McIntosh RP. The importance of timing in hormone and drug delivery. Trends Pharm Sci 1984; 5: 492–501

Meerson FA. Adaptation, stress and prophylaxis. Boston, MA: Springer. 1984: p 86–93

Rege NN, Dahanukar SA, Dahanukar SM. Hepatoprotective effect of Tinospora cardiofolia against carbon tetrachloride induced liver damage. Indian Drugs 1984; 21: 544–580

Singhal GD, Teipathi SN, Chaturredi GN. Fundamental and plastic surgery considerations in ancient Indian surgery, vol. I. Varanasi, India: Singhal Publications. 1981: p 15–16

Srikanta Murthy KR. Clinical methods in Ayurveda. Varanasi: Chaurhambha Orientalia

CHAPTER CONTENTS

35

Botanical medicine – a modern perspective

Michael T. Murray, ND

Joseph E. Pizzorno Jr, ND

INTRODUCTION

The term "herb" refers to a plant used for medicinal purposes. Are herbs effective medicinal agents or is their use merely a reflection of folklore, outdated theories, and myth? To the uninformed, herbs are generally thought of as ineffective medicines used prior to the advent of more effective synthetic drugs. To others, herbs are simply sources of compounds to isolate and then market as drugs. But to some, herbs and crude plant extracts are effective medicines to be respected and appreciated.

For many of the people of the world, herbal medicines are the only therapeutic agents available. In 1985, the World Health Organization estimated that about 80% of the world's population rely on herbs for their primary health care needs.[1] This widespread use of herbal medicines is not restricted to developing countries, as it has been estimated that 70% of all medical doctors in France and Germany regularly prescribe herbal preparations.

Although herbal medicine has existed since the dawn of time, our knowledge of how plants actually affect human physiology remains largely unexplored. Many individuals formulate their view of herbal medicine based on opinion, philosophy, and ideology. This chapter seeks to facilitate an informed view of herbal medicine. The past as well as the future of herbal medicines are discussed. The authors believe that the continued evolution of the tradition of herbal medicine can only be accomplished within the context of continued scientific investigation.

THE REBIRTH OF HERBAL MEDICINE

Throughout the world, but especially in Europe and Asia, there has been a tremendous renaissance in the use and appreciation of herbal medicine. In Germany, estimates show that over $4 billion are spent on herbal products each year. In Japan, the figure is thought to be even higher. Herbal products are a major business in the US as well, with an estimated annual sales of $4 billion for 1996. Annual sales have been increasing for several years. However, it is interesting to note that while annual sales of ginseng products in the US in 1992 was roughly $10 million, over 3 million pounds (roughly $100 million) of American ginseng were exported.[2,3]

The rebirth of herbal medicine, especially in developed countries, is largely based on a renewed interest by the public and scientific researchers. During the last 10–20 years, there has been an explosion of scientific information concerning plants, crude plant extracts, and various substances from plants as medicinal agents. Plants still play a major role in modern pharmacy.

The role of herbs in modern pharmacy

For the past 25 years, about 25% of all prescription drugs in the US have contained active constituents obtained from plants. Digoxin, codeine, colchicine, morphine, vincristine, and yohimbine are some popular examples. Many over-the-counter (OTC) preparations are also composed of plant compounds. Current estimates show that more than $11 billion of plant-based medicines are purchased each year in the US alone and $43 billion worldwide.[4]

Pharmacognosy, the study of natural drugs and their constituents, plays a major role in current drug development. Unfortunately, the standard path of the approval of a drug is a process that typically takes 10–18 years at a total cost of roughly $230 million.

Because a plant cannot be patented, plants are screened for biological activity and then the so-called "active" constituents (compounds) are isolated and, typically, chemically modified to produce unique substances. If the compound is powerful enough, the drug company will begin the process to procure Food and Drug Administration (FDA) approval. Because of the expense and lack of patent protection, very little research has been done during this century on whole plants or crude plant extracts as medicinal agents, per se, by the large American pharmaceutical firms.

In contrast, European regulatory policies and practices have made it economically feasible for companies to research and develop herbs as medicines. For example, in Germany, herbal products can be marketed with drug claims if they have been proven to be safe and effective.[5] Whether the herbal product is available by prescription or OTC is based upon its application and safety of use. Herbal products sold in pharmacies are reimbursed by insurance if they are prescribed by a physician.

The proof required by a manufacturer in Germany to illustrate safety and effectiveness for an herbal product is less (and more appropriate) than the proof required by the FDA for drugs in the US. In Germany, a special commission (Commission E) developed a series of 400 monographs on herbal products similar to the OTC monographs in the US.[6] An herbal product is viewed as safe and effective if a manufacturer meets the quality requirements of the monograph or produces additional evidence of safety and effectiveness that can include data from existing literature, anecdotal information from practicing physicians, as well as limited clinical studies.

The best single illustration of the difference in the regulatory issues of herbal products in the US compared to Germany is *Ginkgo biloba*. In Germany, as well as France, extracts of *Ginkgo biloba* leaves are registered for the treatment of cerebral and peripheral vascular insufficiency.[7] *Ginkgo* products are available by prescription and OTC purchase. *Ginkgo* extracts are among the top three most widely prescribed drugs in both Germany and France, with a combined annual sales of more than $500 million. In contrast, in the US, extracts, which are identical to those approved in Germany and France, are available as "food supplements".

No medicinal claims are allowed for most herbal products, because the FDA requires the same standard of absolute proof as is required for new synthetic drugs. Thus far, the FDA has rejected the idea of establishing an independent "expert advisory panel" for the development of monographs similar to Germany's Commission E monographs, as well as other ideas to create a suitable framework for the marketing of herbal products in the US. Currently, herbal products continue to be sold as "food supplements" and manufacturers are prohibited from making any therapeutic claims for their products.

The German experience: St John's wort extract as an example

Over 25 double-blind controlled trials (15 vs. placebo, 10 vs. standard anti-depressant drugs) have shown St John's wort (*Hypericum perforatum*) extracts standardized for hypericin content to yield excellent results in the treatment in depression with virtually no side-effects.[5] Yet, most American physicians have never heard of St John's wort extract and go on to erroneously state that there is no research to support its use when patients or the media ask them about them.

In contrast, a total of 66 million daily doses of St John's wort preparations were prescribed by German physicians in 1994.[5] The obvious questions is: "Why do so many German MDs know about St John's wort, *Ginkgo*, and other herbal medicines while conventional medical doctors in the US remain ignorant?" The answer: Germany addressed the issue of rational claims for herbal products by developing the Commission E series of monographs (now totaling over 400).

The monograph system allowed companies to market their products according to the guidelines of the Commission E. With the ability to make appropriate claims, many companies achieved success with their products and were then able to then fund the necessary research to gain greater acceptance within mainstream, conventional medicine. The use of St John's wort extract in the treatment of depression is a perfect case in point to illustrate how the Commission E monographs have led to significant documentation of the efficacy of plants with a long history of folk use for depression.

When the Commission E monograph for St John's wort came out in 1984, it identified the constituent hypericin as the active constituent and permitted the medicinal use of the herb (in average doses of 2–4 g of herb, or 0.2–1.0 mg total hypericin) for depression, anxiety, or nervous excitement.

Originally it was thought that hypericin acted as an inhibitor of the enzyme monoamine oxidase, thereby resulting in the increase of CNS monoamines such as serotonin and dopamine. However, newer information indicates that St John's wort does not inhibit MAO in vivo.[8] The anti-depressant activities appear to be related more to inhibiting serotonin reuptake, similar to the SRI drugs like Prozac, Paxil, and Zoloft.[9,10] In addition, it appears that while hypericin is an important marker, there are other compounds such as flavonoids which are thought to play a major role in the pharmacology of St John's wort.

The great fallacy

One of the great fallacies promoted by the US's medical establishment has been that there is no firm scientific evidence for the use of many natural therapies, including herbal medicine. This assertion is simply not true. In fact, during the last 10–20 years there has been an explosion of information concerning plants, crude plant extracts, and nutritional substances as medicinal agents.

Science and medicine now have available the technology and understanding necessary to evaluate herbal medicines properly. Thirty years ago it was impossible to determine exactly how herbs promote their healing effects because analytical science had not advanced to a sufficient level of sophistication. This point is well illustrated by the fact that the main mechanism of action responsible for aspirin's anti-inflammatory effect was not understood until the early 1970s, and its mechanism of action for pain relief has yet to be fully understood.

Since the mechanism of therapeutic action of a particular herb could not be fully elicited, many effective plant medicines were erroneously labeled as possessing no pharmacological activity. Now, researchers equipped with greater understanding and more sophisticated technology are rediscovering the wonder of plants as medicinal agents. Much of the increased understanding is, interestingly, a result of synthetic drug research.

For example, one of the latest classes of so-called "wonder drugs" are the calcium-channel blockers. These agents block the entry of calcium into smooth muscle cells, thereby inhibiting contraction and promoting muscular relaxation. Calcium-channel blocking drugs are currently being used in the treatment of high blood pressure, angina, asthma, and other conditions associated with smooth muscle contraction. They, in many ways, represent the most highly evolved stage of modern drug pharmacy. After calcium channel drugs became better understood, it was discovered that many herbs contain components which possess calcium-channel blocking activity. In most cases, the historical use of these herbs correspond to their calcium-channel blocking activity.

In addition to possessing currently understood pharmacological activity, many herbs possess pharmacological actions that are not consistent with modern pharmacological understanding. For example, many herbs appear to impact on homeostatic control mechanisms to aid normalization of many of the body's processes. When there is a hyper-state the herb will have a lowering effect, and when there is a hypo-state it will have a heightening effect. This action is totally baffling to orthodox pharmacologists, but not to experienced herbalists who have used terms such as alterative, amphiteric, adaptogen, or tonic to describe this effect.

The advantages of herbal medicines

In general, herbal preparations are thought to have three major advantages: lower cost, fewer side-effects and medicinal effects which tend to normalize physiological function. When used most effectively, the mechanism of action of an herb will often correct the underlying cause of a disorder. In contrast, a synthetic drug is often designed to alleviate the symptom or effect without addressing the underlying cause. Interestingly, research has often shown for many plants that the whole plant or crude extract is much more effective than isolated constituents.

Herbal medicine will certainly play a major role in the medicine of the future. As modern medicine gains more knowledge and understanding about health and disease, it is adopting therapies that are more natural and less toxic. Lifestyle modification, stress reduction, exercise, meditation, dietary changes and many other traditional naturopathic therapies are becoming much more popular in standard medical circles. This illustrates the paradigm shift that is occurring in medicine. What was once scoffed at is now becoming generally accepted as an effective alternative. In fact, in most instances these natural alternatives offer significant benefit over standard medical practices.

The difference is due to the growing sophistication of herbal medicine. With the continuing advancement in science and technology, there has been a great improvement in the quality of herbal medicines available and in the understanding of their optimal clinical utilization. Improvements in cultivation techniques coupled with improvements in quality control and standardization of potency will continue to increase the effectiveness of herbal medicines.

The study of herbal medicine

The study of herbal medicine spans the breadth of pharmacology, the study of the history, source, physical and chemical properties, mechanisms of action, absorption, distribution, biotransformation, excretion, and therapeutic uses of "drugs". In many respects, the pharmacological investigation of herbal medicine is just beginning. This textbook is replete with examples of herbs whose historical use is being justified by new investigations into its pharmacology.

THE HISTORY OF HERBAL MEDICINE

The history of the use of plants as medicines is full of interesting stories and fascinating facts. The evolution that has occurred in herbal medicine over the centuries is only beginning to be recognized as more natural medicines gain acceptance. Interestingly, this acceptance is largely a result of increased scientific investigation.

There is a trend towards using substances found in nature, including compounds which are found in the human body such as interferon, interleukin, insulin, and human growth hormone, as well as foods, food components, herbs, and herbal compounds. More and more researchers are discovering the tremendous healing properties of these natural compounds and their advantages over synthetic medicines and surgery in the treatment of many health conditions. Through these scientific investigations, a trend towards natural medicine is emerging. To better appreciate this evolutionary trend, this section presents some of the historical aspects of herbal medicine. Much of the following is derived from Barbara Griggs' *Green Pharmacy: a History of Herbal Medicine*.[11]

In the beginning

Plants have been used as medicines since the dawn of animal life. The initial use of plants as medicines by humans is thought to have been a result of "instinctive" dowsing. Animals in the wild still provide evidence that this phenomena occurs. Animals will, with a few notable exceptions, eat those plants that will heal them and avoid those plants which will do them harm. Presumably humans also possessed this instinct at one time.

As civilizations developed, medicine men and women were responsible for transmitting the information on herbs to their successors. Before the advent of written language, this information was handed down by verbal and experiential means.

Besides instinctive dowsing, it was commonly believed that plants had been signed by the "creator" with some visible or other clue that would indicate its therapeutic use. This concept is commonly referred to as "the doctrine of signatures". Common examples of this doctrine are:

- *Panax ginseng* (ginseng), whose root bears strong resemblance to a human figure and whose general use is as a tonic
- *Caulophyllum thalictroides* blue (cohosh), whose branches are arranged like limbs in spasm indicating its usefulness in the treatment of muscular spasm
- *Sanguinaria canadensis* (bloodroot), whose roots and sap are a beautiful blood color corresponding to its traditional use as a "blood purifier"
- *Lobelia inflata* (lobelia), whose flowers are shaped like a stomach corresponding to its emetic qualities
- *Hydrastis canadensis* (goldenseal), whose yellow-green root signifies its use in jaundice as well as infectious processes.

All of these uses have been confirmed by recent research.

Materia medicas

With the development of written language, materia medicas (books containing prescribing information on herbs) became the vehicle of passing information about the medicinal use of herbs to future herbalists. Materia medicas were recorded in ancient China, Babylon, Egypt, India, Greece, and other parts of the world. From these materia medicas, it is quite obvious that herbal medicines were highly respected therapies in ancient times.

Galen's influence

There was no system, rules, or classification to Western herbal materia medicas until the 1st century AD when Galen, the Greek physician who founded experimental physiology, established his system of rules and classification. Galen's classification was based on Hippocratic medicine, i.e. balance of the four humors – blood, bile, phlegm, and choler – and a profound belief in a beneficent nature. Although his system is considered seriously flawed in the light of modern medical knowledge, Galen is historically considered to be the founder of scientific herbalism.

Galen evaluated and classified each plant according to its relation to Hippocratic medical theory. Although based initially in Hippocratic principles, Galen constructed his own elaborate, and rigid, system of medicine. Galen's work also signified the beginning of a clear division between the professional physician and the traditional healer. As only the well educated could understand Galen's system, and even with the best schooling it remained a mystery to many, all challenges to the professional physician were effectively squelched by dogma.

Galen's system dominated European medical thinking for 1,500 years. Perhaps if the Roman Empire had continued to flourish others would have surfaced to develop alternative theories. Instead, Galenical medicine reigned unchallenged throughout the middle ages. By the 19th century, the "professional" physician, confident in his supposedly superior knowledge, took Galenical philosophy to an extreme probably never imagined by Galen by the adoption of bloodletting, purging, and administering exotic medicines. This was in direct contrast to the traditional healer's patient use of traditional herbs and tremendous faith in the healing power of nature.

The Black Plague and syphilis

Although Galenical medicine dominated the Middle Ages, herbal medicine was still deeply entrenched in Europe culture. The Black Plague of 1348 may have been the beginning of change in medical thought, as conventional medicine was totally useless. As nearly one-third of Europe died as a result of this plague, the public began to lose faith in Galenical medicine. Nearly 150 years later another blow was dealt to Galenical medicine when syphilis became the major medical problem. Unlike the Black Death, patients with syphilis tended to survive longer, giving physicians more time to experiment with treatments. At this time, perhaps the greatest hoax in the history of medicine began. Mercury became the standard medical treatment for syphilis despite the fact that even Galen thought mercury too poisonous to use.

Syphilis did, however, open the door for the use of some new herbs from the Americas. A French physician, Nicholas Monardes, published a comprehensive account of sarsaparilla and several other "new" drugs in the treatment of syphilis in 1574. Many Europeans at the time believed that syphilis had come to Europe from the West Indies with Columbus' sailors, and since there was a general belief that whatever disease was native to a country might be cured by the medicinal herbs growing in that region, it was only natural for sarsaparilla to become a very popular remedy. Since at that time the standard treatment of syphilis was the use of mercury, which often resulted in greater morbidity than did syphilis, sarsaparilla was a welcome alternative. Despite initial excitement, Monardes' sarsaparilla cure eventually lost favor, probably due to other components in the cure; specifically, patients were confined to a warm room for 30 days, and for the following 40 days were required to abstain from both wine and sexual intercourse.

Although the public popularity of sarsaparilla waned, it continued to be used in the treatment of syphilis. During military operations in Portugal in 1812, a British Inspector General of Hospitals noted that the Portuguese soldiers suffering from syphilis who used sarsaparilla recovered much faster and more completely than their British counterparts who were treated with mercury.

Sarsaparilla was also used by the Chinese in the treatment of syphilis. Later clinical observations in China would demonstrate, through the use of blood tests, that sarsaparilla is effective in about 90% of cases of acute syphilis and 50% of cases of chronic syphilis.[11]

Although sarsaparilla was clearly more beneficial than mercury in the treatment of syphilis, mercury was the standard medical treatment of choice for over four and a half centuries. Some historians have stated that "the use of mercury in the treatment of syphilis may have been the most colossal hoax ever perpetrated" in the history of medicine.[11] Mercury represented a new kind of medicine, one formulated and prepared in a laboratory using the new techniques of chemistry. It helped to prepare the way for future synthetic and mineral drugs at the expense of herbal medicines.

Challenges to Galenical medicine

The 1500s also saw a strong challenge to Galenical medicine from within the traditional circles. Specifically, Paracelsus, an alchemist who believed strongly in the doctrine of signatures, was responsible for founding modern pharmaceutical medicine. Paracelsus is probably most remembered for the development of laudanum (tincture of opium). After Paracelsus, Galenical preparations and treatments fell greatly out of favor.

In public circles, herbal medicine was regaining some respect as well. In the early 1600s, Culpepper, an English pharmacist, published his book entitled, *The English Physician*. Instead of requiring patients to purchase expensive exotic or imported drugs, Culpepper recommended the herbs his clients and readers had growing in their own back yards. Although Culpepper's herbal is based on astrological rationalizations, it reinforced a strong English tradition of domestic herbal medicine. This came at a time when professional physicians were beginning to become contemptuous of herbal medicine.

Meanwhile, in the Americas during the 1600 and 1700s, herbs used traditionally by the Native Americans were becoming quite popular, especially in the treatment of malaria and scurvy. Herbal medicine continued to gain even greater respect in the late 1700s, as exemplified by English physician Withering's classic description of digitalis. However, mercury, bleeding, and purging were still the "standard" medical treatments epitomized by George Washington's death from complications incurred during treatment of a sore throat (i.e. he was bled to death).

The Thomsonian and Eclectic movements

During the early 1800s, standard medicine may have been ready to reconsider traditional herbal remedies, but then came the Thomsonian movement. Samuel Thomson (1769–1843) patented a system of herbal medicine that, in 1839, claimed over 3,000,000 faithful followers. Although Thomson brought back to medicine the vitalistic Hippocratic idea of *vis medicatrix naturae* and gained widespread public support for the use of herbal medicine, the Thomsonian movement was probably detrimental to medical reform.

Thomsonians became locked in prejudice and dogma and insisted that all medical knowledge was complete and could be found in Samuel Thomson's works. These and other claims roused scorn, indignation, rage, and resentment in the average North American doctor. Frequently based on purging through the use of herbal emetics, Thomson's treatments often were as harsh as the standard treatments of the times (for further discussion, see Ch. 2).

During the 1800s, the Eclectic movement attempted to bridge the gaps between standard medical thought, Thomsonianism, and traditional herbal medicines. Rather than attack the existing medical system, the Eclectic movement sought to bring about reform by educating physicians about the use of herbal medicines. Several Eclectic medical colleges were established and, for a while, it appeared that the Eclectic movement was making headway in its attempt to reform the medical system from within.

The movement, however, eventually failed. Several factors were probably responsible for the failure of the Eclectic movement: a split in the ranks which diluted the movement; harsh measures like mercury, calomel, and bloodletting were finally discarded by the conventional professional physician due to a decrease in infectious disease as a result of improved sanitation and hygiene; and, perhaps most important, the failure to establish and sustain quality medical schools.

The Flexner report on medical education in 1910 spelled doom for the eclectics: by 1920, seven of the eight that existed prior to the report had closed with the last school closing in 1938. Meanwhile, the standard medical schools, aided by the Rockefeller Foundation, flourished, promoting the growth of the modern pharmaceutical industry and the current near-monopoly of the medical profession.

The growth of the pharmaceutical industry

Since a plant cannot be patented, very little research has been done this century on plants as medicinal agents, per se, by the large American pharmaceutical firms. Instead, plants have been screened for biological activity and then the so-called "active" constituents have been isolated and chemically modified to produce unique, patentable compounds. Much to the dismay of the researchers was the discovery that in many instances the isolated constituents were less biologically active than the crude herb. Since the crude herb provided no economical reward to the American pharmaceutical firm, the crude herb or extract never reached the marketplace. In contrast, European policies on herbal medicines made it economically feasible for companies to research and develop phytopharmaceuticals.

Another of the problems of herbal medicine in the US has been the lack of standardization. The herb which best exemplifies this dilemma is digitalis. One batch of crude digitalis might have a very low level of active constituents, making the crude herb ineffective, while the next batch might be unusually high in active constituents, resulting in toxicity or even death, when standard amounts were used. The lack of standardization made it easier for US pharmaceutical firms to rationalize their economic need to isolate, purify, and chemically modify the active constituents of digitalis so they could market these compounds as drugs. The problem with using the pure active constituent is that the safe dosage range is smaller: digitalis toxicity and death have increased dramatically as a result of purification. Toxicity was less of a factor when using the crude herb because overconsumption of potentially toxic doses resulted in vomiting or diarrhea, thus avoiding the severe heart disturbance and death which now occur with pure digitalis cardiac glycoside drugs.

Fortunately, several European and Asian pharmaceutical firms began specializing in phytopharmaceuticals in the early part of the 20th century. These companies have played a prominent role in researching, developing, and promoting herbal medicines.

Research is demonstrating that crude extracts often have greater therapeutic benefit than the isolated "active" constituent. This has been known for quite some time in other parts of the world, but in this country isolated plant drugs are still thought of as having the greatest therapeutic effect. This myth is gradually being eroded as our knowledge of herbal medicines increases.

If current standardization techniques had been available earlier in this century, it is possible that the majority of our current prescription drugs would be herbal extracts instead of isolated and modified active constituents or synthetic chemicals.

THE FUTURE OF HERBAL MEDICINE

Currently, there is a renaissance occurring in herbal medicine. It is ironic that this renewal is coming not from traditional herbalists but rather from pubic demand for alternatives to the monopolistic conventional medicine and renewed scientific investigation into the use of plant medicines. It seems that science and medicine have finally advanced to a level where nature can be appreciated rather than discounted. The scientific investigation of plant medicines is replacing some of the mystery and romance of herbalism with a greater understanding of the ways in which herbs work. Those herbal traditions willing to learn are being improved by modern scientific research and technology.

Improvements in plant cultivation techniques and the quality of herbal extracts (quality control and standardization) have led to the development of some very effective plant medicines. It is quite apparent that many of the "wonder drugs" of the future will be derived from plants or plant cell cultures and from compounds naturally occurring in the human body produced by cell cultures (e.g. interferon, interleukin-II, various hormones, etc.). Several herbal medicines described in this textbook may in fact already fulfill the role of wonder drug, e.g. *Ginkgo biloba, Hypericum perforatum, Silybum marianum, Panax ginseng,* and *Vaccinium myrtillus.*

The future of herbal medicine looks extremely positive. Many of the previous shortcomings of herbal medicine have been overcome (e.g. lack of scientific support, standardization, quality control, etc.). The future of herbal medicine is dependent on several factors:

- continued research into herbal medicine
- adoption by manufacturers of recognized standards of quality
- continued existence of the naturopathic medical schools teaching herbal medicine at a high level of sophistication
- increased public awareness of the tremendous therapeutic value of herbs.

Herbal medicine will undoubtedly play a major role in the medicine of the 21st century.

HERBAL PREPARATIONS

The clinical application of botanical medicine involves the use of a variety of herbal preparations. That being the case, it is imperative that practitioners and physicians using herbal medicines understand the differences among the various forms. Commercial herbal preparations are as bulk dried herbs, teas, tinctures, fluid extracts, and tablets or capsules. Each of these forms has advantages and disadvantages and varying ways of expressing their medicinal strength. This section reviews the major extraction forms, discusses the benefits of standardized botanical extracts and emphasizes the importance of delivering a clinically effective level of active compounds regardless of the form of the herbal preparation.

Extracts

Extracts defined

An extract is defined as a concentrated form of the herb obtained by mixing the crude herb with an appropriate solvent (such as alcohol and / or water). One of the major advances in the herb industry has been the improvement in extraction and concentration processes.[12]

When an herbal tea bag is steeped in hot water, it is actually a type of herbal extract known as an infusion. The water is serving as a solvent in removing some of the medicinal properties from the herb. Teas often are better sources of bioavailable compounds than the powdered herb, but are relatively weak in action compared to tinctures, fluid extracts, and solid extracts. These forms are commonly used by the lay public and herbal practitioners for medicinal effects.

Tinctures are typically made using an alcohol and water mixture as the solvent. The herb is soaked in the solvent for a specified amount of time, depending on the herb. This soaking is usually from several hours to days; however, some herbs may be soaked for much longer periods of time. The solution is then pressed out, yielding the tincture.

Fluid extracts are similar to, but more concentrated than, tinctures. Although they are most often made from hydroalcoholic mixtures, other solvents may be used (vinegar, glycerin, propylene glycol, etc.). Commercial fluid extracts are usually made by distilling off some of the alcohol, typically by using methods that do not require elevated temperatures, such as vacuum distillation and counter-current filtration. However, some small manufacturers produce fluid extracts in a similar manner to tinctures via a percolation at room temperature.

A solid extract is produced by further concentration of the extract by the mechanisms described above for fluid extracts, as well as by other techniques such as thin layer evaporation. The solvent is completely removed, leaving a viscous extract (soft solid extract) or a dry solid extract depending upon the plant, portion of the plant, solvent and drying process (if any) used. The dry solid extract, if not already in powdered form, can be ground into course granules or a fine powder. A solid extract also can be diluted with alcohol and water to form a fluid extract or tincture.

Strengths of extracts

The potencies or strengths of herbal extracts are generally expressed in two ways. If they contain known active principles, their strengths are commonly expressed in terms of the content of these active principles. Otherwise, the strength is expressed in terms of their concentration. For example, tinctures are typically made at a 1:5 (to 1:10) concentration. This means one part of the herb (in grams) is soaked in five parts solvent (in ml of volume). This means that there is five times the amount of solvent (alcohol / water) in a tincture as there is herbal material. Fluid extracts are typically 1:1.

A 4:1 concentration means that one part of the extract is equivalent to, or derived from, four parts of the crude herb. This is the typical concentration of a solid extract. A quantity of 1 g of a 4:1 extract is concentrated from 4 g of crude herb.

Typically, 1 g of a 4:1 solid extract is equivalent to 4 ml of a fluid extract and 20–40 ml of a tincture. Some solid extracts are concentrated as high as 100:1, meaning it would take nearly 100 g of crude herb, or 100 ml of a fluid extract, or 1 L of a tincture to provide an equal amount of herbal material in 1 g of a 100:1 extract.

Determining quality

In the past, the quality of the extract produced often was difficult to determine as many of the active principles of the herbs were unknown. However, recent advances in extraction processes, coupled with improved analytical methods, have reduced this problem of quality control.[12–14] The concentration method of expressing the strength of an extract does not accurately measure potency since there may be great variation among manufacturing techniques and raw materials. By using a high quality herb (i.e. rich in active compounds), it is possible to have a more potent dried herb, tincture, or fluid extract compared to the solid extract that was made from a lower quality herb. Standardization is the solution to this problem.[14]

Standardized extracts: the best solution

Standardized extracts (also referred to as guaranteed potency extracts) refer to an extract guaranteed to contain a "standardized" level of active compounds or key chemical marker. Stating the content of active compounds or key chemical marker rather than the concentration ratio allows for more accurate dosages to be made.

The best scenario for determining the quality of an herb is the level of active components or key biological markers. Regardless of the form the herb is in, it should be analyzed to ensure that it contains these components at an acceptable standardized level. More accurate dosages can then be given. This form of standardization is generally accepted in Europe and is beginning to be used in the US as well.

This form of standardization, i.e. stating the content of active constituents versus drug concentration ratio, allows for dosage to be based on active constituents.[3] For example, in Europe *Vaccinium myrtillus*, *Silybum marianum*, and *Centella asiatica* extracts dosage levels are based on their active constituent levels rather than drug ratio or total extract weight, e.g. 40 mg anthocyanosides for *Vaccinium myrtillus*, 70 mg silymarin for *Silybum marianum*, and 30 mg triterpenic acids for *Centella asiatica*. This type of dosage recommendation provides the greatest degree of consistency and assurance of quality.

Although referred to in terms of active constituents, it must be kept in mind that these are still whole extracts and not isolated constituents. For example, an *Uva ursi* extract standardized for its arbutin content, say 10%, still contains all of the synergistic factors which enhance the active ingredient's (arbutin) function.

Techniques used in the production of herbal products

There is a tremendous range of sophistication in the processing of herbs – from crude herb to highly concentrated standardized extracts. Nonetheless, there are some common stages. The following describes some of the processes in the production of herbal products and the machines that perform the functions.[15]

Collection/harvesting

When plants are collected from their natural habitat, they are said to be "wild-crafted". When they are grown utilizing commercial farming techniques, they are said to be "cultivated". Collection of plants from cultivated sources ensures that the plant collected is the one that is desired. When an herb is wild-crafted, there is a greater chance that the wrong herb will be picked and greater variation in potency. However, some herbal practitioners believe that wild-crafted herbs are inherently superior, since growth in their natural habitat produces an herb with constituents and properties more consistent with their traditional use. The use of analytical techniques can be employed to guarantee that the plant collected is the one desired and that its concentrations of medicinal constituents are within an acceptable range.

In the US marketplace, herbs from all over the world are marketed. The collectors of the herbs vary from uneducated natives to self-proclaimed "herbalists" to trained botanists.

The mode of harvesting varies from hand labor to very sophisticated equipment. The mode is not as important as the time of year. A plant should be harvested when the part of the plant being used contains the highest possible level of active compounds. Again, this is ensured by the use of analytical techniques.

Drying

After harvesting, most herbs have a moisture content of 60–80% and cannot be stored without drying. Otherwise, important compounds would break down and / or microorganisms would contaminate the material. As many of the desired compounds are heat labile, the majority of herbs require relatively mild conditions for drying. Commercially, most plants are dried within a temperature range of 100–140°F. During drying, the plant constituents must not be damaged or suffer losses that would prevent it from conforming to accepted standards. With proper drying, the herb's moisture content is reduced to less than 14%.

Garbling

Garbling refers to the separation of the portion of the plant to be used from other parts of the plant, dirt, and other extraneous matter. This step is often done during collection. Although there are machines that perform garbling, garbling is usually performed by hand.

Grinding

Grinding or mincing an herb means mechanically breaking down either leaves, roots, seeds, or other parts of a plant into very small pieces ranging from larger course fragments to fine powder. Grinding is employed in the production of crude herbal products as well as in the initial phases of extracts.

Often the material has to be pre-chopped or minced before feeding it into a grinder. In the process of grinding, a number of machines can be used, but the most widely used is the hammer mill. These machines are simple in design. The hammers, arranged radially, follow the rotation of the shaft to which they are attached, breaking up the material that is fed into the machine from above. On the walls of the chamber is a grid, which determines the size of the material that is passed through it. Other types of grinders include knife mills and teeth mills.

Extraction

The process of extraction is used in making tinctures, fluid extracts, and solid extracts. Extraction in the context of this textbook refers to separating by physical or chemical means the desired material from a plant with the aid of a solvent. In the US health food industry, most extracts utilize alcohol and water mixtures as solvents to remove soluble compounds from the herb. The exceptions are liposterolic extracts, which are produced either through the use of lipophilic solvents or with the aid of hypercritical carbon dioxide (CO_2 gas compressed to a liquid by high pressures).

Most extracts that are produced by small manufacturers use maceration procedures. The simplest process consists of soaking the herb in the alcohol/water solution for a period of time and then filtering. For many botanicals this process will yield a lower quantity of active constituents at a higher price because of the cost of the solvent. Since tinctures are 1:5 concentrates, this means that 80% of the bottle is alcohol and water and only 20% is herbal material. In essence, the cost of the alcohol is a major portion of the retail price of tinctures.

Larger manufacturers utilize more elaborate techniques to ensure that the herb is fully extracted and the solvent is reused. For example, counter-current extraction is often used. In this process, the herb enters into a column of a large percolator composed of several columns. The material to be extracted is pumped through the different columns at a specific temperature and flow speed where it continuously mixes with solvent. The extract-rich solvent then passes into another column, while fresh solvent once again comes into contact with herbal material as it is passed into a new chamber. In this process, complete extraction of health-promoting compounds can be performed. The extract-rich solvent is then concentrated by techniques described below.

Concentration

After extraction of the herb, the resulting solutions can be concentrated into fluid extracts or solid extracts. In large manufacturing operations, techniques and machines, such as thin layer evaporators, are utilized to ensure that the extracted plant components are not damaged. These machines work by evaporating the solvent and leaving the plant compounds. The solvent vapors pass into a condenser whereby they return to a liquid and for reuse. The result is separation of the extracted materials from the solvent so that the final product is a pure extract and the solvent can be used again and again.

Drying of extracts

Many practitioners prefer the extract dried to a solid form, since it is more chemically stable and lower in cost (alcohol is often more expensive than the herb). In addition, tinctures and fluid and soft extracts can more easily be contaminated by bacteria and other microorganisms. Liquid forms of extracts also promote reactions which eventually break down some active constituents. A number of drying techniques are employed including freeze-drying and spray-drying (atomization). The result is a dried powdered extract that can then be put into capsules or tablets.

Excipients

The same excipients used in the manufacture of drug preparations and vitamin and mineral supplements are often used in the production of tablets and capsules containing herbs or herbal extracts. Many manufacturers will provide a list of excipients contained in their products.

Analytical methods

Improvements in analytical methods have definitely led to improvements in harvesting schedules, cultivation techniques, storage, stability and concentration of active compounds, and product purity. All of these gains have resulted in tremendous improvements in the quality of herbal preparations now available.

Methods currently utilized in evaluating herbs and their extracts include:

- organoleptic
- microscopic
- physical
- chemical/physical
- biological.

Organoleptic

Organoleptic means the "impression of the organs". Organoleptic analysis involves the application of sight, smell, taste, touch, and occasionally even sound, to identify the plant. Typically, the initial sight of the plant or extract is so specific it is easily recognized. If this is not enough, perhaps the plant or extract has a characteristic odor or taste. Organoleptic analysis represents the simplest, yet the most human, form of analysis.

Microscopic evaluation

Microscopic evaluation is indispensable in the initial identification of herbs, as well as in identifying small fragments of crude or powdered herbs. It is also important in the detection of contaminants and adulterants (e.g. insects, animal feces, mold, fungi, etc.). Every plant possesses a characteristic tissue structure, which can be demonstrated through study of tissue arrangement, cell walls, and configuration when properly mounted in stains reagents and media.

Physical/chemical analysis

In crude plant evaluation, physical methods often are used to determine the solubility, specific gravity, melting point, water content, degree of fiber elasticity, and other physical characteristics. Various chemical/physical methods also are used to determine the percentage of active principles, alkaloids, flavonoids, enzymes, vitamins, essential oils, fats, carbohydrates, protein, ash, acid-insoluble ash, or crude fiber present.

Chromatography

The most sophisticated analytical processes involve more highly technological assays to determine quality. Advanced techniques, such as thin layer chromatography, high-pressure liquid chromatography (HPLC), capillary electrophoresis and nuclear magnetic resonance (NMR), are used to precisely separate, identify and quantify molecules. The readings from these machines provide a chemical "fingerprint" as to the nature of chemicals contained in the plant or extract. These techniques are invaluable in the effort to identify herbs, as well as standardize extracts.

Biological analysis

The plant or extract can also be evaluated by various biological methods, mostly animal tests, to determine pharmacological activity, potency, and toxicity.

Quality control in herbal products

Quality control is a term that refers to processes involved in maintaining the quality or validity of a product. Regardless of the form of herbal preparation, some degree of quality control should exist. Currently, there is no organization or government body that certifies an herb as labeled correctly.

Without quality control, there is no assurance that the herb contained in the bottle is the same as what is stated on the outside. The widespread disregard for quality control in the health food industry has tarnished the reputation of many important medicinal herbs. For example, it has been estimated that because of supplier errors in collection, more than 50% of the Echinacea sold in the US from 1908 through 1991 was actually *Parthenium integrifolium*.[16] This highlights the importance of using the Latin scientific name, since both of the above-mentioned herbs are referred to as "Missouri snakeroot", as well as the need for proper plant identification based upon organoleptic, microscopic, and technological analysis.

Recent chemical analysis of commercially available *Tanacetum parthenium* (feverfew) and *Tabebuia avellanedae* (taheebo) for active components parthenolide and lapachol, respectively, has also shown need for concern. Analysis of over 35 different commercial preparations of feverfew found that the majority of products contained no parthenolide or only traces.[17] Analysis of 12 commercial sources of taheebo could identify lapachol (in trace amounts) in only one product.[18] Perhaps the best example of problems that can result when there is lack of quality control is *Panax ginseng*.

Panax ginseng and quality control

Panax ginseng (Korean ginseng) contains at least 13 different steroid-like compounds, collectively known as ginsenosides, which are believed to be its most important active ingredients. The usual concentration of ginsenosides in mature ginseng roots is between 1 and 3%. Ginsenoside Rg1 is present in significant concentrations in *Panax ginseng*. In contrast, American ginseng (*Panax quinquefolius*) contains primarily ginsenosides Rb1 and very little, if any, Rg1. This difference is extremely important since Rb1 and Rg1 have different effects. In general, Rb1 possesses a sedative effect while Rg1 possesses a stimulatory effect. Since American ginseng is much higher in Rb1 than Rg1, its action is much different than that of Korean ginseng.

Independent research and published studies have clearly documented a tremendous variation in the ginsenoside content of commercial preparations.[19,20] In fact, the majority of products on the market contain only trace amounts of ginsenosides, and many formulations contain no ginseng at all. The lack of quality control has led to several problems, ranging from toxic reactions (discussed below) to absence of medicinal effect. The widespread disregard for quality control in the herbal industry has done much to tarnish the reputation of ginseng, as well as other important botanicals.

The problem of quality control is exemplified by a 1979 article entitled "Ginseng abuse syndrome" which appeared in the *Journal of the American Medical Association*.[21] In this article, a number of side-effects are reported, including hypertension, euphoria, nervousness, insomnia, skin eruptions, and morning diarrhea. Given the extreme variation in quality of ginseng in the American marketplace and the use both of non-official parts of the plant and of adulterants, it is not surprising that side-effects were noted. None of the commercial preparations used in the trial had been subjected to controlled analysis. Furthermore, the species of ginseng used included *Panax ginseng, Panax quinquefolius, Eleutherococcus senticosus,* and *Rumex hymenosepalus* in a variety of different forms, i.e. roots, capsules, tablets, teas, extracts, cigarettes, chewing gum, and candies.

It is virtually impossible to derive any firm conclusions from the data presented in the *JAMA* article, especially in light of the fact that studies performed on standardized extracts of *Panax ginseng* have demonstrated the absence of side-effects, as well as no mutagenic or teratogenic effects.[22,23] These findings further support the superiority of using herbal products that were produced using quality control measures.

The "hairy baby" story

To further illustrate problems that can occur without proper plant identification and standardization, let's examine the case of the "hairy baby". In another *JAMA* article,[24] it was reported that a 30-year-old woman took "Siberian ginseng" (mistakenly identified in the article as *Panax ginseng*) at a dose of two 650 mg tablets twice daily during her 9 months of pregnancy and 2 weeks of breast feeding. She had experienced repeated premature uterine contractions during late pregnancy and had noted increased and thicker hair growth on her head, face, and pubic area. The woman gave birth to a full-term baby boy who was noted to have thick black pubic hair over his entire forehead along with other signs suggestive of androgenization. The authors of the report used this anecdotal evidence to warn physicians of the dangers of ginseng.

At first glance, this case report appears to be quite alarming. However, when examining the scenario more closely, a different picture is presented. First of all, controlled animal and human studies with *Eleutherococcus senticosus* have shown it to be extremely safe. In fact, in the animal studies, eleutherococcus extract actually prevented the teratogenic effects of xenobiotics, and in a human study of 1,770 pregnant women it was shown that eleutherococcus improved pregnancy outcome. There were no signs of androgenic effects in either the animal or human studies.[25]

The *JAMA* article caught the attention of Dr Dennis Awang (then head of the Natural Products Bureau of Drug Research, Health Protection Branch Health and Welfare Canada). Upon examination of the product the woman had taken, Dr Awang discovered that the product did not contain Siberian ginseng, but was a totally different herb, *Periploca sepium*.[26]

Does this mean the woman's reaction was due to *Periploca sepium*? Studies in animals have determined that *Periploca sepium*, like Siberian ginseng, does not produce an androgenic response.[27] The most likely explanation for the "hairy baby" was that it had nothing to with the herbal product being used.

Addressing the quality control problem

The solution to the quality control problem that exists in the US is for manufacturers and suppliers of herbal products to adhere to quality control standards and good manufacturing practices. With improvements in the identification of plants by laboratory analysis, consumers should at least be guaranteed that the right plant is being used. Consumers, health food stores, pharmacists, herbalists and physicians who use or sell herbal products should ask for information from the suppliers of herbal products on their quality control process. What do they do to guarantee the validity of their product? As more consumers, retailers, and professionals begin demanding quality control from the suppliers, more quality control processes will be utilized by manufacturers.

Currently, only a few manufacturers adhere to complete quality control and good manufacturing procedures.

Companies supplying standardized extracts currently offer the greatest degree of quality control, hence these products typically offer the highest quality.

Most standardized extracts are currently made in Europe under strict guidelines set forth by individual members of the European Economic Council (EEC) as well as those proposed by the EEC.[12–15] Also included are guidelines for acceptable levels of impurities, such as parasites (bacterial counts), pesticides, residual solvents, heavy metals, and product stability.

The production of standardized extracts serves as a model for quality control processes for all forms of herbal preparations. In general, it is believed that if the active components of a particular herb are known, whatever the form of the herb product, the herb should be analyzed to ensure that it contains these components at a medicinally appropriate level. More accurate dosages can then be given. Products should also be subjected to bacteriological counts.

Currently, in many countries, numerous standardized extracts fulfill requirements for marketing as drugs. These extracts have typically gone through the quality control steps in Table 35.1.

Standardized extracts vs. tinctures

There are several misconceptions regarding standardized extracts that need to be addressed. One is that standardizing an extract results in the loss of important compounds. This is simply not true for the vast majority of standardized extracts. Chemical analysis of standardized extracts and tinctures, whether it be thin layer chromatography (TLC) or HPLC, have clearly demonstrated that standardized extracts are not only higher in active compounds but also have a broader range of chemical constituents due to more effective extraction.

Another common misconception is that they are more expensive than alcohol-based tinctures and fluid extracts. Calculations based on the cost of delivery of an effective dosage show that the standardized extract is significantly more cost-effective. This is because, as noted above, there is less of the herb in tinctures and fluid extracts, resulting in consumers paying extra for alcohol, bottle, and the cost of shipping.

Table 35.1 List of quality control steps necessary for the registration of plant-based drug formulation

1. Selection of suitable plant material
2. Botanical investigation using organoleptic and microscopic techniques
3. Chemical analysis using appropriate laboratory equipment
4. Screening for biological activity
5. Analysis of active fractions of crude extracts
6. Isolation of active principles
7. Determination of chemical structure of active principles
8. Comparison with compounds of similar structure
9. Analytical method developed for formulation
10. Detailed pharmacological evaluation
11. Studies performed to determine activity and toxicity of formulation
12. Studies on absorption, distribution, and elimination of herbal compounds
13. Clinical trials performed to determine activity in humans
14. Registration by National Drug Authorities

The question of an effective dosage

The effectiveness of any herb or herbal product from a pharmacological perspective is dependent upon providing an effective dosage of active compounds. Regardless of the form of the herbal preparation, clinical effectiveness requires delivery of an active dosage. Standardization or accurate analysis of the content of active constituents or key biological markers is the only real assurance of the delivery of an effective dosage.

This view should not be controversial. Unfortunately, controversy arises from the fact that from a pharmacological perspective it is unlikely that the dosage schedules historically recommended for most herbal tinctures are sufficient to produce significant pharmacological effects. While tinctures of such potentially toxic herbs such as gelsemium, aconite, belladonna, and digitalis often produce a pharmacological effect when given at low dosages, for most common medicinal herbs it is very difficult to produce an adequate and cost-effective response when the herb is administered in tincture form.

The administration of small dosages of herbs in tincture form is an offshoot of the homeopathic and Eclectic use of "mother tinctures" and "specific medicines". The effectiveness of these preparations and their ability to exert pharmacological effects have not been proved for all but a few botanicals.

The questioning of the clinical effectiveness of herbal tinctures by science-based or evidence-based naturopathic physicians is often viewed as heretical and sacrilegious by many professing to be "master herbalists". The opinion of the editors of this textbook is that if a natural medicine, whether it is a tincture, standardized extract, or nutrient, is truly clinically effective it should be able to stand up to scientific scrutiny and rationale.

The systems of herbal medicine that have been proved to a very large extent are based upon delivering much higher levels of herbal compounds than those easily obtained via the use of tinctures. Specifically, we are referring to the use of highly concentrated standardized extracts from Europe and the use of herbal preparations in Traditional Chinese Medicine and Ayurveda. In Traditional Chinese Medicine, the typical daily dosage of prescribed crude herbal material is approximately 20 g. This high level of dosage is in stark contrast to much smaller average amount of the herbal material recommended in the *British Herbal Pharmacopoeia* of 2–4 ml of a 1:5 tincture, which provides less than 1 g of herbal material. This difference in dosage may explain the differences in popularity of herbal medicine in China, Japan, India, and Germany compared with its relative obscurity in England as well as in the US prior to the last decade. The key point is that herbal medicine is not going to be very popular if it is not very effective. The greater the effectiveness, the greater the popularity.

The tremendous growth noted in the US over the past decade is, in our opinion, the result of the influx of high quality standardized extracts into the marketplace. For years, herbal medicine in the US labored and struggled because of inadequate dosages. Now, better clinical results are being achieved with herbal medicines because they are using better products which are able to deliver an effective dosage of active constituents.

SUMMARY

One of the major developments in herbal medicine involves improvements in extraction and concentration processes. These improvements have led to several very effective, clinically proven herbal products. The best assurance of quality and results when using herbal products is to use those products from suppliers who employ quality control standards and good manufacturing practices. Standardized and accurately analyzed extracts which state the level of active compounds provide the greatest benefit due primarily to more accurate and reliable dosages.

While the future looks extremely promising for herbal medicine in the US, ultimately its success will determine by the degree to which reliable herbal products are used by health care providers and consumers.

REFERENCES

1. Farnsworth N et al. Medicinal plants in therapy. Bull World Health Org 1985; 63: 965–981
2. Deveny K. Garlic and ginseng supplements become potent drugstore sellers. The Wall Street Journal 10/1/92: B1, B5
3. Market Report. HerbalGram 1992; 26: 40
4. Principe PP. The economic significance of plants and their constituents as drugs. Econ Med Plant Res 1989; 3: 1–17
5. Keller K. Legal requirements for the use of phytopharmaceutical drugs in the Federal Republic of Germany. J Ethnopharamacol 1991; 32: 225–229
6. Kleijnen J, Knipschild P. Drug profiles – *Ginkgo biloba*. Lancet 1993; 340: 1136–1139
7. Linde K et al. St. John's wort for depression – an overview and meta-analysis of randomized clinical trials. BMJ 1996; 313: 253–258
8. Thiede HM, Walper A. Inhibition of MAO and COMT by hypericum extracts and hypericin. J Geriatr Psychiatry Neurol 1994; 7(1): S54–56
9. Thiele B, Brink I, Ploch M. Modulation of cytokine expression by hypericum extract. J Geriatr Psychiatry Neurol 1994; 7(1): S60–62
10. Perovic S, Muller WEG. Pharmacological profile of hypericum extract. Effect of serotonin uptake by postsynaptic receptors. Arzneim Forsch 1995; 45: 1145–1148
11. Griggs B. Green Pharmacy. A history of herbal medicine. London: Robert Hale. 1981
12. Bonati A. Formulation of plant extracts into dosage forms. In: Wijeskera ROB, ed. The medicinal plant industry. Boca Raton, FL: CRC Press. 1991: p 107–114
13. Karlsen J. Quality control and instrumental analysis of plant extracts. In: Wijeskera ROB, ed. The medicinal plant industry. Boca Raton, FL: CRC Press. 1991: p 99–106
14. Bonati A. How and why should we standardize phytopharmical drugs for clinical validation? J Ethnopharmacol 1991; 32: 195–197
15. Bombardelli E. Technologies for the processing of medicinal plants. In: Wijeskera ROB, ed. The medicinal plant industry. Boca Raton, FL: CRC Press. 1991: p 85–98
16. Awang DVC, Kindack DG. Echinacea. Can Pharm J 1991; 124: 512–516
17. Heptinstall S et al. Parthenolide content and bioactivity of feverfew (*Tanacetum parthenium* (L.) Schultz-Bip.). Estimation of commercial and authenticated feverfew products. J Pharm Pharmacol 1992; 44: 391–395
18. Awang DVC. Commercial taheebo lacks active ingredient. Can Pharm J 1988; 121: 323–326
19. Liberti LE and Marderosian AD. Evaluation of commercial ginseng products. J Pharm Sci 1978; 67: 1487–1489
20. Soldati F, Sticher O. HPLC separation and quantitative determination of ginsenosides from *Panax ginseng*, *Panax quinquefolium* and from ginseng drug preparations. Planta Med 1980; 39(4): 348–357
21. Siegel RK. Ginseng abuse syndrome. JAMA 1979; 241: 1614–1615
22. Hikino H. Traditional remedies and modern assessment. The case of ginseng. In: Wijeskera ROB, ed. The medicinal plant industry. Boca Raton, FL: CRC Press. 1991: p 149–166
23. Shibata S, et al. Chemistry and pharmacology of Panax. Econ Medicinal Plant Res 1985; 1: 217–284
24. Koren GS, et al. Maternal ginseng use associated with neonatal androgenization. JAMA 1990; 264: 2866
25. Farnsworth NR, et al. Siberian ginseng (*Eleutherococcus senticosus*). current status as an adaptogen. Econ Medicinal Plant Res 1985; 1: 156–215
26. Awang DVC. Maternal use of ginseng and neonatal androgenization. JAMA 1991; 265: 1828
27. Waller DP et al. Lack of androgenicity of Siberian ginseng. JAMA 1992; 267: 2329

SUMMARY

CHAPTER CONTENTS

36

Contemporary homeopathy

Allen M. Kratz, PharmD

INTRODUCTION

Homeopathy is a therapeutic approach developed over 200 years ago by a German physician, Dr Samuel Hahnemann. A basic tenet is that symptoms of a "disease" are a natural part of the healing process. They are the body's innate reaction to a challenge and, as such, should be respected and allowed to occur. In fact, the homeopathic practitioner actually seeks to express these symptoms through allopathic means. Assisting the body to heal is the focus of homeopathy.

Homeopathically prepared substances are chosen based on the "law of similarities". Substances that, in large doses, induce similar symptoms in a well person, as determined by a homeopathic "proving", are prescribed in homeopathic form to safely augment or express these same symptoms in an individual who is ill.

The appropriate homeopathic formulation is chosen based on a careful and thorough review and evaluation of symptoms, physical as well as mental. In classical homeopathy, a single, well chosen substance may be all that is needed, particularly in acute clinical conditions. However, in our modern day society, conditions or "diseases" have become more chronic, thus requiring more complex approaches.

One of the primary reasons for the revival of interest in homeopathy has been its contemporization. Since the late 1970s, homeotherapeutics has undergone a change. This change has been necessitated by the impact of modern day lifestyles – ingestion of devitalized, processed foods; higher levels of stress; and the reliance on symptom-suppressing drugs, all of which interfere with the body's inherent ability to heal and self-repair. The accumulated effects of these damaging influences are the primary causes of the dramatic rise in the incidence of chronic, degenerative "disease". The modern practice of homeopathy has contemporized to adapt to these new challenges.

HISTORY

Hippocrates taught "the same things which can cause disease can cure it" as well as "first, do no harm", a definition of contemporary homeopathy from the father of medicine.

"The cause is the cure" is exemplified by the use of homeopathic mercury to treat iatrogenic mercury toxicity during the last century. Conventional physicians of that era were using mercury as a cure-all. It was the wonder drug of its time: a laxative, a diuretic, and an antisyphilitic. As with many wonder drugs, its toxicity caught up with it. In fact, the word "quack" comes from the German word for mercury, *quecksilber*, or our quicksilver, used as a pejorative term to describe those turn of the century conventional physicians who prescribed mercury so indiscriminately. It is interesting how the word "quack" is now being used to disparage the modern unconventional practitioner. In the current Homeopathic Pharmacopoeia of the US, there are 17 different monographs for mercury, all from an earlier time. This confirms the observation that, during the last century, conventionally prescribed mercury was being antidoted by homeopathically prepared mercury – "the cause is the cure". Is history repeating itself with the use of dental amalgam/mercury?

CONTEMPORARY HOMEOTHERAPEUTICS

As mentioned, practitioners of contemporary homeopathy view all symptoms of a condition ("disease") as positive events – signs of adaptation, detoxification and healing. To further assist the healing process, these symptoms are homeopathically expressed rather than suppressed. When symptoms are "relieved" by conventional medications, normal detoxification is suppressed, thereby creating a deeper retoxification of organs/systems. This retoxification can cause more severe conditions. Contemporary homeopathic practitioners recognize three basic types of conditions:

- acute
- chronic
- constitutional.

Acute

Many acute conditions are self-limiting and may be self-treated by informed consumers. Other acute conditions require a diagnosis from a physician and more skilled prescribing. These acute conditions respond to lower potencies (e.g. 3×, 6×) of single or complex homeopathic formulations.

Chronic

Chronic conditions, often associated with toxicity, require the counsel of a practitioner familiar with the effects of clearing, detoxification and support. These chronic conditions respond to middle range potencies (e.g. 9× to 200×) of complex homeopathic or homeovitic formulations.

Constitutional

Constitutional conditions, with both physical and emotional/mental components, require the supervision of a practitioner trained in classical homeopathy. These constitutional conditions respond to high potencies (e.g. above 200×) of single homeopathic formulations.

RECOGNITION OF CONTEMPORARY HOMEOPATHY

Over the years, homeopathy has proven to be very effective in both acute and constitutional conditions. Today's lifestyles and some conventional medical drug treatments have greatly increased the incidence of chronic conditions associated with toxicities. As a result, there has been a significant increase in the use of detoxifying homeopathic formulations. Homeopathy has contemporized to meet these new challenges.

The Homeopathic Pharmacopoeia of the United States (HPUS), the oldest official drug compendium in this country, has been in continuous publication since 1897. In 1982, a supplement to the HPUS was published to respond to changes that had occurred in the practice of homeopathy. The HPUS established two new classes of homeopathic formulations in its General Pharmacy section: allersodes and isodes.

The Homeopathic Pharmacopoeia Revision Service, initiated in 1988, has also embraced contemporary homeopathy by several inclusions in the General Pharmacy section:

- the recognition of the usefulness of complex/combination homeopathic formulations
- the acceptance of contemporary dosage forms, including oral liquids and compressed tablets
- the use of stabilizers other than alcohol in dosage forms
- the inclusion of newer sterilization techniques
- the inclusion of newer analytical procedures for quality control and stability assessment.

The General Pharmacy section of this Homeopathic Revision Service makes the following "statement regarding combinations of homeopathic drugs":

> Whereas, combinations of homeopathic drugs are in general use by many homeopathic physicians of the United States and internationally, and,
>
> Whereas, such combinations of homeopathic medicines are an essential part of their armamentarium and,

Whereas, homeopathic physicians depend upon homeopathic pharmacists for manufacture and preparation of such homeopathic medicines and combinations of such homeopathic medicines and,

Whereas, the Pharmacopoeia Convention of the United States recognizes the necessity for the manufacture, preparation and distribution of combinations of homeopathic medicines to meet the needs of those homeopathic physicians using combination medicines.

Be it therefore resolved: That combination of homeopathic medicines are within the scope and tenants of Homeopathy, provided each component is listed in the Homeopathic Pharmacopoeia of the United States.

Approved this 11th day of February, 1981, by the Directors of the Homoeopathic Pharmacopoeia Convention of the United States.

Definitions

The following definitions of contemporary homeopathic terminology are presented.

Allersodes. Allersodes are homeopathic attenuations of antigens, i.e. substances which under suitable conditions can induce the formation of antibodies.

Isodes. Sometimes called "detoxodes", isodes are homeopathic attenuations of botanical, biological, chemical or synthetic substances, or drugs, including excipients or binders, which have been ingested or otherwise absorbed by the body and are believed to have produced a disease or disorder which interferes with homeostasis.

Anthroposophic homeopathy. This is an etiological approach, utilizing specially prepared single ingredient and multiple ingredient remedies, based upon an understanding of the "essential nature" of a remedy and of its similarity to the "formative influences" ultimately responsible for conditions of illness or imbalance.

Biotherapy. This comprises a variety of therapeutic approaches, including nutritional, manipulative, mechanical and medicinal interventions, which act to stimulate or otherwise facilitate the living system to maintain or regain its healthy functions by means of its own internal health regulatory mechanisms. Homeopathy is one of these biotherapeutic approaches.

Classical homeopathy. This involves election of a single remedy, most similar to the "essence" of the case, based upon a hierarchical evaluation of the "totality of symptoms", with emphasis upon subjective sensations, "strange, rare and peculiar" symptoms, modalities, desires and aversions, and "mental generals". In order for it to be possible to select a remedy in this manner, the remedy must present a delineated symptom "picture" complete with subjective sensations, mental and emotional symptoms, desires, aversions and reactional modalities. Since it is possible for only one remedy to be most similar to the "totality of symptoms," only one remedy at a time is to be used; remedies are never to be alternated or mixed together. The selected single remedy is usually (but by no means always) administered in a medium or high attenuation.

Complexism or combination homeopathy. This is the practice of using two or more remedies at the same time or in combination with each other.

Gemmotherapy involves the use of glycerin/alcohol macerates (made in accordance with processes described in the French Pharmacopoeia) of fresh plant material taken from non-toxic plants during the budding, flowering or early growth cycle of the plant, and given upon organotropic indications in order to stimulate or facilitate the histological vitalization of the organ or tissue for which the plant has an elective affinity.

Homeovitics. This is a contemporary approach that focuses on the problem of cellular toxicity. Formulations are used to clear, destress, detoxify and support the body on a cellular level. This approach holds that toxicity, i.e. chemicals, metals, is a predisposing factor in all chronic conditions.

Isotherapy. As used in modern homeopathic literature, isotherapy refers to the therapeutic administration of isodes upon the basis of etiotropic similarity. The cause is the cure. It is also known as the homeovitic approach (*homeo* = same, *vitic* = energy). This practice is especially popular with many European homeopathic physicians (see also "tautopathy").

Oligotherapy. This refers to trace elements as found in the human body under normal, healthy conditions and which play a role as catalysts in maintaining physiological life functions. Examples are tissue salts and other HPUS minerals or elements.

Organotropic. This pertains to substances which act on the organs of the body; having affinity for the tissues (Plakiston's Medical Directory, 2nd edn); or, as would be said in homeopathy, remedies which have an elective affinity for particular organs or tissues of the body. Another phrase (with the same meaning) found in the older homeopathic literature is "seat of specificity of action".

Potency accord, potency spectrum. This is the mixing of two or more attenuations of the same remedy in one preparation.

Single remedy therapy. This is the use of a single ingredient remedy based on the similarity of that single remedy to the characteristic indications found in a particular, individual case of illness or imbalance.

Tautopathy is the administration of a homeopharmaceutically attenuated preparation of the same substances which caused a state of ill health to develop. This is analogous to the homeovitic or isopathic approach.

Ultramolecular. This refers to the homeopharmaceutical preparation of a remedy which has been attenuated to the 12th centesimal or 24th decimal dilution, or beyond, and in which, therefore, no molecules of the original or base substance of the remedy can statistically be present.

Another term found in the literature which has the same meaning is "submolecular".

Many of these definitions are included in pharmacist Jay Yasgur's *A dictionary of homeopathic medical terminology*.[1] This is a very useful reference text for all homeopathic practitioners, classical as well as contemporary.

RESEARCH

One of the seminal studies in contemporary homeopathy was published in *Human Toxicology* by Cazin et al[2] and was entitled "A study of the effect of decimal and centessimal dilutions of arsenic on the retention and mobilization of arsenic in the rat". This study proved the effectiveness of homeopathic arsenic in helping laboratory rats to detoxify arsenic. Interestingly, the researchers found that middle range potencies (14×) had the strongest effects. They also concluded that decimal dilutions (1–10×) augmented the elimination of arsenic more than centesimals. This is an example of the isopathic or homeovitic approach. This study was cited as part of a comprehensive review of a significant number of studies on detoxification using homeopathically produced substances.[3] After careful review of 105 studies, the authors concluded that this approach was scientifically valid.

Because of their greater popularity in Europe, most reports on clinical trials of these types of formulations have been published in France and Germany. Typical of these studies are two conducted in Germany. One was a randomized, placebo-controlled, double-blind study which demonstrated the efficacy of a combination formulations in the treatment of knee injuries.[4] Another controlled trial demonstrated the clinical efficacy of a complex formulation homeopathic ointment in the treatment of athletic injuries.[5]

Clinical research in contemporary homeopathy has also been conducted in the UK. In 1980, a double-blind clinical trial was conducted of 20 different homeopathic remedies employed in the treatment of rheumatoid arthritis. A significant positive clinical response was found over the placebo-controlled study group.[6]

In 1985, Dr David T. Reilly, a noted Scottish homeopathic physician, and his colleagues began the first of three landmark studies on the effectiveness of contemporary homeopathic therapies over placebo. The first study demonstrated efficacy using isopathic pollens in treating hay fever.[7] Its positive results led to a second study which was published in *The Lancet*.[8] Mixed pollens prepared homeopathically again showed very positive results in the treatment of hay fever as compared with placebo. The reporting of these two trials created quite a stir in conventional medical circles. The results were again replicated in a third trial. On December 10 1994, *The Lancet* published the results of this third positive trial under the title "Is evidence for homeopathy reproducible?"[9] The introduction to this study is quoted below:

> A pilot study specifically designed to answer the question "Is homeopathy a placebo response?" suggested that it was not, a result replicated in a larger trial. As these findings were controversial, the original investigators approached independent colleagues in the University of Glasgow to find out if the result could be replicated in a third trial. The three studies used homeopathic immunotherapy in inhalant allergy as a model, the first two in hay fever, the third in asthma with the same main outcome measure – a visual analogue source of overall symptom intensity. We report the results of this third study and a meta-analysis of all three.

As interest in contemporary homeopathy grows, one can expect more research to be published in medical journals. Clinical studies of combination or complex formulations are now being published in the US. The Office of Alternative Medicine of the National Institutes of Health is currently funding pilot studies on homeopathy.

HOMEOPATHIC ORGANIZATIONS

The Homeopathic Pharmacopoeial Convention of the United States (HPCUS) is responsible for the US Homeopathic Pharmacopoeia, now in its revised eighth edition. HPCUS is composed of representatives from all constituents of the profession: production, clinical practice, distribution and educational organizations.

The American Association of Homeopathic Pharmacists (AAHP) represents the majority of companies that produce homeopathic formulations. It is a trade organization that interacts with the US Food and Drug Administration to preserve the legal status of homeopathy. The American Homeopathic Pharmaceutical Association (AHPA) is a newly formed group representing pharmacists with a special interest in homeopathy.

The National Center for Homeopathy (NCH) is a non-profit public educational organization. It disseminates information to the public about homeopathy and sponsors educational programs on homeotherapeutics to health care providers. The NCH publishes a monthly newsletter, *Homeopathy Today* [(703)548-7790]. It also maintains a directory of practitioners. A similar organization is the International Foundation for Homeopathy (IFH), which publishes *Resonance* [(206)324-8230].

The American Institute of Homeopathy (AIH), founded in 1844, is the oldest medical society in the US. It represents physicians that specialize in homeopathy and publishes the *Journal of the AIH* [(303)898-5477]. The Homeopathic Academy of Naturopathic Physicians (HANP) comprises a membership of naturopathic physicians with an interest in homeopathy. It publishes the journal *Simillimum* [(503)829-5477]. The Chiropractic Academy of Homeopathy (CAH) represents chiropractic physicians with interests in homeopathy. It publishes a journal, *The Prover* [(303)226-1719].

CONCLUSION

Contemporary homeopathy is being used by greater numbers of informed individuals who have become aware of the need to be more responsible for their own health. A person who uses a homeopathic formulation for acute first aid at home will welcome its use in more serious, chronic conditions under the care of a practitioner.

Physicians interested in treating chronic illness in a natural, drugless way will find the use of contemporary homeotherapeutics, particularly for clearing and detoxification, a logical prelude to rebuilding with clinical nutrition and/or botanical medicines.

REFERENCES

1. Yasgur J. A Dictionary of homeopathic medical terminology. 2nd edn. Greenville, PA: Van Hoy. 1994
2. Cozin JC et al. A study of the effect of decimal and centesimal dilutions of arsenic on the retention and mobilization of arsenic in the rat. Human Toxicology 1987; 6: 315–320
3. Linde K, Jonas WB, Melchart D et al. Critical review and meta-analysis of serial agitated dilutions in experimental toxicology. Hum Exp Tox 1994; 13: 481–492
4. Theil BB. The treatment of recent traumatic blood effusions of the knee joint. Biological Therapy 1994; 12: 242–248
5. Bohmer D, Ambrus P. Sports injuries and natural therapy; a clinical double blind study with a homeopathic ointment. Biological Therapy 1992; 10: 290–300
6. Gibson RG et. al. Homeopathic therapy in rheumatoid arthritis: evaluation by double blind clinical therapeutic trial. Br J Clin Pharmac 1980; 9: 453–459
7. Reilly DT, Taylor MA. Potent placebo or potency? A proposed study model with initial findings using homoeopathically prepared pollens in hay fever. Br Hom J 1985; 74: 65–75
8. Reilly DT, Taylor MA, McSharry C, Aitchison T. Is homeopathy a placebo response? Controlled trial of homeopathic potency with pollen in hay fever as a model. Lancet 1986; ii: 881–886
9. Reilly DT, Taylor MA, Beattie NGM et al. Is evidence for homeopathy reproducible? Lancet 1994; 344: 1601–1606

CHAPTER CONTENTS

37

Environmental medicine

Walter J. Crinnion, ND

INTRODUCTION

The 20th century with its promise of "better living through chemistry" has also brought a host of chemical toxin-related illnesses (referred to here as "environmental illnesses"). Recent articles in the medical literature have shown that the rate of cancers not associated with smoking is higher for those born after 1940 than before, and that this increase of cancer is due to environmental factors not related to smoking.[1] We are also experiencing the new medical diagnoses of sick (closed) building syndrome[2,3] and multiple chemical sensitivity (MCS),[4–6] both of which are known to be related to overexposure to environmental contaminants. The environmental toxins which cause the most problems are pesticides, solvents and heavy metals. The primary damage caused by the solvents and major pesticide classes is to disrupt neurological function.[7,8] In addition to being neurotoxic, these compounds are profoundly immunotoxic and are often toxic to the endocrine system as well.[9–12] The adverse health effects are not limited to those systems only, as these compounds can also cause a variety of dermatological, gastrointestinal, genitourinary, respiratory, musculoskeletal, and cardiological problems. Heavy metals poison a diverse range of enzyme function, affecting virtually every system of the body.[6]

ENVIRONMENTAL TOXIC LOAD

Prevalence of environmental toxins in humans

Our environment is currently flooded with chemicals that contaminate our air, our water, our food and ourselves. Since 1976, the Environmental Protection Agency (EPA) has been engaged in the National Human Adipose Tissue Survey (NHATS).[13] In this study, adipose samples are taken from cadavers and elective surgeries from all regions of the country and the levels of toxins are measured. In 1982, they expanded beyond their original list to look for the presence of 54 different environmental chemical toxins. Their results are a cause for great concern. Five of the chemicals – OCDD (a dioxin), styrene, 1,4-dichlorobenzene, xylene, and ethylphenol – were found in 100% of all samples. Another nine chemicals – benzene, toluene, chlorobenzene, ethylbenzene, DDE,* three dioxins and one furan – were found in 91–98% of all samples. In addition, PCBs were found in 83% of all samples and beta-BHC in 87%. A total of 20 toxic compounds were found in 76% or more of all samples! These ongoing assessments have shown quite clearly that it is not a question of *if* we are carrying a burden of toxic xenobiotic compounds, but one of *how much* and how do they affect our health.

Additional studies have shown the same alarming facts. A CDC study of 5,994 persons aged 12–74 found that 99.5% had *p,p*-DDE at levels in the range 1–379 ppb.[14] A study of adipose levels of chemicals in persons from Texas showed the presence of *p,p*-DDE, dieldrin, oxychlordane, heptachlor epoxide and *para*-BHC in 100% of all samples.[15] That study was done on adipose samples taken from autopsies, and was from older subjects. A study of 4-year-olds in Michigan showed the presence of DDT in over 70%, PCB in 50% and PBB in 13–21%.[16] Nursing was the primary source of exposure for these children.

Sources of environmental toxins

This multiple chemical load is due to several decades of chemical exposure from contaminated air, food and water. Both outdoor and indoor air are contaminated with chemicals. The EPA's TEAM study has documented the following chemicals as 'ubiquitous' in the air:

- *p*-xylene
- tetrachloroethylene
- ethylbenzene
- benzene
- 1,1,1-trichloroethane
- *o*-xylene.

Those listed as "often present" were:[17]

- chloroform
- carbon tetrachloride
- styrene
- *p*-dichlorobenzene.

This study found that air samples taken with a personal monitor attached to the study individuals showed higher levels of chemicals in the "personal" air space over a 24-hour period than in outdoor air samples. These elevated personal levels and elevated breath levels were more directly attributable to indoor air pollution. However, they did note that persons who visited a service station or a dry cleaner had elevated personal breath levels of the solvents, as well as those who smoked and drove a vehicle during the day. They also found that certain occupations, such as chemical manufacturing, painting and plastic manufacturing, caused higher levels of exposure.

Testing for chemical residues on food has been routinely employed throughout the world. None of the studies has found food sources free of contamination. On the contrary, multiple contaminants are usually found. The most comprehensive for the United States is the ongoing FDA Total Diet Survey.[18] While the Total Diet Survey looked for the presence of many different chemicals, their findings for chlorinated pesticides, listed in Table 37.1, are alarming. For example, DDE was found in 63% or more of the 42 foods sampled.

The foods with the highest concentrations of DDE were:

- fresh or frozen spinach (mean concentration, 0.0234 ppm)
- butter (mean concentration, 0.0195 ppm)
- collards (0.0126 ppm)
- pork sausage (0.0124 ppm)
- lamb chops (0.0113 ppm)
- canned spinach (0.0109 ppm).

Since DDT and DDE have been banned from use in the US since 1972, it is likely that some of this contamination is from produce imported from other countries where it is still used.

Unfortunately, since toxic chemicals are ubiquitously used throughout the world, they move easily around the globe on the winds. Unless these pesticides are trapped in the soil, tree bark, or other stable materials, persistent volatile pesticides, including DDT and toxaphene, begin a wind-driven leapfrogging around the globe.

The more volatile the chemical, the faster it hops and the less readily it enters the fat of any plant or animal

Table 37.1 Presence of DDT in US food samples

Food	Percentage of samples contaminated
Raisins, spinach (fresh and frozen), chili con carne (beef and bean), beef	100
American processed cheese, hamburger, hot dogs, bologna, collards, chicken, turkey, ice cream	93
Lamb chops, salami, canned spinach, meat loaf and butter	87
Cheddar cheese, pork sausage, quarter pounders, white sauce, creamed spinach	81

*DDE is formed by a partial dechlorination of DDT. This can occur in the human body within 6 months of exposure to DDT. It also occurs in nature, but studies vary as to the half-life ($t_{½}$) of DDT in nature. Previously, the $t_{½}$ of DDT was thought to be 2 years, but recent findings in Yakima, Washington, indicate that it may be decades in certain circumstances. Upon degradation the DDT becomes DDE or DDD.

it contacts. Volatile chemicals applied in tropical regions evaporate into the atmosphere and then condense in cooler climates. As the ambient temperature falls, the compound becomes less volatile, so the periods between hopping of a compound from one place to another tend to lengthen. So, if two forests were exposed to identical amounts of a volatile pesticide, trees in the colder climate would become more heavily contaminated.

DDT and DDE are less volatile than solvents and do not leapfrog as well, and so tend to stay where they land and may be there for a year before jumping again. This global leapfrogging can account for one alarming study of the diet of Arctic indigenous women. The diet of two groups of women (from the eastern and western Canadian Arctic) were found to be very high in organochlorine compounds (OCC). The primary sources of these compounds were the meat and blubber of ringed seal, walrus, mattak and narwhal, as well as caribou, whitefish, inconnu, trout and duck.[19] Since these OCCs were transported in the air, they landed in the Arctic, but due to the low temperature were unable to volatilize again and leapfrog away.

HEALTH EFFECTS OF ENVIRONMENTAL TOXINS

While there is virtually no debate left about whether our world is polluted or not, there is a considerable amount of debate as to whether or not these environmental toxins have adverse health effects on humans. This chapter provides information that supports the concept that accumulation of recurrent low-level exposures to environmental toxins is damaging to health. Enough evidence of a positive association between chemical exposure and disease exists to document that a serious problem exists and that caution is urged.

An article published in *JAMA* in 1994 by Devra Lee Davis et al,[20] entitled "Decreasing cardiovascular disease and increasing cancer among whites in the United States from 1973 through 1987, good news and bad news", showed that while heart disease was declining, cancer mortality for men and women born after 1940 was much higher than for previous generations. These cancers were not linked to smoking, but were relegated to other environmental factors. For men the rate of cancer was 200% of that of previous generations, and for women the rate was 50% higher. Not only are cancer rates rising, but there is currently an alarming rise in the incidence of asthma, especially among children throughout the world. These incidents appear to be associated with ambient pollution levels. Much has also been said about the estrogenic effect of certain environmental chemicals and the devastating effect upon wildlife, and possibly humans as well.

There is, therefore, much evidence to indicate that several chronic health problems appear to be related to environmental chemicals. For the purpose of this chapter, the discussion is confined to the known immunotoxic, neurotoxic and endocrinotoxic effects of these environmental chemicals.

Immunotoxicity

Environmental chemicals have a wide range of damaging effects on the function of the immune system. These range from decreased cell-mediated immunity (with a decrease in infection and tumor fighting) to increased sensitivity (allergy) and increased autoimmunity.[21–23]

Organochlorine compounds

Among the organochlorine compounds (OCCs), DDT has been found to have many damaging effects on the immune system:

- reduced killing capacity of PMNs
- reduced number of plasma responder cells
- increased degranulation of mast cells
- leukopenia
- decreased phagocytic ability
- changes in the spleen, thymus, and lymph glands
- variation in complement
- disturbances in fetal and perinatal immune regulation.

Similar effects have also been found after exposure to hexachlorobenzene (HCB) and the chlordanes (also OCCs).[23] Hexachlorobenzene is a chlorinated pesticide used as a fungicide. It is also found to be present in chlorinated solvents such as perchloroethylene, which is used in dry cleaning and is very elevated in individuals from western Europe. Chlordanes were primarily used as termiticides in the US and Canada until 1978 when they were banned from use in the home. They are still used on certain crops and in some seed treatment.

Studies of thousands of patients at the Environmental Health Center-Dallas have shown that persons with two or more OCCs present in their serum have some form of immunotoxicity.[24]

Polycylic aromatic hydrocarbons

The chemicals produced by combustion, the polycyclic aromatic hydrocarbons (PAHs), have been shown to have similar inhibiting effects on the immune system, including:[25]

- decreased T-cell-dependent antibody response
- decreased splenic activity
- diminished T-cell effector functions
- suppression of T-cytotoxic induction
- lower natural killer cell activity.

They are also highly carcinogenic.

Organophosphate pesticides

The organophosphate pesticides (OPs), which are not as biologically persistent as the OCCs, are also toxic to the immune system. They have been found to cause decreased percentages of CD_4 and CD_5 cells, increased number and percentages of CD_{26} cells, increased incidence of atopy and antibiotic sensitivity, and high rates of autoimmunity. This elevation in autoimmunity is reflected by high levels of antibodies to smooth muscle, parietal cells, brush border, thyroid, myelin and elevated ANA.[26] Similar immunosuppression is also found for the organotins and for the heavy metals.[26]

The mode of exposure to the pesticide appears to have an effect on the persistence of immunotoxicity, as demonstrated by two polybrominated biphenyl (PBB) spills. One exposure took place in Taiwan when rice bran cooking oil was contaminated with PBBs. Those who used this oil for cooking were found to have immune abnormalities. One year after exposure, they were found to have decreased concentrations of IgM and IgA (with normal IgG), low T-suppresser cells, low B-cells and suppression of delayed hypersensitivity to recall antigens. When rechecked 2 years after exposure, the above indices had returned to normal. This was not the case in Michigan, where a massive PBB spill occurred in 1973/74. During that time, a PBB-containing flame retardant called "Firemaster" was inadvertently sold as an animal feed called "Nutrimaster". This mistake was devastating to both the livestock and those who raised them and consumed their products. Exposed individuals were found to have lower levels of circulating T-lymphocytes and reduced lymphoproliferation response, resulting in reduced cell-mediated immunity (CMI). They also had a high prevalence of persistent skin, neurological and musculoskeletal symptoms.[27] These changes have persisted in all subsequent studies. This seems to indicate that when these toxins are concentrated in the food chain before reaching humans, their effect is longer lasting.

(For a good review of numerous studies of the immunotoxicity of pesticides the author recommends Repetto & Baliga[28]).

Autoimmune disease

The development of autoimmunity has been linked with chemical exposure as well. The notion of chemically induced autoimmune states is, of course, not new since many chemicals are known to induce the onset of SLE. Some chemicals, like formaldehyde and other volatile organic compounds, are thought to induce tissue-specific autoimmune reactions by acting as haptens. These low-molecular-weight molecules will bind to various tissues in the body, making a new antigenic combination. The immune system then makes an antibody to this new combination which can attack the parent tissue with or without the chemicals being present. Chemically exposed individuals will often present with elevated antibodies to certain body tissues, including anti-myelin, anti-parietal, anti-brush border, and anti-smooth muscle.[29] The abnormalities found in a study of 298 patients exposed to industrial chemicals are shown in Table 37.2.

Table 37.2 Abnormalities found in patients with exposure to industrial chemicals[30]

- Either very low activity or very high activity when compared with controls
- Lymphocyte blastogenic response to T-cell mitogens (PHA, CONA) and B-cell mitogens were between 30 and 45% lower than controls
- Elevated IgG and IgM levels against formaldehyde, trimellitic anhydride, phthalic anhydride, and benzene ring. These rates were usually higher in persons with elevated T4/T8 ratio, which was found in almost 15% of the exposed patients
- Autoantibodies against their own tissue

Toxin-associated cancers

As mentioned earlier, the Davis et al[20] study showed that men born in the 1940s had twice as many cancers as those born in 1888–1897, and more than twice as many cancers not linked to smoking. Women born in the 1940s had 50% more cancers, and 30% more cancers not linked to smoking (whites). In the following, we present a condensed version of the voluminous amount of information available in the literature associating cancers with environmental toxins.

Breast cancer

One of the cancers that has very clear association with environmental chemicals is breast cancer. Three studies have shown elevated levels of different OCCs in the adipose tissue of breast cancer patients as compared with controls. The chemicals found to be higher in the women with malignancies were DDT, DDE, PCBs and HCH (hexachlorocyclohexane; also known as Lindane or BHC, this is a chlorinated pesticide that is still commonly used to treat lice infestations (Kwell shampoo)).[31–33] Not only are they higher in the adipose tissue of breast cancer patients, but they are actually found in higher concentrations in the malignant tissue than in adjacent healthy tissue.[31]

Serum levels of OCCs have also been associated with an increased risk of breast cancer. Elevated levels of DDE and PCB in the serum can indicate a fourfold increased risk of breast cancer compared with normal risk (which is already too high).[32] The author has found that individuals with breast cancer often have both higher levels and greater numbers of individual OCCs than other patients. If Wolff et al's information is correct,[32] then serum testing of OCCs may provide an easily obtained and reliable means of assessing breast cancer risk. The presumption may then be made that early detection of elevated levels of DDE and PCB, followed by prompt treatment, could conceivably drastically reduce the risk for developing breast cancer in certain individuals.

Childhood cancers

Childhood cancers have also been evaluated for epidemiological association with chemical exposure. In one study, 45 childhood brain cancer patients were compared with 85 friend controls. A significant positive association was found between brain cancer and exposure to no-pest strips, termite treatment, Kwell shampoo (Lindane), flea collars on pets, diazinon use in the garden or orchard, and the use of herbicides in yard (odds ratio [OR], 6.2). When compared with 108 controls, a significant positive association was found with pesticide bombs in the home, termite treatment, flea collars on pets, insecticide use in the garden, carbaryl in garden, and herbicide use in the garden.[33]

Several other studies of childhood chemical exposures found the following associations:

- 2,4-D (a common weed killer) use around the home associated with soft tissue sarcomas (OR, 4.0)[34]
- no-pest strips in the home associated with leukemia (OR, 3.0)
- insecticide use in the home associated with brain tumors for those aged <20 (OR, 2.3)
- household pesticide use associated with leukemia (OR, 4.0)
- garden pesticide use associated with leukemia (OR, 5.6)
- household insecticide use associated with nonlymphocytic leukemia (OR, 3.5).

2,4-D, a chlorophenoxy acid herbicide, gained notoriety from its combination with 2,4,5-T to form a mixture known as "Agent Orange". It is commonly used by municipalities and states to spray roadways and rights-of-way to keep the weeds down. It can be purchased at home stores for home lawn care and is often applied by chemical lawn care companies. It contains several dioxin contaminates and, in my opinion, is quite toxic to animals, children and adults.

For adults, the use of chlorophenoxy acid herbicides (2,4-D) has been strongly associated with an increased incidence of lung cancer, stomach cancer, leukemia, Hodgkin's lymphoma (two studies found a fivefold increased risk), non-Hodgkin's lymphomas (NHL, five- to sixfold increased risk), and soft tissue sarcomas (many studies have shown a five to sevenfold increased risk, with one review study finding a 40-fold increased risk).[35] One study showed Kansas farmers having a sixfold increased risk of lymphomas and soft tissue sarcomas in persons using it 20+ days/year compared with non-exposed individuals. Those who mixed and applied herbicides and were exposed 20+ days/year were eight times as likely to contract NHL.

Factors associated with increased risk of NHL from 2,4-D exposure are:

- increased period of time of exposure
- not using protective equipment
- using backpack or hand sprayers
- employing tractor-mounted or mist blower sprayer
- applying herbicides aerially.

Hematologic malignancies

Several studies have associated exposure to solvents with acute myelogenous leukemia (AML), multiple myeloma, and other forms of leukemia. A retrospective cohort study of 14,457 workers exposed to trichloroethylene between 1952 and 1953 showed that mortality was increased for multiple myeloma and NHL in white women.[36] In a Finnish study, workers exposed to 1,1,1-trichloroethylene showed excess cancers of the cervix uteri and lymphohematopoietic tissues. After 10 years (from the first measurement), excess pancreatic cancer and NHL were seen. At a 20 year follow-up, excess multiple myeloma and cancer of the nervous system were found. Workers exposed to trichloroethylene showed (after a 20 year follow-up) an excess of cancers of the stomach, liver, prostate, and lymphohematopoeitic tissues.[37]

A review article revealed that there have been 280 cases of aplastic anemia associated with pesticide exposure reported in the literature. The majority of these cases were young (average age 34) with a short latency (mean, 5 months) and had a history of occupational exposure to pesticides.[38] Another study which looked at the cancer risk for painters showed increased cancer rates for multiple myeloma (OR, 1.95), bladder tumors (OR, 1.52), as well as kidney and other urothelial tumors (OR, 1.45).[39] A study in Sweden of 275 confirmed diagnoses of multiple myeloma showed a clear association between farming and multiple myeloma. This study revealed that exposures to chlorophenoxy acid herbicides (2,4-D) and DDT were prime risk factors.[40]

Neurotoxicity

The nervous system is a particularly sensitive target for toxic agents for several reasons, as listed in Table 37.3.

Besides the nervous system being such a good target, there are powerful neurotoxic agents available to attack it. Most of the major classes of pesticides kill pests by attacking their nervous system. They are neurotoxins by design. The OCCs affect the nerve by disrupting the ion flow along the axon. The OPs, which came out of nerve

Table 37.3 Reasons for the high sensitivity of the nervous system to toxins

- The adult neuron does not divide, and therefore replacement of lost neurons is not possible. Nerve cells killed by toxins cannot regenerate
- The blood–brain barrier does not block non-polar substances or items that are actively transported
- Since the normal function of the nervous system requires the action of a complex integrated network, damage to even a small portion of the nervous system can sometimes result in marked effects on function
- Neurons are dependent on glucose and oxygen, and some cell bodies exist at borderline levels of O_2. If high-energy demands are placed on the system, and delivery of O_2 is reduced, then cell death may occur
- Because of high lipid content (myelin) there is an accumulation and storage of lipophylic xenobiotics
- Neurons have high surface areas and therefore increased exposure to toxins

gas research, and carbamates affect acetylcholinesterase, resulting in excessive acetylcholine levels in the synapses. Solvents, some of which were originally used as anesthetics, dampen the propagation and transmission of electrical impulses along the nerve axons. All of these agents produce various forms of toxic encephalopathy (either acute or chronic, selective or diffuse toxic encephalopathies), as neuronopathies, axonopathies, myelinopathies or vasculopathies.

Neuronopathies

Neuronopathies can be diffuse or selective, depending on whether specific neurons are affected, or if the damage is more broadly spread throughout the nervous system. The target site of toxic agents producing neuronopathies is the nerve cell body, with the consequence of either axonal or dendritic breakdown.

An example of a neurotoxin causing diffuse neuronopathy is methylmercury which preferentially damages the granule cells of layer IV in the visual cortex, granule cells in the granular layer of the cerebellum, and the sensory neurons of the dorsal root ganglia.[26] This brings about neuronal degeneration, progressing to necrosis with axonal dystrophy and demyelination. Another is aluminum which causes fatal dialysis encephalopathy following 3–7 years of intermittent dialysis. Although brain aluminum levels were elevated, there was no evidence of neurofibrillary tangles in these patients, indicating that the presence of aluminum alone is insufficient to lead to the senile dementia of the Alzheimer's type.

The neuronopathies can also be selective, affecting only certain neurons. Examples of agents causing selective neuronopathies would include adriamycin, which affects the dorsal root ganglia; cisplatin, which affects sensory neurons; and manganese (metal fume fever), which produces a Parkinson-like syndrome.

Manganese-induced damage is found in the substantia nigra, globus pallidus, and caudate nucleus, with depletion of dopamine and serotonin levels. Symptoms begin with psychiatric changes followed by impaired motor activity with muscle rigidity and tremors. Parkinsonism is also caused by MPTP, a contaminant found in synthetic heroin.[41] This compound has brought on sudden Parkinson-like symptoms rapidly after exposure to the heroin. MPTP is metabolized in monoamine-oxidase (MAO) containing tissues to MPP+, "the ultimate neurotoxin to MAO-containing tissues" which is selectively toxic to substantia nigra cells. It effectively blocks dopamine production.[42]

Axonopathies

Axonopathies are differentiated by the area of the axon that is affected. The proximal axon is different in its ability to initiate action potentials and to synthesize protein. Damage to this part of the axon is referred to as proximal axonopathy. This is the type of damage seen in amyotrophic lateral sclerosis (ALS). Proximal axonopathies are often caused by volatile organic compounds – e.g. halomethane, methylene chloride, carbon tetrachloride, and butane – all of which decrease the excitability of the neuron by stabilizing membranes and decreasing ion flux. Distal axonopathies have been shown to be caused by a variety of compounds including Acrylamide (a polymerizing agent to strengthen paper) which primarily affects sensory fibers, and carbon disulfide (a solvent for fats and lacquers and for extraction of oil from olives, palmstones and other oil-bearing fruits) which produces distal axonopathy to both sensory and motor fibers. It also decreases norepinephrine levels. Hexacarbon solvents lead to multifocal distal progressive sensorimotor axonopathy with giant axonal swelling. Paranodal demyelination of swollen axons occurs frequently with exposure to these solvents.

The group of compounds that causes distal axonopathies also includes the OPs (Parathion, malathion, diazinon, etc.) and the carbamates. OPs cause acetylcholinesterase enzymes to be phosphorylated. Exposures may be additive and the effects may last until more acetylcholinesterase is synthesized. Carbamates (carbaryl, sevin, aldicarb) cause the acetylcholinesterase to be carbamylated. This is not a stable bond, and is hydrolyzed fairly easily.

Myelinopathies

Myelinopathies are caused by the organotins, which are used as stabilizers in plastic polymers and catalysts in silicon and epoxy curing. They are also used in wood and textile preservation as fungicides, bactericides and insecticides. Examples of the organotins are TET and TMT. Hexachlorophene (HCP) added to soaps for antimicrobial action also causes damage to the myelin. It is readily absorbed through intact skin and mucous membranes. Like TET and TMT, it causes blurred vision and muscular weakness progressing to paralysis. The optic nerve is particularly susceptible to HCP. The optic nerve is also sensitive to particular solvents, such as ingested methanol and ethanol, inhaled trichlorethylene, toluene, CS_2, and benzene. Other solvents can lead to specific myelinopathies, as the trigeminal nerve is especially sensitive to trichloroethylene (found in dry cleaning fluid). Hearing loss is commonly caused by toluene, styrene, xylene, and trichloroethylene, which causes myelin damage to the vestibulocochlear nerve. Other toxins, such as carbon monoxide and cuprisone (a copper chelating agent used in the treatment of Wilson's disease), are examples of toxins affecting the maintenance of myelin.

Lead, a well-known neurotoxin, brings about encephalopathy by causing vascular changes leading to neuronal degeneration and necrosis as well as by causing neuronal degeneration itself. Early stages of plumbism include headache and nausea. Demyelination of motor nerves is also seen with lead.

Endocrinotoxicity

With the exception of the rodenticide Vacor, agents that affect endocrine function, other than reproduction, tend to be compounds with extensive effects on other organs as well (heavy metals, pesticides, solvents). It would be very unusual to find an endocrine disorder as the sole or primary manifestation of an environmental toxicity.

The most common symptoms of toxic damage to the endocrine system are listed in Table 37.4.

Adrenal gland

In addition to the well documented estrogenic effect of the OCCs, actual damage to the endocrine organs is also noticeable. Aliphatic compounds (3–6 carbons in length with electronegative groups on both ends) cause necrosis of zona fasiculata and zona reticularis of the adrenals, where the glucocorticoids are produced. OCCs and carbamates have caused histologic changes to these areas in animal models.[26,43] Cadmium and CCl_4 have both been shown to cause non-specific inhibition of steroidogenesis. Occupational lead workers showed decreased secretions of corticosteroids, both glucocorticoids (17-hydroxy) and androgenic steroids (17-keto). In these persons, the lesion was apparently at the hypothalamus/pituitary level because normal ACTH response was found with stimulation. Dioxins and mirex (used to treat fire ants) cause direct suppression of glucocorticoid synthesis, resulting in hypoglycemia.

Table 37.4 Common symptoms of toxic damage to the endocrine system

- Sleep disturbances or changes in energy level or mood
- Alterations in weight, appetite and bowel function
- Sexual interest and function change; in females any menstrual change
- Changes in temperature perception, sweating, or flushing
- Alteration of hair growth and skin texture

Thyroid

The thyroid is not immune to environmental toxins, as many chemicals can cause a reduction of both T4 and T3. Thiocyanates, perchlorates and pertechnetates are all competitive inhibitors of iodine transport in the thyroid, causing decreases in T4 and T3 and an increase in TSH. Compounds which inhibit the thyroid peroxidase needed in the second step of thyroid hormone synthesis include:

- thiourea
- thiouracil
- PTU
- carbimazole
- aniline derivatives
- PABA
- substituted phenols like resorcinol
- phloroglucinol.

Iodide and lithium block thyroid hormone release from the gland itself. Depressed levels of thyroid function have been correlated with exposures to lead, carbon disulfide, and PBBs. Lead workers, a heavily studied population, appear to suffer from a decrease in thyroid secondary to problems with the hypothalamus (TRF). In Michigan, PBB-exposed persons showed non-goitrogenic thyroid dysfunction. Less well documented, but suggested to adversely affect the thyroid, are:

- organophosphates
- carbamates
- OCCs
- fungicides
- food coloring
- PCBs
- mercury (animal studies).

Inducers of hepatic cytochrome P450 like phenobarbital, benzodiazepines, calcium-channel blockers, steroids, retinoids, chlorinated hydrocarbons, and polyhalogenated biphenyls will (in addition to inducing P450) cause alteration in thyroid structure, leading to reduction in T4.[25]

Besides causing reduced functioning, some compounds will also cause thyroid cancer. Polycyclic hydrocarbons, nitrosamines, and other compounds are initiators of thyroid carcinogenesis. A common component of permanent hair dye preparations, 2,4-diaminoanisole sulfate (2,4-DAAS), when fed at high doses, caused a 58%

incidence of thyroid neoplasms in male rats and 42% in females, compared with 7–8% in controls.[25]

Reproductive

The effect of environmental chemicals, especially the estrogenic OCCs, are well documented. While many are estrogenic by themselves, when combined together their estrogenicity can increase by a factor of 1,600. Some combinations can also cause previously non-estrogenic compounds to become estrogenic.[44] The facts about environmental estrogens have been cogently set forth in Theo Colborn et al's recent book *Our Stolen Future,* and the reader is directed to that excellent resource for a comprehensive discussion[45]. However, there are also non-estrogenic toxic effects of the OCCs on both male and female reproduction. High levels of OCCs in the serum have been strongly linked to infertility, stillbirths and miscarriages.[46] Urban air pollution has been associated with reduced male fertility.[47] While there appears to be a worldwide decline in the sperm levels of males,[48] males who are organic farmers have very high sperm density.[49] This gives rise to the supposition that exposure to environmental chemicals lowers sperm levels, and that avoidance of such chemicals may help to bring the levels back up. There have been multiple studies on one OCC that is used agriculturally – dibromochloropropane (DBCP) – looking at its effect on sperm levels. These studies have demonstrated that exposure to DBCP leads to azospermia, and severe oligospermia.[50] This may be only associated with DBCP or it may serve as a model of other OCC-induced spermatogenesis problems.

DIAGNOSIS

History

A comprehensive history is the cornerstone of detecting chemically induced health problems. When taking a history, special attention should be paid to both occupational and non-occupational chemical exposures. Occupational exposures are usually the easiest to document, and should always be followed up with a request for the material safety data sheet on each chemical from the employer. Non-occupational exposures are harder to document, but in a family practice are often found to be the main culprit. Specific questions should be asked about the history of residences:

- where the patient lived
- how new the structure is
- age of carpeting
- time of remodel
- type of heating
- use of indoor or outdoor pesticides
- attached garage, etc.

Once the history of residential exposure is garnered and compared with the chronological symptom history, the answer may become quite clear.

Laboratory

Given the ubiquitous nature of the chemicals in question, a history may not always provide a clear picture of exposure. Laboratory tests may be helpful in these cases. The standard CBC and general blood chemistry tests are usually non-remarkable in cases of chronic low-level exposures (although the author has often found leukopenia in his population of toxic patients). In addition, liver enzymes, even when solvents and pesticides are present in the serum, are rarely elevated.[51] Serum tests for the presence of OCCs and solvents are invaluable in detecting such problems. When interpreting these tests, the clinician must keep in mind that the laboratory "normals" generally reflect the average level found in the blood of the most toxic population in the country (the population tested by the laboratory), not the average American. There is no "RDA" for pesticides or solvents, and the presence of any of these compounds should be cause for concern. It should also be kept in mind that serum levels of these compounds are generally lower than tissue levels. This has been demonstrated with DDE in which 1 ppb in the serum will indicate that 5–10 ppb would be found in the brain, 47 ppb in the liver, and 100–300 ppb in the adipose tissue.

If the patient has been exposed to OPs or carbamates, then plasma or RBC cholinesterase levels can be measured. Unfortunately, it is often difficult to assess an OP or carbamate pesticide exposure with this method unless a pre-exposure cholinesterase was obtained for use as a baseline. If that was not done, then a follow-up cholinesterase test may be done after 3 months, provided that the patient does not return to more exposures.

Carbon monoxide exposure can be easily checked with a carboxyhemoglobin level.

If the patient is poisoned by a chemical that cannot be tested for in the serum or urine, then other tests can be considered. Immune panels including T and B subsets, autoantibody panels, chemical antibodies, and NK activity will all indicate that toxin-induced damage to the immune system has occurred.[23]

Neurotoxicity can be diagnosed by SPECT scans,[52] evoked response audiometry,[53] balance testing, and measurement with an iris corder. It can also be indicated when a positive Rhombergism is present.[25]

TREATMENT

The basics of effective treatment for chemically induced illnesses are:

- avoidance of further exposures

- supplementation to support chemical elimination and antioxidant protection mechanisms
- reduction of the body burden of xenobiotics.

Avoidance

Avoidance of further chemical exposure cannot be overlooked, although compliance is often very difficult to obtain. In cases of multiple chemical sensitivity, avoidance is indispensable. Compounds to be avoided include:

- solvents
- paints
- exhaust fumes
- perfumes
- hair sprays
- new furniture
- carpeting, and cabinetry
- plastics
- gas or oil heat, etc.

Since the home is the environment that is most in the patient's control, the home must be made a "safe oasis". If there are building materials that are off-gassing chemicals and these materials cannot be removed, they should be sealed. A number of good books are available to help with this process.[54–56] If the living space has molds present, an ozone generator can be used to clear out the molds. It is very important that no one be present in the home when an ozone generator is being used, as ozone is a potent respiratory sensitizer.

In addition to avoiding environmental chemicals, any foods that cause adverse reactions should be avoided (see Ch. 51). Organically grown foods should be consumed wherever possible as well as purified water. Air purifiers can be used to help reduce the level of chemicals in the indoor air. Charcoal or Hepa filters do the best job of clearing toxins out of the air, but some plants do an admirable job as well. In a study from NASA, five plants were found to be the most effective in cleaning the air:[57]

- Mass cane (Dracaena massangeana)
- Pot mum (Chrysanthemum morifolium)
- Gerbera daisy (Gerbera jamesonii)
- Warnecki (Dracaena deremensis "Warnecki")
- ficus (Ficus benjamina).

If plants are chosen as the preferred method for cleaning the air, then the specific room to be cleaned must have many plants put in it. A single plant in a normal-sized room will have no effect. The author generally tells his patients to "make your home a jungle". Those that have complied with these instructions invariably report that their symptoms decreased after the plants were introduced.

Nutritional support

Nutritional support is aimed at two main areas: critical cofactors for enzymatic biotransformation of xenobiotic compounds, and antioxidants. Additional supplementation will undoubtedly be needed to address the organ systems and tissues that have been damaged by the xenobiotic compounds. However, that is not the focus of this chapter.

Protein

Metabolism of toxic chemicals and drugs has been shown to be impaired by protein deprivation (see Table 37.5). Increased toxicity of chemical compounds and drugs have been reported with protein deficiency. Protein deficiency decreases the activity of liver mixed function oxidase (MFO) systems, which results in an increase in the half-life of numerous toxic chemicals and drugs and potentiates drug action and toxicity. The quantity and quality of protein in the diet alter both phase I and phase II liver drug metabolism processes (a gelatin diet induces very low MFO activity). The toxicity of OCCs, acetylcholinesterase inhibitors, herbicides, and fungicides have all been shown to be increased several-fold by protein deficiency. Reduced clearance and increased half-life of antipyrine are found in Asian vegetarians eating a low-protein diet. This was not found in Caucasian vegetarians with adequate protein intake.

While protein deficiency clearly reduces the ability of the body to adequately metabolize chemicals, the opposite also appears to be true.[58] Isocalorically increasing of the ratio of dietary protein to carbohydrate in well-nourished volunteers has been shown to enhance clearance of antipyrine and theophylline. While it is not clear if the effect of the protein is due to the amino acid content alone, it is known that methionine and cysteine deficiency leads to reduction of intestinal and hepatic MFO enzyme activity. Hepatic MFO activity can also be suppressed by folic and choline deficiency. Low methionine intake also impacts selenium metabolism by making less selenium available for GSH-peroxidase biosynthesis. High sugar intake is also known to reduce the clearance rate of certain chemicals from the liver.

Vitamin E

Vitamin E is a well known stabilizer of membranes and therefore facilitates a suitable environment for the

Table 37.5 Effects of a low-protein diet on detoxification

- Decreased cytochrome P450 content of liver, secondary to decreased quantity of microsomal protein
- Decreased NADPH-cytochrome P-450 (c) reductase
- Decreased cytochrome b5
- Decrease in hepatic GSH
- Increased liver UDP-glucuronlytransferase (phase II)

synthesis and activity of membrane-associated enzymes that protect against toxin damage. In addition, it has antioxidant properties. Although CCl_4 does not cause liver damage via lipid peroxidation, vitamin E partially prevents CCl_4 hepatotoxicity. Pretreatment of animals and humans with vitamin E prior to ozone and nitrous oxide exposure has been shown to provide partial protection against the toxicity of these agents.

Vitamin A and beta-carotene

Beta-carotene is required for epithelial cell differentiation and regulates the stability of biological membranes. It quenches singlet oxygen species non-chemically and is essential for a normal estrogen cycle. Beta-carotene also protects against singlet oxygen-induced damage.

Deficiency of vitamin A is associated with increased binding of benzo(*a*)pyrene to tracheal epithelia. Organophosphates, DDT and PCBs will decrease the vitamin A content in the liver which increases their toxic effect on the body. In another example of how veterinarian nutritional care is more advance then human care, an intramuscular injection of 1,500,000 units of vitamin A is given yearly to cattle to treat organophosphate poisoning. OPs are applied directly to the animals once yearly to take care of insects that would otherwise cause problems with the cattle. The author has not yet heard of the farmers who apply these pesticides by hand to each of their cattle ever getting the vitamin A injection!

Other items that lower vitamin A levels are:

- alcohol
- coffee
- cold weather
- cortisone
- diabetes
- excessive iron
- infections
- laxatives
- liver disease
- mineral oil
- nitrates
- sugar
- tobacco
- vitamin D deficiency
- zinc deficiency.

Thiamin

Thiamin depletion occurs from excess formaldehyde exposure or any other items that increase aldehydes (alcohol, *Candida*, etc.), because the coenzyme of thiamin (TPP) is used to metabolize the aldehyde group. Magnesium is also used in this process. Thiamin also serves as a coenzyme (TPP) for pyruvate dehydrogenase and alpha-ketoglutarate dehydrogenase. Besides being used in the phase II pathways, thiamin is needed to restore oxidized GSH.

Thiamin deficiency increases the toxicity of PCBs, dieldrin, heptachlor and the aniline dyes. These compounds can also lead to thiamin deficiency, which enhances their toxicity.

Treatment of cattle with 100 mg/day of thiamin prevents clinical signs of lead poisoning and death.

Riboflavin

Riboflavin is a component of the coenzymes in various flavoprotein enzymes required for oxidation/reduction reactions. Liver microsomal flavoprotein NADPH-cytochrome reductase supplies reducing equivalents to cytochrome P450. These are essential for proper functioning of the phase I biotransformation pathways. Riboflavin facilitates the destruction of azo dyes in the liver by MFO, thereby protecting against azo dye-induced cancer. Riboflavin is also used in the glutathione reductase pathways, which work with SOD to block free radical damage.

Niacin

Nicotinamide is a component of two related coenzymes NAD and NADP which are oxidized to NAD^+ and $NADP^+$, and are reduced to NADH and NADPH. These are needed for the proper functioning of phase I. This vitamin is used in the deamination of amino acids, fatty acid synthesis, and beta-oxidation of fatty acids. It also participates in steroid formation and drug metabolism.

Pyridoxine

Exposure to carbon disulfide (CS_2), PCBs and penicillamine has been shown to disrupt the normal function of vitamin B_6. Chronic exposure to these compounds can cause B_6 deficiency. Dr Rea has stated that 60% of the chemically sensitive patients at EHC-Dallas are deficient in this nutrient, whether or not they are taking oral supplements.[6]

Low B_6 can lead to low taurine levels. When taurine is low, extreme sensitivities to chlorine, chlorite (bleach), aldehydes, alcohols, solvents, and ammonia can develop. Vitamin B_6 deficiency also results in a poor ability to conjugate epinephrine and serotonin.

Vitamin C

A cellular antioxidant, ascorbic acid scavenges free radical superoxides and hydroxyl radicals. It protects against phenol, phenylqumolin, carboxylic acid and barbiturate toxicity. It protects against ozone-induced pulmonary edema, O_2 toxicity and CCl_4 toxicity. It reduces the toxicity of pesticides, heavy metals, hydrocarbons, PCB, and acetaminophen. It enhances MFO activity (there is decreased cytochrome P450 activity in vitamin C deficiency) and enhances the incorporation of iron into heme. Vitamin C prevents nitrosamine formation from nitrites in the gastrointestinal tract, and protects against lead and cadmium toxicity.

Elevated levels of dietary vitamin C may facilitate metabolic degradation of xenobiotics by liver MFO. Conversely xenobiotics will increase vitamin C excretion in the urine.

Iron

Iron plays a central role in the heme-containing molecules of cytochrome P450 and hemoglobin. However, there is no apparent increase in phase I levels with supplementation of iron. Aniline metabolism is most sensitive to iron deficiency, and increases susceptibility to lead toxicity, yet there is a decrease in MFO activity in iron-overloading states.

Magnesium

A deficiency of magnesium was found in 40% of the chemically sensitive patients at EHC-Dallas.[6] Deficiency of magnesium leads to decreased amounts of cytochrome P450 and NADPH cytochrome reductase, both of which are essential to the proper functioning of phase I. Decreased hydroxylation of aniline, and demethylation of aminopyrene are seen in cases of magnesium deficiency. Fortunately, magnesium supplementation reverses both of these effects.

Selenium

Selenium is a required component of glutathione peroxidase (GSH-PX) which maintains integrity of cellular and subcellular membranes, as well as being one of the main molecules for phase II xenobiotic conjugation. Fortunately selenium supplementation increases GSH-PX levels, something that reduced glutathione supplementation does not appear to do. This feat is also accomplished by supplementation with *N*-acetyl cysteine and L-cysteine. This provides us with a low-cost, reliable method to increase GSH levels. Selenium reduces the toxicity of lead, and increases biliary excretion of cadmium and mercury. It also prevents the typical cadmium-induced decrease of Cyto-P450.

Selenium deficiency increases the toxicity of numerous xenobiotic compounds.

Zinc

Both deficient and excess zinc can influence the metabolism and detoxification of xenobiotics. Zinc deficiency decreases enzyme function, but excess zinc decreases cytochrome P450 levels! Zinc deficiency also causes a reduction of GSH levels.

Glutathione (GSH)

Not only is glutathione crucial to the glutathione conjugation pathway, one of the phase II pathways, but it is also one of the main molecules that quenches the peroxide molecules in the body, especially in the liver. While many naturally minded physicians give reduced glutathione to their patients in the hope of helping to increase their levels, there is insufficient evidence to support this practice at the present time. There is only one human study on oral glutathione absorption, and the subjects showed no increase in their glutathione levels with oral supplementation.[59] All of the other studies reported the use of injectable or food source GSH rather than oral doses. On the other hand, there have been many studies showing that supplementation with selenium, *N*-acetyl cysteine, cysteine, vitamin A and vitamin E can increase GSH levels.[60] Other compounds such as the botanical medicine *Silybum marianum* have also been shown to increase the GSH level. Vitamins E and C, as well as cysteine have all been shown to inhibit GSH depletion and lipid peroxidation after endrin exposure.

Botanical medicines

The two major botanical medicines useful in treating chemical toxicity are *Silybum marianum* (milk thistle) and *Curcuma longa* (turmeric). The reader is referred to the Chapters 111 and 80 further information.

Depuration (cleansing)

The removal of impurities from the body is known as depuration. This is the preferred term for cleansing xenobiotics from the body. The commonly used term "detoxification" means to remove or alter the toxic quality of a compound. Since healing for the toxic person involves removal of the actual xenobiotic from the body, rather than mere alteration of the compound, the word depuration will be used.

There are only two methods of xenobiotic depuration discussed in the scientific literature. Most of the published literature is from one of the Health Med clinics, associated with the Church of Scientology, who are doing the "Hubbard purification rundown". This protocol utilizes exercise, high temperature saunas, increasing doses of niacin, and electrolyte replacement. They have published several studies showing the benefit of this protocol for reducing levels of PCBs, PBBs, and HCBs.[61–63] Their studies, along with unpublished data from William Rea MD at the Environmental Health Center-Dallas have shown that sauna therapy will bring about a reduction of the xenobiotic levels in treated individuals.

The only published treatment besides sauna therapy that has shown benefit in treating poisoned individuals is fasting (see Ch. 47). This has been documented in a study which looked at individuals poisoned by PBB-contaminated rice bran cooking oil in Taiwan.[64] While fasting reduced their symptoms, it increased the level of circulating xenobiotics in their serum. Presumably the elevation of circulating toxins is due to the increased rate of lipolysis in fasting individuals. Thus the fat-soluble PBBs were released from storage into the bloodstream at higher than normal rates. At that point, it would be up to the liver to clear these out of the serum or they would be redeposited into the adipose tissue. More research is obviously needed on the role of fasting in the treatment of environmental overload.

A comprehensive naturopathic protocol for treating environmentally poisoned individuals was developed by the author and has been used for over 10 years. An outcome study on patients who underwent this protocol for a variety of chemically induced ills showed it to be surprisingly effective. Of the subjects (with various problems) treated with the depuration protocol, 83% rated their results as good or great. The two conditions in which 100% of the participants reported great results were asthma ($n = 3$), and addiction recovery ($n = 1$). The problem (chief complaint) categories in which 100% of the participants rated their results as moderate, good or great were autoimmune, dermatological, and GI/liver. The categories with the next highest ratings of moderate, good or great were fatigue, with 92% improvement; allergies, with 85% improvement; and chemical sensitivities, with 84% improvement.[65]

The Crinnion depuration protocol

The Crinnion depuration protocol consists of the following components:

- *Exercise* – daily exercise usually consisting of using an exercycle, rebounder or brisk walking to begin lipolysis and diaphoresis.
- *Thermal chambers*. Up to three 60 minute "sauna" sesions are done with temperatures at a range of 120–135°F with cool-down periods in between. Glass bottled spring water is given along with electrolyte replacement. While the Hubbard clinics use higher temperatures, we find that individuals will put out more toxins (as evidenced by stronger chemical odors) and will experience less adverse symptoms when the lower temperatures are used. The thermal chambers will increase the rate of lipolysis in the adipose tissue throughout the body. When this occurs the lipophilic xenobiotics will be released into the bloodstream. The compounds in the subcutaneous fat pads will be mobilized through sweat as well as into the blood.
- *Constitutional hydrotherapy* – the use of alternating hot and cold towels with sine wave stimulation as done by pioneering naturopaths Drs O. G. Carrol and Harold Dick. This therapy has been used for decades to stimulate the body's own self-healing activity. We have found that it also increased the amount of toxin-laden bile dumped from the liver into the intestines. Also assisting the cholerectic and cholegogue action on the liver is a herbal capsule taken daily consisting of *Chelidonium*, *Chionanthus*, *Taraxacum*, *Arctium lappa*, *Silybum marianum* and *Urtica dioca*.
- *Colonic irrigation*. Gravity-fed machines are used to gently introduce triple-filtered water into the large intestines, providing an avenue for the toxic bile to rapidly leave the body. Individuals will routinely have "liver dumps" of bile that ranges in color from yellow to red, with occasional gray or brown. The color of bile normally ranges from green to yellow to orange to red depending upon the amount of time of exposure to bacterial action in the bowel. However, in this situation we believe that it is dumped from the liver and rapidly passed through the small intestines, similar to what is seen in "gastric dumping" syndrome. We are therefore unable to account for the differences in color of this effluent. In some patients with heavy agricultural exposure, we have seen higher amounts of fluorescent yellow bile. Hence, the color of the bile may be more attributable to the chemical compounds in the bile than the bacterial action upon the bile. We have documented that chlorinated pesticides are present in this effluent that we refer to as "bile dumps".
- *Constitutional homeopathy*. This has been used primarily as a stand-alone treatment with the use of any other supplements or treatments prohibited. However, we have found it to be a valuable component of this protocol and completely compatible with all the other treatment methods involved. It appears most beneficial in those individuals who need a boost for their vital force to facilitate their moving toward healing, and for those who are stuck in emotional issues that they haven't been willing to look at.
- *Body therapies (massage, shiatsu, craniosacral, visceral, spinal and joint adjustment)*. These are done as needed for the individual to treat specific musculoskeletal problems and to assist in mobilizing toxins that were stored in the tissues.
- *Counseling*. Mental and emotional toxins are as big a problem as physical/chemical toxins. When people are exposed to powerful emotional toxins (abuse, etc.) that they have no outlet for handling, they end up "stuffing" the emotional toxins. When this "emotional stuffing" occurs, any physical toxins that they were exposed to at that time are also "stuffed" (stored) rather than being eliminated. Because of this, when they start to mobilize the physical toxins, the old emotional issues will come

back into consciousness. When this occurs and individuals choose once again to suppress the emotional issues (rather than facing them), their physical cleansing will also stop. This is evidenced by the observations that they will stop sweating in the thermal chambers, stop heating the cold towels in the hydrotherapy and stop having good liver releases during the colonic therapy. When the emotional "toxins" are faced and released, these cleansing parameters are returned to former levels. Assisting all of the individuals going through this depuration protocol with their emotional issues helps them to cleanse physically. (See Ch. 4, especially the section "Utilize altered states of consciousness", for a more complete discussion of the role of past emotional states and associations in the development and maintenance of disease.)

This protocol is utilized on a daily basis that usually lasts between 4 and 8 weeks (five sessions weekly). The protocol begins the depuration process which must then be continued once the individual returns home. Most individuals will need to continue regular cleansing (use of home saunas, hydrotherapy and colon therapy) for at least 12 months after completing their intensive in-office cleansing. When testing for serum levels of OCCs and solvents is repeated along with immune parameters after 12 months, improvements are routinely seen. In addition to symptomatic relief, improvements in the laboratory reports (decrease in serum xenobiotics and reduction in autoantibodies, etc.) is clearly evident.

SUMMARY

Environmental chemicals are ubiquitous in our environment. Once they enter the body they bioaccumulate and are stored in adipose tissue throughout the body. They alter the functioning of the immune system, nervous system and endocrine system, leading to a host of chronic problems. The diagnosis of xenobiotic-induced damage can be elucidated by a comprehensive history along with evidence of serum toxin levels and toxin-induced immune system damage.

Treatment overview

- Avoidance of further chemical exposure through air, food and water
- Nutrient support for transformation, elimination, and antioxidant pathways
  —vitamin C: 6,000–12,000 mg/day
  —vitamin E: 400–1,200 units of D-alpha-tocopherol daily
  —B-complex: once daily
  —vitamin A: 25,000–50,000 units/day (unless the person is a menstruating female who is at risk for pregnancy)
  —*N*-acetyl cysteine: up to 1000 mg t.i.d.
  —selenium: 300–600 mcg/day
  —*Silybum marianum* (standardized): 100 mg two to three times/day
  —adequate protein in diet with each meal
  —magnesium: 300–600 mg/day
  —psyllium husks powder: begin with 0.5 tsp in water nightly (to bind bile in the intestines)
- Depuration protocol
  —daily exercise
  —thermal chambers (low temperature saunas)
  —constitutional hydrotherapy
  —colonic irrigations
  —constitutional homeopathy
  —body work
  —counseling

REFERENCES

1. Davis DL, Dinse GE, Hoel DG. Decreasing cardiovascular disease and increasing cancer among whites in the United States from 1973 through 1987. JAMA 1994; 271: 431–437
2. Rogers SA. Diagnosing the tight building syndrome. Env Health Pers 1987; 76: 195–198
3. Godish T. Sick buildings, definition, diagnosis, and mitigation. Boca Raton, Fl: Lewis Pub. 1995
4. Cullen MR, ed. Workers with multiple chemical sensitivities. Occupational Medicine State of the Art Reviews. Phila Hanley & Belfus 1987; 2: 655–661
5. Hileman B. Multiple chemical sensitivity. C&EN 1991; 69: 29
6. Rea WJ. Chemical sensitivity, vols 1, 2 and 3. Boca Raton, Fl: Lewis Pub. 1992, 1994, 1996
7. Chambers JE, Levi PE, eds. Organophosphates, chemistry, fate, and effects. San Diego, CA: Academic Press. 1992
8. Arlien-Soberg P. Solvent neurotoxicity. Boca Raton, FL: CRC Press. 1992
9. Luster MI, Rosenthal GJ. The immunosuppressive influence of industrial and environmental xenobiotics. TIPS; 1986: 408–412
10. Vial T, Nicolas B, Descotes J. Clinical immunotoxicity of pesticides. J Tox Env Med 1996; 48: 215–219
11. Editorial. Diagnostic markers in clinical immunotoxicology and neurotoxicology. J Occup Med Tox 1992; 1: v–ix
12. Rea WJ. Chemical sensitivity, vol. 3. Boca Raton, FL: CRC Press. 1996
13. EPA, Office of Toxic Substances. EPA-560/5-86-035, Broad scan analysis of the FY82 National Human Adipose Tissue Survey specimens. Washington, DC: EPA. 1986
14. CDC. J Tox Env Health 1989; 27: 405–421
15. Adeshina F, Todd EL. Organochlorine compounds in human adipose tissue from north Texas. J Tox Env Health 1990; 29: 147–156
16. Jacobsen JL. Determinants of polychlorinated biphenyls (PCBs). Polybrominated biphenyls (PBBs), and dichlorodiphenyl trichloroethane (DDT) levels in the sera of young children. AJPH 1989; 79: 1401–1404
17. Wallace LA et al. Personal exposures, indoor-outdoor relationships, and breath levels of toxic air pollutants measured for 355 persons in New Jersey. EPA 0589
18. Gunderson EL. FDA total diet survey, April 1982–April 1986, dietary intakes of pesticides, selected elements and other chemicals. Washington, DC: Food and Drug Administration, Division of Contaminants Chemistry

19. Kuhnlein HV, Receveur O, Muir D et al. Arctic indigenous women consume greater than acceptable levels of organochlorines. J Nutr 1995; 125: 2501–2510
20. Davis DL, Dinse GE, Hoel, DG. Decreasing cardiovascular disease and increasing cancer among whites in the United States from 1973 through 1987, good news and bad news. JAMA 1994; 271: 431–437
21. Luster M, Rosenthal GJ. The immunosuppressive influence of industrial and environmental xenobiotics. TIPS 1986; Oct: 408–412
22. Vial T, Nicolas B, Descotes J. Clinical immunotoxicity of pesticides. J Tox Env health 1996; 48: 215–229
23. Hueser G. Diagnostic markers in clinical immunotoxicology and neurotoxicology. J Occ Med Toxicol 1992; 1: v–ix
24. Rea WJ. Presentation at 13th International symposium on man and his environment in health and disease, Dallas. 1995
25. Haschek WM. Rousseaux, CG. Handbook of toxicologic pathology. San Diego, CA: Academic Press. 1991: 442–448
26. Thrasher JO, Madison R, Broughton A. Immunologic abnormalities in humans exposed to chlorpyrifos. preliminary observations. Arch Env Health 1993; 48: 89–93
27. Anderson HA, Lilis R, Selikoff I et al. Unanticipated prevalence of symptoms among dairy farmers in Michigan and Wisconsin. Env Health Persp 1978; 23: 217–226
28. Repetto R, Baliga SS. Pesticides and the immune system; the public health risks. Washington, DC: World Resources Institute. 1996
29. Broughton A, Thrasher JD. Chronic health effects and immunological alterations associated with exposure to pesticides. Comm Toxicol 1990; 4: 59–71
30. Vojdani A, Ghoneum M, Brautbar N. Immune alteration associated with exposure to toxic chemicals. Tox. Indust. Health 1992; 8: 239–253
31. Wasserman, Nogueira D, Tomatis et al. Organochlorine compounds in neoplastic and adjacent apparently normal breast tissue. Bull Env Contam Toxic 1976; 15: 4
32. Mussalo-Rauhamaa H. Occurrence of beta-hexachlorocyclohexane in breast cancer patients. Cancer 1990; 66: 2124–2128
33. Falck F. Pesticides and polychlorinated biphenyl residues in human breast lipids and their relation to breast cancer. Arch Env Health 1992; 47: 2
32. Wolff MS, Toniolo P, Lee E et al. Blood levels of organochlorine residues and risk of breast cancer. J Natl Cancer Inst 1993; 85: 8
33. Davis JR. Family pesticide use and childhood brain cancer. Arch Env Contam Toxicol 1993; 24: 87–92
34. Leiss J, Savitz D. Home pesticide use and childhood cancer. a case control study. AJPH 1995; 85: 249–252
35. Claggett S. 2,4-D Information packet. Northwest Coalition for Alternatives to Pesticides. 1990
36. Spirtas R, Stewart P, Lee J et al. Retrospective cohort mortality study of workers at an aircraft maintenance facility. Br J Indust Med 1991; 48: 515–530
37. Anttila A, Pukkala E, Sallmen M et al. Cancer incidence among Finnish workers exposed to halogenated hydrocarbons. JOEM 1995; 37: 797–806
38. Fleming L, Timmeny Wm. Aplastic anemia and pesticides, an etiologic association? JOEM 1993; 35: 1106–1115
39. Bethwaite PB, Pearce N, Fraser J. Cancer risks in painters. study based on the New Zealand Cancer Registry. Br J Indust. Med 1990; 47: 742–746
40. Eriksson M, Karlsson M. Occupational and other environmental factors and multiple myeloma. a population based case-control study. Br J Indust Med 1992; 49: 95–103
41. Synder SH, D'Amato RJ. Predicting Parkinson's disease. Nature 1985; 317: 198–199
42. Calne DB et al. Positron emission tomography after MPTP. observations relating to the cause of Parkinson's disease. Nature 1985; 317: 246–248
43. Lund B, Bergman A, Brandt I. Metabolic activation and toxicity of a DDT-metabolite, 3-methylsulphonyl-DDE, in the adrenal zona fasciculata in mice. Chem Biol Interaction 1988; 65: 25–40
44. McLachlan JA. Estrogen pairings can increase potency. Science News 1996; 149: 356
45. Colborn T, Myers JP, Dumanoski D. Our stolen future: how we are threatening our fertility, intelligence and survival. A scientific detective story. New York, NY: Dutton Books. 1997
46. Leoni V et al. PCB and other organochlorine compounds in blood of women with or without miscarriage. a hypothesis of correlation. Ecotox Env Safety 1989; 17: 1–11
47. Laino C. City air pollution linked to male infertility. Med Trib 1995; Nov. 9: 14
48. Carlsen E, Givercman A, Skakkebaek NE. Evidence for decreasing quality of semen during past 50 years. Br Med J 1992; 305: 609–613
49. Abell A, Ernst E, Bonde JP. High sperm density among members of Organic Farmers Association. Lancet 1994; 343: 1498
50. Sever LE, Hessol NA. Toxic effects of occupational and environmental chemicals on the testes. Endocrine toxicity. Raven Press 1985: p 211–248
51. Lundberg I, Hakansson M. Normal serum activities of liver enzymes in Swedish paint industry workers with heavy exposure to organic solvents. Br J Indust Med 1985; 42: 596–600
52. Simon TR. Brain SPECT and neurotoxicity. Presentation at 14th international symposium on man and his environment in health and disease. Dallas, TX. 1996
53. Jauman M. Use of evoked response audiometry to assess neurotoxicity. 14th international symposium on man and his environment in health and disease. Dallas, TX. 1996
54. Gorman C. Less toxic living. Dallas: Environmental Health Center-Dallas (tel: 214 368-4132). 1993
55. Golos N. Success in the clean bedroom. Rochester, NY: Pinnacle. 1992
56. Rousseau D. Your home, your health, your well-being. Vancouver, BC: Hartley and Marks. 1988
57. Wolverton BC, Johnson A, Bounds K. Interior landscape plants for indoor air pollution abatement. Stennis Space Center, MS: National Aeronautics and Space Administration. 1989
58. Meydani M. Dietary effects on detoxification processes. In: Hathcock J, ed. Nutritional toxicology, vol. II. New York, NY: Academic Press. 1987
59. Witschi A, Reddy S, Stofer B, Lauterburg BH. The systemic availability of oral glutathione. Eur J Clin Pharm 1992; 43: 667–669
60. Numan IT, Hassan MQ, Stohs SJ. Protective effects of antioxidants against Endrine induced lipid peroxidation, glutathione depletion, and lethality in rats. Arch Env Cont Tox 1990; 19: 302–306
61. Schnare DW, Denk G, Shields M, Brunton S. Evaluation of a detoxification treatment for fat stored xenobiotics. Med Hypothesis 1982; 9: 265–282
62. Schnare DW, Ben M, Shields MG. Body burden reductions of PCBs, PBBs, and chlorinated pesticides in human subjects. Ambio 1984; 13: 378–380
63. Tretjak Z, Shields MG, Beckman SL. PCB reduction and clinical improvement by detoxification. and unexploited approach? Hum Exp Toxicol 1990; 9: 235–244
64. Imamura M, Tung TC. A trial of fasting cure for PCB-poisoned patients in Taiwan. Am J Indust Med 1984; 5: 147–153
65. Crinnion WJ. Results of a decade of naturopathic treatment for environmental illness. J Nat Med, 1977; (7)2: 21–28

CHAPTER CONTENTS

38

The exercise prescription

Bobbi Lutack, MS ND

INTRODUCTION

The publication of Dr Kenneth Cooper's book, *Aerobics*, in 1968, had a profound influence on the exercise habits of Americans. Sedentary men and women all across the country were prompted by the book's message to take up aerobic training programs. Aerobics became the exercise catchword, and the fitness boom had begun. Running was the primary aerobic exercise, and beginning in the mid-1970s, marathon running became popular. More than 20,000 runners now annually participate in the New York, London, and Glasgow marathons.

In 1984, however, running took a giant step backward with the death of Jim Fixx, an internationally known runner and author who died of a massive myocardial infarction while running in Vermont. With him died an exercise myth: marathoner immunity to heart disease.

While a complete description of the physiologic changes induced by exercise is beyond the scope of this chapter, the following review will help provide a basis for understanding the exercise prescription. The basics of exercise physiology will be reviewed, considering the benefits and adverse effects of exercise with regard to the primary and secondary prevention of chronic lifestyle diseases, and the potential contraindications to exercise will be discussed. Special topics are also discussed. The reader is encouraged to peruse the position papers listed in Appendix 1 for additional resources.

EXERCISE PHYSIOLOGY

Exercise places significant metabolic and cardiorespiratory stress on the body. At maximal exertion, skeletal muscle increases its metabolic rate 50-fold, the overall metabolic rate 10-fold, and cardiac output from fourfold to as much as sixfold in the physically fit (due primarily to a threefold increase in heart rate).[1,2] In healthy individuals at submaximal workloads, the relationship between heart rate and oxygen uptake is essentially linear.

The physiological effects of exercise depend on the

intensity, duration and frequency, as well as the type of exercise. Isometric exercise (increase in muscle tension without a shortening in muscle length) increases peripheral vascular resistance without a significant change in cardiac output. Isotonic exercise (shortening of muscle with little increase in tension) increases cardiac output and decreases peripheral vascular resistance. Isometric exercise increases muscle strength and bulk, but has little effect on cardiorespiratory conditioning, while isotonic exercise increases endurance and cardiorespiratory conditioning, the goal of most exercise programs.

Well-conditioned individuals typically have lower heart rates than those who are sedentary. This is thought to be due to increased vagal tone, decreased sympathetic activity (probably due to the drop in beta-adrenergic receptor density), and increased stroke volume.[2] The best overall measurement of physical fitness is $V\text{O}_{2\ max}$, which decreases with age; for example, a 60-year-old has only two-thirds the $V\text{O}_{2\ max}$ of a 20-year-old. This trend is, however, much less apparent in those who exercise regularly. Three weeks of bed rest will cause a 20–25% decline in $V\text{O}_{2\ max}$, while sedentary individuals can increase their $V\text{O}_{2\ max}$ by 30–40% by engaging in a program of moderate exercise.[2]

MUSCLE PHYSIOLOGY

Skeletal muscle is composed of two types of fiber: red fibers (type I) and white fibers (type II). The red fibers are high in myoglobin. content, mitochondria, and oxidative capacity but are low in glycolytic enzymes and slow in contraction time. White fibers are lower in myoglobin content, mitochondria, and oxidative capacity, and high in glycolytic enzymes and myosin ATPase activity, and fast in reaction time.[2] Sprinters have high proportions of white fibers for high-intensity exercise, while long-distance runners have a preponderance of red fibers. It is unclear, however, if training can alter the phenotype of muscle fibers.[3]

As skeletal muscle contains only limited amounts of high-energy phosphate compounds – preformed adenosine triphosphate (ATP) and creatine phosphate (CP) muscle stores are inadequate for a 100 yard dash – energy must be generated during exercise. Three sources of fuel are available to skeletal muscle:

- endogenous muscle glycogen
- blood glucose
- free fatty acids (FFA) derived from muscle triglycerides stores or adipose tissue.

Table 38.1 lists the body's relative proportions of each of these energy stores.

The intensity of exercise determines the substrate utilized. Low-intensity exercise and exercise well within the aerobic limits preferentially utilize free fatty acids (FFAs) first, and muscle glycogen second. Catecholamines, released early in exercise, stimulate adipose lipase, which cleaves triglyceride into glycerol and three FFAs. Serum FFA levels of six times the normal level are rapidly induced during exercise. In muscle, FFAs are metabolized to acetyl CoA, which undergoes oxidative metabolism in the citric acid cycle to produce ATP production during exercise; (see Fig. 38.1 and Fig. 47.2 in Ch. 47).[2,4]

Table 38.1 Energy stores available to skeletal muscle

Body store	Size of store (kcal)	Running distance (miles)
Blood glucose	40	0.5
Liver glycogen	220	2.2
Muscle glycogen	380	3.8
Adipose tissue	100,000	1,000

As the exercise intensity increases, glycogen becomes more important than FFAs, contributing twice the energy at 80% maximal work capacity and virtually all at 100%. While within the aerobic limit, glycogen is metabolized in the cytoplasm to pyruvate, which then enters the citric acid cycle. When sufficient oxygen is not available, in anaerobic metabolism, energy is produced by glycolysis (only 5% as efficient), and pyruvate is reduced to lactate instead of entering the citric acid cycle. The resulting acidosis limits muscular performance, and buffering by bicarbonate generates CO_2, causing tachypnea.[2,4]

THE COMPONENTS OF PHYSICAL FITNESS

There are five components of physical fitness:

- cardiovascular endurance
- muscular strength
- muscular endurance
- flexibility
- body composition.

Cardiovascular endurance

Cardiovascular endurance refers to the ability of the heart, lungs, and blood vessels to function optimally both at rest and during exercise. From the exercise specialist's point of view, it is the most important component. This variable is addressed through the aerobic portion of an exercise program. Aerobic is defined as the ability to process and deliver enough oxygen to meet tissue energy needs. At work loads above 80% of maximum, skeletal muscle demands more oxygen than can be delivered, thus exceeding the aerobic limit.[2] As muscle metabolism becomes anaerobic, energy is produced by glycolysis rather than glucose oxidation. This results in the build-up of lactic acid, requiring the buffering of bicarbonate.

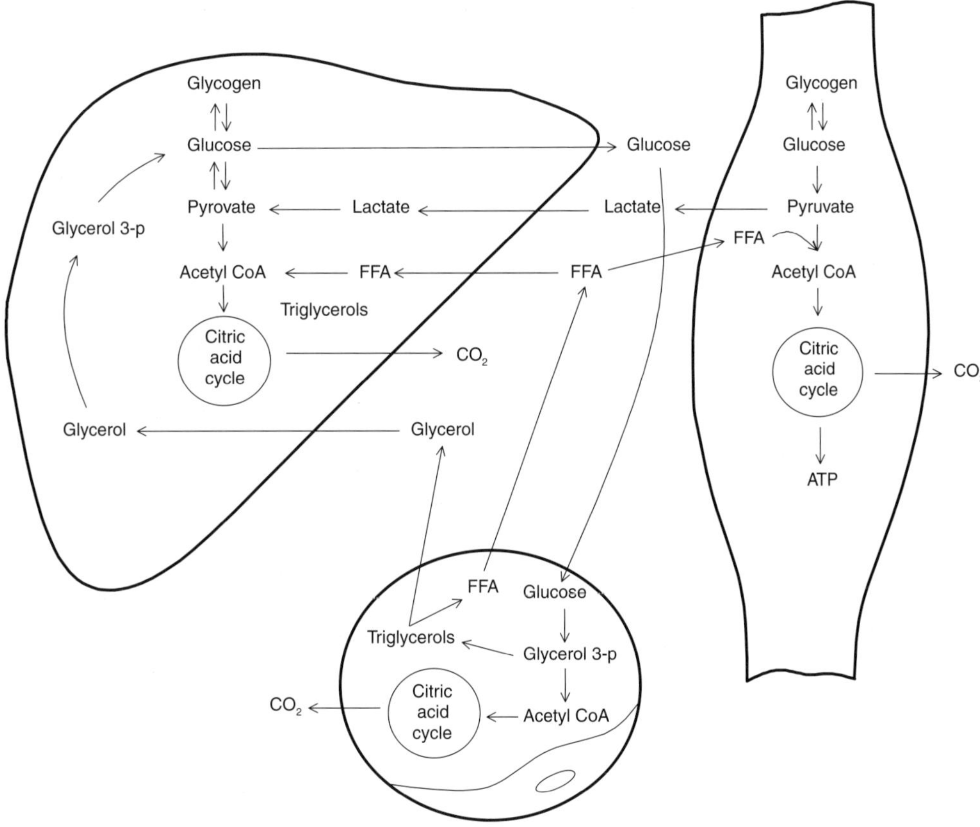

Figure 38.1 Muscle energy metabolism.

The subsequent CO_2 release results in increased respiratory rate, a sensation of dyspnea, and progressively decreased work capacity. (Although some athletes inhale 100% of oxygen after intense activity to hasten recovery and improve subsequent performance, this has proven to be ineffective.[5])

To qualify as an aerobic activity, the exercise must be continuous, rhythmical, use large muscle groups, and be performed at an intensity that significantly increases cardiovascular output. Examples of aerobic exercise include running, cross-country skiing, cycling, swimming, skating, hiking, etc. The aerobic concept, applied to physical fitness, requires following specific training guidelines. If pursued regularly and with proper intensity and duration, this training:[6]

- strengthens the respiratory muscles
- increases breathing efficiency
- stabilizes or lowers blood pressure
- improves tissue capacity to utilize oxygen and dispose of waste products
- increases muscular endurance
- increases heart function and circulation
- controls body weight
- provides increased energy
- promotes psychological well-being.

Cardiovascular endurance can be measured in the physician's office with a graded exercise test on a treadmill or bike, or in the field with, for example, the popular 12-minute walk-run (see Cooper[7] for a detailed description) on a measured course. The distance covered correlates well with maximum oxygen consumption.[7]

Muscular strength

Muscular strength refers to the ability of a muscle to exert force against resistance. Typically, strength is defined relative to maximum force-producing capabilities. A simple, but accurate, estimate of strength, referred to as the "one repetition maximum", is to have an individual lift as much as he or she can lift just one time. Upper and lower body strength can be assessed using exercises like the bench press and the leg press.[8] As a rule of thumb, the ability to bench press one's own body weight indicates good upper body strength.

Muscular endurance

Muscular endurance is the ability of a muscle or muscle group to sustain repeated contractions of a given force over time. This ability is highly correlated with strength.

Push-up and sit-up tests have traditionally been used to determine muscular endurance, although abdominal "crunches" or half sit-ups are actually a better measure of abdominal endurance/strength. An example of good muscular endurance for a 30-year-old male is the ability to perform 35–39 timed (60 second) sit-ups. For a 30-year-old female, 25–39 modified push-ups and 31–35 timed (60 second) sit-ups would indicate good muscular endurance.[8]

Flexibility

Flexibility is the ability to move a muscle through its full range of motion, which involves the interrelationships between muscles, ligaments, tendons, and joints. Range of motion is restricted by a lack of flexibility and the performance of routine movement is hindered. It is difficult to test flexibility as it is joint-specific, but one test that is frequently used to test low back, hamstring, and hip flexibility is the "sit and reach test". This test is described in detail in Appendix 1. A good score is 19–21 inches.[8] An exercise program which incorporates stretching and yoga exercises can increase flexibility.

Body composition

Body composition is the interrelationship between lean body mass (muscle, bones, and connective tissues) and body fat. For optimal fitness, high levels of lean tissue and relatively low levels of body fat (about 20% for women and 15% for men) are desirable. The percentage of body fat can be measured quickly, accurately, and relatively inexpensively in a physician's office through the use of skinfold calipers (we recommend high-quality calipers such as Lange or Harpenden). Several skinfold sites must be measured to maximize accuracy. One set of recommended measurement sites for women comprises the thigh, triceps, and suprailium, and for men the thigh, chest, and abdomen. These measurements are then used in a regression equation or a table (such as the one found in Pollack et al,[8] p. 220) to estimate body fat. The body fat percentages are based on Siri's underwater equation, where percentage fat = $[(4.95/\text{Db}) - 4.5] \times 100$, where Db is the body density. (See Chapter 175 for a discussion of one- and four-site skinfold measurement techniques and interpretive tables.)

THE EXERCISE PRESCRIPTION: BASIC GUIDELINES

Many people are confused about the type and amount of exercise necessary to become fit. Knowledgeable and accurate instructions are important to help prepare an exercise program that meets the specific needs of each individual. The American College of Sports Medicine (ACSM), an internationally recognized expert organization in the field of exercise science, has published a position paper (see Appendix 1) on the proper exercise prescription for healthy adults. This paper, based on existing documentation from throughout the world, summarizes the most widely accepted guidelines for developing and maintaining cardiovascular fitness and optimal body composition. The following is a summary of its content.

Cardiorespiratory conditioning

The essential components of cardiorespiratory exercise

There are four essential components of a sound cardiorespiratory exercise program:

Type of activity. Aerobic (defined previously).

Intensity. The exercise has to be strenuous enough to place an "overload" on the cardiorespiratory system. This corresponds to 60–90% of maximum heart rate. To calculate maximum heart rate (MHR), subtract the individual's age from 220. Multiplying this figure by 0.60 and 0.90 yields the target heart rate (THR), i.e. the range of sufficient intensity to overload the cardiorespiratory system. For example, for a 40-year-old:

- MHR = 220 – 40 = 180 bpm
- 180 bpm × 60% = 108 bpm
- 180 bpm × 90% = 162 bpm
- THR = 108 –162 bpm.

Although the MHR covers a wide range, it is useful as a ball park measure of how to determine the intensity of exercise.

To further increase the accuracy of intensity evaluation, a rating scale of perceived exertion (RPE) can be used. The Borg scale of perceived exertion is a good example.[9] The Borg scale is numerical, ranging from 6 to 20, with corresponding verbal descriptions provided at odd numbers of how hard the exercise feels. For example, a rating of 6–7 corresponds to "very, very easy", while a rating of 19–20 corresponds to "very, very hard". The RPE response to graded exercise correlates closely with cardiorespiratory and metabolic variables such as heart rate. As a valid and reliable indicator of the level of exertion of a given exercise, it can be used to prescribe intensity. A rating of 12–13 (described as "comfortable" to "somewhat hard") corresponds to about 60% of MHR and a rating of 15–16 (expressed as "hard") corresponds to about 90% of MHR.[10] When prescribing an exercise program, a perceived exertion range of "comfortable" to "hard" is the recommended intensity level. When used in conjunction with the THR at the beginning of an exercise program, it helps participants to develop a physical and cognitive "feel" for how hard exercise should be. Once this knowledge is obtained, RPE can be used as the primary indicator of intensity.

Duration. This is inversely related to intensity. Duration of aerobic exercise, exclusive of warm-up and cool-down, typically varies in length from 15 to 60 minutes. A common conditioning phase is 30 minutes. High-intensity exercise requires a shorter duration for the same cardiovascular effect, and vice versa. High-intensity, short-duration exercise is not recommended until good cardiovascular conditioning has been achieved. A good rule of thumb to gauge a proper intensity/duration ratio is the degree of fatigue experienced 1 hour after exercising.

Frequency. Three to five exercise sessions per week are recommended, with no more than 48 hours between workouts. Depending on the level of fitness, intensity, duration, and motivation, sessions can be daily. With less than three sessions per week, improvement in cardiorespiratory endurance is minimal and there is no loss in body fat.[11]

When instructing previously sedentary individuals on how to exercise properly and become conditioned, emphasis should be placed on making progression slowly. People who have been sedentary for years will require time to rebuild their bodies. It is better to do too little than too much. All too often, people who are motivated to "get back in shape" will over-exert themselves their first time out (e.g. by jogging 2 miles instead of combining walking and jogging). When they wake up the next day with sore muscles and unaccustomed pain, they give up on the exercise program. The old adage "no pain, no gain" is an exercise myth (except in strength building, as noted below). The aerobic exercise component of a physical fitness program should feel fairly comfortable. Being able to talk with an exercise partner while working out suggests an appropriate level of exercise, while breathlessness and inability to carry on a conversation indicates excessive intensity. Being able to sing suggests too little intensity.

The three phases of cardiorespiratory exercise

In addition to the components of mode, frequency, intensity and duration, the effective exercise session is divided into three phases:

- warm-up
- cardiorespiratory conditioning
- cool-down.

The warm-up phase should be of 5–10 minutes' duration and should prepare the body for the conditioning activity. Light calisthenics, stretching and/or the conditioning activity performed at a light intensity (approximately 50% of the intensity of the conditioning phase) are suitable warm-up activities. Breaking into "a light sweat" is a sign that the body is warming up. Proper warm-up may also help to prevent exercise-induced muscle pulls, strains and soreness.[12]

The conditioning phase is the 15–60 minutes of aerobic activity described earlier. Vigorous participation in sports is recommended as an enjoyable alternative but only after an adequate level of fitness is achieved. The adage "don't play sports to get in shape, get in shape to play sports" is sound advice.

The recommended cool-down is 5–10 minutes of tapering-off activity, such as slowing the intensity of the exercise performed in the conditioning phase, stretching, and then relaxing for a short period. For most people, the heart rate should be under 100 bpm at the end of the cool-down period.[12] The major purpose of this phase is to keep the primary muscle groups involved in the conditioning phase moving, to prevent peripheral pooling of blood, which can cause a vaso-vagal response. Cooling down can also help to prevent muscle soreness.[8]

Muscular conditioning

Most of the attention for exercise program prescriptions has focused on the cardiovascular component, probably due to the belief of exercise authorities that cardiovascular fitness is the most important component. However, flexibility, strength and muscular endurance also form an important part of any physical fitness program. Sound musculoskeletal function is necessary throughout life to make daily living activities easier to perform, to help prevent low back problems, and to help prevent the inevitable loss of lean body tissue as one ages. As lean body mass is lost, a concomitant decrease in basal metabolic rate and strength occurs.

Individual exercise prescriptions for developing muscular endurance and strength should be tailored to the sport being played or to the individual's goals. Weight loss (fat loss), for example, would necessitate a different prescription from power lifting. For a general overall strength/endurance-building program, the following guidelines may be used:

- *Mode* – free weights, universal, Nautilus, Cybex, calisthenics, etc.
- *Duration* – one to three sets of five to 15 repetitions (optimal strength gains appear to be achieved with five to seven repetitions if the muscle is maximally fatigued). Allow about 1 minute's rest between sets.
- *Intensity* – the intensity (weight lifted) should be such that only five to 15 repetitions can be performed. The adage, "no burn, no gain" has much validity.
- *Frequency* – 3–5 days per week (5 days only after preconditioning). Allow at least a 24 hour rest period between workouts of the same muscle group (i.e. a complete day of rest between workouts).[8]

- Example:
  —Monday: upper body workout
  —Tuesday: lower body workout
  —Thursday: upper body workout
  —Friday: lower body workout.

Proper and safe strength training requires emphasis on form, technique and execution. The following guidelines will help to maximize the effects and minimize the risks of exercise programs:[10]

- *Warm-up*. To prepare the muscles for the intense effort that lies ahead, stretch and perform a few repetitions with about 50% of the weight to be used during the training sets.
- *Controlled movement*. Control all movements to achieve steadiness. Do not "throw" the weight. For maximum strengthening benefits, at the height of the lift or at its fullest extension or flexion, pause briefly before lowering the weight. A good routine is to lift for 2 seconds, pause and then lower for 4 seconds.
- *Muscle group isolation*. Concentrate on isolating the muscle(s) being exercised and moving them through their full range of motion.
- *Fatigue avoidance*. Proceed from major muscle groups to minor muscle groups to minimize fatigue.
- *Proper breathing*. Do not hold the breath or perform the Valsalva maneuver. Exhale as the weight is lifted and inhale as it is lowered.

For additional information, please refer to Appendix 1.

Flexibility conditioning

Flexibility is necessary to ensure maintenance of adequate range of motion of all joints. Decreased flexibility can lead to the common complaint of low back pain (discussed further below).[8] Stretching should be done at least three times per week (ideally before and after each workout) and can be part of the warm-up and cool-down phases of the cardiovascular portion of the fitness program. Stretching should be preceded by a mild warm-up (e.g. light calisthenics), and the exercises tailored to the muscles being worked. Stretches should be performed slowly and progressively, using a dynamic movement followed by a static stretch held for 30–60 seconds. The stretch should cause a feeling of tightness but no pain.[13]

At this point, a note of caution is necessary. The above recommendations and guidelines are designed for apparently healthy, asymptomatic adults. According to the ACSM, apparently healthy individuals under the age of 45 can begin and participate in exercise programs without prior stress testing; however, some screening prior to participation is recommended.[10] The age, health status and type of exercise program the participant will be engaging in determines the degree of evaluation required. Individuals with known cardiac, pulmonary or metabolic disease or who have symptoms suggesting coronary artery disease and/or at least one major coronary risk factor should undergo a maximal exercise tolerance test prior to beginning a vigorous exercise program. The ACSM also recommends such a test for anyone who is 45 or older prior to participation in an exercise program.

EXERCISE AND SPECIFIC DISEASES

(Additional discussion of the current research into the benefit of exercise can be found in the chapters covering most of the following conditions.)

Coronary heart disease

Running was the popular aerobic exercise in the 1970s and was touted to have many beneficial side-effects. During its heyday, Dr Tom Bassler even proposed that marathoners were immune to heart disease.[14,15] The death of Jim Fixx in 1984 laid that theory permanently to rest.

The concept that regular aerobic exercise will provide some protection against the clinical manifestation of coronary heart disease (CHD) is generally accepted today by both the public and health professionals. Regular exercise, in conjunction with other risk-reducing behaviors, is believed to help protect against an initial cardiac event (primary prevention), aid in the recovery following a cardiac event (e.g. myocardial infarction, coronary artery bypass graft surgery, etc.), and help to reduce the risk of recurrent cardiac events (secondary prevention). The exercise conditioning effects that help to prevent CHD are listed in Table 38.2.

Although the etiology and pathogenesis of CHD and atherosclerosis are still not completely understood, multiple research approaches have identified several factors which play causative roles. Although a cause and effect relationship has yet to be definitively demonstrated, there are strong indications that regular exercise leads to reduced risk for CHD and its clinical manifestations of myocardial ischemia, myocardial infarction, and cardiac arrest.

Pioneering observational studies by Morris et al,[18] Paffenbarger et al,[19] and Taylor et al[20] of London bus drivers and postal workers, longshoremen, and US railroad workers, respectively, were among the first to report an inverse correlation between CHD risk and physical activity. Another landmark investigation, the Framingham study, also indicated that moderate exercise was associated with decreased CHD risk.[21]

Table 38.2 Exercise conditioning effects are potentially beneficial for the prevention of CHD[16,17]

Serum lipid effects
- Reduction of serum cholesterol and triglycerides
- Increase of serum high-density lipoproteins (HDL_2)

Metabolic effects
- Lowering of circulating catecholamines – lowering of circulating by exercise
- Reduction of blood clotting – reduction by exercise; tendencies
- Increased fibrinolysis
- Increase of insulin sensitivity – increased by exercise

Cardiac effects
- Augmentation of coronary arterial bed
- Decrease of myocardial work and oxygen demand
- Increase of myocardial function (increased stroke volume)
- Reduction of systolic and diastolic blood pressure – reduction by exercise

Miscellaneous effects
- Improvement of psychological outlook – improvement by exercise
- Reduction of adiposity

More recently, an observational study by Leon found physical inactivity to increase risk of heart attack, and the 7 year MRFIT study showed that moderate exercise reduced both fatal and non-fatal CHD events.[22,23]

Research has shown that higher levels of leisure-time physical activity are associated with increased longevity in college alumni, while Paffenbarger et al[24,25] have shown that it was physical activity as an adult, not college athleticism, that is associated with a decreased risk of death.

In a study conducted at the Cooper clinic in Dallas, Texas, the physical fitness and risk of all-cause and cause-specific mortality were followed in 10,000 men and 3,000 women for an average of 8+ years.[26] The study concluded that poor physical fitness was an important risk factor in both men and women. Higher levels of physical fitness appeared to delay all-cause mortality, primarily due to lowered rates of CHD and cancer. This study is particularly important as it is the first large-scale study to include extensive follow-up, maximal exercise tests, a wide range of physical fitness evaluations, an objective end-point (mortality), and a large enough sample of women to permit meaningful comparative gender analyses. The results of the study are useful from both a clinical and a public health standpoint.

In addition to lowering risk for developing CHD, aerobic exercise training has been shown to help in recovery from cardiac events (cardiac rehabilitation).[27–29]

One additional note of interest: until recently, most exercise scientists believed that only aerobic exercise training was beneficial in reducing CHD risk. Research now shows that weight resistance training also has a beneficial effect on CHD risk by favorably affecting lipoprotein-lipid profiles, insulin response to glucose ingestion, and blood pressure.[30–33]

Hypertension

Exercise training clearly decreases the risk of hypertension. One study of 6,000 healthy adults found a 52% increased risk for hypertension in sedentary individuals compared with those who were fit, while another found a 35% increase.[34,35] Regular exercise produces a sustained decrease in systolic and diastolic blood pressure and catecholamine levels in hypertensive patients.[36] One study of patients with mild hypertension found that half could discontinue their antihypertensive drugs after engaging in a regular aerobic program.[37] A note of caution: as isometric exercises cause an acute increase in blood pressure, static exercise by patients with significant hypertension should be supervised.

Cancer

Lack of regular physical activity has been linked to colon cancer, breast cancer, and lung cancer, with most of the research focusing on the link between fitness and colon cancer.[38–41] Physical activity may reduce the incidence of colon cancer because it reduces intestinal transit time.[42] In the Cooper clinic study, higher levels of physical fitness were associated with delayed mortality partly due to lowered rates of cancer.[26]

Obesity

Physical inactivity may be a major cause of obesity in the US. Indeed, childhood obesity seems to be associated more with inactivity than overeating, and strong evidence suggests that 80–86% of adult obesity begins in childhood. In the adult population, Brownell and Stunkard found that obese adults were less active than their normal-weighted counterparts.[8] However, it is still unclear whether inactivity is a cause of obesity or a result of it. Despite the lack of definitive evidence, regular exercise should be prescribed for the obese due to the following factors:

- When weight loss is achieved by dieting without exercise, a substantial portion of the total weight loss comes from the lean tissue primarily as water loss.[43]
- When exercise is included in a weight-loss program, there is usually an improvement in body composition due to a gain in lean body weight because of an increase in muscle mass and a concomitant decrease in body fat.[44]
- Exercise helps to counter the reduction in basal metabolic rate (BMR) that usually accompanies calorie restriction alone.[45]
- Exercise increases the BMR for an extended period of time following the exercise session.[10]
- Moderate to intense exercise may have an appetite suppressant effect.[10]
- Those subjects who exercise during and after weight

reduction are better able to maintain the weight loss than those who do not exercise.[46]

The concept of "spot reduction" is a myth.[47] Exercise draws from all of the fat stores of the body, not just from local deposits. While aerobic exercise generally enhances weight loss programs, weight training programs can also substantially alter body composition, by increasing lean body weight and decreasing body fat.[48–50] Research into the use of resistance training during energy restriction is limited, but preliminary evidence suggests that calorie restriction does not affect the strengthening or hypertrophic response of muscle.[50] Thus, weight training may be just as, or more, effective than aerobic exercise in maintaining or increasing lean body weight and, therefore, the metabolic rate of individuals undergoing weight reduction.

Generally, aerobic exercise prescriptions for weight loss should emphasize long duration, low intensity, and a frequency of at least 3–4 days/week since, as the discussion of muscle metabolism above indicates, this type of exercise preferentially utilizes fatty acids from adipose stores. Swimming appears less effective than walking or cycling for reducing body fat.[51] It takes 35 miles of walking or jogging to metabolize the calories contained in 1 pound of fat. Table 38.3 lists the metabolic costs of various activities.

Weight loss (combined diet and exercise) should not exceed 2–3 pounds/week.[10] For additional information, refer to the ACSM position statement in Appendix 1.

Diabetes

The current treatment for type II diabetes is exercise, oral hypoglycemics, and dietary modification.[10] Exercise is beneficial to diabetics as it increases insulin sensitivity and enhances the biological effects of endogenous insulin.[52] As mentioned previously, exercise can also help by combating obesity and improving lipoprotein profiles.

Special precautions need to be taken when prescribing exercise for those with insulin-dependent diabetes, as exercise may induce hypoglycemia through its insulin-like effect. An exercising insulin-dependent diabetic needs to reduce insulin intake or increase carbohydrate intake. The following regime is recommended for insulin-dependent diabetics who exercise to maintain blood glucose control:

1. Monitor blood glucose more frequently.
2. Decrease insulin dose (1–2 units or as needed) or increase carbohydrate intake (10–15 g per 0.5 hour of exercise) prior to an exercise session.
3. Inject insulin into a site that will not be active during exercise (e.g. runners might inject into the abdomen).
4. Avoid exercise during peak insulin periods.
5. Eat carbohydrate snacks before and during prolonged exercise sessions.
6. Exercise with a partner (in case of a hypoglycemic reaction).
7. Avoid late evening exercise.[10,53]
8. Wear a medical-alert bracelet.

The exercise prescription needs to be individualized, and in some cases exercise is not advisable due to poor metabolic control and/or frequent hypoglycemic reactions.[53]

For type I diabetics, exercise consistency is most important.[54] Daily exercise helps to maintain a regular pattern of diet and insulin dosage. Intensity can be prescribed in the normal range (i.e. 60–90% of MHR) and duration need only be 20–30 minutes per session, due to the high frequency.

Prescribing exercise for type II diabetics is not as complicated. As obesity is a key contributing factor to this type of diabetes, emphasis should be placed on high frequency (5–7 days/week), long duration (45–60 minutes per session), and low intensity (about 60% of MHR) for maximizing caloric expenditure from fat stores.[10,52]

Diabetic patients with advanced retinopathy should not participate in activities that jar or those that cause marked fluctuations in blood pressure. A non-jarring exercise like swimming is recommended.[10]

Table 38.3 Metabolic costs* of various activities[2]

Occupational	Recreational	Energy used (kcal/min)
Desk work, driving	Standing, walking	2–2.5 kcal/min
Janitor, typing	Level bicycling	2.5–4
Cleaning windows	Cycling, 6 mph; walking, 3 mph	4–5
Painting, paperhanging	Dancing, table tennis	5–6
Digging in garden	Walking, 4 mph; skating	6–7
Shoveling, 10# 10×/min	Cycling, 11 mph; tennis	7–8
Sawing hardwood	Jogging, 5 mph; basketball	8–10
Shoveling, 14# 10×/min	Running, 5.5 mph; handball	10–11
Shoveling, 16# 10×/min	Running, >6 mph	>10

*Includes resting metabolic needs.

Pulmonary disease

In patients with advanced chronic obstructive pulmonary disease (COPD), dyspnea at progressively lower levels of exertion often results in deconditioning, which can lead to further disability. Although aerobic exercise will not improve indices of pulmonary function,[55,56] it may improve endurance and exercise tolerance.[56,57–59] In patients with mild to moderate asthma, 3 months of controlled, submaximal exercise can produce significant improvements in fitness and cardiorespiratory performance.[60]

The effects of exercise are tempered by the severity of airway obstruction, which may vary from mild to severe. Individuals with mild COPD will respond to exercise in a similar way to patients with CHD, so the intensity can also be prescribed by the heart rate method. The recommended duration, frequency, and mode are also the same as for CHD patients.[10]

Individuals suffering from more severe COPD who experience dyspnea with mild exercise will be limited by their dysfunctional respiratory systems. Supplemental oxygen may be used during exercise if a trial shows objective improvement in exercise capacity as a result of oxygen use; however, modifications to the exercise prescription will be required.[10] Duration should be "as tolerated", with perhaps two 10-minute or four 5-minute sessions/day to build up tolerance. As tolerance increases, sessions can gradually be reduced to 3–5 days/week for 20–30 minutes. Intensity should be determined by signs of breathlessness. Lower body aerobic exercise, such as walking or cycling, is preferable to upper body exercise due to the higher ventilation requirement of upper body exercise.

Additional benefits of exercise therapy for pulmonary patients include improved mechanical skills in the trained muscles, particularly in the respiratory muscles, and improved psychological state.[61,62]

End-stage renal disease

Many patients with end-stage renal disease (ESRD) suffer from muscle weakness, fatigue, bone disease, CHD, and multiple psychosocial problems. Attention has recently been directed at rehabilitation of this patient group. Exercise training has been found to be especially beneficial for selected patients undergoing hemodialysis.

The incidence of ESRD in the United States is approximately 1 in 10,000 per annum, and the average age of patients on dialysis is 48.[63] The most common treatment for ESRD patients is hemodialysis.

A major study conducted at the Washington University School of Medicine and the Chromalloy American Kidney Center using an aerobic exercise program on non-dialysis days found:[63]

- a 19% increase in the duration of exercise tolerance
- a 21% increase in $VO_{2\,max}$
- improvements in blood pressure and lipoprotein profiles
- lowered fasting plasma insulin
- a 27% increase in hematocrit
- a reduction of depression.

There were no changes in these parameters in the control group. Positive results were also reported by Squires et al[64] with exercise training following renal transplantation.

Exercise training (specifically cycling) has also been performed during hemodialysis.[65] The benefits are similar to those found with training on non-dialysis days. Because typical hemodialysis patients utilize an artificial kidney machine three times a week for 4–5 hours/session, exercise training could help to alleviate the tediousness of the sessions and provide a supervised setting for exercise in this high-risk group of patients.

The exercise prescription for ESRD patients has to be a low-intensity (use the RPE method to designate intensity), non-weight-bearing (e.g. stationary cycling), interval (i.e. exercise period followed by a rest period) activity. Frequency should be at least 3 days/week and duration should be about 30–45 minutes. Exercise sessions should be monitored and adjustments made to accommodate any complications, e.g. an increase in serum potassium.[63,66]

Chronic pain

Pain is the leading symptom that prompts patients to see physicians. Today, virtually all pain management programs include some type of aerobic and/or weight training exercise program.[67] Pain specialists attribute the positive effects of decreased sensitivity to pain and significant psychological benefit to exercise-induced elevation of endorphins.[68,69] A recent study proposed that prolonged rhythmic exercise activates central opiod systems by triggering increased discharge from mechanosensitive afferent nerve fibers in contracting skeletal muscle and that many of the cardiovascular, analgesic, and behavioral effects of exercise are mediated by this mechanism. The authors also proposed that the same or similar mechanisms are responsible for the central and peripheral effects of acupuncture.[69] Aerobic exercise may also help to reduce pain through promotion of delta sleep, the deepest stage of sleep, during which musculoskeletal renewal takes place.[67] The two most common pain complaints are low back pain (LBP), affecting about 15% of Americans, and headaches.[67]

Low back pain

While 90% of patients with back injuries return to work within 2 months, the remaining 10% account for billions of dollars in medical expenses, lost income and productivity, workers' compensation benefits, and litigation fees.[67,70] It has been postulated that post-injury deconditioning, not the original injury, is the primary cause of the chronic pain condition and is frequently the major impediment to functional restoration.[68] Reversal of post-injury deconditioning through a progressive, active physical exercise program can restore function and decrease pain. While healing may restore structural integrity, it does not restore flexibility, strength, endurance, or coordination. Unrecognized or untreated deconditioning can lead to the recurrence of pain on return to work or resumption of normal activities. It is theorized that high-resistance exercise training helps minimize pain by breaking down existing muscle fiber and stimulating its replacement with stronger and more flexible replacement fiber.[67]

Arthritis

With arthritis, slight pain may have to be tolerated during exercise sessions in order to achieve the pain-alleviating effects of conditioning. Exercise producing excessive stress on osteoarthritic joints should be avoided, but a program designed to improve range of motion and muscle strength should be performed daily to combat the effects of disuse and decrease pain. Exercises of short duration and high frequency help to limit stress on the joints. Weight-bearing activities may have to be limited due to inflammation, but cycling, rowing, swimming, etc. are all acceptable modes of exercise.[10,71] There is no evidence to support the assertion that running causes degenerative joint disease. Since synovial fluid enters cartilage to provide nutrition through exercise-induced compression, it is possible that long-term repetitive exercise is actually beneficial for joints as well as bones.[2] Excessive trauma is, however, associated with joint degeneration (see Ch. 176).

Peripheral vascular disease

Individuals with peripheral vascular disease (PVD) suffer claudication discomfort ranging from excruciating and unbearable pain to definite discomfort. Exercise can help to alleviate the pain. Frequency should be 7 days/week, preferably with two periods of exercise per day. The duration should be at least 20 minutes (exercise might have to be intermittent), and the type of exercise should be aerobic (walking, stationary cycling, warm water exercise, etc.). The intensity will be determined by the level of pain (moderate discomfort or pain from which the patient can be distracted by conversation or other stimuli may have to be tolerated).[10]

Mental health

A considerable body of knowledge attests to the mental health benefits associated with long-term aerobic exercise.[72–75] Improved mood has been observed in both non-hospitalized outpatients and normal individuals, as well as those suffering from psychopathology.[76] Exercise may also help normal individuals as it decreases stress, and emotions such as anxiety, and decreases the sympathoadrenal response to stress found in men with a type A personality.[77–80] An "improved sense of well-being" has been reported by many people following exercise. In general, this has been attributed to a decrease in anxiety and depression.[79] Exercise is almost as effective as antidepressant drug therapy in selected types of anxiety and depression.[69]

Although studies are controversial, the endorphin hypothesis has become widely accepted as a mechanism by which exercise improves mood.[81] The controversy is largely due to the inability of some investigators to block exercise-induced mood elevation with naloxone.[69] Perhaps the dosages were insufficient or other mechanisms are in action. Evidence also indicates that aerobic exercise produces an effect in depressed persons that is similar to the effect caused by tricyclic antidepressants, i.e. it increases the production of the neurotransmitter norepinephrine. This exercise effect is not found in those who are not depressed.[82]

Whatever the relationship, cause and effect, or association, there is sufficient evidence to support regular, vigorous exercise to promote psychological well-being. In general, the principles of exercise prescription described for healthy adults are also appropriate for those who suffer from mental illness.

EXERCISE IN SPECIAL CONDITIONS

Pregnancy

Many physically active women want to continue exercising during pregnancy. The currently accepted view is that this is satisfactory if they take some precautions. In addition to benefits cited earlier, exercising during pregnancy can:[83–85]

- enhance self-esteem
- increase energy
- improve sleep
- decrease backache
- decrease problems with varicose veins
- decrease water retention
- improve posture and appearance
- possibly decrease labor complications
- shorten labor and postpartum recovery.

For trained women, exercise therapists typically recommend continuing the prepregnancy exercise program at the same "perceived level of exertion" (use RPE) during pregnancy. Women who previously have been sedentary and want to exercise while pregnant should begin at a very low intensity and increase gradually.[86]

General and relative contraindications include: hemodynamically significant CHD, toxemia, eclampsia, uncontrolled diabetes mellitus, uncontrolled hypertension, and obesity.[10,87] Pregnant women should avoid participating in sporting activities that involve physical contact or that might induce a fall, e.g. downhill skiing for the inexperienced. As body weight increases, a non-weight-bearing activity might be more suitable, e.g. swimming instead of jogging, and intensity should be decreased to minimize oxygen debt and lactate production. Intensity and duration should also be modified to limit core temperature increases.[87]

Some concerns regarding fetal heart rate during maternal exertion have been raised. Signs of fetal distress include prolonged fetal bradycardia and tachycardia. Several studies have shown no effect on fetal heart rate with maternal exertion at 70–80% of their MHR.[88–90]

With some modifications, continuing a regular exercise program during pregnancy can be both a safe and enjoyable experience for the expectant mother.

Children

The leading causes of mortality in the United States are lifestyle-induced diseases, typically originating in childhood. Risk factors such as smoking, hypertension, obesity, diabetes mellitus, hyperlipidemia and stress are seen in children and youth aged 7–17 years. Studies have also reported high-risk profiles in preschool-age children.[91] According to current statistics, an American child has a one in five chance of developing clinical symptoms of CHD before the age of 16.[91]

Although studies in adults have linked regular exercise to decreased overall risk for mortality, the few studies of children have been equivocal, except those conducted on obesity which confirm that increased daily activity and exercise help to control weight in obese children.[91] As mentioned earlier in the section on obesity, studies suggest that childhood obesity is associated more with inactivity than with overeating.

Encouraging exercise habits at an early age is especially important in light of research indicating that advancing age and elapsed time after initial adaptation of an activity routine are among the most consistent predictors of inactivity.[91] The ACSM currently recommends 20–30 minutes of vigorous exercise every day (see Appendix 1).[92]

As can be seen in Table 38.4, strength training with weights shows differing results in pre- (Tanner stage II) and postpubescent boys and girls.

A special concern that needs to be addressed in exercising children is the still common practice of "making weight" by wrestlers (i.e. losing weight to be certified for a weight class lower than their pre-season weight). Wrestlers typically make weight by a combination of food restriction, fluid deprivation, and sweating induced by thermal or exercise procedures.[96] Dehydration through sweating appears to be the most commonly used method.[96] Misuse of rubber suits, saunas, laxatives, steam rooms, and diuretics, singly or in combination, have all been employed in the practice of making weight.[96] Not only are these practices dangerous, but a recent study looking at repeated weight loss and gain, or weight cycling, in adolescent wrestlers also indicated decreased resting metabolic rate which may result in an increase in body fat.[97] The possibility of future problems with obesity is suggested. Physicians can help to prevent such problems by educating coaches, wrestlers and others, in the same manner as was suggested in the section on steroids.

Table 38.4 Effects of weight training on boys and girls[93–95]

Group	Strength	Muscle mass
Prepubescent		
Boys	Sl increase in only abdomen and back	No change
Girls	No data	No data
Postpubescent		
Boys	Increases	Increases
Girls	Increases	No change, unless anabolic steroids are used

The elderly

From peak function at the age of 30, the functional capacity of most organ systems decreases at a rate of about 0.75–1.0% per year. Physical work capacity, muscle strength and mass, flexibility, cardiac output, maximum heart rate, vital capacity, and renal and liver function all decline approximately 30% between the ages of 30 and 70.[98] Moreover, by the age of 70, women lose 30%, and men about 15%, of their bone mass. Approximately 50% of this decrease in function can be attributed to decreased physical activity.[98]

Exercise training can help to offset the decline in physiological function associated with aging. Elderly males and females can help to maintain bone mass and increase their physical work capacity through improving their cardiorespiratory endurance, strength, flexibility, and body composition.[99] These positive changes are demonstrated regardless of previous exercise patterns and current fitness status. The degree of improvement (expressed in relative terms) is comparable to that demonstrated by younger individuals, although the mechanism for the improvement may differ (i.e. strength may increase through improved recruitment of motor units rather than muscle hypertrophy).[99]

The older individual may need to begin exercising at a lower intensity, and progress more slowly than a younger subject, but with time the benefits will be the same.

Exercise and the immune system

Recently, attention has been focused on the possible effects of exercise on immune function. Early research with experimental animals found that it may enhance resistance to the growth of experimentally induced tumors, suggesting that exercise may stimulate the immunosurveillance function of natural immunity.[100] A recent study in humans indicated that frequent *tai chi quan* induced increases in T-lymphocyte count; exercise increased T-lymphocytes in the body.[101] The research thus far suggests that moderate exercise stimulates the immune system,[102] while intense exercise (e.g. training for the Olympics) can have the opposite effect.[102] The combination of increased stress and intense training that competitive athletics require may explain this phenomenon. The mechanism responsible for exercise-induced suppression or enhancement of immune function may be increased cortisol, catecholamines and/or endorphins, singly or in combination.

ENVIRONMENTAL CONSIDERATIONS

For outdoor exercisers, uncontrolled factors such as heat, cold, air pollution, and altitude will affect the exercise prescription.

Heat and humidity

During exercise, 75% of the metabolic energy of muscle action is converted to heat. Elite marathoners generate heat at 15–18 times the basal rate, which, if no heat were dissipated externally, would result in a 1°C increase in core temperature every 5 minutes.[103]

It is not surprising, then, that a number of deaths have been attributed to exercising in heat coupled with high relative humidity.[104,105] When exercising in hot weather, the body relies on the sweating mechanism for cooling, but in high humidity, evaporation cooling is limited. The amount of sun exposure is also critical as direct radiation is a major source of heat gain. Evaporation is also reduced when air movement is low.

There are a number of ways by which an exercising individual can decrease his/her risk of suffering heat-caused illness (heat cramps, heat exhaustion, heat stroke, or heat syncope) or death while exercising in hot weather.

Adequate hydration is a primary concern, particularly as strenuous exercise in a warm environment can result in water loss of up to 2 L/hour. The thirst mechanism is not a reliable indicator of the need to drink as dehydration will have already begun.[106] Water should be consumed prior (6–8 ounces), regularly during, and after strenuous exercise. Water and a diluted electrolyte solution appear to be the best fluids for quick rehydration.[8] Fluids high in glucose content slow gastric emptying and are not recommended.[106] Salt tablets are also not recommended as they draw water from the cells back into the gastrointestinal system. If necessary, extra salt added to food is more appropriate.[8,105]

Exercising during the cooler part of the day (i.e. early morning or early evening) and avoiding the sun's direct radiation is recommended. Wearing light-colored and minimal clothing (to expose the skin to air) is also recommended, as well as decreasing the intensity and duration of exercise during high-temperature and/or high-humidity days.

Exercisers should be able to recognize the early symptoms of heat injury, which include excessive sweating, headache, nausea, dizziness, and any impairment of consciousness.[105] They should also be aware that some populations are more susceptible than others – the very young and very old, the obese, the unconditioned, the unacclimatized, etc. – and that heat injury can occur under varied conditions: high temperature and low humidity, high humidity and low temperature, high solar radiation, little wind, on a relatively warm day following a bout of cooler weather and, of course, the lethal combination of high temperature and high humidity.[105]

Individuals respond differently to heat, and for those who cannot or do not want to change their routines, acclimatization helps the body to tolerate heat much more effectively. Fourteen days of training in the heat is necessary to become 90% acclimatized.[8] For additional information, refer to Appendix 1. The ACSM recommends against distance races when the wet bulb temperature exceeds 28°C.

Cold

Cold weather exercising presents far fewer problems than exercising in the heat. Temperatures (including wind chill factor) as low as –20°F can be tolerated if an individual is dressed appropriately.[8] Clothing should be worn in layers to allow flexibility in achieving the desired level of heat retention. The inner layer – cotton or silk – should absorb sweat to keep the outermost layer dry. A middle layer of wool will absorb excess sweat and allow evaporation, and an outermost layer of Goretex or polypropylene will protect against wind, rain and snow, yet let the body "breathe". A hat that covers the ears is very important, as 50% of body heat is lost or gained via the head. (On extremely cold days, goggles, a mask and/or petroleum jelly on the face might be necessary.) Gloves or mittens are particularly critical as circulation to the extremities is decreased due to their distance from the heart and limited musculature. Socks should be a wool/cotton mix or a ribbed, woven synthetic material.[8] Overdressing should be avoided; when appropriately dressed, the exerciser should feel slightly chilly at the start of exercise and begin to warm shortly after.

The clinical manifestations of cold injury include chilblains, muscle cramps, frostbite, and/or whole-body hypothermia, i.e. a rectal temperature of less than 35°C.[107] Conditions that increase the risk of cold stress include wet clothing, wind chill, remaining outside while sweating after cessation of the exercise session, and becoming lost while exercising in the cold.

Wind-chill factor, the combined effects of absolute temperature and wind velocity, should be a matter of great concern to the outdoor exerciser. Wind chill can dramatically affect absolute temperature, e.g. a 15 mph wind at 0°F would reduce effective temperature to –32°F.[8] Severe cold such as this can freeze exposed skin within minutes. As the exerciser tires, the metabolic heat production from exercise may decrease (if energy substrates are no longer available) to a point where heat loss to the environment exceeds heat production. After 1–2 hours of exposure, there are potentially fatal consequences.[8]

Some people are uncomfortable breathing cold air (especially cardiac patients susceptible to angina). A scarf draped around the face or a knitted ski mask worn to warm the inhaled air will help to prevent discomfort.[8]

The aforementioned guidelines are for outdoor exercise in cold air. Rapid heat loss is also a serious situation when swimming in a non-heated water environment. Extreme caution is advised.[107]

Air pollution

Recently, air pollution has become another factor to be concerned about when exercising outdoors, particularly in large metropolitan areas.

Carbon monoxide, due to its great affinity for binding with hemoglobin, impedes oxygen transport. High concentrations of carbon monoxide greatly decrease physical work capacity. Ozone has also been shown to have a negative effect on exercise performance.[8] Although only one pollutant in a given area may be identified as having reached an "alert" level, typically other pollutants will also be present, with cumulative detrimental effects on exercising individuals.

Exercisers can decrease air pollution exposure by exercising during the early morning hours before pollution accumulates, during periods of increased air movement (i.e. windy days), in less traveled areas, or indoors when pollution levels are high. The author has found value in wearing a surgical mask while exercising in major metropolitan areas, but has been unable to find any studies that have evaluated the efficacy of this or other more extreme precautionary measures, such as gas masks.

Altitude

As altitude increases, the partial pressure of oxygen is proportionately lower than at sea level. This makes it more difficult to deliver oxygen to the exercising muscles, and so performance is decreased in direct proportion to altitude.[8] As elevation increases, ambient temperature decreases, adding the stressor of cold to the equation.

As a result of this additional stress, exercise intensity should be decreased. If the RPE method for determining exercise intensity is used regularly, exercisers can adjust to maintain a level of exertion at high altitudes comparable to that they experience at sea level. After several weeks at a particular altitude, the body partially acclimatizes, but performance is still compromised. Caution must be exercised by individuals with CHD or abnormal lung function (i.e. emphysema and chronic bronchitis).[8]

SIDE-EFFECTS AND CONTRAINDICATIONS OF EXERCISE

Athlete's heart

While originally a pathologic diagnosis, athlete's heart, or increased heart size, is now known as a normal physiological response to training. Increased heart size may manifest as:[2]

- bradycardia
- a more prominent sinus arrhythmia
- a forceful apical impulse
- third and fourth heart sounds
- systolic flow murmurs.

ECG changes consistent with increased vagal tone (sinus bradycardia and arrhythmia, PR prolongation, and Wenckebach second-degree heart block) and ventricular hypertrophy may also be present.

Sports anemia

A mild decrease in hemoglobin or hematocrit, the so-called sports anemia, is commonly seen in endurance athletes. This, however, is not a true anemia, as red cell mass is normal. Rather, plasma volume is disproportionately increased.[2] Although only a small amount of iron is lost through perspiration, menstruating women who consume a low-iron diet may be at risk.

Exercise-induced hemolysis or gastrointestinal bleeding (occurring in 8–22% of marathon runners) may, however, exist and should be considered. While footstrike can produce intravascular hemolysis in runners, intravascular hemolysis has also been reported in swimmers, suggesting that trauma alone does not explain the phenomenon.[2] Contact activities such as karate, marching and football may produce enough trauma to capillaries to damage normal red blood cells. The effects are typically short-term and chronic anemia is rare. Sickle cell trait may increase risk, but the research is mixed.[2]

Athlete's hematuria and albuminuria

Exercise-induced hematuria and albuminuria are benign, self-limiting conditions occurring in many athletes. Microscopic or gross hematuria and mild albuminuria are most likely in the first urine voided after exercise and should resolve within 48 hours.[2] Severe or slowly resolving hematuria or albuminuria indicate the need for careful urinary tract evaluation.

Exercise-induced asthma

The association between vigorous exercise and asthma has long been recognized. Exercise-induced asthma (EIA) is not a variant form of asthma but rather a non-specific response occurring in approximately 12% of the population. During or immediately after exercise, symptoms and signs of EIA or bronchospasm are recognizable as dyspnea, choking, increased mucous production, fatigue, chest pain, and/or wheezing. The mechanism by which EIA is triggered is still unknown. It has been suggested that the increased loss of heat and/or water from the respiratory tract that results from exercise-induced hyperpnea, may be a trigger.[108] It has also been suggested that exercise intensity is the triggering factor, and that climatic conditions modify the severity of the EIA. In the study by Noriski et al,[109] it was found that the higher the intensity, the more severe the EIA.

Exercise therapy for asthma was not generally accepted as a treatment 10–15 years ago, due to the 40–95% rate of exercise-induced bronchospasm in asthmatic children exercising at school or on a playground.[110] Today, it is recognized that although exercise doesn't change the basic asthmatic condition as objectively measured by spirometry, it does improve physical fitness, develop skills, and help affected individuals to cope with the disease and its emotional component.[111]

EIA is frequently defined as 5–15 minutes of respiratory difficulty following 5–8 minutes of sustained exercise.[111] Running appears to be the most attack-provoking exercise and swimming the least.[111,112] Swimming the backstroke may help to alleviate breathing problems encountered in the water.[110]

The exercise prescription should initially be limited to 5 minute intervals to avoid triggering an attack. Short bursts of activity are tolerated well. The mode of exercise tolerated best appears to be those performed indoors in a controlled environment such as swimming, wrestling or stationary bicycling. Intensity can be high if intervals are short, 2–3 minutes. However, moderate exercises build endurance more effectively.[111] Frequency is the same as recommended for those without EIA. After training regularly for a year, other modes of exercise, even running, may be substituted.[110]

Exercise-induced urticaria and anaphylaxis

Exercise, fever, or a warm bath may induce a hypersensitivity reaction characterized by tiny urticarial lesions surrounded by large areas of erythema. Serum histamine levels are elevated and wheezing may occur[2] (see Ch. 191 for further discussion and therapeutic approach).

Occasionally, exercise may produce a syndrome virtually identical to allergen-induced anaphylaxis. The syndrome begins with a prodrome fatigue, warmth and pruritis, progressing to generalized urticaria and possibly to angioedema. Full-blown attacks result in choking, respiratory distress, abdominal colic, nausea, and syncope.[2] While the cause is unknown, the mechanism includes mast cell activation and elevated levels of histamine. There is a possible link to specific foods,[113] and familial cases have been reported.

Menstrual dysfunction and changes in sex hormones

Delayed menarche has been reported in girls who train heavily before puberty and amenorrhea or oligomenorrhea in highly trained adult female athletes. Nineteen per cent of Olympic marathon runners are amenorrheic. The pathogenesis is unknown, but is most likely multifactorial. Many factors have been associated with athletic menstrual dysfunction (AMD) including:

- weight loss
- intensity of exercise
- energy drain
- quantity and quality of diet
- aberrant nutritional patterns
- chronological age
- gynecological age
- competition stress-induced hypothalamic dysfunction (elevated serum cortisol and catecholamines appear to suppress LH release and possibly FSH, prolactin, and estradiol).

No long-term effects on reproductive function have been noted.[2]

A frequently cited cause is low body fat based on the work of Frisch and McArthur. They suggested that 22% body fat is necessary for onset and maintenance of menstrual function and hypothesized that this amount of body fat is necessary as adipose tissue converts androgens to estrogen. The major criticism of their research is that they used an indirect method, i.e. equations and height/weight tables, to estimate body fat. Other researchers using more direct body fat measurement, i.e. hydrostatic weighing, found no significant association between percentage body fat and AMD.[114] The body fat connection to athletic amenorrhea is controversial. While some studies have found a correlation,[115] several others have not,[114,116–118] suggesting that other factors are involved.

Endurance athletes, especially those who are amenorrheic, may be taking in too few calories to compensate for their energy output. Yet these athletes appear to maintain a stable weight, suggesting that there may be conservation of energy in other areas. As a lower resting metabolic rate has been associated with calorie restriction, it has been proposed that amenorrhea may be an energy-conserving response to a hypocaloric diet. Eating disorders have been found to be prevalent amongst endurance athletes, ballet dancers, and recreational and competitive body builders.[114,119] Research attention is now being focused on the association between diet and athletic activity as the cause of AMD. One recent study found that amenorrheic high-mileage runners seem to have a less adequate diet than eumenorrheic runners, although they appear to maintain an adequate energy balance and stable weight through a reduction in resting metabolic rate.[114]

In men, acute exercise increases, while chronic exercise and weight loss decrease, testosterone. A small number of highly trained marathon runners are also found to have oligospermia.[2]

Osteoporosis

Amenorrheic athletes may be at risk of osteoporosis. Vertebral (but not radius) bone density is reduced in these women, and an increased incidence of fractures has been found.[2] Young ballet dancers with delayed menarche and secondary amenorrhea have an increased risk of scoliosis and stress fractures.[120] Slightly decreasing exercise or increasing body weight usually re-establishes their menstrual cycle. Both menstruating and menopausal physically fit women have higher bone density than sedentary women.

Incontinence

A common, although little known, problem for women is incontinence during exercise. While considerable research has studied the effects of exercise on most of the body's organs and structures, little attention has been paid to the lower urogenital tract until recently. A 1990 study by Nygaard et al[121] found that 47% of participants had some degree of incontinence. This figure correlated with the number of vaginal deliveries. Of these, 30% noted incontinence during at least one type of exercise. Exercises involving repetitive bouncing (i.e. running, high-impact aerobics, tennis, low-impact aerobics, and walking) were associated with the highest incidence of incontinence. Incontinence caused 20% of exercisers to stop an exercise, 18% to change the way a specific exercise was performed, and 55% to wear a pad during exercise. With one in three women experiencing the problem, this study clearly demonstrated that incontinence during exercise is not unusual. Exercise per se is not the cause of incontinence (only one woman was incontinent solely during exercise), but could prove to be a possible obstacle for some women. In this study, women appeared to be very adaptive. Some non-surgical options to ameliorate incontinence include Kegel exercises, weighted vaginal cones, and interferential therapy.[122]

Acute muscle injury

Elevated levels of muscle enzymes usually accompany exercise. Creatine kinase is the most sensitive, rising within minutes of even mild exercise and lasting for days after strenuous exercise. Delayed onset muscle soreness after exercise correlates with CK levels. Strenuous exercise produces mild elevations in serum AST (formerly SGOT) and myoglobin, while high levels of the latter may indicate potentially serious rhabdomyolysis.

Heat stroke

Heat stroke, representing a serious failure of thermoregulation, is a medical emergency. A diminution of sweating is commonly observed prior to the onset of symptoms, which are, typically:

- the abrupt onset of altered consciousness
- prostration
- flushed, dry skin
- tachycardia
- dehydration.

Body temperatures in excess of 41.1°C are common, although some victims have lower temperatures. The primary treatment is intravenous fluids and active cooling, involving the application of ice packs or ice-water baths until core temperature reaches 39°C. Adjunct therapy includes fluids, electrolytes as needed, correction of acidosis, treatment of arrhythmias, and circulatory and respiratory support.[2]

Sudden death

The 1984 death of author and marathon runner, Jim Fixx, raised questions about the safety of vigorous exercise. As exercising increased in popularity in the 1970s and 1980s, several studies were published reporting cardiovascular complications and sudden deaths during or following vigorous exercise.[123–128] However, a report by Koplan[129] estimated that, statistically, 100 deaths per year would occur during jogging, simply by chance.

The cause of death in both young (under 30 years) and old (over 30 years) conditioned subjects who die suddenly during or immediately following vigorous exercise is congenital or acquired CHD in 90% of cases.[130] In those over the age of 30, atherosclerotic heart disease is the primary killer, while in those under 30, congenital coronary artery anomalies and hypertrophic cardiomyopathy are the primary causes.[130–132] Sudden death in young men is often predated by such symptoms as syncope and chest pain.

The data suggests that exercise contributes to sudden death in susceptible persons. This implies that those over the age of 30 who participate in vigorous exercise without also modifying other high-risk factors for CHD (e.g. hypercholesterolemia, smoking, etc.), increase their risk of sudden death during vigorous exercise.[133,134] This is, however, offset by the decreased risk of cardiac mortality induced by fitness.

Steroid use

Anabolic-androgenic steroid use is currently viewed as a serious health problem. At one time, weight lifters were the primary consumers of these drugs, but recently both male and female power athletes, endurance athletes, and even non-athletes are consuming steroids.

While the use of steroids may be accompanied by gains in lean body mass, body weight, and strength, it has also been associated with adverse effects. These include liver, cardiovascular, reproductive, and psychological abnormalities, as well as lowered HDL levels.[2,135,136] Other risks include diseases associated with shared needles, such as hepatitis and AIDS.[137]

Despite the growing awareness of the potential side-effects of steroid use, its popularity is increasing and the consumers are getting younger. A recent study by Windsor & Dumitru[138] found a significant percentage of male and female high school students (particularly male athletes from upper socioeconomic levels) using anabolic steroids obtained illicitly (group I male athletes reported a 10.2% prevalence).

Athletes use steroids in an attempt to improve performance in a variety of sports, most commonly those requiring considerable strength such as football, wrestling, weight lifting, sprinting, shot put, etc. They are also used by swimmers, cyclists, and male and female bodybuilders. One recent study found users among high school students who did not even participate in organized sports.[139]

The use of androgenic steroids began in the 1950s and has increased in the decades since, despite warnings of potential harmful side-effects and their banning by the International Olympic Committee.[135] Education is of vital importance to curb the abuse of steroids. Physicians can contribute to the education effort by providing athletes and other users with timely and accurate information on the health risks and performance enhancement effects of steroid use. For additional information, please refer to the ACSM position statement in Appendix 1.

CONCLUSION

Although many unanswered questions still remain, a sufficient body of data is available to conclude that regular physical activity promotes good health. This may seem an obvious statement to those who believe in the value of exercise, but due to the multifactorial nature of disease, it is a difficult hypothesis to prove. The probable benefits of exercise are many, including prevention of the leading causes of morbidity and mortality in the United States. Exercise therapy plays a major role in naturopathic medicine, which advances the concept that a healthy and fit body promotes a healthy and fit mind.

REFERENCES

1. Astrand PO, Rodahl K. Textbook of work physiology. New York, NY: McGraw-Hill. 1977: p 555–558
2. Rubenstein E, Federman DD. Scientific American medicine. New York, NY: Scientific American. 1991: p CTM: I: 1–32
3. Kuipers H, Janssen GME, Bosman F et al. Structural and ultrastructural changes in skeletal muscle associated with long-distance training and running. Int J Sports Med 1989; 10: S156
4. Orten JM, Neuhaus OW. Human Biochemistry. St Louis: CV Mosby. 1982: p 680–681
5. Winter FD, Snell PG, Stray-Gunderson J et al. Effects of 100% oxygen on performance of professional soccer players. JAMA 1989; 262: 227
6. Weber H. The energy cost of aerobic dance. Fitness for Living 1974; 8: 26–30
7. Cooper K. The aerobics way. New York, NY: Bantam Books. 1977: p 88, 280–283
8. Pollack ML, Wilmore JH, Fox SM. Exercise in health and disease. Philadelphia, PA: WB Saunders. 1984: p 131, 141–147, 219–221, 228–234, 378, 382, 384–385, 457–458
9. Borg GV. Psychophysical bases of perceived exertion. Med Sci Sports Exerc 1982; 14: 377–381
10. American College of Sports Medicine. Guidelines for graded exercise testing and prescription. 3rd edn. Philadelphia, PA: Lea & Febiger. 1986. p 1–4, 22, 36, 48–49, 74–78, 80–83, 456–459
11. Pollack ML, Miller HS, Linnerud AC, Cooper KH. Frequency of training as a determinant for improvement in cardiovascular function and body composition of middle-aged men. Phys Med Rehab 1975; 58: 141–145
12. Getchell B, Marshall MG. The basic guidelines for being fit. In: Strauss RH, ed. Sports medicine. Philadelphia, PA: WB Saunders. 1984: p 457–467

13. Beaulieu JE. Developing a stretching program. Phys Sports Med 1981; 9: 59–65
14. Bassler TJ. Athletic activity and longevity (letter). Lancet 1972; i: 712–713
15. Bassler TJ. Marathon running and immunity to atherosclerosis. Ann NY Acad Sci 1977; 301: 579–592
16. Haskell WL. Cardiovascular benefits and risks of exercise: the scientific evidence. In: Strauss RH, ed. Sports medicine. Philadelphia, PA: WB Saunders. 1984: p 57–75
17. Paffenbarger RS, Jr, Hyde RT, Jung DC, Wing AL. Epidemiology of exercise and coronary heart disease. Clinics in Sports Medicine 1984; 3: 297–315
18. Morris JN, Heady JA, Raffle PAB et al. Coronary heart disease and physical activity of work. Lancet 1953; ii: 1111
19. Paffenbarger RS, Jr, Hale WE, Brand RJ, Hyde RT. Work. energy level, personal characteristics, and fatal heart attack: a birth-cohort effect. Am J Epidemiol 1977; 105: 200–203
20. Taylor HL, Klepetar E, Keys A et al. Death rates among physically active and sedentary employees of the railroad industry. Am J Public Health 1962; 52: 1697–1707
21. Kannel WB, Gordon T, Sorlie P et al. Physical activity and coronary vulnerability: the Framingham study. Cardiol Digest 1971; 6: 28
22. Leon AS. Physical activity levels and CHD. Analysis of epidemiologic and supporting studies. Med Clin N Am 1985; 69: 3–40
23. Leon AS, Connett J, Jacobs DR Jr, Rauramaa R. Leisure-time physical activity levels and risk of CHD and death: the multiple risk factor intervention trial. JAMA 1987; 258: 2388–2395
24. Paffenbarger RS, Jr, Hyde RT, Wing A, Hsieh CC. Physical activity, all-cause mortality and longevity of college alumni. New Engl J Med 1986; 314: 605–613
25. Paffenbarger RS, Jr, Hyde RT, Wing AL, Steinmetz CH. A natural history of athleticism and cardiovascular health. JAMA 1984; 252: 491–495
26. Blair SN, Kohl HW III, Paffenbarger RS, Jr et al. Physical fitness and all-cause mortality. A prospective study of healthy men and women. JAMA 1989; 262: 2395–2401
27. Kallio VH, Hamalainen H, Hakkila J, Luurila OJ. Reduction in sudden deaths by a multifactorial intervention programme after acute myocardial infarction. Lancet 1979; ii: 1091–1098
28. Debusk RF, Houston N, Haskell W et al. Exercise training soon after myocardial infarction. Am J Cardiol 1979; 44: 1223–1229
29. Savin WM, Haskell WL, Houston-Miller N, DeBusk RF. Improvement in aerobic capacity soon after myocardial infarction. J Cardiac Rehab 1981; 1: 337–342
30. Goldberg LE, Elliot DL, Schutz RW, Kloster FE. Changes in lipid and lipoprotein levels after weight training. JAMA 1984; 252: 504–506
31. Miller WJ, Sherman WM, Ivy JL. Effect of strength training on glucose tolerance and post-glucose insulin response. Med Sci Sports Exerc 1984; 16: 539–543
32. Hagberg JM, Ehsani AA, Goldring O et al. Effect of weight training on blood pressure and hemodynamics in hypertensive adolescents. J Ped 1984; 104: 147–151
33. Hurley BF, Hagberg JM, Goldberg AP et al. Resistive training can reduce coronary risk factors w/o altering VO_2MAX or percent body fat. Med Sci Sports Exerc 1988; 20: 150–154
34. Blair SN, Goodyear NN, Gibbons LW et al. Physical fitness and incidence of hypertension in healthy normotensive men and women. JAMA 1984; 252: 487
35. Paffenbarger RS, Jr, Wing AL, Hyde RT et al. Physical activity and incidence of hypertension in college alumni. Am J Epidem 1983; 117: 245
36. Duncan JJ, Farr JE, Upton SJ et al. The effects of aerobic exercise on plasma catecholamines and blood pressure in patients with mild essential hypertension. JAMA 1985; 254: 2609
37. Cade R, Mars D, Wagemaker H et al. Effect of aerobic exercise training on patients with systemic arterial hypertension. Am J Med 1984; 77: 785
38. Powell KE, Caspersen CJ, Koplan JP, Ford ES. Physical activity and chronic diseases. Am J Clin Nutr 1989; 49: 999–1006
39. Vena JE, Graham S, Zielezny M et al. Lifetime occupational exercise and colon cancer. Am J Epidemiol 1985; 122: 357–365
40. Persky V, Dyer AR, Leonas J et al. Heart rate. a risk factor for cancer? Am J Epidemiol 1981; 114: 477–487
41. Paffenbarger RS, Jr, Hyde RT, Wing AL. Physical activity and incidence of cancer in diverse populations. a preliminary report Am J Clin Nutr 1987; 45: 312–317
42. Cordain L, Latin RW, Behnke JJ. The effects of an aerobic running program on bowel transit time. J Sports Med 1986; 26: 101–104
43. American College of Sports Medicine. Position statement on proper and improper weight loss programs. Med Sci Sports Exer 1983; 15: ix–xiii
44. Oscai LB, Holloszy JO. Effects of weight changes produced by exercise, food restriction or overeating on body composition. J Clin Invest 1969; 48: 2124–2128
45. Lennon D, Nagle F, Stratman F et al. Diet and exercise training effects on resting metabolic rate. Int J Obes 1988; 9: 39–47
46. Hill JO, Schlundt DG, Sbrocco T et al. Evaluation of an alternating-calorie diet with and without exercise in the treatment of obesity. Am J Clin Nutr 1989; 50: 238–254
47. Gwinup G, Chelvam R, Steinberg T. Thickness of subcutaneous fat and activity of underlying muscles. Am Int Med 1971; 74: 408–411
48. Fahey TD, Brown CH. The effects of anabolic steroid on strength, body composition and endurance of college males when accompanied by a weight training program. Med Sci Sports 1973; 5: 272–276
49. Wilmore JH. Alterations in strength, body composition and athropometric measurements consequent to a 10-week weight training program. Med Sci Sports 1974; 6: 133–138
50. Ballor DL, Katch VL, Becque MD, Marks CR. Resistance weight training during calorie restriction enhances lean body weight maintenance. Am J Clin Nutr 1988; 47: 19–25
51. Gwinup G. Weight loss without dietary restriction. efficacy of different forms of aerobic exercise. Am J Sports Med 1987; 15: 275
52. Ekoe JM. Overview of diabetes mellitus and exercise. Med Sci Sports Exerc 1989; 21: 353–355
53. Vitug A, Schneider SH, Ruderman NB. Exercise and type I diabetes mellitus. Exerc Sports Sci Rev 1988; 16: 285–304
54. Duda M. The role of exercise in managing diabetes. Phys Sports Med 1985; 13: 164–170
55. Hughes RL, Davison R. Limitation of exercise reconditioning in cold. Chest 1983; 83: 241
56. Swerts PMJ, Kretzers LMJ, Terpstra-Lindeman E et al. Exercise reconditioning in the rehabilitation of patients with chronic obstructive pulmonary disease: a short- and long-term analysis. Arch Phys Med Rehabil 1990; 71: 570–573
57. Unger KM, Moser KM, Hansen P. Selection of an exercise program for patients with chronic obstructive pulmonary disease. Heart Lung 1980; 9: 68–76
58. Pierce AK, Taylor HF, Archer RK et al. Responses to exercise training in patients with emphysema. Arch Int Med 1964; 113: 78
59. Sinclair DJM, Ingram CG. Controlled trial of supervised exercise training in chronic pulmonary bronchitis. Br Med J 1980; 280: 519
60. Cochrane LM, Clark CJ. Benefits and problems of a physical training programme for asthmatic patients. Thorax 1990; 45: 345–351
61. Chester EH, Belman MJ, Bauler RC et al. Multidisciplinary treatment of chronic pulmonary insufficiency. 3. The effect of physical training on cardiopulmonary performance in patients with COPD. Chest 1977; 72: 695
62. Harver A, Mahler DA, Daubenspeck JA. Targeted inspiratory muscle training improves respiratory muscle function and reduces dyspnea in patients with chronic obstructive pulmonary disease. Ann Intern Med 1989; 111: 117
63. Painter PL. Exercise in end-stage renal disease. Exerc Sport Sci Rev 1988; 16: 305–339
64. Squires RW, Brekke JD, Gau GT et al. Early exercise testing and training after renal transplantation (abstract). Med Sci Sports Exerc 1985; 17: 184
65. Painter P, Nelson-Worel JN, Hill MM et al. Effects of exercise training during hemodialysis. Nephron 1986; 43: 87–92
66. Zabetakis PM, Gleim GW, Pasternak FL et al. Long-duration

submaximal exercise conditioning in hemodialysis patients. Clin Neph 1982; 18: 17
67. Raithel KS. Chronic pain and exercise therapy. Phys Sports Med 1989; 17: 203–209
68. Selby DK. Conservative care of non-specific low back pain. Orthop Clin N Amer 1982; 13: 427
69. Thoren P, Flores JS, Hoffman P, Seals DR. Endorphins and exercise, physiological mechanisms and clinical implications. Med Sci Sports Exerc 1990; 22: 417–428
70. Lichter RL, Hewson JK, Radke SJ, Blum M. Treatment of chronic low-back pain. Clin Orthop 1984; 190: 115–123
71. McGain GA, Bell DA, Mai FM et al. A controlled study of the effects of a supervised cardiovascular fitness training program on the manifestations of primary fibromyalgia. Arthritis Rheum 1988; 31: 1135–1141
72. Cureton TK. Improvement of psychological states by means of exercise-fitness programs. J Assoc Phys Mental Rehabil 1963; 17: 14–25
73. McCann L, Holmes DS. Influence of aerobic exercise on depression. J Pers Soc Psychol. 1984; 46: 1142–1147
74. Berger BG, Owen OR. Mood alteration with swimming – swimmers really do "feel better". Psychosom Med 1983; 45: 425–433
75. Farmer ME, Locke BZ, Mosciki EK et al. Physical activity and depressive symptomatology. the NHANES 1 epidemiologic follow-up study. Am J Epidemiol 1988; 1328: 1340–1351
76. Morgan WP. Physical fitness and emotional health. a review. Amer Corr Ther J 1969; 23: 124–127
77. Taylor CB, Sallis JF, Needle R. The relationship between physical activity and exercise and mental health. Public Health Rep 1985; 100: 195–202
78. Raglin JS, Morgan WP. Influence of vigorous exercise on mood state. Behav Ther 1985; 8: 179–183
79. Morgan WP. Affective beneficence of physical activity. Med Sci Sports Exerc 1985; 17: 94–100
80. Blumenthal JA, Fredrickson M, Kuhn CM et al. Aerobic exercise reduces levels of cardiovascular and sympathoadrenal responses to mental stress in subjects without prior evidence of myocardial ischemia. Am J Cardiol 1990; 65: 93
81. Steinberg H, Sykes EA. Introduction to symposium on endorphins and behavioral processes: review of literature on endorphins and exercise. Pharmacol Biochem Behav 1985; 23: 857–862
82. Leer F. Running as an adjunct to psychotherapy. Social Work 1980; Jan: 20–25
83. Kulpa PJ, White BM, Visscher R. Aerobic exercise in pregnancy. Am J Obstet Gynecol 1987; 156: 1395–1403
84. Wallace AM, Boyer DB, Dan A, Holm K. Aerobic exercise, maternal self-esteem and physical discomforts during pregnancy. J Nurse Midwifery 1986; 31: 255–262
85. Hall DC, Kaufmann DA. Effects of aerobic and strength conditioning on pregnancy outcomes. Am J Obstet Gynecol 1987; 157: 1199–1203
86. American College of Sports Medicine. Meeting report. Pregnancy and exercise. Phys Sports Med 1985; 13: 145–147
87. Paisley JE, Mellion MB. Exercise during pregnancy. AFP 1988; 38: 143–150
88. Carpenter MW, Sady SP, Hoegsberg B et al. Fetal heart rate response to maternal exertion. JAMA 1988; 259: 3006–3009
89. Beller JM, Dolny DG. Effect of an aerobic endurance exercise program on maternal and fetal heart rate during the second and third trimester. Med Sci Sports Exerc 1987; 19: 55
90. Dressendorfer RH, Goodlin RC. Fetal heart rate response to maternal exercise testing. Phys Sports Med 1980; 8: 90–93, 96
91. Dishman RK, Dunn AL. Exercise adherence in children and youth: implication for adulthood. In: Dishman RK, ed. Exercise adherence. Champaign, IL: Human Kinetics Books. 1988: p 155–200
92. American College of Sports Medicine. Opinion statement on physical fitness in children and youth. Med Sci Sports Exerc 1988; 20: 422–423
93. Kuland DN, Tottossy M. Warm-up, strength and power. Orthop Clin N Am 1983; 14: 427
94. Vrijens J. Muscle strength development in the pre- and post-pubescent age. Medicine Sport 1978; 11: 152–158
95. American Academy of Pediatrics. Policy statement on weight training and weight lifting. information for the pediatrician. News and Comment 1982; 33: 7
96. American College of Sports Medicine. Position statement on weight loss in wrestlers. Med Sci Sports Exerc 1976; 8: xi–xiii
97. Steen SN, Oppliger RA, Brownell KD. Metabolic effects of repeated weight loss and regain in adolescent wrestlers. JAMA 1988; 260: 47–50
98. Landin RJ, Linnemeir TJ, Rothbaum DA et al. Exercise testing and training of the elderly patient. In: Wenger NK, ed. Exercise and the heart. 2nd edn. Philadelphia, PA: FA Davis. 1985: p 201–218
99. Stamford BA. Exercise and the elderly. Exec Sport Sci Rev 1988; 16: 341–379
100. Makinnon LT. Exercise and natural killer cells: what is their relationship? Sports Med 1989; 7: 141–149
101. Xusheng S, Yugi X, Yunjian X. Determination of E-rosette-forming lymphocytes in aged subjects with tai chi quan exercise. Int J Sport Med 1989; 10: 217–219
102. Fitzgerald L. Exercise and the immune system. Immunol Today 1988; 9: 337–339
103. Nadel ER, Wenger CB, Roberts MF et al. Physiological defenses against hyperthermia of exercise. Ann NY Acad Sci 1977; 301: 98
104. Sutton JR, Bar-or O. Thermal illness in fun running. Am Heart J 1980; 100: 778–771
105. Sutton JR. Heat illness. In: Strauss RH, ed. Sports medicine. Philadelphia, PA: WB Saunders. 1984: p 307–322
106. American College of Sports Medicine. Position Statement on the prevention of thermal injuries during distance running. Med Sci Sports Exerc 1987; 19: 529–533
107. Bangs CC. Cold injuries. In: Strauss RH, ed. Sports Medicine. Philadelphia, PA: WB Saunders. 1984: p 323–343
108. Sheppard D. What does exercise have to do with "exercise-induced" asthma? Am Rev Respir Dis 1987; 136: 547–549
109. Noriski N, Bar-Yishay E, Gur I, Godfrey S. Exercise intensity determines and climatic conditions modify the severity of EIA. Am Rev Respir Dis 1987; 136: 592–594
110. Szentagothai K, Gyene I, Szocska M, Osuath P. Physical exercise program for children with bronchial asthma. Pediatric Pulmonol 1987; 3: 166–172
111. Kennel JH. Sports participation for the child with a chronic health problem. In: Strauss RH, ed. Sports medicine. Philadelphia, PA: WB Saunders. 1984: p 227–228
112. Inbar O, Dotan R, Dlin RA et al. Breathing dry or humid air and exercise-induced asthma during swimming. Eur J Appl Physiol 1980; 44: 43–50
113. Buchbinder EM, Bloch KJ, Moss J et al. Food-dependent, exercise-induced anaphylaxis. JAMA 1983; 250: 2973
114. Myerson M, Gutin B, Warren MP et al. Resting metabolic rate and energy balance in amenorrheic and eumenorrheic runners. Med Sci Sports Exerc 1991; 23: 15–22
115. Bullen BA, Skrinar GS, Beitins IZ et al. Induction of menstrual disorders by strenuous exercise in untrained women. New Engl J Med 1985; 312: 1349
116. Sanborn CF, Albrecht BH, Wagner WW. Athletic amenorrhea: lack of association with body fat. Med Sci Sports Exerc 1987; 19: 207–212
117. Baker ER, Mathur RS, Kirk FR, Williamson HO. Female runners and secondary amenorrhea: correlation with age, parity, mileage and plasma hormonal and sex-hormone-binding globulin concentrations. Fertil Steril 1981; 36: 183–187
118. Wakat DK, Sweeney KA, Rogol AD. Reproductive system function in women runners. Med Sci Sports Exerc 1982; 14: 263–269
119. Walberg JL, Johnston CS. Menstrual function and eating behavior in female recreational weight lifters and competitive body builders. Med Sci Sports Exerc 1991; 23: 30–36
120. Warren MP, Brooks-Gunn J, Hamilton LH et al. Scoliosis and fractures in young ballet dancers. relation to delayed menarche and secondary amenorrhea. New Engl J Med 1986; 146: 39
121. Nygaard I, DeLancy JOL, Arnsdorf L et al. Exercise and incontinence. Obstet Gyn 1990; 75: 848–851

122. Olah KS, Bridges N, Denny J et al. The conservative management of patients with symptoms of stress incontinence: a randomized prospective study comparing weighted vaginal cones and interferential therapy. Am J Obstet Gyn 1990; 162: 87–92
123. Thompson PD, Funk EJ, Carleton RA et al. Incidence of death during jogging in Rhode Island from 1975 through 1980. JAMA 1982; 247: 2535
124. Opie LH. Sudden death and sport. Lancet 1975; i: 263–266
125. Opie LH. Long distance running and sudden death. New Engl J Med 1975; 293: 941–942
126. Vuori I, Makarainen M, Jaaskelianen A. Sudden death and physical activity. Cardiology 1978; 63: 287–304
127. McManus BM, Waller BF, Graboys TB et al. Exercise and sudden death – Part I. Curr Prob Cardiol 1981; 9: 1–89
128. McManus BM, Waller BF, Graboys TB et al. Exercise and Sudden death – Part II. Curr Prob Cardiol 1982; 10: 1–57
129. Koplan JP. Cardiovascular deaths while running. JAMA 1979; 242: 2578–2579
130. Waller B. Exercise-related sudden death in young (age <30 years) and old (age >30 years) conditioned subjects. In: Wenger NK. ed. Exercise and the heart. 2nd edn. Philadelphia, PA: FA Davis. 1985: p 9–73
131. Thompson PD, Stern MP, Williams P et al. Death during running or jogging. A study of 18 cases. JAMA 1979; 242: 1265–1267
132. Maron BJ, Roberts WC, McAllister HA, Jr et al. Sudden death in young athletes. Circulation 1980; 62: 218–229
133. Noakes TD. Heart disease in marathon runners. a review. Med Sci Sports Exerc 1987; 19: 187–194
134. Hellerstein NK, Moir WT. Distance running in the 1980s. cardiovascular benefits and risks. In: Wenger NK, ed. Exercise and the heart. 2nd edn. Philadelphia, PA: FA Davis. 1985: p 75–85
135. American College of Sports Medicine. Position statement on the use of anabolic-androgenic steroids in sports. Med Sci Sports Exerc 1987; 19: 534–539
136. Hallagan JB, Hallagan LF, Snyder MB. Anabolic-androgenic steroid use by athletes (letter). New Engl J Med 1989; 321: 1042–1045
137. Sklarek HM, Mantovani RP, Evens E et al. AIDS in a body builder using anabolic steroids. New Engl J Med 1984; 311: 1701
138. Windsor R, Dumitru D. Prevalence of anabolic steroid use by male and female adolescents. Med Sci Sports Exerc 1989; 21: 494–497
139. Johnson MD, Jay MS, Shoup JB, Richert VI. Anabolic steroid use by male adolescents. Pediatrics 1989; 83: 921–924

CHAPTER CONTENTS

39

Faith: a powerful force for healing

Lara E. Pizzorno, MA (Divinity)

INTRODUCTION

Faith and medical science are not mutually exclusive. In fact, faith's efficacy as a powerful healing force has been scientifically validated by hundreds of experiments exhibiting all the criteria of good science.[1] Research into the healing power of participation in religious activities such as prayer has demonstrated that faith in a supreme being – whether God, Allah, Brahman, the Tao, the Absolute, the Universal Mind – produces significant, beneficial effects on health, including lowering blood pressure, protecting against heart disease, improving surgical outcomes and lessening recovery time, increasing feelings of well-being, ameliorating depression, and improving the ability to cope with stress while lessening its adverse physiological effects. Religious commitment has been shown to help protect children from drug abuse, alcohol abuse, and suicide. Among the elderly, those who live in faith tend to live longer.[2]

In the current medical model, most physicians are led to believe that any consideration of religious commitment is beyond the interest and scope of medical care. The dogma is that faith is not amenable to serious scientific scrutiny, and is merely a relic from earlier less enlightened ages, a crutch for the scientifically disinclined. Medical students and residents get the subliminal message that to personally pursue an active religious faith is to court schizophrenia, traveling simultaneously down the right-brain path of faith, religion, and prayer (read: irrationality and superstition), and the left-brain arterial of logic, analytical diaphoresis, and rational thought (read: science). In modern medical education, devotions are to be paid only to "Science" with a capital "S", which leaves the whole realm of the numinous outside the Venn diagram locus of serious medicine. So, members of the health care professions tend to disassociate their spirituality from their science, both in their training and later in their clinical practice and academic endeavors. Recent scientific research itself, however, has made such an uncritical stance medically irresponsible.

Significant evidence exists that prayer functions at a distance to change physical processes in a variety of organisms, from bacteria to humans. In addition to humans, the subjects in studies have included water, enzymes, bacteria, fungi, yeast, red blood cells, cancer cells, pacemaker cells, seeds, plants, algae, moth larvae, mice and chicks. Processes influenced include the activity of enzymes, the growth rates of leukemic white blood cells, mutation rates of bacteria, germination and growth rates of various seeds, the firing rate of pacemaker cells, healing rates of wounds, the size of goiters and tumors, the time required to awaken from anesthesia, autonomic effects such as electrodermal activity of the skin, rates of hemolysis of red blood cells, and hemoglobin levels.[3] Given the scientific support of prayer's beneficial effects, not praying for the best possible outcome for one's patients may be the equivalent of deliberately withholding an effective drug or surgical procedure.

PRAYER CONCEPTUALIZED

In *Healing Words: the Power of Prayer and the Practice of Medicine,*[1] Larry Dossey MD provides a review of the scientific evidence plus the terminology and conceptual framework with which to discuss and evaluate new studies on prayer.

The word "prayer" is derived from the Latin *precarius* ("obtained by begging") and *precari* ("to entreat – to ask earnestly, beseech, implore"). This suggests the two most common forms of prayer: *petition,* asking something for one's self; and *intercession,* asking something for others. Other types of prayer include:

- *confession* – the repentance of wrongdoing and asking for forgiveness
- *lamentation* – crying in distress and asking for vindication
- *adoration* – giving honor and praise
- *invocation* – summoning the presence of the Almighty
- *thanksgiving* – offering gratitude.

Prayer, in which communication frequently surpasses the limits of language, is often wordless. Theologian Ann Ulanov and Professor Barry Ulanov have termed such prayer "primary speech…the most fundamental, primordial, and important 'language' humans speak".[4] Prayer may be individual or communal, conscious or unconscious, emerging in dreams.

Perhaps most importantly, prayer is a *non-local* event – it is not confined to a specific place and time, but reaches outside the here and now, operating at a distance, and outside the present moment. Since prayer is initiated by a mental action, the implication is that some aspect of ourselves is also non-local. Because a limited non-locality is a contradiction in terms, the non-locality of prayer implies that something of ourselves is infinite in space and time, eternal, immortal. Empirical evidence for the power of prayer is indirect evidence for the soul, and for a relationship with the Divine whose locus is within each of us.

RESEARCH

Despite growing practitioner and patient acceptance of the important role of faith and prayer in health and healing, this area has received relatively little research attention, and health care professionals receive minimal or no formal training. A systematic analysis of 4,306,906 studies indexed on Medline from 1980 to 1996 revealed only 364 abstracts considering faith, religion or prayer. Although all of these case reports involved religious and spiritual issues, only 45 (12%) explicitly mentioned a religious professional. Of these, only eight (2%) indicated any collaboration between health care and religious professionals.[5]

Another study looked at all quantitative studies in the *Journal of Family Practice* published from 1976 to 1986, to determine how often religious variables were included.[6] A total of 1,086 studies were reviewed. More than half measured at least one quantified variable. However, only 21 (3.5%) of those quantified studies measured at least one religious variable. Measures of religious commitment, such as frequency of church attendance, social support, prayer and relationship with God, were found to be beneficial to health 83% of the time, neutral 17% of the time and harmful at no time at all.

A systematic review of major psychiatric journals from 1978 through 1989 found 2,348 studies that included quantified data. Among the quantitative studies, 59 (2.5%) included one or more religious measures. In only three of the studies was a religious measure a central variable.[7] During 12 years, religious commitment measures of ceremony, social support, prayer and relationship with God showed benefit 92% of the time, were neutral 4% of the time, and negative 4% of the time.

Larson et al[8] have identified several factors impeding clinical research in this area:

- conceptual barriers – lack of consensus regarding what constitutes religion and spirituality
- methodological barriers – difficulty in establishing appropriate control groups, and difficulty in controlling for factors which might not be measured
- structural barriers – long history of conflict between science and religion
- professional disincentive – publication bias, possible inhibition of tenure and limited funding.

One interesting investigation found that studies on

alternative approaches are likely to be discriminated against by journals. Using a randomized, double-blind protocol, one researcher submitted a fictional study on obesity treatment to 398 expert peer reviewers. The articles were identical, except for the therapy – one used a conventional drug, the other a homeopathic remedy. The reviewers were three times more likely to recommend publication of the drug study over the homeopathic study.[9]

The paucity of published studies (0.008% of the Medline records) and appalling lack of collaboration between health care and religious professionals demonstrate a serious gap between the public, the health care system and the medical research establishment. This gap must be bridged for the benefit of our patients.

Religious activity is prevalent in society

Religion plays an important role in the lives of the vast majority of patients, especially the elderly. This is well demonstrated in a study that examined the prevalence of religious beliefs and practices among medically ill hospitalized older adults and related them to social, psychological and health characteristics. Consecutive patients age 60 or over admitted to the general medicine cardiology and neurology services of Duke University Medical Center were evaluated for participation in a depression study. As part of the evaluation, information on religious affiliation, religious attendance, private religious activities, intrinsic religiosity and religious coping was collected from 455 cognitively unimpaired patients. Demographic, social, psychological and physical health characteristics were also assessed. Over one-half (53.4%) of the sample reported attending religious services once per week or more often; 58.7% prayed or studied the Bible daily or more often; over 85% of patients held intrinsic religious attitudes; and over 40% spontaneously reported that their religious faith was the most important factor that enabled them to cope. Bivariate and multivariate analysis showed that religious belief and activity were consistently and independently related to race (black), lower education, higher social support and greater life stressors, and religious attendance was associated with a lower medical illness burden. Religious attendance was also related to fewer depressive symptoms, although the association weakened when other covariates were controlled.[10]

Religious commitment and engaging in prayer improve health

The positive benefit of religious commitment is documented by a growing number of studies in the medical literature. Looking at the single religious commitment measure of frequency of attendance at religious services, one review of studies found that those attending services weekly or more had significantly better health across a vast array of illnesses. Attending religious services benefited health 81% of the time, showed no effect 15% of the time, and had a 4% rate of harm. Researchers concluded that given this strikingly positive association, infrequent church attendance could be regarded as a risk factor for greater incidence of disease.[11]

An intriguing large randomized, controlled, double-blind study utilized 90 volunteers (agents) to pray for 406 subjects. The subjects were randomly assigned to three groups: controls, prayed for directly and prayed for indirectly. Agents were randomly assigned to either the directed or non-directed prayer group. In the directed prayer group, prayers had a specific goal, image or outcome in mind; in the non-directed group, no specific outcome was requested. Photographs and names of subjects were used as foci. Prayer was offered for 15 minutes daily for 12 weeks. Three agents prayed for each subject. Five pre-test and post-test objective measures and six post-test subjective measures were taken. Subjects improved significantly on all 11 measures, and the agents themselves improved significantly on 10 measures. A significant positive correlation was found between the amount of prayer the agents did and their scores on the five objective tests. Agents had significantly better scores than did subjects on all objective measures. Subjects' views of the locus of God's action showed significance in three objective measures. Improvement on four objective measures was significantly related to subjects' belief in the power of prayer for others. Improvement on all 11 measures was significantly related to subjects' conviction concerning whether they had been assigned to a control or an experimental group.[12]

However, no differences in outcome were found between the control and experimental conditions, and no differences were found between the directed and non-directed prayer groups. While agents experienced a highly significant relationship between the amount of prayer and health benefits, there was no such correlation with the subjects. Possible explanations suggested by the researchers included:

- Prayer does not work.
- Simply enrolling in the project was a commitment to improvement that overwhelmed the experimental effect.
- The subjects may all have had a specific expectation of improvement causing significant differences.
- All subjects were told that if prayer proved effective, those in the control group would be prayed for at the completion of the study. This could have caused a time-displaced effect.
- Outside prayer "contaminated" the results.

Specific areas in which prayer and religious activity have been shown to be effective

Blood pressure

One study found that people who were both frequent church attendees and rated their religion as very important had lower diastolic blood pressures, an association that held true even for smokers.[13] The analyses were adjusted for other blood pressure risk factors, such as age, socioeconomic status, and weight. Those who rated religion as highly important to them and attended church weekly or more had mean diastolic pressures almost 5 mm lower than those who rated religion as unimportant and infrequently or never attended church.

Smokers who rated religion as very important were 7.1 times less likely to have to have an abnormal diastolic pressure than those smokers who gave a low rating for the personal importance of religion. Furthermore, smokers who attended church weekly or more frequently were four times less likely to have abnormal diastolic pressure than were less frequent attendees or non-attendees. These beneficial findings among smokers who attend church frequently contradict the thesis that religion is clinically beneficial only because it helps people to avoid risk-producing behaviors.

A systematic review of 20 studies published over 30 years on blood pressure and religious activity found an inverse correlation between strong religious commitment and blood pressure.[14] The authors concluded: "Hypertension is a common and serious problem which appears to be mitigated by religion…."

Another study found an inverse association between frequency of religious attendance and rates of arteriosclerotic disease in both men and women.[6] Even after allowing for the effects of smoking, socioeconomic status and water hardness, the risk for the frequent church attendees was only 60% of the risk for men who attended church infrequently. The risk of dying from heart disease among women was about twice as high among infrequent church attendees than among those who attended church weekly or more regularly.

A recent study examined the association between blood pressure, selected health behaviors, and religious activity. Data were obtained on 112 woman who were at least 35 years of age and of the Judeo-Christian faith. Resting blood pressure measures were taken with an automated sphygmomanometer; height and weight were measured to determine body mass index (BMI), and intermediate health variables (e.g. physical activity, smoking, diet, and alcohol consumption) were measured by questionnaire. A multifactorial questionnaire was used to assess various dimensions of religious activity. Multiple regression analysis found a direct inverse effect between both systolic and diastolic blood pressure and the level of religious activity, not mediated by changes in health behaviors.

Alcohol and drug abuse

A review of the literature found 20 studies that examined the relationship between religion and drug use.[15] One study found that religious commitment was a protector against drug abuse:[16]

> Whenever religion is used in an analysis, it predicts those who have not used an illicit drug regardless of whether the religious variable is defined in terms of membership, active participation, religious upbringing, or the meaningfulness of religion as viewed by the person himself.

In a more recent review of the literature, 11 of 12 studies found that drug abuse is correlated with the absence of religious commitment in a person's life.[16] In 10 of 11 studies of alcohol abuse, religious commitment protected against such abuse.[16–19]

Suicide

One community study found that persons who did not attend church were four times more likely to commit suicide than were frequent church attendees. In a review of studies on suicide, 12 out of 12 studies showed that persons with a strong religious commitment were substantially less likely to commit suicide. The religiously committed had fewer suicidal thoughts and more negative attitudes towards taking their own lives.[20]

Delinquency

Twelve of 13 studies summarized in two reviews found that religious commitment – particularly church attendance – played a protective role against delinquency.[20,21] An additional, particularly revealing, study by Freeman[22] showed that those black males who are able to leave the ghetto and avoid falling prey to delinquency or drug abuse are those who attend church on a regular basis.

Surgical outcome

Elderly women recovering from hip surgery who regarded God as a source of strength and comfort and who attended religious services frequently were less depressed and could walk a greater distance at discharge than others. The authors suggested that the ability to walk farther was possibly explained by the lower amount of depression, as the more religious patients were less depressed and thus responded better to physical therapy.[23]

An interesting double-blind intervention study measured the effect of prayer on cardiac surgery outcome. Patients in a care unit in a large general hospital who consented to participate were randomly assigned to receive or not to receive regular intercessory prayers by an interdenominational group of committed Christians unknown to them. The patients themselves, staff, and doctors were unaware as to which patients were assigned to which group. Each intercessor was asked to pray on a daily basis for each of the following clinical issues: rapid recovery, prevention of complications and death, and any other areas they believed would be beneficial to the patient. The patients who received daily intercessory prayer had fewer life-threatening events and complications (congestive heart failure, cardiopulmonary arrests, intubations, and pneumonia) during their stay in the hospital coronary care unit than did those patients who did not receive the prayer.[24]

Length and quality of life

Five community-based studies have shown that the religiously committed person, particularly the church attendee, has a greater chance of living longer than do persons lacking such a commitment.[7] Not only do the religiously committed have a greater chance of living longer, but they are more satisfied with their lives. Another study showed that those who frequently pray and who have a close relationship with God have high levels of life satisfaction, existential well-being, and overall happiness.[21]

EFFECTIVE PRAYER

After spending more than a decade performing simple laboratory experiments that showed that prayer works, the Spindrift organization in Salem, Oregon, investigated which type of prayer strategy works best. Distinguishing essentially two types of prayer – "directed" prayer in which prayers have a specific goal, image or outcome in mind, and "undirected" prayer, in which no specific outcome is requested – researchers found that while both types of prayer produced results, the undirected approach was quantitatively more effective, frequently yielding results twice as great, or more, compared with the directed approach.[25]

Undirected prayer, a letting go and affirmation of trust in the Absolute, is at once a source of release, peace and hope. "Thy will be done" confers its own immediate blessing, regardless of physiological outcome.

Side-effects and contraindications

As with any intervention, misuse or inappropriate usage can cause problems. While the explicit inclusion of faith and prayer in health care can have a significant positive impact on clinical outcomes, this does not mean that these approaches can take the place of effective treatment. Unfortunately, some religious beliefs can be interpreted to prohibit many types of conventional medical interventions. One disconcerting study evaluated the deaths of children from families whose beliefs prohibited certain types of medical intervention. The researchers evaluated the records of 172 of these children who died in the US between 1975 and 1995 and for whom there was sufficient documentation to determine the cause of death. Of these, medical intervention would have resulted in a typical survival rate of 90% in 140, >50% in 18, and all but three of the remainder would likely have had some benefit.[26] While the research was flawed by the design bias, i.e. researchers did not look for positive results, only negative ones, the study gives cause for grave concern.

While it is easy for the clinician and social worker to condemn the belief systems of these children's families, how much does the well-documented unwillingness of most practitioners to consider faith and religious practice as factors in the therapeutic process contribute to these families' extreme position?

ILLNESS, THE GIFT OF SPIRITUAL HEALING

We have typecast illness as our enemy, when, in fact, it is our teacher. In the words of Germany's great poet, Ranier Maria Rilke:[27]

> So you must not be frightened...You must think that...life has not forgotten you, that it holds you in its hand; it will not let you fall. Why do you want to shut out of your life any agitation, any pain, any melancholy, since you really do not know what these states are working upon you? Why do you want to persecute yourself with the question when all this may be coming and whither it is bound? ...just remember that sickness is the means by which an organism frees itself of foreign matter; so one must just help it to be sick, to have its whole sickness and break out with it, for that is its progress...you must be patient as a sick man...there are in every illness many days when the doctor can do nothing but wait. And this it is that you, insofar as you are your own doctor, must now above all do.

Although physicians are taught to banish pain at all costs, and allopathic doctors are trained to eliminate symptoms as quickly as possible with drugs and surgery, failure to effect an immediate physiological cure does not necessarily mean failure to assist in a patient's healing process. Particularly during times of serious illness, we are forced to be quiet, to tune in to our true center. When our stillness is grounded in faith, what we recognize when we search within is God. Prayer at this intersection of quiet and acceptance, where we become truly aware that we are not our disease, but essentially something inviolate, is the type of prayer most frequently associated with miracle cures, radical spontaneous remissions and healings.

On a spiritual level, simply to recognize this dimension of the spiritual, the numinous, is to be healed. As Jung put it: "The approach to the numinous is the real therapy and inasmuch as you attain to the numinous experiences you are released from the curse of pathology. Even the very disease takes on a numinous character."[28]

SUMMARY

Religious faith, as primarily measured by regular attendance at religious services and a personal belief in God, is remarkably effective in the promotion of health. A substantial body of research published in diverse journals documents the efficacy of faith and prayer, for both the person praying and those prayed for, in longevity, recovery from surgery, prevention of disease, and improvement in lifestyle and behaviors. Every practitioner committed to providing the best possible care needs to be aware of, and use, this powerful healing factor.

For further information

For further information on the role of faith in healing, contact:

National Institute for Healthcare Research
6110 Executive Blvd., Suite 680
Rockville, MD 20852

Department of Spirituality in Health and Medicine
Bastyr University
14500 Juanita Drive
Kenmore, WA 98028

REFERENCES

1. Dossey L. Healing words. New York, NY: HarperSanFrancisco/HarperCollins. 1993
2. Oman D, Reed D. Religion and mortality among the community-dwelling elderly. Am J Pub Health 1998; 88: 1469–1475.
3. Benor DJ. Survey of spiritual healing research. Comp Med Res 1990; 4: 9–33
4. Ulanov A, Ulanov B. Primary speech: a psychology of prayer. Atlanta: John Knox Press. 1982: p. vii.
5. Lukoff D, Provenzano R, Lu F, Turner R. Religious and spiritual case reports on MEDLINE: a systematic analysis of records from 1980 to 1996. Altern Ther Health Med 1999; 5: 64–70
6. Craigie FC, Larson DB, Liu IY. References to religion in *The Journal of Family Practice*: dimensions and valence of spirituality. J Family Practice 1990; 30: 477–480
7. Larson DB, Sherrill KA, Lyons JS et al. Associations between dimensions of religious commitment and mental health reported in the *American Journal of Psychiatry* and *Archives of General Psychiatry*: 1978–1989. Am J Psychiatry 1992; 149: 557–559
8. Larson D, Swyers J, McCullough M. Scientific review on spirituality and health. Rockville, MD: National Institute of Health Care Research. 1998
9. Stein L. Is peer review biased on alternative medicine? Med Herald 1997; November: 44
10. Koenig HG. Religious attitudes and practices of hospitalized medically ill older adults. Int J Geriatr Psychiatry 1998; 13: 213–224
11. Levin JS, Vanderpool HY. Is frequent religious attendance really conducive to better health?: toward an epidemiology of religion. Soc Sci Med 1987; 24: 589–600
12. O'Laoire S. An experimental study of the effects of distant, intercessory prayer on self-esteem, anxiety, and depression. Altern Ther Health Med 1997; 3: 38–53
13. Levin JS, Vanderpool HY. Is religion therapeutically significant for hypertension? Soc Sci Med 1989; 29: 69–78
14. Hixson KA, Gruchow HW, Morgan DW. The relation between religiosity, selected health behaviors, and blood pressure among adult females. Prev Med 1998; 27: 545–552
15. Gorsuch RL, Butler MC. Initial drug abuse: a view of predisposing social psychological factors. Psychol Bull 1976; 3: 120–137
16. Gartner J, Larson DB, Allen G. Religious commitment and mental health: a review of the empirical literature. J Psychol Theol 1991; 19: 6–25
17. Argyle M, Beit-Hallahmi B. The social psychology of religion. London: Routledge & Kegan Paul. 1975
18. Walters OS. The religious background of 50 alcoholics. Quart J Stud Alcohol 1957; 18: 405–413
19. Larson DB, Wilson WP. Religious life of alcoholics. Southern Med J 1980; 73: 723–727
20. Comstock GW, Partridge KB. Church attendance and health. J Chron Dis 1972; 25: 665–672
21. Poloma MM, Pendleton BF. The effects of prayer and prayer experiences on measures of general well-being. J Psychol Theol 1991; 19: 71–83
22. Freeman RB. Who escapes? The relation of church-going and other background factors to the socio-economic performance of black male youths from inner-city poverty tracts. Working paper no. 1656. Cambridge, MA: National Bureau of Economic Research. 1985
23 Pressman P, Lyons JS, Larson DB, Strain JJ. Religious belief, depression, and ambulation status in elderly women with broken hips. Am J Psychiatry 1990; 147: 758–760
24. Byrd RB. Positive therapeutic effects of intercessory prayer in a coronary care unit population. Southern Med J 1988; 81: 826–829
25. Owen R. Qualitative research: the early years. Salem, OR: Grayhaven Books. 1988
26. Asser SM, Swan R. Child fatalities from religion-motivated medical neglect. Pediatrics 1998; 101: 625–629
27. Rilke RM. Letters to a young poet (transl. M.D. Herter). New York, NY: Norton Press. 1934
28. Adler G, Jaffé A, eds. Jung's letters, vol. 1. Princeton, NJ: Princeton University Press. 1973: p. 377

FURTHER READING

Dossey L. Prayer is good medicine. New York: HarperSanFrancisco/HarperCollins. 1996.
Moyers B. Healing and the mind. New York: Doubleday. 1993
Justice B Who gets sick. New York: G.P. Putnam's Sons. 1987.
Laskow L. Healing with Love. New York: HarperSanFrancisco/HarperCollins. 1992
Shealy CN, Myss CM. The creation of health. Walpole, NH:Stillpoint Publishing. 1993

CHAPTER CONTENTS

40

Glandular therapy

Michael T. Murray, ND

Joseph E. Pizzorno Jr, ND

INTRODUCTION

For almost as long as historic records have been kept, glandular therapy has been an important form of medicine. The basic concept underlying the medicinal use of glandular substances from animals is that "like heals like". For example, if the liver needs support or a patient is suffering from liver disease then they may benefit from eating beef liver. Modern glandular therapy, however, primarily involves the use of concentrated glandular extracts.

What is a gland?

A gland is defined as a secretory organ. The internal secretory organs of the body are called endocrine glands. These ductless glands secrete hormones directly into the bloodstream. The glands which are known to have endocrine function include the pineal, pituitary, thyroid, parathyroid, thymus, adrenal, pancreas, and gonads (testes or ovaries). Although not technically glands, it is common to refer to other organs of the body as glandulars when they are used in glandular therapy. For example, tissue extracts of heart, spleen, prostate, uterus, brain, and other tissues are often used in glandular or organotherapy.

SCIENTIFIC VALIDATION OF GLANDULAR THERAPY

Science has, without question, confirmed that certain glandular preparations and hormones are quite effective when taken orally. It is well established that a number of glandular preparations are effective orally because of active hormone or enzyme content, e.g. thyroid, adrenal cortex, and pancreatin preparations. There is also a good deal of literature support for pharmaceutical grade liver, aorta, and thymus extracts, and some support for pituitary, spleen, orchic (testes), and ovarian extracts as well. However, despite this scientific support, many people still question the effectiveness of glandular products on human health.

The true question should not be "Are glandulars effective?", but rather "Are the glandulars currently available in the United States effective?". Manufacturers of glandular products will claim their method of production of a glandular extract is the most ideal. However, the majority of their contentions are based on theoretical or philosophical grounds, not on firm scientific evidence or clinical results. There are no quality control procedures or standards enforced in the glandular industry. It is left up to the individual company to adopt quality control and good manufacturing procedures. Nonetheless, many glandular preparations available in the US marketplace appear to be effective.

METHODS OF MANUFACTURE OF GLANDULAR PREPARATIONS

It is critical that properly processed glandular material be used, as the biologically active material such as enzymes, soluble proteins, natural lipid factors, vitamins, minerals and hormone precursors are destroyed or eliminated if the product is not prepared properly.

Most glandular products are derived from beef (bovine) sources, the exception being pancreatic extracts which are most often derived from pork (porcine). The four most widely-known methods of processing are the azeotrophic method, salt precipitation, freeze-drying, and predigesting.

The azeotrophic method

The azeotrophic method begins by quick freezing the material at well below 0°F, and then washing the material with a powerful solvent (ethylene dichloride) to remove the fatty tissue. The solvent is then distilled off and the material is dried and ground into a powder so that it can be placed in tablets or capsules. Although the azeotrophic method eliminates the problem of fat-stored toxins like pesticides and healthy metals, unfortunately it also removes fat-soluble hormones, enzymes, essential fatty acids, and other potentially beneficial materials and there are still traces of the solvent that remain.

The salt precipitation method

This method involves the maceration of fresh glandular material in a salt and water. Because the salt increases the density of the water soluble material, when the mixture is centrifuged the lighter fat-soluble material can be separated out. The material is then dried and powdered. The benefit with the salt precipitation method is that no toxic solvents are used to separate the fatty material. The down side is that most people could do without the remaining salt in the product.

Freeze-drying

The freeze-drying process involves quickly freezing the glandular material at temperatures 40–60° below 0°F and then placing the material into a vacuum chamber which removes the water by direct vaporization from its frozen state – hence the term freeze-drying. The benefit of freeze-drying is that it contains a higher concentration of unaltered protein and enzymes as well as all of the fat-soluble components. Since the fat is not removed, it is critical that the glands are derived from livestock that have grazed on open ranges not sprayed with pesticides or herbicides. The animals must also be free from antibiotics, synthetic hormones, and infection.

Predigestion

The final process to discuss is the predigestion method. This method employs the aid of plant and animal enzymes or some other method to partially digest or hydrolyze the glandular material. The partially digested material is then passed through a series of filtrations to separate out fat-soluble and large molecules. The purified material is then freeze-dried. This method of extraction is ideal for glandulars (such as the liver and thymus) where the polypeptide (small proteins) and other water-soluble fractions are desired.

EVIDENCE FOR INTACT PROTEIN ABSORPTION

Contrary to long-held theories that the healthy intestinal mucosa is an essentially impermeable barrier to proteins and large polypeptides, there is now irrefutable evidence that large macromolecules can and do pass intact from the human gut into the bloodstream under normal conditions. In some instances, the body appears to recognize which molecules it needs to absorb intact and which molecules it needs to break down into smaller units. This phenomenon may help to explain the effectiveness of glandular therapy.

Numerous whole proteins have been shown in human and animal studies to be absorbed intact into the bloodstream following oral administration.[1–7] These include human albumin and lactalbumin, bovine albumin, ovalbumin, lactoglobulin, ferritin (molecular weight, 500,000), chymotrypsinogen, elastase, and other large molecules.

Furthermore, proteins and polypeptides, as well as various hormones that are absorbed intact from the gut, have been shown to exert effects in target tissues. For example, in addition to thyroxine or thyroid hormone and cortisone, several peptide hormones are known to be biologically active when administered orally, including luteinizing hormone-releasing factor and thytropin-releasing hormone.[8,9] Even insulin has been shown to be absorbed orally under certain circumstances (e.g. in the presence of protease inhibitors or hypertonic solutions in the intestines).[10,11]

All of this data indicates that at least some of the larger molecules in glandular products are absorbed intact to induce physiological effects, particularly polypeptides which exert hormone or hormone-like action. Detractors of glandular therapy often claim that when a glandular is consumed, it is immediately digested into smaller building blocks like amino acids. However, these detractors are not up to date with current understanding of normal physiology.

CLINICAL APPLICATIONS

An adequate body of research now exists to support the use of orally administered glandular extracts. The following is a brief discussion of several glandular preparations and their use. Table 40.1 lists the primary conditions responding to glandular therapy.

Adrenal extracts

Oral adrenal extracts have been used in medicine since at least 1931.[12] Adrenal extracts may be made from the whole adrenal or just from the adrenal cortex. Whole adrenal extracts (usually in combination with essential nutrients for the adrenal gland) are most often used in cases of low adrenal function, presenting as fatigue, inability to cope with stress, and reduced resistance. Because extracts made from the adrenal cortex contain small amounts of corticosteroids, they are typically used as a "natural" cortisone in severe cases of allergy and inflammation (asthma, eczema, psoriasis, rheumatoid arthritis, etc.).

Dosage

The dosage of adrenal extract depends upon the quality and potency of the product. The best measure of an

Table 40.1 Therapeutic uses of glandular extracts

Extract	Clinical applications
Adrenal extracts	Chronic fatigue Asthma Eczema Psoriasis Rheumatoid arthritis
Aortic glycosaminoglycans	Cerebral and peripheral arterial insufficiency Venous insufficiency and varicose veins Hemorrhoids Vascular retinopathies, including macular degeneration Post-surgical edema
Liver extracts	Chronic hepatitis Chronic liver disease
Pancreatic extracts	Pancreatic insufficiency Cystic fibrosis Inflammatory and autoimmune diseases such as rheumatoid arthritis, scleroderma, athletic injuries, and tendinitis Cancer Infections
Spleen extracts	After splenecotomy Immune potentiation Infection Cancer Hyposplenia Celiac disease Dermatitis herpetiformis Ulcerative colitis Rheumatoid arthritis Glomerulonephritis Systemic lupus erythematosus Vasculitis Low white cell counts Thrombocytopenia
Thymus extracts	Recurrent and chronic viral infections, such as chronic fatigue syndrome, respiratory infections, AIDS, acute hepatitis B infection Cancer patients with immune depression from chemotherapy or radiation Allergies such as asthma, hayfever, eczema, and food allergies Autoimmune disorders, such as rheumatoid arthritis, lupus erythematosis, and scleroderma
Thyroid extracts	Hypothyroidism

effective dose for a preparation may be the level of stimulation (irritability, restlessness, and insomnia) the patient experiences. When prescribing adrenal extracts, start at one-third the recommended dosage on the label and slowly increase the dosage every 2 days until a stimulatory effect is noted. Once this effect is noticed, reduce the dosage to a level just below the level that will produce stimulation.

Aortic glycosaminoglycans

A mixture of highly purified bovine-derived glycosaminoglycans naturally present in the aorta, including dermatan sulfate, heparan sulfate, hyaluronic acid, chondroitin sulfate, and related hexosaminoglycans, has been shown to protect and promote normal artery and vein function. Over 50 clinical studies have shown an orally administered complex of aortic GAGs to be effective in a number of vascular disorders, including:

- cerebral and peripheral arterial insufficiency
- venous insufficiency and varicose veins
- hemorrhoids
- vascular retinopathies, including macular degeneration post-surgical edema.[13–22]

Significant improvements in both symptoms and blood flow have been noted.

In addition, aortic GAGs have many important effects which interfere with the progression of atherosclerosis, including preventing damage to the surface of the artery, formation of damaging blood clots, migration of smooth muscle cells into the intima, and formation of fat and cholesterol deposits, as well as lowering total cholesterol levels while raising HDL-cholesterol.[23–28]

Dosage

The dosage of the mixture of highly purified bovine-derived glycosaminoglycans naturally present in the aorta is 100 mg daily. Similar, but not nearly as impressive, results in the treatment of atherosclerosis have been noted with chondroitin sulfate at a daily dose of 3 g (1 g with meals, three times daily).[29]

Liver extracts

Hydrolyzed liver extracts have been used to treat chronic liver diseases since 1896. Numerous scientific investigations into the therapeutic efficacy of liver extracts have demonstrated that these extracts improve fat utilization, promote tissue regeneration, and prevent damage to the liver.[30–33] In short, clinical studies have demonstrated that oral administration of hydrolyzed liver extracts can be quite effective in improving liver function.

For example, in one double-blind study, 556 patients with chronic hepatitis were given either 70 mg of liver hydrosylate or a placebo three times daily.[33] At the end of 3 months of treatment, the group receiving the liver extract was shown to have far lower serum liver enzyme levels. Since the level of liver enzymes in the blood reflect damage to the liver, it can be concluded that the liver extract is effective in chronic hepatitis via an ability to improve the function of damaged liver cells as well as prevent further damage to the liver.

Dosage

The dosage is entirely dependent upon the concentration, method of preparation, and quality of the liver extract. The highest quality products are aqueous hydrolyzed extracts because they have had the fat-soluble components removed and typically contain more than 20 times the nutritional content of raw liver, including 3–4 mg of heme-iron per gram.

Liver extracts should not be used in patients suffering from an iron-storage disorder such as hemochromatosis.

Pancreatic extracts

Pancreatic enzymes are most often employed in the treatment of pancreatic insufficiency. Pancreatic insufficiency is characterized by impaired digestion, malabsorption, nutrient deficiencies, and abdominal discomfort. Pancreatic enzymes are also used by physicians in the treatment of:

- cystic fibrosis
- inflammatory and autoimmune diseases like rheumatoid arthritis, scleroderma, athletic injuries, tendinitis, etc.
- cancer
- infections.

For a full discussion of pancreatic enzymes see Chapter 101.

Dosage

Full-strength products are preferred to lower potency pancreatin products because lower potency products are often diluted with salt, lactose, or galactose to achieve desired strength (e.g. 4× or 1×). The dosage recommendation for a 10× USP pancreatic enzyme product is 500–1,000 mg three times a day immediately before meals when used as a digestive aid and at least 20 minutes before meals or on an empty stomach when anti-inflammatory effects are desired.

Pancreatic extracts are generally well tolerated and are not associated with any significant side-effects.

Spleen extracts

As early as the 1930s, orally administered bovine spleen extracts were shown to possess some physiological action in increasing white blood cell counts in patients with extreme deficiencies of white blood cells, as well as being of some benefit in patients with malaria and typhoid fever.[34–36]

Like thymus extracts, pharmaceutical grade bovine spleen extracts are currently quite popular in Germany for the treatment of infectious conditions and as an immune-enhancing agent in cancer. Spleen tissue extracts may be of benefit in enhancing general immune function, as many potent immune system enhancing compounds secreted by the spleen are small molecular weight peptides. For example, the potent immunostimulants tuftsin and splenopentin are composed of only four and five amino acids, respectively.

Both tuftsin and splenopentin have been shown to exert profound immune enhancing activity. Tuftsin stimulates macrophages that have taken up residence in specific tissues like the liver, spleen, and lymph nodes. These large cells engulf and destroy foreign particles, including bacteria, cancer cells, and cellular debris. Macrophages are essential in protecting against invasion by microorganisms as well as cancer. Tuftsin also helps to mobilize other white blood cells to fight against infection and cancer. A deficiency of tuftsin is associated with signs and symptoms of frequent infections.[37]

Splenopentin, like tuftsin, has also demonstrated significant immune-enhancing effects. Its effects are primarily directed towards enhancing the immune system's response to regulating compounds such as colony-stimulating factors.[38] Colony-stimulating factors, such as interleukin-3, and granulocyte/macrophage colony-stimulating factors stimulate the production of white blood cells. Splenopentin is probably the factor responsible for the results noted in those clinical studies during the 1930s with spleen extracts in the treatment of depressed white blood cell counts.

Splenopentin has also been shown to enhance natural killer cell activity.[39] Natural killer cells destroy cells that have become cancerous or infected with viruses and are the body's first line of defense against cancer.

In addition to tuftsin and splenopentin, hydrolyzed (predigested) spleen extracts concentrated for peptides have demonstrated impressive immune restorative properties in mice.[40] In one study, mice were exposed to radiation to significantly damage the immune system. Mice treated with the spleen extract recovered within 6–8 weeks. In contrast, those treated with a placebo recovered after 10 weeks at the earliest.

The primary clinical uses of spleen extracts are after removal of the spleen and conditions associated with low spleen function (hyposplenia) such as:

- celiac disease
- dermatitis herpetiformis
- ulcerative colitis
- rheumatoid arthritis
- glomerulonephritis
- systemic lupus erythematosus
- vasculitis
- thrombocytopenia.

Spleen extracts may also be useful in the treatment of low white blood cell counts, bacterial infections, and as an adjunct in cancer therapy. Individuals who have had splenectomies, who have low tuftsin levels, or autoimmune conditions linked to low RES activity should use spleen extracts.

Since the spleen is difficult to repair, severe spleen trauma usually requires splenectomy to stop the severe hemorrhage. The spleen is also removed in the medical treatment of certain diseases such as idiopathic thrombocytic purpura (ITP) and to determine the extent of Hodgkin's disease.

The removal of the spleen is associated with an increased risk for infection. In children and adults this increased risk of infection makes them particularly susceptible to pneumococcal pneumonia. About 2.5% of patients having their spleen removed will die from pneumococcal pneumonia within 5 years of splenectomy. It is often recommended that a child who has undergone a splenectomy receive a pneumococcal vaccine and receive long-term antibiotic treatment. Use of spleen extracts, especially those rich in tuftsin, may be a natural alternative.

Spleen extracts should probably be viewed as a necessary medicine for people who have had their spleen removed. If the thyroid, adrenals, or ovaries are removed, most patients would be prescribed the corresponding hormone. It only makes sense that if the spleen is removed, the body should be supplied with necessary spleen substances like tuftsin and splenopentin.

The increased risk of infection is attributed primarily to a deficiency of tuftsin.[41,42] Tuftsin is produced only in the spleen; without the spleen there simply is no tuftsin in the circulation. Without tuftsin, the body is without one of its key stimulators of the immune system. Individuals without spleens need an outside source of tuftsin like spleen extracts.

Dosage

Clinically, hydrolyzed (predigested) products concentrated for tuftsin and splenopentin content are preferable to crude preparations. The daily dose should provide 50 mg tuftsin and splenopentin or roughly 1.5 g of total spleen peptides.

No side-effects or adverse effects have been reported with the use of oral spleen preparations.

Thymus extracts

There is a substantial amount of clinical research to support the effectiveness of orally administered thymus extracts. Specifically, numerous clinical trials have shown that oral administration of predigested calf thymus extract rich in thymus-derived polypeptides is effective in:

- preventing recurrent respiratory infections in children
- correcting the T-cell defects in human immunodeficiency virus infections (AIDS)
- treating acute hepatitis B infections
- restoring the number of peripheral leukocytes in cancer patients with chemotherapy-induced depression of WBC counts
- allergies including asthma, hayfever, and food allergies in children.[43,44]

The effectiveness of the thymus extract in these conditions is reflective of broad-spectrum immune system enhancement presumably mediated by improved thymus gland activity. This effect fits in nicely with one of the basic concepts of glandular therapy, i.e. that the oral ingestion of glandular material of a certain animal gland will strengthen the corresponding human gland. The result is a broad general effect indicative of improved glandular function. It is interesting that thymus extracts have been shown to normalize the ratio of T-helper cells to suppressor cells whether the ratio is low, as in AIDS, chronic infections, and cancer, or high, as in allergies, migraine headaches, and autoimmune diseases like rheumatoid arthritis.

Chronic viral infections. Recurrent or chronic infections, including the so-called *chronic fatigue syndrome* and *chronic post-viral syndrome*, are characterized by a depressed immune system. This is a difficult condition to treat due to the repetitive cycle of a compromised immune system leading to infection, which leads to damage to the immune system, further weakening resistance to viral infection. Thymus extracts may provide the answer to chronic infections by restoring healthy immune function.

The ability of thymus extracts to treat and then reduce the number of recurrent infections was studied in groups of children with a history of recurrent respiratory tract infections. Double-blind studies revealed not only that orally administered thymus extracts were able to effectively eliminate infection, but also that treatment over the course of a year significantly reduced the number of respiratory infections and significantly improved numerous immune parameters.[45]

One of the most difficult viral infections for the body to throw off is type B viral hepatitis. Thymus extracts have been shown to be effective in several double-blind studies in both acute and chronic cases. In these studies, therapeutic effect was noted by accelerated decreases of liver enzymes (transaminases), elimination of the virus, and a higher rate of seroconversion to anti-HBe, signifying clinical remission.[46,47]

The most extreme example of a chronic viral infection is AIDS. Although thymus extracts have not been shown to reverse this difficult disease, studies have shown an ability to improve several immune parameters including an ability to raise the T-helper cells, a critical goal in AIDS treatment.[48]

Cancer. The primary application of thymus extracts in cancer has been to counteract the immune-suppressing effects of radiation and chemotherapy. The net effect of thymus extract administration is to prevent the tremendous depression of white blood cell levels and activity that result from chemotherapy or radiation.[44,49]

Allergies. People with allergies typically have derangements in the immune system. Levels of the allergic IgE antibody and eosinophils are typically elevated, while levels of suppressor T-cells are typically depressed. These abnormalities are clear indications of altered immune function.

The oral administration of thymus extracts has been shown in double-blind clinical studies to improve the symptoms and course of hayfever, allergic rhinitis, asthma, eczema, and food allergies.[44,50–52] Presumably this clinical improvement is the result of restoration of proper immune function, as levels of IgE and eosinophils have been reduced while the ratio of helper to suppressor T-cells have improved.

It is interesting to note that, in several double-blind studies, children receiving thymus extracts during food allergy elimination diets are often able to tolerate foods that had previously been allergenic and symptom-producing.[51,52]

Autoimmune disorders. Autoimmune disorders, such as rheumatoid arthritis, are characterized by the body's own antibodies attacking body tissues. Central to this autoimmunity is a high T-helper to suppressor cell ratio. A high T-helper to suppressor cell ratio results in increased antibody formation. The higher the ratio, the higher the number of antibodies being produced to damage body structures. In one clinical study, rheumatoid arthritis patients with a helper to suppressor ratio of 3.3 achieved normal ratios (1.02–2.46) after 3 months of therapy with a thymus extract.[44]

Although use of a thymus extract may not result in substantial clinical improvement, it appears to be useful in restoring proper immune function in autoimmune diseases including rheumatoid arthritis, lupus, and scleroderma.

Dosage

From a practical view, products concentrated and standardized for polypeptide content are preferable to crude preparations. The daily dose should be equivalent to 120 mg pure polypeptides with molecular weights less than 10,000 or roughly 750 mg of the crude polypeptide fraction.

No side-effects or adverse effects have been reported with the use of thymus preparations.

Thyroid extracts

Desiccated natural thyroid is available by prescription according to United States Pharmacopoeia (USP) guidelines. Preparations are derived from porcine thyroid glands. Many naturopathic physicians prefer natural thyroid to isolated synthetic T_4, as it contains both thyroxine (T_4) and tri-iodothyronine (T_3). Typical levels of thyroid hormone contained per grain in USP thyroid are 38 mcg for T_4 and 9 mcg for T_3.

The thyroid extracts sold as "nutritional supplements" are required by the Food and Drug Administration (FDA) to be thyroxine-free. However, it is nearly impossible to remove all the hormone from the gland. In other words, think of these nutritional thyroid preparations as milder forms of desiccated natural thyroid.

The primary use of thyroid preparations is in the medical treatment of hypothyroidism. In all but its most mildest forms, treatment involves the use of desiccated thyroid or synthetic thyroid hormone. For more discussion, see Chapter 162.

Dosage

Dosage is determined by basal body temperature (see Ch. 162 for directions).

SUMMARY

From the scientific data that currently exists, there is enough evidence to support the use of orally administered glandular extracts. For best results, physicians should choose glandular products made by reputable companies that employ established methods of manufacture to produce extracts of known concentration.

REFERENCES

1. Gardener MLG. Gastrointestinal absorption of intact proteins. Ann Rev Nutr 1988; 8. 329–350
2. Gardner MLG. Intestinal assimilation of intact peptides and proteins from the diet – a neglected field? Biol Rev 1984; 59: 289–331
3. Udall JN, Walker WA. The physiologic and pathologic basis for the transport of macromolecules across the intestinal tract. J. Pediatr. Gastroenterol Nutr 1982; 1: 295–301
4. Kleine MW, Stauder GM, Beese EW. The intestinal absorption of orally administered hydrolytic enzymes and their effects in the treatment of acute herpes zoster as compared with those of oral acyclovir therapy. Phytomedicine 1995; 2: 7–15
5. Hemmings WA, Williams EW. Transport of large breakdown products of dietary protein through the gut wall. Gut 1986; 27: 715–723
6. Ambrus JL, Lassman HB, De Marchi JJ et al. Absorption of exogenous and endogenous proteolytic enzymes. Clin Pharmacol Therap 1967; 8: 362–368
7. Kabacoff BB. Absorption of chymotrypsin from the intestinal tract. Nature 1963; 199: 815–817
8. Ormiston BJ. Clinical effects of TRH and TSH after i.v. and oral administration in normal volunteers and patients with thyroid disease. In: Hal R et al, eds. Thytropin Releasing hormone (Frontiers of hormone research, vol. I). Basel: Karger. 1972: p 45–52
9. Amoss MS, Monahan MW, Verlander MS. Release of gonadotrophins by oral administration of synthetic LRF or tripeptide fragment of LRF. J Clin Endocrinol Metab 1977; 35: 175–177
10. Seifert J. Mucosal permeation of macromolecules and particles. Angiology 1966; 17: 505–513
11. Laskowski M. Effect of trypsin inhibitor on passage of insulin across the intestinal barrier. Science 1958; 127: 1115–1116
12. Britton SW, Silvette H. Further experiments on cortico-adrenal extract. Its efficacy by mouth. Science 1931; 74: 440–441
13. Abate G, Berenga A, Caione F et al. Controlled multicenter study on the therapeutic effectiveness of mesoglycan in patients with cerebrovascular disease. Minerva Med 1991; 82(3): 101–105
14. Mansi D, Sinsi L, De Michele G et al. Open trial of mesoglycan in the treatment of cerebrovascular ischemic disease. Acta Neurol 1988; 10: 108–112
15. Laurora G, Cesarone SR, De Sanctis MT et al. Delayed arteriosclerosis progression in high risk subjects treated with mesoglycan. Evaluation of intima-media thickness. J Cardiovasc Surg 1993; 34(4): 313–318
16. Vecchio F, Zanchin G, Maggioni F et al. Mesoglycan in treatment of patients with cerebral ischemia. effects on hemorheologic and hematochemical parameters. Acta Neurol 1993; 15(6): 449–456
17. De Donato G, Sangiuolo P. Instrumental evaluation of the mesoglycan effects in phlebopathic patients. Prospective randomized double-blind study. Min Med 1986; 77: 1927–1931
18. Oddone G, Fiscella GF, De Franceschi T. Assessment of the effects of oral mesoglycan sulphate in patients with chronic venous pathology of the lower extremeties. Gazzetta Medica Italiana 1987; 146: 111–114
19. Prandoni P, Cattelan AM, Carta M. Long-term sequelae of deep venous thrombosis of the legs. Experience with mesoglycan. Ann Ital Med Int 1989; 4(4): 378–385
20. Sangrigoli V. Mesoglycan in acute and chronic venous insufficiency of the legs. Clin Ter 1989; 129(3): 207–209
21. Petruzezellis V, Velon A. Therapeutic action of oral doses of mesoglycan in the pharmacological treatment of varicose syndrome and its complications. Min Med 1985; 76; 543–548
22. Saggioro A, Chiozzini G, Pallini P et al. Treatment of hemorrhoidal syndrome with mesoglycan. Min Diet Gastr 1985; 31: 311–315
23. Stevens RL, Colombo M, Gonzales JJ et al. The glycosaminoglycans of the human artery and their changes in atherosclerosis. J Clin Invest 1976; 58: 470–481
24. Tammi M, Seppala PO, Lehtonen et al. Connective tissue components in normal and atherosclerotic human coronary arteries. Atherosclerosis 1978; 29: 191–194
25. Day CE, Powell JR, Levy RS. Sulfated polysaccharide inhibition of aortic uptake of low density lipoproteins. Artery 1975; 1: 126–137
26. Pernigotti LM et al. Effect of mesoglycan on clotting, fibrinolysis and platelet aggregation in normal subjects and hyperaggregating arteriosclerosis. In: Widhalm K, Sinzinger H, eds. Current aspects of atherosclerosis. Lipids, lipoproteins, platelets, prostaglandins, and experimental findings. Madrich: Verlag Wilhelm. 1983: p 164–175

27. Postiglione A, De Simone B, Rubba P et al. Effect of oral mesoglycan-sulphate on plasma lipoprotein concentration and on lipoprotein concentration in primary hyperlipidemia. Pharmacol Res Commun 1984; 16: 1–8
28. Saba P. Hypolipidemic effect of mesoglycan in hyperlipidemic patients. Current Therap Res 1986; 40: 761–768
29. Nakazawa K, Murata K. The therapeutic effect of chondroitin polysulphate in elderly atherosclerotic patients. J Int Med Res 1978; 6: 217–225
30. Nagai K. A study of the excretory mechanism of the liver – effect of liver hydrolysate on BSP excretion. Jap J Gastroenterol 1970; 67: 633–638
31. Ohbayashi A, Akioka T, Tasaki H. A study of effects of liver hydrolysate on hepatic circulation. J Therapy 1972; 54: 1582–1585
32. Sanbe K. Treatment of liver disease – with particular reference to liver hydrolysates. Jap J Clin Exp Med 1973; 50: 2665–2676
33. Fujisawa K. Therapeutic effects of liver hydrolysate preparation on chronic hepatitis – A double blind, controlled study. Asian Med J 1984; 26: 497–526
34. Minter MM. Agranulocytic angina: treatment of a case with fetal calf spleen. Texas State J Med 1933; 2: 338–343
35. Gray GA. The treatment of agranulocytic angina with fetal calf spleen. Texas State J Med 1933; 29: 366–369
36. Greer AE. Use of fetal spleen in agranulocytosis. Preliminary report. Texas State J Med 1932; 28: 338–343
37. Fridkin M, Najjar VA. Tuftsin. its chemistry, biology, and clinical potential. Crit Rev Biochem Mol Biol 1989; 24: 1–40
38. Diezel W, Weber HA, Maciejewski J et al. The effect of splenopentin (DA SP-5) on in vitro myelopoiesis and on AZT-induced bone marrow toxicity. Int J Immunopharmac 1993; 15: 269–273
39. Rastogi A, Singh VK, Biswas S et al. Augmentation of human natural killer cells by splenopentin analogs. FEBS Lett 1993; 317: 93–95
40. Volk HD, Eckert R, Diamantstein T et al. Immunorestitution by a bovine spleen hydrosylate and ultrafiltrate. Arzniem Forsch 1991; 41: 1281–1285
41. He SW. Effect of splenectomy on phagocytic function of leukocytes. Chung Hua Wai Ko Tsa Chih 1989; 27: 354–356, 381
42. Spirer Z, Zakuth V, Diamant S et al. Decreased tuftsin concentrations in patients who have undergone splenectomy. Br Med J 1977; 2: 1574–1576
43. Cazzola P, Mazzanti P, Bossi G. In vivo modulating effect of a calf thymus acid lysate on human T lymphocyte subsets and CD4+/CD8+ ratio in the course of different diseases. Curr Ther Res 1987; 42: 1011–1017
44. Kouttab NM, Prada M, Cazzola P. Thymomodulin. Biological properties and clinical appliactions. Med Oncol Tumor Pharmacother 1989; 6: 5–9
45. Fiocchi A, Borella E, Riva E et al. A double-blind clinical trial for the evaluation of the therapeutic effectiveness of a calf thymus derivative (Thymomodulin) in children with recurrent respiratory infections. Thymus 1986; 8: 831–839
46. Galli M, Crocchiolo P, Negri C et al. Attempt to treat acute type B hepatitis with an orally administered thymic extract (Thymomodulin). Preliminary results. Drgus Exptl Clin Res 1985; 11: 665–669
47. Bortolotti F et al. Effect of an orally administered thymic derivative, Thymodulin, in chronic type B hepatitis in children. Curr Ther Res 1988; 43: 67–72
48. Valesini G, Barnaba V, Benvenuto R et al. A calf thymus lysate improves clinical symptoms and T-cell defects in the early stages of HIV infection. Second report. Eur. J Cancer Clin Oncol 1987; 23: 1915–1919
49. Kang SD, Lee BH, Yang JH, Lee CY. The effects of calf-thymus extract on recovery of bone marrow function in anticancer chemotherapy. New Med J (Korea) 1985; 28: 11–15
50. Marzari R, Mazzanti P, Cazzola P et al. Perennial allergic rhinitis. prevention of the acute episodes with Thymomodulin. Min Med 1987; 78: 1675–1681
51. Genova R, Guerra A. Thymomodulin in management of food allergy in children. Int J Tiss React 1986; 8: 239–242
52. Cavagni G, Piscopo C, Rigoli E et al. Food allergy in children. An attempt to improve the effects of the elimination diet with an immunomodulating agen (thymomodulin). A double-blind clinical trial. Immunopharmacol Immunotoxicol 1989; 11: 131–142

CHAPTER CONTENTS

41 Homeopathy

Andrew Lange, ND

INTRODUCTION

Homeopathy is a highly systematized method of medical therapeutics and clinical evaluation. The term "homeopathy" is derived from the Greek words *homeos*, meaning similar, and *pathos*, meaning suffering. The medicines used in this system of therapeutics are chosen according to the "law of similars" (the concept of like curing like), a fundamental homeopathic principle based upon the observed relationship between a medicine's ability to produce a specific constellation of signs and symptoms in a healthy individual and the same medicine's ability to cure a sick patient with similar signs and symptoms. This principle was first recognized by Hippocrates, who noticed that herbs given in low doses tended to cure the same symptoms they produced when given in toxic doses.

Homeopathic medicines are derived from a wide variety of plant, mineral, and chemical substances. They are prepared according to the standards of the *United States Homeopathic Pharmacopoeia*, a recently revised version of which has been approved by the Food and Drug Administration, and Congress.

HISTORY

The homeopathic school of medicine was founded by a German physician, Samuel Hahnemann. He had already gained a reputation in chemistry and medicine, having formulated a soluble form of mercury and developed a safer method for its use, and having written a number of works on pharmacology, hygiene and public health, industrial toxicology, and psychiatry. His treatise on arsenic poisoning (1786) is still considered authoritative. A prolific writer, Hahnemann collected, compiled, revised, and edited the existing pharmacological knowledge. The work was well received by the medical profession of the time. In fact, Hahnemann was one of the most learned men of his generation in medicine, chemistry, and pharmacology, making his later criticisms of medicine all the more significant.[1]

Disillusioned with the theories and practice of 18th century medicine, Hahnemann retired from practice in 1782 and spent the next 14 years earning a meager living doing chemical research, writing, and translating English, French, Italian, and Latin works. He wrote of his time of practice:[2]

> It was painful for me to grope in the dark, guided only by books in the treatment of the sick. To prescribe according to this or that (fanciful) view of the nature of diseases, substances that only owed to mere opinion their place in the materia medica; I had conscientious scruples about treating unknown morbid states in my suffering fellow creatures with these unknown medicines which, being powerful substances, may, if they were not exactly suitable (and how could the physician know whether they were suitable or not, seeing that their peculiar special actions were not yet elucidated) easily change life into death, or produce new affections and chronic ailments, which are often more difficult to remove than the original disease.

In his struggle to determine a reliable basis for therapeutics, he was distressed by his inability to provide medical care for the acute illnesses of his own growing family. In 1790, during his translation of William Cullen's (a Scottish physician) *Materia Medica*, he added a footnote disagreeing with Cullen's conclusions that the basis of cinchona bark's effectiveness was its bitter and astringent qualities. *Cinchona officinalis* (Peruvian bark), from which the drug quinine is derived, was known to be clinically effective in malaria and intermittent fevers (then called ague). He argued that there were several drugs in common usage that, in smaller doses, had greater bitter and astringent qualities, yet had no specific action upon fevers. As an experiment, Hahnemann took four drachms of cinchona twice daily, and soon developed the paroxysmal symptoms characteristic of intermittent fevers.

This duplication of symptoms was a revelation to him and ultimately resulted in his formulation of the concept of determining the properties of a medicine by studying its effects on healthy humans.

While homeopathy offers a profoundly deep and unified evaluation in the treatment of chronic diseases (see "Evaluating the case" below), it had gained most of its early reputation in the treatment of acute and epidemic diseases. An uproar was caused in Cincinnati in 1849, when two immigrant German homeopaths, treating cholera with camphor and other homeopathically prescribed remedies, published in the newspapers statistics indicating that only 35 of their 1,116 treated cases had died. During the 19th century, 33–50% of patients with cholera who were given standard medical care, died. In the 1879 epidemic of yellow fever, New Orleans homeopaths treated 1,945, cases with a mortality rate of 5.6%, while the standard medical doctors were losing 16%. These and similar statistics had a profound effect on Congress and public opinion.[3]

Over time, the homeopaths established their own network of treatment facilities. By 1892, they controlled about 110 hospitals, 145 dispensaries, 62 orphan asylums and retirement homes, over 30 nursing homes and sanatoria, and 16 insane asylums.

Constantine Hering established the first homeopathic medical school in the United States in 1835. It later moved from its original site in Allentown, Pennsylvania to Philadelphia, where it remains today as an orthodox medical school: the Hahnemann Medical College and Hospital. Hering's promotion of homeopathy and development of the materia medica was equaled only by Hahnemann himself. His 10 volume work, *The Guiding Symptoms of Our Materia Medica*, remains the definitive work on the clinical verifications of the homeopathic approach. It is unfortunate that, of the many medicines introduced by Hering, only nitroglycerine remains in medical practice as a tribute to his medical genius.

Throughout the world, homeopathy has maintained a consistent tradition. Frederick Harvey Foster Quinn introduced it to England in the 1840s. It has since become a postgraduate medical specialty, recognized by the Department of Health by virtue of an Act of Parliament. Homeopathic hospitals and outpatient clinics are part of the National Health System. Homeopaths have been engaged as personal physicians to the royal family for the past four generations.

Homeopathy is widely practiced in Europe, India, Argentina, and Mexico, and is experiencing a renaissance in the United States.

PHILOSOPHY

Provings

Hahnemann defined his method of testing medicines on healthy people as "provings". He expanded his investigations to include a wide range of substances, using his family, friends, and associates as experimental subjects.

Historically, Hahnemann was not the first to utilize this methodology: in 1760, Anton Stoerck reported testing *stramonium* (datura) by rubbing it on the skin, inhaling the vapors of the freshly crushed leaves, and, finally, ingesting the fresh extract. He theorized that if *stramonium* disturbs the senses and produces mental derangements in healthy people, it might be administered to maniacs for the purpose of restoring the senses by effecting a change of ideas. The recent medical literature has contained examples of inadvertent provings: in 1983, a study in the *New England Journal of Medicine* reported that pyridoxine (vitamin B_6), which is used in the treatment of some types of peripheral neuropathy, was also capable of producing neuropathies when given in very large doses.[4] In 1796, Hahnemann published, in *Hufeland's Journal*, the fruit of his investigations in an article, "Essay on a new principle for ascertaining the curative power of drugs, with a few glances at those hitherto employed".

Like treating like

Hahnemann also recognized the tendency of a natural disease to have a "homeopathic effect", i.e. a preventive or therapeutic effect, on other diseases with similar symptomatology. Although he ascribed this to the stimulation of the organism to eradicate the disease, he felt the deliberate induction of a disease to be difficult, uncertain, and dangerous.[5] This concept has many parallels in modern medical science. Descriptions of viral interference under natural conditions were described in 1937 by G. Findlely and F. MacCallum, who found that monkeys infected with the Raft Valley fever virus were protected from the more fatal yellow fever virus. They adopted the term "virus interference" and believed that when one virus infects a group of cells, a second virus is somehow excluded.[6] This eventually led to the discovery of interferon in 1957 by Alick Isaacs and Jean Lindenmann.

In 1799, Hahnemann gained increased professional acceptance of his ideas by the successful application of *Atropa belladonna* (deadly nightshade) in the prevention and treatment of scarlet fever (which had at that time reached epidemic proportions). In 1860, it was recommended as the treatment of choice in the National Dispensatory, which stated: "as long as persons are under the influence of belladonna ... the liability to contract scarlatina is very much diminished."[7]

The organon of medicine

In 1810, Hahnemann published his *Organon of Medicine*, a book which, through six editions, formed the foundation and definition of the homeopathic practice of medicine. It contains the philosophy, observations, and clinical applications of homeopathy, and citations from the historical and current literature of the time. Hahnemann challenged the reductionistic and mechanistic practices of his time, stating that the nature of disease is dynamic and could not be defined by isolating process, grasping for an explanation. He further asserted that the cause of disease could not be known, and that the categorization of disease states and attempts to manipulate physiology were insufficient, since they did not address the integrity and complexity of organization of the organism as a whole.

He described this organization as spiritual, meaning in accordance with the animating principle of life which is the underlying energetic pattern to which matter conforms.

Disease is therefore addressed descriptively in the context of the whole patient, with the patient's unique symptoms being indicative of that individual's vital response to the condition. For any given disease there may be a long list of remedies which have been clinically effective, but it is the individualization and differentiation between medicines, based on the patient's unique indications, that leads to a successful homeopathic prescription.

Vitalism

Disease, in the homeopathic model, is thought to arise from inherent or developed weaknesses in the patient's defense mechanisms, creating a susceptibility to "morbific influences" (toxic factors in the environment, bacteria, psychological stresses, etc.). This viewpoint is considered "vitalistic" (see Ch. 3 for a more detailed discussion) and, while not denying a corporeal reality, considers pathology to be but a singular focus in a complex net of interactions.

William Boyd, in his *A Textbook of Pathology*, discusses the limitations of the causal approach to disease, currently in vogue in medicine, when he states:[8]

> We must admit, however unwillingly, that we seldom or never really know the cause of anything. Many a beautiful idea has been slain by ugly fact. We merely note a constant association with one thing always following another. We say that the tubercle bacillus is the cause of tuberculosis. That is merely another way of saying that the bacillus is associated with a constant type of lesion; it is no explanation of how the lesions are produced by the bacillus. Nor does it explain why some persons and animals are susceptible to the infection while others are immune.

Vitalism can be better understood in the context of Hahnemann's time, when theories of the causation of disease and its treatment abounded, such as:

- Galen's doctrine that the secondary quality of a medicine, i.e. its action on the disease, can be determined from its primary qualities, such as, its taste or smell
- the evaluation of medicines by the study of their interactions when mixed with human blood in a jar[1]
- iatrochemistry, which had been reduced from the Paracelcean application of spagyric tinctures or oils of metals to dangerous toxic doses
- the classification of drugs according to the Dioscordian approach, which was based on the physiological action (i.e. diuresis, diaphoresis, etc.) and chemical composition
- the "doctrine of signatures," which held that the outer form and color of a plant revealed its inner archetypal action.

Although some studies of the effects of medicinal agents were done with animals, Hahnemann observed that they had different effects on humans: pigs could safely eat *Nux vomica* in quantities that would immediately kill humans; dogs could eat *Aconitum napellus*, a deadly poison to humans, without injury. He also rejected the method of testing drugs by studying their effects on the sick as haphazard and unreliable, particularly since the results being sought were often only symptomatic relief rather than eradication of the disease state.

Hahnemann defined the application of medicines whose purpose was to alter physiology or act as an antagonist to disease as the practice of "allopathy" (*allo-* meaning "contrary" in Greek). The current dominant medical system is heavily influenced by the causalistic and allopathic paradigms. This results in the diagnosis being the focal point of practice, without which appropriate therapy cannot be instituted. This pharmacological approach is limited to the end results of disease rather than the origins of pathogenesis. This causes problems, since only the primary action of the pharmaceutical agent is utilized for treating a specific disease state, while the remaining range of physiological, as well as psychological, effects are ignored or unwanted and therefore classified as side-effects. In the homeopathic model, the side-effects are an important part of the agent's action and the body's response to them, and by ignoring them, a drug's usefulness is greatly limited, while its toxicity is increased.

Hahnemann's empirical investigations led not only to new applications of medicines, but provided a method for integrating the physical, mental, and emotional effects of a drug. This allowed the treatment of the totality of a patient's symptoms as a dynamic pattern of interaction. Vitalists stress the teleological behavior of organisms, i.e. the goal-directedness and design in biological phenomena. Disease is therefore regarded as a positive expression of the organism's self-regulatory process in response to an environmental, or other, stress. This response is not accidental or caused by the stressor, but is rather the effort of the organism to ward off deeper or more internal disorganization. It is the natural wisdom of the body, the *vis medicatrix naturae*, or, using current scientific terminology, the tendency of the body to maintain homeostasis. Medical intervention often acts in conflict with these vital intra- and extracellular regulatory functions.

Karl Menninger, in 1948, commented on this medical dilemma:[9]

> I believe that clinicians have come to think more and more in terms of a disturbance in the total economics of the personality, a temporary overwhelming of the efforts of the organism to maintain a continuous internal and external adaptation to continuously changing relationships, threats, pressures, instinctive needs and reality demands. ... It is the imbalance, the organismic disequilibrium, which is the real pathology, and when that imbalance reaches a degree or duration that threatens the comfort or survival of the individual, it may correctly be denoted disease.

Homeopathy is a method of specific induction of non-specific resistance, which stimulates the body's inherent defense and self-regulatory mechanisms, rather than, by taking over a function of the body, initiating dependency on the medicine itself.

THE CLINICAL APPLICATION OF HOMEOPATHIC PRINCIPLES

The homeopathic clinical, or therapeutic, process consists of three interrelated processes: case-taking, evaluation, and prescribing. The process is comprehensive and engages the observations of the patient as well as those of the doctor. Hahnemann describes the process in paragraphs 84–103 of the *Organon* and stresses the importance of distinguishing between chronic and acute, or self-limiting disease.

The homeopathic interview

The initial history of complaints is elicited from the patient with as little interruption as possible (as long as the patient does not digress unduly) so that the patient's train of thought is not disrupted or directed along lines imposed by the physician's biases. According to Hahnemann:

> The physician elicits further particulars about each of the patient's statements without ever putting words in his mouth, or asking a question that can be answered only by yes or no, which induces the patient to affirm something untrue or half true or else deny something really there to avoid discomfort or out of desire to please, thereby giving a wrong picture of the disease, which would lead to the wrong treatment.

An entire review of symptoms is recorded in descriptive detail, taking into consideration all modalities which affect a symptom. Hahnemann emphasized the general symptoms, i.e. those affecting the entire organism, as the leading indications for the remedy. These key symptoms include mental and emotional affects, the metabolism and its reactions to environmental stimuli, sleep positions, food cravings and aversions, thirst, body type, and all manifestations of unconscious and autonomic regulation.

Unique characteristic symptoms, particularly those regarded as "strange, rare, and peculiar", are important considerations in the selection of the remedy. These might be the expression of a paradoxical or unusual relationship, such as pain ameliorated by pressure or the sensation of the legs being made of wood or glass. The association of the start of a disease or symptom complex with an environmental or emotional event can be very important and emphasizes the importance of an accurate and extensive interview.

Hahnemann emphasizes the importance of taking a comprehensive case, particularly in chronic disease:[5]

> In chronic diseases in women one should pay particular attention to such things as pregnancy, infertility, sexual

desire, confinement, miscarriages, nursing, vaginal discharges, and the condition of the monthly flow, especially noting whether it recurs at intervals that are too short or too long, how many days it lasts, whether or not it is interrupted, the quantity, how dark with color, any leukorrhea before or after the flow. If there is leukorrhea, what it is like, what symptoms accompany it, what is its quantity, under what conditions does it appear, what brings it on?

Since the patient's symptoms are the expressions of the body's attempts to heal itself, symptomatic treatment, i.e. most allopathic therapies, impairs the physician's ability to obtain vital information and complicates the taking of the case. This problem has also been recognized by some medical authors, such as Boyd, who states: "We recognize that the pattern of disease has changed out of recognition during the last thirty to forty years owing to modern drugs, particularly the antibiotics."[8]

Case evaluation

Considering the vitalistic and holistic perspective of the homeopathic approach, a clear definition of cure is necessary in order to establish the treatment goal. Mere palliation or suppression of symptoms at the cost of the overall vitality and function of the individual is considered negligent by the homeopathic practitioner. For example, if a patient's skin disease is treated and appears to resolve, but is followed by asthma, fatigue, and confusion, the treatment is evaluated as having been suppressive. If, upon proper treatment, the more serious lung and systemic disruptions are alleviated and the prior skin lesions return, the patient is considered as progressing towards a cure. When further appropriate therapy results in final alleviation of the skin disease, without any undue stress to the patient, it is then considered a true cure.

This evaluative procedure is part of what is known as "Hering's law of cure", an observation of the principles of curative responses which can be applied to any healing process, regardless of the school of thought. In true healing, according to this set of observations, symptoms follow these patterns:

- from above, down the body to the extremities
- from within to without (often in the form of discharges and other eliminative processes)
- from the most important organs (e.g. the CNS) to the least important organs (typically the skin)
- in reverse order of their appearance, i.e. the chronologically most recent being replaced by those of the earlier stages of the disease, and, in some instances, earlier in the patient's life.

Homeopathy holds that the disease first affects the vital force, and is manifested first by a change in the patient's well-being, long before any objective changes can be observed. Illness is usually first recognized when the patient becomes aware of the early manifestations of the disease.

Disease and cure must also be considered in the context of the belief system and culture of the patient. Much of what we call disease arises from the individual's inability to find meaning and purpose. Many forms of healing are capable of enabling the person to integrate into the fabric of daily life and of providing ways to help the person address personal needs for fulfillment.

In his study of disease, Hahnemann noted that there were inherited predispositions to disease, which he related to the improper treatment, and therefore suppression, of skin eruptions and venereal disease. He called these predispositions miasmas, and in 1828, published his findings in *Chronic Diseases: Their Nature and Homeopathic Cure*. He observed that many people, despite apparently healthy lifestyles, develop degenerative diseases. These often become established in childhood, and continue to plague the person throughout life, despite medical treatment.

More recently, George Vithoulkas, a contemporary homeopathic author and teacher, has defined health on three levels: mental, emotional, and physical. The mind should be capable of functioning with clarity, rationality, coherence, and logical sequence. It should be capable of engaging in creative service for the good of others, as well as for the good of oneself, demonstrating a freedom from selfishness and possessiveness. On the emotional level, there should be a state of serenity free from excessive passion, a state which should not be confused with lack of emotional response generated as a protection against emotional vulnerability. Finally, on the physical level, there should be freedom from pain. The healing person should experience a subjective sense of well-being and a progressive increase in vitality.[10]

Prescription

Since homeopathy is oriented towards the administration of a single medicine at a time (probably due to the fact that there have been few provings of combination remedies, whose interactions can therefore only be assumed, but not known), careful prescribing is important. It is through the application of single medicines that physicians have been able to record clinical verification of the provings and amass an impressive body of literature.

The process of selecting the correct remedy is called "repertorization", and involves both careful study of the patient's symptomatology and medical history, and matching these with the appropriate remedy. This requires a sound understanding of the homeopathic materia medica (see below).

Homeopathic pharmacy and potency selection

This leads to a discussion of what has remained the greatest mystery of homeopathic medicine (and the source of the considerable ridicule and misunderstanding) – the use of "potentized" substances.

As Hahnemann began his research, he found that when treating patients according to the law of similars there was an initial aggravation of the symptoms, the "healing crisis," when using the high dosages typical of that era. He empirically tried using progressive dilutions of the medicines, beginning with tinctures from plants and titurations with milk sugar for metals and salts. He made the dilutions serially by mixing one drop of the tincture to 100 drops of alcohol which were then succussed (shaken by pounding against a resilient surface) vigorously. He found that, with increasing dilution, the severity of the aggravation lessened while the patient continued to improve, often with deeper and more enduring results. He called these diluted remedies "potentized". As an analytical chemist, he was aware of Avogadro's theories (they were contemporaries), but he persisted in evaluating dilutions beyond the point where chemical activity could be detected.

Various techniques have been used to determine if there is a physical difference between the potentized dilution and the unmodified vehicle. These studies have used UV spectroscopy, conductivity measurements, IR spectroscopy, surface tension measurements, Ranian-laser spectroscopy, NMR, and other methods. Much of this work has shown regular peaks and troughs in activity with progressive dilutions, and Heintz has claimed that the peaks correspond to the maximum effects found in the biological studies he has reported.[11]

The most cogent demonstration of the physical properties of homeopathic preparations has been the work of Shui-Yin Lo PhD. Dr Lo, a particle physicist, has demonstrated that stable rigid structures, which he calls IE structures, can be formed in water molecules by the electric dipole moment, which can conform to solutes present in the water.[12,13] IE structures stand for ice formed under electric fields. Although most of Dr Lo's work has been concerned with applications of IE crystals in engine combustion efficiency, when he tested homeopathic preparations by fluorescence spectrophotometry and transmission electron microscopy, he was able to demonstrate unique structures of IE crystals, which were stable at room temperatures and heat-resistant.

Further studies are necessary to confirm and develop the understanding of the mechanisms and validity of homeopathic medicines.

In terms of clinical practice, there have evolved general guidelines for the determination of potency. In the sixth edition of the *Organon*, Hahnemann recommends ascending the scale of potencies gradually. In paragraph 248, he suggests that the medicinal solution be succussed anew with use. In chronic cases, the patient is directed to take 1 teaspoonful daily or every other day, and in acute diseases, as frequently as needed. If the solution is used up before the problem alleviates, the next higher dilution is used (if still indicated by the symptom pattern).[5]

The higher potencies, whose use largely developed in the United States, are given much less frequently, and are generally reserved for the experienced practitioner. The more potentized the remedy, the closer it must meet the law of similars, i.e. the accuracy of the prescription must be high, for a curative effect.

It is important to note however, that the sixth edition was unavailable until 1924, 76 years after Hahnemann's death. The predominant clinical application of homeopathic potencies had developed using an ascending scale. A single dose was used until its action had ceased, when the same potency would be repeated. When that potency seemed to no longer demonstrate an enduring effect, a higher potency was used. The general range of potencies used included 6C, 12C, 30C, 200C, 1M, 10M, and CM ("C" denotes the centesimal scale utilized by Hahnemann).

The study of the materia medica

Constantine Hering once stated:

> A mere acquaintance with the principle symptoms cannot be called studying the materia medica, although we make it the basis of our study. The study of materia medica must be regarded and dealt with in exactly the same manner as that of other natural sciences.

To give a perspective on the way in which homeopathic physicians organize the proving symptoms into clinical pictures, we will draw from an essay on *Sepia* by E. B. Nash:[14]

> This is another of our wonderful remedies of which the dominant school knows nothing, except what they have learned from us. Its chief sphere of action seems to be in the abdomen and pelvis, especially in women. No remedy produces stronger symptoms here. We quote from different but equally good observers.
>
> Sensation of bearing down in the pelvic region, with dragging pains from the sacrum; or feeling of bearing down of all pelvic organs. (Hahnemann)
>
> Labor-like pains accompanied with the feeling as though she must cross her legs and "sit close" to keep something from coming out through the vagina. (Guernsey)
>
> Pain in uterus, bearing down, comes from back to abdomen, causing oppression of breathing; crosses limbs to prevent protrusion of parts. (Hering)
>
> Prolapse of the uterus, of the vagina, with pressure as if everything would protrude. (Lippe)
>
> Experience has shown its value in cases of ulceration and congestion of the os and cervix uteri. Its use supersedes all local applications. (Dunham)

No higher authority than the united testimony of these five of our best observers could be brought to show the action of *Sepia* upon the pelvic organs.

Now when we come to examine the provings in Allen's *Encyclopedia*, we find that these symptoms were mainly produced by Hahnemann and his provers, and Hahnemann advocated proving remedies in the 30th, and some of them were produced by the 200th, especially those most strongly verified by black-faced type.

We confess that we cannot understand how so many question the value of potencies for proving or curing…

Sepia, like *Sulphur*, affects the general circulation in a very marked manner. **Flashes of heat** with **perspiration** and **faintness** is almost as characteristic of this remedy as of *Sulphur*. But there are, with *Sepia*, more apt to be associated with them the pelvic symptoms already given, and they are also more apt to occur in conjunction with the **climacteric**. Indeed, these flashes often seem with *Sepia* to start in the pelvic organs and from thence to spread over the body.

But this irregularity of circulation extends as far as that of *Sulphur*. The hands and feet are hot alternately, that is, if the feet are hot, the hands are cold, and *vice versa*. There is not so much **sensation** of burning with *Sepia* as with *Sulphur*, but there is actual heat, and the venous congestion, which seems to be the real state of the organs where the pressive bearing down et cetera is felt, is also accompanied with much throbbing and beating.

This local congestion to the pelvic organs is not simply sensational. There are actual displacements in consequence of it, and the long continued congestion results in inflammations, ulcerations, leukorrheas and even malignancies or cancerous organizations. Induration with a painful **sense** of stiffness in the uterine region is characteristic.

This pelvic congestion also affects the rectum in a marked degree. The rectum prolapses, there is a sensation of fullness, or of a foreign substance as of a **ball or weight**, and oozing of moisture from the rectum. Indeed, the rectal and anal symptoms are almost as strong as the uterine and vaginal. It is impossible to enumerate all the symptoms connected with the circulatory disturbances of *Sepia* is such a work as this, only a general study of the Materia Medica can do it.

The urinary organs come in for their share of symptoms. The same pressure and fullness consequent upon the portal congestion reaches here. We will now proceed to give what we have found to be particularly valuable symptoms under the various organs in this region. "Pressure on bladder and frequent micturation with tension in lower abdomen." "Sediment in the urine like clay; as if clay burnt on the bottom of the vessel; urine **very offensive** (*Indium*), can't endure to have it in the room, it is reddish or may be bloody." This is found mostly in women. With children there is one peculiar symptom which has often been verified. "The child always wets the bed during its **first sleep**."

Upon the male organs I have found it particularly useful in chronic gleet. There is not much discharge, but a few drops, perhaps, which glue up the orifice of the urethra in the morning; but it is so persistent and the usual remedies will not "dry it up." In my early practice I used to use a weak injection of *Sulphate of Zinc*, but it used to annoy me that I could not use it without resorting to local measures. *Sepia* does it in the majority of cases and *Kali iodatum* will do it in the rest. I have, where there was a thick discharge of long standing and the smarting and burning on urination continued, several times finished the case with *Capsicum*.

As a rule, this long continued slight, passive gleety discharge is a result of weakness of the male genitals, *as is shown by a flaccidity of the organs and frequent seminal emissions. The emissions are thin and watery. Sepia* covers all of this and often sets all to rights in a short time.

The mind symptoms of *Sepia* are like *Pulsatilla*, in that she is sad and cries frequently without knowing the reason why. So if in a tearful mind with uterine disturbances *Pulsatilla* should fail you, the next remedy to be studied is *Sepia*. But there is another condition of mind not found under *Pulsatilla* or any other remedy in the same degree, and that is, that, notwithstanding there is no sign of dementia from actual brain lesion, the patient, contrary to her usual habit, **becomes indifferent to her occupation**, her house work, her family or their comfort, **even to those whom she loves the best**. This is a very peculiar symptom and a genuine keynote for the exhibition of *Sepia*…

I once cured a very obstinate case of entero-colitis (so-called cholera infantum), after the complete failure of two eminent allopaths, with *Sepia*, the leading symptom being, **always worse after taking milk**. Oozing of moisture from the anus finds its remedy here sometimes, but oftener in *Antimonium crudum*. The *Sepia* patient is very weak. A short walk fatigues her very much. She **faints** easily from extremes of cold and heat, after getting wet, from riding in a carriage, while kneeling at church, and on other trifling occasions. This fainting, or sense of sinking faintness, may be found in pregnancy, child bed, or during lactation; or, again, it may come on after hard work, such as "laundry work;" so it has come to be called the "washer woman's" remedy. *Phosphorus* has washer woman's toothache."

As can be seen by this excerpt, the indications for a remedy are complex, requiring study and understanding.

RESEARCH IN HOMEOPATHY

Since homeopathy arose from empirical observations, and operates from phenomenologically descriptive fields rather than causal relationships, its evaluation by the scientific method, as described by Karl Popper, poses unique problems. A recent critical review appeared in *The British Homeopathic Journal* describing the methods utilized in various attempts to verify this school of medicine.[11] The following briefly discusses some of the studies which have been done.

Human studies

Science is based on the premise of non-biased inquiry. Despite antagonism towards homeopathy, researchers have persisted in producing clinical trials, most of which have demonstrated its efficacy. The method of individualization in homeopathic prescribing has challenged study designs, and required several studies to be questioned. However a recent meta-analysis of 119 placebo-controlled trials showed that for every negative study, an average of 2.45 studies were published which demonstrated the efficacy of homeopathy.[15] The *British Journal of Homeopathy* and *The Lancet* remain useful resources for homeopathic research published in English. References for homeopathic research may be found on the internet at www.healthy.net/homeopathicresearch. A few interesting studies follow.

During World War II, isopathic preparations were given prophylactically, and homeopathic therapies were used in mustard gas burns. A statistical analysis shows that these treatments yielded significant results when compared with placebos. The remedies used were mustard gas, *Rhus toxicodendron*, and *Kali bichromium*.[11]

Gibson et al[16] published a double-blind clinical trial of homeopathic treatment in rheumatoid arthritis.[20] The 3-month study was elegantly designed, in that the prescribing was individualized to the patient's symptoms and was controlled, on a double-blind basis, by giving half the patients the correct remedy and the rest a placebo. All patients continued to use conventional, non-steroidal, anti-inflammatory drugs, and the treated group showed significant improvement in subjective pain, articular index, stiffness, and grip strength.

In another study, Shipley et al[17] compared *Rhus toxicodendron* and fenoprofen in the treatment of osteoarthritis. The study demonstrated no effects from the *Rhus toxicodendron*, but it has been deservedly criticized since it lasted only 2 weeks (hardly enough time for the remedy to work since, in chronic diseases, homeopaths typically wait 4–6 weeks before attempting to evaluate the efficacy of the remedy) and the remedy was not individualized for the patient.

Animal studies

Caulophylum (in the 30th centesimal potency) was given to 10 sows to test its efficacy in the control of stillbirths. The results showed a statistically significant drop in the number of stillbirths and led to a larger, uncontrolled study in a whole herd. After4 months of therapy, piglet mortality dropped from 20 to 2.6%.[18]

Cloudhury[19] obtained dramatic results from injecting mice intraperitoneally with *Kali phosphoricum*, *Calcarea phosphorica*, or *Ferrum phosphorica* (in the 30th decimal potency) 12 days after implantation of fibrosarcoma. Of the 77 treated mice, 52% were cured and survived more than 1 year, whereas all of the 77 controls died within 10–15 days.

Scofield,[20] in his review article, discusses numerous experiments with humans, animals, and plants using isopathic treatment for poisoning and experimental liver damage, and various in vitro studies. According to his exhaustive evaluations, although many of the studies demonstrated that homeopathic preparations have effects, even when not applied according to the homeopathic method, most lacked statistical analysis or were poorly designed, making a definitive statement of efficacy impossible at this time.

CONCLUSION

Homeopathy represents an integrated holistic system of natural therapeutics. Its capacity for addressing psychosomatic disease and acute pathology as a dynamic process is unique. It has remained a coherent system, with extensive clinical verification, for over two centuries. Homeopathy is an economical and effective method which has been established as an integral part of the medical system in several countries. With the resurgence of interest in natural medicine, this discipline will undoubtedly be more widely utilized.

Unfortunately, however, homeopathy is also an extremely difficult system to master, requiring both considerable understanding of case-taking and materia medica as well as extensive consultation time with the patient. It has, therefore, often been discarded, even by those aware of its efficacy. Although attempts have been made to reduce it to simpler systems (allergy desensitizations, vaccination, Schuessler's cell salts, and isopathic preparations from diseased tissues and heavy metals, etc.), they are not considered homeopathic unless prescribed according to their effects upon healthy people or the confirmed observations of cured symptoms.

In the context of modern naturopathic medicine, it is important to recognize that Hahnemann did not ignore the importance of lifestyle in the treatment of the patient:

> While taking a case of chronic disease one should examine and weigh the particular conditions of the patient's day to day activities, living habits, diet, domestic situation, and so on. One should ascertain whether there is anything in them which may cause or sustain the disease and remove it to help the cure.

REFERENCES

1. Coulter H. Divided legacy: a history of the schism in medical thought, vol. 2. Washington, DC: Wehawken Book Co. 1977
2. Hahnemann S. Lesser writings. New York, NY: Radde. 1852
3. Coulter H. Divided legacy: a history of the schism in medical thought, vol. 3. Washington, DC: Wehawken Book Co. 1977: p 305
4. Schaumber H, Kaplan J, Windebank A. Sensory neuropathy from pyridoxine abuse. New Engl J Med 1983; 309: 445–448 *See Chapter 122 for a full discussion of this report and an alternative explanation for the phenomenon*
5. Hahnemann S. Organon of medicine. Los Angeles, CA: JP Tarcher. 1980
6. Isaacs A. Interferon. Scientific American 1961; 204: 51–57
7. Harris C. Homeopathic influences in 19th century allopathic therapeutics. Washington, DC: American Institute of Homeopathy. 1973: p 39
8. Boyd W. A textbook of pathology. 8th edn. Philadelphia, PA: Lea & Febinger. 1970: p 3–12
9. Menninger K. Changing concepts of disease. Ann Int Med 1948; 29: 318–325
10. Vithoulkas G. The science of homeopathy. New York, NY: New York Grove Press. 1979

11. Scofield AM. Experimental research in homeopathy – a critical review. Br Homeop J 1984; 73: 161–266
12. Shui-Yin Lo et al. Physical proproperties of water with IE structures. Mod Phys Lett B 1996; 10: 921–930
13. Shui-Yin Lo et al. Anomalous state of ice. Mod Phys Lett B 1996; 10: 909–919
14. Nash EB. Leaders in homeopathic therapeutics. 6th edn. New Dehli, India: Jain. 1982: p 200–206 (reprint, first published in 1926)
15. Linde K, Clausius N, Ramairez G et al. Are the clinical effects of homeopathy placebo effects? A meta-analysis of placebo-controlled trials. Lancet 1997; 350: 834–843
16. Gibson RG, Gibson SL, MacNeil AD, Buchanan WW. Homeopathic therapy in rheumatoid arthritis: evaluation by double-blind clinical therapeutic trial. Br J Clin Pharm 1980; 9: 453–459
17. Shipley M, Berry H, Broster G et al. Controlled trial of homeopathic treatment of osteoarthritis. Lancet 1983; i: 97–98
18. Day C. Control of stillbirths in pigs using homeopathy. Vet Rec 1984; 114: 216
19. Cloudhury H. Cure of cancer in experimental mice with certain biochemic salts. Br Homeop J 1980; 69: 168–170
20. Scofield A. Experimental research in homeopathy – a critical review. Br Hom J 1984; 73: 211–225

FURTHER READING

Books

Boerke W. Pocket Manual of Materia Medica with Repertory. 1936. Reprint: New Delhi, India: Jain. 1982

Clark J. Dictionary of Practical Materia Medica, 3 vols. 1900. Reprint: Essex, England: Health Sciences. 1962

Coulter H. Homeopathic science and modern medicine: the physics of healing with microdoses. Berkely, CA: North Atlantic. 1981

Gibson DM. First aid homeopathy in accidents and injuries. London, England: British Homeopathic Association

Kent JT. Materia Medica. 1900. Reprint: Berkely, CA: North Atlantic. 1979

Nash EB. Leaders in homeopathic therapeutics. 1898. Reprint: New Delhi, India: Jain. 1983

Panos M, Heimlich J. Homeopathic medicine at home. Los Angeles, CA: JP Tarcher. 1980

Roberts HA. The principles and art of cure by homeopathy. Essex, England: Health Sciences. 1942

Vithoulkas G. Homeopathy: medicine of the new man. New York: Arco. 1979

Journals

British Homeopathic Journal

Journal of the American Institute of Homeopathy

CHAPTER CONTENTS

42

Hydrotherapy

Robert Barry, ND

INTRODUCTION

Hydrotherapy may be defined as the use of water, in any of its forms, for the maintenance of health or the treatment of disease. Although one of the oldest known therapies, it has received little attention from the research community, particularly recently. Much of the information presented here is compiled from older works which, although they lack the quantification available with current technology, show a remarkable attention to clinical effects and patient response.

HISTORY

As one of the ancient methods of treatment, hydrotherapy has been used to treat disease and injury by many different peoples, including the Egyptians, Assyrians, Persians, Greeks, Hebrews, Hindus, and Chinese. In the *Rig Veda*, written about 1500 BC, we read that "water cures the fever's glow".

Hippocrates used hydrotherapy extensively around 400 BC. In his writings concerning baths are some of the earliest dictums on the therapeutic uses of water:[1]

> Much will depend on whether the patient, when in good health, was very fond of the bath, and in the custom of taking it: for such persons, especially feel the want of it, and are benefited if they are bathed, and injured if they are not. In general it suits better with cases of pneumonia than in ardent fevers; for the bath soothes the pain in the side, chest and back; cuts the sputum, promotes expectoration, improves the respiration, and allays lassitude; for it soothes the joints and outer skin, and is diuretic, removes heaviness of the head, and moistens the nose. Such are the benefits to be derived from the bath, if all the proper requisites be present; but if one or more be wanting, the bath, instead of doing good, may rather prove injurious; for every one of them may do harm if not prepared by the attendants in the proper manner.

He writes further to explain the specific contraindications to the use of the bath.

As these early writings show, the uses of water had been explored extensively at very early times, with many of the principal effects having been observed and utilized.

The modern history of hydrotherapy begins in the 17th century with the publication, in 1697, of *The history of cold bathing* by Sir John Floyer. Following Floyer were several works which attempted to provide a scientific foundation for the uses of water in medicine. Probably the strongest impetus for its use came from central Europe, where it was advocated by such well known hydropaths as Priessnitz, Rausse, and Father Kneipp. They were able to popularize specific water treatments which quickly became the vogue in Europe during the 19th century. By the end of the 19th century, there were many individuals, both in the US and in Europe, who were actively engaged in practicing hydrotherapy.

Probably the best known American was J. H. Kellogg, a medical doctor who approached hydrotherapy scientifically, performing many and varied experiments on its use and effects. In 1900, he published what may still be considered a definitive treatise on hydrotherapy, entitled *Rational hydrotherapy*,[2] in which he considers the physiological and therapeutic effects of water, along with an extensive discussion of hydrotherapeutic techniques.

The scientific and lay literature of this period shows a wide disparity of thought as to the validity and efficacy of hydrotherapeutic treatments. In Germany the uses of hydrotherapy were openly embraced, whereas in nearby France hydrotherapy was seriously questioned, never becoming as popular or widely used.

During the 20th century, the popularity of hydrotherapy treatments declined, along with the numbers of practitioners and institutions providing treatments. One of the few physicians to maintain an active practice in hydrotherapy was Dr O. G. Carroll, a naturopath practicing for many years in Spokane, Washington. He developed a specific constitutional hydrotherapy treatment which is currently receiving an increased amount of interest from the naturopathic profession.

Although hydrotherapy declined in use for many years, it is rightfully being revived at the present time. It is a highly effective, non-invasive means of treating the sick, which may be used both in the office and in the home, is economical, and involves patients directly in their care. As such, it is an ideal naturopathic treatment modality.

RECENT RESEARCH

The scientific medical literature, although not replete with research concerning hydrotherapy, continues to have occasional articles or books devoted to the subject.

Two articles that clearly demonstrate the disparity of current thought have appeared. The first, an extensive review article from Belgium, states:[3]

> Hydrotherapy is based on the physical properties of water, acting from outside the body mainly during the time of its application. The underlying cause of the disease being treated is not affected, so hydrotherapy must be considered as an adjunct, as a palliative measure facilitating the activity of other remedies or spontaneous healing.

The second article, appearing in 1977 in a German medical journal, would seem to be in counterpoint to the Belgian premise. It states:

> Immunological tests were performed on 34 patients undergoing hydrotherapy according to Kneipp. IgM, alpha-2-macroglobulin and complement factor C_3 concentrations were increased after this treatment but not in 10 health volunteers (controls).

These two articles exemplify the nature of the continuing debate concerning the uses of hydrotherapy. German healers continue to be the most active proponents of hydrotherapy as a significant means of treating disease.

In a review article in *Scientific American*, Edelson & Fink[4] discussed the significant role of the skin in immune function. Although they make no references to topical applications of water having an effect on this mechanism, it certainly provides an impetus for further work in this area and may, at some point, provide the rationale for many of the effects which have been ascribed to hydrotherapeutic procedures.

Two recent studies provide additional documentation of the physiological effects of hydrotherapy. In the first study, 10 healthy subjects who swim regularly in ice cold water during the winter were evaluated before and after their short-term whole body exposure. The researchers found a drastic decrease in uric acid concentration seen during and following the exposure to cold stimulus and an increase in the level of oxidized glutathione and the ratio of oxidized glutathione/total glutathione. Baseline concentration of reduced glutathione was increased and the concentration of oxidized glutathione was decreased in the erythrocytes of winter swimmers as compared with those of non-winter swimmers. These changes were interpreted by the researchers as an adaptation to repeated oxidative stress. This research supports the hydrotherapy concept of "hardening", i.e. the exposure to a natural stimulus, in this case thermal, which results in an increased tolerance to stress and disease.[5]

The other study evaluated the impact of a cold-wet sheet pack on the trunk in patients suffering from chronic cardiac, rheumatic, and metabolic diseases, as well as functional disorders. The control group received a dry sheet pack, but without the stimulus of hydrotherapy. The study showed a significant difference in the outcome of both applications. The mental well-being was affected positively in 18 patients during their real treatment, compared with nine in the control group.[6]

PROPERTIES OF WATER

Water has several unique properties which contribute to its effectiveness as a therapeutic agent. It has an ability to store and transmit heat, which renders it most appropriate for treatment purposes. Water absorbs more heat for a given weight that any other substance – almost twice as much as alcohol or paraffin, 10 times more than copper or iron, and 30 times more than lead or gold. Water is also a good conductor of heat.

The solvent properties of water account for its usefulness in the most common of all hydrotherapy procedures, baths and showers. Water is commonly considered the universal solvent.

Water's non-toxicity allows for its use both internally and externally, even in individuals who are extremely sensitive to their surroundings.

Water also has the ability to change states within a narrow, easily obtainable temperature range. As ice, it is an effective cooling agent. In the liquid state, water may be applied as packs, baths, sprays, compresses, and douches at any desired pressure and temperature. As a vapor, it may be employed in vapor or steam baths or by inhalation.

Since the density of water is near that of the human body, it can be used as an exercise medium for patients with paralysis, inflammations, or atropy.[7] Upon immersion of the body in water, hydrostatic pressure is exerted upon the body surface, which has the effect of increasing venous and lymph flow from the periphery and increasing urine output.

Water is also unique in that it is universally available, readily accessible, and applied with relatively simple and inexpensive equipment.

Physiological effects

The physiological effects of hydrotherapy may be classified as thermal, mechanical, and chemical. Thermal effects are produced by the application of water at temperatures above or below that of the body. The greater the variation from body temperature, the greater the effect produced, other factors being equal. The mechanical effects are produced by the impact of water upon the surface of the body in the form of sprays, douches, frictions, whirlpools, etc. The chemical effects are produced when it is taken by mouth or used to irrigate a body cavity, such as the large colon. The most commonly utilized effect, therapeutically, is the thermal one. It is the only one which will be dealt with in this section.

Heat may be transferred from one object to another in several different ways, including conduction, convection or conversion. In hydrotherapy, the heating and cooling effects are produced by conduction of heat from the water to the body. The contact of water with the body is accomplished by means of baths, showers, sprays, packs, compresses, etc.

The primary variable of concern is temperature, both of the water and of the patient. The temperature of the human body in a state of health is considered to be normal at 98.6°F orally, although it varies throughout the day from a low of near 97°F between 3 and 6 a.m. to a high of over 99°F around 6 p.m. These variations are important to consider when evaluating an individual prior to a hydrotherapy application. There is also a wide range of temperature variation within the healthy human body, as can be seen in Table 42.1.[2]

Body temperature is also a reflection of other factors, such as exercise, fasting, ovulation, etc. In an infant, the temperature may be elevated by 1–3°F during a prolonged crying spell.

During a fever, the temperature is elevated due to any of several factors, including:

- infection
- tissue destruction
- malignancy
- foreign proteins in the blood
- dehydration
- hormonal imbalances
- muscular or chemical activity.

Proper evaluation of the degree and cause of a fever is necessary prior to hydrotherapy treatments.

When we consider water temperature, the terms "hot" and "cold" are related to body temperature. The range of temperatures useful in hydrotherapy applications varies from very cold to very hot. Table 42.2 provides general terminology.

Deep well water is near 53°F. Cold tap water in Seattle varies in temperature throughout the year depending on the depth of the pipes and other exposures to the environment. During the winter it may be as low as 40°F, and in the summer as high as 60°F. This temperature

Table 42.1 Temperature of various tissues

Tissue	Temperature (°F)
Average temp of the skin	93
Average temp of the blood	102
Brain	104
Liver	106
Left ventricle of the heart	107

Table 42.2 Sensations when the forearm is immersed in water of various temperatures

Temperature (°F)	Description	Sensation
>104	Very hot	Can tolerate for only a short period
98–104	Hot	Skin redness if prolonged
95–98	Warm	Comfortably warm
92–95	Neutral	No sensation
80–92	Tepid	Slightly cooling
65–80	Cool	Cool
55–65	Cold	Sensation of coldness
32–55	Very cold	Pain and numbness

variation may be a significant factor in hydrotherapy treatments; therefore, it is advisable to be aware of your water temperature when using hydrotherapy techniques.

Effects of cold applications

Cold applications may be made by means of ice, cold water, or cold air, or by the evaporation of water or other liquids from the surface of the body. Although the applications may vary, the principles and effects remain consistent.

The primary or direct effect of cold applications is depressant in nature, leading to a decrease in function, either locally or systemically, depending on the application. The longer and colder the application, the longer and more intense will be the depressant effect. However, as the body responds to the cold application, there is a return to normal function which may lead to a state of increased activity. This is known as the secondary, or indirect, effect of cold, also termed the "reaction". If the cold application is a short one, the reaction follows quickly, its intensity reflecting the intensity (i.e. coldness) of the application. The secondary effect, or reaction, occurs only when the body has the vitality to respond to the cold, either following its removal from the body, in such applications as showers, sprays, baths, etc., or after the body has warmed the application, in such cases as cold compresses or packs. In general, the colder the application the greater the reaction.

Many hydrotherapy techniques are directed at producing the reaction to the cold application.

Effects of hot applications

Heat may be applied to the body in a variety of ways, including hot packs, fomentations, steam, hot air, baths, showers, etc. All hot applications produce definite physiological responses which are attempts to eliminate heat in order to prevent a rise in local and systemic temperatures. The effects produced by hot applications depend on the mode, temperature, and duration of the application and the condition of the patient.

Water at 98°F or above is generally perceived as hot, and over 104°F it is considered to be very hot. At 120°F, an immersion bath becomes unendurable, although small areas of the body, such as the hand, may be conditioned to endure a temperature 10–15° higher for short periods. The mucous membranes, unlike the skin, may endure temperatures as high as 135°F, which accounts for our ability to drink very hot liquids, such as tea or coffee. Hot air may be tolerated by many individuals for fairly long periods, such as in a sauna, in which the temperature may reach as high as 200°F. Although exposure to the high temperatures of hot tubs and saunas has become quite popular in recent years, repeated and prolonged use may act to weaken the individual, unless counteracted by frequent cold applications, such as showers or ablutions.[2]

A comparison of the effects of hot and cold on several body systems is given in Table 42.3.

PRINCIPLES OF BLOOD MOVEMENT WITH HYDROTHERAPY

In order to promote healing, either locally or systemically, it is important to maximize circulation of well-oxygenated, nutrient-rich, toxin-low blood. Hydrotherapy techniques are one of the most effective means of accomplishing this, if used in conjunction with proper levels of activity, optimal nutritional intake, and adequate detoxification.

There are four basic modifications of blood movement within the body:

- increased rate of blood flow through an organ or area of the body
- decreased rate of blood flow through an organ or area of the body
- increased volume of blood in an anemic area
- decreased volume of blood in a congested area.

Table 42.3 Comparison of the effects of hot and cold on several body systems[2]

System/Organ	Cold		Hot
	Primary	Secondary	
Skin			
—blood vessels	Constriction	Dialation	Dilation
—respiration	Decreased	Increased	Increased
—heat loss	Decreased	Increased	Increased
Blood vessels	Constriction	Dilation	Dilation (constriction if intense)
Heart	Rate increased	Rate decreased	First decreased, then increased
Nerves	Numbed		Excited
Muscles	Volume decreased		Volume increased
Respiration	Slowed and deepened		Rate increased
Stomach	Motility and HCl increased		Motility and HCl decreased

In order to accomplish these modifications there are five relevant physiological principles:

- revulsive effect
- derivative effect
- spinal cord reflex
- collateral circulation
- arterial trunk reflex.

Revulsive effect

The revulsive effect provides a means of increasing the rate of blood flow through an organ or other body part, such as an extremity. The most effective means of accomplishing this is by using alternating hot/cold either as compresses, baths, showers, sprays, etc.

Local, alternating, hot and cold applications produce marked stimulation of local circulation. It has been shown that a 30 minute contrast bath produces a 95% increase in local blood flow when the lower extremities alone are immersed. When all four extremities are immersed at the same time, there is a 100% increase in blood flow in the upper extremities and a 70% increase in the lower extremities.[8]

Several studies have researched the optimal treatment times for revulsive effects. Woodmansey et al[9] found 6 minutes of hot application and 4 of cold to be optimal for the British subjects he studied. Krussen[10] found 4 minutes hot and 1 minute cold to be the best treatment protocol. Moor[11] states that 3 minutes hot, followed by 30–60 seconds of cold, provides satisfactory clinical results. From these variations, we may infer that, due to the variations in procedures and locales, it is best for practitioners to determine their own ideals, based on their observations of clinical results. Basically, the cold application need only be long enough to produce vasoconstriction, and this can be shown to occur in as short a period as 20 seconds.

Repetition of applications is another important variable to be considered when applying revulsive treatments. A series of three hot/cold applications seems to be practical. Most individuals show a decreasing secondary reaction to repeated applications of cold.

Due to the increased blood flow within an area, the revulsive effect is ideal for treating situations presenting primarily as congestion. An example of this effect is the use of alternating hot/cold compresses over the face for sinus congestion. As a powerful decongestant, the revulsive effect also acts as an analgesic for pain resulting from congestion. Because of its marked stimulation of local circulation, the revulsive treatment is an exceptionally effective hydrotherapeutic procedure.

Derivative effect

The derivative effect may be considered the opposite of the revulsive effect. Its primary intent is to alter the volume of blood in an organ or area of the body. This effect is best obtained by the prolonged use of either cold or heat depending on whether one wants to draw blood into an area (hot application) or to drive blood out of an area (cold application). An example of the derivative effect would be the prolonged application of heat to the feet, as with a hot foot bath, in order to decrease congestion in the head. This form of treatment may be quite successful for certain forms of congestive headaches. In general, the greater the area of the body exposed to the application, the more extreme the temperature, and the longer the application, the greater will be the effect.

Spinal reflex effect

The spinal reflex effect provides a means of affecting a distant area of the body through a local application. A sufficiently intense local application of hot or cold not only affects the immediate skin area, but also causes remote physiological changes, mediated through spinal reflex arcs. These effects have been carefully observed over many years, and have led to a mapping which correlates each surface area with its corresponding internal area and/or organ. Most texts on hydrotherapy contain such a diagram (see Kellogg,[2] pp. 721–722).

Some examples of studies dealing with specific reflex effects follow. Hewlett,[12] Stewart[13] and Briscoe[14] all noted changes in blood flow in the opposite arm and hand when one arm and hand were placed in hot or cold water. Ruhmann[15] observed that when cold was applied to the epigastrium, there was a decrease in tone of the stomach, with a quieting of the pylorus. Heat at 50°C applied to the epigastrium produced increased tone in a relaxed stomach and decreased tone in a contracted stomach. Poulton[16] demonstrated that esophageal function could be influenced by irritation of the skin over the sternum. Bing & Tobiassen[17] were able to show reflex relationships between the skin of the abdominal wall and the colon. Bing & Tobiassen also demonstrated a reflex relationship between the lungs and the skin of the chest wall. Kuntz[18] stated that:

> In view of the facility with which cutaneous stimulation elicits reflex visceral reactions, particularly vasomotor changes and changes in the tonic state of the visceral musculature, it must be apparent that many visceral disorders, particularly disorders of the gastrointestinal canal, may be influenced beneficially by appropriate stimulation of the corresponding cutaneous area.

Fisher & Solomon[19] stated: "externally applied heat not only decreased intestinal blood flow, but also diminishes intestinal motility and decreases acid secretion in the stomach, while cold has the opposite effect". This is an example of a contrary effect in which the reflex effect is not the same as that observed in the local reflex

Table 42.4 Reflex effects of prolonged heat

Application location	Effect
One extremity	Vasodilation in contralateral extremity
Abdominal wall	Decreased intestinal blood flow, intestinal motility and acid secretion
Pelvis	Relaxes pelvic muscles, dilates blood vessels, increases menstrual flow
Precordium	Increases heart rate, decreases its force and lowers blood pressure
Chest	Promotes ease of respiration and expectoration
Trunk	Relaxes ureters or bile ducts, relieves renal or gall bladder colic
Over kidney	Increases production of urine

Table 42.5 Reflex effects of prolonged cold

Application location	Effect
Trunk of an artery	Contraction of the artery and its branches
Nose, back of neck and hands	Contraction of the blood vessels of the nasal mucosa
Precordium (ice bag)	Slows the heart rate and increases its stroke volume
Abdomen	Increases intestinal blood flow, intestinal motility and acid secretion
Pelvic area	Stimulates muscles of the pelvic organs
Thyroid gland	Contracts its blood vessels and decreases its function
Hands and scalp	Contraction of brain blood vessels
Acutely inflamed joints or bursae	Vasoconstriction and relief of pain

Table 42.6 Reflex effects of short cold

Application location	Effect
Local application of intense cold as brief as 30 seconds	General peripheral vasoconstriction
Face, hands and head	Increase in mental alertness and activity
Precordial area	Increase in heart rate and stroke volume
Chest, with friction or percussion	Initial increase in respiratory rate, then slower, deeper respiration

skin area, i.e. local heat decreases, rather than increases, intestinal blood flow as one might expect. Prolonged cold has the opposite effect.

Tables 42.4–42.6 show some of the observed reflex effects of hydrotherapeutic procedures.[11]

Collateral circulation effect

The collateral circulation effect may be considered as a special case of the derivative effect.[2] In general use, the derivative effect involves blood volume changes from one area of the body to another, as previously discussed. The collateral circulation effect, on the other hand, more specifically considers the local circulatory effects on deep (rather than superficial) collateral branches of the same artery.

If we consider the circulatory patterns of a large body part, such as the thigh, we see that both superficial and deep areas are supplied by the same artery. A hot application to this area will dilate the surface vessels, drawing blood to the superficial areas and concurrently decreasing the blood flow to the deep areas. A cold application will cause the opposite effect. Local compresses and fomentations are the most commonly used techniques to affect collateral circulatory changes.

Arterial trunk reflex

The arterial trunk reflex effect is a special case of general reflex effects.[2] It has been observed that prolonged cold applied over the trunk of an artery produces contraction of the artery and its branches distal to the application. Prolonged hot applications have the opposite effect of producing dilatation in the distal arterial bed.

An example of this effect would be the application of prolonged cold to the area of the femoral artery in the groin in order to decrease blood flow in a foot or ankle that had sustained an acute injury which resulted in either internal or external hemorrhage. Following the acute phase, prolonged hot applications might be used in like manner in order to increase circulation and speed healing of the injured part.

GENERAL RULES OF HYDROTHERAPY

1. The first rule of hydrotherapy is the same as for any therapy: treat the whole person. This involves considering all aspects, including medical history, current condition, current medications and any other relevant information.

2. Use hydrotherapy treatments in a coordinated and integrated manner with any treatments or medications the individual is receiving.

3. Always measure the person's temperature before beginning a treatment. If their temperature is below normal, apply more heat or leave the hot applications on for a longer time. If body temperature is above normal, use less heat and more intense cold during the treatment.

4. Explain the treatment procedure before beginning, including the technique to be used, the duration, frequency, and any other relevant factors. Try to ensure that the patient feels comfortable with the procedure before beginning.

5. In order to provide as precise a treatment as possible, grade the patient in terms of age, severity of problems, vitality, emotional state, circulatory condition, etc. Be especially careful with young or elderly persons, individuals who are chilly, have cardiac problems, are

weak or debilitated, are obese, or have other severe physical compromises.

For individuals with insulin-dependent diabetes, the application of heat to the extremities is never indicated. Diabetics frequently have arterial disease, which may reduce blood flow to an extremity. The application of heat increases the metabolism of the tissues. Due to impaired circulation, the metabolic needs can very quickly overuse the nutrients and oxygen available from the blood, and cells may die from oxygen depletion simply as the result of hot applications.[20] Therefore, hot foot baths are contraindicated in diabetics.

For diabetics with conditions in which a hot application to the feet would normally be the treatment of choice, you may use instead a large hot compress to the lower abdomen, groin, and thighs in order to get a reflex reaction in the lower extremities.

Diabetics may also display peripheral neuropathies which decrease their ability to sense heat, thereby increasing the possibility of causing a burn with hot applications. Other individuals with neurological injury or disease should also be treated with extreme caution during hot applications.

6. The environment in which the treatments are given should enhance and stimulate the healing forces as much as possible. This may include such considerations as color of the room, light intensity, music, plants, etc.

7. If a patient becomes chilled during a treatment, it may be necessary to stop the treatment and warm the person. Sometimes it may suffice to warm the person (by such means as hot drinks, friction rubs, additional blankets, or a hot water bottle to the feet) while continuing the treatment. If the person fails to warm following these attempts, then stop the treatments and warm them. Never allow a patient to become chilled to the point of shivering.

8. Following a hydrotherapy treatment, avoid excessive heat in the form of overly warm clothing, overly warm rooms, sun exposure, or exercise. Excessive heat may slow or prevent the body reaction to the treatment and negate the benefit of the treatment.

9. It is best to do the treatment at an optimal time of day for that patient. It is best to do treatments before meals, or at least 1 hour after a meal. From Chinese medicine, we learn the relationships between disease and time of day. For those who have this knowledge, it is well to use it when deciding at what time to do hydrotherapy treatments.

As with any therapy, it is important to practice hydrotherapy with a research orientation, noting unusual reactions and physiological effects. Many physiological parameters, such as urine chemistries and microscopic components, specific gravity, body temperature, and blood sugar levels, may be easily monitored and recorded during treatment. This information helps to optimize the treatment protocols, stimulates further research, and validates hydrotherapy as an effective and useful therapeutic modality.

POSSIBLE SIDE-EFFECTS OF HYDROTHERAPY

Although hydrotherapeutic procedures are generally mild, they may in some situations produce unexpected or undesired effects. These effects may be the result of improperly applied treatments, but they may, in some cases, result simply from the individual's reaction to the treatment. They may, in the long term, be beneficial. Any time an individual experiences an undesired effect following a treatment, the therapist should review the treatment's length, intensity, and appropriateness for the individual at this time. If more treatments are considered, they may need to be modified in order to lessen the undesired effects.

Some of the possible side-effects of hydrotherapy treatments are:

- headache (resulting from too long or intense a treatment, or from the release of toxic products in the body)
- vertigo
- nervousness
- aches and pains
- insomnia
- nausea
- palpatations
- faintness
- chilliness.

Following an unpleasant reaction to a hydrotherapy treatment, discontinue the treatment and wait at least 2–3 hours before attempting another treatment. Calming teas, such as catnip or chamomile, may be helpful. In cases of chilliness, always act quickly to warm the person. Coaching the person in deep, slow breathing exercises for several minutes often relaxes the person and decreases the reaction.[20] If you are providing the treatment in your office, reassure yourself that the patient has fully regained his/her balance before allowing him/her to leave.

Although these effects may occur during, or immediately following, treatments, they may also occur as long as 24 hours later. Therefore, it is important for practitioners to be available to patients during off-duty hours.

HYDROTHERAPY TECHNIQUES

The variety of ways in which water may be applied to the human body therapeutically is only limited by the imagination of the practitioner. J. H. Kellogg, in his seemingly exhaustive treatise on hydrotherapy, devotes 541 pages to describing the techniques of hydrotherapy. There are also several other books available which describe in detail specific procedures and techniques.[11,20–25] Those desiring to use these techniques in practice are encouraged to obtain one or several of these reference works.

To successfully use hydrotherapy, one must be familiar enough with the procedure to use it in an efficient and competent manner. Although the equipment required for these techniques is quite simple, it is important that it be clean, easily available, and maintained properly. Care for the comfort and confidence of the patient will greatly increase the effectiveness of the treatments.

Compresses

There are three basic types of compresses: hot, cold, and alternating hot and cold. They are each applied using cloth, or other compress material, which is wrung out to the desired amount of moisture, and then applied to any surface of the body.

A single compress consists only of layers of the wet material, whereas a double compress is one in which the wet cloth is completely covered by dry material, usually wool, which acts to prevent cooling by evaporation or heat loss. This allows the body, in the case of a cold double compress, to warm the area, thereby producing a secondary reaction to the cold.

Compresses are commonly referred to by the area of the body they are applied to, such as the throat, head, joint, trunk, or limb.

Cold compress

A cold compress consists of a cloth wrung from cold or ice water and then applied to the body. The water may contain solutes such as NaCl, baking soda, Epsom salts, boric acid, or cider vinegar. Herbs may also be used to create a more specific effect from the compress. Some commonly used herbs are hayflower, oatstraw, and fenugreek, made as teas into which the compress cloths are dipped.

The *cold single compress* has primarily a vasoconstrictive effect, both locally and distally. Due to this effect, it may be used to prevent or relieve congestion, reduce blood flow to an area, prevent edema following injury, inhibit inflammation, and relieve pain due to congestion. It may also be used to reduce body temperature when applied over a large area of the body.

These compresses are renewed frequently (every 1–5 minutes) in order to maintain the primary cold effect. The temperature of a cold compress will depend on the specific problem being treated, as well as the state of health of the patient. In general, the colder the application, the briefer the period of application.

Cold compresses should not be used locally in a person who is chilly or who has pleurisy, sinusitis, or acute asthma, as these conditions may be seriously aggravated.

The *cold double compress*, also known as the heating compress, consists of a cold compress covered completely by several layers of dry material such as flannel or wool. It is allowed to remain on until warmed by the body. The layers of dry material prevent heat loss by evaporation, thereby permitting accumulation of heat and creating a general heating effect. Cold double compresses are used most commonly in upper respiratory infections, such as sore throats, bronchitis, influenza, pneumonia, and swollen lymph glands in the neck. They may also be applied over the trunk or abdomen, genital area, joints, limbs or feet.

The primary effect of cold double compresses is to increase the local circulation, thereby providing for increased nutrition and oxygenation of the tissues, and increased elimination of metabolic waste from the area. As with cold single compresses, the temperature of the initial application depends on the state of the patient and the condition being treated. In general, the colder the application, the stronger will be the secondary reaction to the cold. As weak and debilitated patients are unable to generate a strong secondary reaction, cool rather than cold application may be indicated. The same general precautions as for a cold single compress should be followed.

Hot compress

The hot compress is a prolonged application of moist heat, generally to a local area of the body. The fomentation is a special case of a hot compress, which provides prolonged exposure at a higher temperature.

Hot compresses and fomentations have several therapeutic effects. In many situations they may create an analgesic effect, thereby decreasing pain. They are generally more effective locally for pain resulting from spasm than for pain due to congestion. They also create a derivative effect, which may be used to increase blood flow to the periphery, thereby decreasing internal congestion. By applying short, intensely hot compresses, a stimulation effect may be obtained. This may be used to increase blood flow to a part, to stimulate certain organ functions, to decrease others, and to produce tissue warming and relaxation. Mildly hot compresses may be beneficial for their sedative effects in treating insomnia, nervous tension, and mild muscular spasms.

Fairly hot compresses may be applied directly to the skin surface, with care taken to not burn or startle the patient. As stated previously, hot applications are contraindicated on the extremities of diabetic individuals.

When treating the elderly, or those with impaired neurological function, edema, or decreased circulation, special caution must also be taken. Fomentations are commonly applied at temperatures which are not tolerated directly on the skin, and therefore must be applied over a bath towel placed on the area.

Baths

Baths are full or partial immersions of the body into water of various temperatures. Bath waters may contain additional substances such as salts, minerals, herbs, or medications and may be in an agitated state, as with a whirlpool.

Hot full immersion baths

These are given within a temperature range of 100–106°F for up to 20 minutes. They are indicated as home treatment for rheumatoid arthritis, to aid in relief of muscular spasms, for cleansing the body, and to induce sweating. Given for brief periods, they may help to reduce fevers by creating peripheral vasodilation, thereby promoting an increased heat loss.

In most instances they are best followed by a brief cool bath, shower, or spray. Prolonged hot tub baths are never appropriate in the very old or very young, weak or anemic persons, individuals with severe organic disease, or in anyone with a tendency to hemorrhage.

Neutral bath

The neutral bath is a full immersion bath given at the average temperature of the skin, 92–95°F, in which the recipient has neither the sensation of being warmed nor that of being cooled. A minor variation in temperature of as little as 2°F may create a totally different therapeutic effect. As the ideal temperature is dependent on the patient's condition and reaction to the water, it is often better to use their sensation, rather than a thermometer, as a guide to adjusting the temperature. The duration of a neutral bath may vary from 15 minutes to 4 hours. If the bath lasts longer than 20 minutes, it will be necessary to add warm water to maintain the temperature.

The primary effect of a neutral bath is to create a state of decreased excitation. This sedative effect, similar to that produced in deprivation tanks, calms the nervous system.

A second effect is activation of the kidneys, creating increased urinary output due to the absorption of water into the body during periods of prolonged immersion.[26] It is aided by the neutral temperature, which provides no stimulus for water loss through sweating. Nephrotic patients display increased phosphate excretion following prolonged immersion; therefore, they warrant special care when given prolonged immersion baths.[27]

Lastly, the neutral bath causes a decrease in the surface temperature of the body due to the lack of the normal heat-producing stimulus of cool air on the skin. As a result, the surface may be cooled as much as 6°F, creating a tendency to chilling following the bath. This effect necessitates special care in keeping the patient warm. When prescribed for home treatment, a neutral bath is best taken just before getting into bed, in order to avoid chilling.

Therapeutically, neutral baths are most commonly used for their calmative effects in cases of insomnia, anxiety, nervous irritability, exhaustion, or chronic pain. By increasing kidney output, they may be appropriate in detoxification programs for substances such as alcohol, tobacco, or coffee, or as an adjunct treatment for peripheral edema. They also serve a valuable role in the control of fevers in individuals who would not be able to react to stronger measures, such as the Brand bath. These patients would include the very young, very old, feeble, or exhausted.

Start the baths at about 98°F and lower the temperature slowly over a period of 5–10 minutes to 92–93°F, until the desired body temperature is reached.[21]

Sitz bath

The sitz bath is a partial immersion bath of the pelvic region. It is more easily given in a specially constructed tub but may also be effectively done in a regular bath tub. Often it is taken with the feet immersed in a separate tub of hot water before or during the bath. A sitz bath may be taken hot, neutral, cold, or contrast hot and cold.

The *hot sitz bath* is generally taken for 3–10 minutes at 105–115°F. The primary effect is analgesic. It may be helpful in cramps of the uterus or ureters, pain from hemorrhoids, ovaries or testicles, sciatica, urinary retention, and after cystoscopy or hemorrhoidectomy. It is followed by cool sponging or effusion of the area. Hot sitz baths are not indicated in cases of acute inflammation, but may be appropriate for chronic PID. Hot applications to the pelvis are also contraindicated during menses in most instances. The hot sitz bath is best taken with a hot foot bath at 110–115°F.

Neutral sitz baths are more appropriate for situations of acute inflammation, such as cystitis and acute PID. They are given at 92–95°F for between 15 minutes and 2 hours. It is necessary to provide adequate coverings during this period to avoid chilling. Neutral sitz baths may also be very effective for pruritis of the anus or vulva. Appropriate herbs, salts or other medications may be added to the water to optimize the treatment.

The *cold sitz bath* is given immediately following a warm-to-hot sitz bath of 1–3 minutes, and lasts (at a temperature of 55–75°F) from 30 seconds to 8 minutes. It is important to ensure that the water level of the hot bath on the body is at least 1 inch above the level of the cold water. This insures adequate warming of the area, thereby preventing chilling. Friction rubs to the hips during the cold sitz bath promote an increased reaction.

The cold sitz bath is used mainly for its tonifying effects. It may be used for subinvolution of the uterus, metrorrhagia, atonic constipation, enuresis, atony of the bladder, and chronic prostatic congestion. Since it increases the tone of the smooth muscles of the uterus, bladder, and colon, it lessens the tendency to bleed from the uterus, the lower bowel and rectum.

Contrast sitz baths are given in groups of three, i.e. three alterations of hot to cold. Two separate tubs are necessary to facilitate this process. The hot is at 105–115°F, the cold at 55–85°F, with the temperatures again dependent on the condition being treated and the strength of the patient. A standard treatment would be 3 minutes hot and 30 seconds cold. The water level in the hot tub is set 1 inch higher than in the cold. Adequate draping is necessary to prevent chilling. As with all hydrotherapy treatments, one always finishes with the cold.

The contrast sitz bath increases pelvic circulation and tone of the smooth muscles of the region. It is indicated in chronic PID, chronic prostatitis, atonic constipation, and other atonic conditions of the pelvis. The strong revulsive effect created increases the blood flow in the pelvic region dramatically.

Cold friction rubs and ablutions

Cold friction rubs, or ablutions, consist of frictioning the body in a predetermined sequence with cold water. They differ from spongings in that they are more tonifying and are done more vigorously with rougher materials. A woolen bath mitt works well, but if this is not available, a coarse washcloth or loofa may also be used.

A *whole body ablution* is carried out with the patient lying supine, covered completely and not chilly. Using cool to cold water the therapist dips the mitt into the water and vigorously frictions a portion of the body. Depending on the cooling effect desired, the mitt may either be saturated or wrung dry prior to the frictioning. The body part is frictioned until reddening occurs. If the patient is weak, it is best to dry the areas as you proceed using a coarse dry towel. If the patient is strong and vigorous, one can wait and dry them at the end of the treatment.

One sequence for an ablution treatment would be, with the patient supine, to proceed from the chest to the arms, and then the legs, then, turning the patient over, to do the back of the legs and feet, the buttocks, and finally the back. Only that part being frictioned is exposed at any time.

The primary effect of a cold ablution is tonic. Therefore, it may be used for any condition in which you desire a tonifying treatment, such as fatigue following illness or surgery or after hot applications, such as saunas, whirlpools, or hot baths. It is an excellent prophylactic hydrotherapy technique when used regularly along with saunas, hot tubs, and massage.

Wet sheet pack

The wet sheet pack is one of the most useful of all hydrotherapy procedures. It may be done either in the office or as a home treatment, if adequate direction is provided. It requires from 1–3 hours, depending on the condition of the patient. The technique is common to most schools of hydrotherapy. It is important to understand the process completely before using this treatment:

1. Using either a bed or treatment table, place two wool blankets lengthwise on the table with a small pillow at the head. The blankets must be large enough to cover the person being treated. If wool is not available, acrylic is the next best choice.
2. The patient must be warm before the pack is applied. If not, they may be warmed by a hot bath or shower, dry blanket pack, diathermy over the back, or any other appropriate technique.
3. Once the patient is ready, a clean white cotton sheet (equal in length to the height of the patient) is wrung as dry as possible after being soaked in cold water. It is much easier if two people are available to wring out the sheet. The sheet is opened and placed lengthwise along the table with equal amounts draped over each side of the table. The sheet should be 1–2 inches below the height of the blankets.
4. The patient now removes all clothing and lies on the wet sheet with shoulders 4 inches below the top of the sheet. Both arms are raised while the attendants quickly wrap one side of the sheet around the body, tucking it in on the opposite side, and carefully molding it to the body. Below the hips, the sheet is wrapped around the leg on the same side.
5. The arms are now lowered and the opposite side of the sheet is drawn over the body, covering both arms. It also wraps the opposite leg. The wet sheet is quickly smoothed over the body to ensure complete contact and is tucked in around the feet. As this is a shocking experience, it should be performed quickly and efficiently.
6. At this point, the blankets are quickly pulled over the body and tucked in firmly, ensuring there are no drafts around the neck or the feet. Additional blanket(s) may be laid over the patient and tucked in as appropriate. A stocking cap may be pulled over the head to increase the heating effect.

While the patient is in the pack, it is necessary to have someone nearby at all times. Sudden attacks of claustrophobia in some individuals can create extreme anxiety. Should this occur, first remove the sheet from the feet, as this may allow enough movement to allay the attack. If this is unsuccessful, it may be necessary to stop the treatment.

Providing hot teas is very helpful throughout the treatment. If the patient complains of chilliness, add blankets, place a hot water bottle to the feet, or provide warm drinks.

The wet sheet pack proceeds through four stages: tonic or cooling, neutral, heating, and eliminative. Depending on the desired effect, the therapist may wish to prolong any one specific stage:

- *Tonic stage.* This stage may last from 2 to 15 minutes and is finished when the patient no longer perceives the sheet as being cold. This phase is intensely alterative to the body, due to the intense thermic reaction induced.

The length of this stage is directly dependent on the amount of water left in the sheet. For weak or exhausted patients, the sheet should be wrung out as completely as possible. For young, strong individuals for whom a more tonifying treatment is desired, more water may be left in the sheet.

- *Neutral stage.* Once the sheet reaches body temperature, the person no longer feels cold. At this time, the neutral phase begins. It may last from 15 minutes to an hour or longer, depending on the vitality of the patient. During this phase, there is a sense of calm which is similar to that experienced during a neutral bath. Very often the patient will fall asleep during this phase. This stage is indicated in cases of insomnia, anxiety, and delirium. In order to prolong the neutral phase, provide only adequate covering to prevent the patient feeling cool. Greater amounts of blankets will trap more heat and the neutral phase will finish sooner.

- *Heating stage.* As heat accumulates beneath the blankets, the patient will gradually sense the warming, and eventually begin to show light perspiration on the forehead. The time between the patient feeling warm and the beginning of perspiration is known as the heating phase. This may last from 15 minutes to 1 hour.

- *Elimination stage.* The final stage begins when the body begins to perspire. In a febrile patient this stage will be reached sooner. This stage is especially beneficial for those patients in a detoxification process such as from alcohol, tobacco, coffee, or other toxins. It my also be used with acute infections, such as colds, flu or bronchitis. Certain skin conditions, such as jaundice, may also benefit from this stage, as well as acute inflammatory conditions, such as arthritis.

During the elimination phase, it is important to provide adequate fluid to the patient. Herb teas, used for either their diaphoretic or therapeutic effects, are most appropriate.

This phase may last up to 1 hour. The treatment should be ended quickly if the patient begins to feel chilled or becomes uncomfortable.

The treatment is ended by quickly removing the patient from the pack, frictioning the skin briskly with a dry towel, and having the patient dress. As this is often an intensive treatment, it should be followed with rest or appropriate activity. Lying in a warm room for an hour is an ideal follow-up to this treatment. If done at home, it is best done in the evening just prior to retiring.

CONCLUSION

Hydrotherapy provides the naturopathic physician with an effective form of treatment for many conditions. In this chapter we have touched on only a few of the many techniques which have been developed over the years. References 2, 11, 20 and 21 provide those who are interested in further study in this area with appropriate information.

REFERENCES

1. Hippocratic Writings in The Great Books. Chicago, Il: William Benton. 1952
2. Kellogg JH. Rational hydrotherapy. 4th edn. Battle Creek, Mn: Modern Medical. 1923
3. Franchimont P, Juchmes J, Lecomte J. Hydrotherapy – mechanisms and indications. Pharmocol Ther 1983; 20: 79
4. Edelson RL, Fink JM. The immunologic function of skin. Sci Am 1985; 252: 46
5. Siems WG, van Kuijk FJ, Maass R et al. Uric acid and glutathione levels during short-term whole body cold exposure. Free Radical Biol Med 1994; 16: 299–305
6. Kuhn G, Buhring M. Physical medicine and quality of life: design and results of a study on hydrotherapy. Comp Ther Med 1995; 3: 138–141
7. Golland A. Basic hydrotherapy. Physiotherapy 1981; 67: 258
8. Engel JP, Watkin G, Erickson DJ, Krussen FH. The effect of contrast baths on the peripheral circulation of patients with R.A. Arch Phys Med 1950; 31: 135
9. Woodmansey A, Collins DH, Ernst MM. Vascular reactions to the contrast bath in health and in rheumatoid arthritis. Lancet 1938; ii: 1350
10. Krussen FH. Physical medicine. Philadelphia: WB Sanders. 1941
11. Moor FB, Peterson S, Manwell E et al. Manual of hydrotherapy and massage. Mountain View, Ca: Pacific Press. 1964: p 964
12. Hewlett AW. The effect of some hydrotherapeutic procedures on the blood flow in the arm. Arch Int Med 1911; 8: 591
13. Stewart GN. The effect of reflex vasomotor excitation on the blood flow in the hand. Heart 1912; 3: 76
14. Briscoe G. Observations on venous and capillary pressures with special reference to the Raynaud Phenomena. Heart 1918; 7: 35
15. Ruhmann W. Reflex irritability of abdominal organs by local application of heat and cold. Munchen Med Wchnschr 1926; 73: 401
16. Poulton EP. An experimental study of certain visceral sensations. Lancet 1928; ii: 1223, 1277

17. Bing HJ, Tobiassen ES. Viscerocutaneous and cutovisceral abdominal reflexes. Acta Med Scand Supp 1936; 78: 824
18. Kuntz A. Autonomic nervous system. Philadelphia: Lea & Febiger. 1945
19. Fisher E, Soloman S. Physiological responses to heat and cold. In: Therapeutic heat and cold. 2nd edn. New Haven, CT: Elizabeth Licht. 1965
20. Thrash AM, Thrash CL. Home remedies. Seale, Al: Thrash. 1981
21. Buchman D. The complete book of water therapy. New York, NY: EP Dutton. 1979
22. Ring J and Teichmann W: Immunologische Veranderungen bei hydrotherpeutischer Kurbehandlung. Deutsche Med Wschr 45: 1625, 1977
23. Bierman W, Licht S. Physical medicine in general practice. New York: Hoeber. 1957
24. Finnerty GB, Corbitt T. Hydrotherapy. New York: Frederick Ungar. 1960
25. Burn Jones W: Mineral springs and medicine in North Carolina, North Carolina Med J 44: 593, 1983
26. Epstein M, Saruta T. Effect of water immersion on renin, aldosterone, and renal sodium handling in normal man. J Appl Physiol 1971; 31: 363
27. Brown C. Renal calcium and magnesium handling in water immersion in nephrotic patients. Nephron 1983; 33: 17

CHAPTER CONTENTS

43

Manipulation

Robert M. Martinez, DC ND

THERAPEUTIC KEYS

- Manipulation is a passive manual maneuver that is performed in such a way that the patient is unable to prevent it and that introduces movement beyond the passive range of motion's elastic barrier but does not exceed the anatomical barrier.[1] Mobilizations are passive stretches with or without oscillations over which the patient can exert control.[2] Spinal adjustments are chiropractic techniques that range in force from a near imperceptible force to high-velocity thrust with joint cavitation (popping noise).
- Initial evaluation of patients for "red flags" of fracture, infection, neoplasm, progressive neurologic deficit, cord pressure or cauda equina syndrome is the prudent starting point.[3,4]
- A correct differential diagnosis is key to the selection of patients, and the functional assessment is key to the selection of appropriate manual medicine techniques.[5]
- If gross signs of inflammation are present in a joint (heat, swelling, redness, and pain), manipulation of that joint most likely will aggravate the condition.
- When a motion causes pain, forcing the motion can result in injury.
- If applying heat for 10 minutes, followed by active and passive motion of the joint, improves the condition, manipulation will usually help. When this causes aggravation, manipulation will usually make the condition worse.
- Relaxation techniques (heat, muscle work, calming environment) prior to a manipulation are very helpful in achieving best results. They are especially indicated in patients complaining of aching and stiffness prior to manipulation.[6]
- If pain is the chief complaint, icing the area for 5 minutes will cause surface anesthesia, and 20 minutes will cause sedation of the actions of the muscle spindle cells. Sedation of a muscle reflex arc prior to manipulation of a fixated painful joint will facilitate the treatment.[2]

• If the patient reports an increase in pain or stiffness after a manipulation, ice the area of treatment for 10–30 minutes after manipulation to reduce spasm and pain.[7,8]

• "The goal of manipulation is to restore maximal pain-free movement of the musculoskeletal system in postural balance."[9]

• Don't treat muscle spasm as a primary condition. Muscle spasm is almost always a response of the body to a noxious stimulus. Find the cause and treat it.[10]

• Trigger points (TPs) are myofascial irritations which are frequently caused by underlying joint fixations. If one manipulates over a TP, it will frequently precipitate a muscle spasm later that day or the next morning.[11]

HISTORICAL PERSPECTIVE

The popularity of manipulation could be likened to the course of a roller coaster – diving up and down and taking many unexpected turns. The literature is replete with references to the use of manipulation. Manipulations are depicted in prehistoric cave drawings and Chinese statues, circa 2700 BC.[12] The early history of manipulation has been researched by Lomax and presented in two papers. She credits Hippocrates with the earliest recorded written physician's prescription of manipulative treatment methods. Worthington notes that Hippocrates in *On Joints* clearly states method and motive for the application of manipulative therapy.[13] Hippocrates advocated many of the premises in use today: judicious use of force, direction of thrust, and proper levering of the joints. Even at this early date, mention is made of the abuse of manipulative therapy.[13]

Until the sixth century, manipulative treatment saw little change. At that time, treatment with open wounds was used by Arab physicians, based on the humoral theory of disease.[13] During the Dark Ages, priests provided medical treatment at their monasteries. Kessler states: "Friar Moultan, of the order of St. Augustine, wrote The Complete Bonesetter. The text, which was revised by John Turner in 1656, suggests that manipulation was practiced in medical settings throughout the Middle Ages and Renaissance."[14]

The course of the history of manipulation in the late 1700s and afterward is colorful and flamboyant. Three main concepts developed during this time still have a major influence on our thoughts regarding manipulation. The first held that vertebral luxation was responsible for spinal deformity. The second was held by the largest group which followed the writings of Percival Pott and maintained that caries of the spine were more common than previously thought. This idea caught hold and was taken to an extreme. This faction of physicians treated spinal deformity by blood-letting and rest, while condemning extension and manipulation as both useless and dangerous. A third group held that muscles were the main cause of problems, and treatment should be complete rest or active exercise, as the case warranted.[13]

Central to the early issues, aside from the political and economic waves the irregulars were creating for the allopaths, were concerns about the potentially disastrous effects of manipulating tuberculous, neoplastic, rheumatic, or fractured joints. More recently, questions of vertebral disc herniation, precipitation of CVAs (cerebral vascular accidents), and the lack of a differential diagnosis by many non-allopathic manipulators has caused concern. To this, add the controversial issues of cost-effectiveness and efficacy of treatment, and one can begin to understand the apprehension with which allopathic practitioners approach manipulative therapy.

It is interesting to note that:

• Hippocrates railed against the abuse of manipulative therapy by physicians and others of his time.

• Physicians of the late 1700s assailed one another's methods of treatment (an example can be found in *The Lancet* December 16, 1826, p. 347, the page banner appropriately reading "THE YELLOW JOURNAL").

• Surgeons held "bonesetters" in great contempt "when they condescend[ed] to speak at all of bonesetters and their works".[12]

• Bonesetters held their secrets and passed them from father to son.

• Financial competition was noted early in the literature. "It is known to most practitioners of surgery, and has been made known to many to their great cost and loss, that a large portion of the cases of impaired mobility or usefulness of limbs after injury fall into the hands of a class of men called 'bonesetters'."[15]

• Although there is a great deal of animosity, and claims of superiority are made by the various practitioners of manipulative treatment even today, "specific conclusions cannot be derived from the scientific literature for or against either the efficacy of spinal manipulative therapy or the pathophysiologic foundations from which it is derived".[16]

There appears to be nothing new in the controversies except the names of the groups and the coined terms they use.

The allopathic group claims the right to control over all the healing arts, and the sole privilege of using the generic terms "physician", "medicine", and "medical treatment".[17] The "unorthodox" groups buck this authority. They seek a physician's position, while not always being willing to accept the accompanying responsibility of adequate differential diagnosis and critical assessment and validation (other than empirical and anecdotal reporting) of their therapeutic regimens. Each group maneuvers politically, judicially, and economically to gain advantage over the other.[18]

SCHOOLS OF THOUGHT IN MANIPULATION

Early history (Oriental, Egyptian, Greek, Indian)

Knowledge of exactly which techniques were used, and with what success, is limited or speculative. It is known that many cultures have used manipulative techniques.[12]

Bone setters of England

They generally held that a bone was out of place and had a "feel" for what was wrong. Hutton described the information gained from a bonesetter as "bring[ing] some spoils out of the camp of the Philistines".[15]

Chiropractic

D. D. Palmer, "the founder", and his son B. J. Palmer, "the developer", of chiropractic added one of the most colorful pages to the history of manipulative treatment. D. D., who "rediscovered" the principle of "lost nerve tone" in a revelation from a deceased friend, Dr Atkinson, re-established this method of healing.

The first chiropractic manipulation was given to a deaf janitor. D.D. learned that the janitor's hearing had been lost when he stooped over and felt something give in his back. D.D. reasoned that if the deafness occurred from something slipping out, restoring the vertebra to its correct position should cure the condition: "With this new objective in view, a half-hour's talk persuaded Mr. Lillard to allow me to replace it."[19]

The stormy history of chiropractic was led by a son who hated his father (and was actually accused of running him down in a parade, causing injuries that lead to his death), who drove chiropractic to a zenith, and who later nearly destroyed the profession. The evolution of chiropractic is well documented by Gibbons. It is worth noting that many early developments in chiropractic were years ahead of their time. B. J. developed the prototype of today's EEG, he started a radiology laboratory only 13 years after Roentgen discovered X-radiation, and he had one of the finest diagnostic centers in the midwest at his school (complete with MDs and PhDs).[20]

A new focus in chiropractic is rehabilitation and incorporation of manual medicine techniques. *Rehabilitation of the Spine, A Practitioner's Manual*, edited by Craig Liebenson,[4] is considered by many in the field a landmark publication. It emphasizes the need for rehabilitation and puts manipulation as a component of the process.

Naturopathic

All naturopathic techniques result from the blending of the thoughts of the other schools of medicine. This is appropriate when one realizes there is little new in manipulation, only refining and relabelling. It is also appropriate that naturopathy doesn't lay claim to originating a school of thought on manipulation, but uses this method of treatment when indicated, not exclusively, but as part of a therapeutic regime.

Several naturopathic schools in the past were associated with chiropractic and eclectic schools of medicine. The genesis of the naturopathic profession is well documented in Chapter 2.

Osteopathic

Andrew Still, three of whose children died from meningitis, in the tradition of Hanneman left the practice of medicine and started the school of osteopathy in Kirksville, Missouri. It is highly probable that D. D. Palmer went to this school and learned some of the techniques, but it is not well documented. The famed "equal but separate" movement of the osteopaths led to a 1921 resolution, submitted at the AOA convention, that allowed entrance of chiropractors with advanced standing into their schools. Still, before his death, saw the defection of his osteopathic profession into the ranks of medical orthodoxy.[20–22] It is interesting to note that manipulation is now only an elective segment in some American osteopathic schools, while in England it is still the mainstay of osteopathic practice.

The resurgence of interest in manual medicine has been brought to the forefront by the Osteopathic College at Michigan State University. Greenman's[1] *Principles of Manual Medicine* adds a useful text to the field of manual medicine. This school has been teaching manual medicine to physical therapists, MDs and DOs.

Allopathic

In the 20th century, the numbers of allopathic practitioners who promote manipulative treatment are growing daily. The individuals mainly responsible for major contributions are James Cyriax, James Mennell, and John Mennell. These brilliant physicians have written valuable texts on manipulative therapy, although they do not agree totally on the effects they achieve with manipulation. Mennell holds to the correction of lost joint play and denies effect on the intervertebral disc,[23] while Cyriax claims reduction of a protruding disc.[10]

Bourdillion, Calliet, McNabb, Maigne, Maitland, Kaltenborn, and Williams are popularizing the treatment modality. Their works are too exhaustive to mention in this brief chapter.

"Controversy and contention" best describe the higher levels of the respective schools of medical thought. The impression one gets in reading through the literature is intolerance of others' ideas expressed in *ad hominem* attacks. The mistake "lay" manipulators and "non-physicians" make is not ineffectiveness but their willingness to seek training outside the fraternal order of the "medical" brotherhood; to address the public directly rather than communicating exclusively within the order; and, worst of all, to openly compete, economically and politically, against the fraternal order (Star, Lomax, Hood).

Donald B. Tower, in the chairman's summary at the NINCDS conference in 1975, noted a physician who has received little credit for his early contribution to the field: J. Evans Riadore, a London physician who wrote a treatise on "Irritation of the spinal nerves" in 1843. He attributed many diseases to this condition, stating: "If any organ is deficiently supplied with nervous energy of blood, its functions immediately, and sooner or later its structure, become deranged." This was a viewpoint subsequently echoed by osteopaths and chiropractors.[24]

Spinal Manipulation (5th edn) by Bourdillion et al,[25] the first author of which was a medical manipulator, has been largely reworked from previous editions and heavily influenced by osteopathic methods.

Over the past 15 years, American awareness of contributions in manual medicine from other countries has been growing. Jirout, Lewit, Janda, Bogduk and many others have been teaching and publishing in the US.

DIFFERENTIAL DIAGNOSIS

The methodology for performing the differential diagnosis of musculoskeletal pain can follow many diverse patterns depending on the approach taken, but the multiple branching pathway[3,26] for patient selection is a very good start. Four basic categories of pathology are described to begin the sorting process: neoplasm, infection, neurologic, and mechanical disorder. The following presents a brief overview in differentiating between these, and is organized to aid the generalist in selecting a starting point for making the final diagnosis. Refer to the texts and articles noted for detailed information.

Four primary categories of spinal disorders

Neoplasm

The patient history or family history may reveal neoplasm. The character of the pain is often described as deep, boring, and usually worse at night. The pain is progressive – sometimes better, sometimes worse – but is usually always present to some degree. Laboratory tests will possibly reveal an elevated sedimentation rate. Most mechanical conditions will show a 50% improvement in 2–4 weeks with appropriate care or the patient should be carefully re-evaluated or referred for a second opinion.

Infection

There will be signs of acute or chronic illness. Laboratory tests will reveal a shift to the left in the WBC count and possibly an elevated sedimentation rate. There will be local joint inflammation.

Neurologic

A routine office neurologic screening examination will often reveal the presence of a lesion. Specific neurologic tests help to determine if a lesion is present and, if so, its location; whether the lesion is life-threatening; and whether the patient will respond to conservative care.

The search pattern for neurologic lesions breaks the system into the following:

Cerebrum. Lesions are discovered during the consultation by the patient's affected cognition, interaction, mannerisms or loss of orientation in time, space, or body part awareness, etc. Nausea, vomiting, seizure, loss of consciousness, visual disturbances and headache are warning signs.

Cerebellar vs. posterior column lesions. Test coordination of movements, with basic differentiation done by repeating acts with the eyes open and eyes closed.

Cerebellar. Actions are jerky with the eyes open or closed; dysarthria, ataxic (drunken) gait, and dysdiadochokinesia may be present.

Posterior columns. The actions are smooth with the eyes open, but cannot be repeated as well with the eyes closed, due to the loss of proprioception. A broad-based, stomping gait may be present.

Brain stem. This area is evaluated by testing the cranial nerves.

Spinal cord lesions and peripheral nerve lesions (differentiation between upper and lower motor neuron lesions). Think of the abnormal reactions by focusing on the words "spastic" and "flaccid". If the superficial reflexes are absent, continue with tests to rule out upper motor neuron lesions (UMNs) and lower motor neuron lesions (LMNs). Table 43.1 lists the key differential considerations.

Muscle stretch reflexes (MSRs). These are often incorrectly called deep tendon reflexes.[27] Communication of results can be confusing, since various practitioners use different notations, e.g. a grade 3 may be listed 3, +3, 3+, +++ or just 3, and do not have a consistent definition. Table 43.2 lists a grading scale that is commonly used.

The main objective is to compare the reflexes side to

Table 43.1 Comparison of neurological signs of upper vs. lower motor neuron disease[28]

Sign/symptom	UMN (spastic)	LMN (flaccid)
Paralysis	Spastic	Flaccid
Deep tendon reflexes	Clonic	Diminished/absent
Muscle tone	Increased	Decreased
Pathologic reflexes	Present	Absent
Superficial reflexes	Absent	Absent
Fasciculations	Absent	Present
Reaction of degeneration	Absent	Present

Table 43.2 Grading of reflexes

Grade	Reflex
0	Absent with reinforcement
1	Hypoactive – less than the expected response
2	Normal – you may note brisk or sluggish
3	Hyperactive – more than the expected response
4	Hyperactive with transient clonus
5	Hyperactive with sustained clonus
Clonus	More than one muscle jerk when the tendon is tapped

Table 43.3 Grading of muscle strength

Grade	Muscle strength
0 (zero)	No trace of muscle contraction
1 (trace)	Evidence of slight contractility, no joint motion
2 (poor)	Complete range of motion with gravity eliminated
3 (fair)	Complete range of motion against gravity
4 (good)	Complete range of motion against gravity with some resistance
5 (normal)	Complete range of motion against full resistance

side and in comparison to Table 43.2. If the reactions are not equal, note according to the scale.

Pathologic reflexes. Toe sign (Babinski), Hoffman's, glabellar (indicating upper motor neuron lesions). Practice on an infant to elicit these abnormal signs.

Painless loss of strength. This is usually neurologic. Use numbers 0–5 to rate muscle strength, according to the scale shown in Table 43.3.

Loss of sensation. If it follows a dermatome, the problem is usually a nerve root; if it follows a named nerve pattern, a peripheral mixed nerve is involved.

Nerve root tension signs. Patients may be bracing themselves when they present (in an effort to decompress the nerve root) and may complain of pain radiating into an extremity. Movement may cause pains shooting into the extremity. Loss of sensation follows the dermatome distribution, MSRs are diminished or lost, and muscle strength in muscles innervated by the affected nerve is lost or diminished.

If neurologic findings are present, other than minor changes in sensation, keep the patient under close observation. Direct nerve root pressure can cause permanent muscle weakness with resultant permanent impairment. Appropriate conservative care is effective.[29] Progressive neurologic deficit is an indication for referral to a neurosurgeon or physiatrist.

Mechanical

A fracture is usually traumatic when presenting in young and middle-aged patients. In older patients, pathologic fractures are a concern. Presentation may be delayed in motor vehicle accidents or athletic injuries, or non-traumatic fractures in the elderly. The cardinal signs of fracture are:

- pinpoint pain over the site
- deformity of the part
- crepitus
- loss of function of the part, usually proportional to the severity of the injury
- abnormal mobility at the site of pain.

Always check for nerve lesions and soft tissue injuries that would complicate the injury before beginning treatment.

Also check for multiple injuries (ring fracture in two places). In particular, look above and below the site of injury, as the force of trauma may be transmitted and cause a fracture some distance from the site of impact.[26]

Note. Don't be deceived by the absence of obvious signs of fracture.

Orthopedic tests

Orthopedic tests are designed to stress the damaged tissue and reproduce the pain of the primary complaint. The examiner is not looking merely for pain to be reported as a result of the maneuver, but rather pain that is specific for the test *and* reproduces the pain of the primary complaint. Therefore:

- The examiner can make the patient worse by forcing tests or performing them incorrectly.
- Do the least stressful tests first. If the first test causes severe pain, most of the other motions will be painful afterward and confuse your findings.
- The test *by definition* has a positive response, that correlates to a *specific condition*, that must be produced when the test is performed for the test to be positive; e.g. Lindner's test and Soto Hall test are performed in the same way, but the findings to report a positive test are different.
- The test must reproduce the pain of the primary complaint and be positive by the test's definition.
- The tests are centered in allopathic medicine to diagnose pathology, fracture, moderate to severe sprain/strain and dislocation and will often be negative in the ambulatory, chronic patient.

When used without an understanding of the mechanism of action of the stress and the tissues the stress will act on, the plethora of tests and maneuvers available usually serve to confuse the practitioner and aggravate the patient's condition. A detailed text that covers this area in detail, such as Magee[30] or Evans[31], is helpful and should be referred to for additional information.

Lumbar spine

The following summarizes the key mechanisms utilized by orthopedic tests of the spine.

Lumbar spine nerve root entrapment. The patient presents with pain radiating into the gluteal muscle, hip, thigh, or possibly to the foot. Flexion and lateral bending with extension will aggravate the pain and reproduce or exacerbate the radiation of pain.

Disc lesion. The position of the patient, leaning towards the side of the leg pain (posteromedial – 60% require surgery), away from the side of leg pain (posterolateral), or forward (central) gives an indication of the direction of the disc lesion.

Straight leg raising (SLR). When the thigh is flexed on the abdomen in the SLR, the initial 30° of motion is primarily in the ipsilateral hip and sacroiliac joint. The 30–60° range stresses the ipsilateral nerve roots and lumbar spine, while the 60–90° range stresses the contralateral sacroiliac and lumbosacral joints.

In the SLR maneuver with a disc protrusion, the nerve root is being stretched over the bulge and causes pain. This effect can be accentuated by internal rotation and dorsiflexion of the foot. Additionally, the Valsalva maneuver may be added at the same time to increase the intrathecal pressure, thus causing swelling of the meninges by decreasing venous drainage. By putting all the stresses on at the same time, the amount of irritation present in the area can be discovered.

Methods of accentuating the signs and symptoms of space-occupying lesions of the spine

Following the principle of "do no harm", test reflexes and sensation first. Then proceed to active tests such as the Valsalva maneuver to test if there is increased intrathecal pressure. If radiating pain results, it is a sign of a space-occupying lesion. Next do light stretch/distraction tests (SLR and add dorsiflexion of the foot with extension of the great toe) and finally compression tests (Milgram's bilateral leg raising and Lindner's test (forcefully flexing the trunk while the patient is supine): this forces the disc posteriorly (if herniated) and causes increased intra-abdominal pressure, resulting in increased intrathecal pressure (Valsalva effect).

Some additional ideas to finding the area of lesion in the lumbar spine are:

- Support Adams (the belt test) – With the patient standing, have him/her bend forward and note the level of pain. The doctor then secures the patient's pelvis by hugging the anterior superior iliac spines with the arms, pressing the patient's sacrum into the doctor's hip. If the patient's pain is decreased, it indicates the lesion is in the pelvis (probably the sacroiliac joint); if pain increases, it is in the lumbar spine (probably the lumbosacral joint).
- Patrick's FABER – **f**lexion, **ab**duction and **e**xternal **r**otation of the hip are blocked; this causes pain over the inguinal fossa and into the thigh when a hip lesion is present.

This is only an introduction to one common problem that may present with many variations. Careful study of the mechanism of action of the tests used will add confirmation, rather than confusion, to a diagnostic impression.

Cervical spine

The cervical spine presents another diagnostic challenge. Although the mechanism of the tests in the lumbar spine are similar, the area is much more delicate and thus requires more careful application. If there is compression of the nerve root or cervical instability, the patient may present holding the head, lifting it cephalically to decompress the root. If there is traction on the brachial plexus, the patient may support the arm in abduction and flexion. Any such presentation is best handled by a neurosurgeon because even passive ranges of motion assessment may cause permanent injury.

If overt signs of nerve root compression are present, mobilization and manipulation must be performed with skill and caution.

Cervical distraction. If distraction of the head from the shoulders causes aggravation of the patient's complaints at 12 pounds of traction (the average weight of the head), stabilization and relaxation techniques are indicated. If distraction of the head from the shoulders causes relief of the radiating pain at 12 pounds of traction, slowly increase the traction to 25 pounds. If this relieves the complaint of neck pain, it is an indication that mobilization and traction are indicated therapies. If it aggravates the complaint, it is an indication of inflammation or instability and suggests caution in using mobilization or traction.

Cervical compression that causes radiating pain to the arms is a sign that stabilization and relaxation techniques are indicated.

MCRC. If rotation, lateral bending and compression (MCRC) cause radiating arm pain, it is a sign of nerve root compression and you should avoid mobilizing in that direction.

Spurling's maneuver. When combined cervical rotation, lateral bending and extension with overpressure (Spurling's maneuver) aggravates or reproduces the complaint or radiating pain to the midback or arm, it indicates nerve root irritation, and manipulation in that direction places the patient at risk for aggravation of their condition. If the pain is local it is a sign of facet irritation that often responds well to manipulation.

After determining that the lesion is not a "hard" orthopedic or neurologic lesion, differential tissue tension tests are used to determine the involved tissue.

THE DIFFERENTIAL DIAGNOSIS OF SOFT TISSUE INJURIES BY MEANS OF ACTIVE AND PASSIVE MOVEMENTS

This is based on the work of James Cryiax,[10] but recent texts give a much improved presentation of the material.[14,30] The process is to assess strain and sprain injuries, and is most appropriate in the early stages of a complaint, but monitoring the capsular patterns of joints will help to guide the rehabilitation process. This brief overview is only intended to give an introduction to the material.

Active movements

First, active ROMs are performed to determine voluntary ROM and patient status. Measuring active ROMs cannot differentiate whether the loss of function is due to pain, weakness or stiffness / lesion, but are helpful to determine patient tolerance to motion and how guarded they are when moving.

Resisted isometric tests

Next, isometric muscle tests are performed to test the contractile tissue (muscle and tendons) with the joint in neutral to avoid involving the non-contractile tissues. The following results may be noted:

- normal – painless and full strength
- minor tear – pain with full strength
- moderate tear – pain with little strength
- neurologic deficit – no pain and little strength.

Passive movements

When the joint is put through passive motion, it reaches an end-point, which has an "end-feel" that helps to determine the status of the soft tissue around the joint. The end-feel of a joint may be:

- normal – the amount of motion and feel of the tissues are appropriate for age
- abnormal – normal end-feels that are not normal for the joint and ROM that are being tested, e.g. the feeling of bone on bone is the normal end-feel at the elbow when extended, but is abnormal when it occurs at the end range of knee extension.
- pathologic – these end-feels are only present in joints that have undergone pathologic changes.

Normal end-feels

Capsular end-feel. This is a firm, "leathery" feeling, felt, for example, when the normal shoulder is at full external rotation. When felt in conjunction with a capsular pattern of restriction, and in the absence of significant inflammation or effusion, it indicates capsular fibrosis.

Bony end-feel. This feels abrupt as when moving the normal elbow into full extension. When accompanying a restriction of movement, it may suggest hypertrophic bony changes, such as those that occur with degenerative joint disease, or possible malunion of bony segments following healing of a fracture.

Soft tissue approximation end-feel. This is a soft end-feel, as when fully flexing the normal elbow or knee. It may accompany joint restriction in the presence of significant muscular hypertrophy.

Muscular end-feel. This more rubbery feel resembles what is felt at the extremes of straight-leg raising from tension on the hamstrings. It is less abrupt than a capsular end-feel.

Pathologic joint end-feels indicate disease; they are limited and are never normal:

- empty – bursitis, space-occupying lesion, neoplasm
- boggy – joint effusion
- spasm – guarding from inflammation
- internal derangement – loose body / torn meniscus.

The tissue involved is determined by the response to the passive ROMs and by moving the joint into closed pack position.

Muscle or tendon. Active and passive movements are limited and / or painful when the muscle is contracting *and* the muscle is being stretched at the same time.

Ligaments. Both active and passive movements are limited and / or painful in the same direction.

Capsular pattern. Only joints that are controlled by muscles will have a capsular pattern. Pain will be caused on both active and passive motions and the limitation of motion is in a specific proportion that is listed in tables in the texts referenced.

Barrier concepts[1]

Joint motion is described from neutral to an end range that is ultimately limited by the anatomical barrier of the surrounding tissues, which if exceeded causes tissue trauma. The extent of the active range of motion can be increased by passive motion to a point at which all of the tissues around the joint have been brought to tension, called by some the elastic barrier. Beyond the elastic barrier is a very small range of motion referred to as the paraphysiologic space.[32] It is within the paraphysiologic space that joint cavitation, the "popping" sound, occurs. It is important to remember that when joints and soft tissues are dysfunctional, alterations of ranges of motion may occur both within the range of motion and at the end of the range of motion. If one focuses only on working in the paraphysiologic space, one severely limits the effects we can have on dysfunction.

TREATMENT CONCEPTS

In the case of injury, treatment with passive therapies is indicated to control pain and inflammation until the tissues heal. Use of passive therapies in chronic conditions is falling into disfavor due to the issues of cost-effectiveness and managed care protocols. Determine the stage of inflammation by comparing the cardinal signs of inflammation (heat, swelling, pain, redness, and loss of function) with the suspected stage of the acute inflammatory process. In reality, the stages overlap and it is a continuum:[33]

1. vasoconstriction – inconsistent, lasting only 3–5 seconds in minor injuries
2. active congestion – caused by vasodilation and increased vessel permeability
3. passive congestion – the venous return is partially dammed by clotting
4. consolidation – fibrinous coagulation at the site of the injury
5. fibrosis – resulting from the formation of scar tissue.

By knowing time frame and pathophysiology of the affected tissues, one can select an appropriate therapy. Manipulation is contraindicated in the first two phases and may be contraindicated in the third. Direct treatment of the tissues according to the level of inflammation. Observe the post-treatment results to see if the signs of inflammation worsen, indicating incorrect application or inappropriate therapy.

During treatment, the patient should be in a position that relieves symptoms. If the patient can't get into such a position, it is probable that the severity of the lesion is such that it won't respond to conservative therapy alone, *or* that the patient's condition is misdiagnosed or misunderstood.

Use the differential tissue tension tests and joint function tests to determine joint lesions, and functional assessment to determine the therapeutic regimen.

Before using manipulation, think about the joint end-feel (the way the joint feels at the end of its range of motion) and determine which pattern is present:

- Edematous and boggy end-feel – indicates joint effusion and possibly inflammation. Remember not to treat muscle spasm as a primary condition, it is almost always a response of the body to a noxious stimulus or pathophysiologic fault. Cryotherapy, positive galvanism, and pulsed ultrasound are indicated in acute conditions.
- Springy and taut end-feel – ligamentous fixations (as felt in the normal knee in lateral bending stress tests and drawer tests). Manipulation will work well on these types of fixations. Surging sinusoidal and interferential current, ultrasound, and moist hot packs will facilitate the treatment. Follow with cryotherapy in the subacute stages.
- Bone on bone end-feel – usually indicative of degenerative joint disease (as felt in the normal elbow in extension). If there is fine crepitus, mild degenerative joint disease (DJD) may be present; coarse crepitus indicates moderate DJD; and joint creaking may be advanced DJD. Diathermy, contrast baths, and other naturopathic therapies indicated in osteoarthritis are helpful.

Develop the habit of looking at the sedimentation rate and WBC differential count to avoid missing a concurrent condition or a difficult diagnosis.

By always starting high on the differential list, one misses few diagnoses. Exhaustive work-ups are infrequently warranted, but if treatment is directed to mechanical relief and the patient can't find a comfortable position which relieves the pain, it is doubtful that satisfactory results will be achieved using a mechanical approach.

General guides for manipulative technique

Texts on manipulative techniques by Liebenson, Lewit, Greenman, McKenzie, Bourdillion, and Maitland are good sources for learning the basics of the art. (Refer to the annotated further reading list for recommendations.)

Personal instruction is invaluable, but unless the rationales of joint mechanics, pathomechanics and pathophysiology are the basis of the teacher's approach it can be confusing and lead to cookbook approaches.

Functional assessment

Often the focus is on injury, pathology and disease, but the majority of musculoskeletal pain is from pathomechanics due to repetitive strain, deconditioning, fatigue and nutritional factors that must be addressed if treatment is to be successful. Once the portion of the patient's condition that is a musculoskeletal problem has been established, the mechanical fault should be determined. Manipulative treatment without correction of the mechanical fault will result in prolonged treatment and recurrence. Detecting this is sometimes easy, while at other times it is a mystery that takes careful investigation, as discussed in Greenman,[1] Lewit,[5] and Liebenson.[4]

Preparation for the manipulation

The patient should be comfortable and relaxed and on a firm but well-padded table. The room should be at a comfortable ambient temperature, and the physician should wear no watches or jewelry that might catch the patient's hair or skin.

The physician must be comfortable and relaxed. Manipulation is an individual art, but in general side posture manipulation of the pelvis and lumbar spine is easiest on a table that is at knee height; prone and supine thoracic manipulation is easiest at mid-thigh height; and cervical manipulation is easiest when seated, kneeling, or on a table at waist height. One may either change the height of the table or simply bend at the knees. Manipulation of the joints of the extremities can be performed in any position that allows the physician control over the joint and body parts.

Notes on the art

Manipulation is an art. Assuming a proper differential diagnosis, one acquires a "feel" that allows recognition of the difference between the three basic types of fixations and knowledge of when to manipulate.

If a movement causes pain, do not perform the movement, unless the diagnosis of the patient's condition is sure and the motion will cause no harm. Frequently, motion in the direction that is free and painless will free other ranges of motion.[34]

Joint motion

Joint motion descriptions can become elaborate, or one may simply say that there are six degrees of freedom of motion (plus long axis extension): flexion, extension, left and right rotation, left and right lateral bending. Not all joints have all six degrees of motion. The normal degrees and range of motion of joints are listed in anatomy and kinesiology texts. If a degree of motion is lost or blocked, determine the type of fixation and which form of manual medicine is indicated.

The fixation

Manipulation of a joint is performed to correct joint fixation, therefore one must:

1. Determine if mobilization or manipulation is the appropriate technique.
2. Identify the location and direction of the fixation.
3. Bring the joint to tension removing the periarticular tissue slack. Mobilization with tissue slack not taken up is safe, but manipulation when tissue slack is present invites injury.
4. Thrust only when the patient is relaxed and the fixation is felt.
5. After the elastic barrier has been stretched, repeated manipulation in the same direction is complicated because the end-feel tension normally felt prior to a manipulation is reduced or absent for at least 20 minutes. The same phenomenon occurs when one "pops" their knuckles. The risk of injury is much greater and changing to mobilization or active muscular relaxation techniques is recommended rather than repeated manipulation.

Stabilization

A point of stabilization is created by one hand and the physician's body weight, while the other hand performs the manipulation. Minor corrections of the position of the stabilized part and/or hand are frequently interpreted by an observer as twisting or wrenching motions. Twisting and wrenching are difficult to control and may cause injury to the patient.

Thrust

The manipulative thrust can be described according to:

- Direction of line of thrust – through the joint space, parallel to joint surfaces or tangential to the point of fixation.
- Velocity – slow for mobilizations. High velocity can correct joint fixations and the speed must be faster than the patient's reaction time, or a strain injury will result if the patient's muscular resistance occurs at the time of the manipulative thrust.
- Amplitude – governed by the quality of the health of the tissue, the quality of the fixation, and the location of the condition on the spectrum of the inflammation response.

Reassess

The condition of the joint fixation should be reassessed after every treatment to determine if the therapy has been successful.

A single manipulation will rarely correct a problem completely. Learning a joint-scanning technique will show one where the problems are that need further evaluation. The goal is to alleviate acute conditions or, if unsuccessful, to turn them into subacute conditions and resolve subacute and chronic conditions before they cause a chronic fatigue response, joint fixation and degeneration, and/or chronic myositis.

Troubleshooting your technique

Common problems blocking successful manipulation can be overcome by:

- learning joint play analysis on the peripheral joints and practicing manipulations of those joints before attempting to manipulate the spinal joints
- practicing the manipulative procedure with repeated light oscillatory movements while modifying the direction to feel the changes in joint tension, thus gaining experience, confidence, and knowledge without inflicting injury
- being sure of the procedure, otherwise the patient may sense the physician's hesitation and guard,

preventing the manipulation and increasing the risk of a poor outcome

- feeling the fixation of the joint as it is brought to tension, otherwise the manipulation will traumatize the tissues unnecessarily or will not gain the desired result
- learning the arthrology of the joint to be manipulated so as not to put the joint in a "locked" or jammed position that will cause the force of the manipulation to be dispersed to the surrounding tissues and joints.

Motion palpation

The following is a short lesson in motion palpation to determine the presence of sacroiliac joint fixation.

Review of anatomy and motion mechanism

Anatomy of the SI joint. The joint is L- or ear-shaped, with the apex of the L facing anteriorly. There can be fixation of the upper fibrous or lower synovial sacroiliac joint, thus altering the normal axis of rotation of the pelvis and causing excess wear on the lumbar spine, hip, knee, and ankle joints.

Sacroiliac gait mechanism. The sacrum and both iliums must be free to move in relation to each other. The sacrum flexes, extends, and nutates (nutation means nodding) in a gyrating figure-of-eight motion.

Effect of position on sacroiliac joint angles. As one sits, there is usually a decreased sacral base angle (slight flexion of the pelvis), and as one stands, the sacral base slightly increases (the pelvis slightly extends).

Mechanism of gait. Analysis of the normal right forward step:

1. The left leg is weight-bearing.
2. The right leg is in swing phase just prior to heel strike.
3. The left gluteus medius contracts to tilt the pelvis right superior, and the right sacrospinalis contracts and is counteracted by contraction of the left psoas muscle.
4. The right knee bends, allowing for foot-drop.
5. The hip rotates internally on the weight-bearing side (left) and rotates externally on the non-weight bearing side (right).

This motion results in right ilium flexion, left ilium extension and a *relative* flexion of the sacrum in relation to the ilium on the left.

In normal gait, the lumbar spine will not deviate to either side. The sacrospinalis will exert a pull on the weight-bearing side, and the psoas group will counter the movement by contracting on the non-weight-bearing side, so the lumbar spine remains in the midline.

Method of motion palpation of the sacroiliac joints

1. Contact the PSIS on the right with the right thumb.
2. Contact the second sacral tubercle with your left thumb.
3. Now ask the patient to flex their right thigh slowly three times up and down to below 90°. This causes flexion of the right innominate, while the sacral prominence will remain relatively stationary. The motion of the PSIS will normally be posterior, toward the floor, and slightly toward the midline. If no motion occurs between the PSIS and second sacral tubercle, there is a fixation of the right upper joint in flexion. Remember, it is the motion *between* the PSIS and second sacral tubercle, not the motion of the joint relative to the floor, that is important.
4. Next, ask the patient to flex their left thigh slowly three times above 90°. The right leg is now weight-bearing and fixed and we are causing the sacrum to flex, which causes a relative extension of the right ilium. If the sacral prominence does not swing medially away from the PSIS as the left thigh flexes above 90°, then the right upper joint is fixed in extension.
5. Now, shift your right thumb to the PIIS and have the patient slowly flex their right thigh three times to below 90° again. The PIIS should move laterally away from the sacral prominence, or there is a flexion fixation of the right lower SI joint.
6. Again, the left thigh is flexed slowly three time above 90° and the sacral prominence should swing medially away from the PIIS, unless there is an extension fixation of the right ilium in the lower joint (after Gillete and Gittleman).

Techniques for correction of these fixations are described in many manipulative texts. I recommend Maigne (pp. 390–395), Bourdillion (pp. 146–173), and Maitland (pp. 314–317).

Psychology

Management of chronic pain and assistance for the patient in dealing with stress are of major importance in the treatment of all conditions, especially NMS injuries. The psychosomatic component of myofascial pain syndromes, and the unique combination of therapies the naturopathic physician can offer, necessitate a thorough understanding of the relaxation response, hypnosis, biofeedback, guided imagery, and personal motivation.

If this area is not developed, some patients seeking help will not find their treatment results satisfactory.

REFERENCES

1. Greenman P. Principles of manual medicine. Baltimore: Williams & Wilkins. 1996: p 39
2. Maitland GD. Peripheral manipulation. 3rd edn. London: Butterworths. 1991
3. Bigos S, Bowyer O, Braen G et al. Acute low back problems in adults. Clinical practice guideline. Rockville, MD: US Department of Health and Human Services, Public Health Service, Agency for Health Care Policy and Research. 1994
4. Liebenson C, ed. Rehabilitation of the spine, a practitioner's manual. Baltimore: Williams & Willikins. 1996: p 355
5. Lewit, K. Manipulative therapy in rehabilitation of the locomotor system. Boston: Butterworths. 1985: p 5
6. Arnell P Beattie S. Heat and cold in the treatment of hypertonicity. J Can Phys Assoc 1972; 24: 61–67
7. Stamford, B. Giving injuries the cold treatment. The Physician and Sportsmedicine 1996; 24: 3 (http://www.physsportsmed.com/issue/mar_96/cold.htm#avoid)
8. Rizzo, TD. Using RICE for injury relief. The Physician And Sportsmedicine 1996; 24: 10 (http://www.physsportsmed.com/issues/oct_96/rizzo.htm)
9. Dvorak J, Dvorak V, Schneider W, eds. Manual medicine. Heidelberg: Springer Verlag. 1985
10. Cyriax J. Textbook of orthopedic medicine, Vol. 1. Diagnosis of soft tissue lesions. 8th edn. Philadelphia, PA: Baillière Tindall. 1982: p 10
11. Travell JG, Simons DG. Myofascial pain and dysfunction, the trigger point manual. Baltimore, MD: Williams & Wilkins. 1983: p 55
12. Schafer R. Chiropractic health care. Foundation of Chiropractic Education and Research. 1976
13. Lomax E. In: Buerger AA, Tobis JS, eds. Approaches to the validation of manipulative therapy. Springfield, IL: CC Thomas. 1977
14. Kessler RM. Management of common musculoskeletal disorders. In: Physical therapy principles and methods. Philadelphia, PA: Harper & Row. 1983: p 129
15. Hood WP. On the so-called "bone-setting," its nature and results. Lancet 1871; i: 304–310; i: 344–349
16. Goldstein M. Introduction, summary and analysis. In: Goldstein M, ed. NINCDS monograph no. 15. The research status of spinal manipulative therapy, a workshop held at the National Institutes of Health, February 2–4, 1975. DHEW Publication No. (NIH) 76-998. Bethesda, MD: US Department of Health Education and Welfare. 1975: p 6
17. Webster's New Collegiate Dictionary. Springfield, MA: GC Merriam. 1975
18. Star P. The social transformation of American medicine, the rise of a sovereign profession and the making of a vast industry. New York, NY: Basic Books. 1982
19. Palmer DD. The science, art and philosophy of chiropractic. Portland, OR: Portland Printing House. 1910: p 18
20. Gibbons R. The evolution of chiropractic: medical and social protest in America. Notes on the survival years and after. In: Haldeman S, ed. Modern developments in the principles and practice of chiropractic. New York: Appleton-Century-Crofts. 1980: p 3–24
21. Northup G. History and development of osteopathic concepts: osteopathic terminology. In: Goldstein M, ed. NINCDS monograph no. 15. The research status of spinal manipulative therapy, a workshop held at the National Institutes of Health, February 2–4, 1975. DHEW Publication No. (NIH) 76–998. Bethesda, MD: US Department of Health Education and Welfare. 1975: p 43–51
22. Wardwell WI. Discussion: the impact of spinal manipulative therapy on the health care system. In: Goldstein M, ed. NINCDS monograph no. 15. The research status of spinal manipulative therapy, a workshop held at the National Institutes of Health, February 2–4, 1975. DHEW Publication No. (NIH) 76–998. Bethesda, MD: US Department of Health Education and Welfare. 1975: p 53–57
23. Mennell JM. History of the development of medical manipulative concepts: medical terminology. In: Goldstein M, ed. NINCDS monograph no. 15. The research status of spinal manipulative therapy, a workshop held at the National Institutes of Health, February 2–4, 1975. DHEW Publication No. (NIH) 76–998. Bethesda, MD: US Department of Health Education and Welfare. 1975: p 20–21
24. Tower DB. Chairman summary: evolution and development of the concepts of manipulative therapy. In: Goldstein M, ed. NINCDS monograph no. 15. The research status of spinal manipulative therapy, a workshop held at the National Institutes of Health, February 2–4, 1975. DHEW Publication No. (NIH) 76–998. Bethesda, MD: US Department of Health Education and Welfare. 1975: p 59
25. Bourdillion JF, Day EA, Bookhout MR. Spinal manipulation. 5th edn. Butterworth-Heinemann. 1992: p ix–x
26. Waddell G. An approach to backache. Br J Hosp Med 1982; Sept: 187–219
27. Haerer A ed. DeJong's the neurologic examination. 5th edn. Philadelphia, PA: J.B. Lippincott. 1992: p 433
28. Wasson J et al. The common symptom guide. 2nd edn. New York, NY: McGraw-Hill. 1984
29. Beneliyahu DJ. Chiropractic management and manipulative therapy for MRI documented cervical disk herniation. J Manipulative Physiol Ther 1994; 17(3): 177–185
30. Magee DJ, Orthopedic physical assessment. 2nd edn. Philadelphia, PA: WB Saunders. 1992
31. Evans RC. Illustrated essential in orthopedic physical assessment. St Louis: Mosby. 1994
32. Sandoz R. Some physical mechanisms and effects of spinal adjustments. Ann Swiss Chirop Assoc 1976; 6: 91
33. Robbins RL, Cotran RS. Pathologic basis of disease. 2nd edn. Philadelphia PA: WB Saunders. 1979: p 55–106
34. Maigne R. Orthopedic medicine, a new approach to vertebral manipulation. Springfield, IL: CC Thomas. 1972: p 137

FURTHER READING

Bourdillion JF, Day EA, Bookhout MR. Spinal manipulation. 5th edn. Butterworth-Heinemann. 1992 *A good text that covers the bases. It is exceeded in many areas by Greenman's text*

Boyling JD, Palastang N. Grieve's modern manaul therapy. 2nd edn. New York, NY: Churchill Livingstone. 1994 *A heavily referenced tome*

Cox JM Low back pain: mechanism, diagnosis and treatment. 5th edn. Baltimore, MD: Williams & Wilkins. 1990 *Addresses aspects of conservative care of low back, especially lumbar disc herniation history, research, diagnosis, and conservative treatment with statistics and research that supports the methods described*

Cryiax J. Textbook of orthopedic medicine, vol. 1. Diagnosis of soft tissue lesions. 8th edn. Philadelphia, PA: Baillière Tindall. 1982 *A difficult text to read that has been translated to a readable format by the other authors listed, but a classic. He was strongly anti-alternative medicine in his approach to certain aspects of physical medicine (especially those who should and should not practice it), and his viewpoints are narrow and limited compared with the more recent publications and journals*

Greenman P. Principles of manual medicine. 2nd edn. Baltimore: Williams & Wilkins. 1996 *One of the best texts that covers the material in a clear, understandable and usable format*

Haldeman S, ed. Principles and practice of chiropractic. 2nd edn. New York: Appleton-Century-Crofts. 1992 *The second edition has major changes, new contributors and is an excellent source of information on history, research, diagnosis and treatment of all phases of manipulation, with special attention to the spine*

Kessler RM. Management of common musculoskeletal disorders,

physical therapy principles and methods. 3rd edn. Philadelphia, PA: Harper & Row. 1996 *A good text for the therapist's approach to treatment, with recap of much of Cryiax's work. Basic concepts of embryology, arthrology, pain and assessment. Techniques of case management, use of hot and cold, manipulative, and relaxation techniques. Ends with detailed discussion of all of the joints of the body. Well worth reading*

Liebenson C, ed. Rehabilitation of the spine, a practitioner's manual. Baltimore: Williams & Wilkins. 1996 *Craig has brought together many fine contributors who address the cutting edge methods of manual medicine. It covers much of what is needed in clinical practice. Very useful and readable. A gold mine of information*

Magee DJ, Orthopedic physical assessment. 2nd edn. Philadelphia, PA: WB Saunders. 1992 *One of the best texts for learning the orthopedic assessment techniques and many of the functional tests*

Maitland GD. Vertebral manipulation. 4th edn. London: Butterworths. 1977 *A physical therapist's approach with emphasis on patient selection, pretreatment assessment, assessment during treatment, assessment after treatment, and therapeutic approach for each area of the spine*

Maitland GD. Peripheral manipulation. 3rd edn. London: Butterworths. 1991 *The same approach as previous book, but for the extremities. The author suggests learning on the extremities before attempting to learn spinal manipulation. After all, a joint is a joint*

Walther DS. Applied kinesiology, vols I and II. Pueblo, CO: Systems DC. 1983 *A chiropractic approach that is in a different realm from physical medicine texts. Treatment approaches that are difficult to find and that are empirically based – often gives a useful solution that defies scientific fact*

CHAPTER CONTENTS

44

Nutritional medicine

Michael T. Murray, ND

Joseph E. Pizzorno Jr, ND

Let your food be your medicine and let your medicine be your food. (Hippocrates)

INTRODUCTION

Nutritional medicine, as described in this textbook, consists of the use of diet and nutritional supplementation as therapeutic modalities. The foundation of nutritional medicine is a health-promoting diet which focuses on the consumption of whole, natural foods. Nutritional supplements are used in the overall context of nutritional medicine as complementary agents, not as sole primary medicines. Diet is always primary, and supplementation secondary.

DIETARY GUIDELINES

There is an ever-growing appreciation of the major role diet plays in determining the level of health. It is now well-established that certain dietary practices cause, as well as prevent, a wide range of diseases. In addition, more and more research is accumulating which indicates that certain diets and foods offer immediate therapeutic benefit. The purpose of this chapter is to initiate the reader into the growing field of nutritional medicine by focusing on 10 key dietary recommendations for a health-promoting diet. These 10 principles are utilized by most naturopathic physicians in their goal of educating and inspiring their patients to attain a higher level of wellness and are as follows:

1. Eat a plant-based, predominantly vegetarian diet
2. Reduce the intake of fat
3. Eliminate refined sugar
4. Reduce exposure to pesticides and herbicides
5. Eliminate the intake of food additives and coloring agents
6. Keep salt intake low, potassium intake high
7. Drink 32–48 ounces of water daily
8. Identify and address food allergies

9. Determine caloric needs to achieve or maintain ideal body weight
10. Use the Healthy Exchange System to construct a health-promoting diet.

A discussion of these 10 recommendations will be followed by a concise description of the role of nutritional supplementation in nutritional medicine.

Eat a plant-based, predominantly vegetarian diet

Based on detailed anatomical and historical evidence, it is thought that humans evolved as "hunter-gatherers", i.e. humans appear to be omnivores capable of surviving on both gathered (plant) and hunted (animal) foods.[1] However, while the human gastrointestinal tract is capable of digesting both animal and plant foods, there are indications that it can accommodate plant foods much easier than animal foods.[2] Specifically, human teeth are composed of 20 molars which are optimal for crushing and grinding plant foods along with eight front incisors which are well-suited for biting into fruits and vegetables. Only the front four canine teeth are designed for meat eating. Human jaws swing both vertically to tear and laterally to crush, while carnivores' jaws only swing vertically. Additional evidence to support the preference for plant foods is the long length of the human intestinal tract. Carnivores typically have a short bowel while herbivores have a bowel length proportionally comparable to humans.

To further examine what humans should eat, many researchers look to other primates, such as chimpanzees, monkeys, and gorillas. Non-human primates are also omnivores – or, as often described, herbivores and opportunistic carnivores. They eat mainly fruits and vegetables but may also eat small animals, lizards, and eggs if given the opportunity. In primates, animal food consumption is inversely related to body weight. The smaller primates eat more animal foods while the larger primates eat much less animal foods. As a percentege of total calories, the gorilla and the orangutan eat only 1 and 2% animal foods, respectively,. The remainder of their diet is from plant foods. Since humans are between the weight of the gorilla and the orangutan, it has been suggested that humans have evolved to eat around 1.5% of their diet as animal foods.[2] Most Americans currently derive well over 50% of their calories from animal foods.[3]

It should also be pointed out that the meat that our ancestors consumed was much different than the meat of modern commerce. Domesticated animals have always had higher fat levels than their wild counterpart, but the desire for tender meat has led to the breeding of cattle which produce meat with a fat content of 25–30% or higher compared with a fat content of lower than 4% for free-living animals or wild game. In addition, the type of fat is considerably different. Domestic beef contains primarily saturated fats and virtually undetectable amounts of omega-3 fatty acids. In contrast, the fat of wild animals contains over five times more polyunsaturated fat per gram and has high levels of the essential omega-3 fatty acids (approximately 4%).[1]

A tremendous amount of evidence now shows that deviating from a predominantly plant-based to a domesticated animal-based diet is a major factor in the development of heart disease, cancer, strokes, arthritis, and many other chronic degenerative disease. It is now the recommendation of many health and medical organizations that the human diet should focus primarily on plant-based foods – vegetables, fruits, grains, legumes, nuts, seeds, etc. Such a diet is thought to offer significant protection against the development of chronic degenerative disease.[3–5]

The health-promoting components of a plant-based diet

One of the key aspects of a predominantly plant-based diet is its high content of dietary fiber. This aspect is thoroughly discussed in Chapter 57. In addition, a predominantly plant-based diet is low in saturated fat, high in essential fatty acids, and high in antioxidant nutrients and phytochemicals.

Many medical experts and departments of the US Government, including the US National Academy of Science, the US Department of Agriculture, the US Department of Health and Human Services, the National Research Council, and the National Cancer Institute, are recommending that Americans consume two to three servings of fruit and three to five servings of vegetables per day in an attempt to reduce the risk of developing heart disease, cancer, and other chronic degenerative diseases. Unfortunately, less than 10% of population are meeting even the lowest recommendation of five servings of a combination of fruits and vegetables.

Numerous population studies have repeatedly demonstrated that a high intake of carotene-rich and flavonoid-rich fruits and vegetables reduces the risk of cancer, heart disease and strokes (see Ch. 67 for a full discussion).[3,5] Carotenes represent the most widespread group of naturally occurring pigments in nature. They are a highly colored (red and yellow) group of fat-soluble compounds. Over 600 carotenoids have been characterized, including 30–50 that the body can transform into vitamin A. Beta-carotene has been termed the most active of the carotenoids, due to its higher provitamin A activity, but several other carotenes exert greater antioxidant effects.

The best dietary sources of carotenes are green leafy vegetables and yellow-orange colored fruits and vegetables, e.g. carrots, apricots, mangoes, yams, and squash.

Red and purple vegetables and fruits – such as tomatoes, red cabbage, berries, and plums – contain a large portion of non-vitamin-A active pigments, including flavonoids. Legumes, grains, and seeds are also significant sources of carotenoids.

The flavonoids are another group of plant pigments providing remarkable protection against cancer, heart disease and strokes. These compounds are largely responsible for the colors of fruits and flowers. Flavonoids act as powerful antioxidants in providing protection against oxidative and free radical damage. Good dietary sources of flavonoids include citrus fruits, berries, onions, parsley, legumes, green tea, and red wine. The average daily intake of flavonoids in the United States is estimated to be somewhere between 150 and 200 mg.

Reduce the intake of fat

There is a great deal of research linking a diet high in fat, particularly a diet high in saturated fat and cholesterol, to numerous cancers, heart disease, and strokes. Both the American Cancer Society and the American Heart Association have recommended a diet containing less than 30% of calories as fat.[3] The easiest way for most people to achieve this goal is to eat less animal products and more plant foods. With the exception of nuts and seeds, most plant foods are very low in fat. With regard to nuts and seeds, while they do contain high levels of fat calories, the calories are derived largely from polyunsaturated essential fatty acids.

In addition to providing the body with energy, the essential fatty acids, linoleic and linolenic acid provided by plant foods function as components of nerve cells, cellular membranes, and prostaglandins. In addition, these polyunsaturated fats, are being shown to be protective and therapeutic against heart disease, cancer, autoimmune diseases like multiple sclerosis and rheumatoid arthritis, many skin diseases, and many others.

Much of the therapeutic benefits in these conditions is related to altering prostaglandin metabolism (see Ch. 85 for a complete discussion of fatty acid metabolism). Prostaglandins and related compounds (e.g. thromboxanes and leukotrienes) are hormone-like molecules derived from 20 carbon chain fatty acids that contain three, four, or five double bonds. Linoleic and linolenic can be converted to prostaglandins through adding two carbon molecules and removing hydrogen molecules (if necessary). The number and position of double bonds in the fatty acid determine the classification of the prostaglandin.

Series 1 and 2 prostaglandins come from the omega-6 fatty acids, with the linoleic acid serving as the starting point. Linoleic acid is changed to gamma-linolenic acid and then dihomo-gamma-linolenic acid, which contains three double bonds and is the precursor to prostaglandin of the 1 series. Dihomo-gamma-linolenic acid (DHGLA) can also be converted to arachidonic acid, which contains four double bonds and is a precursor to the series 2 prostaglandins. However, because the enzyme (delta-5-desaturase) responsible for the conversion of DHGLA to arachidonic acid prefers the omega-3 oils, in humans the greatest source of arachidonic acid is from the diet. Arachidonic acid is found almost entirely in domesticated animal foods along with saturated fats.

Particularly beneficial are the series 3 prostaglandins produced from the omega-3 prostaglandin pathway. This pathway can begin with linolenic acid which can eventually be converted to eicosapentaenoic acid or EPA which is the precursor to the 3 series prostaglandins. Although EPA is found pre-formed in cold-water fish such as salmon, mackerel and herring, certain vegetable oils, such as flaxseed and canola, can, by providing linolenic acid, increase body EPA and 3-series prostaglandin levels.

Prostaglandins of the 1 and 3 series are generally viewed as "good" prostaglandins while prostaglandins of the 2 series are viewed as bad. This is most evident by looking at their effects on platelets. Prostaglandins of the 2 series promote platelet adhesiveness which leads to hardening of the arteries, heart disease, and strokes. In contrast, the 1 and 3 series prostaglandins prevent platelet adhesiveness, improve blood flow, and reduce inflammation. Although the precursor to 2 series prostaglandins can be derived from linoleic acid, in humans the greatest source is directly from the diet. Arachidonic acid is found almost entirely in animal foods along with saturated fats. Prostaglandin metabolism can be manipulated through restricting saturated fat and arachidonic acid intake along with increasing the intake of the other precursors like linolenic, gamma-linolenic, and EPA. Conditions improved through this manipulation include atherosclerosis, multiple sclerosis, psoriasis, eczema, menstrual cramps, rheumatoid arthritis, and many other allergic or inflammatory conditions.

It is important to note that *trans*-fatty acids, which are found primarily in margarines and shortenings, along with alcohol, saturated fats, deficiencies of vitamin C, niacin, B_6, zinc, and magnesium can greatly interfere with prostaglandin metabolism.

Avoid trans*-fatty acids*

For optimal health it appears to be very important to eliminate the intake of margarine and foods containing *trans*-fatty acids and partially hydrogenated oils. The manufacture of margarine and shortening entails the hydrogenation of vegetable oils. This means that a hydrogen molecule is added to the natural unsaturated fatty acid molecules of the vegetable oil to make it more saturated. Hydrogenation results in changing the structure of the natural fatty acid which exists in the *cis-* configuration to the *trans-* configuration. *Trans-*fatty acids interfere with the body's ability to utilize essential fatty acids.

Many researchers and nutritionists have been concerned about the health effects of margarines since they were first introduced. Although many Americans assume they are promoting their health by consuming margarine rather than butter and saturated fats, the reverse appears to be the case. Margarine and other hydrogenated vegetable oils not only raise LDL cholesterol, they also lower the protective HDL cholesterol level, interfere with essential fatty acid metabolism, and are suspected of being causes of certain cancers, such as breast cancer.[6–9]

At the very least, patients should be encouraged to eat less saturated fat and cholesterol, by reducing or eliminating the amounts of animal products in the diet, and to increase the consumption of fiber-rich plant foods (fruits, vegetables, grains, and legumes). Limit the intake of animal protein sources to no more than 4–6 ounces/day and recommend patients choose fish, skinless poultry, and lean cuts rather than fat-ladened choices. Finally, synthetically hydrogenated fats should be eliminated from the diet.

Eliminate refined sugar

Refined sugar and simple sugars in general stress blood sugar control and other homeostatic mechanisms. When high sugar foods are eaten alone, blood sugar levels rise quickly, producing a heightened release of insulin. Eating foods high in simple sugars is usually harmful to blood sugar control – especially in hypoglycemics and diabetics. Sugar, especially when combined with caffeine, also has a detrimental effect on mood, premenstrual syndrome, and many other health conditions.

Currently, more than half of the carbohydrates being consumed by most Americans are in the form of sugars being added to foods as sweetening agents.[3] Encourage patients to read food labels carefully for clues on sugar content. If the words sucrose, glucose, maltose, lactose, fructose, corn syrup, or white grape juice concentrate appear on the label, extra sugar has been added.

Reduce exposure to pesticides and herbicides

In the US each year over 1.2 billion pounds of pesticides and herbicides are sprayed or added to food crops. That is roughly 10 pounds of pesticides for each man, woman, and child. Although the pesticides are designed to act against insects and other organisms, experts estimate that only 2% of the pesticide actually serves its purpose, while over 98% of the pesticide is absorbed into the air, water, soil, or food supply. Most pesticides in use are synthetic chemicals of questionable safety. The major long-term health risks include increased risk of cancer, birth defects and many chronic diseases, while the major health risks of acute intoxication include vomiting, diarrhea, blurred vision, tremors, convulsions, and nerve damage.[10–12]

The health problems of the farmer provide an illustrative example of the problem with agricultural chemicals. The lifestyle of a farmer is generally a healthy one, in that a farmer eats fresh food, breathes clean air, works hard, and doesn't have as high a level of such unhealthy habits as cigarette smoking and alcohol use as city dwellers. Despite this lifestyle, it has been shown in several studies that farmers are at greater risk for several cancers including lymphomas, leukemias, and cancers of the stomach, prostate, brain, and skin.[13]

Large studies of farmers in Canada, Australia, Europe, New Zealand, and the United States have demonstrated that the greater the exposure to agricultual chemicals, the greater is the risk for non-Hodgkin's lymphoma.[11,12] However, because the evidence for the cancer-causing capabilities of pesticides in animals is inadequate, the formal opinion of many "experts" is that they pose no significant risk for the public or the farmer, an apparently untenable position.

The history of pesticide use in the US is riddled with pesticides that were once widely used and then later banned due to health risks. Perhaps the best known example is DDT. Widely used from the early 1940s to 1973, DDT was largely responsible for increasing farm productivity in this country. In 1962, Rachel Carson's classic *Silent Spring* detailed the full range of DDT's hazards, including its persistence in the food chain and its deadly effects, but it was 10 years later before the Federal Government banned the use of this deadly compound. Unfortunately, although DDT has been banned for nearly 20 years, it is still found in the soil and root vegetables such as carrots and potatoes. According to studies performed by the National Resources Defense Council, a public interest environmental group, 17% of the carrots they analyzed still contained detectable levels of DDT.[14]

Widespread environmental contamination has occurred with the halogenated hydrocarbons, DDT, DDE, PCB, PCP, dieldrin, and chlordane. These molecules persist for long periods in the environment, are hard detoxify and accumulate in fat cells. Many of these chemicals mimic estrogen in the body and are thought to be a major factor in the growing epidemics of estrogen-related health problems such as PMS, breast cancer, and low sperm counts[15,16] (see Ch. 37 for an in-depth discussion of this important topic).

Pesticides in use today

The majority of pesticides currently used in the US are

probably less toxic than DDT and other banned pesticides including aldrin, dieldrin, endrin, and heptachlor. However, many pesticides banned from use in the US are shipped to other countries such as Mexico which then in turn sends contaminated food back to the US. Although over 600 pesticides are currently used in the US, most experts are most concerned about relatively few of these. The Environmental Protection Agency has identified 64 pesticides as potential cancer-causing compounds, while the National Research Council found that 80% of US cancer risk from pesticides is due to 13 pesticides used widely on 15 important food crops.[11,14] The pesticides are: linuron, permethrin, chlordimeform, zineb, captafol, captan, maneb, mancozeb, folpet, chlorothalonil, metiram, benomyl, and O-phenylphenol. They are found in many crops, but of greatest concern are the following (in order of decreasing importance):

- tomatoes
- beef
- potatoes
- oranges
- lettuce
- apples
- peaches
- pork
- wheat
- soybeans
- beans
- carrots
- chicken
- corn
- grapes.

Pesticide residue levels in food are monitored by both state and federal regulatory agencies. Such monitoring is used to enforce legal tolerance levels. However, there has been increasing public and governmental concern about the adequacy of the residue monitoring programs. The monitoring system is composed of three collaboration components: the EPA, FDA and a variety of individual state agricultural agencies. The EPA establishes a tolerance level for pesticides in raw or unprocessed foods utilizing key data. The Food and Drug Agency (FDA) is then responsible for enforcing the EPA limits. Individual state organizations, such as the departments of health and agriculture, may also be involved in the monitoring of food safety. Where this system falls short is not simply in the determination of the tolerance level, but in other critical ways:

- less than 1% of the domestic food supply is screened by the FDA
- the FDA does not test for all pesticides
- the FDA does not prevent the marketing of the foods that it finds to contain illegal residues.

A number of pesticide poisoning epidemics have been reported. The largest to date occurred in 1985. It involved aldicarb, an extremely toxic pesticide, and its illegal use on watermelons. Aldicarb is a systemic pesticide, which means it permeates the entire fruit. Over 1,000 people in the western US and Canada were affected. Illness ranged from mild gastrointestinal upset to severe poisoning (vomiting, diarrhea, blurred vision, tremors, convulsions, and nerve damage).[11]

While the EPA and FDA estimate that excessive pesticide residues are found on about 3% of domestic and 6% of foreign produce, and acceptable levels are found in 13% of domestic produce, other organizations report much higher estimates. For example, the National Resources Defense Council conducted a survey of fresh produce sold in San Francisco markets for pesticide residues and found that 44% of 71 fruit and vegetables had detectable levels of 19 different pesticides, with 42% of produce with detectable pesticide residues containing more than one pesticide.[14] The sheer number and amount of pesticides applied to certain foods is alarming. For example, over 50 different pesticides are used on broccoli, 110 on apples, and 70 on bell peppers.[10] As many of the pesticides penetrate the entire fruit or vegetable and cannot be washed off, it is obviously best to buy organic.

Many supermarket chains and produce suppliers are employing their own testing measures for determining the pesticide content of produce and are refusing to stock foods that have been treated with some of the more toxic pesticides such as alachlor, captan, or EBDCs (ethylene bisdithiocarbamates). In addition, many stores are asking growers to disclose all pesticides used on the foods and to phase out the use of the 64 pesticides suspected of being capable of causing cancers. Ultimately it will be pressure from consumers which will influence food suppliers the greatest. Crop yield studies support the use of organic farming if the risk of human health is added to the equation.

Waxes

In addition to pesticides, waxes are applied to many fruits and vegetables to seal in the water contained in the produce, thereby keeping the produce looking fresh. According to FDA law, grocery stores must display a sign noting that waxes or post-harvest pesticides have been applied. Unfortunately, most stores do not comply with the law and the FDA lacks the manpower to enforce it. Currently, the FDA has approved six different waxes for use on produce. Approved compounds include shellac, paraffin, palm oil derivatives, and synthetic resins. These same items are used in furniture, floor, and car waxes. Foods to which these compounds can be applied include apples, avocados, bell peppers, cantaloupes, cucumbers, eggplants, grapefruits, lemons, limes, melons, oranges, parsnips, passion fruits, peaches, pineapples, pumpkins, rutabagas, squashes, sweet potatoes, tomatoes, and turnips.[10]

One of the main reasons the waxes are added is to keep the produce from spoiling during the (often long) period of time from harvest to the grocery store shelves. If grocery store chains bought more local produce, it would not require the chemicals to keep it looking fresh. Instead the large chains sign contracts with large produce suppliers regardless of their location. This is why, for example, a grocery store in New York is stocked with Washington State apples and California broccoli.

The waxes themselves probably pose little health risk. However, most waxes have powerful pesticides or fungicides added to them. Since the waxes cannot be washed off with water, the fungicide or pesticide literally becomes cemented to the produce.

Pesticides exposure can be reduced by:

- Avoiding foods which concentrate pesticides, e.g. animal fat, meat, eggs, cheese, and milk – it makes good sense to avoid these foods
- Buying organic produce. In the context of food and farming, the term organic is used to imply that the produce was grown without the aid of synthetic chemicals including pesticides and fertilizers. In 1973, Oregon became the first state to pass laws that define labeling laws for organic produce. By 1989, 16 other states (California, Colorado, Iowa, Maine, Massachusetts, Minnesota, Montana, Nebraska, New Hampshire, North Dakota, Ohio, South Dakota, Texas, Vermont, Washington, and Wisconsin) had also adopted state laws governing organic agriculture. Highly reputable certification organizations include:
  —California Certified Organic Farmers
  —Demeter
  —Farm Verified Organic
  —Natural Organic Farmers Association
  —the Organic Crop Improvement Association.
  Although under 3% of the total produce grown in the US is grown without the aid of pesticides, organic produce is widely available.
- Encouraging patients, where organic produce is not readily available, to develop a good relationship with the local grocery store produce manager. Have them explain to him or her their desire to reduce the exposure to pesticides and waxes. Ask what measures the store takes to assure pesticide residues are within the tolerance limits. Ask where they get their produce as foreign produce is much more likely to contain excessive levels of pesticides as well as pesticides that have been banned in the US due to suspected toxicity. Try and buy local produce that is in season.
- Removing surface pesticide residues, waxes, fungicides, and fertilizers. This can be done by soaking in a mild solution of additive-free soap like Ivory or pure castille soap from the health food store. There are also all-natural, biodegradable cleansers available at most health food stores. The produce can be sprayed with the cleanser, gently scrubbed, and then rinsed.
- Simply peeling off the skin or removing the outer layer of leaves. This will reduce pesticide levels. The down-side of this is that many of the nutritional benefits are concentrated in the skin and outer layers.

The presence of pesticides in fruits and vegetables should not deter patients from eating a diet high in these foods. The concentrations in fruits and vegetables are much lower than the levels found in animal fats, meat, cheese, whole milk, and eggs. Furthermore, the various antioxidant components in fruits and vegetables help the body to deal with the pesticides.

Eliminate the intake of food additives and coloring agents

Food additives are used to prevent spoiling or enhance flavor and include such substances as preservatives, artificial colors, artificial flavorings, and acidifiers. Although the government has banned many synthetic food additives, it should not be assumed that all the additives currently used in the food supply are safe. There are still a great number of synthetic food additives still in use that are being linked to such diseases as depression, asthma or other allergy, hyperactivity or learning disabilities in children, and migraine headaches.

The FDA has approved the use of over 2,800 different food additives. In 1985, the per capita daily consumption of these food additives was approximately 13–15 g.[17] While an extremist might argue that no food additive is safe, many food additives fulfill important functions in the modern day food supply. Some compounds approved as additives are natural in origin and possess health-promoting properties, while others are synthetic compounds with known cancer-causing effects. Obviously, the most sensible approach is to focus on whole, natural foods and avoid foods which are highly processed.

Coloring agents

The total annual consumption of food colors in the US is approximately 100 million pounds for the entire population. Food color additives are officially designated as either certified or exempt from certification.[18] The food color additives which are exempt from certification are primarily natural in origin. This reflects the popular belief that natural compounds are safer. This contention appears to hold up to scientific scrutiny.

One of the most widely used food colors is FD&C yellow dye #5 or tartrazine. Tartrazine is added to almost every packaged food as well as many drugs, including some antihistamines, antibiotics, steroids, and sedatives.[19] In the United States, the average daily per capita consumption of certified dyes is 15 mg, of which 85% is tartrazine. Among children, consumption is usually much higher.

Although the overall rate of allergic reactions to tartrazine is quite low in the general population, allergic reactions due to tartrazine are extremely common (20–50%) in allergic individuals, especially those sensitive to aspirin.[20,21] Like aspirin, tartrazine is a known inducer of asthma, hives, and other allergic conditions, particularly in children.[21] In addition, tartrazine, as well as benzoate and aspirin, increases the production of the number of mast cells.[22] As mast cells are involved in producing histamine and other allergic compounds, those with increased levels are more prone to allergies. For example, examination of patients with hives shows that greater than 95% have an increase in mast cells.[23]

In studies using provocation tests to determine sensitivity to tartrazine and other food additives in patients with hives, results have ranged from 5 to 46%.[24–37] Diets eliminating tartrazine as well as other food additives in sensitive individuals have in many cases been shown to be of great benefit in patients with hives and other allergic conditions like asthma and eczema.[24–32] Obviously, patinets suffering from allergic conditions should eliminate artificial food colors from their diets.

Antioxidants

The two most widely used antioxidants are butylated hydroxyanisole (BHA) and butylated hydroxytolulene (BHT). These food additives cause cancers in rats. However, there are other studies showing that these antioxidants actually protect against the development of cancers. In fact, many so-called "experts" in life extension have recommended that these substances be taken as food supplements at very high doses (i.e. 2 g/day). Based on extensive research this recommendation is extremely unwise as it is 100 times the estimated acceptable intake of BHA, BHT, or the sum of both as set by the Joint Food and Agriculture Organization of the United Nations/World Health Organization Expert Committee on Food Additives.[38] It is also over 100 times the estimated inhibitory activity and may actually promote cancer. While BHA and BHT may be safe at low levels in foods, in the future they will most likely be replaced by naturally occurring antioxidants.

Preservatives

Preservatives like sodium benzoate, nitrates, nitrites, and sulfites work primarily to prevent spoilage by checking the growth of microorganisms. All of these preservatives have come under attack recently. In the case of nitrates and nitrites, these compounds are known carcinogens. Sulfites and benzoates, on the other hand, are capable of producing allergic reactions.[17,39]

Benzoic acid and benzoates are the most commonly used food preservatives.[17] Although for the general population the rate of allergic response is thought to be less than 1%, the frequency of positive challenges in patients with chronic hives or asthma varies from 4 to 44%.[24–32] Even more of a problem are sulfites, which were once widely used on produce at restaurant salad bars. Since most people were not aware that sulfites were being added, and because most people were unaware they had a sensitivity to sulfites, many unsuspecting people experienced severe allergic or asthmatic reactions. For years the FDA refused to even consider a ban on sulfites, even while admitting these agents provoked attacks in an unknown number of people and in 5–10% of asthma victims. It was not until 1985, when sulfite sensitivity was linked to 15 deaths between 1983 and 1985, that the FDA agreed to review the matter. In 1986, the FDA finally banned sulfite use on produce and required labeling of other foods, such as wine, beer, and dried fruit, that have added sulfites. The average person consumes an average of 2–3 mg/day of sulfites, while wine and beer drinkers typically consume up to 10 mg/day.[39]

The Feingold hypothesis

The hypothesis that food additives can cause hyperactivity in children stemmed from the research of Benjamin Feingold MD and is commonly referred to as the "Feingold hypothesis". According to Feingold, many hyperactive children, perhaps 40–50%, are sensitive to artificial food colors, flavors, and preservatives as well as to naturally occurring salicylates and phenolic compounds.[40] Further discussion on the Feingold hypothesis is given in Chapter 135.

Keep salt intake low, potassium intake high

Excessive sodium chloride consumption, coupled with diminished dietary potassium, greatly stresses the kidney's ability to maintain proper fluid volume. As a result some people are "salt-sensitive", in that high salt intake causes high blood pressure or, in other cases, water retention. However, it is not simply a matter of reducing salt intake, as patients should be encouraged to simultaneously increase the intake of potassium. This is easily done by increasing the intake of high-potassium foods and avoiding high-sodium foods (most processed foods). Instruct patients to read labels carefully in order to keep their total daily sodium intake below 1,800 mg.

Most Americans have a potassium-to-sodium (K:Na) ratio of less than 1:2. This 1:2 ratio means that most people ingest twice as much sodium as potassium. Researchers recommend a dietary potassium-to-sodium ratio of greater than 5:1 to maintain health. This is 10 times higher than the average intake. However, even this may not be optimal. A natural diet rich in fruits and vegetables can produce a K:Na ratio greater than 100:1, as most fruits and vegetables have a K:Na ratio of at least 50:1.

If patients really must have the taste of salt, encourage them to try the so-called salt substitutes such as the popular brands "NoSalt" and "Nu-Salt". These products are composed of potassium chloride which tastes very similar to sodium chloride. Patient compliance can be monitored with the Fantus test (see Ch. 12).

Drink 32–48 ounces of water daily

Adequate water consumption is vital to optimal health. Inadequate water consumption impairs kidney function, increases the concentration of toxins in the urinary tract, increases the risk of gallstones and kidney stones, and impairs immune function.

Unfortunately, there are problems with the water supply. Most of the water supply is full of chemicals, including not only chlorine and fluoride which are intentionally added, but a wide range of toxic organic compounds and chemicals such as PCBs, pesticide residues, nitrates, and heavy metals like lead, mercury, and cadmium.[41] It is estimated that lead alone may contaminate the water of more than 40 million Americans. In an effort to reduce the exposure to these toxic compounds, roughly 2 million home water filtration units are purchased annually.

Identify and address food allergies

The importance of identifying and addressing food allergies and sensitivities is fully discussed in Chapters 15 and 51.

Determine caloric needs to achieve or maintain ideal body weight

In determining calorie needs, it is necessary to first determine ideal body weight. The most popular height and weight charts are the tables of "desirable weight" provided by the Metropolitan Life Insurance Company. The most recent edition of these tables, published in 1983, gives weight ranges for men and women at 1 inch increments of height for three body frame sizes (see Table 44.1).

Table 44.1 1983 Metropolitan height and weight table

Height	Small frame	Medium frame	Large frame
Men			
5'2"	128–134	131–141	138–150
5'3"	130–136	133–143	140–153
5'4"	132–138	135–145	142–156
5'5"	134–140	137–148	144–160
5'6"	136–142	139–151	146–164
5'7"	138–145	142–154	149–168
5'8"	140–148	145–157	152–172
5'9"	142–151	148–160	155–176
5'10"	144–154	151–163	158–180
5'11"	146–157	154–166	161–184
6'0"	149–160	157–170	164–188
6'1"	152–164	160–174	168–192
6'2"	155–168	164–178	172–197
6'3"	158–172	167–182	176–202
6'4"	162–176	171–187	181–207
Women			
4'10"	102–111	109–121	118–131
4'11"	103–113	111–123	120–134
5'0"	104–115	113–126	122–137
5'1"	106–118	115–129	125–140
5'2"	108–121	118–132	128–143
5'3"	111–124	121–135	131–147
5'4"	114–127	124–138	134–151
5'5"	117–130	127–141	137–155
5'6"	120–133	130–144	140–159
5'7"	123–136	133–147	143–163
5'8"	126–139	136–150	146–167
5'9"	129–142	139–153	149–170
5'10"	132–145	142–156	152–173
5'11"	135–148	145–159	155–176
6'0"	138–151	148–162	158–179

*Weights for adults aged 25–59 years based on lowest mortality. Weight are in pounds according to frame size and include indoor clothing (5 pounds for men and 3 pounds for women) and shoes with 1 inch heels.

Determining frame size

Frame size is determined by measuring elbow breadth. Elbow breadth is determined by having the patient bend his or her elbow at a 90° angle and then measuring, with a caliper, the distance between the medial and lateral epicondyles. Table 44.2 lists the elbow breadths of a medium frame size in men and women. A lower reading indicates a small frame, while higher readings indicate a large frame.

Determining appropriate calorie consumption

After the desirable weight has been determined in pounds, convert it to kilograms by dividing it by 2.2. This number is then multiplied by the following calories, depending upon activity level:

- Little physical activity: 30 calories
- Light physical activity: 35 calories

Table 44.2 Elbow breadth of a medium frame size in men and women

Height in 1" heels	Elbow breadth
Men	
5'2"–5'3"	2½"–2⅞"
5'4"–5'7"	2⅝"–2⅞"
5'8"–5'11"	2¾"–3"
6'0"–6'3"	2¾"–3⅛"
6'4"	2⅞"–3¼"
Women	
4'10"–5'3"	2¼"–2½"
5'4"–5'11"	2⅜"–2⅝"
6'0"	2½"–2¾"

- Moderate physical activity: 40 calories
- Heavy physical activity: 45 calories.

Use the Healthy Exchange System to construct a health-promoting diet

The American Dietetic Association (ADA), in conjunction with the American Diabetes Association and other groups, have developed the Exchange System, a convenient tool for the rapid estimation of the calorie, protein, fat, and carbohydrate content of a diet. Originally designed for use in designing dietary recommendations for diabetics, the exchange method is now used in the calculation and design of virtually all therapeutic diets. Unfortunately, the ADA exchange plan does not place a strong enough emphasis on the quality of food choices.

The Healthy Exchange System presented here is a healthier version because it emphasizes better food choices and focuses on unprocessed, whole foods. The diet is prescribed by allotting the number of exchanges allowed per list for 1 day. There are seven exchange lists, although the milk and meat lists should be considered optional:

- List 1: vegetables
- List 2: fruits
- List 3: breads, cereals, and starchy vegetables
- List 4: legumes
- List 5: fats
- List 6: milk
- List 7: meats, fish, cheese, and eggs.

The healthy exchange lists in Appendix 6 can be provided to your patients to facilitate their understanding and adoption of a healthy diet.

Because all food portions within each exchange list provide approximately the same calories, proteins, fats, and carbohydrates per serving, it is easy to construct a diet consisting of the recommended percentages of:

- carbohydrates: 60–70% of total calories
- fats: 15–25% of total calories
- protein: 15–20% of total calories
- dietary fiber: at least 50 g.

Of the carbohydrates ingested, 90% should be complex carbohydrates or naturally occurring sugars. Intake of refined carbohydrate and concentrated sugars (including honey, pasteurized fruit juices, and dried fruit, as well as sugar and white flour) should be limited to less than 10% of the total calorie intake.

Constructing a diet which meets these recommendations is simple using the exchange lists. In addition, the recommendations ensure a high intake of vital whole foods, particularly vegetables, rich in nutritional value. Following are examples of exchange recommendations.

1,500 calorie vegan diet

- List 1 – vegetables: 5 servings
- List 2 – fruits: 2 servings
- List 3 – breads, cereals, and starchy vegetables: 9 servings
- List 4 – beans: 2.5 servings
- List 5 – fats: 4 servings.

This recommendation would result in an intake of approximately 1,500 calories, of which 67% are derived from complex carbohydrates and naturally occurring sugars, 18% from fat, and 15% from protein. The protein intake is entirely from plant sources, but still provides approximately 55 g; this number is well above the recommended daily allowance of protein intake for someone requiring 1,500 calories. At least one-half of the fat servings should be from nuts, seeds, and other whole foods from the Fat Exchange List. The dietary fiber intake would be approximately 31–74.5 g:

- percentage of calories as carbohydrates: 67%
- percentage of calories as fats: 18%
- percentage of calories as protein: 15%
- protein content: 55 g
- dietary fiber content: 31–74.5 g.

1,500 calorie omnivore diet

- List 1 – vegetables: 5 servings
- List 2 – fruits: 2.5 servings
- List 3 – breads, cereals, and starchy vegetables: 6 servings
- List 4 – beans: 1 serving
- List 5 – fats: 5 servings
- List 6 – milk: 1 serving
- List 7 – meats, fish, cheese, and eggs: 2 servings.

- Percentage of calories as carbohydrates: 67%
- Percentage of calories as fats: 18%
- Percentage of calories as protein: 15%

- Protein content: 61 g (75% from plant sources)
- Dietary fiber content: 19.5–53.5 g.

2,000 calorie vegan diet

- List 1 – vegetables: 5.5 servings
- List 2 – fruits: 2 servings
- List 3 – breads, cereals, and starchy vegetables: 11 servings
- List 4 – beans: 5 servings
- List 5 – fats: 8 servings.

- Percentage of calories as carbohydrates: 67%
- Percentage of calories as fats: 18%
- Percentage of calories as protein: 15%
- Protein content: 79 g
- Dietary fiber content: 48.5–101.5 g.

2,000 calorie omnivore diet

- List 1 – vegetables: 5 servings
- List 2 – fruits: 2.5 servings
- List 3 – breads, cereals, and starchy vegetables: 13 servings
- List 4 – beans: 2 servings
- List 5 – fats: 7 servings
- List 6 – milk: 1 serving
- List 7 – meats, fish, cheese, and eggs: 2 servings.

- Percentage of calories as carbohydrates: 66%
- Percentage of calories as fats: 19%
- Percentage of calories as protein: 15%
- Protein content: 78 g (72% from plant sources)
- Dietary fiber content: 32.5–88.5 g.

2,500 calorie vegan diet

- List 1 – vegetables: 8 servings
- List 2 – fruits: 3 servings
- List 3 – breads, cereals, and starchy vegetables: 17 servings
- List 4 – beans: 5 servings
- List 5 – fats: 8 servings.

- Percentage of calories as carbohydrates: 69%
- Percentage of calories as fats: 15%
- Percentage of calories as protein: 16%
- Protein content: 101 g
- Dietary fiber content: 33–121 g.

2,500 calorie omnivore diet

- List 1 – vegetables: 8 servings
- List 2 – fruits: 3.5 servings
- List 3 – breads, cereals, and starchy vegetables: 17 servings
- List 4 – beans: 2 servings
- List 5 – fats: 8 servings
- List 6 – milk: 1 serving
- List 7 – meats, fish, cheese, and eggs: 3 servings.

- Percentage of calories as carbohydrates: 66%
- Percentage of calories as fats: 18%
- Percentage of calories as protein: 16%
- Protein content: 102 g (80% from plant sources)
- Dietary fiber content: 40.5–116.5 g.

3,000 calorie vegan diet

- List 1 – vegetables: 10 servings
- List 2 – fruits: 4 servings
- List 3 – breads, cereals, and starchy vegetables: 17 servings
- List 4 – beans: 6 servings
- List 5 – fats: 10 servings.

- Percentage of calories as carbohydrates: 70%
- Percentage of calories as fats: 16%
- Percentage of calories as protein: 14%
- Protein content: 116 g
- Dietary fiber content: 50–84 g.

3,000 calorie omnivore diet

- List 1 – vegetables: 10 servings
- List 2 – fruits: 3 servings
- List 3 – breads, cereals, and starchy vegetables: 20 servings
- List 4 – beans: 2 servings
- List 5 – fats: 10 servings
- List 6 – milk: 1 serving
- List 7 – meats, fish, cheese, and eggs: 3 servings.

- Percentage of calories as carbohydrates: 67%
- Percentage of calories as fats: 18%
- Percentage of calories as protein: 15%
- Protein content: 116 g (81% from plant sources)
- Dietary fiber content: 45–133 g.

(Note: Use these recommendations as the basis for calculating other calorie diets. For example, for a 4,000 calorie diet add the 2,500 to the 1,500. For a 1,000 calorie diet divide the 2,000 calorie diet by 2.)

NUTRITIONAL SUPPLEMENTATION

The term nutritional supplementation includes the use of vitamins, minerals, and other food factors to support good health as well as preventing or treating illness. The key functions of nutrients like vitamins and minerals in the human body revolve around their role as essential components in enzymes and coenzymes. One of the key concepts in nutritional medicine is to supply the necessary support or nutrients to allow the enzymes of a particular tissue to work at their optimum levels. The concept of "biochemical individuality" was coined by nutritional biochemist Roger Williams in the 1970s to recognize the wide range in enzymatic activity and nutritional needs of humans. These observations also provided the basis for "orthomolecular medicine" as envisioned by two time Nobel laureate Linus Pauling.

Pharmacological aspects

In addition to serving as necessary components in enzymes and coenzymes, many nutrients appear to exert pharmacological effects. Most of these effects appear to be the result of enzyme induction. In other words, when used at supraphysiological levels nutrients can induce the manufacture of enzymes, induce enzymes to become more active, or even inhibit enzyme action. For example, the B vitamin niacin (nicotinic acid) is well known as a lipid-lowering agent when given at high dosages (2–6 g/day in divided dosages). Its mechanism of action is quite diverse, but appears to be via inhibiting enzymes which manufacture of VLDL while simultaneously stimulating the production or activity of enzymes which take up LDL in the liver. The advantage of using nutrients at pharmacological dosages is that they are more recognizable and better metabolized by the body as evident by a broader therapeutic index. Even so, the use of nutrients as pharmacological agents is closely akin to drug therapy. That being the case, it is imperative that they be used and monitored appropriately.

The growing popularity of nutritional supplementation

Growing numbers of Americans are taking nutritional supplements, with one industry source estimating a growth rate of 25% per annum for the past 5 years. Over 100 million Americans now take dietary supplements on a regular basis. Despite the tremendous body of research supporting the use of nutritional supplementation, most medical experts and researchers have still not publicly endorsed nutritional supplementation even though 98% of them take supplements themselves.

Numerous studies have demonstrated that most Americans consume a diet inadequate in nutritional value. Comprehensive studies sponsored by the US government (HANES I and II, Ten State Nutrition Survey, USDA nationwide food consumption studies, etc.) have revealed that marginal nutrient deficiencies exist in a substantial portion of the US population (approximately 50%) and that for some selected nutrients in certain age groups more than 80% of the group consumed less than the RDA.[43]

While most Americans are deficient in many vitamins and minerals, the level of deficiency is usually not severe enough to result in obvious signs and symptoms of nutrient deficiency. A severe deficiency disease like scurvy (lack of vitamin C) is extremely rare, but marginal vitamin C deficiency is thought to be relatively common. The term "subclinical" deficiency is often used to describe marginal nutrient deficiencies. A subclinical or marginal deficiency indicates a deficiency of a particular vitamin or mineral that is not severe enough to produce a classic deficiency sign or symptom. In many instances the only clue of a subclinical nutrient deficiency may be fatigue, lethargy, difficulty in concentration, a lack of well-being, or some other vague symptom. Diagnosis of subclinical deficiencies is an extremely difficult process that involves detailed dietary or laboratory analysis. In most cases it is not worth the cost to perform these tests because they are usually more expensive than a year-long trial of the vitamin thought to be needed.

The RDA is inadequate

Recommended Dietary Allowances (RDAs) for vitamins and minerals have been prepared by the Food and Nutrition Board of the National Research Council since 1941. These guidelines were originally developed to reduce the rates of severe nutritional deficiency diseases such as scurvy (deficiency of vitamin C), pellagra (deficiency of niacin) and beri-beri (deficiency of vitamin B_1), not to promote optimal health. Another problem is that the RDAs were designed to serve as the basis for evaluating the adequacy of diets of groups of people, not individuals. As stated by the Food and Nutrition Board: "Individuals with special nutritional needs are not covered by the RDAs."[43] Finally, the RDAs were designed for normal, "healthy" people experiencing no unusual stressors.

A tremendous amount of scientific research indicates that the "optimal" level for many nutrients, especially the so-called antioxidant nutrients such as vitamins C and E, beta-carotene, and selenium, may be much higher than their current RDA. The RDAs focus only on the prevention of nutritional deficiencies in population groups; they do not define "optimal" intake for an individual.

Other factors the RDAs do not adequately take into consideration are environmental and lifestyle factors which can destroy vitamins and bind minerals. For example, even the Food and Nutrition Board acknowledges that smokers require at least twice as much vitamin C as non-smokers. But, the effect of smoking on other nutrients and the effects of alcohol consumption, food additives, heavy metals (lead, mercury, etc.), carbon monoxide, and other chemicals associated with our modern society are not considered (for a comprehensive discussion of this important topic, see Ch. 108).

Accessory nutrients

In addition to essential nutrients, there are a number of food components and natural physiological agents which have demonstrated impressive health-promoting effects. Many examples are contained in Section V: Pharmacology of Natural Medicines, such as carotenoids, flavonoids, probiotics, carnitine, and coenzyme Q_{10}. These compounds exert significant therapeutic effects with little, if any, toxicity. More and more research indicates that these accessory nutrients, although not considered "essential" in the classical sense, play a major role in preventing illness.

SUMMARY

Nutritional medicine involves the use of dietary therapies and supplementation with naturally occurring compounds to provide an optimal nutritional state for the cellular environment. Nutritional medicine is one of the key foundations of naturopathic medicine and involves adherence to some basic concepts, yet must be tailored for the individual to account for biochemical individuality.

REFERENCES

1. Eaton SB, Konner M. Paleolithic nutrition. A consideration of its nature and current implications. New Engl J Med 1985; 312: 283–289
2. Ryde D. What should humans eat. Practitioner 1985; 232: 415–418
3. National Research Council. Diet and health. Implications for reducing chronic disease risk. Washington, DC: National Academy Press. 1989
4. Trowell H, Burkitt D. Western diseases: their emergence and prevention. Harvard University Press. 1981; Trowell H, Burkitt D, Heaton K. Dietary fibre, fibre-depleted foods and disease. New York, NY: Academic Press. 1985
5. US Dept of Health and Human Services. The Surgeon General's report on nutrition and health. Rocklin, CA: Prima. 1988
6. Willett WC, Stampfer MJ, Manson JE. Intake of trans fatty acids and risk of coronary heart disease among women. Lancet 1993; 341: 581–585
7. Longnecker MP. Do trans fatty acids in margarine and other foods increase the risk of coronary heart disease? Epidemiology 1993; 4: 492–495
8. Booyens J, Van Der Merwe CF. Margarines and coronary artery disease. Med Hypothesis 1992; 37: 241–244
9. Mensink RP, Katan MB. Effect of dietary trans fatty acids on high-density and low-density lipoprotein cholesterol levels in healthy subjects. New Engl J Med 1990; 323: 439–445
10. Quillin P. Safe eating. New York, NY: Evans. 1990
11. Fan AM, Jackson RJ. Pesticides and food safety. Regulatory Toxicol Pharmacol 1989; 9: 158–174
12. Sterling T, Arundel AV. Health effects of phenoxy herbicides. Scand J Work Environ Health 1986; 12: 161–173
13. Wigle DT, Semenciw RM, Wilkins K et al. Mortality study of Canadian male farm operators. Non-Hodgkin's lymphoma mortality and agricultural practices in Saskatchewan. J Nat Canc Inst 1990; 82: 575–582
14. Mott L, Broad M. Pesticides in food. San Francisco, CA: National Resources Defense Council. 1984
15. Falck F, Ricci A, Wolff MS. Pesticides and polychlorinated biphenyl residues in human breast lipids and their relation to breast cancer. Archives of Environmental Health 1992; 47: 143–146
16. Sharpe RM, Skakkebaek NE. Are oestrogens involved in falling sperm counts and disorders of the male reproduction tract. Lancet 1993; 341: 1392–1395
17. Newberne P, Conner MW. Food additives and contaminants. An update. Cancer 1986; 58: 1851–1862
18. Furia T, ed. CRC handbook of food additives, vols 1 and 2. Boca Raton, Fl: CRC Press. 1980
19. Golightly LK, Smolinske SS, Bennett ML. Pharmaceutical excipients. Adverse effects associated with inactive ingredients in drug products. Med Toxicol 1988; 3: 128–165
20. Collins-Williams C. Clinical spectrum of adverse reactions to tartrazine. J Asthma 1985; 22: 139–143
21. Neuman I, Elian R, Nahum H et al. The danger of "yellow dyes" (tartrazine) to allergic subjects. Clin Allergy 1978; 8: 65–68
22. Natbony SF, Phillips ME, Elias JM et al. Histologic studies of chronic idiopathic urticaria. J Allergy Clin Immunol 1983; 71: 177–183
23. Warrington RJ, Sauder PJ, McPhillips S. Cell-mediated immune responses to artificial food additives in chronic urticaria 1986; 16: 527–533
24. Michaelsson G, Juhlin L. Urticaria induced by preservatives and dye additives to food and drugs. Br J Derm 1973; 88: 525–534
25. Thune P, Granhold A. Provocation tests with anti-phlogistic and food additives in recurrent urticaria. Dermatologica 1975; 151: 360–372
26. Ros AM, Juhlin L, Michaelsson G. A follow-up study of patients with recurrent urticaria and hypersensitivity to aspirin, benzoates and azo dyes. Br J Derm 1976; 95: 19–24
27. Warin RP, Smith RJ. Challenge test battery in chronic urticaria. Br J Derm 1976; 94: 401–410
28. Kaaber K. Colouring and preservative agents and chronic urticaria. Value of a provocative trial and elimination diet. Ugeskr Laeger 1978; 140: 1473–1476
29. Meynadier J, Guilhou J, Meynadier J et al. Chronic urticaria. Ann Derm Venereol 1979; 106: 153–158
30. Lindemayr H, Schmidt J. Intolerance to acetylsalicylic acid and food additives in patients suffering from chronic urticaria. Wien Klin Wochenschr 1979; 91: 817–822
31. Gibson A, Clancy R. Management of chronic idiopathic urticaria by the identification and exclusion of dietary factors. Clin Allergy 1980; 10: 699–704
32. Doeglas HMG. Reactions to aspirin and food additives in patients with chronic urticaria, including the physical urticaria. Br J Derm 1975; 93: 135–144
33. Settipane GA, Chafee FH, Postman IM. Significance of tartrazine sensitivity in chronic urticaria of unknown etiology. J Allergy Clin Immunol 1976; 57: 541–549
34. Juhlin L. Recurrent urticaria. clinical investigation of 330 patients. Br J Derm 1981; 104: 369–381
35. Ortolani C et al. Diagnosis of intolerance to food additives. Ann Allergy 1984; 53: 587–591
36. Juhlin L. Additives and chronic urticaria. Ann Allergy 1987; 59: 119–123
37. Supramaniam G, Warner JO. Artificial food additive intolerance in patients with angio-oedema and urticaria. Lancet 1986; ii: 907–909
38. Llaurado JG. The saga of BHT and BHA in life extension myths. J Am Coll Nutr 1985; 4: 481–484
39. Simon RA. Sulfite sensitivity. Annals Allergy 1986; 56: 281–288
40. Feingold N. Why your child is hyperactive. New York, NY: Random House. 1975
41. American Medical Association. Drinking water and human health. Chicago, IL: American Medical Association. 1984
42. National Research Council. Recommended Dietary Allowances. 10th edn., Washington, DC: National Academy Press. 1989

CHAPTER CONTENTS

45

Peat therapeutics and balneotherapy

Mark D. Groven, ND

INTRODUCTION

Balneology refers to the art and science of bathing. Balneotherapy is the use of baths, peloids and other natural substances as well as various climatic elements singly or in combination with each other for the prevention and treatment of disease. The term peloid refers to the pulp of a substance which is applied to the body. Common peloids include peat pulp, lake or sea muds and plant substances to name a few.

For many conditions balneotherapy is a preferable treatment to the pharmacological approach due to the side-effects of synthetic drugs. The combination of balneotherapy and peliodtherapy and the percutaneous absorption of their constituents along with the physiological and psychological effects provide an excellent therapy for those who can no longer tolerate oral or injectable pharmaceuticals and are suffering from chronic degenerative diseases. Life is stressful and our society is aging. We would be wise to utilize the positive benefits of balneotherapy in the conventional treatment of illness along with maintenance and prevention of disease.[1–4] The purpose of this chapter is to describe the general concept of balneotherapy with emphasis on the medicinal application of peat.

BALNEOLOGY

History

Therapeutic bathing is an ancient art and probably the oldest of medical procedures. It enjoyed tremendous popularity until about 75 years ago when, along with other natural techniques, it fell out of favor as conventional medicine produced its modern successes. Since then, the large corpus of empirical wisdom has been expanded upon and much scientific evidence has contributed to the advancement of balneology as a science. Many of balneotherapies' modern day roots lie predominantly in European spas which have some of the longest continuous running histories of any medical institution.

Millions of patients flock to clinics throughout Europe and the world each year for treatment in hydrology departments under the supervision of physicians and their staffs. They provide a variety of balneotherapeutic techniques.[1–23,31]

Regular research continues in this emerging field. Every 4 years a conference of the International Society of Medical Hydrology and Climatology presents new scientific research and validates its findings.

Physiological effects

Balneotherapeutics consider direct and indirect actions on the body. The *direct actions* of balneotherapy take into consideration the physical actions of water on the body such as hydrostatic pressure, buoyancy, viscosity and frictional resistance, as well as thermal effects and the chemical and pharmacological effects of the percutaneous absorption of the substance being used. These substances include hot spring waters of various types such as carbon dioxide, hydrogen sulfide, chloride, sulfate, iron, acid, or radon. Peat muds, plant preparations and mineral-containing muds are also used. In Europe, peat bath and peloids are traditional. These applications are used in combination with exercise, aquatics, steam bath, sauna therapy, climatotherapy, physical therapy and pharmacotherapy, among others, with important consideration during treatment being given to the chronobiological and circadian rhythmic phases of the body.[1–4,22,25]

The *indirect actions* of balneotherapy arise from the repeated application of therapeutic stimulation such as climatic exposure to the elements, training effects of exercises and social and psychological effects arising from changes in environment. These elements act as a complex stimulation in a *non-specific* manner of the physiological function of the organism's central nervous system, autonomic nervous system, endocrine system, immune system, etc. The result of these stimulations is a reactive response by the body leading to activation and improvement of capacity, adaptation, and self-healing potential. In other words balneotherapy has a normalizing effect on the body's systems and rhythms.[2,4,7,11,10,15]

Skin response

The skin is a reflex, metabolic and immune organ. It affects the autonomic, immune and circulatory systems and participates in the biosynthesis of not only vitamin D, but acetylcholine, histamine, and serotonin as well.[2,4,10,15] With baths, significantly higher concentrations of minerals and medicaments can be reached in the epidermis than with systemic flooding via the vascular system.

The primary effects of bath components take place within the skin. For instance hydrogen sulfide acts as a radical trap for oxygen radicals. This functions to reduce inflammation. It is thought that the action comes from the effect of sulfur on the Langerhans cells which play a role in immune presentation and inflammation modulation. In this way, skin responses can act as transmitter activating helping functions. Sulfur-containing peat baths show a pain-reducing and healing effect on rheumatic and degenerative disease. One reason may be because of the reduction in Langerhans cell activity which results from the combination of the components within peat and thermal radiation.[7,15,20,24]

PEAT THERAPEUTICS

History

Peat is a substance that has been used as a medicinal preparation in baths and peloid packs extensively in Europe for the past 200 years. This unique substance contains many chemical constituents which can interact with organic and inorganic compounds. The scientific basis for the physical, chemical and pharmacological effects of peat baths has been long known and used extensively in balneotherapeutic applications in Europe and other parts of the world to treat rheumatic diseases, gynecological disorders, osteoarthritis, lumbago, sciatica, skin diseases, trauma and its sequelae and many other aliments and afflictions. The many substances in peat offer a vast possibility of medicinal cure applications.[6,8–11,17,18,20,23–26,29,31–35]

It is important to consider the region and origin of the peat being used for medicinal purposes. Low moor peat has been shown to contain higher concentrations of nitrous substances, which are thought to contain a higher content of biologically active substances than the high moor peats or peats taken from a shallower depth. It is not just high nitrous content that makes a certain peat more medically useful, but the quality, type and amount of the biologically active substances it contains that is the determining factor on medicinal effect. In Germany these types of peats are now a national resource.[15,16]

Physiological effects

Peat has a structure containing micropores, which accounts for its sponge-like water carrying capacity and its ability to maintain either hot or cold temperatures. When applied, peat produces a gradient rise or fall in temperature which is especially desirable in a therapeutic bath. A peat bath influences the neuromuscular, endocrinological, blood in pulmonary and kidney hemodynamics depending on the consistency volume, partial or full bath.[4,10]

Peat has well documented effects such as tissue dilation, increase in stroke volume and metabolism and immunological stimulation. Peat bath may be preferable to water bath if one considers the gradient rise and fall of temperature, increased buoyancy and prevention of heat loss during a bath and the possible positive chemical and pharmacological effects of the constituents of peat.[1–4,6,8,15,19,21,25,26,32,33]

Peat substances are able to permeate the skin. Their absorption and action has been documented by the comparison of placebo, water, and peat bath using Doppler ultrasound measurement. One study which measured circulation in the uterine artery after bath therapy showed that only the peat bath achieves the physiological effect of prolonged vasodilation and circulation. This effect lasts for several hours after the treatment and is only achieved with the peat bath. It is thought that absorption of peat substances takes place through the hair follicles and apocrine glands by diffusion and partial pinocytosis.[10]

The functions of peat in medicinal applications are antimicrobial, antiviral, anti-inflammatory, and antineoplastic, to name a few.[6,9–11,21] Many biochemical effects have been demonstrated in humans and animals. These include elevation of protein synthesis, estrogen stimulation, reduction of arachidonic acid, and inhibition of inflammatory mediators such as leukotrienes, prostaglandins, and thromboxane. Biological activity is ascribed to peat ingredients such as sulfur compounds, magnesium, manganese, iron and humic acids.[6,7,10,11,16,20,26,33]

CLINICAL APPLICATIONS

Peat has many beneficial applications.

Human papilloma virus

Antiviral effects of peat have been demonstrated on several viruses, including the human papilloma virus. Remission and prevention of implantation of the virus has been described. This is a measure which prevents cancer. The antiviral and antineoplastic effects are thought to be associated with the ability of peat constituents such as humate to bind on lectin binding junctions blocking viral entry into cells.[9,10]

Infertility

A study on infertility due to immature follicle maturation syndrome demonstrated good results with peat therapy in comparison to the group receiving pharmacotherapy. In the peat therapy group, the rate of pregnancy was very good, along with a practically non-existent spontaneous abortion rate, while in the pharmaceutical group the rate of spontaneous abortions was very high.[36]

Ankylosing spondylitis

In the treatment of ankylosing spondylitis, peat therapy has shown a decrease in the level of C-reactive protein and an elevation of hemoglobin with a series of treatments. This coincided with a significant decrease in pain and an increase in function.[26,28]

Hematoma

Organic peat with its intense vasodilating and anti-inflammatory effects, and interactions of its ions and mineral properties, including free iron not transported by macrophages, is an efficient therapy for the treatment of hematomas. Hematomas treated with thermal peat application were resolved 50% faster, with no hemosiderin residue, as compared with treatment with only heat applications which often left residues.[23]

Immune stimulation

Peat bath in combination with hyperthermia shows leukocyte elevation. The immune-stimulating effects of peat bath seen clinically correspond to heamotological changes after baths.[33]

PROCEDURE

The following procedures should be applied with care and forethought as to diagnosis and the skillful administration of the treatment. These procedures are stimulations to the body and the thermal effects should not be taken lightly. Patients must be thoroughly screened for contraindications to treatment before doing full-body immersion hyperthermia.

Hyperthermic medicinal peat bath

The indications and contraindications of this procedure are given in Table 45.1.

Materials

- Peat bath material – the author uses Dr Schirmer's formula
- Tub with water thermometer and safety features like handrails and non-slip floor mats
- Room with table for perspiration time
- Gown or loose-fitting bathing suit
- Two sheets
- Three wool blankets
- Two large towels (one for patient to dry off after treatment and one for head wrap)
- Basin with ice water and a face cloth
- Digital thermometer or otothermometer for patient monitoring (no glass mercury thermometers)

Table 45.1 Indications and contraindications for hyperthermic medicinal peat bath

Indications	Contraindications
Acne	Pre-existing high fever
Arthritis pain	Open wounds
Back pain	Cardiac deficiency
Benign prostatic hypertrophy	Pulmonary deficiency
Bursitis	Respiratory insufficiency
Carpal tunnel syndrome	Lupus
Fibromyalgia	Acute hypertension
Flu	Diabetes
Fractures	Pregnancy
Acute gouty toe	Breast feeding
Chronic gout	Multiple sclerosis
Gynecological disorders	
Headaches	
Hematomas	
Hives	
Insomnia	
Lumbalgia	
Metabolic disorders	
Muscle tension	
Neurological disorders	
Obesity	
Orthopedic disorders	
Osteoarthritis	
Postoperative rehabilitation	
Premenstrual syndrome	
Prostatitis	
Psoriasis	
Rashes	
Rheumatoid arthritis	
Sciatica	
Skin care	
Sprains	
Strains	
Stress relief	
Trauma	
Viral infections	

- Exhaust fan or room air filter
- Foot stool for entering and leaving tub.

The design of the bath area should take into consideration getting patients in and out of the tub and then as directly as possible to a treatment table.

Procedure

1. Patients should be ruled out for cardiovascular risk or any other conditions which do not respond to or are aggravated by thermal therapy before treatments begin.
2. Make sure the tank is clean without a ring. Check log book on last treatment and cleaning. If any evidence of an unclean tank is seen, it must be cleaned and disinfected before use. This is done by using rubber gloves with a scouring sponge and scrubbing tank with disinfectant soap followed by a rinse of first hot and then cold water. Follow this by spraying the surface with 10% bleach solution and wait 10 minutes before rinsing with very hot water.
3. Fill the tank 10 inches from the top with water at a temperature of 105–113°F (41–45°C).
4. The starting temperature and possible duration of treatment are determined by the condition.
5. Straight water bath should not exceed 110°F. With peat additive do not exceed 113°F.
6. Add peat to the bath.
7. Close monitoring during treatment by periodic recording of the patient's pulse, oral temperature, duration of treatment and tank temperature is necessary. A quick spike in pulse above initial pulse within the first minute or minutes is a contraindication to treatment. Any adverse reaction such as fingers and toes tingling, nausea, headache, light-headedness or dizziness should be evaluated closely and treatment terminated. For some patients they may only be able to tolerate a low temperature and short duration for the first treatment. When doing a series of treatments, the first treatment is of shorter duration and lower temperature to see how the patient responds. The ability to tolerate treatments should improve as patients acclimatize through their series of treatments.
8. The patient should enter extremely still water slowly. It will not feel as hot if the water is still.
9. Have them remain still as they become fully immersed to help decrease the sensation of intense heat.
10. To treat the pelvis utilize a sitz bath rather than a full bath to concentrate the effects of the treatment.
11. The water will cool as time passes, although the peat material will help maintain the temperature. If the starting temperature was 105°F, hot water may need to be added.
12. Bath duration is 8–20 minutes and should not exceed 20 minutes.
13. If the patient becomes fatigued or distressed, they should exit the bath to awaiting sheet and wool blankets. Do not wait.
14. As the patient exits the tub, they must have help from two people who provide lifting support from under the arms bilaterally. This is a time to be very careful.
15. Encourage the patient to concentrate on walking on their own.
16. Have them lie down on a fresh sheet and wrap them in both sheets and two or three wool blankets. Cover the head with a towel.
17. Continue to monitor pulse and oral temperature for the duration of the 20 minute perspiration time.
18. Rinse a face cloth in cold water and wipe perspiration from patients face frequently during both bath and perspiration time. This is done every 1 or 2 minutes and is extremely important.
19. Encourage the patient to relax and help them keep their mind on pleasant matters during the bath.
20. After the patient has been wrapped from head to foot in sheet and wool blankets, allow them to go through

hydrotherapy reaction of rise and fall in temperature, pulse and diaphoresis three times before they are removed from sheet and allowed to return to normal activities.

21. Have the patient rest and replace electrolytes after treatment.

22. During the perspiration time, manual traction can be applied to the spine. This is done by grasping the patient's ankles when they are supine and pulling for 30–45 seconds with enough traction that they almost slide on the table. Indications for manual traction are disc problems, scoliosis, impingement.

23. Advise the patient not to shower with soap for up to 12 hours after peat bath as absorption rates continue post-bath if peat additives have been used.

24. Patients should dry thoroughly and remain covered, warm and *out of draft* for 3 hours post-treatment.

25. Clean the tank and room thoroughly after use. Log out time of bath and tank cleaning.

Medicinal peat peloid

The indications and contraindications of this procedure are given in Table 45.2.

Materials

- Peat pulp
- Large towel

Table 45.2 Indications and contraindications for medicinal peat peloid

Indications	Contraindications
Acne	Open wounds
Arthritis pain	Pregnancy
Back pain	Very thin fragile skin
Bursitis	Heat insensitive skin
Carpal tunnel syndrome	Allergies to any of the peloid materials
Fibromyalgia	
Fractures	
Acute gouty toe	
Chronic gout	
Headaches	
Hematomas	
Hives	
Lumbalgia	
Muscle tension	
Molluscum contagiosum	
Orthopedic disorders	
Osteoarthritis	
Postoperative rehabilitation	
Premenstrual syndrome	
Prostatitis	
Psoriasis	
Rashes	
Rheumatoid arthritis	
Sciatica	
Skin care	
Sprains	
Strains	
Stress relief	
Trauma	

- Small towel
- Face cloth
- Small blanket to cover hydrocollator
- Two small stainless basins
- One small paper cup
- Hydrocollator (hot water bottle can alternately be used).

Procedure

This is a thermal peat pack and utilizes Dr Schirmer's technique and medicinal peat formula.

The procedure is as follows:

1. Make a square layer of peat material about 0.25 inches thick, 2 inches bilateral of the spine and 6–8 inches long over the spine. If you are not treating the spinal area, cover the area to be treated. Try to make the area of application flat and level.

2. Cover the peat directly with a warm wet face cloth. Remember borders of peloid exactly by ridging the facecloth around the margins of the peat.

3. Border the wet face cloth-covered peloid with a rolled bath towel, making a quarter turn while folding the towel to match the margin of the peat.

4. Apply one layer of towel over the face cloth and peat material.

5. Put a fresh hydrocollator pack directly over the towel. The hydrocollator should be heated at a gently boil for 1 hour prior to using. *Do not allow any exposed skin to come in contact with the hot pack.*

6. Cover the hydrocollator pack with a towel or small blanket to insulate and prevent heat loss.

7. Have a cup of cold water ready to pour on the wet face cloth-covered peloid if it gets too hot. In a good treatment the peloid pack should get hot enough to require two to three dowsings of water.

8. As soon as the patient tells you that the pack is getting too hot, lift up the hydrocollator pack and towel and pour the water directly over the face cloth-covered peloid until cool. Then replace the hydrocollator and coverings.

9. *Never leave the patient unattended!*

10. Treatment time is approximately 25 minutes.

11. To remove the peat from the skin after treatment, slide a small basin along the skin under the peat, scraping the peat into the bowl. Wipe with a full face cloth wetted with warm water in a gentle twisting motion back and forth to remove peat residue from the skin.

12. Cover the treated area after treatment to maintain warmth for 3 hours.

Partial immersion medicinal peat bath

The indications and contraindications of this procedure are given in Table 45.3.

Table 45.3 Indications and contraindications of partial immersion medicinal peat bath

Indications	Contraindications
Arthritis pain	Open wounds
Bursitis	Pregnancy
Carpal tunnel syndrome	Heat-insensitive area
Eczema	
Fibromyalgia	
Fractures	
Acute gouty toe	
Chronic gout	
Hematomas	
Orthopedic disorders	
Osteoarthritis	
Plantar fascitis	
Postoperative rehabilitation	
Psoriasis	
Rashes	
Rheumatoid arthritis	
Skin care	
Sprains	
Strains	
Tendinitis	
Tenosynovitis	
Trauma	

Materials

- Deep well basin – the tall plastic waste basket size works well for the leg
- Medicinal peat bath
- Water thermometer
- Small towel.

Procedure

1. Fill basin to three-quarters full with 108–114°F water.
2. Add peat to the bath.
3. Have the patient immerse their wrist, ankle, or elbow slowly into the water. Try to immerse the forearm and leg if treating the hand or foot.
4. Keep the body part immersed for 25 minutes.
5. After the treatment, cover the area with a wool sock or clothing and keep covered for 3 hours post-treatment.
6. Often peat material will be sent home with the patient to do home treatments.
7. Clean up the basin by washing with antimicrobial soap. Then disinfect with 10% bleach solution and rinse after 10 minutes.

CONCLUSION

As a physician using Dr Shirmer's technique and peat formula, I have seen accelerated results that would not be achieved with any other method. I have seen excellent results for:

- arthritis
- tenosynovitis
- strains and sprains
- plantar fascitis
- low back pain including sciatica
- scoliosis
- fractures
- gout
- muscle pain
- dermatologic conditions such as eczema.

The combination of medical sophistication in diagnosis and application of various balneological methods provides an excellent tool for the physician to treat in a natural way to the great benefit of their patients.

REFERENCES

1. Praetzel HG. Forty years of medical balneology and climatology. Director Medical Institute of Balneology and Climatology. Germany: Ludwig Maxmillions University. 1990
2. Agishi Y, Ohtsuka Y, Watanabe I et al. Effects of therapeutic elements on physiological funtions in man and balneotherapy recent progress in medical balneology and climatology. Hokkaido University Medical Library Series, Vol. 34. 1995
3. Yuko A, Yoshinori O. Recent progress in medical balneology. Hokkaido University Medical Library Series, Vol 34. 1995
4. Praetzel HG, Schnizer W. Handbook of medical bath. Heidelberg, Germany: Karl F Haug GMBH. 1992
5. Praetzel HG. Preface. Health Resort Medicine. 32nd World Congress of I.S.M.H. Bad Worishofen Germany, April 1994
6. Scheffel KZ, Praetzel HG. Analgesic effects of humic acid bath. Health resort medicine. 32nd World Congress of I.S.M.H. Bad Worishofen, Germany, April 1994
7. Schmidt KL. Sulfur water. Compendium of balneology and cure medicine. Darmstadt: Steinkopff. 1989
8. Magyarosy KL, Resch KH, Krause W et al. Electromyographic research for the efficacy of function of peat packs on musculature of the back. Health resort medicine. 32nd World Congress of I.S.M.H. Bad Worishofen, Germany, April 1994
9. Beer M. Indications for gynecological balneotherapy. Health resort medicine. 32nd World Congress of I.S.M.H. Bad Worishofen Germany, April 1994
10. Goecke C. Efficacy of peat therapy. Health resort medicine. 32nd World Congress of I.S.M.H. Bad Worishofen Germany, April 1994
11. Solovieva VP, Sotnikova EP, Naumova GV, Kosobokova RV. Biologically active peat preparations and their possible applications in medicine. International Peat Society. Proceedings of the 6th International Peat Congress. Duluth, Minnesota, Aug 17–23, 1980
12. Kuhn G, Rohwer J, Buhring M. Balneotherapy for progressive systemic sclerosis. 2nd Symposium, sulfur in health resort medicine. Bad Nenndorf, May 1994
13. Elkayam O, Wigler I, Tishler M et al. Effect of spa therapy in Tiberias on patients with rheumatoid arthritis and osteoarthritis. J Rheumatol 1991; 18: 1799–1803
14. Sukenik S, Nieuman L, Buskila D et al. Dead Sea bath salts for the treatment of rheumatoid arthritis. Clin Exp Rheumatol 1990; 8: 353–357
15. Artmann C, Pratzel HG. Influence on the immune system by sulfur water bath. Sulfur in medicine. International symposium. Bad Nenndorf, Germany, May 1990
16. Bellometti S, Cecchettin M, Lalli L, Galzigna L. Mud pack

treatment increases serum antioxidant defenses in osteoarthrosic patients. Biomed Pharmacother 1996; 50: 37

17. Kotwica S, Split W et al. Spa treatment of sciatic pains at Swieradow. Neurol Neurochir Pol 1976; 10: 719–722
18. Kotwica S, Split W, Rog-Malinowski M, Gredziak B. Spa treatment of shoulder pains at Swieradow. Neurol Neurochir Pol 1976; 10: 715–717
19. Weislaw O, Turowski G, Turowski ZM. The influence of balneotherapy on T-cell populations and direct lymphocytotoxicity in patients with vascular disorders of lower limbs. Health Resort Medicine. 32nd world Congress of I.S.M.H. Bad Worishofen, Germany, April 1994
20. Praetzel HG, Aigner UM, Weinert D, Limbach B. The analgesic effects of sulfur peat baths for non-articular rheumatic afflictions. 2nd Symposium, Sulfur in Health Resort Medicine, Bad Nenndorf, May 1994
21. Ohtsuka Y, Yabunaka N, Watanabe I et al. Platelet antioxidative defense system is modified by balneotherapy and bathing temperature. In: New frontiers in health resort medicine. Japan: Noboribetsu Branch Hospital, Hokkaido University School of Medicine, No. 059–04, 1996
22. Agishi Y, Ohtsuka Y. Chronobiological aspects of cure treatment. In: New frontiers in health resort medicine. Japan: Noboribetsu Branch Hospital, Hokkaido University School of Medicine. No. 059–04, 1996
23. Olivera AP, Schirmer MH, Olivera VM. Treatment of hematomas with peat used in balneotherapy. J Med Esthetics 1997; 3: 1–3
24. Praetzel HG, Aigner UM, Wemert D et al. Therapeutic effects of sulfur-peat baths on patients with rheumatic muscle pain. Phys Rehab Kur Med 1992; 2: 92–97
25. Praetzel HG. Balneologically activated skin functions and their clinical evidence. J Japanese Assoc Phys Med Balneol Climatol 1993; 57: 11–13
26. Peter A. CRProteins of rheumatic afflictions. Physiotherapy 1987; 39: 331–335
27. Dafinova I, Boncheva DV. The effect of mud applications and helium-neon laser irradiation on osteoarthrosis patients with changes in knee joints. 32nd World Congress of the I.S.M.H. Bad Worishofen, Germany, April 1994
28. Tishler M, Yaron M, Brostovski Y. Effect of spa therapy in Tiberias on patients with ankylosing spondylitis. Clin Rheumatol 1995; 14: 21–25
29. Grigor'eva VD, Mamiliaeva DR. The use of low-temperature peloids in treating patients with rheumatoid arthritis(I). Vopr Kurortol Fizioter Lech Fiz Kult 1994; Sept/Oct: 17–21
30. Grigor'eva VD, Mamiliaeva DR. The use of low-temperature peloids in treating patients with rheumatoid arthritis(I). Vopr Kurortol Fizioter Lech Fiz Kult 1995; Jan/Feb: 20–23
31. Gyarmati. Heviz Hungary heilbad (curebath). International symposium. Bad Nenndorf, Germany, May 1990
32. Peter A, Flach R. Changes in immunoglobin G and acute phase proteins in bath cures. Physiother 1974; 26: 357–364
33. Callies R, Kaiser G. Leukocyte evaluation of RA for efficacy of a peat cure. Physiotherapy 1978; 30: 19–26
34. Siderov VD, Mamiliaeva DR. The current aspects of pelotherapy of patients with rheumatoid arthritis. Arthritis Rheum Aug 1994; 37: 1132–1137
35. Levitskii EF, Abdoulkina NG, Zaitsev AA et al. The optimization of the duration of the sanitarium-health resort treatment of patients with neurological manifestations of spinal osteochondrosis (I). Vopr Kurortol Fizioter Lech Fiz Kult 1996; Sep/Oct: 26–28
36. Dietrich J. Endocrinological changes after peat therapy. 32nd World Congress of I.S.M.H. Bad Worishofen, Germany, April 1994

CHAPTER CONTENTS

46

Soft tissue manipulation: diagnostic and therapeutic potential

Leon Chaitow, ND DO

INTRODUCTION

Acupuncture, osteopathy, chiropractic, naturopathic medicine, orthopedic medicine, and physiotherapy all pay attention to the diagnostic and therapeutic potential of the soft tissues of the body. These and other similar therapeutic systems have developed methods of identifying those aspects of soft tissue dysfunction which indicate disease or injury or reflex activity of some type. Regardless of the terms used or the theories propounded, all the systems seem to refer to the same phenomenon: distinct, palpable, usually sensitive areas of soft tissue aberration which are either directly or reflexively related to local or organ dysfunction.[1,2]

The sustained or intermittent adaptive results to the influences listed in Table 46.1 can result in progressive changes, summarized in Table 46.2. These adaptations are discussed fully on p. 391.

Soft tissue manipulation may be utilized to:

- normalize dysfunction preparatory to manipulation of osseous structures[9]
- restore postural or functional integrity – achieving what osseous adjustments can seldom achieve: actual alterations in structural position of musculoskeletal segments[10]

Table 46.1 Soft tissue stressors

- Congenital factors, such as short leg, small hemipelvis
- Birth trauma, such as cranial trauma from forceps delivery which distorts the internal cranial fascia – tentorium cerebelli and falx cerebri – which, because of body-wide fascial continuity, can cause distortions elsewhere
- Overuse, misuse or abuse of the musculoskeletal system in work or recreational settings
- Trauma – either repetitive minor forms or major incidents
- Reflexive factors, including myofascial trigger points
- Chronically held somatization influences generated by negative psychosomatic factors and emotional coping traits, including fear, anger, anxiety, depression, etc.
- Biochemical changes resulting from nutritional, toxic, endocrine, infectious and other influences

Table 46.2 Progressive adaptive changes to soft tissue stressors[3–7]

- An initial "alarm" response will occur in which tissues become hypertonic
- If not short term, localized oxygen deficit is probable, together with retention of metabolic waste products, both of which result in discomfort or pain and the likelihood of an increased hypertonic response
- The constant activity of the neural reporting stations of these tissues leads to increased sensitization and the development of a tendency to hyperreactivity (known in osteopathic medicine as "facilitation")[8]
- Macrophages become activated – along with increased vascularity, fibroblast action and connective tissue production – leading to cross-linkage and shortening of tissues
- Changes in the muscles as a result of hypertonicity which, if sustained, results in progressive fibrotic modification
- Sustained hypertonicity leads to drag on tendinous attachment to the periosteum, and the likelihood of pain and dysfunction in these tissues
- If such stressed tendons or muscles cross joints, they become crowded and their function is modified
- The antagonists of chronically hypertonic muscles will be reciprocally inhibited and, as a result, normal firing sequences of muscles may alter – e.g. where excessive activity of synergist muscles occur in order to take on the tasks of weakened (inhibited) primary movers
- Another possibility is that chronically shortened, hypertonic structures will have a sustained inhibitory effect on their antagonists – an example would be short, tight, erector spinae muscles and weakened (inhibited) abdominal muscles
- Chain reactions of such dysfunction can occur resulting from the shortening over time of postural muscles (type 1 fibers) and the inhibition and weakening (without shortening) of phasic muscles (type 2 fibers)
- Localized areas of hyperreactivity (facilitation) may evolve paraspinally or in particular stress-prone regions of any myofascial structures – trigger points and other reflexively related changes
- These triggers themselves become sources of further dysfunction
- Postural and functional changes will become apparent throughout the body, e.g. in relation to breathing function
- Therapeutic input at these stages involves a need to address the multiple changes which have occurred – reduce hypertonicity, resolve fibrotic changes, lengthen shortened structures, mobilize joints, deactivate trigger points – as well as removal of habitual patterns of use which have added to, or caused, the dysfunctional patterns, including postural and respiratory re-education
- The musculoskeletal changes described above may have components which include biomechanical, biochemical and psychological components, all of which need to be understood and, where possible, modified or removed

- function as part of a comprehensive approach to health care in which the reflex activity, as manifested in surface structures, is used diagnostically and therapeutically.[11]

The distinguished Western acupuncture pioneer, Dr Felix Mann, has stated that, with the vast number of acupuncture and other reflexively active points now charted, there is little, if any, of the body surface left which has not been ascribed therapeutic potential.[12] Thus he maintains that the traditional concept of points and meridians is no longer a valid hypothesis. He concludes that the whole body is, in fact, an acupuncture point. If other systems of identifying discreet areas of reflex potential in the soft tissue, such as Chapman's neurolymphatic reflexes[13] and Bennett's neurovascular reflexes[14] (see below), are examined alongside both traditional and more recently described acupuncture points, Mann's statement becomes readily acceptable.

SOFT TISSUE POINTS

A degree of reductionist thinking is necessary to understand the nature and value of the reflex areas, points, and zones that have been described by the many systems of soft tissue manipulation.

In general, these points can be divided into sensitive soft tissue alterations that result from physical strain or trauma (including the soft tissue effects of emotional stress) and alterations which are the result of reflex activity (e.g. viscerosomatic reflexes). These changes can be considered as adaptive responses to patterns of stress as outlined above.

Methods of identification

There are a variety of methods by which soft tissue changes may be located through palpation. These include:

- traditional massage methods
- specific palpation techniques, such as those developed by osteopathic and other schools[15]
- neuromuscular technique (a method of combined assessment and therapy developed in the 1930s by Stanley Lief, an American-trained naturopathic and chiropractic physician working in Europe)[11]
- skin distraction techniques evolved by the German connective tissue massage (Bindesgewebsmassage)[16] practitioners (see "Hyperalgesic skin zones", p. 397).

All of these, and other methods of palpation, may be utilized in order to identify areas of local soft tissue dysfunction which may be sources of, or results of, reflex activity or other local adaptive responses.[17]

The analysis of the available information present in localized areas of the soft tissues requires consideration of a variety of classifications and systems.

It is necessary to examine some of the systems which have described the same tissue changes in different ways, in order to compare the similarities and differences in the descriptions of "points" (discrete, usually sensitive, areas of altered structure and function in the soft tissue) and the diagnostic and therapeutic significance ascribed to them.

GENERAL SOFT TISSUE MANIPULATIVE TECHNIQUES

Therapeutic effort may be directed toward the diagnosis and correction of the mechanical aspects of dysfunction (trauma, strain, etc.) or toward the use of the available information from such reflex areas in a more wide-ranging, holistic approach to the health of the patient.

General, rhythmic techniques are often employed on the soft tissues to relieve local dysfunction and/or to prepare for subsequent adjustment of osseous structure. They may include all or some of the methods listed in Table 46.3.[9]

In all of these variations, the objectives are the improvement of circulation and drainage, release of contracture, and increased range of movement. Inhibition implies a degree of pressure sufficient to achieve reduction in hepertonia or neurological activity. All of these may be applied in a stimulatory as well as a relaxing manner, but care should be taken to prevent stimulation from becoming irritation.

DISCRETE PALPABLE POINTS RELATED TO TRAUMA OR STRAIN

Researchers and clinicians have used differing terminology to describe similar phenomena, resulting in confusion of what is essentially an uncomplicated pattern.

In the musculature and connective tissues of the body, often in the regions of the origins and insertions of the muscles, there are palpable, sensitive areas of altered structure resulting from injury, irritation, stress, etc. These have been described as "tender" points,[18] "trigger" points,[19] "Ah Shi" points in traditional acupuncture (literally spontaneously tender points'),[19] and "indurated" points,[20] among other descriptions.

Common to these points is their size, which ranges from 0.5 to 1.0 cm across, and their feel, which is described as harder or firmer than surrounding normal tissue, or as having an edematous or stringy feel.[18–21]

It is often noted that these localized areas of altered structure and function occur in bands of stressed fibers, both fascial and muscular. In all cases, such localized areas are, to a greater or lesser degree, sensitive or tender out of proportion to the degree of pressure exerted.[22] All these points are potential "trigger points", but only those which, upon pressure, are noted to refer pain or other symptoms to a distant (target) area are thus classified.[23]

Identification of these points as areas of localized dysfunction is dependent upon palpatory literacy – the ability of the examiner to readily distinguish between the texture and other characteristics of normal and abnormal tissues. Development of such a degree of sensitivity is a matter of practice and is readily acquired by any practitioner willing to spend but a little time touching, feeling, assessing, comparing, and judging what it is that is being felt.[15] In most, but not all, cases, these altered areas of structure and function are found to lie in shortened muscle tissue or fascia.[21,22]

The morphology of acupuncture points has been analyzed and described by various workers. Bossy[23] has noted that all of the maxima points described by Head,[24] the motor points of medical electrotherapy,[25] and fully 70% of Travell's trigger points,[26] are all acupuncture points described in Traditional Chinese Medicine.

As will be noted in the discussion below, there is also a large degree of overlap between these and points described in reflex systems, such as Chapman's neurolymphatic reflexes[13] (which include all the traditional acupuncture alarm points) and Bennett's neurovascular reflexes[14] (which includes all traditional acupuncture "associated" points).

Bossy notes that the common structures found under all acupuncture points include neurovascular structures,

Table 46.3 General soft tissues manipulative techniques

Technique	Description
Articulation	Repetitive passive movements employing leverage through variable ranges of the arc
Effleurage	Superficial drainage technique derived from massage therapy
Inhibition/Ischemic compression	Describes an objective rather than a method; consists of pressure applied for lengthy periods, slowly applied and slowly released, using thumb contact as a rule
Kneading	Deep or superficial rhythmical pressure, usually applied by thenar or hypothenar eminence
Positional release methods	Approaches which instead of acting directly on restricted or shortened structures aim to position these in a state of "ease" by moving away form restriction barriers, allowing a spontaneous normalization to occur involving neural (muscle spindle) resetting and circulatory enhancement. These methods include what in known as strain/counterstrain
Rhythmic traction	Repetitive attempts to separate articulations in order to stretch inter- and periarticular structures
Springing	Repetitive, usually slowly applied, pressure of a gradual nature, often used diagnostically (see viscerosomatic reflex below)
Stretching	Short and long amplitude attempts at separation of muscular attachments, and stretch of ligaments, fascia, and membranes
Vibration	Rapid oscillatory pressure or movement

connective tissues, and subcutaneous fatty tissues. The connective tissues are thought to be vital in producing the acupuncture sensation noted as being essential to effective therapy.[27] These structures impart the "gripping" of the needle, and the manipulation of the needle affects, through localized tissue traction, minute neural reporting stations, such as Meissner corpuscles, muscle spindles, and Golgi tendon organs. Since many of the systems of reflex soft tissue manipulation (strain/counterstrain, etc.) maintain that it is just such neural structures which produce the reflex effects in their methodology,[8] there appears to be common ground between acupuncture and these other systems. This similarity is found in both the identification of the reflex structure (acupuncture point, trigger point, tender point, etc. being the same phenomena in different systems of classification) and, at least in part, the element which acts to convey reflex benefits (e.g. Golgi tendon organs).

In an attempt to make sense of the vast amount of information available from soft tissue changes, a number of systems have been developed that classify variations in significance, role, potential for therapy, etc. Some of these are described below.

All such points are sensitive to pressure, but some also refer symptoms to a distant site when stimulated. The latter are trigger points and the former are potential or latent trigger points. These may be classified in a variety of manners depending upon the system in question.[17,28]

Point classification

Tender points

In the system of soft tissue manipulation named strain/counterstrain, described by Lawrence Jones,[18,29] the tender point lies in a particular area in relation to any strain of a given joint or area. This is often found, not in the area complained of by the patient, but in shortened tissues associated with the strain. Thus, in flexion strains of the low back (strains which occur in a forward bending position), the appropriate tender points will almost always be found on the anterior surface of the body, i.e. around the lateral abdominal region or anterior pelvis, despite the patient reporting back pain. On palpation, these anteriorly located points are reported to be extremely sensitive, although the patient is seldom aware of them prior to their being palpated. Jones's method is to maintain palpatory contact with the tender point while repositioning the patient's body in such a manner as to reduce the reported sensitivity from the point. This position of relative ease is then maintained for some 90 seconds while the neurological reporting stations in the injured tissues re-establish a balanced feedback to the CNS (central nervous system), with resulting release of spasm or contraction. No further therapy is required, since this will usually achieve release of soft tissue dysfunction resulting from strain, and a return to normality.

In many cases the position of ease mimics or exaggerates the position in which the original injury occurred, or the position into which the patient is distorted by the contraction or spasm. Thus, an individual unable to stand erect (due to low back strain, for example), may be placed in a position of increased flexion while the palpation of the tender point is used to "fine tune" the exact position of maximum ease of pain at that point. There is recent evidence confirming the value of these safe methods in bedridden, hospitalized patients.[29]

The points described in this method are similar to those known as Ah Shi points in traditional acupuncture.[19] Almost identical criteria are used to identify spontaneously sensitive Ah Shi points, which are then utilized for acupuncture or acupressure therapy (see below). It is reasonable, therefore, to suppose that the maintenance of inhibitory pressure on the tender point is itself of some therapeutic value, inducing a degree of local and reflex inhibition. Jones denies that this is the intention, stating that he considers the pressure used in his system to be purely diagnostic,[18] but it must remain a strong probability that reflex inhibition of neural activity in the point is occurring as a result of this pressure, since evidence exists supporting the efficacy of pressure techniques in inducing pain relief in such conditions.[30,31]

Indeed, animal studies[30] suggest that pressure techniques have a greater degree of efficacy in promoting endorphin release and ultimate pain relief than does needling. Since Chinese texts describe pressure or needling of points as having the same pain-relieving effect, it is reasonable to assume that endorphin and/or enkephalin release is an important mediating element in such relief.[32] In the experiments mentioned above, artificial CSF was perfused through the lateral ventricle of a donor rabbit while it was receiving finger pressure acupuncture. When this perfusate was injected into a recipient rabbit, a pain threshold increase of 82% was noted. When CSF from a non-treated rabbit was similarly injected, no change was noted in the pain threshold. Highly significant changes were thus noted involving what is assumed to be met-enkephalin. The research group at the Peking Medical College stated:

> From the historical viewpoint, finger pressure was probably the most ancient methods of acupuncture. In our own experience the feeling of soreness and swelling stirred by finger acupuncture was sometimes even keener than that experienced in traditional needling, whereas the local tissue damage was much less with finger-acupuncture.

Trigger points

A trigger point is a localized palpable spot of deep hypersensitivity from which noxious impulses bombard the CNS to give rise to referred pain and other symptoms.

Trigger points as described by Travell and others are responsive to pressure techniques, to spray and stretch methods (see below), to injection with procaine and other anesthetics, and to acupuncture (dry needling).[33] Whichever method is used to obliterate the local trigger point manifestation, several important additional measures are called for. One of these is identification of the cause, since, if it is not resolved, relief is often short-lived. Thus, factors such as posture, use of the body (ergonomics applied to sport or occupational habits, etc.), emotional stress, anatomical abnormalities (short leg, etc.), nutritional status, and inherited elements all require analysis, in this as in all areas of somatic dysfunction.[28]

It is also necessary to normalize the ability of the muscle(s) in which the trigger(s) exists to subsequently reach its normal resting length.[21,30,34] Trigger points are not found in muscles able to stretch to normal lengths. Trigger points are localized foci of neurological disorder. They continue to bombard the CNS and, in reflex, their target tissues until removed by therapy. Without therapy they are self-perpetuating.[17] Once a trigger is dealt with, the muscle in which it lies should be examined for other trigger points, and target tissues should be searched for "satellite" triggers.[17,21]

Travell and others have reported a wide range of symptoms in target tissues associated with trigger point activity, including pain, local vasomotor disturbances (abnormality in pallor, coldness, cyanosis, flushing, etc.), increased or decreased sweat production, and pilomotor activity (all via autonomic nervous system involvement).[35] Gutstein[36] reports trigger point involvement in production of a wide range of symptoms, such as menopausal hot flushes and other pre- and post-menopausal symptoms (triggers noted in occipital, cervical, interscapular, sternal, and abdominal structures) and gastrointestinal symptoms, including pylorospasm, halitosis, regurgitation, heartburn, nausea, distension, constipation, and diarrhea (triggers noted in the lower sternum, epigastrium and parasternal regions).

Direct local pressure starts the process of removing trigger points. It should involve enough pressure to produce the referred symptoms and then be maintained in a make-and-break pattern (5 seconds on and 2–3 seconds reduced by about a third) until symptoms noticeably lessen or tissue changes are palpated.[29,37] This is followed by chilling of both the trigger and target area with fluoromethane spray (or ice) together with simultaneous and subsequent stretching of the involved muscle in order to achieve a normal resting length.[17,21,34,38] Mennell[22] advocates the spray and stretch methods, as does Travell, as part of the method used for obliteration of active trigger points. Many practitioners, such as Gutstein,[36] advocate injection into trigger points of anesthetic substances (procaine, etc.) and some, such as Dittrich,[39] advocate surgical excision. Another alternative, after identifying and ischemically compressing (inhibiting) the point described above, would be to place it into a position of ease (as in the strain/counterstrain methodology discussed earlier) prior to stretching the muscle housing the trigger points.[40,41]

Whichever method is used, stretching of the muscles involved to induce a return to normal resting length is necessary to ensure complete removal of the trigger. To achieve this, a number of methods, apart from standard active and passive stretching techniques, have been developed. Among these is the muscle energy technique.

Muscle energy technique

A potentially stressful physical therapy modality, known as proprioceptive neuromuscular facilitation (PNF), involving full-strength muscular contractions, has evolved into a gentler (very light contractions) method in osteopathic methodology, now called muscle energy technique or hold reflex technique.[42,43] It is aimed at restoring shortened, tight structures to a normal resting length.

A vast amount of research and clinical investigation into the value of this method has been conducted in Europe, mainly in Scandinavia and Czechoslovakia.[1,43] The muscles requiring muscle energy attention are identified by standard orthopedic tests for length and by palpation. Additionally, dysfunctional muscles can be identified by reading the firing sequence of muscles in particular movement patterns. For example, in the prone position, if the leg is elevated (hip extension) the firing sequence when normal is gluteus maximus, hamstrings, contralateral and ipsilateral erector spinae. If this is palpated as anything else, usually hamstring and erector contraction and subsequent gluteal firing, the implication is that there is overactivity in the erectors and hamstrings and inhibition of the gluteals, with a requirement for normalization of the overreactive muscles – using muscle energy procedures or other approaches.[44]

Muscle energy technique involves the use of two physiological phenomena: post-isometric relaxation and reciprocal inhibition. When a muscle is held in isometric contraction, its release is followed by a degree of relaxation not present prior to the contraction.[28] Thus, when muscle fibers contract, but approximation of the origin and insertion is prevented by an exactly equal counterforce, usually provided by the operator (i.e. an isometric contraction), and this contraction is maintained for a specific length of time (typically 7–10 seconds) after which relaxation is allowed, there will occur a marked release of hypertonicity in the tissues. This allows a greater degree of pain-free stretch to take place in the shortened fibers.[1,45] A new, but probably as yet still limited, resting length is then achieved, and this is used as the starting position of the next isometric contraction. This phenomenon of post-isometric relaxation (PIR) is used to sequentially stretch tight musculature in which triggers are found.[1,43] If the tight or shortened tissues are too sensitive to allow active isometric contraction, then their antagonists are contracted isometrically, producing the phenomenon of reciprocal inhibition which is similarly used to gradually increase normal resting length in the shortened structures.[1]

There are a number of variations in muscle energy technique. It is extremely gentle, utilizing only a small percentage of available strength (unlike PNF), which makes it applicable to almost any condition of soft tissue dysfunction, either alone or in combination with pressure or other techniques.[28]

Hartman[1] describes the use of muscle energy techniques in the preparation of a joint for manipulation. The joint is placed in the appropriate position for adjustment, and the patient is then asked to push against the contacting hands of the operator, so that an isometric contraction develops in the tissues surrounding the joint or area being adjusted. After this contraction is released, the degree of "slack" available to the operator will be greater, and the joint will be more easily and effectively adjusted. Indeed, adjustment often occurs during the isometric contraction described (see Table 46.4).

Zones of irritation

Dvorak & Dvorak[17] have described a system which identifies localized areas of spinal sensitivity. In this system, zones of irritation (ZI)[46] are identified by palpation in the paraspinal tissues. These appear in most respects to correspond both with the paraspinal acupuncture points described in the 2nd century AD by Hua Tuo[19,47] and with Jones's tender points.[18] In acupuncture, they are needled or pressed to produce appropriate local and distant effects.

In Dvorak's method, the zones of irritation are used to identify the ideal manipulative direction for adjustment. They are contacted by a palpating thumb or finger (as in Jones's method) and pressure is exerted against the spinous process adjacent to the ZI in such a manner as to reduce their sensitivity. This is considered to be the direction of desirable adjustment. A marked similarity with the method described by Morrison (discussed below) and with strain/counterstrain techniques is recognizable.

Dvorak elaborates on the ZI phenomenon by describing what are termed spondylogenic reflex syndromes,[48] in which ZI in specific paraspinal sites are noted to produce particular patterns of dysfunction in other spinal structures, including muscle groups and vertebral regions.

Induration technique

This method, which describes almost precisely the same technique as that advocated by Dvorak, was developed by Marsh Morrison DC in the 1940s.[20] The sensitive paraspinal point is identified and a push (not an adjustment) is made on the adjacent spinous process until a direction is found in which sensitivity reduces, or tissue release is noted. The pressure is then held for a not less than 20 seconds and no other therapy used. Release of the contracted tissues and lessening of pain on palpation are noted. This is very similar to the Jones's method and is ideal for use by therapists not qualified or licensed to manipulate the osseous structures.[28]

Nimmo's receptor tonus technique

Other workers, such as Raymond Nimmo DC, who developed the receptor/tonus technique, have described similar variations on the theme of identification and normalization of local areas of soft tissue dysfunction using pressure and stretching methods.[49] Nimmo maintained that pressure on such points should last no more than 5–7 seconds and that further pressure was likely to injure tissue. Triggers thus treated would, he maintained, subsequently resolve. He also advocated stretching of the structures. His pressure was delivered by the use of a rubber-tipped wooden instrument, a T-bar, held in the palm of the hand in the interest of reducing stress on the operator's digits.

Different muscle types

In all of these systems, the tissues in which points are found are described as having a characteristic shortened or tight feel, and the work of Lewit[1] and Janda[50] helps to explain why these are found mostly in particular muscles. Janda states that there are two basic muscle activities and types: those which are predominantly postural and others which are mainly phasic in action.

Postural muscles include:

- tibialis posterior
- gastrocnemius-soleus
- rectus femoris
- iliopsoas
- tensor fascia lata
- hamstrings
- short thigh adductors
- quadratus lumborum
- piriformis
- some paravertebral muscles
- pectoralis major (and perhaps minor)
- sternocleidomastoid
- upper trapezius
- levator scapula
- flexors of the upper extremity.

These are all prone to shortening and hypertonia when stressed, abused, or under- or overused.

A number of conditions exist in which specific patterns

Table 46.4 Muscle energy technique: summary of variations

Type of contraction	Indications	Modus operandi	Forces	Duration	Repetitions
Isometric patient direct	Relaxing muscular spasm or contraction. Mobilizing restricted joints. Preparing joint for manipulation	Affected muscle not employed. Antagonists used, therefore shortened muscles relax via reciprocal inhibition. Patient is attempting to push through the barrier of restriction. After the isometric contraction, the tissues are taken to the new restriction barrier (in acute settings) or are stretched through the barrier (in fibrotic settings)	Operator's and patient's forces are matched. Initial effort involves approximately 20% of patient's strength; slow increase to no more than 50% on subsequent contractions. Increase of duration often more effective than increase in force	4–10 seconds initially, increasing to up to 30 seconds in subsequent contractions, in order to recruit additional fibers during the contraction effort	3–5 times
Isometric operator-direct	Relaxing muscular spasm or contraction. Mobilizing restricted joints. Preparing joint for manipulation	Affected muscles used, therefore shortened muscles relax via post-isometric relaxation. Operator is attempting to go through barrier of restriction. After the isometric contraction, the tissues are taken to the new restriction barrier (in acute settings) or are stretched through the barrier (in fibrotic settings)	Operator's and patient's forces are matched. Initial effort involves approximately 20% of patient's strength; slow increase to no more than 50% on subsequent contractions. Increase of duration often more effective than increase in force	4–10 seconds initially, increasing to up t0 30 seconds in subsequent contractions, if greater effort required	3–5 times
Isotonic concentric	Toning weakened musculature	Contracting muscle is allowed to do so, with some resistance from operator	Patient's force is greater than operator resistance. Patient uses maximal effort available but force is built slowly, not via sudden effort	3–4 seconds	5–7 times
Isotonic eccentric (isolytic)	Stretching tight fibrotic musculature	Contracted muscle is prevented from doing so via superior operator effort. Origin and insertion do not approximate. Muscle is taken to, or as close as possible to, full physiological resting length	Operator's force is greater than patient's. Less than maximal patient's force employed at first. Subsequent contractions build towards this, if pain not excessive	2–4 seconds	3–5 times, if pain not excessive
Isokinetic (isotonic and isometric contractions)	Toning weakened musculature. Building strength in all muscles involved in particular joint function. Training effect on muscle fibers	Patient resists with moderate effort at first, progressing to maximal effort subsequently, as operator puts joint through its full range of movements	Operator's force overcomes patient's effort to prevent movement. First mobilization involves moderate force, progressing to full force subsequently		

of dysfunction are associated with shortening of such muscles (e.g. iliopsoas, piriformis, tensor fascia lata, and iliotibeal band), treatment of which is possible using variations of the techniques discussed here (neuromuscular technique, muscle energy technique, etc).[11,28]

The phasic muscles include:

- tibialis anterior
- the vasti
- the glutei
- abdominal muscles (mainly the recti)
- lower stabilizers of the scapula
- some deep neck flexors
- extensors of the upper extremity.

These all tend to hypotonia, weakening, and atrophy under conditions of under- or overuse, or abuse.

Janda asserts that before any attempt is made via exercise, etc. to strengthen weakened musculature, it is critical for the shortened antagonists to be stretched and relaxed. Commencing with exercising of the weakened structures is likely to further increase tone in the already tight musculature. Tight muscles act in an inhibitory way on their antagonists, creating hypotonia. This can be altered by normalization of the tight structures. Whether this stretching is achieved by muscle energy methods or active or passive stretching is a matter of choice.

Summary

In shortened fibers of the soft tissues can be found the palpable and sensitive points discussed above. They may be the result of a combination of structural anomalies, trauma, and/or physical or emotional stress and are always influenced by underlying nutritional and behavioral elements. Some of these may be the source of reflex symptoms and pain (active trigger points). All such soft tissue dysfunctions respond to manual pressure, needling, local anaesthesia, chilling, etc., as well as to release via positional alteration and/or resolution of identifiable underlying or causative factors.

REFLEXES RELATED TO ORGAN OR SYSTEM DYSFUNCTION

Connective tissue massage

The German system of connective tissue massage (CTM)[11,16,28,51] has identified a number of regions or zones which are associated with specific organ or functional problems (e.g. liver zone, constipation zone, arterial disturbance of the legs zone, etc.). Identification of such zones in a patient depends on a method of skin stretching by lifting which indicates the degree of adherence between overlying structures and underlying connective tissue. There is decreased elasticity in areas of dysfunction. Therapy involves a dry contact which lifts and stretches these tissues, producing powerful viscerocutaneous reflex effects. Clinical evidence shows this therapy to be of use in a wide range of problems, as it improves organ, circulatory, and neural dysfunction. A recent hospital study in Scotland indicated CTM to be effective in producing marked reduction in anxiety levels, with resolution of symptoms such as insomnia in patients resistant to drug therapy.[52]

Chapman's neurolymphatic reflexes

Chapman's neurolymphatic reflexes are described in osteopathic literature and involve the use of pairs of reflex points located anteriorly and posteriorly on the body surface.[11,13,28,53,54] The feel of such reflex points is described as similar to that of a nodule, an edematous structure, or a fibrous shotty plaque, depending upon the location.

These reflexes are stated to be the somatic component of lymphatic stasis in associated structures, and treatment of these is felt to assist in resolution of such stasis. A reflex is said to be active if both points of a pair are found to be palpable and sensitive. Treatment is initiated by direct firm rotary pressure, via finger or thumb tip, on the anterior point for 20 seconds to 2 minutes or until decongestion (tissue change) is noted. The posterior point is then similarly treated. Subsequent re-examination of the anterior point of the pair is conducted to ascertain whether sensitivity is still present. If sensitivity is not present, then successful resolution of the associated lymphatic stasis is anticipated. If sensitivity is still noted, however, then it is considered that pathology is too great for this method to be effective and that other therapeutic input is required. This makes the method a useful prognostic indicator, whether or not the reflexes are used therapeutically in the manner described.

When methods such as hydrotherapy, botanical medicine, acupuncture, massage, or nutritional adjustment or supplementation are utilized to treat a particular condition, the activity and sensitivity of Chapman's neurolymphatic reflex points may be monitored in order to assess progress. Also, since these points become active long before symptoms are obvious in associated structures or organs, this method is of significant early diagnostic and prognostic value.

These reflex pairs have been studied in hospitals by the osteopathic profession and were found to be powerful reflex areas. Whether or not the influence is directly on the lymphatic structures is a matter for debate.[55] Points are utilized therapeutically in groups associated with systems, such as the respiratory or gastrointestinal systems, rather than as individual pairs of points. There are some 50 pairs of points, many of which are identical to acupuncture points in location, if not in ascribed areas of influence. Their location and corresponding organ, tissue, system, or symptom are clearly outlined and diagramed in Chaitow[28] (pp. 163–172).

Bennett's neurovascular reflexes

This is a system which utilizes reflex areas, mainly on the abdomen and head.[14,28] It was developed by chiropractic practitioner, Terence Bennett, and involves identification of localized areas of dysfunction (points) which are contracted or indurated, and which display increased sensitivity. These are said to be related to vascular dysfunction. Therapy is via gentle skin distraction over the point, until a pulsation is noted under the palpating digit.[56] Contact is made from a few seconds to several minutes in order to achieve this reflex effect. Many of the points are used purely diagnostically and others are used both diagnostically and therapeutically.

Cross-fertilization of systems

Systems such as applied kinesiology,[57] touch for health,[56] and sacro-occipital technique (SOT)[58] have incorporated into their therapeutic and diagnostic methodology the use of many of the reflex points described by Chapman and Bennett.

Alarm and associated points

In acupuncture there exists a series of specialized points in the meridian system, which are found to become sensitive to pressure when the meridian or organ to which they are reflexively connected is distressed.[59] The points which are sensitive to deep pressure are thought to be involved in excessive energy problems, and those noted on light pressure are related to deficiency problems. Many of the neurolymphatic and neurovascular reflexes described above are found to correlate with these two sets of points in location, and sometimes in ascribed effect (alarm points are found ventrally and associated points dorsally). Treatment of these is by needling as appropriate, or by pressure and by attention to the needs of the system correlated to the dysfunction noted.

Tsubo, G-Jo, judo revival, and other point systems related to Oriental medicine

A number of systems (e.g. Tsubo,[60] G-Jo,[61] and judo revival[62]) with common roots in acupuncture employ reflex points in a variety of ways. Some utilize strong stimulation imparted via the thumbnail to produce rapid reflex effects, while others use more gentle pressures. One recently described method indicates a point on the upper lip (Du26) as an ideal locality for strong stimulation in attempting revival of unconscious children suffering grand or petit mal seizures.[63] It was noted in some hundreds of cases thus treated that termination of the convulsion and full revival of consciousness were achieved in an average of less than 20 seconds. The only failures were in children who were not fully unconscious, for whom the vigorous stimulation was too painful.

Viscerosomatic reflexes

The osteopathic literature describes viscerosomatic reflexes as being localized, sensitive, palpable areas, often found in paraspinal tissues and associated with visceral dysfunction.[64] Beal[65] notes that rigidity is the most common soft tissue manifestation of such a reflex. Initial changes include vasomotor alterations such as increased skin temperature and subtle changes such as increased thickness of the skin, increased subcutaneous fluid, and increased muscular contraction. In chronic conditions, all of these become more evident. There are usually two or more adjacent spinal segments involved in any viscerosomatic reflex, encompassing, as a rule, the costotransverse junction. Areas which are most frequently involved include T1–T5 (associated with viscerosomatic reflexes from the cardiac structures), T5–T10 (esophagus, stomach, small intestine, liver, gall bladder, spleen, and pancreas), and T10–L2 (large bowel, appendix, kidney, ureter, testes, ovaries, adrenal medulla, urinary bladder, and prostate). There is usually some lateralization, e.g. the liver reflex is found on the right.

For assessment, a springing technique is used in which the palpating hand is slid under the supine patient in order to push upwards on the paraspinal regions. Neuromuscular technique is also an excellent method of assessment of such structures.[11,28] Beal suggests that digital pressure may be used to affect local changes and to reflexively influence the involved organs (somaticovisceral reflex). Since this would have only a moderate effect on advanced organic disease, these reflexes are of more diagnostic than therapeutic value. Also, since they are manifested long before other evidence of organ distress is available, they are useful early warnings of developing dysfunction.[65] Regular assessment of the paraspinal tissues, therefore, acts as a monitor of the internal function. This concept is well documented medically and is of potential value in monitoring the efficacy of any type of therapy, since the reflex condition will show improvement in tandem with the organ state.[66,67] The overlap between these reflexes and the points and zones described above should be borne in mind (see Table 46.5).

Hyperalgesic skin zones

Overlying all points and zones involved in reflex activity will be noted skin changes characterized by what may be termed hyperalgesia.

Table 46.5 Summary of ascribed roles of reflexes described in different systems, as found at the 8–10th thoracic inter-spinal and inter-transverse spaces

System	Points/reflexes	Location	Relationship
Hua Tuo		Paravertebral	Diseases of the abdomen and local and lumbar dysfunction
Neurolymphatic reflexes	Posterior reflexes		
	Reflex #12	8/9/10 insterspaces	Small intestine dysfunction (anterior in 8/9/10 intercostal space)
	Reflex #33	10th costotransverse junction	Pyloric stenosis (anterior reflex is on the sternum)
	Reflex #42	9–10 or 10–11 intertransverse	Ovaries (anterior point is on the round ligaments frorm the superior border of the pubic bone inferiorly)
Associated points	Bilaterally bladder point 18	9th–10th interspace	Liver meridian
	Bilaterally bladder point 19	10th–11th interspace	Gall bladder meridian
Tender points			Extension strain at this level
Connective tissue zone		Left side	Stomach zone
		Right side	Liver zone
		Central area	Kidney and part of the head zone
Trigger points		Lower trapezius, multifidus, iliocostalis, and longissimus muscles	Wide distribution of target areas
Zone of irritation		Costotransverse junction	Spondylogenic reflex syndromes involving tissues connected to C2-7, T1–6, L1–5, S1,3,4
Viscerosomatic reflexes		T5–T10	Esophagus, stomach, small intestine, liver, gall bladder, spleen, pancreas

There will be a reduced degree of elasticity noted, and this is diagnostic. Lewit[1] maintains that the introduction of a mild degree of stretch into these hyperalgesic skin areas has a powerful reflex effect on underlying dysfunction (i.e. the trigger or tender point, or zone). Assessment is by gentle distraction of the skin in order to compare it with the surrounding skin and the skin in the same region on the contralateral side of the body. Mapping and confirmation of underlying reflex areas are possible by the use of pressure to ascertain sensitivity and possible referred symptoms. Treatment is by maintaining the degree of distraction in the skin zone (fingers pulling gently apart, or, for larger areas, lateral aspects of the hands doing the same) until a degree of release is noted, as the skin relaxes and is stretched to its normal range. This is all the treatment required to normalize the tissues and to introduce reflex changes into the underlying structures.

The maintenance of the restored elasticity depends upon whether the causative factors have also been dealt with, and the degree of activity in associated reflexes.

A number of other methods of normalization can be utilized, including skin rolling, as described in Western and Oriental massage texts.[11,28,68] Chinese massage techniques include pinch–pull techniques which can be used to tonify or sedate the patient and which have marked similarities with German CTM methods. CTM, as described above, involves far more powerful skin stretching methods than either the pinch–pull techniques or Lewit's distraction and stretch techniques.[16]

Neuromuscular technique

The methods of neuromuscular technique involve the systematic combing of the tissues for the soft tissue changes described above.[11,28,69,70] Its economy of effort and combining of diagnostic and therapeutic procedures have made it popular among practitioners in Europe, where it evolved as a combination of methods derived from Ayurvedic massage,[71] traditional massage, and an American "bloodless surgery" (not to be confused with the Philippine faith-healers' "bloodless surgery") method.[72]

Typically, the thumb tip is used to exert variable pressure on all the accessible origins and insertions and muscle masses in order to identify changes, and, by variations in that pressure, simultaneously treat the recognized abnormalities. This approach is seen as part of an overall assessment rather than as an end in itself. Other methods of traditional massage from both East and West are combined with NMT to normalize those aspects of soft tissue dysfunction which are manifestations of stress, strain, and trauma and to address reflex changes where applicable.

THERAPY AS A STRESS FACTOR

Stress is any added load imposed by forces brought to bear on an individual, organ, or tissue. It may be chemical, toxic, psychic, emotional, or physical.[73] Adaptation denotes the ways in which the organism adjusts itself to intrinsic disturbances or challenges. These responses may be short- or long-term in nature, representing the body's homeostatic mechanisms at work.

Selye, in his classic experiments, noted specific and general responses in disease, observing that "stress can either cure or aggravate a disease, depending upon whether the inflammatory response to a local irritant is necessary or superfluous."[74]

Speransky, in his landmark research in the 1940s, stated:[75]

> It is obvious from this research that the irritation of any point of the complex network of the nervous system can evoke changes not only in adjacent parts but also in remote regions of the organism.

He continues by observing: "There is a rule that only weak degrees of irritation can have useful significance, strong ones inevitably do damage."

Many therapeutic measures involve a degree of stress, whether this be an acupuncture needle, surgery, or intake of toxic substances – even in homeopathic dilutions; applications of heat or cold, or electrotherapy; or, indeed in this consideration, manual pressures and efforts. Attaining the desired response, therefore, will depend upon the therapeutic effort not overwhelming the homeostatic potential of the organism.[20] Therapy may be considered to consist largely of the application of graduated degrees of stress, to which the organism responds according to its unique attributes and potentials. Benefit or harm depends upon the degree of that stimulus and, most importantly, upon the vitality of the patient.

The implications for manual therapists are obvious and call for thoughtful application of the varieties of techniques available.

THE POTENTIAL OF SOFT TISSUE MANIPULATION

The professions within medicine which utilize manual therapy, such as physiotherapy, have tended to discard the tradition of "hands on" treatment in favor of a more technological approach, leaving the soft tissues to massage therapists and sports therapists. Osteopathy (as practiced in Europe where it is not a part of a general medical practice, as it is in the US, but rather a system which addresses structural and functional dysfunction via manipulative methods[9,76]) and chiropractic, which are conceived as being largely concerned with the joints and osseous component of the musculoskeletal system, have in recent years come to recognize the vast importance of the soft tissues in both diagnostic and therapeutic roles. The musculoskeletal system is both the greatest energy consumer of the body and its largest organ of sensory input. While this primary machinery of life has long been unappreciated, in therapeutic terms, the development of methods such as strain/counterstrain, muscle energy technique, and neuromuscular technique and the vast amount of information derived from acupuncture tradition and research, and other reflex systems ensure that the diagnostic and therapeutic potential of the soft tissues are now being recognized and utilized.

Korr,[77] the premier osteopathic researcher of the past three decades, summarizes another vital implication of soft tissue dysfunction – interference with axonal transport mechanisms – thus:

> Any factor that causes derangement of transport mechanism in the axon or that chronically alters the quality or quantity of the axonally transported substances could cause the trophic influences to become detrimental. This alteration in turn would produce aberrations of structure, function and metabolism, thereby contributing to dysfunction and disease. Almost certainly to be included among these harmful factors are the deformation of nerves and roots, such as compression, stretching, angulation and torsion that are known to occur all too commonly in the human being and that are likely to disturb the interaxonal transport mechanisms, intraneural microcirculation and the blood–nerve barrier. Neural structures are especially vulnerable in their passage over highly mobile joints, through bony canals, intervertebral foramina, fascial layers and tonically contracted muscles. Many of these biomechanically induced deformations are of course subject to manipulative amelioration and correction.

This survey has touched on some of the many ways in which soft tissue dysfunction may impinge upon the economy of the body as a whole. Soft tissue manipulation is an important diagnostic and treatment modality and should be considered an integral part of the practice of any physician or practitioner whose intent is to care for the whole person. (Those interested in studying this topic in more depth will find reference 28 very helpful. It thoroughly covers the topics surveyed here and provides useful tables, charts and diagrams and pictures of the various techniques as they are applied to a patient.)

REFERENCES

1. Lewit K (MD). Manipulative therapy in rehabilitation of the motor system. Boston, MA: Butterworths. 1985
2. Baldry P. Acupuncture, trigger points and musculoskeletal pain. London: Churchill Livingstone. 1993
3. Janda V. Introduction to functional pathology of the motor system. Procedings of VII Commonwealth and International conference on sport. Physiother Sport 1982; 3: 39
4. Liebenson C. Rehabilitation of the spine. Baltimore: Williams & Wilkins. 1995
5. DiGiovanna E, ed. An osteopathic approach to diagnosis and treatment. Philadelphia, PA: Lippincott. 1991
6. Greenman P. Principles of manual medicine. Baltimore: Williams & Wilkins. 1996
7. Chaitow L. Palpation skills. London: Churchill Livingstone. 1996
8. Korr I. Neurological mechanisms in manipulative therapy. New York, NY: Plenum Press. 1978

9. Hartman L. Handbook of osteopathic technique. London: Hutchinson. 1985
10. Rolf I. Rolfing: the integration of human structures. New York, NY: Perennial Library, Harper and Row. 1977
11. Chaitow L. Neuromuscular technique. Rochester, VT: Thorsons. 1980
12. Mann F. International conference on acupuncture and chronic pain. New York, September 1983
13. Owens C. An endocrine interpretation of chapman's reflexes. Carmel, CA: Academy of Applied Osteopathy. 1963
14. Bennett T. Dynamics of correction of abnormal function. Sierra Madre, CA: Ralph Martin. 1977
15. Mitchell F. Training and measurement of sensory literacy in relation to osteopathic structural and palpatory diagnosis. Journal of American Osteopathic Association 1976; 75: 874–884
16. Ebner M. Connective tissue massage. Edinburgh: E&S Livingstone. 1962
17. Dvorak J, Dvorak V. Manual medicine: diagnostics. New York, NY: Thieme-Stratton. 1984
18. Jones L. Strain and counterstrain. Colorado Springs, CO: American Academy of Osteopathy. 1981
19. Academy of Traditional Chinese Medicine. An outline of Chinese acupuncture. Peking: Foreign Languages Press. 1975
20. Morrison M. Lecture notes. London: British College of Naturopathy and Osteopathy. 1970
21. Travell J, Simons D. Myofascial pain and dysfunction: the trigger point manual. New York, NY: Williams and Wilkins. 1983
22. Mennell J. The therapeutic use of cold. J Am Osteopath Assoc 1975; 74: 1146–1158
23. Bossy J. Morphological data concerning acupuncture points and channel networks. Acupuncture Electro-Therapeutic Res Int J 1984; 9: 79–106
24. Head H. On disturbances of sensation with especial reference to pain of visceral disease. Brain 1893; 16: 1–133; 1894; 17: 339–480; 1896; 19: 153–276
25. Shestack R. Handbook of physical therapy. New York, NY: Springer. 1956
26. Melzack R, Stillwell D, Fox E et al. Trigger points and acupuncture points for pain. correlations and implications. Pain 1977; 3: 3–27
27. National Symposia of Acupuncture. Moxibustion and acupuncture anaesthesia. Peking, 1–9 June 1979
28. Chaitow L. Soft tissue manipulation. Rochester, VT: Thorsons. 1987
29. Schwartz H. The use of counterstrain in an acutely ill in-hospital population. J Am Ost Assoc 1986; 86: 433–442
30. Scienta Sinica. Peking: Science Press. 1974: p XVII: 112
31. Chaitow L. Acupuncture treatment of pain. Rochester, VT: Thorsons. 1976
32. Kiser RS. Acupuncture relief of chronic pain syndrome correlates with increased plasma met-enkephalin concentrations. Lancet 1983; ii: 1394–1396
33. Melzack E, Stillwell D, Fox E et al. Myofascial trigger points: relation to acupuncture and mechanisms of pain. Arch Phys Med, 1981; 162: 114
34. Lewit K, Simons D. Myofascial pain: relief by post isometric relaxation. Arch Phys Med Rehab 1984; 65: 542–546
35. Travell J, Bigelow N. Role of somatic trigger areas in the patterns of hysteria. Psychosomatic Med 9
36. Gutstein R. A review of myodysneuria (fibrositis). Am Pract Digest Treat 1955; 6: 570–577
37. Chaitow L. Instant pain control. New York, NY: Wallaby Books/Simon & Schuster. 1981
38. Gelb H. Clinical management of head, neck and tmj pain and dysfunction. Philadelphia, PA: Saunders. 1977
39. Dittrich RJ. Somatic pain and autonomic concomitants. Am J Surg 1954
40. Chaitow L. Integrated neuromuscular inhibition technique in treatment of trigger points. Br J Osteopathy 1994; 13: 17–21
41. Chaitow L. Modern neuromuscular techniques. Edinburgh: Churchill Livingstone. 1996
42. Mitchell F, Moran P, Pruzzo N. An evaluation and treatment manual of osteopathic muscle energy procedures. Published by the Authors, Valley Park, MO. 1979
43. Evjenth O, Hamberg J. Muscle stretching in manual therapy: a clinical manual, vols 1 & 2. Alfta, Sweden: Alefta Rehab Vorlag. 1984
44. Jull G, Janda V. Muscle and motor control in low back pain. In: Twomey L, Taylor J, eds. Physical therapy of the low back. New York, NY: Churchill Livingstone. 1987
45. Grieve G. Mobilization of the spine. New York, NY: Churchill Livingstone. 1984
46. Caviezel H. Beitrag zur Kenntnis der Rippenlaisonen. Mannuele Med 1974; 5: 110
47. Ji Xiaoping. Teaching round: sciatica. J Trad Chin Med, 1986; 6: 131–134
48. Sutter M. Wesen, Klinik und Beteutung Spondylogener Reflexsyndrome. Schweiz Rundsch Med, Praxis 1975; 62: 42
49. Nimmo R. Receptor tonus: a neural therapy. London, England: Seminar Notes. 1966
50. Janda V. Muscles, central nervous motor regulation and back problems. In: Korr I, ed. Neurobiologic mechanisms in manipulative therapy. New York, NY: Plenum Press. 1978
51. Bischof I, Elmiger G. Connective tissue massage. In: Licht S, ed. Massage, manipulation and traction. New Haven, CT: Licht. 1960
52. McKechnie A, Wilson F, Watson N, Scott D. Anxiety states: a preliminary report on the value of connective tissue massage. J Psychosomatic Res, 1983; 27: 125–129
53. Arbuckle B. The selected writings of Berly Arbuckle. The National Osteopathic Institute and Cerebral Palsy Foundation. 1977
54. Chaitow L. An introduction to Chapman's reflexes. Br Nat J 1965; Spring: 111–113
55. Mannino DO. The application of neurological reflexes to the treatment of hypertension. J Am Ost Assoc 1979; 79: 225–230
56. Thie J. Touch for health. Santa Monica, CA: DeVorss. 1973
57. Goodheart G. Applied kinesiology research manuals. Detroit. 1964–71 (published by author)
58. De Jarnette M. Sacro occipital. Seminar notes. 1975 (published by author)
59. Pennell R, Heuser G. Seminar of acupuncture for physicians. Independence, MO: IPCI. 1973
60. Serizawa K. Tsubo: vital points for Oriental therapy. Tokyo, Japan: Japan Pub. 1976
61. Blate M. The G-Jo handbook. Davis, FL: Falkynor Books. 1983
62. Lawson-Wood DJ. Judo revival points, athletes points and posture. Santa Barbara, CA: Health Science Press. 1960
63. Pothmann R, Schmitz G. Acupressure in the acute treatment of cerebral convulsions in children. Alt Med, Holland 1985; 1: 63–67
64. Postgraduate Institute of Osteopathic Medicine and Surgery, New York. The Physiological Basis of Osteopathic Medicine. New York: Insight Publishing. 1970
65. Beal M. Palpatory testing for somatic dysfunction in patients with cardiovascular disease. J Am Ost Assoc 1983; 82: 822–831
66. Ward A. Somatic component to myocardial Infarction. Br Med J 1985; 291: 603
67. Ashby E. Abdominal pain of spina origin. Ann Royal Coll Surg, 1977; 59: 242–246
68. Scott J. The treatment of children's diseases. J Chin Med, 1980; 3: 13–22
69. Lief P. Neuromuscular Technique. Br Nat J Ost Rev 1963; 5: 304–324
70. Youngs B. The physiological background of neuromuscular technique. Br Nat J Ost Rev 1963; 5: 176–178
71. Varma D. The human machine and its forces, pranotherapy. London, England: Health for All Publishers. 1937
72. Fielder S, Pyott W. The science and art of manipulative surgery. American Institute of Manipulative Surgery. 1955
73. Wright H. Clinical thinking and practice. New York, NY: Churchill Livingstone. 1979
74. Hoag J. Osteopathic medicine. New York, NY: McGraw Hill. 1969
75. Speransky A. A basis for the theory of medicine. New York, NY: International Publishers. 1943
76. Chaitow L. Osteopathy: a complete health-care system. Rochester, VT: Thorsons. 1982
77. Korr I. The spinal cord as organizer of disease processes. J Am Ost Assoc 1981; 80: 451–458

CHAPTER CONTENTS

47

Therapeutic fasting

Trevor K. Salloum, ND

INTRODUCTION

Fasting is defined as abstinence from all food and drink except water for a specific period of time, usually for a therapeutic or religious purpose.[1] This process spares essential tissue (e.g. vital organs) while utilizing non-essential tissue (e.g. adipose tissue, digestive enzymes, muscle contractile fibers, and glycolytic enzymes) for fuel.

Some medical references use the terms *fasting* and *starvation* interchangeably. Unlike fasting, starvation is a process in which the body uses essential tissue for fuel. During starvation, the body relies on protein as a major fuel source, as most fat stores have been depleted. If an organism does not receive food at the end of the maximum fasting period (several weeks to months depending on fat stores, metabolism, stress, and activity), starvation follows and death will ensue.[2]

Although the term fasting is used loosely in medical literature, the strictest definition (water only) is the focus of this chapter. Some medical studies recommend supplementation with vitamins, fruit and vegetable juices, acaloric fluids (coffee, tea, etc.), and drugs while the patient is "fasting". These practices have not been shown to produce any advantage, and serious problems have sometimes occurred, especially when non-essential medication was permitted. (In special cases it may be necessary to maintain the patient on essential medication while fasting, e.g. thyroid, prednisone, and insulin.)

Although therapeutic fasting is probably one of the oldest known therapies, it has been the object of only limited study by the scientific community. The most recent development in the study and promotion of fasting has been the formation of the International Association of Hygenic Physicians (IAHP).[3] This organization comprises doctors specializing in therapeutic fasting as an integral part of total health care. The section on clinical protocol below reflects the format practiced by the IAHP. Any doctor contemplating the use of therapeutic fasting should receive adequate training. The

IAHP provides guidelines for doctors interested in this training.[3]

Another recent development has been the work of clinical ecologists who use short-term fasting as part of their diagnosis and treatment of food intolerance.[4,5]

HISTORY

Throughout history, people of various cultures and religions have recognized the value of fasting. Numerous references occur in the Bible, Koran, pagan writings, and writings of the ancient Greeks.[6–8]

One of the earliest doctors to use therapeutic fasting in the United States was Isaac Jennings MD (1788–1874). In 1822, Jennings discarded the use of drugs and, through the influence of a Presbyterian preacher, Sylvester Graham (1794–1851), began advocating fasting and other aspects of hygienic treatment (vegetarian diet, pure water, sunshine, clean air, exercise, emotional poise, and rest). This later came to be known as the Natural Hygiene or Hygienic system.[9–11]

Other doctors who followed in the hygienic tradition included: James C. Jackson (1811–1895), Russell T. Trall (1812–1877), William A. Alcott (1798–1859), Mary Grove Nichols (1810–1884), Thomas L. Nichols (1815–1901), Edward H. Dewey (1837–1904), George H. Taylor (1821–1896), Harriet Austin (1826–1891), Charles E. Page (1840–1925), Emmett Densmore (1837–1911), Helen Densmore (?–1904), Susanna W. Dodds (1830–1915), Felix Oswald (1845–1906), Robert Walter (1841–1921), John H. Tilden (1851–1940), and George S. Weger (1874–1935). Most of these physicians graduated as MDs from eclectic medical schools, and they published various works on hygiene.[9–16]

Herbert M. Shelton

The hygienic lineage continued into the mid-1900s, mainly due to Herbert M. Shelton (1895–1985), who developed a stricter protocol for fasting (water only; no enemas, exercise, or treatments; and complete rest) and other aspects of hygiene. Shelton began his study of fasting in 1911 by reading the popular writers of his day: Sinclair, Carrington, Hazzard, Haskell, Purinton, Tilden, and MacFadden. He studied under the fasting authorities of his time at MacFadden's College (Chicago, IL), Crane's Sanatorium (Elmhurst, IL), and Crandall's Health School (York, PA).[9,10] (Among the earliest fasting institutions of this time were MacFadden's Healthatorium, Tilden's Health School, Lindlahr's Nature Cure Sanatoriums, and Lust's Jungborn – operated by Benedict Lust, the founder of naturopathy in the United States.[10]) In 1924, he completed doctorates from the American School of Chiropractic and the American School of Naturopathy in New York.

Shelton was a dynamic lecturer, prolific writer, and publisher. He founded (in 1928) a fasting institution and health school which provided services for over 40 years.[9] In 1949, along with William Esser ND DC, Christopher Gian-Cursio ND DC, and Gerald Benesh ND DC, he formed the American Natural Hygiene Society,[9,16] a lay organization dedicated to preserving the tenets of hygiene. In 1978, a professional branch was formed, the aforementioned International Association of Hygenic Physicians.[3] Today, the IAHP organizes annual meetings, a journal, research and certification for doctors specializing in therapeutic fasting.

CLINICAL RESEARCH

Research into fasting has been reported since 1880. Since then, medical journals have carried articles on the use of fasting in the treatment of:

- diabetes
- mental disease
- skin disease
- obesity
- cardiovascular disease
- gastrointestinal disease
- chemical poisoning
- arthritis
- allergies.

The earliest research was primarily observational; physiologic and metabolic changes were recorded while an individual fasted. These included: Tanner, 40 days (1880);[17] Jacques, 30 days (1887) and 40 days (1888);[18] Penny, 30 days (1905);[19] and Levanzin, 31 days (1912).[20] The earliest record of therapeutic fasting in the medical literature occurred in 1910.

Further investigation into the physiologic changes that accompany fasting was conducted in 1923 at the University of Nebraska by Morgulis. This classic study, *Fasting and undernutrition*, provides an in-depth analysis of animal and human reactions during fasting.[21]

In 1950, Ancel Keys and colleagues at the University of Minnesota compiled two volumes entitled *The biology of human starvation*. Thirty-two volunteers fasted for up to 8 months while detailed observations were made. These findings were compared with food deprivation observations which were made during the Second World War. Through their studies, the researchers found that fasting did not cause vitamin or mineral deficiencies and that diabetes and skin diseases improved.[22]

Diabetes

Guelpa recorded the benefits of fasting in diabetes and gout, as well as in inflammation and surgery.[23] The treatment of diabetes with fasting was further explored by Allen in 1915. He noted that rest and fasting usually stopped glycosuria, and he also observed improvements in gangrene and carbuncles.[24]

Epilepsy

The treatment of seizures through fasting was begun in the early 1900s in France by Guelpa & Marie (cited by Kernt).[25] In 1924, Hoeffel & Moriarty described fasting's beneficial effects in epilepsy.[26] In 1928, Lennox, concurring with other researchers, found that the induction of ketosis via fasting decreased the length, severity, and number of seizures.[27]

Obesity

Fasting for obesity has probably received more attention in the scientific literature than any other aspect. The earliest studies were conducted by Folin & Denis[28] who, in 1915, advocated short fasts as a safe and effective means to lose weight. Bloom,[29] Duncan,[30,31] Drenick,[32,33] and Thompson[34] have published numerous works on the use of short and long fasts in obesity. Perhaps the most famous study on obesity appeared in the *Postgraduate Medical Journal* of 1973, which reported the experience of a 27-year-old male who fasted without complications for 382 days and lost 276 pounds.[35]

In general, weight loss during fasting is initially approximately 0.3% of body weight per day, with a gradual decrease to 0.10%/day after 30 days. The initial weight loss is primarily water and salt. For every pound lost, the body loses approximately 140 g of protein and 250 g of fat.[36]

Although fasting is very effective for weight reduction, fasting alone, without counseling and other lifestyle modifications, does not insure long-term maintenance of the lower weight level. This is well documented in a study of 121 obese patients who were followed for 7.3 years after fasts which had averaged two months. After 2–3 years, 50% had reverted to their pre-fast weight, and by the end of the study 90% had reverted.[102]

Heart disease

Studies of the effects of fasting on patients with heart disease began in the early 1960s. Duncan noted improvements in hypertension and chronic cardiac disease.[28] Others have also found fasting to be beneficial in heart disease, including Gresham,[33] Lawlor,[34] Suzuki,[35] Vessby,[36] and Sorbris.[37] Improvements noted include reduced triglycerides, blood pressure, atheromas, and total cholesterol; increased HDL/cholesterol ratio; and alleviation of congestive heart failure.[28,33–37]

Pancreatitis

In a random trial, in 1984, of 88 patients with acute pancreatitis, fasting was determined to be the treatment of choice. It was suggested that "fasting alone be initially used as the simpler and more economical therapy". The finding was that "neither nasogastric suction nor cimetidine offer any advantage over fasting alone in the treatment of mild to moderate acute pancreatitis of any etiology."[38]

PCB and DDT contamination

A most encouraging use of fasting was published in the *American Journal of Industrial Medicine* in 1984. This study involved patients who had ingested rice oil contaminated with PCBs. All patients reported improvement in symptoms, and some observed "dramatic" relief, after undergoing 7–10 day fasts.[43] This research supports past studies conducted by Inamura of PCB-poisoned patients and indicates the therapeutic effects of fasting. Caution must be used, however, when treating patients known to suffer significant contamination with fat-soluble toxins. DDT is mobilized during a fast and may reach blood levels toxic to the nervous system.[44]

Autoimmune disease

The beneficial effect of fasting in certain autoimmune diseases was reported in *Lancet* in 1958. The researchers found that fasting shortened the early stages of acute glomerulonephritis (reduced glomerular filtration rate, high blood pressure, and edema), thus improving the prognosis. They concluded that "all patients with acute glomerulonephritis should fast".[45] Other autoimmune diseases that have responded to fasting include rosacea, lupus, and chronic uticaria.[46,47]

Arthritis

The subject of arthritis and fasting is receiving greater attention in the scientific literature, with most of the research coming from Scandinavia. Scientists have documented the anti-inflammatory effects of fasting with observations of decreased ESR, arthralgia, pain, stiffness, and need for medication.[48–55] A 1984 US study of 43 patients with definite or classical rheumatoid arthritis found significant improvement in grip strength, pain, PIP swelling, ESR, and functional activity after a fast of 7 days.[52]

A strong link between arthritis and food intolerance has been revealed through fasting (see also Ch. 51). The decrease in symptoms of rheumatoid arthritis during fasting may be due to the decrease in gut permeability which accompanies fasting.[51] This would reduce the absorption of antigenic molecules into the blood from the gastrointestinal tract. In the 1984 *Bulletin on Rheumatic Diseases*, Panush proposes two theories:[56]

- nutritional modification might alter immune responsiveness and thereby affect manifestations of rheumatic diseases
- rheumatic disease may be a manifestation of a food allergy or hypersensitivity.

Food allergy

Fasting, in conjunction with food challenging, is now being used as a diagnostic test to determine food intolerances. Patients are fasted for a minimum of 4 days, and then individual foods are given to determine if a reaction occurs. This method correlates well with skin prick and RAST testing. A letter in the 1984 *Lancet* states:[57]

> When food avoidances prevent headaches, IBS, arthralgia and depression, it is more effective and less costly than traditional treatment and the observation also throws light on the etiology of the disorder.

Other diseases

Other diseases in which the scientific literature indicates that fasting has led to improvement include:

- psychosomatic diseases[39]
- neurogenic bladder[39]
- psoriasis[22,30,31]
- eczema[22,48]
- thrombophlebitis[38]
- varicose ulcers[58]
- neurocirculatory disease[39]
- IBS[39]
- dysorexia nervosa (impaired or deranged appetite)[39]
- bronchial asthma[39]
- lumbago[39]
- depression[39]
- neurosis and schizophrenia[59]
- parasites[60]
- duodenal ulcers[61]
- uterine fibroids.[46]

These diseases are not a complete list of indications for fasting, but rather are those that have been studied in the scientific literature. There has been considerable empirical study of fasting in the treatment of a wide variety of diseases. Records of the results can be found in lay, hygienic, and medical literature published since the early 1900s.[62–70] The vast potential of therapeutic fasting is only beginning to be realized, as recent research reveals such pervasive and important effects as enhancement of immune system function.[53,71–75]

PHYSIOLOGY

The study of the physiology of fasting reveals a highly ordered series of events (see Fig. 47.1) which conserve body energy reserves while maintaining the basal metabolic rate (the BMR decreases by about 1%/day during fasting, until it stabilizes at about 75% of normal[36]). It has been suggested that humans, like other species, have evolved special biochemical pathways to subsist for long periods of time without food.[76] During periods of food scarcity due to climate, injury, illness, etc., animals require adaptive mechanisms to survive. It is now apparent that, in addition to maintaining the BMR, fasting also enhances the healing process.

Research in the early 1990s using MRS indicated that glucogenesis may be responsible for 64% and hepatic glycogenolysis for 36% of fuel requirements in the first 22 hours of fasting. This is a radical departure from biochemistry of the past which suggested that hepatic glycogenolysis represented 65% of fuel requirements in the first 22 hours of fasting. Scientists agree that this preliminary research necessitates further studies before any strong conclusions can be reached.[77–79]

The body's response to the lack of energy input can be divided into three stages: early fasting, fasting, and starvation. Maintaining adequate energy resources for metabolism during fasting involves several adaptations, which change as the body moves from one stage to the next. The following discussion, Tables 47.1–47.4, and

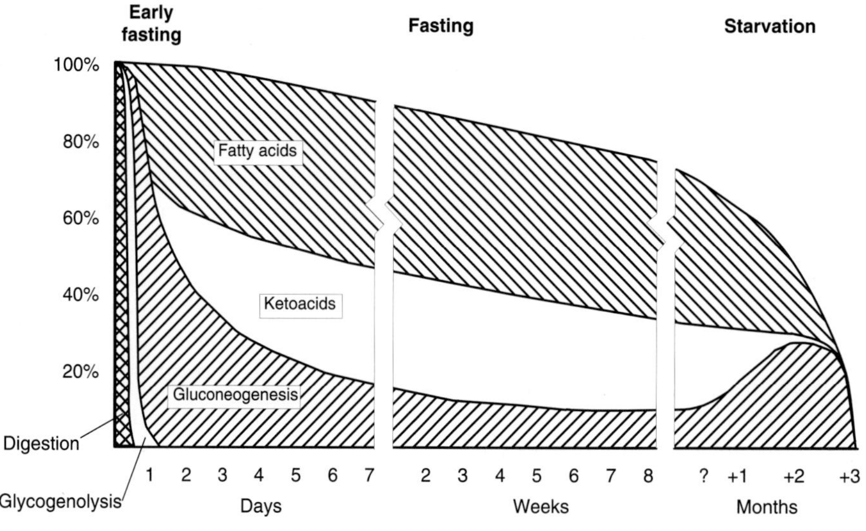

Figure 47.1 Energy reserve utilization during fasting.

Table 47.1 Mobilizable fuel reserves in a 70 kg man[80]

Tissue (weight, kg)	Glucose/glycogen		Protein		Triglyceride	
	g	kcal	g	kcal	g	kcal
Blood (10)	15	60	100	400	5	45
Liver (1)	100	400	100	400	50	450
Intestines (1)	0	0	100	400	0	0
Brain (1.4)	2	8	40	160	0	0
Muscle (30)	300	1,200	4,000	16,000	600	5,400
Adipose (15)	20	80	300	1,200	12,000	108,000
Skin, lung spleen (4)	13	52	240	960	40	360
Total	450	1,800	4,880	19,520	12,695	114,255

Table 47.2 Energy reserve utilization[36,81–83]

Energy source	Reserve*
Glucose	1 hour
Digestion	4–8 hours
Glycogen	12 hours
Amino acids	48 hours
Protein	3 weeks (if protein were the only fuel used for gluconeogenesis) 24 weeks (obligatory loss only)
Triglycerides	8 weeks

*These estimates are based on 100% utilization of each fuel.

Table 47.3 Daily resource utilization of an average 70 kg man during fasting[36]

Resource	Early (g)	Late (g)
Protein	60–84	18–24
Fat	100–140*	160–200*
Glucose	100–180	80
Sodium	3.5–5.8	0.02–0.35
Potassium	1.6–1.8	0.4–0.6

*These values are much higher in obese individuals.

Table 47.4 Summary of metabolic events in early versus late stages of fasting

	Early	Late
Brain	Uses glucose for fuel	Adapts to using ketones and some glucose
Liver glycogen	Breaks down to supply glucose	Slowly regenerates
Amino acids	High demand for making glucose	Significantly reduced demand for making glucose
Glycerol	High demand for making glucose	Significantly reduced demand for making glucose
Fatty acids	Supply energy directly for most tissues	Major source of energy for most tissues, including ketones for brain
Metabolic rate	Slight reduction	Significant reduction
Net effect	High use of protein to supply glucose to the brain	Less need for glucose, conservation of protein, utilization of fat reserved

Figures 47.1 and 47.2 describe these stages and their metabolic significance. First, however, a summary of energy production and utilization is useful.

Energy production and utilization

Glucose, fatty acids, and L-amino acids are the major fuels of the body. Although a complete description of their metabolism is beyond the scope of this chapter (a good resource is *Biochemistry: a case-oriented approach*[82]), their use for energy production can be simplified as follows:

1. Fatty acid catabolism occurs in the mitochondria of virtually all tissues except the brain and red blood cells. In the energy-producing process of beta-oxidation, two-carbon fragments are successively removed from

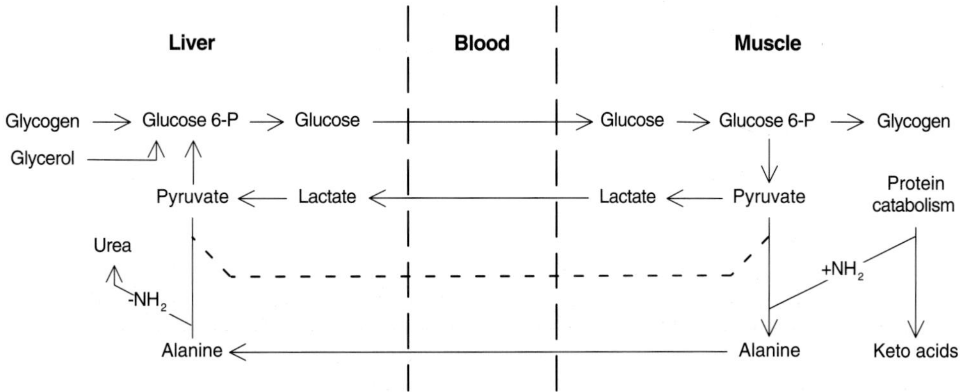

Figure 47.2 Mechanisms of glucose production during fasting.

the fatty acid to form acetyl CoA and ATP. The acetyl CoA enters the Krebs cycle for conversion to more ATP.

2. Energy production from glucose metabolism is primarily through the formation of pyruvate (glycolysis), which is converted to acetyl CoA for entry into the Krebs cycle.

3. When used for energy production, the L-amino acids are, in general, converted to pyruvate, alpha-ketoglutarate, and oxaloacetate, again for entry into the Krebs cycle.

The major form of utilizable energy in all cells is ATP, which is produced by oxidative catabolism of D-glucose, alpha-ketones, fatty acids, and/or L-amino acids.

The energy for resting heart and skeletal muscle is met primarily by oxidation of acetoacetate (produced by the liver from acetyl CoA) and fatty acids, and secondarily by glucose oxidation. Muscle contraction requires a continuous supply of ATP, large amounts of which may be almost instantaneously produced by massive conversion of glycogen to lactate (the primary purpose of muscle glycogen). During extreme muscle activity, other short-term energy sources, such as phosphocreatine, are also used. Neither of these is utilized, however, to maintain energy levels during fasting. Exercise also greatly increases glucose utilization by heart and skeletal muscle, which, as discussed below, is probably why resting is important in fasting, since the major source of glucose during fasting is protein catabolism.

Under the fed condition, the energy requirement of the mature brain is met almost entirely by glucose. Since the glycogen content of the brain is very low (0.1%), there is essentially no brain-glucose reserve. After a few days of fasting, the brain switches to oxidation of beta-hydroxybutyrate (produced by the liver from acetyl CoA) as its primary energy source.

Early fasting

The initial physiological response to the lack of food is the increased synthesis of the glucose by the liver for release into the bloodstream. Glucose is especially needed by the brain, which consumes about 65% of the total circulating glucose (400–600 kcal/day), and the red blood cells.[36,84] Together they consume 100–180 g of glucose per day. Early on in fasting, the liver is the sole source of glucose for the bloodstream. The liver initially synthesizes glucose from glycogen through glycogenolysis. However, liver glycogen stores can only supply enough glucose for a few hours (see Tables 47.1 and 47.2), and glucose production from gluconeogenesis soon becomes necessary. Although muscle actually contains more glycogen than liver, it lacks the enzyme D-glucose-6-phosphatase and therefore cannot convert glycogen to glucose for release into the bloodstream.[85] Later in fasting, the glycogen reserves are restored.[86]

Gluconeogenesis utilizes primarily L-amino acids for glucose synthesis, although glycerol from triglyceride catabolism is also used. Since liver glycogenic amino acid stores are quickly depleted, substrate from other tissues, primarily the muscles, is required. As the fast proceeds, the kidneys become progressively more important in the maintenance of blood glucose levels, and eventually the renal cortex synthesizes more glucose from amino acids than does the liver.[76] If the body continued to require its normal 100–180 g/day of glucose, gluconeogenesis during fasting would quickly use up much body protein, and death would ensue within 3–4 weeks.[81] Early on in fasting, the body catabolizes 60–84 g/day of protein.

Initially, sodium, potassium, and water diuresis occurs and hypovolemia develops. Calcium and magnesium are also lost. Plasma ketones rise, and ketones appear in the urine by the third day.[36]

Fasting

Research using respiratory quotient and urinary nitrogen studies has repeatedly shown that triglycerides are the major fuel during fasting.[2,20,85,87–89] To leave the adipocyte, triglycerides must first be hydrolyzed (lypolysis) to fatty acids and glycerol. The fatty acids are transported in the blood, in a physical complex with albumin, to the liver, muscle, and other tissues.

Although the brain converts to oxidation of beta-hydroxybutyrate after 4–7 days, there is still an obligatory need for approximately 80 g/day of glucose for the brain, red cells, muscles, and other tissues.[85] This requirement increases significantly during exercise. Although much of the lactate produced by anaerobic metabolism of glucose and glycogen is resynthesized to glucose by the liver via the Cori cycle, the need for glucose is increased, since there is a net loss due to urinary excretion of lactic acid and metabolic inefficiency. Approximately 16 g of glucose is synthesized from triglyceride glycerol, with the rest of the glucose requirement (and the other metabolic processes requiring amino acids, e.g. enzyme turnover) being met by the catabolism of 18–24 g/day of protein. In experimental animals, as much as 14% of the energy needed by muscle may come from the oxidation of branched-chain amino acids. Glucose is also recycled by the breakdown of blood cells in the liver.[85,87,88] The mechanisms of glucose production during fasting are summarized in Figure 47.2.

Research has determined that an average 70 kg male has the fat stores to maintain basic caloric requirements for 2–3 months of fasting.[2,20,85,87,88]

Starvation

Starvation occurs when the body's fat reserves are depleted and significant protein catabolism again becomes necessary for energy production.[2] As noted above, unless fat reserves are being utilized for energy production and glucose sparing, the body protein stores are adequate for only a few weeks of gluconeogenesis, after which essential proteins are utilized and death occurs.

Mechanism of ketosis

During fasting, when excessive amounts of fatty acids are being oxidized and inadequate glucose is available, large quantities of ketones are secreted into the bloodstream. Ketone bodies are made in the liver from acetyl CoA.

During adequate energy input, the conversion of fatty acids to acetyl CoA is regulated by the availability of L-glycerol 3-phosphate (derived from glucose through the glycolytic pathway). As the concentration of acetyl CoA rises, it is resynthesized into triglycerides, with L-glycerol 3-phosphate serving as the accepter to which three acyl CoA groups are attached (through esterification). During fasting, there is inadequate glucose to provide the needed glycerol for triglyceride synthesis, resulting in acetyl CoA levels in excess of the oxidative capacity of the Krebs cycle. The excess is then shunted into the synthesis of ketone bodies.[82] These ketone bodies (acetoacetic acid, acetone, and beta-hydroxybutyric acid) are utilized by the heart, and, later in fasting, by the brain for energy production.

Mechanism of acidosis

Since the ketone bodies are acids, their entry into the plasma results in an increase in hydrogen ions. This is buffered by the conversion of bicarbonate into carbonic acid and then to CO_2, which is exhaled. Eventually the buffering capacity is exceeded, and the plasma pH decreases, resulting in mild metabolic acidosis. The body compensates for this by increasing the respiratory rate to promote further elimination of CO_2 and by excreting ketone bodies in the urine. These adaptations may result in some electrolyte imbalance.[82]

Amino acid metabolism

With the exception of leucine, which appears to be a regulator of protein turnover in muscle,[90] all amino acids are glucogenic. However, alanine plays a prominent role in a cycle analogous to the Cori cycle for lactate.[91,92] The alanine cycle provides the mechanism for the recycling of a fixed supply of glucose and the effective transportation to the liver of amino acid nitrogen derived from muscle breakdown. Because muscle, unlike liver, is incapable of synthesizing urea, most of the amino nitrogen from protein breakdown is transferred to pyruvate to form alanine. The alanine enters the blood and is taken up by the liver. The amino groups are removed to form urea, and the resulting pyruvate is converted to glucose. The newly synthesized glucose is secreted into the blood, taken up by the muscle, and catabolized to pyruvate to reseed the alanine cycle.[82]

Electrolyte balance

Serum electrolyte levels usually do not change significantly during fasting and are not good indicators of tissue stores but are considered the most important blood values during fasting.[93] During early fasting the body loses 150–250 mEq (3.5–5.8 g) of sodium and 40–45 mEq (1.6–1.8 g) of potassium a day. Later, these drop to 1–15 mEq (0.02–0.35 g) and 10–15 mEq (0.4–0.6 g), respectively. The total body stores of sodium are 83–97 g (of which 65% is exchangeable) and of potassium are 115–131 g (of which 98% is exchangeable). The typical daily dietary intake of sodium is 3–7 g and of potassium is 3–5 g.[83] Serum potassium usually decreases but may be elevated. Results below 3 mEq/L or above 6 mEq/L may necessitate breaking the fast. Total calcium is usually stable, but ionic calcium often decreases, especially if vomiting is present.[93]

Physical changes during fasting

Physical changes during the fast generally include a decrease in weight, pulse,[20,22,95] and blood pressure.[20,21,22,96] EKG changes may include sinus bradycardia, decreased QRS complex and T-wave amplitude, elongation of the QT interval, and shifts to the right of the QRS and T-wave axes. These changes return to normal after fasting.[22,94–96]

Laboratory changes during fasting

Most laboratory values of the body fluids during fasting do not follow specific patterns, but are unique to the individual and the disease process.[34,94] Assessment of a fasting patient's progress is not based on a sign or symptom, but on the total clinical picture. Although specific predictions of laboratory values during fasting are not possible, some general observations have been made. Some authorities indicate that triglycerides decline with fasting but find elevations if liver damage is present. Serum protein usually declines with fasting. Pancreatic lipase and amylase usually decline with fasting.[93]

Liver enzymes may increase considerably if liver disease is present and may rise even when liver disease is not present. Triglyceride, cholesterol, and uric acid levels usually rise during fasting,[97–99] indicating mobilization of tissue stores. Post-fast values often show a decrease from pre-fast values.[26,40,98] A rise in BUN may occur, but some authors have observed a decrease.[22,27,38,100] Creatinine levels may be elevated[45,97] or may remain stable.[101]

Blood glucose drops in most patients,[24,26,27,48] possibly below 30 mg/dl.[97] If blood glucose is low prior to fasting, it may rise post-fasting.

Complete blood counts usually show no significant change,[102] but decreases in hemoglobin and hematocrit have been observed.[38,99,103] When this occurs, hemolysis or hemorrhage must be ruled out.[93] Hematocrit, hemoglobin, and RBC count may be increased, but this usually indicates inadequate hydration.[75,97,102] Erythrocyte sedimentation rate usually decreases with fasting.[52,53,97] White blood cells are usually unchanged or decrease slightly with fasting; however, infection may cause an increase. An increase may also be observed if levels are low prior to fasting.[93]

Urinalyses may be difficult to interpret during fasting, since the body discards considerable waste via the kidneys.[102] It is not uncommon to see various types of casts, RBCs, WBCs, bilirubin (+1 to +2), protein (trace, +2), and ketones (+4), and, if liver disease is present, urobilinogen elevation. Specific gravity is commonly elevated (possibly to 1.035), which may reflect inadequate hydration.[97]

Hormonal changes during fasting

Hormonal changes during fasting typically include decreases of insulin[76,87,89,94,104] and thyroid hormones.[94,95,105] Increased levels of growth hormone,[94,95,105] cortisol,[75] glucagon,[76,87] plasma norepinephrine,[106] serum melatonin,[106] and certain prostaglandins (in animals) usually occur.[107] By contrast, a decrease in growth hormone is usually found in obese individuals.[94]

In one study conducted on 10 postmenopausal women who underwent short-term fasts, no significant changes in adrenal hormones, androgens, serum and urinary estrogens, plasma epinephrine, or dopamine were recorded.[106]

Effects of fasting on immune function

The immune system undergoes very important changes during the fast, and an increase in various aspects of immune function has been observed. The first evidence of this came from the study in 1923 which found increased resistance to infection during the post-fast period.[21] Changes in the immune system during fasting include:[53,71–75]

- increased macrophage activity
- increased cell-mediated immunity (T-lymphocytes and lymphokines)
- decreased complement factors
- decreased antigen–antibody complexes
- increased immunoglobulin levels
- increased neutrophil bactericidal activity
- depressed lymphocyte blastogenesis
- heightened monocyte killing and bactericidal function
- enhanced natural killer cell activity in animals and humans.

CLINICAL PROTOCOL

Therapeutic fasting of more than 5 days' duration is probably best conducted under supervision at an in-patient facility. Several facilities now exist in the US, Canada, England, and Australia, and these centers follow the standards of care and principles of ethics established by the IAHP.[3]

Consultation standards

- Appropriate case history
- Physical examination
- Evaluation or assessment of the chief complaints
- Explanation and recommendations.

Clinical standards

- Provide an environment conducive to rest and comfort
- Maintain a daily record of progress, including appropriate vital signs
- Supply adequate amounts of water
- Assure the availability of attendants
- Exercise care in terminating a fast and supervising post-fast recuperation, consistent with professional hygienic principles.

Water vs. juice

Only pure water (distilled, spring, reverse osmosis) is recommended while fasting.[65,69] Some authors have recommended juice, but this is considered a restricted diet, not a fast, since juice is a food, and the continued consumption of carbohydrates inhibits the body's conversion to ketotic metabolism. In most cases, the fast is superior to the restricted diet: hunger almost totally disappears;[22,30] ketosis occurs more quickly and efficiently;[22,30] famine edema does not occur;[22] sodium diuresis is more pronounced;[29] weight loss is more dramatic and is from fat rather than protein stores; healing time is shorter; and patient strength may be greater.[69] It is interesting to note that people in developing world countries on protein-deficient diets die sooner than those who fast completely.[76] Restricted diets, however, are often useful before and after fasting, and if a crisis develops or a fast is contraindicated.[68]

Quantity of water

The optimal quantity of water to ingest during fasting is best determined by thirst, but patients should drink at least a few glasses a day. During fasting the need for water decreases, since obligatory water excretion is reduced (due to lower excretion of urea, the major osmotic solute) and water is released from catabolized fat.[76] One cup of water each day is actually sufficient to maintain adequate hydration for most people,[76] although researchers fasting obese individuals often recommend 3 L/day.[36]

Supplements

Loss of minerals or vitamins is usually not a concern, and deficiencies while fasting are rare.[22,29,65,69,108,109] In fact, problems, such as nausea and indigestion, have been reported when these were supplemented during the fast.[32,101] For example, it is well known that nicotinic acid supplementation inhibits the release of free fatty acids from adipose tissue.[36] In one patient in whom vitamin deficiency was reported in the medical literature, the actual fasting protocol was not described. In addition, activity was not restricted and oral medication for intercurrent illness was maintained while fasting.[32] Vitamin and mineral excretion becomes very low after 10 days.

Exercise

Exercise is discouraged while fasting. Fuel conservation is necessary to allow maximal healing and the avoidance of unnecessary gluconeogenesis.[65,69] The body utilizes certain muscle proteins early in a fast, thus initiating the natural restriction of activity. Short walks or light stretching is permissible, but intense exercise will inhibit repair and elimination. In serious chronic disease, an excess of activity has been suspected as cause of death during fasting.[110]

Sunlight

Sunlight is important for general health during fasting, and patients should try to obtain 10–20 minutes/day. An increase in heart rate of 10–15 beats/minute would indicate excessive exposure. Many fasting facilities have solariums in which patients may sunbathe.

Rest

Rest is a most important aspect of the fast, and patients may nap throughout the day. Less sleep is common at night, due possibly to the decreased daily activity and increase in daytime rest.

Laboratory tests

Laboratory tests such as a CBC and chem-screen are usually performed weekly, while others are performed as necessary. Daily urine tests are sometimes performed, and vital signs are checked daily.[97,102]

Enemas

Enemas are not usually necessary and may not offer any added benefit.[49] Some authorities have found that they cause discomfort for the patients.[69] To help prevent constipation, a pre-fast meal of fresh fruit or vegetables will assist in elimination.

Length of fast

The length of a fast is difficult to predict. Factors to consider include size of reserves (see Tables 47.3 and 47.4), individual metabolism, financial limitations, work schedules, degree of disease, age, and sex. This decision is based on all factors, especially the patient's mental state. "The doctor will look for good practical recovery where patient is symptom free and signs of regeneration are present."[111] Although many old texts refer to fasting to completion (i.e. exhaustion of nutrient reserves), this is now uncommon and not usually necessary.[111] Shelton states:[69]

> In most cases, except TB, there can be no sound objection to a fast to completion, although this will seldom be necessary and many patients will not want to fast so long, unless they must.

A positive mental outlook is important for any patient undergoing a fast. It should be emphasized that the benefits are broad and affect all bodily systems. Perhaps the greatest value for patients is the satisfaction of playing a major role in improvement of their own health.

SIDE-EFFECTS

Side-effects from fasting are rarely serious, but fasting may uncover pathology and reveal weaknesses that were previously subclinical.[30] Discomfort during fasting may be due to withdrawal from stimulants, hypoglycemia, acidosis, elimination of wastes, and enhancement of repair. Patients may experience headaches, insomnia, skin irritations, dizziness, nausea, coated tongue, body odor, aching limbs, palpitations, mucous discharge, and visual and hearing disturbances. Hair growth is usually arrested, and dry, scaly skin may develop. Most signs and symptoms are usually brief as the body works to remove the disease.[112]

In certain cases, complications occur which may necessitate breaking the fast early. Examples of such conditions include:

- a sudden drop in blood pressure (possibly due to peripheral circulatory collapse)
- delirium
- prolonged hypothermia
- rapid/slow/feeble/irregular pulse
- extreme weakness
- dyspnea
- vomiting and diarrhea leading to dehydration
- gastrointestinal bleeding
- hepatic decompensation
- renal insufficiency
- severe gout
- cardiac arrhythmias
- emotional distress.

Fasting elevates serum uric acid levels and uric acid

excretion, and if fluid intake is insufficient, gout or renal stones may be precipitated.[36,113]

A few studies have discussed the development of Wernicke's encephalopathy during prolonged fasting, but since this rarely occurs during hygienic fasting, it is difficult to determine whether this is related to methodology. It is important, however, to acknowledge the importance of utilizing B vitamins, especially thiamine, when any fast is broken with i.v. glucose.[114,115]

The decision to terminate the fast should be based on the complete clinical picture and not on an isolated sign or symptom.

CONTRAINDICATIONS

Contraindications to fasting are few, and each case must be judged individually, since no two cases are alike. For example, an inexperienced practitioner may assume that emaciated patients should not fast, while Shelton states:[69]

> Extreme emaciation: In such cases a long fast is impossible. A short fast of 1–3 days may be found beneficial, or a series of such short fasts with longer periods of proper feeding intervening may be found advisable.

Contraindications include severe anemia, porphyria, and serious malnutrition. Individuals with a rare fatty acid deficiency of the enzyme medium-chain acyl-CoA dehydrogenase (MCAD) should also avoid fasting.[46]

The fasting of children and pregnant women is controversial. While a short fast is appropriate for the sick child who does not want to eat, fasting a pregnant women may be seriously contraindicated: ketosis in pregnant diabetic women is known to cause fetal damage. Although this is commonly recognized, the fact that this information has come only from research of diabetic women is not as widely known. There appear to be no studies of the effects of non-diabetic ketosis on fetal development. Doctors (e.g. Shelton, Benesh, Sidwha, and Burton) with considerable experience of fasting pregnant women (during all three trimesters) have found no adverse effects with fasts of a few days to 2–3 weeks. Although the fasting of pregnant women appears, according to clinical observation, to be safe, definitive pronouncement cannot be made until careful research is performed (such as a controlled retrospective analysis of existing cases).[116]

Fasts for children and pregnant women should be shorter and meticulously supervised by an experienced doctor. In *The science and fine art of fasting*, Shelton states: "Few infants require more than 2–3 days of fasting ... I have never hesitated to permit a sick infant to fast and I have yet to see one harmed by it."[69]

Regarding pregnancy he states: "The author would object to a long fast in chronic 'disease' during this period. There can, however, be no objection to a short fast ... "

It is well recognized that fasting during lactation is not generally advised, since milk flow is halted and difficult to resume.[69] Although fasting is considered inappropriate in renal insufficiency,[36] the authors have seen patients with 65% renal function return to normal as a result of fasting and dietary management.

With regard to fasting contraindications in general, Burton stated:[111]

> I have found few health problems which are absolute contraindications to fasting. In my experience, if the need is evident, the only genuine contraindication is fear. ... As for the other conditions often mentioned, e.g. kidney disease, heart impairment, TB, etc., they merely require extreme caution, because of the limits imposed by pathology, but they are not inexorable contraindications.

Supervised fasting as a therapeutic procedure is generally safe and effective. The incidence of death at fasting institutions is low, which is promising, since many of the patients have serious chronic diseases and have exhausted other therapeutic options. Of the hundreds of cases of fasting described in the scientific literature, only seven cases of death have been reported prior to 1985.[58,110,117–120] In all cases, the patients had serious chronic disease prior to fasting, and in five of the seven cases drugs were given to the patients while fasting, while in the other two no description of protocol was provided.

There is no evidence in the scientific literature to suggest that fasting itself can be considered a cause of death. Death during fasting indicates that the remedial efforts of the body have been overpowered by the pathological process. This situation occurs in serious disease, whether eating or fasting. In examining the fallacy of attributing the cause of death to fasting, one researcher in the *Lancet* wrote:[121]

> Fasting short of emaciation is not hazardous, if death results, reasons other than those of the fast should be considered before concluding that all supervised fasts should be discouraged.

CONCLUSION

Therapeutic fasting is a useful protocol for any doctor interested in studying and promoting the inherent ability of the body to heal itself. This fine art and science is generally a safe, economical, and effective therapy for most patients in disease. Those interested in further study should initially direct their attention to the main historical texts and then to the recent hygienic and scientific literature. The references provide a greater depth of information for the topics discussed in this chapter. Internship with a doctor skilled in therapeutic fasting is strongly advised for those interested in providing safe and effective patient care.

REFERENCES

1. Mosby's Medical & Nursing Dictionary. St Louis, MO: CV Mosby. 1983: p 417
2. Lehninger A. Biochemistry. New York, NY: Worth Publishing. 1964: p 841–845
3. IAHP Secretary/Treasurer Atty. Mark A Huberman, 204 Stambaugh Bldg, Youngstown, OH, 44503
4. Randolph TG. Human ecology and susceptibility to the chemical environment. Springfield, IL: CC Thomas. 1962
5. Dickey LD, ed. Clinical ecology. Springfield, IL: CC Thomas. 1976
6. Arbesman R. Fasting and prophecy in pagan and Christian antiquity. Tradition 1951; 7: 1–71
7. MacDermot V. The cult of the seer in the Ancient Middle East. Berkeley, CA: University of California Press. 1971
8. Maulana Mohammad Ali. The religion of Islam: a comprehensive discussion of the sources, principles and practices of Islam. The Ahmadiyya Anjuman Isha'at Islam: Lahore, India. 1936
9. Burns D. The greatest health discovery. Chicago, IL: Natural Hygiene Press. 1972
10. Shelton HM. Some fasting history. Shelton's Hygienic Review 1964; XXV: 12: 291–293
11. Shelton HM. Rubies in the Sand. San Antonio, TX: Shelton's Health School. 1961
12 Numbers RL. Prophetess of health: a study of Ellen G White. New York: Harper and Row. 1976
13. Weiss HB. The great American water cure. New Jersey: Past Times Press. 1967
14. Shelton HM. Natural Hygiene. Man's pristine way of life. San Antonio, TX: Shelton's Health School. 1968
15. Shyrock RH. Medicine in America. Baltimore, MD: Johns Hopkins Press. 1966
16. ANHS, 12816 Race Track Road, Tampa, FL, 33625
17. Dr Tanner's fast. Br Med J 1880; ii: 171
18. Paton DN, Stockman R. Observations of the metabolism of man during starvation. Proc R Soc Edinb 1888–89; 16: 121–131
19. Penny F. Notes on a thirty day's fast. Br Med J 1909; 1: 1414–1416
20. Benedict FG. A study of prolonged fasting, Publication #203. Washington, DC: Carnegie Institute. 1915
21. Morgulis S. Fasting and undernutrition. New York, NY: EP Dutton. 1923
22. Keys A, Brozek J, Henschel A et al. The biology of human starvation, vols 1 and 2. Minneapolis, MN: University of Minnesota Press. 1950
23. Guelpa G. Starvation and purgation in the relief of diabetes. Br Med J 1910; ii: 1050–1051
24. Allen FM. Prolonged fasting in diabetes. Am J Med Sci 1915; 150: 480–485
25. Guelpa, Marie, 1910, cited by Kernt PR, Naughton JL, Driscoll CE et al. Fasting: the history, pathophysiology and complications. West J Med 1981; 137: 379–399
26. Hoeffel G, Moriarty M. The effects of fasting on the metabolism. Am J Dis Child 1924; 28: 16–24
27. Lennox WG, Cobb S. Studies in epilepsy. Arch Neurol Psych 1928; 20: 711–779
28. Folin O, Denis W. On starvation and obesity with special reference to acidosis. J Biol Chem 1915; 21: 183–192
29. Bloom WL. Fasting as an introduction to the treatment of obesity. Metabolism 1959; 8: 214–220
30. Duncan GG, Jenson WK, Cristofori FC, Schless GL. Intermittent fasts in the correction and control of intractable obesity. Am J Med Sci 1963; 245: 515–520
31. Duncan GG, Duncan TG, Schless GL, Cristofori FC. Contraindications and therapeutic results of fasting in obese patients. Ann NY Acad Sci 1965; 131: 632–636
32. Drenick EJ, Swenseid ME, Blahd WH, Tuttle S. Prolonged starvation as a treatment for severe obesity. JAMA 1964; 187: 100–105
33. Drenick EJ. Contraindications to long term fasting. JAMA 1964; 188: 88
34. Thompson TJ, Runcie J, Miller V. Treatment of obesity by total fast for up to 249 days. Lancet 1966; ii: 992–996
35. Stewart WK, Fleming LW. Features of a successful therapeutic fast of 382 days' duration. Postgrad Med J 1973; 49: 203–209
36. Goodhart RS, Shils ME. Modern nutrition in health and disease. 6th edn. Philadelphia, PA: Lea & Febiger. 1980: p 738, 826, 983–986, 1086
37. Gresham GA. Is atheroma a reversible lesion. Atherosclerosis 1976; 23: 379–391
38. Lawlor T, Wells DG. Metabolic hazards of fasting. Am J Clin Nutr 1969; 22: 8: 1142–1149
39. Suzuki J, Yamauchi Y, Horikawa M, Yamagata S. Fasting therapy for psychosomatic disease with special reference to its indications and therapeutic mechanism. Tohoku J Exp Med 1976; 118: 245–259
40. Vessby B, Boberg M, Karlstrom B et al. Improved metabolic control after supplemented fasting in overweight type 2 diabetic patients. Acta Med Scand 1984; 216: 67–74
41. Sorbris R, Aly KO, Nilsson-Ehle P et al. Vegetarian fasting of obese patients. A clinical and biochemical evaluation. Scand J Gastroenterol 1982; 17: 417–424
42. Navarro S, Rose E, Aused R et al. Comparison of fasting, nasogastric suction and cimetidine in the treatment of acute pancreatitis. Digestion 1984; 30: 224–230
43. Imamura M, Tung T. A trial of fasting cure for PCB poisoned patients in Taiwan. Am J Ind Med 1984; 5: 147–153
44. Shakman RA. Nutritional influences on the toxicity of environmental pollutants: a review. Arch Env Health 1974; 28: 105–133
45. Brod J, Pavkova L, Fencl V et al. Influence of fasting on the immunological reactions and course of acute glomerulonephritis. Lancet 1958; i: 760–763
46. Fuhrman J. Fasting and eating for health. New York, NY: St. Martin's Press. 1995
47. Okamoto O, Murakami I, Itami S et al. Fasting diet therapy for chronic urticaria: report of a case. J Derm 1992; 19: 7. 428–431
48. Lithell H, Bruce A, Gustafsson IB et al. A fasting and vegetarian diet treatment trial on chronic inflammatory disorders. Acta Derm Venereol 1983; 63: 397–403
49. Skoldstam L, Larsson L, Lindstrom FD. Rheumatoid arthritis. Scand J Rheumatol 1979; 8: 249–255
50. Skoldstam L, Lindstrom FD, Lindblom B. Impaired con A suppressor cell activity in patients with rheumatoid arthritis shows normalization during fasting. Scand J Rheumatol 1983; 12: 4: 369–373
51. Sundquist T, Lindstrom F, Magnusson K, Skoldstam L. Influence of fasting on intestinal permeability and disease activity in patients with rheumatoid arthritis shows normalization during fasting. Scand J Rheumatol 1982; 11: 33–38
52. Kroker GF, Stroud RM, Marshall R et al. Fasting and rheumatoid arthritis: a multicentre study. Clin Ecology 1984; 2: 3: 137–144
53. Uden AM, Trang L, Venizelos N, Palmblad J. Neutrophil function and clinical performances after total fasting in patients with rheumatoid arthritis. Ann Rheum Dis 1983; 42: 45–51
54. Palmblad J, Hafstrom I, Ringertz B. Antirheumatic effects of fasting. Rheum Dis Clin North Am 1991; 17: 2: 351–362
55. Kjeldsen-Kragh J, Mellbye OJ, Haugen M et al. Changes in laboratory variables in rheumatoid arthritis patients during a trial of fasting and one-year vegetarian diet. Scand J Rheum 1995; 24: 2: 85–93
56. Panush RS. Controversial arthritis remedies. Bull Rheum Dis 1984; 34: 1–10
57. Gerrard JL. Food intolerances. Lancet 1984; ii: 413
58. Spencer IOB. Death during therapeutic starvation for obesity. Lancet 1968; i: 1288–1290
59. Boehme DL. Preplanned fasting in the treatment of mental disease: survey of the current Soviet literature. Schizophr Bull 1977; 3: 2: 288–296
60. Millet V, Spencer MJ, Chapin M et al. Dientamoeba fragilis, a protozoan parasite in adult members of a semicommunal group. Dig Dis Sci 1983; 28: 4: 335–337
61. Johnston DA, Wormsley KG. The effects of fasting on 24-h

gastric secretions of patients with duodenal ulcers resistant to ranitidine. Aliment Pharmacol Ther 1989; 3: 5: 471–479
62. Dewey EH. The no-breakfast plan and the fasting-cure. New York, NY: The Health Culture Co. 1900
63. MacFadden B. Fasting for health. New York, NY: MacFadden. 1923
64. Hazzard LB. Scientific fasting. New York, NY: Grant Publications. 1927
65. Carrington H. Fasting for health and long life. Mokelume Hill, CA: Health Research. 1963
66. Devries A. Therapeutic fasting. Los Angeles, CA: Chandler Book Co. 1963
67. Shelton HM. Fasting can save your life. Chicago, IL: Natural Hygiene Press. 1964
68. Shelton HM. Fasting for renewal of life. Chicago, IL: Natural Hygiene Press. 1978
69. Shelton HM. The science and fine art of fasting. Chicago, IL: Natural Hygiene Press. 1978
70. Oswald JA, Shelton HM. Fasting for the health of it. Pueblo, CO: Nationwide Press. 1983
71. Wing EJ, Boehme SM, Barczynski LK. Effects of acute nutritional deprivation on immune function in mice. Immunology 1983; 48: 543–550
72. Wing EJ, Stanko RT, Winnkelstein A, Adibi SA. Fasting enhanced immune effector mechanism in obese patients. Am J Med 1983; 75: 91–96
73. Friend PS, Fernandes G, Good RA et al. Dietary restrictions early and late. Effects on the nephropathy of NZBxNZW mouse. Lab Invest 1978; 38: 629–632
74. Miller JD. Life extension. N Eng J Med 1985; 313: 760
75. Palmblad J, Cantell K, Holm G et al. Acute energy deprivation in man. Effect on serum immunoglobulins, antibody response, complement factors 3 & 4, acute phase reactants and interferon producing capacity of blood lymphocytes. Clin Exp Immunol 1977; 30: 50–55
76. Young VR, Scrimshaw NS. The physiology of starvation. Sci Am 1971; 225: 4: 14–21
77. Rothman DL, Magnusson I, Katz LD et al. Quantitation of hepatic glycogenolysis and gluconeogenesis in fasting humans with 13C NMR. Science 1991; 254: 573–576
78. Editorial. Insights into fasting. Lancet 1992; 339: 152–153
79. Koff RS, Rapid induction of gluconeogenesis during fasting. Gastroenterology 1992; 102: 6: 2174–2175
80. Elkeles RS, Tavill AS. Biochemical aspects of human disease. Boston, MA: Blackwell. 1983: p 141
81. White A, Handler P, Smith EL et al. Principles of biochemistry. 6th edn. New York, NY: McGraw-Hill. 1978: p 496
82. Montgomery R, Dryer RL, Conway TW, Spector AA. Biochemistry: a case-oriented approach. 4th edn. St Louis, MI: CV Mosby. 1983: p 493–498
83. Nutrition Reviews. Present knowledge in nutrition. 5th edn. Washington, DC: Nutrition Foundation. 1984: p 439–453
84. Reinmuth OM, Scheinberg P, Bourne B. Total cerebral blood flow and metabolism. Arch Neurol 1965; 12: 49–66
85. Saudek C, Felig P. The metabolic events of starvation. Am J Med 1976; 60: 117–126
86. Haro EN, Blum SF, Faloon WW. The glucagon response of fasting obese subjects. Metabolism 1965; 14: 976–984
87. Cahill GF Jr, Owen OE, Morgan AP. The consumption of fuels during prolonged starvation. Adv Enzyme Regul 1968; 6: 143–150
88. Cahill GF, Jr, Owen OE. Starvation and survival. Trans Am Clin Climatol Assoc 1967; 79: 13–20
89. Felig P, Owen OE, Morgan AP, Cahill GF Jr. Utilization of metabolic fuels in obese subjects. Am J Clin Nutr 1968; 21: 1129–1133
90. Buse MG, Reid SS. Leucine, a possible regulator of protein turnover in muscle. J Clin Invest 1975; 56: 1250–1261
91. Felig P, Pozefsky T, Marliss E, Cahill GF Jr. Alanine. Key role in gluconeogenesis. Science 1970; 167: 1003–1004
92. Mallette LE, Exton JH, Park CR. Control of gluconeogenesis from amino acids in the perfused rat liver. J Biol Chem 1969; 244: 5713–5723
93. Cinque R. Hematological changes during fasting. IAHP Newsletter 1993; 7: 1: 6–8
94. Kernt PR, Naughton JL, Driscoll CE, Loxterkamp DA. Fasting: the history, pathophysiology and complications. West J Med 1982; 137: 379–399
95. Theorell T, Kjellberg J, Palmblad J. Electrocardiographic changes during total energy deprivation (fasting). Acta Med Scand 1978; 203: 13–19
96. Consolazio CF, Nelson RA, Johnson HL. Metabolic aspects of acute starvation in normal humans: performance and cardiovascular evaluation. Am J Clin Nutr 1967; 20: 684–693
97. Goldhammer A. Personal communication. 1986
98. Valenta LJ, Elias AN. Modified fasting in the treatment of obesity. Postgrad Med J 1986; 79: 263–267
99. Ende N. Starvation studies with special reference to cholesterol. Am J Clin Nutr 1962; 11: 270–280
100. Immerman AM. Fasting and diet restriction in the treatment of cardiovascular disease. ACA J Chiropractic 1980; 140: S42–S54
101. Rapoport GL, From A, Hudson H. Metabolic studies in prolonged fasting: inorganic metabolism and kidney function. Metabolism 1965; 14: 1: 30–47
102. Scott DJ. Personal communication. 1986
103. Rooth G, Carlstrom S. Therapeutic fasting. Acta Med Scand 1970; 187: 455–463
104. Spark RF, Arky RA, Obrian JT et al. Renin aldosterone and glucagon in the natriuresis of fasting. N Eng J Med 1975; 292: 1335–1340
105. Harrison MT, Harden RM. The long-term value of fasting in the treatment of obesity. Lancet 1966; ii: 1340–1342
106. Beitins IZ, Barkan A, Kiblanski A et al. Hormonal responses to short term fasting in post menopausal women. J Clin Metab 1985; 60: 1120–1126
107. Kim YC, Brodows RG. Starvation stimulates pancreatic PGE content. Prostaglandins 1983; 25: 365–371
108. Cinque R. Personal communication. 1986
109. Benesh G. Personal communication. 1986
110. Kahan A. Death during therapeutic starvation. Lancet 1968; i: 1378–1379
111. Burton A. Fasting too long. Health Science 1979; 2: 144–146
112. Salloum TK. Fasting signs and symptoms. East Palestine, OH: Buckeye Naturopathic Press. 1992
113. Drenick EJ. Hyperuricemia, acute gout, renal insufficiency and urate nephrolithiasis due to starvation. Arth Rheum 1965; 8: 988–997
114. Devathansen G. Wernicke's encephalopathy in prolonged fasting. Lancet 1982; 2: 8307: 1108–1109
115. Falzi G, Ronchi E. Wernicke's lethal encephalopathy in voluntary, total prolonged fasting. Foren Sci Int 1990; 47: 17–20
116. Churchill JA, Berendes HW, Nemore J. Neuropsychological deficits in children of diabetic mothers. Am J Obst Gyn 1969; 105: 257–268
117. Cubberley PT, Polster SA, Schulman CL. Lactic acidosis and death after treatment of obesity by fasting. N Eng J Med 1965; 272: 628–630
118. Garnett ES, Barnard DL, Ford J, Goodbody RA. Gross fragmentation of cardiac myofibrils after therapeutic starvation. Lancet 1969; i: 914–916
119. Norbury FB. Contraindication to long term fasting. JAMA 1964; 188: 88
120. Runcie J, Thompson TJ. Prolonged starvation – a dangerous procedure. Br Med J 1970; 3: 432–435
121. Stewart WK, Fleming LW. Fragmentation of cardiac myofibrils after therapeutic starvation. Lancet 1969; 1: 1154

SECTION 4

Syndromes and special topics

SECTION CONTENTS

Careful study of the various diseases to which humans are heir indicates that a limited number of underlying problems either cause or significantly contribute to most diseases. The reductionist philosophy which underlies most of modern medical research and practice results in better diagnosis and progressively more specific therapies for a given disease, but makes recognition of broad patterns of disease causation extremely difficult.

We believe the reader will find the syndromes discussed in this chapter extremely interesting and a compelling inducement for developing a more holistic approach to patients. Old-fashioned ideas such as “bowel toxemia” and “liver toxicity” are not only intuitively reasonable, but now have solid scientific evidence to support their validity. As one reads the chapters in this section, a compelling concept of medicine emerges:

Poor diet + unhealthy lifestyle + toxin exposure

↓

Nutritional deficiencies + food allergies + toxicity

↓

Metabolic dysfunction + subacute disease

↓

Clinically recognizable diseases which are apparently unrelated to the underlying causes

CHAPTER CONTENTS

48

Chronic candidiasis

Michael T. Murray, ND

Joseph E. Pizzorno Jr, ND

INTRODUCTION

An overgrowth in the gastrointestinal tract of the usually benign yeast *Candida albicans* is now becoming recognized as a complex medical syndrome known as chronic candidiasis or the yeast syndrome.[1,2] Specifically, the overgrowth of *Candida* is believed to cause a wide variety of symptoms in virtually every system of the body, with the gastrointestinal, genitourinary, endocrine, nervous, and immune systems being the most susceptible.[3]

Although chronic candidiasis has been clinically defined for a long time, it was not until Orion Truss published *The Missing Diagnosis* and William Crook published *The Yeast Connection* that the public and many physicians became aware of the magnitude of the problem.[1,2]

GENERAL CONSIDERATIONS

Normally, *Candida albicans* lives harmoniously in the inner warm creases and crevices of the digestive tract (and vaginal tract in women). However, when this yeast overgrows, or immune system mechanisms are depleted, or the normal lining of the intestinal tract is damaged, the body can absorb yeast cells, particles of yeast cells, and various toxins.[3] As a result, there may be significant disruption of body processes, resulting in the development of the "yeast syndrome".

This syndrome is generally characterized by patients saying they "feel sick all over". Fatigue, allergies, immune system malfunction, depression, chemical sensitivities, and digestive disturbances are just some of the symptoms patients with the yeast syndrome may experience.[3]

The typical patient with the yeast is female, as women are eight times more likely to experience the yeast syndrome compared with men due to the effects of estrogen, birth control pills, and the higher number of prescriptions for antibiotics (see Table 48.1).[4]

Table 48.1 Typical chronic candidiasis patient profile

Sex: female

Age: 15–50 years

General symptoms
- Chronic fatigue
- Loss of energy
- General malaise
- Decreased libido

Gastrointestinal symptoms
- Thrush
- Bloating, gas
- Intestinal cramps
- Rectal itching
- Altered bowel function

Genitourinary system complaints
- Vaginal yeast infection
- Frequent bladder infections

Endocrine system complaints
- Primarily menstrual complaints

Nervous system complaints
- Depression
- Irritability
- Inability to concentrate

Immune system complaints
- Allergies
- Chemical sensitivities
- Low immune function

Past history
- Chronic vaginal yeast infections
- Chronic antibiotic use for infections or acne
- Oral birth control usage
- Oral steroid hormone usage

Associated conditions
- Premenstrual syndrome
- Sensitivity to foods, chemicals, and other allergens
- Endocrine disturbances
- Eczema
- Psoriasis
- Irritable bowel syndrome

Other
- Craving for foods rich in carbohydrates or yeast

Causal factors

Chronic candidiasis is a classic example of a "multi-factorial" condition, as shown in Table 48.2. Therefore, the most effective treatment involves addressing and correcting the factors which predispose to *Candida* overgrowth and involves much more than killing the yeast with antifungal agents, whether synthetic or natural.

Table 48.2 Predisposing factors to *Candida* overgrowth

- Decreased digestive secretions
- Dietary factors
- Impaired immunity
- Nutrient deficiency
- Drugs (particularly antibiotics)
- Impaired liver function
- Underlying disease states
- Altered bowel flora
- Prolonged antibiotic use

Antibiotics

Prolonged antibiotic use is believed to be the most important factor in the development of chronic candidiasis in most cases. Antibiotics, through suppressing normal intestinal bacteria which prevent yeast overgrowth and suppression of the immune system, strongly promote the overgrowth of *Candida*.

There is little argument that, when used appropriately, antibiotics save lives. However, there is also little argument that antibiotics are seriously overused. While the appropriate use of antibiotics makes good medical sense, what does not make sense is the reliance on antibiotics for such conditions as acne, recurrent bladder infections, chronic ear infections, chronic sinusitis, chronic bronchitis, and non-bacterial sore throats. Relying on antibiotics in the treatment of these conditions does not make sense, as either the antibiotics rarely provide benefit or these conditions are effectively treated with natural measures.

The growing problem of antibiotic resistance. The widespread use and abuse of antibiotics is becoming increasingly alarming for many reasons besides the epidemic of chronic candidiasis, including the development of "superbugs" that are resistant to currently available antibiotics. According to many experts, as well as the World Health Organization, we are coming dangerously close to arriving at a "post-antibiotic era" where many infectious diseases will once again become almost impossible to treat.[5–7]

Inappropriate use greatly increases the risk of developing complications such as overgrowth of *Candida albicans* and other organisms, as well as increasing the risk of developing a bacterial infection that is resistant to antibiotics.

Antibiotic resistance is probably an inevitable process, as bacteria transfer genetic material both within species and between species to help ensure survival of the organism. It has been well demonstrated that antibiotic resistance is much more common where antibiotics are used more often.[6] This is particularly a problem in hospitals where infections caused by resistant strains of organisms such as *Staphylococcus aureus* and *Pseudomonas aeruginosa* often lead to fatal complications.

Since there is evidence that resistance to antibiotics is less of a problem when antibiotics are used sparingly, reduction in antibiotic prescriptions may be the only significant way to address the problem. According to several authorities, as well as the World Health Organization, antibiotic use must be restricted and the inappropriate use halted if the growing trend towards bacterial resistance to antibiotics is to be stopped or reversed.[5–7] However, prescriptions for antibiotics are not the only source of concern. Antibiotics have also been added to animal nutrition since the 1950s.

In addition to creating antibiotic-resistant microorganisms, it may be several more decades before it is truly known what effects the widespread use of antibiotics is having in many different health conditions. For example, antibiotic exposure is now being linked to Crohn's disease.[8] Prior to the 1950s, Crohn's disease was found in selected groups with a strong genetic component. Since this time, there has been a rapid increase in developed countries, particularly in the United States, and in countries that had previously had virtually no reported cases. In fact, since 1950, Crohn's disease has spread like an epidemic. The annual increase in prescriptions of antibiotics and the fact that there is a parallel increase in the annual incidence of Crohn's disease are causing great concern. Comparative statistics have shown that wherever antibiotics are used early and in large quantities, the incidence of Crohn's disease is now quite high.

Syndromes related to the yeast syndrome

Eventually the yeast syndrome will likely be replaced by a more comprehensive term to include small intestinal bacterial overgrowth and the leaky gut syndrome. Both of these conditions are often associated with *Candida albicans* overgrowth and may produce identical symptoms to the yeast syndrome. For further discussion of small intestinal bacterial overgrowth and leaky gut syndrome, see Chapters 7 and 21.

DIAGNOSIS

Questionnaire

One of the most useful screening methods for determining the likelihood of yeast-related illness is a comprehensive questionnaire (see Appendix 2: *Candida* questionaire).

Although the *Candida* questionnaire can help, the best method for diagnosing chronic candidiasis is clinical evaluation by a physician knowledgeable about yeast-related illness. It is more than likely that the manner in which the doctor will diagnose the yeast syndrome will be based on clinical judgment from a detailed medical history and patient questionnaire. He or she may also employ laboratory techniques such as stool cultures for *Candida* and measurement of antibody levels to *Candida* or *Candida* antigens in the blood. However, while these laboratory exams are useful diagnostic aids, they should be used to confirm the diagnosis. In other words, the diagnosis is best made by evaluation of a patient's history and clinical picture.

The comprehensive stool and digestive analysis

Rather than simply culture a stool sample for the presence of *Candida albicans*, the comprehensive digestive stool analysis (CDSA) is more clinically useful (discussed in detail in Ch. 9). This battery of integrated diagnostic laboratory tests evaluates digestion, intestinal function, intestinal environment, and absorption by carefully examining the stool. It is a very useful tool in determining the digestive disturbance which is likely to be the underlying factor responsible for *Candida* overgrowth. In addition, the CDSA may determine that the symptoms are not related to *Candida* overgrowth but rather to conditions such as small intestinal bacterial overgrowth and the "leaky gut" syndrome.

Antibody and antigen levels

Another laboratory method to confirm the presence of *Candida* overgrowth is measuring the level of antibodies to *Candida* or the level of antigens in the blood.[3,9] However, rarely are these tests really needed, as the results typically only confirm what the patient history, physical examination, and CDSA reveal. Hence, the test does not change the course of action. Nonetheless, some patients and physicians may desire confirmation that *Candida albicans* is a responsible factor in the patient's health equation. In that situation, these blood studies can be quite helpful and can also be used as a way of monitoring therapy.

THERAPEUTIC CONSIDERATIONS

A comprehensive approach is more effective in treating chronic candidiasis than simply trying to kill the *Candida* with a drug or natural anti-*Candida* agent. Drugs like nystatin, ketoconazol, and diflucan as well as various natural anti-*Candida* agents rarely produce significant long-term results because they fail to address the underlying factors which promote *Candida* overgrowth. It is a bit like trying to weed your garden by simply cutting the weed, instead of pulling it out by the roots. Nonetheless, in many cases it is very useful to try to eradicate *Candida albicans* from the system, preferably with the help of natural anti-*Candida* therapies such as timed-release caprylic acid preparations, enteric-coated volatile oil preparations, or fresh garlic preparations. A follow-up stool culture and *Candida* antigen determination will confirm if the *Candida* has been eliminated. If it has and symptoms are still apparent, it is likely that the symptoms they are experiencing are unrelated to an overgrowth of *Candida albicans*. Similar symptoms to those attributed to chronic candidiasis can be caused by small intestinal bacterial overgrowth. In this scenario, pancreatic enzymes and berberine-containing plants like goldenseal can be helpful.

In addition to using natural agents to eradicate *Candida albicans*, it is important to address predisposing factors, recommend a *Candida* control diet, and support various body systems according to the individual patient's need.

Diet

A number of dietary factors appear to promote the overgrowth of *Candida*. The most important factors are a high intake of sugar, milk and other dairy products, foods containing a high content of yeast or mold, and food allergies.

Sugar

Sugar is the chief nutrient of *Candida albicans*. It is well accepted that restriction of sugar intake is an absolute necessity in the treatment of chronic candidiasis. Most patients do well by simply avoiding refined sugar and large amounts of honey, maple syrup, and fruit juice.[1–4]

Milk and dairy products

There are several reasons to restrict or eliminate the intake of milk in patients with chronic candidiasis:

- the high lactose content promotes the overgrowth of *Candida*
- milk is one of the most frequent food allergens
- milk may contain trace levels of antibiotics which can further disrupt the gastrointestinal bacterial flora and promote *Candida* overgrowth.[1–4]

Mold and yeast-containing foods

It is generally recommended by many experts that individuals with chronic candidiasis avoid foods with a high content of yeast or mold, including alcoholic beverages, cheeses, dried fruits and peanuts. Even though many patients with chronic candidiasis may be able to tolerate these foods, I think it is still a good idea to eliminate them from the diet. At the very least they should be avoided until the situation is under control.[1–4]

Food allergies

Food allergies are another common finding in patients with the yeast syndrome.[3] ELISA tests, which determine both IgE- and IgG-mediated food allergies, are often very helpful in identifying food allergies.

Hypochlorhydria

An important step in treating chronic candidiasis in many cases is improving digestive secretions. Gastric hydrochloric acid, pancreatic enzymes, and bile all inhibit the overgrowth of *Candida* and prevent its penetration into the absorptive surfaces of the small intestine. Decreased secretion of any of these important digestive components can lead to overgrowth of *Candida albicans* in the gastrointestinal tract. Therefore, restoration of normal digestive secretions through the use of supplemental hydrochloric acid, pancreatic enzymes, and substances which promote bile flow is critical in the treatment of chronic candidiasis. The comprehensive stool and digestive analysis can provide valuable information in identifying which factor is most important.

Patients on anti-ulcer drugs like Tagamet (cimetidine) and Zantac (ranitidine) actually develop *Candida* overgrowth in the stomach.[10] This occurrence highlights the importance of hydrochloric acid in the prevention of *Candida* overgrowth. Restoring proper levels of gastric acid by supplemental hydrochloric acid is often quite useful in chronic candidiasis.

Pancreatic enzymes can also be quite useful in the treatment of chronic candidiasis. As well as being necessary for protein digestion, the proteases serve several other important functions. The proteases are largely responsible for keeping the small intestine free from parasites (including bacteria, yeast, protozoa, and intestinal worms).[11,12] A lack of proteases or other digestive secretions greatly increases an individual's risk of having an intestinal infection, including chronic *Candida* infections of the gastrointestinal tract.

Enhancing immunity

Recurrent or chronic infections, including chronic candidiasis, are characterized by a depressed immune system. What makes it difficult for these people to overcome chronic candidiasis is a repetitive cycle: a compromised immune system leads to infection, and infection leads to damage to the immune system, further weakening resistance.

The importance of a healthy immune function protecting against *Candida* overgrowth is well known by any physician who has seen a patient suffering from AIDS or taking drugs which suppress the immune system. In either case, severe overgrowth of *Candida albicans* is a hallmark feature. The occurrence of *Candida* overgrowth in these conditions provides considerable evidence that attaining better immune function is absolutely essential in the patient with chronic candidiasis.

In addition, patients with chronic candidiasis often suffer from other chronic infections, presumably due to a depressed immune system. Typically, this depression of immune function is related to decreased thymus function demonstrating primarily as depressed cell-mediated immunity. Although expensive laboratory tests can document this depression, it is better to rely on the history of repeated viral infections (including the common cold), outbreaks of cold sores or genital herpes, and prostatic (men) or vaginal (women) infections.

Causes of depressed immune function in candidiasis

The patient with chronic candidiasis is typically stuck in a vicious cycle (Fig. 48.1). With regard to the immune

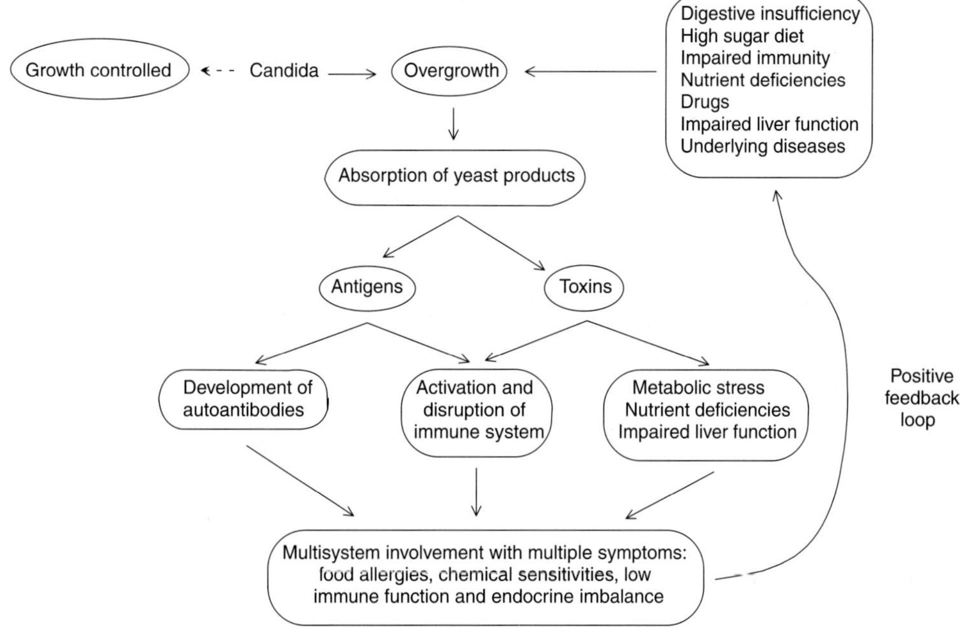

Figure 48.1 The vicious cycle of chronic candidiasis.

Table 48.3 Triggers to impaired immunity in candidiasis

- Antibiotic use
- Corticosteroid use
- Other drugs which suppress the immune system
- Nutrient deficiency
- Food allergies
- High sugar diet
- Stress

system, a triggering event such as antibiotic use or nutrient deficiency (see Table 48.3) can lead to immune suppression allowing *Candida albicans* to overgrow and become more firmly entrenched in the lining of the gastrointestinal tract. Once the organism attaches itself to the intestinal cells, it competes with the cell and ultimately the entire body for nutrition – potentially robbing the body of vital nutrition. In addition, *Candida albicans* secretes a large number mycotoxins and antigens.[13,14] *Candida albicans* is referred to as a "polyantigenic" organism because over 79 distinct antigens have been identified. Because of this tremendous number of antigens, an overgrowth of *Candida albicans* greatly taxes the immune system.

Restoring proper immune function

Restoring proper immune function is one of the key goals in the treatment of chronic candidiasis. There really isn't any single magic bullet which can immediately restore immune function in patients with chronic candidiasis. Instead, a comprehensive approach involving lifestyle, stress management, exercise, diet, nutritional supplementation, glandular therapy, and the use of plant-based medicines is used.

Perhaps the most effective intervention in re-establishing a healthy immune system is employing measures designed to improve thymus function. Promoting optimal thymus gland activity involves:

- prevention of thymic involution or shrinkage by ensuring adequate dietary intake of antioxidant nutrients such as carotenes, vitamin C, vitamin E, zinc, and selenium
- use of nutrients that are required in the manufacture or action of thymic hormones
- using products containing concentrates of calf thymus tissue.

There is a substantial amount of clinical data to support the effectiveness of orally administered calf thymus extracts in restoring and enhancing immune function.[15,16] The effectiveness of thymus extract is reflective of broad-spectrum immune system enhancement presumably mediated by improved thymus gland activity.

The dosage will vary from one manufacturer to another as there are no quality control procedures or standards enforced in the glandular industry; it is left up to the individual company to adopt quality control and good manufacturing procedures.

From a practical view, products concentrated and standardized for polypeptide content are preferable to crude preparations. Based on current clinical research, the daily dose should be equivalent to 120 mg pure polypeptides with molecular weights less than 10,000 or roughly 750 mg of the crude polypeptide fraction. No side-effects or adverse effects have been reported with the use of thymus preparations.

Promoting detoxification

Candida patients usually exhibit multiple chemical sensitivities and allergies, an indicator that detoxification reactions are stressed. Therefore, the liver function of the *Candida* patient needs to be supported. In fact, improving the health of the liver and promoting detoxification may comprise one of the most critical factors in the successful treatment of candidiasis.

Damage to the liver is often an underlying factor in chronic candidiasis as well as chronic fatigue. When the liver is even slightly damaged by chemical toxins, immune function is severely compromised.

The immune system suppressing effect of non-viral liver damage has been repeatedly demonstrated in experimental animal studies and human studies. For example, when the liver of a rat is damaged by a chemical toxin, immune function is severely hindered.[17] Liver injury is also linked to *Candida* overgrowth, as evident in studies in mice demonstrating that when the liver is even slightly damaged, *Candida* runs rampant through the body.[18]

A rational approach to aiding the body's detoxification involves:

- a diet which focuses on fresh fruits and vegetables, whole grains, legumes, nuts, and seeds
- a healthy lifestyle including avoiding alcohol and exercising regularly
- a high potency multiple vitamin and mineral supplement
- lipotropic formulas and silymarin to protect the liver and enhance liver function
- a 3 day fast at the change of each season.

If any of the factors in Table 48.4 apply to the patient, enhancing detoxification is a major therapeutic goal.

Table 48.4 Indications of the need for detoxification

- More than 20 pounds overweight
- Diabetes
- Presence of gallstones
- History of heavy alcohol use
- Psoriasis
- Natural and synthetic steroid hormone use
  —anabolic steroids
  —estrogens
  —oral contraceptives
- High exposure to certain chemicals or drugs
  —cleaning solvents
  —pesticides
  —antibiotics
  —diuretics
  —non-steroidal anti-inflammatory drugs
  —thyroid hormone
- History of viral hepatitis

Lipotropic factors

The nutrients choline, betaine, and methionine are often beneficial in enhancing liver function and detoxification reactions. These nutrients are referred to as "lipotropic agents" – compounds which promote the flow of fat and bile to and from the liver. In essence, they produce a "decongesting" effect on the liver and promote improved liver function and fat metabolism. Formulas containing lipotropic agents are very useful in enhancing detoxification reactions and other liver functions. Lipotropic formulas have been used for a wide variety of conditions by nutrition-oriented physicians, including a number of liver disorders such as hepatitis, cirrhosis, and chemical-induced liver disease. The dosage should provide a daily dose of 1,000 mg of choline and 1,000 mg of either methionine and/or cysteine.

Lipotropic formulas appear to increase the levels of two important liver substances: SAM (S-adenosyl-methionine), the major lipotropic compound in the liver, and glutathione, one of the major detoxifying compounds in the liver.[19,20]

Silymarin

There are a long list of plants which exert beneficial effects on liver function. However, the most impressive research has been done on a special extract of milk thistle (*Silybum marianum*) known as silymarin. Silymarin refers to a group of flavonoid compounds. These compounds exert tremendous effect on protecting the liver from damage as well as enhancing detoxification processes. Silymarin has shown impressive results in double-blind studies.[21–23] The standard dosage for silymarin is 70–210 mg three times daily.

Promoting elimination

In addition to directly supporting liver function, proper detoxification also involves promoting proper elimination. A diet which focuses on high-fiber plant foods should be sufficient to promote proper elimination by supplying an ample amount of dietary fiber. If additional support is needed, fiber formulas can be prescribed. These formulas are composed of natural plant fibers derived from psyllium seed, kelp, agar, pectin, and plant gums like karaya and guar. Alternatively, they can be purified semi-synthetic polysaccharides like methyl-cellulose and carboxymethyl cellulose sodium. Psyllium-containing laxatives are the most popular and usually the most effective. Fiber formulas are the laxatives which approximate most closely the natural mechanism that promotes a bowel movement. In the treatment of candidiasis, recommend 3–5 g of soluble fiber at bedtime – especially if anti-yeast therapies are employed to ensure that dead yeast cells are excreted and not absorbed.

Probiotics

The intestinal flora plays a major role in the health of the host.[24,25] The intestinal flora is intimately involved in the host's nutritional status and affects immune system function, cholesterol metabolism, carcinogenesis, and aging. Due to the importance of *L. acidophilus* and *B. bifidum* to human health, probiotic supplements can be used to promote overall good health. There are, however, several specific uses for probiotics. The four primary areas of uses related to chronic candidiasis are promotion of proper intestinal environment, post-antibiotic therapy, vaginal yeast infections, and urinary tract infections.

The dosage of a commercial probiotic supplement is based upon the number of live organisms. The ingestion of 1–10 billion viable *L. acidophilus* or *B. bifidum* cells daily is a sufficient dosage for most people. Amounts exceeding this may induce mild gastrointestinal disturbances, while smaller amounts may not be able to colonize the gastrointestinal tract.

Natural anti-yeast agents

There are a number of natural agents with proven activity against *Candida albicans*. Rather than relying on these agents as a primary therapy, however, it is still important to address the factors which predispose one to chronic candidiasis, especially lack of either hydrochloric acid or pancreatic enzymes. The four approaches we feel most comfortable in recommending as natural agents against *Candida albicans* are:

- caprylic acid
- berberine-containing plants
- garlic
- enteric-coated volatile oil preparations.

Most patients (but not all) can achieve benefits from the natural agents described here rather than the drug approach. Use of any effective anti-yeast therapy alone will likely result in the Herxheimer ("die-off") reaction due to the rapid killing of the organism and subsequent absorption of large quantities of yeast toxins, cell particles, and antigens. The Herxheimer reaction refers to a worsening of symptoms as a result of this dying off. The Herxheimer reaction can be minimized by:

- following the dietary recommendations for a minimum of 2 weeks before taking an anti-yeast agent
- supporting the liver by following the recommendations given above
- starting any of the above-described anti-yeast medications in low doses and gradually increasing dosages over 1 month to achieve full therapeutic dosage.

Caprylic acid

Caprylic acid is a naturally occurring fatty acid which has been reported to be an effective antifungal compound in the treatment of candidiasis.[26,27] Since caprylic acid is readily absorbed in the intestines, it is necessary to take timed-release or enteric-coated caprylic acid formulas to allow for gradual release throughout the entire intestinal tract.[28] The standard dosage for these delayed-release preparations is 1,000 to 2,000 mg with meals.

Berberine-containing plants

Berberine-containing plants include goldenseal (*Hydrastis canadensis*), barberry (*Berberis vulgaris*), Oregon grape (*Berberis aquifolium*), and goldthread (*Coptis chinensis*). Berberine, an alkaloid, has been extensively studied in both experimental and clinical settings for its antibiotic activity. Berberine exhibits a broad spectrum of antibiotic activity, having shown antibiotic activity against bacteria, protozoa, and fungi, including *Candida albicans*.[29–35]

Berberine's antibiotic action against some of these pathogens is actually stronger than that of antibiotics commonly used for disease these pathogens cause. Berberine-containing plants should be considered in infectious processes involving the above-mentioned organisms. Berberine's action in inhibiting *Candida*, as well as pathogenic bacteria, prevents the overgrowth of yeast which is a common side-effect of antibiotic use.

Diarrhea is a common symptom in patients with chronic candidiasis. Berberine has shown remarkable anti-diarrheal activity in even the most severe cases. Positive clinical results have been shown with berberine in relieving diarrhea in cases of cholera, amebiasis, giardiasis, and other causes of acute gastrointestinal infection (e.g. *E. coli*, *Shigella*, *Salmonella*, and *Klebsiella*) and may also relieve the diarrhea seen in patients with chronic candidiasis.[36–44]

The dosage of any berberine-containing plant should be based on berberine content. As there is a wide range of quality in goldenseal preparations, standardized extracts are preferred. Three times a day dosages are as follows:

- dried root or as infusion (tea), 2–4 g
- tincture (1:5), 6–12 ml (1.5–3 tsp)
- fluid extract (1:1), 2–4 ml (0.5–1 tsp)
- solid (powdered dry) extract (4:1 or 8–12% alkaloid content), 250–500 mg.

Note that the dosage recommendations for berberine would be 25–50 mg three times daily or a daily dosage of up to 150 mg. This dosage is consistent with the dosage range in the positive clinical studies in patients with gastrointestinal infections. For children, a dosage based on body weight is appropriate. The daily dosage would be the equivalent to 5–10 mg of berberine/kg (2.2 pounds) body weight.

Berberine and berberine-containing plants are generally non-toxic at the recommended dosages; however, berberine-containing plants are not recommended for use during pregnancy and higher dosages may interfere with B vitamin metabolism.[45]

Allium sativum

Garlic has demonstrated significant antifungal activity. In fact, its inhibition of *Candida albicans* in both animal and test tube (in vitro) studies have shown it to be more potent than nystatin, gentian violet, and six other reputed antifungal agents.[46–48] The active component is allicin – the pungent and odorous principle of garlic.

The modern clinical use of garlic features the use of commercial preparations designed to offer the benefits of garlic without the odor. These preparations are prepared in such a manner that the allicin is not formed until the enteric-coated tablet is delivered to the small and large intestine.

The treatment of chronic candidiasis requires a daily dose of at least 10 mg allicin or a total allicin potential of 4,000 mcg. This amount is equal to approximately one clove (4 g) of fresh garlic. Going beyond this dosage with these preparations usually results in the odor of garlic being detectable.

Enteric-coated volatile oils

The most recent "new wave" natural anti-*Candida* formulas are enteric-coated volatile oil preparations. Volatile oils from oregano, thyme, peppermint, and rosemary are all effective antifungal agents. A recent study compared the anti-*Candida* effect of oregano oil with that of caprylic acid.[49] While the minimum inhibitory concentration of oregano oil was less than 0.1 mcg/ml and the 0.1% survival of *C. albicans* occurred at a concentration of 45 mcg/ml, the minimum inhibitory concentration of caprylic acid was less than 500 mcg/ml and 0.1% survival occurred at a concentration of 5,000 mcg/ml. These results indicate that the anti-*Candida* activity of oregano oil is greater than 100 times more potent than caprylic acid. Since the volatile oils are quickly absorbed, as well as being associated with inducing heartburn, an enteric coating is recommended to ensure delivery to the small and large intestine. An effective dosage for an enteric-coated volatile oil preparation is 0.2–0.4 ml twice daily between meals.

THERAPEUTIC APPROACH

The following is a comprehensive step by step approach to the successful elimination of chronic candidiasis.

Step 1. Identify and address predisposing factors:

- Eliminate the use of antibiotics, steroids, immune-suppressing drugs, and birth control pills (unless there is an absolute medical necessity)
- Perform a comprehensive stool and digestive analysis
- Follow the specific recommendations if the identifiable predisposing factor is dietary factors, impaired immunity, impaired liver function, or an underlying disease state.

Step 2. Recommend the *Candida* control diet:

- Eliminate refined and simple sugars
- Eliminate milk and other dairy products
- Eliminate foods with a high content of yeast or mold, including alcoholic beverages, cheeses, dried fruits, melons, and peanuts
- Eliminate all known or suspected food allergies.

Step 3. Provide nutritional support:

- A high potency multiple vitamin and mineral formula
- Additional antioxidants
- One tablespoon of flaxseed oil daily.

Step 4. Support immune function:

- Promote a positive mental attitude
- Help patients to deal with stress by teaching positive stress coping techniques
- Recommend avoiding factors like alcohol, sugar, smoking, and elevated cholesterol levels which can impair immune function
- Recommend plenty of rest and good sleep
- Support thymus gland function; prescribe 750 mg of crude polypeptide fractions daily.

Step 5. Promote detoxification and elimination:

- Recommend 3–5 g of a water-soluble fiber source such as guar gum, psyllium seed, or pectin at night
- If necessary, recommend lipotropic factors and silymarin to enhance liver function.

Step 6. Recommend probiotics:

- Dosage: 1–10 billion viable *L. acidophilus* and *B. bifidum* cells daily.

Step 7. Use appropriate anti-yeast therapy:

- Ideally, use the recommended nutritional and/or herbal supplements to help control against yeast overgrowth and promote a healthy bacterial flora
- If necessary, use prescription anti-yeast drug appropriately.

These simple steps should take care of chronic candidiasis in most cases. If a patient follows these guidelines and fails to achieve significant improvement or complete resolution, further evaluation is necessary to determine if chronic candidiasis is the underlying factor. Repeat stool cultures and antigen levels are often helpful in this goal. If the organism has not been eradicated, stronger prescription antibiotics can be used along with the other general recommendations.

REFERENCES

1. Truss O. The missing diagnosis. Birmingham, AL: POB 26508. 1983
2. Crook WG. The yeast connection. 2nd edn. Jackson, TN: Professional Books. 1984
3. Kroker GF. Chronic candidiasis and allergy. In: Brostoff J, Challacombe SJ, eds. Food allergy and intolerance. Philadelphia, PA: WB Saunders. 1987: p 850–872
4. Crook WG. The Yeast Connection and the Woman. Jackson, TN: Professional Books. 1995
5. Woodhead M. Antibiotic resistance. Brit J Hosp Med 1996; 56: 314–315
6. Cohen M. Epidemiology of drug resistance. Implications for a post antibiotic era. Science 1992; 257: 1050–1055
7. World Health Organization. Fighting disease, fostering development. Report of the Director General. London: HMSO. 1996
8. Demling L. Is Crohn's disease caused by antibiotics. Hepato-Gastroenterol 1994; 41: 549–551
9. Bauman DS, Hagglund HE. Correlation between certain polysystem chronic complaints and an enzyme immunoassay with antigens of *Candida albicans*. J Advancement Med 1991; 4: 5–19
10. Boero M, Pera A, Andriulli A et al. Candida overgrowth in gastric juice of peptic ulcer subjects on short- and long-term treatment with H_2-receptor antagonists. Digestion 1983; 28: 158–163
11. Rubinstein E et al. Antibacterial activity of the pancreatic fluid. Gastroenterology 1985; 88: 927–932
12. Sarker SA, Gyr R. Non-immunological defense mechanisms of the gut. Gut 1990; 33: 1331–1337
13. Iwata K. Toxins produced by *Candida albicans*. Contr Microbiol Immunol 1977; 4: 77–85
14. Axelson NH. Analysis of human *Candida precipitins* by quantitative immunoelectrophoresis. Scand J Immunol 1976; 5: 177–190
15. Cazzola P, Mazzanti P, Bossi G. In vivo modulating effect of a calf thymus acid lysate on human T lymphocyte subsets and CD4+/CD8+ ratio in the course of different diseases. Curr Ther Res 1987; 42: 1011–1017
16. Kouttab NM, Prada M, Cazzola P. Thymomodulin. Biological properties and clinical applications. Med Oncol Tumor Pharmacother 1989; 6: 5–9
17. Klein A, Paffas SC, Gordon P et al. The effect of nonviral liver damage on the T-lymphocyte helper/suppressor ratio. Clin Immunol Immunopathol 1988; 46: 214–220
18. Abe F, Nagata S, Hotchi M. Experimental candidiasis in liver injury. Mycopathologica 1987; 100: 37–42
19. Barak AJ, Beclaenhauer HC, Junnila M et al. Dietary betaine promotes generation of hepatic S-adenosylmethionine and protects the liver from ethanol-induced fatty infiltration. Alcohol Clin Exp Res 1993; 17: 552–555
20. Zeisel SH, Da Costa KA, Franklin PD et al. Choline, an essential nutrient for humans. FASEB J 1991; 5: 2093–2098
21. Salmi HA, Sarna S. Effect of silymarin on chemical, functional, and morphological alteration of the liver. A double-blind controlled study. Scand J Gastroenterol 1982; 17: 417–421
22. Boari C, Raffi GB, Gennari P et al. Occupational toxic liver diseases. Therapeutic effects of silymarin. Min Med 1985; 72: 2679–2688
23. Ferenci P et al. Randomized controlled trial of silymarin treatment in patients with cirrhosis of the liver. J Hepatol 1989; 9: 105–113
24. Hentges DJ. Human intestinal microflora. In: Hentges DJ, ed. Health and disease. New York: Academic Press. 1983
25. Shahani KM, Friend BA. Nutritional and therapeutic aspects of lactobacilli. J Appl Nutr 1984; 36: 125–152
26. Keeney EL. Sodium caprylate. A new and effective treatment of moniliasis of the skin and mucous membrane. Bull Johns Hopkins Hosp 1946; 78: 333–339
27. Neuhauser I, Gustus EL. Successful treatment of intestinal moniliasis with fatty acid resin complex. Arch Intern Med 1954; 93: 53–60
28. Scwhabe AD, Bennett LR, Bowman LP. Octanoic acid absorption and oxidation in humans. J Applied Physiol 1964; 19: 335–337
29. Hahn FE, Ciak J. Berberine. Antibiotics 1976; 3: 577–588
30. Amin AH, Subbaiah TV, Abbasi KM. Berberine sulfate. Antimicrobial activity, bioassay, and mode of action. Can J Microbiol 1969; 15: 1067–1076
31. Johnson CC, Johnson G, Poe CF. Toxicity of alkaloids to certain bacteria. Acta Pharmacol Toxicol 1952; 8: 71–78
32. Kaneda Y et al. In vitro effects of berberine sulfate on the growth of *Entamoeba histolytica, Giardia lamblia* and *Tricomonas vaginalis*. Annals Trop Med Parasitol 1991; 85: 417–425
33. Subbaiah TV, Amin AH. Effect of berberine sulfate on *Entamoeba histolytica*. Nature 1967; 215: 527–528
34. Ghosh AK. Effect of berberine chloride on *Leishmania donovani*. Ind J Med Res 1983; 78: 407–416
35. Majahan VM, Sharma A, Rattan A. Antimycotic activity of berberine sulphate. An alkaloid from an Indian medicinal herb. Sabouraudia 1982; 20: 79–81
36. Gupta S. Use of berberine in the treatment of giardiasis. Am J Dis Child 1975; 129: 866
37. Bhakat MP et al. Therapeutic trial of Berberine sulphate in non-specific gastroenteritis. Ind Med J 1974; 68: 19–23
38. Kamat SA. Clinical trial with berberine hydrochloride for the control of diarrhoea in acute gastroenteritis. J Assoc Physicians India 1967; 15: 525–529
39. Desai AB, Shah KM, Shah DM. Berberine in the treatment of diarrhoea. Ind Pediatr 1971; 8: 462–465
40. Sharma R, Joshi CK, Goyal RK. Berberine tannate in acute diarrhea. Ind Pediatr 1970; 7: 496–501
41. Choudry VP, Sabir M, Bhide VN. Berberine in giardiasis. Ind Pediatr 1972; 9: 143–146
42. Kamat SA. Clinical trial with berberine hydrochloride for the control of diarrhoea in acute gastroenteritis. J Assoc Physicians India 1967; 15: 525–529
43. Gupte S. Use of berberine in treatment of giardiasis. Am J Dis Child 1975; 129: 866
44. Rabbani GH, Butler T, Knight J et al. Randomized controlled trial of berberine sulfate therapy for diarrhea due to enterotoxigenic *Escherichia coli* and *Vibrio cholerae*. J Infect Dis 1987; 155: 979–984
45. Hladon B. Toxicity of berberine sulfate. Acta Pol Pharm 1975; 32: 113–120
46. Moore GS, Atkins RD. The fungicidal and fungistatic effects of an aqueous garlic extract on medically important yeast-like fungi. Mycologia 1977; 69: 341–348
47. Sandhu DK, Warraich MK, Singh S. Sensitivity of yeasts isolated from cases of vaginitis to aqueous extracts of garlic. Mykosen 1980; 23: 691–698
48. Prasad G, Sharma VD. Efficacy of garlic (*Allium sativum*) treatment against experimental candidiasis in chicks. Br Vet J 1980; 136: 448–451
49. Stiles JC. The inhibition of *Candida albicans* by oregano. J Applied Nutr 1995; 47: 96–102

CHAPTER CONTENTS

49

Chronic fatigue syndrome

Michael T. Murray, ND

Joseph E. Pizzorno Jr, ND

DIAGNOSTIC SUMMARY

- Mild fever
- Recurrent sore throat
- Painful lymph nodes
- Muscle weakness
- Muscle pain
- Prolonged fatigue after exercise
- Recurrent headache
- Migratory joint pain
- Depression
- Sleep disturbance (hypersomnia or insomnia).

INTRODUCTION

The chronic fatigue syndrome (CFS) is a newly established syndrome that describes varying combinations of symptoms including recurrent fatigue, sore throats, low-grade fever, lymph node swelling, headache, muscle and joint pain, intestinal discomfort, emotional distress and/or depression, and loss of concentration.

Although newly defined and currently popular, CFS is not a new disease at all. References to a similar condition in the medical literature go back as far as the 1860s. In the past, chronic fatigue syndrome has been known by a variety of names including, among many others:

- chronic mononucleosis-like syndrome or chronic EBV syndrome
- Yuppie flu
- postviral fatigue syndrome
- post-infectious neuromyasthenia
- chronic fatigue and immune dysfunction syndrome (CFIDS)
- Iceland disease
- Royal Free Hospital disease.

In addition, symptoms of chronic fatigue syndrome mirror symptoms of neurasthenia, a condition first described in 1869.

Definition

In response to the growing interest, chronic fatigue syndrome was formally defined in 1988 by a consensus panel convened by the Centers for Disease Control (CDC) in an attempt to establish a guide for evaluating patients with chronic fatigue of unknown cause by clinical physicians and researchers.[1]

A formal (and controversial) set of diagnostic criteria were established by the CDC (see Table 49.1). These criteria are controversial for many reasons including the fact that psychological symptoms are both a minor criterion and potential grounds for exclusion. One of the major complaints from physicians about the CDC definition is that it appears better suited for research than for clinical purposes. A major problem with the CDC criteria is that they ignore many of the common symptoms reported by patients with CFS (see Table 49.2).

The British and Australian criteria for the diagnosis of CFS are less strict than the CDC definition.[2] In particular, the minor diagnostic criteria are not required and the major diagnostic criteria are not as strict. For example, in the Australian definition the major criterion is simply fatigue at a level which causes disruption of daily activities in the absence of other medical conditions associated with fatigue.

Using the CDC criteria, the prevalence of CFS in individuals suffering from chronic fatigue in the United States is thought to be about 11.5%, using British criteria it is about 15%, and using the Australian criteria it is about 38%.[2]

Table 49.1 CDC diagnostic criteria for chronic fatigue syndrome

Major criteria
- New onset of fatigue causing 50% reduction in activity for at least 6 months
- Exclusion of other illnesses that can cause fatigue

Minor criteria
- Presence of eight of the 11 symptoms listed below, or six of the 11 symptoms and two of the three signs

Symptoms
1. Mild fever
2. Recurrent sore throat
3. Painful lymph nodes
4. Muscle weakness
5. Muscle pain
6. Prolonged fatigue after exercise
7. Recurrent headache
8. Migratory joint pain
9. Neurological or psychological complaints
   —sensitivity to bright light
   —forgetfulness
   —confusion
   —inability to concentrate
   —excessive irritability
   —depression
10. Sleep disturbance (hypersomnia or insomnia)
11. Sudden onset of symptom complex

Signs
1. Low-grade fever
2. Non-exudative pharyngitis
3. Palpable or tender lymph nodes

Table 49.2 Frequency of symptoms in CFS

Symptom/sign	Frequency (%)
Fatigue	100
Low-grade fever	60–95
Muscle pain	20–95
Sleep disorder	15–90
Impaired mental function	50–85
Depression	70–85
Headache	35–85
Allergies	55–80
Sore throat	50–75
Anxiety	50–70
Muscle weakness	40–70
Post-exercise fatigue	50–60
Premenstrual syndrome (women)	50–60
Stiffness	50–60
Visual blurring	50–60
Nausea	50–60
Dizziness	30–50
Joint pain	40–50
Dry eyes and mouth	30–40
Diarrhea	30–40
Cough	30–40
Decreased appetite	30–40
Night sweats	30–40
Painful lymph nodes	30–40

ETIOLOGY

Epstein–Barr virus

Many research studies have focused on identifying an infectious agent as the cause of CFS. The Epstein–Barr virus (EBV) emerged as the leading, yet controversial, candidate.[3–7] EBV is a member of the herpes group of viruses, which includes herpes simplex types 1 and 2, varicella zoster virus, cytomegalovirus, and pseudorabies virus. A common aspect of these viruses is their ability to establish a life-long latent infection after the initial infection. This latent infection is kept in check by a normal immune system. When the immune system is compromised in any way, these viruses can become active as viral replication and spread is increased. This is commonly observed with herpes virus infections, especially in immunocompromised individuals such as those with AIDS, cancer, or drug-induced immunosuppression.

Infection with EBV is inevitable among humans. By the end of early adulthood, almost all individuals demonstrate detectable antibodies in their blood to the Epstein–Barr virus, indicating past infection. When the primary infection occurs in childhood, there are usually no symptoms, but when it occurs in adolescence or early adulthood, the clinical manifestations of infectious mononucleosis develop in approximately 50% of the cases.

Although reports of a prolonged or recurrent mononucleosis-like syndrome began appearing in the 1940s and 1950s, it wasn't until the 1980s that evidence had implicated EBV in this broad clinical spectrum of chronic fatigue and associated symptoms. Numerous studies have now demonstrated persistently elevated titers (levels) of serum antibodies against the Epstein–Barr virus (specifically, anti-EBV capsid antibody titers > 1:80) in a number of patients presenting with the symptom pattern of this syndrome.

A careful study of 134 patients who had undergone EBV antibody testing because of suspected chronic mononucleosis-like syndrome found mixed results about the importance of EBV infection.[8] Fifteen patients identified as having severe, persistent fatigue of unknown origin were compared with the remaining 119 with less severe illness and with 30 age- and race-matched controls. The more seriously ill patients generally had higher levels of EBV antibodies than did the comparison groups, and, interestingly, they also demonstrated higher antibody titers to cytomegalovirus, herpes simplex viruses types 1 and 2, and measles. This led the researchers to conclude that "some patients with these illnesses (syndromes of chronic fatigue) may have an abnormality of infectious and/or immunologic origin", and that there remain "questions concerning the relationship between CFS and EBV".

Current knowledge about EBV infection can be summarized as follows:

- EBV and the herpes group of viruses produce latent life-long infections.
- The host's immune system (T-lymphocytes, interferon, and other lymphokines) normally holds the latent infection in check.
- Any compromise in the immune system can lead to the reactivation of the virus and recurrent infection.
- The infection itself can compromise and/or disrupt immunity, thereby leading to other diseases.
- Elevated EBV antibody levels are observed in a significant number of diseases characterized by immunological dysfunction.
- Elevated antibody titers to the herpes group viruses, measles, and other viruses have also been observed in patients with chronic fatigue syndrome.

EBV antibody testing (and antibody testing for other herpes group viruses and measles) may be useful as a measure of immune function and overall host resistance, but should not be relied upon for diagnosis of CFS.

Other infectious agents

In addition to EBV, a number of other viruses have been investigated as possible causes of EBV. This search for a viral agent is consistent with the mainstream medical approach to focus on the infectious organism rather than on reducing susceptibility and supporting the individual's immune system to deal with the organism effectively.[3–5] Table 49.3 lists the organisms currently proposed as causative agents in CFS.

Table 49.3 Organisms proposed as causative agents in CFS

- Epstein–Barr virus
- Human herpes virus-6
- Inoue–Melnich virus
- *Brucella*
- *Borrelia burgdorferi*
- *Giardia lamblia*
- Cytomegalovirus
- Enterovirus
- Retrovirus

Immune system abnormalities

There is little argument that a disturbed immune system plays a central role in CFS. A variety of immune system abnormalities have been reported in CFS patients (see Table 49.4). While no specific immunological dysfunction pattern has been recognized, the most consistent abnormality is a decreased number or activity of natural killer (NK) cells.[3,4,9,10] NK cells received their name because of their ability to destroy cells that have become cancerous or infected with viruses. In fact, for a time, CFS was also referred to as low natural killer cell syndrome (LNKS).

Other consistent findings include a reduced ability of lymphocytes, key in the battle against viruses, to respond to stimuli.[10] One of the reasons for this lack of response may be a reduced activity or decreased production of interferon. While both low and high levels of interferon have been reported in CFS, levels are depressed in most cases. When interferon levels are low, reactivation of latent viral infection is likely. Conversely, when interferon (as well as other chemical mediators like interleukin-1) levels are high, many of the symptoms may be related to the physiological effects of interferon. When interferon is used as a therapy in cancer and viral hepatitis, the side-effects produced are quite similar to the symptoms of CFS.

Table 49.4 Immunologic abnormalities reported for CFS

- Elevated levels of antibodies to viral proteins
- Decreased natural killer cell activity
- Low or elevated antibody levels
- Increased or decreased levels of circulating immune complexes
- Increased cytokine (e.g. interleukin-2) levels
- Increased or decreased interferon levels
- Altered helper/suppressor T-cell ratio

Chronic fatigue syndrome, fibromyalgia and multiple chemical sensitivities

Fibromyalgia (FM) and multiple chemical sensitivities (MCS), like CFS, are recently recognized disorders with a substantial overlap of symptomatology.[3,4,11,12] The only difference in diagnostic criteria for fibromyalgia and CFS is the requirement of musculoskeletal pain in fibromyalgia and fatigue in CFS. The likelihood of being diagnosed as having fibromyalgia or CFS is dependent upon the type of physician consulted. Specifically, if a rheumatologist or orthopedic specialist is consulted, the patient is much more likely to be diagnosed with fibromyalgia (Table 49.5 presents the diagnostic criteria for fibromyalgia).

One group of researchers carefully compared the symptomatology of 90 patients who had been diagnosed as having CFS, MCS or FM (30 in each category).[12] Utilizing the same questionnaire for all 90 patients, 70% of the patients diagnosed with FM and 30% with MCS met the Centers for Disease Control criteria for CFS. Particularly significant was the observation that 80% of both the FM and MCS patients met the CFS criteria of fatigue lasting more than 6 months with a 50% reduction in activity. More than 50% of the CFS and FM patients reported adverse reactions of various chemicals.

Other causes of chronic fatigue

Chronic fatigue can be caused by a variety of physical and psychological factors. Table 49.6 lists the major causes of chronic fatigue in an order of importance that is representative of how common the cause is among sufferers of chronic fatigue in the general population. The list is based on the findings of several large studies as well as the authors' clinical experience (chronic fatigue syndrome is listed under a broader category of impaired immune function).

Table 49.5 Diagnostic criteria for fibromyalgia. Diagnosis requires fulfillment of all three major criteria and four or more minor criteria

Major criteria
- Generalized aches or stiffness of at least three anatomic sites for at least 3 months
- Six or more typical, reproducible tender points
- Exclusion of other disorders which can cause similar symptoms

Minor criteria
- Generalized fatigue
- Chronic headache
- Sleep disturbance
- Neurological and psychological complaints
- Joint swelling
- Numbing or tingling sensations
- Irritable bowel syndrome
- Variation of symptoms in relation to activity, stress, and weather changes

Table 49.6 Causes of chronic fatigue

- Pre-existing physical condition
  —diabetes
  —heart disease
  —lung disease
  —rheumatoid arthritis
  —chronic inflammation
  —chronic pain
  —cancer
  —liver disease
  —multiple sclerosis
- Prescription drugs
  —antihypertensives
  —anti-inflammatory agents
  —birth control pills
  —antihistamines
  —corticosteroids
  —tranquilizers and sedatives
- Depression
- Stress/low adrenal function
- Impaired liver function and/or environmental illness
- Impaired immune function
  —chronic fatigue syndrome
  —chronic *Candida* infection
  —other chronic infections
- Food allergies
- Hypothyroidism
- Hypoglycemia
- Anemia and nutritional deficiencies
- Sleep disturbances
- Cause unknown

DIAGNOSIS

A great number of factors must be considered when evaluating a patient with chronic fatigue. A detailed medical history and review of body systems goes a long way to identifying important factors. The goal is to identify as many factors as possible which may be contributing to the patient's feeling of fatigue. For example, if a patient has heart disease, diabetes, or some other health condition, and the condition or the drug they are taking is clearly responsible for their fatigue, the treatment of their fatigue becomes secondary to the treatment of their underlying health condition.

In many cases of chronic fatigue, further evaluation is needed. The next steps can include a complete physical examination and laboratory studies. In the physical examination, look for any possible clues which may indicate the cause for the chronic fatigue. For example, swollen lymph nodes may indicate a chronic infection; and the presence of a diagonal crease on both ear lobes usually indicates impaired blood flow to the brain, a significant cause of fatigue in the elderly.

Avoid ordering expensive laboratory tests unless they are absolutely necessary. A complete blood count (CBC) and a chemistry panel (including serum ferritin in menstruating women) are useful as screening tools for other diseases. Avoid ordering laboratory tests to confirm a diagnosis that is not going to affect treatment. For example, if it is quite obvious that the patient has impaired immunity, it does not make much sense to perform elaborate and expensive blood tests on immune function because the results of these tests are not likely to influence the method of treatment.

Of particular value are assessment of liver detoxification function, bowel dysbiosis and gastrointestinal permeability (see Chs 9, 16 and 21).

THERAPEUTIC CONSIDERATIONS

Since chronic fatigue and the CFS are generally multifactorial conditions, the therapeutic approach typically involves multiple therapies which address different facets of the clinical picture.

A person's energy level, as well as their emotional state, is determined by an interplay between two primary factors – internal focus and physiology. Many people with chronic fatigue focus on how tired they are. They repeatedly reaffirm their fatigue to themselves and to anyone who will listen. Their physiology includes not only the chemicals and hormones floating around in the body, but also the way they hold their body (usually slouched) and the way they breathe (shallow). In most patients with chronic fatigue, both the mind and the body need to be addressed. The most effective treatment is a comprehensive program that is designed to help the use of their mind, attitude, and physiology to fuel higher energy levels.

Underlying health problems

Depression

The first factor to address is any underlying depression. Depression is one of the major causes of chronic fatigue and it is one of the common features of CFS. In the absence of a pre-existing physical condition, depression is generally regarded as the most common cause of chronic fatigue. However, it is often difficult to determine whether the depression preceded the fatigue or vice versa. Depression is fully discussed in Chapter 126.

Stress

Stress is another factor to consider in the patient with chronic fatigue or CFS. Stress can be the underlying factor in the patient with depression, low immune function, or other cause of chronic fatigue (see Ch. 60 for guidelines for assessing the role of stress in chronic fatigue and CFS).

One of the tools we recommend to rate stress levels is the "Social Readjustment Rating Scale" developed by Holmes & Rahe.[13] The scale was originally designed to predict the likelihood of a person getting a serious disease due to stress. Various life-change events are numerically rated according to their potential for causing disease. Even events commonly viewed as positive, such as an outstanding personal achievement, carry with them stress.

Impaired liver function and/or environmental illness

Exposure to food additives, solvents (cleaning materials, formaldehyde, toluene, benzene, etc.), pesticides, herbicides, heavy metals (lead, mercury, cadmium, arsenic, nickel, and aluminum), and other toxins can greatly stress liver and detoxification processes. This exposure can lead to a condition labeled by many naturopathic and nutrition-oriented physicians as the "congested liver" or "sluggish liver" or the more recently coined "impaired hepatic detoxification". These terms signify a reduced ability of the liver to detoxify. The congested or sluggish liver is characterized by a diminished bile flow, a condition known in medical terms as cholestasis, while impaired hepatic detoxification refers to decreased phase I and/or phase II enzyme activity. Phase I detoxification rates in excess of phase II activity will also cause toxicity problems due to excessive accumulation of activated intermediates (see Ch. 16). In addition to exposure to toxic chemicals, impairment of bile flow within the liver can be caused by a variety of other agents and conditions, as listed in Table 49.7.

Although many of the conditions listed in the table are typically associated with alterations in laboratory tests of liver function (serum bilirubin, AST, ALT, LDH, GGTP, etc.), relying on these tests alone to evaluate liver function may not be adequate, as these tests are elevated only when the liver has been significantly damaged and many of these conditions in the initial or "subclinical" stages may have normal laboratory values.

Table 49.7 Causes of cholestasis

- Dietary factors
  —saturated fat
  —refined sugar
  —low fiber intake
- Obesity
- Diabetes
- Presence of gallstones
- Alcohol
- Endotoxins and other gut-derived bacterial toxins
- Hereditary disorders such as Gilbert's syndrome
- Pregnancy
- Natural and synthetic steroid hormones
  —anabolic steroids
  —estrogens
  —oral contraceptives
- Certain chemicals or drugs
  —cleaning solvents
  —pesticides
  —antibiotics
  —diuretics
  —non-steroidal anti-inflammatory drugs
  —thyroid hormone
  —viral hepatitis

Although there are more sensitive tests to determine the functional activity of the liver, such as the serum bile acid assay and various clearance tests (see Ch. 16), clinical judgment based on medical history remains the major diagnostic tool for the "sluggish liver" or impaired hepatic detoxification enzymes, the presence of chronic fatigue being the hallmark symptom.

People with a sluggish liver may also complain of, among other things:

- depression
- general malaise
- headaches
- digestive disturbances
- allergies and chemical sensitivities
- premenstrual syndrome
- constipation.

Not surprisingly, these are the same types of symptoms that people exposed to toxic chemicals often complain of. Many toxic chemicals (especially solvents) and heavy metals (see Ch. 18) have an affinity to nervous tissue, giving rise to a variety of psychological and neurological symptoms, such as:[14,15]

- depression
- headaches
- mental confusion
- mental illness
- tingling in extremities
- abnormal nerve reflexes
- other signs of impaired nervous system function.

A hair mineral analysis is a good screening test for heavy metal toxicity. If the hair mineral analysis is inconclusive, a more sensitive indicator is the 8 hour lead mobilization test. This test employs the chelating agent EDTA (edetate calcium disodium) and measures the level of lead excreted in the urine for a period of 8 hours after the injection of EDTA.

An interesting multiclinic research study of chronically ill patients, many of whom were diagnosed as suffering from CFIDS, evaluated the efficacy of a comprehensive detoxification program. Patients were placed on a hypoallergenic diet and provided a dietary food supplement rich in nutrients that facilitate liver detoxification. The patients reported a 52% reduction in symptoms after 10 weeks and symptom improvement was mirrored by normalization of hepatic phase I and phase II detoxification.[16]

Excessive gastrointestinal permeability

Excessive gastrointestinal permeability, as measured by the lactulose/mannitol absorption test (see Ch. 21), is a common finding in CFS.[17] A treatment program utilizing food allergy control, nutrients to stimulate gastrointestinal regeneration and to support hepatic phase I and II detoxification, and an oligoantigenic rice protein food replacement formula was provided to 22 patients who fulfilled the classic CDC/NIH criteria for CFS. The patients' average duration of CFS was 4.6 years. The treatment resulted in symptom reduction in 81.2% of the patients, with clinical improvement being paralleled by normalization of gastrointestinal permeability and hepatic detoxification function.[18]

Impaired immune function and/or chronic infection

When the immune system is impaired, infections can linger and fatigue persist. There is a good reason for fatigue during an infection – fatigue is the body's response mechanism to infection because the immune system works best when the body is at rest.

In order to determine the role that the immune system is playing in patients with chronic fatigue, the series of questions listed in Table 49.8 can be utilized during the patient interview to indicate an impaired immune system. Chapter 20 describes in substantial detail the laboratory methodologies for assessing immune function.

Chronic Candida *infection*

One of the most common findings in individuals with impaired immune function is gastrointestinal overgrowth of *Candida albicans*. Candidal overgrowth is now becoming recognized as a complex medical syndrome also known as "the yeast syndrome" and "chronic candidiasis". This overgrowth is believed to cause a wide variety of symptoms in virtually every system of the body, with the gastrointestinal, genitourinary, endocrine, nervous, and immune systems being the most susceptible. Table 49.9 lists the typical chronic candidiasis patient profile (see Ch. 48 for a comprehensive discussion).

The diagnosis of chronic candidiasis is often quite difficult as there is no single specific diagnostic test. Stool cultures and elevated antibody levels to *Candida* are useful diagnostic aids, but they should not be relied upon for diagnosis. The best method for diagnosing chronic candidiasis in most cases is a detailed medical history and patient questionnaire (see Appendix 2). Table 49.10 lists the factors that typically predispose a patient to candidal overgrowth.

Table 49.8 Questionnaire for recognition of impaired immune function

- Do you get more than two colds per year?
- When you catch a cold, does it take more than 5–7 days to get rid of the symptoms?
- Have you ever had infectious mononucleosis?
- Do you have herpes?
- Do you suffer from chronic infections of any kind?

Table 49.9 Typical chronic candidiasis patient profile

- Sex: female
- Age: 15–50 years

General symptoms
- Chronic fatigue
- Loss of energy
- General malaise
- Decreased libido

Gastrointestinal symptoms
- Thrush
- Bloating, gas
- Intestinal cramps
- Rectal itching
- Altered bowel function

Genitourinary system complaints
- Vaginal yeast infection
- Frequent bladder infections

Endocrine system complaints
- Primarily menstrual complaints

Nervous system complaints
- Depression
- Irritability
- Inability to concentrate

Immune system complaints
- Allergies
- Chemical sensitivities
- Low immune function

Past history
- Chronic vaginal yeast infections
- Chronic antibiotic use for infections or acne
- Oral birth control usage
- Oral steroid hormone usage

Associated conditions
- Premenstrual syndrome
- Sensitivity to foods, chemicals, and other allergens
- Endocrine disturbances
- Psoriasis
- Irritable bowel syndrome

Other
- Craving for foods rich in carbohydrates or yeast

Table 49.10 Factors predisposing to *Candida* overgrowth

- Impaired immune function
- Anti-ulcer drugs
- Broad-spectrum antibiotics
- Cellular immunodeficiency
- Corticosteroids
- Diabetes mellitus
- Excessive sugar in the diet
- Intravascular catheters
- Intravenous drug use
- Lack of digestive secretions
- Oral contraceptive agents

Food allergies

As far back as 1930, chronic fatigue was recognized as a key feature of food allergies.[19] Originally, Rowe & Rowe[19] used the term "allergic toxemia" to describe a syndrome that included the symptoms of fatigue, muscle and joint aches, drowsiness, difficulty in concentration, nervousness, and depression. Around the 1950s, this syndrome began to be referred to as the "allergic tension-fatigue syndrome".[20] With the popularity of CFS, many physicians and others are forgetting that food allergies can lead to chronic fatigue. Furthermore, between 55 and 85% of individuals with CFS have allergies. For more information on food allergies, see Chapter 15.

Hypothyroidism

Hypothyroidism is a common cause of chronic fatigue. However, the condition is often overlooked. The reason for this may be the reliance on standard blood measurements of thyroid hormone levels as the method of diagnosis.[21–23] Undiagnosed hypothyroidism is a serious concern as failure to treat such a critical and underlying problem will reduce the effectiveness of every other measure designed to increase energy levels. For more information, see Chapter 162.

Hypoglycemia

The association between hypoglycemia and fatigue is well known. What is not as well known is the role that hypoglycemia plays in contributing to depression. Numerous studies have shown that depressed individuals suffer from hypoglycemia.[24–27] Since depression is the most common cause of chronic fatigue, hypoglycemia must always be ruled out (see Ch. 161).

Hypoadrenalism

Adrenal exhaustion was first proposed as a cause of chronic fatigue over 50 years ago by Tintera.[28] A small, but growing, body of evidence now supports the role of a disruption of the hypothalamic–pituitary–adrenal axis (HPA) in CFS.[29]

One of the major symptoms of glucocorticoid deficiency is debilitating fatigue. Glucocorticoid insufficiency is also characterized by a stressing event followed by feverishness, arthralgias, myalgias, adenopathy, post-exertional fatigue, exacerbation of allergic responses and disturbances of mood and sleep, i.e. the typical presentation of CFS. These symptoms are seen in partial or subclinical adrenal insufficiency, which may only be detected by the ACTH stimulation test or other endocrine testing. Glucocorticoids have a very profound endogenous immunosuppressive effect. In subclinical adrenal insufficiency, this may allow for the symptoms of chronic fatigue, including exacerbation of allergic responses, enhanced antibody titers to a variety of viral antigens, and elevations in cytokine levels. A group of CFS researchers believe that these patients form a heterogenous group with a variety of infectious and non-infectious antecedents.[29] They feel that chronic fatigue syndrome does not represent a discrete disease with a singular cause, but rather a clinical condition. Chronic fatigue syndrome is analogous to a number of complex medical conditions such as hypertension in which a variety of direct and indirect factors lead to the development of the clinical syndrome.

The researchers hypothesize that in chronic fatigue syndrome, specific pathophysiological antecedents, such as acute infection, stress, and pre-existing or concurrent psychiatric illness, may ultimately converge in a final common biological pathway resulting in the clinical syndrome of chronic fatigue syndrome. They believe that their data and others suggest that a reduction in adrenal cortical secretion is an important pathophysiological component in the development of many of the biological and behavioral features of the syndrome.

For example, in one of their studies, 30 patients with classically defined chronic fatigue syndrome were compared with 72 normal volunteers and patients.[30] The CFS patients were found to have significantly reduced evening cortisol levels and low 24 hour urinary free cortisol excretion. The CFS patients also had elevated basal ACTH concentrations and increased adrenal cortical sensitivity to ACTH, but a reduced maximal response, and showed attenuated net integrated ACTH response to corticotrophin-releasing hormone. These results are most compatible with a mild, central, adrenal insufficiency, secondary to either a deficiency of CRH or some other central stimulus to the pituitary–adrenal axis. The authors feel that the hyperresponsiveness of the adrenal cortex to ACTH in patients with chronic fatigue syndrome may reflect a secondary adrenal insufficiency in which adrenal ACTH receptors have become hypersensitive due to inadequate exposure to ACTH. The reduction in response to large doses of ACTH might suggest overall adrenal atrophy. The evidence suggests that the mild hypocortisolism in these patients reflects a defect at or above the level of the hypothalamus, resulting in deficiency in the release of CRH and/or other secretagogs that serve to activate the pituitary–adrenal axis.

Mind and attitude

The mind and attitude play a critical role in determining the status of the immune system and energy levels. Many patients with chronic fatigue (including CFS) are either depressed or just seem to have lost a sense of real enthusiasm for life. Of course, it is not easy to have a lot of enthusiasm when you do not have much energy. But the two usually go hand in hand.

The first step is to convey to CFS patients that they can get better. Many patients with CFS are told it is "something they will have to live with" and "there is no cure". Achieving or maintaining a positive mental attitude is critical to good health and high energy levels, especially in patients with CFS. In order to achieve a positive mind, a person needs to exercise or condition the attitude, similar to the way in which one would condition the body. In order to help patients, prescribe mental exercises such as visualizations, goal setting, affirmations, and empowering questions as detailed in Chapter 126.

Diet

Energy level appears to be directly related to the quality of the foods routinely ingested. Have patients adhere to the dietary guidelines given in Chapter 44. It is especially important to eliminate or restrict caffeine and refined sugar.

Although acute caffeine consumption provides stimulation, regular caffeine intake may actually lead to chronic fatigue. While mice fed one dose of caffeine demonstrated significant increases in their swimming capacity, when the dose of caffeine was given for 6 weeks, a significant decrease in swimming capacity was observed.[31]

It is also interesting to note that several studies have found caffeine intake to be extremely high in individuals with psychiatric disorders. Another interesting finding is that the degree of fatigue experienced is often related to the quantity of caffeine ingested. In one survey of hospitalized psychiatric patients, 61% of those ingesting at least 750 mg/day (at least five cups of coffee) complained of fatigue, compared with 54% of those ingesting 250–749 mg/day, and only 24% of those ingesting less than 250 mg/day.[32]

Be aware that in patients who routinely drink coffee, abrupt cessation of coffee drinking will probably result in symptoms of caffeine withdrawal, including fatigue, headache, and an intense desire for coffee.[33,34] Fortunately, this withdrawal period does not last more than a few days.

Nutritional supplements

Nutritional supplementation is essential in the treatment of chronic fatigue. A deficiency of virtually any nutrient can produce the symptoms of fatigue as well as render the body more susceptible to infection. Individuals with chronic fatigue require, at the bare minimum, a high potency multiple vitamin–mineral formula, along with extra vitamin C (3,000 mg/day in divided doses) and magnesium (500–1,200 mg/day in divided doses).

Magnesium

An underlying magnesium deficiency, even if subclinical, can result in chronic fatigue and symptoms similar to CFS. In addition, low red blood cell magnesium levels, a more accurate measure of magnesium status than routine blood analysis, have been found in many patients with chronic fatigue and CFS. Several studies have shown good results with magnesium supplementation.

For example, in one double-blind, placebo-controlled trial, 32 CFS patients received an intramuscular injection of either magnesium sulfate (1 g in 2 ml injectable water) or a placebo (2 ml injectable water) for 6 weeks. At the end of the study, 12 of the 15 patients receiving magnesium reported, based on strict criteria, significantly improved energy levels, better emotional state, and less pain. In contrast, only three of the 17 placebo patients reported that they felt better and only one reported improved energy levels.[35]

This study seems to confirm some impressive results obtained in clinical trials during the 1960s on patients suffering from chronic fatigue.[36–39] These studies utilized oral magnesium and potassium aspartate (1 g each) rather than injectable magnesium. Between 75 and 91% of the nearly 3,000 patients studied experienced relief of fatigue during treatment with the magnesium and potassium aspartate. In contrast, the number of patients responding to a placebo was between 9 and 26%. The beneficial effect was usually noted after only 4–5 days, but sometimes 10 days were required. Patients usually continued treatment for 4–6 weeks; afterwards fatigue frequently did not return.

Injectable magnesium is not necessary to restore magnesium status.[40] Absorption studies indicate that magnesium is easily absorbed orally when it is bound to aspartate or citrate. In addition, both of these compounds may also help fight off fatigue. Aspartate feeds into the Krebs cycle, the final common pathway for the conversion of glucose, fatty acids, and amino acids to chemical energy (ATP), while citrate is itself a component of the Krebs cycle. Krebs cycle components including aspartate, citrate, fumarate, malate, and succinate usually provide a better mineral chelate, as evidence suggests that minerals chelated to the Krebs cycle intermediates are better absorbed, utilized, and tolerated compared with inorganic or relatively insoluble mineral salts, including magnesium chloride, oxide, or carbonate.[40,41]

Other therapies

Breathing, posture, and bodywork

Proper care of the body is critical to high energy levels. Breathing with the diaphragm, good posture, and bodywork (massage, spinal manipulation, etc.) are all important in helping to relieve the stress that is a common contributor to fatigue.

Exercise

Exercise alone has been demonstrated to have a tremendous impact on improving mood and the ability to handle stressful life situations.[42] Regular exercise has also been shown to lead to improved immune status. For CFS patients, regular exercise has been shown to lead to a significant increase (up to 100%) in natural killer cell activity.[43,44] Although more strenuous exercise is required to benefit the cardiovascular system, light to moderate exercise may be best for the immune system. One study found that immune function was significantly increased by the practice of t'ai chi exercises.[45] T'ai chi is a martial art technique which features the movement from one posture to the next in a flowing motion that resembles dance. The research thus far suggests that light to moderate exercise stimulates the immune system, while intense exercise (e.g. training for the Olympics) can have the opposite effect.[46]

Botanical medicine

Eleutherococcus senticosus

In addition to supporting adrenal function and acting as a non-specific adaptogen, Siberian ginseng has been shown to exert a number of beneficial effects on immune function that may be useful in the treatment of CFS. In one double-blind study, 36 healthy subjects received either 10 ml of a fluid extract of *Eleutherococcus senticosus* or placebo daily for 4 weeks.[47] The group receiving the Siberian ginseng demonstrated significant improvements in a variety of immune system parameters. Most notable were a significant increase in T-helper cells and an increase in natural killer cell activity – both of which are of value in the treatment of CFS.

Glycyrrhiza glabra

Considering the possible roles of viral infection and hypoadrenalism in CFS, licorice root with its antiviral and glucocorticoid potentiating properties (see Ch. 90 for documentation of these properties) would seem to be an ideal botanical for this condition.[48] Unfortunately, this has not been rigorously evaluated, although an excellent response in a single patient has been reported.[49] The whole root must be used as DGL has had the glucocorticoid potentiating glycyrrhizic and glycyrrhetinic acids removed.

THERAPEUTIC APPROACH

Successful treatment of CFS requires a comprehensive diagnostic and therapeutic approach. Especially important is identifying underlying factors which may be impacting energy levels or the immune system. The strong correlation between chronic fatigue syndrome, fibromyalgia and multiple chemical sensitivities suggests that all may respond to hepatic detoxification, food allergy control, and a gut restoration diet.[16–18, 50] Special attention should be paid to the advice on immune support in Chapter 53.

Diet

Identify and control food allergies. Increase the consumption of water while eliminating consumption of caffeine-containing drinks and alcohol. Strongly suggest a diet of whole, organically grown foods. Control hypoglycemia through the elimination of sugar and other refined foods and the regular consumption of small meals and snacks. To speed the detoxification process, consider prescribing a course lasting for several weeks of a medical food replacement such as one of the UltraClear products.

Lifestyle

Teach the patient diaphragmatic breathing and a proper posture. Prescribe a regular exercise program; low intensity activities may produce greatest benefits.

Supplementation

- High potency multiple vitamin and mineral formula according to guidelines given in Chapter 44
- Vitamin C: 500–1,000 mg three times/day
- Vitamin E: 200–400 IU/day
- Thymus extract: 750 mg of the crude polypeptide fraction once or twice daily
- Magnesium bound to citrate or Krebs cycle intermediates: 200–300 mg three times/day
- Pantothenic acid: 250 mg/day.

Botanical medicines

- *Eleutherococcus senticosus*
  —dried root: 2–4 g
  —tincture (1:5): 10–20 ml
  —fluid extract (1:1): 2.0–4.0 ml
  —solid (dry powdered) extract (20:1 or standardized to contain greater than 1% eleutheroside E): 100–200 mg
- *Glycyrrhiza glabra*
  —powdered root: 1–2 g
  —fluid extract (1:1): 2–4 ml
  —solid (dry powdered) extract (4:1): 250–500 mg

Counseling

Either counsel the patient directly or refer him or her to a professional counselor to establish a regular pattern of mental, emotional, and spiritual affirmations.

REFERENCES

1. Holmes GP, Kaplan J, Gantz N et al. Chronic fatigue syndrome: a working case definition. Ann Intern Med 1988; 108: 387–389
2. Bates DW et al. Prevalence of fatigue and chronic fatigue syndrome in a primary care practice. Arch Int Med 1993; 2759–2765
3. Shafran SD. The chronic fatigue syndrome. Am J Med 1991; 90: 731–739
4. Kyle DV, Deshazo RD. Chronic fatigue syndrome. A conundrum. Am J Med Sci 1992; 303: 28–34
5. Komaroff AL. Chronic fatigue syndromes: relationship to chronic viral infections. J Virol Meth 1988; 21: 3–10
6. Jones JF, Ray C, Minnich L et al. Evidence for active Epstein-Barr virus infection in patients with persistent unexplained illness: elevated anti-early antigen antibodies. Ann Intern Med 1985; 102: 1–7
7. Straus SE, Tosato G, Armstrong G et al. Persisting illness and fatigue in adults with evidence of Epstein-Barr virus infection. Ann Intern Med 1985; 102: 7–16
8. Holmes GP, Kaplan J, Stewart J et al. A cluster of patients with a chronic mononucleosis-like syndrome. Is Epstein-Barr virus the cause? JAMA 1987; 257: 2297–2302
9. Caligiuri M, Murray C, Buchwald D et al. Phenotypic and functional deficiency of natural killer cells in patients with chronic fatigue syndrome. J Immunol 1987; 139: 3306–3313
10. Gupta S, Vayuvegula B. A comprehensive immunological analysis in chronic fatigue syndrome. Scand J Immunol 1991; 33: 319–327
11. Komaroff AI, Goldenberg D. The chronic fatigue syndrome. Definition, current studies and lessons for fibromyalgia research. J Rheumatol 1989; 16: 23–27
12. Buchwald D, Garrity DL. Comparison of patients with chronic fatigue syndrome, fibromyalgia and multiple chemical sensitivities. Arch Int Med 1994; 154: 2049–2053
13. Holmes TH, Rahe RH. The social readjustment scale. J Psychosomatic Res 1967; 11: 213–218
14. Seaton A, Jeelinek EH, Kennedy P. Major neurological disease and occupational exposure to organic solvents. Quart J Med 1992; 305: 707–712
15. Rutter M, Russell-Jones R, eds. Lead versus health: sources and effects of low level lead exposure. New York, NY: John Wiley. 1983
16. Bland JS, Barrager E, Reedy RG, Bland K. A medical food-supplemented detoxification program in the management of chronic health problems. Alt Ther 1995; 1: 62–71
17. Rigden S. Entero-hepatic resuscitation program for CFIDS. CFIDS Chron 1995; Spring: 46–49
18. Rigden S. Entero-hepatic resuscitation as a therapeutic strategy in CFIDS patients. Unpublished
19. Rowe AH, Rowe A, Jr. Food allergy. Its manifestations and control and the elimination diets. A compendium. Springfield, IL: CC Thomas. 1972
20. Breneman JC. Basics of food allergy. Springfield, IL: CC Thomas. 1977
21. Barnes BO, Galton L. Hypothyroidism: the unsuspected illness. New York, NY: Thomas Crowell. 1976
22. Langer SE, Scheer JF. Solved: the riddle of illness. New Canaan, CT: Keats. 1984
23. Gold M, Pottash A, Extein I. Hypothyroidism and depression, evidence from complete thyroid function evaluation. JAMA 1981; 245: 1919–1922
24. Winokur A, Maislin G, Philips J et al. Insulin resistance after glucose tolerance testing in patients with major depression. Am J Psychiatry 1988; 145: 325–330
25. Wright JH, Jacisin J, Radin N et al. Glucose metabolism in unipolar depression. Br J Psychiatry 1978; 132: 386–393
26. Schauss AG. Nutrition and behavior: complex interdisciplinary research. Nutr Health 1984; 3: 9–37

27. Jenkins DJ, Wolever TM, Taylor RH et al. Glycemic index of foods. a physiological basis for carbohydrate exchange. Am J Clin Nutr 1981; 24: 362–366
28. Tinera JW. The hypoadrenocortical state and its management. NY State Ned H 1955; 55: 1869–1876
29. Demitrack MA. Chronic fatigue syndrome: a disease of the hypothalamic-pituitary-adrenal axis? Ann Med 1994; 26: 1–3
30. Demitrack MA et al. Evidence for impaired activation of hypothalamic-pituitary-adrenal axis in patients with chronic fatigue syndrome. J Clin Endocrinol Metab 1991; 73: 1224–1234
31. Estler CJ, Ammon HP, Herzog C. Swimming capacity of mice after prolonged treatment with psychostimulants. I. Effects of caffeine on swimming performance and cold stress. Psychopharmacolo 1978; 58: 161–166
32. Greden JF, Fontaine P, Lubetsky M et al. Anxiety and depression associated with caffeinism among psychiatric inpatients. Am J Psychiatry 1978; 135: 963–966
33. Chou T. Wake up and smell the coffee. Caffeine, coffee, and the medical consequences. West J Med 1992; 157: 544–553
34. Hughes JR, Higgins ST, Bickel WK et al. Caffeine self-administration, withdrawal, and adverse effects among coffee drinkers. Arch Gen Psych 1991; 48: 611–617
35. Cox IM, Campbell MJ, Dowson D. Red blood cell magnesium and chronic fatigue syndrome. Lancet 1991; 337: 757–760
36. Ahlborg H, Ekelund LG, Nilsson CG. Effect of potassium-magnesium aspartate on the capacity for prolonged exercise in man. Acta Physiologica Scandinavica 1968; 74: 238–245
37. Hicks JT. Treatment of fatigue in general practice: a double blind study. Clin Med 1964; Jan: 85–90
38. Friedlander HS. Fatigue as a presenting symptom: management in general practice. Curr Ther Res 1962; 4: 441–449
39. Shaw DL. Management of fatigue: a physiologic approach. Am J Med Sci 1962; 243: 758–769
40. Gullestad L, Oystein Dolva L, Birkeland K et al. Oral versus intravenous magnesium supplementation in patients with magnesium deficiency. Magnes Trace Elem 1991; 10: 11–16
41. Lindberg JS, Zobitz MM, Poindexter JR et al. Magnesium bioavailability from magnesium citrate and magnesium oxide. J Am Coll Nutr 1990; 9: 48–55
42. Farmer ME, Locke BZ, Moscicki EK et al. Physical activity and depressive symptomatology. The NHANES 1 epidemiologic follow-up study. Am J Epidemiol 1988; 1328: 1340–1351
43. Fiatarone MA, Morley JE, Bloom ET et al. The effect of exercise on natural killer cells activity in young and old subjects. J Gerontol 1989; 44: M37–45
44. Makinnon LT. Exercise and natural killer cells: what is their relationship? Sports Med 1989; 7: 141–149
45. Xusheng S, Yugi X, Yunjian X. Determination of E-rosette-forming lymphocytes in aged subjects with tai chi quan exercise. Int J Sport Med 1989; 10: 217–219
46. Fitzgerald L. Exercise and the immune system. Immunol Today 1988; 9: 337–339
47. Bohn B, Nebe CT, Birr C. Flow-cytometric studies with *Eleutherococcus senticosus* extract as an immunomodulatory agent. Arzniem Forsch 1987; 37: 1193–1196
48. Brown D. Licorice root – potential early intervention for chronic fatigue syndrome. Quart Rev Nat Med 1996; Summer: 95–96
49. Baschetti R. Chronic fatigue syndrome and liquorice (letter). New Zealand Med J 1995; 108: 156–157
50. Bell DS. Chronic fatigue syndrome update. Postgrad Med 1994; 96: 73–81

CHAPTER CONTENTS

50

Detoxification

Michael T. Murray, ND

Joseph E. Pizzorno Jr, ND

INTRODUCTION

The concepts of internal cleansing and detoxifying have been integral to naturopathic philosophy since the profession's inception over a century ago. The problem of "toxicity" has grown as the number and quantity of poisonous compounds in the air, water, and food have increased. A substantial and growing body of research now supports the significant impact on health of acute and chronic exposure to endogenous and exogenous toxins and the efficacy of an individual's detoxification mechanisms (see Ch. 37).

Toxins damage the body in an insidious and cumulative way. Once the detoxification system becomes overloaded, toxic metabolites accumulate, and sensitivity to other chemicals, some of which are not normally toxic, becomes progressively greater. This accumulation of toxins can wreak havoc on normal metabolic processes.

This chapter identifies "toxins" and natural ways to support their detoxification and elimination, with particular focus on enhancing the function of the liver, the body's primary organ for neutralization of undesirable chemicals.

TOXINS

A toxin is defined as any compound that has a detrimental effect on cell function or structure. The discussion of toxins in this chapter is organized into the four areas:

- heavy metals
- chemical toxins
- microbial compounds
- breakdown products of protein metabolism.

Heavy metals

The heavy metals most commonly causing problems in humans are:

- lead
- mercury
- cadmium

- arsenic
- nickel
- aluminum.

These metals tend to accumulate within the brain, kidneys, and immune system where they can severely disrupt normal function.[1–6] It is conservatively estimated that up to 25% of the US population suffer to some extent from heavy metal poisoning. Hair mineral analysis is a good screening test for heavy metal toxicity (see Ch. 18).[1]

Most of the heavy metals in the body are a result of environmental contamination due to industry. For example, in the United States alone, industrial sources contribute more than 600,000 tons/year of lead into the atmosphere to be inhaled or – after being deposited on food crops, in fresh water, and soil – to be ingested.[1]

Common sources of heavy metals, in addition to industrial sources, include lead from the solder in tin cans and copper pipes, pesticide sprays, and cooking utensils; cadmium and lead from cigarette smoke; mercury from dental fillings, contaminated fish, latex paints and cosmetics; and aluminum from antacids and cookware.[1] Some professions with extremely high exposure include battery makers, gasoline station attendants, printers, roofers, solderers, dentists, and jewelers.[1] Unfortunately, arsenic and mercury have now also been found as contaminants or intentional additions to imported Chinese and Ayurvedic herbal medicines.

Early signs of heavy metal poisoning are vague or associated with other problems. Early symptoms can include:

- headache
- fatigue
- muscle pains
- indigestion
- tremors
- constipation
- anemia
- pallor
- dizziness
- poor coordination.

The person with even mild heavy metal toxicity will experience impaired ability to think or concentrate. As toxicity increases, so do the severity of signs and symptoms.[1–6]

Numerous studies have demonstrated a strong relationship between childhood learning disabilities (and other disorders including criminal behavior) and body stores of heavy metals, particularly lead[7–12] (see Ch. 135).

Chemical toxicants

This category of toxins, primarily dealt with by the liver, includes:

- toxic chemicals
- solvents, e.g. cleaning materials, formaldehyde, toluene, benzene, etc.
- drugs
- alcohol
- formaldehyde
- pesticides
- herbicides
- food additives.

Exposure or toxicity to toxic chemicals can give rise to a number of symptoms. Most common are psychological and neurological symptoms such as depression, headaches, mental confusion, mental illness, paresthesia, abnormal nerve reflexes, and other signs of impaired nervous system function. Respiratory tract allergies and increased rates for many cancers are also found in people chronically exposed to chemical toxins.[13–19]

Microbial compounds

The waste products and cellular debris from bacteria and yeast in the gut can be absorbed, causing significant disruption of body functions. Examples include:

- endotoxins
- exotoxins
- toxic amines
- toxic derivatives of bile
- various carcinogenic substances.

Gut-derived microbial toxins have been implicated in a wide variety of diseases, including liver diseases, Crohn's disease, ulcerative colitis, thyroid disease, psoriasis, lupus erythematosus, pancreatitis, allergies, asthma, and immune disorders.

In addition to toxic substances being produced by microorganisms, antibodies formed against microbial antigens can cross-react with the body's own tissues, thereby causing autoimmunity. The list of autoimmune diseases which have been linked to cross-reacting antibodies includes rheumatoid arthritis, myasthenia gravis, diabetes, pernicious anemia, and autoimmune thyroiditis.

The immune system and the liver are responsible for dealing with the toxic substances that are absorbed from the gut.

Breakdown products of protein metabolism

The end-products of protein metabolism – ammonia, urea, etc. – cause significant problems if allowed to accumulate. Most are eliminated by the kidneys.

DETOXIFICATION MECHANISMS

The body eliminates toxins either by directly neutralizing them or by excreting them in the urine or feces (and to

Table 50.1 Major detoxification systems

Organ	Method	Typical toxin neutralized
Skin	Excretion through sweat	Fat-soluble toxins such as DDT and heavy metal such as lead and mercury
Liver	Filtering of the blood	Bacteria and bacterial products, immune complexes
	Bile secretion	Cholesterol, hemoglobin breakdown products, extra calcium
	Phase I detoxification	Many prescription drugs (e.g. amphetamine, digitalis, pentobarbital), many over-the-counter drugs (acetaminophen, ibuprofen), caffeine, histamine, hormones (both internally produced and externally supplied), benzopyrene (carcinogen from charcoal-broiled meat), aniline (the yellow dyes), carbon tetrachloride, insecticides (e.g. Aldrin, Heptachlor), arachidonic acid
	Phase II detoxification	
	Glutathione conjugation	Acetaminophen, nicotine from cigarette smoke, organophosphates (insecticides), epoxides (carcinogens)
	Amino acid conjugation	Benzoate (a common food preservative), aspirin
	Methylation	Dopamine (neurotransmitter), epinephrine (hormone from adrenal gland), histamine, thiouracil (cancer drug)
	Sulfation	Estrogen, aniline dyes, coumarin (blood thinner), acetaminophen, methyl-dopa (used for Parkinson's disease)
	Acetylation	Sulfonamides (antibiotics), mescaline
	Glucuronidation	Acetaminophen, morphine, diazepam (sedative, muscle relaxant), digitalis
	Sulfoxidation	Sulfites, garlic compounds
Intestines	Mucosal detoxification	Toxins from bowel bacteria
	Excretion through feces	Fat-soluble toxins excreted in the bile
Kidneys	Excretion through urine	Many toxins, after they are made water-soluble by the liver

a lesser degree from the mucous membranes, lungs and skin). Toxins that the body is unable to eliminate build up in the tissues, typically in the fat stores and bone. The liver, intestines, and kidneys are the primary organs of detoxification (see Table 50.1).

EXPOSURE DIAGNOSIS

Both recognition of exposure and assessment of the efficacy of the detoxification mechanisms are essential for effective detoxification of the patient. Exposure assessment is discussed here, while description of assessment of liver detoxification efficacy is integrated into the discussion of the liver's detoxification pathways.

While an accurate and exhaustive history and physical examination will probably always be the mainstay of diagnosis of toxin exposure and build-up, a number of useful laboratory techniques have been developed for detecting toxins in the body.

Heavy metal assessment

For heavy metals, the most reliable measure of chronic exposure is the hair mineral analysis. Reliable results of hair analysis is dependent upon (1) a properly collected, cleaned, and prepared sample of hair, and (2) the test being performed by experienced personnel using appropriate analytical methods in a qualified laboratory. This procedure is discussed thoroughly in Chapter 18.

Chemical exposure

For determining exposure to toxic chemicals, a detailed medical history is essential. When appropriate, the laboratory analysis for this group of toxins can involve measuring blood and fatty tissue for suspected chemicals. Table 50.2 lists common indications for suspecting chemical exposure.

Recently, innovative laboratory assessment methodologies for the assessment of chemical exposure have become commercially available. Perhaps the most promising is urinary organic acid analysis. Traditionally only used to assess and define inborn errors of metabolism that cause death within the first year of life or severe mental retardation, metabolic profiling has now become useful for identifying enzyme impairment due not only to genetic diseases but also to nutritional deficiencies and chemical poisoning (see Ch. 29 for a full discussion of this useful methodology).

Table 50.2 Common indications for suspecting chemical exposure

- More than 20 pounds overweight
- Diabetes
- Presence of gallstones
- History of heavy alcohol use
- Psoriasis
- Natural and synthetic steroid hormone use
  —anabolic steroids
  —estrogens
  —oral contraceptives
- High exposure to certain chemicals or drugs
  —cleaning solvents
  —pesticides
  —antibiotics
  —diuretics
  —non-steroidal anti-inflammatory drugs
  —thyroid hormone
- History of viral hepatitis

Microbial compounds

A number of laboratory techniques are available to determine the presence of microbial compounds. Those most commonly used include tests for the presence of abnormal microbial concentrations and disease-causing organisms in the stool (see Ch. 9), microbial by-products (see Ch. 31), endotoxins (erythrocyte sedimentation rate is a rough estimator), and bacterial overgrowth in the small intestine (see Ch. 7).

Breakdown products of protein metabolism

The determination of the presence of high levels of breakdown products of protein metabolism and kidney function involves both blood and urine measurement of these compounds (see Ch. 31).

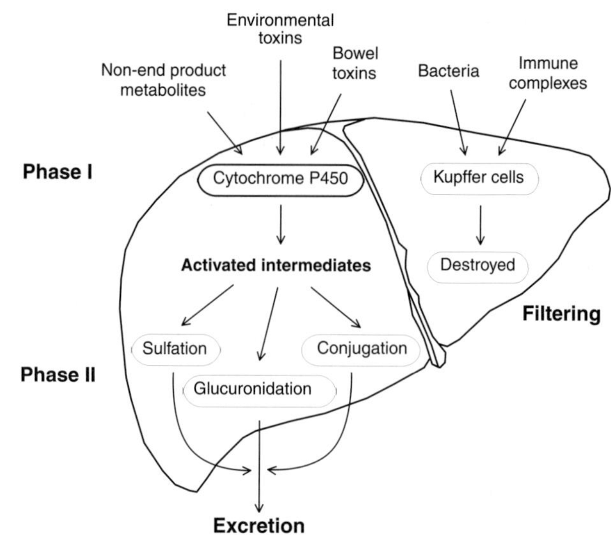

Figure 50.1 The liver's detoxification pathways.

LIVER DETOXIFICATION

Overview

The liver is a complex organ that plays a key role in most metabolic processes, especially detoxification. The liver neutralizes a wide range of toxic chemicals, both those produced internally and those coming from the environment. The normal metabolic processes produce a wide range of chemicals and hormones for which the liver has evolved efficient neutralizing mechanisms. However, the level and type of internally produced toxins increases greatly when metabolic processes go awry, typically as a result of nutritional deficiencies. These non-end-product metabolites have become a significant problem in this age of conventionally grown foods and poor diets (see Ch. 108).

Many of the toxic chemicals the liver must detoxify come from the environment: the content of the bowels and the food, water, and air. The polycyclic hydrocarbons (e.g. DDT, dioxin, 2,4,5-T; 2,4-D, PCB, and PCP), which are components of various herbicides and pesticides, are one example of chemicals that are now found in virtually all adipose tissues measured. Even those eating unprocessed organic foods need an effective detoxification system because all foods contain naturally occurring toxic constituents.

The liver plays several roles in detoxification: it filters the blood to remove large toxins, synthesizes and secretes bile full of cholesterol and other fat-soluble toxins, and enzymatically disassembles unwanted chemicals. This enzymatic process usually occurs in two steps referred to as phase I and phase II. Phase I either directly neutralizes a toxin, e.g. caffeine, or modifies the toxic chemical to form activated intermediates which are then neutralized by one or more of the several phase II enzyme systems. These processes are summarized in Figure 50.1.

Proper functioning of the liver's detoxification systems is especially important for the prevention of cancer. Up to 90% of all cancers are thought to be due to the effects of environmental carcinogens, such as those in cigarette smoke, food, water, and air, combined with deficiencies of the nutrients the body needs for proper functioning of the detoxification and immune systems. The level of exposure to environmental carcinogens varies widely, as does the efficiency of the detoxification enzymes, particularly phase II. High levels of exposure to carcinogens coupled with slow detoxification enzymes significantly increases susceptibility to cancer.

The link between the detoxification system's effectiveness and susceptibility to environmental toxins, such as carcinogens, is exemplified in a study in Italy of Turin chemical plant workers who had an unusually high rate of bladder cancer. When the liver detoxification enzyme activity of all the workers was tested, those with the most dysfunctional detoxification system were the ones who developed bladder cancer.[20]

Filtering the blood

One of the liver's primary functions is filtering the blood. Almost 2 quarts of blood pass through the liver every minute for detoxification. Filtration of toxins is absolutely critical as the blood from the intestines contains high levels of bacteria, bacterial endotoxins, antigen–antibody complexes, and various other toxic substances. When working properly, the liver clears 99% of the bacteria and other toxins during the first pass. However, when the liver is damaged, such as in alcoholics, the passage of toxins increases by over a factor of 10.

Bile excretion

The liver's second detoxification process involves the synthesis and secretion of bile. Each day the liver manufactures approximately 1 quart of bile, which serves as a carrier in which many toxic substances are dumped into the intestines. In the intestines, the bile and its toxic load are absorbed by fiber and excreted. However, a diet low in fiber results in inadequate binding and reabsorption of the toxins. This problem is magnified when bacteria in the intestine modify these toxins to more damaging forms.

Phase I detoxification

The liver's third role in detoxification typically involves a two-step enzymatic process for the neutralization of unwanted chemical compounds (Table 50.3). These not only include drugs, pesticides, and toxins from the gut, but also normal body chemicals such as hormones and inflammatory chemicals (e.g. histamine) which become toxic if allowed to build up. Phase I enzymes directly neutralize some chemicals, but most are converted to intermediate forms that are then processed by phase II enzymes. These intermediate forms are much more chemically active and therefore more toxic. If the phase II detoxification systems are not working adequately, these intermediates can cause substantial damage, including the initiation of carcinogenic processes.

Phase I detoxification of most chemical toxins involves a group of enzymes which, collectively, have been named cytochrome P450. Some 50–100 enzymes make up the cytochrome P450 system. Each enzyme works best in detoxifying certain types of chemicals, but with considerable overlap in activity among the enzymes.

Table 50.3 Chemicals detoxified by phase I

Drugs
- Phenytoin
- Erythromycin
- Codeine
- Warfarin
- Amitryptyline
- Phenobarbital
- Prednisone
- Steroids

OTCs
- Acetaminophen
- Ibuprofen
- Salicylates

Foods
- Caffeine
- Vanillin

Nutrients
- Arachidonic acid
- Fatty acids

Environmentals
- Alcohol
- Insecticides
- CCl_4
- Benzopyrenes (cigarette smoke, charcoal-broiled meat)

The activity of the various cytochrome P450 enzymes varies significantly from one individual to another, based on genetics, the individual's level of exposure to chemical toxins, and his or her nutritional status. Since the activity of cytochrome P450 varies so much, so does an individual's risk for various diseases. For example, as highlighted in the study of chemical plant workers in Turin discussed above, those with underactive cytochrome P450 are more susceptible to cancer.[21] This variability of cytochrome P450 enzymes is also seen in the variability of people's ability to detoxify the carcinogens found in cigarette smoke and helps to explain why some people can smoke with only modest damage to their lungs, while others develop lung cancer after only a few decades of smoking.

Patients with underactive phase I detoxification will experience caffeine intolerance, intolerance to perfumes and other environmental chemicals, and an increased risk for liver disease, while those with an overactive system will be relatively unaffected by caffeine drinks. One way of objectively determining the activity of phase I is to measure how efficiently a person detoxifies caffeine. Using this test, a surprising fivefold difference in the detoxification rates of apparently healthy adults has been discovered.[22]

When cytochrome P450 metabolizes a toxin, it chemically transforms it to a less toxic form, makes it water-soluble, or converts it to a more chemically active form. Caffeine is an example of a chemical directly neutralized by phase I. Making a toxin water-soluble allows its excretion by the kidneys. Transforming a toxin to a more chemically reactive form makes it more easily metabolized by the phase II enzymes.

A significant side-effect of phase I detoxification is the production of free radicals as the toxins are transformed – for each molecule of toxin metabolized by phase I, one molecule of free radical is generated. Without adequate free radical defenses, every time the liver neutralizes a toxin exposure, it is damaged by the free radicals produced.

The most important antioxidant for neutralizing the free radicals produced in phase I is glutathione. In the process of neutralizing free radicals, however, glutathione (GSH) is oxidized to glutathione disulfide (GSSG). Glutathione is required for one of the key phase II detoxification processes. When high levels of toxin exposure produce so many free radicals from phase I detoxification that the glutathione is depleted, the phase II processes dependent upon glutathione stop.

Another potential problem occurs because the toxins transformed into activated intermediates by phase I are substantially more reactive. Unless quickly removed from the body by phase II detoxification mechanisms, they can cause widespread problems, especially carcinogenesis. Therefore, the rate at which phase I produces activated intermediates must be balanced by the rate at which phase II finishes their processing. People with a very active phase I detoxification system coupled with slow or inactive phase II enzymes are termed "pathological detoxifiers". These people suffer unusually severe toxic reactions to environmental poisons.

An imbalance between phase I and phase II can also occur when a person is exposed to large amounts of toxins or exposed to toxins for a long period of time. In these situations, the critical nutrients needed for phase II detoxification are depleted, which allows the highly toxic activated intermediates to build up.

Recent research shows that the cytochrome P450 enzyme systems are also found in other parts of the body, especially the brain cells. Inadequate antioxidants and nutrients in the brain result in an increased rate of neuron damage, such as seen in Alzheimer's and Parkinson's disease patients.

As with all enzymes, the cytochrome P450s require several nutrients, listed in Table 50.4, in order to function.

A considerable amount of research has found that various substances activate cytochrome P450 (see Table 50.5) while other substances inhibit it (see Table 50.6).

Table 50.4 Nutrients needed by phase I detoxification

- Copper
- Magnesium (deficiency substantially increases toxicity of many drugs)
- Zinc
- Vitamin C

Table 50.5 Substances that activate phase I detoxification

Drugs
- Alcohol
- Nicotine in cigarette smoke
- Phenobarbital
- Sulfonamides
- Steroids

Foods
- Cabbage, broccoli, and brussels sprouts
- Charcoal-broiled meats (due to their high levels of toxic compounds)
- High-protein diet
- Oranges and tangerines (but not grapefruits)

Nutrients
- Niacin
- Vitamin B_1 (thiamin)
- Vitamin C

Herbs
- Caraway and dill seeds

Environmental toxins
- Carbon tetrachloride
- Exhaust fumes
- Paint fumes
- Dioxin
- Pesticides

Table 50.6 Inhibitors of phase I detoxification

Drugs
- Benzodiazepines (e.g. Halcion, Centrax, Librium, Valium, etc.)
- Antihistamines (used for allergies)
- Cimetidine and other stomach-acid secretion blocking drugs (used for stomach ulcers)
- Ketoconazole
- Sulfaphenazole

Foods
- Naringenin from grapefruit juice
- Curcumin from the spice turmeric
- Capsaicin from red chili pepper
- Eugenol from clove oil
- Quercetin from onions

Botanicals
- *Curcuma longa* (curcumin)
- *Capsicum frutescens* (capsaicin)
- *Eugenia caryophyllus* (eugenol)
- *Calendula officinalis*

Other
- Aging
- Toxins from inappropriate bacteria in the intestines

Inducers of phase I detoxification

Cytochrome P450 is induced by some toxins and by some foods and nutrients. Obviously, it is beneficial to improve phase I detoxification in order to eliminate toxins as soon as possible. This is best accomplished by providing the needed nutrients and non-toxic stimulants while avoiding those substances that are toxic. However, stimulation of phase I is contraindicated if the patient's phase II systems are underactive.

All of the drugs and environmental toxins listed in Table 50.5 activate P450 to combat their destructive effects, and in so doing, not only use up compounds needed for this detoxification system but contribute significantly to free radical formation and oxidative stress.

Among foods, the brassica family, i.e. cabbage, broccoli, and brussels sprouts, contains chemical constituents that stimulate both phase I and phase II detoxification enzymes. One such compound is indole-3-carbinol, which is also a powerful anti-cancer chemical. It is a very active stimulant of detoxifying enzymes in the gut as well as the liver.[23] The net result is significant protection against several toxins, especially carcinogens. This helps to explain why consumption of cabbage family vegetables protects against cancer.

Oranges and tangerines (as well as the seeds of caraway and dill) contain limonene, a phytochemical that has been found to prevent and even treat cancer in animal models.[24] Limonene's protective effects are probably due to the fact that it is a strong inducer of both phase I and phase II detoxification enzymes that neutralize carcinogens.

Inhibitors of phase I detoxification

Many substances inhibit cytochrome P450. This situation can cause substantial problems as it makes toxins potentially more damaging because they remain in the body longer before detoxification. For example, grapefruit juice decreases the rate of elimination of drugs from the blood and has been found to substantially alter their clinical activity and toxicity.[25] Eight ounces of grapefruit juice contains enough of the flavonoid naringenin to decrease cytochrome P450 activity by a remarkable 30%. The common inhibitors of phase I detoxification are listed in Table 50.6.

Curcumin, the compound that gives turmeric its yellow color, is interesting because it inhibits phase I while stimulating phase II. This effect can be very useful in preventing certain types of cancer. Curcumin has been found to inhibit carcinogens, such as benzopyrene (the carcinogen found in charcoal-broiled meat), from inducing cancer in several animal models. It appears that the curcumin exerts its anti-carcinogenic activity by lowering the activation of carcinogens while increasing the detoxification of those that are activated. Curcumin has also been shown to directly inhibit the growth of cancer cells.[26]

As most of the cancer-inducing chemicals in cigarette smoke are only carcinogenic during the period between activation by phase I and final detoxification by phase II, curcumin in the turmeric can help to prevent the cancer-causing effects of tobacco. In one human study, 16 chronic smokers were given 1.5 g/day of turmeric while six non-smokers served as a control group.[27] At the end of the 30 day trial, the smokers receiving the turmeric demonstrated significant reduction in the level of mutagens excreted in the urine. These results are quite significant as the level of urinary mutagens is thought to correlate with the systemic load of carcinogens and the efficacy of detoxification mechanisms. Those exposed to smoke, aromatic hydrocarbons, and other environmental carcinogens will probably benefit from the frequent use of curry or turmeric.

The activity of phase I detoxification enzymes decreases in old age. Aging also decreases blood flow though the liver, further aggravating the problem. Lack of the physical activity necessary for good circulation combined with the poor nutrition commonly seen in the elderly add up to a significant impairment of detoxification capacity, which is typically found in aging individuals. This helps to explain why toxic reactions to drugs are seen so commonly in the elderly.

Phase II detoxification

Phase II detoxification typically involves conjugation in which various enzymes in the liver attach small chemicals to the toxin. This conjugation reaction either neutralizes the toxin or makes the toxin more easily excreted through the urine or bile. Phase II enzymes act on some toxins directly, while others must first be activated by the phase I enzymes. There are essentially six phase II detoxification pathways:

- glutathione conjugation
- amino acid conjugation
- methylation
- sulfation
- acetylation
- glucuronidation.

Table 50.1 provides examples of toxins neutralized by each of these pathways. Some toxins are neutralized through several pathways.

In order to work, these enzyme systems need nutrients both for their activation and to provide the small molecules they add to the toxins. In addition, they utilize metabolic energy to function and to synthesize some of the small conjugating molecules. Thus, mitochondrial dysfunction, such as found in chronic fatigue syndrome, a magnesium deficiency or physical inactivity, can cause phase II detoxification to slow down, allowing the build-up of toxic intermediates. Table 50.7 lists the key nutrients needed by each of the six phase II detoxification systems. Table 50.8 lists the activators and Table 50.9 the inhibitors of phase II enzymes.

Glutathione conjugation

A primary phase II detoxification route is conjugation with glutathione (a tripeptide composed of three amino

Table 50.7 Nutrients needed by phase II detoxification enzymes

Phase II system	Required nutrients
Glutathione conjugation	Glutathione, vitamin B_6
Amino acid conjugation	Glycine
Methylation	S-adenosyl-methionine
Sulfation	Cysteine, methionine, molybdenum
Acetylation	Acetyl-CoA
Glucuronidation	Glucuronic acid

Table 50.8 Inducers of phase II detoxification enzymes

Phase II system	Inducer
Glutathione conjugation	Brassica family foods (cabbage, broccoli, and brussels sprouts), limonene-containing foods (citrus peel, dill weed oil, and caraway oil)
Amino acid conjugation	Glycine
Methylation	Lipotropic nutrients (choline, methionine, betaine, folic acid, and vitamin B_{12})
Sulfation	Cysteine, methionine, taurine
Acetylation	None found
Glucuronidation	Fish oils, cigarette smoking, birth control pills, phenobarbital, limonene-containing foods

Table 50.9 Inhibitors of phase II detoxification enzymes

Phase II system	Inhibitor
Glutathione conjugation	Selenium deficiency, vitamin B_2 deficiency, glutathione deficiency, zinc deficiency
Amino acid conjugation	Low protein diet
Methylation	Folic acid or vitamin B_{12} deficiency
Sulfation	Non-steroidal anti-inflammatory drugs (e.g. aspirin), tartrazine (yellow food dye), molybdenum deficiency
Acetylation	Vitamin B_2, B_5, or C deficiency
Glucuronidation	Aspirin, probenecid

Table 50.10 Phase II glutathione conjugation

Detoxifies	Acetaminophen, nicotine, organophosphates (insecticides), epoxides (carcinogens)
Nutrients needed	Glutathione, B_6
Activators	Brassica family foods (cabbage, broccoli, brussels sprouts), limonene-containing foods (citrus peel, dill weed, and caraway oil)
Inhibitors	Deficiency of vitamin B_2, glutathione, selenium, zinc
Clinical indicators of dysfunction	Chronic exposure to chemical toxins, chronic alcohol consumption
Laboratory assessment	Acetaminophen clearance shows low urine acetaminophen mercaptuates

acids – cysteine, glutamic acid, and glycine) (Table 50.10). Glutathione conjugation produces water-soluble mercaptates which are excreted via the kidneys. The elimination of fat-soluble compounds, especially heavy metals like mercury and lead, is dependent upon adequate levels of glutathione, which in turn is dependent upon adequate levels of methionine and cysteine.

When increased levels of toxic compounds are present, more methionine is utilized for cysteine and glutathione synthesis. Methionine and cysteine have a protective effect on glutathione and prevent depletion during toxic overload. This, in turn, protects the liver from the damaging effects of toxic compounds and promotes their elimination.

Glutathione is also an important antioxidant. This combination of detoxification and free radical protection results in glutathione being one of the most important anticarcinogens and antioxidants in our cells, which means that a deficiency is cause of serious liver dysfunction and damage.[28]

Exposure to high levels of toxins depletes glutathione faster than it can be produced or absorbed from the diet. This results in increased susceptibility to toxin-induced diseases, such as cancer, especially if phase I detoxification system is highly active.[29]

Disease states due to glutathione deficiency are not uncommon. A deficiency can be induced either by diseases that increase the need for glutathione, deficiencies of the nutrients needed for synthesis, or diseases that inhibit its formation. For example, patients with idiopathic pulmonary fibrosis, adult respiratory distress syndrome, HIV infection, hepatic cirrhosis, cataract formation, and advanced AIDS have been found to have a deficiency of glutathione, probably due to their greatly increased need for glutathione, both as an antioxidant and for detoxification.[30] Smoking increases the rate of utilization of glutathione, both in the detoxification of nicotine and in the neutralization of free radicals produced by the toxins in the smoke.

Glutathione is available through two routes: diet and synthesis. Dietary glutathione (found in fresh fruits and vegetables, cooked fish, and meat) is absorbed well by the intestines and does not appear to be affected by the digestive processes. Dietary glutathione in foods appears to be efficiently absorbed into the blood.[31] However, the same may not be true for glutathione supplements.

In one study, seven healthy subjects were given a single dose of up to 3,000 mg of glutathione. Blood values indicated that the concentration of glutathione did not increase significantly, suggesting the systemic availability of a single dose of up to 3,000 mg of glutathione is negligible.[32] The authors of the study concluded: "It is not feasible to increase circulating glutathione to a clinically beneficial extent by the oral administration of a single dose of 3 g of glutathione."[32]

In contrast, in healthy individuals, a daily dosage of 500 mg of vitamin C may be sufficient to elevate and maintain good tissue glutathione levels. In one double-blind study, the average red blood cell glutathione concentration rose nearly 50% with 500 mg/day of vitamin C.[33] Increasing the dosage to 2,000 mg only raised RBC glutathione levels by another 5%.

Vitamin C raises glutathione by increasing its rate of synthesis. In addition, to vitamin C, other compounds which can help increase glutathione synthesis include *N*-acetylcysteine (NAC), glycine, and methionine.

In an effort to increase antioxidant status in individuals with impaired glutathione synthesis, a variety of antioxidants have been used. Of these agents, only vitamin C and NAC have been able to offer some possible benefit. To determine the relative effectiveness of vitamin C vs. NAC, a 45-month-old girl with an inherited deficiency of glutathione synthesis was followed before and during treatment with vitamin C or NAC. High doses of vitamin C (500 mg/day or 3 g/day) or NAC (800 mg/day) were given for 1–2 weeks. Measurements of glutathione (GSH) levels indicated that 3 g/day of vitamin C increased white blood cell GSH fourfold and plasma GSH levels eightfold. NAC also increased white blood cell (3.5-fold) and plasma (two- to fivefold) GSH. Based on these results, it was decided that vitamin C would be given for 1 year at the 3 g/day dosage. At the end of a year, glutathione levels remained elevated and the hematocrit increased from a baseline 25.4 to 32.6% and the reticulocyte count decreased from 11 to 4%. These results indicate that vitamin C can decrease cellular damage in patients with hereditary glutathione deficiency and is more effective than the more expensive NAC.[34]

Over the past 5–10 years the use of NAC and glutathione products as antioxidants has become increasingly popular among nutritionally oriented physicians and the public. While supplementing the diet with high doses of NAC may be beneficial in cases of extreme oxidative stress (e.g. AIDS, cancer patients going through chemotherapy, or drug overdose), it may be an unwise practice in healthy individuals. One study indicated that when NAC was given orally to six health volunteers at a dosage of 1.2 g/day for 4 weeks, followed by 2.4 g/day for an additional 2 weeks, it actually increased oxidative damage by acting as a pro-oxidant.[35] Compared with controls, the concentration of glutathione in NAC-treated subjects was reduced by 48% and the concentration of oxidized glutathione was 80% higher. Oxidative stress increased by 83% in those receiving NAC.

Amino acid conjugation

Several amino acids (glycine, taurine, glutamine, arginine, and ornithine) are used to combine with and neutralize toxins (Table 50.11). Of these, glycine is the most commonly utilized in phase II amino acid detoxification. Patients suffering from hepatitis, alcoholic liver disorders, carcinomas, chronic arthritis, hypothyroidism, toxemia of pregnancy, and excessive chemical exposure are commonly found to have a poorly functioning amino acid conjugation system. For example, using the benzoate clearance test (a measure of the rate at which the body detoxifies benzoate by conjugating it with glycine to form hippuric acid, which is excreted by the kidneys), the rate of clearance in those with liver disease is 50% of that in healthy adults.[36]

Even in apparently normal adults, a wide variation exists in the activity of the glycine conjugation pathway. This is due not only to genetic variation, but also to the availability of glycine in the liver. Glycine and the other amino acids used for conjugation become deficient on a low-protein diet and when chronic exposure to toxins results in depletion.

Table 50.11 Phase II amino acid conjugation

Detoxifies	Benzoate, aspirin
Nutrients needed	Glycine
Activators	Glycine
Inhibitors	Low protein diet
Clinical indicators of dysfunction	Intestinal toxicity Toxemia of pregnancy
Laboratory assessment	Acetylsalicylic acid clearance shows low urine salicyluric acid

Table 50.12 Phase II methylation

Detoxifies	Dopamine, epinephrine, histamine, thiouracil
Nutrients needed	S-adenosylmethionine
Activators	Lipotropic nutrients (choline, methionine, betaine, folic acid, and vitamin B_{12})
Inhibitors	Folic acid or vitamin B_{12} deficiency
Clinical indicators of dysfunction	Premenstrual syndrome, estrogen excess, cholestasis,OCA use
Laboratory assessment	

Methylation

Methylation involves conjugating methyl groups to toxins (Table 50.12). Most of the methyl groups used for detoxification come from S-adenosylmethionine (SAM). SAM is synthesized from the amino acid methionine, a process which requires the nutrients choline, vitamin B_{12}, and folic acid.

SAM is able to inactivate estrogens (through methylation), supporting the use of methionine in conditions of estrogen excess, such as PMS. Its effects in preventing estrogen-induced cholestasis (stagnation of bile in the gall bladder) have been demonstrated in pregnant women and those on oral contraceptives.[37] In addition to its role in promoting estrogen excretion, methionine has been shown to increase the membrane fluidity that is typically decreased by estrogens, thereby restoring several factors that promote bile flow. Methionine also promotes the flow of lipids to and from the liver in humans. Methionine is a major source of numerous sulfur-containing compounds, including the amino acids cysteine and taurine.

Sulfation

Sulfation is the conjugation of toxins with sulfur-containing compounds (Table 50.13). The sulfation system is important for detoxifying several drugs, food additives, and, especially, toxins from intestinal bacteria and the environment.

In addition to environmental toxins, sulfation is also used to detoxify some normal body chemicals and is the main pathway for the elimination of steroid and thyroid

Table 50.13 Phase II sulfation

Detoxifies	Aniline dyes, coumarin, acetaminophen, methyl-dopa, estrogen, testosterone, thyroid
Nutrients needed	Cysteine, methionine, molybdenum
Activators	Cysteine, methionine, taurine
Inhibitors	Tartrazine dye, non-steroidal anti-inflammatory drugs (e.g. aspirin) Molybdenum deficiency
Clinical indicators of dysfunction	Intestinal toxicity, Parkinson's disease, Alzheimer's disease, rheumatoid arthritis
Laboratory assessment	Acetaminophen clearance shows low urine acetaminophen sulfates

hormones. Since sulfation is also the primary route for the elimination of neurotransmitters, dysfunction in this system may contribute to the development of some nervous system disorders.

Many factors influence the activity of sulfate conjugation. For example, a diet low in methionine and cysteine has been shown to reduce sulfation.[38] Sulfation is also reduced by excessive levels of molybdenum or vitamin B_6 (over about 100 mg/day).[39] In some cases, sulfation can be increased by supplemental sulfate, extra amounts of sulfur-containing foods in the diet, and the amino acids taurine and glutathione.

Acetylation

Conjugation of toxins with acetyl-CoA is the primary method by which the body eliminates sulfa drugs (Table 50.14). This system appears to be especially sensitive to genetic variation, with those having a poor acetylation system being far more susceptible to sulfa drugs and other antibiotics. While not much is known about how to directly improve the activity of this system, it is known that acetylation is dependent on thiamin, pantothenic acid, and vitamin C.[40]

Glucuronidation

Glucuronidation, the combining of glucuronic acid with toxins, requires the enzyme UDP-glucuronyl transferase (UDPGT) (Table 50.15). Many of the commonly prescribed drugs are detoxified through this pathway. It also helps to detoxify aspirin, menthol, vanillin (synthetic vanilla), food additives such as benzoates, and some hormones. Glucuronidation appears to work well, except for those with Gilbert's syndrome – a relatively common syndrome characterized by a chronically elevated serum bilirubin level (1.2–3.0 mg/dl). Previously considered rare, this disorder is now known to affect as much as 5% of the general population. The condition is usually without serious symptoms, although some patients do complain about loss of appetite, malaise, and fatigue (typical symptoms of impaired liver function). The main way this condition is recognized is by a slight yellowish tinge to the skin and white of the eye due to inadequate metabolism of bilirubin, a breakdown product of hemoglobin.

The activity of UDPGT is increased by foods rich in the monoterpene limonene (citrus peel, dill weed oil, and caraway oil). Methionine administered as SAM has been shown to be quite beneficial in treating Gilbert's syndrome.[41]

Table 50.14 Phase II acetylation

Detoxifies	Sulfonamides, mescaline
Nutrients needed	Acetyl-CoA
Inhibitors	Vitamin B_2, B_5, or C deficiency

Table 50.15 Phase II glucuronidation

Detoxifies	Acetaminophen, morphine, diazepam, digitalis, aspirin, vanillin, benzoates
Nutrients needed	Glucuronic acid
Activators	Fish oils, limonene-containing foods, birth control pills, cigarette smoking, phenobarbital
Inhibitors	Aspirin, probenecid
Clinical indications of dysfunction	Gilbert's disease, yellow discoloration of eyes and skin, not due to hepatitis
Laboratory assessment	Acetaminophen clearance shows low urine acetaminophen glucuronide

Sulfoxidation

Sulfoxidation is the process by which the sulfur-containing molecules in drugs (such as chlorpromazine) and foods (such as garlic) are metabolized (Table 50.16). It is also the process by which the body eliminates the sulfite food additives used to preserve many foods and drugs. Various sulfites are widely used in potato salad (as a preservative), salad bars (to keep the vegetable looking fresh), dried fruits (sulfites keep dried apricots orange), and some drugs (such as those used in the past for asthma). Normally, the enzyme sulfite oxidase metabolizes sulfites to safer sulfates, which are then excreted in the urine. Those with a poorly functioning sulfoxidation system, however, have an increased ratio of sulfite to sulfate in their urine.

The strong odor in the urine after eating asparagus is an interesting phenomenon because, while it is unheard of in China, 100% of the French have been estimated to experience such an odor (about 50% of adults in the US notice this effect). This situation is an excellent example of genetic variability in liver detoxification function.

Those with a poorly functioning sulfoxidation detoxification pathway are more sensitive to sulfur-containing drugs and foods containing sulfur or sulfite additives. This is especially important for asthmatics, who can react to these additives with life-threatening attacks. Dr Jonathan Wright discovered several years ago that providing molybdenum to asthmatics with an elevated

Table 15.16 Sulfoxidation

Detoxifies	Sulfites, garlic compounds, chlorpromazine
Nutrients needed	Molybdenum
Activators	Molybdenum
Clinical indicators of dysfunction	Adverse reactions to sulfite food additives, garlic; asthma reactions after eating at a restaurant; eating asparagus results in a strong urine odor
Laboratory assessment	Elevated urine sulfite/sulfate ratio

ratio of sulfites to sulfates in their urine resulted in a significant improvement in their condition. Molybdenum helps because sulfite oxidase is dependent upon this trace mineral. Although most nutrition textbooks believe it to be an uncommon deficiency, an Austrian study of 1,750 patients found that 41.5% were molybdenum-deficient.[42]

Bile excretion

One of the primary routes for the elimination of modified toxins is through the bile. However, when the excretion of bile is inhibited (i.e. cholestasis), toxins stay in the liver longer. Cholestasis has several causes, including obstruction of the bile ducts and impairment of bile flow within the liver. The most common cause of obstruction of the bile ducts is the presence of gallstones. Currently, it is conservatively estimated that 20 million people in the US have gallstones. Nearly 20% of the female and 8% of the male population over the age of 40 are found to have gallstones on biopsy and approximately 500,000 gall bladders are removed because of stones each year in the US. The prevalence of gallstones in this country has been linked to the high-fat, low-fiber diet consumed by the majority of Americans.

Impairment of bile flow within the liver can be caused by a variety of agents and conditions, as listed in Table 50.17. These conditions are often associated with alterations of liver function in laboratory tests (serum bilirubin, alkaline phosphatase, SGOT, LDH, GGTP, etc.) signifying cellular damage. However, relying on these tests alone to evaluate liver function is not adequate, since, in the initial or subclinical stages of many problems with liver function, laboratory values remain normal. Among the symptoms people with enzymatic damage may complain of are:

- fatigue
- general malaise
- digestive disturbances
- allergies and chemical sensitivities
- premenstrual syndrome
- constipation.

Table 50.17 Causes of cholestasis

- Presence of gallstones
- Alcohol
- Endotoxins
- Hereditary disorders such as Gilbert's syndrome
- Hyperthyroidism or thyroxine supplementation
- Viral hepatitis
- Pregnancy
- Certain chemicals or drugs
  - —natural and synthetic steroidal hormones: anabolic steroids, estrogens, oral contraceptives
  - —aminosalicylic acid
  - —chlorothiazide
  - —erythromycin estolate
  - —mepazine
  - —phenylbutazone
  - —sulphadiazine
  - —thiouracil

Perhaps the most common cause of cholestasis and impaired liver function is alcohol ingestion. In some especially sensitive individuals, as little as 1 ounce of alcohol can produce damage to the liver, which results in fat being deposited within the liver. All active alcoholics demonstrate fatty infiltration of the liver.

Methionine administered as SAM has been shown to be quite beneficial in treating two common causes of stagnation of bile in the liver – estrogen excess (due to either oral contraceptive use or pregnancy) and Gilbert's syndrome.[41,43]

Liver detoxification support

Nutritional factors

Antioxidant vitamins like vitamin C, beta-carotene, and vitamin E are obviously quite important in protecting the liver from damage as well as helping in the detoxification mechanisms, but even simple nutrients like B vitamins, calcium, and trace minerals are critical in the elimination of heavy metals and other toxic compounds from the body.[44–46]

The lipotropic agents, choline, betaine, methionine, vitamin B_6, folic acid, and vitamin B_{12}, are useful as they promote the flow of fat and bile to and from the liver. Lipotropic formulas have been used for a wide variety of conditions by nutrition-oriented physicians including a number of liver disorders such as hepatitis, cirrhosis, and chemical-induced liver disease.

Lipotropic formulas appear to increase the levels of SAM and glutathione. Although SAM is not currently available in the United States, methionine, choline, and betaine have been shown to increase the levels of SAM.[47–49]

Botanical medicines

There is a long list of plants which exert beneficial effects on liver function. However, the most impressive research has been done on silymarin, the flavonoids extracted from *Silybum marianum* (milk thistle). These compounds exert a substantial effect on protecting the liver from damage as well as enhancing detoxification processes. Silymarin prevents damage to the liver through several mechanisms: by acting as an antioxidant, by increasing the synthesis of glutathione and by increasing the rate of liver tissue regeneration.[50–52]

Silymarin is many times more potent in antioxidant activity than vitamin E and vitamin C. The protective effect of silymarin against liver damage has been demonstrated in numerous experimental studies. For example, silymarin has been shown to protect the liver from the damage produced by such liver-toxic chemicals as carbon tetrachloride, amanita toxin, galactosamine, and praseodymium nitrate.[50–52]

One of the key mechanisms by which silymarin enhances detoxification is by preventing the depletion of glutathione. Silymarin not only prevents the depletion of glutathione induced by alcohol and other toxic chemicals, but has been shown to increase the level of glutathione of the liver by up to 35%, even in normals.[53]

In human studies, silymarin has been shown to have positive effects in treating liver diseases of various kinds, including cirrhosis, chronic hepatitis, fatty infiltration of the liver (chemical- and alcohol-induced fatty liver), and inflammation of the bile duct.[54–58] The standard dosage for silymarin is 70–210 mg three times/day.

HEAVY METAL DETOXIFICATION

Nutritional factors which combat heavy metal poisoning include:[1,59–69]

- a high potency multiple vitamin and mineral supplement
- minerals such as calcium, magnesium, zinc, iron, copper, and chromium
- vitamin C and B-complex vitamins
- sulfur-containing amino acids (methionine, cysteine, and taurine) and high sulfur-containing foods like garlic, onions, and eggs
- water-soluble fibers such as guar gum, oat bran, pectin, and psyllium seed.

Heavy metal toxicity and detoxification are discussed in detail in Chapters 18 and 37.

SYSTEMIC DETOXIFICATION

Over the millennia, several traditional systemic detoxification procedures have evolved: fasting, saunas, and hydrotherapy. Recent research has now not only documented their efficacy for many of the common toxins but also helped refine our understanding of how to better apply them.

Fasting

Fasting is often used as a detoxification method as it is one of the quickest ways to increase elimination of wastes and enhance the healing processes of the body. Fasting is defined as "abstinence from all food and drink except water for a specific period of time, usually for a therapeutic or religious purpose" (see Ch. 47 for a full discussion of this useful therapy and specific instructions on its utilization).

Although therapeutic fasting is probably one of the oldest known therapies, it has been largely ignored by the medical community despite a substantial body of published research. Fasting has been studied in the treatment of:

- obesity
- chemical poisoning
- rheumatoid arthritis
- allergies
- psoriasis
- eczema
- thrombophlebitis
- leg ulcers
- the irritable bowel syndrome
- impaired or deranged appetite
- bronchial asthma
- depression
- neurosis
- schizophrenia.

One of the most significant studies regarding fasting and detoxification involved patients who had ingested rice oil contaminated with polychlorinated-biphenyls (PCBs). All patients reported improvement in symptoms, and some observed "dramatic" relief, after undergoing 7–10 day fasts.[70] This documented efficacy with fat-soluble toxins also indicates the need for care when fasting patients with high levels of these toxins and impaired detoxification mechanisms. For example, the pesticide DDT has been shown to be mobilized during a fast and may reach blood levels toxic to the nervous system.[6]

Another challenge with fasting is the depletion of liver glutathione, which occurs after approximately 24 hours. This leads to impairment of free radical quenching from phase I and impaired glutathione conjugation. This has led to the development of "modified food fasts".

Several products are now on the market to help aid the detoxification process. When used properly as part of a fast, these products initiate the same detoxification processes, albeit at a lower rate, while ensuring the availability of the critical nutrients needed to maintain energy and the liver's detoxification processes. Especially important are glutathione, antioxidants, and botanicals like *Silybum marianum*.

Saunas

Saunas are an age-old detoxification therapy. They are based on the concept that as the body sweats, toxins are released through the skin. Prolonged saunas (over an hour at a lower temperature) are thought to increase the excretion of fatty acids through the skin and thus fat-soluble toxins. There is some research that documents this method of detoxification. One group of researchers studied 14 firemen who had been exposed to highly toxic polychlorinated biphenyls in a transformer fire and

Table 50.18 Effects of extended time, modest temperature saunas[72–75]

- Increases excretion of heavy metals (cadmium, lead)
- Increases excretion of fat-soluble chemicals (PCBs, PBBs, and HCBs)
- Increases excretion of trace minerals
- Increases lipolysis, growth hormone

explosion and who subsequently developed neuropsychological problems 6 months after the fire. They underwent 2–3 weeks of experimental detoxification, which was a medically supervised diet, exercise, and sauna program. They were compared with firemen from the same department who did not participate in the detoxification program. Those who followed the detoxification program showed significant improvement in scores in three memory tests as compared with those who did not.[71] Self-appraisal for depression, anger, and fatigue, however, did not improve. This was a very short period of time for eliminating such toxins, but the results do suggest potential benefit. Table 50.18 lists the detoxification benefits of extended time, modest temperature saunas. Note, however, that this procedure also increases the secretion of essential trace minerals.[72]

As valuable as saunas are, they must be used with care as greatly elevating body temperature can cause problems in some situations. Specifically, they are contraindicated in pregnant women in their first trimester, young children, adults with heart disease or seizure disorders, immediately after intense exercise, and after drinking alcohol or ingesting cocaine.[76]

Hydrotherapy

Hydrotherapy, the application of hot and/or cold water to the various surfaces of the body, has been used for health promotion and detoxification throughout recorded history (see Ch. 42 for a full discussion). Some research is now documenting its efficacy in increasing the elimination of toxins, specifically lead.

A very interesting retrospective and experimental study evaluated the efficacy of the historic Bath General Hospital in treating lead poisoning. The hospital was established in 1741 to both treat patients suffering from lead poisoning (and other maladies) and objectively evaluate the efficacy of the therapies. Meticulous records were kept, and, considering the clear clinical picture of lead poisoning (*colica pictonum*), the diagnosis and evaluation, which were made by teams of doctors to limit bias, appear reliable. The researchers analyzed 120 years of documents which recorded the efficacy of the baths in 3,377 patients with lead poisoning. Their success was remarkable: 45.4% cured and 93% improved. As a control, they analyzed several other diseases for which the baths were used and found far lower success rates. The treatment protocol was composed of full-body (standing) immersion in 35°C water for at least 1.5 hours at least three times per week. In addition, the patients drank 1–1.5 pints of the Bath mineral waters a day. The average stay was 150 days.

The same researchers then conducted physiological experiments to determine if a rationale for this efficacy could be established. They found that full immersion increased cardiac output by 50% and increased urinary excretion of lead a remarkable 250%. The peak lead excretion was reached at 2.5 hours.[77]

SUMMARY

Detoxification of harmful substances is a continual process in the body. The ability to detoxify and eliminate toxins largely determines an individual's health status. A number of toxins (heavy metals, solvents, pesticides, microbial toxins, etc.) are known to cause significant health problems and their concentration in the environment continues to increase. Optimal functioning of the detoxification systems combined with periodic systemic detoxification are important tools for the health promotion-oriented physician.

REFERENCES

1. Passwater RA, Cranton EM. Trace elements, hair analysis and nutrition. New Canaan, CT: Keats. 1983
2. Rutter M, Russell-Jones R, eds. Lead versus health: sources and effects of low level lead exposure. New York, NY: John Wiley. 1983
3. Yost KJ. Cadmium, the environment and human health. An overview. Experentia 1984; 40: 157–164
4. Gerstner BG, Huff JE. Clinical toxicology of mercury. J Toxicol Environ Health 1977; 2: 471–526
5. Nation JR, Hare MF, Baker DM et al. Dietary administration of nickel: effects on behavior and metallothionein levels. Physiol Behavior 1985; 34: 349–353
6. Editorial. Toxicologic consequences of oral aluminum. Nutr Rev 1987; 45: 72–74
7. Marlowe M, Cossairt A, Welch K, Errara J. Hair mineral content as a predictor of learning disabilities. J Learn Disabil 1984; 17: 418–421
8. Pihl R, Parkes M. Hair element content in learning disabled children. Science 1977; 198: 204–206
9. David O, Clark J, Voeller K. Lead and hyperactivity. Lancet 1972; ii: 900–903
10. David O, Hoffman S, Sverd J. Lead and hyperactivity. Behavioral response to chelation: a pilot study. Am J Psychiatry 1976; 133: 1155–1188
11. Benignus VA, Otto DA, Muller KE, Seiple KJ. Effects of age and body lead burden on CNS function in young children. EEG spectra. EEG and Clin Neurophys 1981; 52: 240–248
12. Rimland B, Larson G. Hair mineral analysis and behavior: an analysis of 51 studies. J Learn Disabil 1983; 16: 279–285
13. Hunter B. Some food additives as neuroexcitors and neurotoxins. Clini Ecol 1984; 2: 83–89

14. Cullen MR, ed. Workers with multiple chemical sensitivities. Philadelphia, PA: Hanley & Belfus. 1987
15. Stayner LT, Elliott L, Blade L et al. A retrospective cohort mortality study of workers exposed to formaldehyde in the garment industry. Am J Ind Med 1988; 13: 667–681
16. Kilburn KH, Warshaw R, Boylen CT et al. Pulmonary and neurobehavioral effects of formaldehyde exposure. Archiv Environ Health 1985; 40: 254–260
17. Sterling TD, Arundel AV. Health effects of phenoxy herbicides. Scand J Work Environ Health 1986; 12: 161–173
18. Dickey L, ed. Clinical ecology. Springfield, IL: CC Thomas. 1976
19. Lindstrom K, Riihimaki H, Hannininen K. Occupational solvent exposure and neuropsychiatric disorders. Scan J Work Environ Health 1984; 10: 321–323
20. Talska G. Genetically based n-acetyltransferase metabolic polymorphism and low-level environmental exposure to carcinogens. Nature 1994; 369: 154–156
21. Gallagher JE, Everson RB, Lewtas et al. Comparison of DNA adduct levels in human placenta from polychlorinated biphenyl exposed women and smokers in which CYP 1A1 levels are similarly elevated. Terato Carcino Mutagen 1994; 14: 183–192
22. Campbell ME, Grant DM, Inaba T, Kalow W. Biotransformation of caffeine, paraxanthine, theophylline, and theobromine by polycyclic aromatic hydrocarbon-inducable cytochrome P-450 in human liver microsomes. Drug Metab Disp 1987; 15: 237–249
23. Beecher CWW. Cancer preventive properties of varieties of Brassica oleracea. A review. Am J Clin Nutr 1994; 59(suppl): 1166S–1170S
24. Crowell PL, Gould MN. Chemoprevention and therapy of cancer by d-limonene. Critical Rev Oncogenesis 1994; 5: 1–22
25. Yee GC, Stanley DL, Pessa LJ et al. Effect of grapefruit juice on blood cyclosporin concentration. Lancet 1995; 345: 955–956
26. Nagabhushan M, Bhide SV. Curcumin as an inhibitor of cancer. J Am Coll Nutr 1992; 11: 192–198
27. Polasa K, Raghuram TC, Krishna TP, Krishnaswamy K. Effect of turmeric on urinary mutagens in smokers. Mutagenesis 1992; 7: 107–109
28. Hagen TM, Wierzbicka GT, Bowman BB et al. Fate of dietary glutathione. Disposition in the gastrointestinal tract. Am J Physiol 1990; 259: G524–529
29. Ketterer B, Harris JM, Talaska G et al. The human glutathione S-transferase supergene family: its polymorphism, and its effects on susceptibility to lung cancer. Env Health Persp 1992; 98: 87–94
30. White AC. Glutathione deficiency in human disease. J Nutr Biochem 1994; 5: 218–226
31. Peristeris P, Clark BD, Gatti S et al. N-acetylcysteine and glutathione as inhibitors of tumor necrosis factor production. Cell Immunol 1992; 140: 390–399
32. Witschi A, Reddy S, Stofer B, Lauterburg BH. The systemic availability of oral glutathione. Eur J Clin Pharmacol 1992; 43: 667–669
33. Johnston CJ, Meyer CG, Srilakshmi JC. Vitamin C elevates red blood cell glutatione in healthy adults. Am J Clin Nutr 1993; 58: 103–105
34. Jain A, Buist NR, Kennaaway NG et al. Effect of ascorbate or N-acetylcysteine treatment in a patient with hereditary glutathione synthetase deficiency. J Pediatr 1994; 124: 229–233
35. Kleinveld HA, Demacker PNM, Stalenhoef AFH. Failure of N-acetylcystein to reduce low-density lipoprotein oxidizability in healthy subjects. Eur J Clin Pharmacol 1992; 43: 639–642
36. Quick AJ. Clinical value of the test for hippuric acid in cases of disease of the liver. Arch Int Med 1936; 57: 544–556
37. Frezza M, Pozzato G, Chiesa L et al. Reversal of intrahepatic cholestasis of pregnancy in women after high dose S-adenosyl-L-methionine (SAMe) administration. Hepatology 1984; 4: 274–278
38. Gregus S, Oguro T, Klaassen CD. Nutritionally and chemically induced impairment of sulfate activation and sulfation of xenobiotics in vivo. Chem-Biol Interactions 1994; 92: 169–177
39. Barzatt R, Beckman JD. Inhibition of phenol sulfotransferase by pyridoxal phosphate. Biochem Pharmacol 1994; 47: 2087–2095
40. Skvortsova RI, Pzniakovskii VM, Agarkova IA. Role of vitamin factor in preventing phenol poisoning. Vopr Pitan 1981; 2: 32–35
41. Bombardieri G. Effects of S-adenosyl-methionine (SAMe) in the treatment of Gilbert's syndrome. Curr Ther Res 1985; 37: 580–585
42. Birkmayer JGD, Beyer W. Biological and clinical relevance of trace elements. Arztl Lab 1990; 36: 284–287
43. Di Padova C, Triapepe T, Di Padova F et al. S-adenosyl-L-methionine antagonizes oral contraceptive-induced bile cholesterol supersaturation in healthy women: preliminary report of a controlled randomized trial. Am J Gastroenterol 1984; 79: 941–944
44. Flora SJS, Singh S, Tandon SK. Prevention of lead intoxication by vitamin B complex. Z Ges Hyg 1984; 30: 409–411
45. Shakman RA. Nutritional influences on the toxicity of environmental pollutants: a review. Arch Env Health 1974; 28: 105–133
46. Flora SJS, Jain VK, Behari JR, Tandon SK. Protective role of trace metals in lead intoxication. Toxicol Lett 1982; 13: 51–56
47. Wisniewska-Knypl J, Sokal JA, Klimczark J et al. Protective effect of methionine against vinyl chloride-mediated depression of non-protein sulfhydryls and cytochrome P-450. Toxicol Lett 1981; 8: 147–152
48. Barak AJ, Beckenhauer HC, Junnila M, Tuma DJ. Dietary betaine promotes generation of hepatic S-adenosylmethionine and protects the liver from ethanol-induced fatty infiltration. Alcohol Clin Exp Res 1993; 17: 552–555
49. Zeisel SH et al. Choline, an essential nutrient for humans. FASEB J 1991; 5: 2093–2098
50. Hikino H, Kiso Y, Wagner H, Fiebig M. Antihepatotoxic actions of flavonolignans from *Silybum marianum* fruits. Planta Medica 1984; 50: 248–250
51. Vogel G, Trost W. Studies on pharmacodynamics, site and mechanism of action of silymarin, the antihepatotoxic principle from *Silybum marianum* (L.) Gaert. Arzneim.-Forsch 1975; 25: 179–185
52. Wagner H. Antihepatotoxic flavonoids. In: Cody V, Middleton E, Harbourne JB, eds. Plant flavonoids in biology and medicine: biochemical, pharmacological, and structure-activity relationships. New York, NY: Alan R. Liss. 1986: p 545–558
53 Valenzuela A, Aspillaga M, Vial S, Guerra R. Selectivity of silymarin on the increase of the glutathione content in different tissues of the rat. Planta Med 1989; 55: 420–422
54. Sarre H. Experience in the treatment of chronic hepatopathies with silymarin. Arzneim.-Forsch 1971; 21: 1209–1212
55. Canini F, Bartolucci, Cristallini E et al. Use of silymarin in the treatment of alcoholic hepatic steatosis. Clin Ter 1985; 114: 307–314
56. Salmi HA, Sarna S. Effect of silymarin on chemical, functional, and morphological alteration of the liver. A double-blind controlled study. Scand J Gastroenterol 1982; 17: 417–421
57. Boari C, Gennari P, Violante FS et al. Occupational toxic liver diseases. Therapeutic effects of silymarin. Min Med 1985; 72: 2679–2688
58. Ferenci P, Dragosics H, Frank H et al. Randomized controlled trial of silymarin treatment in patients with cirrhosis of the liver. J Hepatol 1989; 9: 105–113
59. Flora SJS, Jain VK, Behari JR, Tandon SK. Protective role of trace metals in lead intoxication. Toxicol Lett 1982; 13: 51–56
60. Hsu HS. Interaction of dietary calcium with toxic levels of lead and zinc in pigs. J Nutrit 1975; 105: 112–168
61. Petering HG. Some observations on the interaction of zinc, copper and iron metabolism in lead and cadmium toxicity. Environ Health Perspect 1978; 25: 141–145
62. Papaioannou R, Sohler A, Pfeiffer CC. Reduction of blood lead levels in battery workers by zinc and vitamin C. J Orthomol Psychiatry 1978; 7: 94–106
63. Flora SJS, Singh S, Tandon SK. Role of selenium in protection against lead intoxication. Acta Pharmacol et Toxicol 1983; 53: 28–32
64. Tandon SK, Flora SJ, Behari JR, Ashquin M. Vitamin B complex in treatment of cadmium intoxication. Annals Clin Lab Sci 1984; 14: 487–492
65. Bratton GR, Zmudzki J, Bell MC, Warnock LG. Thiamin (vitamin B_1) effects on lead intoxication and deposition of lead in tissue. Therapeutic potential. Toxicol Appl Pharmacol 1981; 59: 164–172
66. Flora SJS, Singh S, Tandon SK. Prevention of lead intoxication by

vitamin B complex. Z Ges Hyg 1984; 30: 409–411
67. Ballatori N, Clarkson TW. Dependence of biliary excretion of inorganic mercury on the biliary transport of glutathione. Biochem Pharmacol 1984; 33: 1093–1098
68. Murakami M, Webb MA. A morphological and biochemical study of the effects of L-cysteine on the renal uptake and nephrotoxicity of cadmium. Br J Exp Pathol 1981; 62: 115–130
69. Cha CW. A study on the effect of garlic to the heavy metal poisoning of rat. J Korean Med Sci 1987; 2: 213–223
70. Imamura M, Tung T. A trial of fasting cure for PCB poisoned patients in Taiwan. Am J Ind Med 1984; 5: 147–153
71. Kilburn K, Warsaw RH, Shields MG. Neurobehavioral dysfunction in firemen exposed to polychlorinated biphenyls (PCBs). Possible improvement after detoxification. Arch Envir Health 1989; 44: 345–350
72. Cohn JR, Emmett EA. The excretion of trace metals in human sweat. Ann Clin Lab Sci 1978; 8: 270–275
73. Schnare DW, Robinson PC. Reduction of the body burdens of hexachlorobenzene and polychlorinated biphenyls. IARC Sci Publ 1986; 77: 597–603
74. Tretjak Z, Shields M, Beckmann SL. PCB reduction and clinical improvement by detoxification: an unexploited approach? Hum Exp Toxicol 1990; 9: 235–244
75. Lammintausta R, Syvalahti E, Pekkarinen A. Change in hormones reflecting sympathetic activity in Finnish sauna. Ann Clin Res 1976; 8: 266–271
76. Press E. The health hazards of saunas and spas and how to minimize them. Am J Publ Health 1991; 81: 1034–1037
77. Heywood A. A trial of the Bath waters: the treatment of lead poisoning. Med Hist Supl 1990; 10: 82–101

51

Food allergies

Stephen Barrie, ND

CHAPTER CONTENTS

INTRODUCTION

Food and environmental allergies have been implicated in a wide range of medical conditions affecting virtually every part of the body – from mildly uncomfortable symptoms such as indigestion and gastritis, to severe illnesses such as celiac disease, arthritis, and chronic infection. Allergies have also been linked to numerous disorders of the central nervous system, including depression, anxiety, and chronic fatigue.

Food allergy causes the immune system to synthesize and release reactive chemical agents, such as cytokines, lymphokines, and interferons. These hormone-like substances can dramatically influence cellular physiology, producing far-reaching effects on the immune, endocrine and nervous systems. Because toxins can initiate a very similar set of reactions, food allergy and toxicity are considered intimately connected in a clinical sense (see Ch. 50).

An allergic response to food or environmental inhalants may be the culprit lurking behind a "mysterious" set of symptoms which are not readily diagnosable using conventional methods of testing. Not being able to effectively pinpoint the cause of these symptoms can create profound frustration for the physician and the patient alike.

Testing for specific allergies (covered in Ch. 15) is one of the ways to uncover foundation causes of illness. Armed with the knowledge provided by approach, the physician can design a specific treatment program to reduce or eliminate exposure to antigenic substances, and thus effectively help to alleviate the patient's symptoms.

Allergy testing is also valuable as a preventive measure for patients who are not currently experiencing overt symptoms related to allergic reactions. It can reveal unsuspected food sensitivities which, if ignored, could result in cumulative stress on the immune and other systems over time – a condition that may eventually lead to severe illnesses.

History of food allergy

The recognition of food sensitivity was first recorded by Hippocrates, who observed that milk could cause gastric upset and urticaria. In 200 AD, Galen described a case of allergy to goat's milk, and in 1679 Willis observed that the ingestion of wine could precipitate asthma.

Soon after the start of the 20th century, Shloss described several cases that established a strong correlation between food allergy and the pathogenesis of atopic dermatitis.[1] Duke was one of the first to make extensive observations of foods causing allergic responses. In the early 1920s, he published several papers linking food ingestion to bladder pain, Ménière's syndrome, colitis, GI upset, and diarrhea.[2,3] Not long afterwards, Walzer and his colleagues[4,5] performed experiments clearly demonstrating that ingested food antigens could penetrate the GI barrier and be transported through the bloodstream to mast cells in the skin.

In the 1930s, Rinkel[6] first described food sensitivities that differed from the classic immediate anaphylactic reactions. The symptoms he described occurred hours or even days subsequent to ingestion and could be masked or unmasked by the offending food. Rinkel's discovery has been borne out by recent research confirming that delayed-type food allergies play a primary role in the immune system's response to ingestants.[7]

Allergies today

The incidence of food and environmental allergies and the number of atopic individuals have increased dramatically in recent times. Hypersensitivities involving bronchial symptoms and asthma, for example, have nearly doubled in the last decade.[8] It is estimated that atopic dermatitis alone now affects between 10–15% of the population at some time during their lives, and that this condition is often directly provoked by food antigens.[9,10]

Adverse reactions to food are now reported in about 25% of younger children.[11] Some physicians even claim that food allergies are a leading cause of most undiagnosed symptoms. As one investigator noted: "The management of allergic diseases involves considerable financial and other costs. In industrialized countries, atopic disease is the commonest cause of morbidity and a significant factor in mortality."[8]

The primary causes for the increased incidence of allergy appears to be excessive, regular consumption of a limited number of foods (often hidden as ingredients in commercially prepared foods) and the high level of preservatives, stabilizers, artificial colorings and flavorings, as well as medicinal drugs such as penicillin, now added to foods.[12] Some researchers and clinicians believe that the increased chemical pollution in our air, water, and food is to blame. Foods can easily become contaminated following the use of insecticides in farming.

Other possible reasons for increased food hypersensitivity include:

- earlier weaning and earlier introduction of solid foods to infants
- genetic manipulation of plants, resulting in food components which cross-react with normal tissues
- impaired digestion (especially hypochlorhydria)
- less diversity in the average diet – leading to repeated exposure to food substances and the subsequent development of hypersensitivities.

Probably all of these and more have contributed to the increased frequency and severity of allergic symptoms.

Causes and development

It is well documented that food allergy is an expression of an inherited genetic predisposition.[13] Hence allergic histories can often be found in both parents and siblings. One study discovered that when both parents are allergic, 67% of the children are also allergic. When only one parent is allergic, 33% are allergic.[14]

Inadequate digestion of food products due to hypochlorhydria and/or pancreatic enzyme deficiency is also thought to be a significant cause of food allergies. When proteins are not digested to amino acids, dipeptides, or short-chain polypeptides, they retain their antigenic properties. These antigenic molecules are then exposed to the immune system, or absorbed through a "leaky gut", creating a state of chronic immune hypersensitivity.

Signs and symptoms

Food and environmental allergies have been linked to a wide range of medical conditions affecting virtually every part of the body. They have been shown to cause migraine headache, eczema, thrombophlebitis, arthritis, colitis, enuresis, ear infections, gall bladder disease, childhood hyperactivity, hypotension, urticaria, asthma, glaucoma, and many other pathological conditions.[15–25] Table 51.1 lists symptoms and diseases that should make the clinician suspect possible food allergies. Gastrointestinal dysfunctions such as peptic ulcer, dyspepsia, gastroduodenitis, and hiatal hernia may promote some of these adverse reactions to food.[26]

THE ROLE OF THE IMMUNE SYSTEM IN THE ALLERGIC RESPONSE

The immune system is a complex molecular network with specific functions that defend the human host against invading organisms and cancer cells. While the

Table 51.1 Symptoms and diseases commonly associated with food allergy

System	Symptoms and diseases
Gastrointestinal	Canker sores, celiac disease, chronic diarrhea, duodenal ulcer, gastritis, irritable colon, malabsorption, ulcerative colitis
Genitourinary	Bed-wetting, chronic bladder infections, nephrosis
Immune	Chronic infections, frequent ear infections
Mental/emotional	Anxiety, depression, hyperactivity, inability to concentrate, insomnia, irritability, mental confusion, personality change, seizures
Musculoskeletal	Bursitis, joint pain, low back pain
Respiratory	Asthma, chronic bronchitis, wheezing
Skin	Acne, eczema, hives, itching, skin rash
Miscellaneous	Arrhythmia, edema, fainting, fatigue, headache, hypoglycemia, itchy nose or throat, migraines, sinusitis

system normally performs well, indeed is essential to maintaining health, under certain circumstances it goes awry.

Overview of the immune system

There are two types of immunity the body develops to protect itself: innate immunity and acquired immunity.

Innate immunity

When functioning properly, the immune system has the ability to resist almost all types of organisms and toxins that damage human tissue. This system includes:

- phagocytosis of bacteria and other invaders by white blood cells and cells of the macrophage system
- destruction of organisms by the acid secretion of the stomach
- integumentary defense
- destruction of foreign organisms or toxins by chemical compounds in the bloodstream (lysozyme, complement complex, polypeptides, natural killer cells).

Acquired immunity

Acquired immunity is the human body's ability to develop extremely powerful specific immunity against individual invading agents such as lethal bacteria, viruses, toxins, etc. There are two basic types of acquired immunity:

- humoral, or B-cell, immunity, which is the production of circulating antibodies
- cell-mediated, or T-cell, immunity, which is the formation of large numbers of activated lymphocytes specifically designed to destroy the foreign agent.

There are five major classes of immunoglobulins: IgE, IgD, IgG, IgM, and IgA. IgE defends against parasitic infection and is known as the reaginic antibody for its major role in instigating immediate allergic responses. The other immunoglobulins seem to be more involved in delayed reactions. Of these, IgG is the most abundant, comprising about 80% of all circulating antibodies.[27]

Types of immune reactions

Although the function of the immune system is to protect the host from foreign antigens, abnormal immune responses can lead to tissue injury and disease. Food allergy reactions are just one expression of this type of immune-mediated damage. The mechanisms of immune tissue injury have been classified into four distinct types:[28]

- *Type I – immediate hypersensitivity*. These reactions occur less than 2 hours after contact with allergens. Antigens bind to pre-formed IgE antibodies already attached to the surface of the mast cell or the basophil and cause the release of chemical mediators such as histamine and the eosinophilic chemotactic factor. A variety of allergic symptoms may result, depending on the location of the mast cell: in the nasal passages there may be sinus congestion; in the bronchioles, constriction (asthma); in the skin, hives and eczema; in the synovial cells, arthritis; in the intestinal mucosa, inflammation with resulting malabsorption; and in the brain, headaches, loss of memory and inability to concentrate.
- *Type II – cytotoxic reactions*. These reactions involve the binding of either IgG or IgM antibodies to cell-bound antigen. The antigen–antibody binding activates the complement cascade, resulting in the destruction of the cell to which the antigen is bound.
- *Type III – immune complex-mediated reactions*. Immune complexes are formed when antigens bind to antibodies. They are usually cleared from circulation by the phagocytic system. However, deposition of these complexes in tissues or in vascular endothelium can produce immune complex-mediated tissue injury. This tissue damage is further enhanced by the presence of vasoactive amines, which increase vascular permeability and promote the deposition of more immune complexes. Type III responses are usually delayed, occurring hours or even days after exposure. They have been shown to involve both IgG and IgG immune complexes.[29,30]

- *Type IV – T-cell-dependent*. This delayed-type reaction is mediated primarily by T-lymphocytes, after an allergen makes contact with a mucosal surface. By stimulating sensitized T-cells, inflammation may result within 36–72 hours of contact. A type IV reaction does not involve antibodies.

The allergic reaction

Acquired immunity is extensively involved in allergic reactions. Substances that initiate immune response are known as antigens. Generally, antigens are proteins or large polysaccharides having a high molecular weight (8,000 Da or greater).

Food represents the largest antigenic challenge confronting the human immune system.[28] The surface area of the GI tract is greater than the area of a tennis court, making it the largest, most active immune-reacting surface in the body. Immunologically mediated food hypersensitivity is the result of interactions among ingested food antigens, the digestive tract, tissue mast cells and circulating basophils, and food antigen-specific immunoglobulins.

Role of IgE and IgG_4 in allergy

Repeated exposure to an antigen can eventually produce allergy-like responses, or hypersensitivities. IgE antibodies are believed to trigger allergic reactions when they cross-link on the surface of gastrointestinal mast cells, stimulating the release and production of chemical mediators such as histamine, proteoglycans, and leukotrienes. These potent reactors instigate a barrage of effects on surrounding intestinal tissue, such as increased intestinal permeability, which may allow passage of food antigens into the bloodstream. When this happens, other organs in the body can then also become involved in the allergic reaction. Involvement of other cell types in the body may result in the creation of a chronic, perpetual autoimmune response.

Since most severe, immediate allergy symptoms are IgE-mediated, many conventional practitioners have limited their testing to this class of immunoglobulins. Certainly, an abundance of medical literature supports using the IgE assay as a means of diagnosing type I allergic reactions.[31–35] There is also considerable evidence, however, underscoring the significance of IgG as a marker in allergy testing as well. In fact, it is estimated that IgG and IgG complex mediators are involved in 80% of all food allergy reactions.[36]

These reactions are usually delayed, with symptoms that may not surface until hours, or even days, after the initial exposure. One study found that nearly 60% of patients with food intolerance exhibited late (delayed), rather than immediate or early, reactions to provoking foods.[37] Although IgE may be involved, it is theorized that the delayed reactions are primarily mediated by IgG. Specific IgE has a half-life in circulation of 1–2 days, and a half-life on the mast cell of about 14 days. IgG, on the other hand, appears to have a circulating half-life of 21 days with a residual time on the mast cells that can last as long as 2–3 months.[38] Thus an IgG assay is an essential tool for diagnosing the possible causes of delayed, non-anaphylactic responses, the so-called "hidden" allergies, which cannot be detected with conventional IgE tests such as RAST or skin testing.

A greater clinical significance is attached to the IgG_4 subclass than to IgG alone. Several studies indicate a role for IgG_4 in non-IgE, mast-cell mediated diseases.[39–43] IgG_4 is most commonly associated with high antigen levels, particularly food antigens. When antigen levels increase, more IgG_4 is produced by the body in response. After chronic antigenic exposure, IgG_4 concentrations reach much higher levels than do other IgG subclasses, particularly in atopic individuals.[35,44–46] Since antigen–antibody complexes trigger allergic responses, the measurement of IgG_4 is considered critical for a comprehensive assessment of antigen activity.

IgG_4 is also unique in that it is the only IgG subclass that induces basophil degranulation. This action triggers the release of histamine and other potent chemical mediators upon exposure to specific antigens – a common mechanism of allergic reactions.[39–41]

IgE/IgG and physiological function

Besides providing a means for diagnosing suspected antigens, IgE and IgG can have crucial implications for gastrointestinal and immune function. In experimental models, IgG antibodies have been shown to increase intestinal permeability.[47,48] This increased permeability is believed to be caused by a selective transport mediated by Fc receptors on epithelial surfaces.[49] By increasing intestinal permeability, elevated levels of IgG could result in increased exposure to antigens.

Production of IgG_4 and IgE is controlled by at least two cytokines, interleukin-4 (IL-4) and interferon-g (IFN-gamma). Since there is evidence that increased synthesis of IgG_4 and IgE is a result of decreased inhibitory effect of IFN-gamma,[50,51] it is postulated that defective immunoregulation involving IL-4 and IFN-gamma both sustains and increases the synthesis of IgG_4 and IgE antibodes.[46]

FOOD ALLERGY TESTING

Skin testing, RAST and IgG_4

Although many food allergy experts believe that oral challenge testing provides the most accurate and reliable results for diagnosing immediate food hypersensitivities, it can be costly, time-consuming, and potentially dangerous.[52] Moreover, using an oral challenge test to diagnose delayed sensitivities can be an extremely difficult and complicated process. In patients with a defined history of allergic reaction to a particular food, measurement of the combination of food-specific IgE and IgG_4 has been shown to correspond more closely with the history than the actual challenge itself.[38]

Since RAST and skin testing only measure IgE-mediated reactions, they cannot guide physicians as to the potential for delayed, non-IgE-mediated reactions.[38] In one study, researchers surmised that because IgG_4 was involved in late-onset reactions, patients exhibiting delayed bronchial allergic reactions failed to show positive skin test reactions or RAST results to a specific allergen.[53] In addition, there are clinical situations where skin testing is unfeasible and may inadvertently trigger life-threatening symptoms.[54] Food allergy testing is more completely discussed in Chapter 15.

Follow-up testing

The immune system is a highly sensitive, reactive molecular network that is constantly changing and adapting in response to myriad stimuli. Because of this ongoing state of flux, food sensitivities in the same individual may vary over the course of time. In one study, 580 patients with pathological reactions to foods were examined after a period of 9 years. Researchers found a dramatic shift in the patients' antigenic responses to different food groups, with many individuals exhibiting sensitivities to foods they had not reacted to 9 years earlier, perhaps due to changes in food consumption patterns and preparation methods.[12] This underscores the need for ongoing, consistent follow-up testing as time progresses, to carefully monitor the patient's immune response and to modify therapeutic interventions, as needed.

Related tests to consider

Intestinal permeability

A healthy intestinal tract provides an effective barrier against excessive absorption of food antigens. With increased gut permeability, greater quantities of antigens are allowed to penetrate the GI barrier, resulting in an overly sensitized, reactive immune system in some individuals. Increased permeability has been implicated in type I, type II, and type IV allergies.[55] Contact between an allergen and the digestive tract significantly increases intestinal absorption of macromolecules, leading the researchers to conclude that: "evaluation of intestinal permeability ... provides an objective means of diagnosing food allergy and assessing the effectiveness of anti-allergic agents".[56,57] Intestinal permeability testing evaluates the small intestine's effectiveness as a macromolecule barrier, monitors changes in mucosal permeability, and determines underlying causes of systemic problems linked to GI function (see Ch. 21 for a complete discussion of this important topic).

Comprehensive digestive stool analysis (CDSA)

Maldigestion of food products is considered a significant cause of food allergy. When proteins are not digested properly to amino acids, dipeptides, or short-chain polypeptides, they retain their antigenic properties. This can trigger repeated allergic responses by the immune system, possibly leading to a state of chronic hypersensitivity. The comprehensive digestive stool analysis can provide clues about the possible cause of food allergies by closely examining the digestion and absorption status of the gastrointestinal tract.

Some researchers have suggested that food allergy is not an immunological disease but a disorder of bacterial fermentation in the colon. According to this theory, food intolerance is caused by a combination of factors, including reduced gut enzyme concentrations, imbalanced bacterial flora, and increased intestinal permeability (also known as "leaky gut syndrome";[58] see Ch. 9 for a more complete discussion).

Fecal sIgA

Secretory IgA (sIgA) is the predominant immunoglobulin in intestinal secretions, the first-line defender against bacteria, parasites, fungi, toxins, and viruses. Found abundantly in saliva and other mucosal fluids, sIgA works by forming immune complexes with pathogenic microorganisms, allergenic food proteins, and carcinogens, preventing them from binding to the surface of absorptive cells. If sIgA response is impaired, mucosal tissue repair may be compromised, leading to reduced mucosal integrity and immunity against foreign invaders. Fecal sIgA testing uses sIgA as a clinical marker to evaluate the status of mucosal immunity. Low sIgA levels can signal the presence of a previously unsuspected allergy or other autoimmune disorder.

Adrenocortex stress and melatonin profiles

Since the etiology of food and environmental allergy involves interaction between numerous chemical mediators in the immune system, including serotonin, many sensitized individuals commonly exhibit various endocrine dysfunctions. Moreover, the severity of allergy symptoms often follow a chronobiotic pattern, highly influenced by circadian hormone rhythms.

THERAPEUTIC CONSIDERATIONS

Allergy testing reveals whether certain food and environmental substances may be antigenic, providing the clinician with clear, specific results to use in designing an effective therapeutic program. Treatment involves five essential components:

- avoidance of identified allergens
- rotation diet until sensitivity is decreased
- re-establishment of proper microbial milieu
- healing of the damaged intestinal mucosa
- correction of underlying causative factors, such as maldigestion.

Since the body's immunological response involves a very complex series of molecular relationships that are still not fully understood, it is important that each patient's case be carefully evaluated using a variety of criteria. Antibody test results, a detailed medical history, and a thorough physical examination are all important factors to consider when diagnosing a suspected adverse reaction to food or inhalants. Additional challenge tests may also be necessary, once certain antigen candidates have been ruled out as unlikely by preliminary diagnostic tests.

Diet

Oligoantigenic diet

An oligoantigenic diet has been proven, in a large number of studies, to be highly effective in treating many types of food allergies. Children with attention deficit disorder show a marked improvement in their hyperactive behavior following the removal of provoking foods from their diets.[59] In another study, 93% of 88 children with severe frequent migraine recovered on an oligoantigenic diet, even in instances when the migraines were provoked by additional factors such as blows to the head, exercise, or flashing lights.[60] A low-allergen diet also significantly reduced symptoms of colic in infants and chronic urticaria with arthralgia in adult patients.[49,61]

Rotation diet

Diversified rotation diets are often used to prevent new allergies from developing and to give the immune system a rest and the intestines a chance to heal (see Ch. 58). Once the intestines are damaged and a food allergy susceptibility established, virtually any food eaten regularly will eventually establish an antibody response.

This diet consists of eating tolerated foods at regularly spaced intervals of 4–7 days.[62] This approach is based on the principle that infrequent consumption of tolerated foods is not likely to induce new sensitivities or increase any mild sensitivities, even in highly sensitized and immune-compromised individuals. As tolerance for eliminated foods returns, they may be added back into the rotation schedule without reactivation of the allergy. Professional nutritional counseling should be provided to a person attempting to design a rotation diet, in order to ensure proper nutritional intake and classification of foods by related taxanomical groupings. An excellent aid (*The rotation game* by Sally Rockwell, available at PO Box 31065, Seattle, WA, 98103) is available to assist patients in following such a diet.

Re-establishing a healthy bowel microflora

Fundamental to correction of gastrointestinal dysfunction is re-establishment of the appropriate microbial flora of the intestine. The health-inducing bacteria are especially important because they suppress the growth of toxic bacteria. Reseeding the intestines is done through the use of probiotics and prebiotics. Probiotics are the normal bacteria found in the healthy intestines. Prebiotics are indigestible substances that help the healthful bacteria grow. Prebiotics also help by increasing the production of secretory IgA in the intestines, which also helps protect against bacteria and food allergens.[63]

The primary beneficial organisms used to reseed the intestines are *Lactobacilli* and *Bifidobacteria*. They play many important roles, a crucial one of which is inhibiting the growth of toxic bacteria, viruses, fungi, yeasts, and parasites.[64] An important part of reseeding the intestines is to ensure that the food the health-promoting bacteria need to live on is easily available. One of the best ways to do this is with oligosaccharides, especially fructooligosaccharides. Fructooligosaccharides are short-chain carbohydrates composed of three to 10 molecules of sugars, at least two of which are fructose. This molecule is essentially indigestible by humans. However, the *Bifidobacteria* and *Lactobacilli* preferentially utilize fructooligosaccharides to grow and multiply. In contrast, toxic bacteria are unable to use these short-chain carbohydrates.[65] Foods rich in fructooligosaccharides include onions, asparagus, bananas, and maple syrup.

Healing the damaged gut

Re-establishing a healthy intestine is critical for the elimination of food allergies because a leaky gut will continue to expose food antigens to the immune system. Healing the damaged intestinal mucosa requires a comprehensive approach that includes eliminating all factors that injure the intestine (such as toxic bacteria), re-establishing the normal bowel flora, removing toxins from the intestines, improving digestion, decreasing inflammation, and promoting the metabolism and repair of the intestinal-lining cells.

Decreasing the gut inflammatory reaction

Several nutrients help decrease the local inflammatory reaction. Quercetin is a natural bioflavonoid that inhibits the release of inflammatory chemicals from sensitized mast cells, an especially useful effect for the sensitized gut. Quercetin and other bioflavonoids have been shown to inhibit the release of inflammatory chemicals from mast cells, scavenge free radicals, and inhibit irritability of the muscles of the intestines. It has been used in clinical trials to reduce the intestinal damage caused by ingestion of a food allergens.[66] A typical dosage of quercetin is 250 mg three times a day along with vitamin C.

Also of value are fish oils which have now been utilized for a wide variety of inflammatory and allergic diseases. Fish oil is rich in the polyunsaturated N-3 fatty acids, and eicosapentaenoic (EPA) and docosahexaenoic acids (DCHA). EPA competes with arachidonic acid (AA) for metabolism by the cyclooxygenase and lipoxygenase pathways. Metabolites derived from EPA have reduced inflammatory activities as compared with their AA-derived counterparts. Dietary supplementation with EPA leads to incorporation of EPA into membrane phospholipids, inhibition of 5-lipoxygenase pathway activity, and a reduction of the elaboration of platelet-activating factor. Neutrophil chemotaxis and the capacity of these cells to adhere to endothelial cells are also substantially attenuated. Clinical trials in rheumatoid arthritis, psoriasis, atopic dermatitis, and bronchial asthma have shown beneficial effects.[67] The typical dosage is 1–3 grams per day of EPA.

Stimulating regeneration of the gut mucosa

Several nutrients help heal the intestines. Of particular value is glutamine, the most abundant amino acid in the blood. As one of the principal fuels used by the intestinal lining cells, it accounts for 35% of their energy production. While readily available in the diet and synthesized in the body, supplementation improves the energy metabolism of the gastrointestinal mucosa, thus stimulating regeneration.[68] Glutamine prevents intestinal mucosal damage and has been shown to decrease bacterial leakage across the intestines after they are damaged, presumably by stimulating repair.[69] A typical dosage of glutamine is 100 mg three times a day (see Ch. 54 for a more comprehensive discussion of intestinal repair).

Re-establishing normal digestion

The Heidelberg gastric analysis test should be performed if achlorhydria or hypochlorhydria is suspected (see Ch. 19). Hypochlorhydria can be treated with oral betaine HCl supplementation (see Appendix 7).

Pancreatic insufficiency can be treated with exogenous pork or beef pancreatin (see Ch. 101) or microbial-derived digestive enzymes such as those extracted from *Aspergillus oryzae* (see Ch. 66).

SUMMARY

Food allergies are a widespread, often unrecognized cause of chronic ill health and disease. Substantial experience has shown remarkable clinical response when the offending foods are recognized and eliminated from the diet. The primary challenge is the difficulty in making an accurate diagnosis.

REFERENCES

1. Shloss OM. Allergy to common foods. Trans Am Pediatr Soc 1918; 27: 62–68
2. Duke WW. Food allergy as a cause of abdominal pain. Arch Intern Med 1921; 28: 151
3. Duke WW. Ménière's syndrome caused by allergies. JAMA 1923; 81: 2179
4. Brunner M, Walzer M. Absorption of undigested proteins in human beings: the absorption of unaltered egg protein in infants. Arch Intern Med 1928; 42: 173–179
5. Wilson SJ, Walzer M. Absorption of undigested proteins in human beings. IV. Absorption of unaltered egg protein in infants. Am J Dis Child 1935; 50: 49–54
6. Rinkel HJ. Food Allergy. J Kansas Med Soc 1936; 37: 177
7. Breneman JC. Immunology of delayed food allergy. Otolaryngol Head Neck Surg 1995; 113: 702–704
8. Chandra RK. Food allergy and food intolerance. Lessons from the past and hopes for the 21st century. In: Somoyogi JC, Muller HR, Ockhuizen T, eds. Food allergy and food intolerance. Nutritional aspects and developments. Bibl Nutr Dieta 1991; 48: 149–156
9. Sampson HA. Eczema and food hypersensitivity. In: Metcalfe DD, Sampson HA, Simon RA, eds. Food allergy: adverse reactions to foods and food additives. Boston: Blackwell Scientific. 1991: p 113–128
10. Sampson HA. Food hypersensitivity and dietary management in atopic dermatitis. Ped Dermatol 1992; 9: 376–379
11. Kjellman, NI. Natural history and prevention of food sensitivity. In: Metcalfe DD, Sampson HA, Simon RA, eds. Food allergy: adverse reactions to foods and food additives. Boston: Blackwell Scientific. 1991: p 319–331
12. Andre F, Andre C, Colin L et al. Role of new allergens and of allergens consumption in the increased incidence of food sensitizations in France. Toxicology 1994; 93: 77–83
13. Gerrard JW, Ko CG, Vickers P. The familial incidence of allergic disease. Ann All 1976; 36: 10
14. Taub EL. Food allergy and the allergic patient. Springfield, MA: Thomas. 1978
15. Monro J, Carini C, Brostoff J, Zilkha K. Food allergy in migraine. Lancet 1980; 2: 1
16. Atherton DJ, Sewell M, Soothill JF, Wells RS. A double-blind controlled crossover trial of an antigen-avoidance diet in atopic eczema. Lancet 1978; 1: 402
17. Rea WJ, Peters DW, Smiley RE et al. Recurrent environmentally triggered thrombophlebitis: a five year follow-up. Ann Allergy 1981; 47: 338–344
18. Andresen AFR. Ulcerative colitis – an allergic phenomenon. Amer J Dig Dis 1942; 9: 91

19. Ader R, ed. Psychoneuroimmunology. New York: Academic Press. 1981
20. Egger J, Graham PJ, Carter CM, Gumley D. Controlled trial of oligoantigenic treatment in the hyperkinetic syndrome. Lancet 1985; 1: 540
21. Edwards AM. Food-allergic disease. Clin Exp Allergy 1995; 25(1): 16–19
22. Michaelson G, Juhlin L. Urticaria induced by preservatives and dye additives in food and drugs. Br J Dermatol 1973; 88: 525–532
23. Warin RP, Smith RJ. Challenge test battery in chronic urticaria. Br J Dermatol 1976; 94: 401–406
24. Rowe AH, Young EJ. Bronchial asthma due to food allergy alone in 95 patients. JAMA 1959; 169: 1158
25. Raymond LF. Allergy and chronic simple glaucoma. Ann All 1964; 22: 146
26. Ciprandi C, Canonica GW. Incidence of digestive diseases in patients with adverse reactions to foods. Ann Allergy 1988; 61: 334–336
27. Buckley RH, Metcalfe D. Food allergy. JAMA 1982; 248: 2627–2631
28. Spencer MJ. Immunologic methods useful in the diagnosis of infectious disease. In: Lawlor GJ, Jr, Fischer TJ, eds. Manual of allergy and immunolgy. Boston: Little Brown. 1981: p 365–392
29. Perlmutter L. Non-IgE mediated atopic disease. Ann All 1984; 52: 640
30. Paganelli F, Levinsky RJ, Atherton DJ. Detection of specific antigen within circulating immune complexes. Lancet 1979; 1: 1270
31. Kaczmarski M, Malinowska I, Stasiak A et al. IgE in children with adverse reactions to food. Pneumonologia I Alergologia Polska 1992; 60(1): 9–15
32. Edwards AM. Food allergic disease. Clin Exp Allergy 1995; 25(1): 16–19
33. Businco L, Falconieri P, Giempietro P, Bellioni B. Food allergy and asthma. Ped Pulmonol 1995; 11: 59–60
34. Moneret-Vautrin DA, Kanny G, Halpern G. Detection of antifood IgE by in vitro tests and diagnosis of food allergy. Allergie et Immunologie 1993; 25: 198–204
35. Shakib F, McLaughlan P, Stanworth DR et al. Elevated serum IgE and IgG4 in patients with atopic dermatitis. Br J Dermatol 1977; 97: 59–63
36. Hamburger R. Proceedings of the First International Symposium on Food Allergy;Vancouver, BC. 1982
37. Vatn MH, Grimstad IA, Thorsen L et al. Adverse reaction to food. Assessment by double-blind placebo-controlled food challenge and clinical, psychosomatic and immunologic analysis. Digestion 1995; 56: 421–428
38. El Rafei A, Peters SM, Harris N, Bellanti JA. Diagnostic value of IgG4 measurement in patients with food allergy. Ann Allergy 1989; 62: 94–99
39. Vijay HM, Perlmutter L. Inhibition of reagin-mediated PCA reactions in monkeys and histamine release from human leukocytes by human IgG4 subclass. Int Arch Allergy Appl Immunol 1977; 53: 78–87
40. Vijay HM, Perlmutter L, Berstein JL. Possible role of IgG4 in discordant correlation between intracutaneous skin tests and RAST. Int Arch Allergy Appl Immunol 1978; 56: 517–522
41. Fagan DL, Slaughter CA, Capra JD, Sullivan TJ. Monoclonal antibodies to immunoglobulin G4 induce histamine release from human basophils in vitro. J Allergy Clin Immunol 1982; 70: 399–404
42. Nakagawa T, Stadler BM, Heiner DC et al. Flow-cytometric analysis of human basophil degranulation. II. Degranulation induced by anti-IgE, anti-IgG4, and the calcium ionophone A231187. Clin Allergy 1981; 2: 21–30
43. Parrish WE. The clinical relevance of heat stable, short term, sensitizing anaphylactic Ig G antibodies and of related acitivites of Ig G4 and Ig G2. Br J Dermatol 1981; 105: 223–231
44. Kemeny DM, Urbanke R, Ewan P et al. The subclass of IgG antibody in allergic disease. II. The IgG subclass of antibodies produced following natural exposure to dust mite and grass pollen in atopic and non-atopic individuals. Clin Exp Allergy 1989; 19: 545–549
45. Morgan JE, Daul CB, Lehrer SB. The natural history of shrimp-specific immunity. J Allergy Clin Immunol 1990; 86: 88–93
46. Barnes RM, Lewis-Jones MS, Allan S et al. Development and isotype diversity of antibodies to inhalant and dietary antigens in childhood atopic eczema. Clin Exp Dermatol 1993; 18: 211–216
47. Tolo K, Brandtzaeg P, Jonsen J. Mucosal penetration of antigen in the presence or absence of serum-derived antibody. Immunology 1977; 33: 733
48. Quinti I, Papetti C, D'Offizi et al. IgG subclasses to food antigens. Allergie Imunol 1988; 20: 41
49. Paganelli R, Fagiolo U, Cancian M, Scala E. Intestinal permeability in patients with chronic urticaria-angioedema with and without arthralgia. Ann Allergy 1991; 66: 181–184
50. Romagnani S. Regulation and deregulation of human IgE synthesis. Immunology Today 1990; 11: 316–321
51. Schultz CL, Coffman RL. Control of isotype switching by T cells and cytokines. Current Opinion Immunology Today 1990; 11: 316–321
52. Van Arsdel PP Jr, Larson EB. Diagnostic tests for patients with suspected allergic disease. Ann Intern Med 1989; 110: 304–312
53. Gwynn CM, Ingram J. Bronchial provocation tests in atopic patients with allergen specific IgG4 antibodies. Lancet 1982; 1: 254–256
54. Sampson HA, Metcalfe DD. Food allergies. JAMA 1992; 268: 2840–2844
55. Hunter JO. Food allergy – or enterometabolic disorder? Lancet 1991; 338: 495–496
56. Carter CM, Urbanowicz M, Hemsley R et al. Effects of a few food diet in attention deficit disorder. Arch Dis Child 1993; 564–568
57. Egger J, Carter CM, Wilson J et al. Is migraine food allergy? A double-blind controlled trial of oligoantifenic diet treatment. Lancet 1983; 2: 865–869
58. Hill DJ, Hudson IL, Sheffield LJ et al. A low allergen diet is a significant intervention in infantile colic. Results of a community-based study. J Allergy Clin Immunol 1995; 96: 886–892
59. Butkus SN, Mahan LK. Food allergies. Immunological reactions to food. J Am Dietetic Assoc 1986; 86: 601–608
60. Andre F, Andre C, Feknous M et al. Digestive permeability to different-sized molecules and to sodium cromoglycate in food allergy. Allergy Proc 1991; 12: 293–298
61. Andre C, Andre F, Colin L, Cavagna S. Measurement of intestinal permeability to mannitol and lactulose as a means of diagnosing food allergy and evaluating therapeutic effectiveness of disodium cromoglycate. Ann Allergy 1987; 59: 127–130
62. Rinkel RJ. Food Allergy IV. The function and clinical application of the rotary diversified diet. J Pediat 1948; 32: 266
63. Roberfroid MG, Gibson GR. Dietary modulation of the human colonic microbiota. Introducing the concept of prebiotics. J Nutr 1995; 125: 140 1–12
64. Lee Y-K, Salminen S. The coming of age of probiotics. Trends Food Sci Technol 1995; 6: 2415
65. Hidaka H et al. The effects of undigestible fructo-oligosaccharides on intestinal microflora and various physiological new functions in human health. I. In: Furda I, Brine CJ, eds. New developments in dietary fiber. New York: Plenum Press. 1990: p 105–117
66. Ci Carlo G, Mascolo N et al. Effects of quercetin on the gastrointestinal tract in rats and mice. Phytotherapy Res 1994; 8: 42–45
67. Lee TH, Arm JP, Horton CE et al. Effects of dietary fish oil lipids on allergic and inflammatory diseases. Allergy Proc 1991; 12: 299–303
68. Scoba WW. Glutamine. A key substrate for the splanchnic bed. Ann Rev Nutr 1991; 11: 285–308
69. Klimberg VS, Salloum RM, Kasper M et al. Oral glutamine accelerates healing of the small intestine and improves outcome after whole abdominal radiation. Arch Surg 1990; 125: 1040–1045

CHAPTER CONTENTS

52

Homocysteine metabolism: nutritional modulation and impact on health and disease*

Alan L. Miller, ND

Gregory S. Kelly, ND

INTRODUCTION

Homocysteinuria, an autosomal disease with considerable genetic heterogeneity, is the second most common inborn error of amino acid metabolism. While the full genetic disorder affects only 1:200,000 live births, abnormal homocysteine metabolism – due to enzyme dysfunction, lifestyle or nutritional deficiencies – appears to be surprisingly common.

Hyperhomocysteinemia has received increasing attention during the past decade and has joined smoking, dyslipidemia, hypertension, and obesity as a significant independent risk factor for cardiovascular disease. In addition to its possible role in cardiovascular disease, increased homocysteine levels have been implicated in several other clinical conditions, including neural tube defects, spontaneous abortion, placental abruption, renal failure, non-insulin-dependent diabetes and complications of diabetes, rheumatoid arthritis, alcoholism, osteoporosis, and neuropsychiatric disorders.

HOMOCYSTEINE METABOLISM

Homocysteine metabolism is greatly impacted by enzyme function, lifestyle choices, and nutritional status. Following is a discussion of the role of gender, genetics, lifestyle, and key nutrients in homocysteine metabolism.

Gender and genetics

Studies of healthy men and women indicate that certain acquired and genetic determinants may impact total plasma homocysteine. Women tend to have lower basal levels than men,[1] and neither contraceptives nor hormone replacement therapy seem to alter their levels significantly.[2] However, in postmenopausal women, hormone replacement therapy might slightly decrease elevated homocysteine concentrations. No significant lowering effect was observed in women with low homocysteine

*Reprinted with permission from *Alternative Medicine Review* 1997; 2(4): 234–254

levels.[3] Generally, homocysteine concentrations are significantly higher in postmenopausal women than in pre-menopausal women; however, the above-mentioned sex differences in homocysteine concentrations persist even in elderly populations.[4–6] The anti-estrogen drug tamoxifen, used in the long-term treatment of breast cancer patients, is reported to decrease homocysteine levels in postmenopausal women with breast cancer.[7]

Epidemiological evidence has shown homocysteine levels to be over 45% lower in Westernized adult black Africans than in age-matched white adults, revealing racial genetic differences in homocysteine metabolism.[8]

Lifestyle

An association between coffee consumption and the concentration of total homocysteine in plasma has been reported. A marked positive dose–response relation between coffee consumption and plasma homocysteine levels was observed. The relationship was most marked in males and females consuming greater than eight cups of coffee per day. The combination of cigarette smoking and high coffee intake was associated with particularly high homocysteine concentrations.[9] Chronic ingestion of alcohol has also been associated with increased homocysteine levels.[10,11]

Nutritional considerations

Nutrition impacts homocysteine concentrations in both men and women. For example, those individuals in the lowest quartiles for serum folate and vitamin B_{12} (nutrients which significantly impact homocysteine metabolism) have significantly higher concentrations of homocysteine, and men in the lowest quartile of serum pyridoxal 5′-phosphate (P5P – the bioactive form of vitamin B_6) also have increased homocysteine concentrations.[2]

Methionine

Metabolism of the amino acid methionine, a limiting amino acid in the synthesis of many proteins, affects several biochemical pathways involving the production of nutrients which are essential to the optimal functioning of the cardiovascular, skeletal, and nervous system.

Homocysteine is an intermediate product of methionine metabolism and is itself metabolized by two pathways: the re-methylation pathway which regenerates methionine, and the trans-sulfuration pathway which degrades homocysteine into cysteine and then taurine. In essence, the intermediate metabolite homocysteine is located at a metabolic crossroads, so it directly and indirectly impacts all methyl and sulfur group metabolism occurring in the body. Experiments have demonstrated that high levels of L-homocysteine and adenosine in the cell inhibit all methylation reactions.[12]

The re-methylation pathway (see Fig. 52.1) comprises two intersecting biochemical pathways and results in the transfer of a methyl group (CH_3) to homocysteine by either methylcobalamin or betaine (trimethylglycine). Methylcobalamin originally receives its methyl group from S-adenosylmethionine (SAM) or 5-methyltetrahydrofolate (5-methylTHF), an active form of folic acid. After re-methylation, methionine can be re-utilized to produce SAM, the body's "universal methyl donor", which participates in several key metabolic pathways, including methylation of DNA and myelin, synthesis of carnitine, coenzyme Q_{10}, creatine, epinephrine, melatonin, methylcobalamin, and phosphatidylcholine, as well as phase II methylation detoxification reactions.

The trans-sulfuration pathway of methionine/homocysteine degradation (see Fig. 52.1) produces the amino acids cysteine and taurine, which are important nutrients for cardiac health, hepatic detoxification, cholesterol excretion, bile salts formation, and glutathione production. This pathway is dependent on adequate dietary intake and hepatic conversion of vitamin B_6 into its active form, P5P. Also necessary is the amino acid serine, a down-line metabolite generated from betaine via the homocysteine-remethylation pathway.

In addition to 5-methylTHF, methylcobalamin, betaine, and P5P, *N*-acetylcysteine has been reported to significantly lower homocysteine levels.[13]

Methyltetrahydrofolate

Folates function as carbon donors in the synthesis of serine from glycine, directly in the synthesis of purines and pyrimidine bases, indirectly in the synthesis of transfer RNA, and as a methyl donor to create methylcobalamin which is used for re-methylation of homocysteine to methionine. Dietary folic acid is a mixture of folates in the form of polyglutamates, which are readily destroyed by cooking.

Synthesis of the active forms of folic acid is a complex process requiring several enzymes as well as adequate supplies of niacin, P5P, and serine as cofactors (see Fig. 52.2). In plants, folic acid is formed from a heterobicyclic pteride ring, *para*-aminobenzoic acid (PABA), and glutamic acid. Folate is initially deconjugated in the cells of the intestinal wall to the monoglutamate form. This is then reduced to dihydrofolate and then to tetrahydrofolate (THF) via folate and dihydrofolate reductase. Both of these enzymes require NADPH (niacin-dependent) as a cofactor. Serine combines with P5P to transfer a hydroxymethyl group to THF. This results in the formation of 5,10-methylenetetrahydrofolate (5,10-methyleneTHF) and glycine. This molecule is of central importance, being the precursor of the metabolically active 5-methylTHF, which is involved in homocysteine metabolism, and methylidynetetrahydrofolate (involved

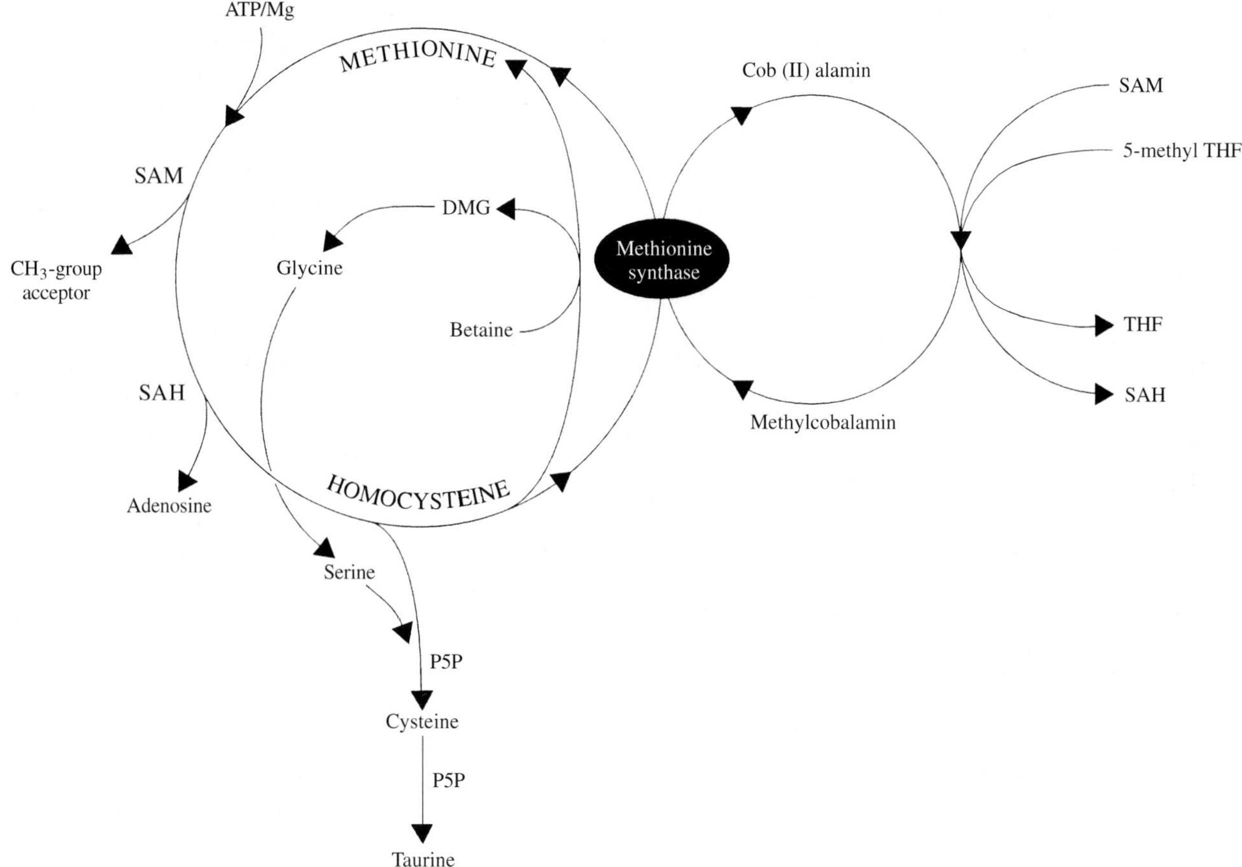

Figure 52.1 Homocysteine metabolism. SAM, S-adenosylmethionine; SAH, S-adenosylhomocysteine; 5-methylTHF, 5-methyltetrahydrofolate; THF, tetrahydrofolate; DMG, dimethylglycine; P5P, pyridoxal 5′-phosphate (vitamin B_6).

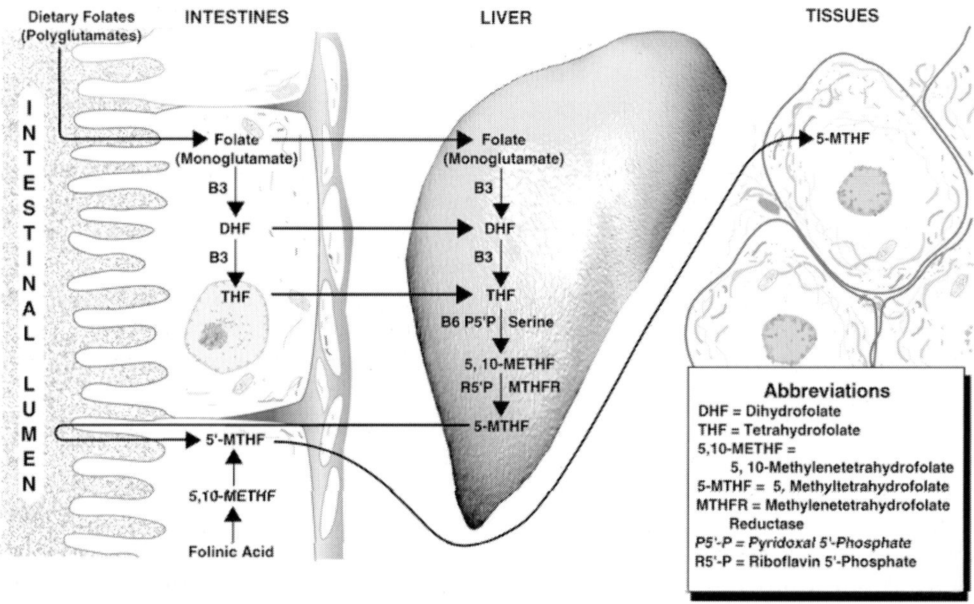

Figure 52.2 Absorption and activation of folic acid. DHF, dihydrofolate; THF, tetrahydrofolate; 5,10-METHF, 5,10-methylenetetrahydrofolate; 5-MTHF, 5-methyltetrahydrofolate; MTHFR, methylenetetrahydrofolate reductase; P5′-P, pyridoxal 5′-phosphate; R5′-P, riboflavin 5′-phosphate.

in purine synthesis), as well as functioning on its own in the generation of thymine side chains for incorporation into DNA.

The following may contribute to a deficiency of folic acid:

- a deficient food supply
- a defect in utilization, as in alcoholics
- malabsorption
- increased needs in pregnant women and in cancer patients
- metabolic interference by drugs
- folate losses in hemodialysis
- enzyme or cofactor deficiency needed for generation of active folic acid.

Individuals using supplements or consuming either breakfast cereals or green leafy vegetables have significantly greater plasma folate and lower homocysteine levels than non-users.[1]

Folinic acid (5-formylTHF), available supplementally as calcium folinate (also known as leucovorin calcium), is an immediate precursor to 5,10-methyleneTHF and 5-methylTHF. Folinic acid can correct deficiencies of the active forms of folic acid, is more stable than folic acid and has a longer half-life in the body. Folinic acid also readily crosses the blood–brain barrier and is slowly cleared, compared with folic acid, which is poorly transported into the brain, and once in the CNS is rapidly cleared.[14]

Methylcobalamin

The coenzyme form of vitamin B_{12} is a very complex molecule containing cobalt bound to five nitrogens and one carbon. The metal–carbon bond found on this coenzyme is the only known biological example of this type of linkage. Surrounding the cobalt is a corrin ring, which structurally resembles the porphyrin ring found in hemoglobin, the cytochromes and chlorophyll. The use of cobalt in the two biologically active forms of cobalamin, adenosyl- and methylcobalamin, is the only known function of this metal in biological systems.

In humans, the cobalt in cobalamin exists in a univalent oxidation state, designated as cob(I)alamin. The compound commonly referred to as vitamin B_{12} has a cyanide molecule at the metal-carbon position and the oxidation state of the cobalt is +3 instead of the biologically active +1. In order to be utilized in the body, the cyanide molecule must be removed. It is thought that glutathione may be the compound that performs this function. Other available forms of vitamin B_{12} include hydroxocobalamin, and the two active forms, adenosylcobalamin (cobamamide) and methylcobalamin.

The absorption of dietary cobalamin requires the formation of a complex between dietary B_{12} and R-proteins and the secretion, by the stomach mucosa, of intrinsic factor. The B_{12} complex is split by pancreatic proteases and the released B_{12} attaches to intrinsic factor and is absorbed in the distal ileum. The amount of cobalamin required in the diet is very low and even people with pernicious anemia can generally absorb sufficient amounts if the coenzyme is supplemented at a high enough dosage.

Although the basic cobalamin molecule is only synthesized by microorganisms, all mammalian cells can convert this into the coenzymes adenosylcobalamin and methylcobalamin. Adenosylcobalamin is the major form in cellular tissues, where it is retained in the mitochondria. Methylcobalamin predominates in blood plasma and certain other body fluids, and in cells is found in the cytosol.

Adenosylcobalamin functions in reactions in which hydrogen groups and organic groups exchange places. In humans, adenosylcobalamin is required in only two reactions: the catabolic isomerization of methylmalonyl-CoA to succinyl-CoA, and interconversion of alpha- and beta-leucine. After its formation from methylmalonyl-CoA, succinyl-CoA is either involved in the synthesis of porphyrin molecules (along with glycine) or transfers its coenzyme A to form acetyl coenzyme A. The latter reaction is magnesium-dependent and the remaining succinate is fed into the citric acid cycle. Deficiencies in this coenzyme form of vitamin B_{12} result in increased amounts of methylmalonyl-CoA and generally an increase in glycine levels.

Methylcobalamin's only known biological function in humans is in the re-methylation of homocysteine to methionine via the enzyme methionine synthase, also known as 5-methyltetrahydrofolate-homocysteine methyltransferase. In order to originally form methylcobalamin from cyanocobalamin or other Cob(III)alamin or Cob(II)alamin precursors, SAM must be available to supply a methyl group. Once methylcobalamin is formed, it functions in the regeneration of methionine by transferring its methyl group to homocysteine. Methylcobalamin can then be regenerated by 5-methylTHF (see Fig. 52.3). The cell's ability to methylate important compounds such as proteins, lipids, and myelin will be compromised by a deficiency of either folate or vitamin B_{12}.[15] Shortages of active folic acid, SAM, or a dietary deficiency of cobalamin will lead to a decrease in the generation of methylcobalamin and a subsequent impairment of homocysteine metabolism. Since lack of methylcobalamin leads to depressed DNA synthesis, rapidly dividing cells in the brain and elsewhere are affected.

At least 12 different inherited inborn errors of metabolism related to cobalamin are known. Abnormalities are detectable by urine and plasma assays of methylmalonic acid and homocysteine, and plasma and erythrocyte analysis of cobalamin coenzymes, which can reveal

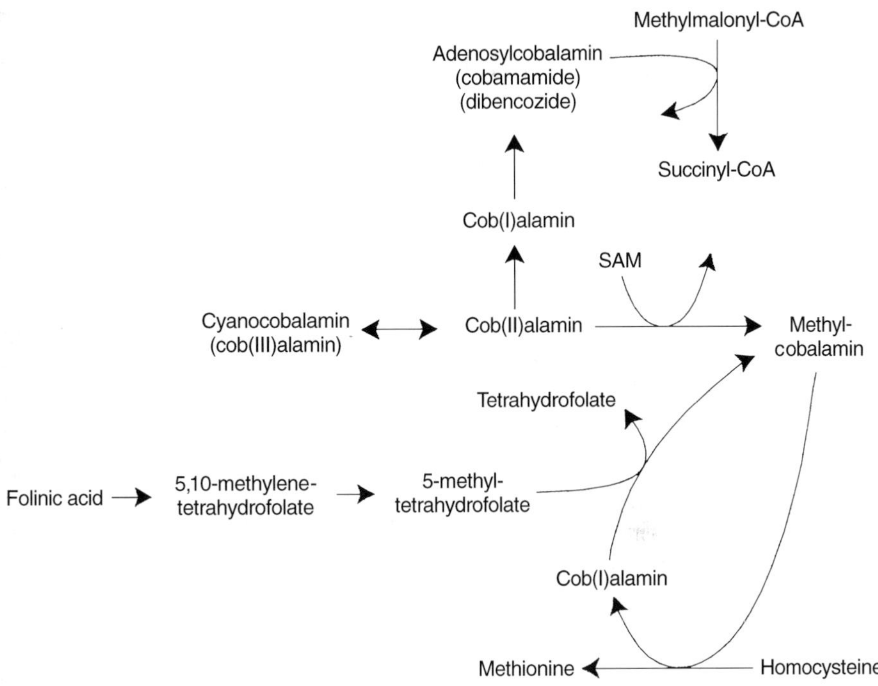

Figure 52.3 Cobalamin metabolism.

deficiencies of methylcobalamin or adenosylcobalamin[16] (see Ch. 29 for further discussion).

Betaine

The metabolic pathways of betaine, methionine, methylcobalamin and methylTHF are interrelated, intersecting at the regeneration of methionine from homocysteine. This regeneration is accomplished in one of two ways. One involves the generation in the cytosol of 5-methylTHF from methylene tetrahydrofolate and the transfer of its methyl group to regenerate methylcobalamin, which then acts as a coenzyme in the regeneration of methionine. Since tetrahydrofolate and its derivatives can only cross the mitochondrial membrane very slowly, inside the mitochondria regeneration of methionine relies on recovery of a methyl group from betaine.

Betaine donates one of its three methyl groups, via the enzyme betaine:homocysteine methyltransferase, to homocysteine resulting in the regeneration of methionine. After the donation of the methyl group, one molecule of dimethylglycine (DMG) remains. This molecule is oxidized to glycine and to two molecules of formaldehyde, by riboflavin-dependent enzymes. The formaldehyde can combine with tetrahydrofolate within the mitochondria to generate one of the active forms of folic acid, methylenetetrahydrofolate, which can be converted to 5-methylTHF and subsequently used as a methyl donor (see Fig. 52.4).

In animal studies, a disturbance in the metabolism of either of the two methyl-donor pathways, due to limited availability of either betaine, or folates and vitamin B_{12}, has a direct impact on levels of nutrients in the coexisting pathway, since more of a drain will be placed on the other pathway as a source of methyl groups. Rats fed diets deficient in choline and methionine have hepatic folate concentrations half that of controls after 5 weeks.[17] During choline deficiency, hepatic SAM concentrations have also been shown to decrease by as much as 50%.[18] Similarly, THF deficiency results in decreased hepatic total choline levels.[19]

Patients with a congenital deficiency of the enzyme methyltetrahydrofolate reductase (MTHFR), which is needed for the formation of 5-methylTHF, have reduced levels of both methionine and SAM in the cerebrospinal fluid and show demyelination in the brain and degeneration of the spinal cord. Methionine is effective in the treatment of some of these patients; however, betaine was shown to restore CSF SAM levels to normal and to prevent the progress of neurological symptoms in all patients in whom it was tried.[20]

Betaine supplementation has been shown to reduce homocysteine levels while resulting in modest increases of plasma serine and cysteine levels.[21] Stimulation of betaine-dependent homocysteine re-methylation causes a commensurate decrease in plasma homocysteine that can be maintained as long as supplemental betaine is taken.[22]

Serine levels are depressed in some individuals with excess homocysteine who are treated with folic acid, cobalamin, and vitamin B_6.[23] Because serine is required: (1) for the conversion of folic acid to its active form, (2) as a shuttle for methyl groups between the cytosol and

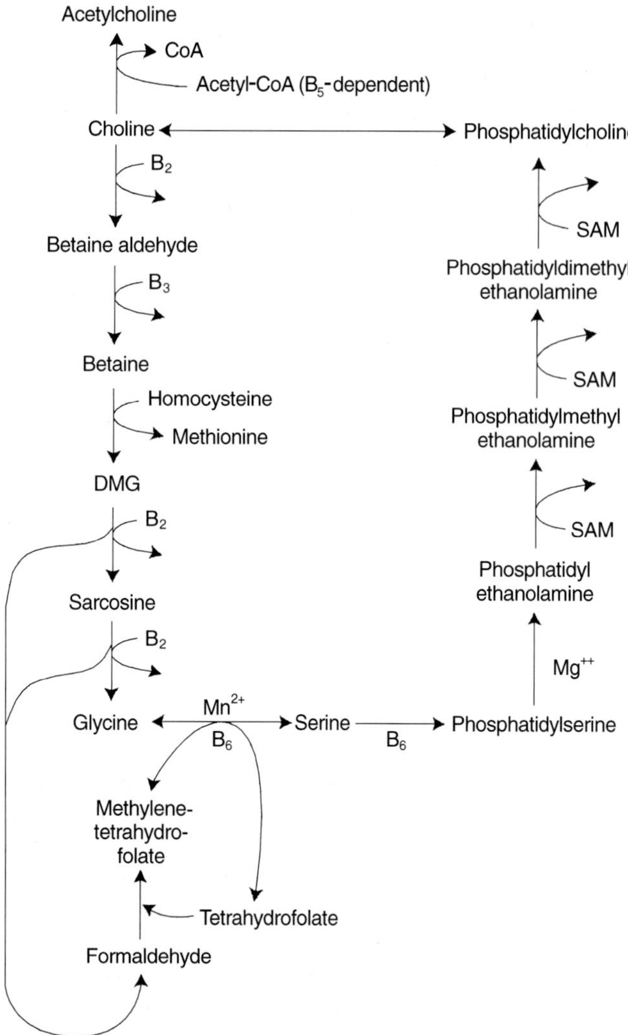

Figure 52.4 Phosphatidylcholine metabolism.

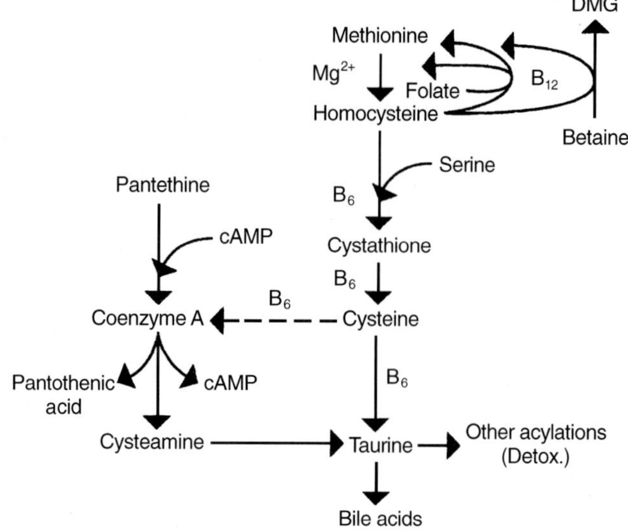

Figure 52.5 Synthesis of taurine.

the mitochondria, and (3) as a cofactor in the trans-sulfuration pathway of methionine/homocysteine metabolism, supplementation with betaine should be included with folic acid, cobalamin, and P5P in order to optimize the interrelated pathways of homocysteine metabolism.

Pyridoxal 5′-phosphate

P5P is the active coenzyme form of vitamin B_6. This cofactor is involved in a myriad biological processes, including the trans-sulfuration pathway of homocysteine. This degradation pathway involves a two-step process, resulting in the formation of cystathionine and its subsequent cleavage to cysteine. Both of the enzymes involved, cystathionine synthase and cystathioninase, require P5P as a cofactor, and the committed first step in the degradation of homocysteine, cystathionine synthase, also requires serine, a downstream metabolite of betaine (see Fig. 52.5).

Once cysteine is generated, it can be directed into several different pathways, including synthesis of glutathione, acetyl-CoA, and taurine. There are three known pathways from cysteine to taurine; all require P5P.

IMPACT OF HOMOCYSTEINE ON KEY NUTRIENTS

Because of its central role in sulfur and methyl group metabolism, elevated levels of homocysteine would be expected to negatively impact the biosynthesis of all of the following: SAM, carnitine, chondroitin sulfates, coenzyme A, coenzyme Q_{10}, creatine, cysteine, dimethylglycine, epinephrine, glucosamine sulfate, glutathione, glycine, melatonin, pantethine, phosphatidylcholine, phosphatidylserine, serine, and taurine.

S-Adenosylmethionine

Methionine is a component of many proteins and cannot be manufactured from other dietary amino acids. It serves as a source of available sulfur for the synthesis of both cysteine and taurine, and, as SAM, it is the most important methyl-group donor in cellular metabolism.

SAM is formed by the transfer of an adenosyl group from ATP to the sulfur atom of methionine. This reaction requires magnesium as a cofactor. When methyl groups are transferred from SAM, S-adenosylhomocysteine is formed. This is then hydrolyzed to release the adenosine, and results in the formation of homocysteine.

SAM is known to be utilized in the synthesis of the following compounds: carnitine, coenzyme Q_{10}, creatine, methylcobalamin from cob(III)alamin, 1-methylnicotinamide, *N*-methyltryptamine, phosphatidylcholine, and polyamines. It is also utilized in methylation reactions as part of hepatic phase II detoxification.

Carnitine

A trimethylated amino acid roughly similar in structure to choline, carnitine is a cofactor for transformation of free long-chain fatty acids into acyl-carnitines, and their transport into mitochondrial matrix, where they undergo beta-oxidation for cellular energy production. Mitochondrial fatty acid oxidation is the primary fuel source in heart and skeletal muscle. Synthesis of carnitine begins with the methylation of the amino acid L-lysine by SAM. Methionine, magnesium, vitamin C, iron, P5P, and niacin, along with the cofactors responsible for regenerating SAM from homocysteine (5-methylTHF, methylcobalamin, and betaine), are required for optimal carnitine synthesis (see Fig. 52.6).

A pivotal enzyme in carnitine synthesis, betaine aldehyde dehydrogenase, is the same enzyme responsible for synthesis of betaine from choline. Two recent studies suggest that this enzyme has a preference for the choline–betaine conversion, and that choline supplementation may decrease carnitine synthesis; therefore, it may be of greater benefit to supplement with betaine rather than its precursor, choline.[24,25]

Chondroitin sulfates, glucosamine sulfate and other sulfated proteoglycans

Proteoglycans are amino sugars found in all tissues, but which are highest in cartilage, tendons, ligaments, synovial fluid, skin, finger, and toenails, heart valves, and the basement membrane of all blood vessels. Perhaps the most widely known of the amino sugars are the chondroitin sulfates and glucosamine sulfate (see Ch. 89 for further discussion).

Chondroitin sulfates are primarily composed of alternating residues of *N*-acetyl-D-galactosamine and D-glucuronate. Sulfate residues are present on C-4 of the galactosamine residues in one type of chondroitin and on C-6 in another. Glucosamine sulfate is a simple molecule composed of glucose, the amino acid glutamine, and a sulfate group. Other sulfated proteoglycans include dermatan sulfates, keratan sulfates, and heparan sulfates.

High levels of homocysteine are likely to negatively impact the formation of the sulfated amino sugars because, although some sulfates are present in the diet, the sulfoxidation of cysteine is an important source of sulfate molecules. The sulfoxidation pathway proceeds through the toxic intermediate sulfite and requires molybdenum as a cofactor.

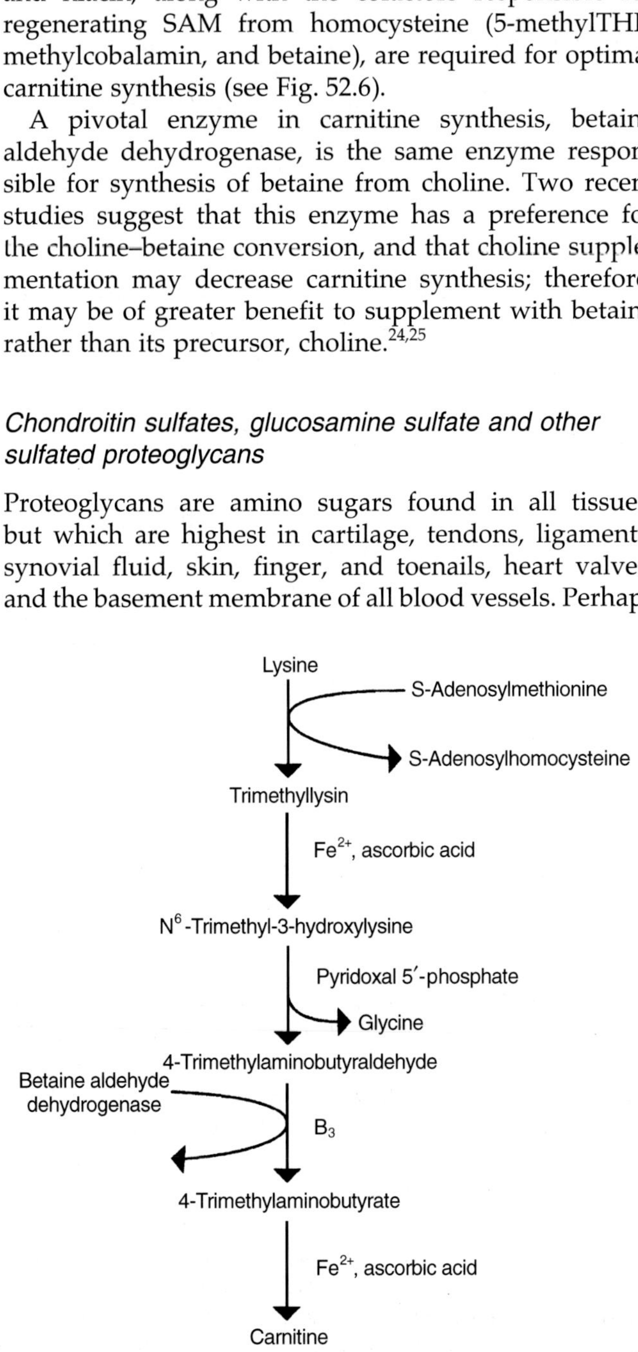

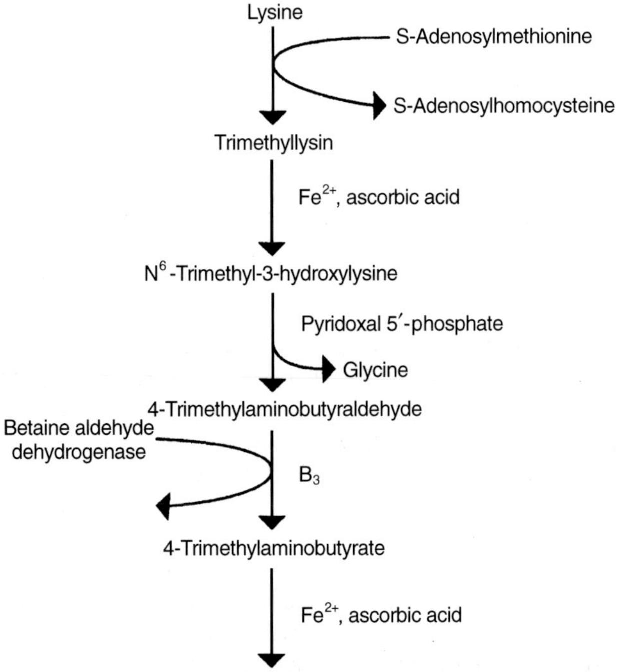

Figure 52.6 Synthesis of carnitine.

Coenzyme A

Coenzyme A consists of an adenine nucleotide and phosphopantetheine. Contained within the structure of this coenzyme is pantothenic acid; however, the reactive component of the molecule is a sulfhydryl group which is not contained within the vitamin. In order to form the sulfhydryl-containing molecule (pantotheine), pantothenic acid must combine with cysteamine. Cysteamine is formed through conjugation and decarboxylation reactions of cysteine. As was previously discussed, the metabolic stagnation implied with elevated homocysteine levels indicates that the body has suboptimal levels of cysteine. Because of this, even in the presence of adequate levels of pantothenic acid, it is possible to have inadequate biosynthesis of acetyl coenzyme A. The disulfate form of pantetheine, known as pantethine, as opposed to pantothenic acid, bypasses cysteine conjugation and decarboxylation. This might account for some of the clinical benefits seen with pantethine supplementation which have not been reproduced with the supplementation of pantothenic acid (see Fig. 52.7A–D for the chemical structures of pantotheine, pantothine, pantothenic acid, and cysteamine).

$$-O-CH_2-C(CH_3)^2-CH(OH)-CO-NH-CH_2-CH_2-CO-NH-CH_2-CH_2-SH$$

A

$$[HO-CH_2-C(CH_3)^2-CH(OH)-CO-NH-CH_2-CH_2-CO-NH-CH_2-CH_2-S-]^2$$

B

$$-O-CH_2-C(CH_3)^2-CH(OH)-CO-NH-CH_2-CH_2-CO$$

C

$$-NH-CH_2-CH_2-SH$$

D

Figure 52.7 A: Pantotheine. B: Pantothine. C: Pantothenic acid. D: Cysteamine.

Coenzyme Q_{10}

Coenzyme Q_{10} (CoQ_{10}) is a fat-soluble quinone occurring in the mitochondria of every cell (see Ch. 76 for a full discussion). The primary biochemical action of CoQ_{10} is as a cofactor in the electron transport chain, the biochemical pathway that generates adenosine triphosphate (ATP). Since most cellular functions are dependent on an adequate supply of ATP, CoQ_{10} is essential for the health of virtually all human tissues and organs. CoQ_{10} also functions as an antioxidant, assisting in the recycling of vitamin E.[26,27]

Biosynthesis of CoQ_{10} begins with the amino acid tyrosine. Pantothenic acid, P5P and vitamin C are all required for the initial steps in its synthesis. An isoprenyl side chain from farnesyl diphosphate, an intermediate in cholesterol synthesis between 3-hydroxy-3-methylglutaryl-CoA (HMG-CoA) and squalene, is then added. An inadequate supply of this intermediate, which can be caused by HMG-CoA reductase inhibitors (cholesterol-lowering drugs of the statin family) results in decreased levels of CoQ_{10}.[28]

In two of the final steps in the synthesis of CoQ_{10}, methyl groups are provided by SAM (see Fig. 52.8). Adequate dietary methionine and a sufficient supply of the nutrients required for the re-methylation of homocysteine to methionine (5-methylTHF, methylcobalamin, and betaine) are required to generate sufficient SAM. Suboptimal amounts of SAM may negatively impact on the ability of the body to synthesize sufficient CoQ_{10}. This relationship between SAM and CoQ_{10} has been suggested in various animal studies.[29,30]

Creatine

In humans, over 95% of the total creatine content is located in skeletal muscle, of which approximately one-third is in its free form as creatine, also known as methylguanidinoacetic acid, while the remainder is present in a phosphorylated form as creatine phosphate (also called phosphocreatine). Creatine phosphate is utilized within skeletal muscle as a means for storing high-energy phosphate bonds.

Creatine is formed in the liver, kidney and pancreas, beginning with the combination of arginine and glycine to produce guanidinoacetate. A methyl group from SAM is then transferred, resulting in the formation of creatine. The by-product of this reaction, S-adenosylhomocysteine, is subsequently hydrolyzed into homocysteine and adenosine. In order to optimize endogenous production of creatine, the amino acids arginine, glycine, and methionine must be available as substrates. Additionally, cofactors needed to optimize re-methylation of homocysteine to form methionine are required to recycle the homocysteine to methionine for reuse as SAM (see Fig. 52.9). Serum creatine levels have been positively correlated with plasma homocysteine levels, i.e. as creatine levels rise, so do homocysteine levels.[31]

Epinephrine and melatonin

Derivatives of the aromatic amino acids, L-tyrosine and L-tryptophan, require methylation for the biosynthesis of their down-line metabolites.

The biosynthesis of catecholamines begins with the amino acid L-tyrosine and proceeds through dopa and dopamine, resulting in the formation of norepinephrine, the neurotransmitter substance found in the majority of sympathetic nerve terminals, as well as in some synapses of the central nervous system. In the chromaffin cells of the adrenal medulla, a methyl group is provided by SAM, resulting in the formation of epinephrine from norepinephrine. A number of metabolites are formed from the degradation of both norepinephrine and epinephrine.

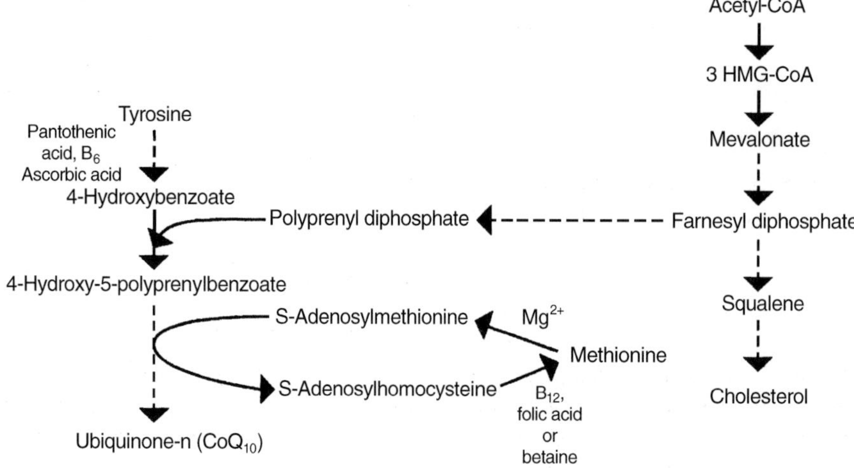

Figure 52.8 Synthesis of coenzyme Q_{10}.

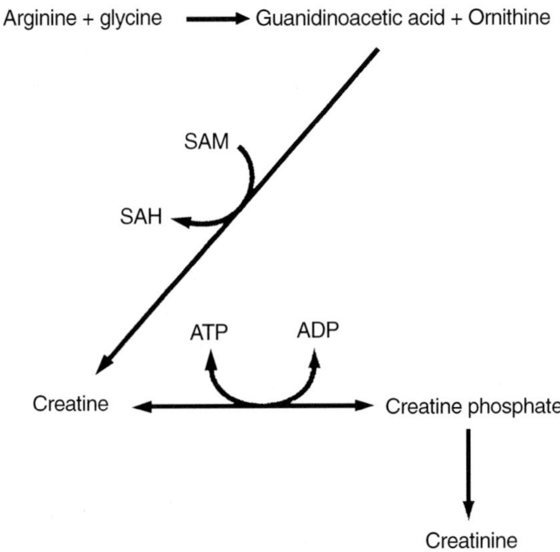

Figure 52.9 Synthesis of creatine, creatine phosphate and creatinine.

Catecholamine degradation proceeds independently, in addition to conjunction with monoamine oxidase, by catechol-O-methyltransferase. This enzyme catalyzes the transfer of a methyl group donated by SAM and, depending on the substrate, results in the formation of homovanillic acid, normetanephrine, and metanephrine.

The formation of melatonin from L-tryptophan proceeds through 5-hydroxytryptophan, serotonin, and *N*-acetylserotonin. Melatonin is then formed in the pineal gland by the donation of a methyl group. 5-Methoxytryptamine, an alternate metabolite of serotonin, also requires the addition of a methyl group.

Since elevated homocysteine results in suboptimal synthesis of SAM, some impact on aromatic amino acid derivatives will occur. The exact nature of the impact on catecholamine metabolites is still unclear due to SAM's role in both synthesis and degradation. It appears likely that the biochemical stagnation associated with elevated levels of homocysteine would negatively impact the synthesis of melatonin.

Phosphatidylcholine

Phosphatidylcholine (PC) is a primary component of lecithin. It is the most frequently encountered phospholipid in animals and is structurally related to phosphatidylserine and phosphatidylethanolamine. PC consists of a glycerol backbone that is esterified with fatty acids on carbon atoms 1 and 2, and with a phosphoric acid/choline complex in position 3. Although phosphatidylcholine is usually referred to as if it were a single compound, it is actually a group of related compounds which vary depending upon the fatty acid composition at position C-1 and C-2.

Dietary choline is derived primarily from PC, which after absorption by the intestinal mucosa is metabolized to choline in the liver by the enzyme phospholipase D. Most choline is re-phosphorylated to PC; however, a small amount is carried to the brain via the bloodstream, where it is converted to the neurotransmitter acetylcholine. If PC or choline are lacking in the diet, they can be synthesized from phosphatidylserine and phosphatidylethanolamine (see Fig. 52.4). Synthesis of PC is dependent on the availability of SAM as a methyl donor, since synthesis involves the transfer of methyl groups from three SAM molecules to phosphatidylethanolamine in order to generate one molecule of PC.

The metabolic pathways of phosphatidylcholine, methionine, methylcobalamin and 5-methylTHF are interrelated, intersecting at the regeneration of methionine from homocysteine by betaine (see Fig. 52.1). The use of choline molecules as methyl donors in this process is probably the main factor that determines how rapidly a diet deficient in choline will induce pathological changes.[18]

Taurine

Taurine is a unique amino acid because it carries a sulfonic acid group (-SO_3H) instead of a carboxyl group (-CO_2H). Taurine is biosynthesized from methionine or from cysteine via the trans-sulfuration pathway (see Fig. 52.5). As discussed previously, homocysteine can be re-methylated to form methionine; however, it can also be degraded to form cysteine. Once cysteine is generated, it can be directed into several different pathways including synthesis of glutathione, acetyl-CoA, 3′-phosphate 5′-phosphosulfate (PAPS), and taurine. Degradation involves a two-step process resulting in the formation of cystathionine and its subsequent cleavage to cysteine. Both of the enzymes involved require P5P as a cofactor, and the committed first step in the degradation of homocysteine, cystathionine synthase, also requires serine. In humans, defects in both of these enzymatic reactions occur. Homocysteinuria, resulting from an absence of cystathionine synthase, can lead to mental retardation. Low levels of this enzyme can also lead to abnormally high levels of homocysteine, especially when remethylation cofactors are also deficient.

CLINICAL APPLICATIONS

Phase II detoxification

Because homocysteine is a critical intermediate in both methyl and sulfur group metabolism, elevated levels could indicate nutrient deficiencies which might compromise function in virtually all of the hepatic phase II detoxification reactions (see Ch. 50).

Amino acid conjugation reactions require either glycine, glutamine, or taurine. Glycine functions in the conjugation of aromatic acids (e.g. benzoic acid to hippuric acid). Elevated levels of homocysteine might indicate reduced nutritional levels of betaine and subsequently its downline metabolite glycine. Taurine functions in acylations (e.g. bile conjugation). As discussed, optimal taurine synthesis requires proper movement of homocysteine into its degradation pathway. There are no known interactions between glutamine and homocysteine.

Sulfur conjugation requires *N*-acetylcysteine (NAC), glutathione (GSH), PAPS, or methionine/cysteine. NAC is used for mercapturic acid synthesis and is involved in detoxification of a wide variety of compounds including aromatic hydrocarbons, some phenols, halides, esters, epoxides, and caffeine. GSH is involved in dismutation reactions of organic nitrates (e.g. nitroglycerin). PAPS is utilized in sulfate ester synthesis, mostly with phenols, and some aliphatic alcohols (e.g. ethanol) and aromatic amines. Methionine and cysteine are used in cyanide-thiocyanate detoxification. A portion of the inorganic sulfur needed for the formation of all of these compounds passes through the homocysteine cycle.

Alkylation reactions require SAM, methylcobalamin, or 5-methylTHF. These compounds provide methyl groups to detoxify compounds containing OH, SH, or NH_2 groups. Examples of these reactions include norepinephrine to epinephrine, epinephrine to metanephrine, guanidoacetic acid to creatine, and *N*-acetylserotonin to melatonin.

Other phase II detoxification reactions which might be impacted by elevated homocysteine as a biological marker of reduced nutrient formation include acetylation by acetylcoenzyme A, which requires cysteine as a source of its cysteamine component; and the use of carnitine for the conversion of valproic acid to valpropylcarnitine.

Heart disease

A significant component in the pathogenesis, prevention, and treatment of heart disease involves the amino acid homocysteine. Increased blood levels of homocysteine are correlated with significantly increased risk of coronary artery disease (CAD),[32–35] myocardial infarction,[36,37] peripheral occlusive disease,[38–41] cerebral occlusive disease,[38,41] and retinal vascular occlusion.[42]

It has been known for over 25 years that inborn errors of homocysteine metabolism result in high levels of homocysteine in the blood and severe atherosclerotic disease. We now know that, even within the range which is considered normal (4–16 μmol/L), there is a graded increase in risk for CAD. In a study of 304 patients with CAD vs. controls, the odds ratio for CAD increased as plasma homocysteine increased, even within the normal range. A 5 μmol/L increase in plasma homocysteine was correlated with an increase in the odds ratio of 2.4 ($P < 0.001$), with no "threshold effect".[35]

A review of a number of studies found that mild hyperhomocysteinemia after a methionine load test occurs in 21%, 24%, and 32% of patients with CAD, cerebrovascular disease, and peripheral vascular disease, respectively.[43] Another group of researchers found the incidence of hyperhomocysteinemia (> 14 μmol/L by their definiion) in a group of 1,160 elderly (ages 67–96) individuals, in the Framingham Heart Study, to be 29.3%. The study also indicated that plasma homocysteine levels increase with age.[38]

Homocysteine facilitates the generation of hydrogen peroxide.[44] By creating oxidative damage to LDL cholesterol and endothelial cell membranes, hydrogen peroxide can then catalyze injury to vascular endothelium.[44,46]

Nitric oxide and other oxides of nitrogen released by endothelial cells (also known as endothelium-derived relaxing factor, or EDRF) protect endothelial cells from damage by reacting with homocysteine, forming S-nitrosohomocysteine, which inhibits hydrogen peroxide formation. However, as homocysteine levels increase, this protective mechanism can become overloaded, allowing damage to endothelial cells to occur.[45–47] Because of the role of sulfate compounds in the formation of amino sugars needed to form the basement membrane of blood vessels, high levels of homocysteine are likely to contribute to the formation of blood vessels which are more susceptible to oxidative stress.[47] The end result of the combination of oxidative damage and endothelial collagen instability can be the formation of atherosclerotic plaques.

Decreased plasma folate levels are correlated with increased levels of homocysteine, and a subsequent increased incidence of CAD. In a 15 year Canadian study of CAD mortality in 5,056 men and women aged 35–79 years, lower serum folate levels were correlated with a significantly increased risk of fatal CAD.[48] In a cohort from the Framingham Heart Study, concentrations of folate and P5P were inversely correlated with homocysteine levels and the risk of extracranial carotid-artery stenosis.[38] Low P5P and low vitamin B_{12} have also been linked with hyperhomocysteinemia and a significantly increased risk of CAD.[35]

Re-methylation of homocysteine and the subsequent formation of SAM is critical for biosynthesis of L-carnitine, CoQ_{10}, and creatine. Similarly, the trans-sulfuration pathway must be functioning properly for optimal biosynthesis of cysteine, GSH, pantethine, and taurine. All of these nutrients are used clinically to reduce oxidative stress, improve risk factor markers, or treat heart disease.

Peripheral vascular disease

Elevated homocysteine levels have been established as an independent risk factor for intermittent claudication

(IC) and deep vein thrombosis. Elevated homocysteine levels corresponded with an increased incidence of intermittent claudication and decreased serum folate levels in a study of 78 patients with IC.[49] A fourfold increase in risk of peripheral vascular disease was noted in individuals with hyperhomocysteinemia compared with those with normal homocysteine levels.[50] A group of researchers in the Netherlands found high homocysteine levels to be a significant risk factor for deep-vein thrombosis, with a stronger relationship among women than men.[51]

An increased risk of peripheral vascular occlusion has been noted in women taking oral contraceptives, which might be linked to the significantly increased homocysteine levels in women so affected. It is already known that oral contraceptives can cause declines or deficiencies in vitamins B_6, B_{12}, and folate, nutrients integral to the processing of homocysteine. Laboratory assessment of plasma homocysteine levels may be helpful to detect women who may be predisposed to peripheral vascular occlusion while on oral contraceptives.[52]

Stroke

Stroke patients have significantly elevated homocysteine levels compared with age-matched controls,[53] with a linear relationship between risk of stroke and homocysteine levels,[54] and a significant decrease in blood folate concentrations in those with elevated homocysteine.[55]

Pregnancy

Biochemical enzyme defects and nutritional deficiencies are receiving increasing attention for their role in causing neural tube defects (NTD) as well as other negative pregnancy outcomes, including spontaneous abortion, placental abruption (infarct), pre-term delivery, and low infant birth weight. Recent evidence has suggested that derangement of methionine-homocysteine metabolism could be the underlying mechanism of pathogenesis of neural tube defects and might be the mechanism of prevention observed with supplementation of folic acid.[56,57] It has been firmly established that a low dietary intake of folic acid increases the risk for delivery of a child with a NTD, and that periconceptional folic acid supplementation reduces the occurrence of NTD.[58–64] Research also indicates that supplemental folic acid intake results in increased infant birth weight and improved Apgar scores, along with a concomitant decreased incidence of fetal growth retardation and maternal infections.[65–68] A derangement in methionine-homocysteine metabolism has also been correlated with recurrent miscarriage and placental infarcts (abruption).[69]

The amino acid homocysteine, when elevated, might be a teratogenic agent contributing to congenital defects of the heart and neural tube. Evidence from experimental animals lends support to this belief. When avian embryos were fed homocysteine to raise serum homocysteine to over 150 nmol/ml, dysmorphogenesis of the heart and neural tube, as well as of the ventral wall, was observed.[70]

Because homocysteine metabolism, through the remethylation and trans-sulfuration pathways, affects several biochemical pathways involving the production of nutrients which are essential to the optimal functioning of the cardiovascular, skeletal, and nervous systems, it is not surprising that these other nutrients have been linked to complications of pregnancy in animal models and humans. Low plasma vitamin B_{12} levels have been shown to be an independent risk factor for NTD.[71,72] Methionine has been shown to reduce the incidence of NTD by 41% in an animal model when administered on days 8 and 9 of pregnancy.[73,74] This evidence indicates that a disturbance in the remethylation pathway with a subsequent decrease in SAM may be a contributing factor to these complications of pregnancy.

Phosphatidylcholine, due to its role as a precursor to acetylcholine and choline, is acknowledged as a critical nutrient for brain and nerve development and function.[75–77] Since the metabolic pathways of choline (via betaine), methionine, methylcobalamin and 5-methylTHF are interrelated, intersecting at the regeneration of methionine from homocysteine, a disturbance in the metabolism of either of these two methyl-donor pathways, due to limited availability of key nutrients or decreased enzyme activity, will have a direct impact on the body's ability to optimize levels of SAM.

Evidence suggests that women with a history of NTD-affected pregnancies have altered folic acid metabolism.[78–81] Patients with a severe congenital deficiency of the enzyme MTHFR, which is needed for the formation of 5-methylTHF, have reduced levels of both methionine and adenosylmethionine in the cerebrospinal fluid and show demyelination in the brain and degeneration of the spinal cord.[2,82] Because of its direct impact in the activation of folic acid to its methyl derivative, a milder version of this enzyme defect is also strongly suspected to increase the incidence of NTD.[83]

It is established that high vitamin A intake during the first 2 months of pregnancy is associated with a several-fold higher incidence of birth defects.[84,85] Although the mechanism of action remains to be elicited, in an animal model the activity of hepatic MTHFR is suppressed with high vitamin A levels, suggesting that its teratogenic effect during early pregnancy may be associated with a subsequent derangement in the remethylation of homocysteine.[86]

Since a more significant correlation has been found between high homocysteine levels in women experiencing placental abruption, infarction, and spontaneous abortion than in control women, and since homocysteine and CoQ_{10} synthesis are both dependent upon the methionine-SAM-homocysteine pathway, it is possible that low CoQ_{10} and elevated homocysteine independently found in complicated pregnancy may also in fact be found to be related conditions.[87,88]

Nutritional intervention with the cofactors required for optimal metabolism of the methionine-homocysteine pathways offers a new integrated possibility for primary prevention of NTD and several other complications of pregnancy. Supplementation with betaine, and the active forms of cobalamin and folic acid, such as methylcobalamin and folinic acid, along with riboflavin-5′-phosphate (because of its role as a cofactor for the MTHFR enzyme), may play a significant role in reducing or preventing these emotionally devastating outcomes.

Neurological and mental disorders

In addition to the known impact of homocysteine on the cardiovascular system and micronutrient biochemical pathways, numerous diseases of the nervous system are correlated with high homocysteine levels and alterations in B_{12}, folate, or B_6 metabolism, including depression, schizophrenia, multiple sclerosis, Parkinson's disease, Alzheimer's disease, and cognitive decline in the elderly.

Methylation reactions via SAM, including methylation of DNA and myelin, are vitally important in the CNS. The neurologic complications of vitamin B_{12} deficiency are thought to be due to a reduction of activity of the B_{12}-dependent enzyme methionine synthase, and the subsequent reduction of SAM production. The CNS lacks the alternate betaine pathway of homocysteine remethylation; therefore, if methionine synthase is inactivated, the CNS has a greatly reduced methylation capacity.[89] Other causes of reduced methionine synthase activity include folic acid deficiency and nitrous oxide anesthesia exposure.[90]

Homocysteine has also been found to be a neurotoxin, especially in conditions in which glycine levels are elevated, including head trauma, stroke, and B_{12} deficiency.[91] Homocysteine interacts with the *N*-methyl-D-aspartate receptor, causing excessive calcium influx and free radical production, resulting in neurotoxicity.[91] The neurotoxic effects of homocysteine and/or reduced methylation reactions in the CNS contribute to the mental symptomatology seen in B_{12} and folate deficiency. Increased homocysteine levels can also be seen in schizophrenics.[92]

Significant deficiencies in B_{12} and folate are common in the elderly population, and can contribute to a decline in cognitive function.[93–95] An investigation of cognitive ability in older men (aged 54–81) found poorer spatial copying skills in those individuals with higher homocysteine levels. Better memory performance was correlated with higher vitamin B_6 levels.[96]

B_{12} deficiency and increasing severity of cognitive impairment have been seen in Alzheimer's disease (AD) patients compared with controls and patients with other dementias.[97] In a study of 52 AD patients, 50 hospitalized non-demented controls, and 49 elderly subjects living at home, patients with AD were found to have the highest homocysteine levels and the highest methylmalonic acid (an indicator of B_{12} deficiency) levels.[98] In a study of 741 psychogeriatric patients, high plasma homocysteine levels were found in demented and non-demented patients; however, only demented patients also had lower blood folate concentrations compared with controls. Patients with concomitant vascular disease had significantly higher plasma homocysteine than those without diagnosed vascular disease. Significantly higher homocysteine levels, compared with controls, have also been found in Parkinson's patients.[99]

Homocysteine's effects on neurotransmitter metabolism, along with its potential reduction of methylation reactions, could be a contributing factor to the etiology of depression. Folate and B_{12} deficiency can cause neuropsychiatric symptoms including dementia and depression. Although no studies have been performed to date investigating depression, folate and B_{12} deficiency and homocysteine levels, with what is known about these deficiencies and methionine synthase inhibition, it is suggestive that this connection will be revealed in the future. We do know that SAM is used therapeutically as an antidepressant in Europe and is the third most popular antidepressant treatment in Italy in 1995.[100,101] As yet, SAM is not available as a supplement in the US.

Methylation of myelin basic protein is vital to the maintenance of the myelin sheath. The worst-case scenario of folate and B_{12} deficiency includes demyelination of the posterior and lateral columns of the spinal cord, a disease process called subacute combined degeneration of the spinal cord (SCD).[89] SCD can also be precipitated by nitrous oxide anesthesia, which causes an irreversible oxidation of the cobalt moiety of the B_{12} molecule and the subsequent inhibition of methionine synthase activity, a decrease in homocysteine remethylation, and decreased SAM production.[90] This has been treated using supplemental methionine, which further supports the theory of a nitrous oxide-induced biochemical block at methionine synthase.[102] Particularly at risk for this condition are B_{12}-deficient individuals who then visit their dentist and receive nitrous oxide.[90,103]

Abnormal methylcobalamin metabolism is one of the proposed mechanisms for the pathophysiology of the demyelinating disease multiple sclerosis. Deficiency of vitamin B_{12} has been linked to some cases of multiple sclerosis, and it is suggested that dietary deficiency, or more likely, a defect in R-protein-mediated absorption or methylation of B_{12}, might be a significant contributor to the pathogenesis of MS.[104]

Diabetes mellitus

Homocysteine levels appear to be lower in individuals with type 1 diabetes mellitus. Forty-one type 1 diabetic subjects (age 34.8 ± 12 years, duration of illness: 10.7 ± 11.1 years) were compared with 40 age-matched control subjects (age 34.2 ± 9.1 years). Following an overnight fast, homocysteine was significantly ($P = 0.0001$) lower in the diabetic group (6.8 ± 2.2) than in the controls (9.5 ± 2.9). This difference was apparent in male and female subgroups.[105] However, increased levels of homocysteine have been reported in type 1 diabetics with proliferative retinopathy[106] and nephropathy.[106,107]

Evidence to date suggests that metabolism of homocysteine is impaired in patients with non-insulin-dependent diabetes mellitus (NIDDM). Following a methionine load, hyperhomocysteinemia occurred with significantly greater frequency in patients with NIDDM (39%) as compared with age-matched controls (7%). The area under the curve over 24 hours, reflecting the total period of exposure to increased homocysteine, was also elevated with greater frequency in patients with NIDDM and macrovascular disease (33%) as compared with controls (0%). The authors concluded that hyperhomocysteinemia is associated with macrovascular disease in a significant proportion of patients with NIDDM.[108] Other researchers have reported a correlation between increased homocysteine levels and the occurrence of macroangiopathy in patients with NIDDM. Intramuscular injection of 1,000 μg methylcobalamin daily for 3 weeks reduced the elevated plasma levels of homocysteine in these individuals.[109]

Elevated homocysteine levels appear to be a risk factor for diabetic retinopathy in individuals with NIDDM. This might be due to a point mutation on the gene for the enzyme MTHFR.[110,111] A significantly higher percentage of diabetics with retinopathy exhibit this mutation.[112] Elevated homocysteine levels cause cell injury to the small vessels, which may contribute to the development of retinopathy as well as macroangiopathy in the cardiovascular system.[110]

Rheumatoid arthritis

Elevated total homocysteine levels have been reported in patients with rheumatoid arthritis. Twenty-eight patients with rheumatoid arthritis and 20 healthy age-matched control subjects were assessed for homocysteine levels, while fasting and in response to a methionine challenge. Fasting levels were 33% higher in rheumatoid arthritis patients than in controls. Four hours following the methionine challenge, the increase in plasma homocysteine concentration was also higher in patients with rheumatoid arthritis.[112] Another study found statistically significant increases in homocysteine in RA patients ($P = 0.003$), with 20% of the patients having homocysteine levels above the reference range.[113] A mechanism for this increased homocysteine in RA patients has not been elucidated. Penicillamine, a common sulfhydryl-containing arthritis treatment, has been found to lower elevated homocysteine levels in vivo.[114] Further investigation into both the prevalence of hyperhomocysteinemia and the mechanism of action impacting rheumatoid arthritis is needed.

Kidney failure

Because homocysteine is cleared by the kidneys, chronic renal failure, as well as absolute or relative deficiencies of 5-methylTHF, methylcobalamin, P5P, or betaine, results in increased homocysteine levels. In 176 patients with end-stage renal disease on peritoneal or hemodialysis, homocysteine concentrations averaged 26.6 ± 1.5 μmol/L in patients with renal failure as compared with 10.1 ± 1.7 μmol/L in normals. Abnormal values exceeded the 95th percentile for normal controls in 149 of the patients with renal failure.[115] Data also indicate that plasma homocysteine values represent an independent risk factor for vascular events in patients on peritoneal and hemodialysis. Patients with a homocysteine concentration in the upper two quintiles (> 27.8 μmol/L) had an independent odds ratio of 2.9 (CI, 1.4–5.8; $P = .007$) of vascular complications. Vitamin B levels were also lower in patients with vascular complications than in those without.[116]

Alcoholism and ethanol ingestion

Chronic alcoholism is known to interfere with one-carbon metabolism. Because of this, it is not surprising to find that mean serum homocysteine levels are two times higher in chronic alcoholics than in non-drinkers ($P < 0.001$). Beer consumers have lower concentrations of homocysteine compared with drinkers of wine or spirits ($P = 0.05$). In chronic alcoholics, serum P5P and red blood cell folate concentrations have been shown to be significantly lower than in control subjects.[10] Plasma homocysteine is significantly higher, compared with controls, in 42 active alcoholics hospitalized for detoxication. In another group of 16 alcoholics, abstaining from ethanol ingestion, plasma homocysteine did not deviate from that of controls.[11]

Feeding ethanol to rats produces prompt inhibition of methionine synthase as well as a subsequent increase in activity of betaine homocysteine methyltransferase. Despite the inhibition of methionine synthase, the enhanced betaine homocysteine methyltransferase pathway utilizes hepatic betaine pools to maintain levels of SAM.[117] Results indicate that ethanol feeding produces a significant loss in SAM in the first week, with a return to normal SAM levels in the second week. Betaine feeding enhances hepatic betaine pools in control as well as ethanol-fed animals; attenuates the early loss of SAM in ethanol-fed animals; produces an early increase in betaine homocysteine methyltransferase activity; and generates increased levels of SAM in both control and ethanol-fed groups.[118] It has been shown that minimal supplemental dietary betaine at the 0.5% level increases SAM twofold in control animals and fivefold in ethanol-fed rats. Concomitant with the betaine-generated SAM, ethanol-induced hepatic fatty infiltration was ameliorated.[117] Betaine supplementation also reduces the accumulation of hepatic triglyceride produced after ethanol ingestion.[118]

Gout

Although homocysteine levels have been positively correlated with increased uric acid levels,[2,119,120] no studies exist to date which have investigated homocysteine levels in gout patients. It is possible the increased uric acid levels in gout are due to decreased SAM production because of the reduction in homocysteine recycling. The excess adenosine, which would have reacted with methionine to form SAM, is degraded to form uric acid as its end product.

Niacin is contraindicated in gout, as it competes with uric acid for excretion.[121] Animal studies have shown that increased levels of S-adenosylhomocysteine (SAH), and thus homocysteine, cause significant reductions in SAM-dependent methylation reactions.[12] Therefore, since degradation of the niacin-containing coenzyme nicotinamide adenine dinucleotide (NAD) is dependent on methylation by SAM, and SAM activity is severely reduced in hyperhomocysteinemia, niacin levels might be higher in these people, resulting in less uric acid excretion, higher uric acid levels and increased gout symptoms in susceptible individuals. This possibility and its mechanism need further investigation.

Osteoporosis

Homocystinuria due to cystathionine synthase deficiency is an autosomal recessive error of sulfur amino acid metabolism characterized clinically by lens dislocation, mental retardation, skeletal abnormalities and thromboembolic phenomena.[122] Individuals with this enzyme deficiency have decreased concentrations of cysteine and its disulfide form, cystine. In children with homocystinuria, osteoporosis is a common presenting symptom.[123] Because of the role of sulfur compounds in the formation of sulfated amino sugars, disturbed cross-linking of collagen has been proposed as a possible mechanism of action. One group of researchers studying 10 patients with homocystinuria found normal synthesis of collagen, but a significant reduction of cross-links.[124]

Because of the correlation between homocystinuria and osteoporosis in children with this amino acidopathy, and because of the increase in homocysteine concentrations in postmenopausal women, several authors have implied that elevated homocysteine levels contribute to postmenopausal osteoporosis. To date, no evidence is available which demonstrates that homocysteine levels are higher in postmenopausal women with osteoporosis than in age-matched controls.

DIAGNOSTIC CONSIDERATIONS

Many of the studies cited herein have used a reference range, with 12–16 μmol/L being the upper limit of the normal range. We will probably see this level drop, as we did with cholesterol testing, as researchers have found a highly significant increase in relative risk of atherosclerotic cardiovascular disease and other disease processes as homocysteine levels increase, even within the "normal" range. A number of clinical laboratories currently perform plasma homocysteine determinations, by itself or within a cardiovascular panel.

THERAPEUTIC CONSIDERATIONS

If a dietary deficiency or an increased demand, resulting from genetic biochemical individuality exists for 5-methylTHF, methylcobalamin, P5P, or betaine, treatment with these micro-nutrients should reduce homocysteine levels. Several studies utilizing folic acid, B_6, B_{12}, and betaine, either alone or in combination, have demonstrated the ability of these nutrients to normalize homocysteine levels.[21,39,41,125,126] In a recent placebo-controlled clinical study of 100 men with hyperhomocysteinemia, oral therapy with 650 mcg folic acid, 400 mcg vitamin B_{12}, 10 mg vitamin B_6, or a combination of the three nutrients was given daily for 6 weeks. Plasma homocysteine was reduced 41.7% ($P < 0.001$) during folate therapy and 14.8% ($P < 0.01$) during B_{12} therapy, while 10 mg B_6 did not reduce plasma homocysteine significantly. The combination worked synergistically to reduce homocysteine levels by 49.8%.[127] In 68 patients with recent myocardial infarction, 18% had increased plasma homocysteine. Oral folate therapy (2.5 mg) reduced this hyperhomocysteinemia in 94% of treated patients (mean decrease 27%).[36]

In a group of 48 patients with peripheral atherosclerotic vascular disease, 50% had abnormally high fasting plasma homocysteine levels, while 100% had abnormal plasma homocysteine after a methionine load. Treatment with 5 mg folic acid and 250 mg pyridoxine for 12 weeks normalized 95% of the fasting levels and 100% of post-load homocysteine levels.[39] Other studies confirm that oral folate supplementation will almost always lower high homocysteine, while B_6 and B_{12} will lower homocysteine only in those with a genetic metabolic defect and / or dietary deficiency in those nutrients.[125,128]

A deficiency of the P5P dependent enzyme cystathione synthase is the most common genetic abnormality affecting the trans-sulfuration pathway of homocysteine breakdown. Fortunately, B_6 supplementation stimulates this enzyme and, in combination with betaine, corrects the hyperhomocysteinemia in these individuals.[21,125]

Therapeutic approach

Supplements

- Folinic acid: 800 mcg t.i.d.
- Methylcobalamin: 800 mcg t.i.d.
- Pyridoxal 5′-phosphate: 20 mg t.i.d.
- Betaine (trimethylglycine): 1,200 mg t.i.d.
- *N*-acetylcysteine: 500 mg t.i.d.

REFERENCES

1. Tucker KL, Selhub J, Wilson PW, Rosenberg IH. Dietary intake pattern relates to plasma folate and homocysteine concentrations in the Framingham Heart Study. J Nutr 1996; 126: 3025–3031
2. Lussier-Cacan S, Xhignesse M, Piolot A et al. Plasma total homocysteine in healthy subjects. sex-specific relation with biological traits. Am J Clin Nutr 1996; 64: 587–593
3. van der Mooren MJ, Wouters MG, Blom HJ et al. Hormone replacement therapy may reduce high serum homocysteine in postmenopausal women. Eur J Clin Invest 1994; 24: 733–736
4. Wouters MGAJ, Moorrees MTEC, van der Mooren MJ et al. Plasma homocysteine and menopausal status. Eur J Clin Invest 1995; 25: 801–805
5. Brattstrom L, Lindgren A, Isrealsson B et al. Homocysteine and cysteine. Determinants of plasma levels in middle-aged and elderly subjects. J Intern Med 1994; 236: 633–641
6. Nygard O, Vollset SE, Refsum H et al. Total plasma homocysteine and cardiovascular risk profile – the Hordaland homocysteine study. JAMA 1995; 274: 1526–1533
7. Anker G, Lonning PE, Ueland PM et al. Plasma levels of the atherogenic amino acid homocysteine in post-menopausal women with breast cancer treated with tamoxifen. Int J Cancer 1995; 60: 365–368
8. Vermaak WJ, Ubbink JB, Delport R et al. Ethnic immunity to coronary heart disease? Atherosclerosis 1991; 89: 155–162
9. Nygard O, Refsum H, Ueland PM et al. Coffee consumption and plasma total homocysteine. The Hordaland Homocysteine Study. Am J Clin Nutr 1997; 65: 136–143
10. Cravo ML, Gloria LM, Selhub J et al. Hyperhomocysteinemia in chronic alcoholism. Correlation with folate, vitamin B-12, and vitamin B-6 status. Am J Clin Nutr 1996; 63: 220–224
11. Hultberg B, Berglund M, Andersson A, Frank A. Elevated plasma homocysteine in alcoholics. Alcohol Clin Exp Res 1993; 17: 687–689
12. Duerre JA, Briske-Anderson M. Effect of adenosine metabolites on methyltransferase reactions in isolated rat livers. Biochim Biophys Acta 1981; 678: 275–282
13. Wiklund O, Fager G, Andersson A et al. N-acetylcysteine treatment lowers plasma homocysteine but not serum lipoprotein(a) levels. Atherosclerosis 1996; 119: 99–106
14. Spector R. Cerebrospinal fluid folate and the blood-brain barrier. In: Botez MI, Reynolds EH, eds. Folic acid in neurology, psychiatry, and internal medicine. New York, NY: Raven Press. 1979: p 187
15. Scott JM, Weir DG, Molloy A et al. Folic acid metabolism and mechanisms of neural tube defects. Ciba Found Symp 1994; 181: 180–187
16. Linnell JC, Bhatt HR. Inherited errors of cobalamin metabolism and their management. Baillière's Clin Haematol 1995; 8: 567–601
17. Horne DW, Cook RJ, Wagner C. Effect of dietary methyl group deficiency on folate metabolism in rats. J Nutr 1989; 119: 618–621
18. Zeisel SH, Zola T, daCosta K et al. Effect of choline deficiency on S-adenosylmethionine and methionine concentrations in rat liver. Biochem J 1989; 1117: 333–339
19. Zeisel SH, Epstein MF, Wurtman RJ. Elevated choline concentration in neonatal plasma. Life Sci 1980; 26: 1827–1831
20. Hyland K, Smith I, Bottiglieri T et al. Demyelination and decreased S-adenosylmethionine in 5, 10-methylenetetrahydrofolate reductase deficiency. Neurology 1988; 38: 459–462
21. Wilcken DE, Dudman NP, Tyrrell PA. Homocystinuria due to cystathionine beta-synthase deficiency – the effects of betaine treatment in pyridoxine-responsive patients. Metabolism 1985; 12: 1115–1121
22. Dudman NP, Guo XW, Gordon RB et al. Human homocysteine catabolism. Three major pathways and their relevance to development of arterial occlusive disease. J Nutr 1996; 126: 1295S–1300S
23. Dudman NP, Tyrrell PA, Wilcken DE. Homocysteinemia. Depressed plasma serine levels. Metabolism 1987; 20: 198–201
24. Daily JW 3rd, Sachan D. Choline supplementation alters carnitine homeostasis in humans and guinea pigs. J Nutr 1995; 125: 1938–1944
25. Dodson W, Sachan D. Choline supplementation reduces urinary carnitine excretion in humans. Am J Clin Nutr 1996; 63: 904–910
26. Thomas S, Neuzil J, Stocker R. Cosupplementation with coenzyme Q prevents the prooxidant effect of alpha-tocopherol and increases the resistance of LDL to transition metal-dependent oxidation initiation. Arterioscler Thromb Vasc Biol 1996; 16: 687–696
27. Weber C, Sejersgard Jakobsen T, Mortensen S et al. Antioxidative effect of dietary coenzyme Q_{10} in human blood plasma. Int J Vitam Nutr Res 1994; 64: 311–315
28. Bargossi A, Grossi G, Fiorella P et al. Exogenous CoQ_{10} supplementation prevents plasma ubiquinone reduction induced by HMG-CoA reductase inhibitors. Mol Aspects Med 1994; 15: S187–S193
29. Kang D, Fujiwara T, Taheshige K. Ubiquinone biosynthesis by mitochondria, sonicated mitochondria, and mitoplasts of rat liver. J Biochem 1992; 111: 371–375
30. Donchenko GV, Kruglikova AA, Shavchko LP et al. The role of vitamin E in the biosynthesis of ubiquinone (Q) and ubichromenol (QC) in rat liver. Biokhimiia 1991; 56: 354–360
31. Silberberg J, Crooks R, Fryer J et al. Fasting and post-methionine homocyst(e)ine levels in a healthy Australian population. Aust N Z J Med 1997; 27: 35–39
32. Hopkins P, Wu L, Wu J et al. Higher plasma homocyst(e)ine and increased susceptibility to adverse effects of low folate in early familial coronary artery disease. Arterioscler Thromb Vasc Biol 1995; 15: 1314–1320
33. Loehrer F, Angst C, Haefeli W et al. Low whole-blood S-adenosylmethionine and correlation between 5-methyltetrahydrofolate and homocysteine in coronary artery disease. Arterioscler Thromb Vasc Biol 1996; 16: 727–733
34. Boushey C, Beresford S, Omenn G, Motulsky A. A quantitative assessment of plasma homocysteine as a risk factor for vascular disease. Probable benefits of increasing folic acid intakes. JAMA 1995; 274: 1049–1057
35. Robinson K, Mayer E, Miller D et al. Hyperhomocysteinemia and low pyridoxal phosphate. Common and independent reversible risk factors for coronary artery disease. Circulation 1995; 92: 2825–2830
36. Landgren F, Israelsson B, Lindgren A et al. Plasma homocysteine in acute myocardial infarction. homocysteine-lowering effect of folic acid. J Int Med 1995; 237: 381–388
37. Chasan-Taber L, Selhub J, Rosenberg I et al. A prospective study

of folate and vitamin B6 and risk of myocardial infarction in US physicians. J Am Coll Nutr 1996; 15: 136–143
38. Selhub J, Jacques P, Bostom A et al. Association between plasma homocysteine concentrations and extracranial carotid-artery stenosis. N Engl J Med 1995; 332: 286–291
39. van den Berg M, Boers G, Franken D et al. Hyperhomocysteinaemia and endothelial dysfunction in young patients with peripheral arterial occlusive disease. Eur J Clin Invest 1995; 25: 176–181
40. van den Berg M, Stehouwer C, Bierdrager E, Rauwerda J. Plasma homocysteine and severity of atherosclerosis in young patients with lower-limb atherosclerotic disease. Arterioscler Thromb Vasc Biol 1996; 16: 165–171
41. Franken D, Boers G, Blom H et al. Treatment of mild hyperhomocysteinaemia in vascular disease patients. Arterioscler Thromb Vasc Biol 1994; 14: 465–470
42. Wenzler E, Rademakers A, Boers G et al. Hyperhomocysteinemia in retinal artery and retinal vein occlusion. Am J Ophthalmol 1993; 115: 162–167
43. Boers G. Hyperhomocysteinaemia. A newly recognized risk factor for vascular disease. Neth J Med 1994; 45: 34–41
44. Starkebaum G, Harlan JM. Endothelial cell injury due to copper-catalyzed hydrogen peroxide generation from homocysteine. J Clin Invest 1986; 77: 1370–1376
45. Stamler J, Loscalzo J. Endothelium-derived relaxing factor modulates the atherothromogenic effects of homocysteine. J Cardiovasc Pharmacol 1992; 12: S202–S204
46. Stamler J, Osborne J, Jaraki O et al. Adverse vascular effects of homocysteine are modulated by endothelium-derived relaxing factor and related oxides of nitrogen. J Clin Invest 1993; 91: 308–318
47. Stamler J, Slivka A. Biological chemistry of thiols in the vasculature-related disease. Nutr Rev 1996; 54: 1–30
48. Morrison H, Schaubel D, Desmeules M, Wigle D. Serum folate and risk of fatal coronary heart disease. JAMA 1996; 275: 1893–1896
49. Molgaard J, Malinow MR, Lassvik C et al. Hyperhomocyst(e)inaemia. An independent risk factor for intermittent claudication. J Intern Med 1992; 231: 273–279
50. Cheng SW, Ting AC, Wong J. Fasting total plasma homocysteine and atherosclerotic peripheral vascular disease. Ann Vasc Surg 1997; 11: 217–223
51. den Heijer M, Koster T, Blom HJ et al. Hyperhomocysteinemia as a risk factor for deep-vein thrombosis. N Engl J Med 1996; 334: 759–762
52. Beaumont V, Malinow MR, Sexton G et al. Hyperhomocyst(e)inemia, anti-estrogen antibodies and other risk factors for thrombosis in women on oral contraceptives. Atherosclerosis 1992; 94: 147–152
53. Brattstrom L, Lindgren A, Israelsson B et al. Hyperhomocysteinaemia in stroke. Prevalence, cause, and relationships to type of stroke and stroke risk factors. Eur J Clin Invest 1992; 22: 214–221
54. Perry IJ, Refsum H, Morris RW et al. Prospective study of serum total homocysteine concentration and risk of stroke in middle-aged British men. Lancet 1995; 346: 1395–1398
55. Hultberg B, Andersson A, Lindgren A. Marginal folate deficiency as a possible cause of hyperhomocystinaemia in stroke patients. Eur J Clin Chem Clin Biochem 1997; 35: 25–28
56. Eskes TK. Possible basis for primary prevention of birth defects with folic acid. Fetal Diagn Ther 1994; 9: 149–154
57. Steegers-Theunissen R, Boers G, Trijbels FJ, Eskes TK. Neural-tube defects and derangement of homocysteine metabolism. N Engl J Med 1991; 324: 199–200 [letter]
58. MRC Vitamin Study Research Group. Prevention of neural tube defects. Results of the Medical Research Council Vitamin Study. Lancet 1991; 338: 131–137
59. Vergel RG, Sanchez LR, Heredero BL et al. Primary prevention of neural tube defects with folic acid supplementation. Cuban experience. Prenat Diag 1990; 10: 149–152
60. Milunsky A, Jick H, Jick SS et al. Multivitamin/folic acid supplementation in early pregnancy reduces the prevalence of neural tube defects. JAMA 1989; 262: 2847–2852
61. Czeizel AE, Dudas I. Prevention of the first occurrence of neural-tube defects by periconceptional vitamin supplementation. N Engl J Med 1992; 327: 1832–1835
62. Bower C, Stanley FJ. Dietary folate as a risk factor for neural tube defects. evidence from a case-controlled study in Western Australia. Med J Aust 1989; 150: 613–619
63. Werler MM, Shapiro S, Mitchell AA. Periconceptional folic acid exposure and risk of occurrent neural tube defects. JAMA 1993; 269: 1257–1261
64. Shaw GM, Schaffer D, Velie EM et al. Periconceptional vitamin use, dietary folate, and the occurrence of neural tube defects. Epidemiology 1995; 6: 219–226
65. Tamura T, Goldenberg R, Freeberg L et al. Maternal serum folate and zinc concentrations and their relationships to pregnancy outcome. Am J Clin Nutr 1992; 56: 365–370
66. Scholl TO, Hediger ML, Schall JI et al. Dietary and serum folate: their influence on the outcome of pregnancy. Am J Clin Nutr 1996; 63: 520–525
67. Frelut ML, deCoucy GP, Christides JP et al. Relationship between maternal folate status and foetal hypotrophy in a population with a good socio-economical level. Int J Vitamin Nutr Res 1995; 65: 267–271
68. Goldenberg RL, Tamura T, Cliver SP et al. Serum folate and fetal growth retardation: a matter of compliance? Obstet Gynecol 1992; 79: 719–722
69. Goddijn-Wessel TA, Toos AW et al. Hyperhomocysteinemia. A risk factor for placental abruption or infarction. Eur J Obst Gyn Reprod Biol 1996; 66: 23–29
70. Rosenquist TH, Ratashak SA, Selhub J. Homocysteine induces congenital defects of the heart and neural tube. Effect of folic acid. Proc Natl Acad Sci 1996; 93: 15 227–15 232
71. Kirby PN, Molloy AM, Daly LE et al. Maternal plasma folate and vitamin B12 are independent risk factors for neural tube defects. Q J Med 1993; 86: 703–708
72. Mills JL, Scott JM, Kirke PN et al. Homocysteine and neural tube defects. J Nutr 1996; 126: 756S–760S
73. Essien FB, Wannberg SL. Methionine but not folinic acid or vitamin B-12 alters the frequency of neural tube defects in Axd mutant mice. J Nutr 1993; 123: 973–974
74. Potier de Courcy G, Bujoli J. Effects of diets with or without folic acid, with or without methionine, on fetus development, folate stores and folic acid-dependent enzyme activities in the rat. Biol Neonate 1981; 39: 132–140
75. Zeisel SH. Choline and human nutrition. Annu Rev Nutr 1994; 14: 269–296
76. Garner SC, Mar MH, Zeisel SH. Choline distribution and metabolism in pregnant rats and fetuses are influenced by the choline content of the maternal diet. J Nutr 1995; 125: 2851–2858
77. Meck WH, Smith RA, Williams CL. Pre- and postnatal choline supplementation produces long-term facilitation of spatial memory. Dev Psychobiol 1988; 21: 339–353
78. Wild J, Seller MJ, Schorah CJ, Smithells RW. Investigation of folate intake and metabolism in women who have had two pregnancies complicated by neural tube defects. Br J Obstet Gynaecol 1994; 101: 197–202
79. Wild J, Schorah CJ, Sheldon TA, Smithells RW. Investigation of factors influencing folate status in women who have had a neural tube defect-affected infant. Br J Obstet Gynaecol 1993; 100: 546–549
80. Yates JR, Ferguson-Smith MA, Shenkin A et al. Is disordered folate metabolism the basis for the genetic predisposition to neural tube defects? Clin Genet 1997; 31: 279–287
81. Lucock MD, Wild J, Schorah CJ et al. The methylfolate axis in neural tube defects. In vitro characterisation and clinical investigation. Biochem Med Metabol Biol 1994; 52: 101–114
82. Kluijtmans LAJ, Van den Heuvel LPWJ et al. Molecular genetic analysis in mild hyperhomocysteinemia. A common mutation in the methylenetetrahydrofolate reductase gene is a genetic risk factor in cardiovascular disease. Am J Hum Genet 1996; 58: 35–41
83. Whitehead AS, Gallagher P, Mills JL. A genetic defect in 5,10 methylenetetrahydrofolate reductase in neural tube defects. QJM 1995; 88: 763–766
84. Kubler W. Nutritional deficiencies in pregnancy. Bibl Nutr Dieta 1981; 30: 17–29

85. Martinez-Frias ML, Salvador J. Epidemiological aspects of prenatal exposure to high doses of vitamin A in Spain. Eur J Epidemiol 1990; 6: 118–123
86. Fell D, Steele RD. Modification of hepatic folate metabolism in rats fed excess retinol. Life Sci 1986; 38: 1959–1965
87. Noia G, Littarru GP, De Santis M et al. Coenzyme Q_{10} in pregnancy. Fet Diag Ther 1996; 11: 264–270
88. Noia G, Lippa S, Di Maio A et al. Blood levels of coenzyme Q_{10} in early phase of normal or complicated pregnancies. In: Folkers K, Yamamura Y. Biomedical and clinical aspects of coenzyme Q. Amsterdam: Elsevier. 1991: p 209–213
89. Weir DG, Scott JM. The biochemical basis of the neuropathy in cobalamin deficiency. Baillière's Clin Haematol 1995; 8: 479–497
90. Flippo TS, Holder WD Jr. Neurologic degeneration associated with nitrous oxide anesthesia in patients with vitamin B12 deficiency. Arch Surg 1993; 128: 1391–1395
91. Lipton SA, Kim WK, Choi YB et al. Neurotoxicity associated with dual actions of homocysteine at the N-methyl-D-aspartate receptor. Proc Natl Acad Sci 1997; 94: 5923–5928
92. Regland B, Johansson BV, Grenfeldt B et al. Homocysteinemia is a common feature of schizophrenia. J Neural Transm Gen Sect 1995; 100: 165–169
93. Metz J, Bell AH, Flicker L et al. The significance of subnormal serum vitamin B12 concentration in older people. A case control study. J Am Geriatr Soc 1996; 44: 1355–1361
94. Quinn K, Basu TK. Folate and vitamin B12 status of the elderly. Eur J Clin Nutr 1996; 50: 340–342
95. Fine EJ, Soria ED, eds. Myths about vitamin B12 deficiency. South Med J 1991; 84: 1475–1481
96. Riggs KM, Spiro A 3rd, Tucker K, Rush D. Relations of vitamin B-12, vitamin B-6, folate, and homocysteine to cognitive performance in the Normative Aging Study. Am J Clin Nutr 1996; 63: 306–314
97. Levitt AJ, Karlinsky H. Folate, vitamin B12 and cognitive impairment in patients with Alzheimer's disease. Acta Psychiatr Scand 1992; 86: 301–305
98. Joosten E, Lesaffre E, Riezler R et al. Is metabolic evidence for vitamin B-12 and folate deficiency more frequent in elderly patients with Alzheimer's disease? J Gerontol A Biol Sci Med Sci 1997; 52: M76–M79
99. Allain P, Le Bouil A, Cordillet E et al. Sulfate and cysteine levels in the plasma of patients with Parkinson's disease. Neurotoxicology 1995; 16: 527–529
100. Reynolds EH, Carney MW, Toone BK. Methylation and mood. Lancet 1984; 2: 196–198
101. Arpino C, Da Cas R, Donini G et al. Use and misuse of antidepressant drugs in a random sample of the population of Rome, Italy. Acta Psychiatr Scand 1995; 92: 7–9
102. Stacy CB, Di Rocco A, Gould RJ. Methionine in the treatment of nitrous-oxide-induced neuropathy and myeloneuropathy. J Neurol 1992; 239: 401–403
103. Schilling RF. Is nitrous oxide a dangerous anesthetic for vitamin B12-deficient subjects? JAMA 1986; 28; 255: 1605–1606
104. Reynolds EH, Bottiglieri T, Laundy M et al. Vitamin B12 metabolism in multiple sclerosis. Arch Neurol 1992; 49: 649–652
105. Robillon JF, Canivet B, Candito M et al. Type 1 diabetes mellitus and homocyst(e)ine. Diabete Metab 1994; 20: 494–496
106. Hultberg B, Agardh E, Andersson A et al. Increased levels of plasma homocysteine are associated with nephropathy, but not severe retinopathy in type 1 diabetes mellitus. Scand J Clin Lab Invest 1991; 51: 277–282
107. Agardh CD, Agardh E, Andersson A, Hultberg B. Lack of association between plasma homocysteine levels and microangiopathy in type 1 diabetes mellitus. Scand J Clin Lab Invest 1994; 54: 637–641
108. Munshi MN, Stone A, Fink L, Fonseca V. Hyperhomocysteinemia following a methionine load in patients with non-insulin-dependent diabetes mellitus and macrovascular disease. Metabolism 1996; 45: 133–135
109. Araki A, Sako Y, Ito H. Plasma homocysteine concentrations in Japanese patients with non-insulin-dependent diabetes mellitus. effect of parenteral methylcobalamin treatment. Atherosclerosis 1993; 103: 149–157
110. Vaccaro O, Ingrosso D, Rivellese A et al. Moderate hyperhomocysteinaemia and retinopathy in insulin-dependent diabetes. Lancet 1997; 349: 1102–1103 [letter]
111. Neugebauer S, Baba T, Kurokawa K, Watanabe T. Defective homocysteine metabolism as a risk factor for diabetic retinopathy. Lancet 1997; 349: 473–474
112. Roubenoff R, Dellaripa P, Nadeau MR et al. Abnormal homocysteine metabolism in rheumatoid arthritis. Arthritis Rheum 1997; 40: 718–722
113. Krogh Jensen M, Ekelund S, Svendsen L. Folate and homocysteine status and haemolysis in patients treated with sulphasalazine for arthritis. Scand J Clin Lab Invest 1996; 56: 421–429
114. Kang SS, Wong PW, Glickman PB et al. Protein-bound homocyst(e)ine in patients with rheumatoid arthritis undergoing D-penicillamine treatment. J Clin Pharmacol 1986; 26: 712–715
115. Dennis VW, Robinson K. Homocysteinemia and vascular disease in end-stage renal disease. Kidney Int 1996; 57: S11–S17
116. Robinson K, Gupta A, Dennis V et al. Hyperhomocysteinemia confers an independent increased risk of atherosclerosis in end-stage renal disease and is closely linked to plasma folate and pyridoxine concentrations. Circulation 1996; 94: 2743–2748
117. Barak AJ, Beckenhauer HC, Tuma DJ. Betaine, ethanol, and the liver. A review. Alcohol 1996; 13: 395–398
118. Barak AJ, Beckenhauer HC, Tuma DJ. Betaine effects on hepatic methionine metabolism elicited by short-term ethanol feeding. Alcohol 1996; 13: 483–486
119. Malinow MR, Levenson J, Giral P et al. Role of blood pressure, uric acid, and hemorheological parameters on plasma homocyst(e)ine concentration. Atherosclerosis 1995; 114: 175–183
120. Coull BM, Malinow MR, Beamer N et al. Elevated plasma homocyst(e)ine concentration as a possible independent risk factor for stroke. Stroke 1990; 21: 572–576
121. Gershon SL, Fox IH. Pharmacologic effects of nicotinic acid on human purine metabolism. Lab Clin Med 1974; 84: 179–186
122. Tamburrini O, Bartolomeo-De Iuri A, Andria G et al. Bone changes in homocystinuria in childhood. Radiol Med 1984; 70: 937–942
123. Kaur M, Kabra M, Das GP et al. Clinical and biochemical studies in homocystinuria. Indian Pediatr 1995; 32: 1067–1075
124. Lubec B, Fang-Kircher S, Lubec T et al. Evidence for McKusick's hypothesis of deficient collagen cross-linking in patients with homocystinuria. Biochim Biophys Acta 1996 1315: 159–162
125. Dudman N, Wilcken D, Wang J et al. Disordered methionine/homocysteine metabolism in premature vascular disease. Its occurrence, cofactor therapy, and enzymology. Arterioscler Thromb 1993; 13: 1253–1260
126. Wilcken DE, Wilcken B, Dudman NP, Tyrrell PA. Homocystinuria – the effects of betaine in the treatment of patients not responsive to pyridoxine. N Engl J Med 1983; 309: 448–453
127. Ubbink J, Vermaak W, van der Merwe et al. Vitamin requirements for the treatment of hyperhomocysteinemia in humans. J Nutr 1994; 124: 1927–1933
128. Mason J, Miller J. The effects of vitamins B12, B6, and folate on blood homocysteine levels. Ann NY Acad Sci 1992; 669: 197–203

CHAPTER CONTENTS

53

Immune support

Michael T. Murray, ND

Joseph E. Pizzorno Jr, ND

INTRODUCTION

The immune system is a complex integration of synergistic segments that are continuously barraged by stimuli. Immunology is a rapidly developing field with concepts being continually devised and revised. For the physician interested in assessing and maintaining a patient's health, the development of a thorough understanding of the immune system and the many factors which enhance and/or inhibit normal function is essential. The immune system is truly "wholistic", as evidenced by the close association of psychological, neurological, nutritional, environmental, and endocrinologic factors with immune function.

Supporting the immune system is critical to good health. Conversely, good health is critical to supporting the immune system. The best approach to supporting immune function is a comprehensive plan involving lifestyle, stress management, exercise, diet, nutritional supplementation, glandular therapy, and the use of plant-based medicines.

PSYCHONEUROIMMUNOLOGY

Psychoneuroimmunology is a term used to describe the interactions between the emotional state, nervous system function, and the immune system. The growing body of knowledge documenting the mind's profound influence on physiology in health and disease necessitates a fundamental change in the way physicians perceive their patients. An important step is the study of nervous system response to environmental or intra-psychic perceptions that activate endocrine processes which, in turn, influence the immune system.

A complete and detailed account of the many facets of psychoneuroimmunology (PNI), or behavioral immunology, is beyond the scope of this chapter. Instead, we will concentrate on the effects of stress and neurotransmitters on the immune response.

Stress

The term stress-induced illness is certainly not a misnomer, since many clinical and experimental studies have clearly demonstrated that stress, personality, attitude, and emotion are etiologic or contributory in many diseases.[1] Reaction to stressful stimuli is entirely individual, reinforcing the fact that people differ significantly in their perceptions and responses to various life events. The variations in response help to account for the wide diversity of stress-induced illnesses. Stress-induced increases in corticosteroids and catecholamines lead to an immunosuppressed state, leaving the host susceptible to infectious and carcinogenic illnesses. This immunosuppression is proportional to the level of stress and, although the effects are numerous, they appear to involve a common mechanism: an increase in intracellular cyclic AMP. Other mechanisms are also significant, with thymic involution and suppressed lymphopoiesis being perhaps the most important.

Cyclic nucleotides and immune function

In many systems of the body, cholinergic and beta-adrenergic stimulation mediate diametrically opposed actions. On the cellular level, this antagonism is mediated via cyclic AMP and cyclic GMP. Beta-adrenergic stimulation of responsive target tissues causes a rise in intracellular cAMP, whereas acetylcholine acting on muscarine receptors leads to increased levels of cGMP. The immune system is also affected by this yin–yang balance, although it appears to be much more complex than in other systems.

Cyclic AMP and GMP have shown antagonistic effects in all immune functions studied to date. The immune effects of cGMP include: [2–7]

- enhanced lymphocyte mediated cytotoxicity
- stimulation of T-cell rosette formation (a measure of thymus-derived lymphocyte activity) with inhibition of B-cell rosette formation
- enhanced lymphoid cell and lymphocyte proliferation
- increased lymphocyte lysosomal enzyme release
- increased leukocyte chemotaxis.

From this information, it is apparent that cGMP usually serves to enhance immune function during infection and carcinogenesis. In contrast, cAMP appears to inhibit white cell proliferation and functional response, thus possibly serving to modulate the immune system.

While there are many conditions where enhancing cGMP activity and inhibiting cAMP activity is contraindicated (e.g. autoimmune disease, atopy, gout, and psoriasis), in acute or chronic infection the cGMP:cAMP ratio should be enhanced. Although many exogenous compounds alter the cGMP:cAMP ratio, paramount in any treatment plan is adequate rest and elimination of stressful activity. This promotes an increase in cholinergic activity while concurrently lowering beta-adrenergic activity. In addition, other cAMP promoting factors should be eliminated (e.g. caffeine and its analogs) while increasing cGMP stimulators (e.g. ascorbic acid).[6,7]

Table 53.1 Lifestyle practices associated with higher natural killer cell activity

- Not smoking
- Increased intake of green vegetables
- Regular meals
- Proper body weight
- More than 7 hours of sleep
- Regular exercise
- A vegetarian diet

LIFESTYLE

A healthy lifestyle goes a long way in establishing a healthy immune system. This benefit is perhaps most obvious when looking at the effects of lifestyle on natural killer cell activity.[8,9] Table 53.1 lists the lifestyle practices which are associated with higher natural killer cell activity.

NUTRITIONAL FACTORS

The health of the immune system gland is greatly impacted by a person's nutritional status. Dietary factors which depress immune function include nutrient deficiency, excess consumption of sugar, consumption of allergic foods and high cholesterol levels in the blood. Dietary factors which enhance immune function include all essential nutrients, antioxidants, carotenes, and flavonoids.

Consistent with good health, optimal immune function requires a healthy diet that:

- is rich in whole, natural foods, such as fruits, vegetables, grains, beans, seeds, and nuts
- is low in fats and refined sugars
- contains adequate, but not excessive, amounts of protein.

On top of this, individuals are encouraged to drink five or six 8-ounce glasses of water per day (preferably pure). These dietary recommendations along with a positive mental attitude, a good high potency multivitamin-mineral supplement, a regular exercise program, daily deep breathing and relaxation exercises (meditation, prayer, etc.), and at least 7 hours of sleep daily will go a long way in helping the immune system function at an optimum level.

Nutrient deficiency

Nutrient deficiency is the most frequent cause of a depressed immune system. Although, historically, research relating nutritional status to immune function has concerned itself with severe malnutrition states (i.e. kwashiorkor and marasma), attention is now shifting towards marginal deficiencies of single or multiple nutrients and the effects of overnutrition. The plethora of clinical and experimental data has made inevitable the conclusion that a single nutrient deficiency can profoundly impair the immune system.

Given the widespread problem of subclinical nutrient deficiency in Americans, it can be concluded that many are suffering from impaired immunity amenable to nutritional supplementation. This statement is particularly true in the elderly. Numerous studies have shown that most elderly Americans are deficient in at least one nutrient. Likewise, there are numerous studies which show that taking a multiple vitamin and mineral supplement enhances immune function in elderly subjects (whether they suffer from overt nutritional deficiency or not).

General factors

Protein

The importance of adequate protein intake to proper immune function has been extensively studied.[10] The most severe effects of protein-calorie malnutrition (PCM) are on cell-mediated immunity, although all facets of immune function are ultimately affected. PCM is not, however, usually a single nutrient deficiency. It is normally associated with multiple nutrient deficiencies, and some immune dysfunctions attributed to PCM are most likely due to these other factors. Partial deficiencies of dietary vitamins produce a comparatively greater depression in the natural and inducible levels of cytotoxic activities than do partial protein deficiencies. Nonetheless, adequate protein is essential for optimal immune function.

Sugar

The oral administration of 100 g portions of carbohydrate as glucose, fructose, sucrose, honey, and orange juice all significantly reduces neutrophil phagocytosis, while starch has no effect. As can be seen in Figure 53.1, effects start within less than 30 minutes, last for over 5 hours, and typically show a 50% reduction in phagocytic activity at the peak of inhibition (usually 2 hours after ingestion).[11,12] Since PMNs constitute 60–70% of the total WBC and are a major portion of the defense mechanism, impairment of phagocytic activity leads to an immune-compromised state. Oral administration of increasing amounts of glucose progressively lowers neutrophil phagocytosis, with maximal inhibition corresponding to maximal blood glucose levels.

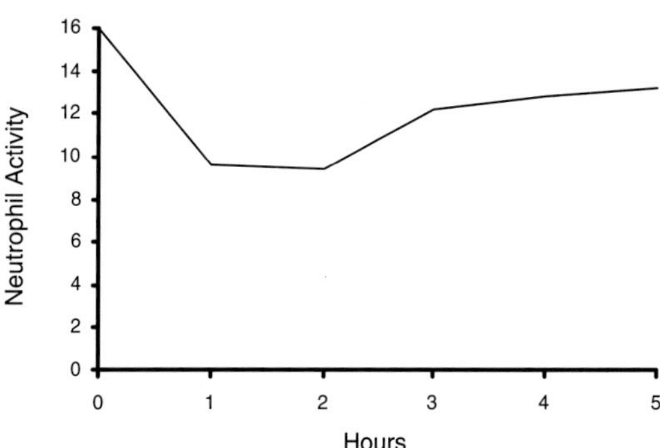

Figure 53.1 The effects of sugar on white cell phagocytic activity.

Oral ingestion of 75 g of glucose has also been shown to depress lymphocyte response to mitogens, apparently due to the elevation of insulin levels.[13] Other parameters of immune function are also undoubtedly affected by sugar consumption.

It has been hypothesized that the ill effects of high glucose levels are a result of elevation of insulin levels and competition with vitamin C for membrane transport sites.[14,15] This is based on evidence that vitamin C and glucose appear to have opposite effects on immunological function and the fact that both require insulin for membrane transport into many tissues.

Considering that the average American consumes 125 g of sucrose, plus 50 g of other refined simple sugars, each day, the inescapable conclusion is that most Americans have chronically depressed immune systems. It is clear, particularly during an infection, that the consumption of simple sugars, even in the form of fruit juice, is deleterious to the host's immune status.

Short-term fasting could be encouraged, particularly during the first 24–48 hours of an acute infectious illness, since this results in a significant (up to 50%) increase in phagocytic index.[11] The fast should not be continued for an excessive period, since eventually the leukocyte's energy sources will become depleted.

Obesity

Obesity is associated with decreased immune status, as evidenced by the decreased bactericidal activity of leukocytes, and increased morbidity and mortality from infections.[16] Cholesterol and lipid levels are usually elevated in obese individuals, which may explain their impaired immune function (see below).

Lipids

Increased levels of cholesterol, free fatty acids, triglycerides, and bile acids inhibit various immune functions, including:[17–20]

- lymphoproliferation
- response to mitogens
- antibody response
- PMN chemotaxis
- phagocytosis.

Optimal immune function is therefore dependent on control of these serum components. Interestingly, L-carnitine, even at minimal concentrations, has been shown to neutralize lipid-induced immunosuppression.[20] This is probably due to carnitine's role as a rate-limiting factor in the removal of fat emulsion from the blood.[21]

Alcohol

Alcohol increases the susceptibility to experimental infections in animals; and alcoholics are known to be more susceptible to pneumonia. Studies of human polymorphonuclear leukocytes show a profound depression in the rate of mobilization into the traumatized skin of nutritionally normal people. Alcohol does not, however, alter phagocytosis or cytotoxic activity.[22]

Vitamins

Vitamin A

Vitamin A plays an essential role in maintaining the integrity of the epithelial and mucosal surfaces and their secretions. These systems constitute a primary nonspecific host defense mechanism. Vitamin A has been shown to stimulate and/or enhance numerous immune processes, including:[23–26]

- induction of cell-mediated cytotoxicity against tumors
- natural killer cell activity
- lymphocyte blastogenesis
- mononuclear phagocytosis
- antibody response.

These effects are not due simply to reversal of vitamin A deficiency, since many of them are further enhanced by the administration of (supposedly) excessive levels of vitamin A.[26] In addition, vitamin A prevents and reverses stress-induced thymic involution, while added vitamin A can actually promote thymus growth.[27] Retinol also demonstrates potent viricidal activity.[28]

Carotenes

Carotenes have demonstrated a number of immune-enhancing effects.[29] In addition to being converted into vitamin A, carotenes function as antioxidants. Since the thymus gland is so susceptible to free radical damage, beta-carotene may be more advantageous in enhancing the immune system than retinol. For more information, see Chapter 121.

Vitamin C

Vitamin C (ascorbic acid) plays an important role in the natural approach to immune enhancement. Although vitamin C has been shown to be antiviral and antibacterial, its main effect is via improvement in host resistance. Many different immunostimulatory effects have been demonstrated, including enhancing lymphoproliferative response to mitogens and lymphotrophic activity and increasing interferon levels, antibody responses, immunoglobulin levels, secretion of thymic hormones, and integrity of ground substance.[23–30] Vitamin C also has direct biochemical effects similar to interferon.[31]

Numerous clinical studies support the use of vitamin C in the treatment of infectious conditions. In addition to its well-known effects in reducing the frequency, duration, and severity of the common cold, vitamin C has also been shown to be useful in other infectious conditions.[30,32–36] Vitamin C levels are quickly depleted during the stress of an infection.[37]

It is useful to supplement vitamin C concurrently with flavonoids since these compounds raise the concentration of vitamin C in some tissues and potentiate its effects, as well as exerting their own effects.[38]

Vitamin E

Vitamin E enhances both humoral and cell-mediated immunity. A vitamin E deficiency results in lymphoid atrophy and decreased lymphoproliferative response to mitogens, splenic plaque-forming colonies, antibody response, and monocyte function.[23,24] Vitamin E supplementation (30–150 IU) has been shown to:[39]

- increase lymphoproliferative response to mitogens
- prevent free radical-induced thymus atrophy
- enhance helper T-cell activity
- increase splenic plaque-forming colonies, serum immunoglobulins, antibody response, PMN phagocytosis, and reticuloendothelial system activity.

Elderly subjects may benefit from even higher dosages of vitamin E. A recent study sought to determine the effect of vitamin E supplementation at different dosages on immune function in 88 patients over the age of 65 years.[40] To determine the effect of vitamin E on immune function, the researchers measured T-cell function by assessing delayed-type hypersensitivity (DTH) skin response; antibody response to hepatitis B, tetanus, and diphtheria, and pneumococcal vaccines; and autoantibodies to DNA and thyroglobulin.

Vitamin E was given at either 60, 200, or 800 IU for

235 days. While the placebo group only experienced an 8% increase in DHT, the 60 IU group had a 20% increase in DTH; the 200 IU group had a 58% increase in DTH; and the 800 IU group had a 65% increase in DTH. With regard to antibody production, the best results were observed in the patients receiving 200 IU daily. No effect was noticed on autoimmune antibodies. No adverse effects were observed at any of the three dosage schedules of vitamin E.

Pyridoxine

A pyridoxine deficiency results in depressed cellular and humoral immunity, lymphoid tissue atrophy, leukopenia, reduction in quantity and quality of antibody production, depressed lymphoproliferative response to mitogens, and decreased thymic hormone activity.[23,24] Factors predisposing to deficiency are low dietary intake, excess protein intake, consumption of hydralazine (yellow) dyes, and alcohol and oral contraception use.

Folic acid and vitamin B_{12}

The megaloblastic state induced by a deficiency of vitamin B_{12} and/or folate results in improper WBC production and abnormal lymphocyte responses. Folic acid deficiency (the most common vitamin deficiency in the US) has been shown to result in lymphoid atrophy and decreased lymphoproliferative response to mitogens, splenic plaque-forming colonies, and antibody production. A B_{12} deficiency, besides producing a deficiency in folate conversion to its active tetrahydrofolate form, leads to impaired PMN phagocytosis and bactericidal action.[23,24]

Other B vitamins

Thiamin, riboflavin, and pantothenic acid deficiencies lead to reduced antibody response, decreased splenic plaque-forming colonies, and lymphoid atrophy.[25]

Minerals

Iron

Iron deficiency is a commonly encountered isolated nutritional deficiency which causes immune dysfunction in large numbers of patients. Marginal iron deficiency, even at levels that do not lower hemoglobin values, can influence the immune system. Lymphoid tissue atrophy, decreased lymphoproliferative response to mitogens, defective macrophage and neutrophil function, and decreased proportion of T-cell to B-cell ratios are common experimental and clinical findings.[23,24]

Iron is an important nutrient to bacteria as well as humans. During infection, one of the body's non-specific defense mechanisms to limit bacterial growth is to reduce plasma iron, and in vitro studies have shown that the bacteriostatic and some of the bactericidal effects of serum are eliminated by the addition of iron to the serum.[41] As temperature rises, plasma iron levels drop, and when temperature is raised to fever levels, the growth of bacteria is inhibited, but not at high iron concentrations.

These observations lead us to the conclusion that iron supplementation is probably contraindicated during acute infection, especially in patients with low transferrin levels. However, in patients with impaired immune function, chronic infections, and subnormal iron levels, adequate supplementation is essential.

Trace minerals

Trace minerals primarily function as activators of enzyme-metal-substrate complexes in which they are loosely bound cofactors. The role of these elements in these metaloenzymes is either structural, in which they influence the reactivity of the protein by stabilizing strained configurations of binding ligands about the metal atom, or catalytic, in which they act as centers of positive charge.

Zinc

The hereditary zinc deficiency disease, acrodermatitis enteropathica (AE), offers an excellent model for understanding the role of zinc in immunity. In AE, the number of T-cells is reduced, lymphoproliferative response to mitogens is reduced, thymic hormone levels are lower, delayed cutaneous hypersensitivity is decreased, and PMN phagocytosis, chemotaxis, and cytotoxic activities are impaired. All of these effects are reversible upon adequate zinc administration and absorption.[42]

Zinc serves a vital role in many immune system reactions, e.g. it promotes the binding of complement (C1q) to immune complex, acts as a protectant against iron-catalyzed free radical damage, acts synergistically with vitamin A, is required for lymphocyte transformation, acts independently on lymphocytes as a mitogen, and is a necessary cofactor in activating serum thymic factor.[43,44] Zinc inhibits, in vitro, the growth of several viruses including rhino, picorna and toga viruses, and herpes simplex and vaccinia virus.[45]

Adequate zinc nutriture is particularly important in the elderly, and zinc supplementation in elderly subjects results in increased numbers of T-cells and enhanced cell-mediated immune responses.[46]

Throat lozenges containing zinc became popular in the treatment of the common cold as a result of a double-blind clinical trial in 1984 which demonstrated that zinc-containing lozenges significantly reduced the average duration of common colds by 7 days.[47] The lozenges used in this study contained 23 mg of elemental zinc, which the patients were instructed to dissolve in their mouths every 2 waking hours after an initial double dose. After 7 days, 86% of the 37 zinc-treated subjects were symptom-free, compared with 46% of the 28 placebo-treated subjects. Additional studies have confirmed these results.[48] Because high doses of zinc can actually impair immune function, a daily intake of greater than 150 mg of zinc for longer than 1 week cannot be recommended.

Selenium

Selenium in its vital role in glutathione peroxidase affects all components of the immune system including the development and expression of all white blood cells. Selenium deficiency results in depressed immune function, whereas selenium supplementation results in augmentation and / or restoration of immune functions. Selenium deficiency has been shown to inhibit resistance to infection as a result of impaired white blood cell and thymus function, while selenium supplementation (200 mcg/day) has been shown to stimulate white blood cell and thymus function.[49–51]

The ability of selenium supplementation to enhance immune function goes well beyond simply restoring selenium levels in selenium-deficient individuals. For example, in one study selenium supplementation (200 mcg/day) to individuals with normal selenium concentrations in their blood resulted in a 118% increase in the ability of lymphocytes to kill tumor cells and an 82.3% increase in the activity of natural killer cells.[50] These effects were apparently related to the ability of selenium to enhance the expression of the immune-enhancing compound interleukin-2 and, consequently, the rate of white blood cell proliferation and differentiation into forms capable of killing tumor cells and microorganisms. The supplementation regimen did not produce significant changes in the blood selenium levels of the participants. The results indicated that the immune-enhancing effects of selenium in humans require supplementation above the normal dietary intake.

ENHANCING THYMUS FUNCTION

Perhaps the most effective method in re-establishing a healthy immune system is employing measures to improve thymus function. Promoting optimal thymus gland activity involves:

- prevention of thymic involution or shrinkage by ensuring adequate dietary intake of antioxidant nutrients
- use of nutrients that are required in the manufacture or action of thymic hormones
- using botanical medicines or glandular products containing concentrates of calf thymus tissue to enhance thymus activity.

Antioxidants

The thymus gland shows maximum development immediately after birth. During the aging process, the thymus gland undergoes a process of shrinkage or involution. The reason for this involution is that the thymus gland is extremely susceptible to free radical and oxidative damage caused by stress, radiation, infection, and chronic illness.

Many patients with impaired immune function as well as conditions associated with impaired immunity (e.g. chronic fatigue syndrome, cancer, AIDS, etc.) suffer from a state of oxidative imbalance characterized by a greater number of pro-oxidants in their system than antioxidants. This situation is quite detrimental to thymus function. One of the primary ways in which antioxidants impact the immune system, particularly cell-mediated immunity, may be via protecting the thymus gland from damage. The antioxidant nutrients most important for protecting the thymus include the carotenes, vitamin C, vitamin E, zinc, and selenium.

Nutrients

Many nutrients function as important cofactors in the manufacture, secretion and function of thymic hormones. A deficiency of any one of these nutrients results in decreased thymic hormone action and impaired immune function. Zinc, vitamin B_6, and vitamin C are perhaps the most critical. Supplementation with these nutrients has been shown to increase thymic hormone function and cell-mediated immunity.

Zinc is perhaps the critical mineral involved in thymus gland function and thymus hormone action. Zinc is involved in virtually every aspect of immunity. When zinc levels are low, the number of T-cells is reduced; thymic hormone levels are lower, and many white blood functions critical to the immune response are severely lacking. All of these effects are reversible upon adequate zinc administration and adsorption.[52,53]

Thymus extracts

A substantial amount of clinical data now supports the effectiveness of orally administered calf thymus extracts in restoring and enhancing immune function.[54,55] The effectiveness of thymus extracts is reflective of broad-spectrum immune system enhancement presumably mediated by improved thymus gland activity. This effect fits in nicely with one of the basic concepts of glandular therapy, i.e. that the oral ingestion of glandular material of a certain animal gland will strengthen the corresponding human gland. The result is a broad general effect indicative of improved glandular function.

Thymus extracts may provide the answer to chronic viral infections and low immune function. The ability of thymus extracts to treat and then reduce the number of recurrent infections was studied in groups of children with a history of recurrent respiratory tract infections. Double-blind studies revealed not only that orally administered thymus extracts were able to effectively eliminate infection, but also that treatment over the course of a year significantly reduced the number of respiratory infections and significantly improved numerous immune parameters.[56]

Thymus extract has been shown to normalize the ratio of T-helper cells to suppressor cells whether the ratio is low or high.[54,55]

BOTANICALS

Many herbs have been shown to have antibacterial, antiviral, and immunostimulatory effects, and a complete discussion is outside the scope of this chapter (several immune-enhancing botanicals are discussed in depth in Section 5). This chapter focuses on two of the most popular immune-enhancing botanicals – *Echinacea* and *Astragalus*. These two herbs were selected based on their ability to exert broad-spectrum effects on immune functions. They stimulate the body's natural defense mechanisms via slightly different mechanisms and are in many ways the prototypes of the hundreds of plants with known antimicrobial and immunological activity.

Echinacea *sp.*

Perhaps the most widely used Western herb for enhancement of the immune system is echinacea. The two most widely used species are *Echinacea angustifolia* and *Echinacea purpurea*. Both have been shown to exert profound immune-enhancing effects. Several classes of constituents contribute to this action.[57]

One of the most important immune-stimulating components of *Echinacea* are large polysaccharides, such as inulin, that activate the alternative complement pathway (one of the immune system's non-specific defense mechanisms) and increase the production of immune chemicals that activate macrophages. The result is increased activity of many key immune parameters: production of T-cells, macrophage phagocytosis, antibody binding, natural killer cell activity, and levels of circulating neutrophils.[57]

Echinacea strengthens the immune system even in healthy people. For example, oral administration of an *E. purpurea* root extract (a dose of 30 drops three times daily) to healthy males for 5 days resulted in a remarkable 120% increase in leukocyte phagocytosis.[58] In another study of healthy volunteers aged 25–40 years, the fresh-pressed juice of *E. purpurea* extract was found to increase the phagocytosis of *Candida albicans* by 30–40%; it also increased the migration of white cells to the scene of battle by 30–40%.[59]

Besides immune support, *Echinacea* also exerts direct antiviral activity and helps prevent the spread of bacteria by inhibiting a bacterial enzyme called hyaluronidase. This enzyme is secreted by bacteria in order to break through the body's first line of defense, the protective membranes such as the skin or mucous membranes, so that the organism can enter the body.

Echinacea is discussed fully in Chapter 82.

Astragalus membranaceus

The root of *Astragalus* is a traditional Chinese medicine used for viral infections. Clinical studies in China have shown it to be effective when used prophylactically against the common cold.[60] It has also been shown to reduce the duration and severity of symptoms in acute treatment of the common cold as well as to raise white blood cell counts in chronic leukopenia.

Research in animals has shown that *Astragalus* apparently works by stimulating several factors of the immune system, including enhancing phagocytic activity of monocytes and macrophages, increasing interferon production and natural killer cell activity, enhancing T-cell activity, and potentiating other antiviral mechanisms.[60,61] *Astragalus* appears particularly useful in cases where the immune system has been damaged by chemicals or radiation. In immunodepressed mice, astragalus has been found to reverse the T-cell abnormalities caused by cyclophosphamide, radiation, and aging.[62] Like *Echinacea*, the polysaccharides contained in the root of *Astragalus membranaceus* contribute to the immune-enhancing effects.

THERAPEUTIC APPROACH

A major challenge to the discerning clinician is to determine which of the above factors is the key to reactivating or supporting a patient's immune system. The regimen listed below is meant as a general approach and must be tailored to the patient's specific needs in order to maximize the desired effects and limit unnecessary treatment.

General measures

- Rest (bed rest better)
- Drink large amount of fluids (preferably diluted vegetable juices, soups, and herb teas)
- Limit simple sugar consumption (including fruit sugars) to less than 50 g a day.

Supplements

- High potency multiple vitamin and mineral formula
- Vitamin C – 500 mg every 2 hours
- Bioflavonoids – 1,000 mg/day

- Vitamin A – 5,000 IU/day; or beta-carotene – 25,000 IU/day
- Zinc – 30 mg/day
- Thymus extract – the equivalent to 120 mg pure polypeptides with molecular weights less than 10,000 or roughly 500 mg of the crude polypeptide fraction.

Botanicals

All dosages to be three times/day.

Echinacea *sp.*

- Dried root (or as tea): 0.5–1 g
- Freeze-dried plant: 325–650 mg
- Juice of aerial portion of *E. purpurea* stabilized in 22% ethanol: 2–3 ml
- Tincture (1:5): 2–4 ml
- Fluid extract (1:1): 2–4 ml
- Solid (dry powdered) extract (6.5:1 or 3.5% echinacoside): 150–300 mg.

Astragalus membranaceus

- Dried root (or as decoction): 1–2 g
- Tincture (1:5): 2–4 ml
- Fluid extract (1:1): 2–4 ml
- Solid (dry powdered) extract (0.5% 4-hydroxy-3-methoxy isoflavone): 100–150 mg.

REFERENCES

1. Rose R. Endocrine responses to stressful psychological events. Psych Clin N Amer 1980; 3: 251–275
2. Strom T, Carpenter C. Cyclic nucleotides in immunosuppression – Neuroendocrine pharmacologic manipulation and in vivo immunoregulation of immunity acting via second messenger systems. Transplant Proc 1980; 12: 304–310
3. Ferriera G, Massuda H, Javierre et al. Rosette formation by human T and B lymphocytes in the presence of adrenergic and cholinergic drugs. Experientia 1976; 32: 1594–1596
4. Singh U. In vitro lymphopoiesis in fetal thymic organ cultures. Effect of various agents. Clin Exp Immunol 1980; 41: 150–155
5. Grieco M, Siegel I, Goel Z. Modulation of human T lymphocyte rosette formation by autonomic agonists and cyclic nucleotides. J Allergy Clin Immunol 1976; 58: 149–159
6. Gallin J, Sandler J, Clyman R et al. Agents that increase cyclic AMP inhibit accumulation of cGMP and depress human monocyte locomotion. J Immunol 1978; 120: 492–496
7. Stephens C, Snyderman R. Cyclic nucleotides regulate the morphologic alterations required for chemotaxis in monocytes. J Immunol 1982; 128: 1192–1197
8. Kusaka Y, Kondou H, Morimoto K. Healthy lifestyles are associated with higher natural killer cell activity. Prev Med 1992; 21: 602–615
9. Nekachi K, Imai K. Environmental and physiological influences on human natural killer cell activity in relation to good health practices. Jap J Cancer Res 1992; 83: 789–805
10. Chandra R, Newberne R. Nutrition, Immunity, and Infection. New York: Pleneum Press. 1977
11. Sanchez A, Reeser J, Lau H et al. Role of sugars in human neutrophilic phagocytosis. Am J Clin Nutr 1973; 26: 1180–1184
12. Ringsdorf W, Cheraskin E, Ramsay R. Sucrose, neutrophil phagocytosis and resistance to disease. Dent Surv 1976; 52: 46–48
13. Bernstein J, Alpert S, Nauss K, Suskind R. Depression of lymphocyte transformation following oral glucose ingestion. Am J Clin Nutr 1977; 30: 613
14. Mann G. Hypothesis. The role of vitamin C in diabetic angiopathy. Pers Biol Med 1974; 17: 210–217
15. Mann G, Newton P. The membrane transport of ascorbic acid. Ann N Y Acad Sci 1975; 258: 243–251
16. Palmblad J, Hallberg D, Rossner S. Obesity, plasma lipids and polymorphonuclear (PMN) granulocyte functions. Scand J Heamatol 1977; 19: 293–303
17. Waddell C, Tauton D, Twomey J. Inhibition of lymphoproliferation by hyperlipoproteinemic plasma. J Clin Invest 1976; 58: 950–954
18. Gianni L, Padova F, Zuin M, Podda M. Bile acid-induced inhibition of the lymphoproliferative response to phytohemagglutinin and pokeweed mitogen. An in vitro study. Gastroenterol 1980; 78: 231–235
19. Dianzani M, Torriella M, Canuto R et al. The influence of enrichment with cholesterol on the phagocytic activity of rat macrophages. J Path 1976; 118: 193–199
20. Simone C, Ferrari M, Lozzi A et al. Vitamins and immunity. II Influence of L-carnitine on the immune system. Acta Vit Enz 1982; 4: 135–140
21. Simone D, Ferrari M, Meli D et al. Reversibility by l-carnitine of immunosuppression induced by an emulsion of soya bean oil, glycerol and egg lecithin. Arzneim Forsch 1982; 32: 1485–1488
22. Brayton R, Stokes P, Schwartz M, Louria D. Effect of alcohol and various diseases on leukocyte mobilization, phagocytosis and intracellular bacterial killing. New Engl J Med 1970; 282: 123–128
23. Beisel W, Edelman R, Nauss K, Suskind R. Single-nutrient effects of immunologic functions. JAMA 1981; 245: 53–58
24. Dowd P, Heatley R. The influence of undernutrition on immunity. Clin Sci 1984; 66: 241–248
25. Tachibana K, Sone S, Tsubura E, Kishino Y. Stimulation effect of vitamin A on tumoricidal activity of rat alveolar macrophages. Br J Cancer 1984; 49: 343–348
26. Semba RD. Vitamin A, immunity, and infection. Clin Inf Dis 1994; 19: 489–499
27. Seifter E, Rettura G, Seiter J et al. Thymotrophic action of vitamin A. Fed Proc 1973; 32: 947
28. Reinhardt A, Auperin D, Sands J. Mechanism of viricidal activity of retinoids. Protein removal from bacteriophage 6 envelope. Antimicrob Agents Chemother 1980; 17: 1034–1037
29. Bendich A. Beta-carotene and the immune response. Proc Nutr Soc 1991; 50: 263–274
30. Bendich A. Vitamin C and immune responses. Food Technol 1987; 41: 112–114
31. Scott J. On the biochemical similarities of ascorbic acid and interferon. J Theor Biol 1982; 98: 235–238
32. Hemila H. Vitamin C and the common cold. Br J Nutr 1992; 67: 3–16
33. Hemila H and Herman ZS. Vitamin C and the common cold. A retrospective analysis of Chalmers' review. J Am Coll Nutr 1995; 14: 116–123
34. Hunt C et al. The clinical effects of vitamin C supplementation in elderly hospitalized patients with acute respiratory infections. Int J Vit Nutr Res 1994; 64: 212–219
35. Cathcart RF. The third face of vitamin C. J Orthomol Med 1992; 7: 197–200
36. Baur H, Staub H. Treatment of hepatitis with infusions of ascorbic acid. Comparison with other therapies. JAMA 1954; 156: 565
37. Ginter E. Optimum intake of vitamin C for the human organism. Nutr Health 1982; 1: 66–77
38. Havsteen B. Flavonoids, a class of natural products of high pharmacological potency. Biochem Pharmacol 1983; 32: 1141–1148

39. Kelleher J. Vitamin E and the immune response. Proceedings Nutr Soc 1991; 50: 245–249
40. Meydani SN, Meydani M, Blumberg JB et al. Vitamin E supplementation and in vivo immune response in healthy elderly subjects. A randomized controlled trial. JAMA 1997; 277: 1380–1386
41. Stockman J. Infections and iron. Too much of a good thing? Am J Dis Child 1981; 135: 18–20
42. Prasad A. Clinical, biochemical and nutritional spectrum of zinc deficiency in human subjects. An update. Nutr Rev 1983; 41: 197–208
43. Eaterbrook-Smith S. Activation of the binding of C1q to immune complexes by zinc. FEBS Lett 1983; 162: 117–119
44. Hadden JW. The treatment of zinc deficiency is an immunotherapy. Int J Immunopharmac 1995; 17: 697–701
45. Katz E, Margalith E. Inhibition of vaccinia virus maturation by zinc chloride. Antimicrobial Agents Chemother 1981; 19: 213–217
46. Gershwin M, Beach R, Hurley L. Trace metals, aging, and immunity. J Am Ger Soc 1983; 31: 374–378
47. Eby GA, Davis DR, Halcomb WW. Reduction in duration of common colds by zinc gluconate lozenges in a double-blind study. Antimicrob Agents Chemother 1984; 25: 20–24
48. Mossad SB, Macknin ML, Medendorp SV et al. Zinc gluconate lozenges for treating the common cold. A randomized, double-blind, placebo-controlled study. Annals Intern Med 1996; 125: 81–88
49. Kiremidjian-Schumacher L, Stotsky G. Selenium and immune responses. Environmental Res 1987; 42: 277–303
50. Kiremidjian-Schumacher L et al. Supplementation with selenium and human immune cell functions. II. Effect on cytotoxic lymphocytes and natural killer cells. Biol Trace Elem Res 1994; 41: 115–127
51. Roy M. Supplementation with selenium and human immune cell functions. I. Effect on lymphocyte proliferation and interleukin 2 receptor expression. Biol Trace Elem Res 1994; 41: 103–114
52. Dardenne M, Pleau M, Nabarra B et al. Contribution of zinc and other metals to the biological activity of the serum thymic factor. Proc Natl Acad Sci 1982; 79: 5370–5373
53. Bogden JD, Oleske JM, Munves EM et al. Zinc and immunocompetence in the elderly. Baseline data on zinc nutriture and immunity in unsupplemented subjects. Am J Clin Nutr 1987; 46: 101–109
54. Cazzola P, Mazzanti P, Bossi G. In vivo modulating effect of a calf thymus acid lysate on human T lymphocyte subsets and CD4+/CD8+ ratio in the course of different diseases. Curr Ther Res 1987; 42: 1011–1017
55. Kouttab NM, Prada M, Cazzola P. Thymomodulin. Biological properties and clinical applications. Med Oncol Tumor Pharmacother 1989; 6: 5–9
56. Fiocchi A et al. A double-blind clinical trial for the evaluation of the therapeutic effectiveness of a calf thymus derivative (Thymomodulin) in children with recurrent respiratory infections. Thymus 1986; 8: 831–839
57. Bauer R, Wagner H. Echinacea species as potential immunostimulatory drugs. Econ Med Plant Res 1991; 5: 253–321
58. Erhard M et al. Effect of echinacea, acontium, lachesis, and apis extracts, and their combinations on phagocytosis of human granulocytes. Phytother Res 1994; 8: 14–77
59. Wildfeuer A, Meyerhofer D. Study of the influence of phytopreparation on the cellular function of bodily defense. Arzneim Forsch 1994; 44: 361–366
60. Chang HM, But PPH eds. Pharmacology and applications of Chinese Materia Medica. Singapore: World Scientific. 1987: p 1041–1046
61. Zhao KS, Mancini C, Doria G. Enhancement of the immune response in mice by *Astragalus membranaceus*. Immunopharmacol 1990; 20: 225–233
62. Chu DT, Wong WL, Mavlight GM. Immunotherapy with Chinese medicinal herbs. J Clin Lab Immunol 1988; 25: 119–129

CHAPTER CONTENTS

54

Intestinal dysbiosis and dysfunction

Michael T. Murray, ND

Joseph E. Pizzorno Jr, ND

INTRODUCTION

Overgrowth of inappropriate bacteria in the various segments of the intestines is becoming recognized as a significant, but rarely recognized, cause of chronic disorders not only of the intestines but also of other systems of the body. Although widespread, it is frequently unsuspected because its symptoms often mimic other disorders. Environmental exposure, widespread antibiotic use and a low-fiber diet, as well as digestive disorders, have resulted in increasing incidence of intestinal dysbiosis and dysfunction with age.

Further discussion of the substantive role of the digestive tract in health and disease can be found in Chapters 7, 9, 19, 21, 23, 31, 57, 131, 163 and 165. The length of the list in itself indicates the wide-ranging effects of intestinal dysbiosis. This chapter provides some overview and fills in the gaps between the above listed chapters.

SMALL INTESTINE

Bacterial overgrowth

The upper portion of the human small intestine is normally relatively free of bacteria. Overgrowth of organisms in this area results in carbohydrate fermentation which produces excessive gas, bloating, and abdominal distention, and protein putrefaction which produces vasoactive amines.[1] For example, bacteria and yeast contain decarboxylases which can convert the amino acids histidine to histamine and tyrosine to tyramine, ornithine to putrescine and lysine to cadaverine. All of these compounds cause constriction and relaxation of blood vessels by acting on their smooth muscle. In the intestinal tract, excessive vasoactive amine synthesis can lead to increased gut permeability (i.e. the "leaky gut" syndrome), abdominal pain, altered gut motility, and pain (see Ch. 21).

Diagnosis of small intestinal overgrowth involves comprehensive digestive and stool analysis (see Ch. 9) and breath tests which measure the hydrogen and methane after the administration of lactulose and glucose (see Ch. 7).

Symptoms of small intestinal bacterial overgrowth are similar to those generally attributed to achlorhydria and pancreatic insufficiency – indigestion and sense of fullness (bloating) – but may also include symptoms generally associated with *Candida* overgrowth (discussed below), nausea, diarrhea, and arthritis. This latter association is quite important as many patients with rheumatoid arthritis exhibit small intestinal bacterial overgrowth, the degree of which correlates with the severity of symptoms and disease activity.[2]

Several protective measures prevent bacterial overgrowth in the small intestine: digestive enzymes, liver secretions, peristalsis and immunological factors.[3–7] Hydrochloric acid, bile and pancreatic enzymes play a critical role in preventing significant numbers of bacteria from transiting through the stomach or migrating up the small intestine.[4,5] Decreased motility of the small intestine due to a motility disorder (e.g. systemic sclerosis) or a meal high in refined sugar can also contribute to small intestinal bacterial overgrowth.[6,7] The mechanism by which a high sugar meal decreased mobility is simple: when blood sugar levels rise too rapidly, the feedback system inhibits gastrointestinal peristalsis. Since glucose is primarily absorbed in the duodenum and jejunum, inhibition of this portion of the gastrointestinal tract is the strongest. Low immune function, food allergies, stress, and other factors which reduce the level of secretory IgA can also contribute to bacterial overgrowth in the small intestine (Table 54.1). Finally, a weak ileocecal can lead to overpopulation of the small intestinal tract with bacteria from the colon. A weak ileocecal valve is most often the consequence of long-term constipation or straining excessively at defecation. In both of these cases, a low-fiber diet is most often responsible.

An overgrowth in the gastrointestinal tract of the usually benign yeast *Candida albicans* is now becoming recognized as a complex medical syndrome known as the yeast syndrome or chronic candidiasis (see Ch. 48).

Table 54.1 Factors associated with small intestinal bacterial overgrowth

- Decreased digestive secretions
  —achlorhydria
  —hypochlorhydria
  —drugs which inhibit hydrochloric acid
  —pancreatic insufficiency
  —decreased bile output due to liver or gall bladder disease
- Decreased motility
  —scleroderma (progressive systemic sclerosis)
  —systemic lupus erythematosus
  —intestinal adhesions
  —sugar-induced hypomotility
  —radiation damage
- Low secretory IgA
- Weak ileocecal valve

The overgrowth of *Candida* is believed to cause a wide variety of symptoms in virtually every system of the body, with the gastrointestinal, genitourinary, endocrine, nervous, and immune systems being the most susceptible. Eventually this syndrome will be replaced by a more comprehensive term to include small intestinal bacterial overgrowth and the leaky gut syndrome.

Treatment

Obviously, addressing the cause of the small intestinal bacterial overgrowth is the first step. The subject of decreased digestive secretions is discussed in Chapter 55. The decreased motility is usually addressed by decreasing sugar consumption while increasing dietary fiber (see Ch. 57 for more in-depth discussion).[7]

Restoring secretory IgA to normal levels involves eliminating food allergies (see Ch. 51) and enhancing immune function (see Ch. 53). Stress is particularly detrimental to secretory IgA. This effect offers an additional explanation as to why stressful events tend to worsen gastrointestinal function and food allergies.

Pancreatic enzymes and botanical medicines containing berberine can be used to inhibit the bacteria growing in the small intestinal overgrowth. In addition to exerting broad-spectrum antibiotic activity (including activity against *Candida albicans*), berberine has been shown to inhibit the bacterial decarboxylase enzyme which converts amino acids into vasoactive amines.[8] Pancreatic enzymes, in addition to enhancing protein digestion, are largely responsible for keeping the small intestine free from bacteria as well as parasites (pathogenic bacteria, yeast, protozoa, and helminths).[9] A lack of proteases or other digestive secretions greatly increases an individual's risk of having an intestinal infection including chronic *Candida* infections of the gastrointestinal tract.

COLON

The large intestine is not significantly involved in digestion but does play a role in the absorption of water and electrolytes and provides temporary storage for waste products and the formation of stool. The health of the colon is largely determined by amount of dietary fiber and the proper elimination of waste products. (Irritable bowel syndrome is discussed in Ch. 165, and Crohn's disease and ulcerative colitis are fully covered in Ch. 163.)

Constipation

An old-time naturopathic belief was that "disease begins in the colon". There appears to be great wisdom in that statement: improper elimination of waste products has

Table 54.2 Causes of constipation

Dietary	Highly refined and low-fiber foods, inadequate fluid intake
Physical inactivity	Inadequate exercise, prolonged bed rest
Pregnancy	
Advanced age	
Drugs	Anesthetics, antacids (aluminum and calcium salts), anticholinergics (bethanechol, carbachol, pilocarpine, physostigmine, ambenonium), anticonvulsants, antidepressants (tricyclics, monoamine oxidase inhibitors), antihypertensives, anti-Parkinsonism drugs, antipsychotics (phenothiazines), beta-adrenergic blocking agents (propanolol), bismuth salts, diuretics, iron salts, laxatives and cathartics (chronic use), muscle relaxants, opiates, toxic metals (arsenic, lead, mercury)
Metabolic abnormalities	Low potassium stores, diabetes, kidney disease
Endocrine abnormalities	Low thyroid function, elevated calcium levels, pituitary disorders
Structural abnormalities	Abnormalities in the structure or anatomy of the bowel
Bowel diseases	Diverticulosis, irritable bowel syndrome (alternating diarrhea and constipation), tumor
Neurogenic abnormalities	Nerve disorders of the bowel (aganglionosis, autonomic neuropathy), spinal cord disorders (trauma, multiple sclerosis, tabes dorsalis), disorders of the splanchnic nerves (tumors, trauma), cerebral disorders (strokes, Parkinsonism, neoplasm)
Enemas (chronic use)	

serious health repercussions. Constipation regularly affects over 4 million people in the United States.[10] This high incidence translates to over $500 million in annual sales of laxatives. There are a number of possible causes of constipation, but the most common cause is a low-fiber diet (Table 54.2).

Treatment

While constipation will usually respond to a high-fiber diet, plentiful fluid consumption, and exercise, many sufferers of chronic constipation do not avail themselves of these healthful approaches and use laxatives instead.

It is well accepted that increasing dietary fiber is an effective treatment of chronic constipation. High levels of dietary fiber increase both the frequency and quantity of bowel movements, decrease the transit time of stools, decrease the absorption of toxins from the stool, and appear to be a preventive factor in several diseases. Particularly effective in relieving constipation are bran and prunes. The typical recommendation for bran (oat preferable to wheat) is half a cup of bran cereal, increasing to 1.5 cups over several weeks. Whole prunes as well as prune juice possess good laxative effects. Eight ounces is usually an effective dose. Be sure that patients are consuming enough liquids. Prescribe the drinking of at least six to eight glasses per day. In addition, recommend the consumption of 25–35 g of fiber.

When patients need additional support, consider using fiber formulas. These formulas act as bulking agents. They can be composed of natural plant fibers derived from psyllium seed, kelp, agar, pectin, and plant gums like karaya and guar. They can also be made from purified semi-synthetic polysaccharides like methyl-cellulose and carboxymethyl cellulose sodium. Psyllium-containing laxatives are the most popular and usually the most effective.

If patients have been using stimulant laxatives, even natural ones like *Cascara sagrada* (*Rhamnus purshiana*) or senna (*Cassia senna*), they will need to "retrain" their bowels. Table 54.3 lists the recommended rules for re-establishing bowel regularity. The recommended procedure will take 4–6 weeks.

Diverticular disease

Most often the presence of diverticula is without symptoms; however, if the diverticula becomes inflamed, perforated, or impacted, symptomatic diverticulitis results. Only about 20% of people with diverticulosis develop diverticulitis. Symptoms of diverticulitis include episodes of lower abdominal pain and cramping, changes in bowel habits (constipation or diarrhea), and

Table 54.3 Rules for bowel retraining

- Find and eliminate known causes of constipation
- Never repress an urge to defecate
- Eat a high-fiber diet, particularly fruits and vegetables
- Drink six to eight glasses of fluid per day
- Sit on the toilet at the same time every day (even when the urge to defecate is not present), preferably immediately after breakfast or exercise
- Exercise for at least 20 minutes, three times per week
- Stop using laxatives (except as discussed below to re-establish bowel activity) and enemas
- Week 1: Every night before bed take a stimulant laxative containing either cascara or senna. Take the lowest amount necessary to reliably ensure a bowel movement every morning
- Weekly: Each week decrease dosage by 50%. If constipation recurs, go back to the previous week's dosage. Decrease dosage if diarrhea occurs

a sense of fullness in the abdomen. In more severe cases, fever may be present along with tenderness and rigidity of the abdomen over the area of the intestine involved.

Treatment

Treatment of diverticular disease involves the recommendation of a high-fiber diet. In severe cases of diverticulitis, an antibiotic may be warranted.

Dysbiosis

The microecology of the human gastrointestinal tract is an incredibly complex ecosystem as there are at least 500 different species of microflora that are part of the "normal" intestinal flora.[11] There are nine times as many bacteria in the gastrointestinal tract as there are cells in the human body. The type and number of gut bacteria play an important role in determining health and disease. A state of altered bacterial flora in the gut has become popularly known as "dysbiosis". The term was first used by noted Russian scientist Elie Metchnikoff to reflect a state of living with intestinal flora that has harmful effects. He theorized that toxic compounds produced by the bacterial breakdown of food were the cause of degenerative disease.[12] There is a growing body of evidence that is supporting and refining Metchnikoff's theory. The major causes of dysbiosis are listed in Table 54.4.

Obviously, treatment begins with addressing these major causes. In addition, it is important to re-seed the gastrointestinal tract with probiotics. The most important healthful bacteria are *Lactobacillus acidophilus* and *Bifidobacterium bifidum* (see Ch. 105 for a full discussion).

The symbiosis or pathogenicity of the 500 normal microbial inhabitants of the human digestive tract is largely determined by the environment in which they live and the balance between the various types. *Candida albicans* is an example of an organism that, under normal circumstances, lives in harmony with the host, but if *Candida* overgrows and is out of balance with other gut microbes it can result in problems. In general, parasites cause most of their problems by interfering with digestion and/or damaging the intestinal lining, either of which can lead to increased mucous secretion and/or diarrhea.

One of the most intriguing hypotheses explaining the balance and growth of the various organisms is the type of level of digestion of carbohydrates in the diet. The research in this area and clinical applications of modification of dietary carbohydrates are covered in a very interesting book, *Breaking the Vicious Cycle*, by nutritionist Elaine Gottschall.[13] The presence of undigested and unabsorbed carbohydrates within the small intestine and/or colon result in increased fermentation and overgrowth of certain, toxic species of bacteria. Not only is the production of gas increased, but so also is the production of short-chain organic acids, such as lactic acid, which are damaging to the intestinal mucosa. The damage to the intestinal mucosa aggravates the problem by decreasing the level of disaccharides (lactase, sucrase, isomaltase and, less often, maltase) in the lining cells, thus further increasing the levels of undigested disaccharides. As the gastrointestinal tissues become more damaged, mucous secretion increases, further separating complex carbohydrates from their digestive sites.

Treatment involves the "specific carbohydrate diet", which breaks the vicious cycle by only allowing carbohydrates that are either predigested or easily digested and virtually totally absorbed in the duodenum, making them unavailable to more distal bacteria. Basically, all disaccharides (e.g. lactose, sucrose), all grain starches (e.g. wheat, rice, corn syrup), and starchy vegetables (e.g. potatoes) are eliminated, as are most legume starches. Simple sugars such as glucose and fructose (found in honey, fruits, and some vegetables) and lactose-hydrolyzed milk products are allowed.

Interestingly, although not acknowledged (all historic references are to conventional medical practitioners), several of these concepts were first promulgated by

Table 54.4 Causes of intestinal dysbiosis

- Dietary disturbances
  —high protein
  —high sugar
  —high fat
  —low fiber
  —food allergies
- Lack of digestive secretions
- Stress
- Antibiotic/drug therapy
- Decreased immune function
- Malabsorption
- Intestinal infection
- Altered pH

Table 54.5 Common protozoa and helminths

Protozoa
- Ameba
- *Giardia*
- *Trichomonas*
- *Cryptosporidium*
- *Dientamoeba fragilis*
- *Iodamoeba butschlii*
- *Blastocystis*
- *Balantidium coli*
- *Chilomastix*

Helminths
- Roundworm (*Ascaris lumbricoides*)
- Pinworm (*Enterobius vermicularis*)
- Hookworm (*Necator americanus*)
- Threadworm (*Strongyloides stercoralis*)
- Whipworm (*Trichuris trichiura*)
- Tapeworms (various species)

Table 54.6 Incidence of parasites in 200,000 stool samples[14]

Organism	Incidence	Notes
Protozoa		
Giardia lamblia	7.2%	Significant increase from the 4% found in 1979; more than 9% of the specimens were located around the Great Lakes or in the north-west of the United States
Entamoeba coli and *Endolimax nana*	4.2%	
Blastocystis hominis	2.6%	
Entamoeba histolytica	0.9%	
Cryptosporidium species	0.2%	
Nematodes		
Hookworm	1.5%	
Trichuris trichiura	1.2%	
Ascaris lumbricoides	0.8%	
Clonorchis and *Opisthorchis* species	0.6%	
Strongyloides stercoralis	0.4%	
Hymenolepis nana	0.4%	
Enterobius vermicularis	0.4%	Tape tests positive for 11.4% of 9,597 specimens
Taenia species	0.1%	

"Professor" Arnold Erhardt at the turn of the century in his book *The Mucousless Diet*.

Parasites

Diarrheal diseases caused by parasites still constitute the greatest single worldwide cause of illness and death. The problem is more severe in underdeveloped countries with poor sanitation, but even in the United States diarrheal diseases are the third major cause of sickness and death. Furthermore, the ease and frequency of worldwide travel and increased migration to the United States is resulting in growing numbers of parasitic infections. In addition to normal inhabitants of the gastrointestinal system acting as parasites, there are also significant diarrheal diseases associated with protozoa and helminths (Table 54.5). (One parasite, *Ascaris lumbricoides* is discussed in more detail in Ch. 131.)

The apparent incidence of the various parasites are listed in Table 54.6. These data come from state diagnostic laboratories which evaluated over 200,000 stool specimens in 1987. Parasites were found in 20.1% of the stool samples.

While the most commonly reported symptoms of parasitic infection are diarrhea and abdominal pain, these symptoms do not occur in every case (Table 54.7). In fact, there appears to be a growing number of individuals experiencing milder than usual gastrointestinal symptoms due to parasitic infections and/or symptoms not traditionally considered to be linked to parasitic infections. For example, in many cases of the irritable bowel syndrome, indigestion, and poor digestion, parasites may be causing the symptoms. In addition, parasitic infections are often an unsuspected cause of chronic illness and fatigue.

Table 54.7 Signs and symptoms of parasitic infections

- Abdominal pain and cramps
- Constipation
- Depressed secretory IgA
- Diarrhea
- Fatigue
- Fever
- Flatulence
- Food allergy
- Foul-smelling stools
- Gastritis
- Headaches
- Hives
- Increased intestinal permeability
- Indigestion
- Irregular bowel movements
- Irritable bowel syndrome
- Loss of appetite
- Low back pain
- Malabsorption
- Weight loss

Treatment

A number of natural compounds can be useful in helping the body rid itself of parasites. However, before selecting a natural alternative to an antibiotic in parasitic infections, the underlying factors which may have been responsible for setting up the internal terrain for a parasitic infection, e.g. achlorhydria, decreased pancreatic enzyme output, etc., must be controlled. Proper treatment with either an antibiotic or a natural alternative requires monitoring by repeating multiple stool samples 2 weeks after therapy (see Ch. 131 for a more detailed therapy).

The treatment of parasitic infections typically utilizes high dosages of pancreatic enzymes (10 × USP 750–1,000 mg, 10–20 minutes before meals) and berberine-containing plants such as *Hydrastis canadensis*, *Berberis vulgaris*, *Berberis aquifolium*, and *Coptis chinensis*. When using these plants, the dosage should be based on berberine content. As there is a wide range of quality, standardized extracts are preferred. Three times a day dosages are as follows:

- dried root or as infusion (tea): 2–4 g
- tincture (1:5): 6–12 ml (1.5–3 tsp)
- fluid extract (1:1): 2–4 ml (0.5–1 tsp)
- solid (powdered dry) extract (4:1 or 8–12% alkaloid content): 250–500 mg.

These dosage recommendations result in a berberine dosage of 25–50 mg three times daily or a daily dosage of up to 150 mg. This dosage is consistent with the dosage range in the positive clinical studies in various parasitic infections (see Ch. 91). For children a dosage based on body weight is appropriate. The daily dosage would be the equivalent to 5–10 mg of berberine/kg body weight.

REFERENCES

1. Sawada Y, Periera SP, Murphy GM, Dowling RH. Polyamines in the intestinal lumen of patients with small bowel bacterial overgrowth. Biochem Soc Trans 1994; 22: 392(S)
2. Henriksson AEK, Blomquist L, Nord CE et al. Small intestinal bacterial overgrowth in patients with rheumatoid arthritis. Ann Rheum Dis 1993; 52: 503–510
3. Sarker SA, Gyr R. Non-immunological defense mechanisms of the gut. Gut 1990; 33: 1331–1337
4. Saltzman JR, Kowdley KV, Pederosa MC et al. Bacterial overgrowth without clinical malabsorption in elderly hypochlorhydric subjects. Gastroenterol 1994; 106: 615–623
5. Rubinstein E, Mark Z, Hasple J et al. Antibacterial activity of the pancreatic fluid. Gastroenterol 1985; 88: 927–932
6. Husebye E. Gastrointestinal motility disorders and bacterial overgrowth. J Intern Med 1995; 237: 419–427
7. Russo A, Fraser R, Horowitz M. The effect of acute hyperglycemia on small intestinal motility in normal subjects. Diabetologia 1996; 39: 984–989
8. Watanabe A, Obata T, Nagashima H. Berberine therapy of hypertyraminemia in patients with liver cirrhosis. Acta Med Okayama 1982; 36: 277–281
9. Rubinstein E, Mark Z, Hasple J et al. Antibacterial activity of the pancreatic fluid. Gastroenterol 1985; 88: 927–932
10. Sonnenberg A, Koch TR. Epidemiology of constipation in the United States. Dis Colon Rectum 1989; 32: 1–8
11. Hentges DJ, ed. Human intestinal microflora. In: Health and disease. New York, NY: Academic Press. 1983
12. Metchnikoff E. The prolongation of life. New York, NY: Arna Press. 1908 (1977 reprint)
13. Gotschall E. Breaking the vicious cycle. Kirkton, Ontario: Kirkton Press. 1994
14. Results of testing for intestinal parasites by state diagnostic laboratories, United States, 1987. Morbid Mortal Weekly Rep 1992; 40(SS-4): 25–30

CHAPTER CONTENTS

55

Maldigestion

Michael T. Murray, ND

Joseph E. Pizzorno Jr, ND

INTRODUCTION

Proper digestion, absorption, and elimination are necessary in order to gain the nutritional benefits from foods. Any disruption of these processes causes substantial, and usually progressive, health problems throughout the body. As discussed in several chapters in this textbook (e.g. Chs 7, 21, 31, 57, 131, 163, and 165), intestinal dysfunction is a common, yet inadequately recognized, problem.

This chapter provides some overview of digestive dysfunction and ways to improve digestion. Intestinal dysfunction, independent of digestive dysfunction, is discussed in Chapter 54. A full discussion of the various laboratory procedures for evaluation of digestive function can be found in Chapters 9, 19, and 23.

THERAPEUTIC CONSIDERATIONS

Indigestion

The term indigestion is often used by patients to describe a feeling of gaseousness or fullness in the abdomen. It can also be used to describe "heartburn". Indigestion can be attributed to a great many causes, including not only increased secretion of acid but also decreased secretion of acid and other digestive factors and enzymes.

Indigestion is commonly treated with antacids and histamine (H_2)-receptor antagonists either self-prescribed by patients or prescribed by medical practitioners. The use of these agents will typically raise the gastric pH above 3.5, effectively inhibiting the action of pepsin, the enzyme involved in protein digestion that can be irritating to the stomach. Although raising the pH can reduce symptoms, it also substantially impairs protein digestion and mineral disassociation. In addition, the change in pH can adversely effect gut microbial flora including the promotion of an overgrowth of *Helicobacter pylori*. Finally, most nutrition-oriented physicians believe that lack of acid, not excess, is the true culprit for most patients.

According to surveys, most people use antacids to relieve symptoms of reflux esophagitis.[1] However, reflux esophagitis is most often caused by *overeating*, not excessive acid production. Other common causes include:

- obesity
- cigarette smoking
- chocolate
- fried foods
- carbonated beverages
- alcohol
- coffee.

These factors either increase intra-abdominal pressure or they decrease the tone of the esophageal sphincter.

Chronic heartburn may also be a sign of a hiatal hernia. However, while 50% of people over the age of 50 have hiatal hernias, only 5% of patients with hiatal hernias actually experience reflux esophagitis.

Perhaps the most effective treatment of chronic reflux esophagitis and symptomatic hiatal hernias is to utilize gravity. The standard recommendation is to simply place 4-inch blocks under the bedposts at the head of the bed. This elevation of the head is very effective in many cases. Another recommendation to heal the esophagus, is using deglycyrrhizinated licorice (DGL).

Hypochlorhydria

In the patient with chronic indigestion, rather than focus on blocking the digestive process with antacids, the natural approach to indigestion focuses on aiding digestion. Although much is said about hyperacidity conditions, a more common cause of indigestion is a lack of gastric acid secretion. There are many symptoms and signs that suggest impaired gastric acid secretion, and a number of specific diseases have been found to be associated with insufficient gastric acid output.[2–12] These are listed in Tables 55.1 and 55.2.

Several studies have shown that the ability to secrete gastric acid decreases with age.[13–16] Some studies found low stomach acidity in over half of those over the age of 60. The best method of diagnosing a lack of gastric acid is the Heidelberg gastric analysis (Ch. 19).[17] It has been suggested by Wright[18] that the response to a bicarbonate challenge during Heidelberg gastric analysis, not simply resting pH, is the true test of the functional ability of the stomach to secrete acid.

Table 55.1 Common signs and symptoms of low gastric acidity

- Bloating, belching, burning, and flatulence immediately after meals
- A sense of "fullness" after eating
- Indigestion, diarrhea, or constipation
- Multiple food allergies
- Nausea after taking supplements
- Itching around the rectum
- Weak, peeling, and cracked fingernails
- Dilated blood vessels in the cheeks and nose
- Acne
- Iron deficiency
- Chronic intestinal parasites or abnormal flora
- Undigested food in stool
- Chronic candida infections
- Upper digestive tract gassiness

Table 55.2 Diseases associated with low gastric acidity

- Addison's disease
- Asthma
- Celiac disease
- Dermatitis herpetiformis
- Diabetes mellitus
- Eczema
- Gall bladder disease
- Graves' disease
- Chronic autoimmune disorders
- Hepatitis
- Chronic hives
- Lupus erythematosus
- Myasthenia gravis
- Osteoporosis
- Pernicious anemia
- Psoriasis
- Rheumatoid arthritis
- Rosacea
- Sjögren's syndrome
- Thyrotoxicosis
- Hyper- and hypothyroidism
- Vitiligo

Since the Heidelberg gastric acid analysis is not widely available, a clinical trial of HCl supplements can be used as described in Appendix 7.

Etiology

Like peptic ulcer disease, achlorhydria and hypochlorhydria have been linked to the overgrowth of the bacteria *Helicobacter pylori*. Approximately 90–100% of patients with duodenal ulcers, 70% with gastric ulcers, and about 50% of people over the age of 50 test positive for *H. pylori*.[19] The presence of *H. pylori* is determined by measuring the level of antibodies to *H. pylori* in the blood or saliva, or by culturing material collected during an endoscopy as well as measuring the breath for urea. More recently, a breath test has become available for assessment of current *H. pylori* activity.

Low gastric output is thought to predispose to *H. pylori* colonization and *H. pylori* colonization increases gastric pH, thereby setting up a positive feedback scenario and increasing the likelihood for the colonization of the stomach and duodenum with other organisms.[20] Interestingly, there has been only scant research into the effects of antacids and H_2-receptor antagonists on promoting *H. pylori* overgrowth.[21]

Although the typical conventional medicine approach is to focus only on the infective agent, as usual host defense factors are equally or more important. Unfortunately, the research has focused on eradicating the organism and there is little information on protective factors against infectivity. Proposed protective factors against *H. pylori*-induced intestinal damage are maintaining a low pH and ensuring adequate antioxidant defense mechanisms.[22–24] Low levels of vitamin C and vitamin E and other antioxidant factors in the gastric juice not only appear to lead to the progression of *H. pylori* colonization, but also contribute to the ulcer formation since the mechanism by which *H. pylori* damages the stomach and intestinal mucosa is via oxidative damage.[25] Furthermore, antioxidant status and gastric acid output appear to explain the observation that most people infected with *H. pylori* do not develop peptic ulcer disease or gastric cancer.

Deglycyrrhizinated licorice

Deglycyrrhizinated licorice (DGL) may prove useful for both eradicating the organism and stimulating increased host defense factors. DGL has shown good results in healing both duodenal ulcers and gastric ulcers (discussed more fully in Ch. 180). Rather than inhibit the release of acid, DGL stimulates the normal defense mechanisms that prevent ulcer formation. Specifically, DGL:[26,27]

- improves both the quality and quantity of the protective substances which line the intestinal tract
- increases the life span of the intestinal cell
- improves blood supply to the intestinal lining.

The active components of DGL are believed to be flavonoid derivatives. These compounds have demonstrated impressive protection against chemically induced ulcer formation in animal studies. Several similar flavonoids have also been shown to inhibit *H. pylori* in a concentration-dependent manner.[28] In addition, unlike antibiotics, the flavonoids were also shown to augment natural defense factors which prevent ulcer formation. The activity of flavone, the most potent flavonoid in the study, was shown to be similar to that of bismuth subcitrate.

Bismuth

Bismuth is a naturally occurring mineral that can act as an antacid as well as exert activity against *H. pylori*.[29] The best known and most widely used bismuth preparation is bismuth subsalicylate (e.g. Pepto-Bismol). However, bismuth subcitrate has produced the best results against *H. pylori* and in the treatment of non-ulcer-related indigestion as well as peptic ulcers.[30,31] In the United States, bismuth subcitrate preparations are available through compounding pharmacies (contact the International Academy of Compounding Pharmacists: 1-800–927–4227).

One of the key advantages of bismuth preparations over standard antibiotic approaches to eradicating *H. pylori* is that while the bacteria may develop resistance to various antibiotics it is very unlikely to develop resistance to bismuth.

The usual dosage for bismuth subcitrate is 240 mg twice daily before meals. For bismuth subsalycilate the dosage is 500 mg four times daily.

Bismuth preparations are safe when taken at prescribed dosages. Bismuth subcitrate may cause a temporary and harmless darkening of the tongue and/or stool. Bismuth subsalicylate should not be given to children recovering from the flu, chickenpox, or any other viral infection as it may mask the nausea and vomiting associated with Reye's syndrome, a rare but serious illness.

Pancreatic insufficiency

Both physical symptoms and laboratory tests can be used to assess pancreatic function. Common symptoms of pancreatic insufficiency include abdominal bloating and discomfort, gas, indigestion, and the passing of undigested food in the stool. For laboratory diagnosis, the comprehensive stool and digestive analysis (discussed in Ch. 9) is quite useful.

The most severe level of pancreatic insufficiency is seen in cystic fibrosis. Although cystic fibrosis is quite rare, mild pancreatic insufficiency is thought to be a relatively common condition, especially in the elderly.

Pancreatic enzyme supplements

Pancreatic enzyme products are an effective treatment for pancreatic insufficiency and are widely used. Most commercial preparations are prepared from fresh hog pancreas (i.e. pancreatin) (see Ch. 101 for a full discussion).

The dosage of pancreatic enzymes is based on the level of enzyme activity of the particular product as defined by the *United States Pharmacopoeia* (USP). A 1× pancreatic enzyme (pancreatin) product has in each milligram not less than 25 USP units of amylase activity, not less than 2.0 USP units of lipase activity, and not less than 25 USP units of protease activity. Pancreatin of higher potency is given a whole number multiple indicating its strength. For example, a full-strength undiluted pancreatic extract that is 10 times stronger than the USP standard would be referred to as 10× USP. Full-strength products are preferred to lower potency pancreatin products because lower potency products are often diluted with salt, lactose, or galactose to achieve desired strength (e.g. 4× or 1×). The dosage recommendation for a 10× USP pancreatic enzyme product is typically 350–1,000 mg three times/day immediately before meals when used as a digestive aid and 10–20 minutes before meals or on an empty stomach when anti-inflammatory effects are desired.

Enzyme products are often enteric-coated. However, numerous studies have shown that non-enteric-coated enzyme preparations actually outperform enteric-coated products if they are given prior to a meal (for digestive purposes) or on an empty stomach (for anti-inflammatory effects).

For vegetarians, bromelain, papain and enzymes extracted from *Aspergillus oryzae* can substitute for pancreatic enzymes.

REFERENCES

1. Graham DY, Smith JL, Patterson DJ. Why do apparently healthy people use antacid tablets. Am J Gastroenterol 1983; 78: 257–260
2. Bray GW. The hypochlorhydria of asthma in childhood. Br Med J 1930; i: 181–197
3. Rabinowitch IM. Achlorhydria and its clinical significance in diabetes mellitus. Am J Dig Dis 1949; 18: 322–333
4. Carper WM, Butler TJ, Kilby JO, Gibson MJ. Gallstones, gastric secretion and flatulent dyspepsia. Lancet 1967; i: 413–415
5. Rawls WB, Ancona VC. Chronic urticaria associated with hypochlorhydria or achlorhydria. Rev Gastroent 1950; Oct: 267–271
6. Gianella RA, Broitman SA, Zamcheck N. Influence of gastric acidity on bacterial and parasitic enteric infections. Ann Int Med 1973; 78: 271–276
7. De Witte TJ, Geerdink PJ, Lamers CB. Hypochlorhydria and hypergastrinaemia in rheumatoid arthritis. Ann Rheum Dis 1979; 38: 14–17
8. Ryle JA, Barber HW. Gastric analysis in acne rosacea. Lancet 1920; ii: 1195–1196
9. Ayres S. Gastric secretion in psoriasis, eczema and dermatitis herpetiformis. Arch Derm 1929; Jul: 854–859
10. Dotevall G, Walan A. Gastric secretion of acid and intrinsic factor in patients with hyper and hypothyroidism. Acta Med Scand 1969; 186: 529–533
11. Howitz J, Schwartz M. Vitiligo, achlorhydria, and pernicious anemia. Lancet 1971; i: 1331–1334
12. Howden CV, Hunt RH. Relationship between gastric secretion and infection. Gut 1987; 28: 96–107
13. Rafsky HA, Weingarten M. A study of the gastric secretory response in the aged. Gastroent 1946; May: 348–352
15. Davies D, James TG. An investigation into the gastric secretion of a hundred normal persons over the age of sixty. Br J Med 1930; i: 1–14
16. Baron JH. Studies of basal and peak acid output with an augmented histamine meal. Gut 1963; 3: 136–144
17. Mojaverian P, Ferguson RK, Vlasses PH et al. Estimation of gastric residence time of the Heidelberg capsule in humans. Gastroenterology 1985; 89: 392–397
18. Wright J. A proposal for standardized challenge testing of gastric acid secretory capacity using the Heidelberg capsule radiotelemetry system. J John Bastyr Col Nat Med 1979; 1: 2: 3–11
19. Berstad K, Berstad A. *Helicobacter pylori* infection in peptic ulcer disease. Scand J Gastroenterol 1993; 28: 561–567
20. Sarker SA, Gyr K. Non-immunological defense mechanisms of the gut. Gut 1992; 33: 987–993
21. Stockbruegger RW, Seeberg S, Hellner L et al. Intragastric nitrites, nitrosamines, and bacterial overgrowth during cimetidine therapy. Gut 1982; 23: 1048–1054
22. Shibata T, Imoto I, Taguchi Y et al. High acid output may protect the gastric mucosa from injury caused by *Helicobacter pylori* in duodenal ulcer patients. J Gastroenterol Hepatol 1996; 11: 674–680
23. Rokkas T, Papatheodorou G, Karameris A et al. *Helicobacter pylori* infection and gastric juice vitamin C levels. Digestive Dis Sci 1995; 40: 615–621
24. Phull PS, Price AB, Thorniley MS et al. Vitamin E concentrations in the human stomach and duodenum – correlation with *Helicobacter pylori* infection. Gut 1996; 39: 31–35
25. Baik SC et al. Increased oxidative DNA damage in *Helicobacter pylori*-infected human gastric mucosa. Cancer Res 1996; 56: 1279–1282
26. van Marle J, Aarsen PN, Lind A, van Weeren-Kraner J. Deglycyrrhizinised liquorice (DGL) and the renewal of rat stomach epithelium. Eur J Pharmacol 1981; 72: 219–225
27. Johnson B, McIssac R. Effect of some anti-ulcer agents on mucosal blood flow. Br J Pharmacol 1981; 1: 308
28. Beil W, Birkholz C, Sewing KF. Effects of flavonoids on parietal cell acid secretion, gastric mucosal prostaglandin production and *Helicobacter pylori* growth. Arzneim Forsch 1995; 45: 697–700
29. Kang JY, Tay HH, Wee A et al. Effect of colloidal bismuth subcitrate on symptoms and gastric histology in non-ulcer dyspepsia. A double blind placebo controlled study. Gut 1990; 31: 476–480
30. Marshall BJ, Valenzuela JE, McCallum RW et al. Bismuth subsalicylate suppression of *Helicobacter pylori* in non-ulcer dyspepsia: a double-blind placebo-controlled trial. Dig Dis Sci 1993; 38: 1674–1680
31. Lambert JR, Midolo P. The actions of bismuth in the treatment of *Helicobacter pylori* infection. Aliment Pharmacol Ther 1997; 11(suppl 1): 27–33

CHAPTER CONTENTS

56

Non-pharmacological control of pain

Richard Kitaeff, MA ND DAc

INTRODUCTION

Pain in its myriad forms is one of the most common symptoms for which patients seek relief. Acute pain is an unpleasant experience primarily associated with tissue injury, and the protective response patients have to pain provides the clinician with valuable diagnostic information.

The reaction to pain is highly subjective and, as a function of higher centers, is extremely variable. It is influenced by many factors depending on the individual patient and his or her situation. When pain becomes chronic, the multifactorial influences (e.g. anxiety; depression; social, cultural, and economic factors; and secondary gain) play an even larger role.

When treating a patient for pain, it is essential first to determine the primary cause, the pathogenesis, and secondary or contributing factors. The relief of pain may then be achieved by removal of the primary cause (e.g. cure of an infection), neutralization of the effect of the stimulus (e.g. emollients for an ulcer), relief of discomfort (e.g. biofeedback), suppression of the disease process (e.g. anti-inflammatory agents), and dulling or obliterating the sense of pain (e.g. analgesics or acupuncture).[1]

Although the medical profession has chosen to emphasize the pharmacological methods of pain control, many non-pharmacological options are available. Their applicability and efficacy are documented below. (Although this chapter liberally utilizes childbirth pain control, the examples and concepts are generalizable to any situation involving acute and/or chronic pain.)

THE EXPERIENCE OF PAIN

A psychological model

Pain is generally acknowledged to be a complex physiological/psychological phenomenon. It involves motivational and emotional components and conceptual interpretation, which may or may not have their basis in actual nociception. Verbal reports of pain and associated behavioral responses are controlled, at least in part, by psychological, cultural, and situational factors.

For acute pain, such as that of childbirth, in which the painful experience can be directly related to nociceptive input, a multiprocess feedback model can be considered. However, one must keep in mind the complexity of the psychological processes intervening between sensory event and observable response, ranging from the physiological to the social aspects of personality. These include:

- elements of information processing
- performance ability
- attention
- memory
- expectancy
- attitudes and beliefs
- secondary gain
- self-concept
- designated sick roles.

In the psychological model, the brain infers information from bodily signs and integrates this with existing personal and situational variables to direct behavior. When consideration must also be given to the interactions with interested observers, such as physicians, family members and birth attendants, who influence the interpretation with their own experiences and attitudes about pain, the complexity becomes even greater.

According to this model, which does not differ in essence from a general model of stress, a primary appraisal of the personal danger or threat posed by the painful stressor is followed by a secondary appraisal of one's ability to cope, based on emotional feedback, and contributions of situational and sociocultural response factors. On this basis, a woman in labor could choose to consider pain as "positive", "functional", or "creative"; "pain with a purpose"; or, alternatively, "part of a process involving injury".[2] This conceptualization of painful stress suggests that intervention could be successful at several levels: cognitive patterning, physiological arousal associated with emotional stress, and control of environmental stimuli. Examples of appropriate strategies could be: cognitive coping skills such as restructuring and utilization of preparatory information and attention shifts; muscular relaxation, physical or electrical stimulation, and biofeedback techniques; and structuring of the environment in a way conducive to effective coping (such as by making it non-threatening and comfortable).[3]

Neuropsychological mechanisms of pain

According to research on the mechanisms of pain, pain can be treated not only by anesthetic blocks, surgical intervention and the like, but also by influencing the motivational-affective and cognitive factors as well.[4] The traditional specificity theory of pain, first enunciated by Descartes in the 17th century, holds that pain messages are conducted from specific pain receptors at the periphery through discrete pathways to pain centers in the brain. However, there are individual differences in pain responses, pain is not consistently stopped by cutting or blocking the "pain pathway", and it is now known that non-painful types of stimulation will activate the A-delta and C fibers that are associated with pain. Therefore, later modifications of pain theory took into account patterning of nerve impulses over time to reflect differences in degree and intensity of stimuli and summation of signals from an extended area.[5]

The currently accepted view of pain is the gate control theory of Melzack & Wall[6], which they formulated in 1965. Based on neurological data and a categorization of the words used to describe pain, this theory conceptualizes the pain experience as having sensory-discriminative, motivational-affective, and cognitive-evaluative components or modalities, corresponding to different patterns of nervous impulses. Neurologically, a specialized cluster of nerve cells in the substantia gelatinosa of the spinal column is thought to operate like a valve or gate, controlling nerve signals before they evoke the perception of, and response to, pain. Besides this monitoring of sensory data in the central nervous system, gating is also influenced by the relative amount of activity in large-diameter (A-beta) and small-diameter (A-delta and C) nerve fibers. The large fibers tend to inhibit transmission, or close the gate, preventing pain, and the small fibers tend to facilitate transmission, or open the gate, resulting in pain. The fact that large fibers are activated by pressure, touch, massage, and vibration suggests a mechanism for such pain control techniques as acupressure, acupuncture, and transcutaneous electrical nerve stimulation (TENS). Such stimulation apparently closes the spinal gate via the large-fiber system. Melzack & Casey[4] expanded this theory by proposing the possibility of a higher level gate, in the reticular or limbic structures of the brain, that probably mediates the drive to escape from unpleasant stimuli.

At central nervous system levels, the biochemical mechanisms of gate control may involve the endorphins, natural morphine-like substances that have been implicated in the pain-controlling effects produced by acupuncture.[7]

Pain in childbirth

A psychological/social learning approach to pain emphasizes control of motivation, expectation, focus of attention, stress, and feelings of anxiety, depression and helplessness. Factors specifically operative in labor pain include these as well as social support and the physiological factors of hunger, rest, and muscular tension.[8]

All of these can contribute to the interpretation of pain being placed on the nociceptive message provided by uterine contractions. The influence of motivation on labor pain was effectively demonstrated in a prospective study of maternal attitudes toward pregnancy in 8,000 American women. One of the factors found to be strongly related to maternal attitude toward having a baby was the need for analgesics in labor.[9]

Cultural conditioning may also be fundamental to the labeling of childbirth as painful. Throughout most of the world, analgesics are not required for labor; in fact, a Japanese anesthesiologist suggests that the idea of "painless delivery" is a strange one to his culture.[10] American women, on the other hand, "live through a largely self-fulfilling prophecy of birth as a painful, terrifying ordeal, and/or as a medical, drugged process over which they have no control".[8] This relates to body fantasies of injury, brought about in a hospital environment where distress is an expected response to the expulsive reflex.[2]

PAIN CONTROL

Moderating variables and psychological techniques

Psychological strategies

The psychological strategies recommended for control of labor pain, many of them part of prepared childbirth programs, generally aim to provide control, communication, relaxation, attention focus, and support, as well as physical counter-stimuli. There is considerable psychological research supporting the use of these in the development of pain tolerance.

The significance of various characteristics of an individual's psychological profile has been studied by evaluating the effects on pain perception of such parameters as:

- introversion-extroversion[11–13]
- augmenters-reducers[14]
- field dependence[15,16]
- repression-sensitization.[17–19]

For example, on the repression-sensitization axis, repressors may be characterized as those who avoid having to cope with pain, while sensitizers have an obsessive need to cope. They like to be informed in advance about the situation and to have control over it. The superior initial tolerance exhibited by repressors in response to heat and pressure stimuli disappears in repeated trials, showing that the sensitizers' predilection for challenge enables them to endure long-term pain better.

The importance of individual difference variables is also illustrated by the observation that one-third of patients undergoing surgical operations do not request pain-killing medication.[20] This common ability to suppress pain indicates that not all surgical patients consider themselves passive victims. In fact, during the postoperative period, pain persists longer for those who accept medication.

Cognitive strategies

The impetus for devising cognitive strategies to promote tolerance of pain has been particularly supported by investigations showing that pain tolerance increases with greater predictability and perception of control.[21–25] Similarly, preparatory communications and information received prior to the onset of experimental or surgical pain consistently decreases the subjects' perception of pain.[26–29] Animal studies have demonstrated higher rates of instrumental responses when painful shocks are signaled than when they are unsignaled.[30] Kanfer & Seidner[31] found that subjects who could advance slides of travel pictures at their own rate tolerated ice-water immersion of the hand longer than yoked subjects whose slides were changed by the experimenter.

When surgery patients are given a sense of control by providing them with preparatory information concerning postsurgery discomforts and operative care, in combination with training in rehearsal of realistic, positive aspects of the surgical experience, they showed a significant reduction in postsurgical anxiety (as indicated by nurses' observations), requests for sedatives, and length of hospital stay.[32] Furthermore, preparation for repeated peridontal surgery by auditory and visual messages classified as "control enhancement" was associated with reduction of pain after a second surgery.[33] Subjects who could cognitively redefine a threat of electric shocks as interesting new physiological sensations also reduced stress to a greater extent than subjects not provided with this coping strategy.[34]

Meichenbaum and Turk developed a procedure utilizing "stress inoculation".[35] It begins with an educational phase (in which subjects are given a conceptual framework for understanding the nature of their stressful reactions), followed by rehearsal of behavioral and cognitive coping skills, based on a set of coping self-statements generated by the client in collaboration with the therapist. Such cognitive-behavioral techniques, sometimes in combination with EMG biofeedback control, have been found successful in treatment of chronic low back pain.[36–38] Also, cognitive-behavioral strategies have been effective in alleviating the pain of irritable bowel syndrome,[39] temporomandibular joint syndrome,[40] cancer,[41] migraine headaches,[42] and rheumatic conditions.[43] This emphasis on conceptualization, preparatory information, and cognitive transformation seems to have been incorporated into the Read method of natural childbirth, which replaces fear with knowledge about birth.[8] Sheila

Kitzinger,[2] in her method of prepared childbirth, similarly emphasizes the necessity of "acquiring knowledge and understanding of what labor involves, the terminology used by obstetricians and midwives, and information about what happens in hospitals".

A study by Stevens & Heide[35] conducted at the University of Wisconsin used ice-water to test perception and endurance of pain in subjects who had been taught methods used in childbirth education classes. The controls for this training and an additional control group offered only distraction during the tests. Those who had been taught the techniques reported only about half the pain of the controls and endured it 2.5 times longer. The prepared childbirth strategies improved with practice, were effective for pain lasting longer than most contractions in labor, and were more effective than distraction techniques.[44] However, this later finding introduces some confusion, since some prepared childbirth methods include either distraction techniques or some other deliberate disposition of one's attention.

Attention-focusing

Distraction of focused attention, mostly utilizing the rhythms of the breath, is essential to the Lamaze method, the most popular prepared childbirth program in America, and important in the Bradley and other methods. Sheila Kitzinger describes the controlled attention focusing as:[2]

> ... concentration on what is happening, one's response to it as a task, and visualization of what is being achieved by the work of the uterus during contractions. The focus may be on the fantasy of the contractions as a shape provided by actual objects (furniture, architectural details, flowers, a painting) in the room, or a combination of these factors.

Stevens & Heide[44] found that attention-focusing functions effectively as an analgesia for labor pain. Such strategies are strongly supported by much psychological research. The focus may be on a competing response, as in the Kanfer & Goldfoot[45] study showing that when attention was directed to self-presented external slides, individuals were able to increase their tolerance of the pain of cold water. Focus on a competing response is also shown in the use of hypnosis as an analgesic and in the meditative states of Raj yogis, who pinpoint attention on the tip of their nose or a point on the back of their skull, and then do not react physiologically to cold water, bright lights, or sudden sounds.[46,47] Other adepts in unusual feats of pain tolerance, such as having spikes stuck through their skin, either maintain an unfocused attitude, without evaluation, or pinpoint attention totally on the pain, but without evaluation.[48] In such cases, the attitude of detachment from the pain can be reflected by an undisturbed EEG pattern of alpha or beta waves throughout performance of the feat.

Relaxation training

Relaxation training is another essential element of pain control, and is found in all childbirth training programs. A considerable body of literature supports its importance in pain control, since a state of lowered autonomic arousal is incompatible with anxiety. While progressive muscular relaxation, systematic desensitization, and autogenic training are all well-established physiological approaches to muscular relaxation, meditation traditions provide quicker methods to achieve what Benson[49] has called, the "relaxation response". One of the simplest meditation practices – maintaining a focal awareness of the flow of the breath – is taught by Rahima Baldwin in *Special Delivery* and is identical to the ancient Buddist practice of *vipassana* or insight meditation.

Hypnosis

Hypnosis or auto-hypnosis is another method utilized to induce deep relaxation for pain control. It incorporates many of the therapeutic elements already referred to – focused attention, positive expectation, and a supportive or permissive attitude – in making suggestions that alleviate anxiety. Thus, its success in pain management may be viewed from a cognitive-behavioral perspective.[50] In one technique, "glove anesthesia" is induced in one hand and the "numb, heavy wooden feeling" so produced is transferred to the other hand, the face, and eventually to the abdomen in order to "relieve the discomfort" of uterine contractions (the word "pain" is never used, as this would be countersuggestive).[51]

Control of environmental stress

Kitzinger[2] cites animal research to show how environmental stress can interfere with the physiological processes of labor and delivery. Education for childbirth therefore promotes verbal and non-verbal support from husband, obstetrician, midwife or anyone else who is part of the birthing environment. Touch relaxation and coaching techniques combine the essential elements of relaxation, massage counter-stimulus, and the direct supportive communication of a partner.[8]

Several studies agree that comfort in labor is also enhanced by a more vertical position such as the squatting posture that is adopted in many other cultures.[52–54]

Counter-stimulus methods: massage, acupuncture, TENS

The hand reflexology method of grasping combs during labor to activate points on the fingertips and balls of the hand that relate to uterine functioning is one example of counter-stimulus strategy.[8] Foot reflexology, acupressure, acupuncture and transcutaneous electrical nerve stimulation (TENS) might also share a common autonomic nervous mode of operation.

Transcutaneous electrical nerve stimulation (TENS)

The use of TENS to control pain during delivery has been evaluated by several studies. The method used in a Swedish study, which was subsequently replicated in Germany and Britain, was originally developed in the US by Shealy for the control of acute and chronic pain.[55,56] Generally, the electrodes are placed over the painful area in order to stimulate the cutaneous nerves in that area. For use in labor, four electrodes are placed on either side of the midline of the spine to stimulate the posterior primary rami of the spinal segments (T11–L1 and S2–S4) receiving the painful stimuli during labor (it is interesting to note that these are the loci of acupuncture points (BL-20, BL-27, and BL-28) which are traditionally thought to reflect female reproductive function).

The selection of this area for stimulation is based on Bonica's account of the neurological mechanism of delivery pain.[57] During the first stage, pain receptors are assumed to be activated by contractions of the uterus and dilation of the cervix. The evoked impulses are mediated in afferents which run in the hypogastric nerves and reach the spinal cord via the dorsal roots T10–L1. The pain is referred to large areas of the abdomen and back. During the second stage, pain is also caused by distension and stretching of the delivery canal, the pelvic floor, the vulva, and the perineum. The pain is localized, and the impulses reach the spinal cord mainly via the pudendal nerves and the dorsal roots S2–S4. The pain during the first stage is characterized as an ache considered to be mediated in small-diameter C fibers. During the second stage, the pain has the more localized intensive nature usually identified with the delta-afferent fibers.[57,58]

In the typical application of this technique for control of pain during labor, low-intensity stimulation is given continuously and a high-intensity stimulation could be initiated by the parturient herself whenever pain increased. Stimulation via the thoracic electrodes is maintained throughout the delivery at an amplitude that is maximal for a pleasant sensation, whereas sacral stimulation is added from the later part of the first stage. Table 56.1 summarizes the uniformly good results which have been reported.

It has been especially appreciated by those patients who complained of backache. An Austrian study compared the analgesic effects of TENS, pethidine and placebos on labor pain in 30 parturient women during the first stage of labor. No significant difference was found between the placebo, unspecific TENS, and control groups in the increase in pain during the test period.

Table 56.1 The results of the use of TENS for pain control in labor

Study	*n*	Good (%)	Moderate (%)	None (%)
Augustinsson et al[55]	147	44	44	12
Andersson et al[59]	27	48	37	15
Kanfer & Goldfoot[45]	35	20	62	18
Stewart[60]	67	31	56	13
Kubista et al[61]	102	55	24	21
Bundsen et al[62]	347	47	42	11

Patients who had received pethidine and those who had been given TENS experienced considerable relief of pain.[63] It is curious that apart from a passing reference by Shealy to its use in labor, no research on its obstetric application appeared for many years in any of the US literature. A 1996 review of 30 studies on TENS stimulation of acupuncture points in labor substantiated the conclusions of earlier research.[64]

In view of the relatively good results and lack of complications, the consensus of all the above studies is that the TENS method is recommended as a primary pain-relieving measure, to which conventional methods can be added as needed. Robson[65] comments that TENS is non-invasive and is believed to be safe for both mother and baby. It is easy to apply and can be operated throughout labor by doctor, midwife, father, or mother. Augustinsson et al[55] were most impressed by the lack of complications, since the conventional methods, including analgesic and sedative drugs, N_2O inhalation, epidural anesthesia and local blockades, all possess a varying degree of potential risks.[55] Another advantage is that TENS, since it does not give complete analgesia, does not eliminate pain as a diagnostic tool; it can be interrupted whenever needed for clinical evaluation. More importantly, perhaps, from the point of view of the woman in labor is the fact that her consciousness is not altered to the point of excluding her own active participation in, and experience of, the delivery.

Both Stewart[60] and Augustinsson et al[55] reported the method to be inadequate alone for analgesia in the second stage of labor. Augustinsson et al see this difference as possible support for the assumption that C-fiber-mediated pain is more amenable to blocking by electrical stimulation than is A fiber-mediated pain. Stewart mentions simply that many patients did not wish to use the stimulator at that time as it proved a distraction from their efforts to bear down. In this connection, it is interesting to note that "those who were well prepared and keen on natural childbirth were not always the most enthusiastic and, in fact, two of the early failures were patients who had been to relaxation classes."[60] Robson[65] explains that TENS could distract some patients from their breathing or other focus of attention learned in courses.

A related issue in the TENS literature is introduced by the comment of Andersson et al[59] that there was a correlation between the degree of hypnotisability and pain relief in their subjects. Such a correlation may, of course, imply only a susceptibility to any type of therapeutic effect. Neumark et al[63] tested this effect by including a placebo group that was given no current through the electrodes, and found that the result for the placebo group was not different from TENS applied non-specifically (i.e. incorrectly), but was significantly different from the effect of TENS placed over the relevant nerve distribution and from that of pethidine. Robson,[65] while making no attempt to assess a patient's degree of susceptibility to hypnosis, switched off the machine for at least two contractions. All patients asked for it to be switched on again, indicating that the technique was providing pain relief. Augustinsson et al[55] consider the suggestive effect, if it occurs, to be of minor significance, since several investigators have found the pain-reducing effect of TENS to be achieved through demonstrable neurophysiological mechanisms. Stewart[60] points out that the increased personal contact between patient and attendant essential to the use of this method may introduce an element of suggestibility or distraction affecting the pain experience.

Acupuncture

Hundreds of studies have investigated the efficacy and mechanisms of acupuncture analgesia for acute and chronic pain, in surgical operations, and in childbirth. In a review article of 24 studies, Lewith & Machin[66] found that the typical clinical trial showed a 70% efficacy when compared with placebo treatment. Reichmanis & Becker[67] found similar results in a review of 17 studies of acupuncture analgesia in experimentally induced pain. At the same time, somatosensory EEG-evoked potential studies have provided objective evidence of the analgesic effect of acupuncture.[68–70]

Hyodo & Gega[10] of the Osaka Medical College have reviewed the literature (summarized in Table 56.2) on acupuncture anesthesia and analgesia in normal delivery and found mixed results. For example, Wallis et al[72] reported that while 19 of the 21 volunteer parturients considered acupuncture unsuccessful in providing analgesia for labor, one-third of them indicated that they would choose acupuncture analgesia in labor again. Some authors criticize the technique as being inconsistent, unpredictable, incomplete, time-consuming, and interfering with movement and electronic monitoring.

Table 56.2 Results of acupuncture analgesia in the control of labor pain

Study	*n*	Good (%)	Poor or none (%)
Hyodo & Gega[10]			
Primapara	16	62.5	37.5
Multipara	16	93.7	7.3
Ito[71]	80	85	15
Wallis et al[72]		9–33	67–91
Abouleish & Depp[73]		80.5	19.5

In their own study, Hyodo & Gega[10] tested 32 patients, equally divided between primaparas and multiparas. Low-frequency electrical current was introduced through needles at LI-4, ST-36, and SP-6, a standard therapeutic repertory for sedation of the reproductive organs. The result, as assessed by relief noted by the patient as well as by the obstetrician's observation, was 62.5% finding good or excellent effect on the subjective scale, and 62.6% good or excellent on the objective scale among the primapara; and 93.8% subjective relief, and 93.7% objective relief among the multipara. Overall, 90% of the cases experienced relief of pain within 20 minutes of initiation of acupuncture anesthesia. They noted the considerable disparity in reports of effectiveness of acupuncture from Japan and America, and explained it as a novelty effect:

> It is natural that in Japan, where no analgesic methods are normally used, the scoring in favor of acupuncture will be high compared with that in America.

They concluded that it is useful for delivery, especially because of its safety, despite more erratic and less potent results than conventional anesthetic techniques.[10]

A considerable amount of research has focused on determining a mechanism for acupuncture analgesia. A 1995 review of studies on acupuncture effects in pain and disease pointed out that, like exercise, acupuncture produces rhythmic discharges in nerve fibers and causes the release of endogenous opioids and oxytocin. Furthermore, "experimental and clinical evidence suggests that acupuncture may affect the sympathetic system via mechanisms of the hypothalamic and brain-stem levels".[74] Animal studies continue to demonstrate that acupuncture analgesia is mediated in the central and peripheral nervous systems by opioid peptides.[75–77] The cortex and hippocampus appear to participate in the modulation of chronic pain, and the analgesic action of electroacupuncture seems to operate along this pathway.[76] A study carried out on dogs seems to verify the traditional theory of points of tonification and sedation, by differential production of sympathomimetic and parasympathomimetic effects on the cardiovascular system upon stimulation of different points.

In a study of labor induction and inhibition by electroacupuncture, Tsuei et al[78] utilized SP-6 and SP-4 points, located in the territory of the L-4 dermatome. The spleen meridian, to which these loci belong, runs across the dermatomes of L-4, L-5, L-2, and L-1, and then upward from T-12 to T-5. Since the sympathetic nerve controlling the uterus through the pelvic plexus receives preganglionic fibers from T-5 to L-4, Tsuei et al concluded that it is highly possible that stimulation of the electropermeable loci within this area may alter the physiologic function of the uterus.[78] The LI-4 points of the upper extremities, often added to the spleen meridian points in the acupunctural control of labor pain, perhaps represent the central approach to the autonomic nervous system, since these loci control pain to the head and neck. It should be noted, however, that Motoyama[79] has attempted to verify the traditional subtle anatomy of meridian pathways through tests of electrocutaneous resistance at meridian points, and claims that these effects cannot be adequately explained in terms of the conventional sympathetic dermatomes, but imply an alternative bioelectric transmission system.

The discovery of the Head McKenzie sensory zones has shown the possible mediation of the invisible meridians and points of traditional Eastern medicine between internal organs and corresponding skin areas. Nakatani[80] was able to detect the electropermeable line as an apparent viscerocutaneous autonomic nerve reflex when organic diseases are involved. Hyodo[81] has explained acupuncture stimulation as the transmission of impulses centrally from the reactive electropermeable loci, via a sympathetic afferent fiber, and the autonomic nerve in the viscera is stimulated to response by the reverse of the McKenzie theory.

CONCLUSION

This chapter has presented many of the current non-pharmacological strategies for control of pain. Since the mechanism of pain perception has been shown to involve both physiological and psychological components, the optimal treatment might combine psychological factors of preparatory information, attention focus, relaxation, and supportive communication, in conjunction with the physical stimuli of transcutaneous electrical nerve stimulation or acupuncture. In fact, such a multidisciplinary approach to patients with chronic back pain was evaluated following a 4 week program which included back schooling, psychological intervention, and treatment by acupuncture, chiropractic, the Alexander technique and a pain specialist. Significant improvement was maintained for a period of 6 months.[82] The selection, balance, and application of these treatment components should be based on consideration of an individual's coping styles. Such a treatment program could be developed to provide a more consistently effective analgesia than the individual components can provide separately. Relieving the pain of childbirth, for example, without diminishing or distorting the full consciousness of the experience for the mother, would be consistent with the goals of the contemporary physician of natural medicine.

REFERENCES

1. Krupp MA, Chatton MJ. Current medical diagnosis and treatment. Los Altos, CA: Lange Medical. 1984: p 1–5
2. Kitzinger S. Pain in childbirth. J Med Ethics 1978; 4: 119–121
3. Kitaeff R. Cognitive strategies for control of painful stress. Unpublished. 1979
4. Melzack R, Casey KC. Sensory, motivational and central control of pain. In: Kenshalo DL, ed. The skin senses. Springfield IL: CC Thomas. 1968: p 423–443
5. Feurerstein M, Skjei E. Mastering pain. New York, NY: Bantam. 1979: p 17–21
6. Melzack R, Wall PD. Pain mechanisms: a new theory. Science 1965; 150: 971–979
7. Cheng R, Pomerantz B. Electroacupuncture analgesia could be mediated by at least two pain-relieving mechanisms. endorphin and non-endorphin systems. Life Sci 1979; 25: 1957–1962
8. Baldwin R. Special delivery. Millbrae, CA: Les Femmes. 1979
9. Laukaran V, Van Den Berg B. The relationship of maternal attitude of pregnancy outcomes and obstetric complications. Am J Ob Gyn 1980; 136: 374–379
10. Hyodo M, Gega O. Use of acupuncture anesthesia for normal delivery. Am J Chin Med 1977; 5: 63–69
11. Davidson P, McDougall E. The generality of pain tolerance. J Psychosom Res 1969; 13: 83–89
12. Eysenck S. Personality and pain assessment in childbirth of married and unmarried mothers. J Mental Sci 1961; 107: 417–429
13. Levine F, Tursky B, Nichols D. Tolerance for pain, extroversion and neuroticism: failure to replicate results. Percept Motor Skills 1966; 23: 847–850
14. Morgan A, Lezard R, Prytulak S, Hilgard E. Augmenters, reducers and their reaction to cold-pressor pain in waking and suggested hypnotic analgesia. J Person Soc Psych 1970; 16: 5–11
15. Mumford J, Newton A, Ley P. Personality, pain perception and pain tolerance. Br J Psych 1973; 64: 105–107
16. Sweeney D, Fine B. Pain reactivity and field dependence. Percept Motor Skills 1965; 21: 757–758
17. Andrew J. Coping style, stress-relevant learning and recovery from surgery. Dissert Abstr 1968; 28: 1182–1183
18. Davidson P, Bobey M. Repressor sensitizer differences on repeated exposure to pain. Percept Motor Skills 1970; 31: 711–714
19. Cohen F, Lazarus R. Active coping processes, coping dispositions, and recovery from surgery. Psycho Med 1973; 35: 375–389
20. Chapman CR. Lecture. University of Washington. October, 1979
21. Bowers K. The effects of UCS temporal uncertainty on heart rate and pain. Psychophysiol 1973; 8: 382–389
22. Bandler R Jr, Madaras G, Bem D. Self-observation as a source of pain perception. J Person Soc Psych 1968; 9: 205–209
23. Geer J, Davison G, Gatchel R. Reduction of stress in humans through non-veridical perceived control of aversion stimulation. J Person Soc Psych 1970; 16: 731–738
24. Pervin L. The need to predict and control under conditions of threat. J Person Soc Psych 1963; 31: 570–585
25. Staub E, Tursky B, Schwartz G. Self-control and predictability: their effects on reactions to aversive stimulation J Person Soc Psych 1971; 18: 157–162
26. Bobey M, Davidson P. Psychological factors affecting pain tolerance. J Psychos Res 1970; 14: 371–376
27. Johnson J. Effects of accurate expectations about sensations on the sensory and distress components of pain. J Person Soc Psych 1973; 25: 381–389
28. Neufeld R, Davidson P. The effects of vicarious and cognitive rehearsal on pain tolerance. J Psychos Res 1971; 15: 329–335
29. Staub E, Kellett D. Increasing pain tolerance by information about aversive stimuli. J Person Soc Psych 1972; 21; 198–203
30. Seligman M, Maier S, Solomon R. Unpredictable and

uncontrollable aversive events. In: Brush F, ed. Aversive conditioning and learning. New York, NY: Academic Press. 1969
31. Kanfer F, Seidner M. Self-control factors enhancing and tolerance of noxious stimulation. J Person Soc Psych 1973; 25: 381–389
32. Langer E, Janis I, Wolfer J. Effects of cognitive device and preparatory information on psychological stress in surgical patients. Unpublished manuscript. Yale University. 1973
33. Croog SH, Baume RM, Nalbandian J. Pain response after psychological preparation for repeated periodontal surgery. J Am Dent Assoc 1994; 125: 1353–1360
34. Holmes DS, Houston BK. Effectiveness of situation redefinition and affective isolation in coping with stress. J Person Soc Psych 1974; 29: 212–218, 1974
35. Stevens R J, Heide F. Paper at Congress on Psychosomatic Medicine and Gynaecology. Rome, 1977
36. Newton-John TR, Spence SH. Cognitive-behavioral therapy versus EMG biofeedback in the treatment of chronic low back pain. Behav Res Ther 1995; 33: 691–697
37. Vlaeyen JW, Huazen JW, Schwerman JA et al. Behavioral rehabilitation of chronic low back pain. Br J Clin Psycho 1995; 34: 95–118
38. Turner JA, Jensen MP. Efficacy of cognitive therapy for chronic low back pain. Pain 1993; 52: 169–177
39. van Delmen AM, Fennis JF, Bleijenberg G. Cognitive-behavioral group therapy for irritable bowel syndrome. Psychosom Med 1996; 58: 508–514
40. Dworkin SF. Behavioral and educational modalities. Oral Surg Med Pathol Oral Radiol Endod 1997; 83: 128–133
41. Arathuzi KD. Effects of cognitive-behavioral strategies on pain in cancer patients. Cancer News 1994; 17: 207–214
42. Osterhaus SO, Passchier J, van der Helm-Hylkeema H et al. Effects of behavioral psychophysiological treatment on school children with migraine in a nonclinical setting. J Pediatr Psychol 1993; 18: 697–715
43. Basler HD. Group treatment for pain and discomfort. Patient Educ Couns 1993; 20: 167–175
44. Stevens R J, Heide F. Analgesic characteristics of childbirth techniques. J Psychos Res 1977; 21: 429–438
45. Kanfer F, Goldfoot D. Self-control and tolerance of noxious stimulation. Psych Reports 1966; 18: 79–85
46. Evans M, Paul G. Effects of hypnotically suggested analgesia on physiological and subjective responses to cold stress. J Consul Clin Psych 1970; 35: 362–371
47. Anand BK, Chhina ES, Singh B. Some aspects of electroencephalographic studies in yogis. EEG Clin Neurophysio 1961; 13: 452–456
48. Pelletier K, Peper E. The Chutzpah factor in altered states of consciousness. J Humanis Psych 1977; 17: 63–73
49. Benson H. The relaxation response. New York, NY: Avon. 1976
50. Chaves JF. Recent advances in the application of hypnosis to pain management. Am J Clin Hypn 1994; 37: 117–129
51. Kroger WS. Clinical and experimental hypnosis. Philadelphia, PA: Lippincott. 1963: p 197–198
52. Dunn PM. Obstetric delivery today, for better or for worse? Lancet 1976; i: 790–793
53. Flynn A, Kelly J. Continuous fetal monitoring in the ambulatory patient in labour. Br Med J 1986; 2: 842–843
54. Liu Y-C. Effects of an upright position during labor. Am J Nurs 1974; 74: 2203–2205
55. Augustinsson LE, Bohlin P, Bundsen P. Pain during delivery by transcutaneous electrical nerve stimulation. Pain 1977; 4: 59–65
56. Shealy CN, Maurer D. Transcutaneous nerve stimulation for control of pain. Surg Neurol 1974; 2: 45–57
57. Bonica JJ. Principles and practice of obstetric analgesia and anesthesia, vol I. Fundamental considerations. Philadelphia, PA: Davis. 1967
58. Bonica JJ. The nature of pain in parturition. Clin Obs Gyn 1975; 2: 499–516
59. Andersson SA, Block E, Holmgren E. Lagfrekvent transkutan elektrisk stimulering for smartlindring vid forlassning. Lakartidringen 1976; 73: 2421–2423
60. Stewart P. Transcutaneous nerve stimulation as a method of analgesia in labour. Anaesthesia 1979; 34: 361–364
61. Kubista E, Kucera H, Riss P. The effect of transcutaneous nerve stimulation on labor pain. Geburtsh.u.Frauenheilk 1978; 38: 1079–1084
62. Bundsen P, Carlsson CA, Forssman L, Tyreman NO. Pain relief during delivery by transcutaneous electrical nerve stimulation. Prakt Anasth 1978; 13: 20–27
63. Neumark J, Pausner G, Scherzer W. Pain relief in childbirth. an analysis of the analgesic effects of transcutaneous nerve stimulation (TNS), pethidine and placebos. Prokt Anasth 1978; 13: 13–20
64. Kemp T. The use of transcutaneous electrical nerve stimulation on acupuncture points in labor. Midwives 1996; 109: 318–320
65. Robson JE. Transcutaneous nerve stimulation for pain relief in labor. Anesthesia 1979; 34: 357–360
66. Lewith GT, Machin D. On the evaluation of the clinical effects of acupuncture. Pain 1983; 16: 111–127
67. Reichmanis M, Becker RO. Relief of experimentally-induced pain by stimulation at acupuncture loci. a review. Comp Med East West 1977; 5: 281–288
68. Chapman CR, Colpitts YM, Benedetti C et al. Evoked potential assessment of acupunctural analgesia. Pain 1980; 9: 183–197
69. Kumar A, Tandon OP, Bhattarcharya A et al. Somatosensory evoked potential changes following electroacupuncture therapy in chronic pain patients. Anaesthesia 1995; 50: 411–414
70. Xu X, Shibaski H, Shindo K. Effects of acupuncture on somatosensory evoked potentials: a review. J Clin Neurophys 1993; 10: 370–377
71. Ito T. Painless labor with acupuncture anesthesia. The Japan J Anesth 1974; 23: 10–16
72. Wallis L et al. An evaluation of acupuncture analgesia in obstetrics. Anesthes 1974; 41: 596–601
73. Abouleish E, Depp R. Acupuncture in obstetrics. Anesthes Analges. 1975; 51: 1 83
74. Anderson S, Lundeberg T. Acupuncture – from empiricism to science. Med Hypoth 1995; 45: 271–281
75. Wu GC, Shu J, Coo X. Involvement of opioid peptides of the preoptic area during electroacupuncture analgesia. Acupunc Electro-Therap Res 1995; 20: 1–6
76. Xhu L, Li C, Ji C, Li W. The role of opiate-like substances in peripheral acupuncture analgesia in arthritic rats. Chen Tzu Yen Chiu Acupunc Res 1993; 18: 214–218
77. Xhou L, Jiang JG, Wu GC, Cao XD. Changes of endogenous opioid peptides content in RPGL during acupuncture analgesia. Shangli Hsueh Pao (Acta Physiologica Sinica) 1993; 45: 36–43
78. Tsuei J J, Facog Y-F L, Sharma S. The influence of acupuncture stimulation during pregnancy. J Obs Gyn 1977; 50: 479–488
79. Motoyama H. How to measure and diagnose the functions of meridians and corresponding internal organs. Tokyo: The Institute for Religious Psychology. 1976
80. Nakatani Y. A guide for application of Ryodoraku autonomous nerve regulatory therapy. Tokyo: Japanese Society of Ryodoraku Autonomic Nervous System. 1972
81. Hyodo M. New management of pain. Tokyo: Chiyugai Igakushiya. 1970
82. Eikayam O, Ben Itzhak S, Avrahami E. Multidisciplinary approach to chronic back pain. Clin Exp Rheumatol 1996; 14: 281–288

CHAPTER CONTENTS

57

Role of dietary fiber in health and disease

Michael T. Murray, ND

Joseph E. Pizzorno Jr, ND

INTRODUCTION

The appreciation of the role of diet in determining the level of health continues to grow. A substantial body of research has now well established that certain dietary practices cause, as well as prevent, a wide range of diseases. In addition, the research is now showing that certain diets and foods can provide immediate therapeutic benefit.

This chapter discusses the major diseases of Western society and how they relate to one key component of the diet: dietary fiber. The dietary fiber hypothesis has two basic components:

- a diet rich in foods which contain plant cell walls (i.e. whole grains, legumes, fruits, and vegetables) is protective against a wide variety of diseases, in particular those that are prevalent in Western society
- a diet providing a low intake of plant cell walls is a causative factor in the etiology of these diseases and provides conditions under which other etiological factors are more active.

The term "Western diet" is used throughout this chapter, as well as in many other parts of the textbook. It refers to the typical diet of Western peoples, also referred to as "foods of commerce". It consists of a high intake of refined carbohydrates, saturated fats, processed foods, salt and cholesterol, and an extremely low intake of dietary fiber.

The primitive diet

Detailed anatomical and historical evidence suggests that humans evolved as "hunter-gatherers" i.e. humans appear to be omnivores capable of surviving on both gathered (plant) and hunted (animal) foods.[1] However, while the human gastrointestinal tract is capable of digesting both animal and plant foods, there are indications that it functions better with plant foods.[2] There is a tremendous amount of evidence showing that deviating from a predominantly plant-based diet is a major factor in the development of heart disease, cancer, strokes, arthritis, and many other chronic degenerative diseases. It is now the recommendation of many health and medical organizations that the human diet should focus primarily on plant-based foods – vegetables, fruits, grains, legumes, nuts, seeds, etc. Such a diet is thought to offer significant protection against the development of chronic degenerative disease.[3–5]

DIETARY FIBER AND CHRONIC DEGENERATIVE DISEASE

The belief in the beneficial effects of fiber in the diet goes back to at least 1585. However, the link between dietary fiber and chronic disease in the medical literature originated to a great extent from the work of two medical pioneers, Denis Burkitt MD and Hugh Trowell MD, authors of *Western diseases: their emergence and prevention*, which was first published in 1981.[3] Based on extensive studies examining the rate of diseases in various populations (epidemiological data) and his own observations of primitive cultures, Burkitt formulated the following sequence of events:

- *First stage*. The primal diet of plant eaters contains large amounts of unprocessed starch staples; there are few examples of chronic degenerative diseases like osteoarthritis, heart disease, diabetes, and cancer.
- *Second stage*. Commencing Westernization of diet, obesity and diabetes commonly appear in privileged groups.
- *Third stage*. With moderate Westernization of the diet, constipation, hemorrhoids, varicose veins, and appendicitis become common complaints.
- *Fourth stage*. Finally, with full Westernization of the diet, chronic degenerative diseases like osteoarthritis, rheumatoid arthritis, gout, heart disease, cancer, etc. are extremely common.

Although now extremely well-recognized, the work of Burkitt and Trowell is actually a continuation of the landmark work of Weston A. Price, a dentist and author of *Nutrition and physical degeneration*.[6] In the early 1900s, Dr Price traveled the world observing changes in teeth and palate (orthodontic) structure as various cultures discarded traditional dietary practices in favor of a more "civilized" diet. Price was able to follow individuals as well as cultures over periods of 20–40 years, and carefully documented the onset of degenerative diseases as their diets became more Westernized.

It is now well documented that diet is the major factor responsible for many chronic degenerative diseases. In 1984, the National Research Council's Food and Nutrition Board established the Committee on Diet and Health and undertook a comprehensive analysis on diet and major chronic diseases.[5] It is the Food and Nutrition Board which develops the Recommended Dietary Allowance (RDA) guidelines on the desirable amounts of essential nutrients in the diet. Their findings, as well as those of the US Surgeon General and other research groups, have brought to the forefront the need for Americans to change their eating habits to reduce their risk for chronic disease. Table 57.1 lists diseases with convincing links to a diet low in dietary fiber and plant foods. Many of these now common diseases were extremely rare before the 20th century.

Table 57.1 Diseases highly associated with a low-fiber diet

Metabolic	Obesity, gout, diabetes, kidney stones, gallstones
Cardiovascular	Hypertension, cerebrovascular disease, ischemic heart disease, varicose veins, deep vein thrombosis, pulmonary embolism
Colonic	Constipation, appendicitis, diverticulitis, diverticulosis, hemorrhoids, colon cancer, irritable bowel syndrome, ulcerative colitis, Crohn's disease
Other	Dental caries, autoimmune disorders, pernicious anemia, multiple sclerosis, thyrotoxicosis, dermatological conditions

Trends in US food consumption

During this century, food consumption patterns have changed dramatically: total dietary fat intake has increased from 32% of the calories in 1909 to 43% in 1985; overall carbohydrate intake dropped from 57 to 46%; and protein intake has remained fairly stable at about 11%.[5] Compounding these detrimental changes are the individual food choices accounting for the changes. There has been a rise in the consumption of meat, fats and oils, and sugars and sweeteners, in conjunction with the decreased consumption of non-citrus fruits, vegetables, potatoes, and grain products. These changes have resulted in the percentage of calories from starches or complex carbohydrates, as found naturally occurring in grains and vegetables, to drop from 68% in 1909 to 47% in 1980. Currently, more than half of the carbohydrates being consumed are in the form of sugars (sucrose, corn syrup, etc.) being added to foods as sweetening agents. High consumption of refined sugars is linked to many chronic diseases, including obesity, diabetes, heart disease, and cancer.

DEFINITION AND COMPOSITION OF DIETARY FIBER

Generally, the term "dietary fiber" refers to the components of plant cell wall and non-nutritive residues. Originally, the definition was restricted to substances that are not digestible by the endogenous secretions of the human digestive tract. This latter definition is specious, since it depends on an exact understanding of what exactly is not digestible.

Table 57.2 Dietary fiber constituents of the food groups

Food group	Main dietary fibers
Fruits and vegetables	Cellulose, hemicellulose, lignin, pectic substances, cutin, waxes
Grains	Cellulose, hemicellulose, lignin, phenolic esters
Seeds (other than grains)	Cellulose, hemicellulose, pectic substances, guar endosperm
Seed husk of *Plantago ovata*	Arabinogalacturonosyl-phamno-xylan (mucilage)
Food additives	Gum arabic, alginate, carrageenan, carboxymethylcellulose

Table 57.3 Classification of dietary fiber

Fiber class	Chemical structure	Plant part	Food sources	Physiological effect
I. Cellulose	Unbranched 1-4-beta-D-glucose polymer	Principal plant wall component	Wheat bran	Increases fecal weight and size
II. Non-cellulose polysaccharides				
A. Hemicelluloses	Mixture of pentose and hexose molecules in branching chains	Plant cell walls	Oat bran	Increases fecal weight and size, binds bile acids
B. Gums	Branched chain uronic acid containing polymers		Karaya, gum arabic	Laxative
C. Mucilages	Similar to hemicelluloses	Endosperm of plant seeds	Guar, legumes, psyllium	Hydrocolloids that bind steroids and delay gastric emptying, heavy metal chelation
D. Pectins	Mixture of methyl esterified galacturan, galactan, and arabinose in varying proportions		Citrus rind, apple, onion skin	As above
E. Algal polysaccharides	Polymerized D-mannuronic acid and L-glucuronic acid		Algin, agar, carrageenan	As above
III. Lignins	Non-carbohydrate polymeric phenylpropene	Woody part of plant	Wood (40–50%), wheat (25%), apple (25%), cabbage (6%)	Antioxidants, anti-carcinogenic

The composition of the plant cell wall varies according to the species of plant. Typically, the dry cell wall contains 35% cellulose, 45% non-cellulose polysaccharides, 17% lignins, 3% protein, and 2% ash.[7–9] It is important to recognize that dietary fiber is a complex of these constituents, and supplementation of a single component does not substitute for a diet rich in high-fiber foods. However, in some clinical conditions the use of specific components is a useful adjunct to a healthy diet. Tables 57.2 and 57.3 summarize the classifications of dietary fibers.

Cellulose

The best known dietary fiber component is cellulose. This unbranched 1-4-beta-D-glucose polymer ranges in size from 3,000 to 100,000 glucose units. It is a relatively insoluble, hydrophilic material. This ability to bind water accounts for its effect of increasing fecal size and weight. Although undigestible by humans, it is partially degraded by the microflora of the gut. This anaerobic process (fermentation) occurs in the colon, results in the degradation of about 50% of the cellulose, and is an important source of short-chain fatty acids (SCFAs).[7,8] SCFAs have very important properties in the colon, as discussed below.

Non-cellulose polysaccharides

The majority of polysaccharides in the plant cell wall are a non-cellulose type, i.e. they are water-soluble and posses diverse properties. Included in this class are hemicelluloses, gums, mucilages, algal polysaccharides, and pectin substances.[7–9]

Hemicelluloses

These compounds contain a mixture of pentose and hexose molecules in branched-chain configurations of much smaller size than cellulose. Their ability to increase fecal weight is dependent on the pentose fraction. The hemicelluloses are also an important source of SCFAs via bacterial degradation.[7–9]

Pectin and pectin-like substances

Pectins are found in all plant cell walls as well as in the outer skin and rind of fruits and vegetables. For example, the rind of an orange contains 30% pectin; an apple peel 15%; and onion skins 12%. The gel-forming properties of pectin are well known to anyone who has made a jelly or jam. These same gel-forming qualities are responsible for the cholesterol-lowering effects of pectins. Pectins lower cholesterol by binding the cholesterol and bile acids in the gut and promoting their excretion.[7–9]

Gums

Plant gums are a complex group of water-soluble, branched-chain, uronic acid-containing polymers. They are produced by the plant in response to injury, and are commercially produced by incising a plant or tree and collecting the fluid extract. Gums are used as emulsifiers, thickeners, and stabilizers by the food industry and as laxatives in pharmaceuticals.[7–9]

Mucilages

Structurally, mucilages resemble the hemicelluloses, but they are not classed as such due to their unique location in the seed portion of the plant. They are generally mixed with the endosperm of the plant seeds, where they retain water, preventing seed desiccation.

Guar gum, found in leguminous plants, is the most widely studied mucilage. It is isolated from the endosperm of *Cyamopsis tetragonolobus*, a plant cultivated in India for livestock feed. It is used commercially as a protective colloid, stabilizer, thickening and film-forming agent for paper sizing, cheese, salad dressings, ice cream, soups, toothpaste, pharmaceutical jelly, lotion, skin cream, and tablets. It is also used as a laxative. Guar gum and other mucilages are perhaps the most potent cholesterol-lowering agents of the gel-forming hydrocolloids, including pectin and glucomannan. Guar gum has been shown to reduce fasting and postprandial glucose and insulin levels in both healthy and diabetic subjects; and it has decreased body weight and hunger ratings when taken with meals by obese subjects. Psyllium seed husk (*Plantago ovata*) is another example of a mucilage which is widely used as a bulking and laxative agent.[7,8]

Algal polysaccharides

Included in this category are alginic acid, agar, and carrageenan. Marine-derived polysaccharides are used extensively by the food industry. Alginate has been shown to inhibit heavy metal uptake in the gut, as do other gel-forming fibers. Agar is used as a thickening agent and as a gel for holding microbiological media. It has laxative and fecal bulk-increasing activity.[7,8]

Carrageenan is used in milk and chocolate products due to its ability to react with milk proteins. However, unlike other plant polysaccharides, it adversely affects the intestinal mucosa.[7,8] It has been shown in rats to induce ulcer formation in the cecum, due to the promotion of mucosal macrophage release of lysosomal enzymes. Other rat studies have shown carrageenan to enhance carcinogen induction of neoplasia, colerectal carcinoma, birth defects, and hepatomegaly.[10]

Lignins and lignans

Lignins are composed of aromatic polymers of conyiferyl, para-coumaryl, and sinapyl alcohols in varying ratios. Vanillin (artificial vanilla) and other aromatic chemicals are synthesized from lignins. Lignans are fiber compounds related to lignins that are typically composed of cinnamic acid, cinnamyl alcohol, propenylbenzene, and allylbenzene precursor units. Many plant lignans show important properties, such as anticancer, antibacterial, antifungal, and antiviral activity. Plant lignins are metabolized by the gut flora into the animal lignins enterolactone and enterodiol, both of which posses anti-estrogenic activity and are believed to be protective against cancer.[11]

Phytic acid

In the plant, phytic acid (inositol hexaphosphoric acid) is responsible for storing minerals such as calcium, phosphorus, magnesium, and potassium. There is some concern that phytates can adversely affect the uptake and utilization of many minerals, including calcium, iron, and zinc. The major sources of phytate in the diet are cereal grains and legumes (see Table 57.4). Phytate is destroyed by heat and by the enzyme phytase during the leavening of bread.[7,8]

Phytic acid exerts impressive antioxidant and antitumor effects.[12–14] When administered in drinking water or injected, phytic acid has demonstrated a consistent antitumor effect in animals against colon cancer and fibrosarcomas. Clinical trials in humans are in preparation.

Table 57.4 Occurrence of phytic acid in plant tissues

Plant phytic acid	Percentage dry weight
Soybeans	1.4
Wheat	0.9
Corn	1.1
Rice	0.9
Peanuts	1.9
Sesame seeds	5.4
Lima beans	2.5
Barley	1.0
Oats	0.8

Table 57.5 Beneficial effects of dietary fiber

- Decreased intestinal transit time
- Delayed gastric emptying resulting in reduced postprandial hyperglycemia
- Increased satiety
- Increased pancreatic secretion
- Increased stool weight
- More advantageous intestinal microflora
- Increased production of short-chain fatty acids
- Decreased serum lipids
- More soluble bile

PHYSIOLOGICAL EFFECTS OF DIETARY FIBER

It is beyond the scope of this chapter to detail all known effects of dietary fiber on humans. Instead, we will cover effects of greatest clinical significance (stool weight, transit time, digestion, colon function, short-chain fatty acids, and colon flora). Beneficial effects of dietary fiber are given in Table 57.5.

Stool weight and transit time

Fiber has long been used in the treatment of constipation. Dietary fiber, particularly the water-insoluble, hydrophilic fibers such as cellulose (e.g. bran), increases stool weight as a result of their water-holding properties.[7–9] Transit time, the time taken for passage of material from the mouth to the anus, is greatly reduced on a high-fiber diet. Cultures consuming a high-fiber diet (100–170 g/day) usually have a transit time of 30 hours and a fecal weight of 500 g. In contrast, Europeans and Americans who eat a typical, low-fiber diet (20 g/day) have a transit time of greater than 48 hours and a fecal weight of only 100 g.[3,15] Interestingly, when fiber is added to the diet of subjects with abnormally rapid transit times (less than 24 hours) it causes slowing of the transit time.[7,8]

Dietary fiber's effect on transit time is apparently directly related to its effect on stool weight and size. A larger, bulkier stool passes through the colon more easily, requires less intraluminal pressure, and subsequently less straining.[1–4] It has been hypothesized that the decreased intraluminal pressure (due to the greater leverage the colon mucosa has on a larger stool) results in less hydrostatic stress on the colon wall and therefore avoids the ballooning effect, which results in diverticuli.

The increased intestinal transit time associated with the Western diet allows prolonged exposure of various compounds, both natural and man-made, to the intestinal flora, resulting in increased conversion to potential carcinogens.[3,4,7,8]

Digestion

Although dietary fiber increases the rate of transit through the GI tract, it slows gastric emptying, thus reducing postprandial hyperglycemia in both normal and diabetic subjects.[7,8] Pancreatic enzyme secretion and activity also increase in response to fiber, although excessive levels of fiber (greater than 10% of the meal by weight) have a converse effect.[16] A number of research studies have examined the effects of fiber on mineral absorption. Although the results have been somewhat contradictory, it now appears that large amounts of dietary fiber may result in impaired absorption and/or negative balance of some minerals. While fiber as a dietary component does not appear to interfere with the minerals in other foods, supplemental fiber, especially hemicelluloses, may result in a negative mineral balance.[2–4]

Short-chain fatty acids (SCFAs)

The fermentation of dietary fiber by the intestinal flora produces three main end products:

- short-chain fatty acids
- various gases
- energy.

The SCFAs, acetic, proprionic, and butyric acids, are the main anions in the large intestine and have many important physiological functions. For every 20 g of fiber consumed each day, approximately 200 mmol of SCFAs will be produced, of which 62 will be acetate, 25 proprionate, and 16 butyrate.[8]

Proprionate and acetate are transported directly to the liver and utilized for energy production, while butyrate provides an important energy source for the colonic mucosa. In fact, butyrate is the preferred substrate for energy metabolism in the distal colon.[7,8] Butyrate production may also be responsible for the anti-cancer properties of dietary fiber.[7,8,17] Even at extremely low concentrations, butyrate has been shown, in vitro, to profoundly affect gene expression and other nucleic processes, such as DNA synthesis, resulting in suppressed cell proliferation in both normal and malignant cells. Butyrate causes trophic effects on normal colonocytes, stops the growth of neoplastic colonocytes, inhibits the pre-neoplastic hyperproliferation induced by certain tumor promoters in vitro, inhibits the expression of certain protooncogenes and causes differentiation of colon cancer cell lines.[18] Some of these effects are due to the acetylation of histones and the stabilization of the chromatin structure. Short-chain fatty acids are exhibiting impressive anti-cancer results in both animal and human experiments.[17] Butyrate is also being used in enemas in the treatment of ulcerative colitis.

Certain fibers appear to be more effective than others in increasing the levels of SCFAs in the colon. Pectins (both apple and citrus, guar gum and other legume fibers) and vegetable fiber isolates produce more SCFAs than wheat fiber, corn fiber or oat bran.[7,8]

Intestinal bacterial flora

Dietary fiber appears to improve all aspects of colon function. Of central importance is the role it plays in maintaining a "suitable" colonic bacterial flora. A low-fiber intake is associated with both an overgrowth of Enterobacteriaceae and other endotoxin-producing bacteria and a lower percentage of *Lactobacillus* and other acidophilic bacteria.[7,8] A diet high in dietary fiber promotes acidophilic bacteria through the increased synthesis of colonic SCFAs, which reduces the colon pH, a condition conducive to the growth of beneficial bacteria.

DISEASES ASSOCIATED WITH A LOW-FIBER DIET

Because of the important physiological effects of dietary fiber, a diet low in dietary fiber will obviously lead to altered physiology or disease. The diseases with the strongest correlation with a lack of dietary fiber are diseases of the colon and gastrointestinal tract, heart disease and gallstones, obesity, and diabetes. Each of these will be briefly discussed below.

Diseases of the colon and gastrointestinal disorders

The epidemiological and experimental data documenting the protective effect of dietary fiber on colon cancer are overwhelming. There is evidence for similar strong links with other common diseases of the colon – diverticulitis, diverticulosis, irritable bowel syndrome, ulcerative colitis, and appendicitis as well as hemorrhoids, peptic ulcers, and hiatal hernia.[3,4,7,8] Furthermore, these very same diseases will often respond to a high fiber diet.

Heart disease and gallstones

Dietary fiber has been shown to be quite protective against heart disease and gallstones. A diet high in dietary fiber is known to reduce total cholesterol and triglyceride levels while increasing HDL-cholesterol levels and the production and storage of less saturated bile acids.[3,4,7,8]

The binding of bile acids and micellar components to various grains, food fibers, and isolated fiber compounds results in the reduction of the enterohepatic circulation of bile salts and cholesterol. Loss of cholesterol and bile salts through the feces is the major pathway for elimination of these compounds from the body. Dietary fiber also decreases cholesterol biosynthesis and increases the conversion of cholesterol to the bile acids via activation of the vitamin C-dependent enzyme 7-alpha-hydroxylase, the rate-limiting step in bile acid synthesis.[7,8] This enhancement of bile acid synthesis and excretion is the result of dietary fiber's preferential binding of deoxycholic acid, resulting in a compensatory increase in circulating levels of chenodeoxycholic acid. Chenodeoxycholic acid has been shown to inhibit cholesterol absorption and synthesis at its rate-limiting enzyme HMG-CoA reductase.[8] Binding of chenodeoxycholic acid by dietary fiber results in an increase in the taurocholate to glycocholate ratio. The ultimate result of these alterations in bile salt concentrations and ratios is a less saturated bile which solubilizes cholesterol more effectively and is resistant to stone formation.

Obesity

A dietary fiber-deficient diet is an important etiological factor in the development of obesity.[3,4,7,8] Dietary fiber plays a role in preventing obesity by:

- increasing the amount of necessary chewing, thus slowing the eating process
- increasing fecal caloric loss
- altering digestive hormone secretion
- improving glucose tolerance
- inducing satiety by increased gastric filling, stimulation of cholecystokinin release, and intestinal bulking action.

Other effects of dietary fiber on obesity are discussed below under diabetes mellitus – 60–90% of type II diabetics are obese.

Diabetes mellitus

Epidemiological and experimental data show diabetes mellitus to be one of the diseases most clearly related to inadequate dietary fiber intake.[3,4,7,8] Clinical trials that have demonstrated the beneficial therapeutic effect of dietary fiber on diabetes have further substantiated this association (discussed below). Dietary fiber's prevention and modulation of diabetes is due to its effects on glucose and, subsequently, insulin levels. A high-complex carbohydrate, high-fiber diet reduces postprandial hyperglycemia (largely by delaying of gastric emptying and thereby reducing insulin secretion) and increases tissue sensitivity to insulin (how, or if, this relates to chromium uptake and metabolism has not been determined).[7,8] Fermentation products of fiber, chiefly SCFAs, enhance hepatic glucose metabolism and may further contribute to the ameliorating effects of dietary fiber on diabetes.

CLINICAL USE OF DIETARY FIBER

The best and most cost-effective way of using dietary fiber in a clinical setting is via encouraging a diet rich in plant foods (see Table 57.6 for the dietary fiber content of selected foods). A good goal for dietary fiber intake

Table 57.6 Dietary fiber content of selected foods

Food	Serving	Calories	Grams of fiber
Fruits			
Apple (with skin)	1 medium	81	3.5
Banana	1 medium	105	2.4
Cantaloupe	¼ melon	30	1.0
Cherries (sweet)	10	49	1.2
Grapefruit	½ medium	38	1.6
Orange	1 medium	62	2.6
Peach (with skin)	1	37	1.9
Pear (with skin)	½ large	61	3.1
Prunes	3	60	3.0
Raisins	¼ cup	106	3.1
Raspberries	½ cup	35	3.1
Strawberries	1 cup	45	3.0
Vegetables (raw)			
Bean sprouts	½ cup	13	1.5
Celery (diced)	½ cup	10	1.1
Cucumber	½ cup	8	0.4
Lettuce	1 cup	10	0.9
Mushrooms	½ cup	10	1.5
Pepper (green)	½ cup	9	0.5
Spinach	1 cup	8	1.2
Tomato	1 medium	20	1.5
Vegetables (cooked)			
Asparagus (cut)	1 cup	30	2.0
Beans (green)	1 cup	32	3.2
Broccoli	1 cup	40	4.4
Brussels sprouts	1 cup	56	4.6
Cabbage (red)	1 cup	30	2.8
Carrots	1 cup	48	4.6
Cauliflower	1 cup	28	2.2
Corn	½ cup	87	2.9
Kale	1 cup	44	2.8
Parsnip	1 cup	102	5.4
Potato (with skin)	1 medium	106	2.5
Potato (without skin)	1 medium	97	1.4
Spinach	1 cup	42	4.2
Sweet potatoes	1 medium	160	3.4
Zucchini	1 cup	22	3.6
Legumes			
Baked beans	½ cup	155	8.8
Dried peas (cooked)	½ cup	115	4.7
Kidney beans (cooked)	½ cup	110	7.3
Lima beans (cooked)	½ cup	64	4.5
Lentils (cooked)	½ cup	97	3.7
Navy beans (cooked)	½ cup	112	6.0
Rice, breads, pastas, and flour			
Bran muffins	1 muffin	104	2.5
Bread (white)	1 slice	78	0.4
Bread (whole wheat)	1 slice	61	1.4
Crisp bread, rye	2 crackers	50	2.0
Rice, brown (cooked)	½ cup	97	1.0
Rice, white (cooked)	½ cup	82	0.2
Spaghetti (reg. cooked)	½ cup	155	1.1
Spaghetti (whole wheat, cooked)	½ cup	155	3.9
Breakfast cereals			
All-Bran	⅓ cup	71	8.5
Bran Chex	⅔ cup	91	4.6
Corn Bran	⅔ cup	98	5.4
Cornflakes	1¼ cup	110	0.3
Grape Nuts	¼ cup	101	1.4
Oatmeal	¾ cup	108	1.6
Raisin Bran-type	⅔ cup	115	4.0
Shredded Wheat	⅔ cup	102	2.6
Nuts			
Almonds	10 nuts	79	1.1
Filberts	10 nuts	54	0.8
Peanuts	10 nuts	105	1.4

is 25–35 g daily. This can easily be achieved if the dietary focus is on whole, unprocessed, plant foods.

In addition to the well-known use of dietary fiber as a laxative, the principle use of supplemental dietary fiber is in the treatment of irritable bowel syndrome and other functional disturbances of the colon, elevated cholesterol levels, and obesity.

The best fiber sources for non-laxative effects are psyllium, guar gum, glucomannan, gum karaya, and pectin, because they are rich in water-soluble fibers. While there are many fiber supplements to choose from, the most clinically effective are those that are rich in water-soluble fiber and low in added sugar or other sweeteners.

Irritable bowel syndrome

The treatment of irritable bowel syndrome (IBS) by increasing the intake of dietary fiber has a long, although irregular, history. In general, consuming a diet rich in complex carbohydrates and dietary fiber while avoiding sugar and refined foods is effective in many cases. The most effective fiber supplements are the water-soluble forms. However, the type of fiber often used in both research and clinical practice is wheat bran.[1] As wheat is among the most commonly implicated foods in malabsorptive and allergic conditions, the use of wheat bran is usually not indicated in individuals with symptoms of IBS since food allergy is a significant causative factor in this condition. In addition, while patients with constipation are likely to respond to wheat bran, those with diarrhea may actually worsen their symptoms.

Elevated cholesterol levels

A recent review article concluded that soluble-fiber supplementation was very effective in lowering cholesterol levels.[19] Specifically, a significant reduction in the level of serum total cholesterol was found in 68 of the 77 (88%) studies reviewed. The effect of soluble fiber supplementation was clearly dose-dependent. In other words, the higher the intake of soluble fiber, the greater the reduction in serum cholesterol. The average doses and reductions noted in clinical trials are shown in Table 57.7.

Many of the studies utilized oat bran or oatmeal as

Table 57.7 Cholesterol-lowering effects of various fibers

Fiber	Dosage (g)	Typical reduction in total cholesterol
Oat bran (dry)	50–100	20%
Guar gum	9–15	10%
Pectin	6–10	5%
Psyllium	10–20	10–20%
Vegetable fiber	27	10%

the source of fiber. The overwhelming majority of these studies demonstrated that individuals with high cholesterol levels will experience significant reductions with frequent oatmeal or oat bran consumption. In contrast, individuals with normal or low cholesterol levels will experience little change. In individuals with high cholesterol levels (above 220 mg/dl) the consumption of the equivalent of 3 g of soluble oat fiber lowers total cholesterol by 8–23%. This is highly significant as with each 1% drop in serum cholesterol level there is a 2% decrease in the risk of developing heart disease. Three grams of fiber would be provided by approximately one bowl of ready-to-eat oat bran cereal or oat meal. Although oatmeal's fiber content (7%) is less than that of oat bran (15–26%), it has been determined that the polyunsaturated fatty acids contribute as much to the cholesterol-lowering effects of oats as the fiber content. Although oat bran has a higher fiber content, oatmeal is higher in polyunsaturated fatty acids. In practical terms, the dosage level for dry oat bran would be ⅓–1 cup; for dry oatmeal 1–1⅔ cups.[19,20]

Obesity

When taken with water before meals, water-soluble fiber sources bind to the water in the stomach to form a gelatinous mass that makes an individual feel full. As a result, they will be less likely to overeat. However, the benefits of fiber go well beyond this mechanical effect. Fiber supplements have been shown to enhance blood sugar control and insulin effects, as well as actually reduce the number of calories absorbed by the intestines.[7] In some of the clinical studies demonstrating weight loss, fiber supplements were shown to reduce the number of calories absorbed by 30–180 calories/day. Over the course of a year, this could result in a reduction of 3–18 pounds.

The most impressive results in weight loss studies have been achieved with guar gum, a water-soluble fiber obtained from the Indian cluster bean (*Cyamopsis tetragonoloba*). In one study, nine women weighing between 160 and 242 pounds were given 10 g of guar gum immediately before lunch and dinner. They were told not to consciously alter their eating habits. After 2 months, the women reported an average weight loss of 9.4 pounds – over 1 pound/week. Reductions were also noted for cholesterol and triglyceride levels.[21] It is estimated that a person will lose 50–100% more weight by supplementing their diet with fiber than by simply restricting calories alone (see Table 57.8 for information on clinical studies of the treatment of obesity with dietary fiber supplements).

Cancer prevention

The body of research documenting the cancer-preventing effects of a high-fiber diet has continued to accumulate. In addition to the epidemiological associations, researchers have now also performed prospective and supplementation studies. Virtually every study has shown a significant protective effect of dietary fiber for a wide range of cancers.

Several recent studies have shown benefit for prevention of breast cancer. One representative study evaluated the association between breast cancer and dietary intake in two Chinese populations (Shanghai and Tianjin) who are at low risk for breast cancer. These populations have one-fifth the rate of breast cancer of US white women. There were two case-controlled studies. In the 834 women studied, the intake of crude fiber, carotene and vitamin C showed a strong significant inverse association with breast cancer risk. The effect was closely associated with the intake of green vegetables. The women in the lowest tertile intake of crude fiber intake and the highest tertile intake of fat intake had a 2.9-fold increased risk for breast cancer relative to those in the highest tertile of crude fiber intake and the lowest tertile of fat intake.[33]

The same protective effect has also been found in

Table 57.8 Clinical studies of the treatment of obesity with dietary fiber supplements

Fiber	Number of subjects	Length of study	Dosage (g/day)	Calorie Restriction	Average weight loss (fiber) (lbs)	Average weight loss (placebo)	Reference
Guar	9	2 months	20	None	9.4	No placebo group	21
Guar	7	1 year	20	None	61.9	No placebo group	22
Guar	21	2.5 months	20	None	15.6	No placebo group	23
Guar	33	2.5 months	15	None	5.5	0.9 lbs	24
Glucomannan	20	2 months	3	None	5.5	Weight gain of 1.5 lbs	25
Glucomannan	20	2 months	3	None	8.14	0.44 lbs	26
Citrus Pectin	14	4 weeks	5.56	Yes	12.8	No placebo group	27
Mixture A	60	12 weeks	5	Yes	18.7	14.7 lbs	28
Mixture A	89	11 weeks	10	Yes	13.9	9.2 lbs	29
Mixture B	45	3 months	7	Yes	13.6	9 lbs	30
Mixture B	97	3 months	7	Yes	10.8	7.3 lbs	31
Mixture B	52	6 months	7	Yes	12.1	6.1 lbs	32

Mixture A, 80% fiber from grains/20% fiber from citrus; mixture B, 90% insoluble/10% soluble fiber from beet, barley, and citrus fibers.

fibrocystic disease of the breast. In a study of the diet of 354 women with benign proliferative epithelial disorders of the breast who were compared with 354 matched controls and 189 unmatched controls, an inverse association between dietary fiber and the risk of benign, proliferative, epithelial disorders of the breasts was observed.[34]

The protective effects of supplemental dietary fiber have now been demonstrated, even in those with previous colon cancer. A total of 411 patients with colorectal adenomas were placed on a 25% fat content diet, supplemented with 25 g of wheat bran daily, and a capsule of 20 mg of beta-carotene daily. Patients with the combination of a low-fat diet and added wheat bran had zero large adenomas at both 2 and 4 years, a statistically significant effect compared to the control group.[35]

DOSAGE RECOMMENDATIONS

When using dietary fiber supplements, encourage patients to start out with a small dosage and increase gradually. Since water-soluble fibers are fermented by intestinal bacteria, a great deal of gas can be produced. If the patient is not accustomed to a high-fiber diet, an increase in dietary fiber can lead to increased flatulence and abdominal discomfort. Start out with a dosage between 1 and 2 g before meals and at bedtime and gradually increase the dosage to 5 g.

POSSIBLE ADVERSE EFFECTS

Mineral malabsorption

A number of research studies have examined the effects of fiber on mineral absorption. Although the results have been somewhat contradictory, it now appears that large amounts of dietary fiber may result in impaired absorption and/or negative balance of some minerals. Fiber as a dietary component does not appear to interfere with the minerals in other foods. However, supplemental fiber, especially wheat bran, may result in a mineral deficiencies. Fiber supplements may also inhibit the absorption of certain drugs. A good recommendation would be for the patient to take the fiber supplement away from medications.

Safety

If a patient has a disorder of the esophagus, fiber supplements in a pill form are contraindicated as they may expand in the esophagus and lead to obstruction.[36] Fiber supplements in capsules appear to be slightly better tolerated than tablets, but should still be used with caution. The difference is in how the tablets and capsules interact with water. One study showed that fiber (glucomannan) tablets swelled to seven times their original size within 1 minute of coming into contact with water.[37] In contrast, fiber-filled gelatin capsules took 6 minutes to begin to swell. One very important recommendation is to consume amounts of water with the fiber supplement.

SUMMARY

A diet high in plant foods is associated with a decreased incidence of most of the degenerative diseases of Western society. While this is largely due to increased levels of dietary fiber, such a diet is also high in other important nutrients, most of which are also deficient in the Western diet. It is clear from the literature that the best source of dietary fiber is from whole foods, although fiber supplements do have a place in the treatment phase of specific diseases.

It must be stressed that even with a diet high in dietary fiber, when as little as 18% of the total calories are in the form of refined carbohydrates, many of the beneficial effects of dietary fiber are greatly reduced. There is no substitute for a healthy diet, i.e. a diet composed of foods as close to their original form as possible.

REFERENCES

1. Eaton SB, Konner M. Paleolithic nutrition. A consideration of its nature and current implications. New Engl J Med 1985; 312: 283–289
2. Ryde D. What should humans eat? Practitioner 1985; 232: 415–418
3. Trowell H, Burkitt D. Western diseases: their emergence and prevention. Harvard University Press. 1981; Trowell H, Burkitt D, Heaton K. Dietary fibre, fibre-depleted foods and disease. New York, NY: Academic Press. 1985
4. US Dept of Health and Human Services. The Surgeon General's report on nutrition and health. Rocklin, CA: Prima. 1988
5. National Research Council. Diet and health. Implications for reducing chronic disease risk. Washington, DC: National Academy Press. 1989
6. Price W. Nutrition and physical degeneration. La Mesa, CA: Price-Pottinger Foundation. 1970
7. Spiller GA. Dietary fiber in health and nutrition. Boca Raton, FL: CRC Press. 1994
8. Vahouny G, Kritchevsky D. Dietary fiber in health and disease. New York, NY: Plenum Press. 1982
9. Selvendran RR. The plant cell wall as a source of dietary fiber: chemistry and structure. Am J Clin Nutr 1984; 39: 320–337
10. Watt J, Marcus R. Harmful effects of carrageenan fed to animals. Canc Det Prev 1981; 4: 129–134
11. Setchell KDR. Discovery and potential clinical importance of mammalian lignans. In: Flaxseed in human nutrition. Chaimpaign, IL: AOCS Press. 1995: p 83–98
12. Graf E, Empson KL, Eaton JW. Phytic acid. A natural antioxidant. J Biol Chem 1987; 262: 11 647–11 650
13. Vucenik I, Tomazic VJ, Fabian D et al. Antitumor activity of phytic acid (inositol hexaphosphate) in murine transplanted and metastatic fibrosarcoma, a pilot study. Cancer Lett 1992; 65: 9–13
14. Graf, Eaton JW. Suppression of colonic cancer by dietary phytic acid. Nutr Cancer 1993; 19: 11–19

15. Physicians Committee for Responsible Medicine, P.O. Box 6322, Washington, DC, 20015
16. Sommer H, Kasper H. Effect of long-term administration of dietary fiber on the exocrine pancreas in the rat. Hepato-gastroenterology 1984; 31: 176–179
17. Royall D, Wolever TM, Jeejeebhoy KN et al. Clinical significance of colonic fermentation. Am J Gastroenterol 1990; 85: 1307–1312
18. Velazquez OC, Lederer HM, Rombeau JL. Butyrate and the colonocyte. implications for neoplasia. Dig Dis Sci 1996; 41: 727–739
19. Glore SR, Van Treeck D, Knehans AW et al. Soluble fiber and serum lipids. A literature review. J Am Diet Assoc 1994; 94: 425–436
20. Ripsin CM, Keenan JM, Jacobs DR et al. Oat products and lipid lowering, a meta-analysis. JAMA 1992; 267: 3317–3325
21. Krotkiewski M. Effect of guar on body weight, hunger ratings and metabolism in obese subjects. Clin Sci 1984; 66: 329–326
22. Krotkiewski M, Smith U. Dietary fibre in obesity. In: Leeds AR, Avenell A, eds. Dietary fiber perspectives. Reviews and bilbiography. London: John Libbey. 1985: p 61
23. Krotkiewski M. Effect of guar gum on body-weight, hunger ratings and metabolism in obese subjects. Br J Nutr 1984; 52: 97–105
24. Anonymous. Better than oat bran. Science News 1994; 145: 28
25. Walsh DE, Yaghoubian V, Behforooz A. Effect of glucomannan on obese patients. A clinical study. Int J Obesity 1984; 8: 289–293
26. Biancardi G, Palmiero L, Ghirardi PE. Glucomannan in the treatment of overweight patients with osteoarthrosis. Curr Ther Res 1989; 46: 908–912
27. El-Shebini SM. The role of pectin as a slimming agent. J Clini Biochem Nutr 1988; 4: 255–262
28. Solum TT, Ryttig KR, Solum E et al. The influence of a high-fibre diet on body weight, serum lipids and blood pressure in slightly overweight persons. A randomized, double-blind, placebo-controlled investigation with diet and fibre tablets (DumoVital). Int J Obesity 1987; 11(1): 67–71
29. Ryttig KR, Larsen S, Haegh L. Treatment of slightly to moderately overweight persons. A double-blind placebo-controlled investigation with diet and fibre tablets (DumoVital). Tidsskr Nor Laegeforen 1984; 104: 989–991
30. Rossner S, von Zweigbergk D, Ohlin A et al. Weight reduction with dietary fibre supplements. Results of two double-blind studies. Acta Med Scand 1987; 222: 83–88
31. Ryttig KR, Tellnes G, Haegh L et al. A dietary fibre supplement and weight maintenance after weight reduction. A randomized, double-blind, placebo-controlled long-term trial. Int J Obesity 1989; 14: 763–769
32. Rigaud D, Ryttig KR, Angel LA et al. Mild overweight treated with energy restriction and a dietary fiber supplement. A 6-month randomized, double-blind, placebo-controlled trial. Int J Obesity 1990; 14: 763–769
33. Yuan JM, Wang QS, Ross RK et al. Diet and breast cancer in Shanghai and Tianjin, China. Br J Cancer 1995; 71: 1353–1358
34. Baghurst PA, Rohan TE. Dietary fiber and risk of benign proliferative epithelial disorders of the breast. Int J Cancer 1995; 63: 481–485
35. MacLennan R, Macrae F, Bain C et al. Randomized trial of intake of fat, fiber, and beta-carotene to prevent colorectal adenomas. J Natl Cancer Inst 1995; 87: 1760–1766
36. Halama WH, Maudlin JL. Distal esophageal obstruction due to a guar gum preparation. South Med J 1992; 85: 642–646
37. Henry DA, Mitchell AS, Aylward J et al. Glucomannan and risk of oesophageal obstruction. Br Med J 1986; 292: 591–592

CHAPTER CONTENTS

58

Rotation diet: a diagnostic and therapeutic tool

Sally J. Rockwell, PhD CNN

INTRODUCTION

Food allergy/intolerance is a common component of many chronic diseases (see Ch. 51). However, it is often not recognized as problematic because conventional laboratory diagnosis is not very sensitive for food allergies and most allergists dismiss the concept of delayed hypersensitivity reactions to foods (see Chs 10 and 15). A time-honored effective approach to both diagnosis and treatment of food sensitivities is an elimination/rotation diet. This approach has the advantage of being low-cost, but the techniques must be followed assiduously to ensure clinical efficacy. Table 58.1 lists the typical indications for an elimination diet.

THE ELIMINATION DIET

The first step in the elimination diet is to remove from the diet all of the most common allergenic foods – i.e. wheat and other glutinous grains, dairy products, eggs, corn, soy and tofu, peanuts, citrus fruits, yeast and refined sugars – and other often problematic substances such as highly processed foods, chemicals, additives, preservatives, artificial colorings, flavorings, caffeine (coffee, tea, cola drinks, chocolate), and alcohol.

The object is to avoid all suspect foods and substances for at least 5 days, or long enough to clear all traces of those foods from the digestive tract. The omitted foods are then reintroduced into the diet one at a time. By keeping an accurate food and symptom diary, the offending foods can be identified and eliminated; then,

Table 58.1 Indications for the use of the elimination diet

- Documented or suspected food allergies/intolerances
- Chronic complaints that have not subsided with treatment
- Symptomatic patients whose tests results are all "normal"
- Patients suspected of mental health problems due to lack of significant progress
- Children and teens who are labeled ADD, hyperactive, or autistic, or who have behavior problems

depending upon the severity of the initial test response, the foods can be retested and added back into the diet within 3–6 months.

While some recommend eliminating only one food at a time, clinicians in this area have found that multiple allergies are the rule, not the exception. Eliminating only one allergen may not improve symptoms enough to allow the improvement to be recognized. The advantages of eliminating all major allergens in the beginning include rapid clearing, minimal adverse reactions, and accurate test results. When symptoms clear rapidly, the patient is inspired and eager to continue with the testing.

As Dr Doris Rapp explains:

> If there are several tacks in the bottom of a shoe, the whole foot hurts; removing only one tack will make little or no difference. But remove all the tacks, let the foot heal, then add back one tack at a time and the source of pain is isolated and easily identified. If only one tack (or food) is removed, no significant difference will be noted.

Variations of the elimination diet range from the most stringent plan – i.e. elimination of all the major allergens, refined foods and toxic substances – to a more lenient approach – elimination of only wheat, dairy and refined sugars. Consideration of the patient's lifestyle, age, weight, general health, food preferences, attitude and family system will determine the approach. For children and pregnant or lactating women, the amount of calories or carbohydrates should not be restricted; simply omit the major allergens.

Variations of the elimination diet

As can be seen in Table 58.2, all elmination/challenge diets are simply variations on the same theme:

1. Eliminate suspect foods for at least 5 days
2. Introduce/test by challenge ingestion
3. Carefully record reactions
4. Rotate foods, avoiding those shown to cause disagreeable reactions.

Table 58.2 Elimination diet variants

Type	Protocol
Water fast	Water-only fast for 5 days, reintroduce foods
Dilute juice fast	Dilute fruit juice fast for 5 days, reintroduce omitted foods
Fruit, melon and vegetable plan	Only fruits, melons and vegetables for 5 days, reintroduce omitted foods
Cave man (person) plan	Proteins, nuts, seeds, legumes, fruits and vegetables for 5 days – reintroduce omitted foods. Eat only natural, unprocessed foods

Water fast

Water fast should only be done under the close guidance of a health professional experienced in supervising fasts. A lifetime of accumulated toxins can be released in a short period of time, creating unwarranted discomfort and complications which overwhelm the patient and interfere with testing (see Ch. 47 for a complete description of fasting methodologies).

The dilute juice fast

Less severe than water fasting, and more acceptable to patients, is the dilute juice fast. The diluted juices provide a modest amount of calories, stabilize blood sugar levels and decrease the adverse detoxification–withdrawal reactions which may occur while eliminating all common allergens. The basic procedure is to use three parts distilled or mineral water to one part of fresh, sugar-free juice. The dilute juices are sipped throughout the day. Ideally, a different juice is used each day: celery, carrot, papaya, cranberry, berry, apple, pineapple, and other fruits or vegetables that have not been consumed on a daily basis. Citrus fruits should be avoided. Low-allergen protein supplements, e.g. Ultra Clear, Medi Pro Protein Powder, pure free-form amino acids, N Foods, or Vivonex, may be added after the third day. In addition, liberal amounts of pure water should be consumed throughout the day in order to dilute and flush out toxic substances.

Note. This works for most *Candida* patients as the juice is so dilute that it rarely creates a problem. However, commercially prepared juices (especially tomato and citrus juice) often contain molds which can be problematic.

Fruit and/or vegetable plan

The patient consumes unlimited amounts of clean fresh fruit and melons and raw, steamed, or baked vegetables throughout the day. If *Candida* overgrowth is severe, or if weight loss is desired, vegetables should be emphasized over fruits.

The cave man (person) plan

When the major allergenic foods are eliminated, what's left are the basic foods that the cave man consumed: vegetables, fruits, berries, honey, nuts, seeds, beans, peas, sprouts, roots, gourds, poultry, fish, seafood, and wild game.

Procedure

Beginning the elimination diet

An ideal elimination diet begins with:

1. 2 days of the dilute juice, then
2. Fruits and vegetables for the next 2 days, then

3. 2 days of the cave person diet, or until symptoms clear.

Any one, or combination of, the above elimination plans will clear the patient of allergenic substances. If after 5 days the patient's symptoms have not diminished (or disappeared), continue for another 5 days. If not clear in 10 days, begin to rotate, as they may be reacting to a food or substance they are consuming every day. (Unsuspected environmental allergens may be contributing to the symptoms also – see "Helpful hints and suggestions", p. 52.)

Testing by challenge ingestion

Introduce one suspect food every other day. The object is to provide the patient with sufficient calories, build a reliable list of safe foods, and delay unpleasant reactions for as long as possible. Begin with rarely ingested foods as they are least likely to cause adverse reactions. Do not test foods which are known to cause severe reactions.

Suggested testing sequence

Reintroduce back into the diet in the following order whenever possible: vegetables, fruits, melons, beans, nuts and seeds, yeasts, dairy products and finally grains. When adding dairy, test goat products first: plain yogurt, cheeses, and then milk. Repeat the same process with cow's milk. Test grains in the following order: quinoa, amaranth, buckwheat, wild rice, brown rice, millet, *barley, spelt, kamut, teff, oats, rye,* corn and *wheat* last (gluten-containing grains are in *italics*). Also test dietary supplements one at a time.

Food and symptom diary

Have the patient record chronologically in a notebook all foods, liquids, supplements, moods, symptoms and reactions. The foods eaten throughout the day should be noted in pencil, or blue or black ink. Highlight or circle symptoms using colored ink so that those adverse reactions will stand out clearly. In 2–3 weeks a repetitive pattern of symptoms will be clearly visible, which allows for identification and elimination of the problematic foods or food combinations causing symptoms.

In the beginning, a patient may not be able to describe in exact words how he or she feels, and so a numbering system may be useful to note general moods throughout the day. Number from 1 (poor) to 10 (excellent). Feeling sort of medium, neither poor nor excellent, would be recorded as a 5. In general, depending on the patient's health and motivation, foods causing a mild reaction should be avoided for 3 months, and those causing a severe reaction are best avoided for at least 6 months before being reintroduced.

Testing children

Play a game with children – make testing fun. Have them draw a picture of how they feel or write their name before and after testing a substance. Note the differences.

THE DIVERSIFIED ROTATION DIET

The basic concept of the diversified rotation diet is to:

- eliminate all major allergenic substances
- eat the remaining foods once every 4 days
- allow 2 or 4 days between food families.

Rotation can be simplified by using a template – the "master chart" – with foods correctly arranged according to their botanical family classifications. The spacing of the foods, and food families, are pre-organized into four columns, one for each day, so the patient simply chooses foods from the appropriate column each day. A color-coding system further simplifies the process of choosing the correct foods.

The master chart, plan I (see Appendix 10) is the most liberal of the two plans. It provides 4 days between specific foods and only 2 days between food families.

The master chart, plan II is used for severely sensitive individuals (see Appendix 10). It incorporates 4 days between specific foods and 4 days between food families. If necessary, it can be easily adapted to a 7 day rotation.

Using the master charts

Use a pencil to cross out the major allergens, plus any known or suspected problem foods, in each of the four columns. The patient may eat the remaining foods from the appropriate column throughout the day. The foods which are not crossed out are what they are allowed to eat.

The arrows on the chart (↔) indicate a food which is essentially the only food of a family and which is not cross-reactive with other foods. Therefore, it is not restricted to any one particular day, and can be moved to another column if additional food choices are needed.

Those who will be rotating for any length of time will welcome the benefits of using the color-coding system. A color is assigned to each day. Each column represents a day – day 1: green, column one; day 2: yellow, column two; day 3: blue, column three; and day 4: red, column four. After day 4, rotate back to day 1 and repeat the process. Food containers are labeled and color-coded to coordinate with the color of the day. The color-coding system enables the entire family to see at a glance which foods are permitted on each of the days.

Example. The first column of the master chart is day 1, green day; place green labels, green twist-ties or green rubber bands on all appropriate food containers for day 1, and so on.

Modifications for vegans

The master charts can be used for vegans by simply crossing out all foods of animal origin. After the initial elimination phase, proceed with the food challenges. Legumes (beans and peas) are generally an important part of the vegan diet; so test each legume, one at a time, beginning with the least allergenic, rarely eaten beans, then soy and tofu, and test peanuts last. Depending upon the allergic response to legumes, the patient may be able to tolerate legumes daily, as long as a different legume is eaten each day. In other words, while the *four days between foods* rule continues to be honored, the *one day between food families* rule may be safely ignored for some patients.

Food preparation

For testing purposes, use fresh, organic foods whenever possible. Otherwise frozen or dehydrated foods are a better choice than canned goods. Most vegetables are best raw, steamed, or baked. Fish, poultry, and meat are best poached, steamed, sautéed, baked or simmered in a crock pot. Soups and stews are fine. Use only sea salt for seasoning; all spices and flavorings need to be avoided until they are individually tested.

Stabilize blood sugar levels by advising the patient to eat small, frequent meals throughout the day. Using hypoallergenic foods, prepare four mixtures of "trail mix" – nuts and dried fruits – for each day. Refer to the master chart for specific food choices. Maintain a supply of healthy snacks everywhere: home, school, office and automobile.

Helpful hints and suggestions

Control of withdrawal symptoms and allergenic reactions. Ascorbates buffered with calcium, potassium and/or magnesium are suggested as a daily source of vitamin C for allergenic individuals. They help to balance an acidic body pH, and are valuable for neutralizing unpleasant allergic reactions. Stabilizing pH eases the symptoms of withdrawal from allergenic foods, and the cravings which occur when breaking an addiction – whether it's sugar, wheat, coffee, cigarettes, alcohol or a drug.

For *daily use,* determine an individual's requirement for vitamin C. Begin with ⅛ tsp of buffered ascorbate in ½ glass of water 3 times a day (between meals and at bedtime). Gradually increase by an additional ⅛ tsp per dose every 2 days until they reach bowel tolerance: loose stool, gas or diarrhea. Reduce dosage. As the patient improves, their vitamin C requirement will likely decrease and the dosage may need to be decreased again.

Note. Buffered C should not be taken with meals as it will neutralize stomach acid, which is often deficient in patients with food allergy/intolerance (see Ch. 19).

For *temporary* relief of symptoms or to neutralize an adverse reaction, mix and drink a ½ teaspoon of buffered vitamin C in ½ glass of water or dilute juice. Available commercial products include Klaire Labs Bi-carbs, Cardiovascular's Tri-salts and Alka Seltzer Gold label (not the blue label). If all of the above are unavailable, ½ teaspoon of baking soda in ½ glass of water can be useful.

Environmental allergies. If the patient doesn't respond in a timely fashion, and all other possibilities have been ruled out, suspect environmental and/or chemical sensitivities. Step one is to eliminate all scented toiletries, room sprays and cleaning solutions in the home and work place.*

Ensure adequate protein intake. As the most allergenic foods also tend to be those highest in protein, care must be taken to ensure the patient is consuming enough protein. Patients with large numbers of food allergies should be referred to a competent nutritionist to help them develop an adequately balanced diet.

Be patient. Be especially patient and supportive of those who have experienced long-term conventional treatment only. You may be the first physician to remind them that symptoms are the body's way of communicating and that learning to pay attention to what they eat and drink, and the possible adverse symptoms, is a vital part of getting well again.

Allergy-free cook books. Recipes, plus dozens of helpful hints and suggestions can be found in specialty cook books. The author has published several self-help books and tapes, including *The rotation game,* complete with instructions, colored visual aids, recipes, etc.

Utilization of the rotation diet can be greatly assisted through the use of a commercial product developed by the author: *The rotation game* (see address in footnote, below; a free copy of *Allergy Alert* newsletter is available on request).

*Contact S. J. Rockwell at the following address for a patient "how-to" checklist: PO Box 31065, Seattle, WA 98013 (tel: (206) 547 1814; fax: 547 7696; e-mail: docrock@accessone.com).

CHAPTER CONTENTS

59

Sports nutrition

*Gregory S. Kelly, ND**

INTRODUCTION

The increased focus on fitness and subsequent research in the exercise field have expanded the role of nutrition in sports performance. Because there is widespread belief among athletes that special nutritional practices will enhance their achievements in competition, the use of supplements has become common. This chapter reviews the efficacy of some of supplements currently promoted to athletes. The topic has been divided into two broad categories: sports nutrition for strength athletes; and sports nutrition for endurance athletes. This division is to a degree arbitrary, so some of the supplements discussed might be applicable for athletes in both of these categories.

SPORTS NUTRITION FOR STRENGTH ATHLETES

Creatine monohydrate

Creatine monohydrate has become one of the most popular supplements in the history of body-building. It is used primarily to increase strength and lean body mass and has shown consistent results in promoting these effects in experimental subjects.

In humans, over 95% of the total creatine content is located in skeletal muscle. Approximately one-third is in its free form as creatine, also known as methylguanidinoacetic acid, while the remainder is present in a phosphorylated form as creatine phosphate (also called phosphocreatine). Creatine phosphate is utilized within skeletal muscle storing high energy phosphate bonds.

Creatine is formed in the liver, kidney, and pancreas. Initially, arginine and glycine combine to produce guanidinoacetate. A methyl group from S-adenosylmethionine (SAM) is then transferred, resulting in the formation of creatine. The by-product of this reaction, S-adenosylhomocysteine, is subsequently hydrolyzed into homo-

*Reprinted with permission from *Alternative Medicine Review* 1997; 2(4): 282–295

cysteine and adenosine. In order to optimize endogenous production of creatine, the amino acids arginine, glycine, and methionine must be available as substrates. Additionally, magnesium is required as a cofactor to form SAM from methionine, and B_{12}, folic acid and betaine are required to recycle the homocysteine to methionine for reuse as SAM.

While creatine can be synthesized endogenously as described above, it is also found in a variety of foods in varying concentrations. The richest source is considered to be wild game, but in domesticated animals, beef (lean red meat) is the richest source; 1.1 kg of fresh uncooked steak contains about 5 g of creatine.[1] Fish is also a good source, especially herring, salmon, and tuna. However, it is believed that creatine in foods may be destroyed or reduced significantly by cooking.

Creatine is transported to muscle tissue where it exists in equilibrium with creatine phosphate. Creatine phosphate spontaneously converts to creatinine (estimated to be at a rate of about 2 g/day for a 150 pound male) and is then excreted in the urine.[2] While part of this turnover can be replaced through dietary sources of creatine, especially meat and fish, the remainder must be supplied by endogenous synthesis. Because of this, there is a constant drain on arginine, glycine, methionine, and nutritional cofactors to maintain a supply of creatine and creatine phosphate. In vegetarians, daily needs must be met exclusively by endogenous synthesis. When dietary creatine is high, the synthetic pathway is correspondingly regulated downward.[3]

In addition to its use in skeletal muscle, some creatine is used by cardiac muscle. Chronic heart failure patients might have decreased stores of creatine and have been shown to have improved exercise capacity following administration of creatine.[4] One week of creatine (20 g/day) supplementation to patients with chronic heart failure increased skeletal muscle energy-rich phosphagens and performance for both strength and endurance.[4]

Creatine phosphate produces energy in the form of ATP in muscle cells for about 10 seconds of activity. After it is depleted, the muscle shifts to anaerobic glycolysis for fuel. It is thought skeletal muscles are capable of storing significantly more creatine than is generally supplied by the diet and by endogenous synthesis. Because of this, increased serum creatine, following an oral dose of creatine monohydrate, will be available for storage in muscle tissue. Over time, this increased dietary consumption can allow the muscle to become saturated with creatine. When the muscle has this extra creatine, it should theoretically be able to delay fatigue and refuel itself more quickly during high-intensity, short-duration exercise, and so should be capable of greater work.

When muscle absorbs creatine, it is hypothesized that it also brings water intracellularly with it, so the muscle becomes more "hydrated". It is estimated that muscles are about 70% water, so this results in a larger, fuller muscle. Evidence suggests when a cell is well hydrated it might accelerate its synthesis of new proteins and might also minimize protein degradation.[5]

One gram of creatine monohydrate or less in water produces only a modest rise in plasma creatine concentration; however, a 5 g oral dose has been shown to significantly increase plasma creatine concentration. Repeated dosing with 5 g of creatine monohydrate every 2 hours sustains the plasma concentration at around 1,000 mmol/L.[1]

Recent studies have shown that feeding large amounts of creatine (typically 20–30 g/day for 5 days) increases muscle total creatine (and phosphocreatine) content.[1,6] The extent of the increase normally observed is inversely related to the pre-supplementation level.[1,6] Vegetarians, because they have a very low dietary creatine intake and low to normal total creatine content, would be expected to show large increases.[1] Muscle creatine uptake appears to be augmented substantially in individuals adhering to a program of repeated high-intensity exercise during the period of supplementation.[1] Resynthesis of phosphocreatine following 1 minute of recovery from intense muscular contraction is accelerated in individuals consuming creatine.[6] Adequate vitamin E status might also be needed to optimize creatine uptake.[7]

In one study of eight subjects, biopsy samples were taken after 5 days of ingestion of 20 g creatine/day. In five of the eight subjects, there was substantially increased muscle total creatine concentration and creatine phosphate resynthesis during recovery. In the remaining subjects, creatine supplementation slightly increased total creatine concentration but did not increase creatine phosphate resynthesis.[6] In three subjects measured, uptake into muscle was greatest during the first 2 days of supplementation, accounting for 32% of the total 30 g of creatine monohydrate given orally per day. In these subjects, renal excretion was 40, 61 and 68% of the creatine dose over the first 3 days, respectively. Approximately 20% or more of the creatine taken up was measured as phosphocreatine, while no changes were observed in the muscle ATP content.[1]

Oral creatine monohydrate supplementation has also been shown, in a patient with extrapyramidal movement disorder and extremely low creatinine concentrations in serum and urine, to significantly increase brain creatine levels. Phosphorus magnetic resonance spectroscopy of the brain revealed no detectable creatine phosphate before oral substitution of creatine and a significant increase afterward. Partial restoration of cerebral creatine concentrations was accompanied by improvement of the patient's neurologic symptoms. Oral substitution of arginine, a substrate for creatine synthesis, was unable to elevate cerebral creatine levels.[8]

Creatine supplementation has been shown to improve performance in situations where the availability of creatine phosphate is important, such as very high-intensity exercise, especially where repeated bursts of energy are required with short recovery periods.[9–13] Several studies have documented creatine monohydrate's effect on muscle size and strength. Typically, after a 5–7 day loading dose, there is an increase in the amount of work done in repeated bouts of maximal exercise and a gain in body mass of between 0.5 and 1.0 kg.[10,12] One group of researchers reported 28 days of supplementation (20 g/day) producing a fat-free mass increased by 1.7 kg.[9]

While creatine supplementation increased performance in sprint-trained cyclists, it does not appear to improve endurance performance.[14] One study actually reported a worsening in performance during prolonged continuous exercise following creatine supplementation. This finding remains unexplained, although the authors believe the increase in body mass due to supplementation might be a contributing factor.[15] Research shows that creatine supplementation has no measurable effect on respiratory gas exchange and blood lactate concentrations during either incremental submaximal exercise or recovery, suggesting that creatine phosphate produces energy in the form of ATP in muscle cells for about 10 seconds of activity. After it is depleted, the muscle must shift to anaerobic glycolysis for fuel. Creatine supplementation does not influence substrate utilization during and after this type of exercise.[16]

Results from an unpublished human trial indicate that insulin might be a potent upregulator of a muscle's ability to take in creatine. This has resulted in many users supplementing creatine monohydrate with a simple carbohydrate (such as glucose, dextrose, or maltose) which simultaneously causes a release in insulin. In a 4 week trial, a large increase in speed, anaerobic power, and lean body mass, along with a decrease in body fat, was reported in individuals receiving doses of 20 g/day of creatine for the first 5 days, followed by 10 g/day for the remainder of the 4 weeks. An even greater response in these parameters was reported in the athletes using a creatine/carbohydrate mix, which contained creatine monohydrate, dextrose, taurine, disodium phosphate, magnesium phosphate, and potassium phosphate.

Dosage

Typically, dosing of creatine monohydrate follows a loading and a maintenance cycle. During the loading period, larger doses of creatine monohydrate are ingested for 5–7 days. A typical dose for individuals weighing less than 225 pounds is 5 g q.i.d, while heavier individuals might take up to six doses per day. The maintenance dose would be 0.03 g/kg body weight.[17,18] Larger doses are probably not of any greater benefit since the capability of muscle to take in and store creatine is finite.[1] In fact, this dosing schedule might exceed the ability of most individuals to incorporate creatine into muscle tissue, as evidenced by the renal excretion rate of creatine (40–68% of the supplemented dose) reported in individuals given 30 g/day.[1] A recent study supports the possible use of lower oral doses. One study reported that 3 g/day for 28 days increased muscle creatine and creatine phosphate stores to a level comparable to a loading phase.[17]

Most of the gains in size and strength occur within the first month, after which muscles are generally saturated with creatine. Evidence indicates that these gains will remain while supplementation continues, but will gradually disappear over time when the supplement is discontinued. Typically, levels of creatine drop back to pre-supplementation levels about 1 month after discontinuing supplementation. The size and strength increase resulting from improved muscle cell hydration also disappear over this same time interval. However, actual gains in muscle mass due to increased work capacity while on creatine will remain.

Anecdotal reports suggest that 20–30% of individuals who take creatine do not respond with increased muscle mass or strength. Presently, this finding is unexplained; however, individuals with lower initial tissue levels are most likely to benefit.[1] Because of the success of creatine monohydrate, several other forms have become available, including creatine phosphate and creatine citrate. These are claimed to produce similar results; however, creatine monohydrate is the only form shown, to date, to increase strength, lean body mass, and tissue creatine phosphate levels.

Toxicity

Reported side-effects from creatine supplementation include gastric disturbance, headaches, clenched teeth, and the sound of blood rushing in the ear. Creatine supplementation might cause serum creatinine levels to increase. This is due to the increase in muscle creatine phosphate and its subsequent spontaneous conversion to creatinine. Since most of the studies have only supplemented creatine for short periods of time, and in the single study reporting long-term supplementation only 1 g/day was utilized,[19] it is not currently known whether long-term, high-dose supplementation has adverse side-effects.

Some concern exists that caffeine use (0.5 mg/kg per day) can have a negative impact on the effectiveness of creatine. However, in at least one study, participants were instructed to dissolve the creatine monohydrate in tea or coffee before ingestion. Body weight increase was still observed in seven of eight subjects and all subjects had increased muscle total creatine and phosphocreatine resynthesis.[6] Although these results suggest caffeine does not negate the effects of creatine supplementation, until more is known it might be best to minimize caffeinated substances, or drink them several hours away from supplementation, if seeking optimal results.

Creatine supplementation is widely practiced by athletes in many sports and does not contravene current doping regulations.[3] Since creatine supplementation does not enhance performance in endurance athletes and evidence suggests an actual decline in performance, endurance athletes should avoid creatine supplementation. In athletes concerned with improving strength, body composition, or short-duration repetitive high-intensity exercise, I recommend creatine monohydrate be incorporated into any supplementation protocol. Although quicker results will be seen following a loading dose, the cost-effectiveness of the 3 g/day dose might be a more appealing option for many athletes.

HMB

HMB (beta-hydroxy beta-methylbutyrate) is a new product which has only been available in limited supply since the end of 1995. The nutritional use of HMB for nitrogen retention has been patented by the Iowa State University Research Foundation and is licensed to Metabolic Technologies.

HMB is a leucine metabolite. It has not yet been established how HMB is synthesized from leucine in humans; however, in animals evidence suggests that the majority of circulating HMB is formed following the transamination of leucine to alpha-ketoisocaproate with its subsequent oxidation to HMB.[20] It has not been determined either to what extent HMB is normally produced in vivo or which specific cofactors might influence its production.

While the mechanism of action of HMB is still equivocal, it is hypothesized that HMB decreases muscle protein turnover and might work primarily by minimizing protein degradation. Suggestive evidence of HMB's blocking of catabolism is based on its ability to decrease urinary 3-methylhistidine (a marker of muscle breakdown), and to decrease plasma levels of creatine phosphokinase and lactic dehydrogenase.[21] Anecdotal reports indicate that individuals who work out more often and most intensely get the best results with HMB. This is important since typically the more an individual works out, the more muscle catabolism also occurs; so at a certain point, the anabolic gains achieved by stimulating the muscles through training are offset by the catabolic effects of frequent, high-intensity workouts. HMB's anti-catabolic effects might move this balance point further in the direction of anabolic growth, allowing an individual to train more often and still receive positive results in strength and mass gains.

In a human study conducted over a 3 week period, 3 g/day of oral HMB supplementation was shown to decrease body fat, increase lean mass and strength, and reduce muscle damage in individuals beginning resistance-training exercises. In this trial, participants also consumed either 117 or 175 g/day of protein. While protein intake did not seem to impact strength, participants with higher protein intakes, independent of HMB supplementation, appeared to have greater increases in lean body mass.[21] Because these results came from individuals who had not previously engaged in weight training, doubt existed as to whether they would be reproducible in body-builders or other athletes who had already engaged in long-term resistance training. However, in a subsequent study, not yet published as a full paper, researchers have indicated that HMB feeding resulted in equal increases in strength, body composition, and decreased fat in both trained and untrained individuals.[22]

Dosage

The recommended dosage for HMB is 3 g/day. Since relatively high protein intake was reported in the study demonstrating HMB's efficacy, and because it is unknown whether the same results will occur while on a low-protein diet, a similar protein intake of between 120 and 175 g/day for athletes supplementing with HMB might produce best results.

Toxicity

At this point, the primary concern regarding HMB is anecdotal evidence which indicates that many individuals have not experienced expected results with this supplement. Since HMB is thought to function primarily as an anti-catabolic substance, it is possible these individuals did not train with enough intensity to optimize its effect. The other possibility is that, similar to creatine monohydrate, HMB might be ineffective in some individuals. Since this is such a new supplement, no information is available on its long-term safety.

Whey protein

Whey protein, often referred to as lactalbumin, is currently the supplemental protein source of choice for many body-builders and strength athletes. Whey proteins represent the major proteins in human breast milk, as opposed to bovine milk which is comprised primarily of casein with lesser amounts of whey. Whey is comprised of alpha-lactoglobulin, beta-lactoglobulin, bovine serum albumin (BSA), and immunoglobulins (IgG1, IgG2, secretory IgA, and IgM). Other components of the lactalbumin fraction include: enzymes, iron binding proteins, calcium, potassium, sodium, phosphorous, and vitamins A, C, B_1, B_2, B_3, B_5, B_{12}, folic acid, and biotin. Whey is a balanced source of essential amino acids and peptides with a high protein efficiency ratio. It is considered to be an excellent source of sulfur amino acids (methionine and cysteine), as well as the branched-chain amino acids (leucine, isoleucine and valine), and glutamine (see sections on branched-chain amino acids and glutamine for information on their potential benefits).

Whey transits the stomach quickly and is rapidly absorbed from the human intestine. The beta-lactoglobulin component remains soluble in the stomach and empties rapidly as an intact protein needing further hydrolysis by pancreatic enzymes. Casein, on the other hand, transits the stomach slowly.[23]

No studies exist comparing the impact on nitrogen balance, body composition, or performance of different protein sources in trained athletes. However, whey has been shown to promote growth and enhance nitrogen balance in experimental animals, low-birth-weight infants, and burn victims.[24–26]

Whey protein is rich in substrates for glutathione synthesis,[27] and contains substantially more cysteine, which is considered to be a rate-limiting step in glutathione synthesis, than does casein. Whey also contains high amounts of glutamine and glycine.

Glutathione is a powerful antioxidant and is involved in metabolic detoxification pathways. The role free radicals play in the development of exercise-induced tissue damage, or the protective role antioxidants might play, remains to be completely elucidated. Research has indicated that free radical production and subsequent lipid peroxidation are normal sequelae to the rise in oxygen consumption with exercise.[28] However, physical training has been shown to result in an augmented antioxidant system and a reduction in lipid peroxidation. Supplementation with antioxidants appears to further reduce lipid peroxidation but has not been shown to enhance exercise performance.[29]

Glutathione levels have been shown to decrease with exercise.[30] Additionally, running a marathon causes a large increase in the tissue content of oxidized glutathione (189%) at the expense of reduced glutathione.[31] While no information is available on the effects of resistance exercise and glutathione levels, it is hypothesized that an increased intake of antioxidants might protect against minor muscle injuries.[32]

Whey protein is more efficient at inducing supernormal glutathione levels than a cysteine-enriched casein diet.[33] A whey-rich diet has been shown to increase heart and liver tissue glutathione content in rats. The whey protein diet appeared also to increase longevity when fed at the onset of senescence.[33] Whey-based formula enhances cysteine retention and results in greater taurine excretion, thought to be a reflection of greater taurine stores.[34] Whey protein fed to three HIV-seropositive individuals over a period of 3 months, at doses increasing progressively from 8.4 to 39.2 g/day, resulted in progressive weight gain and increased glutathione levels in all three.[35]

Experimental studies suggest that the whey protein component of milk might exert an inhibitory effect on the development of several types of tumor. It is thought that the rich supply of substrates for glutathione synthesis contributes to this inhibitory effect.[36] In experimental animals, a diet consisting of 20 g of whey/100 g diet has been shown to be more protective than similar diets utilizing casein, soybean, or red meat against dimethylhydrazine-induced intestinal cancers.[37] Peptides from whey protein have also been shown to have antithrombotic[38] and immunoenhancing activities.[38,39]

Dosage

The routine use of a post-workout shake might be the most important nutritional supplementation habit for enhancing body composition. It is probably in this manner that whey can be best utilized by athletes concerned with maximizing lean body mass and strength.

Amino acid availability following a workout regulates protein synthesis and degradation. Because of the anabolic effects of insulin on protein synthesis and protein degradation, a rapid synergistic response occurs when both amino acids and insulin increase after a protein-containing meal.[40] It is thought that the body is highly insulin-sensitive after exercise and preferentially shuttles carbohydrates and protein into muscle cells rather than fat cells. Experts think this sensitivity gradually declines post-workout for about 2 hours until it again reaches normal sensitivity.

A carbohydrate-whey protein supplement has been shown to be more effective in generating a plasma insulin response than either a carbohydrate or a protein supplement alone during recovery from prolonged exhaustive exercise. The rate of muscle glycogen storage was also significantly faster during the carbohydrate-protein treatment. The participants in this study ingested 112.0 g of carbohydrate and 40.7 g of protein immediately after each exercise bout.[41]

Whey is an excellent choice as a protein source for the post-workout shake because of its rapid transit into the small intestine and because of its high levels of branched-chain amino acids and glutamine. Glucose polymers or maltodextrins are considered to be the best form of carbohydrates to use because of their ability to stimulate an insulin response. Fat should not be added because it might slow transit and decrease the insulin response.

Toxicity

The primary concerns about supplementing whey protein are the possibility of food allergies, its lactose content, and proposed links to insulin-dependent diabetes mellitus (IDDM). While the possibility of food allergies from whey has to be considered, it is probable it is no more, and possibly less, antigenic than soy, casein, or egg-based protein supplements. A significant concern might be the method of processing of the whey protein, since high temperatures during heating or drying can generate browning reaction products by covalent interaction of proteins and lactose. Browned proteins have lowered digestibility and are thought to result in greater uptake of intact protein through intestinal mucosa. All whey protein available contains some degree of lactose, although many have very low amounts.

The BSA component of whey has been implicated as a possible trigger for IDDM in children. A similarity exists between the amino acid sequence of the beta-cell protein, found on the insulin-secreting beta cells of the pancreas, and BSA. Because elevated levels of anti-BSA antibodies have been found in sera from children developing IDDM, it has been proposed that absorption of BSA, or partially digested fragments of BSA, stimulate the immune system which then incorrectly destroys beta cells.[42] One study reported the prevalence of anti-BSA antibodies as 52% in children with less than 1 year of IDDM, 47% in children with greater than 1 year of IDDM, and 28% in the control group. The researchers concluded that the prevalence of anti-BSA antibodies is higher in IDDM subjects than in control subjects; however, because of the large overlap of antibody titers observed in patients and control subjects, anti-BSA antibodies were neither sensitive nor specific markers of IDDM.[43] Others have found that IgG antibodies to BSA were not significantly increased at the onset of IDDM.[44] Currently, the exact nature of the relationship between BSA and IDDM remains unclear.

Phosphatidylserine

Phosphatidylserine is becoming widely used by individuals engaged in resistance training, primarily due to its presumed ability to prevent muscle tissue degradation. Phosphatidylserine has been shown to have an effect on the body's production of glucocorticoids. While the mechanism of action of phosphatidylserine is still unknown, it has been proposed that it exerts an effect on the hypothalamic–pituitary–adrenal axis.[45]

Phosphatidylserine is formed by adding a serine to a phosphatidyl group. This requires pyridoxal 5′-phosphate (active B_6), and occurs in the same biochemical loop involved with phosphatidylcholine, choline, betaine, and dimethylglycine metabolism.

Physical exercise induces a significant increase in plasma epinephrine, norepinephrine, adrenocorticotropic hormone (ACTH), cortisol, growth hormone (GH), and prolactin (PRL). It is theorized that preventing the increase in cortisol subsequent to intense exercise would prevent the excess muscle tissue breakdown. Pretreatment of eight healthy men with both 50 and 75 mg of intravenous brain cortex-derived phosphatidylserine within 10 minutes of the start of exercise blunted the ACTH and cortisol responses to physical stress.[46] Oral administration of phosphatidylserine derived from brain cortex, 800 mg/day for 10 days, significantly blunted the ACTH and cortisol responses to physical exercise ($P = 0.003$ and $P = 0.03$, respectively), without affecting the rise in plasma GH and PRL. Although participants also experienced reductions in plasma cortisol concentrations at a dose of 400 mg/day of phosphatidylserine, the area under the curve of plasma cortisol was significantly lower after the higher dose of 800 mg/day.[45]

While the results of this preliminary work appear promising, to date no trials have reported an increase in strength or an improvement in body composition after phosphatidylserine supplementation. Until these results are determined, claims of phosphatidylserine's ability to decrease muscle tissue catabolism should be considered unsubstantiated.

Arginine

Arginine is an amino acid which is used occasionally by body-builders to stimulate growth hormone secretion. It was very popular in the mid-1980s; however, interest in it has since waned. Several studies have shown its ability to stimulate growth hormone and insulin-like growth factor I secretion and improve nitrogen balance after i.v. administration; however, equivocal results have been obtained following oral supplementation.

Oral arginine/lysine (3 g/day of each) is apparently not a practical means of chronically enhancing GH secretion in older men.[47] Additionally, it is debatable whether increasing growth hormone levels in people not already deficient has an anabolic effect.

Arginine is required for creatine synthesis and some believe it will enhance synthesis if supplemented. In rats, arginine and glycine supplementation increased muscle creatine.[48]

One study reported that individuals receiving arginine and ornithine, 5 days a week for 5 weeks, had higher gains in strength and enhancement of lean body mass when compared with controls. Dosages amounted to 2 or 1 g each of L-arginine and L-ornithine taken orally, and 600 mg of calcium and 1 g of vitamin C as placebos. Subjects taking the arginine and ornithine also had significantly lower urinary hydroxyproline, a marker of tissue breakdown, than subjects receiving placebo. The authors concluded that arginine and ornithine, in conjunction with a high-intensity strength training program, can increase strength and lean body mass, and minimize tissue breakdown.[49]

Dosage

The typical dosage is 2 g/day. Based upon the results of Elam et al,[49] it appears that a combination of arginine and ornithine might exert a positive impact on body composition and strength; however, no additional research has substantiated these findings.

Branched-chain amino acids

Leucine, isoleucine, and valine are considered as branched-chain amino acids (BCAAs) because of their similar chemical structures and interlocking methyl groups. Exercise results in marked alterations in amino acid metabolism within the body. The branched-chain amino acids, especially leucine, are particularly important since they contribute as energy substrates and as nitrogen donors in the formation of alanine, glutamine and aspartate. Calculations indicate that the recommended dietary intake of leucine is inadequate, since it is lower than the measured whole-body rates of leucine oxidation. This inadequacy is exacerbated in individuals who are physically active.[50]

An increased supply of BCAAs appears to have a sparing effect on muscle glycogen degradation during exercise.[51] Short-term (3–4 hours) infusion of branched-chain amino acids has been shown to suppress muscle protein breakdown.[52] In humans nourished parenterally, provision of balanced amino acid solutions or of only the three BCAAs cause similar improvements in nitrogen balance for several days.[40]

Administration of BCAAs can greatly increase their concentration in plasma and subsequently their uptake by muscle during exercise.[51] Long-term exercise following BCAA administration results in significantly greater muscle NH_3, alanine and glutamine production, as well as lower lactate production, than is observed during exercise without BCAA supplementation.[53]

While evidence indicates that BCAAs might be significant in enhancing protein synthesis or minimizing protein degradation, supplementation with these amino acids has not produced significant changes in body composition. If whey or another top-quality protein formula is being used, adequate amounts of BCAAs are provided.

Glutamine

Glutamine is the most abundant amino acid in the blood and in the free amino acid pool of skeletal muscle. Glutamine stimulates the synthesis and inhibits the degradation of proteins, is an important vehicle for the transport of nitrogen and carbon within the tissues, stimulates the synthesis of hepatic glycogen, and is an energy source for cell division.[54] Because glutamine deficiency can occur during periods of metabolic stress, it has led to the reclassification of glutamine as a conditionally essential amino acid.[55] Glutamine is also a precursor for the synthesis of amino acids, proteins, nucleotides, glutathione, and other biologically important molecules.

Glutamine is considered to have an anabolic effect on skeletal muscle. It stimulates the synthesis and inhibits the degradation of proteins. Experiments with various animal models have demonstrated that glutamine supplementation can result in better nitrogen homeostasis, with conservation of skeletal muscle.[55] The mechanism by which glutamine affects skeletal muscle protein turnover, and thus muscle protein balance, is unknown. However, glutamine has an anabolic effect of promoting protein synthesis and also might reduce protein breakdown.[56]

Glutamine was shown to increase cell volume, while insulin and glutamine together seem to work synergistically to enhance cellular hydration. The effects of glutamine in skeletal muscle include the stimulation of protein synthesis, which occurs in the absence or presence of insulin, the response being greater with insulin.[57]

During various catabolic states, such as infection, surgery, burns, and trauma, glutamine homeostasis is placed under stress, and glutamine reserves, particularly in the skeletal muscle, are depleted. In these conditions, the body requirements of glutamine appear to exceed the individual's muscle deposits, resulting in a loss of muscle mass.[58] In critically ill patients, parenteral glutamine reduces nitrogen loss and causes a reduction in mortality.[54]

With regard to glutamine metabolism, exercise stress can be viewed in a similar light to other catabolic stresses. Plasma glutamine concentrations increase during prolonged, high-intensity exercise. However, during the post-exercise recovery period, plasma concentrations decrease significantly. Several hours of recovery are required before plasma levels are restored to pre-exercise levels. If recovery between exercise bouts is inadequate, the acute effects of exercise on plasma glutamine concentrations can be cumulative. It has been observed that overtrained athletes appear to maintain low plasma glutamine levels for months or years.[59] Some experts believe that reduced concentration of plasma glutamine can provide a good indication of severe exercise stress.[60] Research suggests that, after exercise, increased availability of glutamine promotes muscle glycogen accumulation by mechanisms possibly including diversion of glutamine carbon to glycogen.[61]

Following trauma there is a loss of nitrogen, with a concomitant reduction of skeletal muscle protein synthesis. This is accompanied by a decrease in the stores of muscle free glutamine. Nutritional support with either glutamine or its carbon skeleton, alpha-ketoglutarate, has been shown to counteract the postoperative fall of muscle free glutamine and of muscle protein synthesis.[62]

Evidence suggests that oral glutamine supplementation results in an increased release of growth hormone. An oral glutamine load (2 g) was administered to nine healthy subjects to determine the effect on plasma glutamine, bicarbonate, and circulating growth hormone concentrations. Eight of nine subjects responded with an increase in plasma glutamine at 30 and 60 minutes before returning to the control value at 90 minutes. Ninety minutes after the glutamine administration load, both plasma bicarbonate concentration and circulating plasma growth hormone concentration were elevated.[63]

Dosage

Although some advocates recommend as much as 30 g, it is likely that only marginal benefits are found at supplementary levels higher than 2–3 g/day.

Ornithine alpha-ketoglutarate (OKG)

Ornithine alpha-ketoglutarate (OKG) is a salt formed of two molecules of ornithine and one molecule of alpha-ketoglutarate. OKG has been successfully used by the enteral and parenteral route in burn, traumatized, and surgical patients, and in chronically malnourished subjects. According to the metabolic situation, OKG treatment decreases muscle protein catabolism and/or increases synthesis. In addition, OKG promotes wound healing. The mechanism of action of OKG is not fully understood, but the secretion of anabolic hormones (insulin, human growth hormone), and the synthesis of metabolites (glutamine, polyamines, arginine, ketoacids) might be involved.[64]

This supplement has been available for several years. It has been used successfully in hospitalized burn victims to slow protein loss. Only one study appears to have evaluated its effect on performance. In this study, OKG (10 g/day with 75 g of carbohydrates) was given for 6 weeks. The OKG group experienced a significant increase in bench-press strength and biceps circumference. Body weight and percentage fat were not different between groups. No differences in growth hormone levels were seen between groups. Body composition changes were seen among several individuals in the OKG group, but no significance was found either within or between experimental groups.[64]

Anecdotal reports from some individuals supplementing with OKG indicate increased appetite and better disposition to train. Some anecdotal reports claim great results while others experience no results.

Dosage

The recommended dosage of OKG is 10 g along with a 75 g carbohydrate drink.

Vitamin C

There have been several investigations during the past four decades of the potential effect of high-dose vitamin C supplementation on physical performance. However, the results have been equivocal. Most studies could not demonstrate an effect. On the other hand, a suboptimal vitamin C status results in an impaired working capacity which can be normalized by restoring vitamin C body pools.[65]

A potent antioxidant required for collagen synthesis, ascorbic acid might help protect muscles from excessive damage due to training or trauma. Data suggests prior vitamin C supplementation might exert a protective effect against exercise-induced muscle damage.[66]

Ascorbic acid might decrease cortisol production.[67] It has also been suggested that ascorbic acid might have a role in facilitating an adequate response to stress.[68]

Dosage

Because of ascorbic acid's potential for minimizing muscle damage and cortisol-induced muscle catabolism, 1–3 grams should be supplemented daily.

Boron

Recently, a proliferation of athletic supplements has been marketed touting boron as an ergogenic aid capable of increasing testosterone. While this might to be true in some populations under specific conditions, boron's impact on testosterone is still equivocal.

Boron appears to increase testosterone levels in rats in a time- and dose-dependent manner.[69] In postmenopausal women, increasing dietary intake of boron from 0.25 to 3.25 mg/day has been reported to more than double plasma testosterone.[70] In a subsequent study of healthy men, boron supplementation resulted in an increase in the concentrations of both plasma estrogen and testosterone.[71] However, one study reported that changing boron intake had no impact on testosterone levels in postmenopausal women.[72]

The effect of boron supplementation was investigated in 19 male body-builders aged 20–27 years. Ten were given a 2.5 mg boron supplement, while nine were given a placebo every day for 7 weeks. Both groups demonstrated significant increases in total testosterone, lean body mass, and one-repetition maximum squat and bench-press. However, analysis of variance indicated no significant effect of boron supplementation on any of the dependent variables. The authors concluded that the gains were a result of 7 weeks of body-building, not of boron supplementation.[73]

Dosage

It is prudent to supplement the diet with 3 mg/day of boron to ensure against deficiency; however, an expectation of increased strength and improved body composition is unrealistic.

Chromium

Chromium is highly promoted in body-building circles as a fat-burning supplement and as an aid in increasing lean mass. Available research does not support either of these claims.

Changes in body weight, a sum of three body circumferences, a sum of three skinfolds, and the one-repetition maximum for the squat and bench-press were examined in 59 college-age students over a 12 week weight-lifting program. Half of the students were given 200 mcg/day elemental chromium as chromium picolinate, while the other half received a placebo. No treatment effects were seen for the strength measurements. The only significant treatment effect found was an increase in body weight observed in the females supplementing with chromium.[74]

The effects of 9 weeks of daily chromium supplementation (200 mcg chromium as picolinate) were investigated in a double-blind design in football players during sprint training. Chromium picolinate supplementation was ineffective in bringing about changes in body composition or strength.[75]

The same results were shown in another study of 200 mcg of chromium supplemented to untrained males (23 ± 4 years), in conjunction with a progressive, resistive exercise training program. Chromium supplementation was not found to promote a significant increase in strength or lean body mass, or a significant decrease in percentage body fat.[76]

Increasing dosage and length of supplementation also did not help. A double-blind, placebo-controlled protocol for 16 weeks provided 400 mcg of chromium as picolinate or a placebo. At the end of 16 weeks, the chromium group failed to show a significantly greater reduction in either percentage body fat or body weight, or a greater increase in lean body mass, than did the placebo group. It was concluded that chromium picolinate was ineffective in enhancing body fat reduction in this group.[77]

In yet another study, this one involving 8 weeks of daily chromium supplementation in 36 men in a double-blind design, it was found that strength, mesomorphy, fat-free mass, and muscle mass increased with resistance training independently of chromium supplementation ($P < 0.0001$). These findings suggest that routine chromium supplementation has no beneficial effects on body composition or strength gain in men, although it must be noted that the placebo group received a trace level of chromium.[78]

Evidence strongly indicates that supplementation of chromium will not enhance strength or body composition. Similar to boron, chromium-rich foods or a supplement containing chromium should be included in the diet to avoid deficiency; however, it is unrealistic to expect gains in strength or improvement in body composition.

Selenium

Selenium is a trace mineral which is utilized as a cofactor in several enzymes. It is commonly found in antioxidant formulas because of its role as a cofactor in the enzyme glutathione peroxidase. Evidence suggests that the administration of organic selenium partially compensates for and decreases the intensity of oxidative stress in athletes.[79] While optimal antioxidant status is critical to athletes, selenium might have an additional role in the determination of body composition. Selenium deficiency can affect the metabolism of thyroid hormones. Iodothyronine 5′-deiodinase, which is mainly responsible for peripheral T_3 production, has been demonstrated to be a selenium-containing enzyme.[80] In rats fed a selenium-deficient diet, hepatic iodothyronine 5′-deiodinase is decreased by 47%. Lower concentrations of T_3 and T_4 have also been demonstrated in selenium-deficient animals.[81] Reduced peripheral conversion of T_4 to T_3 secondary to a selenium deficiency might create a functional hypothyroidism which would be expected to adversely impact body composition.

Toxicity

There is data suggesting that ingesting more than 750–1,000 ug/day of selenium over an extended period of time may be harmful.

Vanadium (vanadyl sulfate)

Vanadium as vanadyl sulfate is widely utilized by athletes seeking to improve body composition. It is generally promoted as having an anabolic effect which enhances the transport of amino acids into cells. Several studies have indicated its ability to reduce fasting glucose and improve hepatic and peripheral insulin sensitivity in non-insulin-dependent diabetic humans.[82–84] However, vanadyl sulfate does not appear to alter insulin sensitivity in non-diabetic subjects.[84] A single study reported the effect of oral vanadyl sulfate (0.5 mg/kg per day) on anthropometry, body composition, and performance in a 12 week, double-blind, placebo-controlled trial involving 31 weight-training volunteers. No significant treatment effects for anthropometric parameters and body composition were observed. Both groups had similar improvements in performance in most exercises; however, a significant improvement in one repetition-maximum leg extension was found in the treatment group. The authors concluded that although vanadyl sulfate was ineffective in changing body composition in weight-training athletes, its performance-enhancing effect required further investigation.[85]

Toxicity

Anecdotal reports indicate that body-builders often supplement 15 mg t.i.d.; however, this practice is ill-advised due to both the lack of demonstrated efficacy and the lack of information regarding long-term toxicity of high doses of vanadium. Dietary concentrations of 25 mg of vanadium per kg cause mild diarrhea and growth suppression in rats and up to 50 mg/kg severely depressed growth and caused increased diarrhea and mortality. When 12 humans were fed 13.5 mg/day of vanadium for 2 weeks and then 22.5 mg/day for 5 months, five patients developed cramps and diarrhea at the high dosage.[86]

Zinc

Dietary deficiency of zinc is prevalent. Because of this, zinc supplements have been widely advocated for athletes. While it might not be wise to indiscriminately administer zinc, suggestive evidence indicates that zinc might impact body composition due to its interaction with a variety of hormones.

It is thought that intense exercise can result in changes in zinc metabolism. Zinc has been demonstrated to be lowered in trained adolescent gymnasts and even lower in females in the general population. This reduction might play a role in abnormalities of puberty, growth, or muscular performance.[87]

Some investigators have concluded zinc might play an important role in modulating serum testosterone levels in normal men. Dietary zinc restriction in normal young men is associated with a significant decrease in serum testosterone concentrations, while zinc supplementation of marginally zinc-deficient normal elderly men resulted in an increase in serum testosterone from 8.3 ± 6.3 to 16.0 ± 4.4 nmol/L (P = 0.02).[88] However, although zinc deficiency might inhibit testosterone production, zinc supplementation to an individual with adequate levels has not been shown to produce excess testosterone.

Zinc deficiency might result in reduced production of growth hormone (GH) and/or insulin-like growth factor I (IGF-I).[89] Oral zinc replacement has normalized growth hormone levels and increased growth rate in teenagers found to be GH-deficient.[90] Zinc supplementation causes a significant increase in liver synthesis of IGF-I (somatomedin C). In chronic zinc deficiency, reduced liver production of IGF-I is responsible for reduced physical growth; moreover, in this situation, receptor resistance to IGF-I (in addition to GH) has been demonstrated. Receptor sensitivity is re-established after supplementation with zinc. Zinc might also play a role in increasing the number of receptors.[91]

Zinc deficiency might affect the metabolism of thyroid hormones. The structure of nuclear thyroid hormone receptors contains zinc ions, crucial for the functional properties of the protein.[80] In experimental animals, zinc deficiency decreases concentrations of triiodothyronine (T_3) and free thyroxine (fT_4) in serum by approximately 30% when compared with zinc-adequate controls. The concentration of thyroxine (T_4) in serum was not affected by zinc deficiency. In these animals, zinc deficiency also decreased the activity of hepatic iodothyronine 5′-deiodinase by 67%.[81]

Toxicity

Zinc supplementation is generally safe if maintained at levels within two to eight times the RDA. Symptoms of zinc toxicity include gastrointestinal irritation, vomiting, adverse changes in HDL/LDL cholesterol ratios, and impaired immunity. The latter develops when levels above 180 mg/day are consumed for more than several weeks. Excess intake of zinc may either lower copper levels or aggravate an existing marginal copper deficiency.

Because of the multiple interactions of zinc with hormones critical to strength and body composition, it is recommended that athletes get a determination of zinc nutriture and supplement if required.

Summary

Based upon available information, strength athletes are likely to obtain improved results by following a supplementation routine which includes:

- creatine monohydrate (at least 3 g/day)
- a post-workout protein shake (40 g of protein)
- vitamin C (1–3 g/day)
- a multivitamin/mineral formulation containing approximately
  - — 3 mg of boron
  - — 200 mcg of chromium
  - — 200 mcg of selenium
  - — 100 mcg of vanadium
  - — 15 mg of zinc.

The published results to date on HMB are impressive. For athletes utilizing HMB, the recommended dosage is 3 g/day. While a theoretical argument can be made for the inclusion of phosphatidylserine in a supplement routine, the high cost and the lack of information on bottom-line results of improved strength or body composition make it difficult to justify its use. Although compelling evidence could be used to make an argument for many of the isolated amino acids, a high-quality protein supplement, such as whey, provides adequate levels of all of the amino acids for the majority of athletes. Because of the correlation of low glutamine levels and overtraining, supplementing 2 g/day of glutamine in addition to a protein supplement, in individuals whose training regimen places them at risk for overtraining, seems prudent.

SPORTS NUTRITION FOR ENDURANCE ATHLETES

Panax ginseng

Panax ginseng, also known as *Panax schinseng*, is a member of the family Araliaceae. In Mandarin Chinese it is called *Ren Shen* but is commonly referred to as Korean or Chinese ginseng. Several closely related species are also often sold as ginseng. These include *Panax quinquefolium* (American ginseng); *Panax notoginseng,* also known as *Panax pseudoginseng* (Himalayan ginseng), and *Panax japonicum* (Japanese ginseng). Ginseng was used traditionally as a tonic for a broad range of medical conditions. It was believed to be a revitalizing agent capable of enhancing health and promoting longevity (for a more detailed discussion, see Ch. 100).

Soviet scholars, beginning in the early 1950s, were the first to establish the fact that many Araliaceae family plants, especially *Panax ginseng,* are adaptogens.[92] Adaptogens, among their many properties, are thought to promote regeneration of the body after stress or fatigue and to rebuild strength. Because of its reputation as an adaptogen, *Panax ginseng* is among the most popular botanical supplements used by athletes.

Many animal studies with *Panax ginseng,* or its active components, have demonstrated an enhanced response to physical or chemical stress.[93–97] In rats, the aqueous suspensions of roots of *Panax ginseng* were tested for anti-stress activity by the "mice swimming endurance test" and anabolic activity by noting gain in body weights and muscle. A significant increase in mice swimming time was shown by ginseng-fed rats as compared with the control group.[98]

In animal models, administration of ginseng has been shown to impact several hormones which might impact performance. High doses of ginseng have been reported to increase blood testosterone level.[99] Experiments indicate that the binding of corticosteroid to certain brain regions is increased in adrenalectomized rats given ginseng saponin.[100] Ginseng saponin has also been reported to act on the hypothalamus and/or hypophysis, stimulating ACTH secretion which results in increased synthesis of corticosterone in the adrenal cortex.[101]

While studies with animals have been compelling, ginseng's value as an ergogenic aid in humans is still equivocal.[102] Extracts of *Panax ginseng* are reported to increase plasma total and free testosterone, dihydrotestosterone, and FSH and LH levels in infertile males.[103] The addition of ginseng root extract to a multivitamin base is reported to have improved subjective parameters in a population exposed to the stress of high physical and mental activity.[104] In a double-blind, randomized, crossover study, 50 healthy males received two capsules of a preparation containing ginseng extract, dimethylaminoethanol bitartrate, vitamins, minerals, and trace elements, or two capsules of placebo every day for 6 weeks. The total workload and maximal oxygen consumption during exercise were significantly greater after the ginseng preparation than after placebo. The authors also noted decreased plasma lactate levels, carbon dioxide production, and heart rate during exercise in participants receiving the ginseng preparation.[105] Others evaluated the impact on performance of a ginseng saponin extract (8 or 16 mg/kg body weight) ingested daily for 7 days. Although time to exhaustion was significantly less during the pre-supplementation control trial than during the placebo and ginseng trials, no significant difference was found between the placebo and the ginseng trials.[106] It should be noted that the duration of the supplementation period was only 1 week in this trial. Since, historically, ginseng, as a tonic, is used for prolonged time periods and since positive results have been reported following 6 weeks of supplementation, a longer trial might have demonstrated an ergogenic effect.

Research in support of the use of *Panax ginseng* as an ergogenic aid, although equivocal, is promising. Because of the anecdotal reputation and allure this plant holds, it is likely to continue to be utilized by many athletes.

Dosage

The quality of available ginseng preparations can vary greatly, so it is imperative to use *Panax ginseng* with documented potency. A typical dose for general tonic effect would contain at least 25 mg of the saponin ginsenoside.[107] *Panax ginseng* contains 2–3% ginsenosides, so a dose of 8–12 g of crude herb, assuming it is of high quality, will provide adequate saponin content. Because of the variability in quality of *Panax ginseng* available, utilizing a preparation standardized for ginsenoside content may be preferable. The dosage for a product standardized to 5% ginsenosides would be 500 mg/day, and to 14% ginsenosides would be about 180 mg.[107] If utilizing ginseng for a prolonged period of time, some authors have recommended discontinuing supplementation periodically for 2 week intervals.

Toxicity

The problem of quality control makes toxicology difficult to address. Studies have been performed on standardized extracts of ginseng which demonstrate the absence of side-effects and mutagenic or teratogenic effects. However, toxicity has been reported with products of uncertified constituents.

Eleutherococcus senticosus

Eleutherococcus senticosus, also known botanically as *Acanthopanax senticosus,* is a member of the Araliaceae family which also contains *Panax ginseng*. In China, the plant is called *Ci Wu Jia*; however, it is most commonly referred to as Siberian ginseng. Because of its wide availability and lower cost, the dried root and rhizome is commonly used as a ginseng substitute; however, ginsenosides, characteristic of *Panax* sp., are not found in the roots of *Eleutherococcus senticosus*.[107] (For a more detailed discussion, see Ch. 83.)[9]

Eleutherococcus senticosus is classified as an adaptogen and is believed to promote recovery and improve endurance. It has a long history of use in Chinese herbal medicine where it was used to enhance general health, longevity, appetite and memory. Soviet scientists, beginning in the late 1950s, because of the rarity of *Panax ginseng*, shifted the focus of their research to other members of the Araliaceae family in order to find suitable substitutes. Four adaptogenic plants were identified, studied and finally introduced into therapeutic practice, between 1955 and 1964. *Eleutherococcus senticosus* was considered to be the most important of these substitutes.[108] Reports indicate that *Eleutherococcus* was used routinely by both Soviet Olympic athletes and military officers.

Extracts of *Eleutherococcus* prolong the exercise time to exhaustion in swimming rats,[109] and modulate changes of the hypophyseo-adrenal system in rats under extreme conditions.[110] Farnsworth et al[111] reviewed the results of clinical trials of *Eleutherococcus* in humans. The data they gathered indicated that ingestion of extracts from the plant increased the ability to accommodate to adverse physical conditions, improved mental performance, and enhanced the quality of work under stressful conditions such as during athletic performance.[111]

Others, however, have concluded that supplementation of *Eleutherococcus senticosus* had no ergogenic effect on the measured parameters associated with submaximal and maximal aerobic exercise tasks. The effect on performance during submaximal and maximal aerobic exercise was measured in 20 highly trained distance runners randomly assigned to matched pairs. Participants consumed either 3.4 ml of extract or placebo daily for 6 weeks. During the 8 week double-blind study, subjects completed five trials of 10 minute runs on a treadmill at their 10 km race pace and a maximal treadmill test. No significant differences were observed between *Eleutherococcus*- and placebo-supplemented groups for heart rate, oxygen consumption, respiratory exchange ratio, and rating of perceived exertion during the 10 km and maximal treadmill tests.[112]

Recently, *Eleutherococcus senticosus* has received attention in the popular press under the name of *Ci Wu Jia*. Trials of its effect on performance have been sponsored by PacificHealth Laboratories, Inc., which is the manufacturer of a standardized extract and the holder of a patent for the use of Ci Wu Jia to enhance stamina and physical performance during, and enhance recovery following cessation of, exercise. All reports on Ci Wu Jia's impact on performance have been based on information provided by this manufacturer.

Ci Wu Jia reportedly has a carbohydrate-sparing action, shifting metabolism to a higher utilization of fat for energy. The carbohydrate shift is also reported to delay the lactic acid build-up associated with muscle fatigue. Reports indicate that Ci Wu Jia might slightly reduce heart rate during exercise and recovery. Participants have usually consumed 800 mg/day of the standardized extract for 2 weeks.

Overall, the evidence for an ergogenic affect from *Eleutherococcus senticosus* is fair. The reported benefits Russian athletes received from supplementation remain the most compelling evidence to date on the ergogenic potential of this plant.

Dosage

Recommended doses vary depending on the form of *Eleutherococcus* utilized. The dose of a 1:1 fluid extract (33% ethanol) is usually between 2.0 and 4.0 ml one to three times per day; however, doses up to 16.0 ml have been used. A standardized 20:1 solid concentrate, is also available. In this form, a minimum recommended dosage would be 300 mg/day, equivalent to 6 g of powdered root. Better results might be experienced at higher doses. In order to avoid accommodation, *Eleutherococcus* should be used for no longer than 60 consecutive days, followed by a period of 2–3 weeks of abstinence before again beginning supplementation.[111]

Toxicity

Toxicity studies in animals have demonstrated that *Eleutherococcus* extracts are virtually non-toxic. In human clinical studies it was demonstrated that in the recommended dosage range, they (33% ethanol) are well tolerated and side-effects are infrequent. A few studies found mild side-effects at higher dosages (4.5–6.0 ml three times/day) when used for long periods (60 days). The symptoms included insomnia, irritability, melancholy, and anxiety.

Carnitine

Carnitine is promoted as a supplement needed to improve the body's ability to use stored fat as fuel. Supplementation purportedly enhances lipid oxidation, increases Vo_{2max}, and decreases plasma lactate accumulation during exercise.

Carnitine is a tri-methylated amino acid, roughly similar in structure to choline. The synthesis of carnitine begins with the methylation of lysine by S-adenosylmethionine. Cofactors required for optimal synthesis include:

- magnesium
- iron
- ascorbic acid
- folic acid

- methylcobalamin
- betaine
- pyridoxal 5′ phosphate
- niacin.

Carnitine is located in the mitochondrial membrane and is a cofactor needed for the transformation of free long-chain fatty acids (LCFAs) into acyl-carnitines for subsequent transport into the mitochondrial matrix. Inside the mitochondria, LCFAs are metabolized into energy by the process of beta-oxidation.

Several investigators have suggested that L-carnitine supplementation might benefit athletes. One study investigated the effect of giving 2 g/day of L-carnitine for 6 weeks to seven male marathon athletes. Improved running speed of 5.68% and decreased average oxygen consumption and heart rate in the treadmill test followed supplementation. The authors suggest that for carnitine to be effective as an ergogenic aid, several preconditions must be met: having an adequate supply of lipids available as fuel, shifting metabolism towards the utilization of fats as an energy source, and having a relative shortage of available endogenous carnitine. Because the average free and total plasma carnitine levels were below the normal ranges prior to supplementation, the L-carnitine might have helped to overcome a relative endogenous deficiency for the participants involved in this study.[113]

In a double-blind cross-over study of 10 moderately trained male subjects, either 2 g of L-carnitine or placebo are provided orally 1 hour prior to exercise. Supplementation with L-carnitine induced a significant post-exercise decrease of plasma lactate and pyruvate and a concurrent increase of acetylcarnitine.[114] Another study gave 2 g of L-carnitine or a placebo to subjects 1 h before they began exercise. At the maximal exercise intensity, treatment with L-carnitine increased both maximal oxygen uptake and power output. The authors also reported that, at similar exercise intensities, oxygen uptake, carbon dioxide production, pulmonary ventilation and plasma lactate were reduced in participants receiving L-carnitine.[115]

While some of the results with L-carnitine supplementation have been promising, not all research is in agreement. One review of carnitine and physical exercise came to the following, among other, conclusions regarding carnitine supplementation:[116]

- its impact on performance in athletes is equivocal
- it does not enhance fatty acid oxidation, spare glycogen or postpones fatigue during exercise
- it does not stimulate pyruvate dehydrogenase activity
- it does not reduce body fat or help with weight loss.

One research group found chronic carnitine supplementation, 6 g/day, resulted in no differences in $\dot{V}O_2$, respiratory exchange ratio, heart rate, or carbohydrate and fat utilization. They also reported that muscle carnitine concentration at rest was unaffected by supplementation.[117] Similar results were reported with carnitine supplementation at 4 g/day for 14 days, which, while effective at increasing plasma total acid-soluble and free carnitine concentrations, had no significant effect on muscle carnitine concentrations.[118] Another group found that loading of athletes with L-carnitine for the 10 days prior to a marathon, while abolishing the exercise-induced fall in plasma-free carnitine and increasing the production of acetylcarnitine, resulted in no detectable improvement in performance.[119]

Still another study investigated the effects of L-carnitine supplementation on metabolism and performance of endurance-trained athletes during and after a marathon run. In a double-blind cross-over field study, seven male subjects received 2 g of L-carnitine 2 hours before the start of a marathon run and again after 20 km of running. Although the administration of L-carnitine was associated with a significant increase in the plasma concentration of all analyzed carnitine fractions, significant changes in running time, plasma concentrations of carbohydrate metabolites (glucose, lactate, and pyruvate), of fat metabolites (free fatty acids, glycerol, and beta-hydroxybutyrate), of hormones (insulin, glucagon, and cortisol); and of enzyme activities (creatine kinase and lactate dehydrogenase) were not observed.[120]

Although available data on L-carnitine as an ergogenic aid is not compelling, under some experimental conditions pretreatment has favored aerobic processes. It is possible that L-carnitine might only exert a beneficial effect when there are actual deficiencies. Availability of fat as a substrate for fuel might also impact on the ability of carnitine to act as an ergogenic aid.

Dosage

Supplementation of 2 g 1 hour prior to intensive exercise might provide some benefits; however, based on the mixed results and the cost of the supplement, chronic administration of L-carnitine is difficult to justify.

Toxicity

See above.

Choline

Choline supplements have been advocated as a means of preventing the decline in choline reported to occur during exercise. Choline in the diet primarily consists of phosphatidylcholine, which after absorption by the intestinal mucosa, is metabolized to choline in the liver. Most choline is re-phosphorylated to phosphatidylcholine; however, a small amount of choline is carried to the brain via the bloodstream, where it is converted to acetylcholine, a chemical messenger required for adequate nerve impulses and memory storage and retrieval.

Running a 26 km marathon reduced plasma choline by approximately 40% according to one study.[121] The decline has been proposed to reduce acetylcholine levels, resulting in a reduction in the transmission of contraction-generating impulses across skeletal muscle.[122] It has been proposed that this reduction might negatively affect endurance performance.[121,122]

One study investigated the effect of lecithin on the plasma choline concentrations during continuous strain in 10 top level triathletes (four women and six men). The participants received either a placebo or 0.2 g lecithin/kg body mass 1 hour before each exercise. Bicycle exercise without lecithin supply decreased plasma choline concentrations in all the triathletes, on average by 16.9%. When lecithin was given before exercise, average plasma choline concentrations remained at the same level as the initial values. In trial II, with 13 adolescent runners (three girls and 10 boys), mean plasma choline concentrations remained stable when running without supplementation of lecithin.[123]

However, another research group found that trained cyclists do not deplete choline during supramaximal brief or prolonged submaximal exercise, nor do they benefit from choline supplementation, as choline bitartrate (2.43 g), to delay fatigue under these conditions.[124]

No evidence to date provides compelling justification for the supplementation of choline as an ergogenic aid. Its potential efficacy for improving physical performance remains largely theoretical.

Coenzyme Q_{10} (ubiquinone)

Coenzyme Q_{10} (CoQ_{10}), because of its role in mitochondrial energy production, is reputed to enhance performance; however, no studies have demonstrated a significant improvement in any aspect of athletic performance.

Biopsy of muscle found that CoQ_{10} levels were positively correlated to exercise capacity and marathon performance.[125] Providing 150 mg/day of CoQ_{10} orally for 2 months to a group of middle-aged men resulted in increased circulating blood levels of CoQ_{10} and improved perceived level of vigor; no improvement in aerobic capacity was found.[126] Supplementing cyclists with 100 mg/day of CoQ_{10} for 8 weeks produced no measurable effect on performance, $VO_{2\,max}$, submaximal physiological parameters, or lipid peroxidation.[127] Others have found that oral ubiquinone was ineffective as an ergogenic aid in both young and older trained men.[128]

Based upon available research, CoQ_{10} appears to have no value as an ergogenic aid.

Pyridoxal-alpha-ketoglutarate (PAK)

Pyridoxal-alpha-ketoglutarate (PAK) consists of pyridoxine (about 54%) and alpha-ketoglutarate (about 46%). It is thought to improve the generation of high-energy phosphate bonds, such as ATP or GTP. In addition, an increased level of alpha-ketoglutarate, along with pyridoxal 5′-phosphate, in the mitochondria might enhance the transamination of pyruvate to alanine, which may prevent or reduce lactic acid formation.[129]

Administration of PAK has been shown to decrease the plasma concentration of lactate in response to isometric exercise in a group of insulin-independent non-ketotic diabetic patients.[130] The administration of 30 mg/kg of PAK for 30 days has been reported to increase $VO_{2\,max}$ (a measurement of maximal aerobic power) and to decrease lactic acid accumulation during short supramaximal workloads. The administration of alpha-ketoglutarate or pyridoxine separately did not alter $VO_{2\,max}$ significantly.[129]

Individually and in combination, the use of PAK and sodium bicarbonate on short-term maximal exercise capacity was studied in eight cyclists. Oral tablets of sodium bicarbonate and PAK were given in doses of 200 and 50 mg/kg, respectively. The investigators found no significant differences between treatments in the ability to sustain maximum power during the exercise trial; however, the best results obtained were from individuals utilizing both PAK and bicarbonate. PAK supplemented by itself did not improve participants' ability to sustain maximum power.[131]

Dosage

The typical dose is 1800–3000 mg/day, depending upon body weight. While PAK might be complementary to athletic training, particularly in conjunction with sodium bicarbonate, available information is limited. PAK supplementation appears to positively influence some physiological parameters associated with enhanced aerobic performance; however, to date this supplement has not been shown to produce a "bottom line" result of improving actual performance.

Pyruvate

Supplementation of pyruvate is becoming popular with athletes due to reports of its endurance and weight loss-enhancing effects. Pyruvate is a stable salt form of pyruvic acid, the naturally occurring end-product of the metabolism of carbohydrates. It is stabilized by the addition of either sodium, potassium, calcium, or magnesium to pyruvic acid. Pyruvic acid occurs naturally in the diet, with fruits and vegetables being good sources. Red apples are possibly the best source with an estimated 450 mg of pyruvic acid per apple.

Pyruvate is a three-carbon compound containing a carboxylic acid and a ketone group. During the process of glycolysis, glucose is converted to pyruvate. Pyruvate is then either converted to acetylCoA, for entry into the citric acid cycle under aerobic conditions, or to lactate under anaerobic conditions. Pyruvate's mechanism of action for weight loss and for enhancing endurance is unknown.

In published research, pyruvate has usually been given in conjunction with dihydroxyacetone. This combination has been reported to be useful in weight loss routines, where it is partially, isocalorically substituted for glucose in obese women. Participants were placed on severely restrictive hypocaloric diets for 21 days while housed in a metabolic ward. In one study, participants fed dihydroxyacetone and pyruvate (DHAP) showed greater weight loss (6.5 ± 0.3 kg, vs. 5.6 ± 0.2 kg for the placebo) and fat loss (4.3 ± 0.2 kg, vs. 3.5 ± 0.1 kg for placebo).[132] In another trial, pyruvate and dihydroxyacetone, given as approximately 20% of energy intake, reduced the reaccumulation of body weight (1.8 ± 0.2 vs. 2.9 ± 0.1 kg) and fat (0.8 ± 0.2 vs. 1.8 ± 0.2 kg) associated with refeeding after a calorie restricted diet.[133]

Pyruvate alone has been reported to be an effective addition to a weight loss program. In one study, participants were obese women housed in a metabolic ward consuming a 4.25 MJ/day liquid diet for 21 days with or without pyruvate partially, isoenergetically substituted for glucose. Participants fed pyruvate showed greater weight loss (5.9 ± 0.7 kg, vs. 4.3 ± 0.3 kg for placebo) and fat loss (4.0 ± 0.5 kg, vs. 2.7 ± 0.2 kg for placebo).[40] The reports indicate that pyruvate had no impact on enhancing nitrogen balance, serum protein concentrations or lean body mass in these subjects.[132–134]

Since the published studies were conducted on obese women consuming restricted calorie diets of either 500 or 1,000 calories/day, these weight losses should not be extrapolated to athletes or other populations on normal or high-calorie diets. Additionally, in the published trials pyruvate has been substituted for glucose, a substance which impacts fat metabolism in overweight individuals because of its role in insulin secretion. It is possible, under similar circumstances, that partially, isocalorically substituting protein or fat for glucose might have produced similar, if not better, results.

Pyruvate has been reported to increase the time required to reach exhaustion and to decrease perceived exertion. In the published studies, pyruvate was again given in relatively high amounts in conjunction with dihydroxyacetone. In both studies, untrained males received either 100 g of pyruvate and dihydroxyacetone or 100 g of a glucose polymer derived from the hydrolysis of corn starch as a placebo for 7 days. Arm endurance was 133 ± 20 minutes after placebo and 160 ± 22 minutes after DHAP.[135] Leg endurance was 66 ± 4 minutes after placebo and 79 ± 2 minutes after DHAP.[136] Muscle glycogen, determined by biopsy, at rest and exhaustion did not differ between placebo and DHAP subjects.[136] Plasma free fatty acids, glycerol, and beta-hydroxybutyrate were similar during rest and exercise for placebo and DHAP subjects in both studies.[135,136] Supplementation of a DHAP mixture has also been reported to decrease the perceived level of exertion.[137]

Feeding DHAP for 7 days appears to increase submaximal endurance in untrained athletes; however, it is unresolved whether similar results would be obtained with trained athletes. In the published studies 25 g/day of pyruvate were given along with 75 g/day of dihydroxyacetone; however, in the lay press Stanko has been quoted as saying: "We see a linear response between 2 and 5 g a day and then the response plateaus. In other words, the response with 10 or 15 g or more is the same as with 5 g." Supporting documentation for this assertion has apparently not been published in scientific literature to date, nor has any research been published on the endurance effects of the supplementation of pyruvate without dihydroxyacetone.

Dosage

Dosage recommendations are 2–5 g/day, taken with food. Better results might be obtained by spreading the 5 g into two or three divided doses.

Since the reported results on endurance were obtained in trials comparing DHAP against a glucose polymer, the only justifiable conclusion is that subjects consuming 100 g of DHAP rather than 100 g of hydrolyzed corn starch, a substance with no nutritional value, experienced better endurance. Research evaluating the performance effects of adding 2–5 g of pyruvate to the diet of trained athletes still needs to be published. The available evidence suggesting that pyruvate acts as an ergogenic aid in high dosages in combination with dihydroxyacetone is questionable. No evidence exists in support of claims of ergogenic action for pyruvate supplementation at the recommended dose of between 2 and 5 g.

Performance drinks

Performance drinks are commonly consumed as an ergogenic aid during endurance sports activities. These drinks are designed to maintain normal hydration, electrolyte balance and blood glucose levels during exercise. Current evidence indicates that ingestion of performance drinks during exercise enhances athletic performance and normalizes markers of thermoregulation. A variety of beverages formulated to provide fluid, carbohydrates, and electrolytes during and following exercise are commercially available. These beverages commonly contain 4–8%

carbohydrate (as glucose, fructose, sucrose or maltodextrins) and small amounts of electrolytes (most often sodium, potassium, and chloride). Contrary to popular belief, rates of sweating and urine flow are not influenced by fluid ingestion during exercise.[138]

Studies have shown that 5–10% solutions of glucose, glucose polymers (maltodextrins) and other simple sugars all have suitable gastric-emptying characteristics for the delivery of fluid and moderate amounts of carbohydrate substrate. The optimal concentration of electrolytes, particularly sodium, remains unknown. Most currently available sports drinks provide a low level of sodium (10–25 mmol/L) in recognition of the fact that sodium intake can promote intestinal absorption of fluid as well as assist in rehydration.[139]

Exercise and dehydration result in increases in core temperature, body fluid osmolality, and heart rate; losses of plasma and other body fluid volumes; and depletion of glycogen. All of these homeostatic disturbances can be ameliorated by fluid consumption during exercise.[140]

During exercise, water and electrolytes are lost from the body in sweat. Sweat rate is determined primarily by the metabolic rate and the environmental temperature and humidity. Under some conditions, the sweat rate can exceed the maximum rate of gastric emptying of ingested fluids. If this occurs, some degree of dehydration is observed. Excessive replacement of sweat losses with plain water or fluids with a low sodium content following prolonged exercise has resulted in hyponatraemia, so sodium replacement is considered essential for post-exercise rehydration.[141]

For moderate-intensity exercise, water ingestion 30–60 minutes prior to exercise seems to minimize homeostatic disturbances; however, at higher intensities of athletic performance, it probably has little effect.[140] During exercise, ingestion of both water and carbohydrate beverages has been shown to minimize homeostatic disturbances. Subjects allowed to drink a carbohydrate-electrolyte beverage (4.85% polycose, 2.65% fructose) or distilled water ad libitum during 3 hours of continuous exercise in the heat (31.5°C) showed no significant differences between drinks for rectal temperature, heart rate, or sweat rate during exercise.[142] No differences in thermoregulatory responses in individuals consuming either carbohydrate beverages or water have been observed.[143]

The efficacy of a given drink is limited by the rate of absorption of fluid from the intestines, which is in turn limited by gastric emptying. Several factors influence gastric emptying, including exercise intensity and the carbohydrate composition of the solution.[144] The gastric-emptying rate might also be influenced by the caloric content, volume, osmolality, temperature, and pH of the ingested fluid; metabolic state and biochemical individuality of the athlete; and the ambient temperature.[145]

The caloric content of the ingested fluid might be the most important variable governing gastric-emptying rate. At rest and during running, water has a faster gastric-emptying time than all other drinks. Gastric emptying is progressively slowed as the caloric content of the fluid increases.[144] During moderate exercise, gastric emptying occurs at a rate similar to that during rest; however, more intense exercise appears to inhibit gastric emptying. Evidence indicates that beverages containing below 10% carbohydrate have gastric-emptying rates closest to that of water.[146] Drinks containing less than or equal to 8–10% carbohydrate are absorbed into the body at similar rates and should behave similarly in replenishing body fluids lost in sweat during exercise.[147]

Several other factors have been shown to impact gastric emptying. Isotonic drinks appear to empty quickly throughout exercise, whereas the gastric-emptying rate of hypertonic drinks has been shown to decrease over time.[148] Fat is believed to delay gastric emptying; however, medium-chain triglycerides (MCTs) might not inhibit gastric emptying as most fat does. Research indicates that MCT-containing drinks have faster gastric-emptying times than drinks containing 100% maltodextrins.[149]

It has been suggested that maltose might be a superior source of carbohydrate for endurance athletes. Some researchers have suggested that ingestion of an 8% solution of maltodextrin or sucrose every 15 minutes during exercise might provide optimal fluid and carbohydrate replacement.[150] The rates of gastric emptying and the peak rates of exogenous carbohydrate oxidation are not significantly different between maltose and glucose.[151]

While ingestion of 13 g carbohydrate per hour did not improve performance during prolonged moderate intensity cycling in one study,[152] most studies report that ingestion of carbohydrate beverages has a beneficial effect on performance. Carbohydrate ingested during exercise appears to be readily available as a fuel for the working muscles, at least when the exercise intensity does not exceed 70–75% of maximum oxygen uptake.[153] Rating of perceived exertion is reported to be higher in athletes consuming water than in athletes consuming carbohydrate drinks.[154] For exercise leading to exhaustion in less than 30 minutes, carbohydrate ingestion is not effective in minimizing homeostatic perturbations or improving exercise performance;[140] however, for exercise of longer duration, ingestion of performance beverages appears to enhance performance. Research has shown that 275 ml of a 6% carbohydrate-electrolyte beverage consumed every 20 minutes maintained blood glucose and enhanced performance better than water during endurance cycling.[155] One study compared the effects of orange flavored drinks containing 0, 6.4, and 10% carbohydrate. The solutions, 3 ml/kg body weight, were given double-blind and counter-balanced at time 0 and every 20 minutes during exercise. Blood glucose and lactate, and temperature were similar for all solutions; however, performance improved with consumption of a carbohydrate drink during exercise. The best results were obtained with ingestion of a 10% carbohydrate drink.[156]

Eight well-trained men cycled for up to 255 minutes at a power output corresponding to $\dot{V}O_2$ at lactate threshold (approximately 68% $\dot{V}O_{2\,max}$) on three occasions separated by at least 1 week. Subjects drank 5 ml/kg body weight of either a water placebo or a liquid beverage containing a moderate (6% carbohydrate) or high (12% carbohydrate) concentration of carbohydrate, beginning at minute 14 of exercise and every 30 minutes thereafter. Exercise time to fatigue was shorter in subjects receiving placebo (190 minutes) as compared with 6% carbohydrate (235 minutes) and 12% carbohydrate (234 minutes) beverages.[157]

In another study, 12 subjects were exercised to exhaustion on a cycle ergometer at a workload corresponding to 70% of maximum oxygen uptake. In one trial, no drinks were given, and in the other trials subjects drank 100 ml every 10 minutes. Median exercise time was greatest (110.3 minutes) for individuals receiving a hypotonic glucose-electrolyte solution (90 mmol/L glucose; 60 mmol/L Na^+; 240 mosmol/kg), followed by individuals receiving an isotonic glucose-electrolyte solution (I: 200 mmol/L glucose; 35 mmol/L Na^+; 310 mosmol/kg) (107.3 min), water (93.1) and no drink (80.7). Significant treatment effects were also observed for heart rate, rectal temperature and serum osmolality.[158]

Twelve highly trained male runners ran 15 km at self-selected pace on a treadmill in warm conditions to demonstrate differences in physiological responses, fluid preferences, and performance when ingesting sports drinks or plain water before and during exercise. One hour prior to the start of running, an equal volume (1,000 ml) of either water or a 6 or 8% carbohydrate-electrolyte drink was ingested. Blood glucose was significantly higher 30 minutes following ingestion of the 6 and 8% carbohydrate-electrolyte beverages compared with water, significantly lower at 60 minutes post-ingestion with both sports drinks than with water, but similar after 7.5 km of the run for all beverages. During the first 13.4 km, oxygen uptake and run times were not different between trials; however, the final 1.6 km performance run was faster with both carbohydrate-electrolyte drinks than with water.[159]

Research indicates that a sugar drink immediately prior to exercise can impair performance. Carbohydrates will invoke an insulin response which increases the likelihood of hypoglycemia occurring during exercise. A fall in blood glucose will result from the ingestion of glucose solutions fed 15–45 minutes before prolonged exercise; however, the consumption of 18–50% solutions of glucose or glucose polymers 5 minutes before prolonged exercise has potential for improving endurance performance.[140]

Many experts recommend consuming a beverage high in carbohydrates within 1 hour after exercise. Exercise-induced depletion of muscle glycogen levels can be rapidly restored by glucose ingestion. Provided adequate carbohydrate is consumed, it appears that the frequency of intake, the form (liquid vs. solid) and the presence of other macronutrients does not affect the rate of glycogen storage.[160] During the post-exercise recovery period, ingesting a carbohydrate-electrolyte beverage is effective in minimizing physiological disturbances. Subjects drink more; plasma volume increases to a higher level; plasma osmolality, glucose, and potassium are greater; and body weight increases more with the ingestion of carbohydrate beverages than with pure water.[161]

Dosage

The optimum frequency, volume and composition of drinks will vary widely depending on the intensity and duration of the exercise, the environmental conditions and the physiology of the individual. However, in general, isotonic beverages, with either glucose, glucose polymers, or maltodextrins as the carbohydrate source, produce the best results. Prior to exercise, only water should be consumed. Drinking carbohydrate solutions 15–60 minutes prior to exercise should be avoided since it can impair performance; however, ingestion immediately prior to beginning exercise might be beneficial. This is because once endurance exercise is started, insulin is generally not increased, so the carbohydrates will likely be available as energy substrates. The staggered ingestion of performance drinks will be beneficial when exercise duration exceeds 30 minutes; however, during shorter duration exercise and especially weight-lifting, there appears to be no additional benefit in ingesting anything other than water.

SUMMARY

Based upon available information, evidence remains mixed but promising on the supplementation of *Panax ginseng* and *Eleutherococcus senticosus*. L-Carnitine's role as an ergogenic aid remains something of a mystery. The mixed results reported in the literature and the high cost of the supplement make it difficult to justify chronic administration of 2 g/day. No evidence to date supports the supplementation of choline as an ergogenic aid. CoQ_{10}'s failure in several studies to demonstrate any performance-enhancing effect should end any debate or recommendations concerning routine administration of this nutrient as an ergogenic aid. Although PAK supplementation has been shown to enhance certain parameters associated with aerobic exercise, it has not yet demonstrated improved performance. Although evidence suggests that pyruvate acts as an ergogenic aid in high dosages in combination with dihydroxyacetone, available evidence does not support claims of an ergogenic action for pyruvate supplementation at a dose of between 2 and 5 g. The staggered ingestion of isotonic, 6–10% carbohydrate performance drinks should be a routine practice in endurance exercise activities of greater than 30 minutes' duration.

REFERENCES

1. Harris RC, Söderlund K, Hultman E. Elevation of creatine in resting and exercised muscle of normal subjects by creatine supplementation. Clin Sci 1992; 83: 367–374
2. Walker JB. Creatine biosynthesis, regulation and function. Adv Enzymol 1979; 50: 117–242
3. Maughan RJ. Creatine supplementation and exercise performance. Int J Sport Nutr 1995; 5: 94–101
4. Gordon A, Hultman E, Kaijser L et al. Creatine supplementation in chronic heart failure increases skeletal muscle creatine phosphate and muscle performance. Cardiovasc Res 1995; 30: 413–418
5. Haussinger D, Roth E, Lang F, Gerok W. Cellular hydration state: an important determinant of protein catabolism in health and disease. Lancet 1993; 341: 1330–1332
6. Greenhaff PL, Bodin K, Soderlund K, Hultman E. Effect of oral creatine supplementation on skeletal muscle phosphocreatine resynthesis. Am J Physiol 1994; 266: E725–730
7. Gerber GB, Gerber G, Koszalka TR et al. Creatine metabolism in vitamin E deficiency in the rat. Am J Physiol 1962; 202: 453–460
8. Stöckler S, Holzbach U, Hanefeld F et al. Creatine deficiency in the brain: a new, treatable inborn error of metabolism. Pediatr Res 1994; 36: 409–413
9. Earnest CP, Snell PG, Rodriguez R et al. The effect of creatine monohydrate ingestion on aerobic power indices, muscular strength and body composition. Acta Physiol Scand 1995; 153: 207–209
10. Balsom PD, Söderlund K, Sjödin B, Ekblom B. Skeletal muscle metabolism during short duration high-intensity exercise. influence of creatine supplementation. Acta Physiol Scand 1995; 154: 303–310
11. Dawson B, Cutler M, Moody A et al. Effects of oral creatine loading on single and repeated maximal short sprints. Aust J Sci Med Sport 1995; 27: 56–61
12. Greenhaff PL, Casey A, Short AH et al. Influence of oral creatine supplementation of muscle torque during repeated bouts of maximal voluntary exercise in man. Clin Sci 1993; 84: 565–571
13. Birch R, Noble D, Greenhaff PL. The influence of dietary creatine supplementation on performance during repeated bouts of maximal isokinetic cycling in man. Eur J Appl Physiol 1994; 69: 268–276
14. Cooke WH, Grandjean PW, Barnes WS. Effect of oral creatine supplementation on power output and fatigue during bicycle ergometry. J Appl Physiol 1995; 78: 670–673
15. Balsom PD, Harridge SD, Söderlund K et al. Creatine supplementation per se does not enhance endurance exercise performance. Acta Physiol Scand 1993; 149: 521–523
16. Stroud MA, Holliman D, Bell D et al. Effect of oral creatine supplementation on respiratory gas exchange and blood lactate accumulation during steady-state incremental treadmill exercise and recovery in man. Clin Sci 1994; 87: 707–710
17. Hultman E, Söderlund K, Timmons JA et al. Muscle creatine loading in men. J Appl Physiol 1996; 81: 232–237
18. Balsom PD, Söderlund K, Ekblom B. Creatine in humans with special reference to creatine supplementation. Sports Med 1994; 18: 268–280
19. Sipila I, Rapola J, Simell O et al. Supplementary creatine as a treatment for gyrate atrophy of the choroid retina. N Engl J Med 1981; 304: 867–870
20. van Koevering M, Nissen S. In vivo conversion of alpha-ketoisocaproate to beta-hydroxy beta-methyl butyrate in vivo. Am J Physiol 1992; 262: 27–31
21. Nissen S, Sharp R, Rathmacher JA et al. The effect of the leucine metabolite beta-hydroxy-beta-methyl butyrate on muscle metabolism during resistance-exercise training. J Appl Physiol 1996; 81: 2095–2104
22. Nissen S, Panton L, Wilhelm R, Fuller JC. Effect of beta-hydroxy-beta-methyl butyrate (HMB) supplementation on strength and body composition of trained and untrained males undergoing intense resistance training. FASEB 10: A287, 1996 [Abstract]
23. Mahe S, Roos N, Benamouzig R et al. Gastrojejunal kinetics and the digestion of (15N) beta-lactoglobulin and casein in humans. the influence of the nature and quality of the protein. Am J Clin Nutr 1996; 63: 546–552
24. Melichar V, Mikova M. Feminar with whey (serum) proteins prepared by thermal denaturation. Nitrogen and lipid balance in neonates with a low birthweight. Cesk Pediatr 1989; 44: 1–5
25. Mahan DC. Efficacy of dried whey and its lactalbumin and lactose components at two dietary lysine levels on postweaning pig performance and nitrogen balance. J Anim Sci 1992; 70: 2182–2187
26. Alexander JW, Gottschlich MM. Nutritional modulation in burn patients. Crit Care Med 1990; 18: S149–153
27. Bounous G, Gervais F, Amer V et al. The influence of dietary whey protein on tissue glutathione and the diseases of aging. Clin Invest Med 1989; 12: 343–349
28. Kanter MM. Free radicals, exercise, and antioxidant supplementation. Int J Sport Nutr 1994; 4: 205–220
29. Clarkson PM. Antioxidants and physical performance. Crit Rev Food Sci Nutr 1995; 35: 131–141
30. Leeuwenburgh C, Leichtweis S, Hollander J et al. Effect of acute exercise on glutathione deficient heart. Mol Cell Biochem 1996; 156: 17–24
31. Cooper MB, Jones DA, Edwards RH et al. The effect of marathon running on carnitine metabolism and on some aspects of muscle mitochondrial activities and antioxidant mechanisms. J Sports Sci 1986; 4: 79–87
32. Shephard RJ, Shek PN. Heavy exercise, nutrition and immune function: is there a connection? Int J Sports Med 1995; 16: 491–497
33. Bounous G, Batist G, Gold P. Immunoenhancing property of dietary whey protein in mice; role of glutathione. Clin Invest Med 1989; 12: 154–161
34. Kashyap S, Okamoto E, Kanaya S et al. Protein quality in feeding low birthweight infants. a comparison of whey-predominant versus casein-predominant formulas. Pediatrics 1987; 79: 748–755
35. Bounous G, Baruchel S, Falutz J, Gold P. Whey proteins as a food supplement in HIV-seropositive individuals. Clin Invest Med 1993; 16: 204–209
36. Bounous G, Batist G, Gold P. Whey proteins in cancer prevention. Cancer Lett 1991; 57: 91–94
37. McIntosh GH, Regester GOP, Le Leu RK et al. Dairy proteins protect against dimethylhydrazine-induced intestinal cancers in rats. J Nutr 1995; 125: 809–816
38. Fiat AM, Migliore-Samour D, Jolles P et al. Biologically active peptides from milk proteins with emphasis on two examples concerning antithrombotic and immunomodulating activities. J Dairy Sci 1993; 76: 301–310
39. Wong CW, Watson DL. Immunomodulatory effects of dietary whey proteins in mice. J Dairy Res 1995; 62: 359–368
40. May ME, Buse MG. Effects of branched-chain amino acids on protein turnover. Diabetes Metab Rev 1989; 5: 227–245
41. Zawadzki KM, Yaspelkis BB 3d, Ivy JL. Carbohydrate-protein complex increases the rate of muscle glycogen storage after exercise. J Appl Physiol 1992; 72: 1854–1859
42. Karjalainen J, Martin JM, Knip M et al. A bovine albumin peptide as a possible trigger of insulin-dependent diabetes mellitus. N Engl J Med 1992; 327: 302–307
43. Pardini VC, Vieira JG, Miranda W et al. Antibodies to bovine

serum albumin in Brazilian children and young adults with IDDM. Diabetes Care 1996; 19: 126–129
44. Ivarsson SA, Mansson MU, Jakobsson IL. IgG antibodies to bovine serum albumin are not increased in children with IDDM. Diabetes 1995; 44: 1349–1350
45. Monteleone P, Maj M, Beinat L et al. Blunting by chronic phosphatidylserine administration of the stress-induced activation of the hypothalamo-pituitary-adrenal axis in healthy men. Eur J Clin Pharmacol 1992; 42: 385–388
46. Monteleone P, Beinat L, Tanzillo C et al. Effects of phosphatidylserine on the neuroendocrine response to physical stress in humans. Neuroendocrinology 1990; 52: 243–248
47. Corpas E, Blackman MR, Roberson R et al. Oral arginine-lysine does not increase growth hormone or insulin-like growth factor-I in old men. J Gerontol 1993; 48: M128–133
48. Minuskin ML, Lavine ME, Ulman EA, Fisher H. Nitrogen retention, muscle creatine and orotic acid excretion in traumatized rats fed arginine and glycine enriched diets. J Nutr 1981; 111: 1265–1274
49. Elam EP, Hardin DH, Sutton RA, Hagen L. Effect of arginine and ornithine on strength, lean body mass and urinary hydroxyproline in adult males. J Sports Nutr 1989; 29: 52–56
50. Hood DA, Terjung RL. Amino acid metabolism during exercise and following endurance training. Sports Med 1990; 9: 23–35
51. Blomstrand E, Ek S, Newsholme EA. Influence of ingesting a solution of branched-chain amino acids on plasma and muscle concentrations of amino acids during prolonged submaximal exercise. Nutrition 1996; 12: 485–490
52. Louard RJ, Barrett EJ, Gelfand RA. Effect of infused branched-chain amino acids on muscle and whole-body amino acid metabolism in man. Clin Sci 1990; 79: 457–466
53. MacLean DA, Graham TE, Saltin B. Stimulation of muscle ammonia production during exercise following branched-chain amino acid supplementation in humans. J Physiol 1996; 493: 909–922
54. Fraga Fuentes MD, de Juana Velasco P, Pintor Recuenco R. Metabolic role of glutamine and its importance in nutritional therapy. Nutr Hosp 1996; 11: 215–225
55. Hall JC, Heel K, McCauley R. Glutamine. Br J Surg 1996; 83: 305–312
56. Rennie MJ, MacLennan PA, Hundal HS et al. Skeletal muscle glutamine transport, intramuscular glutamine concentration, and muscle-protein turnover. Metabolism 1989; 38: 47–51
57. Rennie MJ, Tadros L, Khogali S et al. Glutamine transport and its metabolic effects. J Nutr 1994; 124: 1503S–158S
58. Balzola FA, Boggio-Bertinet D. The metabolic role of glutamine. Minerva Gastroenterol Dietol 1996; 42: 17–26
59. Rowbottom DG, Keast D, Morton AR. The emerging role of glutamine as an indicator of exercise stress and overtraining. Sports Med 1996; 21: 80–97
60. Keast D, Arstein D, Harper W et al. Depression of plasma glutamine concentration after exercise stress and its possible influence on the immune system. Med J Aust 1995; 162: 15–18
61. Varnier M, Leese GP, Thompson J, Rennie MJ. Stimulatory effect of glutamine on glycogen accumulation in human skeletal muscle. Am J Physiol 1995; 269: E309–315
62. Vinnars E, Hammarqvist F, von der Decken A, Wernerman J. Role of glutamine and its analogs in post-traumatic muscle protein and amino acid metabolism. JPEN 1990; 14: 125S–129S
63. Welbourne TC. Increased plasma bicarbonate and growth hormone after an oral glutamine load. Am J Clin Nutr 1995; 61: 1058–1061
64. Cynober L. Ornithine alpha-ketoglutarate in nutritional support. Nutrition 1991; 7: 313–322
65. Gerster H. The role of vitamin C in athletic performance. J Am Coll Nutr 1989; 8: 636–643
66. Jakeman P, Maxwell S. Effect of antioxidant vitamin supplementation on muscle function after eccentric exercise. Eur J Appl Physiol 1993; 67: 426–430
67. Kodama M, Kodama T, Murakami M et al. Autoimmune disease and allergy are controlled by vitamin C treatment. In Vivo 1994; 8: 251–257
68. Kallner A. Influence of vitamin C status on the urinary excretion of catecholamines in stress. Hum Nutr Clin Nutr 1983; 37: 405–411
69. Lee IP, Sherins RJ, Dixon RL. Evidence for induction of germinal aplasia in male rats by environmental exposure to boron. Toxicol Appl Pharmacol 1978; 45: 577–590
70. Nielsen FH, Hunt CD, Mullen LM et al. Effect of dietary boron on mineral, estrogen, and testosterone metabolism in postmenopausal women. FASEB J 1987; 1: 394–397
71. Naghii MR, Lyons PM, Samman S. The boron content of selected foods and the estimation of its daily intake among free-living subjects. J Amer Col Nutr 1996; 15: 614–619
72. Beattie JH, Peace HS. The influence of a low-boron diet and boron supplementation on bone, major mineral and sex steroid metabolism in postmenopausal women. Br J Nutr 1993; 69: 871–874
73. Green NR, Ferrando AA. Plasma boron and the effects of boron supplementation in males. Environ Health Perspect 1994; 102: 73–77
74. Hasten DL, Rome EP, Franks BD, Hegsted M. Effects of chromium picolinate on beginning weight training students. Int J Sports Nutr 1992; 2: 343–350
75. Clancy SP, Clarkson PM, DeCheke ME et al. Effects of chromium picolinate supplementation on body composition, strength, and urinary chromium loss in football players. Int J Sport Nutr 1994; 4: 142–153
76. Hallmark MA, Reynolds TH, DeSouza CA et al. Effects of chromium and resistive training on muscle strength and body composition. Med Sci Sports Exerc 1996; 28: 139–144
77. Trent LK, Thieding-Cancel D. Effects of chromium picolinate on body composition. J Sports Med Phys Fitness 1995; 35: 273–280
78. Lukaski HC, Bolonchuk WW, Siders WA et al. Chromium supplementation and resistance training. effects on body composition, strength, and trace element status of men. Am J Clin Nutr 1996; 63: 954–965
79. Olinescu R, Talaban D, Nita S, Mihaescu G. Comparative study of the presence of oxidative stress in sportsmen in competition and aged people, as well as the preventive effect of selenium administration. Rom J Intern Med 1995; 33: 47–54
80. Olivieri O, Girelli D, Stanzial AM et al. Selenium, zinc, and thyroid hormones in healthy subjects. Low T3/T4 ratio in the elderly is related to impaired selenium status. Biol Trace Elem Res 1996; 51: 31–41
81. Kralik A, Eder K, Kirchgessner M. Influence of zinc and selenium deficiency on parameters relating to thyroid hormone metabolism. Horm Metab Res 1996; 28: 223–226
82. Boden G, Chen X, Ruiz J et al. Effects of vanadyl sulfate on carbohydrate and lipid metabolism in patients with non-insulin-dependent diabetes mellitus. Metabolism 1996; 45: 1130–1135
83. Cohen N, Halberstam M, Shlimovich P et al. Oral vanadyl sulfate improves hepatic and peripheral insulin sensitivity in patients with non-insulin-dependent diabetes mellitus. J Clin Invest 1995; 95: 2501–2509
84. Halberstam M, Cohen N, Shlimovich P et al. Oral vanadyl sulfate improves insulin sensitivity in NIDDM but not in obese nondiabetic subjects. Diabetes 1996; 45: 659–666
85. Fawcett JP, Farquhar SJ, Walker RJ et al. The effect of oral vanadyl sulfate on body composition and performance in weight-training athletes. Int J Sport Nutr 1996; 6: 382–390
86. Harland BF and Harden-Williams BA. Is vanadium of human nutritional importance yet? J Am Dietetic Assoc 1994; 94: 891–895
87. Brun JF, Dieu-Cambrezy C, Charpiat A et al. Serum zinc in highly trained adolescent gymnasts. Biol Trace Elem Res 1995; 47: 273–278
88. Prasad AS, Mantzoros CS, Beck FWJ et al. Zinc status and serum testosterone levels of healthy adults. Nutrition 1996; 12: 344–348
89. Nishi Y. Zinc and growth. J Am Coll Nutr 1996; 15: 340–344
90. Collipp PJ, Castro-Magana M, Petrovic M et al. Zinc deficiency. improvement in growth and growth hormone levels with oral zinc therapy. Ann Nutr Metab 1982; 26: 287–290
91. Ripa S, Ripa R. Zinc and the growth hormone system. Minerva Med 1996; 87: 25–31
92. Baranov AI. Medicinal uses of ginseng and related plants in the Soviet Union: recent trends in the Soviet literature. J Ethnopharmacol 1982; 6: 339–353

93. Banerjee U, Izquierdo JA. Antistress and antifatigue properties of *Panax ginseng*: comparison with piracetam. Acta Physiol Lat Am 1982; 32: 277–285
94. Saito H, Yoshida Y, Takagi K. Effect of *Panax ginseng* root on exhaustive exercise in mice. Jpn J Pharmacol 1974; 24: 119–127
95. Takahashi M, Tokuyama S, Kaneto H. Anti-stress effect of ginseng on the inhibition of the development of morphine tolerance in stressed mice. Jpn J Pharmacol 1992; 59: 399–404
96. Bittles AH, Fulder SJ, Grant EC, Nicholls MR. The effect of ginseng on lifespan and stress responses in mice. Gerontology 1979; 25: 125–131
97. Tadano T, Aizawa T, Asao T et al. Pharmacological studies of nutritive and tonic crude drugs on fatigue in mice. Nippon Yakurigaku Zasshi 1992; 100: 423–431
98. Grandhi A, Mujumdar AM, Patwardhan B. A comparative pharmacological investigation of Ashwagandha and Ginseng. J Ethnopharmacol 1994; 44: 131–135
99. Fahim MS, Fahim Z, Harman JM et al. Effect of *Panax ginseng* on testosterone level and prostate in male rats. Arch Androl 1982; 8: 261–263
100. Fulder SJ. Ginseng and the hypothalamic-pituitary control of stress. Am J Chin Med 1981; 9: 112–118
101. Hiai S, Yokoyama H, Oura H, Yano S. Stimulation of pituitary-adrenocortical system by ginseng saponin. Endocrinol Jpn 1979; 26: 661–665
102. Bahrke MS, Morgan WP. Evaluation of the ergogenic properties of ginseng. Sports Med 1994; 18: 229–248
103. Salvati G, Genovesi G, Marcellini L et al. Effects of *Panax Ginseng* C.A. Meyer saponins on male fertility. Panminerva Med 1996; 38: 249–254
104. Caso Marasco A, Vargas Ruiz R, Salas Villagomez A, Begona Infante C. Double-blind study of a multivitamin complex supplemented with ginseng extract. Drugs Exp Clin Res 1996; 22: 323–329
105. Pieralisi G, Ripari P, Vecchiet L. Effects of a standardized ginseng extract combined with dimethylaminoethanol bitartrate, vitamins, minerals, and trace elements on physical performance during exercise. Clin Ther 1991; 13: 373–382
106. Morris AC, Jacobs I, McLellan TM et al. No ergogenic effect of ginseng ingestion. Int J Sport Nutr 1996; 6: 263–271
107. Pizzorno JE, Murray MT. A textbook of natural medicine. Seattle, WA: Bastyr University Publications. 1996
108. Baranov AI. Medicinal uses of ginseng and related plants in the Soviet Union. recent trends in the Soviet literature. J Ethnopharmacol 1982; 6: 339–353
109. Nishibe S, Kinoshita H, Takeda H, Okano G. Phenolic compounds from stem bark of *Acanthopanax senticosus* and their pharmacological effect in chronic swimming stressed rats. Chem Pharm Bull 1990; 38: 1763–1765
110. Golotin VG, Gonenko VA, Zimina VV et al. Effect of ionol and eleutherococcus on changes of the hypophyseo-adrenal system in rats under extreme conditions. Vopr Med Khim 1989; 35: 35–37
111. Farnsworth NR, Kinghorn AD, Soejarto D, Waller DP. Siberian ginseng (*Eleutherococcus senticosus*). Current status as an adaptagen. Econ Med Plant Res 1985; 1: 156–215
112. Dowling EA, Redondo DR, Branch JD et al. Effect of *Eleutherococcus senticosus* on submaximal and maximal exercise performance. Med Sci Sports Exerc 1996; 8: 482–489
113. Swart I, Rossouw J, Loots JM, Kruger MC. The effect of L-carnitine supplementation on plasma carnitine levels and various performance parameters of male marathon athletes. Nutr Res 1997; 17: 405–414
114. Siliprandi N, Di Lisa F, Pieralisi G et al. Metabolic changes induced by maximal exercise in human subjects following L-carnitine administration. Biochim Biophys Acta 1990; 1034: 17–21
115. Vecchiet L, Di Lisa F, Pieralisi G et al. Influence of L-carnitine administration on maximal physical exercise. Eur J Appl Physiol 1990; 61: 486–490
116. Heinonen OJ. Carnitine and physical exercise. Sports Med 1996; 22: 109–132
117. Vukovich MD, Costill DL, Fink WJ. Carnitine supplementation. effect on muscle carnitine and glycogen content during exercise. Med Sci Sports Exerc 1994; 26: 1122–1129
118. Barnett C, Costill DL, Vukovich MD et al. Effect of L-carnitine supplementation on muscle and blood carnitine content and lactate accumulation during high-intensity sprint cycling. Int J Sport Nutr 1994; 4: 280–288
119. Cooper MB, Jones DA, Edwards RH et al. The effect of marathon running on carnitine metabolism and on some aspects of muscle mitochondrial activities and antioxidant mechanisms. J Sports Sci 1986; 4: 79–87
120. Colombani P, Wenk C, Kunz I et al. Effects of L-carnitine supplementation on physical performance and energy metabolism of endurance-trained athletes: a double-blind crossover field study. Eur J Appl Physiol 1996; 73: 434–439
121. Conlay LA, Sabounjian LA, Wurtman RJ. Exercise and neuromodulators: choline and acetylcholine in marathon runners. Int J Sports Med 1992; 13: S141–142
122. Kanter MM, Williams MH. Antioxidants, carnitine, and choline as putative ergogenic aids. Int J Sport Nutr 1995; 5: S120–131
123. von Allworden HN, Horn S, Kahl J, Feldheim W. The influence of lecithin on plasma choline concentrations in triathletes and adolescent runners during exercise. Eur J Appl Physiol 1993; 67: 87–91
124. Spector SA, Jackman MR, Sabounjian LA et al. Effect of choline supplementation on fatigue in trained cyclists. Med Sci Sports Exerc 1995; 27: 668–673
125. Karlsson J, Lin L, Sylven C, Jansson E. Muscle ubiquinone in healthy physically active males. Mol Cell Biochem 1996; 156: 169–172
126. Porter DA, Costill DL, Zachwieja JJ et al. The effect of oral coenzyme Q_{10} on the exercise tolerance of middle-aged, untrained men. Int J Sports Med 1995; 16: 421–427
127. Braun B, Clarkson PM, Freedson PS et al. Effects of coenzyme Q_{10} supplementation on exercise performance, Vo_{2max}, and lipid peroxidation in trained cyclists. Int J Sport Nutr 1991; 1: 353–365
128. Laaksonen R, Fogelholm M, Himberg JJ et al. Ubiquinone supplementation and exercise capacity in trained young and older men. Eur J Appl Physiol 1995; 72: 95–100
129. Marconi C, Sassi G, Cerretelli P. The Effect of an a-Ketoglutarate-Pyridoxine Complex on Human Maximal Aerobic and Anaerobic Performance. Eur J Appl Physiol 1982; 49: 307–317
130. Dall'Aglio E, Zavaroni I, Alpi O et al. The effect of pyridoxine-alpha-ketoglutarate (PAK) on exercise-induced increase of blood lactate in patients with type I diabetes. Int J Clin Pharmacol Ther Toxicol 1982; 20: 147–150
131. Linderman J, Kirk L, Musselman J et al. The effects of sodium bicarbonate and pyridoxine-alpha-ketoglutarate on short-term maximal exercise capacity. J Sports Sci 1992; 10: 243–253
132. Stanko RT, Tietze DL, Arch JE. Body composition, energy utilization, and nitrogen metabolism with a severely restricted diet supplemented with dihydroxyacetone and pyruvate. Am J Clin Nutr 1992; 55: 771–776
133. Stanko RT, Arch JE. Inhibition of regain in body weight and fat with addition of 3-carbon compounds to the diet with hyperenergetic refeeding after weight reduction. Int J Obes Relat Metab Disord 1996; 20: 925–930
134. Stanko RT, Tietze DL, Arch JE. Body composition, energy utilization, and nitrogen metabolism with a 4.25-MJ/d low-energy diet supplemented with pyruvate. Am J Clin Nutr 1992; 56: 630–635
135. Stanko RT, Robertson RJ, Spina RJ et al. Enhancement of arm exercise endurance capacity with dihydroxyacetone and pyruvate. J Appl Physiol 1990; 68: 119–124
136. Stanko RT, Robertson RJ, Galbreath RW et al. Enhanced leg exercise endurance with a high-carbohydrate diet and dihydroxyacetone and pyruvate. J Appl Physiol 1990; 69: 1651–1656
137. Robertson RJ, Stanko RT, Goss FL et al. Blood glucose extraction as a mediator of perceived exertion during prolonged exercise. Eur J Appl Phys 1990; 61: 100–105
138. Terrados N, Maughan RJ. Exercise in the heat. strategies to minimize the adverse effects on performance. J Sports Sci 1995; 13: S55–62

139. Burke LM, Read RS. Dietary supplements in sport. Sports Med 1993; 15: 43–65
140. Lamb DR, Brodowicz GR. Optimal use of fluids of varying formulations to minimise exercise-induced disturbances in homeostasis. Sports Med 1986; 3: 247–274
141. Maughan RJ, Noakes TD. Fluid replacement and exercise stress. A brief review of studies on fluid replacement and some guidelines for the athlete. Sports Med 1991; 12: 16–31
142. Carter JE, Gisolfi CV. Fluid replacement during and after exercise in the heat. Med Sci Sports Exerc 1989; 21: 532–539
143. Hickey MS, Costill DL, Trappe SW. Drinking behavior and exercise-thermal stress. role of drink carbonation. Int J Sport Nutr 1994; 4: 8–21
144. Rehrer NJ, Beckers E, Brouns F et al. Exercise and training effects on gastric emptying of carbohydrate beverages. Med Sci Sports Exerc 1989; 21: 540–549
145. Murray R. The effects of consuming carbohydrate-electrolyte beverages on gastric emptying and fluid absorption during and following exercise. Sports Med 1987; 4: 322–351
146. Neufer PD, Costill DL, Fink WJ et al. Effects of exercise and carbohydrate composition on gastric emptying. Med Sci Sports Exerc 1986; 18: 658–662
147. Davis JM, Burgess WA, Slentz CA, Bartoli WP. Fluid availability of sports drinks differing in carbohydrate type and concentration. Am J Clin Nutr 1990; 51: 1054–1057
148. Rehrer NJ, Brouns F, Beckers EJ et al. Gastric emptying with repeated drinking during running and bicycling. Int J Sports Med 1990; 11: 238–243
149. Beckers EJ, Jeukendrup AE, Brouns F et al. Gastric emptying of carbohydrate – medium chain triglyceride suspensions at rest. Int J Sports Med 1992; 13: 581–584
150. Wagenmakers AJ, Brouns F, Saris WH, Halliday D. Oxidation rates of orally ingested carbohydrates during prolonged exercise in men. J Appl Physiol 1993; 75: 2774–2780
151. Hawley JA, Dennis SC, Nowitz A et al. Exogenous carbohydrate oxidation from maltose and glucose ingested during prolonged exercise. Eur J Appl Physiol 1992; 64: 523–527
152. Burgess WA, Davis JM, Bartoli WP, Woods JA. Failure of low dose carbohydrate feeding to attenuate glucoregulatory hormone responses and improve endurance performance. Int J Sport Nutr 1991; 1: 338–352
153. Maughan RJ, Noakes TD. Fluid replacement and exercise stress. A brief review of studies on fluid replacement and some guidelines for the athlete. Sports Med 1991; 12: 16–31
154. Carter JE, Gisolfi CV. Fluid replacement during and after exercise in the heat. Med Sci Sports Exerc 1989; 21: 532–539
155. Davis JM, Lamb DR, Pate RR et al. Carbohydrate-electrolyte drinks. effects on endurance cycling in the heat. Am J Clin Nutr 1988; 48: 1023–1030
156. Bacharach DW, von Duvillard SP, Rundell KW et al. Carbohydrate drinks and cycling performance. J Sports Med Phys Fitness 1994; 34: 161–168
157. Davis JM, Bailey SP, Woods JA et al. Effects of carbohydrate feedings on plasma free tryptophan and branched-chain amino acids during prolonged cycling. Eur J Appl Physiol 1992; 65: 513–519
158. Maughan RJ, Bethell LR, Leiper JB. Effects of ingested fluids on exercise capacity and on cardiovascular and metabolic responses to prolonged exercise in man. Exp Physiol 1996; 81: 847–859
159. Millard-Stafford M, Rosskopf LB, Snow TK, Hinson BT. Water versus carbohydrate-electrolyte ingestion before and during a 15-km run in the heat. Int J Sport Nutr 1997; 7: 26–38
160. Burke LM. Nutrition for post-exercise recovery. Aust J Sci Med Sport 1997; 29: 3–10
161. Carter JE, Gisolfi CV. Fluid replacement during and after exercise in the heat. Med Sci Sports Exerc 1989; 21: 532–539

CHAPTER CONTENTS

60

Stress management

Michael T. Murray, ND

Joseph E. Pizzorno Jr, ND

INTRODUCTION

Stress is defined as any disturbance – heat or cold, chemical toxin, microorganisms, physical trauma, strong emotional reaction, etc. – that can trigger the "stress response". How an individual handles stress plays a major role in determining their level of health. Comprehensive stress management involves a truly wholistic approach designed to counteract the everyday stresses of life. Most often the stress response is so mild it goes entirely unnoticed. However, if stress is extreme, unusual, or long-lasting, the stress response can be overwhelming and quite harmful to virtually any body system.

Before discussing methods on how to help patients deal effectively with stress, it is important to understand the stress response. Ultimately, the success of any stress management program is dependent on its ability to improve an individual's immediate and long-term response to stress.

THE GENERAL ADAPTATION SYNDROME

The stress response is actually part of a larger response known as the "general adaptation syndrome", a term coined by the pioneering stress researcher Hans Selye. To fully understand how to combat stress, it is important to understand the general adaptation syndrome. The general adaptation syndrome is composed of three phases: alarm, resistance, and exhaustion.[1] These phases are largely controlled and regulated by the adrenal glands.

The initial response to stress is the alarm reaction which is often referred to as the "fight or flight response". The fight or flight response is triggered by reactions in the brain which ultimately cause the pituitary gland to release adrenocorticotropic hormone (ACTH), which causes the adrenals to secrete adrenaline and other stress-related hormones.

The fight or flight response is designed to counteract danger by mobilizing the body's resources for immediate physical activity. As a result, the heart rate and force of contraction of the heart increases to provide blood to areas necessary for response to the stressful situation. Blood is shunted away from the skin and internal organs, except the heart and lung, while at the same time the amount of blood supplying required oxygen and glucose to the muscles and brain is increased. The rate of breathing increases to supply necessary oxygen to the heart, brain, and exercising muscle. Sweat production increases to eliminate toxic compounds produced by the body and to lower body temperature. Production of digestive secretions is severely reduced since digestive activity is not critical for counteracting stress. Blood sugar levels increase dramatically as the liver converts stored glycogen into glucose for release into the bloodstream.

While the alarm phase is usually short-lived, the next phase – the resistance reaction – allows the body to continue fighting a stressor long after the effects of the fight or flight response have worn off. Other hormones, such as cortisol and other corticosteroids secreted by the adrenal cortex, are largely responsible for the resistance reaction. For example, these hormones stimulate the conversion of protein to energy, so that the body has a large supply of energy long after glucose stores are depleted, and promote the retention of sodium to keep blood pressure elevated.

As well as providing the necessary energy and circulatory changes required to deal effectively with stress, the resistance reaction provides the changes required for meeting emotional crisis, performing strenuous tasks and fighting infection. However, while the effects of adrenal cortex hormones are quite necessary when the body is faced with danger, prolongation of the resistance reaction or continued stress increases the risk of significant disease (including diabetes, high blood pressure, and cancer) and results in the final stage of the general adaptation syndrome, i.e. exhaustion.

Exhaustion may manifest as a partial or total collapse of a body function or specific organ. Two of the major causes of exhaustion are loss of potassium ions and depletion of adrenal glucocorticoid hormones like cortisone. Loss of potassium results in cellular dysfunction and, if severe, cell death. Adrenal glucocorticoid store depletion decreases glucose control, resulting in hypoglycemia.

Another cause of exhaustion is weakening of the organs. Prolonged stress places a tremendous load on many organ systems, especially the heart, blood vessels, adrenals, and immune system and is associated with many common diseases, as listed in Table 60.1.

Table 60.1 Diseases strongly linked to stress[1]

- Angina
- Asthma
- Autoimmune disease
- Cancer
- Cardiovascular disease
- Common cold
- Diabetes (adult onset – type II)
- Depression
- Headaches
- Hypertension
- Immune suppression
- Irritable bowel syndrome
- Menstrual irregularities
- Premenstrual tension syndrome
- Rheumatoid arthritis
- Ulcers
- Ulcerative colitis

STRESS: A HEALTHY VIEW

The father of modern stress research was Hans Selye MD. Having spent many years studying stress, Dr Selye developed valuable insights into the role of stress in disease. According to Dr Selye, stress in itself should not be viewed in a negative context. It is not the stressor that determines the response; instead it is the individual's internal reaction which then triggers the response. This internal reaction is highly individualized. What one person may experience as stress, the next person may view entirely differently. Selye perhaps summarized his view best in a passage in his book *The Stress of Life*:[2]

> No one can live without experiencing some degree of stress all the time. You may think that only serious disease or intensive physical or mental injury can cause stress. This is false. Crossing a busy intersection, exposure to a draft, or even sheer joy are enough to activate the body's stress mechanisms to some extent. Stress is not even necessarily bad for you; it is also the spice of life, for any emotion, any activity causes stress. But, of course, your system must be prepared to take it. The same stress which makes one person sick can be an invigorating experience for another.

The key statement Selye made may be "your system must be prepared to take it". A significant body of knowledge has now accumulated delineating methodologies for assisting patients in developing healthful, rather than disease-facilitating, responses to both short-term and long-term stress.

DIAGNOSTIC CONSIDERATIONS

Many people who are "stressed out" may not be able to identify exactly what is causing them to feel stressed. Typical presenting symptoms include insomnia, depression, fatigue, headache, upset stomach, digestive disturbances, and irritability.

To determine the role that stress may play, the "social readjustment rating scale" developed by Holmes & Rahe[3] may be utilized (see Table 60.2). The scale was originally designed to predict the risk of a serious disease due to stress. Various life-changing events are numerically

Table 60.2 The social readjustment rating scale

Rank	Life event	Mean value
1	Death of spouse	100
2	Divorce	73
3	Marital separation	65
4	Jail term	63
5	Death of a close family member	63
6	Person injury of illness	53
7	Marriage	50
8	Fired at work	47
9	Marital reconciliation	45
10	Retirement	45
11	Change in health of family member	44
12	Pregnancy	40
13	Sex difficulties	39
14	Gain of a new family member	39
15	Business adjustment	39
16	Change in financial state	38
17	Death of a close friend	37
18	Change to different line of work	36
19	Change in number of arguments with spouse	35
20	Large mortgage	31
21	Foreclosure of mortgage or loan	30
22	Change in responsibilities at work	29
23	Son or daughter leaving home	29
24	Trouble with in-laws	29
25	Outstanding personal achievement	28
26	Wife begins or stops work	26
27	Beginning or end of school	26
28	Change in living conditions	25
29	Revision of personal habits	24
30	Trouble with boss	23
31	Change in work hours or conditions	20
32	Change in residence	20
33	Change in schools	20
34	Change in recreation	19
35	Change in church activities	19
36	Change in social activities	18
37	Small mortgage	17
38	Change in sleeping habits	16
39	Change in number of family get-togethers	15
40	Change in eating habits	15
41	Vacation	13
42	Christmas	12
43	Minor violations of the law	11

rated according to their potential for causing disease. Notice that even events commonly viewed as positive, such as an outstanding personal achievement, carry with them stress.

If a person is under a great deal of immediate stress or has endured a fair amount of stress over a few months time or longer, it is appropriate to more accurately assess adrenal dysfunction by utilizing laboratory methods.

Interpretation

The standard interpretation of the social readjustment rating scale is that a total of 200 or more units in 1 year is considered to be predictive of a high likelihood of experiencing a serious disease. However, rather than using the scale solely to predict the likelihood of serious disease, the scale can be used to evaluate a person's level of stressor exposure, as everyone reacts differently to stressful events.

THERAPEUTIC APPROACH

Whether the patient is currently aware of it or not, they have developed a pattern for coping with stress. Unfortunately, most people have found patterns and methods that ultimately do not support good health. Negative coping patterns must be identified and replaced with positive ways of coping. Try to identify any negative or destructive coping patterns listed in Table 60.3 that the patient may have developed and replace the pattern with more positive measures for dealing with stress.

Stress management can be substantially improved by assisting the patient in five equally important areas:

- techniques to calm the mind and promote a positive mental attitude
- lifestyle factors
- exercise
- a healthful diet designed to nourish the body and support physiological processes
- dietary and botanical supplements designed to support the body as a whole, but especially the adrenal glands.

Calming the mind and body

Learning to calm the mind and body is extremely important in relieving stress. Among the easiest methods for the patient to learn are relaxation exercises. The goal of relaxation techniques is to produce a physiological response known as a "relaxation response" – a response that is exactly opposite to the stress response. Although an individual may relax by simply sleeping, watching television, or reading a book, relaxation techniques are designed specifically to produce the "relaxation response".

The relaxation response was a term coined by Harvard professor and cardiologist Herbert Benson MD in the early 1970s to describe a physiological response that is just the opposite of the stress response.[1] With the stress response (see Table 60.4), the sympathetic nervous

Table 60.3 Negative coping patterns

- Dependence on chemicals
  —drugs, legal and illicit
  —alcohol
  —smoking
- Overeating
- Too much television
- Emotional outbursts
- Feelings of helplessness
- Overspending
- Excessive behavior

Table 60.4 The stress response

- The heart rate and force of contraction of the heart increase to provide blood to areas necessary for response to the stressful situation
- Blood is shunted away from the skin and internal organs, except the heart and lung, while at the same time the amount of blood supplying required oxygen and glucose to the muscles and brain is increased
- The rate of breathing increases to supply necessary oxygen to the heart, brain, and exercising muscle
- Sweat production increases to eliminate toxic compounds produced by the body and to lower body temperature
- Production of digestive secretions is severely reduced since digestive activity is not critical for counteracting stress
- Blood sugar levels are increased dramatically as the liver dumps stored glucose into the bloodstream

system dominates. With the relaxation response (see Table 60.5), the parasympathetic nervous system dominates. The parasympathetic nervous system controls bodily functions such as digestion, breathing, and heart rate during periods of rest, relaxation, visualization, meditation, and sleep. While the sympathetic nervous system is designed to protect against immediate danger, the parasympathetic system is designed for repair, maintenance, and restoration of the body.

The relaxation response can be achieved through a variety of techniques. The methodology should be determined by patient interest, as all produce the same physiological effect – a state of deep relaxation. The most popular techniques are meditation, prayer, progressive relaxation, self-hypnosis, and biofeedback. To produce the desired long-term health benefits, the relaxation technique should be utilized at least 5–10 minutes each day.

Breathing

Producing deep relaxation with any technique requires learning how to breathe. One of the most powerful methods of producing less stress and more energy in the body is by breathing with the diaphragm. Diaphragm breathing activates the relaxation centers in the brain. Table 60.6 lists a 10 step technique for teaching diaphragmatic breathing.

Table 60.5 The relaxation response

- The heart rate is reduced and the heart beats more effectively. Blood pressure is reduced
- Blood is shunted towards internal organs, especially those organs involved in digestion
- The rate of breathing decreases as oxygen demand is reduced during periods of rest
- Sweat production decreases, as a person who is calm and relaxed does not experience nervous perspiration
- Production of digestive secretions is increased, greatly improving digestion
- Blood sugar levels are maintained in the normal physiological range

Table 60.6 Instructions to assist patients in learning diaphragmatic breathing

1. Find a comfortable and quiet place to lie down or sit
2. Place your feet slightly apart. Place one hand on your abdomen near your navel. Place the other hand on your chest
3. You will be inhaling through your nose and exhaling through your mouth
4. Concentrate on your breathing. Note which hand is rising and falling with each breath
5. Gently exhale most of the air in your lungs
6. Inhale while slowly counting to 4. As you inhale, slightly extend your abdomen, causing it to rise about 1 inch. Make sure that you are not moving your chest or shoulders
7. As you breathe in, imagine the warmed air flowing in. Imagine this warmth flowing to all parts of your body
8. Pause for 1 second, then slowly exhale to a count of 4. As you exhale, your abdomen should move inward
9. As the air flows out, imagine all your tension and stress leaving your body
10. Repeat the process until a sense of deep relaxation is achieved

Progressive relaxation

One of the most popular techniques for producing the relaxation response is progressive relaxation. The technique is based on a very simple procedure of comparing tension with relaxation. Many people are not aware of the sensation of relaxation. In progressive relaxation an individual is taught what it feels like to relax by comparing relaxation with muscle tension.

The basic technique is to have the patient contract a muscle forcefully for a period of 1–2 seconds and then give way to a feeling of relaxation. The procedure systematically goes through all the muscles of the body, progressively producing a deep state of relaxation. The procedure begins with contracting the muscles of the face and neck, then the upper arms and chest, followed by the lower arms and hands. The process is repeated progressively down the body, i.e. the abdomen, the buttocks, the thighs, the calves, and the feet. This whole practice is repeated two or three times. This technique is often used in the treatment of anxiety and insomnia.

Progressive relaxation, deep breathing exercises, or some other stress reduction technique form an important component of a comprehensive stress management program.

Lifestyle factors

A patient's lifestyle is a major determinant in their stress levels. The two primary areas of concern (other than addressing negative coping patterns) are time management and relationship issues.

One of the biggest stressors for most people is time. They simply do not feel they have enough of it. Table 60.7 provides tips on time management for patients.

Another major cause of stress for many people is interpersonal relationships. Interpersonal relationships

Table 60.7 Patient tips for improved time management

- Set priorities. Realize that you can only accomplish so much in a day. Decide what is important, and limit your efforts to that goal
- Organize your day. There are always interruptions and unplanned demands on your time, but create a definite plan for the day based on your priorities. Avoid the pitfall of always letting the "immediate demands" control your life
- Delegate authority. Delegate as much authority and work as you can. You can't do everything yourself. Learn to train and depend on others
- Tackle tough jobs first. Handle the most important tasks first, while your energy levels are high. Leave the busy work or running around for later in the day
- Minimize meeting time. Schedule meetings to bump up against the lunch hour or quitting time; that way they can't last forever
- Avoid putting things off. Work done under pressure of an unreasonable deadline often has to be redone. That creates more stress than if it had been done right the first time. Plan ahead
- Don't be a perfectionist. You can never really achieve perfection anyway. Do your best in a reasonable amount of time, then move on to other important tasks. If you find time, you can always come back later and polish the task some more

can be divided into three major categories: marital, family, and job-related. The quality of any relationship ultimately comes down to the quality of the communication. Learning to communicate effectively goes a very long way in reducing the stress and occasional (or frequent) conflicts of interpersonal relationships. Table 60.8 lists seven tips for effective communication, regardless of the type of interpersonal relationship.

Exercise

The immediate effect of exercise is stress on the body. However, with a regular exercise program, the body adapts and exercise becomes an effective stress reduction technique. With regular exercise, the body becomes stronger, functions more efficiently, and has greater endurance. Exercise is a vital component of a comprehensive stress management program and overall good health.

People who exercise regularly are much less likely to suffer from fatigue and depression. Tension, depression, feelings of inadequacy, and worries diminish greatly with regular exercise.

Exercise alone has been demonstrated to have a tremendous impact on improving mood and the ability to handle stressful life situations. This effect is seen in adolescents, as well as adults. For example, 2,223 boys and 2,838 girls (mean age, 16.3 years) from 10 teams and 25 different individual sports were studied for the relationship between emotional and psychological well-being. The sport and vigorous recreational activity index was positively associated with emotional well-being independently of other variables.[4]

Dietary guidelines

Individuals suffering from stress or anxiety need to support the biochemistry of the body by following some important dietary guidelines. Specifically, they must:

- eliminate or restrict the intake of caffeine
- eliminate or restrict the intake of alcohol
- eliminate refined carbohydrates from the diet
- eat a diverse range of whole foods
- increase the potassium to sodium ratio
- eat regular planned meals in a relaxed environment
- control food allergies.

According to Selye, the difference between stress being harmful or not is based upon the strength of the system. From a purely physiological perspective, it can

Table 60.8 Keys to assist patients in improving communication

- The first key to successful communication is the most important. Learn to be a good listener. Allow the person you are communicating with to really share their feelings and thoughts uninterrupted. Empathize with them, put yourself in their shoes. If you first seek to understand, you will find yourself being better understood
- Be an active listener. This means that you must be truly interested in what the other person is communicating. Listen to what they are saying instead of thinking about your response. Ask questions to gain more information or clarify what they are telling you. Good questions open lines of communication
- Be a reflective listener. Re-state or reflect back to the other person your interpretation of what they are telling you. This simple technique shows the other person that you are both listening and understanding what they are saying. Re-stating what you think is being said may cause some short-term conflict in some situations, but it is certainly worth the risk
- Wait to speak until the person or people you want to communicate with are listening. If they are not ready to listen, no matter how well you communicate your message will not be heard
- Don't try to talk over somebody. If you find yourself being interrupted, relax, don't try and out-talk the other person. If you are courteous and allow them to speak, eventually (unless they are extremely rude) they will respond likewise. If they don't, point out to them that they are interrupting the communication process. You can only do this if you have been a good listener. Double-standards in relationships seldom work
- Help the other person become an active listener. This can be done by asking them if they understood what you were communicating. Ask them to tell you what is was that they heard. If they don't seem to be understanding what it is you are saying, keep trying until they do
- Don't be afraid of long silences. Human communication involves much more than human words. A great deal can be communicated during silences; unfortunately in many situations silence can make us feel uncomfortable. Relax. Some people need silence to collect their thoughts and feel safe in communicating. The important thing to remember during silences is that you must remain an active listener

be strongly argued that delivery of high-quality nutrition to the cells of the body is the critical factor in determining the strength of the system.

When the eating habits of Americans are examined as a whole, it is little wonder that so many people are suffering from stress, anxiety, and fatigue. Most Americans are not providing their body with the high quality nutrition it deserves. Instead of eating foods rich in vital nutrients, most Americans focus on refined foods high in calories, sugar, fat, and cholesterol.

Caffeine

The average American consumes 150–225 mg of caffeine daily, or roughly the amount of caffeine in two cups of coffee. Although most people can handle this amount, some people are more sensitive to the effects of caffeine than other people, due to decreased activity of phase I detoxification (see Ch. 16). Even small amounts of caffeine can affect sensitive people, while those with normal sensitivity will respond to large amounts. Excessive caffeine consumption can produce "caffeinism characterized by symptoms of depression, nervousness, irritability, recurrent headache, heart palpitations, and insomnia". People prone to feeling stress and anxiety tend to be especially sensitive to caffeine.[5,6]

Alcohol

Alcohol produces chemical stress on the body. It also increases adrenal hormone output, interferes with normal brain chemistry, and interferes with normal sleep cycles. While many people believe that alcohol has a calming effect, a study of 90 healthy male volunteers given either a placebo or alcohol demonstrated significant increases in anxiety scores after drinking the alcohol.[6]

Refined carbohydrates

Refined carbohydrates (e.g. sugar and white flour) are known to contribute to problems in blood sugar control, especially hypoglycemia. The association between hypoglycemia and impaired mental function is well-known. Unfortunately, most patients experiencing depression, anxiety, or other psychological condition are rarely tested for hypoglycemia, nor are they prescribed a diet which restricts refined carbohydrates.

Numerous studies have shown a high percentage of hypoglycemia in depressed patients.[7,8] As depression is one of the most frequent causes of anxiety, this provides a link between hypoglycemia and feelings of stress. Simply eliminating refined carbohydrate from the diet is occasionally all that is needed for effective therapy in patients that have depression or anxiety due to hypoglycemia.

Potassium to sodium ratio

One of the key dietary recommendations to support the adrenal glands is to ensure adequate potassium levels within the body. This can best be done by consuming foods rich in potassium and avoiding foods high in sodium. Most Americans have a dietary potassium-to-sodium (K:Na) ratio of less than 1:2. In contrast, most researchers recommend a dietary potassium-to-sodium ratio of greater than 5:1 for health. However, even this may not be optimal. A natural diet rich in fruits and vegetables can produce a K:Na ratio greater than 50:1, as most fruits and vegetables have a K:Na ratio of over 100:1.

Meal planning

Mealtimes should be spent in a relaxed environment. As noted above, digestion is a process largely controlled by the parasympathetic nervous system. Eating in a rushed manner, in a noisy or hurried environment is not conducive to good digestion or good health.

Food allergies

People with symptoms of anxiety or chronic fatigue need to be concerned about food allergies. As far back as 1930, pioneering allergist Albert Rowe began noticing that anxiety and fatigue were key features of food allergies.[9] Originally, Rowe described a syndrome known as "allergic toxemia" to describe a syndrome that included the symptoms of anxiety, fatigue, muscle and joint aches, drowsiness, difficulty in concentration, and depression. Around the 1950s, this syndrome began to be referred to as the "allergic tension-fatigue syndrome". With the popularity of the new chronic fatigue syndrome, many physicians and other people are forgetting that food allergies can lead to anxiety as well as chronic fatigue.

Nutritional and botanical support

Nutritional and botanical support for the individual experiencing signs and symptoms of stress largely involves supporting the adrenal glands. Long-term stress and corticosteroids cause the adrenal glands to shrink and become dysfunctional, aggravating the stress symptoms of anxiety, depression, or chronic fatigue.

An abnormal adrenal response, either deficient or excessive hormone release, significantly alters an individual's response to stress. Often the adrenals become "exhausted" as a result of constant demands placed upon it. An individual with adrenal exhaustion will usually suffer from chronic fatigue and may complain of feeling "stressed out" or chronically anxious. They will typically have a reduced resistance to allergies and infection.

Nutritional supplements

The nutrients especially important for supporting adrenal function include vitamin C, vitamin B_6, zinc, magnesium, and pantothenic acid. All of these nutrients play a critical role in the health of the adrenal gland as well as the manufacture of adrenal hormones. During stress, the levels of these nutrients in the adrenals decreases substantially.

For example, during chemical, emotional, psychological, or physiological stress, the urinary excretion of vitamin C is increased. Examples of chemical stressors include cigarette smoke, pollutants, and allergens. Extra vitamin C in the form of supplementation and an increased intake of vitamin C-rich foods is often recommended to keep the immune system working properly during times of stress.

Equally important during high periods of stress or in individuals needing adrenal support is pantothenic acid (B vitamin). Pantothenic acid deficiency results in adrenal atrophy characterized by fatigue, headache, sleep disturbances, nausea, and abdominal discomfort. Pantothenic acid is found in whole-grains, legumes, cauliflower, broccoli, salmon, liver, sweet potatoes, and tomatoes. In patients suffering from chronic stress or a history of corticosteroid (prednisone) use, the typical level of supplementation is 100–500 mg daily.

The appropriate daily doses of vitamin B_6 is 50–100 mg; of zinc is 20–30 mg; and of magnesium should be 250–500 mg.

Botanical medicines

Several botanical medicines support adrenal function. Most notable are the ginsengs. Both Chinese ginseng (*Panax ginseng*) and Siberian ginseng (*Eleutherococcus senticosus*) exert beneficial effects on adrenal function and enhance resistance to stress. These ginsengs are often referred to as "general tonics" or "adaptogens".

The term "general tonic" implies that an herb will increase the overall tone of the whole body. The ginsengs are also often referred to as "adrenal tonics" in that they increase the tone and function of the adrenal glands. Chinese and Siberian ginseng can be used to:

- restore vitality in debilitated and feeble individuals
- increase feelings of energy
- increase mental and physical performance
- prevent the negative effects of stress and enhance the body's response to stress
- offset some of the negative effects of cortisone
- enhance liver function
- protect against radiation damage.

All of these applications are backed up by good clinical research.[10–12]

The modern term "adaptogen" is a more descriptive term used to describe the general tonic effects of Siberian and Chinese ginseng. An adaptogen is defined as a substance that:

- must be innocuous and cause minimal disorders in the physiological functions of an organism
- must have a non–specific action (i.e. it should increase resistance to adverse influences by a wide range of physical, chemical, and biochemical factors
- usually has a normalizing action irrespective of the direction of the pathologic state.

According to tradition and scientific evidence, both Siberian and Chinese ginsengs possess this kind of equilibrating, tonic, anti-stress action, and so the term adaptogen is quite appropriate in describing its general effects.

The ginsengs have been shown to enhance the ability to cope with various stressors, both physical and mental.[10–12] Presumably this anti-stress action is mediated by mechanisms which control the adrenal glands. Ginseng delays the onset and reduces the severity of the alarm phase response of the general adaptation syndrome.

People taking either of the ginsengs typically report an increased sense of well-being. Clinical studies have confirmed that both Siberian and Chinese ginsengs significantly reduce feelings of stress and anxiety. For example, in one double-blind clinical study, nurses who had switched from day to night duty rated themselves for competence, mood, and general well-being, and were given a test for mental and physical performance along with blood cell counts and blood chemistry evaluation.[13] The group administered *Panax ginseng* demonstrated higher scores in competence, mood parameters, and mental and physical performance when compared with those receiving placebos. The nurses taking the ginseng felt more alert, yet more tranquil, and were able to perform better than the nurses not taking the ginseng.

In addition to these human studies, several animal studies have shown the ginsengs to exert significant anti-anxiety effects. In several of these studies, the stress-relieving effects were comparable to diazepam (Valium); however, while diazepam causes behavior changes, sedative effects, and impaired motor activity, ginseng produces none of these negative effects.[14]

Based on the clinical and animal studies, it appears that ginseng offers significant benefit to people suffering from stress and anxiety. *Panax ginseng* is generally regarded as being more potent than *Eleutherococcus senticosus*. *Panax ginseng* is probably better for the patient who has experienced a great deal of stress, is recovering from a long-standing illness, or has taken corticosteroids like prednisone for a long period of time. For the patient under mild to moderate stress and experiencing less obvious impaired adrenal function, *Eleutherococcus senticosus* may be the best choice.

REFERENCES

1. Benson H. The relaxation response. New York, NY: William Morrow. 1975
2. Selye H. The stress of life. New York, NY: McGraw Hill. 1978
3. Holmes TH, Rahe RH. The social readjustment scale. J Psychosomatic Res 1967; 11: 213–218
4. Steptoe A, Butler N. Sports participation and emotional wellbeing in adolescents. Lancet 1996; 347: 1789–1792
5. Chou T. Wake up and smell the coffee. Caffeine, coffee, and the medical consequences. West J Med 1992; 157: 544–553
6. Montiero MG et al. Subjective feelings of anxiety in young men after ethanol and diazepam infusions. J Clin Psychiatry 1990 51: 12–16
7. Winokur A et al. Insulin resistance after glucose tolerance testing in patients with major depression. Am J Psychiatry 1988; 145: 325–330
8. Wright JH et al. Glucose metabolism in unipolar depression. Br J Psychiatry 1978; 132: 386–393
9. Rowe AH, Rowe A, Jr. Food Allergy. Its manifestations and control and the elimination diets. A compendium. Springfield, IL: CC Thomas. 1972
10. Farnsworth NR et al. Siberian ginseng (*Eleutherococcus senticosus*): current status as an adaptogen. Econ Med Plant Res 1985; 1: 156–215
11. Hikino H. Traditional remedies and modern assessment: the case of ginseng. In: Wijeskera ROB, ed. The medicinal plant industry. Boca Raton, FL: CRC Press. 1991: p 149–166
12. Shibata S et al. Chemistry and pharmacology of Panax. Econ Med Plant Res 1985; 1: 217–284
13. Hallstrom C, Fulder S, Carruthers M. Effect of ginseng on the performance of nurses on night duty. Comp Med East & West 1982; 6: 277–282
14. Bhattacharya SK, Mitra SK. Anxiolytic activity of *Panax ginseng* roots: an experimental study. J Ethnopharmacol 1991; 34: 87–92

SECTION 5

Pharmacology of natural medicines

SECTION CONTENTS

Careful review of the scientific literature reveals a considerable amount of impressive information documenting the efficacy, pharmacological activity, and toxicology of numerous "natural" medicines. An important purpose of this section is the substantiation, from a scientific standpoint, of the historical use of botanical medicine. Although plants have been used as medicines since antiquity, appreciation of them as effective medicinal agents has greatly diminished during recent times. Hopefully, this section will further revive the appreciation and use of botanical medicines. Although some plant constituents are discussed as separate entities, and in many situations may be the most appropriate therapeutic substances, it is the authors' opinion that the whole herb should be used whenever possible. It has been amply demonstrated that, in many instances, physiological and pharmacological effects of a particular plant constituent are diminished when it is given as an isolated component rather than in its naturally occurring environment. Furthermore, besides synergistic and enhancing effects, there appear to be factors in many plants that prevent many of the side-effects of isolated plant constituents. In understanding the pharmacology, pharmacognosy and historical use of plants, the student of natural medicine is once again inspired by the miracle of nature, and the intuition and empiricism that ancient herbalists possessed.

It is the hope of the authors that this section will help better inform our readers of the impressive uses, and potential dangers, of these natural medicines. We also want to stress that they should not be used simply as substitutes for the drugs commonly used to treat disease. The true physician of natural medicine will use them as part of the treatment of the whole person and in the context of removing the causes of the disease and promoting health, not simply treating symptoms.

Glossary of some terms used in Section 5

Abortifacient – a substance which induces abortion.
Acrid – a pungent biting taste which causes irritation.
Adaptogen – a substance which is safe, increases resistance to stress, and has a balancing effect on body functions.
Adjuvant – a substance which enhances the effect of the medicinal agent or increases the antigenicity of a cancer cell.
Alkaloids – naturally occurring amines, arising from heterocyclic and often complex structures, that display pharmacological activity. Their trivial names usually end in -ine. They are usually classified according to the chemical structure of their main nucleus: phenylalkylamines (e.g. ephedrine), pyridine (e.g. nicotine), tropine (e.g. atropine, cocaine), quinoline (e.g. quinine), isoquinolone (e.g. papaverine), phenanthrene (e.g. morphine), purine (e.g. caffeine), imidazole (e.g. pilocarpine), and indole (e.g. physostigmine, yohimbine).
Alterative – a substance which produces a balancing effect on a particular body function.
Analgesic – a substance which reduces the sensation of pain.
Androgen – hormones which stimulate male characteristics.
Anthelminthic – a substance which causes the elimination of intestinal worms.
Anthocyanidin – a particular class of flavonoids which gives plants, fruits, and flowers colors ranging from red to blue.
Antidote – a substance which neutralizes or counteracts the effects of a poison.
Aphrodisiac – a substance which increases sexual desire.
Astringent – an agent which causes the contraction of tissue.
Balm – a soothing or healing medicine applied to the skin.
Beta-carotene – pro-vitamin A. A plant carotene which can be converted to two vitamin A molecules.
Carminative – a substance which promotes the elimination of intestinal gas.
Carotene – fat-soluble plant pigments, some of which can be converted into vitamin A by the body.
Cathartic – a substance which stimulates the movement of the bowels, more powerful than a laxative.
Cholagogue – a compound which stimulates the contraction of the gall bladder.
Choleretic – a compound which promotes the flow of bile.
Cholestasis – the stagnation of bile within the liver.
Cholinergic – pertaining to the parasympathetic portion of the autonomic nervous system and the release of acetylcholine as a transmitter substance.
Coenzyme – a necessary non-protein component of an enzyme, usually a vitamin or mineral.
Compress – a pad of linen applied under pressure to an area of skin and held in place.
Decoctions – dilute aqueous extracts prepared by boiling the botanical material with water for a specified period of time, followed by straining or filtering.
Demulcent – a soothing substance to irritated mucous membranes.
Emulsify – the dispersement of large fat globules into smaller uniformally distributed particles that can remain in suspension in water.
Enteric-coated – a special way of coating a tablet or capsule to ensure that it does not dissolve in the stomach, so it can reach the intestinal tract.
Enzymes – an organic catalyst which speeds chemical reactions.
Essential oils – also known as volatile oils, ethereal oils or essences. They are usually complex mixtures of a wide variety of organic compounds (e.g. alcohols, ketones, phenols, acids, ethers, esters, aldehydes, oxides, etc.) that evaporate when exposed to air. They generally represent the odoriferous principles of plants.
Extracts – concentrated forms of natural products obtained by treating crude materials containing these substances with a solvent and then removing the solvent completely or partially from the preparation. The most commonly used extracts are fluid extracts, solid extracts, powdered extracts, tinctures and native extracts.
Flavonoid – a generic term for a group of flavone-containing compounds that are found widely in nature. They include many of the compounds that account for plant pigments (anthocyanins, anthoxanthins, apigenins, flavones, flavonols, bioflavonols, etc.). These plant pigments exert a wide variety of physiological effects in the human body.
Fluid extracts – these extracts are typically hydroalcoholic solutions with a strength of one part solvent to one part herb. The alcohol content varies with each product. They are, in essence, concentrated tinctures, constructed to represent 1 grain of the crude drug to 1 minim of fluid extract.
Glycosides – sugar-containing compounds composed of a glycone (sugar component) and an aglycone (non-sugar-containing component) that can be cleaved on hydrolysis. The glycone portion may be glucose, rhamnose, xylose, fructose, arabinose or any other sugar. The aglycone portion can be any kind of organic compound, e.g. sterols, triterpenes, anthraquinones, hydroquinones, tannins, carotenoids, and anthocyanidins.
Infusions – teas produced by steeping the botanical in hot water.

Laxative – a substance which promotes the evacuation of the bowels.

LD_{50} – the dosage which will kill 50% of the animals taking the substance.

Lipotropic – promoting the flow of lipids to and from the liver.

Menstrums – solvents used for extraction, e.g. water, alcohol, acetone, etc.

Metalloenzyme – an enzyme which contains a metal at its active site.

Native extracts – high potency extracts prepared via concentrating under reduced pressure at low temperatures until all solvent is removed.

Oleoresins – primarily mixtures of resins and volatile oils. They either occur naturally or are made by extracting the oily and resinous materials from botanicals with organic solvents (e.g. hexane, acetone, ether, alcohol). The solvent is then removed under vacuum, leaving behind a viscous, semi-solid extract which is the oleoresin. Examples of prepared oleoresins are paprika, ginger, and capsicum.

Powdered extract – a solid extract which has been dried to a powder.

Putrefaction – the process of breaking down protein compounds by rotting.

Recommended dietary allowance (RDA) – recommended dietary allowance.

Resins – complex oxidative products of terpenes that occur naturally as plant exudates, or are prepared by alcohol extraction of botanicals that contain resinous principles.

Saponins – non-nitrogenous glycosides, typically with sterol or triterpenes as the aglycone, that possess the common property of foaming, or making suds, when strongly agitated in aqueous solution.

Solid extracts – thin to thick, viscous liquids or semi-solids prepared from native extracts by adjusting the latter to the specific strength with suitable diluents. Typically, these extracts are 4:1, i.e. one part extract is equivalent to, or derived from, four parts of crude herb.

Strength of an extract – the potencies or strengths of botanical extracts are generally expressed in two ways. If they contain known active principles, their strengths are commonly expressed in terms of their content of active principles. Otherwise their strength is expressed in terms of their concentration of the crude drug. Thus a strength of 4:1 means one part of extract is equivalent to, or derived from, four parts of crude drug. A strength of 1:5 represents one part of extract is comparable to 0.2 parts of the crude drug. This ratio method of expressing drug strength does not accurately measure potency since there may be wide variation between manufacturers.

Tincture – alcoholic or hydro-alcoholic solutions usually containing the active principles of botanicals in low concentrations. They are usually prepared by maceration, percolation or by dilution of their corresponding fluid or native extracts. The strengths of tinctures are typically 1:10 or 1:5. Alcohol content will vary.

Tonic – a substance which exerts a gentle strengthening effect on the body.

CHAPTER CONTENTS

61

Alkylglycerols

Peter T. Pugliese, MD

INTRODUCTION

Sharks have existed, virtually unchanged, for some 450 million years. Some scientists attribute this long staying power to the well developed immune system in the shark, an immune system which is quite similar to our own. Sharks have both a humoral and a cellular component to their immune system, and therefore have both B-cells and T-cells. Sharks also have a spleen and a thymus gland just as we do, although they possess large quantities of akylglycerols found mainly in the liver. In this chapter we shall explore the use of alkylglcyerols from the shark both as immune stimulants and as powerful agents in the treatment of neoplastic disorders.

HISTORY

Alkylglycerols are ether-linked biological compounds that have a long and fascinating history. Much of the early history is found in the literature of histochemistry and is related to methods of staining specific cellular components. One of the greatest histologists of all time was Robert Feulgen (1884–1955), a German physiological chemist to whom we owe the Feulgen reaction. (The Feulgen reaction, or test, is a method to detect animal nucleic acids. It involves an acid hydrolysis with HCL followed by a 1% solution of decolorized rosaniline, which yields a red color in the presence of nucleic acids.) Robert Feulgen and K. Voit discovered plasmalogens in 1924.[1] At the time they thought they had discovered an aldehyde, which they called *plasmal*. The origin of plasmal was believed to be an unknown substance, which they called *plasmalogen*. They were able to demonstrate the presence of this compound in many tissues, from protozoa to humans.

Plasmalogens, it was learned later, were ether lipid compounds that are formed in the metabolic pathway of phosphoglycerides. They differ from phosphoglycerides in that they contain an ether linkage on the C-1 of the glycerol molecule. Intensive work on the structure and formation of the plasmalogens continued over the next 35 years. It was many years, however, before a formula for plasmalogens was finally agreed upon, yet the biological function of plasmalogens remained unknown until after 1960 when their role in organisms was finally discovered.

As in many discoveries there are always unsung heroes: scientists who work quietly in some obscure laboratory, publish a paper and are seen no more. Such was the case with research on the alkylglycerols. The work of Kossel & Edbacher[2] on the starfish *Astropecten aurantiacus* was unknown until 1943 when Bergmann & Stansbury[3] compared their preparation of batyl alcohol, a natural alkylglcyerol obtained from the starfish, to the original work of Kossel & Edbacher[2] and found similar physical and chemical properties of both compounds. From 1915 the story jumps to the 1920s, after the First World War, and to Japan where Tsujimoto & Toyama[4] were working on unsaponifiable compounds from liver extracts. (Unsaponifiable fractions are those fatty compounds that do not form soaps when shaken with strong bases such as potassium or sodium hydroxide. Steroids are an example of this class of compounds.) It was the work of these two investigators that identified two major alkylglycerols in shark and ray liver oil. They called the first compound *selachyl alcohol* from the family name for sharks, Selachoidei, and *batyl alcohol* from the ray family Batoidei. They were uncertain of the exact chemical structure at the time, due to questions about the role of an oxygen atom in the molecules.

In 1924, Toyama[5] isolated a third compound from the liver oils of the ratfish, *Chimera monstrosa*, which he called *chimyl alcohol*. Four years later Heilbron & Owens[6] described the crucial role of the oxygen atom as an ether linkage. They refluxed batyl alcohol with hydroiodic acid and obtained octodecyl iodide, which was conclusive evidence of a glyceryl ether structure.

At about this time, a great deal of work was being conducted on shark liver oil in an attempt to isolate the fat-soluble vitamins A and D. Ether lipids consisting mainly of batyl, chimyl and selachyl alcohols were purified from shark liver oil as a side product of this isolation. This material provided a ready source for further investigation of the ether lipids. This was fortuitous because the first therapeutic use of ether lipids was in 1930 when Giffin & Watkins[7] employed yellow bone marrow to treat a patient with leukopenia. At the time they did not know that the active principle in the marrow was batyl alcohol. Eight years later Marberg & Wiles[8] isolated batyl alcohol from the unsaponifiable fraction of yellow marrow.

The biological function of the ether lipids was not fully elucidated until after 1960, although many investigators ascribed certain biological functions to these compounds, e.g. the antileukopenic effect described above, a central depressant action described by Berger[9] in 1948, an erythopoietic effect reported by Sandler[10] in 1949, a tuberculostatic effect reported by Emmerie et al[11] in 1952, a wound healing action reported by Bodman & Maisin[12] in 1958 and a radioprotective effect reported by Brohult[13] in 1960. The alkyl glycerol ethers were found to be widespread in nature, in fact almost universal, although no clear physiological role was defined for them. Current research has opened many investigative channels for these compounds and new information is now available that is beginning to shed light on the molecular action of the ether lipids. A review of the chemistry of the alkyl glyceryl ethers will help to prepare the reader to understand the physiological action and the potential therapeutic applications.

BASIC CHEMISTRY OF THE ALKYL GLYCERYL ETHERS FROM SHARK LIVER OIL

Some definitions

Lipid chemistry is often viewed as an impenetrable complexity by the student. The terminology is indeed not easy to master at first, but with time and repetition it becomes easier. Part of this problem rests with the lipid chemists who have some difficulty is agreeing on nomenclature. In the case of the ether lipids, we shall limit this discussion to only a few naturally occurring compounds, specifically those occurring in shark liver oil. *Lipids may be broadly defined as a class of organic compounds that are water-insoluble.* They can then be further divided into simple lipids and complex lipids. For example, simple lipids are esters of fatty acids and an alcohol, such as palmitic acid and glycerol to form a monoglyceride. Another example of a simple lipid is a cholesterol ester.

Complex lipids are esters which contain phosphorus and/or nitrogen bases and/or sugars as well as fatty acids and an alcohol. Lecithin, which is phosphotidyl choline, is an important complex lipid. The plasmalogens, which we shall discuss later, are lipid compounds that contain an ether linkage along with both a phosphorus and a nitrogen group, so they are classified as complex lipids.

We also speak of neutral lipids which are not ionically charged, and ionic lipids, or charged lipids. Fats such as common triglycerides found in lard, are neutral lipids, while phospholipids are charged lipids. There are a few other terms that must be defined so that we are all talking the same language. The term *alkoxyl* refers to an organic group RO, which is part of an ether group ROR. Recently the term has been shortened to alkyl, so we denote ether lipid as alkylglycerides. Note that there is no other oxygen atom associated with the R components. The term *acyl* refers to a R – C = O. The term *carbonyl* refers to a C = O group, and the term *carboxyl* refers to a –COOH group, where one oxygen has a double bond to the carbon atom.

The ether bond is the key to understanding the unique functioning of the alkylglycerol. This bond, C–O–C, is found throughout nature in many important biological compounds, the most familiar of which is thyroxin from the thyroid gland. In the plant world, guaicol is another familiar ether-linked substance. Glycerol ethers are quite widespread, having been isolated from many life forms and in many different molecular arrangements. The basic structure of these compounds consists of a glycerol molecule with one or more of the hydroxyl groups being replaced by long-chain fatty acids. The bonding of three fatty acid molecules to the glycerol molecule with an ester linkage is known as a triglyceride, or common fat. The ester linkage is characterized by the –COO group where one oxygen is linked in a double bond to a carbon atom. A typical triglyceride and alkylglycerol are shown in Figures 61.1 and 61.2.

While the chemistry of the alkylglycerols in many animals and plants has been studied quite extensively, we shall limit our discussion to the main ether lipids found in shark liver oil. A note, however, on the composition of shark liver oil is in order. Shark liver oil contains high levels of vitamins A and D along with other constituents besides the ether lipids. In commercial preparations of the alkylglycerols extracted from shark liver oil, all of these components are removed in the extraction process.

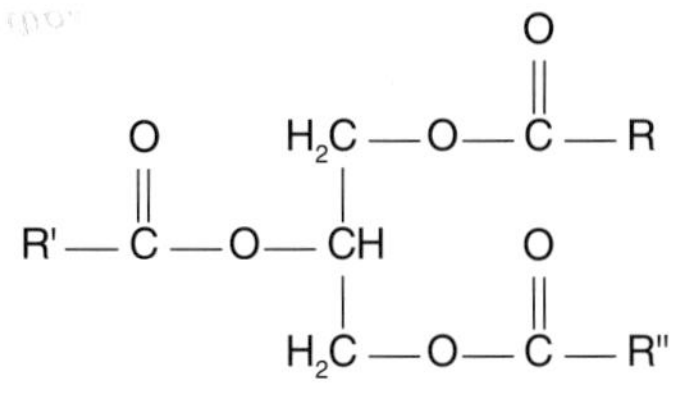

Figure 61.1 Trigylceride.

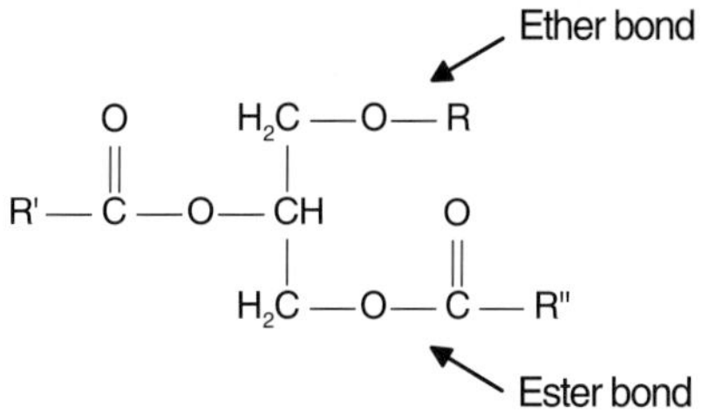

Ether bond

Ester bond

Figure 61.2 Alkylglycerol.

In this article, therefore, when we speak of shark liver-derived alkylglycerols we are referring to a highly refined end product containing only the alkylglycerols.

One of the major sources of natural alkylglycerols is obtained from the Greenland shark, *Somniosus microcephalus*, which contains up to 50% of alkylglycerols. Other sources include the elasmobranch fish such as the small shark, *Chimaera monstrosa*, and the dogfish, *Squalus acanthias*. Cod liver oil and certain mollusks are additional sources of alkylglycerols.[14] These compounds are found in various organs of the animals studied, including bone marrow fat, spleen liver, plasma and erythrocytes, and in milk.[15,16] These compounds are found in the unsaponifiable fraction of the oils obtained from the animals. Tsujimoto & Toyama[4] were the first investigators to report the presence of ether lipids in shark liver oil. Three major natural alkylglycerols obtained from the Greenland shark are batyl alcohol, chimyl alcohol and selachyl alcohol. The chemical structure of these compounds is given in Fig. 61.3. Note that while chimyl and batyl alcohol are saturated chains, selachyl alcohol contains one unsaturated bond. Note also that all the ether bonds are on the number 3 carbon of glycerol. In the natural state these compounds are usually present as ester compounds, with carbons 1 and 2 esterified with C_{16} or C_{18} saturated fatty acids. A fourth natural compound is a

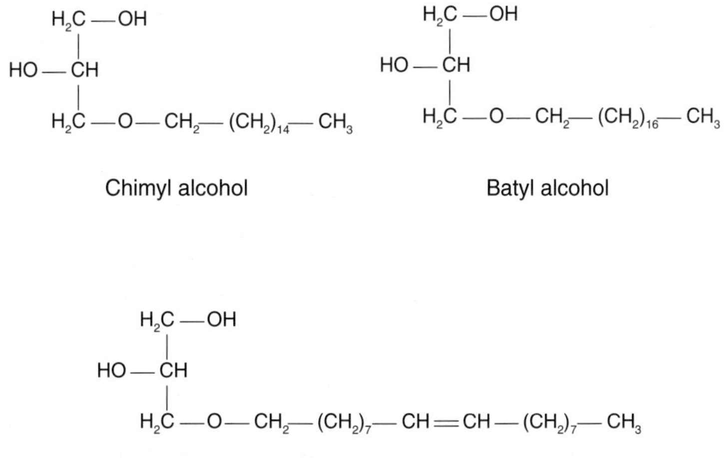

Chimyl alcohol

Batyl alcohol

Selachyl alcohol

Figure 61.3 Batyl alcohol, chimyl alcohol and selachyl alcohol.

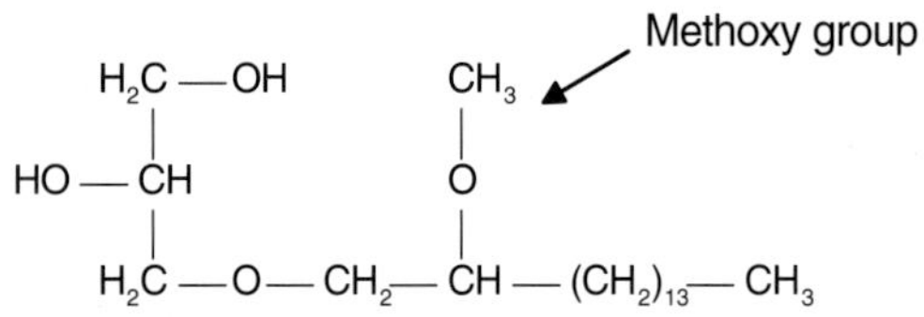

Figure 61.4 Methoxy-substituted alkylglycerol.

methoxy-substituted alkylglycerol, shown in Fig. 61.4, which is quite an active compound, but comprises only a small percentage of natural shark liver oil-derived alkylglycerols, about 3%.

The biological synthesis of the lipid ethers has been well worked out. Most cells in the human body contain lipid ethers but only in small quantities. The following synthesis scheme has been published and is summarized by Mangold & Paltauf [17] as follows:

- *Step 1*. Coenzyme A derivatives of long-chain fatty acids are reduced to alkyl and alkenyl chains via their alcohols, through an aldehyde.
- *Step 2*. The ether bond is formed by reaction of these alcohols with acyldihydroxyacetone phosphates, resulting in the formation of alkylacyldihydroxyacetone phosphates.
- *Step 3*. Reduction of the alkylacydihydroxyacetone phosphates leads to the formation of alkylglycerophosphates.

This may be further summarized as:

fatty acid ⇒ aldehyde ⇒ alcohol ⇒ alkyl ether
⇒ 1-alkenyl ether

It is unlikely that ether lipids exist in nature as free forms; rather, they are esterified. Being ether compounds, they react as aliphatic ethers, i.e. they are stable to most oxidizing and reducing substances, but undergo only one general, non-enzymatic reaction, which is acid hydrolysis.

It is not the purpose of this chapter to discuss the isolation and identification of the alkylglycerols. The scheme for this work is well developed and may be found in references by Mangold & Weber.[18] We shall devote our coverage in this chapter instead to the naturally occurring alkylglcyerols from shark liver oil and relate the structure and fate of these compounds to their physiological effects and potential therapeutic use.

Absorption, fate and excretion

After oral ingestion of ether lipids, absorption occurs from the intestine. About 95% of radioactive (C_{14}-labeled) chimyl alcohol is absorbed in the intestine, with 5% being excreted in the feces in one study.[19] In the gastrointestinal tract a large proportion of the ingested ether lipid in the form of 1-O-alkylglycerols are cleaved at the ether bond with the alkyl moieties giving rise to fatty acids. The remainder is incorporated into 1-O-alkyl 2,3-diacyl-*sn*-glycerols and 1-O-alky-l-2-acyl-*sn*-glycerol and 1-O-alkyl-2-acyl-*sn*-glycerol-3-phosphoethanolamines.[20] Ether lipids are only minor components of human diet, so that the major portion of ether lipids in the body is synthesized in the body.[20] Absorption of the intact ether lipid is the rule since ether lipids are not subject to the action of lipase, which is specific for the ester bond. This means that the "fat" is absorbed rather than the fatty acids. After feeding chimyl alcohol to rats, analysis of the lymph fluid shows that 2–4% of the ether lipids is found as fatty acids combined in phospholipids, about 50% is found in the triglyceride fraction, while another 40% is found as the free chimyl alcohol, or as an esterified alcohol. In the triglyceride fraction, most of the original compound is found as palmitic acid, which indicates that the ether bound in the chimyl alcohol was split during the absorption process. The cetyl alcohol (a C 15 fatty alcohol) moiety of chimyl alcohol is oxidized to palmitic acid (a C 16 fatty acid) during its passage through the intestinal mucosa.

TOXICOLOGY OF THE ALKYLGLYCEROLS

Toxicity in animals

Oral toxicity studies with alkylglcyerols have been conducted on rats, mice and dogs. Alexander et al[21] reported that mice given a diet containing 18% alkyldiacylglycerols showed not ill effects after 2 years. Work by Brohult,[22] Peifer et al,[23] Carlson,[24] Berger[9] and Bandi[25] on oral feeding of alkyglycerols to rats has shown that they are relatively non-toxic. Carlson[24] tested dogs with chimyl batyl and selachyl alcohols by feeding levels of 2.4 g/kg of body weight and found no ill effects.

Subcutaneous injections of batyl alcohol in mice by Berger[9] found that a dose of 3 g/kg was needed to obtain a subcutaneous LD_{50}. Peritoneal injections of batyl alcohol in rats at levels of 5–10 mg/kg of body weight had no effect on the thymus gland or on the production of adenosine triphosphate.

Toxicity in humans

Brohult[22] observed that a healthy human being consumes about 10–100 mg/day of alkylglcyerols in an average diet. Sandler[10] gave healthy adult males 45 mg/day of batyl alcohol for 10 days with no ill effects. This was a relatively low dose compared with that consumed by people who eat shark meat and shark by-products. Only the consumption of shark liver has been reported to produce ill effects, mainly diarrhea, due to the high squalene content. Alkylglycerols from the Greenland shark have been used for over 30 years without undesirable side-effects.

BIOLOGICAL EFFECTS

Bacteriostatic effects

As early as 1952 the bacteriostatic effects of alkylglycerols on tubercle bacillus (*Mycobacterium tuberculosis*) in vitro were reported.[11] This material was isolated from cod liver oil and consisted of the unsaponifiable fraction. There is very little published data on the antimicrobial effects of the alkylglcyerols from natural sources, but a more recent report using a synthetic product, racemic *sn*-1(3)-dodecylglycerol, showed some activity against *Streptococcus mutans* BHT.[26] These investigators found that substantial decreases in the viability of this organism were associated with an accumulation of phosphatidic acid. Current research shows that antibiotic resistance in bacteria is associated with the lipid content of the bacteria in both Gram-positive and Gram-negative organisms.[27] The action of the alkylglycerol was to inhibit the synthesis of lipids in the microbial cell.

Hemopoietic effects

Bone marrow was found to be a useful therapy in treating secondary anemia over 60 years ago. Later it was found that the unsaponifiable fraction of the marrow lipids was responsible for this action, i.e. the stimulation of erythrocyte production. Sandler[10] found that batyl alcohol had a beneficial effect on erythrocyte production in rats. Further studies with subcutaneous injections in humans showed an increase in reticulocycte levels in the blood. The erythropoietic, thrombpoietic and granulopoietic stimulatory activities of 1-octadecylglycerol ethers was confirmed by several investigators.[28–30] It is interesting that chimyl alcohol is able to stimulate hemopoiesis, but selachyl alcohol is not.[31]

Protection against radiation damage

The effects of 1-alkylglycerols in the treatment of radiation-induced leukopenia have been studied extensively. Some investigators have confirmed these benficial effects,[32,33] while others have not.[34,35] Work by Lorenz et al[36] found that lethal irradiation in mice and guinea pigs was counteracted by post-irradiation injection of bone marrow. It was thought by Sandler[10] that batyl alcohol might be the active factor in bone marrow that prevented irradiation leukopenia. His observations, however, noted an increase mainly in erythropoiesis. Additional studies by Arturson & Linback[37] using intraperitioneal injections of batyl alcohol in mice showed an increase in the production of both erythrocytes and reticulocytes.

Other studies have confirmed the positive effect of the alkoxyglycerols on post-irradiation damage. The work of Brohult & Homberg[28] showed that lethal irradiation is counteracted by post-irradiation injections of batyl alcohol. In 1963 Brohult published a thesis on the use of alkylglycerols in radiation treatment. A summary of the major findings in this paper is as follows:

- The post-irradiation decrease in thrombocytes and white cell is notably less in patients treated with alkylgycerols than in those not given alkyglycerols.
- Patients with low thrombocyte counts due to radiation treatment or chemotherapy had increased counts after treatment with alkylglycerols.
- In irradiated rats pretreated with alkylglycerols there was less of a decrease in megacaryocytes and nucleated cells in the bone marrow compared with untreated irradiated controls.
- Selachyl alcohol was more effective than batyl alcohol in preventing megacaryocyte decrease.
- There was a dose-related response with a maximum response at a certain level and then a decreased response when that level was exceeded.
- The alkylglycerols increase the growth rate of rats after treatment and irradiation compared with untreated irradiated rats.
- Batyl alcohol has a greater effect than selachyl alcohol on increasing growth rate in rats.
- In a series of 350 patients with cervical cancer treated with alkylglycerol and given radiation therapy, there was a greater survival rate for 1 year and 5 years than in untreated irradiated controls (we shall discuss this topic in more detail when we discuss the clinical uses of the alkylglycerols).

IMMUNOLOGICAL ASPECTS OF AKYLGLYCEROLS

An overview of the immune system

Early in the investigation and study of ether lipids it was evident that there was an augmentation of the immune system seen in animals that ingested these compounds. It was also apparent that the macrophage was the key cell in this reaction. A brief introduction to the immune system will acquaint the reader with the relationship of the macrophage to other immune active cells and to the immune system in general. The immune system comprises a set of physiological responses used by the body to destroy or neutralize foreign matter, either living or non-living. Included in this system is a process of maintaining an immune surveillance of the body's own cells to detect and destroy malignant cells.

The essential role of the immune system, therefore, is one of recognition of the components of "the self" and protection from "non-self entities". Our own cellular constituents make up a vast array of complex molecules to identify and classify. Adding additional complex biochemicals from bacteria, viruses and parasites of all kinds increases the complexity of the system manifold.

There are two basic responses of the immune system: a *non-specific response* that protects non-selectively against foreign matter, or cells, without the need for recognition of specific identities – examples of this response include the barrier provided by the skin, the inflammatory response to injury, and the complement system; and a *specific response* which depends on recognition of a specific substance prior to an attack by the immune system. The specific response involves highly specialized cells and the formation of specific chemical substances employed in the attack. One of these substances, known collectively as *antibodies*, are *adapter molecules* that identify foreign organisms and interact with the other components of the immune system. Each of these components has three main regions, two of which communicate with complement and the phagocytic cells, known as the biological part, and the other serving to recognize and bind to microorganisms, known as the external recognition function. The body makes millions of these antibodies. The most common antibodies are the immunoglobulins known as IgG, IgA, IgM, IgE and IgD. Chemically, the antibody molecule consists of two active regions, known as the Fc, or constant, part, and the Fab, or variable antigen-specific, part. There are two heavy chains and two light chains in each antibody molecule. The Fc part consists only of heavy chains while the Fab part consist of light and heavy chains.

Complement

A family of proteins known as complement provides a direct means of killing microbes without the need for phagocytosis; however, it plays an important role in phagocytosis as will become apparent in our discussion of alkylglycerols and macrophage activation. A brief review of the major steps in the complement reaction is outlined. Complement is so named because it complements and amplifies the action of the antibodies. Some of the components of the complement system circulate constantly in the bloodstream in an inactive form and are activated in the presence of infection or tissue damage. A cascade reaction results in which some 20 proteins are involved in generating the active moieties. However, we need not discuss all of these, only the major components. Five of the active proteins resulting from the cascade form a complex known as the *membrane attack group complex* or *MAC*. This MAC invades the microbial plasma membrane and disrupts it by creating a leaky channel. Other cascade-generated proteins cause vasodilatation and increased vascular permeability.

The major action of the complement proteolytic cascade is to cleave a component known as C_3 into two active units C_{3a} and C_{3b} Complement C_{3b} is an *opsonin*, a material that helps to attach phagocytes to the microbe. Antibodies are required to activate complement in the classic system, but our concern here is with another complement activation pathway that does not require antibodies, the so-called *alternate complement pathway*. This system is triggered by certain carbohydrates on the bacterial surface which initiate the cascade at a point about halfway through the classic system to generate C_{3b}. The interaction of complement with macrophages is a key step in many immune reactions, as complement enhances the ability of macrophages to bind, ingest, and destroy microorganisms.[38]

The macrophage

The macrophage is an extremely versatile and highly regulated cellular system. Besides their microbicidal activity, macrophages are equipped to recognize and destroy both intracellular and extracellular replicating invaders, whether or not these invaders are prokaryotic or eukaryotic types. They are important scavengers for effector cells and molecules of host origin, as well as for exogenous compounds which they can take up, degrade and detoxify or contain. They are known to regulate a large number of body functions including iron and lipid metabolism. The large number of secretory products generated by the macrophage helps to regulate other cells, including the fibroblasts and cells involved in the formation of myeloid component in the bone marrow.

Obviously such powerful cells need to be tightly controlled, and so they are. The resident macrophages in the tissues are usually downregulated to a high degree. The process of *activation*, which we shall discuss in detail, comes from a variety of extracellular stimuli. We have learned over the years that the macrophage is a multipotential cell with the capacity to develop in many ways, depending on the specific signal it receives. This system is far from being fully understood, but the control of this delicate balance of activities is essential to life, so it has become a prime area of intensive investigation.

The macrophages originate from precursor cells in the bone marrow and pass into the circulation as *monocytes*. They remain in the bloodstream for several hours and then migrate to various tissues where they are transformed into macrophages. The macrophage is an activated monocyte, and is easily distinguished from the smaller neutrophil by its size and characteristic nucleus. While both cells are phagocytic, the macrophage has a far greater potential for killing bacteria. A greater cytoplasmic volume and more cytoplasmic organelles are present in the macrophage, including more lysosomes, microtubles, microfilaments and Golgi membranes. After leaving the bloodstream, the macrophage will enter the peritoneal cavity, other serous cavities, and the red pulp of the spleen and the lymph nodes.

Macrophages possess receptors for the Fc pieces of the immunoglobulins and for the C_{3b} complement fraction discussed above. The adherence of a particle to the macrophage is mediated by complement or by complement plus antibody. Either IgM or IgG is required for this reaction to take place along with C_3. If IgG is bound to the particle it can be ingested without the addition of complement C_3.

The concept of immune activation is quite comprehensive in that it embodies many intercellular and molecular events.[39] The lymphocytes play a key role in activating the macrophage, particularly the T-helper lymphocytes. Macrophages are usually downregulated with respect to their surface active receptors when they are resident in most tissues (resident macrophages are usually not activated). They may be fully activated in several stages, e.g. an inflammatory response in tissues will evoke a reaction that changes the C_3 complement on the surface of the macrophage to fully empower the cell to engulf and destroy bacteria or red cells. They are then further activated to a high killer state by secretions from T-lymphocytes, one of which includes gamma interleukin.

Macrophage activation by alkylglycerols

Inflamed cancerous tissue releases alkyl-lysophospholipids and other alkylglycerols which are degradation products of alkyl phospholipids and alkyl neutral lipids. These compounds are found in cancerous tissue in high concentration, but are in a very low concentration in normal tissues. One of these products, dodecylglycerol (DDG), is one of the most potent macrophage activators known.[40–43] The use of the natural *sn*-3-octylglycerol, or batyl alcohol, found in shark liver oil produced the same effect as DDG.[44] The mechanism of macrophage activation by the natural akylglycerols is most likely identical to the action of lysophospholipids. Keeping in mind that activated macrophages exhibit increased phagocytosis, one method of assaying substances for activation potency is to measure the ingestion of various particles. Erythrocytes coated with IgG are common target particles used in this assay.

Lysophosphotidylcholine has been shown to be effective in increasing macrophage ingestion of IgG-coated erythrocytes.[40,41] Mice were treated with intraperitoneal injections of batyl alcohol in saline and the macrophages were harvested 4–5 days later. Sheep erythrocyte coated with IgG showed a greatly increased ingestion of erythrocytes. There was no increased ingestion when the cells were coated with IgM or complement, which suggests that batyl alcohol activates the macrophages for Fc-mediated ingestion only. It was interesting that batyl alcohol was more effective at a lower dose than the synthetic compound.[42]

There is evidence that oral intake of natural alkylglycerols results in higher levels of plasmalogens in the erythrocytes in human subjects. (Plasmalogens are ether compounds that are formed in the metabolic pathway of phosphoglycerides. They differ from phosphoglycrides in that they contain an ether linkage on the C-1 of the glycerol molecule.) It is know that plasmalogens protect animal cell membranes against oxidative stress. In rat studies, batyl alcohol is incorporated into all tissues except brain tissue and this action is a stereospecific incorporation.[45] It has been shown that alkylglycerols are present in human and cow's milk,[44,46] along with other immunological factors.[47] Since the neonate has not developed a mature immune system,[48] the prospect of transmitting immune functional components in the milk is a practical way to provide some protection for the newborn.[49] In one study, lactating rats were fed alkylglcyerols dissolved in corn oil; the composition of the alkylglycerols was similar to that found in shark liver oil, in that batyl alcohol, chimyl alcohol and selachyl alcohol were the major constituents.[49] The findings from this study showed that while peripheral blood granulocytes were elevated there was no elevation of peripheral lymphocytes. Plasma levels of immunoglobulins were elevated in those pups whose dams were fed alkylglycerols, but not in the controls. Both IgG and IgM were elevated to a significant degree.

CLINCIAL USES OF AKYLGLYCEROLS

Akylglcyerols have been used primarily to treat various types of cancer, usually as adjunct therapy combined with radiation. We shall present in detail the work of Brohult et al[50] on cervical cancer tumor regression and on the decrease of complications resulting from irradiation therapy. Finally we shall discuss a new akylglycerol, a methoxy-substituted alkylglcyerol that occurs naturally at only 3% in shark liver oil, but may be available as a synthetic compound.

Tumor regression with alkylglycerol treatment

Patient selection was determined by stages with the stages being defined as follows:

- Stage I – carcinoma strictly confined to the cervix (early stage)
- Stage IA – cases of early stromal invasion
- Stage IB – all other cases of stage I
- Stage IIA – the carcinoma extends beyond the cervix but has not extended onto the pelvic wall; the carcinoma involves the vagina, but not the lower third; no parametrial involvement
- Stage IIB – the carcinoma extends beyond the cervix but has not extended onto the pelvic wall; the carcinoma involves the vagina, but not the lower third; parametrial involvement is noted
- Stage III – the carcinoma has extended onto the

pelvic wall; on rectal examination there is no cancer-free space between the tumour and the pelvic wall; the tumour involves the lower third of the vagina
- Stage IV – the carcinoma has extended beyond the true pelvis or has involved the mucosa of the bladder or rectum.

(These definitions are from the International Federation of Gynecology and Obstetrics.)

Treatment

Patients were treated with shark liver oil-derived alkylglycerol continuing 100 mg of alkylglycerol, given as two capsules three times a day for a total dose of 600 mg/day. The treated group received 600 mg/day for 7 days prior to irradiation and for 1–3 months after radiation therapy. The study covered three time periods: period 1, from 1 September 1964 to 15 February 1964, comprising 458 patients; period 2, from 1970 to 1973, comprising 137 patients in a double-blind study; period 3, from late 1973 to 1975, comprising 245 patients who were treated with alkylglycerols on as "every second patient".

The control group consisted of all patients who received radiation therapy for cervical cancer but did not receive alkylglycerols.

Findings

The control group in this study consisted of 4,404 patients treated during the same periods, while the total treated group was 841 patients. The mortality after 5 years was 31.0% for the group treated with alkyglycerols and 39.6% for the control group. The difference is statistically significant ($P < 0.001$).[50]

Protection against radiation injuries

Studies of patients treated in 1963–1966 and in 1970–1972 by Brohult et al[51] were aimed at evaluating further the protective effects of ether lipids against irradiation injuries in patients with cancer of the cervix of the uterus. Alkylglycerols derived from Greenland shark liver oil were administered to one group of patients at a level of 600 mg/day during the radiation treatment and 300 mg/day for 1–3 months after treatment. Another group of patients was treated the same way during and after radiation, but was also treated prophylactically 8 days before radiation with 600 mg/day of alkylglycerols. The patients receiving alkylglycerols during and after radiation treatment are referred to as the non-prophylactic group, and the patients also given alkylglycerols before the radiation as the prophylactic group. The system proposed by Kottmeier & Gray[52] was used for evaluation of the radiation injuries that had occurred in the bladder, rectum, uterus, and intestine. Radiation injuries of grade I, with minimal objective changes in the mucosa, were excluded. Patients with radiation injuries of grades II–IV were treated as a single group: "patients with radiation injuries". Grade II was characterized by moderate to severe changes, such as necroses, ulcerations, moderate stenoses, and/or reactions with lengthy bleeding. Radiation complications of grade III included injuries to the bladder, radiation fistulas from the ureters, and rectal and intestinal stenoses of such severity that colostomy or resection was needed. Grade IV was characterized by rectal and intestinal fistulas. Complications included patients with clinical features of radiation injury in whom the symptoms were found to be caused by tumor growth or a combination of tumor growth and radiation injury. These complications were termed "complex injuries" and represented a very serious situation. All patients with complex injuries were dead after 5 years.

The incidence of radiation injuries varies with the spread of the cancer and the radiation technique. The incidence is higher in the more advanced tumor stages than in the less advanced ones. It is also higher after ^{60}Co three-beam treatment of combined high-voltage and X-ray treatment than after conventional X-rays or radium alone. When comparing the groups statistically, standardized proportions have been used in order to cancel out differences with regard to stage distribution and radiation technique.

The total incidence of injuries was lower in the groups that had received alkylglycerols (18.1% in the prophylactic group and 24.4% in the non-prophylactic group) than in the controls (37.1%). The prophylactic group had a considerably lower incidence of complex injuries and multiple injuries than both the controls and the non-prophylactic groups. The differences were highly significant ($P < 0.001$). Analysis of the patients divided into groups according to tumor stage or radiation technique showed that the incidence of complex injuries was lower in all subgroups of prophylactically treated patients than in the corresponding control groups. A double-blind study in 1970–1972 showed a pronounced protective effect of prophylactic treatment against injuries after radiation therapy.[51] The use of increased doses of radium in intracavitary irradiation was followed by a high incidence of radiation injuries, which was considerably reduced by treatment with alkylglycerols, especially when these compounds were administered prophylactically.[53]

The alkylglycerols in other medical conditions

While there are few studies to support the use of natural aklylglycerols in disease states other than cancer it seems appropriate to consider this agent in any condition that would benefit from stimulation of an immune component. Currently the alkylglycerols are viewed as adjunct therapy rather than primary therapeutic agents, except for the methoxy-substituted alkylglycerols. Newer forms of the alkylglycerols have been synthesized and are being tested successfully with a wide range of tumor types. Conditions that are characterized by a hyperproliferative state may benefit from treatment with alkylglycerol.

Considering that one possible effect of the alkylglycerols is competitive inhibition of diacylglycerol, it is plausible that protein kinase C would also be inhibited by this same action since diacylglycerol is a stimulator of protein kinase C. Protein kinase C is essential to the oxidative burst in neutrophils, and agents that inhibit protein kinase C will inhibit this action.[54] The work by Yamamoto et al[42] supports the role of ether analogues as activators of macrophages and as primary cytotoxic agents. This dual role would suggest a wider application of alkyglycerol as adjunct therapy. It has been observed by Oth & Jadhav[55] that alkylglycerols given to lactating mice will increase the peripheral granulocyte count as well as the serum immunoglobulins in the pups. This action suggests the possible use of alkylglycerols in most infectious disorders.

Experimental antitumor activity with methoxy-substituted alkyglycerol

About 3% of the alkylglycerols in the Greenland shark liver oil consists of methoxy-substituted alkylglycerols. The methoxy-substituted alkylglycerols have been found to inhibit tumor growth in cultured cells. Two cell lines were used, a methylchol-anthrene-induced murine sarcoma (MCGI-SS) and a juvenile osteogenic sarcoma (2T). Marked growth inhibition was noted for the mixture of 2-methoxyalkylglycerols from Greenland shark liver oil, different single components derived from this oil (2-methoxyhexadecylglycerol, 2-methoxyhexadecenylglycerol, and 2-methoxyoctadecenylglycerol), and various synthetic compounds including, for example, 2-ethoxyhexadecylglycerol, 2-methoxyhexadecenylglycerol, and 3-methoxyhexadecylglycerol.[56]

In several tumor–host systems, including solid tumors, leukemias, and lymphomas, the methoxy-substituted alkylglycerols were incorporated into the feed in different concentrations (0.1–2%, w/w). Growth inhibition was noted for melanoma B16, for a methylcholanthrene-induced sarcoma (MCG101) and Lewis lung tumor (LLT) in C57BL/6J mice, for lymphoma LAA in A/Sn mice with synthetic 2-methoxyhexadecylglycerol, and for a spontaneous mammary carcinoma in C3H mice with methoxy-substituted alkylglycerols from Greenland shark liver oil. The survival time of DBA/2J mice transplanted with lymphatic leukemia P1534 was increased by synthetic 2-methoxyhexedecylglycerol.[56,57] Metastases induced by the injection of MCG1-SS cells into a tail vein or into the portal vein were inhibited in the liver by methoxy-substituted alkylglycerols from Greenland shark liver oil.[57] Spontaneous metastasis formation from a methylcholanthrene-induced sarcoma (MCG1-SS) in lymph nodes and lungs of CBA mice was inhibited by methoxy-substituted alkylglycerols derived from Greenland shark liver oil as well as by synthetic 2-methoxyhexadecylglycerol.[56] Spontaneous metastasis formation from melanoma B16 was inhibited by synthetic 2-methoxyhexadecylglycerol.[57]

It is notable that the same substance can both stimulate the immune system and inhibit tumors. This has also be shown to be true for alkyllysophospholipids synthesized with a methoxy group in the 2-position of the glycerol part of the molecule, These substances have been studied at the Max-Planck Institute for Immunobiology at Freiburg and at the Department of Haematology and Oncology of the University of Munich.

The German research groups have shown that even alkyllysophospholipids without the 2-methoxy group in the glycerol part can activate macrophages in the bone marrow. This shows that ordinary glycerol ethers, after incorporation into phospholipids, can activate the body's immune defense system. These investigators think that the macrophage-stimulating effects of alkyllysophospholipids explain the effects of these substances on tumors and tumor spread. Tumor cells have only a low activity of enzymes which can break down ethers. This means that alkyl ethers are incorporated into the cell membrane's phospholipids which are then recognized and attacked by macrophages which have a high activity of ether catabolic enzymes.

In experiments performed at the University of Stockholm,[58] it has been shown that both types of methoxy-substituted alkylglycerols (methoxy group in the 1-position and methoxy group in the 2-position of the glycerol part of the molecule) inhibit growth of two tumour cell lines (neuroblastoma from mice and glioma cells from rats), while alkylglycerols without methoxy groups did not have any growth-inhibiting effects on the tumor cell line studied.

Interactions between different types of alkylglycerols and human neutrophil granulocytes have been studied by Palmblad et al.[59] Platelet-activating factor (PAF) was the most potent with regard to the ability to produce an oxidative response, followed by the methoxy-substituted alkylglycerols. The study shows that there is a dissociation between the ability of an alkylglycerol to initiate oxidative and calcium responses, indicating strict structure–activity relationships for the different alkylglycerols studied.

INDICATIONS AND DOSAGE

At present, there are no medical conditions for which shark liver oil-derived alkylglycerols are used as specific therapy; however, they may be used as ancillary, auxiliary or augmentative agents in many disorders. In cancer chemotherapy or irradiation therapy, they are not only protective but also additive in the overall therapeutic effect. Any disorder that has a proliferative component, and that would include most inflammatory disorders, will respond to alkylglycerols. Immune disorders in particular, can be treated effectively with alkyglycerols. In the prevention of infection or neoplastic diseases, 50 mg of alkylglcyerol three times a day is suggested. For aggressively treated disorders, 300 mg/day or more may be needed. The use of the methoxy-derived alkylglcyerols must await further research and availability of this powerful akylglycerol.

CONCLUSIONS

Ether lipids are well known as a new class of tumoricidal compounds, producing strong biological signals. While many new compounds have been synthesized, natural compounds have been known for a long time, beginning with the work of Hanahan on platelet-activating factor, a 1-O-alkyl glycerol. This class of compound, know as plasmalogens, is known to inhibit phosphorylation reactions, particularly those catalyzed by protein kinase C. The dual action of alkylglycerols on both the physical structure of the cell, such as the cell membrane, and the complex biochemical pathways makes them extremely interesting as modulators of cell functions.

The biological action of the alkyglycerols suggests they may have both prophylactic and inhibitory properties against tumors. This action is highly selective and appears to be related mainly to the chemical structure of the alkylglycerol. Most clinical trials with alkyglycerols have been with very advanced cases, but these results are encouraging. The mechanisms involved in antitumor activity are many and include macrophage activation, immune cytotoxicity, NK cell activation, enzyme inhibition and activation, and cell membrane disturbances. Other actions include the anti-infective properties as well as the radiation protective properties of these agents.

Two areas which hold promise with the use of alkylglycerols are the suppression of autoimmune disorders and the selective destruction of leukemic cells. Much of this work is covered in a report of the First International Symposium on Ether Lipids in Oncology published by The American Oil Chemist Society in 1987.[60] The outlook for the use of alkylglycerols in medical treatment and in the maintenance of health is very optimistic.

REFERENCES

1. Feulgen R, Voit K. Gesamte Physiol. Menschen Tiere. Pfluegers Arch 1924; 206: 389
2. Kossel A, Edbacher S. Hoppe-Seyler's. Z Physiol Chem 1915; 94: 277
3. Bergman W, Stanbury HA. Contributions to the study of marine products. J Org Chem 1943; 8: 283
4. Tsujimoto M, Toyama Y. Uber die unverseifbaren Bestandteile (hoheren Alkohole) der Haifisch und Rochenleberole. Chem Umschau 1922; 29: 35–43
5. Toyama Y. Chem Umsch. Geb Fette, Oele, Wachse, Harze 1924; 31: 13
6. Heilbron IM, Owens WM. The unsaponifiable matter from the oils of the elasmobranch fish. Part IV. The establishment of the structure of selachyl and batyl alcohols as monglyceryl ethers. J Chem Soc, Lond 1928; 942
7. Giffin HZ, Watkins C. Treatment of secondary anemia. J Am Med Assoc 1930; 95: 587
8. Marberg CM, Wiles HO. Yellow bone marrow extracts in granulocytopenia. J Am Med Assoc 1937; 109: 1965
9. Berger FM. The relationship between chemical structure and central depressant action of a-substituted ethers of glycerol. J Pharmacol Exp Ther 1948; 93: 470
10. Sandler OE. Some experimental studies on the erythropoietic effect of yellow bone marrow extracts and batyl alcohol. Acta Med Scand 133: 1949; 225: 72
11. Emmerie A, Engel C, Klip W. J Sci Food Agr 1952; 3: 264
12. Bodman J, Maisin J H. The a-glyceryl ethers. Clin Chim Acta 1958; 3: 253
13. Brohult A. Alkoxyglycerols as growth stimulating substances. Nature (London) 1960; 188: 591
14. Tsujimoto M. The liver oils of Elasmobranch fish. J Soc Chem Ind SI 1932; 317
15. Holmberg J, Mysen G, Persson G. Component lipids of some food raw materials. Sixth Congress of the International Society for Fat Research (London). 1962
16. Hallgren B, Larsson S. The glyceryl ethers in the liver oils of elasmobrach fish. Lipid Res 1962; 3: 31–38
17. Mangold HR, Paltauf F. Ether lipids: biochemical and biomedical aspects. New York: Academic Press. 1983, Ch. 11
18. Mangold HR, Weber N. Biosynthesis and biotransformation of ether lipids. Lipids 1987; 22: 789–799
19. Bergstrom S, Blomstrand R. The intestinal absorption and metabolism of chimyl alcohol in the rat. Acta Physiol Scand 1956; 38: I66
20. Blomstrand R, Ahrens E H, Jr. Absorption of chimyl alcohol in man. Proc Soc Exp Biol Med 1959; 100, 802–805
21. Alexander P, Connel T, Brohult A et al. Reduction of radiation induced shortening of life-span by a diet augmented with alkylglycerols and essential fatty acids. Gerontologia 1959; 3: 147
22. Brohult A. Alkylglycerols and their use in radiation. Acta Radiol 1963; 223(Suppl): 7
23. Peifer JJ, Lundberg WO, Ishio S et al. Arch Biochem Biophys 1965; 110: 270
24. Carlson WE. MSc thesis. Vancouver, Canada: University of British Columbia. 1966
25. Bandi ZT, Mangold HK, Holmer G et al. Substrate specificity of enzymes catalyzing interconversions of long-chain acids and alcohols in the rat. FEPS 1 1971; 12: 217
26. Brissette JL, Cabacungan A, Pieringer RA. Studies on the antibacterial activity of dodecylglycerol. J Biol Chem 1986; 261: 6338–6346.
27. Hugo WB, Stretton RJ. The role of cellular lipid in the resistance of some Gram-positive bacteria to penicillins. J Gen Microbiol 1966; 42: 133–138
28. Brohult A, Holmberg J. Alkylglycerols in the treatment of leucopenia caused by irradiation. Nature (London) 1954; 174, 1102
29. Linman JW. Hemopoietic effects of batyl alcohol. J Clin Invest 1958; 37: 913
30. Osmond DG, Roylance PJ, Webb AJ et al. Acta Haematol 1963; 29: 180
31. Suki WN, Grollman A. The effect of batyl alcohol and related alkylglycerols on hemopoiesis in the rat. Tex Rep Biol Med 1960; 18: 662

32. Alexander P, Connel DI, Brohult A et al. Reduction of radiation induced shortening of life-span by a diet augmented with alkoxyglycerols esters and essential fatty acids. Gerontologia 1959; 3: 147
33. Sviridov NK, Ahaturova AV, Shubina AV et al. Moscow Med Sb 1964: 254
34. Ghys H. Effets des alkoxyglycerols (Kaby 700) sur la leucopenie consecutive à la radiotherapie. Laval Med 1962; 30: 331
35. Snyder F, Piantadosi C, Malone B. The participation of 1- and 2-isomers of O-alkylglycerides as acyl acceptors in cell-free systems. Biochim Biophys Acta 1970; 202: 244
36. Lorenze E, Congdon C, Uphoff D. Modification of acute irradiation injury in mice and guineapigs by bone marrow injections. Radiology 1952; 8: 863
37. Arturson G, Lindhack M. Experiments on the effects of batyl alcohol on the number of erythrocytes and reticulocytes in white mice. Acta Soc Med Upsal 1951; 56: 19
38. Cohn ZA. The macrophage – versatile element of inflammation. Harvey Lect 1982; 77: 63
39. Elsbach P. Cell surface changes in phagocytosis. In: Nicolson GL, Poste G, eds. Cell surface reviews, vol. IV. Amsterdam: North-Holland. 1977: p 363
40. Ngwenya BZ, Yamamoto N. Activation of peritoneal macrophages by lysophosphatidylcholine. Biochim Biophs Acta 1985; 839: 9–15
41. Ngwenya BZ, Yamamoto N. Effects of inflammation products on immune systems: lysophosphatidylcholine stimulates macrophages. Cancer Immunol Immunother 1986; 21: 174–182
42. Yamamoto N, St Clair DA, Homma S et al. Activation of mouse macrophages by alkylglycerols, inflammation products of cancerous tissues. Cancer Res 1988; 48: 6044–6049
43. Adams DO, Hamilton TA. The cell biology of macrophage activation. Ann Rev Imunnol 1984; 2: 283–316
44. Hallgren B, Niclasson A, Stallberg G et al. On the occurrence of 1-O-alkylglycerols and 1-O-(2-methoxy alkyl) glycerols in human colostrum, human milk, cow's milk, sheep's milk, human red bone marrow, red cells, blood plasma and a uterine carcinoma. Acta Chem Scand 1974; B28: 1029–1034
45. Das AK, Homes RD, Wilson GN et al. Dietary ether lipid incorporation in tissue plasmalogens of humans and rodents. Lipids 1992; 27: 401–405
46. Hallgren B, Larsson S. The glyceryl ethers in man and cow. J Lipid Res 1962; 3: 39
47. Orga SS, Weintraub D,, Orga PL. Immunologic aspects of human colostrum and milk. J Immunol 1977; 119: 245–248
48. Quie PG. Antimicrobial defenses in the neonate. Semin Perinatol 1990; 14: 2–9
49. Migliore-Samour D, Jolles P. Casein. A prohormone with an immunomodulating role for the newborn? Experientia 1988; 44: 188–193
50. Brohult A, Brohult J, Brohult S et al. Reduced mortality in cancer patients after administration of alkoxygylycerols. Acta Obs Gynecol Scand 1986; 65: 779–785
51. Brohult A, Brohult J, Brohult S et al. Effect of alkyoxyglycerols on the frequency of injuries following radiation therapy for carcinoma of the uterine cervix. Acta Obs Gynecol Scand 1979; 58: 203–207
52. Kottmier HL, Gray MJ. Rectal and bladder injuries in relation to radiation dosage in carcinoma of the cervix. Am J Obs Gynecol 1961; 82: 74
53. Brohult A, Brohult J, Brohult S, Joesson I. Effect of alkyoxyglycerols on the frequency of injuries following radiation therapy for carcinoma of the uterine cervix. Acta Obs Gynecol Scand 1977; 56: 441–448
54. Wilson E, Olcott MC, Bell RM et al. J Biol Chem 1986; 261: 12 616–12 623
55. Oh SK, Jadhav LA. Effects of dietary alkylglcyerols in lactating rats on immune response in pups. Pediat Res 1994; 36: 300–305
56. Hallgren B, Stallgren G, Boeryd B. Occurrence, synthesis and biological effects of methoxy substituted glycerol ethers. Prog Chem Fats Lipids 1978; 16: 45–58
57. Boeryd B, Hallgren B. The influence of the lipid composition of the feed given to mice on the immunocompetence and tumor resistance of the progeny. Int J Cancer 1980; 26: 241–246
58. Brohult J, Personal communication
59. Palmblad J, Samuelsson J, Brohult J. Interaction between alkylglycerols and human neutrophil granulocytes. Scand J Lab Invest 1990; 225: 133
60. Baumann WJ. Ether lipids in oncology. Editor Lipids 1987; 25: 775–980

CHAPTER CONTENTS

62

Allium cepa (onion)

Michael T. Murray, ND

Joseph E. Pizzorno Jr, ND

Allium cepa (family: Amarylladaceae or Liliaceae)
Common name: onion

GENERAL DESCRIPTION

There are numerous forms and varieties of onion as this perennial or biennial herb is cultivated worldwide. The part used is the fleshy bulb. Common varieties are white globe, yellow globe and red globe.

CHEMICAL COMPOSITION

Onion, like garlic, contains a variety of organic sulfur compounds, including:

- S-methylcysteine sulfoxide
- trans-S-(1-propenyl)cysteine sulfoxide
- S-propylcysteine sulfoxide
- dipropyl disulfide.

Onion also has the enzyme alliinase, which is released when the onion is cut or crushed, causing conversion of trans-S-(1-propenyl)cysteine sulfoxide to the so-called lacrimatory factor (propanethial S-oxide). Other constituents include:[1,2]

- flavonoids (primarily quercetin)
- phenolic acids (e.g. caffeic, sinapic, and p-coumaric)
- sterols
- saponins
- pectin
- volatile oils.

HISTORY AND FOLK USE

Although not as valued a medicinal agent as garlic, onion has been used almost as widely. Like garlic (*Allium sativum*), onion has been used as an antispasmodic, carminative, diuretic, expectorant, stomachic, anthelmintic, and anti-infective agent. Externally it has been used as a rubefacient and poultice, giving relief in skin diseases and insect bites.[1–3]

PHARMACOLOGY

Onion and garlic, due to their similar constituents, have many of the same pharmacological effects. There are, however, some significant differences that make one more advantageous than the other in certain conditions.

Antimicrobial activity

Although onion does exhibit some antibacterial, antifungal, and anthelmintic activity, it is not nearly as potent as garlic. Although this suggests that garlic may be better indicated in cases of infection,[2–4] onion can usually be consumed in larger quantities than garlic, which may increase the concentration of antimicrobial constituents in vivo to approximate those of garlic.

Cardiovascular effects

Like garlic, onions and onion extracts have been shown to decrease blood lipid levels, increase fibrinolysis, decrease platelet aggregation, and lower blood pressure in several clinical studies.[5–7] Onion oil, compared with garlic oil, is a stronger inhibitor of the enzymes cyclooxygenase and lipoxygenase, which mediate eicosanoid metabolism (prostaglandins, thromboxanes and leukotrienes).[8] This suggests that onions would also have a greater effect on inhibition of platelet aggregation and other events mediated by eicosanoids. Garlic and onion consumption is associated with lower levels of cholesterol and triglycerides, and an increase in fibrinolytic activity[9] (see Ch. 63 for details). As the quantity of onion consumed in the study cited was so much larger than that of garlic (600 g of onion/week compared with 50 g of garlic), an argument could be made that onion consumption was the major determinant.

Diabetes

Onions have been shown to have significant oral hypoglycemic action, comparable to that of the prescription oral hypoglycemic agents tolbutamide and phenformin.[10,11] The active hypoglycemic principle in onions is believed to be allyl propyl disulphide (APDS), although other constituents, such as quercetin and anthocyanidins, may play a significant role as well. Experimental and clinical evidence suggests that APDS lowers glucose by competing with insulin (also a disulfide) for degradation sites, thereby increasing the half-life of insulin. Other mechanisms, such as increased hepatic metabolism of glucose or increased insulin secretion, have been proposed.

Anti-asthmatic action

Onion has historically been used as an anti-asthmatic agent.[2,3] Its action in asthma, as well as in other conditions associated with increased lipoxygenase derivatives (leukotrienes), such as psoriasis and atopic dermatitis, appears to be greater than that of garlic. (As mentioned previously, onion oil is a much greater inhibitor of cyclooxygenase and lipoxygenase.)[8] The net effect is similar to that of cortisol, which inhibits all eicosanoid metabolism via inhibition of phospholipase. Inhibition of leukotriene formation and onion's quercetin and isothiocyanates content are probably the primary factors responsible for onion's anti-asthmatic effects. These effects have been confirmed in experimental studies.[12,13]

Antitumor effects

An onion extract was found to be cytotoxic to tumor cells in vitro and to arrest tumor growth when tumor cells were implanted in rats.[14] The onion extract was shown to be unusually non-toxic, since a dose as high as 40 times that of the cytotoxic dose for the tumor cells had no adverse effect on the host. Another species of allium, *Allium ascalonicum* (shallots), has been shown to exhibit significant antileukemic activity in mice.[15]

One human study evaluated onion consumption and stomach cancer in over 120,000 men and women between 55 and 69 years of age. After a 3.3 year follow-up, 139 stomach cancers were diagnosed. The researchers found a strong inverse association between onion consumption and stomach cancer incidence, but no association with the use of leeks or garlic.[16]

DOSAGE

Onion can be eaten liberally as part of a nutritious diet. Therapeutic dosages in the various forms are typically 50–150 g/day.

TOXICOLOGY

There have been virtually no reports of toxicity. However, those with heartburn may note an aggravation of symptoms. One study evaluated symptoms of acid reflux in 16 normal subjects and 16 heartburn patients. Subjects were studied with an esophageal pH probe for 2 hours after eating a plain hamburger and a glass of ice water, then on another day an identical meal with a slice of raw onion. In the normal patients, ingestion of onions did not increase any of the variables measured (number of reflux episodes, pH < 4, time of pH < 4, heartburn episodes and belches). In contrast, heartburn subjects experienced a significant increase in all. While the authors of the study conclude that onions can be a potent and long-lasting reflexogenic agent in heartburn patients,[17] an alternative explanation may be that onion simply improved digestive acid secretion, making the symptoms of reflux more noticeable.

SUMMARY

The above discussion on the onion highlights its medicinal value, particularly in cardiovascular disease, diabetes mellitus, and inflammatory conditions. As onion is chiefly regarded as a food or seasoning, this chapter, and the other chapters in this section about common foods and seasonings (e.g. Chs 63, 80 and 124) raise questions about the medicinal effects of other common vegetables and / or seasonings. They also may have significant pharmacological effects that have not been investigated. A diet rich in such foods, spices or seasonings may offer protection and possibly treatment for a wide variety of diseases. Once again, the importance of a relatively natural, unprocessed diet to long-term health is supported. The liberal use of the *Allium* species appears particularly indicated considering the major disease processes of the 20th century.

REFERENCES

1. Leung A. Encyclopedia of common natural ingredients used in food, drugs, and cosmetics. New York, NY: John Wiley. 1980: p 246–247
2. Raj KP, Patel NN. Onion – the vegetable drug. Ind Drugs 1977; 14: 156–160
3. Vahora SB, Rizwan M, Khan JA. Medicinal uses of common Indian vegetables. Planta Med 1973; 23: 381–393
4. Elnima EI, Ahmed SA, Mekkawi A, Mossa JS. The antimicrobial activity of garlic and onion extracts. Pharmazie 1983; 38: 747–748
5. Louria DB, McAnnally JF, Lasser N et al. Onion extract in treatment of hypertension and hyperlipidemia. A preliminary communication. Curr Ther Res 1985; 37: 127–131
6. Mittal MM, Mittal S, Sarin JC, Sharma ML. Effects of feeding onion on fibrinolysis, serum cholesterol, platelet aggregation and adhesion. Ind J Med Sci 1972; 24: 144–148
7. Menon IS. Fresh onions and blood fibrinolysis. Br Med J 1969; i: 845
8. Norwell DY, Tarr RS. Garlic, vampires, and CHD. Osteopath Ann 1983; 11: 546–549
9. Sainani GS, Desai DB, Gohre NH et al. Effect of dietary garlic and onion on serum lipid profile in Jain community. Ind J Med Res 1979; 69: 776–780
10. Bever BO, Zahnd GR. Plants with oral hypoglycemic action. Quart J Crude Drug Res 1979; 17: 139–196
11. Sharma KK, Gupta RK, Gupta S, Samuel KC. Antihyperglycemic effect of onion. effect on fasting blood sugar and induced hyperglycemia in man. Ind J Med Res 1977; 65: 422–429
12. Dorsch W, Adam O, Weber J, Ziegeltrum T. Antiasthmatic effects of onion extracts – detection of benzyl- and other isothiocyanates in mustard oils as antiasthmatic compounds of plant origin. Eur J Pharmacol 1985 107: 17–24
13. Dorsch W, Weber J. Prevention of allergen-induced bronchial constriction in sensitized guinea pigs by crude alcohol onion extract. Agents Action 1984; 14: 626–630
14. Nepkar DP, Chander R, Bandekar JR et al. Cytotoxic effect of onion extract on mouse fibrosarcoma 180 A cells. Ind J Exp Biol 1981; 19: 598–600
15. Caldes G, Prescott B. A potential antileukemic substance present in Allium ascalonicum. Planta Medica 1973; 23: 99–100
16. Dorant E, van den Brandt PA, Goldbohm RA et al. Consumption of onions and a reduced risk of stomach carcinoma. Gastroenterology 1996; 110: 12–20
17. Allen ML, Mellow MH, Robinson MG et al. The effect of raw onions on acid reflux and reflux symptoms. Am J Gastroent 1990; 85: 377–380

CHAPTER CONTENTS

63

Allium sativum (garlic)

Michael T. Murray, ND

Joseph E. Pizzorno Jr, ND

Allium sativum (family: Amaryllidaceae or Liliaceae)
Common names: garlic, allium

GENERAL DESCRIPTION

Garlic, a member of the lily family, is a perennial plant that is cultivated worldwide. The garlic bulb is composed of individual cloves enclosed in a white skin. It is the bulb, either fresh or dehydrated, that is used as a spice or medicinal herb.

CHEMICAL COMPOSITION

Garlic contains 0.1–0.36% of a volatile oil composed of sulfur-containing compounds:

- allicin
- diallyl disulfide
- diallyl trisulfide
- others.

The garlic oil is obtained by steamed distillation of the crushed fresh bulbs.[1] These volatile compounds are generally considered to be responsible for most of the pharmacological properties of garlic. Other constituents of garlic include:[1,2]

- alliin (S-allyl-L-cysteine sulfoxide)
- S-methyl-L-cysteine sulfoxide
- protein (16.8%, dry weight basis)
- high concentrations of trace minerals (particularly selenium)
- vitamins
- glucosinolates
- enzymes (alliinase, peroxidase, and myrosinase).

Allicin is mainly responsible for garlic's pungent odor. It is formed by the action of the enzyme alliinase on the compound alliin. The essential oil of garlic yields approximately 60% of its weight in allicin after exposure to alliinase. The enzyme is inactivated by heat, which accounts for the fact that cooked garlic produces neither as strong an odor as raw garlic nor nearly as powerful physiological effects.[1]

HISTORY AND FOLK USE

Garlic has been used throughout history for the treatment of a wide variety of conditions. Its usage predates written history. Sanskrit records document the use of garlic remedies approximately 5,000 years ago, while the Chinese have been using it for at least 3,000 years. The *Codex Ebers*, an Egyptian medical papyrus dating to about 1550 BC, mentions garlic as an effective remedy for a variety of ailments, including hypertension, headache, bites, worms, and tumors. Hippocrates, Aristotle and Pliny cited numerous therapeutic uses for garlic. In general, garlic has been used throughout the world to treat coughs, toothache, earache, dandruff, hypertension, atherosclerosis, hysteria, diarrhea, dysentery, diphtheria, vaginitis, and many other conditions.[1–3]

Stories, verse and folklore (such as its alleged ability to ward off vampires) give historical documentation to garlic's power. Sir John Harrington in *The Englishman's doctor*, written in 1609, summarized garlic's virtues and faults:[3]

Garlic then have power to save from death
Bear with it though it maketh unsavory breath,
And scorn not garlic like some that think
It only maketh men wink and drink and stink.

In 1721, during a widespread plague in Marseilles, four condemned criminals were recruited to bury the dead. The gravediggers proved to be immune to the disease. Their secret was a concoction they drank consisting of macerated garlic in wine. This became known as *vinaigre des quatre voleurs* (four thieves' vinegar), and it is still available in France today.

Garlic's antibiotic activity was noted by Pasteur in 1858. Garlic was used by Albert Schwietzer in Africa for the treatment of amebic dysentery, and as an antiseptic in the prevention of gangrene during the two World Wars.

PHARMACOLOGY

Although garlic has a wide range of well-documented effects, its most important clinical uses are in the areas of infection, cancer prevention, and cardiovascular disease.

Antimicrobial activity

Garlic has been shown to have broad-spectrum antimicrobial activity against many genera of bacteria, viruses, worms, and fungi, as summarized in several works.[4–6] These findings support the historical use of garlic in the treatment of a variety of infectious conditions.

Antibacterial activity

As far back as 1944, studies have demonstrated that both garlic juice and allicin inhibited the growth of *Staphylococcus, Streptococcus, Bacillus, Brucella*, and *Vibrio* species at low concentrations.[7,8] In more recent studies using serial dilution and filter paper disk techniques, fresh and vacuum-dried powdered garlic preparations were found to be effective antibiotic agents against many bacteria, as listed in Table 63.1. In these studies, the antimicrobial effects of garlic were compared with commonly used antibiotics, including penicillin, streptomycin, chloramphenicol, erythromycin, and tetracyclines. Besides confirming garlic's well-known antibacterial effects, the studies demonstrated its efficacy in inhibiting the growth of some bacteria which had become resistant to one or more of the antibiotics.

Garlic administration has also been shown to significantly reduce the number of coliforms and anaerobes in the feces.[11]

Antifungal activity

Garlic has demonstrated significant antifungal activity in many in vitro and in vivo studies.[4,12–17] From a clinical perspective, inhibition of *Candida albicans* has the most significance, as both animal and in vitro studies have shown garlic to be more potent than nystatin, gentian violet, and six other reputed antifungal agents.[4,13–15] Aqueous garlic extracts have been shown in vivo to be very effective, even at a dilution of 1:100, against the very common tinea corporis, capitis and cruris fungal skin infections.[13]

In one study at a major Chinese hospital, garlic therapy alone was used effectively in the treatment of cryptococcal meningitis, one of the most serious fungal infections imaginable.[16]

Table 63.1 Microbes inhibited by garlic[4–6,9,10]

- Bacteria
  - —alpha- and beta-hemolytic *Streptococcus*
  - —*Citrobacter* sp.
  - —*Escherichia coli*
  - —*Klebsiella pneumoniae*
  - —*Mycobacteria*
  - —*Proteus vulgaris*
  - —*Salmonella enteritidis*
  - —*Staphylococcus aureus*
- Fungi
  - —*Candida albicans*
  - —*Cryptococcus neoformans*
- Helminths
  - —*Ascaris lumbricoides*
  - —hookworms
- Viruses
  - —*Herpes simplex* types 1 and 2
  - —*Human rhinovirus* type 2
  - —*Parainfluenza virus* type 3
  - —*Vaccinia virus*
  - —*Vesicular stomatitis* virus

Anthelmintic effects

Garlic extracts have been shown to have anthelmintic activity against common intestinal parasites, including *Ascaris lumbricoides* (roundworm) and hookworms.[11,18]

Antiviral effects

Garlic's antiviral effects have been demonstrated by its protection of mice from infection with intranasally inoculated influenza virus, and by its enhancement of neutralizing antibody production when given with influenza vaccine.[19]

The in vitro virus-killing effects of fresh garlic, allicin, and other sulfur components of garlic were determined against *Herpes simplex* types 1 and 2, *Parainfluenza virus* type 3, *Vaccinia virus*, *Vesicular stomatitis* virus, and *Human rhinovirus* type 2. The order for virucidal activity was:

ajoene > allicin > allyl methyl thiosulfinate > methyl allyl thiosulfinate

Ajoene was found in oil-macerates of garlic but not in fresh garlic extracts. No antiviral activity was found for alliin, deoxyalliin, diallyl disulfide, or diallyl trisulfide. Fresh garlic extract was virucidal against all viruses tested. Virucidal activity of commercial products was dependent upon their preparation processes. Those products producing the highest level of allicin and other thiosulfinates had the best virucidal activity.[20]

Immune-enhancing effects

A large amount of research has shown that garlic has many immune-potentiating properties, most of which are thought to be due to volatile factors composed of sulfur-containing compounds: allicin, diallyl disulfide, diallyl trisulfide and others. Fresh garlic, commercial products containing allicin, and aged garlic preparations have all shown these properties. Garlic has been shown to enhance the pathogen-attacking activity of T-cells, neutrophils and macrophages, to increase the secretion of interleukin, and to increase natural killer cell activity.[21–24] The increase in killer cell activity was a remarkable 140% in those eating the equivalent of two bulbs a day and 156% in those consuming 1,800 mg of odorless aged garlic.

Anti-cancer effects

The famous Greek physician Hippocrates prescribed eating garlic as a treatment for cancer. Animal research and some human studies suggest this advice may have been well-founded. Several garlic components have displayed significant anti-cancer effects.[25–27]

Human studies showing garlic's anti-cancer effects are largely based on epidemiological studies.[25–28] These studies show an inverse relationship between cancer rates and garlic consumption. In China, a study comparing populations in different regions found that death from gastric cancers in regions where garlic consumption was high was significantly less than in regions with lower garlic consumption.[28]

Garlic extracts and allicin have displayed potent antitumor effects in animal studies.[29–38] Human studies have shown that garlic inhibits the formation of nitrosamines (powerful cancer-causing compounds formed during digestion).[39,40]

Cardiovascular effects

Garlic appears to be an important protective factor against heart disease and strokes via its ability to impact the process of atherosclerosis at many steps. As there is substantial clinical information on garlic's beneficial effects on the cardiovascular system, the pharmacology is discussed in the section on "clinical applications" below.

Other effects

Anti-inflammatory effects

Garlic extract has demonstrated significant anti-inflammatory activity in experimental models of inflammation.[2,11] This activity is probably a result of garlic's inhibition of the formation of inflammatory compounds.

Hypoglycemic action

Garlic (and onions) has often been used in the treatment of diabetes. Allicin has been shown to have significant hypoglycemic action. This effect is thought to be due to increased hepatic metabolism, increased release of insulin and/or insulin-sparing effect.[41] The latter mechanism appears to be the major factor, as allicin and other sulfhydryl compounds in garlic and onions compete with insulin (also a disulfide protein) for insulin-inactivating compounds, which results in an increase in free insulin.

Miscellaneous effects

Garlic possesses diuretic, diaphoretic, emmenagogue, and expectorant action.[1,9] It is also a carminative, antispasmodic and digestant, making it useful in cases of flatulence, nausea, vomiting, colic, and indigestion.[11,42]

CLINICAL APPLICATIONS

Although garlic has long been used in infectious conditions, a use supported by its antimicrobial and immune-enhancing properties, the primary clinical use of garlic has focused on its role in cardiovascular disease. Specifically, garlic is recommended primarily for its ability to lower cholesterol and blood pressure in the attempt to reduce the risk of dying prematurely from a heart attack or stroke.

Cardiovascular disease

The majority of studies showing a positive effect of garlic and garlic preparations in reducing the risk of cardiovascular mortality are those which use products that deliver a sufficient dosage of allicin. Since allicin is the component in garlic that is responsible for its easily identifiable odor, several manufacturers have developed highly sophisticated methods in an effort to provide the full benefits of garlic without odor. These "odorless" garlic products concentrate for alliin because alliin is relatively "odorless" until it is converted to allicin in the body. Products concentrated for alliin and other sulfur components and stabilized in enteric-coated tablets provide all the benefits of fresh garlic but are more "socially acceptable".

In addition to the use of garlic preparations, garlic consumption as a food should be encouraged, despite its odor, in patients with high cholesterol levels and high blood pressure.

Garlic and garlic preparations should also be encouraged in patients with diabetes, candidiasis, asthma, infections (particularly respiratory tract infections), and gastrointestinal complaints.

Cholesterol-lowering activity

Foremost in garlic's ability to offer significant protection against heart disease and strokes is its ability to lower blood cholesterol levels, even in apparently healthy individuals.[43–47] According to the results from numerous double-blind, placebo-controlled studies in patients with initial cholesterol levels greater than 200, supplementation with commercial preparations providing a daily dose of at least 10 mg alliin or a total allicin potential of 4,000 mcg can lower total serum cholesterol levels by about 10–12%; LDL cholesterol will decrease by about 15%; HDL cholesterol levels will usually increase by about 10%; and triglyceride levels will typically drop by 15%.[47–51]

Although the effects of supplemental garlic preparations on cholesterol levels are modest, the combination of lowering LDL and raising HDL can greatly improve the HDL to LDL ratio, a significant goal in the prevention of heart disease and strokes. Garlic preparations standardized for alliin content exert several other beneficial effects in preventing heart disease and strokes (discussed below).

In addition to taking a garlic supplement, individuals with high cholesterol levels should eat more garlic and onions, as increased dietary intake of garlic and onion can also lower cholesterol levels.[43–46,52] In a 1979 population study, researchers studied three populations of vegetarians in the Jain community in India who consumed differing amounts of garlic and onions.[53] Numerous favorable effects on blood lipids, as shown in Table 63.2, were observed in the group that consumed the largest amount. Blood fibrinogen (discussed below) levels were highest in the group eating no onions or garlic. The study is quite significant because the subjects had nearly identical diets, except in garlic and onion ingestion.

Table 63.2 Effects of garlic and onion consumption on serum lipids under carefully matched diets

Garlic/onion	Cholesterol	Triglyceride
None	208 mg/dl	109 mg/dl
10/200 g/week	172 mg/dl	75 mg/dl
50/600 g/week	159 mg/dl	52 mg/dl

Hypertension

Garlic has demonstrated hypotensive action in both experimental animal models and humans with hypertension.[43–46,54–56] A meta-analysis of published and unpublished randomized controlled trials of garlic preparations was conducted to determine the effect of garlic on blood pressure relative to placebo.[54] Eight trials (seven double-blind, one single-blind) were identified as meeting analytical criteria. A total of 415 subjects were included in the analysis.

All trials used a dried garlic powder standardized to contain 1.3% alliin at a dosage of 600 to 900 mg daily (corresponding to 7.8 and 11.7 mg of alliin or the equivalent of approximately 1.8–2.7 g of fresh garlic daily).

The meta-analysis concluded that garlic preparations designed to yield allicin can lower systolic and diastolic blood pressures over a 1–3 month period. The typical drop from pooled data was 11 mmHg in the systolic and 5.0 mmHg in the diastolic. This degree of blood pressure reduction in hypertensives can be quite significant. It is estimated that if the blood pressure-lowering effects of garlic can be maintained, the risk of stroke may be reduced by 30–40% and the risk of heart attack by 20–25%.

Platelet aggregation inhibition

Excessive platelet aggregation is strongly linked to atherosclerosis, heart disease, and strokes. Garlic preparations standardized for alliin content as well as garlic oil have demonstrated significant inhibition of platelet aggregation.[43–46,57] In one study, 120 patients with increased platelet aggregation were given either 900 mg/day of a dried garlic preparation containing 1.3% alliin or a placebo for 4 weeks.[57] In the garlic group, spontaneous platelet aggregation disappeared, the microcirculation of the skin increased by 47.6%, plasma viscosity decreased by 3.2%, diastolic blood pressure dropped from an average of 74 to 67 mmHg, and fasting blood glucose concentration dropped from an average of 90 to 79 mg/dl.

Fibrinolytic activity

Epidemiological studies have suggested that excessive fibrinogen formation is a major primary risk factor for cardiovascular disease.[58] Fibrinogen is an "acute phase" protein involved in the clotting system. However, it plays many other roles, including several which promote atherosclerosis, such as acting as a cofactor for platelet aggregation, determining the viscosity of blood, and stimulating the migration and proliferation of smooth muscle cells in the intima of the artery walls.

Early clinical studies stimulated detailed population studies on the possible link between fibrinogen levels and cardiovascular disease. The first such study was the Northwick Park Heart Study in the UK. This large study involved 1,510 men aged 40–64 years who were randomly recruited and tested for a range of clotting factors, including fibrinogen. At 4 years follow-up, a stronger association was found between cardiovascular deaths and fibrinogen levels than for cholesterol. This association has been confirmed in five other prospective epidemiological studies.[58]

The clinical significance of these findings can be summarized as follows:

1. Fibrinogen levels should be determined and monitored in patients with, or at high risk for, coronary heart disease or stroke.
2. Garlic and other natural therapies which promote fibrinolysis (e.g. omega-3 oils, bromelain, capsicum, etc.) may offer significant benefit in the prevention of heart attacks, strokes, and other thromboembolic events.

Garlic preparations standardized for alliin content as well as garlic oil, and both fried and raw garlic have been shown to significantly increase serum fibrinolytic activity in humans.[59,60] This increase occurs within the first 6 hours after ingestion and continues for up to 12 hours.

Prevention of LDL oxidation

There is growing evidence that lipoprotein (LDL) oxidation plays a significant role in the development of atherosclerosis. Accordingly, substances which prevent oxidation of LDL slow down atherosclerosis. Antioxidants vitamin E, vitamin C, and beta-carotene have all been shown to offer protection against LDL oxidation and heart disease.

Garlic is known to exert antioxidant activity, but until recently, there were no studies examining its effects on LDL oxidation. Healthy human volunteers given 600 mg/day of a garlic preparation providing 7.8 mg alliin for 2 weeks had a 34% lower susceptibility to lipoprotein oxidation compared with controls.[61] These results are quite significant given the short amount of time they took to produce coupled with the importance of reducing lipoprotein oxidation.

In another study, a placebo-controlled double-blind trial of 23 subjects with coronary artery disease who had one to three major coronary arteries that were 75% blocked or higher, 300 mg of garlic powder, 2 and 4 hours after a single dose, showed the atherogenicity of the patients' sera to be markedly decreased. There was less cholesterol accumulation and lower levels of oxidized LDL in human aortic smooth muscle cells cultured with patients sera after treatment compared with those cultured with sera obtained prior to the administration of the garlic. After 3 weeks of therapy at 300 mg, three times daily, blood serum atherogenicity was decreased twofold compared with initial levels.[62]

DOSAGE

The modern use of garlic features the use of commercial preparations designed to offer the benefits of garlic without the odor. The marketplace is swamped with garlic products with each manufacturer claiming their product is the best.

Preparations standardized for alliin content provide the greatest assurance of quality. However, American consumers must be aware of the subtle techniques manufacturers of garlic products use to disguise the quality of their products.

Based on a great deal of clinical research, the dosage of a commercial garlic product should provide a daily dose equal to at least 4,000 mg of fresh garlic. This dosage translates to at least 10 mg alliin or a total allicin potential of 4,000 mcg.

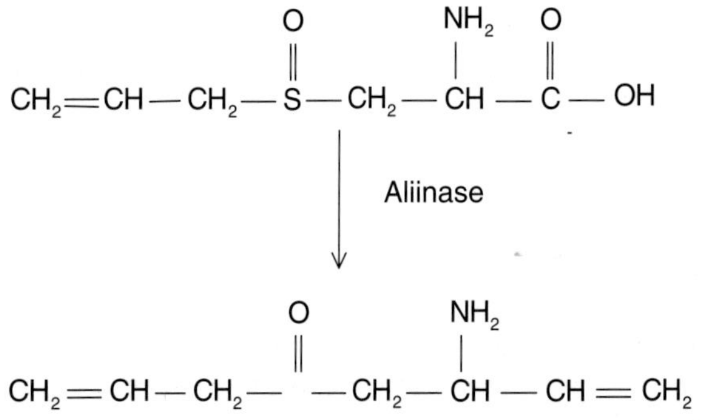

$CH_2{=}CH{-}CH_2{-}S(=O){-}CH_2{-}CH(NH_2){-}C(=O){-}OH$

Aliinase

$CH_2{=}CH{-}CH_2{-}\ (=O)\ {-}CH_2{-}CH(NH_2){-}CH{=}CH_2$

Figure 63.1 Conversion of alliin to allicin.

TOXICITY

For the vast majority of individuals, garlic is non-toxic at the dosages commonly used. For some, however, it can cause irritation to the digestive tract, while others are apparently unable to effectively detoxify allicin and other sulfur-containing components. Prolonged feeding of very large amounts of raw garlic to rats results in anemia, weight loss and failure to grow.[63] Although the exact toxicity of garlic has yet to be definitively determined, side-effects are rare at the dosage recommended above.

REFERENCES

1. Leung A. Encyclopedia of common natural ingredients used in food, drugs, and cosmetics. New York, NY: John Wiley. 1980: p 176–178
2. Raj KP, Parmar RM. Garlic – condiment and medicine. Ind Drugs 1977; 15: 205–210
3. Block E. The chemistry of garlic and onions. Scientific American 1985; March: p 114–118
4. Adetumbi MA, Lau BH. *Allium sativum* (garlic) – A natural antibiotic. Med Hypothesis 1983; 12: 227–237
5. Koch HP. Garlicin – Fact or fiction? Phytother Res 1993; 7: 278–280
6. Hughes BG, Lawson L. Antimicrobial effects of *Allium sativum* L. (Garlic), *Allium ampeloprasum* L. (elephant garlic, and *Allium cepa* L. (onion), garlic compounds and commercial garlic supplement products. Phytother Res 1991; 5: 154–158
7. Huddleson IF et al. Antibacterial substances in plants. J Am Vet Med Assoc 1944; 105: 394–397
8. Cavallito CJ, Bailey JH. Allicin, the antibacterial principle of *Allium sativum*. I. Isolation, physical properties and antibacterial action. J Am Chem Soc 1944; 66: 1950–1951
9. Sharma VD, Sethi MS, Kumar A et al. Antibacterial property of *Allium sativum* Linn. in vivo & in vitro studies. Ind J Exp Biol 1977; 15: 466–468
10. Elnima EI, Ahmed SA, Mekkawi AG et al. The antimicrobial activity of garlic and onion extracts. Pharmazie 1983; 38: 747–748
11. Vahora SB, Rizwan M, Khan JA. Medicinal uses of common Indian vegetables. Planta Med 1973; 23: 381–393
12. Amer M, Taha M, Tosson Z. The effect of aqueous garlic extract on the growth of dermatophytes. Int J Dermatol 1980; 19: 285–287
13. Venugopal P, Venugopal T. Antidermatophytic activity of garlic (*Allium sativum*) in vitro. In J Derm 1995; 34: 278–279
14. Sandhu DK, Warraich MK, Singh S. Sensitivity of yeasts isolated from cases of vaginitis to aqueous extracts of garlic. Mykosen 1980; 23: 691–698
15. Prasad G, Sharma VD. Efficacy of garlic (*Allium sativum*) treatment against experimental candidiasis in chicks. Br Vet J 1980; 136: 448–451
16. Hunan Hospital. Garlic in cryptococcal meningitis. A preliminary report of 21 cases. Chinese Med J 1980; 93: 123–126
17. Fromtling R, Bulmer G. In vitro effect of aqueous extract of garlic (*Allium sativum*) on the growth and viability of Cryptococcus neoformans. Mycologia 1978; 70: 397–405
18. Bastidas GJ. Effect of ingested garlic on Necator americanus and Ancylostoma canium. Am J Trop Med Hyg 1969; 18: 920–923
19. Nagai K. Experimental studies on the preventive effect of garlic extract against infection with influenza virus. Jpn J Infect Dis 1973; 47: 321
20. Weber ND, Anderson DO, North JA et al. In vitro virucidal effects of *Allium sativum* (Garlic) extract and compounds. Planta Med 1992; 58: 417–423
21. Morioka N, Morton DL, Irie RF. A protein fraction from aged garlic extract enhances cytotoxicity and proliferation of human lymphocytes mediated by interleukin-2 and conconavalin. Proc Ann Meet Am Assoc Cancer 1993; 34: A3297
22. Lau BH, Yamasaki T, Gridley DS. garlic compounds modulate macrophage and T-lymphocyte functions. Mol Biother 1991; 3: 103–107,
23. Kandil OM et al. Garlic and the immune system in humans. Its effect on natural killer cells. Fed Proc 1987; 46: 441
24. Hirao Y et al. Activation of immunoresponder cells by the protein fraction from aged garlic extract. Phytotherapy Res 1987; 1: 161–164
25. Lau BH, Yamasaki T, Teel RW. *Allium sativum* (garlic) and cancer prevention. Nutr Res 1990; 10: 937–948
26. Dorant E, van den Brandt PA, Goldbohm RA et al. Garlic and its significance for the prevention of cancer in humans. a critical review. Br J Cancer 1993; 67: 424–429
27. Dausch JG, Nixon DW. Garlic. A review of its relationship to malignant disease. Prev Med 1990; 19: 346–61
28. You WC, Blot WJ, Chang YS et al. Allium vegetables and reduced risk of stomach cancer. J Natl Cancer Inst 1989; 81: 162–164
29. Choy YM, Kwok TT, Fund KP et al. Effect of garlic, Chinese medicinal drugs and amino acids on growth of Erlich ascites tumor cells in mice. Am J Chinese Med 1982; 11: 69–73
30. Weisberger AS, Pensky J. Tumor inhibition by a sulfhydryl-blocking agent related to an active principle of garlic (*Allium sativum*). Cancer Res 1958; 18: 1301–1308
31. Lin X, Liu J, Milner J. Dietary garlic powder suppresses in vivo formation of DNA adducts induced by N-nitroso compounds in liver and mammary tissues. FASEB J 1992; 6: A1392
32. Nagabhushan M, Line D, Polverini PJ et al. Anticarcinogenic action of diallyl sulfide in hamster buccal pouch and forestomach. Cancer Lett 1992; 6: 207–216
33. Meng C, Shyu K. Inhibition of experimental carcinogenesis by painting with garlic extract. Nutr Cancer 1990; 14: 207–217
34. Niukian K, Schwartz J, Shklar G et al. Effects of onion extract on the development of hamster buccal pouch carcinomas as expressed in tumor burden. Nutr Cancer 1987; 9: 171–6
35. Wargovich MJ. Diallyl sulfide, a flavor compound of garlic, inhibits diamethylhydrazine-induced colon cancer. Carcinogenesis 1987; 3: 487–489
36. Belman S. Onion and garlic oils inhibit tumor promotion. Carcinogenesis 1983; 4: 1063–1065
37. Criss WE et al. Inhibition of tumor growth with low dietary protein and with dietary garlic extracts. Fed Proc 1982; 41: 281
38. Kroning F. Garlic as an inhibitor for spontaneous tumors in mice. Acta Unio Intern Contra Cancrum 1964; 20: 855
39. Mei X. The blocking effect of garlic on the formation of N-nitrosoproline in the human body. Acta Nutr Sin 1989; 11: 144–145
40. Xing M. Garlic and gastric cancer – the effect of garlic on nitrite and nitrate in gastric juice. Acta Nutri Sinica 1982; 4: 53–55
41. Bever BO, Zahnd GR. Plants with oral hypoglycemic action. Quart J Crude Drug Res 1979; 17: 139–196
42. Barowsky H, Boyd LJ. The use of garlic (Allistan) in gastrointestinal disturbances. Rev Gastroenterol 1944; 11: 22–26
43. Ali M, Thomson M. Consumption of a garlic clove a day could be beneficial in preventing thrombosis. Prostagl Leukotr Essen Fatty Acids 1995; 53: 211–212
44. Lau BH, Adetumbi MA, Sanchez A. *Allium sativum* (garlic) and atherosclerosis. A review. Nutri Res 1983; 3: 119–128
45. Kendler BS. Garlic (*Allium sativum*) and onion (*Allium cepa*). A review of their relationship to cardiovascular disease. Prev Med 1987; 16: 670–685
46. Ernst E. Cardiovascular effects of garlic (*Allium sativum*). A review. Pharmatherapeutica 1987; 5: 83–89
47. Kleijnen J, Knipschild P, ter Riet G et al. Garlic, onions and cardiovascular risk factors. A review of the evidence from human experiments with emphasis on commercially available preparations. Br J Clin Pharmacol 1989; 28: 535–544
48. Warshafsky S, Kamer RS, Sivak SL. Effect of garlic on total serum cholesterol. Ann Intern Med 1993; 119: 599–605

49. Jain AK, Vargas R, Gotzkowsky S et al. Can garlic reduce levels of serum lipids? A controlled clinical study. Am J Med 1993; 94: 632–635
50. Rotzch W, Richter V, Rassoul F, Walper A et al. Postprandial lipaemia under treatment with *Allium sativum*. Controlled double-blind study in healthy volunteers with reduced HDL_2- cholesterol levels. Arzneim Forsch 1992; 42: 1223–1227
51. Mader FH. Treatment of hyperlipidemia with garlic-powder tablets. Arzneim Forsch 1990; 40: 1111–1116
52. Bordia A. Effect of garlic on blood lipids in patients with coronary heart disease. Am J Clin Nutr 1981; 34: 2100–2103
53. Sainani GS, Desai DB, Gorhe NH, Sainani GS, Desai DB, Gorhe NH et al. Effect of dietary garlic and onion on serum lipid profile in the Jain community. Ind J Med Res 1979; 69: 776–780; Sainani GS et al. Dietary garlic, onion and some coagulation parameters in Jain community. J Assoc Phys Ind 1979; 27: 707–712
54. Silagy CA, Neil AW. A meta-analysis of the effect of garlic on blood pressure. J Hyperten 1994; 12: 463–468
55. Petkov V. Plants with hypotensive, antiatheromatous and coronary dilating action. Am J Chin Med 1979; 7: 197–236
56. Foushee DB, Ruffin J, Banerjee U. Garlic as a natural agent for the treatment of hypertension. A preliminary report. Cytobios 1982; 34: 145–162
57. Kiesewetter H, Jung P, Pindur G et al. Effect of garlic on thrombocyte aggregation, microcirculation, and other risk factors. Int J Clin Pharmacol Ther Toxicol 1991; 29: 151–155
58. Ernst E. Fibrinogen. An important risk factor for atherothrombotic diseases. Annals Med 1994; 26: 15–22
59. Chutani SK, Bordia A. The effect of fried versus raw garlic on fibrinolytic activity in man. Atherosclerosis 1981; 38: 417–21
60. Legnani C, Frascaro M, Guazzaloca G et al. Effects of dried garlic preparation on fibrinolysis and platelet aggregation in healthy subjects. Arzneim Forsch 1993; 43: 119–121
61. Phelps S, Harris WS. Garlic supplementation and lipoprotein oxidation susceptibility. Lipids 1993; 28: 475–477
62. Orekhov AN, Tertov VV, Sobenin IA et al. Garlic powder tablets reduce atherogenicity of low density lipoprotein. A placebo-controlled double-blind study. Nutr Metab Cardiovascular Dis 1996; 6: 21–31
63. Nakagawa S, Masamoto K, Sumiyoshi H et al. Effect of raw and extracted-aged garlic juice on growth of young rats and their organs after perioral administration. J Toxicol Sci 1980; 5: 91–112

CHAPTER CONTENTS

64

Aloe vera (Cape aloe)

Michael T. Murray, ND

Joseph E. Pizzorno Jr, ND

Aloe vera (family: Lilaceae)
Common name: Cape aloe

GENERAL DESCRIPTION

There are more than 300 species of aloe plants, but the most popular medicinal variety is currently *Aloe vera.* The nomenclature of *Aloe vera* has been somewhat confused as the plant has been known by a variety of names, most notably *Aloe barbadensis* and *Aloe vulgari.* The geographical origination of the plant is unclear. Historical records indicate that it may have originated from Egypt or the Middle East. Aloe has been introduced and naturalized throughout most of the tropics and warmer regions of the world, including the Caribbean, the southern US, Mexico, Latin America, the Middle East, India and other parts of Asia.[1]

Aloe vera is a perennial plant with yellow flowers and tough fleshy triangular or spear-like leaves arising in a rosette configuration. The leaves are up to 20 inches long and 5 inches across at the base, tapering to a point. There may be as many as 30 leaves per plant. The margins of the leaf are characterized by saw-like teeth. Inside, the meaty leaf is filled with gel that arises from a clear central mucilaginous pulp. Mature aloe measures 1.5–4 feet long and has a base of 3 inches or greater in diameter.

The leaf is composed of three distinct layers: an outer layer of tough tissue; a corrugated lining just beneath the outer layer; and the major portion of the leaf, the inner layer consisting of parenchymal cells containing large vacuoles of a semi-solid, gelatinous transparent gel. The bitter latex of the corrugated layer protects the plants from predators. Should an animal bite the leaf, the sap causes irritation. The dried latex (juice) derived from the corrugated layer is the source of the laxative properties of aloe. The parenchymal tissue or gel is the portion of the aloe used in other applications.[2]

Aloe vera *terminology*

- *Aloe vera gel* – naturally occurring, undiluted parenchymal tissue obtained from the decorticated leaves of *Aloe vera*
- *Aloe vera concentrate* – *Aloe vera* gel from which the water has been removed
- *Aloe vera juice* – an ingestible product containing a minimum of 50% *Aloe vera* gel
- *Aloe vera latex* – the bitter yellow liquid derived from the pericyclic tubules of the rind of *Aloe vera*, the primary constituent of which is aloin.

CHEMICAL COMPOSITION

Aloe vera contains numerous compounds possessing biological activity. While many botanical medicines suffer from substantial geographical variation in content, commercial aloe is quite consistent. One study found that the composition of the major compounds is remarkably invariable, with aloeresin A, aloesin, and aloin (both epimers A and B) contributing between 70 and 97% of total dry weight, in a ratio of approximately 4:3:2, respectively. Minor compounds were less evenly distributed, with aloinoside A and aloinoside B being found in higher concentrations in Western Countries. The aloin content of the exudate did vary but there were no distinct geographical discontinuities.[3]

Anthraquinones

In 1851, it was discovered that the cathartic action of aloe was due to aloin, a lemon yellow powder formed from drying of the bitter latex. From this material several anthracenes have been isolated, the major anthraquinone being barbaloin. Barbaloin and aloin are often referred to synonymously. Although aloe contains other anthraquinone derivatives, including the anthracene known as aloe-emodin, barbaloin is considered the most potent cathartic. As a whole, the anthraquinone compounds are water-soluble glycosides easily separated from the water-insoluble resinous material.[1–5]

Saccharides

Recent research on *Aloe vera* has focused on the glycoprotein, mucopolysaccharide, and polysaccharide constituents. Aloe contains polysaccharides galactose, xylose, arabinose, and acetylated mannose. This latter polysaccharide, which is similar to guar and locust bean, has received considerable clinical research attention as an antiviral and immunopotentiating agent, especially in the treatment of AIDS. Acemannan, a water-soluble, long-chain polydispersed beta-(1,4)-linked mannan polymer interspersed with O-acetyl groups, is discussed below.

Prostanoids

Several prostanoid compounds have been discovered in *Aloe vera* extracts.[6] The conversion of essential fatty acids to prostanoids by the enzyme cyclooxygenase in a plant such as *Aloe vera* is quite rare. The major unsaturated fatty acid in the plant is gamma-linolenic acid (C18:3) which can be converted to eicosatrienoic acid, the precursor to prostaglandins of the 1 series. The 1 series prostaglandins are known to exert more favorable effects on inflammation, allergy, platelet aggregation, and wound healing. The presence of gamma-linoleic acid and/or prostaglandins in a stable medium, along with inhibitors of thromboxane synthesis, may be another of the important chemical characteristics of aloe responsible for its wound healing effects.

Superoxide dismutase

Extracts from the parenchymatous leaf gel and the rind of aloe (*Aloe barbadensis* Miller) have been shown to contain seven electrophoretically identifiable superoxide dismutases (SODs). Two of these seven are mangano-SODs, while the other five activities are cupro-zinc SODs.[7]

Other constituents

Other biological active compounds found in *Aloe vera* include:

- a serine carboxypeptidase
- salicylates
- minerals
- vitamins
- sterols
- amino acids.

Table 64.1 provides a partial listing of the remarkably diverse range of compounds isolated from *Aloe vera*.[2–5]

HISTORY AND FOLK USE

Aloe vera has a storied history of use. Mesopotamian clay tablets dated 1750 BC indicate that *Aloe vera* was being used for medicinal purposes. Egyptian records from 550 BC also mentioned aloe for infections of the skin. The ancient Greeks were also aware of aloe's medicinal effects as both Pliny (23–79 AD) and Dioscorides (first century AD) wrote of aloe's ability to treat wounds and heal infections of the skin. *Aloe vera* is still widely used in many traditional systems of medicine. In India, for example, in addition to external applications, aloe (whole leaves, the exudate, and the fresh gel) is used as a cathartic, stomachic, and anthelmintic. *Aloe vera* has been adopted into the materia medicas by many cultures of the world.[1]

Table 64.1 Chemical composition of *Aloe vera*[5]

Anthraquinones	Aloin, barbaloin, isobarbaloin, anthranol, aloetic acid, anthracene, ester of cinnamic acid, aloe-emodin, emodin, chrysophanoic acid, ethereal oil, resistannol
Saccharides	Cellulose, glucose, mannose, L-rhamnose, aldopentose
Prostanoids	Gamma-linolenic acid
Enzymes	Oxidase, amylase, catalase, lipase, alkaline phosphatase
Amino acids	Lysine, threonine, valine, methionine, leucine, isoleucine, phenylalanine
Vitamins	Vitamins B_1, B_2, B_6, C, and E, folic acid, choline, β-carotene
Minerals	Calcium, sodium, manganese, magnesium, zinc, copper, chromium
Miscellaneous	Cholesterol, triglycerides, steroids, uric acid, lignins, β-sitosterol, gibberellin, salicylic acid

In the United States, the history of aloe can be traced as far back as the *United States Pharmacopoeia* of 1820, where a number of aloe preparations were described. Most of these preparations were designed to take advantage of aloe's laxative effects. By the early 1900s, more than 27 different aloe preparations were in popular use. In 1920, aloe began being cultivated for pharmaceutical use.[4]

A major development in the modern use of aloe occurred in 1935 when a group of physicians successfully used the fresh juice to treat a patient suffering from facial burns due to X-rays.[8] The relief offered by aloe in the topical treatment of burns, minor irritations, skin ulcers, and other skin disorders is a major reason why companies supplying dermatologic and cosmetic products have incorporated aloe in many of their formulations.

Although more and more of aloe's medicinal effects are being confirmed, aloe is still predominantly administered without direct medical supervision. Therefore, the history and folk use of aloe are continuing to evolve.

PHARMACOLOGY

Gastrointestinal effects

The pharmacology of aloe is surprisingly diverse – laxative, immune potentiation, antimicrobial and wound-healing activities help explain its wide ranging folk and clinical applications.

Laxative effects

Although physicians have prescribed the whole aloe leaf as a cathartic for more than 2,000 years, it was not until 1851 that the active principle aloin was discovered.[1] In small doses, aloin acts as a tonic to the digestive system, giving tone to the intestinal muscle. At higher dosages, it becomes a strong purgative. Its actions are most obvious on the large intestine where it increases colonic secretions and peristaltic contractions. In combination with strychnine and belladonna, aloin became one of the most popular laxatives for chronic constipation for many years. Since aloin often causes painful contraction, other anthraquinone laxatives like cascara and senna are now much more popular.[9,10]

A substantial amount of research activity continues in an effort to understand the laxative effects of aloe. Research using the rat large intestine shows that the increase in water content of the large intestine induced by barbaloin precedes the stimulation of peristalsis, attended by diarrhea. Therefore, it is suggested that the increase in water content is a more important factor than the stimulation of peristalsis in the diarrhea induced by barbaloin.[11] Further studies by the same researchers suggests that aloe-emodin-9-anthrone (AE-anthrone), produced from barbaloin in the rat large intestine may be the actual chemical mediator of this effect. AE-anthrone not only caused an increase in the intestinal water content, but also stimulated mucus secretion.[12]

Bowel detoxification

In 1985, Bland[13] reported the effect of orally consumed *Aloe vera* juice on urinary indican, gastrointestinal pH, stool culture, and stool specific gravity in a semi-controlled study of 10 (five men and five women) healthy human subjects.[13] Urinary indican (see Ch. 31) is used as an indicator of the degree to which either dietary protein is malabsorbed or intestinal bacteria are engaged in putrefactive processes. After one full week of drinking 6 ounces of *Aloe vera* juice three times daily, urinary indican levels decreased one full unit. This suggests that regular *Aloe vera* juice consumption can lead to improved protein digestion and assimilation and/or reduced bacterial putrefaction.

Inhibition of gastric acid secretion

With Heidelberg gastric analysis, the *Aloe vera* juice was shown to increase gastric pH by an average of 1.88 units. This supports the findings of other researchers that *Aloe vera* gel can inhibit the secretion of hydrochloric acid. The Heidelberg test also demonstrated that *Aloe vera* juice can slow down gastric emptying, possibly leading to improved digestion.

Six of the 10 subjects showed marked alterations in stool cultures after the week long study. This implies that *Aloe vera* juice may exert some bacteriostatic or fungistatic activity. In the four subjects with positive cultures for yeast, there was a reduction in the number of yeast colonies.

Stool specific gravity was reduced after the week of *Aloe vera* juice. This implies improved water retention, yet none of the subjects complained of diarrhea or loose stools while taking the *Aloe vera* juice.

Immune-enhancing and antimicrobial activity

Antibacterial and antifungal activity

Aloe has demonstrated activity against many common bacteria and fungi in several studies. In the most detailed of these studies, Robson et al[14] assayed the antimicrobial properties of an *Aloe vera* extract and reviewed the work of others.[15–17] Both mean inhibitory and mean lethal concentrations were determined and compared with silver sulfadiazine, a potent antiseptic used in the treatment of extensive burns. As shown in Table 64.2, the antimicrobial effects of *Aloe vera* compare quite favorably with those of silver sulfadiazine. A 60% *Aloe vera* extract was found to be bactericidal against *Pseudomonas aeruginosa, Klebsiella pneumoniae, Serratia marcescens, Citrobacter* sp., *Enterobacter cloacae, Streptococcus pyogenes*, and *Strep. agalacticae*. Seventy per cent concentrations of aloe were bactericidal for *Staphylococcus aureus*, 80% for *E. coli*, and 90% for *Streptococcus faecalis* and *Candida albicans*. Organisms inhibited in other studies include *Mycobacterium tuberculosis, Trichophyton* sp., and *Bacillus subtilis*.[2,4,5] The antimicrobial activity against common skin pathogens of *Aloe vera* gel in a cream base was shown to be slightly better than silver sulfadiazine in agar well diffusion studies.[14]

Antiviral effects

Acemannan (acetylated mannose) in injectable form has been approved for veterinary use in fibrosarcomas and feline leukemia. Its action in feline leukemia is quite impressive. Feline leukemia, like AIDS, is caused by a retrovirus (feline leukemia virus or FeLV). The virus is so lethal that once cats develop clinical symptoms they are usually euthanized. Typically over 70% of cats will die within 8 weeks of the onset of clinical signs. In a study of 44 cats with clinically confirmed feline leukemia, acemannan was injected (2 mg/kg) weekly for 6 weeks and re-examined 6 weeks after termination of treatment.[18] At the end of the 12 week study, 71% of the cats were alive and in good health.

Acemannan has demonstrated significant antiviral activity against several viruses, including the feline AIDS, human immunodeficiency virus type 1 (HIV-1), influenza virus and measles virus.[19–21]

Table 64.2 Antimicrobial effects of *Aloe vera* extract in cream base compared with silver sulfadiazine in agar well (6 mm) diffusion[14]

Organism	*Aloe vera*	AgSD
Gram-negative		
E. coli	16	12
Enterobacter cloacae	14	12
K. pneumoniae	14	6
P. aeruginosa	17	12
Gram-positive		
S. aureus	18	12
S. pyogenes	16	12
S. agalactiae	16	12
S. faecalis	6	11
B. subtilis	19	14

Inhibition zones measured in mm.

Immune enhancement

Acemannan is a potent immunostimulant.[18,22–25] Among the effects noted for acemannan include the enhancement of macrophage release of interleukin-1-alpha, cytokines, tumor necrosis factor, nitric oxide release, as well as phagocytosis and non-specific cytotoxicity. Acemannan also enhances T-cell function and interferon production, although these actions may also be due to enhanced macrophage function. Macrophage production of cytokines IL-6 and TNF-alpha were dependent on the dose of acemannan provided. These effects can be quite substantial. For example, in one study, acemannan has been shown to enhance the macrophage respiratory burst (twofold increase above the media controls), phagocytosis (45% compared with 25% in controls), and killing of *Candida albicans* (38% killing of *Candida albicans* compared with 0–5% killing in controls).[26]

Hematopoetic effects

Several complex carbohydrates have been found to significantly stimulate hematopoiesis. CARN 750, a polydispersed beta-(1,4)-linked acetylated mannan isolated from the *Aloe vera* plant, has been shown to have hemato-augmenting properties. Subcutaneous injections of 1 mg/mouse of CARN 750 optimally increased hematopoietic progenitors, measured as interleukin-3-supported colony forming units-culture (CFU-C) and high proliferative potential colony-forming cells (HPP-CFC) assays in the spleen. Providing 2 mg/animal of CARN 750 optimally increased bone marrow cellularity, frequency and absolute number of HPP-CFCs and CFU-Cs. The hematopoietic activity of CARN 750 increased with the frequency of administration. The greatest increase in activity in mice myelosuppressed with radiation.[27]

Anti-inflammatory activity

Aloe vera has been shown to exert a number of anti-inflammatory actions, including blocking of the generation of inflammatory mediators like thromboxanes and bradykinin, reducing neutrophil infiltration during inflammation, and reducing edema.[2,4,5,14,28–31] There are several compounds in aloe responsible for these actions. The most important are glycoproteins, which inhibit and actually break down bradykinin, a major mediator of pain and inflammation; various anthraquinones; and salicylates. These anti-inflammatory substances may be of significance in both topical (discussed below) and oral applications.

One comprehensive study evaluated the effects of aqueous, chloroform, and ethanol extracts of *Aloe vera* gel on carrageenan-induced edema in the rat paw, and neutrophil migration into the peritoneal cavity stimulated by carrageenan. Also evaluated was the capacity of the aqueous extract to inhibit cyclooxygenase activity. The aqueous and chloroform extracts decreased the edema induced in the hind paw and the number of neutrophils migrating into the peritoneal cavity, whereas the ethanol extract only decreased the number of neutrophils. The aqueous extract was also found to inhibit prostaglandin E_2 production from arachidonic acid, demonstrating an inhibitory action on cyclooxygenase. The aqueous extract contained anthraglycosides, reductor sugars and cardiotonic glycosides, while the ethanol extract contained saponins, carbohydrates, naftoquinones, sterols, triterpenoids and anthraquinones, and the chloroform extract contained sterols and anthraquinones.[32]

Another useful aspect of aloe is its ability to inhibit lipid peroxidation and scavenge free radicals. One study measured the activity of seven anthraquinones and four anthrones against non-enzymatic and enzymatic lipid peroxidation in vitro and their ability to scavenge free radicals. Using rat hepatocytes exposed to strong oxidizing agents, dithranol and anthrone provided the strongest inhibition of non-enzymatic peroxidation. Rhein anthrone and aloe-emodin showed the highest inhibitory activity against peroxidation of linoleic acid catalyzed by lipoxygenase. Anthrone, dithranol and rhein anthrone were the most effective free radical scavengers.[33]

Other effects

Wound healing

The topical effects of *Aloe vera* appear to be due to a combination of enhancement of wound healing along with anti-inflammatory, moisturizing, emollient, and antimicrobial actions.[2,4,5,14,34–39] *Aloe vera* contains a number of compounds necessary for wound healing, including vitamin C, vitamin E and zinc. Unlike many other anti-inflammatory substances, *Aloe vera* has been shown to stimulate fibroblast and connective tissue formation, thereby promoting wound repair. Finally, aloe appears to stimulate the epidermal growth and repair process, presumably due to its polysaccharides. Mannose-6-phosphate, the major sugar in the *Aloe vera* gel, may its most active growth substance.[40]

Another interesting effect of aloe in wound healing is its ability to counteract the wound healing suppression effects of cortisone. In one study, *Aloe vera* at doses of 100 and 300 mg/kg daily for 4 days blocked the wound healing suppression of hydrocortisone acetate up to 100% using the wound tensile strength assay. The authors suggested this response was because of the growth factors present in *A. vera* masking the wound healing inhibitors.[41]

Alcohol detoxification

Oral administration of aloin (300 mg/kg) given 12 hours prior to the administration of alcohol (3.0 g/kg) significantly decreases the blood alcohol area under the curve by a remarkable 40%. This suggests an increase in the rate of blood alcohol elimination from the body of 45–50%. Analysis of hepatic triglyceride (TG) levels revealed that both ethanol and the aloin given alone significantly increased the TG levels in a comparable manner. However, the level obtained by the combined treatment of aloin and ethanol was not statistically different from that produced by either treatment alone. The levels of serum L-aspartate:2-oxoglutarate aminotransferase (AST) and L-alanine:2-oxoglutarate aminotransferase (ALT) activities were not increased by acute alcohol intoxication, aloin alone, or the combined treatment of alcohol and aloin.[42]

CLINICAL APPLICATIONS

Burns, frost bite, and other tissue damage

Despite growing consumer awareness of *Aloe vera*'s soothing effects on burns and wound healing during the past 40 years, few human studies have been carried out. Most of the studies on *Aloe vera* have utilized different animals in various models of inflammation and wound healing. Virtually all of the studies support the topical use of *Aloe vera* gel, especially in minor burns or skin inflammation. Some recent research is now supporting its use even for more severe tissue damage.

While limited, the human research has been promising. For example, one study found *Aloe vera* gel quite successful in three patients with chronic leg ulcers of 5, 7, and 15 years' duration.[43] The gel was applied to the ulcers on gauze bandages. Rapid reduction in ulcer size was noted in all three subjects and complete resolution occurred in two. Encouraging results were also reported for acne and seborrhea.

In a study of 27 patients with a partial-thickness burn wound, treatment with *Aloe vera* gel was compared with vaseline gauze. The average time of healing in the aloe gel area was a statistically significant and dramatic 1 week shorter: 11.9 days compared with 18.2 days for the vaseline gauze treated wound. Histological evaluation showed early epithelialization in the *Aloe vera* gel treated area.[44]

Another study compared the therapeutic effects of systemic pentoxifylline with topical *Aloe vera* cream in the treatment of frostbite. The frostbitten ears of 10 New Zealand white rabbits were assigned to one of four treatment groups: untreated controls, those treated with *Aloe vera* cream, those treated with pentoxifylline, and those treated with *Aloe vera* cream and pentoxifylline. The control group had a 6% tissue survival. Tissue survival was notably improved with pentoxifylline (20%), better with *Aloe vera* cream (24%), and the best with the combination therapy (30%).[45]

Aloe appears to be effective even in particularly severe tissue injuries, such as those seen in necrotizing fasciitis. Necrotizing fasciitis usually manifests as a low grade cellulitis that quickly deteriorates to a limb and life-threatening soft tissue infection. Immediate surgical debridement is essential followed by aggressive wound management. An interesting report describes excellent results in two cases. Case #1 was a 72-year-old female who, upon presenting to the ER with a "sore bottom", was diagnosed with five problems:

- anal-rectal abscess
- Fournier's gangrene
- ulcerative enterocolitis
- chronic blood loss/anemia
- protein caloric malnutrition.

After debridement, her anal-rectal wound extended from the labia to the left buttock. Care was multidisciplinary and included applying a water-based aloe gel and saline-soaked gauze twice a day. After 45 days, the wound exhibited a pink base with granulation tissue and contraction of the wound edges.

Case #2 was a 48-year-old male with seroma of the left leg secondary to a crush injury. Within 3 days he developed deep vein thrombosis in that leg as well as two large seroma cavities on either side of the thigh. Care included packing with aloe gel and saline soaked sponges. Two weeks after admission, the anterior wound was covered with a split thickness skin graft, while partial closure of the lateral cavity was attempted unsuccessfully with retention sutures. After 5 weeks, healing was complete for the anterior wound and 95% complete for the posterior wound.[46]

Radiation burns

Research into the topical applications of *Aloe vera* gel began in the 1930s in the treatment of radiation burns. During the 1930s, X-rays were used therapeutically for cancer, eczema and other skin complaints, and as a depilatory agent. In 1935, Collins & Collins[8] reported the success of *Aloe vera* gel in one single case, a woman with a patch of severe X-ray dermatitis on her forehead. The woman had tried various medical treatments for 8 months, only to have her condition worsen. The Collins were going to perform a skin graft, but as a temporary measure applied a preparation of fresh whole *Aloe vera* leaves to reduce the itching. The result was that "Twenty-four hours later she reported that the sensation of itching and burning had entirely subsided", and by 5 weeks "there was complete regeneration of the skin of the forehead and scalp, new hair growth, complete restoration of sensation, and absence of scar". Five months after treatment was started there was complete healing. Other case reports followed which, although not as positive as this initial study, clearly indicated that *Aloe vera* was effective in some cases.

Up until the 1940s most of the studies on aloe were reported case histories.[4] In order to substantiate these case studies, animal studies began to appear in the literature. Rowe and colleagues performed several studies in rats with radiation-induced ulcers and determined that fresh aloe pulp was effective while dried aloe powder was not effective.[4,37,38]

In 1953, Lushbaugh & Halé,[39] working for the US Atomic Energy Commission, produced one of the most convincing studies of the efficacy of *Aloe vera* gel. Twenty albino rats were exposed to beta-radiation and different treatments were used on quadrants of the affected area of each animal. The treatments used were fresh *Aloe vera* leaf, a commercial *Aloe vera* ointment, application of a dry gauze bandage, and an untreated control. Both fresh *Aloe vera* and the *Aloe vera* ointment produced clear improvements. At the end of 2 months the *Aloe vera*-treated areas were completely healed while the other two areas had still not healed at the end of 4 months.

However, a recent, large, placebo-controlled, double-blind study has cast doubt on the efficacy of aloe for severe radiation burns. Two phase III randomized trials were reported in this study. The first one was double-blind, utilized a placebo gel, and involved 194 women receiving breast or chest wall irradiation. The second trial randomized 108 such patients to *Aloe vera* gel vs. no treatment. Skin dermatitis was scored weekly during both trials both by patients and by health care providers. Skin dermatitis scores were virtually identical on both treatment arms during both of the trials.[47]

This surprising result might be explained by a another recent study which compared the efficacy of commercially available gels with an acemannan-rich extract from aloe leaves in the treatment of irradiated mice. Male C3H mice received graded single doses of gamma radiation ranging from 30 to 47.5 Gy to the right leg. In most experiments, the gel was applied daily, beginning immediately after irradiation. To determine the timing of application for best effect, gel was applied beginning on days –7, 0, or +7 relative to the day of irradiation (day 0) and continuing for 1, 2, 3, 4, or 5 weeks. The right inner thigh of each mouse was scored on a scale of 0 to 3.5 for severity of radiation reaction from the seventh to the 35th day after irradiation. Dose–response curves were obtained by plotting the percentage of mice that reached or exceeded a given peak skin reaction as a function of dose. The researchers found that while the acemannan-rich extract gel was highly effective, the commercially available gel showed no improvement over the control. They also found that the aloe gel had to applied immediately after irradiation and continued for at least 2 weeks. There was no effect if the aloe gel was applied only before irradiation or beginning 1 week after irradiation. Clearly, the quality and concentration of aloe constituents are crucial if clinical results are to be obtained.[48]

Psoriasis

A recent double-blind, placebo-controlled study evaluated the clinical efficacy and tolerability of topical *Aloe vera* extract 0.5% in a hydrophilic cream and obtained very impressive recults. Sixty patients (36 male/24 female) aged 18–50 years (mean 25.6) with slight to moderate chronic plaque-type psoriasis and PASI (psoriasis area and severity index) scores between 4.8 and 16.7 (mean 9.3) were enrolled and randomized to two groups. The mean duration of the disease prior to enrollment was 8.5 years (range 1–21). Patients self-administered trial medication topically at home three times daily for 5 consecutive days/week (maximum 4 weeks active treatment). Patients were examined on a weekly basis and those showing a progressive reduction of lesions, desquamation followed by decreased erythema, infiltration and lowered PASI score were considered healed. The study was scheduled for 16 weeks with 12 months of follow-up on a monthly basis. The treatment was well tolerated by all the patients, with no adverse drug-related symptoms and no drop-outs. By the end of the study, the *Aloe vera* extract cream had cured 25/30 patients (83.3%) compared with the placebo cure rate of only 2/30 (6.6%), resulting in significant clearing of the psoriatic plaques (328/396 (82.8%) vs. placebo 28/366 (7.7%), and a decreased PASI score to a mean of 2.2.[49]

Gastric ulcers

The use of *Aloe vera* gel internally to treat peptic ulcers was studied in 1963.[50] Twelve patients with X-ray-confirmed duodenal ulcers were given 1 tablespoon of an emulsion of *Aloe vera* gel in mineral oil once daily. At the end of 1 year, all patients demonstrated complete recovery and no recurrence. Based on experimental evidence, the following factors were thought to be responsible for the effectiveness:

- *Aloe vera* gel inactivates pepsin in a reversible fashion. When the stomach is devoid of food, pepsin is inhibited by *Aloe vera* gel; however, in the presence of food, pepsin is released and allowed to digest the food.
- The gel inhibits the release of hydrochloric acid via interference with histamine binding to the parietal cells.
- *Aloe vera* gel is an extremely good demulcent which heals and prevents aggravating irritants from reaching the sensitive ulcer.

AIDS

Although acemannan has demonstrated some direct antiviral activity against HIV-1 by inhibiting glycosylation of viral glycoproteins, its main promise in treating AIDS and HIV may be to enhance the action of azidothymidine (AZT), the antiviral drug used in AIDS. In vitro studies have shown that acemannan combined with suboptimal non-cytotoxic concentrations of AZT or acyclovir acts synergistically to inhibit the replication of HIV and herpes simplex type 1 (HSV-1).[21] Based on these studies, as well as preliminary human studies, researchers believe that the use of acemannan may reduce the amount of AZT required by as much as 90%.[51] This is quite significant. In addition to AZT being extremely expensive, AZT's use is often associated with severe side-effects, including anemia and granulocytopenia due to bone marrow suppression.

Preliminary clinical studies are suggesting that acemannan and *Aloe vera* may be beneficial when administered orally in HIV-positive individuals.[52,53] In one study, 14 HIV patients prescribed oral acemannan (800 mg/day) demonstrated significant increases in circulating monocytes/macrophages. In particular, there were significant increases in the number of large circulating monocytes, indicating improvement in phagocytizing, processing, and presenting cells in the blood.[53] In another study of 15 AIDS patients receiving an oral dose of acemannan (800 mg/day), the average scores of Modified Walter Reed Clinical (MWR) scoring, absolute T-4, absolute T-8, and p24 core antigen levels all improved in those surviving (see Table 64.3) at the end of 900 days. Two patients died of AIDS, and another committed suicide. From this study, as well as others, it

Table 64.3 Acemannan in the treatment of AIDS[52]

Test	Pretreatment	After 900 days
Modified Walter Reed Clinical (MWR)	65	2.0
Absolute T-4	322/mm^3	324/mm^3
Absolute T-8	469/mm^3	660/mm^3
p24 core antigen	5 of 15	4 of 12

has been suggested that prognostic criteria to determine the most responsive patients are those with an absolute T-4 count greater than 150/mm^3 and p24 levels less than 300.[52]

In another study, *Aloe vera* juice (0.6 L/day) was used in conjunction with essential fatty acids and a multiple vitamin, mineral and amino acid supplement to treat 30 patients. The 15 AIDS, 12 ARC and two HIV-seropositive patients continued with regular medication, including AZT. After 180 days, all patients showed clinical improvement according to modified Karnofsky Quality Of Life Assessment scores and the Modified Walter Reed Clinical Evaluation; 25% of those positive for the p24 core antigen converted to non-reactive; anemia induced by AZT showed improvement in all patients; and the patients gained an average of 7%.

Unfortunately, a more recent study does not reproduce these early promising results. A comprehensive study assessed the safety and efficacy of acemannan as an adjunctive to antiretroviral therapy among 63 male patients (mean age, 39 years) with advanced HIV disease receiving zidovudine (ZDV) or didanosine (ddI).[54] The randomized, double-blind, placebo-controlled trial provided a large dose of acemannan (400 mg orally four times daily). Eligible patients had CD4 counts of 50–300/µl twice within 1 month of study entry and had received 26 months of antiretroviral treatment (ZDV or ddI) at a stable dose for the month before entry. CD4 counts were made every 4 weeks for 48 weeks. p24 antigen was measured at entry and every 12 weeks thereafter. Sequential quantitative lymphocyte cultures for HIV and ZDV pharmacokinetics were performed in a subset of patients.

The mean baseline CD4 counts were 165 and 147/µl in the placebo and acemannan groups, respectively; 90% of the patients were receiving ZDV at entry. Six patients in the acemannan group and five in the placebo group developed AIDS-defining illnesses. There was no statistically significant difference between the groups at 48 weeks with regard to the absolute change or rate of decline at CD4 count. Among ZDV-treated patients, the median rates of CD4 change (ACD4) in the initial 16 weeks were –121 and –120 cells/year in the placebo and acemannan groups, respectively; ACD4 decline from week 16 to 48 was 0 and –61 cells/year in the acemannan and placebo groups ($P = 0.11$), respectively. There was no statistical difference between groups with regard to adverse events, p24 antigen, quantitative virology, or pharmacokinetics. Twenty-four patients, 11 receiving placebo and 13 receiving acemannan, discontinued study therapy prematurely, none due to serious adverse reactions. The decreased, but not statistically significant, rate of loss of CD4 cells in the acemannan group from weeks 16 to 48, provides a possible ray of hope that long-term use, such as reported above, may be of value and should be investigated.

Asthma

Oral administration of an extract of *Aloe vera* for 6 months was shown to produce good results in the treatment of asthma in some individuals of various ages.[55] The exception to this was the fact that the *Aloe vera* extract was not effective at all in patients dependent upon corticosteroids. The mechanism of action is thought to be via restoration of protective mechanisms followed by augmentation of the immune system.

The extract used in the study was produced from the supernatant of fresh leaves stored in the dark for 7 days at 4°C. The dosage was 5 ml of a 20% solution of the aloe extract in saline twice daily for 24 weeks. Eleven of 27 patients (40%) without corticosteroid dependence reported significant improvement at the study's conclusion.

Studies indicate that subjecting the leaves to dark and cold results in an increase in the polysaccharide fraction. One gram of the crude extract obtained from leaves stored in the cold and dark produced 400 mg of neutral polysaccharide, as compared with only 30 mg produced from leaves not subjected to cold or dark.

Diabetes

Aloe vera also exhibits a hypoglycemic effect in both normal and alloxan-induced diabetic mice.[56] A small human study shows benefit in diabetics. Five patients with non-insulin dependent diabetes ingested half a teaspoonful of aloe 4 times daily for 14 weeks. Fasting blood sugar in every patient fell from a mean of 273 to 151 mg/dl with no change in body weight. The authors concluded that aloe lowers blood glucose levels by an unknown mechanism.[57] A more recent and larger study (49 men and 23 women) now provides more support for the efficacy of aloe in combination with glibenclamide in diabetes. While there was no response to glibenclamide alone, the combination was very effective.[58] The patients were provided with 1 tablespoon of aloe gel and 5 mg of glibenclamide twice a day, with 5 mg twice a day of glibenclamide serving as the control. After 2 weeks, fasting blood sugar decreased significantly in the treated group, and by day 42 had decreased from an average of 289 mg% to a remarkable 148 mg%. While the drop in serum cholesterol was not significant, serum triglycerides decreased from 223 mg% to (again remarkable) 128 mg% by day 42. No adverse effects were noted using standard blood chemistries.

Contraception

An interesting new application of aloe is as a spermicide. Twenty samples of fresh ejaculate from healthy human volunteers between 20 and 30 years of age were treated in vitro with a 1% concentration of zinc acetate combined with lyophilized *Aloe barbadensis* (at concentrations of 7.5–10%). The combination of zinc acetate with lyophilized *Aloe barbadensis* was shown to possess powerful spermicidal and antiviral effects which were thought to be due to their concentration of minerals (boron, barium, calcium, chromium, copper, iron, potassium, magnesium, manganese, phosphorus, and zinc), which were toxic to the sperm tail, causing instant immobilization. Studies with rabbit vaginal epithelium showed no irritation. This is important because nonoxynol-9, the active spermicidal ingredient used in vaginal contraception for over 30 years, appears to cause cell membrane damage in vaginal and cervical epithelium and may possibly have teratogenic effects.[59]

Cancer prevention

The antigenotoxic and chemopreventive effect of *Aloe barbadensis* on benzo[*a*]pyrene (B[*a*]P)–DNA adducts was investigated in vitro and in vivo in an animal model. Aloe showed a time-course and dose-dependent inhibition of [3H]B[*a*]P–DNA adduct formation in primary rat hepatocytes, inhibited cellular uptake of [3H]B[*a*]P in a dose-dependent manner, and significantly inhibited adduct formation in various organs (liver, kidney, forestomach and lung). When mice were pretreated with aloe for 16 days before B[*a*]P treatment, inhibition of BPDE-I–DNA adduct formation and persistence was enhanced. Phase II glutathione-*S*-transferase activity was slightly increased in the liver, but phase I cytochrome P450 activity was not affected.[60]

This translates into animal cancer studies as protection from Norman murine sarcoma in mice[61] and efficacy in treatment of spontaneous neoplasms in dogs and cats.[62]

TOXICOLOGY

Although rare, hypersensitivity reactions manifesting as generalized nummular eczematous and papular dermatitis as a result of topically applied *Aloe vera* preparations have been reported. It should be noted that *Aloe vera* gel has been shown to delay wound healing in cases of surgical wounds such as those produced during laparotomy or cesarean delivery.[63] Topical aloe preparations are not therefore useful for treating deep vertical wounds.

DOSAGE

Aloe vera gel can be applied liberally for topical applications. A wide range of products are available on the market; however, simple pure *Aloe vera* gel is sufficient.

Aloe vera juice can be consumed orally as a beverage or tonic. As detailed information is currently lacking as to the optimal dose for these types of products, it is recommended that no more than 1 quart be consumed in any one day.

The dose of acemannan being used in HIV/AIDS patients is 800–1,600 mg/day. This would correspond to a dose of approximately 0.5–1 L/day for most *Aloe vera* juice products. However, it appears that there may be great variation in the amount of acemannan in various products.

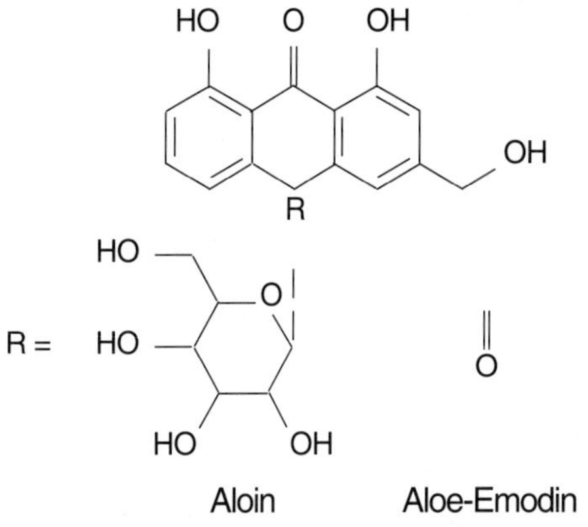

HO O OH
OH
R
R = HO HO HO OH O
Aloin Aloe-Emodin

Figure 64.1 Aloin and aloe-emodin.

REFERENCES

1. Haller JS. A drug for all seasons, medical and pharmacological history of aloe. Bull NY Acad Sci 1990; 66: 647–657
2. Klein AD, Penneys NS. *Aloe vera.* J Am Acad Dermatol 1988; 18: 714–719
3. van Wyk BE, van Rheede, van Oudtshoorn MC, Smith GF. Geographical variation in the major compounds of Aloe ferox leaf exudate. Planta Med 1995; 61: 250–253
4. Grindlay D, Reynolds T. The *Aloe vera* leaf phenomena: a review of the properties and modern use of the leaf parenchyma gel. J Ethnopharm 1986; 16: 117–151
5. Shelton RW. *Aloe vera*, its chemical and therapeutic properties. Int J Dermatol 1991; 30: 679–683
6. Afzal M, Ali M, Hassan RAH et al. Identification of some prostanoids in *Aloe vera* extracts. Planta Med 1991; 57: 38–40
7. Sabeh F, Wright T,, Norton SJ. Isozymes of superoxide dismutase from *Aloe vera.* Enzyme Protein 1996; 49: 212–221
8. Collins CE, Collins C. Roentgen dermatitis treated with fresh whole leaf *Aloe vera.* Am J Roentenol 1935; 33: 396–397
9. Godding EW. Therapeutics of laxative agents with special reference to anthraquinones. Pharmacol 1976; 14(suppl 1): 78–101
10. Anton R, Haag-Berrurier MH. Therapeutic use of natural anthraquinones for other than laxative actions. Pharmacol 1976; 14(suppl 1): 104–112
11. Ishii Y, Tanizawa H,, Takino Y. Studies of aloe. IV. Mechanism of cathartic effect. Biol Pharm Bull 1994; 17: 495–497
12. Ishii Y, Tanizawa H,, Takino Y. Studies of aloe. V. Mechanism of cathartic effect. Biol Pharm Bull 1994; 17: 651–653
13. Bland J. Effect of orally-consumed *Aloe vera* juice on human gastrointestinal function. Natural Foods Network Newsletter 1985; August
14. Robson MC, Heggers JP, Hagstron WJ. Myth, magic, witchcraft, or fact? *Aloe vera* revisited. J Burn Care Rehab 1982; 3: 157–162

15. Fly LB, Keim I. Tests of *Aloe vera* for antibiotic activity. Econ Botany 1963; 17: 46–48
16. Lorenzetti LJ, Salisburg R, Beal J et al. Bacteriostatic property of *Aloe vera*. J Pharm Sci 1964; 53: 1287
17. Heggers JP, Pineless GR, Robson MC. Dermaide *Aloe/Aloe vera* gel: comparison of the antimicrobial effects. J Am Med Technol 1979; 41: 293–294
18. Sheets MA, Unger BA, Giggleman GF, Tizard IR. Studies of the effect of acemannan on retrovirus infections: clinical stabilization of feline leukemia virus-infected cats. Mol Biother 1991; 3: 41–45
19. Kemp MC, Kahlon JB, Chinnah AD et al. In-vitro evaluation of the antiviral effects of acemannan on the replication and pathogenesis of HIV-1 and other enveloped viruses: modification of the processing of glycoprotein precursors. Antiviral Research 1990; suppl 1: 83
20. Kahlon JB, Kemp MC, Carpenter RH et al. Inhibition of AIDS virus replication by acemannan in vitro. Mol Biother 1991; 3: 127–135
21. Kahlon JB, Kemp MC, Yawei N et al. In vitro evaluation of the synergistic antiviral effects of acemannan in combination with azidothymidine and acyclovir. Mol Biother 1991; 3: 214–223
22. Hart LA, Nibbering PH, van den Barselaar MT et al. Effects of low molecular constituents from *Aloe vera* gel on oxidative metabolism and cytotoxic and bactericidal activities of human neutrophils. Int J Immunol Pharmac 1990; 12: 427–434
23. Womble D, Helderman JH. Enhancement of allo-responsiveness of human lymphocytes by acemannan (CarrisynTM). Int J Immunopharmac 1988; 10: 967–974
25. Zhang L, Tizard IR. Activation of a mouse macrophage cell line by acemannan: the major carbohydrate fraction from *Aloe vera* gel. Immunopharmacology 1996; 35: 119–128
26. Stuart RW, Lefkowitz DL, Lincoln JA et al. Upregulation of phagocytosis and candidicidal activity of macrophages exposed to the immunostimulant acemannan. Int J Immunopharmacol 1997; 19: 75–82
27. Egger SF, Brown GS, Kelsey LS et al. Studies on optimal dose and administration schedule of a hematopoietic stimulatory beta-(1,4)-linked mannan. Int J Immunopharmacol 1996; 18: 113–126
28. Davis RH, Shapiro E, Agnew PS. Topical effect of aloe with ribonucleic acid and vitamin C on adjuvant arthritis. J Am Pod Med Assoc 1985; 75: 229–237
29. Yagi A, Harada N, Yamada H et al. Antibradykinin active material in *Aloe saponaria*. J Pharmaceut Sci 1982; 71: 1172–1174
30. Davis RH, Parker WL, Samson RT, Murdoch DP. Isolation of a stimulatory system in an *Aloe* extract. J Am Pod Med Assoc 1991; 81: 473–478
31. Davis RH, Leitner MG, Russo JM, Byrne ME. Anti-inflammatory activity of *Aloe vera* against a spectrum of irritants. J Am Pod Med Assoc 1989; 79: 263–266
32. Vazquez B, Avila G, Segura D, Escalante B. Anti-inflammatory activity of extracts from *Aloe vera* gel. J Ethnopharmacol 1996; 55: 69–75
33. Malterud KE, Farbrot TL, Huse AE,, Sund RB. Antioxidant and radical scavenging effects of anthraquinones and anthrones. Pharmacology 1993; 47(suppl 1): 77–85
34. Henry R. An updated review of *Aloe vera*. Cosmet Toilet 1979; 94: 42–50
35. Shida T, Yagi A, Nishimura H, Nishioka I. Effect of *Aloe* extract on peripheral phagocytosis in adult bronchial asthma. Planta Medica 1985; 51: 273–275
35a. Davis RH, Kabbani JM, Maro NP. *Aloe vera* and wound healing. J Am Pod Med Assoc 1987; 77: 165–169
36. Davis RH, Leitner MG, Russo JM. *Aloe vera*, a natural approach for treating wounds, edema, and pain in diabetes. J Am Pod Med Assoc 1988; 78: 60–68
37. Rowe TD. Effect of fresh *Aloe vera* gel in the treatment of third-degree Roentgen reactions on white rats. J Am Pharm Assoc 1940; 29: 348–350
38. Rowe TD, Lovell BK, Parks LM. Further observations on the use of *Aloe vera* leaf in the treatment of third-degree X-ray reactions. J Am Pharm Assoc 1941; 30: 266–269
39. Lushbaugh CC, Hale DB. Experimental acute radiodermatitis following beta radiation. V. Histopathological study of the mode of action of therapy with *Aloe vera*. Cancer 1953; 6: 690–698
40. Davis RH, Donato JJ, Hartman GM, Haas RC. Anti-inflammatory and wound healing activity of a growth substance in *Aloe vera*. J Am Podiatr Med Assoc 1994; 84: 77–81
41. Davis RH, DiDonato JJ, Johnson RW, Stewart CB. *Aloe vera*, hydrocortisone, and sterol influence on wound tensile strength and anti-inflammation. J Am Podiatr Med Assoc 1994; 84: 614–621
42. Chung JH, Cheong JC, Lee JY et al. Acceleration of the alcohol oxidation rate in rats with aloin, a quinone derivative of Aloe. Biochem Pharmacol 1996; 52: 1461–1468
43. El Zawahry M, Hegazy MR, Helal M. Use of aloe in treating leg ulcers and dermatoses. Int J Dermatol 1973; 12: 68–73
44. Visuthikosol V, Chowchuen B, Sukwanarat Y et al. Effect of *Aloe vera* gel to healing of burn wound. A clinical and histologic study. J Med Assoc Thai 1995; 78: 403–409
45. Miller MB, Koltai PJ. Treatment of experimental frostbite with pentoxifylline and aloe vera cream. Arch Otolaryngol Head Neck Surg 1995; 121: 678–680
46. Ardire L. Necrotizing fasciitis. case study of a nursing dilemma. Ostomy Wound Manage 1997; 43: 30–34
47. Williams MS, Burk M, Loprinzi CL et al. Phase III double-blind evaluation of an *Aloe vera* gel as a prophylactic agent for radiation-induced skin toxicity. Int J Radiat Oncol Biol Phys 1996; 36: 345–349
48. Roberts DB, Travis EL. Acemannan-containing wound dressing gel reduces radiation-induced skin reactions in C3H mice. Int J Radiat Oncol Biol Phys 1995; 32: 1047–1052
49. Syed TA, Ahmad SA, Holt AH et al. Management of psoriasis with *Aloe vera* extract in a hydrophilic cream: a placebo-controlled, double-blind study. Trop Med Int Health 1996; 1: 505–509
50. Blitz JJ, Smith JW, Gerard JR. *Aloe vera* gel in peptic ulcer therapy: preliminary report. J Am Osteo Soc 1963; 62: 731–735
51. Anonymous. *Aloe vera* may boost AZT. Med Tribune 1991; August 22: 4
52. McDaniel HR, Carpenter RH, Kemp M et al. Extended survival and prognostic criteria for acemannan (ACE-M) treated HIV-1 patients. Antiviral Res 1990; suppl 1: 117
53. McDaniel HR, Combs C, McDaniel R et al. An increase in circulating monocyte/macrophages (MM) is induced by oral acemannan (ACE-M) in HIV-1 patients. Am J Clin Pathol 1990; 94: 516–517
54. Montaner JS, Gill J, Singer J et al. Double-blind placebo-controlled pilot trial of acemannan in advanced human immunodeficiency virus disease. J Acquir Immune Defic Syndr Hum Retrovirol 1996; 12: 153–157
55. Yagi A, Nishirnura H, Nishioka I. Effect of Aloe extract on peripheral phagocytosis in adult bronchial asthma. Planta Medica 1985; 51: 273–275
56. Ajabnoor MA. Effect of aloes on blood glucose levels in normal and alloxan diabetic mice. J Ethnopharmacol 1990; 28: 215–220
57. Gnhannam N, Kingston M, Al-Meshaal IA et al. The antidiabetic activity of Aloes. Hormone Research 1986; 24: 288–294
58. Bunyapraphatsara N, Yongchaiyudha A, Rungpitarang S, Chokechaijaroenporn O. Antidiabetic activity of *Aloe vera* juice II. Clinical trial in diabetes meelitus patients in combination with glibenclamide. Phytomed 1996; 3: 245–248
59. Fahim MS, Wang M. Zinc acetate and lyophilized *Aloe barbadensis* as vaginal contraceptive. Contraception 1996; 53: 231–236
60. Kim HS, Lee BM. Inhibition of benzo[a]pyrene-DNA adduct formation by *Aloe barbadensis* Miller. Carcinogenesis 1997; 18: 771–776
61. Peng SY, Norman J, Curtin G et al. Decreased mortality of Norman murine sarcoma in mice treated with the immunomodulator, acemannan. Mol Biother 1991; 3: 79–87
62. Harris C, Pierce K, King G et al. Efficacy of acemannan in treatment of canine and feline spontaneous neoplasms. Mol Biother 1991; 3: 207–213
63. Schmidt JM, Greenspoon JS. *Aloe vera* dermal wound gel is associated with a delay in wound healing. Obstet Gynecol 1991; 78: 115–117

CHAPTER CONTENTS

65

Angelica species

Michael T. Murray, ND

Joseph E. Pizzorno Jr, ND

Angelica sinensis or *polymorpha* (family: Umbelliferae or Apiaceae)
Common names: Chinese angelica, tang-kuei (dong-quai)

Angelica acutiloba (family: Umbelliferae or Apiaceae)
Common name: Japanese angelica

Angelica archangelica (family: Umbelliferae or Apiaceae)
Common name: European angelica

Angelica atropurpurea (family: Umbelliferae or Apiaceae)
Common name: American angelica

Angelica sylvestris (family: Umbelliferae or Apiaceae)
Common name: wild angelica

GENERAL DESCRIPTION

Angelica spp. are biennial or perennial plants with hollow fluted stems that rise to a height of 3–7 feet. The umbel of greenish-white flowers bloom from May to August. The plants are found in damp mountain ravines and meadows, on river banks, and in coastal areas; angelica is also a widely cultivated species. In Asia, it is grown primarily for its medicinal action, while in the US and Europe, it is cultivated for use as a flavoring agent in most major categories of food products, including alcoholic (e.g. bitters, liqueurs, and vermouths) and non-alcoholic beverages, ice cream, candy, gelatins, and puddings. With all species, the roots and rhizomes are the most extensively used portions of the plant.

Angelica sinensis *and* A. acutiloba

In Asia, the authentic and original medicinal angelica is *Angelica sinensis* (dong-quai), native to China. While at least nine other angelica species are used in China, dong-quai is by far the most highly regarded. For several thousand years, dong-quai has been cultivated for medicinal use in the treatment of a wide variety of disorders, in particular, "female" disorders. Several hundred years ago, when the supply of Chinese angelica was scarce, the

Japanese began to cultivate *A. acutiloba*, an angelica species indigenous to Japan, as a substitute.[1] The two species appear to have very similar therapeutic effects, although it is interesting to note that in China, the Japanese angelica is thought to have no therapeutic value, while in Japan, Chinese angelica is thought of as being without effect. Experimentally, both species exhibit very similar therapeutic effects, so each country's claim to produce a superior dong-quai appears to be based more on emotion than scientific investigation.

Angelica archangelica *and* A. atropurpurea

Historical usage suggests that European angelica (*A. archangelica*) and American angelica (*A. atropurpurea*) have properties different from the Asian species. This difference has not, however, been evaluated by chemical analysis.

CHEMICAL COMPOSITION

Angelica sinensis *and* A. acutiloba

No comprehensive data could be found listing the concentration of the chemical constituents. It is assumed that Chinese and Japanese angelica are similarly composed of various coumarins and flavonoids which are responsible for their medicinal actions. The essential oil of oriental angelica contains:[2]

- *n*-butylphthalide
- cadinene
- carvacrol
- *n*-dodecanal
- isosafrole
- linoleic acid
- palmitic acid
- safrole
- sequiterpene
- *n*-tetradecanol.

Angelica archangelica

Also very rich in coumarins, this species of angelica is particularly phototoxic. Coumarins, including osthole, angelicin, osthenol, umbelliferone, archangelicine, bergapten, and ostruthol, are found in significant concentrations, with osthole composing nearly 0.2% of the root. The root is also a good source of flavonoids, including archangelenone and caffeic acids. The root contains 0.3–1.0% volatile oil that is composed mainly of beta-phyllamdrene, alpha-pinene, borneol, limonene, and four macrocylic lactones.[2,3]

HISTORY AND FOLK USE

Angelica sinensis *and* A. acutiloba

In Asia, angelica's reputation is perhaps second only to ginseng. Predominantly regarded as a "female" remedy, angelica has been used in such conditions as dysmenorrhea, amenorrhea, metrorrhagia, menopausal symptoms, and to assure a healthy pregnancy and easy delivery. Angelica is also used in the treatment of abdominal pain, anemia, injuries, arthritis, migraine headache, and many other conditions.[2,4]

Angelica archangelica

One of the most highly praised herbs in old herbal texts, archangelica was used by all north European countries as:

> ... a protection against contagion, for purifying the blood, and for curing every conceivable malady: it was held a sovereign remedy for poisons, agues and all infectious maladies.

According to one legend, archangelica was revealed in a dream as a cure for the plague. One explanation for the name is related to its blooming near May 8, the feast day of Michael the Archangel. It was therefore seen as a "protector against evil spirits and witchcraft".[5]

Archangelica has been used for a wide variety of conditions, including flatulent dyspepsia, pleurisy, respiratory catarrh, and bronchitis. The plant was believed to possess carminative, spasmolytic, diaphoretic, expectorant, and diuretic activity.[5]

Angelica atropurpurea

American angelica's therapeutic use mirrors that of European angelica. Its most common use is for heartburn and flatulent colic.[6]

PHARMACOLOGY

The pharmacology of *Angelica* spp. relates to their high coumarin content. However, unlike other scientific investigations of botanical medicines, much of the research done on *Angelica* spp. has been done on plant extracts, rather than isolated constituents. The overwhelming majority of the studies have been done on the Asian species. Some of the pharmacological activities demonstrated include:

- phytoestrogen activity
- analgesic activity
- cardiovascular effects
- smooth muscle-relaxing effects
- anti-allergy and immunomodulating activity
- antimicrobial activity.

Phytoestrogen effects

Plant estrogenic substances or phytoestrogens are components of many medicinal herbs with an historic use in conditions which are now treated by synthetic estrogens. Chinese and Japanese angelica contain highly active phytoestrogens, although these compounds are much lower in activity than animal estrogens (1:400 as active). This helps to explain why angelica was used in both excessive and deficient estrogen conditions. Phytoestrogens demonstrate an alterative effect by competing with estrogen for binding sites. When estrogen levels are low they are able to exert some estrogenic activity; when estrogen levels are high they reduce overall estrogenic activity by occupying estrogen receptor sites. This alterative action of angelica's phytoestrogens is probably the basis of much of the plant's use in amenorrhea and menopause.

Japanese angelica has demonstrated uterine tonic activity, causing an initial increase in uterine contraction followed by relaxation.[7,8] In addition, administration of Japanese angelica to mice resulted in an increase of uterine weight, increase of the DNA content of the uterus and liver, and increase of glucose utilization by the liver and uterus.[1,7] Because of these and other effects, angelica has been referred to as a uterine tonic.

Cardiovascular effects

Although not used historically for these purposes, angelica does possess significant hypotensive action.[1,7] This is largely due to its vasodilator activity. Dihydropyranocoumarins and dihydro-furanocoumarins from Umbelliferous plants have been shown to possess significant coronary vasodilatory, spasmolytic, and cyclic-AMP-phosphodiesterase inhibitory properties.[9] The mechanism of action appears to be largely a result of calcium channel antagonism. Agents that interact with calcium channels (calcium channel blockers) are quickly coming into prominence in the treatment of a wide variety of conditions, including hypertension and angina. Umbelliferous plants such as angelica may offer similar effects.

Other cardiovascular effects noted for angelica are negative inotropic and anti-arrhythmic action.[1]

Smooth muscle-relaxing activity

Calcium channel blocking compounds are also capable of relaxing the smooth muscles of visceral organs. Angelica (essential oil) has demonstrated relaxing action on the smooth muscles of the intestines and uterus, while the water extract produces an initial contraction and then prolonged relaxation.[1,7,8] This confirms its historical use in the treatment of intestinal spasm and uterine cramps. Its action on other smooth muscles could explain its hypotensive action (vascular smooth muscle) and historical use in asthma (bronchial smooth muscle).

Analgesic activity

Both Chinese and Japanese angelica have demonstrated pain-relieving and mild tranquilizing effects in experimental studies in animals.[1,7,10,11] Angelica's analgesic action was 1.7 times that of aspirin in one study.[11] Its analgesic activity, combined with its smooth muscle-relaxing activity, supports its historical use in such conditions as uterine cramps, trauma, headaches, and arthritis.

Anti-allergy and immunomodulating activity

Angelica has a long history of use by Chinese and Japanese herbalists in the prevention and treatment of allergic symptoms in individuals who are sensitive to a variety of substances (pollen, dust, animal dander, food, etc.).[1,12] Its action is related to its ability to inhibit the production of IgE in a selective manner. Since IgE levels in patients with atopic conditions are typically 3–10 times greater than the upper limit of normal, angelica may offer some benefit by reducing these elevated antibodies.

Coumarin compounds have demonstrated immune-enhancing activity in both healthy and cancer patients.[13,14] Coumarins have been shown to stimulate macrophages and increase phagocytosis.[13] Such activity is thought to offer significant protection against metastasis and growth of tumor cells. Upon coumarin administration, macrophages are said to be "activated" and thus capable of entering the tumor, where a specific destruction of the tumor cells may occur.[13.14]

Coumarin compounds of angelica and the polysaccharides of the water extract of Japanese angelica have immune-modulating activity. They have been shown to possess mitogenic activity to B-lymphocytes, interferon-producing activity, antitumor activity, and complement-activating (both the classical and alternative pathway) activity.[15–18] Chinese angelica has been shown to increase murine IL-2 production, stimulate the reticuloendothelial system, and increase tumor necrosis factor production.[19,20] These effects on the immune system by coumarins, polysaccharides, and extracts of *Angelica* sp. would seem to support their historical anti-cancer effects and their use as adjuncts to current cancer therapy.

Antibacterial activity

Extracts of Chinese angelica have been shown to possess antibacterial activity against both Gram-negative and Gram-positive bacteria, while extracts of Japanese angelica exhibited no antibacterial action.[7] The inconsistency could be due to different essential oil concentrations of the extracts used in the studies. The oil of *A. archangelica* has also exhibited significant antifungal and anthelmintic properties but virtually no antibacterial activity.[3,21,22] As other herbs have much greater antimicrobial activity, *Angelica* sp. would be considered a less than optimum agent if this effect is desired.

CLINICAL APPLICATION

Angelica spp. have been used throughout the world in the treatment of a wide variety of conditions. At this time, it appears that *A. archangelica* and *A. atropurpurea* are most indicated as expectorants, antispasmodics, and carminatives in the treatment of such conditions as respiratory ailments, gas, and abdominal spasm. Chinese angelica (*A. sinensis* or *polymorpha*) and Japanese angelica (*A. acutiloba*) appear most useful in the treatment of disorders of menstruation, menopause (especially hot flashes), atopic conditions, smooth muscle spasm (e.g. uterine cramps, migraines, abdominal spasm, etc.), and possibly as an immunostimulatory adjunct in cancer therapy. Further human research is needed to document the degree clinical of efficacy of *Angelica* spp.

DOSAGE

- Dried root or rhizome: 1–2 g orally, or by infusion, three times/day
- Tincture (1:5): 3–5 ml, three times/day
- Fluid extract (1:1): 0.5–2 ml, three times/day.

TOXICOLOGY

Angelica is generally considered to be of very low toxicity. However, it does contain many photoreactive substances which may induce photosensitivity. This should be kept in mind when using any Umbelliferous plant. This activity can be used therapeutically in the treatment of vitiligo and psoriasis.

REFERENCES

1. Hikino H. Recent research on Oriental medicinal plants. Econ Med Plant Res 1985; 1: 53–85
2. Duke JA. Handbook of medicinal herbs. Boca Raton, FL: CRC Press. 1985: p 43–44
3. Leung AY. Encyclopedia of common natural ingredients used in food, drugs, and cosmetics. New York, NY: John Wiley. 1980: p 28–29
4. Duke JA and Ayensu ES. Medicinal plants of China. Algonac, MI: Reference Publications. 1985: p 74–77
5. Grieve M. A Modern herbal. New York, NY: Dover. 1971: p 35–40
6. Lust J. The Herb Book. New York, NY: Bantam Books. 1974: p 97–99
7. Yoshiro K. The physiological actions of tang-kuei and cnidium. Bull Oriental Healing Arts Inst USA 1985; 10: 269–78
8. Harada M, Suzuki M, Ozaki Y. Effect of Japanese angelica root and peony root on uterine contraction in the rabbit in situ. J Pharm Dyn 1984; 7: 304–311
9. Thastrup O, Fjalland B, Lemmich J. Coronary vasodilatory, spasmolytic and cAMP-phosphodiesterase inhibitory properties of dihydropyranocoumarins and dihydrofuranocoumarins. Acta Pharmacol et Toxicol 1983; 52: 246–53
10. Tanaka S, Ikeshiro Y, Tabata M, Konoshima M. Anti-nociceptive substances from the roots of Angelica acutiloba. Arzneim Forsch 1977; 27: 2039–45
11. Tanaka S, Kano Y, Tabata M, Konoshima M. Effects of "Toki" (*Angelica acutiloba* Kitawaga) extracts on writhing and capillary permeability in mice (analgesic and anti-inflammatory effects). Yakugaku Zassh 1071; 91: 1098–1104
12. Sung CP, Baker AP, Holden DA et al. Effects of Angelica polymorpha on reaginic antibody production. J Natural Products 1071; 45: 398–406
13. Casley-Smith JR. The actions of benzopyrenes on the blood-tissue-lymph system. Folia Angiol 1976; 24: 7–22
14. Berkarda B, Bouffard-Eyuboglu H, Derman U. The effect of coumarin derivatives on the immunological system of man. Agents Actions 1983; 13: 50–52
15. Ohno N, Matsumoto SI, Suzuki I et al. Biochemical characterization of a mitogen obtained from an oriental crude drug, tohki (Angelica acutiloba Kitawaga). J Pharm Dyn 1983; 6: 903–912
16. Yamada H, Kiyohara H, Cyong JC et al. Studies on polysaccharides from Angelica acutiloba. Planta Medica 1984; 48: 163–167
17. Yamada H, Kiyohara H, Cyong JC et al. Studies on polysaccharides from Angelica acutiloba – IV. Characterization of an anti-complementary arabinogalactan from the roots of Angelica acutiloba Kitagawa. Mol Immunol 1985; 22: 295–304
18. Kumazawa Y, Mizunoe K, Otsuka Y. Immunostimulating polysaccharide separated from hot water extract of *Angelica acutiloba* Kitagawa (Yamato Tohki). Immunology 1982; 47: 75–83
19. Weng XC, Zhang P, Gong SS, Xiai SW. Effect of immuno-modulating agents on murine IL-2 production. Immunol Invest 1987; 16: 79–86
20. Haranaka K, Satomi N, Sakurai A, Karanaka R, Okada N, Kobayashi M. Antitumor activities and tumor necrosis factor producibility of traditional Chinese medicines and crude drugs. Cancer Immunol Immunother 1985; 20: 1–5
21. Rhee JK, Woo KJ, Baek BK, Ahn BJ. Screening of the wormicidal Chinese raw drugs on Clonorchis sinesis. Am J Chin Med Winter 1981; 9: 277–284
22. Opdyke DLJ. Angelica root oil. Food Cosmet Toxicol 1975; 13: 713–714

CHAPTER CONTENTS

66

Aspergillus oryzae enzyme therapy

Corey Resnick, ND

INTRODUCTION

Enzymes derived from *Aspergillus oryzae* and other fungal species are effective in the treatment of a broad range of human diseases. In certain cases, fungal enzymes are significantly more effective than animal-derived enzymes or other available therapies. Some fungal enzyme preparations are particularly well suited for human use because of their ability to hydrolyze physiologically and/or pathologically important substrates over a wide pH range.

Although new to many clinicians in the US, fungal enzymes have been used in ethnic food production for many centuries, and in clinical practice and research for about 50 years. In Japan, *Aspergillus oryzae* has been used in the fermentation of soybeans to produce soy sauce, tamari and miso. (It is interesting to note that the traditional method of adding hot water to miso, rather than boiling the miso, preserves some of the activity of *Aspergillus* enzymes, which are remarkably heat stable.)

Clinically, enzyme preparations have typically been used in oral administration at mealtimes to assist digestion by hydrolyzing dietary substrates such as gluten, casein or lactose. Of possibly greater interest, however, is the use of fungal enzymes administered orally between meals. Based on the theory that some portion of the enzyme is absorbed intact into the bloodstream, enzymes can hydrolyze substrates of therapeutic importance (e.g. fibrin). Indirect evidence in support of this theory is presented later in this chapter.

Beginning around the 1950s, published research in Europe and Scandinavia reported on the therapeutic use of purified, concentrated preparations of enzymes from *A. oryzae* and other fungal species. Bergkvist was among the first to report on the isolation and purification of individual enzymes produced by *A. oryzae.* Wolf and Ransberger studied the effects of enzymes from *Aspergillus* and other species (e.g. *Lens esculenta* and *Pisum sativum*) along with animal enzymes (e.g. trypsin, chymotrypsin) in the treatment of cancer. Roschlau and others studied the effectiveness of intravenously administered proteolytic enzymes from *A. oryzae* in the treatment of vascular disease in humans and animals.

Recent research has studied increasingly diverse types and sources of fungal enzymes, including various protease, lipase, carbohydrase, and cellulase preparations. Controlled in vivo studies using enteral and parenteral routes and in vitro studies have examined the effectiveness of these enzymes in a wide range of conditions including:

- maldigestion
- malabsorption
- pancreatic insufficiency
- steatorrhea
- celiac disease
- lactose intolerance
- arterial obstruction
- thrombotic disease.

Anecdotal reports indicate that plant enzymes are being used in an even broader spectrum of clinical conditions.

This chapter reviews published clinical and experimental research in the emerging field of fungal enzyme therapy. Theoretical discussions are presented regarding the oral administration of fungal enzymes for therapeutic purposes, with suggested areas for further research.

PHARMACOLOGY

Intact protein absorption

Contrary to long held theories that the healthy intestinal mucosa is an essentially impermeable barrier to proteins and large polypeptides, there is now irrefutable evidence that macromolecules can and do pass intact from the human gut into the bloodstream under normal conditions.[1–7] This may help to explain the apparent effectiveness of enzyme therapy in the nutritional management of a number of conditions, including vascular disease, maldigestion/malabsorption, food allergies, inflammatory bowel disease, immune dysfunction and certain inflammatory disorders.[1,2,8–17]

Evidence for intestinal absorption of intact proteins

Numerous whole proteins, including plant and animal enzymes, have been shown in human and animal studies to be absorbed intact into the bloodstream following oral administration. These include human albumin and lactalbumin, bovine albumin, ovalbumin, lactoglobulin, ferritin (MW, 500,000), chymotrypsinogen, elastase, and other large molecules, such as botulism toxin (MW, 1,000,000).[1–3,18,19–21] Even inert particles, such as carbon particles from India ink[1] and whole viruses,[22] can cross the healthy intestine.

Immunoglobulins have been detected in peripheral tissues following oral administration. In a study done in rats, 5% of an oral dose of bovine IgG was found substantially intact in peripheral tissues.[6] Studies have demonstrated the intact absorption of plant enzymes, such as bromelain derived from pineapple and peroxidase (MW, 40,000) from horseradish. An in vivo study in fish showed that 0.7% of a dose of horseradish peroxidase was detected intact in examined peripheral tissues following oral administration.[23]

Proteins and polypeptides absorbed intact from the gut can exert pharmacological effects in target tissues. Several peptide hormones are known to be biologically active when administered orally, including luteinizing hormone-releasing factor and thytropin-releasing hormone.[24,25] Even insulin can cross the intestinal mucosa intact and produce significant hypoglycemia under limited circumstances (e.g. in the presence of protease inhibitors or hypertonic solutions in the intestinal lumen).[26,27]

It now appears probable that enzymes such as acid-stable protease from *Aspergillus oryzae* (molecular weight ~ 35,000) are absorbed intact following oral administration. To the extent that such absorption does occur, *Aspergillus*-derived proteases may exhibit properties in the bloodstream which they are known to possess in other applications. This may include the ability to hydrolyze dietary proteins and polypeptides which have leaked into the bloodstream as food antigens. Protease from *Aspergillus* is also known to possess thrombolytic, fibrinolytic and anti-inflammatory properties,[28–34] and has been shown to be effective when administered intravenously in re-establishing circulation through chronically obstructed arteries in humans (see below).[35,36]

Mechanism for intestinal absorption of macromolecules

Two general types of mechanisms have been suggested to account for the intact absorption of macromolecules and particles.[1,2] In the "transcellular route" macromolecules are believed to penetrate the brush-border membrane of intestinal mucosal cells by:

- diffusion through aqueous "pores" or through lipid regions in the membrane
- pinocytosis (endocytosis) or phagocytosis
- carrier-mediated transport systems
- some combination of these routes.

A "paracellular" or intercellular route also appears likely, in which molecules pass between mucosal cells. This route includes passage through so-called "extrusion zones" which occur as old cells are displaced by new ones in the rapidly proliferating mucosal tissue.

A specialized cell type has recently been identified overlying Peyer's patches (subepithelial lymphoid tissue) throughout the small intestine. These so-called "M" cells permit subepithelial tissue lymphocytes to come extremely close to the intestinal lumen, apparently facilitating lymphocyte "sampling" of luminal antigens and thereby stimulating an immune response.

A number of studies have shown rapid passage through M cells (by pinocytosis) of macromolecules such as horseradish peroxidase and solid particles such as viruses.[1,2,37–39]

Pancreatic recycling of enzymes

There is strong evidence that the body seeks to conserve its digestive enzymes by absorbing intact endogenous and exogenous enzymes. Several human studies have shown that exogenous pancreatic enzymes, trypsin and chymotrypsin, are absorbed intact into the bloodstream in an enzymatically active form following oral administration.[40–44]

Even more dramatic is the finding that both endogenous and exogenous pancreatic enzymes are not only absorbed intact from the gut, but also transported through the bloodstream, taken up intact by pancreatic secretory cells, and re-secreted into the intestinal lumen by the pancreas, co-mixed with newly synthesized pancreatic enzymes.[45] The existence of this enteropancreatic circulation of proteolytic enzymes is closely analogous to the recycling of bile salts by the liver.

Of further interest is the possibility that oral supplementation with enzymes may have a sparing effect on the body's own digestive enzymes, perhaps aiding organ regeneration, by hydrolyzing substrates (foods) for which endogenous enzyme would otherwise be required. Support for this hypothesis may also be found in the phenomenon of adaptive secretion by which the pancreas, stomach and possibly other organs secrete specific digestive enzymes in direct response to the type and amount of food substrate present.[46,47]

COMPARISON OF FUNGAL LIPASE AND PANCREATIN

pH range

Many of the enzymes derived from *A. oryzae* and related fungal species possess unusually high stability and activity under a broad range of pH conditions. These properties distinguish them from animal enzymes such as pepsin, pancreatin, trypsin, chymotrypsin, pancrelipase and pancreatic amylase which require pH conditions often lacking in those with impaired health. For example, pepsin is active only below a pH of about 4.5, while pancreatin has digestive activity only in an alkaline medium. In contrast, some preparations of *A. oryzae* enzymes are stable and active at pH values of 2–12.

Enzyme replacement therapy

Human and animal studies have compared the effectiveness of acid-stable lipase from various fungal species with that of pancreatin in the treatment of malabsorption and steatorrhea due to pancreatic insufficiency. Administered orally at mealtime, fungal lipase has been found to be effective in these conditions and to offer certain advantages over both conventional and enteric-coated pancreatic enzyme replacement therapy.

Treatment of steatorrhea using pancreatic enzyme replacement therapy is often unsatisfactory due to several factors. Gastric acid destroys up to 90% of the lipase content of exposed pancreatic enzymes (i.e. conventional pancreatin administered in powder, capsule or tablet form).[48–50] This necessitates large dosages for efficacy and contributes to increased expense, number of tablets or capsules required, and poor patient compliance.[51,52] Furthermore, pancreatin can cause hyperuricosuria and renal damage in large doses due to its high purine content.[53] Although H_2 receptor antagonists such as cimetidine are often used along with pancreatin to lessen intragastric inactivation,[54,55] this is unsuccessful at increasing lipid digestion in many patients[56] and carries the risk of possible adverse side-effects.

Various forms of enteric-coated pancreatin (i.e. enteric-coated capsules, tablets, granules and microspheres) are formulated to dissolve above pH 5.5–6.0 and are intended to protect exogenous pancreatin against gastric acidity.[54,57] These are seldom completely effective, however, as, while the capsules or tablets usually remain intact in the stomach, they often fail to dissolve in the duodenum due to hyperacidity; most patients with pancreatic insufficiency also have decreased bicarbonate secretion. Similarly, jejunal acidification can occur, preventing activation of enteric-coated enzyme preparations designed to release in the jejunum.[58] In addition, chemical excipients required for enteric coating can be problematical in sensitive individuals.

By contrast, a lipase preparation from *Aspergillus oryzae* is resistant to inactivation by gastric acidity and is enzymatically active from pH 2 to 10. It digests dietary fat, beginning in the stomach and continuing in the small intestine.[51,59] It is water-soluble, heat-stable, nontoxic and free from some of the potential drawbacks of pancreatin replacement therapy.[51]

CLINICAL APPLICATIONS

Malabsorption and steatorrhea

Chronic pancreatitis and cystic fibrosis are the most common causes of pancreatic exocrine insufficiency.

Pancreatogenic steatorrhea results from failure of fat digestion, leading to lipid malabsorption, impaired nutrition, weight loss, and considerable social embarrassment.[48,60] Lipase preparations from *Aspergillus oryzae* have been shown to be highly effective in treating malabsorption and steatorrhea under a wide variety of conditions.

A 1985 cross-over study in Germany compared the effectiveness of 10 teaspoons of a conventional pancreatic enzyme preparation (360,000 lipase units) with that of 10 capsules of enteric-coated pancreatin (100,000 lipase units) and 10 capsules of acid-stable fungal enzymes from *Rhizopus arrhizus* (75,000 lipase units) in human patients with chronic pancreatitis, severe pancreatic exocrine insufficiency and steatorrhea.[59] Seventeen patients in the study were divided into two treatment groups based on surgical status.

Nine patients had received Whipple's procedure (bowel resection with partial duodenopancreatectomy) 3–8 months prior to the study (group A). This group had shown a pre-operative reduction in stimulated pancreatic enzyme secretion to less than 10% of normal. In the remaining eight, non-surgical patients (group B), stimulated secretion was reduced to between 4 and 28% of normal.

All patients were placed on a diet containing 100 g fat/day and stools were collected for 72 hours, 5 days after discontinuing all medications (pancreatic enzymes, antacids, and H_2 receptor antagonists). Thereafter, each group was placed on identical 2 week periods of treatment using enteric-coated pancreatin first, then conventional pancreatin and, finally, acid-stable fungal enzymes.

Stools were collected for the last 3 days of each treatment period and analyzed for stool weight, fat concentration, and total fecal fat excretion. Prior to treatment, all fecal parameters were pathologically elevated in all 17 patients, diarrhea and characteristic abdominal symptoms were present, and the patients had a tendency to lose weight.

All three treatment protocols led to a significant reduction in total daily stool weight and total daily fecal fat excretion as compared with controls in both groups. Perhaps more importantly, all patients in both groups became virtually symptom-free on each of the three treatment protocols. Table 66.1 shows fecal fat excretion and stool weight for controls and under each treatment protocol in group A and group B. Individual patient results in each group have been averaged together.

A 1988 placebo-controlled, randomized, cross-over study in England compared the effectiveness of 400 mg (4800 lipase units) of acid-stable lipase from *A. oryzae* with that of 10,000 mg (60,000 lipase units) of pancreatin in the treatment of chronic pancreatic exocrine insufficiency in dogs.[51]

Eleven dogs (weighing 15–21 kg) used in the study underwent total pancreatectomy to produce pancreatic exocrine insufficiency. All animals received intrasplenic autografts of islet of Langerhans tissue to preserve pancreatic endocrine function. Animals served as their own controls by the use of pre-surgical data.

Table 66.1 Stool weight and fecal fat in patients with steatorrhea

Treatment protocol	Fecal fat (g/day)		Stool weight (g/day)	
	Group A	Group B	Group A	Group B
Placebo	180	82	906	675
Enteric-coated pancreatin	75	39	494	324
Pancreatin	55	48	437	345
Fungal lipase	87	48	519	316

The upper limit of the normal range for fecal fat excretion is 7 g/day and for stool weight is 250 g/day

The dogs were maintained on fixed diets containing 46 g/day fat. Each treatment protocol lasted 3 weeks, beginning and ending with weighing of animals and 3 day specimen collections for determination of fecal fat excretion and stool volume.

Dogs in the untreated placebo group experienced significant weight loss ($P < 0.01$) due to malabsorption averaging 0.9 kg over a 3 week period. Dogs receiving either 400 mg/day of *A. oryzae* lipase or 10,000 mg/day of pancreatin did not show significant weight loss.

Similarly, both fecal fat excretion and stool volume were pathologically elevated in the placebo group. Significant reductions occurred in both fecal fat and stool volume, with no significant difference between fungal lipase and pancreatin treated animals.

The most significant finding of the English study was the fact that a small dose of acid-stable lipase from *A. oryzae* (400 mg) was as effective as a dosage of conventional pancreatin 25 times larger (10,000 mg) in the treatment of malabsorption, malnutrition and steatorrhea due to pancreatic exocrine insufficiency in dogs. In the German study, an acid-stable fungal lipase from *R. arrhizus* produced largely the same effect as 1.3 times greater lipase activity from enteric-coated pancreatin and 4.8 times greater lipase activity from conventional pancreatin in the treatment of severe pancreatogenic steatorrhea in humans.[59]

Unlike pancreatin, *A. oryzae* lipase delivers enzyme activity in the broad range from pH 2 to 10. It safely digests dietary fat, beginning in the stomach and continuing in the small intestine, and is more effective than pancreatin in the abnormal acidic conditions commonly found in the duodenum and jejunum of pancreatic insufficiency patients.

Lactose intolerance

Lactose intolerance produces symptoms such as abdominal pain, bloating, cramping, flatulence, belching and diarrhea.[61] Maldigestion of lactose is a common problem in children and adults, occurring in 76% of apparently healthy children in one study, and 56% in another single-blind, controlled trial.[62] Lactose maldigestion can result from genetic non-persistence of intestinal lactase activity at some time after weaning as well as from secondary lactase deficiencies. It may or may not produce symptoms of lactose intolerance.[61]

A lactase enzyme derived from *Aspergillus oryzae* is effective in the treatment of lactose maldigestion and lactose intolerance when taken orally at the time of milk ingestion.[62–67] Moreover, this enzyme aids in the in vivo digestion of milk sugar even in healthy individuals classified as normal lactose digesters. Furthermore, the *A. oryzae*-derived lactase is more effective in the digestion of lactose than a similar enzyme derived from the yeast, *Kluyveromyces lactis*.[62]

It is known that milk pre-hydrolyzed in vitro by incubating it under refrigeration with lactase is effective in the prevention of lactose intolerance in susceptible individuals. A 1986 single-blind, controlled study was designed to determine whether ingestion of lactase at mealtime was equally as effective in the treatment of lactose intolerance as pre-hydrolyzed milk, since the latter requires refrigeration which is difficult to obtain in "underdeveloped" parts of the world. The hydrogen breath test was used as an accurate and sensitive measurement of lactose digestion in vivo (see Ch. 23).

The study included 48 healthy Guatemalan pre-school children. The ability of participants to digest lactose from ingested whole cow's milk was tested against four treatment protocols as follows (each protocol included 240 ml of whole cow's milk containing 12 g. of lactose):

1. whole, intact cow's milk
2. milk pre-hydrolyzed in vitro with lactase enzyme
3. varying amounts of lactase from *K. lactis* administered orally with milk
4. varying amounts of lactase from *A. oryzae* administered orally with milk.

Twenty-seven of the children (56%) proved to be maldigesters of lactose from the ingestion of intact milk. Twenty-five of these lactose maldigesters (93%) were found to show no lactose maldigestion (i.e. successfully treated) after the ingestion of milk pre-hydrolyzed with lactase in vitro for 24 hours. Pre-hydrolyzed milk was used as the standard for successful treatment in comparing the effectiveness of lactase enzymes derived from *A. oryzae* and *K. lactis*.[62]

All experimental dosages of in vivo lactase from both *A. oryzae* and *K. lactis* significantly reduced the volume of post-challenge hydrogen excretion as compared with intact milk ($P < 0.05$). However, lactase from *A. oryzae* was found to be equally as effective as pre-hydrolyzed milk, while *K. lactis* lactase was only 82% as effective.

This research supports the addition of microbial beta-galactosidase (lactase) to milk at mealtimes as effective in the prevention of signs and symptoms of lactose maldigestion. Ingestion of lactase with milk at mealtime avoids the inconvenience of refrigerated 24 hour incubation as well as the sweeter flavor produced when milk is pre-hydrolyzed.

In a somewhat surprising result, *A. oryzae* lactase was also found to increase the degree of lactose digestion in the 21 children classified as normal, complete digesters. This demonstrates that the capacity for lactose digestion is actually a continuum, even in lactase-persistent subjects, rather than an all-or-none phenomenon.

The efficacy of these enzymes in lactose-intolerant children and adults has now been replicated in several studies.[61,68]

Vascular disease

Numerous cross-over, single-blind and placebo-controlled studies have confirmed the effectiveness of a proteolytic enzyme derived from *Aspergillus oryzae* in treating chronically obstructed arteries in humans.[28–32,35,36,69–73]

In fact, intravenous therapy with fungal protease from *A. oryzae* is dramatically more effective than anticoagulant therapy (e.g. heparin, warfarin) at recanalizing obstructed arteries and improving blood flow through stenosed arterial segments.[35,36,73]

A 1978 controlled, single-blind cross-over study evaluated the effectiveness of protease from *A. oryzae* versus anticoagulant therapy and placebo in 18 patients (ages 63–75) with stable intermittent claudication of at least 6 months' duration.[35] Patients were divided into two groups, and a full assessment of each patient was carried out prior to testing. Translumbar aortogram, Doppler ultrasound scanning and peripheral systolic blood pressure were used to assess the patency of eight different arterial segments in each patient (a total of 72 segments in each group). Anticoagulation therapy with warfarin was introduced following assessment and continued throughout an observation period of 3 months and subsequent trial periods. Assessment of peripheral circulation was repeated after the 3 month observation period on anticoagulant therapy. Thereafter, a series of six intravenous infusions of fungal protease and normal saline was given to experimental and control groups, respectively, at regular intervals over the next 2 weeks. Assessment of peripheral circulation was repeated at the end of the protease infusion treatment. No other form of therapy was given, except warfarin for anticoagulation. On admission to the study, the first group of patients receiving fungal protease therapy showed 27 obstructed segments (completely obstructed), 34 stenosed segments (partially obstructed) and only 11 patent arterial segments. The nine patients receiving

Table 66.2 Changes in patency of 72 arterial segments after placebo or fungal enzyme treatment

Arterial status	Placebo		Treated	
	Initial	Final	Initial	Final
No. patent	21	21	11	27
No. stenosed	26	23	34	35
No. obstructed	25	28	27	10

saline (placebo) showed 25 obstructed, 26 stenosed and 21 patent arterial segments prior to treatment (see Table 66.2).

At the end of the 3 month observation period (anticoagulation therapy only), no changes in Doppler ultrasound scanning or ankle/arm blood pressure ratios were found in either group.

At the end of the 2 week trial period, the saline group showed that three of the 72 arterial segments had progressed to increased obstruction (i.e. 4% worse). In contrast, treatment with the fungal protease infusion resulted improved patency of 33 of 72 arterial segments (i.e. a 46% improvement). These changes were significant at the 0.1% level ($P < 0.001$).

The saline group was offered the opportunity to receive a further course of treatment without disclosing a change in regimen from saline to fungal protease infusion. Five placebo patients declined further treatment, while four patients with 32 arterial segments subsequently received the cross-over fungal protease infusion protocol. After treatment, five completely obstructed segments became recanalized.

This research demonstrated that 3 months of anticoagulant therapy produced no improvement whatsoever in peripheral circulation;[35] and neither did subsequent infusions of saline (placebo) during a 2 week period. Six intravenous infusions of a fungal protease derived from *A. oryzae* given within 2 weeks significantly improved peripheral circulation in over half of the chronically obstructed arterial segments in these patients.

Furthermore, detailed analysis of study results suggested that an increase in the number and/or dosage of protease infusions might have resulted in even greater improvement in obstructed and stenosed arterial segments.

Other studies have shown fungal protease to be effective in the treatment of arterial obstruction in patients with more advanced conditions, such as gangrene and other severe ischemic disease.[36,70,72]

Celiac disease

It has been known since the 1950s that the gluten found in wheat, rye and other grains is the cause of intestinal damage in celiac disease, with the gliadin fraction of gluten being the source of its toxicity.[74,75] By the 1970s, fractionation studies had succeeded at identifying the components of gliadin involved in the toxic mechanism. The carbohydrate moiety, consisting mainly of glucose, galactose, xylose and arabinose, is the source of gluten's gastrointestinal toxicity in the celiac patient, rather than the protein fraction as had been previously suspected.[76–78]

Amylytic enzymes from *Aspergillus* species are effective in vitro in the treatment of celiac disease, as they enzymatically cleave the toxic carbohydrate portion of gliadin. Fungal carbohydrase preparations render grains like wheat and rye virtually harmless to individuals with gluten enteropathy.[76,77]

A 1977 study attempting to identify the source of gliadin toxicity used a preparation of amylytic enzymes from *Aspergillus niger* to remove the carbohydrate portion of gliadin in vitro.[76]

To be certain of the variables being tested, native gliadin was chromatographed showing that carbohydrate was associated with four main protein bands. When the carbohydrase-treated gliadin was chromatographed, no alteration was detected in the protein pattern, but carbohydrate was completely absent.

To further establish that the protein make-up remained unchanged as compared with native gliadin, peptide mapping of the treated gliadin was carried out using electrophoresis followed by chromatography. Peptide maps showed no difference between the treated and untreated gliadin, confirming that no alteration had occurred in the primary structure of the protein.

Gliadin treated in this manner was baked into loaves of bread made with gluten-free flour. The study compared the effect of bread with treated versus untreated gliadin on four patients with previously diagnosed celiac disease. All four patients had been on gluten-free diets for at least 3 months prior to the study and were virtually symptom-free. Previously, their clinical and physical signs and symptoms had included the diarrhea, malabsorption, decreased body weight and height, anemia, tetany, impaired D-xylose absorption, decreased intestinal mucosal enzyme secretion, flattened mucosal brush-border and subepithelial tissue lymphocytosis typical of celiac disease.

During the test period, patients 1, 2 and 3 received a total of 50 g of treated gliadin baked into loaves of bread (10 g gliadin/450 g loaf). Xylose absorption tests and intestinal biopsies from jejunal villi were performed before and after each test period.

The celiac patient receiving untreated gliadin (patient no. 4) experienced a return of signs and symptoms of celiac disease – diarrhea, abdominal pain, low values on xylose absorption studies, decreased mucosal enzyme secretion (alkaline phosphatase, lactase, sucrase) and characteristic histological damage (mucosal lymphocytosis and loss of enterocyte height). The patients who received the treated gliadin remained symptom-free during the test period and showed no abnormalities in histological parameters (i.e. general morphology, epithelial cell height, tissue lymphocytes were normal in these patients).

This study demonstrated that carbohydrate-digesting enzymes from *Aspergillus* sp. can be used in vitro to remove the toxicity of gluten to celiac patients and supports the hypothesis that carbohydrate components of gliadin are responsible for its toxicity, rather than protein components as had been widely suspected. It appears that no controlled studies have been done to evaluate the effectiveness of amylytic fungal enzymes at reducing gluten toxicity to celiac patients in vivo by administering these enzymes with gluten-containing foods at mealtime.

It should be noted that although celiac patients show intolerance to the carbohydrate portion of gliadin, this is likely not the only source of gluten-induced pathology. A number of studies suggest that protein components of gluten produce systemic allergic manifestations in some patients.[1,2,8,9,13,79,80] It appears that both gastrointestinal intolerance and immunological hypersensitivity are capable, either individually or in concert, of producing disease symptoms in susceptible individuals. Future studies may also show that both pathological mechanisms are amenable to treatment by hydrolysis of the offending portions of gluten with the appropriate orally administered fungal enzymes. This, however, remains to be proven.

Food allergies

Antigen sampling by subepithelial immune tissue in the gut helps under normal conditions to program the body's defenses and protect against exposure to "foreign" dietary proteins and polypeptides. Under pathological conditions, food allergies can be caused by several factors, including the increased supply of dietary antigens which leak into the bloodstream a a result of inadequate protein digestion.[1,2,4, 8–11,21]

By digesting dietary protein, fungal enzymes administered orally at mealtime work to decrease the supply of antigenic macromolecules available to leak into the bloodstream. In addition, orally administered fungal enzymes which have themselves been absorbed intact may help to "digest" antigenic dietary proteins which they encounter in the bloodstream. Further research is needed to evaluate the role of fungal enzymes in the treatment of food allergies.

SUMMARY

Although the intact absorption of orally administered protein, including enzymes, can no longer be reasonably denied, the quantitative significance of this process will require additional study. While it appears unlikely that this route of absorption is significant from the standpoint of overall nutritional status, considerable evidence exists supporting the biological and therapeutic importance of intact protein absorption and the role of fungal enzyme therapy.

The emerging field of fungal enzyme therapy holds promise as an effective therapy or adjunct in a wide range of conditions, including maldigestion, malabsorption, pancreatic insufficiency, steatorrhea, celiac disease, lactose intolerance, arterial obstruction, and thrombotic disease.

REFERENCES

1. Gardener MLG. Gastrointestinal absorption of intact proteins. Ann Rev Nutr 1988; 8: 329–350
2. Gardner MLG. Intestinal assimilation of intact peptides and proteins from the diet – a neglected field? Biol Rev 1984; 59: 289–331
3. Warshaw AL, Walker WA, Isselbacher KJ. Protein uptake by the intestine: evidence for absorption of intact macromolecules. Gastroenterology 1974; 66: 987–992
4. Udall JN, Walker WA. The physiologic and pathologic basis for the transport of macromolecules across the intestinal tract. J Pediatr Gastroenterol Nutr 1982; 1: 295–301
5. Leohry CA, Axon AT, Hilton PJ et al. Permeability of the small intestine to substances of different molecular weight. Gut 1970; 11: 466–470
6. Hemmings WA, Williams EW. Transport of large breakdown products of dietary protein through the gut wall. Gut 1986; 27: 715–23
7. Menzies IS. Transmucosal passage of inert molecules in health and disease. In: Skahauge E, Heintze K, eds. Intestinal absorption and secretion. Lancaster, PA: MTP Press. 1984: p 527–543
8. Gerguson A, Caldwell F. Precipitins to dietary proteins in serum and upper intestinal secretions of coeliac children. Br Med J 1972; 1: 75–77
9. Husby S, Foged N, Host A et al. Passage of dietary antigens into the blood of children with coeliac disease. Quantification and size distribution of absorbed antigens. Gut 1987; 28: 1062–1072
10. Husby S, Jensenius JC, Svehag SE. Passage of undegraded dietary antigen into the blood of healthy adults: further characterization of the kinetics of uptake and the size distribution of the antigen. Scand J Immunol 1986; 4: 447–455
11. Walker WA. Antigen absorption from the small intestine and gastrointestinal disease. Pediatr Clin North Am 1975; 22: 731–746
12. Hamilton I, Fiarris GM, Rothwell J et al. Small intestinal permeability in dermatological disease. Q J Med 1985; 56: 559–567
13. Lambert MT, Bjarnason I, Connelly J et al. Small intestine permeability in schizophrenia. Br J Psychiatry 1989; 155: 619–622
14. Heatley RV et al. Inflammatory bowel disease, In: Losowsky MS, Heatley RV, eds. Gut defenses in clinical practice. Edinburgh: Churchill Livingstone. 1986: p 255–277
15. Shorter, RG, Huizenga KA, Spencer RJ et al. A working hypothesis for the etiology and pathogenesis of nonspecific inflammatory bowel disease. Am J Dig Dis 1972; 17: 1024–1032
16. Jackson, PG, Lessof MH, Baker RW et al. Intestinal permeability in patients with eczema and food allergy. Lancet 1981; i: 1285–1286
17. Hemmings WA. The absorption of large breakdown products of dietary proteins into the body tissues including the brain. In: Hemmings G, Hemmings WA, eds. The biological basis of schizophrenia. Lancaster, PA: MTP Press. 1978: p 239–257

18. Jakobsson I, Lindberg T, Lothe L et al. Human beta-lactalbumin as marker of macromolecular absorption. Gut 1986; 27: 1029–1034
19. Bockman DE, Winborn WB. Light and electron microscopy of intestinal ferritin absorption: observations in sensitized and non-sensitized hamsters. Anat Res 1968; 155: 603–622
20. Andre C, Lambert R, Bazin H et al. Interference of oral immunization with the intestinal absorption of heterologous albumin. Eur J Immunol 1974; 4: 701–704
21. Dannaeus A, Inganas M, Johansson SG et al. Intestinal uptake of ovalbumin in malabsorption and food allergy in relation to serum lgG antibody and orally administered sodium chromoglycate. Clin Allergy 1979; 9: 263–270
22. Wolf JL, Rubin DH, Finberg R et al. Intestinal M Cells: a pathway for entry of retrovirus into the host. Science 1981; 212: 471–472
23. McLean E, Ash R. The time-course of appearance and net accumulation of horseradish peroxidase presented orally to juvenile carp, cyprinus carpio. Comp Biochem Physiol 1987; 88A: 507–510
24. Ormiston BJ. Clinical effects of TRH and TSH after i.v. and oral administration in normal volunteers and patients with thyroid disease. In: R Hal et al, eds. Thytropin releasing hormone (Frontiers of hormone research, vol. I). Basel: Karger. 1972: p 45–52
25. Amoss M, Rivier J and Guillemin R. Release of gonadotrophins by oral administration of synthetic LRF or tripeptide fragment of LRF. J Clin Endocrinol Metab 1972; 35: 175–177
26. Seifert J. Mucosal permeation of macromolecules and particles. Angiology 1966; 17: 505–513
27. Laskowski M. Effect of trypsin inhibitor on passage of insulin across the intestinal barrier. Science 1958; 127: 1115–1116
28. Bergkvist R, Svard PO. Studies on the thomobolytic effect of a protease from Aspergillus oryzae. Acta Physiol Scand 1964; 60. 363–371
29. Verstraefe M, Verhaege R. Clinical study of brinase, a proteolytic enzyme from *Aspergillus oryzae*. 19th Annual Congr Intern Coll Angiology. Dublin, Ireland. 1977
30. Kiessling H, Svensson R. Influence of an enzyme from *Aspergillus oryzae*, Protease I, on some components of the fibrinolytic system. Acta Chem Scand 1970; 24: 569–574
31. Larsson LJ, Frisch EP, Torenke K et al. Properties of the complex between alpha-2-macro-gobulin and brinase, a proteinase from Aspergillus oryzae with thrombolytic effect. Thrombosis Res 1988; 49: 55–68
32. Vanhove P, Donati MB, Claeys H et al. Action of brinase on human fibrinogen and plasminogen. Thrombos Haemostas 1979; 42: 571–581
33. Kiessling H. Some properties of a complex between alpha-2-macroglobulin and brinase. Protides of Biological Fluids 1975; 23: 47–52
34. Bergkvist R. The proteolytic enzymes of *Aspergillus oryzae* II: properties of the proteolytic enzymes. Acta Chem Scand 1963; 17: 1541–1551
35. Fitzgerald DE, Frisch EP, Milliken JC. Relief of chronic arterial obstruction using intravenous brinase. Scand J Thor Cardiovasc Surg 1979; 13: 327–332
36. Verhaege R, Verstraete M, Schetz J. Clinical trial of brinase and anticoagulants as a method of treatment for advanced limb ischemia. Eur J Clin Pharmacol 1979; 16: 165–170
37. Keljo DJ, Hamilton JR. Quantitative determination of macromolecular transport rate across intestinal Peyer's patches. Am J Physiol 244: G637–644
38. Wolf JL, Bye WA. The membranous epithelial (M) cell and the mucosal immune system. Ann Rev Med 1984; 35: 95–112
39. Bjarnson I, Peters TJ. Helping the mucosa make sense of macromolecules. Gut 1987; 28: 1057–1061
40. Ambrus, JL, Lassman HB, DeMarchi JJ. Absorption of exogenous and endogenous proteolytic enzymes. Clin Pharmacol Therap 1967; 8: 362–368
41. Kabacoff, BB et al. Absorption of chymotrypsin from the intestinal tract. Nature 1963; 199: 815–817
42. Martin GJ et al. Further *in vivo* observations with radioactive trypsin. Am J Pharm 1964; 129: 386–392
43. Avakian S. Further studies on the absorption of chymotrypsin. Clin Pharmacol Therap 1964; 5: 712–715
44. Miller JM. An investigation of trypsin I in patients. Exper Med Surg 1960; 18: 352–370
45. Liebow, C, Rothman SS. Enteropancreatic circulation of digestive enzymes. Science 1975; 189: 472–474
46. Guyton AC, ed. Textbook of medical physiology. 4th edn. Philadelphia, PA: WB Saunders. 1971: p 761
47. Borel P, Armand M, Senft M et al. Gastric lipase: evidence of an adaptive response to dietary fat in the rabbit. Gastroenterology 1991; 100: 1582–1589
48. DiMagno EP, Go VL, Summerskill WH. Relations between pancreatic enzyme outputs and malabsorption in severe pancreatic insufficiency. New Engl J Med 1973; 228: 813–815
49. Heizer WD, Cleaveland FL. Gastric inactivation of pancreatic supplements. Bull Johns Hopkins Hosp 1965; 116: 210–216
50. Go VL, Poley JR, Hofman AF, Summerskill WH. Disturbances in fat digestion induced by acidic jejunal pH due to gastric hypersecretion in man. Gastroenterology 1970; 58: 638–645
51. Griffin SM, Alderson D, Farndon JR. Acid resistant lipase as replacement therapy in chronic exocrine insufficiency: a study in dogs. Gut 1989; 30: 1012–1015
52. DiMagno EP. Controversies in the treatment of pancreatic exocrine insufficiency. Dig Dis Sci 1982; 27: 481–484
53. Stapleton FB. Hyperuricosuria due to high dose pancreatic extract therapy in cystic fibrosis. New Engl J Med 1976; 295: 246–251
54. Gow R, Bradbear R, Francis P et al. Comparative study of varying regimens to improve steatorrhea and creatorrhea in cystic fibrosis: effectiveness of an enteric-coated preparation with and without antacids and cimetidine. Lancet 1981; ii: 1071–1074
55. Graham DY. Pancreatic enzyme replacement. the effect of antacids or cimetidine. Dig Dis Sci 1982; 27: 485–490
56. Staub JL, Sarles H, Soule JC et al. No effect of cimetidine on the therapeutic response to oral enzymes in severe pancreatic insufficiency. New Engl J Med 1981; 304: 1364–1365
57. Regan PT, Malagelada JR, Di Magno EP et al. Comparative effects of antacids, cimetidine and enteric coating on the therapeutic response to oral enzymes in severe pancreatic insufficiency. New Engl J Med 1977; 297. 854–858
58. Zentler-Munro PL, Fitzpatrick WJ, Batten JC et al. Effect of intra-jejunal acidity and aqueous bile acid and lipid concentrations in pancreatic steatorrhea due to cystic fibrosis. Gut 1984; 25: 500–507
59. Schneider, MU, Knoll-Ruzicka ML, Domschke S et al. Pancreatic enzyme replacement therapy: comparative effects of conventional and enteric-coated microspheric pancreatin and acid-stable fungal enzyme preparations on steatorrhea in chronic pancreatitis. Hepatogastroenterol 1985; 32: 97–102
60. Ladas SD, Giorgiotis K, Raptis SA. Complex carbohydrate malabsorption in exocrine pancreatic insufficiency. Gut 1993; 34: 984–987
61. Medow MS, Thek KD, Newman LJ et al. β-Galactosidase tablets in the treatment of lactose intolerance in pediatrics., Arch Am J Dis Child 1990; 144: 1261–1264
62. Barillas C, Solomons NW. Effective reduction of lactose maldigestion in preschool children by direct addition of beta-galactosidases to milk at mealtime. Pediatrics 1987; 79: 766–772
63. Rosado JL, Solomons NW, Lisker et al. Enzyme replacement therapy for primary adult lactase deficiency: effective reduction of lactose malabsorption and milk intolerance by direct addition of beta-galactosidases to milk at mealtime. Gastroenterology 1984; 87: 1072–1082
64. Rosado JL, Deodhar AD, Bourges H et al. The effect of digestion products of lactose (glucose and galactose) on its intraintestinal in vivo hydrolysis by exogenous microbial beta-D-galactosidase. J Am Coll Nutr 1986; 5: 218–290
65. Corazza GR, Benati G, Sorge M et al. beta-Galactosidase from *Aspergillus niger* in adult lactose malabsorption: a double-blind crossover study. Aliment Pharmacol Ther 1992; 6:61–66
66. O'Keefe S. The use of lactase enzyme in feeding malnourished lactose intolerant patients. XIII International Congress of Nutrition, Brighton, England. 1985: p 190
67. Rand AG, Jr. Enzyme technology and the development of lactose-hydrolyzed milk. In: Parge DM, Bayless TM, eds. Lactose digestion: clinical and nutritional implications. Baltimore, MD: Johns Hopkins University Press. 1981: p 219–230

68. Editorial. Lactose intolerance. Lancet 1991; ii: 663–664
69. Fitzgerald DE, Fisch EP. Relief of chronic peripheral artery obstruction by intravenous brinase. Irish Med Ass 1973; 66: 3
70. Lund F, Ekestrom S, Frisch EP et al. Thrombolytic treatment with iv. brinase in advanced arterial obliterate disease. Angiology 1975; 26: 534
71. Frisch EP, Blomback M, Ekestrom S. Dosage of i.v. brinase in man based on brinase inhibitor capacity and coagulation studies. Angiology 1975; 26: 557
72. Roschlau HE, Fisher AM. Thrombolytic therapy with local perfusions of CA-7 (fibrinolytic enzyme from *Aspergillus oryzae*) in the dog. Angiology 1966; 17: 670–682
73. Frisch EP, Blomback M. Blood coagulation studies in patients treated with brinase. In: Davidson JF, ed. Progess in chemical fibrinolysis and thrombolysis. vol. IV. Edinburgh, Churchill Livingstone. 1979: p 184–187
74. Dicke WK. An investigation into the injurious constituents of wheat in connection with their action on patients with Coeliac disease. Acta Pediatr 1953; 42: 223–231
75. Van De Kamer JH, Weijers HA. Coeliac disease: some experiments on the cause of the harmful effect of the gliadin. Acta Pediatr 1955; 44: 465–469
76. Phelan JJ, Stevens FM, McNicholl B et al. Coelic disease: the abolition of gliadin toxicity by enzymes from Aspergillus niger. Clin Sci Molec Med 1977; 53: 35–43
77. McCarthy CF. Nutritional defects in patients with malabsorption. Proc Nutr Soc 1976; 35: 37–40
78. Pehlan JJ. The nature of gliadin toxicity in coeliac disease. Biochem Soc Trans 1974; 2: 1368–1370
79. Hekkens WTJM. Antibodies to gliadin in serum of normals, coeliac patients and schizophrenics. Nature 1963; 199: 259–261
80. Hekkens, WTJM et al. Antibodies to wheat proteins in schizophrenia. Relationship or coincidence. In: Hemmings G, ed. The biochemistry of schizophrenia and addiction. Lancaster, PA: MTP Press. 1980: p 125–33

CHAPTER CONTENTS

67

Beta-carotene and other carotenoids

Michael T. Murray, ND

Joseph E. Pizzorno Jr, ND

INTRODUCTION

The carotenoids represent the most widespread group of naturally occurring pigments in nature. They are a highly colored (red and yellow) group of fat-soluble compounds, composed of hydrocarbons (carotenes) and their oxygenated derivatives (oxycarotenoids or xanthophylls). The basic carotenoid structure consists of eight isoprenoid units with a series of conjugated double bonds. All photosynthetic organisms, whether bacteria or plants, contain carotenoid pigments. These compounds not only function as auxiliary pigments in photosynthesis, but also play a crucial role in protecting the organism or plant against photosensitization by its own chlorophyll.

Over 600 carotenoids have been characterized, but only about 30–50 are believed to have vitamin A activity. Biological activity of a carotenoid has historically been considered synonymous with its corresponding vitamin A activity. However, recent research suggests that this function of carotenoids has been overemphasized, as carotenoids have been found to exhibit many other very important physiological activities. For a carotenoid to have vitamin A activity, it must have an unaltered beta-ionone ring with an attached polyene side chain containing 11 carbon atoms. Beta-carotene has been termed the most active of the carotenoids, due to its higher provitamin A activity (see Fig. 67.1).

Apocarotenoids are compounds that have been shortened by the removal of at least one end of the molecule beyond a designated location (e.g. beta-Apo-8′-carotenal has been cleaved at the 8′ carbon). Apocarotenes and xanthophylls have reduced or no vitamin A activity.[1,2]

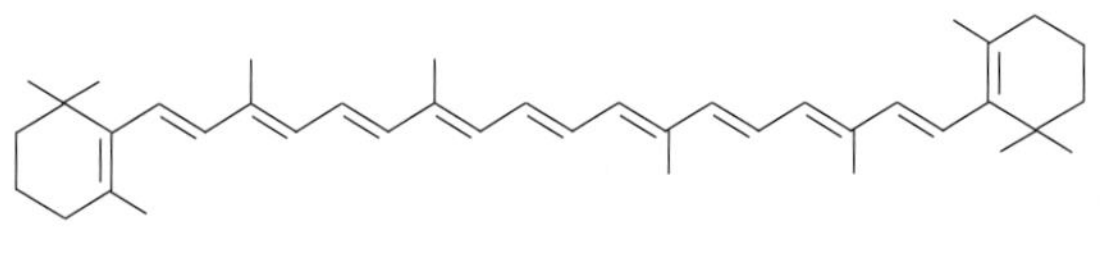

Figure 67.1 Beta-carotene.

DIETARY SOURCES

The carotenoids present in green plants are found in the chloroplasts with chlorophyll, usually in complexes with a protein or lipid. Beta-carotene is the predominant form in most green leaves and, in general, the greater the intensity of the green color, the greater the concentration of beta-carotene. Orange-colored fruits and vegetables, e.g. carrots, apricots, mangoes, yams, squash, etc., typically have higher concentrations of provitamin A carotenoids, the provitamin A content again paralleling the intensity of the color. Yellow vegetables have higher concentrations of xanthophylls, and hence a lowered provitamin A activity. In the orange and yellow fruits and vegetables, beta-carotene concentrations are high, but other provitamin A carotenoids typically predominate. The red and purple vegetables and fruits, such as tomatoes, red cabbage, berries, and plums, contain a large portion of non-vitamin A-active pigments, including flavonoids. Legumes, grains, and seeds are also significant sources of carotenoids. Carotenoids are also found in various animal foods, such as salmon and other fish, egg yolks, shellfish, milk, and poultry. Carotenoids are frequently added to foods as colorants. Table 67.1 lists carotenoids with provitamin A activity found in common food sources, while Table 67.2 lists some important carotenoids that have no vitamin A activity.[1,2] The structures of two of these, lycopene and zeaxanthin, are illustrated in Figures 67.2 and 67.3.

Table 67.2 Non-provitamin A carotenoids and food sources

Carotenoid	Food source
Lycopene	Tomatoes, carrots, green peppers, apricots, pink grapefruit
Zeaxanthin	Spinach, paprika, corn, fruits
Lutein	Green plants, corn, potatoes, spinach, carrots, tomatoes, fruits
Canthaxanthin	Mushrooms, trout, crustaceans
Crocetin	Saffron
Capsanthin	Red peppers, paprika

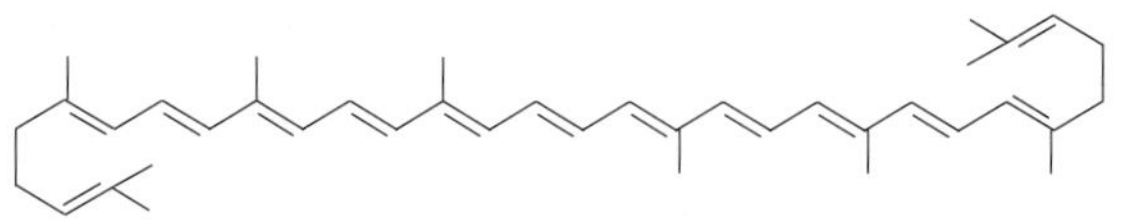

Figure 67.2 Lycopene.

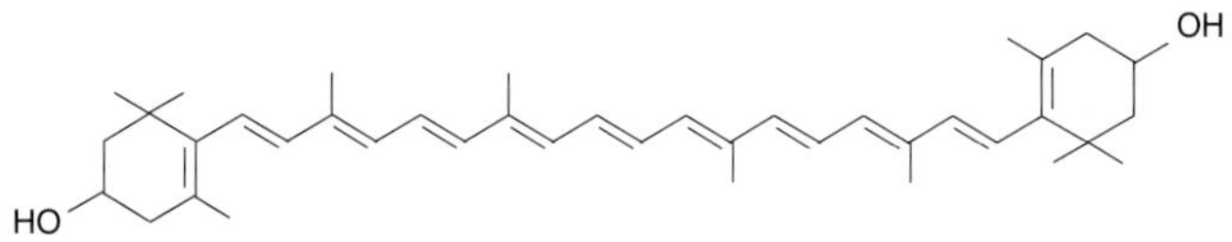

Figure 67.3 Zeaxanthin.

METABOLISM

Absorption

A variety of factors are known to influence the absorption efficacy of vitamin A and carotenoids. Although retinol does not require bile acids to facilitate absorption, carotenoids do. Other factors that affect vitamin A and carotenoid absorption include:

- the presence of fat, protein, and antioxidants in the food
- the presence of bile and a normal complement of pancreatic enzymes in the intestinal lumen
- and the integrity of the mucosal cells.

The absorption efficiency of dietary vitamin A is usually quite high (80–90%), with only a slight reduction in efficiency at high doses. In contrast, beta-carotene's absorption efficiency is much lower (40–60%), and it decreases rapidly with increasing dosage.[1,3] Carotene supplements are better absorbed than the carotenes from foods.[4]

Transformation in the intestinal mucosa

As stated above, of the more than 600 carotenoids that have been reasonably well characterized, only about 30–50 are believed to have provitamin A activity. Yet carotenoids provide the majority of dietary vitamin A. Provitamin A carotene conversion to vitamin A is dependent on diverse factors:[5]

- protein status
- thyroid hormones
- zinc
- vitamin C.

Table 67.1 Provitamin A carotenoids and food sources

Carotenoid	Activity (%)	Food sources
Beta-carotene	100%	Green plants, carrots, sweet potatoes, squash, spinach, apricots, green peppers
Alpha-carotene	50–54	Green plants, carrots, squash, corn, watermelons, green peppers, potatoes, apples, peaches
Gamma-carotene	42–50	Carrots, sweet potatoes, corn, tomatoes, watermelons, apricots
Beta-zeacarotene	20–40	Corn, tomatoes, yeast, cherries
Cryptoxanthin	50–60	Corn, green peppers, persimmons, papayas, lemons, oranges, prunes, apples, apricots, paprika, poultry
Beta-apo-8′-carotenal	72	Citrus fruit, green plants
Beta-apo-12′-carotenal	120	Alfalfa meal

The conversion diminishes as carotene intake increases and when serum retinol levels are adequate.[6] Beta-carotene and other provitamin A carotenes were originally believed to be cleaved by carotene dioxygenase at the 15,15′ double bond, which would yield two molecules of all-*trans* retinal. It is currently believed, however, that the dioxygenase enzyme non-specifically attacks any one of the double bonds of the beta-carotene, resulting in the formation of a corresponding apo-beta-carotenal or retinal.[7] The apocarotenal formed can either be degraded to retinal or absorbed. The retinal formed is then converted to retinol by retinaldehyde reductase.

Uncleaved provitamin A carotenoids, apocarotenoids, and non-provitamin A carotenoids, like retinol, are transported in the chylomicra.

Transport, storage, and excretion

No specific carrier protein exists in the plasma for carotenoids. These compounds are typically transported in human plasma in association with the plasma lipoproteins, particularly by LDL. As a consequence, patients with high serum cholesterol or LDL levels tend to have high serum carotene levels. The concentrations found in the plasma usually reflect the dietary concentration, with beta-carotene typically comprising only 20–25% of the total serum carotene level.[8]

Carotenes may be stored in adipose tissue, the liver, other organs (the adrenals, testes, and ovaries have the highest concentrations), and the skin (see Table 67.3). Deposition in the skin results in carotenodermia. This is a benign (and probably beneficial) state. Carotenodermia not directly attributable to dietary intake or supplementation, however, may be indicative of a deficiency in a necessary conversion factor, i.e. zinc, thyroid hormone, vitamin C, or protein.[1,2]

PHYSIOLOGICAL ROLES

Reproduction

Beta-carotene has also been reported to have a specific effect in fertility distinct from its role as a precursor to vitamin A.[9–11] In bovine nutritional studies, cows fed beta-carotene-deficient diets exhibited delayed ovulation and an increase in the number of follicular and luteal cysts.[9,10] The corpus luteum has the highest concentration of beta-carotene of any organ measured.[11] The carotene cleavage activity changes with the ovulation cycle, with the highest activity occurring during the midovulation stage. It has been speculated that a proper ratio of carotene to retinol must be maintained to ensure proper corpus luteum function.

Table 67.3 Distribution of carotenoids in some human tissues (mcg/kg)

Tissue	Carotenoids	Beta-carotene
Adrenal	20.1 ± 11.9	10.8 ± 5.5
Liver	8.3 ± 21.3	
Testis	5.0 ± 7.7	4.7 ± 2.0
Fat	3.9 ± 6.0	1.3 ± 1.1
Pancreas	2.3 ± 1.2	1.1 ± 1.0
Spleen	1.6 ± 2.2	1.2 ± 0.5
Lung	0.6 ± 1.0	
Thyroid	0.6 ± 0.4	

As the corpus luteum produces progesterone, inadequate corpus luteum function could have significant deleterious effects. Inadequate corpus luteum secretory function is one of the characteristic features of infertile and/or irregular menstrual cycles.[12] Furthermore, an increased estrogen to progesterone ratio has been implicated in a variety of clinical conditions, including ovarian cysts, premenstrual tension syndrome, fibrocystic breast disease, and breast cancer.[13] Since supplemental beta-carotene given to cows significantly reduced the incidence of ovarian cysts (42% in control group vs. 3% in the beta-carotene group), it may have a similar effect in humans.[10,11] Another bovine condition that benefited from increased dietary beta-carotene levels is cystic mastitis.[12] It appears that farmers have a greater appreciation of beta-carotene than do many nutritionists. Of course, there are significant financial reasons as the annual monetary loss from bovine mastitis in the US has been estimated to be at least $1.5–2.0 billion and ovarian cysts represent the major cause of infertility in cattle.

Immune system

Some of these effects are probably related to vitamin A's ability to prevent stress-induced thymic involution as well as promote thymus growth. As carotenes are better antioxidants, they may turn out to be even better at protecting the thymus gland than vitamin A, since the thymus gland is particularly susceptible to free radical and oxidative damage. The clinical use of vitamin A and beta-carotene in infectious diseases is discussed below.

Beta-carotene's primary effects appear to enhance thymus gland function (discussed below) and increase interferon's stimulatory action on the immune system.[14] Interferon is a powerful immune-enhancing compound that plays a central role in protection against viral infections.

Antioxidant activity

In general, carotenes exert significant antioxidant activity, while the antioxidant activity of vitamin A is relatively minor in comparison.[15] The antioxidant activity of carotenes are thought to be the factor responsible for their anti-cancer effects noted in population studies (discussed below). Since aging is associated with free radical damage, a hypothesis developed that carotenes may also protect against aging as well. There is evidence that seems to support this hypothesis. It appears that tissue carotenoid content is the most significant factor in determining maximal life span potential (MLSP) of mammalian species ($r = 0.835$ for 12 mammalian species, and for primates alone, $r = 0.939$!).[16] For example, human MLSP of approximately 90 years correlates with a serum carotene level of 50–300 mcg/dl, while other primates, such as the rhesus monkey, have a MLSP of approximately 34 years, correlating with a serum carotene level of 6–12 mcg/dl.

While beta-carotene has received most of the attention, many carotenes which have either low or no vitamin A activity exert much greater protection compared with beta-carotene. For example, while beta-carotene generates vitamin A much more efficiently than alpha-carotene, alpha-carotene is approximately 38% stronger as an antioxidant and 10 times more effective in suppressing liver, skin, and lung cancer in animals compared with beta-carotene.[17] Even more powerful is lycopene.[18] Studies have shown lycopene to exhibit the highest overall singlet oxygen quenching of the carotenoids thus far studied. Its activity is roughly double that of beta-carotene. Furthermore, lycopene may exert even more impressive anti-cancer effects.

To evaluate the role of lycopene as a protective factor in digestive tract cancers, a case–control study was conducted in northern Italy, where tomato intake is high, but also heterogenous, in that some people eat a lot of tomatoes while others eat very few if any. Tomatoes are a perfect food to study as they are quite high in lycopene, but very low in carotene.

The data were obtained from a series of hospital-based studies on various cancers of the digestive tract between 1985 and 1991.[19] Frequency of consumption of raw tomatoes was divided into four levels: less than two; three to four; four; five to six; and greater than seven servings per week. Results showed a consistent pattern of protection by high intake of raw tomatoes in all examined cancer sites of the digestive tract. The degree of protection was similar to, but somewhat more marked than, those afforded by green vegetables and fruit studies carried on in the same areas. The results support the findings of other researchers who found, for example, a 40% reduction in the risk of esophageal cancer by simply consuming one serving of raw tomatoes per week and a 50% reduced rate for cancers of all sites among elderly Americans reporting a high tomato intake. These results suggest that increasing dietary lycopene levels may be a significant protector against cancer.

According to a detailed analysis of the levels of carotenoids in 120 fruits and vegetables, lycopene is found in very few.[20] Table 67.4 provides a list of the foods which contained lycopene.

Table 67.4 Lycopene content of common foods

Food	Lycopene (mg/100 g)
Apricot, canned	0.06
Apricot, dried	0.8
Grapefruit (pink and raw)	3.4
Guava juice	3.3
Tomato, raw	3.1
Tomato juice, canned	8.6
Tomato paste, canned	6.5
Tomato sauce, canned	6.3
Watermelon, raw	4.1

These values indicate that lycopene levels are retained in food processing.

CLINICAL APPLICATIONS

There are three primary sources of carotenes on the market:

- synthetic all-*trans* beta-carotene
- beta- and alpha-carotene from the algae *Dunaliella*
- mixed carotenes from palm oil.

Of these three, palm oil carotenes seem to be the best form (see Table 67.5).

Palm oil carotenes appear to give much better antioxidant protection. The carotene complex of palm oil closely mirrors the pattern in high carotene foods. In particular, unlike the synthetic version which only provides the *trans* configuration of beta-carotene, natural carotene sources provide beta-carotene in both a *trans* and *cis* configuration:

- 60% beta-carotene (both *trans* and *cis* isomers)
- 34% alpha-carotene
- 3% gamma-carotene
- 3% lycopene.

Palm oil carotenes have been shown to be about 4–10 times better absorbed than synthetic all-*trans* beta-carotene.[21–23] Carotenes from *Dunaliella* have also been shown to be well absorbed.[24]

The widespread health concerns concerning the use of "tropical oils" like palm and coconut do not apply to carotene products extracted from palm oil as the fat content is minimal. In addition, the real problem with palm oil occurs when it is processed, i.e. partially hydrogenated.

Prevention of cancer

Epidemiological studies have clearly demonstrated a strong inverse correlation between dietary carotene intake and a variety of cancers involving epithelial tissues (lung, skin, uterine cervix, gastrointestinal tract, etc).[25,26] The epidemiological association is much stronger for

Table 67.5 Antioxidant potential of different carotene products (per 25,000 IU of vitamin A activity)

Source	Carotenoid	Quenching rate	% in source	mg/25,000 IU	Antioxidant potential
Palm oil	Alpha-carotene	1.9	33	7.36	2.60
	Beta-carotene	1.4	63	14.04	3.66
	Gamma-carotene	2.5	2.5	0.56	0.26
	Lycopene	3.1	0.1	0.02	0.01
	Total				6.54
Algal	Alpha-carotene	1.9	4.0	0.61	0.22
	Beta-carotene	1.4	96.0	14.69	3.83
	Total				4.05
Synthetic	Beta-carotene	1.4	100	14.97	3.90
	Total				3.90

carotene than for vitamin A. This may reflect carotene's superior antioxidant, immune potentiating activity, and anticarcinogenic activity.[27]

While there is no argument that a diet high in carotenes is protective against cancer, the big question is: "Can beta-carotene supplementation reduce the risk of cancer?" The answer appears to be that synthetic beta-carotene supplementation does not. Three highly publicized reports on cancer prevention trials featuring synthetic all-*trans* beta-carotene in high-risk groups have produced negative results. It is important to take a close look at each of these studies to help put things into perspective.

The Alpha-tocopherol, Beta-carotene Cancer Prevention Study Group

This study's population was 29,000 men in Finland who smoked and drank alcohol.[28] The men were given beta-carotene (20 mg daily) and/or vitamin E. The results of this study indicated an 18% increase in lung cancer in the beta-carotene group. This result was not totally unexpected as studies in primates demonstrated that when animals were fed alcohol and beta-carotene, they experienced an increase in liver damage as a result of oxidative damage.[29] Other researchers have pointed out that beta-carotene is very susceptible to oxidative damage.[30] The protection against oxidative damage of beta-carotene is the presence of other antioxidant nutrients.[31] Absence of these protective nutrients could result in the formation of cancer-causing compounds, stressing the importance of relying on foods and broader-spectrum nutritional antioxidant support. Adding support to this statement is the fact that the group that received both beta-carotene and vitamin E did not show an increase in cancer, and in the group not receiving beta-carotene supplements there was a strong protective effect of high dietary beta-carotene and blood carotene levels against lung cancer. All together, this data strongly suggests that the protection offered by beta-carotene is only apparent when other important antioxidant nutrients are provided and may not be provided by the synthetic forms.

The CARET study

The second trial reporting on the role of beta-carotene in a high-risk group is the Carotene and Retinol Efficacy Trial (CARET).[32] This study was composed of over 18,000 US men and women smokers and asbestos workers. This study was halted 21 months prematurely on 13 January 1996 after 4 years of intervention indicated that beta-carotene supplementation (30 mg daily) increased lung cancer by 28% and overall deaths by 17%. While this appears dramatic, a closer look at the numbers and percentages puts them in their proper perspective. Among active smokers, the risk of lung cancer during the CARET study was 5 out of every 1,000. The 28% increase found with beta-carotene supplementation increased this number to roughly 6 out of 1,000.[32]

Interestingly, once again, in the group not taking beta-carotene, the lowest rate of cancer was found among individuals with the highest blood beta-carotene levels; and in former smokers, beta-carotene supplementation actually reduced cancer risk by 20%.

The Physician's Health Study

The Physician's Health Study is composed of 22,071 US male physicians taking either 50 mg of beta-carotene or a placebo every other day for 12 years. Results demonstrated no significant effect – positive or negative – on cancer or cardiovascular disease, even in the group (11%) who smoked.[33]

General comments on the "negative" studies

The results of these three studies indicate that synthetic beta-carotene supplementation may have adverse effects in high-risk groups for cancer and cardiovascular disease. These studies do not invalidate the hundreds of studies showing the preventive effect of a diet rich in carotenes and nutritional antioxidants against cancer and cardiovascular disease. These results seem to indicate the need for a diet high in carotenes and, if carotene supplementation is desired, people should not smoke, natural forms should be used, and the beta-carotene needs to be protected against the formation of toxic derivatives by taking extra vitamin C and E, and selenium.

Other prospective studies

In addition to these three highly publicized studies, there have been several prospective and double-blind studies showing promising results. In particular, beta-carotene supplementation has been shown to be especially effective in the treatment of early cancerous lesions of the oral cavity and esophagus.[34,35] Although beta-carotene has been shown to exert these benefits on its own (in dosages ranging from 15 to 180 mg/day), one of the most positive studies showing a reduction in cancer risk with supplemental beta-carotene to date is one that featured a broader supplement program. The Linxian Cancer Chemoprevention Study is a prospective study of 30,000 rural Chinese adults. In one of the substudies, subjects received one of four supplement programs:

- retinol and zinc
- riboflavin and niacin
- vitamin C and molybdenum
- beta-carotene, vitamin E, and selenium (dosages 1–3 times greater than the US RDA).

The latter group demonstrated 13% fewer cancer deaths and a reduction of 9% in overall deaths.[36,37] These results again support the notion that a combination of antioxidants is superior to high levels of any single antioxidant.

Prevention of cardiovascular disease

As in cancer, a high dietary carotene intake is also associated with lowering the risk of cardiovascular disease.[38] Like other antioxidants, beta-carotene may inhibit damage to cholesterol and the lining of the arteries.[39] However, it appears that beta-carotene is less effective in protecting against cardiovascular disease than vitamin E, probably because vitamin E protects against oxidative damage to cholesterol better than beta-carotene.[40]

Immune enhancement

Carotenes have demonstrated a number of immune-enhancing effects in recent studies.[14] However, the immune-enhancing effects were demonstrated as far back as 1931 when it was found that a diet rich in carotenes, as determined by blood carotene levels, was inversely related to the number of school days missed by children.[41] Originally it was thought that the immune-enhancing properties of carotenes were due to their conversion to vitamin A. We now know that carotenes exert many immune system-enhancing effects independent of any vitamin A activity.[14]

One of the most impressive studies was conducted on normal human volunteers.[42] Results demonstrated that oral beta-carotene (180 mg/day, approximately 300,000 IU) significantly increased the frequency of OKT4+ (helper/inducer T-cells) by approximately 30% after 7 days, and of OKT3+ (all T-cells) after 14 days.[32] As T4+ lymphocytes play a critical role in determining host immune status, this study indicates that oral beta-carotene may be effective in increasing the immunological competence of the host in conditions that are characterized by a selective diminution of the T4 subset of T-cells, such as the acquired immunodeficiency syndrome (AIDS) and cancer.

However, rather than supplementing the diet with synthetic beta-carotene, it may be more advantageous to use natural carotene sources or to increase the intake of carotene-rich foods. In another study, 126 healthy college students were randomly assigned to one of the following groups:

- group A, the control group
- group B, a group that used a 15 mg (25,000 IU) beta-carotene supplement daily
- group C, a group that consumed approximately 15 mg beta-carotene per day from carrots.

Better results, i.e. increase in white blood cell number and function, were achieved in the group eating the carrots.[43]

As the absorption studies have shown supplemental beta-carotene to be much better absorbed than the carotenes from carrots and other vegetables, the differences are likely the result of form, i.e. natural is better than synthetic.[4]

Vaginal candidiasis

It is a well-established fact that women are more susceptible to vaginal candidiasis when the immune system is depressed, a depression which may be due to low carotene levels. Beta-carotene levels were determined in exfoliated vaginal cells in 22 women with vaginal candidiasis and compared to vaginal cells from 20 controls. The beta-carotene level/1 million cells in the women with vaginal candidiasis was 1.46 ng compared with 8.99 ng in the control group, i.e. one-sixth that of normal.[44]

These results, coupled with beta-carotene's known effects on enhancing the immune system, suggest that a low tissue level of beta-carotene is associated with vaginal candidiasis, and a high dietary or supplemental intake of beta-carotene may be protective against vaginal candidiasis.

Photosensitivity disorders

Beta-carotene has become the treatment of choice for photosensitivity disorders. It is most effective in the treatment of erythropoietic protoporphyria (EPP), while its effectiveness in other photosensitivity disorders, such as polymorphous light eruption, solar urticaria, and discoid lupus erythematosus is significant, but not as great.[45–53] Beta-carotene also has a small but significant effect in increasing the exposure at which manifestations of sunburn begin, thus allowing some subjects the opportunity to stay in the sun long enough to get a "tan" for the first time.[53]

Patients with EPP are characterized by elevated levels of porphyrins in blood, feces, and skin and by sensitivity to visible light. This sensitivity manifests itself after exposure to sunlight by a burning sensation followed by swelling and redness. Topical sunscreens are of no value. The photosensitivity is due to excitation of the porphyrin molecule by ultraviolet radiation, resulting in the production of free radicals that are very deleterious to the skin. Direct cell damage results in the release of chemical mediators which in turn damage other cells, resulting in the manifestations of itching, burning, redness, and swelling.

In EPP, it appears that carotene levels must be maintained in the blood at 600–800 mcg/dl for optimum effects and that the protective effect is not usually observed until after 4–6 weeks of therapy. The actions of beta-carotene and other carotenes in human tissue are similar to their action in plant cells, i.e. they function as a cellular screen against sunlight-induced free radical damage.

DOSAGES

For carotenes, a daily dosage of 25,000 IU (15 mg of beta-carotene) appears to be reasonable for general health. For the treatment of pre-cancerous lesions and immune enhancement, the dosage range is 25,000–300,000 IU. In the treatment of EPP, the dosage is based on maintaining blood carotene levels between 600 and 800 mcg/dl. For the best clinical impact, it appears the natural mixed forms of carotene should be used in conjunction with a broad range of other natural antioxidants (see Ch. 99).

TOXICITY

Supplementing the diet with beta-carotene has not been shown to possess any significant toxicity despite its use in very high doses in the treatment of numerous photosensitive disorders (see above). Occasionally patients will complain of loose stools, which usually clears spontaneously and does not necessitate stopping treatment. Elevated carotene levels in the blood do not lead to vitamin A toxicity, nor do they lead to any other significant disturbance besides a yellowing of the skin (carotenodermia). The ingestion of large amounts of carrots or carrot juice (0.45–1.0 kg/day of fresh carrots for several years) has, however, been shown to cause neutropenia as well as menstrual disorders.[54,55] Although the blood carotene levels of these patients did reach levels (221–1,007 mcg/dl) similar to those of patients taking high doses of beta-carotene (typically 800 mcg/dl), the disturbances are due to some other factor in carrots, as neither of these effects nor any others have been observed in subjects consuming very high doses of pure beta-carotene, e.g. 300,000–600,000 IU/day (180–360 mg beta-carotene, which is equivalent to 4–8 pounds of raw carrots) over long periods of time.[56–60] Doses up to 1,000 mg/kg have been given to rats and rabbits for long periods of time with no signs of embryotoxicity, toxicity, tumorigenicity, or interference in reproductive functions.[61]

REFERENCES

1. Underwood B. Vitamin A in animal and human nutrition. In: Sporn M, Roberts A, Goodman S, eds. The retinoids. Vol 1. Orlando, FL: Academic Press. 1984: p 282–392
2. Simpson KL, Chichester CO. Metabolism and significance of carotenoids. Ann Rev Nutr 1981; 1: 351–374
3. Olson R, ed. Nutrition reviews' present knowledge in nutrition. 6th edn. Washington, DC: Nutrition Foundation. 1989: p 96–107
4. Brown ED, Micozzi MS, Craft NE et al. Plasma carotenoids in normal men after a single ingestion of vegetables or purified beta-carotene. Am J Clin Nutr 1989; 49: 1258–1265
5. Brubacher GB, Weiser H. The vitamin A activity of beta-carotene. Int J Vit Nutr Res 1984; 55: 5–15
6. Selhorst JB, Waybright EA, Jennings S et al. Liver lover's headache. Pseudotumor cerebri and vitamin A intoxication. JAMA 1984; 252: 3365
7. Ganguly J, Sastry PS. Mechanism of conversion of beta-carotene into vitamin A – central cleavage versus random cleavage. Wld Rev Nutr Diet 1985; 45: 198–220
8. Olson JA. Serum levels of vitamin A and carotenoids as reflectors of nutritional status. J Natl Cancer Inst 1984; 73: 1439–1444
9. Folman Y, Rosenberg M, Ascarelli I et al. The effect of dietary and climatic factors on fertility, and on plasma progesterone and oestradiol-17B levels in dairy cows. J Steroid Biochem 1983; 19: 863–868
10. Editor. Metabolism of beta-carotene by the bovine corpus luteum. Nutr Rev 1983; 41: 357–358
11. Lotthammer KH. Importance of beta-carotene for the fertility of dairy cattle. Feedstuffs 1979; 51: 16–19
12. O'Fallon JV, Chew BP. The subcellular distribution of β-carotene in bovine corpus luteum. Proc Soc Exp Biol Med 1984; 177: 406–411
13. Sherman BM, Korenman SG. Inadequate corpus luteum function. A pathophysiological interpretation of human breast cancer epidemiology. Cancer 1974; 33: 1306–1312
14. Bendich A. Beta-carotene and the immune response. Proc Nutr Soc 1991; 50: 263–274
15. Krinsky NI. Antioxidant function of carotenoids. Free Rad Biol Med 1989; 7: 627–635
16. Cutler RG. Carotenoids and retinol. Their possible importance in determining longevity of primate species. Proc Natl Acad Sci 1984; 81: 7627–7631
17. Murakoshi M, Nishino H, Satomi Y et al. Potent preventive action of alpha-carotene against carcinogenesis. Cancer Res 1992; 52: 6583–6587
18. Di Mascio P, Kaiser S, Sies H. Lycopene as the most efficient biological carotenoid singlet oxygen quencher. Arch Biochem Biophysics 1989; 274: 532–538

19. Franceschi S, Bidoli E, LaVecchia C et al. Tomatoes and risk of digestive-tract cancers. Int J Cancer 1994; 59: 181–184
20. Manges AR, Holden JM, Beecher GR et al. Carotenoid content of fruits and vegetables. An evaluation of analytic data. J Am Diet Assoc 1993; 93: 284–286
21. Ben-Amotz, A, Mokady S, Edelstein et al. Bioavailability of a natural isomer mixture as compared with synthetic all-trans-beta-carotene in rats and chicks. J Nutr 1989; 119: 1013–1019
22. Mokady S, Avron M, Ben-Amotz A. Accumulation in chick livers of 9-cis versus all-trans beta-carotene. J Nutr 1990; 120: 889–892
23. Carughi A, Hooper FG. Plasma carotenoid concentrations before and after supplementation with a carotenoid mixture. Am J Clin Nutr 1994; 59: 896–899
24. Morinobu T, Tamai H, Murata T et al. Changes in beta-carotene levels by long-term administration of natural beta-carotene derived from Dunaliella bardawil in humans. J Nutr Sci Vitaminol 1994; 40: 421–430
25. Ziegler RG. A review of the epidemiologic evidence that carotenoids reduce the risk of cancer. J Nutr 1989; 119: 116–122
26. National Research Council. Diet and Health. Implications for Reducing Chronic Disease Risk. Washington, DC: National Academy Press. 1989: p 313–314
27. Gerster H. Anticarcinogenic effect of common carotenoids. Internat J Vit Nutr Res 1993; 63: 93–121
28. The Alpha-tocopherol, Beta-carotene Cancer Prevention Study Group. The effect of vitamin E and beta-carotene on incidence of lung cancer and other cancers in male smokers. N Engl J Med 1994; 330: 1029–1035
29. Leo MA, Kim C, Lowe N et al. Interaction of ethanol with beta-carotene. Delayed blood clearance and enhanced hepatotoxicity. Hepatology 1992; 15: 883–891
30. Krinsky NI. The biological properties of carotenoids. Pure Appl Chem 1994; 66: 1003–1010
31. Krinsky NI. Antioxidant functions of carotenoids. Free Rad Biol Med 1989; 7: 617–635
32. Omenn GS, Goodman G, Thornquist M et al. The beta-carotene and retinol efficacy trial (CARET) for chemoprevention of lung cancer in high risk populations. Smokers and asbestos-exposed workers. Cancer Res 1994; 54: 2038S–2043S
33. Rowe PM. Beta-carotene takes a collective beating. Lancet 1996; 347: 249
34. Garewal H, Shamdas GJ. Intervention trials with beta-carotene in precancerous conditions of the upper aerodigestive tract. In: Bendich A, Butterworth CE, eds. Micronutrients in health and disease prevention. New York: Marcel Dekker. 1991: p 127–140
35. Toma S, Benso S, Albanese et al. Treatment of oral leukoplakia with beta-carotene. Oncology 1992; 49: 77–81
36. Blot WJ, Li JY, Taylor PR et al. The Linxian trials: mortality rates by vitamin-mineral intervention group. Am J Clin Nutr 1995; 62: 1424S–1426S
37. Blot WJ, Li JY, Taylor PR et al. Nutrition intervention trials in Linxian, China. Supplementation with specific vitamin/mineral combinations, cancer incidence, and disease-specific mortality in the general population. J Nat Canc Inst 1993; 85: 1483–1491
38. Street DA, Comstock GW, Salkeld RM et al. Serum antioxidants and myocardial infarction. Circulation 1994; 90: 1154–1161
39. Hennekens CH, Gaziano JM. Antioxidants and heart disease. Epidemiology and clinical evidence. Clin Cardiol 1993; 16: 10–15
40. Reaven PD, Khouw A, Beltz WF et al. Effect of dietary antioxidant combinations in humans. Protection of LDL by vitamin E but not by beta-carotene. Arteriosscl Thrombosis 1993; 13: 590–600
41. Clausen SW. Carotenemia and resistance to infection. Trans Am Pediatr Soc 1931; 43: 27–30
42. Alexander M, Newmark H, Miller RG. Oral beta-carotene can increase the number of OKT4+ cells in human blood. Immunol Letters 1985; 9: 221–224
43. Brevard PB. Beta-carotene affects white blood cells in human peripheral blood. Nutr Rep Internat 1989; 40: 139–150
44. Mikhail MS, Palan PR, Basu J et al. Decreased beta-carotene levels in exfoliated vaginal epithelial cells in women with vaginal candidiasis. Am J Reproductive Immunol 1994; 32: 221–225
45. Mathews-Roth MM, Pathak UA, Fitzpatrick TB et al. Beta-carotene as an oral photoprotective agent in erythropoietic protoporphyria. JAMA 1974; 228: 1004–1008
46. Mathews-Roth MM, Pathak UA, Fitzpatrick TB et al. Beta-carotene therapy for erythropoietic protoporphyria and other photosensitivity diseases. Arch Dermatol 1977; 113: 1229–1232
47. Mathews-Roth MM. Photosensitization by porphyrins and prevention of photosensitization by carotenoids. J Natl Cancer Inst 1982; 69: 279–285
48. Mathews-Roth MM. Treatment of erythropoietic protoporphyria with beta-carotene. Photodermatol 1984; 1: 318–321
49. Wennersten G. Carotenoid treatment for light sensitivity. A reappraisal and six years experience. Acta Dermatovener 1980; 60: 251–255
50. Swanback G, Wennersten G. Treatment of polymorphous light eruptions with beta-carotene. Acta Dermatovener 1972; 52: 462–466
51. Newbold PC. Beta-carotene in the treatment of discoid lupus erythematosus. Br J Dermatol 1976; 100: 187–188
52. Fusaro RM, Johnson JA. Hereditary polymorphic light eruption in American Indians – photoprotection and prevention of streptococcal pyoderma and glomerulonephritis. JAMA 1980; 244: 156–159
53. Mathews-Roth MM, Pathak MA, Parrich J et al. A clinical trial of the effects of oral beta-carotene on the responses of human skin to solar radiation. J Invest Dermatol 1972; 59: 349–353
54. Shoenfeld Y, Shaklai M, Ben-Baruch N et al. Neutropenia induced by hypercarotenemia. Lancet 1982; 1: 1245
55. Kemmann E, Pasquale SA, Skaf R. Amenorrhea associated with carotenemia. JAMA 1983; 249: 926–929
56. Mathews-Roth MM. Neutropenia and beta-carotene. Lancet 1982; ii: 222
57. Stampfer MJ, Willett W, Hennekens CH. Carotene, carrots, and neutropenia. Lancet 1982; ii: 615
58. Mathews-Roth MM, Abraham AA, Gabuzda TG. Beta-carotene content of certain organs from two patients receiving high doses of beta-carotene. Clin Chem 1976; 22: 922–924
59. Mathews-Roth MM. Amenorrhea associated with carotenemia. JAMA 1983; 250: 731
60. Poh-Fitzpatrick MB, Barbera LG. Absence of crystalline retinopathy after long-term therapy with B-carotene. J AM Acad Dermatol 1984; 11: 111–113
61. Heywood R, Palmer AK, Gregson RL et al. The toxicity of beta-carotene. Toxicology 1985; 36: 91–100

CHAPTER CONTENTS

68

Boron

*Gregory S. Kelly, ND**

INTRODUCTION

Boron is an ubiquitous constituent of man's external environment. It typically occurs in nature as borates hydrated with varying amounts of water. Boric acid and borax are important boron-containing compounds.[1]

In trace amounts, boron is essential for the growth of many plants, and is found in animal and human tissues at low concentrations.[1] Although it has yet to be recognized as an essential nutrient for humans, recent data from animal and human studies suggest that boron may be important for mineral metabolism, brain function and performance, and prevention of both osteoporosis and osteoarthritis.

SOURCES

Because boron in plants is dependent on the availability of boron in the soil, the same food crop can vary greatly in boron content depending on where and how it is grown. In general, soils exposed to high degrees of precipitation have decreased levels of boron.[2] Food processing results in additional loss of boron.[3] Foods of plant origin, such as leafy vegetables, non-citrus fruits, nuts, legumes, and sea vegetables are considered to be the best sources of boron.[1,4] Wine has also been shown to contribute appreciable amounts of boron to the diet.[5] A diet containing an abundance of these items would provide 2–6 mg/day of boron.[4,6]

Daily intake of boron is dependent upon several variables. Concentration of boron in water varies considerably according to geographic source. In some areas, boron in drinking water and water-based beverages may account for most of the total dietary boron intake. Individual food preference greatly influences daily intake of boron. Fruits, vegetables, tubers, and legumes have higher concentrations of boron than do cereal grains or animal tissues. Boron has also been determined to be a notable contaminant or major ingredient of many

*Reprinted with permission from *Alternative Medicine Review* 1997; 2(1): 48–56

personal care products and it is occasionally used (boric acid) as a food preservative.[7]

In a recently published study, 32 subjects from Sydney, Australia, aged 20–53, were assessed over a 7 day period for their dietary intake of boron. The average boron intake in male and female subjects was found to be 2.28 ± 1.3 and 2.16 ± 1.1 mg/day respectively.[5] The boron content of selected Australian foods has been found to correlate with values in Finnish and US Food and Drug Administration tables and is presented in Table 68.1.[5]

METABOLISM

Chemical properties

Elemental boron was first isolated in 1808. It is the first member (atomic number 5) of the metalloid or semiconductor family of elements, which include silicon and germanium, and is the only non-metal of the group IIIA elements. Like carbon, boron has a tendency to form double bonds and macromolecules.[8] Boron, as boric acid, acts as a Lewis acid, accepting hydroxyl (OH-) ions and leaving an excess of protons.[9] Because boron complexes with organic compounds containing hydroxyl groups, it interacts with sugars and polysaccharides, adenosine-5-phosphate, pyridoxine, riboflavin, dehydroascorbic acid, and pyridine nucleotides.[10] Borate cross-links with polysaccharides, most likely as borate di-esters, to form gels with unique properties. These gels are very plastic in nature and quickly reassemble in response to externally applied stress.[9] Five naturally occurring boron ester compounds have been identified as antibiotics.[11]

Table 68.1 Concentration of boron in selected Australian foods

Food	Boron (mg/100 g)
Almond	2.82
Apple (red)	0.32
Apricots (dried)	2.11
Avocado	2.06
Banana	0.16
Beans (red kidney)	1.40
Bran (wheat)	0.32
Brazil nuts	1.72
Broccoli	0.31
Carrot	0.30
Cashew nuts (raw)	1.15
Celery	0.50
Chick peas	0.71
Dates	1.08
Grapes (red)	0.50
Hazel nuts	2.77
Honey	0.50
Lentils	0.74
Olive	0.35
Onion	0.20
Orange	0.25
Peach	0.52
Peanut butter	1.92
Pear	0.32
Potato	0.18
Prunes	1.18
Raisins	4.51
Walnut	1.63
Wine (Shiraz Cabernet)	0.86

Biochemistry

Boron in food, sodium borate and boric acid are well absorbed from the digestive tract.[12] These compounds are also absorbed through damaged skin and mucous membranes; however, they do not readily penetrate intact skin.[13]

No accumulation of boron has been observed in soft tissues of animals fed chronic low doses of boron; however, in acute poisoning incidents, the amount of boric acid in brain and liver tissue has been reported to be as high as 2,000 ppm. Within a few days of consumption of large amounts of boron, levels in blood and most soft tissues quickly reach a plateau.[14] Tissue homeostasis is maintained by the rapid elimination of excess boron primarily in the urine; with bile, sweat, and breath also contributing as routes of elimination.[10] In humans, urinary boron excretion increases over time in all boron-supplemented subjects who have been studied.[15]

Evidence suggests that supplemental boron does accumulate in bone; however, cessation of exposure to dietary boron results in a rapid drop in bone boron levels. The half-life of boric acid in animals is estimated to be about 1 day.[14]

Biological functions

Boron contributes to living systems by acting indirectly as a proton donor and by exerting an influence on cell membrane structure and function.[16] Although the absolute essentiality of boron for plants is well documented, studies to date have not shown it to be unequivocally essential for either animals or humans. However, boron supplementation has been shown to affect certain aspects of animal physiological function. Experimental animals supplemented with boron demonstrate a high degree of variability in their response. In general, supplemental dietary boron has most marked effects when the diet is deficient in known nutrients.[17]

Evidence suggests that boron might have a slight effect on decreasing fasting serum glucose concentrations in postmenopausal women.[11]

Life span

Boron in an animal model has been shown to have an effect upon life span, although the process is undefined. Extremes in dietary boron, both a deficiency and an excess, decreased the median life span of *Drosophilia* by 69%, while supplementing the diet with low levels of boron increased life span by 9.5%.[18]

Brain function

Brain electrophysiology and cognitive performance were assessed in response to dietary manipulation of boron (approximately 0.25 vs. approximately 3.25 mg boron/ 2,000 kcal per day) in three studies with healthy older men and women. A low boron intake was shown to result in a decrease in the proportion of power in the alpha band and an increase in the proportion of power in the delta band. Other changes in left–right symmetry and brain wave coherence were noted in various sites, indicating an influence on brain function. When contrasted with the high boron intake, low dietary boron resulted in significantly poorer performance ($P < 0.05$) on tasks emphasizing manual dexterity, eye–hand co-ordination, attention, perception, encoding and short- and long-term memory. Collectively, the data from these studies indicate that boron may play a role in human brain function, alertness and cognitive performance.[19]

Hematological

Boron supplementation to human subjects, who had previously followed a dietary regimen deficient in boron, increased blood hemoglobin concentrations, mean corpuscular hemoglobin, and mean corpuscular hemoglobin concentration; and lowered hematocrit, red cell count, and platelet count.[20]

Mineral metabolism

Boron also impacts mineral metabolism and has been shown to impact levels of certain hormones in human subjects. In the first nutritional study with humans involving boron,[13] postmenopausal women first were fed a diet that provided 0.25 mg boron/2,000 kcal for 119 days, and then were fed the same diet with a boron supplement of 3 mg boron/day for 48 days. The boron supplementation reduced the total plasma concentration of calcium and the urinary excretions of calcium and magnesium, and elevated the serum concentrations of 17 beta-estradiol and testosterone.[4]

In a study designed to determine the effects of boron supplementation on blood and urinary minerals in athletic subjects on Western diets, findings suggested that boron supplementation modestly affected mineral status.[15]

DEFICIENCY SIGNS AND SYMPTOMS

Information on boron deficiency is very limited, especially in humans. It is thought that insufficient intake of boron becomes obvious only when the body is stressed in a manner that enhances the need for it. When the diets of animals and humans are manipulated to cause functional deficiencies in nutrients such as calcium, magnesium, vitamin D, and methionine, a large number of responses to dietary boron occur.[21] There is evidence to suggest that more than 21 days on a boron-deficient diet are required to demonstrate detectable effects in humans.[22] The variables that are changed, due to a boron-deficient diet, abruptly improve about 8 days after boron supplementation is introduced.[4] Evidence indicates that hemodialysis results in an excessive decrease in serum boron as compared with controls.[23] While by no means being pathognomonic for a boron deficiency, blood urea nitrogen has been found to be slightly elevated during boron depletion.[24]

NUTRIENT INTERACTIONS

Vitamin D

There is considerable evidence that dietary boron alleviates perturbations in mineral metabolism that are characteristic of vitamin D_3 deficiency.[25] After 26 days, chicks fed on a diet inadequate in vitamin D exhibited decreased food consumption and plasma calcium concentrations and increased plasma concentrations of glucose, beta-hydroxybutyrate, triglycerides, triiodothyronine, cholesterol, and alkaline phosphatase activity. Supplemental boron returned plasma glucose and triglycerides to concentrations exhibited by chicks fed on a diet adequate in vitamin D.[26]

In rachitic chicks, boron elevated the numbers of osteoclasts and alleviated distortion of the marrow sprouts of the proximal tibial epiphysial plate, a distortion characteristic of vitamin D_3 deficiency.[25,27] Higher apparent-balance values of calcium, magnesium, and phosphorus have been observed for rats fed on a vitamin D-deprived diet if the diet is supplemented with boron.[17]

After supplementation with 3.25 mg boron daily, plasma levels of D_2 increased in men over 45 and postmenopausal women on low magnesium and copper diets.[28]

Calcium

Boron supplementation may have a favorable impact on calcium metabolism. A boron supplement of 3 mg/ day affected several indices of mineral metabolism of seven women consuming a low-magnesium diet and five women consuming a diet adequate in magnesium; the women had consumed a conventional diet supplying about 0.25 mg boron/day for 119 days. Boron supplementation modestly reduced the urinary excretion of calcium when dietary magnesium was low.[4]

In men over 45 and postmenopausal women, changes caused by boron supplementation include increased concentration of plasma ionized and total calcium as well as reduced serum calcitonin concentration and urinary excretion of calcium.[28] A 1993 study demonstrated that a low boron diet elevated urinary calcium excretion. The high level of calcium excretion was maintained throughout the 6 week study; however, it remained elevated even after boron supplementation began.[29]

Copper

Supplemental boron acts to increase serum levels of both copper and copper-dependent enzymes in humans. Boron supplementation (3 mg/day), to five men over the age of 45, four postmenopausal women, and five postmenopausal women on estrogen therapy who had been fed a low boron diet (0.23 mg/2,000 kcal) for 63 days, resulted in higher erythrocyte superoxide dismutase, serum enzymatic ceruloplasmin, and plasma copper.[28] In a subsequent study, these same variables were again found to be higher during boron repletion than while subjects were fed on a diet low in boron.[30]

Magnesium

When magnesium deprivation is severe enough to cause typical signs of deficiency, a significant interaction between boron and magnesium is found.[8] A combined deficiency of boron and magnesium causes detrimental changes in the bones of animals. Supplemental boron elevates plasma Mg concentrations and enhances growth.[27]

Boron supplementation has resulted in increased serum magnesium concentrations in human female subjects studied.[14] Boron supplementation increases red blood cell magnesium concentrations.[31] It has been shown that serum magnesium concentrations are greater in sedentary females whose diets are supplemented with boron than in exercising female athletes who are supplemented with boron.[32] This finding, while unexplained to date, may indicate an increased loss of boron through urine and perspiration during exercise.

Phosphorous

Supplemental boron seems to lower serum phosphorus concentrations in female subjects ages 20–27.[32] However, exercise training diminishes these changes,[14] again possibly indicating increased losses or an increased need for boron as a result of exercise. A low magnesium status along with supplementation of boron may depress the urinary excretion of phosphorus. This does not occur in women with an adequate magnesium intake.[4]

Methionine and arginine

In experimental animals, a beneficial impact is consistently observed after boron supplementation when the diet contains marginal methionine and excessive arginine. Among the signs exhibited by rats fed on a diet marginal in methionine and magnesium are depressed growth and bone magnesium concentration, and elevated spleen weight/body weight and kidney weight/body weight ratios. Findings indicate that the severity of these symptoms is alleviated with boron supplementation.[33]

HORMONE INTERACTIONS

In rats, supplemental dietary boron substantially depressed plasma insulin, plasma pyruvate concentrations, and creatine kinase activity and increased plasma thyroxine (T4) concentrations. Boron supplementation also decreased plasma aspartate transaminase activity.[34] In animal experiments, boron supplementation offsets the elevation in plasma alkaline phosphatase caused by vitamin D deficiency.[24]

One researcher has hypothesized that boron might be required for the synthesis of steroid hormones as well as vitamin D. Since the biosynthesis of steroids such as vitamin D, testosterone, and 17 beta-estradiol involves one or more hydroxylation steps, and because of boron's ability as a Lewis acid to complex with hydroxyl groups, boron may facilitate the addition of hydroxyl groups to the steroid structures.[4] It has also been suggested that boron may act in an unspecified manner to protect hormones from rapid inactivation.[4]

An increase in dietary intake of boron from 0.25 to 3.25 mg/day has been reported to increase plasma 17 beta-estradiol by more than 50% and to more than double plasma testosterone levels in postmenopausal women. The elevation seemed more marked when dietary magnesium was low.[4] In a subsequent study of healthy men, boron supplementation resulted in an increase in the concentrations of both plasma estrogen and testosterone; however, not all published trials support these observations.[5]

Ten male bodybuilders, aged 20–26, were given a 2.5 mg boron supplement, while nine male bodybuilders, aged 21–27, were given a placebo for 7 weeks. Because both groups demonstrated significant increases in total testosterone ($P < 0.01$), lean body mass ($P < 0.01$), one repetition maximum squat ($P < 0.001$) and bench press ($P < 0.01$), the authors concluded that the gains were a result of 7 weeks of bodybuilding, not of boron supplementation.[35]

Table 68.2 lists boron's impact on selected hormones in either animals or humans. Some of these interactions have only been demonstrated in animal models (*) while others have not been demonstrated unequivocally to date in all age and gender segments of a human population (**).

Table 68.2 Boron's observed impact on selected hormones

Hormone	Increases	Decreases
Alkaline phosphatase		+
Aspartate transaminase*		+
Calcitonin		+
Cholecalciferol		+
Creatine kinase*	+	
17 beta-estradiol**	+	
Insulin*		+
Super oxide dismutase		+
Testosterone**		+
Thyroxine*		+

CLINICAL APPLICATIONS

Osteoporosis

A considerable body of evidence has shown that both compositional and functional properties of bone are affected by boron status.[36] In experimental animals, histologic findings suggest that supplemental boron enhances maturation of the growth plate.[24] Boron is also found at the highest concentrations in growing and calcifying areas of long bones.[4] In two human studies, boron deprivation caused changes in indices associated with calcium metabolism in a manner that could be construed as being detrimental to bone formation and maintenance; these changes were enhanced by a diet low in magnesium.[4,24] The author concluded that boron and magnesium are apparently needed for optimal calcium metabolism and are thus needed to prevent the excessive bone loss which often occurs in postmenopausal women and older men.[24]

Osteoarthritis and rheumatoid arthritis

A dietary boron deficiency may be a contributing factor in some cases of arthritis.[37] In areas of the world where boron intake routinely is 1.0 mg/day or less, the estimated incidence of arthritis ranges from 20 to 70%, whereas in areas of the world where boron intake ranges from 3–10 mg/day, the estimated incidence of arthritis ranges from 0 to 10%.[37]

Analytical evidence indicates that persons with arthritis have lower boron concentrations in femur heads, bones, and synovial fluid when compared with persons without this disorder. There have also been observations that bones of patients using boron supplements are much harder to cut than those of patients not supplementing with boron.[3]

In 1961, the first anecdotal evidence suggesting that boron may be beneficial for osteoarthritis was presented when one patient had reduction of swelling and stiffness and remained symptom free for 1 year following supplementation with 3 mg of elemental boron twice daily for 3 weeks. A human study also offers evidence that boron supplementation may be beneficial in the treatment of this condition. In a double-blind placebo-controlled trial of 20 subjects with osteoarthritis, 50% of subjects receiving a daily supplement containing 6 mg of boron noted a subjective improvement in their condition. Only 10% of those receiving the placebo improved during the same time interval. There was greater improvement in the condition of all joints ($P < 0.01$) as well as less pain on movement ($P < 0.001$) in subjects receiving the boron supplementation.[38]

Clinical observations indicate that children with juvenile arthritis (Still's disease) improve with boron supplementation (6–9 mg/day) in 2–3 weeks, while adults with osteoarthritis may require 2–4 months of supplementation before benefits are detected. Persons with rheumatoid arthritis may experience an aggravation of symptoms (Herxheimer response) for 1–3 weeks, but generally notice improvement within 4 weeks of beginning boron supplementation.[3]

DOSAGE

The optimal dose of boron for prevention of osteoporosis and proper physiological function appears to be 3–6 mg/day. While it is best to obtain boron by means of a diet with an abundance of fruits, vegetables, legumes, and nuts, persons whose diet is limited in these items may need a supplement containing 3 mg of elemental boron. In patients with arthritis, a trial period of 2–4 months with a dose of 3 mg of boron t.i.d. seems to be indicated.

TOXICOLOGY

Although boron is potentially toxic to all organisms, and, as boric acid and borax, has been used as a pesticide and food preservative, higher animals usually do not accumulate boron because of their ability to rapidly excrete it.[9] Authenticated cases of poisoning in humans have been few and have primarily been the result of accidental ingestion of insecticides and household products containing borates, or use of large amounts of boric acid in the treatment of burns.[39]

The improper use of boric acid-containing antiseptics is still one of the most common causes of toxic accidents in newborns and infants. Since boric acid is readily absorbed through damaged skin, it should not be applied topically to extensive wounds.[12]

In animals, chronic low-level boron exposure has been shown to cause reduced growth, cutaneous disorders, and suppression of male reproductive system function.[40] Studies indicate that male rodents suffer testicular atrophy with dietary exposure to boric acid above 4,500 ppm and have decreased sperm motility at all exposure levels above 1,000 ppm.[41]

Goats orally dosed with toxic but sublethal amounts of

boron show significant increases in packed cell volume, hemoglobin, inorganic phosphate, creatine phosphokinase, conjugated bilirubin, sodium, glucose, cholesterol, and aspartate transaminase. Several serum components were significantly decreased after boron dosing, including alkaline phosphatase, magnesium, glutamyltransferase and potassium. There was also an elevation of cerebrospinal fluid monoamine metabolites.[42]

Humans given 100 mg of boron intravenously or 270 mg of boric acid orally reported no discomfort and showed no obvious signs of toxicity.[43,44] Airborne exposures to boron oxide and its hydration product, boric acid, have been reported to cause respiratory and eye irritation.[45] A fatal outcome has been reported following ingestion of 1 g of boric acid by a child; however, adults have survived acute intakes of nearly 300 g.[46]

Common signs and symptoms of acute boron toxicity include nausea, as well as vomiting and diarrhea which are blue-green in color.[46] Other symptoms seen with acute exposure are abdominal pain, an erythematous rash involving both the skin and mucous membranes, stimulation or depression of the central nervous system, convulsions, hyperpyrexia, renal tubular damage, abnormal liver function, and jaundice.[12] Increased urinary riboflavin excretion has also been reported subsequent to acute boric acid ingestion.[47] Symptoms of chronic intoxication include anorexia, gastrointestinal disturbances, debility, confusion, dermatitis, menstrual disorders, anemia, convulsions, and alopecia.[12]

Because of its ability to increase the excretion of boron, in cases of toxicity, *N*-acetylcysteine is the preferred intervention.[48]

SUMMARY

Although the skeletal response to boron is modified by other nutritional variables such as calcium, magnesium, vitamin D, methionine, and arginine, there is considerable evidence that both compositional and functional properties of bone are affected by boron status.

Findings suggest that boron is an important nutrient not only for mineral metabolism but also for varied aspects of optimal health in humans. While all published trials are not in agreement on the impact of boron supplementation on levels of 17 beta-estradiol and testosterone, evidence strongly suggests that boron deficiency results in decreased levels in postmenopausal women, while supplementation tends to normalize levels in these same women. Boron's impact on sex hormones in other segments of the population is still equivocal. No evidence exists to suggest boron supplementation will act pharmaceutically to increase levels of either 17 beta-estradiol or testosterone above normal physiological levels.

Based on available information, boron appears to offer benefits in the prevention of osteoporosis and arthritis. It is also a safe and potentially effective mineral to consider in any treatment regimen for rheumatoid and osteoarthritis.

REFERENCES

1. Naghii MR, Samman S. The role of boron in nutrition and metabolism. Prog Food Nutr Sci 1993; 17: 331–349
2. Houng K-H. The physiology of boron and molybdenum in plants. In: Okajima H, Uritani I, Houng H-K, eds. The significance of minor elements on plant physiology. Taiwan: ASPAC. 1975: p 61–66
3. Newnham RE. The role of boron in human nutrition. J Appl Nutr 1994; 46: 81–85
4. Nielsen FH, Hunt CD, Mullen LM et al. Effect of dietary boron on mineral, estrogen, and testosterone metabolism in postmenopausal women. FASEB J 1987; 1: 394–397
5. Naghii MR, Lyons PM, Samman S. The boron content of selected foods and the estimation of its daily intake among free-living subjects. J Amer Col Nutr 1996; 15: 614–619
6. McBride J. Banishing brittle bones with boron? Agric Res 1987; Nov/Dec: 12–13
7. Hunt CD, Shuler TR, Mullen LM. Concentration of boron and other elements in human foods and personal-care products. J Am Diet Assoc 1991; 91: 558–568
8. Nielsen FH. Boron – an overlooked element of potential nutritional importance. Nutr Today 1988; 23: 4–7
9. Loomis WD, Durst RW. Chemistry and biology of boron. BioFactors 1992; 3: 229–239
10. Zittle CA. Reaction of borate with substances of biological interest. Adv Enzymol 1951; 12: 493–527
11. Hunt CD. Biochemical effects of physiological amounts of dietary boron. J Trace Elem Exp Med 1996; 9: 185–213
12. Nielsen FH. Ultratrace minerals: Boron. In: Shils ME, Young VR, eds. Modern nutrition in health and disease. Philadelphia: Lea & Febiger. 1988: p 281–283
13. Reynolds JEF, ed. Martindale – the extra pharmacopoeia. London. 1996: p 1680
14. Moseman RF. Chemical disposition of boron in animals and humans. Environ Health Perspect 1994; 102: 113–117
15. Meacham SL, Taper LJ, Volpe SL. Effect of boron supplementation on blood and urinary calcium, magnesium, and phosphorus, and urinary boron in athletic and sedentary women. Am J Clin Nutr 1995; 61: 341–345
16. Barr RD, Barton SA, Schull WJ. Boron levels in man: preliminary evidence of genetic regulation and some implications for human biology. Med Hypotheses 1996; 46: 286–289
17. Dupre JN, Keenan MJ, Hegsted M et al. Effects of dietary boron in rats fed a vitamin D-deficient diet. Environ Health Perspect 1994; 102: 55–58
18. Massie HR, Whitney SJ, Aiello VR et al. Changes in boron concentration during development and ageing of Drosophila and effect of dietary boron on life span. Mech Ageing Dev 1990; 53: 1–7
19. Penland JG. Dietary boron, brain function, and cognitive performance. Environ Health Perspect 1994; 102: 65–72
20. Nielsen FH, Mullen LM, Nielsen EJ. Dietary boron affects blood cell counts and hemoglobin concentrations in humans. J Trace Elem Exp Med 1991; 4: 211–223
21. Nielsen FH. New essential trace elements for the life sciences. Biol Trace Elem Res 1990; 26–27: 599–611
22. Nielsen FH. Facts and fallacies about boron. Nutr Today 1992; May–June: 6–12
23. Usuda K, Kono K, Iguchi K et al. Hemodialysis effect on serum

boron level in the patients with long term hemodialysis. Sci Total Environ 1996; 191: 283–290
24. Nielsen FH. Studies on the relationship between boron and magnesium which possibly affects the formation and maintenance of bones. Mag Trace Elem 1990; 9: 61–69
25. Hunt CD. The biochemical effects of physiologic amounts of dietary boron in animal nutrition models. Environ Health Perspect 1994; 102: 35–43
26. Hunt CD, Herbel JL, Idso JP. Dietary boron modifies the effects of vitamin D3 nutrition on indices of energy substrate utilization and mineral metabolism in the chick. J Bone Miner Res 1994; 9: 171–182
27. Hunt CD. Dietary boron modified the effects of magnesium and molybdenum on mineral metabolism in the cholecalciferol-deficient chick. Biol Trace Elem Res 1989; 22: 201–220
28. Nielsen FH, Shuler TR, Gallagher SK. Effects of boron depletion and repletion on blood indicators of calcium status in humans fed a magnesium-low diet. J Trace Elem Exp Med 1990; 3: 45–54
29. Beattie JH, Peace HS. The influence of a low-boron diet and boron supplementation on bone, major mineral and sex steroid metabolism in postmenopausal women. Br J Nutr 1993; 69: 871–884
30. Nielsen FH. Biochemical and physiologic consequences of boron deprivation in humans. Environ Health Perspect 1994; 102: 59–63
31. Hunt CD, Herbel JL, Nielsen FH. Metabolic responses of postmenopausal women to supplemental dietary boron and aluminum during usual and low magnesium intake: boron, calcium, and magnesium absorption and retention and blood mineral concentrations. Am J Clin Nutr 1997; 65: 803–813
32. Meacham SL, Taper LJ, Volpe SL. Effects of boron supplementation on bone mineral density and dietary, blood, and urinary calcium, phosphorus, magnesium, and boron in female athletes. Environ Health Perspect 1994; 102: 79–82
33. Nielsen FH, Shuler TR, Zimmerman TJ et al. Magnesium and methionine deprivation affect the response of rats to boron deprivation. Biol Trace Elem Res 1988; 17: 91–107
34. Hunt CD, Herbel JL. Boron affects energy metabolism in the streptozotocin-injected, vitamin D3-deprived rat. Magnes Trace Elem 1991; 92: 374–386
35. Ferrando AA, Green NR. The effect of boron supplementation on lean body mass, plasma testosterone levels, and strength in male bodybuilders. Int J Sport Nutr 1993; 3: 140–149
36. McCoy H, Kenney MA, Montgomery C et al. Relation of boron to the composition and mechanical properties of bone. Environ Health Perspect 1994; 102: 49–53
37. Newnham RE. Agricultural practices affect arthritis. Nutr Health 1991; 7: 89–100
38. Travers RL, Rennie GC, Newnham RE. Boron and arthritis: the result of a double-blind pilot study. J Nutr Med 1990; 1: 127–132
39. Locatelli C, Minoia C, Tonini M et al. Human toxicology of boron with special reference to boric acid poisoning. G Ital Med Lav 1987; 9: 141–146
40. Minoia C, Gregotti C, Di Nucci A et al. Toxicology and health impact of environmental exposure to boron. A review. G Ital Med Lav 1987; 9: 119–124
41. Chapin RE, Ku WW. The reproductive toxicity of boric acid. Environ Health Perspect 1994; 102: 87–91
42. Sisk DB, Colvin BM, Merrill A et al. Experimental acute inorganic boron toxicosis in the goat: effects on serum chemistry and CSF biogenic amines. Vet Hum Toxicol 1990; 32: 205–211
43. Jansen JA, Anderson J, Schou JS. Boric acid single dose pharmokinetics after intravenous administration to man. Arch Toxicol 1984; 55: 64–67
44. Aas Jansen J, Schou JS, Aggerbeck B. Gastro-intestinal absorption and in vitro release of boric acid from water-emulsifying agents. Fd Chen Toxic 1894; 22: 49–53
45. Garabrant DH, Bernstein L, Peters JM et al. Respiratory and eye irritation from boron oxide and boric acid dusts. J Occup Med 1984; 26: 584–586
46. Von Burg R. Boron, boric acid, and boron oxide. L Appl Toxicol 1992; 12: 149–152
47. Pinto J, Huang YP, McConnell RJ et al. Increased urinary riboflavin excretion resulting from boric acid ingestion. J Lab Clin Med 1978; 92: 126–134
48. Banner W Jr, Koch M, Capin DM et al. Experimental chelation therapy in chromium, lead, and boron intoxication with N-acetylcysteine and other compounds. Toxicol Appl Pharmacol 1986; 83: 142–147

CHAPTER CONTENTS

69

Bromelain

Michael T. Murray, ND

Joseph E. Pizzorno Jr, ND

Proteolytic enzyme of *Ananas comosus* (family: Bromeliaceae)
Synonyms: bromelin, plant protease concentrate

GENERAL DESCRIPTION

Bromelains are sulfhydryl proteolytic enzymes obtained from the pineapple plant. Commercial bromelain is usually derived from the stem, which differs from the bromelain derived from the fruit. Commercial bromelain is a mixture of several proteases (including carboxypeptidase) and small amounts of several non-proteolytic enzymes (acid phosphatase, peroxidase and cellulase), polypeptide protease inhibitors, and organically bound calcium. Japan, Taiwan, and Hawaii are the major suppliers of commercial bromelain.[1]

CHEMICAL COMPOSITION

Stem bromelain (in its purified form) is a basic glycoprotein with one oligosaccharide moiety and one reactive sulfhydryl group per molecule. It has a molecular weight of 28,000, and its isoelectric point is pH 9.55. It exhibits activity over the pH range of 3–10, with optimal activity being between 5 and 8, depending on the substrate.[1]

Fruit bromelain is an acidic protease (isoelectric point pH 4.6). Its status as a glycoprotein is still in dispute and its molecular weight has been reported as 18,000 by one group of investigators and 31,000 by another.[1]

HISTORY

Bromelain was introduced as a therapeutic agent in 1957, and since that time over 200 scientific papers on its therapeutic applications have appeared in the medical literature.[2,3] Many of the early studies were with Ananase (Rorer), an enteric-coated bromelain tablet. Later studies implied that the failure of bromelain in some of these early studies was due to the enteric coating and inadequate dosages.

PHARMACOLOGY

Commercial bromelain has been reported to exert a wide variety of pharmacological effects:[1–3]

- digestion assistance
- anti-inflammatory activity
- burn debridement
- prevention of induced pulmonary edema
- smooth muscle relaxation
- inhibition of blood platelet aggregation
- enhancement of antibiotic absorption
- cancer prevention and remission
- ulcer prevention
- sinusitis relief
- appetite inhibition
- shortening of labor
- enhanced wound healing.

Most of these are discussed below.

Activating and deactivating factors

Being sulfhydryl proteases, like papain and ficin, both stem and fruit bromelains are inhibited by oxidizing agents, such as hydrogen peroxide, methyl bromide, and iodoacetate, and by certain metallic ions, such as lead, mercury, cadmium, copper, and iron. Bromelain is also inhibited by human serum both in vivo and in vitro. Magnesium and cysteine are activators of commercial bromelain.[1]

Activity

The activity of bromelain is expressed in a variety of enzyme units. The use of milk clotting units (mcu) is the officially recognized method in the Food Chemistry Codex (FCC). Different grades of bromelain are available based on mcu.

Absorption

Bromelain has been shown to be absorbed via a number of routes, and has been effectively administered orally, parenterally, and through intravenous infusion.[4–6] Experiments with dogs have shown oral administration to result in peak levels at 10 hours, while detectable levels are still apparent at 48 hours. Intravenous infusion peaks in 50 minutes and remains detectable for 5 hours.[5] There is definite evidence that, in both animals and humans, up to 40% of the absorbed orally administered bromelain can be absorbed intact.[4–6]

Digestive activity

Bromelain is quite effective as a substitute for trypsin or pepsin in cases of pancreatic insufficiency and post-pancreatectomy.[2] Because of bromelain's wide pH activity, it can act on substrates in the low pH of the stomach as well as in the high pH of the small intestine. The combination of bromelain with pancreatin and ox bile has been demonstrated via double-blind studies to be highly effective in the treatment of patients with pancreatic insufficiency.[7]

Anti-inflammatory activity

Several mechanisms may account for bromelain's anti-inflammatory effects:

- activation of proteolytic activity at sites of inflammation (although bromelain's proteolytic actions are inhibited by serum factors)
- fibrinolysis activity via the plasminogen-plasmin system
- depletion of kininogen
- inhibition of biosynthesis of pro-inflammatory prostaglandins and induction of prostaglandin E_1 accumulation (which tends to inhibit the release of PMN lysosomal enzymes).[3,8,9]

The first hypothesis has not been substantiated, while the latter three may be part of the same mechanism of action. After tissue injury the kinin, complement, fibrinolytic, and clotting systems are activated. These systems are closely interrelated via activation of the Hageman factor (XII) and feedback mechanisms.

Fibrin's role in promotion of the inflammatory response is to form a matrix that walls off the area of inflammation, resulting in blockage of blood vessels and inadequate tissue drainage and edema; while the kinin system cascade causes the production of kinins (e.g. bradykinin and kallidin), which increase vascular permeability, causing edema as well as evoking pain. Bromelain activates fibrinolysis by stimulating plasmin production (see Fig. 69.1), resulting in depolymerization of fibrin and thereby preventing fibrin-clogged venous stasis and localized edema.[8–11] Plasmin has been shown to block the mobilization of endogenous arachidonic acid by phospholipases, thereby reducing platelet aggregation and possibly other prostaglandin-mediated phenomena.[12] Bromelain has also been shown to reduce plasma kininogen, resulting in inhibition in the production of kinins.[13] The depletion of kininogen has been demonstrated to significantly reduce edema.

These actions, the activation of plasmin and the reduction of kinin levels, are probably the main pharmacological effects of bromelain. Bromelain's ability to reduce inflammation has been documented in a variety of experimental models and clinical studies.

Inhibition of platelet aggregation

Bromelain has been demonstrated to be a potent inhibitor of platelet aggregation, both in vitro and in vivo.[14]

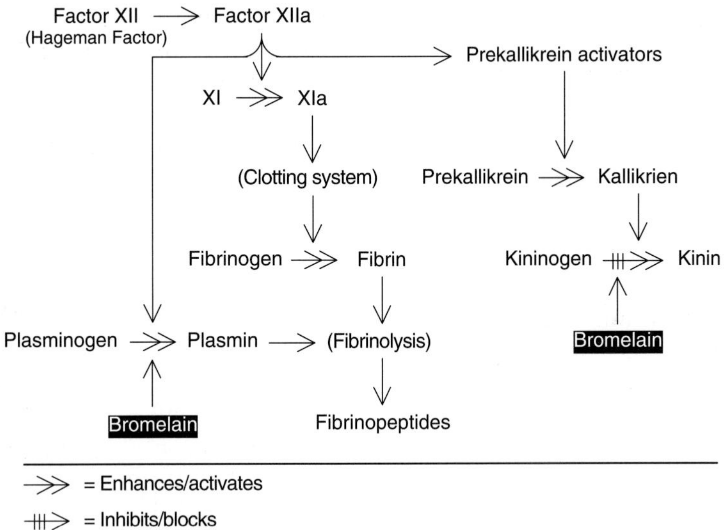

Figure 69.1 Bromelain's effects on the fibrin and kinin pathways.

Again, this is probably due to its plasmin-increasing effects. Plasmin is known to inhibit platelet aggregation by blocking the mobilization of arachidonic acid from membrane-bound phospholipid pools.[12] Platelet aggregation is a major factor in atherogenesis (see Ch. 133). Bromelain supplementation (in conjunction with potassium and magnesium) has been reported to be quite effective in treating angina (see also Table 69.1).[15]

Antibiotic, mucolytic, and permeability-modifying activities

Bromelain has been shown in clinical studies to increase serum levels of a variety of antibiotics (e.g. amoxycillin, tetracycline, and penicillin) in many different tissues and body fluids (e.g. cerebral spinal fluid, sputum, mucus, blood, urine, uterus, salpinx, ovary, gall bladder, appendix, and epithelial tissue).[16–18] In these studies the researchers concluded that bromelain itself possesses significant effects. Bromelain was as effective as antibiotics in treating a variety of infectious processes, i.e. pneumonia, perirectal abscess, cutaneous staphylococcus infection, pyelonephritis, and bronchitis.[16]

Table 69.1 Diseases and conditions in which bromelain has documented clinical efficacy[1–34]

- Angina
- Maldigestion
- Arthritis
- Pancreatic insufficiency
- Athletic injury
- Phytobezoar
- Bronchitis
- Pneumonia
- Burn debridement
- Scleroderma
- Cellulitis
- Sinusitis
- Dysmenorrhea
- Staphylococcal infection
- Ecchymosis
- Surgical trauma
- Edema
- Thrombophlebitis

CLINICAL APPLICATIONS

As is evident, bromelain has wide-ranging clinical utility. Bromelain is particularly effective in virtually all inflammatory conditions, regardless of etiology, including those resulting from physical trauma, infectious agents, surgical procedures, immunological reactions, and prostaglandin metabolism.

Respiratory tract diseases

It appears that bromelain's mucolytic activity is responsible for its particular effectiveness in respiratory tract diseases.[19] In the treatment of chronic bronchitis, bromelain was shown to have an antitussive effect and to reduce the viscosity of sputum. Spirometric examination of patients before and after treatment indicated increased vital capacity and FEV_1, while the residual volume was reduced. These favorable effects were believed to be the results of enhanced resolution of respiratory congestion, due to bromelain's ability to fluidify and decrease bronchial secretions.

Acute sinusitis has also responded to bromelain therapy. Good-to-excellent results were obtained in 87% of bromelain-treated patients, compared with 68% of the placebo group.[20]

Thrombophlebitis

Numerous investigators have demonstrated that orally administered bromelain has a potent favorable effect on acute thrombophlebitis, deep vein thrombosis, cellulitis, ecchymosis, and edema.[15,21–23] In a double-blind study involving 73 patients with acute thrombophlebitis, bromelain, as an adjunct to analgesics, was shown to reduce all the symptoms of inflammation: pain, edema, redness, tenderness, elevated skin temperature, and disability.[21] In this study and others, the common daily dose of bromelain was 60–160 mg of 1,200 mcu bromelain. According to some researchers, doses of 400–800 mg are needed to achieve consistent results in patients with thrombophlebitis; this probably holds true for most other conditions.[15]

Surgical procedures and athletic injuries

The effect of orally administered bromelain on the reduction of edema, bruising, healing time, and pain following various surgical procedures has been demonstrated in several clinical studies.[24–27] Tassman's studies of patients undergoing oral surgery concluded that, while post-surgical medication alone is effective, a regimen of pre- and post-surgical medication is recommended.[24,25] In a double-blind study of patients undergoing oral surgery, bromelain was found to be significantly superior to placebo: swelling decreased in 3.8 days with bromelain, compared with 7 days for the placebo; and the duration of pain was reduced to 5.1 days in the bromelain group, compared with 8.1 in the placebo.[25] Similar observations were made in studies of episiotomy cases. Bromelain reduced edema, inflammation, and pain, and pre-operative administration potentiated the effects.[26]

Bromelain has been used in a variety of sports-related injuries. A 1960 study involving boxers highlights its effects.[27] Among the 74 boxers receiving bromelain, in 58 all signs of bruising cleared completely within 4 days. In the remainder, complete clearance took 8–10 days. Among the 72 controls, at the end of 4 days only 10 showed bruises completely cleared, the remainder taking 7–14 days. It is important to recognize that, while bromelain has been shown to effectively reduce pain, this probably is the result of a reduction in tissue inflammation and edema, rather than a direct analgesic effect.

In a recent open clinical trial, 59 patients with blunt injuries to the musculoskeletal system (e.g. contusions, muscle strains, ligament tears) were given 500 mg of bromelain three times daily, 30 minutes before meals. Swelling, pain at rest and during motion, signs of inflammation, and tenderness to palpation all rapidly improved.[28]

Dysmenorrhea

Bromelain and papain have been used successfully in the treatment of dysmenorrhea.[29] Bromelain is believed to be a smooth muscle relaxant, since it decreases the spasms of the contracted cervix in these patients. Failure of the bromelain protease, when used alone (purified by adsorption), to produce this effect was the first indication that the pharmacologically important factor is not the main protease. The muscle-relaxing effects of bromelain on the uterus are believed to be a result of decreasing prostaglandins of the 2-series, e.g. $PGF_{2\alpha}$ and PGE_2, while increasing levels of PGE_1-like compounds.[3]

DOSAGE

Unless bromelain is being used as a digestive aid, administration should be on an empty stomach (between meals). The dosage depends largely on the potency of the bromelain preparation. Most currently available bromelain is in the 1,800–2,000 mcu range, with the typical dosage being 125–450 mg t.i.d. between meals.

TOXICITY

Very large doses of bromelain (nearly 2.0 g) have been given with no side-effects.[30] It is virtually non-toxic, as no LD_{50} exists up to 10 g/kg. Chronic use appears to be well tolerated. Although no significant side-effects have been noted, as with most therapeutic agents, allergic reactions may occur in sensitive individuals or with prolonged occupational exposure.[31,32]

Bromelain can induce IgE-mediated respiratory and gastrointestinal allergic reactions, as well as cross-react with papain, wheat flour, rye flour, grass pollen, and birch pollen.[31,32] While side-effects are seldom observed, sensitivity manifested by urticaria or skin rash has occurred. There are no reported cases of anaphylactoid reactions. Other possible, but unconfirmed, reactions include nausea, vomiting, diarrhea, metrorrhagia, and menorrhagia.[33]

REFERENCES

1. Jeung A. Encyclopedia of common natural ingredients used in foods, drugs, and cosmetics. New York, NY: John Wiley. 1980: p 74–76
2. Taussig SJ, Batkin S. Bromelain, the enzyme complex of pineapple (*Ananas comosus*) and its clinical application. An update. J Ethnopharma 1988; 22: 191–203
3. Felton G. Does kinin released by pineapple stem bromelain stimulate production of prostaglandin E1-like compounds? Hawaii Med J 1977; 36: 39–47
4. Miller J, Opher A. The increased proteolytic activity of human

blood serum after oral administration of bromelain. Exp Med Surg 1964; 22: 277–280
5. Izaka K, Yamada M, Kawano T, Suyama T. Gastrointestinal absorption and anti-inflammatory effect of bromelain. Jap J Pharmacol 1972; 22: 519–534
6. Seifert J, Ganser R, Brendel W. Absorption of a proteolytic enzyme of plant origin from the gastrointestinal tract into the blood and lymph of adult rats. Z Gastroenterol 1979; 17: 1–18
7. Baakrishnan V, Hareendran A, Nair C. Double-blind cross-over trial of an enzyme preparation in pancreatic steatorrhoea. J Assoc Phys Ind 1981; 29: 207–209
8. Lotz-Winter H. On the pharmacology of bromelain. An update with special regard to animal studies on dose-dependent effects. Plant Med 1990; 56: 249–253
9. Taussig S. The mechanism of the physiological action of bromelain. Med Hypothesis 1980; 6: 99–104
10. Pirotta F, de Giuli-Morghen C. Bromelain – A deeper pharmacological study. Note I – Anti-inflammatory and serum fibrinolytic activity after oral administration in the rat. Drugs Exp Clin Res 1978; 4: 1–20
11. de Giuli-Morghen C, Pirotta F. Bromelain – A deeper pharmacological study. Note II – Interaction with some protease inhibitors and rabbit specific antiserum. Drugs Exp Clin Res 1978; 4: 21–37
12. Schafer A, Adelman B. Plasmin inhibition of platelet function and of arachidonic acid metabolism. J Clin Invest 1985; 75: 456–461
13. Katori M, Ikeda K, Harada Y et al. A possible role of prostaglandins and bradykinin as a trigger of exudation in carrageenin-induced rat pleurisy. Agents Actions 1978; 8: 108–112
14. Heinicke R, van der Wal L, Yokoyama M. Effect of bromelain (*Ananase*) on human platelet aggregation. Experentia 1972; 28: 844–845
15. Taussig S, Nieper H. Bromelain: its use in prevention and treatment of cardiovascular disease present status. J Int Assoc Prev Med 1979; 6: 139–151
16. Neubauer R. A plant protease for the potentiation of and possible replacement of antibiotics. Exp Med Surg 1961; 19: 143–160
17. Luerti M, Vignali M. Influence of bromelain on penetration of antibiotics in uterus, salpinx and ovary. Drugs Exp Clin Res 1978; 4: 45–48
18. Tinozzi S, Venegoni A. Effect of bromelain on serum and tissue levels of amoxycillin. Drugs Exp Clin Res 1978; 4: 39–44
19. Rimoldi R, Ginesu F, Giura R. The use of bromelain in pneumological therapy. Drugs Exp Clin Res 1978; 4: 55–66
20. Ryan R. A double-blind clinical evaluation of bromelains in the treatment of acute sinusitis. Headache 1967; 7: 13–17
21. Seligman B. Oral bromelains as adjuncts in the treatment of acute thrombophlebitis. Angiology 1969; 20: 22–26
22. Seligman B. Bromelain. An anti-inflammatory agent. Angiology 1962; 13: 508–510
23. Felton G. Fibrinolytic and antithrombotic action of bromelain may eliminate thrombosis in heart patients. Med Hypothesis 1980; 6: 1123–1133
24. Tassman G, Zafran J, Zayon G. Evaluation of a plant proteolytic enzyme for the control of inflammation and pain. J Dent Med 1964; 19: 73–77
25. Tassman G, Zafran J, Zayon G. A double-blind crossover study of a plant proteolytic enzyme in oral surgery. J Dent Med 1965; 20: 51–54
26. Howat R, Lewis G. The effect of bromelain therapy on episiotomy wounds – A double blind controlled clinical trial. J Ob Gyn Brit Commonwealth 1972; 79: 951–953
27. Blonstein J. Control of swelling in boxing injuries. Practitioner 1960; 203: 206
28. Masson M. Bromelain in the treatment of blunt injuries to the musculoskeletal system. A case observation by an orthopedic surgeon in private practice. Fortschr Med 1995; 113: 303–306
29. Hunter RG, Henry GW, Henicke RM. The action of papain and bromelain on the uterus. Am J Ob Gyn 1957; 73: 867–880
30. Gutfreund A, Taussig S, Morris A. Effect of oral bromelain on blood pressure and heart rate of hypertensive patients. Hawaii Med J 1978; 37: 143–146
31. Baur X. Studies on the specificity of human IgE-antibodies to the plant proteases papain and bromelain. Clinical Allergy 1979; 9: 451–457
32. Baur X, Fruhman G. Allergic reactions, including asthma, to the pineapple protease bromelain following occupational exposure. Clinical Allergy 1979; 9: 443–450
33. Physicians Desk Reference. Ananase (Rorer). Medical Economics Company. 1982: p 1645
34. Ballard T. Bromelain. J John Bastyr Col Nat Med 1979; 1: 37–41

CHAPTER CONTENTS

70

Camellia sinensis (green tea)

Michael T. Murray, ND

Joseph E. Pizzorno Jr, ND

Camellia sinensis (family: Theaceae)
Common names: green tea

GENERAL DESCRIPTION

Both green tea and black tea are derived from the same plant, the tea plant (*Camellia sinensis*). The tea plant originated in China, but is now grown and consumed worldwide. The tea plant is an evergreen shrub or tree that can grow up to a height of 30 feet, but is usually maintained at a height of 2–3 feet by regular pruning. The shrub is heavily branched with young hairy leaves. Parts used are the leaf bud and the two adjacent young leaves together with the stem, broken between the second and third leaves. Older leaves are considered of inferior quality.

Green tea vs. black tea

Green tea is produced by lightly steaming the freshly cut leaf, while black tea is produced by allowing the leaves to oxidize. During oxidation, enzymes present in the tea convert many polyphenolic therapeutic substances to compounds with much less activity. With green tea, oxidation is not allowed to take place because the steaming process inactivates these enzymes. Green tea is very high in polyphenols with potent antioxidant and anti-cancer properties. Oolong tea is a partially oxidized tea.

Of the nearly 2.5 million tons of dried tea that are produced each year, only 20% are green tea. India and Sri Lanka are the major producers of black tea. Green tea is produced and consumed primarily in China, Japan, and a few countries in North Africa and the Middle East.

CHEMICAL COMPOSITION

The chemical composition of green tea varies with climate, season, horticultural practices, and age of the leaf (position of the leaf on the harvested shoot). The major components of interest are the polyphenols.[1,2] The major polyphenols in green tea are flavonoids, e.g.:

- catechin
- epicatechin
- epicatechin gallate
- epigallocatechin gallate
- proanthocyanidins.

Epigallocatechin gallate is viewed as the most significant active component. The leaf bud and the first leaves are richest in epigallocatechin gallate. The usual concentration of total polyphenols in dried green tea leaf is around 8–12%.

Other compounds of interest in dried green tea leaf include:

- caffeine (3.5%)
- an unusual amino acid known as theanine (one-half of the total amino acid content which is usually 4%)
- lignin (6.5%)
- organic acids (1.5%)
- protein (15%)
- chlorophyll (0.5%).

One cup of green tea usually contains about 300–400 mg of polyphenols and between 50 and 100 mg of caffeine.

Commercial preparations are available that have been decaffeinated and concentrated for polyphenols to between 60 and 80% total polyphenols.

PHARMACOLOGY

Most of the epidemiological and experimental studies on tea have focused on the cancer-causing and cancer-protective aspects. Green tea polyphenols are potent antioxidant compounds which have demonstrated greater antioxidant protection than vitamin C and E in experimental studies.[3]

In addition to exerting antioxidant activity on its own, green tea may increase the activity of antioxidant enzymes. In mice, oral feeding of a polyphenolic fraction isolated from green tea in drinking water for 30 days resulted in significantly increased activities of antioxidant and detoxifying enzymes (glutathione peroxidase, glutathione reductase, glutathione-*S*-transferase, catalase, and quinone reductase) in the small intestine, liver, and lungs, and in small bowel and liver.[4]

With regard to cancer, a number of in vitro and experimental models of cancer have shown that green tea polyphenols may offer significant protection.[5–8] Specifically, green tea polyphenols inhibit cancer by blocking the formation of cancer-causing compounds like nitrosamines, suppressing the activation of carcinogens, and increasing detoxification or trapping of cancer-causing agents. Numerous studies have shown that green tea (including green tea polyphenols and extracts) exert significant inhibitory effects on the formation of nitrosamines in various animal and human models. For example, when human volunteers ingest green tea along with 300 mg sodium nitrate and 300 mg proline, nitrosoproline formation is strongly inhibited.[9]

CLINICAL APPLICATION

The primary clinical application for green tea is in the prevention of cancer. Epidemiological studies have demonstrated that green tea consumption may be one of the major reasons why the rate of cancer is so low in Japan. In contrast, however, black tea consumption appears associated with a substantial increase in the risk of several forms of cancer. Green tea also appears to be of value in several chronic diseases, especially those of the heart and liver.

Cancer

Green tea

The forms of cancer which appear to be best prevented by green tea are those of the gastrointestinal tract, including cancers of the stomach, small intestine, pancreas, and colon; the lung; and estrogen-related cancers, including most breast cancers.[10]

A study in Shanghai, China, found a strong inverse association between green tea consumption and various cancers.[11] For men, compared with non-regular green tea drinkers, the group with the highest green tea consumption had an 18% reduced risk for colon cancer; 28% for rectal cancer; and 37% for pancreatic cancer. In women, the highest group of green tea consumers had a reduced risk of 33% for colon, 43% for rectal, and 47% for pancreatic cancer.

In preventing breast cancer, in vitro studies have shown that green tea extracts have inhibitory effects on the growth of mammary cancer cell lines.[8] The main anti-cancer action is inhibiting the interaction of estrogen with its receptors. Polyphenol compounds in green tea extracts block the interaction of tumor promoters, hormones and growth factors with their receptors – a kind of sealing-off effect. The sealing-off effect would account for the reversible growth arrest noted in the in vitro studies.

In animal studies, green tea has been shown to very effectively inhibit the lung carcinogenesis induced by injections of asbestos and benzo(*a*)pyrene. Rats consuming water with 2% green tea experienced a cancer rate of only 16% compared with 46% for those consuming water without green tea extract.[12]

Black tea

In contrast to green tea's protective effects, population studies seem to indicate that black tea consumption may increase risk for certain cancers (e.g. cancer of the rectum, gall bladder, and endometrium).[12,13]

For example, in one study, the relationship between black tea consumption and cancer risk was analyzed using data from an integrated series of case-control studies conducted in northern Italy between 1983 and 1990.[11] The data set included 119 biopsy-confirmed cancers of the oral cavity and throat, 294 of the esophagus, 564 of the stomach, 673 of the colon, 406 of the rectum, 258 of the liver, 41 of the gall bladder, 303 of the pancreas, 149 of the larynx, 2,860 of the breast, 567 of the endometrium, 742 of the ovary, 107 of the prostate, 365 of the bladder, 147 of the kidney, 120 of the thyroid, and a total of 6,147 controls admitted to hospital for acute non-cancerous conditions. The risk of developing cancer due to tea consumption was derived after allowance for age, sex, area of residence, education, smoking, and coffee consumption. Results indicated an increased risk with tea consumption for cancers of the rectum, gall bladder, and endometrium. There was no association with cancers of the oral cavity, esophagus, stomach, bladder, kidney, prostate, or any other site considered.

In another study, men of Japanese ancestry were clinically examined, beginning during the period 1965–1968.[12] For 7,833 of these men, data on black tea consumption habits were recorded. Since 1965, newly diagnosed cancer incidence cases have been identified: 152 colon, 151 lung, 149 prostate, 136 stomach, 76 rectum, 57 bladder, 30 pancreas, 25 liver, 12 kidney and 163 at other (miscellaneous) sites. Compared with "almost-never" drinkers, men who habitually drink black tea more than once a day had a four times greater chance of developing rectal cancer.[14]

Cardiovascular and liver disease

A prospective epidemiological study begun in 1986 by researchers in Japan evaluated the relationship between diet and chronic disease in Japanese men aged 40 and older.[15] As daily green tea intake increased from less than three, to four to nine, to greater than 10 cups/day, significant increases in serum HDL and decreases in LDL lipoproteins were found. In addition, green tea consumption was found to significantly improve liver profiles, with aspartate aminotransferase and alanine aminotransferase levels decreasing significantly with increasing green tea consumption.

DOSAGE

The normal amount of green tea consumed by Japanese and other green tea drinking cultures is about three cups daily or about 3 g of soluble components providing roughly 240–320 mg of polyphenols. For a green tea extract standardized for 80% total polyphenol and 55% epigallocatechin gallate content, this would mean a daily dose of 300–400 mg.

Note. When selecting commercial products, it is important to look for the level of epigallocatechin gallate, as well as total polyphenol content.

TOXICITY

Green tea is not associated with any significant side-effects or toxicity. As with any caffeine-containing beverage, overconsumption may produce a stimulant effect (nervousness, anxiety, insomnia, irritability, etc.).

Table 70.1 World tea production by type

Type	Dry weight (×1000 tons)
Black	1,940
Green	515
Oolong	60
Total	2,515

REFERENCES

1. Graham HN. Green tea composition, consumption, and polyphenol chemistry. Prev Med 1992; 21: 334–350
2. Min Z, Peigen X. Quantitative analysis of the active constituents in green tea. Phytother Res 1991; 5: 239–240
3. Ho C, Chen Q, Shi H et al. Antioxidative effect of polyphenol extract prepared from various Chinese teas. Prev Med 1992; 21: 520–525
4. Khan SG, Katiyar SK, Agarwal R et al. Enhancement of antioxidant and phase II enzymes by oral feeding of green tea polyphenols in drinking water to SKH-1 hairless mice. Possible role in cancer chemoprevention. Cancer Res 1992; 52: 4050–4052
5. Katiyar SK, Agarwal R and Mukhtar H. Green tea in chemoprevention of cancer. Compr Ther 1992; 18: 3–8
6. Mukhtar H, Wang ZY, Katiyar SK et al. Tea components. Antimutagenic and anticarcinogenic effects. Prevent Med 1992; 21: 351–360
7. Wang ZY, Khan WA, Bickers DR et al. Protection against polycyclic aromatic hydrocarbon-induced skin tumor initiation in mice by green tea polyphenols. Carcinogenesis 1989; 10: 411–415
8. Komori A, Yatsumi J, Okabe S et al. Anticarcinogenic activity of green tea polyphenols. Jpn J Clin Oncol 1993; 23: 186–190
9. Stich HF. Teas and tea components as inhibitors of carcinogen formation in model systems and man. Prevent Med 1992; 21: 377–384
10. Yang CS and Wang ZY. Tea and cancer. J Natl Cancer Inst 1993; 85: 1038–1049
11. Ji HT, Chow WH, Hsing A et al. Green tea consumption and the risk of pancreatic and colorectal cancer. Int J Can 1997; 7: 255–258
12. Luo SQ, Liu XZ, Wang CJ. Inhibitory effect of green tea extract on the carcinogenesis induced by asbestos plus benzo(a)pyrene in rat. Biomed Environ Sci 1995; 8: 54–58
13. La Vecchia C, Negri E, Franceschi S et al. Tea consumption and cancer risk. Nutr Cancer 1992; 17: 27–31
14. Heilbrun LK, Nomura A, Stemmermann GN. Black tea consumption and cancer risk: a prospective study. Br J Cancer 1986; 54: 677–683
15. Imai K, Nakachi K. Cross sectional study of effects of drinking green tea on cardiovascular and liver disease. Br Med J 1995; 310: 693–696

CHAPTER CONTENTS

71

Capsicum frutescens (cayenne pepper)

Michael T. Murray, ND

Joseph E. Pizzorno Jr, ND

Capsicum frutescens (family: Solanacea)
Common names: cayenne pepper, capsicum, chili pepper, red pepper, American pepper

GENERAL DESCRIPTION

Cayenne pepper (also known as chili or red hot pepper) is the fruit of *Capsicum annuum*, a shrubby, tropical plant which can grow to a height of up to 3 feet. The fruit is technically a berry. Paprika is a milder and sweeter tasting fruit produced from a different variety of *Capsicum*. Although cayenne pepper is native to tropical America, it is now cultivated in tropical locations throughout the world and has found its way into the cuisine of many parts of the world, particularly south-east Asia, China, southern Italy, and Mexico.

CHEMICAL COMPOSITION

The most important constituents of cayenne pepper are the pungent compounds, with capsaicin being the most prominent (see Fig. 71.1). Typically, cayenne pepper contains about 1.5% capsaicin and related principles. Other active constituents present include carotenoids, vitamins A and C, and volatile oils.

HISTORY AND FOLK USE

The folk use of cayenne pepper is quite extensive. It has been used for:

- asthma
- fever

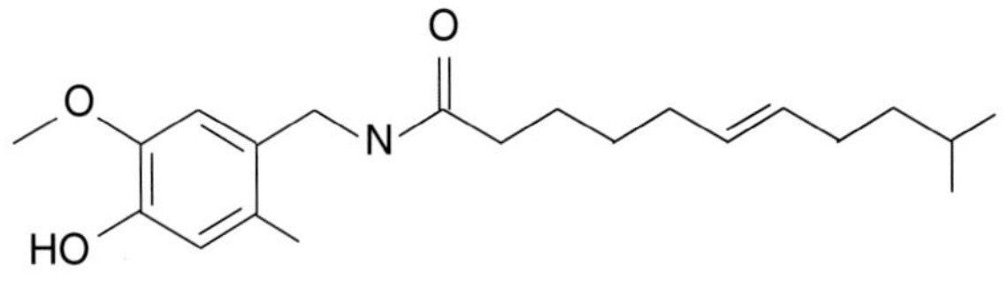

Figure 71.1 Capsaicin.

- sore throats and other respiratory tract infections
- digestive disturbances
- poultices
- cancers.

It was also used as a counter-irritant in the topical treatment of arthritis and neuralgia.

PHARMACOLOGY

The pharmacology of cayenne pepper centers around its capsaicin content. When topically applied to the skin or mucous membranes, capsaicin is known to stimulate and then block small-diameter pain fibers by depleting them of the neurotransmitter substance P. Substance P is thought to be the principal chemomediator of pain impulses from the periphery. In addition, substance P has been shown to activate inflammatory mediators into joint tissues in osteoarthritis and rheumatoid arthritis.[1]

When taken internally, cayenne pepper exerts a number of beneficial effects on the cardiovascular system. In addition to possessing several antioxidant compounds, studies have shown that cayenne pepper reduces the likelihood of developing atherosclerosis by reducing blood cholesterol and triglyceride levels, and platelet aggregation as well as increasing fibrinolytic activity[2–4] (for the significance of these effects see Ch. 133). Cultures consuming large amounts of cayenne pepper have a much lower rate of cardiovascular diseases.

CLINICAL APPLICATIONS

Cayenne pepper should be recommended as a food for its beneficial antioxidant and cardiovascular effects. Although people with active peptic ulcer may be bothered by "spicy" foods containing cayenne pepper, spicy foods in normal individuals do not cause ulcers. In fact, cayenne pepper exerts several beneficial effects on gastrointestinal function, including acting as a digestant and carminative.[5]

Interestingly, capsaicin, although hot to the taste, has actually been shown to lower body temperature by stimulating the cooling center of the hypothalamus.[6] The ingestion of cayenne peppers by cultures native to the tropics appears to offer a way for these people to deal with high temperatures.

The modern clinical use of cayenne pepper has focused on the use of topical capsaicin-containing preparations. Commercial ointments containing 0.025 or 0.075% capsaicin are available over the counter. These preparations may offer significant benefit in a number of conditions, including the pain associated with pain disorders, diabetic neuropathy, cluster headache, osteoarthritis, and rheumatoid arthritis. In addition, topically applied capsaicin may be useful in psoriasis.

Post-herpetic neuralgia

The first studies and approved use for topically applied capsaicin was in relieving post-herpetic neuralgia. Numerous studies now document this FDA approved application. For example, in one study 39 patients with chronic post-herpetic neuralgia (average duration 24 months) were treated with 0.025% capsaicin cream for 8 weeks. During therapy, the patients rated their pain. Nineteen patients (48.7%) substantially improved after the 8 week trial; five (12.8%) discontinued therapy due to side-effects such as intolerable capsaicin-induced burning sensations (four) or mastitis (one); and 15 (38.5%) reported no benefit. The decrease in pain ratings was significant after 2 weeks of continuous application. Of the responders, 72.2% were still improved 10–12 months after the study; with most continuing to apply the cream regularly.

In general, the results of this study are consistent with other studies, i.e. about 50% of people with post-herpetic neuralgia respond to topically applied capsaicin (0.025%).[7–11] Although this may not be a great response, it is better than the 10% response noted in the placebo group. Higher concentration (0.075 vs. 0.025%) may produce better results (as high as 75% response).[12]

Trigeminal neuralgia

Topically applied capsaicin may be effective in reducing the pain of trigeminal neuralgia.[13] In one study, 12 patients were followed up for 1 year after the topical application over the painful area of capsaicin three times a day for several days. Six patients had complete and four patients had partial relief of pain; the remaining two patients had no relief of pain. Of the 10 patients who were responsive to therapy, four had relapses of pain within 95–149 days. There were no relapses following the second therapy for the remainder of the year. These results are quite promising for a condition that usually does not respond to any therapy short of surgery.

Post-mastectomy pain

Topically applied capsaicin may help in the relief of pain after breast reconstruction or mastectomy. In one double-blind study, 23 patients with post-mastectomy pain syndrome (PMPS) applied either capsaicin (0.075%) or vehicle-only cream four times daily for 4–6 weeks.[14] There was a significant difference in jabbing pain, in category pain severity scales, and in overall pain relief scales in favor of capsaicin. Five of 13 patients on capsaicin were categorized as good-to-excellent responses, with eight (62%) having 50% or greater improvement. Only one of 10 cases had a good response to vehicle, with three rated as 50% or better.

In another study, 14 patients with post-mastectomy pain had significant pain relief following application of 0.025% capsaicin cream four times daily for 4–6 weeks.[15] Unpleasant or painful sensations to light touch or pressure in the painful area (hyperaesthesia, allodynia) were also improved.

Mouth pain due to chemotherapy or radiation

In a study conducted at the Yale Pain Management Center, capsaicin was shown to dramatically reduce the pain from mouth sores as a result of chemotherapy or radiation treatment.[16] The interesting feature in this study was the vehicle used to deliver the capsaicin – taffy. The researchers chose taffy because it could be held in the mouth long enough to desensitize the neurons, its sugar decreased the initial burning sensation, and its soft edges would not aggravate sore mouths like a hard candy. All 11 patients in the Yale study said their pain decreased – in two cases stopping entirely – after eating the capsaicin-laced candy.

Diabetic neuropathy

Topically applied capsaicin has been shown to be of considerable benefit in relieving the pain of diabetic neuropathy in numerous double-blind studies.[17–22] In one large double-blind 8 week study, investigators at 12 sites enrolled 277 men and women with painful diabetic neuropathy of the hands and feet; 69.5% of the group applying the capsaicin cream (0.075%) showed improvement compared with 53.4% in those applying only the vehicle cream.

In another study, 40 patients applied either 0.075% capsaicin cream or placebo to their affected extremities daily. After 4 weeks, 76% of treated patients had some pain relief, compared with 50% of placebo patients. In addition, those responding to capsaicin said their pain was cut in half, while those on placebo averaged between 15 and 20% relief.

Cluster headaches

Several studies have found that intranasal application of capsaicin ointment by a physician may relieve cluster headaches. In one double-blind study, patients in acute cluster were randomized to receive either capsaicin or placebo in the nostril for 7 days.[23] Patients recorded the severity of each headache for 15 days. Headaches on days 8–15 of the study were significantly less severe in the capsaicin group versus the placebo group. There was also a significant decrease in headache severity in the capsaicin group on days 8–15 compared with days 1–7, but not in the placebo group. Episodic patients appeared to benefit more than chronic patients.

Arthritis

Topically applied capsaicin may be effective in relieving the pain of osteoarthritis and rheumatoid arthritis. While one study showed it to be more effective in osteoarthritis, another study showed just the opposite.

In the double-blind study showing more effect in osteoarthritis, seven patients with rheumatoid arthritis and 14 patients with osteoarthritis who had painful involvement of the hands applied either capsaicin 0.075% or vehicle-only cream to the hands four times daily. Capsaicin reduced tenderness and pain associated with osteoarthritis, but not rheumatoid arhtritis.[24]

In the study showing greater benefit for rheumatoid arthritis, 70 patients with osteoarthritis and 31 with rheumatoid arthritis received capsaicin or placebo for 4 weeks.[25] The patients were instructed to apply 0.025% capsaicin cream or its vehicle (placebo) to painful knees four times daily. Significantly more relief of pain was reported by the capsaicin-treated patients than the placebo patients throughout the study; after 4 weeks of capsaicin treatment, rheumatoid and osteoarthritis patients demonstrated mean reductions in pain of 57 and 33%, respectively. These reductions in pain were statistically significant compared with those reported with placebo. According to overall evaluations, 80% of the capsaicin-treated patients experienced a reduction in pain after 2 weeks of treatment.

Psoriasis

Excessive substance P levels in the skin have been linked to psoriasis. This finding prompted researchers to study the effects of topically applied capsaicin. In one double-blind study, 44 patients with symmetrically distributed psoriasis lesions applied topical capsaicin to one side of their body and a placebo to the other side.[26] After 3–6 weeks, significantly greater reductions in scaling and redness were observed on the capsaicin side. Burning, stinging, itching, and skin redness were noted by nearly half of the patients initially, but these diminished or vanished upon continued application.

In a more recent study, 197 patients applied capsaicin 0.025% cream or placebo cream four times a day for 6 weeks.[27] Efficacy was based on a physician's evaluation and a combined psoriasis severity score including scaling, thickness, erythema, and pruritus. Capsaicin-treated patients demonstrated significantly greater improvement in physician's evaluation and in pruritus relief, as well as a significantly greater reduction in combined psoriasis severity.

DOSAGE

Cayenne pepper can be used liberally in the diet. Creams containing 0.025 or 0.075% capsaicin can be applied to affected areas up to four times daily.

TOXICITY

Cayenne pepper is generally recognized as safe (GRAS) in the US. Topically applied capsaicin may produce a local burning sensation; however, this effect will go away with time and rarely is severe enough to mean that use of the cream cannot be continued. This was the only adverse effect noted.

REFERENCES

1. Cordell GA, Araujo OE. Capsaicin: identification, nomenclature, and pharmacotherapy. Ann Pharmacother 1993; 27: 330–336
2. Kawada T, Hagihara K, Iwai K. Effects of capsaicin on lipid metabolism fed a high fat diet. J Nutr 1986; 116: 1272–1278
3. Wang JP, Hsu MF, Teng CM. Antiplatelet effect of capsaicin. Thrombosis Res 1984; 36: 497–507
4. Visudhiphan S, Poolsuppasit S, Piboonnukarintr et al. The relationship between high fibrinolytic activity and daily capsicum ingestion in Thais. Am J Clin Nutr 1982; 35: 1452–1458
5. Horowitz M, Wishart J, Maddox A et al. The effect of chilli on gastrointestinal transit. J Gastroenterol Hepatol 1992; 7: 52–56
6. Dib B. Effects of intrathecal capsaicin on autonomic and behavioral heat loss responses in the rat. Pharmacol Biochem Behavior 1987; 28: 65–70
7. Peikert A, Hentrich M, Ochs G. Topical 0.025% capsaicin in chronic post-herpetic neuralgia. Efficacy, predictors of response and long-term course. J Neurol 1991; 238: 452–456
8. Bjerring P, Arendt-Nielsen L, Soderberg U. Argon laser induced cutaneous sensory and pain thresholds in post-herpetic neuralgia. Quantitative modulation by topical capsaicin. Acta Derm Venereol (Stockh) 1990; 70: 121–125
9. Bernstein JE, Korman NJ, Bickers DR et al. Topical capsaicin treatment of chronic postherpetic neuralgia. J Am Acad Dermatol 1989; 21: 265–270
10. Watson CP, Evans RJ, Watt VR. Post-herpetic neuralgia and topical capsaicin. Pain 1988; 33: 333–340
11. Watson CP, Evans RJ, Watt VR et al. Post-herpetic neuralgia. 208 cases. Pain 1988; 35: 289–297
12. Bernstein JE, Bickers DR, Dahl MV et al. Treatment of chronic postherpetic neuralgia with topical capsaicin. A preliminary study. J Am Acad Dermatol 1987; 17: 93–96
13. Fusco BM, Alessandri M. Analgesic effect of capsaicin in idiopathic trigeminal neuralgia. Anesth Analg 1992; 74: 375–377
14. Watson CP, Evans RJ. The postmastectomy pain syndrome and topical capsaicin: a randomized trial. Pain 1992; 51: 375–379
15. Watson CP, Evans RJ, Watt VR et al. The post-mastectomy pain syndrome and the effect of topical capsaicin. Pain 1989; 38: 177–186
16. Nelson C. Heal the burn. Pepper and lasers in cancer pain therapy. J Nat Canc Inst 1994; 86: 1381
17. The Capsaicin Study Group. Effect of treatment with capsaicin on daily activities of patients with painful diabetic neuropathy. Diabetes Care 1992; 15: 159–165
18. David Chad, associate professor of neurology and pathology, Univ. of Massachusetts at Worcester – reported in Med World News 1989; February 27
19. Tandan R, Lewis GA, Krusinski PB et al. Topical capsaicin in painful diabetic neuropathy. Controlled study with long-term follow-up. Diabetes Care 1992; 15: 8–14
20. Tandan R, Lewis GA, Badger GB et al. Topical capsaicin in painful diabetic neuropathy. Effect on sensory function. Diabetes Care 1992; 15: 15–18
21. Basha KM, Whitehouse FW. Capsaicin: a therapeutic option for painful diabetic neuropathy. Henry Ford Hosp Med J 1991; 39: 138–140
22. Pfeifer MA, Ross DR, Schrage JP et al. A highly successful and novel model for treatment of chronic painful diabetic peripheral neuropathy. Diabetes Care 1993; 16: 1103–1115
23. Marks DR, Rapoport A, Padla D et al. A double-blind placebo-controlled trial of intranasal capsaicin for cluster headache. Cephalalgia 1993; 13: 114–116
24. McCarthy GM, McCarty DJ. Effect of topical capsaicin in the therapy of painful osteoarthritis of the hands. J Rheumatol 1992; 19: 604–607
25. Deal CL, Schnitzer TJ, Lipstein E et al. Treatment of arthritis with topical capsaicin: a double-blind trial. Clin Ther 1991; 13: 383–395
26. Bernstein JE, Parish LC, Rapaport M et al. Effects of topically applied capsaicin on moderate and severe psoriasis vulgaris. J Am Acad Dermatol 1986; 15: 504–507
27. Ellis CN, Berberian B, Sulica VI et al. A double-blind evaluation of topical capsaicin in pruritic psoriasis. J Am Acad Dermatol 1993; 29: 438–442

72

Carnitine

Michael T. Murray, ND

Joseph E. Pizzorno Jr, ND

INTRODUCTION

Carnitine is an essential nutrient for the transport of long-chain fatty acids into the mitochondrial matrix. Carnitine (beta-hydroxy / gamma-butyrobetaine) was originally isolated from meat extracts in 1905 and its exact chemical structure was determined in 1932 (see Fig. 72.1). However, despite extensive physiological and pharmacological studies in the 1930s, no physiological role for carnitine could be determined.[1–3] Carnitine's role in human physiology remained a mystery until nearly 50 years after its discovery.

The compound was virtually forgotten until Carter et al[4] created new interest in carnitine in 1952 when they established it as a growth factor for the meal worm *Tenebrio molitor* (hence carnitine's other name vitamin BT). When other species of organisms were also shown to be dependent on carnitine, researchers began to re-examine its role in humans.

Researchers soon found that carnitine was essential in the oxidation of lipids.[1–3] When the first carnitine-deficient human subjects were described in 1973, it stimulated greater investigation.[5] It had always been assumed that an individual could synthesize adequate amounts of carnitine, ingest adequate amounts of dietary carnitine, or meet needs by a combination of both. The discovery that some individuals required supplemental carnitine to maintain normal energy metabolism has resulted in the need to consider carnitine as a vitamin or essential.[6]

Since carnitine can be synthesized (as described below)

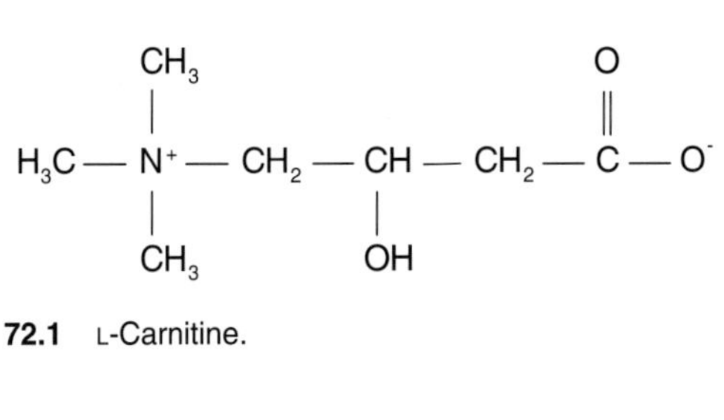

$$H_3C—N^+(CH_3)_2—CH_2—CH(OH)—CH_2—C(=O)—O^-$$

Figure 72.1 L-Carnitine.

from the essential amino acid lysine, many nutritionists and researchers have argued that it should not be considered a vitamin. Others argue that if niacin, which can be synthesized from the essential amino acid tryptophan, can be labelled a vitamin then so should carnitine.

BIOSYNTHESIS

Carnitine is synthesized in humans from lysine with the aid of another essential amino acid, methionine. In non-mammalians, carnitine synthesis begins with stepwise methylation of free lysine by S-adenosyl-methionine to produce trimethyllysine. In mammals, however, protein bound trimethyllysine, rather than free lysine, appears to be the major precursor for carnitine synthesis.[1–3]

Trimethyllysine is then converted through a series of enzymatic reactions to butyrobetaine. This can occur in the liver, kidney, brain, heart, and skeletal muscle. However, the conversion of butyrobetaine to carnitine can only occur in the liver, kidney, and brain, as the enzyme required, butyrobetaine hydroxylase, is only present in these tissues.[1–3]

The synthesis of carnitine is largely controlled by the activity of butyrobetaine hydroxylase. This enzyme appears to be age-dependent. In infancy, the activity of butyrobetaine hydroxylase has been shown to be only 12% of the normal adult mean. By 2.5 years, the activity is 30% of the adult mean, and by 15 years the level is within the standard deviation of the adult mean.[1–3] This data would seem to indicate the importance of preformed-carnitine in breast milk.

As is apparent from Figure 72.2, two essential amino acids (lysine and methionine), three vitamins (ascorbate, niacin, and vitamin B_6), and a metal ion (reduced iron) are required for the synthesis of carnitine. Obviously, a deficiency of any one of these nutrients would result in significantly impaired carnitine synthesis.[1–3]

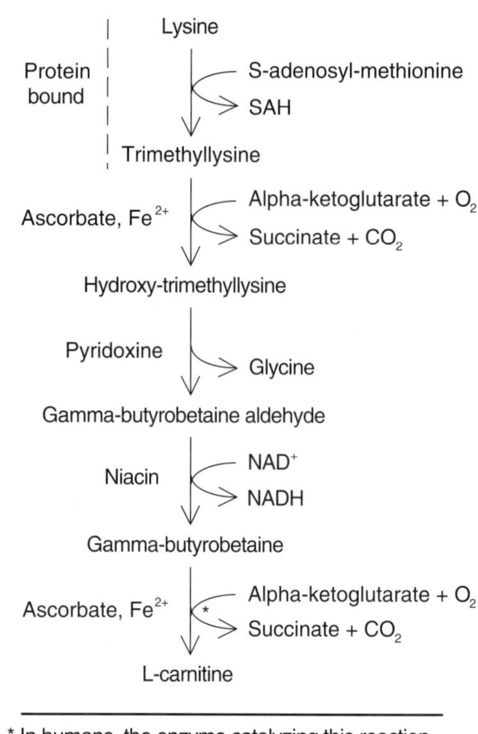

Figure 72.2 Biosynthesis of carnitine.

METABOLISM

Transportation into tissues

The heart and skeletal muscles, as well as many other tissues, depend primarily on fatty acid oxidation as a source of energy. Since they cannot synthesize carnitine, its transport into these tissues is of critical importance.

Specific carnitine binding transport proteins have been identified for several tissues, e.g. cardiac muscle, skeletal muscle, epididymis, liver, and kidney.[1,3] The transport proteins facilitate the transfer of carnitine from the serum into the cells via carrier-mediated transport mechanisms. This active transport mechanism allows the tissues to concentrate carnitine at levels 10 times greater than those found in the plasma.

Excretion and degradation

Urinary excretion of unchanged carnitine is the major route of elimination of carnitine. As the tubular reabsorption of carnitine by the kidneys is extremely efficient, the daily turnover of carnitine is estimated to be only 4–6% of the total body pool of the healthy individual.[1–3] Factors which increase carnitine excretion and degradation are discussed below under causes of carnitine deficiency.

PHYSIOLOGICAL FUNCTIONS

Carnitine's basic function is in the transport of long-chain fatty acids into the mitochondrial matrix and the facilitation of beta-oxidation.[1–3] As acyl-CoA formed in the endoplasmic reticulum or outer mitochondrial membrane cannot penetrate the inner mitochondrial membrane to the site of fatty acid beta-oxidation, the acyl group must be transferred from CoA to carnitine. The acyl-carnitine molecule then transports the fatty acid molecule to the mitochondrial surface of the inner mitochondrial membrane and releases the fatty acid into the matrix where beta-oxidation occurs. This process is summarized in Figure 72.3.

Carnitine has several other physiological functions, including oxidation of the ketoacid analogues of the branched chain amino acids valine, leucine, and isoleucine.[1–3] This function is extremely important during fasting, starvation, and exercise.

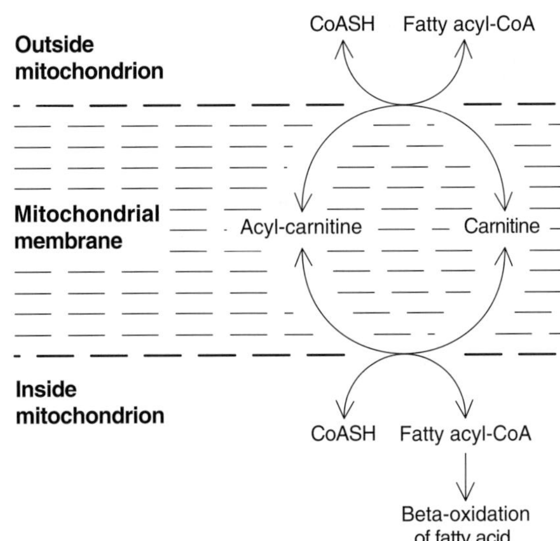

Figure 72.3 Role of carnitine in the transport of long-chain fatty acids through the inner mitochondrial membrane.

Carnitine concentrations are extremely high in the epididymis and spermatozoa, suggesting a role for carnitine in male reproductive function.[1–3] The epididymis derives the majority of its energy requirements from lipids, as do the spermatozoa, during transport through the epididymis. After ejaculation, spermatocytes depend on glycolysis of glucose and fructose and on oxidation of lactate and pyruvate. Carnitine (in the form of acetylcarnitine which is derived from pyruvate) serves as a readily available substrate. The motility of ejaculated sperm correlates positively with acetylcarnitine content.[1,3]

DEFICIENCY

Carnitine deficiency may arise from several causes, as listed in Table 72.1.

Carnitine deficiency states have been classified into two major groups:

- systemic carnitine deficiency
- myopathic deficiency.

Diagnosis of systemic carnitine deficiency can be made using serum or 24 hour urine samples. Total, free, and esterified carnitine levels should be determined. In myopathic carnitine deficiency, diagnosis requires skeletal muscle biopsy.[7]

To date, no patients with primary systemic carnitine deficiency have been identified. The systemic deficiency has always been secondary to some other factor rather than a defect in carnitine synthesis.[1–3,7,8]

The consequences of systemic carnitine deficiency are impaired lipid metabolism and lipid accumulation in the skeletal muscles, myocardium, and liver. Progressive muscle weakness with lipid storage myopathy is found in all patients.[1–3,7] In adults, auxiliary non-mitochondrial oxidation mechanisms are apparently stimulated, resulting in some degree of adaptation. This adaptation occurs in starvation, diabetes, high fat diets, and other causes of secondary carnitine deficiency. Systemic carnitine deficiencies usually respond dramatically to orally administered supplemental L-carnitine.[7,8]

Children are apparently unable to adapt to low carnitine levels as well as adults.[7] Several cases of carnitine deficiency in children, presenting a clinical picture resembling Reye's syndrome (acute encephalopathy associated with altered liver function due to lipid accumulation), have been reported.[8–10]

The clinical presentation of secondary carnitine deficiency in children includes hypotonia, failure to thrive, recurrent infections, encephalopathy, nonketotic hypoglycemia, and cardiomyopathy.[7] Several fatal cases of systemic carnitine deficiency have been reported.[8,11]

In primary myopathic carnitine deficiency, there is an inborn error of carnitine metabolism that is limited to skeletal muscle.[7,8] The defect appears to be in the transport of carnitine into the skeletal muscle as serum carnitine, and the carnitine levels in other tissues are normal. Severe lipid-storage myopathy is the result.

Supplemental carnitine is generally of no value in myopathic carnitine deficiency. Rather, improvements have been noted using diets high in medium-chain triglycerides and low in long-chain triglycerides.[7]

CARNITINE AS A NUTRIENT

Carnitine in the infant diet

It is well known that oxidation of long-chain fatty acids, which requires carnitine, is critical to the survival and

Table 72.1 Causes of carnitine deficiency

- Dietary deficiency of the precursor amino acids lysine and methionine
- Deficiency of any cofactor (such as iron, ascorbic acid, pyridoxine and niacin) required by the enzymes of the lysine to carnitine pathway
- Genetic defect of carnitine biosynthesis
- Defective intestinal absorption of carnitine
- Liver or kidney dysfunction which impairs carnitine synthesis
- Increased metabolic losses of carnitine due to catabolism, impaired tubular resorption, or genetic defect
- Defective transport of carnitine from tissues of synthesis to tissues where it is maximally utilized
- Increased carnitine requirement due to a high fat diet, drugs (e.g. valproic acid), metabolic stress, or disease

normal development of the newborn.[3] Carnitine concentrations in fetal and umbilical cord blood are higher than in maternal blood, suggesting the placenta may actively transport carnitine to the fetus since carnitine synthesis is not fully developed.[3] The initial carnitine concentration in the newborn is dependent upon maternal carnitine concentration.

Supplementation of carnitine during pregnancy may be needed to ensure adequate tissue concentrations in the fetus as well as the mother. Serum carnitine levels are typically lower in pregnant women than non-pregnant women, presumably due to increased excretion.[12,13]

The newborn infant is almost entirely dependent on external sources of carnitine.[3] Breast-fed infants have the best chance of achieving optimal carnitine concentrations. The bioavailability of carnitine from breast milk is significantly greater than that in cow's milk-based formulas,[14] and soy-based infant formulas contain no detectable carnitine.[3] Formula feeding may necessitate supplemental carnitine to achieve normal carnitine concentrations in these infants.

Carnitine administration to preterm infants has potentiated weight gain and growth.[15] In preterm infants, serum values of carnitine decrease dramatically due to limited storage capacity coupled with a decreased ability to synthesize carnitine. Administration of L-carnitine to preterm infants is thought to be very important.

Dietary carnitine content

Analysis of several hundred foods for carnitine content indicates that meat and dairy products are the major dietary sources of carnitine.[3] In general, the redder the meat, the higher the carnitine content. Cereals, fruits, and vegetables contain little or no carnitine. Preliminary studies indicate that the daily diet contains 5–100 mg of carnitine.[3]

CLINICAL APPLICATIONS

Many disease states, in addition to classical as well as secondary carnitine deficiency, may benefit from carnitine administration. There is good evidence to support the assertion that supplemental carnitine may benefit the conditions listed in Table 72.2 and discussed below.

Carnitine is available in several different forms. Always be sure that the form being used is L-carnitine alone or bound to either acetic or propionic acid. Never use the D form of carnitine (discussed below under safety issues). As to which form is best, it really depends upon the objective. For Alzheimer's disease and brain effects, it appears that L-acetylcarnitine (LAC) may provide the greatest benefit. For angina, L-propionylcarnitine (LPC) may be the best choice because the myocardium appears to prefer it to L-acetylcarnitine followed by L-carnitine

Table 72.2 Conditions which may benefit from carnitine supplementation

- Cardiovascular diseases
- Angina pectoris
- Acute myocardial infarction
- Myocardial necrosis
- Arrhythmias and cardiotoxicity induced by drugs
- Familial endocardial fibroelastosis
- Cardiac myopathy
- Idiopathic mitral valve prolapse
- Elevated cholesterol levels
- Elevated triglyceride levels
- Enhancing physical performance
- Alzheimer's disease, senile depression, and age-related memory defects
- Kidney disease and hemodialysis
- Diabetes
- Liver diseases
- Alcohol-induced fatty liver disease
- Liver cirrhosis
- Muscular dystrophies
- Low sperm counts and decreased sperm motility
- Chronic obstructive pulmonary disease
- AIDS
- Inborn errors of amino acid metabolism
- Organic acidurias
- Glutaric aciduria
- Isovaleric acidemia
- Propionicacidemia
- Methylmalonic aciduria
- Toxicity from various drugs

(LC).[16,17] L-Carnitine is, however, the most widely available, least expensive, and best studied form of carnitine.

Cardiovascular disease

Normal heart function is critically dependent on adequate concentrations of carnitine. A deficiency of carnitine in the heart would be similar to trying to run an automobile without a fuel pump. There may be plenty of fuel, but there is no way to get it to the engine. While the normal heart stores more carnitine than it needs, if the heart does not have a good supply of oxygen, carnitine levels quickly decrease. This lack of oxygen leads to decreased energy production in the heart and increased risk for angina and heart disease.

Carnitine is useful in angina due to its ability to improve oxygen utilization and energy metabolism by the myocardium. As a result of improving fatty acid utilization and energy production, carnitine also prevents the production of toxic fatty acid metabolites.[18] These compounds are extremely damaging as they disrupt cellular membranes. Changes in the properties of cell membranes throughout the heart are thought to contribute to impaired contraction of the heart muscle and increased susceptibility to irregular beats, and eventual death of heart tissue. Supplementing the diet with carnitine increases heart carnitine levels and has been shown to prevent the production of fatty acid metabolites which can damage the heart. In addition to angina, all of these effects make carnitine beneficial in recovery from a heart attack, arrhythmias, and congestive heart failure.[19]

Carnitine also exerts a beneficial effect on blood lipids by lowering triglycerides and total cholesterol levels while raising HDL-cholesterol. After 4 months of therapy with L-carnitine in patients with elevated blood lipids, typical changes observed are a 20% reduction for total cholesterol, a 28% decrease in triglycerides, and a 12% increase in HDL levels.[20,21] Due to the higher cost of carnitine compared with other natural agents (e.g. inositol hexaniacinate, garlic, and gugulipid), its use should be reserved for those cases unresponsive to these more cost-effective measures.

Carnitine has also been shown to be of benefit in the treatment of intermittent claudication, which is a condition like angina but instead of the pain occurring in the heart it occurs usually in the calf muscle. Like angina, the pain is described as a cramp or tightness. The cause of the pain is reduced oxygen delivery along with an increase in the production of toxic metabolites and cellular free radicals. Its benefits in peripheral vascular disease are the result of improved energy production during ischemia rather than any effect on blood flow. Nonetheless, good results have been obtained in intermittent claudication and other peripheral vascular diseases (discussed below).

Angina

Numerous clinical trials have demonstrated that carnitine improves angina and heart disease (note that all three commercial forms have been used).[19,22–28] Supplementation with carnitine normalizes heart carnitine levels and allows the heart muscle to utilize its limited oxygen supply more efficiently. This translates to an improvement in cases of angina. Improvements have been noted in exercise tolerance and heart function. The results indicate that carnitine is an effective alternative to drugs in cases of angina.

L-Propionylcarnitine (LPC) may offer the greatest benefit in angina, as well as in other cardiovascular conditions. LPC is taken up by myocardial cells much more rapidly than other forms of carnitine.[16] In one study, LPC (15 mg/kg intravenously) significantly diminished myocardial ischemia as demonstrated by a significant 12 and 50% reduction in ST-segment depression and left ventricular end-diastolic pressure, respectively, during the atrial pacing test.[29] Left ventricular ejection fraction increased by 18%. Recovery of heart function after exercise occurred much quicker in the LPC group compared with the placebo group.

L-Carnitine and LAC have also shown very good results. In one of the larger studies, 200 patients with exercise-induced stable angina received either standard therapy alone (e.g. nitroglycerine, calcium channel blockers, beta-blockers, antihypertensives, diuretics, digitalis, antiarrhythmics, anticoagulants, and hypolipidemics) or in combination with 2,000 mg a day of L-carnitine over a 6 month period.[30] Compared with the control group, the patients on L-carnitine exhibited a significant reduction in premature ventricular contractions at rest, as well as an increased tolerance to exercise as demonstrated by an increased maximal cardiac frequency, increased maximal systolic blood pressure, cardiac output, and reduced ST-segment depression (70% reduction in the L-carnitine group vs. no change in the control group). Reductions in LDL-cholesterol (8%) and triglycerides (12%) were also noted. These results are highly significant and provide a strong rationale for the inclusion of carnitine in patients using standard medical therapy.

Recovery from myocardial infarction

In addition to benefiting angina patients, carnitine has also been shown to be useful in helping individuals recover more quickly from a heart attack.[19] In one double-blind study of 160 patients who had been released from a hospital after a heart attack, the group receiving 4 g of L-carnitine daily showed significant improvements in heart rate, blood pressure, angina attacks, rhythm disturbances, and clinical signs of impaired heart function compared to the control group.[31]

In Italy, a larger study involving 472 patients showed additional benefits.[32] The study was performed to evaluate the effects of L-carnitine administration on long-term left ventricular dilation in patients with acute anterior myocardial infarction. Placebo or L-carnitine was given at a dose of 9 g/day intravenously for the first 5 days and then 6 g/day orally for the next 12 months. Left ventricular volumes and ejection fraction were evaluated on admission, at discharge from hospital and at 3, 6 and 12 months after acute myocardial infarction. A significant attenuation of left ventricular dilation in the first year after acute myocardial infarction was observed in patients treated with L-carnitine compared with those receiving placebo. The percent increase in both end-diastolic and end-systolic volumes from admission to 3, 6 and 12 month evaluation was significantly reduced in the L-carnitine group.

Arrhythmias

In double-blind trials, reductions in the use of conventional antiarrhythmic drugs have occurred in patients with angina who have received carnitine.[19]

Congestive heart failure

Several double-blind clinical studies have shown that carnitine (again, LPC appears to be more effective than LC or LAC) improves cardiac function in patients with congestive heart failure.[19] In one double-blind study of LPC versus placebo in a group of 60 patients with mild to moderate (II and III NYHA class) congestive heart failure LPC produced demonstrable benefit.[33] The group was made up of men and women aged between 48 and 73 years in chronic treatment with digitalis and diuretics for at least 3 months and who still displayed symptoms. Thirty of these patients were chosen randomly and for 180 days received 500 mg of LPC three times a day in addition to their usual treatment. At basal conditions and after 30, 90 and 180 days, the maximum exercise time was evaluated using an exercise tolerance test performed on an ergometer bicycle and the left ventricular ejection fraction was tested by means of echocardiography. After 1 month of treatment, the patients treated with LPC, compared with the control group, showed significant increases in the values of both tests, increases which became even more evident after 90 and 180 days. At the stated times, the increases in the maximum exercise time were 16.4, 22.9, and 25.9%, respectively. The ventricular ejection fraction increased by 8.4, 11.6 and 13.6%, respectively.

In another double-blind study in similar patients, at the end of 6 months of treatment, maximum exercise time on the treadmill increased 16.4% and the ejection fraction increased by 12.1% after 180 days in the group treated with PLC at a dosage of 1 g twice daily.[34]

Peripheral vascular disease

All three forms of carnitine (2–4 g daily) have been shown to improve the walking distance without pain in patients with intermittent claudication. Presumably this improvement is the result of improved energy metabolism within the muscle, as carnitine was not shown to improve blood flow to the calf. LPC appears to offer better effects than either L-carnitine or LAC.[35,36] However, in one double-blind study, L-carnitine at a dosage of 2 g twice daily demonstrated a 75% increase in walking distance after only 3 weeks of therapy.[37]

Enhancing physical performance

The ability to enhance exercise tolerance and physical performance with carnitine may not be limited to patients with cardiovascular disease, as carnitine supplementation has also been shown to be of benefit in healthy subjects and athletes. Efficient utilization of fatty acids by skeletal muscle, like the myocardium, is also dependent upon adequate supply of carnitine.

Carnitine supplementation (usually 2 g two to three times daily) has resulted in significant improvements in cardiovascular function in response to exercise in several double-blind studies in both athletes and normal subjects.[38–40] Compared to control groups, the subjects on carnitine have shown not only improvements in exercise intensity or time, but also evidence of improved energy metabolism within the muscle (lowered blood lactic acid and free fatty acid levels). Obviously, the improved production of energy by the exercising muscle as well as improved heart function could be responsible for carnitine's ability to enhance physical performance.

Although at least three studies showed the benefits of carnitine on exercise performance to be no more of value than a placebo, carnitine supplementation should still be viewed as beneficial, especially in endurance-related events.[41–43] The reason behind this statement is the fact that studies have demonstrated that carnitine improves energy producing enzymes levels in long distance runners.[44] These athletes received either a placebo or 2 g of L-carnitine twice daily for 4 weeks. Runners receiving the L-carnitine showed a significant increase in enzymes involved in energy production (cytochrome c reductase and cytochrome oxidase). In contrast, there were no changes in the placebo group.

It is interesting to note that normal subjects taking carnitine have improved cardiovascular function and a more rapid return of heart rate to the resting rate after exercise.[45] The significance of these improvements is that it appears that carnitine is able to mimic the benefits in heart and vascular function produced by regular exercise training without working up a sweat.

Alzheimer's disease, senile depression, and age-related memory defect

A great deal of research has been conducted over the last decade with L-acetylcarnitine (LAC) in the treatment of Alzheimer's disease, senile depression, and age-related memory defects. As described above, LAC is a molecule composed of acetic acid and L-carnitine bound together. This reaction occurs naturally in the human brain, and therefore it is not exactly known how much greater an effect is noted with LAC vs. L-carnitine or PAC. However, LAC is thought to be substantially more active than these other forms of carnitine in conditions involving the brain.[46,47]

LAC is structurally related to acetylcholine, a major neurotransmitter responsible for memory and proper brain function. In Alzheimer's disease, and to a lesser extent the normal aging human brain, there is a defect in the utilization of acetylcholine. The close structural similarity between LAC and acetylcholine led researchers to begin testing LAC in Alzheimer's disease. The results have been encouraging.

Researchers have now shown that LAC does indeed mimic acetylcholine and is of benefit not only in patients with early-stage Alzheimer's disease, but also in elderly patients who are depressed or who have impaired memory.[47] It has also been shown to act as a powerful antioxidant within the brain cell, to stabilize cell membranes, to improve energy production within the brain cell as well as enhancing or mimicking the function of acetylcholine.[48]

The results in delaying the progression of Alzheimer's disease have been outstanding. The studies have been well controlled and extremely thorough.[46,49–51] For example, in one study, LAC (2 g twice daily) or placebo was given to 130 patients with Alzheimer's disease over the course of 1 year.[51] The patients were evaluated by 14 different outcome measures such as assessment scales, cognitive function tests, memory tests, and physician evaluations. The group receiving the LAC had better outcome scores in all cases.

The memory impairment need not be as severe as in Alzheimer's disease in order for LAC to demonstrate benefit.[52–54] In one double-blind study of 236 elderly subjects with mild mental deterioration, as evident by detailed clinical assessment, the group receiving 1,500 mg of LAC daily demonstrated significant improvement in mental function, particularly in memory and constructional thinking.[54]

Many of the elderly suffer from depression not only as a result of experiencing a great deal of loss in their lives, but also because of the biochemical changes in the brain associated with aging. LAC has been shown to improve depression in elderly subjects in double-blind studies using assessment scales standard to scientific research of antidepressant drugs (e.g. Hamilton Depression Scale, Clinical Global Impression, Sandoz Clinical Assessment, etc.). The usual dosage has been 500 mg three times daily. Those elderly subjects with the highest depression scores are usually the ones who benefit the most from acetyl-L-carnitine.[55,56]

Down syndrome

Given that both Down syndrome and Alzheimer's disease are characterized by a deficit in cholinergic transmission, a study was conducted to assess the effect of a 90 day treatment with L-acetylcarnitine (LAC) in individuals with Down syndrome.[57] Findings were evaluated statistically and compared to three further groups of subjects: untreated Down syndrome, mental deficiency due to other cases treated and not treated with LAC. Treated Down syndrome patients showed statistically significant improvements of visual memory and attention both in absolute terms and in comparison with the other groups. No improvement was found in mentally deficient non-Down subjects, so that the favorable effect of LAC appears to be specific for Down patients. An effective dosage is 20 mg of LAC for every 2 pounds of body weight. It is suggested that the action of LAC in these pathologies is related to its direct and indirect cholinomimetic effect.

Kidney disease and hemodialysis

Carnitine supplementation is very much indicated in kidney diseases because the kidney is a major site of carnitine synthesis. Damage to the kidney or reduced kidney function has a profound effect on carnitine metabolism. It is well established that patients undergoing hemodialysis suffer from carnitine deficiency due to the loss of considerable quantities of carnitine during dialysis as well as decreased synthesis. Serum carnitine levels drop nearly 80% during hemodialysis.[1–3]

Carnitine supplementation has been extensively studied in patients undergoing hemodialysis due to chronic renal failure. These studies indicated that L-carnitine supplementation is effective in reducing triglyceride levels while raising HDL-cholesterol levels and thus helps to decrease the risk of heart disease in dialysis patients.[58–61] Carnitine-treated dialyzed patients have also shown additional benefits, including:[62–64]

- disappearance of angina pectoris and arrhythmias occurring during dialysis
- reduction of muscle symptoms including muscle cramps
- increased muscle mass
- significant improvement of the chronic anemia seen in these patients as demonstrated by an increased hematocrit, hemoglobin, and red blood cell count.

In the last decade, a major advancement in the treatment of the anemia associated with hemodialysis is recombinant human erythropoietin (EPO) therapy. However, this therapy is expensive and is not without side-effects. In a recent study, L-carnitine (1 g intravenously after every dialysis session) administered for 6 months led to a significant reduction in dosage as well as improvements in membrane fragility and endogenous EPO secretion.[65] Given the high cost of EPO, if doctors are unwilling to follow this procedure, insurance companies should get involved and force dialysis units to employ L-carnitine.

Diabetes

Patients with diabetes have been reported to have reduced serum carnitine concentrations but normal skeletal muscle carnitine levels. Due to the increased risk of atherosclerotic cardiovascular disease and reduced kidney and liver function found in diabetic patients, supplementation with L-carnitine appears warranted.

Carnitine (especially LPC) has also been shown to greatly improve peripheral vascular function, as well as nerve function, in patients with diabetes.[66] The improvement in nerve conduction is largely due to significantly increased conduction velocity.[67]

Liver disease

Carnitine plays an extremely important role in the utilization and metabolization of fatty acids in the liver. There is some evidence that carnitine deficiency within the liver promotes fatty infiltration (also known as steatosis or liver congestion).[68]

Alcohol ingestion is a common cause of fatty infiltration of the liver. It has been suggested that chronic alcohol consumption results in a functional deficiency of carnitine. A functional deficiency means that there is plenty of carnitine around, but its function is inhibited just as if there was a deficiency. Many commonly used agents for fatty infiltration, such as choline, niacin, and cysteine, appear to have little value in relieving alcohol-induced fatty liver. However, carnitine significantly inhibits, and reverses, alcohol-induced fatty liver disease.[69]

Since carnitine normally facilitates fatty acid transport and oxidation in the mitochondria, a high liver carnitine level may be needed to handle the increased fatty acid load produced by alcohol consumption or other liver injury.[70] Supplemental carnitine has been shown to reduce free fatty acid levels in patients with liver cirrhosis, and to reduce serum triglycerides and liver enzyme levels while elevating HDL-cholesterol in alcohol-induced fatty liver disease.[68–70]

Carnitine's use in liver disorders associated with fatty infiltration appears warranted, especially when these changes are due to the ingestion of alcohol or exposure to xenobiotics (man-made chemicals toxic to biological processes such as pesticides and herbicides).

Muscular dystrophies

Patients with various muscular dystrophies have reduced levels of carnitine in their skeletal muscles.[71–73] Although levels were not as low as those observed in patients with classical myopathic carnitine deficiency, the low carnitine levels are thought to contribute to the muscular weakness experienced by these patients. Unfortunately, for some reason it has not been determined if supplemental carnitine would be of any value in patients with muscular dystrophy.

Low sperm counts and decreased sperm motility

In the human sperm, high carnitine concentrations are critical to sperm energy metabolism. Several studies have shown that the level of free carnitine in the seminal fluid is inversely correlated with sperm count and motility.[74,75] The lower the carnitine content, the more likely it is that a man is infertile.

Given the known physiological role of carnitine in sperm function and its link to male infertility, a recent study was designed to assess the therapeutic effect of carnitine in men with low sperm counts and depressed sperm motility.[76] One hundred men selected from infertility clinics participated in the "Italian Study Group on carnitine and male infertility". Each subject was given 3,000 mg of L-carnitine daily for 4 months.

The results of the study indicated that L-carnitine was able to increase sperm counts and sperm motility, in both a qualitative and a quantitative manner:

- the number of ejaculated sperm increased from 142 to 163 billion
- the percentage of motile sperm increased from 26.9 to 37.7%
- the percentage of sperm with rapid linear progression increased from 10.8 to 18%
- the mean sperm velocity increased from 28.4% to 32.5%.

The results are even more impressive if only the patients with the poorest sperm motility are studied. This subgroup saw even more significant gains on all parameters. For example, the percentage of motile sperm increased from 19.3 to 40.9% and the percentage of sperm with rapid linear progression increased from 3.1 to 20.3%.

Chronic obstructive pulmonary disease

Patients with chronic respiratory insufficiency are often severely affected by even the simplest physical activity. Treatment with L-carnitine (2 g three times/day) resulted in significant improvements in exercise capability.[77]

AIDS

Several reports indicate that systemic carnitine deficiency may be a problem in patients with AIDS. Reduced levels of serum carnitine are most often found in AIDS patients. However, more important is the carnitine depletion in peripheral blood mononuclear cells (PBMC). In fact, even AIDS patients with normal serum carnitine levels demonstrate low levels of carnitine in white blood cells.[78] Increasing the carnitine content of the PWBC strongly improved lymphocyte function and highlights the importance of carnitine to immune function.

L-Carnitine has been shown to prevent the toxicity of the drug AZT on the mitochondria of the muscle cells.[79] AZT poisons the mitochondria of the muscle, leading to abnormal energy production within the muscle which manifests clinically as muscle fatigue and pain. If L-carnitine is able to prevent this negative effect of AZT in human patients with AIDS, it would be a major improvement in the clinical management of AIDS.

Preliminary studies indicate that L-carnitine supplementation can improve immune function and reduce the level of HIV-induced immune suppression. When AIDS patients being treated with AZT were given 6 g of L-carnitine/day, it led to significant increased PBMC proliferation and reduced blood levels of triglycerides and circulating tumor necrosis factor.[80] Given the suspected systemic carnitine deficiency along with the tremendous safety of use, carnitine supplementation appears to be warranted in AIDS.

Inborn errors of amino acid metabolism

The use of carnitine in the treatment of inborn errors of metabolism involving the urea acid cycle appears to be well justified. Preliminary studies have shown impressive therapeutic response to L-carnitine supplementation in cases of glutaric aciduria, isovaleric acidemia, propionicacidemia, and methylmalonic aciduria.[81–84]

Protection against drug toxicity

Carnitine has been shown to protect against the damaging effects on the heart produced by the chemotherapy drug adriamycin.[85] Carnitine has also been shown to improve the symptoms attributed to anticonvulsant medications such as valproic acid (trade names: Depa, Depakene, Depakote, and Deproic) and carbamazepine (trade names: Epitol and Tegretol).[86,87] However, the most recent study has challenged the need to administer carnitine prophylactically since no significant differences were noted in well-being scores between the carnitine group and the placebo group.[88]

DOSAGE

The daily dosage of L-carnitine in all of its forms has typically been between 1,500 and 4,000 mg in divided doses. Given the safety of carnitine, it appears to be better to err on the side of taking too much rather than too little. The exception is in patients undergoing hemodialysis. A paradoxical effect on triglyceride levels and platelet aggregation in patients on hemodialysis has been reported.[89] Slightly higher doses were used (3 g/day) compared with other studies of supplementation in chronic renal failure (typical dose 20 mg/kg body weight or 2 g/day). In addition, the study size was extremely small, and the results are in conflict with other studies using similar doses. However, it appears wise to reduce the risk of this effect by using lower doses and carefully monitoring patients with impaired renal function.

TOXICOLOGY

L-Carnitine is extremely safe, with no significant side-effects ever being reported in any of the human clinical studies. Again, it is important to mention that only L-carnitine should be used. The D form, the mirror image of the L form, has produced side-effects indicating that it interferes with the natural L form of carnitine. Patients undergoing hemodialysis given a mixture containing D,L-carnitine for 45 days experienced muscle pain and loss of muscle function presumably due to lack of energy.[90] The symptoms disappeared upon cessation of D,L-carnitine supplementation. Subsequent studies showed that D-carnitine produces an L-carnitine deficiency in cardiac and skeletal muscle.[91] While L-carnitine results in significant improvement in exercise tolerance in angina patients, D,L-carnitine actually dangerously reduces exercise tolerance in these patients.[92]

Interactions

There are no known adverse interactions between carnitine and any drug or nutrient. Carnitine and coenzyme Q_{10} appear to work synergistically when combined.[93] The same is true for pantethine.[94]

Perhaps the most important interaction is the one with choline. In young adult women, daily choline supplementation (20 mg/kg body weight) resulted in a 75% lower urinary carnitine excretion than in controls, without significantly altering plasma carnitine concentrations. Studies in guinea pigs demonstrated that choline supplementation resulted in a significantly lower urinary excretion and higher skeletal muscle carnitine concentrations. These studies indicate that choline supplementation results in a conservation of carnitine and may increase intracellular carnitine levels.[95]

REFERENCES

1. Bremer J. Carnitine – metabolism and function. Physiol Rev 1983; 63: 1420–1480
2. Bamji MS. Nutritional and health implications of lysine carnitine relationship. Wld Rev Nutr Diet 1984; 44: 185–211
3. Borum PR. Carnitine. Ann Rev Nutr 1983; 3: 233–259
4. Carter HE, Bhattacharyya PK, Weidman KR et al. Chemical studies on vitamin BT isolation and characterization as carnitine. Arch Biochem Biophys 1952; 38: 405–416
5. Engel AG, Angelini C. Carnitine deficiency of human skeletal muscle with associated lipid storage myopathy: a new syndrome. Science 1973; 179: 899–902
6. Borum PR, Bennett SG. Carnitine as an essential nutrient. J Am Coll Nutr 1986; 5: 177–182
7. Gilbert EF. Carnitine deficiency. Pathology 1985; 17: 161–169
8. Winter SC, Szabo-Aczel S, Curry CJR et al. Plasma carnitine deficiency, clinical observations in 51 pediatric patients. AJDC 1987; 141: 660–665
9. Glasgow AM, Eng G, Engel AG. Systemic carnitine deficiency simulating recurrent Reye syndrome. J Pediatr 1980; 96: 889–891
10. Chapoy PR, Angelini C, Brown WJ et al. Systemic carnitine deficiency. A treatable inherited lipid storage disease presenting as Reye's syndrome. New Engl J Med 1980; 303: 1389–1394
11. Rebouche CJ, Engel AG. Carnitine metabolism and deficiency syndromes. Mayo Clin Proc 1983; 58: 533–540

12. Scholte HR, Stinis JT, Jennekens FGI. Low carnitine levels in serum of pregnant women. New Engl J Med 1979; 299: 1079–1080
13. Cederblad G, Fahraeus L, Lindgren K. Plasma carnitine and renal-carnitine clearance during pregnancy. Am J Clin Nutr 1986; 44: 379–383
14. Warshaw JB, Curry E. Comparison of serum carnitine and ketone body concentrations in breast and in formula-fed infants. J Pediatr 1980; 97: 122–125
15. Ardissone P, Baccolla D, Berberis L et al. The effects of treatment with L-carnitine of hypoglycemia in pre-term AGA infants. Curr Ther Res 1985; 38: 256–264
16. Siliprandi N et al. Transport and function of L-carnitine and L-propionylcarnitine. Relevance to some cardiac myopathies and cardiac ischemia. Z Cardiol 1987; 76: 34–40
17. Paulson DJ, Traxler J, Schmidt M. Protection of the ischaemic myocardium by L-propionylcarnitine. Effects on the recovery of cardiac output after ischaemia and repurfusion, carnitine transport, and fatty acid oxidation. Cardiovasc Res 1986; 20: 336–341
18. Opie LH. Role of carnitine in fatty acid metabolism of normal and ischemic myocardium. Am Heart J 1979; 97: 373–378
19. Goa KL, Brogden RN. L-carnitine – A preliminary review of its pharmacokinetics, and its therapeutic use in ischemic cardiac disease and primary and secondary carnitine deficiencies in relationship to its role in fatty acid metabolism. Drugs 1987; 34: 1–24
20. Pola P. Statistical evaluation of long-term L-carnitine therapy in hyperlipoproteinemias. Drugs Exp Clin Res 1983; 9: 925–934
21. Pola P. Carnitine in the therapy of dyslipidemic patients. Curr Ther Res 1980; 27: 208–215
22. Silverman NA, Schmitt G, Vishwanath M et al. Effect of carnitine on myocardial function and metabolism following global ischemia. Ann Thor Surg 1985; 40: 20–25
23. Cherchi A, Lai C, Angelinno F et al. Effects of L-carnitine on exercise tolerance in chronic stable angina. A multicenter, double-blind, randomized, placebo controlled crossover study. Int J Clin Pharm Ther Toxicol 1985; 23: 569–572
24. Orlando G, Rusconi C. Oral L-carnitine in the treatment of chronic cardiac ischemia in elderly patients. Clin Trials J 1986; 23: 338–344
25. Kamikawa T, Suzuki Y, Kobayaashi A et al. Effects of L-carnitine on exercise tolerance in patients with stable angina pectoris. Jap Heart J 1984; 25: 587–597
26. Kosolcharoen P, Nappi J, Peruzzi P et al. Improved exercise tolerance after administration of carnitine. Curr Ther Res 1981; 30: 753–764
27. Pola P, Savi L, Serricchio M et al. Use of physiological substance, acetyl-carnitine, in the treatment of angiospastic syndromes. Drugs Exp Clin Res 1984; X: 213–217
28. Lagioia R, Scrutinio D, Mangini SG. Propionyl-L-carnitine. a new compound in the metabolic approach to the treatment of effort angina. Int J Cardiol 1992; 34: 167–172
29. Bartels GL, Remme WJ, Pillay M. Effects of L-propionylcarnitine on ischemia-induced myocardial dysfunction in men with angina pectoris. Am J Cardiol 1994; 74: 125–130
30. Cacciatore L, Cerio R, Ciarimboli M. The therapeutic effect of L-carnitine in patients with exercise-induced stable angina. A controlled study. Drugs Exp Clin Res 1991; 17: 225–335
31. Davini P, Bigalli A, Lamanna F. Controlled study on L-carnitine therapeutic efficacy in post-infarction. Drugs Exp Clin Res 1992; 18: 355–365
32. Iliceto S, Scrutinio D, Bruzzi P. Effects of L-carnitine administration on left ventricular remodeling after acute anterior myocardial infarction. The L-Carnitine Ecocardiografia Digitalizzata Infarto Miocardico (CEDIM) Trial. J Am Coll Cardiol 1995; 26: 380–387
33. Mancini M, Rengo F, Lingetti M. Controlled study on the therapeutic efficacy of propionyl-L-carnitine in patients with congestive heart failure. Arzneim Forsch 1992; 42: 1101–1104
34. Pucciarelli G, Mastursi M, Latte S. The clinical and hemodynamic effects of propionyl-L-carnitine in the treatment of congestive heart failure. Clin Ter 1992; 141: 379–384
35. Brevetti G, Perna S, Sabba C. Superiority of L-propionylcarnitine vs L-carnitine in improving walking capacity in patients with peripheral vascular disease. An acute, intravenous, double-blind, cross-over study. Eur Heart J 1992; 13: 251–255
36. Sabba C, Berardi E, Antonica G. Comparison between the effect of L-propionylcarnitine, L-acetylcarnitine and nitroglycerin in chronic peripheral arterial disease. A haemodynamic double blind echo-Doppler study. Eur Heart J 1994; 15: 1348–1352
37. Brevetti G, Chiariello M, Ferulano G. Increases in walking distance in patients with peripheral vascular disease treated with L-carnitine. A double-blind, cross-over study. Circulation 1988; 77: 767–773
38. Dragan AM et al. Studies concerning some acute biological changes after exogenous administration of 1 g L-carnitine in elite athletes. Physiologie 1987; 24: 231–234
39. Dragan GI, Vasiliu A, Georgescu E. Studies concerning acute and chronic effects of L-carnitine on some biological parameters. Physiologie 1987; 24: 23–28
40. Dragan GI, Wagner W, Ploesteaunu E. Studies concerning the ergogenic value of protein supply and L-carnitine in elite junior cyclists. Physiologie 1988; 25: 129–132
41. Soop M, Bjorkman O, Cederblad G. Influence of carnitine supplementation on muscle substrate and carnitine metabolism during exercise. J Appl Physiol 1988; 64: 2394–2399
42. Greig C, Finch KM, Jones DA. The effect of oral supplementation with L-carnitine on maximum and submaximum exercise capacity. Eur J Appl Physiol 1985; 54: 131–135
43. Marconi C, Sassi G, Carpinelli A. Effects of L-carnitine loading on the aerobic and anaerobic performance of endurance athletes. Eur J Appl Physiol 1985; 54: 131–135
44. Huertas R, Campos Y, Diaz E. Respiratory chain enzymes in muscle of endurance athletes. Effect of L-carnitine. Biochem Biophys Res Commun 1992; 188: 102–107
45. Dal Negro R et al. Changes in physical performance of untrained volunteers: effects of L-carnitine. Clin Trials J 1986; 23: 242–248
46. Bowman B. Acetyl-carnitine and Alzheimer's disease. Nutrition Reviews 1992; 50: 142–144
47. Carta A, Calvani M, Bravi D. Acetyl-L-carnitine and Alzheimer's disease. Pharmacological considerations beyond the cholinergic sphere. Ann NY Acad Sci 1993; 695: 324–326
48. Calvani M, Carta A, Caruso G. Action of acetyl-L-carnitine in neurodegeneration and Alzheimer's disease. Ann NY Acad Sci 1993; 663: 483–486
49. Pettegrew JW, Klunk WE, Panchalingam K. Clinical and neurochemical effects of acetyl-L-carnitine in Alzheimer's disease. Neurobiol Aging 1995; 16: 1–4
50. Sano M, Bell K, Cote L. Double-blind parallel design pilot study of acetyl levocarnitine in patients with Alzheimer's disease. Arch Neurol 1992; 49: 1137–1141
51. Spagnoli A, Lucca U, Menasce G. Long-term acetyl-L-carnitine treatment in Alzheimer's disease. Neurology 1991; 41: 1726–1732
52. Passeri M, Cucinotta D, Bonati PA et al. Acetyl-L-carnitine in the treatment of mildly demented elderly patients. Int J Clin Pharmacol Res 1990; 10: 75–79
53. Salvioli G, Neri M. L-acetylcarnitine treatment of mental decline in the elderly. Drugs Exp Clin Res 1994; 20: 169–176
54. Cipolli C, Chiari G. Effects of L-acetylcarnitine on mental deterioration in the aged: initial results. Clin Ter 1990; 132: 479–510
55. Garzya G, Corallo D, Fiore A. Evaluation of the effects of L-acetylcarnitine on senile patients suffering from depression. Drugs Exptl Clin Res 1990; 16: 101–106
56. Tempesta E, Casella L, Pirrongelli C. L-acetylcarnitine in depressed elderly subjects. A cross-over study vs. placebo. Drugs Exptl Clin Res 1987; 8: 417–423
57. De Falco FA, D'Angelo E, Grimaldi G. Effect of the chronic treatment with L-acetylcarnitine in Down's syndrome. Clin Ter 1994; 144: 123–127
58. Gjuarnieri GF, Ranieri F, Toiga G et al. Lipid-lowering effect of carnitine in chronically uremic patients treated with maintenance hemodialysis. Am J Clin Nutr 1980; 33: 1489–1492
59. Lacour B, Di Giulio S, Chanard J et al. Carnitine improves lipid abnormalities in haemodialysis patients. Lancet 1980; ii: 763–765
60. Bertoli M, Battistella PA, Vergam L et al. Carnitine deficiency induced during hemodialysis and hyperlipidemia. Effect of replacement therapy. Am J Clin Nutr 1981; 34: 1496–1500

61. Vacha GM, Giorcelli G, Siliprandi N et al. Favorable effects of L-carnitine treatment on hypertriglyceridemia in hemodialysis patients. Decisive role of low levels of high-density lipo-protein cholesterol. Am J Clin Nutr 1983; 38: 532–540
62. Bellinghieri G, Savica V, Mallamace A et al. Correlation between increased serum and tissue L-carnitine levels and improved muscle symptoms in hemodialyzed patients. Am J Clin Nutr 1983; 38: 523–531
63. Donatelli M, Terrizzi C, Zummo G et al. Effects of L-carnitine on chronic anemia and erythrocyte adenosine triphosphate concentration in hemodialyzed patients. Curr Ther Res 1987; 41: 620–624
64. Golper TA et al. Multicenter trial of L-carnitine in maintenance hemodialysis. Kidney International 1990; 38: 904–918
65. Labonia D. L-carnitine effects on anemia in hemodialyzed patients treated with erythropoietin. Am J Kidney Dis 1995; 26: 757–764
66. Greco AV, Mingrone G, Bianchi M. Effect of propionyl-L-carnitine in the treatment of diabetic angiopathy. Controlled double blind trial versus placebo. Drugs Exp Clin Res 1992; 18: 69–80
67. Morabito E, Serafini S, Corsico N. Acetyl-L-carnitine effect on nerve conduction velocity in streptotocin-diabetic rats. Arzneim Forsch/Drug Res 1993; 43: 343–346
68. Sachan DS, Rhew TH, Ruark RA. Ameliorating effects of carnitine and its precursors on alcohol-induced fatty liver. Am J Clin Nutr 1984; 39: 738–744
69. Sachan DA, Rhew TH. Lipotropic effect of carnitine on alcohol-induced hepatic stenosis. Nutr Rep Int 1983; 27: 1221–1226
70. Noto R, Maugeri A, Grasso R et al. Free fatty acids and carnitine in patients with liver disease. Curr Ther Res 1986; 40: 35–39
71. Borum PR, Broquist HP, Roelofs RI. Muscle carnitine levels in neuromuscular disease. J Neurol Sci 1977; 34: 279–286
72. Carrier HN, Berthiller G. Carnitine levels in normal children and adults and in patients with diseased muscle. Muscle Nerve 1980; 3: 326–334
73. Bresolin N, Freddo L, Tegazzin V et al. Carnitine and acyltransferase in experimental neurogenic atrophies. Changes with treatment. J Neurol 1984; 231: 170–175
74. Bornman MS, du Toit D, Otto B. Seminal carnitine, epididymal function and spermatozoal motility. S Afr Med J 1989; 75: 20–21
75. Menchini-Fabris GF, Canale D, Izzo PL. Free L-carnitine in human semen: its variability in different andologic pathologies. Fertil Steril 1984; 42: 263–267
76. Costa M, Canale D, Filicori M. L-carnitine in idiopathic asthenozoospermia: a multicenter study. Andrologia 1994; 26: 155–159
77. Dal Negro R, Soccatelli D, Pomari C et al. L-carnitine and physiokinesiotherapy in chronic respiratory insufficiency. Clinical Trials J 1985; 22: 353–360
78. De Simone C, Famularo G, Tzantzoglou S. Carnitine depletion in peripheral blood mononuclear cells from patients with AIDS. Effect of oral L-carnitine. AIDS 1994; 8: 655–660
79. Semino-Mora MC et al. Effect of L-carnitine on the zidovudine-induced destruction of human myotubes. Lab Invest 1994; 71: 102–112
80. De Simone C, Tzantzoglou S, Famularo G. High dose L-carnitine improves immunologic and metabolic parameters in AIDS patients. Immunopharmacol Immunotoxicol 1993; 15: 1–12
81. Seccombe DW, James L, Booth F. L-carnitine treatment in glutaric aciduria type I. Neurology 1986; 36: 264–267
82. Sousa CD, Chalmers RA, Stacey TE et al. The response to L-carnitine and glycine therapy in isovaleric acidemia. Eur J Pediatr 1986; 144: 451–456
83. Roe CR, Bohon TP. L-carnitine therapy in propionicacidemia. Lancet 1982; i: 1411–1412
84. Roe CR, Hoppel CL, Stacey TE et al. Metabolic response to carnitine in methylmalonic aciduria. Arch Dis Child 1983; 58: 916–920
85. Furitano G, Paterna S, Perricone R et al. Polygraphic evaluation of effects of carnitine in patients on adriamycin treatment. Drugs Exp Clin Res 1984; 10: 107–111
86. O'Conner JE, Costell M, Miguez MP et al. Influence of the route of administration on the protective effect of L-carnitine on acute hyperammonemia. Biochem Pharmacol 1986; 18: 3173–3176
87. Matsuda I, Ohtani Y, Ninomiya N. Renal handling of carnitine in children with carnitine deficiency and hyperammonemia associated with valproate therapy. J Pediatr 1986; 109: 131–134
88. Freeman JM. Does carnitine administration improve the symptoms attributed to anticonvulsant medications? A double-blinded, crossover study. Pediatrics 1994; 93: 893–895
89. Weschler A, Aviram M, Levin M et al. High dose of L-carnitine increases platelet aggregation and plasma triglyceride levels in uremic patients on hemodialysis. Nephron 1984; 38: 120–124
90. Bazzato G, Mezzina C, Ciman M et al. Myasthenia-like syndrome associated with carnitine in patients on long-term dialysis. Lancet 1979; i: 1041–1042
91. Paulson DJ, Shug AL. Tissue specific depletion of L-carnitine in rat heart and skeletal muscle by D-carnitine. Life Sci 1981; 28: 2931–2938
92. Watanabe S, Ajisaka R, Masuoka T. Effects of L- and DL-carnitine on patients with impaired exercise tolerance. Jpn Heart J 1995; 36: 319–331
93. Bertelli A, Ronca F, Ronca G. L-carnitine and coenzyme Q_{10} protective action against ischaemia and reperfusion of working rat heart. Drugs Exptl Clin Res 1992; 18: 431–436
94. Gleeson JM, Wilson DE, Chan IF et al. Effect of carnitine and pantethine on the metabolic abnormalities of acquired total lipodystrophy. Curr Ther Res 1987; 41: 83–88
95. Daily JW 3rd, Sachan DS. Choline supplementation alters carnitine homeostasis in humans and guinea pigs. J Nutr 1995; 125: 1938–1944

CHAPTER CONTENTS

73

Catechin [(+)-cyanidanol-3]

Michael T. Murray, ND

Joseph E. Pizzorno Jr, ND

INTRODUCTION

This naturally occurring flavonoid has been widely used in Europe in the treatment of hepatic disease and other conditions. It is found in high concentrations in *Acacia catechu* (black catechu, black cutch) and *Uncaria gambier* (pale catechu, gambier).[1]

PHARMACOKINETIC STUDIES IN HUMANS

Studies of radiolabeled catechin demonstrate that 55% of the oral dose administered to human volunteers is excreted in the urine.[2] Of this excreted catechin, 70% was excreted within 12 hours and 90% within 24 hours. Urinary excretion of unchanged catechin was quite low (0.1–1.4% of oral dose). The major urinary metabolites (composing three-quarters of the total urinary excretion) are glucuronides of catechin, and 3'-O-methyl-catechin and its sulphate. The majority of metabolites retained the flavanol ring structure. Ring scission is a minor metabolic pathway and results in the excretion of benzoic, hippuric, and phenylpropionic acids.

Unchanged catechin is detected in the plasma between 30 minutes and 12 hours after ingestion, while metabolites persist for at least 120 hours. Researchers have concluded that the rapid rate of absorption, coupled with relatively low plasma levels of the unchanged catechin molecule, suggests that hepatic extraction and localization are extremely efficient, a desirable trait considering catechin's hepatoprotective properties.[1,2]

PHARMACOLOGY

Antiviral and immunostimulatory effects

Many flavonoids have been shown to possess antiviral activity, with quercetin being perhaps the most effective. Catechin has, however, been shown to inhibit infectivity by human viruses (e.g. polio virus, parainfluenza virus type 3, respiratory synctial virus, and herpes simplex type 1).[3] This appears to be due to a direct flavonoid virus interaction.

Perhaps more important, however, are its immune stimulation properties.[4] Catechin and 3′-O-methylcatechin, its major derivative, have been shown to significantly increase spontaneous, pokeweed mitogen- and *Staphylococcus aureus*-induced lymphocyte transformation, and immunoglobulin synthesis. Catechin has also been shown to increase T-cell rosette formation;[5] stimulate cell-mediated immune response (as measured by the leukocyte migration inhibition test); and promote antigen-induced proliferative response in patients with HBsAg-positive chronic active hepatitis.[6]

Many of the immunostimulatory effects of flavonoids may be due to their ability to inhibit the catabolism of cGMP in leukocytes,[7] an action known to augment many immune responses (see Ch. 53 for further discussion concerning cyclic nucleotides' effects on immune functions).

Antioxidant

Catechin has been shown, in vitro and in vivo, to be a powerful free radical scavenger and antioxidant, preventing both environmental chemical- and normal metabolism-induced oxidative damage.[8] Catechin has a sparing effect on glutathione metabolism as well.

Anti-endotoxin effects

The role of endotoxins (lipopolysaccharide cell wall components of Gram-negative bacteria) in the pathogenesis of liver diseases (particularly all types of hepatitis, and alcohol-induced cirrhosis) and associated systemic disorders has been demonstrated by many investigators (see Ch. 54 for a complete discussion).

Under normal conditions, endotoxins, produced by intestinal Gram-negative bacteria, are absorbed into the portal venous circulation and detoxified by Kuppfer cells. Impairment of the reticuloendothelial system (RES), phagocytic function, or the portal-sinusoidal blood flow – i.e. interference of normal endotoxin clearance mechanisms – amplifies the biologic activities of endotoxins (e.g. activation of the alternative complement pathway, lipid peroxidation, and promotion of such calcium-mediated phenomena as smooth muscle contraction and mast cell degranulation).

Catechin's anti-endotoxin effects are both direct – degradation of endotoxin and prevention of free radical-induced damage by the lipid portion of the endotoxin molecule – and indirect – stabilization of biomembranes and interference with the liver adenylate cyclase system (this latter is significant since exotoxins, such as cholera toxin from *Vibrio cholerae,* cause their symptoms by excessive activation of adenylate cyclase which disturbs the cyclic AMP/ATP balance in the cells).[9]

Collagen effects

Catechin affects collagen metabolism in various ways. These include:

- an increase in cross-linkage formation in normal[10] and lathyritic[11] collagen (covalent binding of seven catechin residues per collagen alpha-chain)
- a reduction in prolyl and lysyl hydroxylase activities[12]
- an accelerated conversion of soluble to insoluble collagen in lathyritic,[13] diabetic,[14] and genetically abnormal[15] collagen.

Collagen synthesized in the presence of catechin has been shown to be resistant to the action of collagenase[10] and pepsin.[16] Collagen biosynthesis has variously been reported to be decreased,[12] unaffected,[17] and, in the case of adjuvant arthritis,[18] increased in the presence of catechin. The significance of these effects is discussed below.

Histidine decarboxylase

This enzyme is responsible for converting histidine to histamine. Catechin and other flavonoids have been shown to be potent inhibitors of histidine decarboxylase in vitro[19] and in vivo.[20] This action has wide clinical application, e.g. allergic conditions, peptic ulcers, inflammatory processes, and other conditions where histamine is involved.

CLINICAL AND EXPERIMENTAL STUDIES

Hepatitis

An international workshop in 1981 on the use of catechin in diseases of the liver concluded that the flavonoid has much promise for the treatment of many types of hepatic disease, particularly both acute and chronic viral hepatitis.[1] Catechin has been shown, in numerous double-blind clinical studies, to decrease serum bilirubin levels in patients with all types of acute viral hepatitis (i.e. types A, B, and non-A, non-B).[1,21–27] Furthermore, there is a more rapid relief of clinical symptoms (i.e. anorexia, nausea, asthenia, pruritus, and abdominal discomfort), a more accelerated clearance of HBsAg from the blood, and a greater reduction of SGPT and SGOT levels than in control groups. The hepatoprotective effect of catechin is related to its free radical and antioxidant properties, its anti-endotoxin effects, and its ability to stabilize membranes.

The most recent double-blind study utilizing catechin involved 338 patients with chronic hepatitis B as confirmed by the presence of hepatitis B e antigen (HBeAg).[27] Patients were given either catechin at a daily dose of 1.5 g for 2 weeks, followed by 2.25 g for a further 14 weeks, or a placebo. The HBeAg titer decreased by at least 50% in 44 of 144 cases treated with catechin compared with 21 of 140 cases treated with placebo. The HBeAg disappeared in 16 of the catechin cases and four of the placebo, and a seroconversion was observed in six catechin patients and three placebo patients. The mean HBeAg titer in the catechin group was significantly lower than that in the placebo group at the end of the 16 weeks of therapy. The patients whose HBeAg titers were lowered were largely those with chronic active hepatitis, and they had higher initial values of SGPT, SGOT, and gamma-globulin than the patients whose HBeAg titers remained unchanged. The mean values for these liver function tests also fell significantly in the former subgroup. Catechin was well tolerated, the only notable side-effect being a transient febrile reaction in 13 patients.

Alcohol-induced liver disease

Elevated hepatic NADH:NAD ratios and decreased ATP concentrations are found during ethanol intoxication. These metabolic disturbances, along with the increased production of acetate (as a result of ethanol detoxification), produce cholestasis and induce hepatic lipid accumulation by decreasing fatty acid oxidation and favoring incorporation of fatty acids into triglycerides.[28]

In animal studies, catechin has been shown to correct these aberrations.[28–30] However, clinical studies in humans have failed to show convincing evidence that catechin is of benefit in alcohol-related liver disease.[31,32] This could be a result of insufficient dosage. In the animal studies, the dose is usually 200 mg/kg, compared with 20–40 mg/kg in human studies. Furthermore, the high rate of patient drop-out in long-term studies has prevented adequate evaluation. A recent long-term clinical trial (6 months) demonstrated that 2 g of catechin gave some protection against ethanol-induced hepatic damage, as evidenced by lowering of hepatic enzymes (SGOT, SGPT, and gamma GT).[32]

Peptic ulcer

Catechin, via its ability to inhibit histidine decarboxylase, offers anti-ulcer activity. Experimental studies in guinea pigs and rats have demonstrated that catechin has significant anti-ulcer activity in various models.[19,20,33] In a human clinical study, oral administration (1,000 mg five times a day) resulted in reduced histamine levels in the gastric tissue (determined by biopsy) of normal patients and those with gastric and duodenal ulcers and acute gastritis.[20] It was also demonstrated that the histamine levels, which significantly increase in patients with urticaria and food allergy after the local application of the antigen to the gastric mucosa, could be decreased by the prior administration of catechin.

Postoperative complications

The formation of adhesions is a common and severe problem in surgery, particularly in abdominal surgery. Lower abdominal surgery, particularly appendectomies and gynecological procedures, are often followed by adhesions which may result in pain and obstruction. The incidence of postoperative peritoneal adhesions varies from 67 to 92%.[34] It has been assumed that surgery leads to the stimulation of connective tissue formation, resulting in an overproduction of procollagen and collagen and increased deposition around the damaged or ischemic area.

In rats, catechin, when administered within the first 5 days following the procedure, substantially inhibits adhesion formation following experimental adhesion induction.[35] Catechin, via its inhibition of procollagen and collagen biosynthesis, should also reduce adhesion formation in humans. Intraperitoneal administration was significantly more effective than the oral administration in the experimental study. However, in humans, oral administration may result in sufficient tissue concentrations. Catechin has also been shown, in a double-blind study, to significantly reduce postoperative edema.[35]

Osteogenesis imperfecta (OI)

This heterogenous autosomal dominant bone disease is characterized by defective synthesis of collagen, resulting in impaired connective tissue and bone matrix formation. Prior to the use of catechin for this disorder, treatment was based solely upon orthopedic measures, as no effective medical treatment was available.[36] The main clinical problems in OI are multiple fractures of the long bones in children and progressive collapse of the vertebral bodies in adulthood. Catechin has been shown to reduce fractures. There is also histological, electron microscopic, and biochemical evidence of improvement after treatment.[36,37] Catechin's role in improving collagen defects in OI probably centers around its ability to:

- reduce, by its reduction of lysyl hydroxylase activity, the increased level of hydroxylysine reported in the collagen of many patients with type I OI
- increase the number of cross-links in the collagen matrix (which may be deficient or exhibit delayed maturation in OI)
- improve the supramolecular organization and stability of the collagen fibers
- possibly increase the reduced collagen production occurring in OI.

Rheumatoid arthritis and scleroderma

The effects that catechin has on collagen suggest that the flavonoid would have therapeutic benefit in rheumatoid arthritis and scleroderma, as well as in other collagen diseases. Inflammation and collagen are linked in several ways. Pre-existing collagen is destroyed during the initial stages of inflammation, whereas its biosynthesis is increased in the later stages. Catechin appears to be an ideal agent due to its ability to inhibit the breakdown of collagen caused by either free radicals or enzymes (hyaluronidase, collagenase, and pepsin), coupled with its ability to cross-link with collagen fibers and inhibit pro-collagen biosynthesis.[12]

Catechin was included in a long-term treatment program of 115 patients with generalized scleroderma that brought about arrest of progression in 89% of the patients, and a subtotal or total recovery in more than 40%.[38] Although a number of combinations of collagen inhibitors were used in the study, the combination of catechin with D-penicillamine and L-glutamine was the most effective. Unfortunately, catechin was not used alone.

Cancer

Several epidemiological studies have now shown an inverse correlation between tea consumption and the incidence of several cancers. For example, people in Japan smoke more cigarettes than those in Western countries, yet their incidence of lung cancer is lower. Other studies show a lower incidence of colonic polyps in humans drinking green tea. This protection has been attributed in part to their high tea consumption. This is consistent with laboratory research showing a preventive effect of tea in animal models of lung cancer. In mice models, drinking green tea resulted in lung tumor induction being inhibited by 50%. Green and black tea reduced the incidence of cancer of the lung, forestomach, esophagus, and liver in rats and mice when these were induced by carcinogens. These anti-cancer effects appear to be due to catechin's potent antioxidant activity of tea, lowering the modification of DNA in the tissues by hydroxyl radicals and similar active oxygen compounds.[39]

DOSAGE

Typically, the dosages used have been:

- 1 g three times a day for hepatic disease
- 1 g five times a day for peptic ulcers
- 500 mg three times a day for osteogenesis imperfecta.

TOXICOLOGY

Catechin was initially regarded as being remarkably free from side-effects. However, soon after its introduction in France, rare but serious side-effects began to be linked with catechin. Chief among the serious side-effects were autoimmune hemolysis, febrile reactions, and urticaria. Catechin must be used with extreme caution.

Two different series of case reports highlight the seriousness of side-effects. In the first, six patients who developed hemolysis while receiving catechin were studied.[40] The disorder was episodic in all patients and resolved after discontinuation. The causative antibodies could be demonstrated in all six cases, even when the hemolytic episode had preceded analysis by more than 1 year. It seems that the stable association of catechin with RBC generates antigenic sites against which a heterogeneous immune response is elicited, giving rise to long-lasting drug-dependent antibodies as well as autoantibodies.

In the other series of patients, five patients who received catechin for 4–36 months were presented.[41] Three developed both hemolytic anemia and thrombocytopenia, while two had only thrombocytopenia. After suspending the catechin, the hematological values returned to normal in all of the patients. Catechin-dependent platelet antibodies were detected in four of the five patients, and catechin-dependent red blood cell antibodies were present in three.

REFERENCES

1. Conn H, ed. International workshop on (+)-cyanidanol-3 in diseases of the liver. Royal Society of Medicine International Symposia Series, #47. London: Academic Press. 1981
2. Hackett A, Griffiths L, Broillet A, Wermeille M. The metabolism and excretion of (+)-[14C]cyanidanol-3 in man following oral administration. Xenobiotica 1983; 13: 279–286
3. Kaul T, Middleton E, Ogra P. Antiviral effect of flavonoids on human viruses. J Med Virol 1985; 15: 71–79
4. Brattig N, Diao G, Berg P. Immunoenhancing effect of flavonoid compounds on lymphocyte proliferation and immunoglobulin synthesis. Int J Immunopharm 1984; 6: 205–215
5. Sipos J, Gabor V, Toth Z, Bartok K, Ribiczey P. In vitro effect of (+)-cyanidanol-3 on rosette formation. In: Conn H, ed. International workshop on (+)-cyanidanol-3 in diseases of the liver. Royal Society of Medicine International Symposia Series, #47. London: Academic Press. 1981: p 113–115
6. Vallotton J, Frei P. Influence of (+)-cyanidanol-3 on the leukocyte migration inhibition test carried out in the presence of purified protein derivative and hepatitis B surface antigen. Inf Immun 1981; 32: 432–437
7. Ruckstuhl M, Beretz A, Anton R, Landry Y. Flavonoids are selective cyclic GMP phosphodiesterase inhibitors. Biochem Pharmacol 1979; 28: 535–538
8. Chen H, Tappell AL. Vitamin E, selenium, Trolox C, ascorbic acid palmitate, acetylcysteine, co-enzyme Q, B-carotene, canthaxanthin, and (+)-catechin protect against oxidative damage to kidney, heart, lung and spleen. Free Rad Res 1995; 22: 177–186
9. Scevola D, Magliulo E, Barbarini G et al. Possible antiendotoxin activity of (+)-cyanidanol-3 in experimental hepatitis in the rat. Hepato-gastroenterol 1982; 29: 178–182
10. Pontz B, Krieg T, Muller P. (+)-Cyanidanol-3 changes functional properties of collagen. Biochem Pharmacol 1982; 31: 3581–3589

11. Orloff S, Rao V, Bose S. Effect of certain flavonoids on the crosslinking of lathyritic collagen. Indian J Biochem Biophys 1974; 11: 314–317
12. Blumenkrantz N, Asboe-Hansen G. Effect of (+)-catechin on connective tissue. Scand J Rheumatol 1978; 7: 55–60
13. Ronziere M, Herbage D, Garrone R, Frey J. Influence of some flavonoids on reticulation of collagen fibrils in vitro. Biochem Pharmacol 1981; 30: 1771–1776
14. Tenni R, Tavella D, Donnelly P et al. Cultured fibroblasts of juvenile diabetics have excessively soluble pericellular collagen. Biochem Biophys Res Comm 1980; 92: 1071–1075
15. Francis G, Donnelly P, Di Ferrante N. Abnormally soluble collagen produced in fibroblast cultures. Experientia 1976; 32: 691–692
16. De Luca G, Tenni R, Rindi S, Cetta G, Zanaboni G, Castellani A. (+)-Catechin can improve collagenous protein recovery from growth medium of cultured fibroblasts from normal and osteogenesis imperfecta affected subjects. Ital J Biochem 1980; 29: 305–306
17. Rao C, Rao V, Steinman B. Influence of bioflavonoids on the metabolism and cross-linking of collagen. Ital J Biochem 1981; 30: 259–270
18. Rao C, Rao V, Steinman B. Influence of bioflavonoids on the collagen metabolism in rats with adjuvant arthritis. Ital J Biochem 1981; 30: 54–62
19. Parmar N, Ghosh M. Gastric anti-ulcer activity of (+)-cyanidanol-3, a histidine decarboxylase inhibitor. Eur J Pharmacol 1981; 69: 25–32
20. Wendt P, Reiman H, Swoboda K, Hennings G, Blumel G. The use of flavonoids as inhibitors of histidine decarboxylase in gastric diseases. Experimental and clinical studies. Naunyn-Schmiedeberg's Arch Pharma 1980; 313: 238
21. Blum A, Doelle W, Kortum K et al. Treatment of acute viral hepatitis with (+)-cyanidanol-3. Lancet 1977; ii: 1153–1155
22. Berengo A, Esposito R. A double-blind trial of (+)-cyanidanol-3 in viral hepatitis. In: New trends in the therapy of liver diseases. Karger; Basel 1975: p 177–181
23. Theodoropoulos G, Dinos A, Dimitriou P, Archimandritis A. Effect of (+)-cyanidanol-3 in acute viral hepatitis. In: Conn H, ed. International workshop on (+)-cyanidanol-3 in diseases of the liver. Royal Society of Medicine International Symposia Series, #47. London: Academic Press. 1981: p 89–91
24. Demeulenaere F, Desmet V, Dupont E et al. Study of (+)-cyanidanol-3 in chronic active hepatitis. Results of a controlled multicentre study. In: Conn H, ed. International workshop on (+)-cyanidanol-3 in diseases of the liver. Royal Society of Medicine International Symposia Series, #47. London: Academic Press. 1981: p 135–141
25. Laverdant C. Treatment of polyphasic hepatitis with (+)-cyanidanol-3. In: Conn H, ed. International workshop on (+)-cyanidanol-3 in diseases of the liver. Royal Society of Medicine International Symposia Series, #47. London: Academic Press. 1981: p 131–134
26. Piazza M, Guadagnino V, Picciotto L et al. Effect of (+)-cyanidanol-3 in acute HAV, HBV, and non-A, non-B viral hepatitis. Hepatology 1983; 3: 45–49
27. Suzuki H, Yamamoto S, Hirayama C et al. Cianidanol therapy for HBe-antigen-positive chronic hepatitis: a multicentre, double-blind study. Liver 1986; 6: 35–44
28. Gajdos A, Gajdos-Torok M, Horn R. The effect of (+)-catechin on the hepatic level of ATP and the lipid content of the liver during experimental steatosis. Biochem Pharmacol 1972; 21: 595–600
29. Ryle P, Chakraborty J, Thomson A. Biochemical mode of action of a hepatoprotective drug. Observations on (+)-catechin. Pharmacol Biochem Behavior 1983; 18: 473–478
30. Ryle P, Chakraborty J, Shaw G, Thomson A. The effect of (+)-cyanidanol-3 on alcoholic fatty liver in the rat. In: Conn H, ed. International workshop on (+)-cyanidanol-3 in diseases of the liver. Royal Society of Medicine International Symposia Series, #47. London: Academic Press. 1981: p 185–193
31. Editorial. (+)-Cyanidanol-3. Lancet 1982; i: 549
32. World M, Aps E, Shaw G, Thomson A. (+)-Cyanidanol-3 for alcoholic liver disease: results of a six month clinical trial. Alcohol 1984; 19: 23–29
33. Parmar N, Hennings G, Gulati O. Histidine decarboxylase inhibition. A novel approach towards the development of an effective and safe anti-ulcer drug. Agents Actions 1984; 15: 494–501
34. Rivkind A, Marshood M, Durst A, Becker Y. Cianidanol ([+]-Cyanidanol-3) prevents the development of abdominal adhesions in rats. Arch Surg 1983; 118: 1431–1433
35. Baruch J. Effect of Endotelon in postoperative edema. Results of a double-blind study versus placebo in 32 female patients. Ann Chir Plast Esthet 1984; 29: 393–395
36. Jones C, Cummings C, Ball, Beihgton P. A clinical and ultrastructural study of osteogenesis imperfecta after flavonoid (Catergen) therapy. S Afr Med J 1984; 66: 907–910
37. Cetta G, Lenzi L, Rizzotti M et al. Osteogenesis imperfecta, morphological, histochemical and biochemical aspects. Modifications induced by (+)-catechin. Connective Tissue Res 1977; 5: 51–58
38. Asboe-Hansen G. Treatment of generalized scleroderma with inhibitors of collagen synthesis. Int J Derm 1982; 21: 159–161
39. Exploring the chemopreventive properties of tea. Primary Care and Cancer. American Health Foundation Update 1995; 15: 30–31
40. Salama A, Mueller-Eckhardt C. Cianidanol and its metabolites bind tightly to red cells and are responsible for the production of auto- and/or drug-dependent antibodies against these cells. Br J Haematol 1987; 66: 263–266
41. Gandolfo GM, Girelli D, Conti L et al. Hemolytic anemia and thrombocytopenia induced by cyanidanol. Acta Haematol 1992; 88: 96–99

CHAPTER CONTENTS

74

Centella asiatica (gotu kola)

Michael T. Murray, ND

Joseph E. Pizzorno Jr, ND

Centella asiatica (family: Umbelliferae or Apiaceae)
Synonym: *Hydrocotyle asiatica* L.
Common names: gotu kola, Indian pennywort, South African pennywort, mandukaparni

GENERAL DESCRIPTION

Centella asiatica is an herbaceous perennial plant native to India, China, Indonesia, Australia, the South Pacific, Madagascar, and southern and middle Africa. This slender, creeping plant flourishes in and around water. Although it grows best in damp, swampy areas, centella is often observed growing along stone walls or other rocky, sunny areas at elevations of approximately 2,000 feet in India and Ceylon.[1]

Depending on the environment, the form and shape of centella can change dramatically. In shallow water, centella will form floating leaves, while in dry locations, the leaves are small and thin, and numerous roots are formed.[1]

Typically, the constantly growing roots give rise to reddish stolons. The round-to-reniform, smooth-surfaced leaves, found on furrowed petioles, can reach a width of 1 inch and a length of 6 inches. The leaf margin may be smooth, crenate, or slightly lobed. Usually three to six red flowers arise in a sessile manner or on very short pedicels in axillary umbels at the end of 0.08–0.3 inches long peduncles. The fruit, formed throughout the growing season, is approximately 0.2 inches long with seven to nine ribs and a curved, strongly thickened pericarp.[1]

Historically, the entire plant is used medicinally, with harvesting occurring at any time during the year.[1]

CHEMICAL COMPOSITION

Although the primary pharmacologically active constituents of *Centella asiatica* are known to be triterpenoid compounds,[2] the exact chemical profile of centella is difficult to determine due to duplicate names and contradictory findings. In addition, centella samples from

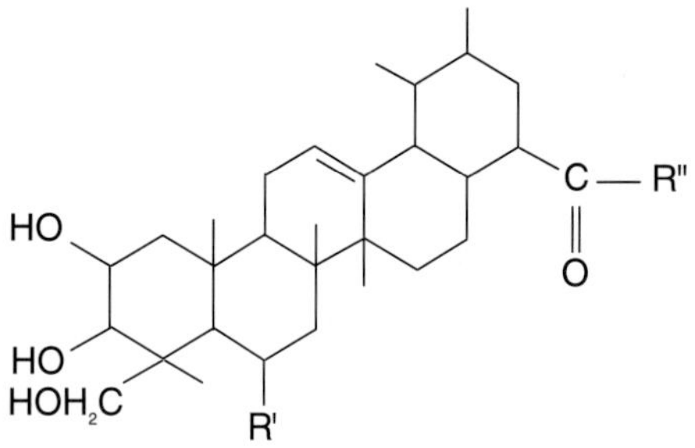

Compound	R′	R″
Asiatic acid	H	OH
Madecassic acid	OH	OH
Asiaticoside	H	O-glucose-glucose-rhamnose
Madecassoside	OH	O-glucose-glucose-rhamnose

Figure 74.1 The triterpene compounds of *Centella asiatica*.

India, Sri Lanka, and Madagascar apparently do not contain the same constituents.[3,4] In India, three (and possibly more) chemically different subspecies of *Centella asiatica* have been found.[5]

The concentration of triterpenes in centella can vary between 1.1 and 8%, with most samples yielding a concentration between 2.2 and 3.4%.[5]

Figure 74.1 below illustrates the major triterpenoid components of *Centella asiatica*:

- asiatica acid
- madecassic acid
- asiaticoside
- madecassoside.

The Madagascar variety is most commonly used to produce standardized extracts and yields triterpene concentrations of asiatic acid (29–30%), madecassic acid (29–30%), asiaticoside (40%), and madecassoside (1–2%).[2]

Centella also contains a green, volatile oil which is composed of an unidentified terpene acetate (which accounts for 36% of the total oil), camphor, cineole, and other essential oils. Centella oil also contains glycerides of fatty acids, various plant sterols such as campesterol, stigmasterol, and sitosterol, and various polyacetylene compounds.[1,2]

Other notable compounds isolated from centella include the flavonoids keampferol, quercetin, and their glycosides, myoinositol, sugars, a bitter substance (vellarin), amino acids, and resins.[1,2]

HISTORY AND FOLK USE

Centella has been utilized as a medicine in India since prehistoric times and is thought to be identical to the plant mandukaparni, listed in the *Susruta Samhita*. Centella was also used extensively as a medicine, both internally and externally, by the people of Java and other islands of Indonesia. The medicinal use of centella in India and Indonesia centered around its ability to heal wounds and relieve leprosy.[1]

In the 19th century, centella and its extracts were incorporated into the Indian pharmacopeia, where in addition to being recommended for wound healing, it was recommended in the treatment of skin conditions such as leprosy, lupus, varicose ulcers, eczema, and psoriasis. It was also used to treat diarrhea, fever, amenorrhea, and diseases of the female genitourinary tract.[1]

In China, the leaves are prescribed for turbid leukorrhea and toxic fevers, while the shoots are used for boils and fevers. The plant is also used in the treatment of fractures, contusions, strains, and snakebites.[1] Centella was also used in China to delay senescence. One of the reported "miracle elixirs of life", centella's reputation as a promoter of longevity stems from the report of Chinese herbalist, LiChing Yun, who reportedly lived 256 years. LiChing Yun's longevity was supposedly a result of his regular use of an herbal mixture chiefly composed of centella.[6,7]

Centella asiatica was first accepted as a drug in France in the 1880s. Since then, extracts of centella have been used in the treatment of many of the same conditions listed above along with those described in "Clinical applications" (p. 653).

Centella, or gotu kola, has aroused much curiosity in American consumers. Many confuse gotu kola with kolanuts and assume gotu kola's rejuvenating activity is nothing more than the stimulant effect of caffeine. However, gotu kola is not related to the kolanut (*Cola nitida* or *Cola acuminata*), nor does it contain any caffeine.

PHARMACOLOGY

Centella asiatica, specifically the triterpenes, exerts remarkable wound-healing activity. Although the exact mechanism of action has not yet been fully determined, a number of interesting observations have been made.

In one of the early pharmacological investigations of centella, Boiteau & Ratsimamanga[8] demonstrated that asiaticoside substantially hastened the healing of experimentally induced wounds. These authors concluded that asiaticoside works selectively in stimulating the rapid and healthy activity of the reticuloendothelial system.

Additional studies on the mechanisms of action of centella's enhancing wound-healing have shown that asiaticoside given orally, by intramuscular injection, or by implantation to rats, mice, guinea pigs, and rabbits produces a wide range of effects, as shown in Table 74.1.

The efficacy of centella in stimulating collagen synthesis has now been demonstrated in human tissue cultures.[13] Interestingly, this research also demonstrated an added benefit when vitamin C was added to the experimental cultures.

The outcome of centella's complex actions is a balanced

Table 74.1 Physiological effects of *Centella asiatica*

- Stimulates hair and nail growth[1,8–10]
- Increases vascularization of connective tissue[1,8–10]
- Increases the formation of mucin and structural glycosaminoglycans like hyaluronic acid and chondroitin sulfate[1,8–10,12]
- Increases the tensile integrity of the dermis[1,8–10]
- Increases keratinization of epidermis through stimulation of the stratum germinativum[1,10,12–14]
- Possesses a eutrophic or balancing effect on connective tissue[1,10]

multiphasic effect on cells and tissues participating in the process of healing, particularly connective tissues. Enhanced development of normal connective tissue matrix is perhaps the prime therapeutic action of *Centella asiatica*.

CLINICAL APPLICATIONS

Obviously, from the brief description of centella's pharmacological activity given above, it is a valuable agent for the healing of wounds. Table 74.2 provides an abridged list of documented clinical applications of *Centella asiatica*. The more popular uses of this valuable plant are discussed below.

Burns

The standardized extract from *Centella asiatica* has been effectively used in the treatment of patients with second- and third-degree burns caused by boiling water, electrical current, or gas explosion. Daily local application and/or intramuscular injections of the extract resulted in excellent results when the treatment was begun immediately after the accident. The extract prevented or limited the shrinking and swelling of the skin caused by skin infection, and it inhibited scar formation, increased healing, and decreased fibrosis.[18,19]

Table 74.2 Clinical applications of *Centella asiatica*

Conditions	References
Anal fissure	15
Bladder ulcers	16, 17
Burns	18, 19
Cellulite	20–25
Cirrhosis	26–28
Dermatitis	20, 29
Fibrocystic breast	30
Hemorrhoids	31
Keloids	32–34
Leprosy	11, 19, 35, 36
Lupus erythematosus	37
Mental retardation	38
Mycosis fungiodes	37
Peptic ulcer	39, 40
Perineal lesions	41
Periodontal disease	42
Retinal detachment	43
Scleroderma	44–47
Skin ulcers	48–55
Surgical wounds	8, 43, 49, 56–61
Tuberculosis	8, 62
Venous disorders	63–75
Wound healing	8, 43, 49, 56–61

Cellulite

Standardized extracts of *Centella asiatica* have demonstrated good results in the treatment of cellulite in a number of clinical studies.[10,20–25] Bourguignon[20] observed the action of the extract on several types of cellulite in 65 patients who had undergone other therapies without success. Over a period of 3 months, very good results were produced in 58% of the patients and satisfactory results in 20%. Other investigations have shown a similar success rate (~80%).[21–24]

The effect of centella in the treatment of cellulite appears to be related to its ability to enhance connective tissue structure and reduce sclerosis by acting directly on fibroblasts (see Ch. 141 for further discussion.)

Cirrhosis of the liver

Darnis et al[26] reported on the therapeutic use of an extract of *Centella asiatica* in alcohol-induced cirrhosis (six patients), cirrhosis of unknown etiology (two patients), and chronic hepatitis. In the cirrhosis patients, improvement in the histological findings and regression of inflammatory infiltration were observed. No effect was observed in the patients with chronic hepatitis. Other reports have supported the use of centella in fibrotic conditions of the liver.[27,28]

Keloids

The standardized extract of *Centella asiatica* has demonstrated impressive clinical results in the treatment of keloids and hypertrophic scars.[32–34] Its mechanism of action appears to be multifaceted, but is basically due to reducing the inflammatory phase of scar formation while simultaneously enhancing the maturation phase of scar formation.

Keloids and hypertrophic scars are characterized by a prolonged inflammatory phase which may go on for months or even years without progressing to the maturation phase. The inflammatory phase is characterized histologically by large numbers of immature, swollen collagen bundles intermingled with inflammatory debris, while the maturation phase is characterized by mature fibrocytes, normal collagen fibers, and few inflammatory cell elements.

In one study, a total of 227 patients with keloids or hypertrophic scars were treated by oral administration with a standardized centella extract (effective dosage 60–90 mg). The centella extract was used alone in 139 patients (the curative group) and 88 used the extract along with surgical scar revision (preventive group).[32]

In the curative group, 116 patients (82%) were found

after 2–18 months to have benefited from the extract, either by relief of their symptoms or by disappearance of the inflammatory phase. In a double-blind substudy of 46 of the 139 patients, 22 out of 27 receiving the extract improved, while only nine of 19 given a placebo improved.

In the preventive group, the centella extract also demonstrated significant positive effect. The therapeutic course in these patients was started a few weeks prior to surgery. If a positive response was observed, the patient was brought to surgery and kept on the centella extract for 3 months. (This method of preselection allowed the researchers to offer other forms of therapy to unresponsive patients.) Clinical improvement was observed in 72 of the 88 patients (79%).

Leprosy

Several investigators have reported impressive clinical results using *Centella asiatica* and its extracts (oral, intramuscular, and/or topical) in the treatment of leprosy in both uncontrolled and controlled studies.[11,19,35,36] The therapeutic response is comparable to that of dapsone, the standard allopathic drug used in the treatment of leprosy.

In addition to its wound-healing activity, it appears that oxyasiaticoside, an oxidized form of asiaticoside, inhibits the growth of the tubercle bacillus in vitro and in vivo by dissolving the waxy coating of *Mycobacterium leprae*.[8]

Improving mental function

Appa Rao et al[38] reported a significant increase in the mental abilities of 30 developmentally disabled children treated with *Centella asiatica*. After a 12 week period, the children were more attentive and better able to concentrate on assigned tasks.

Centella's triterpenes have demonstrated mild tranquilizing, anti-stress, and anti-anxiety action via enhancement of cholinergic mechanisms.[76] Presumably this mechanism is responsible for the enhancement of mental function as well.

Scleroderma

The standardized extract of *Centella asiatica* has been tested in several trials in the treatment of scleroderma (including systemic sclerosis).[44–47] In addition to decreasing skin induration, patients have noticed a lessening of arthralgia and improved finger motility. Presumably the positive therapeutic response is a result of centella's eutrophic effect on connective tissue, thereby preventing the excessive collagen synthesis observed in scleroderma.

Venous disorders

Numerous studies have demonstrated that standardized extracts of *Centella asiatica* are effective in the treatment of venous insufficiency. This appears to be due to centella's ability to enhance the connective tissue structure of the perivascular sheath, reduce sclerosis, and improve blood flow through the affected limbs.[1,10,63–75]

Significant improvement in symptomatology (such as feelings of heaviness in the lower legs, paresthesias, nocturnal cramps, etc.), physical findings (edema, telangiectasias, trophic ulcers, vein distensibility, etc.), and functional capacity (improved venous flow) was observed in approximately 80% of patients in the clinical trials[1,10,63–75] (for further discussion, see Ch. 193).

Wound healing

Standardized extracts of *Centella asiatica* have been shown, in a large number of clinical studies, to greatly aid wound repair.[1,8,10,43,48–61] The types of wounds healed include:

- surgical wounds such as episiotomies and ENT surgeries
- skin ulcers due to arterial or venous insufficiency
- traumatic injuries to the skin
- gangrene
- skin grafts
- schistosomiasis lesions
- perineal lesions produced during childbirth.

DOSAGE

The majority of clinical studies on *Centella asiatica* utilized proprietary formulas available in Europe (e.g. Madecassol, TECA, and Centelase). These standardized extracts contain asiaticoside (40%), asiatic acid (29–30%), madecassic acid (29–30%), and madecassoside (1–2%).

Since the concentration of triterpenes in centella can vary between 1.1 and 8%, it is difficult to calculate an appropriate dosage when simply using the crude plant material. However, since most samples yield a concentration between 2.2 and 3.4%, approximately 2–4 g/day of crude plant material would contain an appropriate quantity of triterpenes, although it is not known if this correlates with the clinical efficacy of the standardized extracts.

Daily dosages of the various forms of centella are as follows:

- Standardized extract (40% asiaticoside, 29–30% asiatic acid, 29–30% madecassic acid, and 1–2% madecassoside): 60–120 mg/day
- Crude dried plant leaves: 2–4 g/day
- Tincture (1:5): 10–20 ml/day
- Fluid extract (1:1): 2.0–4.0 ml/day.

TOXICOLOGY

Centella asiatica and its extracts are very well-tolerated, especially orally.[1] However, the topical application of a salve containing centella has been reported to cause contact dermatitis, although quite infrequently.[1]

While the oral administration of asiaticoside at a dose of 1 g/kg body weight has not proved toxic in toxicology studies, the toxic dose of asiaticoside by intramuscular application to mice and rabbits is reported as 40–50 mg/kg body weight.[1]

Asiaticoside has been implicated as a possible skin carcinogen where repeated applications are used in an experimental animal model.[77] Teratological studies using the extract in rabbits have proved negative.[32]

REFERENCES

1. Kartnig T. Clinical applications of *Centella asiatica* (L.) Urb. Herbs Spices Med Plants 1988; 3: 146–173
2. Castellani C, Marai A, Vacchi P. The *Centella asiatica*. Boll Chim Farm 1981; 120: 570–605
3. Battacharya SC. Constituents of *Centella asiatica*. I. Examination of the Ceylonese variety. J Ind Chem Soc 1956; 33: 579–586
4. Battacharya SC. Constituents of *Centella asiatica*. I. Examination of the Indian variety. J Ind Chem Soc 1956; 33: 893–898
5. Rao PS, Seshadri TR. Variation in the chemical composition of Indian samples of *Centella asiatica*. Curr Sci 1969; 38: 77–79
6. Duke JA. *Handbook of Medicinal Herbs*. Boca Raton, FL: CRC Press. 1985
7. Tyler V, Brady L, Robbers J. *Pharmacognosy*, 8th edn. Philadelphia, PA: Lea & Febiger. 1981
8. Boiteau P, Ratsimamanga AR. Asiaticoside extracted from *Centella asiatica*, its therapeutic uses in the healing of experimental or refractory wounds, leprosy, skin tuberculosis, and lupus. Therapie 1956; 11: 125–149
9. Boiteau P, Nigeon-Dureuil M, Ratsimamanga AR. Action of asiaticoside on reticuloendothelial tissue. Acad Sci Compt Rend 1951; 232: 760–762
10. Monograph. *Centella asiatica*. Milan: Indena S.p.A. 1987
11. Abou-Chaar CI. New drugs from higher plants recently introduced into therapeutics. Lebanese Pharm J 1963; 8: 15–37
12. Lawrence JC. The morphological and pharmacological effects of asiaticoside upon skin *in vitro* and *in vivo*. Europ J Pharmacol 1967; 1: 414–424
13. Bonte F, Dumas M et al. Influence of asiatic acid, madecassic acid, and asiaticoside on human collagen I synthesis. Planta Med 1994; 60: 133–135
14. May A. The effect of asiaticoside on pig skin in organ culture. Europ J Pharmacol 1968; 4: 177–181
15. Bensaude A. The treatment of anal fissure. Phleobologie 1980; 33: 683–688
16. Aziz-Fam A. Use of titrated extract of *Centella asiatica* (TECA) in bilharzial bladder lesions. Int Surg 1973; 58: 451–452
17. Etrebi A, Ibrahim A, Zaki K. Treatment of bladder ulcer with asiaticoside. J Egypt Med Assoc 1975; 58: 324–327
18. Gravel JA. Oxygen dressings and asiaticoside in the treatment of burns. Laval Med 1965; 36: 413–415
19. Boiteau P, Ratsimamanga AR. Important cicatrizants of vegetable origin and the biostimulins of Filatov. Bull Soc Sci Bretagne 1959; 34: 307–315
20. Bourguignon D. Study of the action of titrated extract of *Centella asiatica*. Gaz Med Fr 1975; 82: 4579–4583
21. Bonnett GF. Treatment of localized cellulitis with asiaticoside Madecassol. Progr Med 1974; 102: 109–110
22. Grosshans E, Keller F. Cellulite: reality or imposter? J Med Strasbourg 1983; 14: 563–567
23. Keller F, Grosshans E. Cellulitis: reality or fraud? Med Hyg 1983; 1: 1513–1518
24. Tenailleau A. On 80 cases of cellulitis treated with the standard extract of *Centella asiatica*. Quest Med 1978; 31: 919–924
25. Carraro Pereira I. Treatment of cellulitis with *Centella asiatica*. Folha Med 1979; 79: 401–414
26. Darnis F, Orcel L, de Saint-Maur PP, Mamou P. Use of a titrated extract of *Centella asiatica* in chronic hepatic disorders. Sem Hosp Paris 1979; 55: 1749–1750
27. El Zawahry MD, Khalil AM, El Banna MH. Madecassol, a new therapy for hepatic fibrosis. Bull Soc Int Chir (Belgium) 1975; 34: 296–297
28. El Zawahry MD, Khalil AM, El Banna MH. Madecassol, a new therapy for hepatic fibrosis. Bull Soc Int Chir (Belgium) 1975; 34: 573–577
29. Fincato M. On the treatment of cutaneous lesions with extract of *Centella asiatica*. Minerva Chir 1960; 15: 1235–1238
30. Sterkers Desagnat M, Philbert M, Moreau L. Medical treatments for benign disease of the breast. Therapeutique 1975; 51: 121–124
31. Guarnerio F, Sansonetti G, Donzelli R, Marelli C. Treatment of hemorrhoids with *Centella asiatica*. G Ital Angiol 1986; 6: 46–52
32. Bosse JP, Papillon J, Frenette G et al. Clinical study of a new antikeloid drug. Ann Plast Surg 1979; 3: 13–21
33. Basset A, Ullmo A, Maleville J, Alt J. Treatment of keloids with Madecassol. Bull Soc Fr Dermatol Syph 1970; 77: 826–827
34. Ippolito F. Medical treatment of keloids. G Ital Dermatol 1977; 112: 377–381
35. Chakrabarty T, Deshmukh S. *Centella asiatica* in the treatment of leprosy. Science Culture 1976; 42: 573
36. Chudhuri S, Ghosh S, Chakrabarty T, Kundu S, Hazra SK. Use of a common Indian herb "Mandukaparni" in the treatment of leprosy. J Ind Med Assoc 1978; 70: 177–180
37. Wolram VS. Erfahrungern mit Maddecassol bei der behandlung ulzereroserser hautveranderungen. Wien Med Wschr 1965; 115: 439–442
38. Appa Rao MVR, Srinivasan K, Koteswara RTL. The effect of *Centella asiatica* on the general mental ability of mentally retarded children. Ind J Pschiatry 1977; 19: 54–59
39. Kyoo WC. Medical treatment of peptic ulcer. J Korean Med Assoc 1980; 23: 31–35
40. Pergola F. Treatment of peptic ulcer with a titrated extract of *Centella asiatica*. Med Chir Dig 1974; 36: 445–448
41. Baudon-Glanddier B. Perineal lesions and asiaticoside. Gaz Med Fr 1963; 70: 2463–2464
42. Benedicenti A, Galli D, Merlini A. The clinical therapy of periodontal disease. The use of potassium hydroxide and the water-alcohol extract of *Centella asiatica* in combination with laser therapy in the treatment of severe periodontal disease. Parodontol Stomatol 1985; 24: 11–26
43. Abou-Shousha ES, Khalil HA. Effect of asiaticoside (Madecassol) on the healing process in cataract surgical wounds and retinal detachment operations (clinical and experimental study). Bull Ophthalmol Soc Egypt 1967; 60: 451–470
44. Bletry O. Comment on the treatment of scleroderma. Gazz Med Fr 1980; 87: 1989–1990
45. Fontan I, Rommel A, Geniaux M, Maleville J. Localized scleroderma. Concours Med 1987; 109: 498–504
46. Sasaki S, Shinkai H, Akashi Y, Kishihara Y. Experimental and clinical effects of asiaticoside (Madecassol) on fibroblasts, granulomas, and scleroderma. Jap J Clin Dermatol 1971; 25: 585–593
47. Sasaki S, Shinkai H, Akashi Y, Kishihara Y. Studies on the mechanism of action of asiaticoside (Madecassol) on experimental granulation tissue and cultured fibroblasts and its clinical application in systemic scleroderma. Acta Diabetol Lat 1972; 52: 141–150
48. Balina LM, Cardama JE, Gatti JC et al. Clinical results of an asiaticoside in cutaneous ulcerous lesions. Dia Med 1961; 33: 1693–1696
49. Bazex J, Nogue J, Peyrot J. Periulcerous eczema type cutaneous reaction during and after ulcers of the leg. Rev Med Toulouse 1982; 18: 171–174

50. Dulauney MM. Postphlebitic leg ulcers and indications for therapy. Bordeaux Med 1979; 12: 1807–1810
51. Hanna LK, Amin L, El Serafy I. Trophic ulcers and their treatment with Madecassol. Afr Med 1969; 8: 315–318
52. Huriez CL. Action of the titrated extract of *Centella asiatica* on cicatrization of leg ulcers (10 mg tablets). Apropos of 50 cases. Lille Med 1972; 17: 574–579
53. Sarteel AM, Merlen JF. Treatment of leg ulcers. Phlebologie 1983; 36: 375–379
54. Thiers H, Fayolle J, Boiteau P, Ratsimamanga AR. Asiaticoside, the active principle of *Centella asiatica*, in the treatment of cutaneous ulcers. Lyon Med 1957; 197: 389–395
55. Vittori F. The treatment of ulcus cruris. J Med Lyon 1982; 63: 429–432
56. Castellani C, Gillet JY, Lavernhe G, Dellenbach P. Asiaticoside and cicatrization of episiotomies. Bull Fed Soc Gynecol Obstet 1966; 18: 184–186
57. Collonna d'Istria J. Research on the healing action of Madecassol in cervical and laryngeal surgery after ionizing radiations. J Fr Otorhinolaryngol 1970; 19: 507–510
58. O'Keeffe P. A trial of asiaticoside on skin graft donor areas. Brit J Plast Surg 1974; 27: 194–195
59. Pignataro O, Teatini GP. Clinical research on the cicatrizing action of Madecassol in comparison of oropharyngeal mucosa. Minerva Med 1965; 56: 2683–2686
60. Riu R, Alavoine J, Auriault A, Le Mouel C. Clinical study of Madecassol in otorhinology. J Med Lyon 1966; 47: 693–706
61. Sevin P. Some observations on the use of asiaticoside (Madecassol) in general surgery. Progr Med (France) 1962; 90: 23–24
62. King DS. Tuberculosis. New Engl J Med 1950; 243: 530–536, 565–571
63. Allegra C. Comparative capillaroscopic study of certain bioflavonoids and total triterpenic fractions of *Centella asiatica* in venous insufficiency. Clin Terap 1984; 110: 555–559
64. Allegra C, Pollari G, Criscuolo A et al. *Centella asiatica* extract in venous disorders of the lower limbs. Comparative clinico-instrumental studies with a placebo. Clin Terap 1981; 99: 507–513
65. Barletta S, Borgioli A, Corsi C. Results with *Centella asiatica* in chronic venous insufficiency. Gazz Med Ital 1981; 140: 33–35
66. Basellini A, Agus GB, Antonucci E, Papacharalambus D. Varicose disease in pregnancy. Ann Obstet Gyn Med Perinat 1985; 106: 337–341
67. Boely C. Indications of titrated extract of *Centella asiatica* in phlebology. Gazz Med Fr 1975; 82: 741–744
68. Bolgert M, Gautron G. An extract from *Centella asiatica* in phlebology. Progr Med (France) 1972; 100: 31–32
69. Cappelli R. Clinical and pharmacological study on the effect of an extract of *Centella asiatica* in chronic venous insufficiency of lower limbs. G Ital Angiol 1983; 3: 44–48
70. Cospite M, Ferrara F, Milio G, Meli F. Study about pharmacologic and clinical activity of *Centella asiatica* titrated extract in the chronic venous deficiency of the lower limbs. Valuation with strain gauge plethysmography. G Ital Angiol 1984; 4: 200–205
71. Frausini G, Rotatori T, Oliva S. Controlled trial on clinical-dynamic effects of three treatments in chronic venous insufficiency. G Ital Angiol 1985; 5: 147–151
72. Marastoni F, Baldo A, Redaelli G, Ghiringhelli L. *Centella asiatica* extract in venous pathology of the lower limbs and its evaluation as compared with tribenoside. Minerva-Cardioangiol 1982; 30: 201–207
73. Mariani G, Patuzzo E. Treatment of venous insufficiency with extract of *Centella asiatica*. Clin Eur (Italy) 1983; 22: 154–158
74. Mazzola C, Gini MM. *Centella asiatica* extract in treatment of chronic venous insufficiency. Clin Eur (Italy) 1982; 21: 160–166
75. Pointel JP, Boccalon H, Cloarec M et al. Titrated extract of *Centella asiatica* (TECA) in the treatment of venous insufficiency of the lower limbs. Angiology 1987; 38: 46–50
76. Ramaswamy AS, Periyasamy SM, Basu N. Pharmacological studies on *Centella asiatica* L. (Brahma manduki) (N.O. Umbelliferae). J Res Ind Med 1970; 4: 160–175
77. Laerum OD, Iversen OH. Reticuloses and epidermal tumors in hairless mice after topical skin applications of cantharidin and asiaticoside. Cancer Res 1972; 32: 1463–1469

CHAPTER CONTENTS

75

Cimicifuga racemosa (black cohosh)

Michael T. Murray, ND

Joseph E. Pizzorno Jr, ND

Cimicifuga racemosa (family: Ranunculaceae)
Common names: black cohosh, macrotys, rattleweed, black snake root

GENERAL DESCRIPTION

Cimicifuga racemosa is a perennial herb native to North America that grows on hillsides and in woods at higher elevations from Maine and Ontario to Wisconsin, Georgia, and Missouri. The large, creeping rhizome produces stems up to 9 feet high. The ovate or oblong leaflets are 1–6 inches long and 4 inches wide, while the smaller leaflets are ternate, then pinnate, and sometimes even further divided. Small, white, fetid flowers grow in long racemes from May to August. The rhizome is the portion of the plant used for medicinal purposes.

CHEMICAL COMPOSITION

The components of cimicifuga which have garnered the most attention are the triterpene glycosides:

- actein
- cimicifugoside (aglycone cimegenol)
- 27-deoxyactein.

Other compounds of interest include flavonoids (formononetin) and caffeic acid derivatives (isoferulic acid) (see Figs 75.1 and 75.2).

HISTORY AND FOLK USE

The generic name *Cimicifuga* comes from the Latin *cimex*,

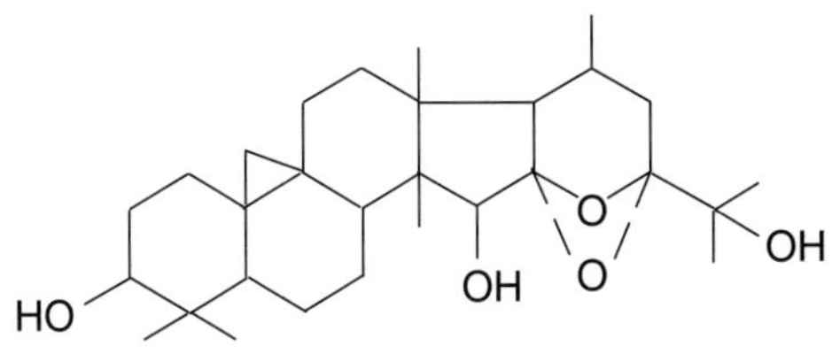

HO OH O O OH

Figure 75.1 Cimigenol.

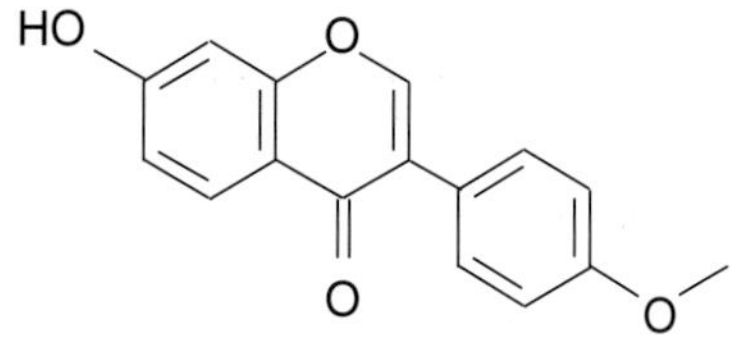

Figure 75.2 Formononetin.

a bug, and *fugo*, to drive away, alluding to its use as a vermifuge. Native Americans used cimicifuga rhizomes for the relief of pain during menses and childbirth as well as snakebite. The rhizome of *Cimicifuga racemosa* was listed in the National Formulary from 1936 to 1950, and in the United States Pharmacopeia from 1820 to 1936. Eclectic physicians in the early part of the 20th century used cimicifuga in gynecological disorders as well as rheumatoid and myalgic pain.

While use in the US declined dramatically from 1950 to 1995, cimicifuga preparations have been used extensively in Europe during this same period primarily as a natural alternative to hormone replacement therapy during menopause. This popularity is based upon substantial empirical and clinical evidence.

PHARMACOLOGY

The primary pharmacological effects of cimicifuga appear to revolve around its ability to impact endocrine regulatory mechanisms.[1–4] Much of this activity may be related to various phytoestrogenic components of cimicifuga, with formononetin perhaps being the most significant.[5] However, the activity of phytoestrogens is substantially less than endogenous estrogens, indicating they exert more of an anti-estrogen than pro-estrogen effect. The estrogenic action of cimicifuga goes well beyond its phytoestrogen content. For example, the isoflavonoid formononetin has been identified as being the chief phytoestrogen of cimicifuga; however, it is much less active than many other phytoestrogens (e.g. genestein), as its relative binding affinity for estrogen receptors is only one-hundredth as strong as 17-beta-estradiol.[5]

In addition, cimicifuga's action appears to be more closely related to estriol than to estradiol. While estradiol is associated with an increased risk for breast, ovarian, and endometrial cancers, estriol is actually associated with offering some protection against these cancers.[6,7] The reason may be that estriol is much weaker in action and has a shorter dwelling time on receptors on the surface of the cells compared with the more potent estradiol. Estrogen-dependent tumors are not stimulated by the weak-acting estriol, as it is acting as a partial antagonist to estradiol. Physiologically, estriol exerts its effects primarily on the vaginal lining, while estradiol exerts its effects primarily on the uterine lining. This action appears to mirror the effects with extracts of cimicifuga noted in clinical studies in menopausal women concerning its effect on the vaginal epithelium.

Cimicifuga's primary effect on endocrine regulatory mechanisms appears to be the result of complex synergistic actions of its key ingredients – the triterpenes and flavone derivatives. Evidence suggests that these compounds act on both the hypothalamus and vasomotor centers to produce significant clinical benefits in menopause. For example, one study involved in determining the endocrinological actions of cimicifuga extract involved treating 110 women with either cimicifuga extract (supplying a total daily dosage of 8 mg of 27-deoxyactein) or placebo.[4] After 2 months of treatment, LH decreased by 20% in the cimicifuga group compared with the placebo group. Unlike estrogens, cimicifuga does not affect the release of prolactin and follicle-stimulating hormone (FSH). Researchers then divided the extract into three distinct types of active compounds based upon their ability to reduce LH secretion in ovariectomized rats and to compete in vitro with 17-beta-estradiol for estrogen receptor binding sites, as follows:

- constituents that did not bind to estrogen receptors, but that did suppress LH secretion
- constituents able to bind to estrogen receptor sites and to inhibit LH secretion
- compounds able to bind to estrogen receptors, but which did not inhibit LH secretion.

The authors concluded that: "the LH suppressive effect of *Cimicifuga racemosa* extracts observed in menopausal women and ovariectomized rats is caused by at least three different synergistically acting compounds."

In summary, one of cimicifuga's key pharmacological effects is inhibition of the secretion of luteinizing hormone (LH) by the pituitary. This effect is accomplished equally by components which do and do not bind to estrogen receptors. If cimicifuga was simply mimicking the effects of estrogen, it would certainly alter the secretion of other pituitary hormones just like estrogen, but it does not.

CLINICAL APPLICATIONS

A special extract of *Cimicifuga racemosa* standardized to contain 1 mg of triterpenes calculated as 27-deoxyacteine per tablet (trade name = Remifemin) is the most widely used and thoroughly studied natural alternative to hormone replacement therapy in menopause. In 1996, nearly 10 million monthly units of this extract were sold in Germany, the US, and Australia. Clinical studies have shown this cimicifuga extract to relieve not only hot flashes, but also depression and vaginal atrophy.[4,8–11]

While there is also some evidence that cimicifuga may provide benefit in other gynecological complaints such as premenstrual syndrome, amenorrhea (both primary

Table 75.1 Cimicifuga in the treatment of menopause

Symptom	Percentage no longer present (%)	Percentage improved %	Total percentage improved (%)
Hot flashes	43.3	43.3	86.6
Profuse perspiration	49.9	38.6	88.5
Headache	45.7	36.2	81.9
Vertigo	51.6	35.2	86.8
Heart palpitation	54.6	35.2	90.4
Ringing in the ears	54.8	38.1	92.9
Nervousness/irritability	42.4	43.2	85.6
Sleep disturbances	46.1	30.7	76.8
Depressive moods	46.0	36.5	82.5

and secondary), dysmenorrhea, polymenorrhea, uterine fibroids, and fibrocystic breast disease, its primary clinical application is menopause.[12–14]

Menopause

In a large open study involving 131 doctors and 629 female patients, cimicifuga extract (two tablets twice daily providing a daily dosage of 4 mg 27-deoxyactein) produced clear improvement of menopausal symptoms in over 80% of patients within 6–8 weeks.[8] As shown in Table 75.1, both physical and psychological symptoms improved.

Most patients reported noticeable benefits within 4 weeks after the onset of cimicifuga therapy. After 6–8 weeks, complete resolution of symptoms were achieved in a large percentage of patients. Cimicifuga was very well tolerated as there was no discontinuation of therapy and only 7% of patients reported mild transitory stomach complaints.

In a double-blind study, 60 patients were given cimicifuga extract (two tablets twice daily providing a daily dosage of 4 mg 27-deoxyactein), conjugated estrogens (0.625 mg daily), or diazepam (2 mg daily) for 12 weeks.[9] Results from standard indexes of menopausal symptoms indicated a clear advantage of cimicifuga extract over both drugs. Cimicifuga's effect on relieving the depressive mood and anxiety associated with menopause was far superior to either diazepam or conjugated estrogens, as shown in Table 75.2.

One of the most utilized assessments in clinical studies in menopause is the Kupperman Menopausal Index. This quantitative assessment of menopausal symptoms is achieved by grading in severity: severe = 3, moderate = 2, mild = 1, not present = 0. The symptoms assessed are:

Table 75.2 Effect on Kupperman Menopausal Index of cimicifuga compared with conjugated estrogens and diazepam

Treatment group	Beginning	At 12 weeks
Cimicifuga	35	14
Conjugated estrogens	35	16
Diazepam	35	20

- hot flashes
- depressive moods
- profuse perspiration
- feelings of vertigo
- sleep disturbances
- loss of concentration
- headache
- joint pain
- nervousness/irritability
- heart palpitation.

The results on the Kupperman Menopausal Index from this trial clearly demonstrate cimicifuga extract's superiority over conjugated estrogens and diazepam, especially when safety and side-effects are taken into consideration.

In another double-blind study, 80 patients were given cimicifuga extract (two tablets twice daily providing a daily dosage of 4 mg 27-deoxyactein), conjugated estrogens (0.625 mg daily), or placebo for 12 weeks.[10] Cimicifuga produced better results in the Kupperman Menopausal Index, the Hamilton anxiety test, and the vaginal lining than estrogens or placebo. The number of hot flashes experienced each day dropped from an average of five to less than one in the cimicifuga group. In comparison, the estrogen group only dropped from five to 3.5. Even more impressive was the effect of cimicifuga on the vaginal lining. While both conjugated estrogens and the placebo produced little effect, a dramatic increase in the number of superficial cells was noted in cimicifuga group.

In a double-blind study of 110 women, cimicifuga extract (two tablets twice daily providing a daily dosage of 4 mg 27-deoxyactein) was shown to exert significant improvements in menopausal symptoms.[4] In addition to providing relief of hot flashes, cimicifuga once again demonstrated impressive results on the vaginal lining as confirmed by vaginal smear.

In a study of 60 women under the age of 40 who had hysterectomies leaving at least one intact ovary, the women were given either cimicifuga extract (two tablets twice daily providing a daily dosage of 4 mg 27-deoxyactein), estriol (1 mg daily), conjugated estrogens (1.25 mg daily), or estrogen-progestin combination (Trisequens, one tablet daily).[11] Although the hormone therapies produced better results as determined by a modified Kupperman's Menopausal Index, cimicifuga still displayed significant effects in relieving the symptoms of "surgical menopause". These results indicate that cimicifuga can be a suitable alternative to estrogens in women having partial, and possibly even complete, hysterectomies.

Effects on bone resorption

One of the most publicized effects of estrogen is its role in maintaining bone health and preventing osteoporosis. While there is experimental and epidemiological evidence that phytoestrogens prevent osteoporosis and reduce bone resorption, there are currently no long-term studies demonstrating cimicifuga can prevent or improve osteoporosis. However, based on cimicifuga's mechanism of action and long-term clinical experience, many experts believe it will be shown to positively influence bone resorption. In patients at high risk for osteoporosis or those with confirmed low bone density, physicians should monitor therapy with cimicifuga by using the Osteomark-NTX or other suitable indicator of bone resorption.

DOSAGE

The dosage of cimicifuga is based on its content of 27-deoxyactein, which serves as an important biochemical marker to indicate therapeutic effect. The dosage of the cimicifuga extract used in the majority of clinical studies has been 2 mg of 27-deoxyacteine twice daily. Here are the approximate dosage recommendations using other forms (non-standardized) of *Cimicifuga racemosa*:

- 27-deoxyacteine: 2 mg b.i.d.
- powdered rhizome: 1–2 g
- tincture (1:5): 4–6 ml
- fluid extract (1:1): 3–4 ml (1 tsp)
- solid (dry powdered) extract (4:1): 250–500 mg.

The German Commission E has recommended that treatment with cimicifuga be limited to 6 months (which is also the standard recommendation for hormone replacement therapy); however, this recommendation was made prior to the detailed toxicology studies discussed below. Based on currently available data, cimicifuga is appropriate for long-term continued use.

TOXICOLOGY

The standardized extract of *Cimicifuga racemosa* providing 1 mg of 27-deoxyactein per approximately 40 mg of extract per tablet known as Remifemin has been used in Germany since 1956 and has a remarkable safety record. No serious side-effects have ever been reported. The BGA, the German equivalent to the FDA in the US, includes no contraindications or limitations of use for cimicifuga. Therefore, cimicifuga offers a suitable natural alternative to hormone replacement therapy for menopause, especially where hormone replacement therapy is contraindicated, e.g. in women with a history of cancer, unexplained uterine bleeding, liver and gall bladder disease, pancreatitis, endometriosis, uterine fibroids or fibrocystic breast disease.

Since cimicifuga extract shows some, albeit weak, estrogenic activity, researchers have sought to determine Remifemin's effect on established breast tumor cell line whose growth in vitro depends on the presence of estrogens. The results from these experiments show no stimulatory effects, but rather inhibitory effects.[15] Furthermore, combining Remifemin with tamoxifen was shown to potentiate the inhibitory effects of tamoxifen.

Detailed toxicology studies have also been performed on Remifemin. No teratogenic, mutagenic, or carcinogenic side-effects have been noted. The no-effect dosage in studies in a 6 month chronic toxicity study in rats was at 1,800 mg/kg body weight – or roughly 90 times the therapeutic dose.[16] A 6 month toxicological study in rats is comparable to an unlimited treatment time in humans.

REFERENCES

1. Harnischfeger G, Stolze H. Proven active substances from natural materials. Black snake root. Notabene Medici 1980; 10: 446–450
2. Jarry H, Harnischfeger G. Studies on the endocrine efficacy of the constituents of *Cimicifuga racemosa*. I. Influence on the serum concentration of pituitary hormones in ovariectomied rats. Planta Med 1985; 51: 80–83
3. Jarry H, Harnischfeger G, Duke E. Studies on the endocrine efficacy of the constituents of *Cimicifuga racemosa*. II. In vitro binding of compounds to estrogen receptors. Planta Med 1985; 51: 291–296
4. Duker EM et al. Effects of extracts from *Cimicifuga racemosa* on gonadotropin release in menopausal women and ovariectomized rats. Planta Medica 1991; 57: 420–424
5. Miksicek RJ. Commonly occurring plant flavonoids have estrogenic activity. Molecular Pharmacology 1993; 44: 37–43
6. Tzingounis VA, Aksu MF, Greenblatt RB. Estriol in the management of the menopause. JAMA 1978; 239: 1638–1641
7. Lemon HM. Pathophysiologic considerations in the treatment of menopausal symptoms with oestrogens; the role of oestriol in the prevention of mammary carcinoma. Acta Endocrinol 1980; 233: 17–27
8. Stolze H. An alternative to treat menopausal complaints. Gynecology 1982; 3: 14–16
9. Warnecke G. Influencing menopausal symptoms with a phytotherapeutic agent. Med Welt 1985; 36: 871–874
10. Stoll W. Phytopharmacon influences atrophic vaginal epithelium. Double-blind study – Cimicifuga vs. estrogenic substances. Therapeuticum 1987; 1: 23–31
11. Lehmann-Willenbrock E et al. Clinical and endocrinologic examinations of climacteric symptoms following hysterectomy with remaining ovaries. Zent Gynakol 1988; 110: 611–618

12. Bruker A. Essay on the phytotherapy of hormonal disorders in women. Med Welt 1960; 44: 2331–2333
13. Schildge E. Essay on the treatment of premenstrual and menopausal moods swings and depressive states. Rigelh Biol Umsch 1964; 19(2): 18–22
14. Gorlich N. Treatment of ovarian disorders in general practice. Arztl Prax 1962; 14: 1742–1743
15. Nesselhut T, Borth S, Kuhn W. Influence of *Cimicifuga racemosa* extracts with estrogen-like activity on the in vitro proliferation of mammary carcinoma cells. Arch Gynecol Obstet 1993; 254: 817–818
16. Korn WD. Six-month oral toxicity study with Remifemin-granulate in rats followed by an 8-week recovery period. Hannover: International Bioresearch. 1991

CHAPTER CONTENTS

76

Coenzyme Q_{10}

Alan R. Gaby, MD

INTRODUCTION

Coenzyme Q_{10} (CoQ_{10}) is a compound found naturally in the human body. Because of its ubiquitous presence in nature and its quinone structure (similar to that of vitamin K), CoQ_{10} is also known as ubiquinone (Fig. 76.1). The primary biochemical action of CoQ_{10} is as a cofactor in the electron-transport chain, the series of redox reactions that are involved in the synthesis of ATP. Since most cellular functions are dependent on an adequate supply of ATP, CoQ_{10} is essential for the health of virtually all human tissues and organs.

Although CoQ_{10} can be synthesized in vivo, situations may arise in which the body's synthetic capacity is insufficient to meet CoQ_{10} requirements. Susceptibility to CoQ_{10} deficiency appears to be greatest in cells that are the most metabolically active (such as those in the heart, immune system, gingiva, and gastric mucosa), since these cells presumably have the highest requirements for CoQ_{10}. Tissue deficiencies or subnormal serum levels of CoQ_{10} have been reported to occur in a wide range of medical conditions, including cardiovascular disease, hypertension, periodontal disease, and acquired immunodeficiency syndrome (AIDS). In addition, CoQ_{10} levels decline with advancing age, and this decline might contribute in part to some of the manifestations of aging.

A need for supplemental CoQ_{10} could theoretically result from:

- impaired CoQ_{10} synthesis due to nutritional deficiencies
- a genetic or acquired defect in CoQ_{10} synthesis or utilization

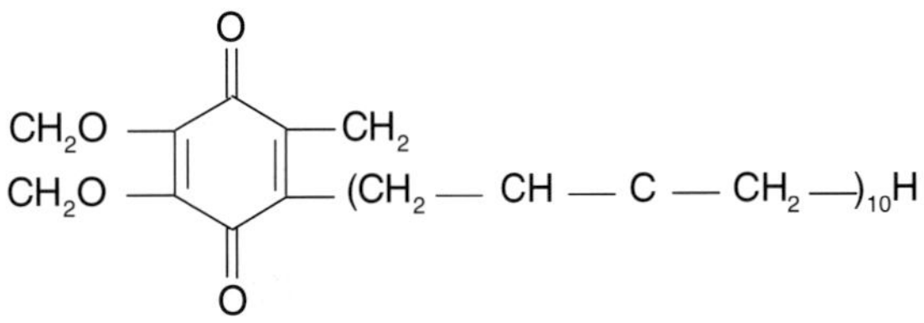

O
CH_2O — CH_2
CH_2O — $(CH_2 — CH — C — CH_2 —)_{10}H$
O

Figure 76.1 Coenzyme Q_{10}.

- increased tissue needs resulting from a particular illness
- the requirement to prevent the side-effects of a medical intervention.

Since oral administration of CoQ_{10} can increase tissue levels of the nutrient, it is possible to correct CoQ_{10} deficiency and its associated metabolic consequences by supplementation.[1]

Detection of CoQ_{10} deficiency

CoQ_{10} participates in the citric acid cycle (Krebs cycle) enzyme known as succinate dehydrogenase-CoQ_{10} reductase. An assay of the activity of this enzyme has been used to detect deficiencies of CoQ_{10}.[2] If the enzyme is fully saturated with CoQ_{10} in vivo, then addition of exogenous CoQ will not increase enzyme activity. On the other hand, exogenous CoQ will increase activity appreciably when tissue levels of CoQ_{10} are low. More recently, measurements of serum CoQ_{10} levels have been used to detect deficiencies.

CLINICAL APPLICATIONS

Immune function

Cells and tissues that play a role in immune function are highly energy-dependent and therefore require an adequate supply of CoQ_{10} for optimal function. Several studies have demonstrated immune-enhancing effects of CoQ_{10} or its analogues.[3–5] These effects included increased phagocytic activity of macrophages, increased proliferation of granulocytes in response to experimental infections, and prolonged survival in mice infected with *Pseudomonas aeruginosa, Staphylococcus aureus, Escherichia coli, Klebsiella pneumoniae*, or *Candida albicans*. Inoculation of animals with Friend leukemia virus reduced CoQ_{10} levels in the blood and spleen,[6] whereas treatment of infected animals with CoQ_{10} increased the survival rate and decreased the severity of hepatomegaly and splenomegaly.[7]

Immune function tends to decline with advancing age. In a study of elderly mice, suppression of the immune response was associated with a marked decline of CoQ_{10} levels in thymic tissue.[8] This immune suppression was partly reversed by treatment with CoQ_{10}.[9] In a study of eight chronically ill patients, administration of 60 mg/day of CoQ_{10} was associated with significant increases in serum levels of immunoglobulin G (IgG) after 27–98 days of treatment.[10] These studies suggest that CoQ_{10} may help to prevent or reverse the immunosuppression that is associated with aging or chronic disease.

Acquired immunodeficiency syndrome (AIDS)

AIDS is a complex disease that is associated with a wide range of nutritional deficiencies and immunological disorders. While correction of nutritional deficiencies will not cure AIDS, appropriate nutritional interventions may help to prevent weight loss and enhance overall immune function. In addition, since oxidative stress is believed to be involved in the pathogenesis of AIDS-related diseases, the antioxidant activity of CoQ_{10} may be of value for individuals with AIDS.[11]

In one study, blood levels of CoQ_{10} were significantly lower in patients with AIDS-related complex (ARC) than in a control group and were significantly lower in patients with AIDS than in those with ARC.[12] Six patients with AIDS or ARC were treated with 200 mg/day of CoQ_{10}. T-cell helper/suppressor ratios increased in three patients, becoming normal in one case. Five patients reported symptomatic improvement, which was dramatic in some cases. Furthermore, none of the patients developed opportunistic infections during a 4–7 month follow-up period. This study demonstrates that CoQ_{10} deficiency is common in patients with HIV infection, and that supplementation with CoQ_{10} may improve immune function and reduce the incidence of opportunistic infections.

Cancer

Because of its role in enhancing immune function, CoQ_{10} has been considered as a possible anti-cancer agent. Administration of CoQ_{10} reduced tumor size and increased survival in mice exposed to a chemical carcinogen.[13] Preliminary studies in humans, though uncontrolled, are promising. In one study, 32 women with breast cancer who were classified as "high risk" because of tumor spread to the axillary lymph nodes received 90 mg/day of CoQ_{10}, along with vitamin C, vitamin E, beta-carotene, and essential fatty acids. In six of these women, the tumor became smaller. During the 18 month treatment period, none of the patients died (the expected number of deaths was four) and none showed signs of further distant metastases. Six patients had an apparent partial remission. In addition, patients receiving CoQ_{10} required fewer pain killers.[14]

In another report, two women with metastatic breast cancer received 390 mg/day of CoQ_{10}. One was a 44-year-old woman with numerous liver metastases. After treatment with CoQ_{10} for 11 months, all of the liver metastases had disappeared and the patient was reported to be in excellent health. The other patient was a 49-year-old woman with breast cancer that had metastasized to the pleural cavity. After 6 months of CoQ_{10} therapy, the pleural fluid had completely resolved and the patient was reported to be in excellent health.[15]

Although these reports are anecdotal, the results are far better than would normally be expected. Considering that CoQ_{10} is virtually free of side-effects, empirical treatment of breast cancer with CoQ_{10} seems justified.

Periodontal disease

Periodontal disease affects about 60% of young adults and 90% of individuals over the age of 65. Although proper oral hygiene is helpful, many people suffer from intractable gingivitis, often requiring surgery and resulting in eventual loss of teeth. Because periodontal disease is so common, the costs of periodontal surgery and other treatments contribute a significant amount to the overall cost of health care in the United States.

Healing and repair of periodontal tissues require efficient energy production, which depends on an adequate supply of CoQ_{10}. However, gingival biopsies revealed subnormal tissue levels of CoQ_{10} in 60–96% of patients with periodontal disease and low levels of CoQ_{10} in leukocytes in 86% of cases.[16–19] These findings indicate that periodontal disease is frequently associated with CoQ_{10} deficiency.

Eighteen patients with periodontal disease received either 50 mg/day of CoQ_{10} or a placebo in a 3 week double-blind trial.[20,21] Results were assessed according to a "periodontal score", which included gingival-pocket depth, swelling, bleeding, redness, pain, exudate, and looseness of teeth. All eight patients receiving CoQ_{10} improved, compared with only three of 10 receiving the placebo ($P < 0.01$). The treating dentists, who were unaware that a study was being conducted, consistently remarked about the "very impressive" rate of healing in patients treated with CoQ_{10}. One prosthodontist commented that the amount of healing that took place in 3 weeks in patients receiving CoQ_{10} would normally require about 6 months.

In an open trial, administration of CoQ_{10} produced "extraordinary post-surgical healing" (two to three times as fast as usual) in seven patients with advanced periodontal disease.[22] The beneficial effect of CoQ_{10} has also been confirmed in dogs, where it reduced the severity of experimentally induced periodontal disease.[23]

Gastric ulcer

Susceptibility to gastric ulceration is related to the balance between ulcer-promoting factors (such as excessive gastric acidity and infection with *Helicobacter pylori*) and resistance factors (such as tissue integrity, production of protective mucus, and repair mechanisms). Free radical damage is believed to be one of the primary mechanisms by which external factors induce gastric injury and peptic ulceration.[24,25] Since CoQ_{10} possesses antioxidant activity, it may be capable of preventing ulceration by reducing the amount of free radical damage. In addition, the production of protective mucus and the rapid cell turnover of gastric mucosa are highly energy-dependent processes, which require the presence of adequate amounts of CoQ_{10}.

The efficiency of these protective and reparative processes may be compromised in some patients with gastric ulcers. With advancing age, the fundic mucosa and its rich blood supply are gradually replaced by pyloric tissue, which has poor vascularity. This change in cell type may result in hypoxia in certain portions of the stomach. The hypoxic state of gastric tissue could explain why gastric ulcers frequently become intractable in elderly patients or in those with chronic heart or lung disease.

The importance of CoQ_{10} for healing of gastric ulcers has been demonstrated in animals.[26] Gastric ulcers were induced in mice by the application of acetic acid. The mice were then maintained either in room air (20% oxygen) or under mild hypoxic conditions (17% oxygen). Ulcers healed normally in mice exposed to room air, but increased in size under hypoxic conditions. However, in hypoxic mice treated with CoQ_{10} (50 mg/kg per day) the ulcers healed normally.

This study demonstrates that hypoxia has an adverse effect on the healing of gastric ulcers in animals, and that the effect of hypoxia can be prevented by administration of CoQ_{10}. Although human studies have not been done, empirical use of CoQ_{10} seems to be a reasonable option for elderly patients with intractable gastric ulcers, particularly those who also have diseases likely to produce hypoxia.

Obesity

The tendency to become overweight is associated in some cases with impaired energy production. This abnormality may be in part genetically determined. Individuals with a family history of obesity have a 50% reduction in their thermogenic response to meals, suggesting the presence of an hereditary defect in energy output. Since CoQ_{10} is an essential cofactor for energy production, it is possible that CoQ_{10} deficiency is a contributing factor in some cases of obesity.

Serum levels of CoQ_{10} were found to be low in 14 (52%) of 27 morbidly obese patients.[27] Nine of these 27 individuals (five with low CoQ_{10} levels) received 100 mg/day of CoQ_{10} along with a 650 kcal/day diet. After 8–9 weeks, the mean weight loss in the CoQ_{10}-deficient group was 13.5 kg, compared with 5.8 kg in those with normal levels of CoQ_{10}.

One possible interpretation of this study is that about 50% of obese individuals are deficient in CoQ_{10} and that replacement therapy accelerates weight loss during calorie restriction. However, it is also possible that CoQ_{10} treatment had nothing to do with the accelerated weight loss. Obese individuals with low CoQ_{10} levels may have other metabolic abnormalities which are more directly related to their obesity. A low CoQ_{10} level might therefore have been an effect, rather than a cause, of the abnormalities that caused obesity. Until a controlled study is done to evaluate the effectiveness of this therapy, the potential value of CoQ_{10} as a treatment for obesity remains speculative.

Physical performance

Because CoQ_{10} is involved in energy production and its concentration in muscle is correlated with performance, it is possible that supplementation could enhance aerobic capacity and muscle performance. In one study, six healthy sedentary men (mean age, 21.5 years) performed a bicycle ergometer test before and after taking CoQ_{10} (60 mg/day) for 4–8 weeks.[28] CoQ_{10} treatment improved certain performance parameters, including work capacity at submaximal heart rate, maximal work load, maximal oxygen consumption, and oxygen transport. These improvements ranged from 3 to 12% and were evident after about 4 weeks of supplementation. This study suggests that administration of CoQ_{10} improves physical performance in sedentary individuals. The effect of CoQ_{10} on the performance of trained athletes has not shown benefit (see Ch. 59 for a more complete discussion).

Muscular dystrophy

Biochemical evidence of CoQ_{10} deficiency was found in cardiac and skeletal muscle of animals with hereditary muscular dystrophy.[29] In addition, treatment with CoQ_{10} or its analogues increased survival and improved the performance of dystrophic mice, rabbits, and monkeys, as determined by a reduction of creatinuria, regaining of righting reflex, and weight gain.[30–33]

Deficiency of CoQ_{10} has been found in muscle mitochondria of humans with muscular dystrophy.[34] This deficiency could conceivably be involved in the pathogenesis of cardiac disease, which occurs in virtually every form of muscular dystrophy and myopathy. In a double-blind study, 100 mg of CoQ_{10} was given daily for 3 months to 12 patients with progressive muscular dystrophy. CoQ_{10} treatment resulted in significant improvements in cardiac output and stroke volume, as well as increased physical well-being in four of eight patients.[35] Subjective improvements included increased exercise tolerance, reduced leg pain, better control of leg function, and less fatigue. The mechanism of action of CoQ_{10} is probably related to improved energy production in muscle cells.

Allergy

When passively sensitized guinea pig lung tissue was preincubated with CoQ_{10}, release of both histamine and slow-reacting substance of anaphylaxis induced by antigen challenge was markedly inhibited.[36] This study raises the possibility that CoQ_{10} may be of value in the treatment of various allergy-related disorders. However, no clinical trials have been performed in this area.

Cardiovascular disease – general considerations

Enhancing myocardial function is an important, though frequently overlooked, component of the overall prevention and treatment of cardiovascular disease. CoQ_{10} plays a key role in energy production, and is therefore essential for all energy-dependent processes, including heart muscle contraction. CoQ_{10} deficiency has been documented in patients with various types of cardiovascular disease. It is not clear whether a decline in CoQ_{10} levels is a primary cause or a consequence of heart disease. However, given the fundamental involvement of CoQ_{10} in myocardial function, it is not unlikely that CoQ_{10} deficiency would exacerbate heart disease and that correction of such a deficiency would have therapeutic value.

In addition, CoQ_{10} has been shown to be a potent antioxidant. In fact, ubiquinol-10, the reduced form of CoQ_{10}, protected human low-density lipoproteins (LDL) more efficiently against lipid peroxidation than did vitamin E.[37] Since oxidation of LDL is believed to be an initiating factor in the development of atherosclerosis, CoQ_{10} would appear to be a preventive factor.

Cardiac disease

Circulating levels of CoQ_{10} are significantly lower in patients with ischemic heart disease and in those with dilated cardiomyopathy (mostly New York Heart Association [NYHA] functional class III or IV) than in healthy controls.[38,39] In another study, CoQ_{10} levels in myocardial tissue (estimated by enzymatic methods) were low in approximately 75% of patients undergoing cardiac surgery. Concentrations of CoQ_{10} declined progressively in both blood and myocardial tissue with increasing severity of heart disease.[40] Myocardial deficiencies of CoQ_{10} were also found in the majority of patients with aortic stenosis or insufficiency, mitral stenosis or insufficiency, diabetic cardiomyopathy, tetralogy of Fallot, atrial septal defects and ventricular septal defects.[41] In patients with cardiomyopathy and myocardial deficiency of CoQ_{10}, oral administration of 100 mg/day of CoQ_{10} for 2–8 months resulted in an increase in myocardial CoQ_{10} levels, ranging from 20 to 85%.[42] These findings suggest that CoQ_{10} deficiency is common in patients with various types of cardiovascular disease, and that oral administration of CoQ_{10} can increase tissue levels of this nutrient.

Cardiomyopathy

In one study, 126 patients with dilated cardiomyopathy (98% of whom were in NYHA functional class III or IV) received 100 mg/day of CoQ_{10} for periods of up to 66 months. After 6 months of treatment, the mean ejection fraction increased from 41% to 59% ($P < 0.001$), and remained stable thereafter with continued treatment. After 2 years 84% of the patients were still alive, and at 5.5 years 52% were alive.[43] These survival rates are considerably better than the published survival statistics of patients given conventional therapy (i.e. 2-year survival rate of 50% for symptomatic cardiomyopathy, and 1-year survival rate of 50% for decompensated cardiomyopathy).

In another study, 88 patients with cardiomyopathy received 100 mg/day of CoQ_{10} for periods of 1–24 months. Significant improvements in at least two of three cardiac parameters (ejection fraction, cardiac output, and NYHA class) were seen in 75–85% of the patients. Approximately 80% of the patients improved to a lower (i.e. more favorable) NYHA functional class.[44]

In a double-blind, cross-over trial, 19 patients with cardiomyopathy (NYHA classes III and IV) received 100 mg/day of CoQ_{10} or a placebo, each for 12 weeks. Compared with placebo, CoQ_{10} treatment significantly increased cardiac stroke volume and ejection fraction. Eighteen patients reported improvement in activity while taking CoQ_{10}.[45]

Congestive heart failure

The potential of CoQ_{10} as a treatment for congestive heart failure (CHF) was suggested as early as 1967 by Japanese researchers.[46] In 1976, these same investigators administered 30 mg/day of CoQ_{10} to 17 patients with CHF. All of the patients improved, and nine (53%) became asymptomatic after 4 weeks of treatment.[47]

In an open trial of 34 patients with refractory NYHA class IV CHF, administration of 100 mg/day of CoQ_{10} resulted in sustained improvement in cardiac function in 28 cases (82%). The survival rate after 2 years was 62%, compared with an expected 2-year survival rate of less than 25% for similar patients.[48]

In another study, 12 patients with advanced CHF who had failed to respond adequately to digitalis and diuretics received 100 mg/day of coenzyme Q_{10} for 7 months. Two-thirds of the patients showed definite clinical improvement after a mean treatment period of 30 days. In these patients, dyspnea at rest disappeared and energy level and tolerance for activity increased. Objective improvements included decreased hepatic congestion, reductions in heart rate and heart volume, and a decline in systolic time intervals (suggesting improved myocardial performance). Withdrawal of coenzyme Q_{10} was followed by severe clinical relapse, with subsequent improvement upon resumption of treatment.[49]

In a large multicenter trial, 1,113 CHF patients received 50–150 mg/day of CoQ_{10} for 3 months (78% of the patients received 100 mg/day). The proportion of patients with improvements in clinical signs and symptoms were as follows:[50]

- cyanosis, 81%
- edema, 76.9%
- pulmonary rales, 78.4%
- enlargement of the liver area, 49.3%
- jugular reflux, 81.5%
- dyspnea, 54.2%
- palpitations, 75.7%
- sweating, 82.4%
- arrhythmia, 62%
- insomnia, 60.2%
- vertigo, 73%
- nocturia, 50.7%.

The results of these uncontrolled studies were confirmed more recently in a double-blind trial. Some 641 patients with CHF (NYHA classes III or IV) were randomly assigned to receive placebo or CoQ_{10} (2 mg/kg per day) for 1 year. Conventional therapy was continued in both groups. The number of patients requiring hospitalization during the study for worsening heart failure was 38% less in the CoQ_{10} group than in the placebo group ($P < 0.001$). Episodes of pulmonary edema were reduced by about 60% in the CoQ_{10} group, compared with the placebo group ($P < 0.001$).[51]

Angina

Twelve patients with stable angina pectoris were randomly assigned to receive 150 mg/day of CoQ_{10} or a placebo in a 4 week double-blind cross-over trial. CoQ_{10} treatment significantly increased exercise tolerance on a treadmill (time before onset of chest pain), and significantly increased the time until ST-segment depression occurred. Compared with placebo, there was a 53% reduction in the frequency of anginal episodes and a 54% reduction in the number of nitroglycerin tablets needed during CoQ_{10} treatment; however, these differences were not statistically significant.[52]

These results suggest that CoQ_{10} is a safe and effective treatment for angina pectoris. Although the amelioration of anginal attacks was not statistically significant, the magnitude of the effect was large. It would therefore be worthwhile to perform a similar study with a larger number of patients.

Arrhythmias

Twenty-seven patients with ventricular premature beats (VPBs) and no evidence of organic heart disease received a placebo for 3–4 weeks, followed by 60 mg/day of CoQ_{10} for 4–5 weeks. The reduction in VPBs was significantly greater after CoQ_{10} than after placebo. The beneficial effect of CoQ_{10} was seen primarily in diabetics, in whom the mean reduction in VPB frequency was 85.7%. A significant reduction in VPBs also occurred in one (11%) of nine otherwise healthy patients and in four (36%) of 11 patients with hypertension.[53]

Prevention of adriamycin toxicity

The clinical value of adriamycin as an anti-cancer agent is limited by its toxicity, which includes cardiomyopathy and irreversible heart failure. Adriamycin-induced cardiotoxicity is believed to be caused, at least in part, by a reduction in CoQ_{10} levels and by inhibition of CoQ_{10}-dependent enzymes. In rats treated with adriamycin, administration of CoQ_{10} restored the levels of this nutrient to normal and prevented adriamycin-induced morphologic changes in the heart.[54] Treatment with CoQ_{10} also prevented adriamycin-induced cardiotoxicity in rabbits.[55]

Cancer patients receiving adriamycin had lower myocardial levels of CoQ_{10} than did controls. The magnitude of CoQ_{10} depletion was directly related to the severity of cardiac impairment.[56] To determine the effect of CoQ_{10} supplementation on adriamycin cardiotoxicity, seven patients receiving adriamycin were also given 100 mg/day of CoQ_{10}, beginning 3–5 days before adriamycin was started. Another seven patients (control group) received adriamycin without CoQ_{10}. Cardiac function deteriorated significantly in the control group, whereas patients given CoQ_{10} had little or no cardiotoxicity, even though the cumulative dose of adriamycin in the CoQ_{10} group was 50% greater than that in the control group.[57] Despite the small number of patients in this study, the results are highly encouraging. Since administration of CoQ_{10} does not appear to affect the antitumor activity of adriamycin, CoQ_{10} prophylaxis seems appropriate for all patients receiving adriamycin.[58]

Protection during cardiac surgery

Postoperative low cardiac output is a major cause of early death following cardiac surgery. Fifty patients undergoing cardiac surgery for acquired valvular lesions were randomly assigned to receive 30–60 mg/day of CoQ_{10} for 6 days prior to surgery or to a control group that did not receive CoQ_{10}. Postoperatively, a state of severe low cardiac output developed in 48% of the patients in the control group, compared with only 12% of those in the CoQ_{10} group. These results suggest that pre-operative administration of CoQ_{10} increases the tolerance of the heart to ischemia during aortic cross-clamping.[59]

Mitral valve prolapse

Cardiac performance was evaluated using an isometric hand-grip test in 194 children with symptomatic mitral valve prolapse. Prior to treatment, all patients had an abnormal hand-grip test. Sixteen children received 2 mg/kg per day of CoQ_{10} or a placebo for 6 weeks, in a single-blind trial. Hand-grip strength became normal in seven of the patients receiving CoQ_{10} and in none of the placebo-treated patients.[60]

However, the relevance of this study to the treatment of mitral valve prolapse in adults is doubtful. Aside from the study's inadequate blinding, isometric hand-grip may not be a reliable test of cardiac function. Furthermore, impaired cardiac function is not typical of mitral valve prolapse in adults, and the symptoms associated with this condition do not appear to be caused by diminished cardiac function. While the symptoms associated with mitral valve prolapse may respond to magnesium supplementation,[61] the role of CoQ_{10} in the treatment of this disorder is unclear.

Hypertension

Enzymatic assays revealed a deficiency of CoQ_{10} in 39% of 59 patients with essential hypertension, compared with only 6% of healthy controls. In animal models of hypertension, including spontaneously hypertensive rats, uninephrectomized rats treated with saline and deoxycorticosterone, and experimentally hypertensive dogs, orally administered CoQ_{10} significantly lowered blood pressure.[62–65]

Twenty-six patients with essential hypertension received 50 mg of CoQ_{10} twice a day. After 10 weeks of treatment, mean systolic blood pressure decreased from 164.5 to 146.7 mmHg and mean diastolic blood pressure decreased from 98.1 to 86.1 mmHg ($P < 0.001$). The fall in blood pressure was associated with a significant reduction in peripheral resistance, but there were no changes in plasma renin activity, serum and urinary sodium and potassium, and urinary aldosterone. These results suggest that treatment with CoQ_{10} decreases blood pressure in patients with essential hypertension, possibly because of a reduction in peripheral resistance.[66]

In another study, 109 patients with essential hypertension received CoQ_{10} (average dose, 225 mg/day) in addition to their usual antihypertensive regimen. The dosage of CoQ_{10} was adjusted according to clinical response and blood CoQ_{10} levels (the aim was to attain blood levels greater than 2.0 mcg/ml). The need for antihypertensive medication declined gradually, and after a mean treatment period of 4.4 months, about half of the patients were able to discontinue between one and three drugs.[67] Similar results have been reported by others.[68]

It should be noted that the effect of CoQ_{10} on blood pressure was usually not seen until after 4–12 weeks of therapy. That observation is consistent with the delayed increase in enzyme activity that results from administration of CoQ_{10}. Thus, CoQ_{10} is not a typical antihypertensive drug; rather, it seems to correct some metabolic abnormality that is involved in the pathogenesis of hypertension.

Diabetes mellitus

Diabetes mellitus is a multifactorial disease that is associated with a number of different metabolic abnormalities. The electron transport chain, of which CoQ_{10} is a component, plays a major role in carbohydrate metabolism. A deficiency of CoQ_{10} might therefore have an adverse effect on glucose tolerance.

Decreased levels of CoQ_{10} (measured as total CoQ) were found in rats with experimentally induced diabetes. Administration of CoQ_7 (an analog of CoQ_{10}) partially corrected abnormal glucose metabolism in alloxan-diabetic rats. (Before CoQ_{10} became commercially available, some therapeutic trials were done with CoQ_7. These two compounds are considered to be nutritionally equivalent.)

Thirty-nine diabetics received 120 mg/day of CoQ_7 for 2–18 weeks. Fasting blood sugar levels fell by at least 30% in 31% of the patients and the concentration of ketone bodies declined by at least 30% in 59% of the patients. One patient who was poorly controlled on 60 units/day of insulin showed a marked fall in fasting blood sugar and ketone bodies after receiving CoQ_7.[69]

Infertility

Because sperm production and function are highly energy-dependent processes, CoQ_{10} deficiency could presumably be a contributing factor to infertility in men. In one study, administration of 10 mg/day of CoQ_7 resulted in a considerable increase in sperm count and motility in a group of infertile men.[70] Additional research is needed to determine whether CoQ_{10} therapy has a role in the treatment of infertility.

Drug interactions

Cholesterol-lowering drugs such as lovastatin and pravastatin inhibit the enzyme 3-hydroxy-3-methylglutaryl(HMG)-CoA reductase, which is required for biosynthesis of both cholesterol and CoQ_{10}. Thus, administration of these drugs might compromise CoQ_{10} status by decreasing its synthesis. Supplementation of the diet of rats with lovastatin (400 mg/kg of diet) for 4 weeks reduced the concentration of CoQ_{10} in the heart, liver, and blood.[71] In another study, administration of lovastatin to five patients receiving CoQ_{10} for heart failure was followed by a reduction in blood levels of CoQ_{10} and a significant deterioration of clinical status. Some of these patients improved after the dosage of CoQ_{10} was increased or the lovastatin was discontinued.[72]

These results suggest that people who have low CoQ_{10} levels and suboptimal cardiac function might develop clinically significant CoQ_{10} depletion after taking an HMG-CoA reductase inhibitor. Although individuals with high CoQ_{10} levels and good cardiac function can probably tolerate these drugs better, a case can be made that all patients being treated with HMG-CoA reductase inhibitors should also receive CoQ_{10} prophylactically.

The beta-blockers propranolol and metaprolol have been shown to inhibit CoQ_{10}-dependent enzymes.[73] The antihypertensive effect of these drugs might therefore be compromised in the long run by the development of CoQ_{10} deficiency. In one study, administration of 60 mg/day of CoQ_{10} reduced the incidence of drug-induced malaise in patients receiving propranolol.[74]

A number of phenothiazines and tricyclic antidepressants have also been shown to inhibit CoQ_{10}-dependent enzymes. It is therefore possible that CoQ_{10} deficiency may be a contributing factor to the cardiac side-effects that are frequently seen with these drugs. In two clinical studies, supplementation with CoQ_{10} improved electrocardiographic changes in patients on psychotropic drugs.[75]

DOSAGE

The optimal dose of CoQ_{10} is not known and probably varies according to the severity of the condition being treated. For example, 30 mg/day of CoQ_{10} was reportedly effective in the treatment of mild congestive heart failure, 90 mg/day resulted in improvements in some cases of cancer, and 390 mg/day was associated with complete regression of liver metastases in a patient with breast cancer.

The usual dosage of CoQ_{10} is 30 mg/day, with a range of 20–100 mg/day. Although higher doses were used in some studies, it is not clear that these larger amounts are necessary for most clinical situations. The dosage of CoQ_{10} should be adjusted according to the response of the patient. Larger doses (up to 100 mg/day) may be needed in cases of severe cardiac disease. Because of the serious nature of the cardiotoxicity induced by adriamycin, CoQ_{10} prophylaxis should follow the reportedly effective dosage schedule (100 mg/day, beginning 3–5 days prior to the start of adriamycin therapy). Some cases of muscular dystrophy may require large doses of CoQ_{10}; the dosage in these cases should be assessed according to clinical response.

Since the synthesis of new CoQ_{10}-dependent enzymes is a slow process, a clinical response might not occur until 8 or more weeks after therapy is begun.[76]

TOXICOLOGY

Coenzyme Q_{10} is generally well tolerated, and no serious adverse effects have been reported with long-term use. Because safety during pregnancy and lactation has not been proven, CoQ_{10} should not be used during these times unless the potential clinical benefit outweighs the risks. CoQ_{10} is contraindicated in cases of known hypersensitivity. In a series of 5,143 patients treated with 30 mg/day of CoQ_{10}, the following incidence of side-effects was reported:[59]

- epigastric discomfort, 0.39%
- loss of appetite, 0.23%
- nausea, 0.16%
- diarrhea, 0.12%.

REFERENCES

1. Kitamura N, Yamaguchi A, Otaki M et al. Myocardial tissue level of coenzyme Q_{10} in patients with cardiac failure. In: Folkers K, Yamamura Y, eds. Biomedical and clinical aspects of coenzyme Q, vol. 4. Amsterdam: Elsevier. 1984: p 243–252
2. Nakamura R, Littarru GP, Folkers K, Wilkinson EG. Study of Co Q_{10}-enzymes in gingiva from patients with periodontal disease and evidence for a deficiency of coenzyme Q_{10}. Proc Natl Acad Sci 1974; 71: 1456
3. Mayer P, Hamberger H, Drews J. Differential effects of ubiquinone Q7 and ubiquinone analogs on macrophage activation and experimental infections in granulocytopenic mice. Infection 1980; 8: 256–261
4. Saiki I, Tokushima Y, Nishimura K, Azuma I. Macrophage activation with ubiquinones and their related compounds in mice. Int J Vitam Nutr Res 1983; 53: 312–320
5. Bliznakov E, Casey A, Premuzic E. Coenzymes Q stimulants of the phagocytic activity in rats and immune response in mice. Experientia 1970; 26: 953–954
6. Bliznakov E, Casey A, Kishi T et al. Coenzyme Q deficiency in mice following infection with Friend leukemia virus. Int J Vitam Nutr Res 1975; 45: 388–395
7. Bliznakov EG. Effect of stimulation of the host defense system by coenzyme Q_{10} on dibenzpyrene-induced tumors and infection with Friend leukemia virus in mice. Proc Natl Acad Sci 1973; 70: 390–394
8. Bliznakov EG, Watanabe T, Saji S, Folkers K. Coenzyme Q deficiency in aged mice. J Med 1978; 9: 337–346
9. Bliznakov EG. Immunological senescence in mice and its reversal by coenzyme Q_{10}. Mech Ageing Dev 1978; 7: 189–197
10. Folkers K, Shizukuishi S, Takemura K et al. Increase in levels of IgG in serum of patients treated with coenzyme Q_{10}. Res Commun Chem Pathol Pharmacol 1982; 38: 335–338
11. Sugiyama S, Kitazawa M, Ozawa K et al. Anti-oxidative effect of coenzyme Q_{10}. Experientia 1980; 36: 1002–1003
12. Folkers K, Langsjoen P, Nara Y et al. Biochemical deficiencies of coenzyme Q_{10} in HIV infection and exploratory treatment. Biochem Biophys Res Commun 1988; 153: 888–896
13. Bliznakov EG. Effect of stimulation of the host defense system by coenzyme Q_{10} on dibenzpyrene-induced tumors and infection with Friend leukemia virus in mice. Proc Natl Acad Sci 1973; 70: 390–394
14. Lockwood K, Moesgaard S, Hanioka T, Folkers K. Apparent partial remission of breast cancer in 'high risk' patients supplemented with nutritional antioxidants, essential fatty acids and coenzyme Q_{10}. Molec Aspects Med 1994; 15: S231–240
15. Lockwood K, Moesgaard S, Yamamoto T, Folkers K. Progress on therapy of breast cancer with vitamin Q_{10} and the regression of metastases. Biochem Biophys Res Commun 1995; 212: 172–177
16. Nakamura R, Littarru GP, Folkers K, Wilkinson EG. Study of CoQ_{10}-enzymes in gingiva from patients with periodontal disease and evidence for a deficiency of coenzyme Q_{10}. Proc Natl Acad Sci 1974; 71: 1456–1460
17. Hansen IL, Iwamoto Y, Kishi T, Folkers K. Bioenergetics in clinical medicine. IX. Gingival and leucocytic deficiencies of coenzyme Q_{10} in patients with periodontal disease. Res Commun Chem Pathol Pharmacol 1976; 14: 729–738
18. Littarru GP, Nakamura R, Ho L et al. Deficiency of coenzyme Q_{10} in gingival tissue from patients with periodontal disease. Proc Natl Acad Sci 1971; 68: 2332–2335
19. Nakamura R, Littarru GP, Folkers K, Wilkinson EG. Deficiency of coenzyme Q in gingiva of patients with periodontal disease. Int J Vitam Nutr Res 1973; 43: 84–92
20. Wilkinson EG, Arnold RM, Folkers K. Bioenergetics in clinical medicine. VI. Adjunctive treatment of periodontal disease with coenzyme Q_{10}. Res Commun Chem Pathol Pharmacol 1976; 14: 715–719
21. Wilkinson EG, Arnold RM, Folkers K. Treatment of periodontal and other soft tissue diseases of the oral cavity with coenzyme Q. In: Folkers K, Yamamura Y, eds. Biomedical and clinical aspects of coenzyme Q, vol. 1. Amsterdam: Elsevier/North-Holland Biomedical Press. 1977: p 251–265
22. Wilkinson EG, Arnold RM, Folkers K et al. Bioenergetics in clinical medicine. II. Adjunctive treatment with coenzyme Q in periodontal therapy. Res Commun Chem Pathol Pharmacol 1975; 12: 111–124
23. Shizukuishi S, Inoshita E, Tsunemitsu A et al. Therapy by coenzyme Q_{10} of experimental periodontitis in a dog-model supports results of human periodontitis therapy. In: Folkers K, Yamamura Y, eds. Biomedical and clinical aspects of coenzyme Q, vol. 4. Amsterdam: Elsevier. 1984: p 153–162
24. Salim AS. Removing oxygen-derived free radicals stimulates healing of ethanol-induced erosive gastritis in the rat. Digestion 1990; 47: 24–28
25. Salim AS. Oxygen-derived free radicals and the prevention of duodenal ulcer relapse: a new approach. Am J Med Sci 1990; 300: 1–6
26. Kohli Y, Suto Y, Kodama T. Effect of hypoxia on acetic acid ulcer of the stomach in rats with or without coenzyme Q_{10}. Jpn J Exp Med 1981; 51: 105–108
27. van Gaal L, de Leeuw ID, Vadhanavikit S, Folkers K. Exploratory study of coenzyme Q_{10} in obesity. In: Folkers K, Yamamura Y, eds. Biomedical and clinical aspects of coenzyme Q, vol. 4. Amsterdam: Elsevier. 1984: p 369–373
28. Vanfraecchem JHP, Folkers K. Coenzyme Q_{10} and physical performance. In: Folkers K, Yamamura Y, eds. Biomedical and clinical aspects of coenzyme Q, vol. 3. Amsterdam: Elsevier. 1981: p 235–241
29. Littarru GP, Jones D, Scholler J, Folkers K. Deficiency of coenzyme Q_{10} in mice having hereditary muscular dystrophy. Biochem Biophys Res Commun 1970; 41: 1306–1313
30. Farley TM, Scholler J, Smith JL, Folkers K. Hematopoietic activity of hexahydrocoenzyme Q4 in the monkey. Arch Biochem Biophys 1967; 121: 625–632
31. Smith JL, Scholler J, Moore HW et al. Studies on the mechanism of vitamin-like activity of coenzyme Q. Arch Biochem Biophys 1966; 116: 129–137
32. Dinning JS, Fitch CD, Shunk CH, Folkers K. The response of the anemic and dystrophic monkey to treatment with coenzyme Q. J Am Chem Soc 1962; 84: 2007–2008
33. Wagner AF, Stopkie RJ, Folkers K. Coenzyme Q. LIII. Novel finding of activity for hexahydrocoenzyme Q4 in the dystrophic rabbit. Arch Biochem Biophys 1964; 107: 184–186
34. Folkers K, Wolaniuk J, Simonsen R et al. Biochemical rationale and the cardiac response of patients with muscle disease to therapy with coenzyme Q_{10}. Proc Natl Acad Sci 1985; 82: 4513–4516

35. Folkers K, Wolaniuk J, Simonsen R et al. Biochemical rationale and the cardiac response of patients with muscle disease to therapy with coenzyme Q_{10}. Proc Natl Acad Sci 1985; 82: 4513–4516
36. Ishihara Y, Uchida Y, Kitamura S, Takaku F. Effect of Coenzyme Q_{10}, a quinone derivative, on guinea pig lung and tracheal tissue. Arzneimittelforsch 1985; 35: 929–933
37. Stocker R, Bowry VW, Frei B. Ubiquinol-10 protects human low density lipoprotein more efficiently against lipid peroxidation than does alpha-tocopherol. Proc Natl Acad Sci 1991; 88: 1646–1650
38. Hanaki Y, Sugiyama S, Ozawa T, Ohno M. Ratio of low-density lipoprotein cholesterol to ubiquinone as a coronary risk factor. N Engl J Med 1991; 325: 814–815
39. Langsjoen PH, Langsjoen PH, Folkers K. Long-term efficacy and safety of coenzyme Q_{10} therapy for idiopathic dilated cardiomyopathy. Am J Cardiol 1990; 65: 521–523
40. Littarru GP, Ho L, Folkers K. Deficiency of coenzyme Q_{10} in human heart disease. Part I. Int J Vitam Nutr Res 1972; 42: 291–305
41. Folkers K, Littarru GP, Ho L et al. Evidence for a deficiency of coenzyme Q_{10} in human heart disease. Int J Vitam Nutr Res 1970; 40: 380–390
42. Folkers K, Vadhanavikit S, Mortensen SA. Biochemical rationale and myocardial tissue data on the effective therapy of cardiomyopathy with coenzyme Q_{10}. Proc Natl Acad Sci 1985; 82: 901–904
43. Langsjoen PH, Langsjoen PH, Folkers K. Long-term efficacy and safety of coenzyme Q_{10} therapy for idiopathic dilated cardiomyopathy. Am J Cardiol 1990; 65: 521–523
44. Langsjoen PH, Folkers K, Lyson K et al. Effective and safe therapy with coenzyme Q_{10} for cardiomyopathy. Klin Wochenschr 1988; 66: 583–590
45. Langsjoen PH, Vadhanavikit S, Folkers K. Effective treatment with coenzyme Q_{10} of patients with chronic myocardial disease. Drugs Exptl Clin Res 1985; 11: 577–579
46. Yamamura Y, Ishiyama T, Yamagami T et. al. Clinical use of coenzyme-Q for treatment of cardiovascular disease. Jpn Circ J 1967; 31: 168. *In this study, CoQ7 was used; however, this compound is apparently converted by the body into* CoQ_{10}.
47. Ishiyama T, Morita Y, Toyama S et al. A clinical study of the effect of coenzyme Q on congestive heart failure. Jpn Heart J 1976; 17: 32–42
48. Anonymous. Coenzyme aids cardiomyopathy. Med World News 1985; 8/12: 69
49. Mortensen SA, Vadhanavikit S, Baandrup U, Folkers K. Long-term coenzyme Q_{10} therapy. A major advance in the management of resistant myocardial failure. Drugs Exptl Clin Res 1985; 11: 581–593
50. Baggio E, Gandini R, Plancher AC et al. Italian multicenter study on the safety and efficacy of coenzyme Q_{10} as adjunctive therapy in heart failure (interim analysis). Clin Invest 1993; 71: S145–149
51. Morisco C, Trimarco B, Condorelli M. Effect of coenzyme Q_{10} in patients with congestive heart failure: a long-term multicenter randomized study. Clin Invest 1993; 71: S134–136
52. Kamikawa T, Kobayashi A, Yamashita T et al. Effects of coenzyme Q_{10} on exercise tolerance in chronic stable angina pectoris. Am J Cardiol 1985; 56: 247–251
53. Fujioka T, Sakamoto Y, Mimura G. Clinical study of cardiac arrhythmias using a 24-hour continuous electrocardiographic recorder (5th report) – antiarrhythmic action of coenzyme Q_{10} in diabetics. Tohoku J Exp Med 1983; 141: 453–463
54. Ogura R, Toyama H, Shimada T, Murakami M. The role of ubiquinone (coenzyme Q_{10}) in preventing adriamycin-induced mitochondrial disorders in rat heart. J Appl Biochem 1979; 1: 325–335
55. Domae N, Sawada H, Matsuyama E et al. Cardiomyopathy and other chronic toxic effects induced in rabbits by doxorubicin and possible prevention by coenzyme Q_{10}. Cancer Treat Rep 1981; 65: 79–91
56. Karlsson J, Folkers K, Astrum H et al. Effect of adriamycin on heart and skeletal muscle coenzyme Q (CoQ_{10}) in man. In: Folkers K, Yamamura Y, eds. Biomedical and clinical aspects of coenzyme Q, vol. 5. Amsterdam: Elsevier. 1986
57. Judy WV, Hall JH, Dugan W et al. Coenzyme Q_{10} reduction of adriamycin cardiotoxicity. In: Folkers K, Yamamura Y, eds. Biomedical and clinical aspects of coenzyme Q, vol. 4. Amsterdam: Elsevier. 1984: p 231–241
58. Cortes EP, Gupta M, Chou C et al. Adriamycin cardiotoxicity: early detection by systolic time interval and possible prevention by coenzyme Q_{10}. Cancer Treat Rep 1978; 62: 887–891
59. Tanaka J, Tominaga R, Yoshitoshi M et al. Coenzyme Q_{10}: the prophylactic effect on low cardiac output following cardiac valve replacement. Ann Thorac Surg 1982; 33: 145–151
60. Oda T, Hamamoto K. Effect of coenzyme Q_{10} on the stress-induced decrease of cardiac performance in pediatric patients with mitral valve prolapse. Jpn Circ J 1984; 48: 1387
61. Gaby AR. Magnesium. New Canaan: Keats Publishing. 1994
62. Yamagami T, Iwamoto Y, Folkers K, Blomqvist CG. Reduction by coenzyme Q_{10} of hypertension induced by deoxycorticosterone and saline in rats. Int J Vitam Nutr Res 1974; 44: 487–496
63. Igarashi T, Nakajima Y, Tanaka M, Ohtake S. Effect of coenzyme Q_{10} on experimental hypertension in rats and dogs. J Pharmacol Exp Ther 1974; 189: 149–156
64. Iwamoto Y, Yamagami T, Folkers K, Blomqvist CG. Deficiency of coenzyme Q_{10} in hypertensive rats and reduction of deficiency by treatment with coenzyme Q_{10}. Biochem Biophys Res Commun 1974; 58: 743–748
65. Okamoto H, Kawaguchi H, Togashi H et al. Effect of coenzyme Q_{10} on structural alterations in the renal membrane of stroke-prone spontaneously hypertensive rats. Biochem Med Metabol Biol 1991; 45: 216–226
66. Digiesi V, Cantini F, Oradei A et al. Coenzyme Q_{10} in essential hypertension. Molec Aspects Med 1994; 15: S257–263
67. Langsjoen P, Langsjoen P, Willis R, Folkers K. Treatment of essential hypertension with coenzyme Q_{10}. Molec Aspects Med 1994; 15: S265–272
68. Digiesi V, Cantini F, Brodbeck B. Effect of coenzyme Q_{10} on essential hypertension. Curr Ther Res 1990; 47: 841–845
69. Shigeta Y, Izumi K, Abe H. Effect of coenzyme Q7 treatment on blood sugar and ketone bodies of diabetics. J Vitaminol 1966; 12: 293–298
70. Tanimura J. Studies on arginine in human semen. Part III. The influences of several drugs on male infertility. Bull Osaka Med School 1967; 12: 90–100
71. Willis RA, Folkers K, Tucker JL et al. Lovastatin decreases coenzyme Q levels in rats. Proc Natl Acad Sci 1990; 87: 8928–8930
72. Folkers K, Langsjoen P, Willis R et al. Lovastatin decreases coenzyme Q levels in humans. Proc Natl Acad Sci 1990; 87: 8931–8934
73. Kishi T, Kishi H, Folkers K. Inhibition of cardiac CoQ_{10}-enzymes by clinically used drugs and possible prevention. In: Folkers K, Yamamura Y, eds. Biomedical and clinical aspects of coenzyme Q, vol. 1, Amsterdam: Elsevier/North-Holland Biomedical Press. 1977: p 47–62
74. Hamada M, Kazatani Y, Ochi T et al. Correlation between serum CoQ_{10} level and myocardial contractility in hypertensive patients. In: Folkers K, Yamamura Y, eds. Biomedical and clinical aspects of coenzyme Q, vol. 4. Amsterdam: Elsevier Science. 1984: p 263–270
75. Kishi T, Makino K, Okamoto T et al. Inhibition of myocardial respiration by psychotherapeutic drugs and prevention by coenzyme Q. In: Yamamura Y, Folkers K, Ito Y, eds. Biomedical and clinical aspects of coenzyme Q, vol. 2. Amsterdam: Elsevier/North-Holland Biomedical Press. 1980: p 139–154
76. Kishi T, Makino K, Okamoto T. Metabolism of exogenous coenzyme Q_{10} in vivo and the bioavailability of coenzyme Q_{10} preparations in Japan. In: Folkers K, Yamamura Y, eds. Biomedical and clinical aspects of coenzyme Q, vol. 4. Amsterdam: Elsevier Science. 1984: p 131–142

CHAPTER CONTENTS

77

Coleus forskohlii

Michael T. Murray, ND

Joseph E. Pizzorno Jr, ND

Coleus forskohlii (family: Labiatae)
Synonyms: *Coleus barbatus, Plectranthus barbatus, P. forskohlii*
Common name: coleus

GENERAL DESCRIPTION

Coleus forskohlii is a small member of the mint (Labiatae) family. It grows as a perennial on the sun-exposed, dry hill slopes between an altitude of 1,000 to 6,000 feet on the mountains in the subtropical, temperate climactic zone of India, Nepal, Sri Lanka, and Thailand. Its Latin name comes from the word *coleos,* which means "sheath" and refers to the fused filaments that form a sheath around the stylus of the flower. The epithet, *forskohlii,* was given to commemorate the Finnish botanist Forskal, who traveled extensively in Egypt and Arabia in the 18th century.

The radially spread rootstock is the portion of the plant that has been used for medicinal purposes. The rootstock is also the source of a compound of unique biological importance, forskolin. No other species of *Coleus* contains forskolin.

CHEMICAL COMPOSITION

The primary chemical of clinical interest contained in *C. forskohlii* is the diterpine forskolin (Fig. 77.1). In 1974, forskolin was discovered during a large-scale screening of medicinal plants by the Indian Central Drug Research Institute. The screening revealed the presence of a hypo-

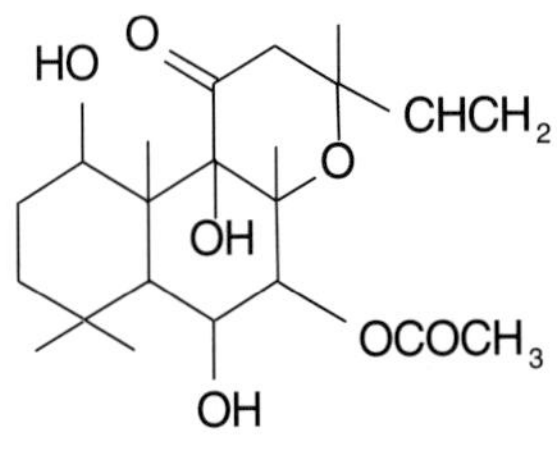

Figure 77.1 Forskolin.

tensive and spasmolytic component which was initially named coleanol.[1] Additional investigation determined the exact chemical structure and the name was changed to forskolin. Between 1981 and 1994, forskolin was investigated in over 5,000 in vitro research studies designed to understand better the cellular processes governed by cAMP (discussed below). While most of these studies have used this isolated constituent, there is evidence that other components within the plant extract enhance the absorption and biological activity of forskolin. However, no detailed analysis of the chemical composition of *C. forskohlii* could be found.

HISTORY AND FOLK USE

Coleus forskohlii has a long history of use in Ayurvedic, Siddha, and Unani systems of medicine. Studies of the pharmacological activity of forskolin substantiate the traditional uses of *C. forskohlii* in such conditions as:[1]

- cardiovascular disease
- eczema
- abdominal colic
- respiratory disorders
- painful urination
- insomnia
- convulsions.

PHARMACOLOGY

The basic mechanism of action of forskolin is the activation of adenylate cyclase, which increases cyclic adenosine monophosphate (cAMP) in cells.[2] Cyclic AMP is perhaps the most important cell-regulating compound. Once formed, it activates many other enzymes involved in diverse cellular functions.

Under normal situations, cAMP is formed when an activating hormone (e.g. epinephrine) binds to a receptor site on the cell membrane and stimulates the activation of adenylate cyclase. This enzyme is found in all cellular membranes and only the specificity of the receptor site determines which hormone will activate it in a particular cell. In contrast, forskolin appears to directly activate adenylate cyclase, bypassing hormonal transmembrane activation of adenylate cyclase.

The physiological and biochemical effects of a raised intracellular cAMP level include:

- inhibition of platelet activation and degranulation
- inhibition of mast cell degranulation and histamine release
- increased force of contraction of heart muscle
- relaxation of the arteries and other smooth muscles
- increased insulin secretion
- increased thyroid function
- lipolysis.

Recent studies have found forskolin to possess additional mechanisms of action independent of its ability to directly stimulate adenylate cyclase and cAMP-dependent physiological responses.[3] Specifically, forskolin has been shown to inhibit a number of membrane transport proteins and channel proteins through a mechanism that does not involve the production of cAMP. The result is again a transmembrane signaling that results in activation of other cellular enzymes. Research is underway to determine the exact receptors to which forskolin is binding.

Another action of forskolin is the inhibition of platelet-activating factor (PAF) by interfering with PAF binding to receptor sites.[4] PAF plays a central role in many inflammatory and allergic processes, including neutrophil activation, increasing vascular permeability, smooth muscle contraction including bronchoconstriction, and reduction in coronary blood flow. Treatment of platelets with forskolin prior to PAF exposure results in a 30–40% decrease in PAF binding. This decrease in PAF binding caused by forskolin was concomitant with a decrease in the physiological responses of platelets induced by PAF. However, this forskolin-induced decrease in PAF binding was not a consequence of cAMP formation, as the addition of a cAMP antagonist did not inhibit the action of forskolin. In addition, the inactive analog of forskolin, dideoxyforskolin, which does not activate adenyl cyclase, also reduced PAF binding to its receptor. Researchers speculate that the action of forskolin on PAF binding is due to a direct effect of this molecule and its analog on the PAF receptor itself or to components of the post-receptor signaling for PAF.

CLINICAL APPLICATIONS

The therapeutic ramifications of *C. forskohlii* based on the pharmacology of forskolin are immense. There are many conditions where a decreased intracellular cAMP level is thought to be a major factor in the development of the disease process. At present, *C. forskohlii* appears to be especially well indicated in these types of conditions which include:

- atopic dermatitis
- asthma
- psoriasis
- angina
- hypertension.

Although *C. forskohlii* can be used alone, it may prove to be most useful when combined with other botanicals and / or other measures in the treatment of these disorders.

Inflammatory conditions

Allergic conditions such as asthma and eczema are characterized by a relative decrease in cAMP in both the bronchial smooth muscle and the skin. As a result, mast cells degranulate and smooth muscle cells contract more readily. In addition, these allergic conditions are also characterized by excessive levels of PAF.

Asthma and eczema

Current drug therapy for allergic conditions like asthma and eczema is largely designed to increase cAMP levels by using substances which either bind to receptors to stimulate adenylate cyclase (e.g. corticosteroids) or inhibit the enzyme phosphodiesterase which breaks down cAMP once it is formed (e.g. methylxanthines). These actions are different than forskolin's ability to increase the production of cAMP via transmembrane activation of adenylate cyclase. The cAMP-elevating action of forskolin supports the use of *C. forskohlii* extracts alone or in combination with standard drug therapy in the treatment of virtually all allergic conditions.

Coleus forskohlii extracts may be particularly useful in asthma, as increasing intracellular levels of cAMP results in relaxation of bronchial muscles and relief of respiratory symptoms. Forskolin has been shown to have remarkable effects in relaxing constricted bronchial muscles in asthmatics.[5,6,7] This type of smooth muscle is also found in the gastrointestinal tract, uterus, bladder, and arteries. Forskolin has been shown to have tremendous antispasmodic action on these various smooth muscles. This antispasmodic action of forskolin supports the folk medicine use of *C. forskohlii* in the treatment of not only asthma, but also intestinal colic, uterine cramps (menstrual cramps), painful urination, angina, and hypertension. In addition to forskolin's ability to relax smooth muscle, its other anti-allergic activities, such as inhibiting the release of histamine and synthesis of allergic compounds, are also of benefit in the treatment of asthma.[8]

One double-blind clinical study sought to compare the anti-asthmatic effects of forskolin with the drug fenoterol. Sixteen patients with asthma were studied using three different preparations:

- single inhalation doses of fenoterol
- dry powder capsules of fenoterol (0.4 mg)
- metered doses of fenoterol (0.4 mg), and forskolin dry powder capsules (10.0 mg).

All three caused a significant improvement in respiratory function and bronchodilation. However, while the fenoterol preparations caused tremors and decreased blood potassium levels, no such negative effects were seen with forskolin.

In another study, the bronchodilating effect (after 5 minutes) of forskolin was as good as that produced by fenoterol in 12 healthy volunteers (non-smokers), as determined by whole body plethysmography.[9] Both substances were administered by metered dose inhalers. At the beginning (after 3 and 5 minutes), the protective effect of forskolin against inhaled acetylcholine was as good as that produced by fenoterol, while later on (after 15 and 30 minutes), fenoterol provided stronger protection.

Whether orally administered forskolin in the form of *C. forskohlii* extract would produce similar bronchodilatory effects is yet to be determined. However, based on the plant's historical use and additional mechanisms of action, it appears likely.

Psoriasis

Psoriasis is a common skin disorder that seems to be caused by a relative decrease in cAMP as compared with cyclic guanine monophosphate (cGMP). The result is a tremendous increase in cell division. In fact, cells divide in psoriasis at a rate 1,000 times greater than the normal. Preliminary studies have indicated that forskolin may be of great benefit to individuals with psoriasis via its ability to re-establish the normal balance between cAMP and cGMP.[1]

Cardiovascular effects

Perhaps the most useful clinical applications of *C. forskohlii* extracts will turn out to be for cardiovascular diseases such as hypertension, congestive heart failure, and angina. The cardiovascular effects of *C. forskohlii* and its components have been studied in great detail.[1,10,11] Its basic cardiovascular actions involve lowering of blood pressure along with improving contractility of the heart. Again, this is related to increasing cAMP levels throughout the cardiovascular system which results in relaxation of the arteries and increased force of contraction. The net effect is significant improvement of cardiovascular function.

Hypertension and cardiac failure

Several clinical and animal studies have supported the use of forskolin in hypertension and cardiac failure.[10–13] In one human study involving seven patients with dilated cardiomyopathy, forskolin was shown to improve left ventricular function primarily via reduction of preload and without raising metabolic costs.[12] This study confirmed earlier animal studies showing forskolin increases the contractile force of heart muscle.[11]

In another human study, the hemodynamic effects of intravenous (3 mcg/kg per minute) forskolin given to patients with dilated cardiomyopathy was evaluated.[13] Although systemic vascular resistance and diastolic pressure fell, forskolin had no effect on cardiac index, ejection fraction, or myocardial oxygen consumption at this very low dosage. However, when a small dosage of dobutamine was given along with the forskolin, an increase of all four parameters was observed. At a higher dosage (4 mcg/kg per minute), forskolin increased heart function by 19% and produced a 16% rise in heart rate. However, these changes were associated with symptomatic flush syndromes. These results indicate that forskolin may best be used in congestive heart failure in combination with other botanicals such as *Crataegus* (see Ch. 79).

Forskolin has also been shown to be a direct cerebral vasodilator, indicating that it may prove to be useful in cerebral vascular insufficiency and post-stroke recovery.[14]

An additional mechanism of action particularly beneficial in a wide range of cardiovascular conditions is inhibition of platelet aggregation. In this area, the evidence indicates that the standardized *C. forskohlii* extract is superior to pure forskolin.[15] In an animal model for evaluating in vivo inhibition of platelet aggregation, rats were divided into four groups: group 1 received *C. forskohlii* extract (480 mg/kg supplying 20 mg/kg of forskolin); group 2 received forskolin (20 mg/kg); group 3 received dipyridamole; and group 4 served as the control. All treatments were given orally once daily. ADP-induced platelet aggregation was measured on odd days 1 through 15. All three treatments produced significant inhibition of platelet aggregation. On day 15, the inhibitions were approximately 42% for group 1, 37% for group 2, and 52% for group 3. Hence, the extract of *C. forskohlii* produced greater inhibition than the pure forskolin.

OTHER CLINICAL APPLICATIONS

Coleus forskohlii extracts concentrated and standardized for forskolin content may prove to be useful in a number of other clinical applications, including:

- weight-loss programs
- hypothyroidism
- malabsorption and digestive disorders
- depression
- prevention of cancer metastases
- immune system enhancement.

Glaucoma

In clinical studies, forskolin has been shown to greatly reduce intraocular pressure (IOP) when it is applied directly to the eyes.[16–19] This effect indicates that topical forskolin preparations may turn out to be of benefit in the treatment of glaucoma. Unlike current drug therapy, forskolin actually increases intraocular blood flow, has no side-effects, and does not induce miosis.

Weight-loss programs

Lipolysis, the breakdown of stored fat, is regulated by cAMP. Forskolin has been shown to stimulate lipolysis as well as inhibit the synthesis of fat in adipocytes.[20–23] Forskolin has also been shown to counteract the age-related decreased response of fat cells to lipolytic hormones like epinephrine.[24]

Hypothyroidism

Forskolin has been shown to increase thyroid hormone production as well as stimulate thyroid hormone release.[25]

Malabsorption and digestive disorders

Forskolin stimulates digestive secretions including the release of hydrochloric acid, pepsin, amylase, and pancreatic enzymes.[26,27] Forskolin has been shown to promote nutrient absorption in the small intestine.[28] *C. forskohlii* extracts may prove to be quite useful in treating dry mouth, as forskolin increases salivation.[29]

Depression

Forskolin has been shown to exert antidepressant activity in animal studies.[30]

Cancer metastases

Forskolin has been shown to be a potent inhibitor of cancer metastasis in mice injected with malignant cells.[31] As little as 82 mcg administered to mice inhibited metastasis by over 70%.

Immune system enhancement

Forskolin exhibits potent immune system enhancement (primarily through activation of macrophages and lymphocytes) in several models.[32–34]

DOSAGE

The recommended dosage should be based upon the level of forskolin. As the forskolin content of *Coleus* root is typically only 0.2–0.3%, crude *Coleus* products may not be sufficient to produce a pharmacological effect and the safety of the whole root at high dosages is not as well studied. It is best to use standardized extracts which have known forskolin content.

Daily dosages are as follows:

- forskolin: 5–10 mg two to three times daily
- standardized extract (18% forskolin): 50 mg two to three times daily
- dried root: 2–5 g two to three times daily.

TOXICOLOGY

The animal studies on forskolin indicate low toxicity. The pharmacology of forskolin suggests it would be wise to restrict the use *C. forskohlii* preparations in patients with low blood pressure and peptic ulcers. *C. forskohlii* preparations should be used with caution in patients on prescription medications, especially anti-asthmatics and antihypertensives, due to its ability to potentiate these and other drugs' effects.

REFERENCES

1. Ammon HPT, Muller AB. Forskolin. from Ayurvedic remedy to a modern agent. Planta Medica 1985; 51: 473–477
2. Seamon KB, Daly JW. Forskolin. A unique diterpene activator of cAMP-generating systems. J Cyclic Nucleotide Research 1981; 7: 201–224
3. Laurenza A, Sutkowski EM, Seamon KB. Forskolin. A specific stimulator of adenyl cyclase or a diterpene with multiple sites of action? Trends Pharmacol Sci 1989; 10: 442–447
4. Wong S, Mok W, Phaneuf S. Forskolin inhibits platelet-activating factor binding to platelet receptors independently of adenylyl cyclase activation. Eur J Pharmacol 1993; 245: 55–61
5. Wong S, Mok W, Phaneuf S. Forskolin inhibits platelet-activating factor binding to platelet receptors independently of adenylyl cyclase activation. Eur J Pharmacol 1993; 245: 55–61
6. Lichey J, Friedrich T, Priesnitz M et al. Effect of forskolin on methacholine-induced bronchoconstriction in extrinsic asthmatics. Lancet 1984; ii: 167
7. Bauer K, Dietersdorfer F, Sertl K. Pharmacodynamic effects of inhaled dry powder formulations of fenoterol and colforsin in asthma. Clin Pharmacol Ther 1993; 53: 76–83
8. Marone G, Columbo M, Triggiani M. Forskolin inhibits the release of histamine from human basophils and mast cells. Agents Actions 1986; 18: 96–99
9. Kaik G, Witte PU. Protective effect of forskolin in acetylcholine provocation in healthy probands. Comparison of 2 doses with fenoterol and placebo. Wien Med Wochenschr 1986; 136: 637–641
10. Dubey MP, Srimal RC, Nityand S, Dhawan BN. Pharmacological studies on coleonol, a hypotensive diterpene from *Coleus forskohlii*. J Ethnopharmacology 1981; 3: 1–13
11. Lindner E, Dohadwalla AN, Bhattacharya BK. Positive inotropic and blood pressure lowering activity of a diterpene derivative isolated from *Coleus forskohlii*. Forskolin. Arzneim Forsch 1978; 28: 284–289
12. Kramer W, Thormann J, Kindler M. Effects of forskolin on left ventricular function in dilated cardiomyopathy. Arzneim Forsch 1987; 37: 364–367
13. Schlepper M, Thormann J, Mitrovic V. Cardiovascular effects of forskolin and phosphodiesterase-III inhibitors. Basic Res Cardiol 1989; 84: 197–212
14. Wysham DG, Brotherton AF, Heistad DD. Effects of forskolin on cerebral blood flow. Implications for a role of adenylate cyclase. Stroke 1986; 17: 1299–1303
15. Wysham DG, Brotherton AF, Heistad DD. Effects of forskolin on cerebral blood flow. Implications for a role of adenylate cyclase. Stroke 1986; 17: 1299–1303
16. Potter DE, Burke JA, Temple JR. Forskolin suppresses sympathetic neuron function and causes ocular hypotension. Current Eye Research 1985; 4: 87–96
17. Caprioli J, Sears M. Forskolin lowers intraocular pressure in rabbits, monkeys, and man. Lancet 1983; i: 958–960
18. Meyer BH, Stulting AA, Muller FO. The effects of forskolin eye drops on intraocular pressure. S Afr Med J 1987; 71: 570–571
19. Seto C, Eguchi S, Araie M. Acute effects of topical forskolin on aqueous humor dynamics in man. Jap J Ophthalmol 1986; 30: 238–244
20. Allen DO, Quesenberry JT. Quantitative differences in the cyclic AMP-lipolysis relationships for isoproterenol and forskolin. J Pharmacol Exp Ther 1988; 244: 852–858
21. Allen DO, Ahmed B, Naseer K. Relationships between cyclic AMP levels and lipolysis in fat cells after isoproterenol and forskolin stimulation. J Pharmacol Exp Ther 1986; 238: 659–664
22. Okuda H, Morimoto C, Tsujita T. Relationship between cyclic AMP production and lipolysis induced by forskolin in rat fat cells. J Lipid Res 1992; 33: 225–231
23. Bianco AC, Kieffer JD, Silva JE. Adenosine 3',5'-monophosphate and thyroid hormone control of uncoupling protein messenger ribonucleic acid in freshly dispersed brown adipocytes. Endocrinology 1992; 130: 2625–2633
24. Hoffman BB, Chang H, Reaven GM. Stimulation and inhibition of lipolysis in isolated rat adipocytes. Evidence for age-related changes in responses to forskolin and PGE1. Horm Metab Res 1987; 19: 358–360
25. Saunier B et al. Cyclic AMP regulation of Gs protein. Thyrotropin and forskolin increase the quantity of stimulatory guanine nucleotide-binding proteins in cultured thyroid follicles. J Biol Chem 1990; 265: 19 942–19 946
26. Roger PP, Servais P, Dumont JE. Regulation of dog thyroid epithelial cell cycle by forskolin, an adenylate cyclase activator. Exp Cell Res 1990; 172: 282–292
27. Haye B, Aublin JL, Champion S. Chronic and acute effects of forskolin on isolated thyroid cell metabolism. Mol Cell Endocrinol 1990; 43: 41–50
28. Reymann A, Braun W, Woermann C. Proabsorptive properties of forskolin. Disposition of glycine, leucine and lysine in rat jejunum. Naunyn Schmiedebergs Arch Pharmacol 1986; 334: 110–115
29. Larsson O, Detsch T, Fredholm BB. VIP and forskolin enhance carbachol-induced K+ efflux from rat salivary gland fragments by a Ca2(+)-sensitive mechanism. Am J Physiol 1990; 259: C904–910
30. Wachtel H, Loschmann PA. Effects of forskolin and cyclic nucleotides in animal models predictive of antidepressant activity. Interactions with rolipram. Psychopharmacol 1986; 90: 430–435
31. Agarwal KC, Parks RE. Forskolin. A potential antimetastatic agent. Int J Cancer 1983; 32: 801–804
32. Schorlemmer HU. Forskolin for immune stimulation. Chem Abstr 1985; 102: 1009
33. Krall JF, Fernandey EI, Connolly-Filtingoff M. Human aging. Effect on the activation of lymphocyte cyclic AMP-dependent protein kinase by forskolin. Proc Soc Exp Biol Med 1987; 184: 396–402
34. Chang J, Cherney ML, Moyer JA. Effect of forskolin on prostaglandin synthesis by mouse resident peritoneal macrophages. European J Pharmacology 1984; 103: 303–312

CHAPTER CONTENTS

78

Commiphora mukul (mukul myrrh tree)

Michael T. Murray, ND

Joseph E. Pizzorno Jr, ND

Commiphora mukul (family: Burseraceae)
Common name: mukul myrrh tree

GENERAL DESCRIPTION

Commiphora mukul is a small thorny tree 4–6 feet tall that is native to Arabia and India. In its natural setting, the tree remains essentially free of foliage for most of the year. Its bark is ash-colored and comes off in rough flakes, exposing the under-bark that also peels off. Upon injury, the tree exudes a yellowish gum resin that has a balsamic odor. This oleoresin is referred to as "gum guggul" or "guggulu". It is this resin which is used for medicinal purposes. When tapped during the winter, the average tree yields 1.5–2 lb of resin.[1]

CHEMICAL COMPOSITION

Guggulu contains a mixture of diverse chemical constituents which can be separated into several fractions.[1] The first step in the fractionation process involves mixing guggulu with ethyl acetate, yielding a soluble and an insoluble fraction (see Fig. 78.1). The insoluble fraction, containing the carbohydrate constituents, is regarded as toxic and is the major reason why extracts of the soluble portion are preferred to crude gum guggul for medical use. The insoluble portion has no demonstrable pharmacological activity other than toxicity.[1]

In contrast, the soluble portion possesses significant cholesterol-lowering and anti-inflammatory activity. The soluble portion can be further separated into base, acid, and neutral fractions. The neutral portion possesses almost all of the cholesterol lowering activity while the acid portion possesses the anti-inflammatory components.[1]

Upon further purification of the neutral portion, it was determined that the ketone fraction contains the most potent cholesterol-lowering components. The ketone fraction is composed of C_{21} or C_{27} steroids, with the major components being Z- and E-guggulsterone (see Fig. 78.2).

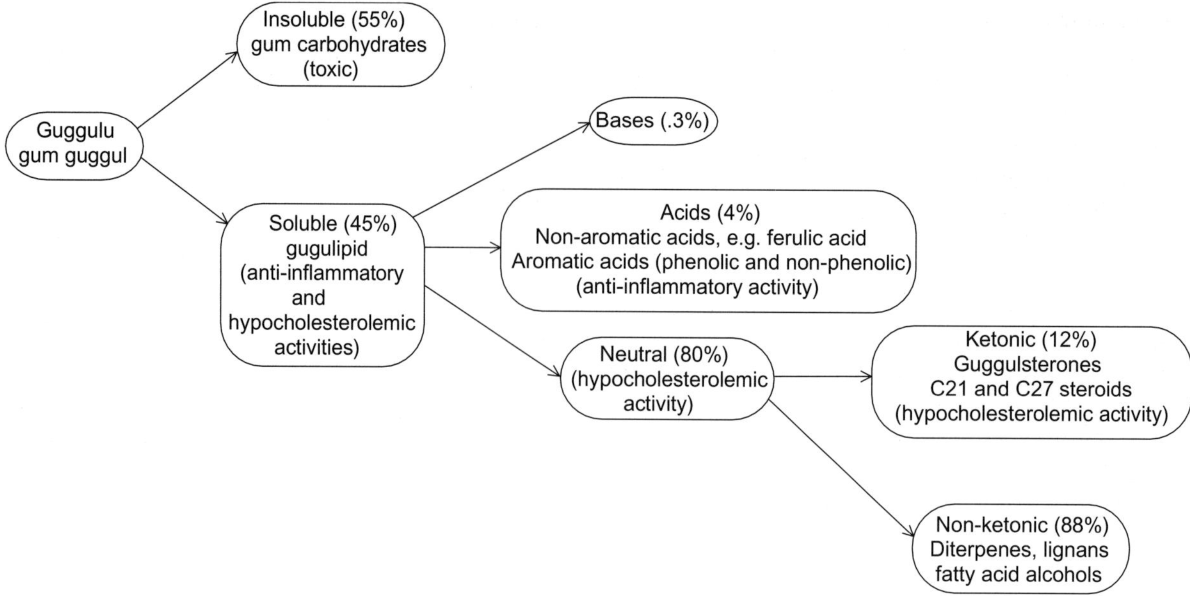

Figure 78.1 Chemical segregation of gum guggulu.

Figure 78.2 E-Guggulsterone.

These compounds are considered the major active components of gum guggul and its extracts.[1]

For medicinal purposes, a standardized extract known as gugulipid, which is standardized to contain a minimum of 50 mg of guggulsterones/g, is regarded as the most beneficial in terms of safety and effectiveness.[1,2] In addition to guggulsterones, gugulipid contains various diterpenes, sterols, esters, and fatty alcohols. These accessory components appear to exert a synergistic effect.[1,2]

HISTORY AND FOLK USE

Guggulu is a highly valued botanical medicine in the Indian system of medicine, Ayurveda. It is included in formulas for a variety of health conditions including rheumatoid arthritis and lipid disorders. The classic Ayurvedic medical text, the *Sushrutasamhita*, describes in detail the usefulness of guggul in the treatment of obesity and other disorders of fat metabolism, including "coating and obstruction of channels".[1,2]

Inspired by this description, researchers began studying, in well-designed scientific studies, the clinical effectiveness of gum guggul and its extracts in disorders of lipid metabolism – specifically, its ability to lower cholesterol and triglyceride levels and promote weight loss. This research resulted in the development of a natural cholesterol-lowering substance that is safer and more effective than many cholesterol-lowering drugs, including niacin. Gugulipid was granted approval in India for marketing as a lipid-lowering drug in 1986.[1,2]

PHARMACOLOGY

Lipid disorders

Numerous studies in humans and animals have shown that gum guggul (both crude and purified alcohol extract),[3–7] its petroleum ether extract (referred to as fraction A),[8–11] and gugulipid (standardized ethyl acetate extract)[12,13] all exert effective lipid-lowering activity. All lower both elevated cholesterol and triglyceride levels. The effect on cholesterol is particularly beneficial as guggul lowers VLDL and LDL cholesterol while simultaneously elevating HDL-cholesterol, thus offering protection against heart disease due to atherosclerosis.

Guggul preparations appear most indicated in type IIb (increased LDL, VLDL, and triglycerides) and type IV (increased VLDL and triglycerides) hyperlipidemias. In the human clinical trials using gugulipid, cholesterol levels typically dropped 14–27% in a 4–12 week period while triglyceride levels dropped from 22 to 30%.[12–14]

As seen in Table 78.1, the effect of gugulipid on serum

Table 78.1 Serum lipid effects of gugulipid compared with standard drugs

Agent	Total cholesterol	HDL cholesterol	Triglycerides
Gugulipid	–24%	+16%	–23%
Cholestyramine	–14%	+8%	+10%
Clofibrate	–10%	+11%	–22%
Lovastatin	–34%	+8%	–25%

cholesterol and triglycerides is comparable to that of conventional lipid lowering drugs. Clofibrate, niacin, and cholestyramine lower cholesterol levels 6–12%, 10–17% and 20–27%, respectively, but are associated with some degree of toxicity. In contrast, appropriate extracts of gugulipid are without reported side-effects. In addition to the excellent safety demonstrated in the human studies, safety studies in animals have demonstrated gugulipid to be non-toxic (see "Toxicology" below).

The primary mechanism of action for gum guggul and gugulipid's cholesterol-lowering action is stimulation of liver metabolism of LDL cholesterol, i.e. guggulsterones increase the uptake of LDL cholesterol from the blood by the liver.[14,15] However, another action of guggulsterone which also affects lipid levels is its ability to stimulate thyroid function.[16] This thyroid-stimulating effect may be responsible for some of gugulipid's weight loss activity.

In addition to lowering lipid levels, gum guggul and its extracts, including gugulipid, have been shown to prevent the formation of atherosclerosis and aid in the regression of pre-existing atherosclerotic plaques in animals. This implies that it may have a similar effect in humans.

Gum guggul and gugulipid have also been shown to prevent the heart from being damaged by free radicals and to improve the metabolism of the heart.[9,14] Gum guggul and its extracts have a mild effect in inhibiting platelet aggregation and promoting fibrinolysis, implying that it may also prevent the development of a stroke or embolism.[2,14]

This research indicates that gugulipid offers considerable benefit for preventing and treating atherosclerotic vascular disease, the leading cause of death in the US.

Anti-inflammatory effects

The guggulsterone fraction of gum guggul has been shown to exhibit significant anti-inflammatory action in experimental models of inflammation (e.g. raw paw edema and adjuvant arthritis method).[17–19] Its activity in models of acute inflammation is comparable to approximately one-fifth that of hydrocortisone, and equal to phenylbutazone and ibuprofen.[17] In models of chronic inflammation, it was shown to be more effective than hydrocortisone, phenylbutazone, and ibuprofen in reducing the severity of secondary lesions. The anti-inflammatory action is thought to be due to inhibition of delayed hypersensitivity reactions.[18,19]

DOSAGE

While the crude oleoresin (gum guggul), alcohol extract, and petroleum ether extract all exert lipid-lowering and anti-inflammatory action, they are associated with side-effects (skin rashes, diarrhea, etc.) at the doses required to produce a clinical effect. It is interesting to note that in classic Ayurvedic texts, the purification of crude guggul in Triphala kashaya is recommended to eliminate these side-effects.[2]

Gugulipid, the standardized ethyl acetate extract of the gum guggul, has demonstrated not only greater clinical efficacy, but also much greater patient tolerance than crude or purified gum guggul. The dosage of gugulipid is based on its guggulsterone content. Clinical studies have demonstrated that 25 mg of guggulsterone three times per day is an effective treatment for elevated cholesterol levels, elevated triglyceride levels, or both. For a 5% guggulsterone content extract, this translates to an effective dose of 500 mg three times per day.

For comparison, the daily dosage of the other forms would be:

- crude gum guggul – 10 g
- alcoholic extract – 4.5 g
- petroleum ether extract – 1.5 g.

TOXICOLOGY

The side-effects of crude gum guggul, alcoholic and petroleum ether extracts are discussed above. In clinical studies, gugulipid has not displayed any untoward side-effects, nor has it adversely affected liver function, blood sugar control, kidney function, or hematological parameters.[11–13]

Safety studies in rats, rabbits, and monkeys have demonstrated gugulipid to be non-toxic.[14] It does not possess any embryotoxic, fetotoxic effects and is therefore considered safe to use in pregnancy. In mice, the oral and intraperitoneal LD_{50} values are 1,600 mg/kg.[1]

REFERENCES

1. Satyavati GV. Gugulipid. A promising hypolipidaemic agent from gum guggul (*Commiphora wightii*). Econ Med Plant Res 1991; 5: 47–82
2. Satyavati GV. Gum guggul (*Commiphora mukul*) – The success story of an ancient insight leading to a modern discovery. Ind J Med Res 1988; 87: 327–335
3. Satyavati GV, Dwarakanath C, Tripathi SN. Experimental studies of the hypocholesterolemic effect of *Commiphora mukul*. Ind J Med Res 1969; 57: 1950–1962
4. Khana DS, Agarwal OP, Gupta SK, Arora RB. A biochemical approach to anti-atherosclerotic action of *Commiphora-mukul*. An Indian indigenous drug in Indian domestic pigs. Ind J Med Res 1969; 57: 900–906
5. Nityand S, Kapoor NK. Hypocholesterolemic effect of *Commiphora mukul* resin. Ind J Exp Biol 1971; 9: 376–377
6. Kuppurajan K, Rajagopalan SS, Koteswara RT, Sitaraman R. Effect of guggul on serum lipids in obese hypercholesterolemic and hyperlipidemic cases. J Assoc Phys India 1978; 26: 367–371

7. Baldwa VS, Bhasin V, Ranka PC, Mathur KM. Effects of *Commiphora mukul* (Guggul) in experimentally induced hyperlipidemia and atherosclerosis. JAPI 1981; 29: 13–17
8. Malhotra SC, Ahuja MMS. Comparative hypolipidaemic effectiveness of gum guggulu (*Commiphora mukul*) fraction "A", ethyl-p-chlorophenoxyisobutyrate and Ciba-13437-Su. Ind J Med Res 1971; 10: 1621–1632
9. Arora RB, Das D, Kapoor SC, Sharma RC. Effect of some fractions of *Commiphora mukul* on various serum lipid levels in hypercholesterolemic chicks and their effectiveness in myocardial infarction in rats. Ind J Exp Biol 1973; 11: 166–168
10. Malhotra SC, Ahuja MMS, Sundaram KR. Long term clinical studies on the hypolipidaemic effect of *Commiphora mukul* (guggulu) and clofibrate. Ind J Med Res 1977; 65: 390–395
11. Verna SK, Bordia A. Effect of *Commiphora mukul* (gum guggulu) in patients of hyperlipidemia with special reference to HDL-cholesterol. Ind J Med Res 1988; 87: 356–360
12. Agarwal RC, Singh SP, Saran RK et al. Clinical trial of gugulipid: a new hypolipidemic agent of plant origin in primary hyperlipidemia. Ind J Med Res 1986; 84: 626–634
13. Nityanand S, Srivastava JS, Asthana OP. Clinical trials with gugulipid, a new hypolipidaemic agent. J Assoc Phys India 1989; 37: 321–328
14. Gugulipid. Drugs of the Future 1988; 13: 618–619
15. Singh V, Kaul S, Chander R, Kapoor NK. Stimulation of low density lipoprotein receptor activity in liver membrane of guggulsterone treated rats. Pharmacol Res 1990; 22: 37–44
16. Tripathi YB, Tripathi P, Malhorta P, Tripathi SN. Thyroid stimulatory action of (Z)-guggulsterone. Mechanism of action. Planta Medica 1988; 54: 271–277
17. Arora RB, Kapoor V, Gupta SK, Sharma RC. Isolation of a crystalline steroidal compound from *Commiphora mukul* and its anti-inflammatory activity. Ind J Exp Biol 1971; 9: 403–404
18. Arora RB, Taneja V, Sharma RC, Gupta SK. Anti-inflammatory studies on a crystalline steroid isolated from *Commiphora mukul*. Ind J Med Res 1972; 60: 929–931
19. Sharma JN, Sharma JN. Comparison of the anti-inflammatory activity of *Commiphora mukul* (an indigenous drug) with those of phenylbutazone and ibuprofen in experimental arthritis induced by mycobacterial adjuvant. Arzneim Forsch 1977; 27: 1455–1457

79

Crataegus oxyacantha (hawthorn)

Michael T. Murray, ND

Joseph E. Pizzorno Jr, ND

Crataegus oxyacantha (family: Rosacea)
Common names: hawthorn, may bush, whitethorn, haw

GENERAL DESCRIPTION

Crataegus oxyacantha is a spiny tree or shrub that is native to Europe. It may reach a height of 30 feet, but is often grown as a hedge plant. Its common name, hawthorn, is actually a corruption of "hedgethorn", as it was used in Germany to divide plots of land. Its botanical name, *Crataegus oxyacantha,* is from the Greek *kratos,* meaning hardness (of the wood), *oxus* meaning sharp, and *akantha* meaning a thorn. The fruit and blossoms are used medicinally.[1]

Other species of crataegus, e.g. *C. monogyna* and *C. pentagyna,* have similar pharmacological actions to *C. oxyacantha* and may be suitable alternatives.[2,3]

CHEMICAL COMPOSITION

Hawthorn leaves, berries, and blossoms contain many biologically active flavonoid compounds, particularly anthocyanidins and proanthocyanidins (polymers of anthocyanidins, also known as biflavans or procyanidins) (see Fig. 79.1).[4,5] These flavonoids are responsible for

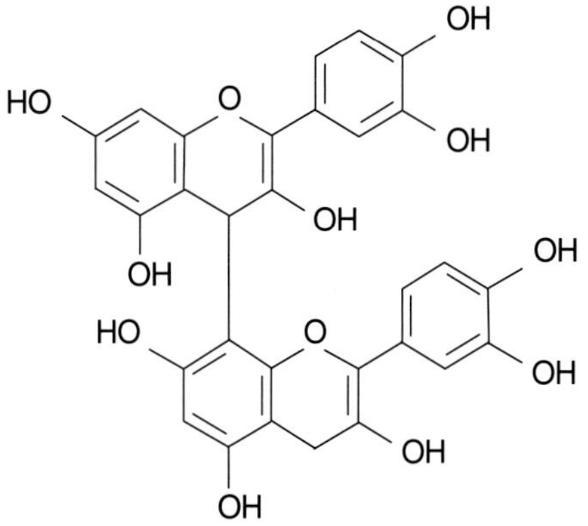

Figure 79.1 Proanthocyanidin B_2.

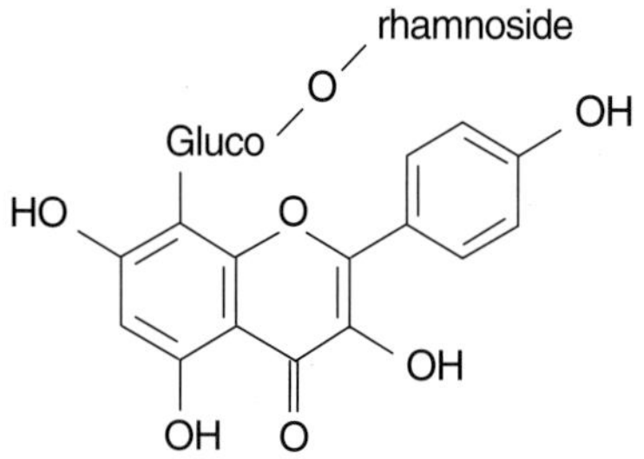

Figure 79.2 Vitexin-4′-rhamnoside.

the red to blue colors not only of hawthorn berries, but also of blackberries, cherries, blueberries, grapes, and many flowers as well. These compounds are highly concentrated in hawthorn berry and flower extracts.

High-performance liquid chromatography and thin layer chromatography (of crataegus extracts) have demonstrated that extracts of the flowers are particularly rich in flavonoids (quercetin, quercetin-3-galactoside, vitexin, vitexin-4′-rhamnoside, etc.) and proanthocyanidins (see Fig. 79.2).[5,6]

In addition to flavonoids, crataegus extracts also contain:[7]

- cardiotonic amines (e.g. phenylethylamine, o-methoxyphenylethylamine, tyramine, isobutylamine)
- choline and acetylcholine
- purine derivatives (e.g. adenosine, adenine, guanine, and caffeic acid)
- amygdalin
- pectins
- triterpene acids (ursolic, oleonolic, and crategolic acids).

HISTORY AND FOLK USE

Crataegus flowers and berries have been utilized primarily as cardiac tonics and mild diuretics in organic and functional heart disorders. They were also utilized for their astringent qualities for relief of the discomfort of sore throats.[1]

PHARMACOLOGY

The pharmacology of crataegus centers on its flavonoid components. The proanthocyanidins in crataegus are largely responsible for its cardiovascular activities.

Synergism with vitamin C

As stated above, crataegus is particularly rich in anthocyanidins and proanthocyanidins. These flavonoids have very strong "vitamin P" activity. Included in their effects are an ability to increase intracellular vitamin C levels, stabilize vitamin C (by protecting it from oxidation), and decrease capillary permeability and fragility.[4,8,9]

Collagen-stabilizing action

Crataegus' flavonoid components possess significant collagen-stabilizing action. Collagen is the most abundant protein of the body and is responsible for maintaining the integrity of ground substance, tendons, ligaments, and cartilage. Collagen is destroyed during inflammatory processes that occur in rheumatoid arthritis, periodontal disease, and other inflammatory conditions involving bones, joints, cartilage, and other connective tissue. Anthocyanidins, proanthocyanidins and other flavonoids are remarkable in their ability to prevent collagen destruction. They affect collagen metabolism in many ways, including:

- the unique ability to actually cross-link collagen fibers, resulting in reinforcement of the natural cross-linking of collagen that forms the collagen matrix of connective tissue (ground substance, cartilage, tendon, etc.)[4,8,9]
- the prevention of free radical damage, due to potent antioxidant and free radical scavenging action[4,8–10]
- the inhibition of enzymatic cleavage by enzymes secreted by leukocytes during inflammation[4,8,9]
- the prevention of the release and synthesis of compounds that promote inflammation, such as histamine, serine proteases, prostaglandins, and leukotrienes.[9–12]

These effects on collagen and their potent antioxidant activity make hawthorn extracts extremely useful in the treatment of a wide variety of inflammatory conditions. Hawthorn berries, like cherries,[13] are particularly effective in the treatment of gout, as their flavonoid components are able to reduce uric acid levels as well as reduce tissue destruction.

Cardiovascular effects

Crataegus extracts are effective in reducing blood pressure, angina attacks, and serum cholesterol levels, preventing the deposition of cholesterol in arterial walls and improving cardiac function.[2,14,15] Hawthorn extracts are widely used in Europe for their antihypertensive and cardiotonic activity. The beneficial pharmacological effects of crataegus in the treatment of these conditions appear to be a result of the following actions:

- improvement of the blood supply to the heart by dilating the coronary vessels[2,14,16–19]
- improvement of the metabolic processes in the heart which results in an increase in the force of

contraction of the heart muscle and elimination of some types of rhythm disturbances[2,14,20–22]
- inhibition of angiotensin-converting enzyme (ACE).[23]

Crataegus' ability to dilate coronary blood vessels has been repeatedly demonstrated in experimental studies.[2,14,16–19] This effect appears to be due to relaxation of vascular smooth muscle. Various flavonoid components in crataegus have been shown to inhibit vasoconstriction by a variety of substances, including hypophysin, histamine, and acetylcholine.[2,8,9] In addition, procyanidins have been shown to inhibit angiotensin converting enzyme (discussed below).[23]

Improvement in cardiac metabolism has been demonstrated in humans and animals to whom crataegus extracts have been administered.[2,14,20,21] The improvement is not only a result of increased blood and oxygen supply to the myocardium, but also a result of flavonoid–enzyme interactions. In particular, crataegus extracts and various flavonoid components in crataegus have been shown to inhibit cyclic AMP phosphodiesterase (cAMP-PDE).[22] This results in increased levels of cAMP within the myocardium, leading to a positive inotropic effect, i.e. an increase in the force of contraction. This is particularly beneficial in cases of congestive heart failure (discussed below).

Recently, several proanthocyanidins have demonstrated a specific inhibition of angiotensin-converting enzyme similar to that of captopril.[23] Captopril (D-2-methyl-3-mercaptopropanoyl-L-proline, SQ 14,225) is a synthetic ACE inhibitor widely used in the treatment of essential and renal hypertension. The proanthocyanidins that appear to have the highest activity are proanthocyanidins B-5 3,3′-di-O-gallate and C-1 3,3′,3″-tri-O-gallate. It is not surprising that these proanthocyanidins are found in relatively high concentrations in hawthorn berries, flowers, and their extracts.[4,5]

CLINICAL APPLICATIONS

The clinical use of crataegus revolves around its cardiovascular effects. Its use in atherosclerosis, hypertension, congestive heart failure, and arrhythmias is discussed below:

Atherosclerosis

Crataegus preparations, although in a supplement form, should be thought of as a necessary food in the prevention and treatment of atherosclerosis. Increasing the intake of flavonoid compounds by taking crataegus extracts has numerous health-promoting effects, including reducing cholesterol levels and decreasing the size of existing atherosclerotic plaques.[15] This again is probably a result of collagen stabilization.

A decrease in the integrity of the collagen matrix of the artery results in cholesterol deposition. Many researchers feel that if the collagen matrix of the artery remains strong, the atherosclerotic plaque will never develop. Crataegus flavonoids, by increasing the integrity of collagen structures, may offer significant protection against atherosclerosis. In addition, feeding proanthocyanidin extracts to animals has resulted in reversal of atherosclerotic lesions, as well as decreases in serum cholesterol levels.[15]

Flavonoids contained in hawthorn extracts appear to offer significant prevention, as well as potential reversing effects, in the treatment of atherosclerotic processes, which are still the major causes of death in the US.

Hypertension

Crataegus exerts a mild antihypertensive effect, which has been demonstrated in many experimental and clinical studies. Its action in lowering blood pressure is quite unique, in that it does so through a number of diverse pharmacological effects. Specifically, it dilates the coronary vessels, inhibits ACE, acts as an inotropic agent, and possesses mild diuretic activity.

Crataegus' effects generally require prolonged administration, and in many instances it may take up to 2 weeks before adequate tissue concentrations are achieved.

It should be kept in mind that as beta-blockers (e.g. Inderal) lower blood pressure by reducing cardiac output, crataegus administration to patients on these drugs may produce a mild hypertensive response.

Congestive heart failure

Crataegus has a long history of use in the treatment of congestive heart failure, particularly in combination with digitalis or other herbs containing cardiac glycosides (e.g. *Cereus grandifloris,* also known as *Cactus grandifloris,* and *Convallaria majalis*). It potentiates the action of the cardiac glycosides, presumably via its ability to inhibit cAMP-PDE and to interact with calcium channels.

Because of this enhancing effect, lower doses of cardiac glycosides can be used. In addition, magnesium has also been shown to augment digitalis action. For mild to moderate cases of CHF, crataegus extract used alone may be sufficient, but for moderate to severe CHF, it should be used in combination with other cardiac glycosides.

In early or mild stages of CHF, the effectiveness of crataegus has been repeatedly demonstrated in double-blind studies.[24–27] In one of the most recent studies, 30 patients with congestive heart failure (NYHA stage II) were assessed in a randomized double-blind study.[26] Treatment consisted of a crataegus extract standardized to contain 15 mg procyanidin oligomers per 80 mg capsule. Treatment duration was 8 weeks, and the substance was administered at a dose of one capsule taken twice a day. The group receiving the crataegus extract showed a statistically significant advantage over placebo in terms of changes in heart function as determined by standard testing procedures. Systolic and diastolic blood pressures were also mildly reduced. Like all other studies with crataegus extracts, no adverse reactions occurred.

In another study, 78 patients with CHF (NYHA stage II) were given either 600 mg of standardized crataegus extract or placebo daily.[27] The parameter used to measure effectiveness was the patient's working capacity on a bicycle ergometer. After 56 days of treatment, the crataegus group had a mean increase of 25 W compared with the placebo group's increase of only 5 W. In addition, the crataegus group also experienced a mild, but significant, reduction in systolic blood pressure (from 171 to 164 mmHg) and heart rate (from 115 to 110 beats/minute). There was no change in blood pressure or heart rate in the placebo group.

DOSAGE

The dosage depends on the type of preparation and source material. Standardized extracts, similar to those used in Europe and Asia as prescription medications, are available commercially. The doses listed for the various crataegus formulas are for use three times a day:

- berries or flowers (dried): 3–5 g or as infusion
- tincture (1:5): 4–5 ml (alcohol may elicit pressor response in some individuals)
- fluid extract (1:1): 1–2 ml
- freeze dried berries: 1–1.5 g
- flower extract (standardized to contain 1.8% vitexin-4′-rhamnoside): 100–250 mg.

TOXICOLOGY

Crataegus has been shown to have low toxicity. In rats, the typical acute LD_{50} of the tincture is about 25 ml/kg for oral administration; toxicity for chronic administration is found at about 5 ml/kg.[14] Similar results, adjusted for concentration, are found with other forms of crataegus.

Although some studies have shown that proanthocyanidins may be carcinogenic, more careful evaluation has indicated that the carcinogenicity was probably due to nitrosamines found in the extracts used.[28] Purified proanthocyanidins have been found to be non-mutagenic, according to the *Salmonella* mutagenicity assay system.[24]

REFERENCES

1. Grieve M. A modern herbal, vol 1. New York, NY: Dover. 1971: p 385–386
2. Petkov V. Plants with hypotensive, antiatheromatous and coronarodilating action. Am J Chin Med 1979; 7: 197–236
3. Thompson EB, Aynilian GH, Gora P, Farnsworth NR. Preliminary study of potential antiarrhythmic effects of *Crataegus monogyna*. J Pharm Sci 1974; 63: 1936–1937
4. Kuhnau J. The flavonoids: a class of semi-essential food components. Their role in human nutrition. Wld Rev Nutr Diet 1976; 24: 117–191
5. Ficarra P, Ficarra R, Tommasini A et al. High-performance liquid chromatography of flavonoids in *Crataegus oxyacantha*. Il Farmaco Ed Pr 1983; 39: 148–157
6. Wagner H, Bladt S, Zgainski EM. Plant drug analysis. New York, NY: Springer-Verlag. 1984: p 166, 178, 179
7. Wagner H, Grevel J. Cardiotonic drugs IV, cardiotonic amines from *Crataegus oxyacantha*. Planta Medica 1982; 45: 98–101
8. Gabor M. Pharmacologic effects of flavonoids on blood vessels. Angiologica 1972; 9: 355–374
9. Havsteen B. Flavonoids, a class of natural products of high pharmacological potency. Biochem Pharm 1983; 32: 1141–1148
10. Middleton E. The flavonoids. Trends Pharm Sci 1984; 5: 335–338
11. Amella M, Bronner C, Briancon F et al. Inhibition of mast cell histamine release by flavonoids and bioflavonoids. Planta Medica 1985; 51: 16–20
12. Busse WW, Kopp DE, Middleton E. Flavonoid modulation of human neutrophil function. J Allergy Clin Immunol 1984; 73: 801–809
13. Blau LW. Cherry diet control for gout and arthritis. Tex Rep Biol Med 1950; 8: 309–311
14. Ammon HPT, Handel M. Crataegus, toxicology and pharmacology. Planta Medica 1981; 43: 101–120, 318–322
15. Wegrowski J, Robert AM, Moczar M. The effect of procyanidolic oligomers on the composition of normal and hypercholesterolemic rabbit aortas. Biochem Pharm 1984; 33: 3491–3497
16. Mavers VWH, Hensel H. Changes in local myocardial blood flow following oral administration to a crataegus extract to non-anesthetized dogs. Arzniem Forsch 1974; 24: 783–785
17. Roddewig VC, Hensel H. Reaction of local myocardial blood flow in non-anesthetized dogs and anesthetized cats to oral and parenteral application of a crataegus fraction (oligomere procyanidins). Arzneim Forsch 1977; 27: 1407–1410
18. Rewerski VW, Piechocki T, Tyalski M, Lewak S. Some pharmacological properties of oligomeric procyanidin isolated from hawthorn (*Crataegus oxyacantha*). Arzniem Forsch 1967; 17: 490–491
19. Hammerl H, Kranzl C, Pichler O, Studlar M. Klinixch-experimentelle toffwechseluntersuchungen mit einem crataegus-extrakt. Arzniem Forsch 1971; 21: 261–263
20. Vogel VG. Predictability of the activity of drug combinations – yes or no? Arzniem Forsch 1975; 25: 1356–1365
21. O'Conolly VM, Jansen W, Bernhoft G, Bartsch G. Treatment of cardiac performance (NYHA stages I to II) in advanced age with standardized crataegus extract. Fortschr Med 1986; 104: 805–808
22. Petkov E, Nikolov N, Uzunov P. Inhibitory effect of some flavonoids and flavonoid mixtures on cyclic AMP phosphodiesterase activity of rat heart. Planta Medica 1981; 43: 183–186
23. Uchida S, Ikari N, Ohta H et al. Inhibitory effects of condensed tannins on angiotensin converting enzyme. Jap J Pharmacol 1987; 43: 242–245
24. O'Conolly VM, Jansen W, Bernhoft G, Bartsch G. Treatment of cardiac performance (NYHA stages I to II) in advanced age with standardized crataegus extract. Fortschr Med 1986; 104: 805–808
25. O'Conolly VM, Jansen W, Bernhoft G, Bartsch G. Treatment of cardiac performance (NYHA stages I to II) in advanced age with standardized crataegus extract. Fortschr Med 1986; 104: 805–808

26. Leuchtgens H. Crataegus special extract WS 1442 in NYHA II heart failure. A placebo controlled randomized double-blind study. Fortschr Med 1993; 111: 352–354
27. Schmidt U, Kuhn U, Ploch M, Hubner WD. Efficacy of the hawthorn (Crataegus) preparation LI 132 in 78 patients with chronic congestive heart failure defined as NYHA functional class II. Phytomed 1994; 1: 17–24
28. Yu CI, Swaminathan B. Mutagenicity of proanthocyanidins. Food Chem Toxicol 1987; 25: 135–139

CHAPTER CONTENTS

80

Curcuma longa (turmeric)

Michael T. Murray, ND

Joseph E. Pizzorno Jr, ND

Curcuma longa (family: Zingiberaceae)
Common names: turmeric, curcuma, Indian saffron

GENERAL DESCRIPTION

Curcuma longa, a perennial herb of the ginger family, is extensively cultivated in India, China, Indonesia, and other tropical countries. It has a thick rhizome from which arise large, oblong, and long-petioled leaves. The rhizome is the part used; it is usually cured (boiled, cleaned, and sun-dried) and polished.[1]

CHEMICAL COMPOSITION

Turmeric contains:[1,2]

- 4–14% of an orange-yellow volatile oil that is composed mainly of turmerone, atlantone, and zingiberone
- 0.3–5.4% curcumin
- sugars (28% glucose, 12% fructose, 1% arabinose)
- resins
- protein
- vitamins
- minerals.

Its chemical structure is shown in Figure 80.1.

HISTORY AND FOLK USE

Turmeric is the major ingredient of curry powder and is also used in prepared mustard. It is extensively used in foods for both its color and flavor. In addition, turmeric is used in both the Chinese and Indian (Ayurvedic)

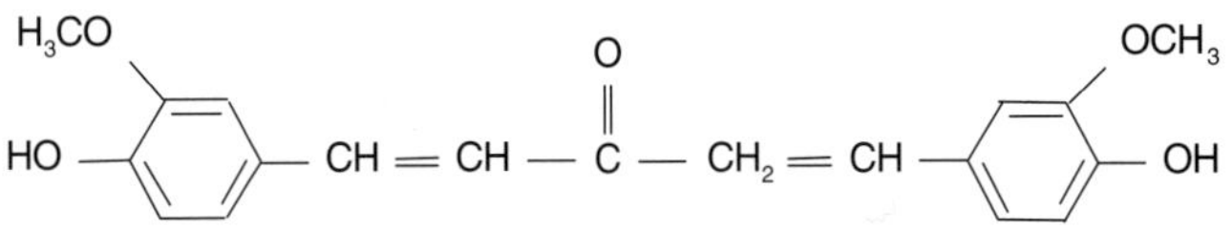

H_3CO O OCH_3

HO — [ring] — CH = CH — C(=O) — CH_2 = CH — [ring] — OH

Figure 80.1 Curcumin.

systems of medicine as an anti-inflammatory agent and in the treatment of numerous conditions, including flatulence, jaundice, menstrual difficulties, bloody urine, hemorrhage, toothache, bruises, chest pain, and colic.[1] Turmeric poultices are often applied locally to relieve inflammation and pain.

PHARMACOLOGY

Turmeric and its derivatives have a great deal of pharmacological activity.[2] Although a number of components have demonstrated activity, the volatile oil components and curcumin are believed to be the most active components. Turmeric has been found to be:

- an effective antioxidant
- anticarcinogenic
- anti-inflammatory
- cardiovascular
- hepatic
- gastrointestinal
- an antimicrobial agent.

Antioxidant effects

Turmeric extracts exert significant antioxidant activity. Although both water- and fat-soluble extracts have been shown to be effective antioxidants in various in vitro and in vivo models, curcumin is the most potent component.[3–6] The antioxidant activity of curcumin is comparable to standard antioxidants like vitamins C and E, and butylated hydroxyanisole (BHA) and butylated hydroxytoluene (BHT).[3,7] Because of its bright yellow color and antioxidant properties against lipid peroxidation, curcumin is used in butter, margarine, cheese, and other food products.

For active oxygen species, curcumin is slightly weaker than vitamin C, but stronger than vitamin E and superoxide dismutase. Against hydroxyl radicals, curcumin offers greater effectiveness than these vitamins.[3,4,7] Not all of the antioxidant properties of turmeric are due to curcumin alone, as the aqueous extract of turmeric is more effective against superoxide than curcumin and is much stronger in inhibiting oxidative damage to DNA.[5,6]

Anticarcinogenic effects

The anti-neoplastic effects of turmeric and curcumin have been demonstrated at all steps of carcinogenesis: initiation, promotion, and progression. In addition to inhibiting the development of cancer, several studies suggest that curcumin can also promote cancer regression.

Turmeric and curcumin are non-mutagenic and have been shown to suppress the mutagenicity of several common mutagens (cigarette smoke condensates, benzopyrene, DMBA, etc.), as do chili and capsaicin.[8–10] Turmeric and curcumin have also demonstrated impressive anticancer effects against a number of chemical carcinogens on a wide range of cell types in both in vitro and in vivo studies.[11–18] Curcumin has demonstrated an impressive ability to reduce the levels of urinary mutagens.[19,20]

The protective effects of turmeric and its derivatives are only partially explained by its direct antioxidant and free radical scavenging effects. It also inhibits nitrosamine formation, enhances the body's natural antioxidant system, increases the levels of glutathione and other non-protein sulfhydryls, and acts directly on several enzymes and gene loci.

Anti-inflammatory effects

The volatile oil fraction of *Curcuma longa* has been demonstrated to possess anti-inflammatory activity in a variety of experimental models, e.g. Freund's adjuvant-induced arthritis, formaldehyde- and carrageenan-induced paw edema, and cotton pellet and granuloma pouch tests.[21,22] Its effects in these studies were comparable to cortisone and phenylbutazone.

Even more potent in acute inflammation is curcumin.[23–25] Curcumin is as effective as cortisone or phenylbutazone in models of acute inflammation, but only half as effective in chronic models. However, while phenylbutazone and cortisone are associated with significant toxicity, curcumin displays virtually no toxicity (see "Toxicology", p. 692).

The rank in order of potency of curcumin analogues, cortisone, and phenylbutazone in carrageenan-induced paw edema is:[24,25]

sodium curcuminate > tetrahydrocurcumin > curcumin > cortisone > phenylbutazone > triethylcurcumin

Sodium curcuminate can be produced by mixing turmeric with slaked lime. This mixture, applied as a poultice, is an ancient household remedy for sprains, muscular pain, and inflamed joints.[25]

Curcumin's counter-irritant effect may also be a major factor in its topical anti-inflammatory action.[24] Capsaicin, a similar pungent principle from *Capsicum frutescens* (cayenne pepper), has been shown to be quite effective as a topical pain reliever in cases of post-herpetic neuralgia and arthritis. Both capsaicin and curcumin deplete nerve endings of the neurotransmitter of pain, substance P.[26]

Used orally, curcumin exhibits many direct anti-inflammatory effects including:[2,23,24,27–29]

- inhibition of leukotriene formation
- inhibition of platelet aggregation
- promotion of fibrinolysis
- inhibition of neutrophil response to various stimuli involved in the inflammatory process
- stabilization of lysosomal membranes.

In addition to its direct anti-inflammatory effects, curcumin also appears to exert some indirect effects. In models of chronic inflammation, curcumin is much less active in adrenalectomized animals. Possible mechanisms of action include:

- stimulation of the release of adrenal corticosteroids
- "sensitizing" or priming cortisol receptor sites, thereby potentiating cortisol action
- increasing the half-life of endogenous cortisol through alteration of hepatic degradation.

Cardiovascular effects

The effects of turmeric and curcumin on the cardiovascular system include the lowering of cholesterol levels[30,31] and the inhibition of platelet aggregation.[32,33] This is of great significance in preventing atherosclerosis and its complications.

Adding as little as 0.1% curcumin to a high cholesterol rat diet decreases cholesterol levels to one-half of those found in rats fed cholesterol but no curcumin.[30] This indicates that even at small doses, curcumin may be effective.

Curcumin's cholesterol-lowering actions include interfering with intestinal cholesterol uptake; increasing the conversion of cholesterol into bile acids by increasing the activity of hepatic cholesterol-7-alpha-hydroxylase, the rate-limiting enzyme of bile acid synthesis; and increasing the excretion of bile acids via its choleretic effects.[30,31,34]

Turmeric and curcumin's action on inhibiting platelet aggregation appears mediated by inhibiting the formation of thromboxanes (a promoter of aggregation) while simultaneously increasing prostacyclin (an inhibitor of aggregation).[32,33]

Hepatic effects

Curcumin has exhibited hepatoprotection similar to that of glycyrrhizin and silymarin (see Chs 90 and 111 for further discussion) against carbon tetrachloride and galactosamine-induced liver injury.[2,35] This protection is largely a result of its potent antioxidant activity. Similar results are seen with Javanese turmeric (*Curcuma xanthorriza*). Mice given intraperitoneal injections of the hepatoxic drugs carbon tetrachloride (32 mg/kg) and acetaminophen (600 mg/kg) experienced significantly decreased liver damage, as measured by SGOT and SGPT when treated with 100 mg/kg of turmeric.[36]

The antioxidant and hepatoprotective effects alone would support turmeric's historical use in liver disorders; however, turmeric and curcumin also exert anti-inflammatory and choleretic effects. The increases of SGOT and SGPT commonly seen in experimental models of inflammation have been prevented by curcumin.[23]

Curcumin is an active choleretic, increasing bile acid output by over 100%.[2] In addition to increasing biliary excretion of bile salts, cholesterol, and bilirubin, curcumin also increases the solubility of the bile.[34] This suggests a benefit in the prevention and treatment of cholelithiasis.

Gastrointestinal effects

Turmeric and its components exert a number of beneficial effects on the gastrointestinal system. Turmeric's long use as a carminative has significant research support.[2] Specifically, curcumin has been shown to inhibit gas formation by *Clostridium perfringens* and in rats given diets rich in flatulence-producing foods. In addition, sodium curcuminate has been shown to inhibit intestinal spasm, and another compound from turmeric, *p*-tolymethylcarbinol, has been shown to increase the secretion of secretin, gastrin, bicarbonate, and pancreatic enzymes.[2]

As a component of curries and spicy foods, there is some concern that turmeric may be irritating to the stomach. However, several studies have shown turmeric to be beneficial to gastric integrity. Turmeric and curcumin have been shown to increase the mucin content of the stomach and exert gastroprotective effects against ulcer formation induced by stress, alcohol, indomethacin, pyloric ligation, and reserpine.[2,37] However, at high doses, curcumin or turmeric may be ulcerogenic (see "Toxicology", p. 692).

Antimicrobial effects

Alcohol extracts and the essential oil of *Curcuma longa* have been shown in one study to inhibit the growth of most organisms occurring in cholecystitis, i.e. *Sarcina, Gaffkya, Corynebacterium,* and *Clostridium*.[2] Other microorganisms which are inhibited include *Staphylococcus, Streptococcus, Bacillus, Entamoeba histolytica,* and several pathogenic fungi.[2,38] The concentrations used in these studies were relatively high: 0.5–5.0 mg/ml of the alcohol extract and essential oil, and 5–100 ug/ml of curcumin.

CLINICAL APPLICATIONS

Turmeric and curcumin have several clinical applications. Most notable are:

- cancer prevention and treatment adjunct
- inflammation
- atherosclerosis
- liver disorders
- cholelithiasis
- irritable bowel syndrome.

Cancer prevention and treatment adjunct

As discussed above, turmeric and curcumin have demonstrated significant protective effect against cancer development in experimental studies in animals. There is also some human research showing similar results.

In one human study, 16 chronic smokers were given 1.5 g of turmeric daily while a control group of six non-smokers served as a control group.[19] At the end of the 30 day trial, the smokers receiving the turmeric demonstrated significant reduction in the level of mutagens excreted in the urine. These results are quite significant as the level of urinary mutagens is thought to correlate with the systemic load of carcinogens and the efficacy of detoxification mechanisms. Due to widespread exposure to smoke, aromatic hydrocarbons, and other environmental carcinogens, the frequent use of turmeric as a spice appears warranted.

Turmeric extracts and curcumin have demonstrated direct antitumor results in a number of experimental models of skin, epithelial, stomach and liver cancers.[15,39,40] This effect has also been substantiated in a human study.[41] Sixty-two patients with either ulcerating oral or cutaneous squamous cell carcinomas who had failed to respond to the standard treatments of surgery, radiation, and chemotherapy were given either an ethanol extract of turmeric (for oral cancers) or an ointment containing 0.5% curcumin in Vaseline. The ointment or extract was applied topically three times daily. At the end of the 18 month study, the treatment was found to have been effective in reducing the smell of the lesion (90%), itching, exudate (70%), pain (50%), and size of the lesion (10%). Although these are not spectacular results, it must be pointed out that this patient population had failed to respond to standard medical treatment.

While more human studies are needed on the use of turmeric and curcumin in cancer, there is ample evidence to support their use in cancer prevention and as an adjunct in an overall cancer treatment plan.

Inflammation

Curcuma longa has been used in Ayurvedic medicine, both locally and internally, in the treatment of sprains and inflammation. This use seems to be substantiated not only by the experimental studies described above, but also by clinical investigations.[42,43]

In one double-blind crossover clinical trial in patients with rheumatoid arthritis, curcumin (1,200 mg/day) was compared to phenylbutazone (300 mg/day). The improvements in the duration of morning stiffness, walking time, and joint swelling were comparable in both groups.[42] However, while phenylbutazone is associated with significant adverse effects, curcumin has not been shown to produce any side-effects at the recommended dosage level.

In another study which used a new human model for evaluating NSAIDs, the postoperative inflammation model, curcumin was again shown to exert comparable anti-inflammatory action to phenylbutazone.[43] While curcumin has an anti-inflammatory effect similar to phenylbutazone and various NSAIDs, it does not possess direct analgesic action.

The results of these studies indicate that turmeric or curcumin may provide benefit in the treatment of inflammation. Furthermore, the safety and excellent tolerability of curcumin compared with standard drug treatment is a major advantage.

TOXICOLOGY

Toxicity has not been reported at standard dosage levels. The oral LD_{50} levels for turmeric, its alcohol extracts, and curcumin have not been determined, as 2.5 g/kg fed to mice, rats, guinea pigs, and monkeys, and 3.0 g/kg sodium curcuminate fed to rats resulted in neither mortality nor chromosomal aberrations in teratology tests.[2,44–46] At very high doses, curcumin or turmeric may damage the gastrointestinal system, as curcumin, with doses of 100 mg/kg body weight, is ulcerogenic in rats.[2]

DOSAGE

Based on the evidence presented above, turmeric should be consumed liberally in the diet. When specific medicinal effects are desired, higher doses of turmeric can be given or extracts of *Curcuma longa* or curcumin can be used.

The recommended dosage for curcumin as an anti-inflammatory is 200–400 mg three times a day. To achieve a similar amount of curcumin using turmeric would require a dosage of 4,000–40,000 mg.

Because the absorption of orally administered curcumin may be limited (pharmacokinetic studies in animals show that 40–85% of an oral dose of curcumin passes through the gastrointestinal tract unchanged[44,45]), curcumin is often formulated in conjunction with bromelain to possibly enhance absorption. In addition, bromelain also has anti-inflammatory effects (see Ch. 69).

A curcumin–bromelain combination is best taken on an empty stomach 20 minutes before meals or between meals.

Providing curcumin in a lipid base such as lecithin, fish oils, or essential fatty acids may also increase absorption. This combination is probably best absorbed when taken with meals.

REFERENCES

1. Leung A. Encyclopedia of Common Natural Ingredients Used in Food, Drugs, and Cosmetics. New York, NY: John Wiley. 1980: p 313–314
2. Ammon HPT, Wahl MA. Pharmacology of *Curcuma longa*. Planta Medica 1991; 57: 1–7
3. Toda S, Miyase T, Arich H et al. Natural antioxidants. Antioxidative compounds isolated from rhizome of Curcuma longa L. Chem Pharmacol Bull 1985; 33: 1725–1728
4. Zhao B, Li X, He R et al. Scavenging effect of extracts of green tea and natural antioxidants on active oxygen radicals. Cell Biophysics 1989; 14: 175–185
5. Shalini VK, Srinivas L. Lipid peroxide induced DNA damage: protection by turmeric (*Curcuma longa*). Mol Cell Biochem 1987; 77: 3–10
6. Srinivas L, Shalini VK. DNA damage by smoke. Protection by turmeric and other inhibitors of ROS. Free Radical Biol Med 1991; 11: 277–283
7. Sharma OP. Antioxidant properties of curcumin and related compounds. Biochem Pharmacol 1976; 25: 1811–1825
8. Jensen NJ. Lack of mutagenic effect of turmeric oleoresin and curcumin in the salmonella/mammalian microsome test. Mut Res 1982; 105: 393–396
9. Nagabhushan M, Amonkar AJ, Bhide SV. In vitro antimutagenicity of curcumin against environmental mutagens. Fd Chem Toxic 1987; 25: 545–547
10. Nagabhushan M, Bhide SV. Nonmutagenicity of curcumin and its antimutagenic action versus chili and capsaicin. Nutr Cancer 1986; 8: 201–210
11. Jiang TL, Salmon SE, Liu RM. Activity of camptothecin, harrington, catharidin and curcumae in the human tumor stem cell assay. Eur J Cancer Clin Oncol 1983; 19: 263–270
12. Mehta RG, Moon RC. Characterization of effective chemopreventive agents in mammary gland in vitro using an initiation-promotion protocol. Anticancer Res 1991; 11: 593–596
13. Kuttan R, Bhanumathy P, Nirmala K, George MC. Potential anticancer activity of turmeric (*Curcuma longa*). Cancer Lett 1985; 29: 197–202
14. Soudamini NK, Kuttan R. Inhibition of chemical carcinogenesis by curcumin. J Ethnopharmacol 1989; 27: 227–233
15. Azuine M, Bhide S. Chemopreventive effect of turmeric against stomach and skin tumors induced by chemical carcinogens in Swiss mice. Nutr Cancer 1992; 17: 77–83
16. Nagabhushan N, Bhide SV. Curcumin as an inhibitor of cancer. J Am Coll Nutr 1992; 11: 192–198
17. Azuine MA, Kayal JJ, Bhide SV. Protective role of aqueous turmeric extract against mutagenicity of direct-acting carcinogens as well as benzopyrene-induced genotoxicity and carcinogenicity. J Cancer Res Clin Oncol 1992; 118: 447–452
18. Boone CW, Steele VE, Kelloff GJ. Screening of chemopreventive (anticarcinogenic) compounds in rodents. Mut Res 1992; 267: 251–255
19. Polasa K, Raghuram TC, Krishna TP, Krishnaswamy K. Effect of turmeric on urinary mutagens in smokers. Mutagenesis 1992; 7: 107–109
20. Polasa K, Sesikaran B, Krishna TP, Krishnaswamy K. Turmeric (*Curcuma longa*)-induced reduction in urinary mutagens. Fd Chem Toxic 1991; 29: 699–706
21. Chandra D, Gupta S. Anti-inflammatory and anti-arthritic activity of volatile oil of curcuma longa (Haldi). Ind J Med Res 1972; 60: 138–142
22. Arora R, Basu N, Kapoor V, Jain A. Anti-inflammatory studies on *Curcuma longa* (turmeric). Ind J Med Res 1971; 59: 1289–1295
23. Srimal R, Dhawan B. Pharmacology of diferuloyl methane (curcumin), a non-steroidal anti-inflammatory agent. J Pharm Pharmac 1973; 25: 447–452
24. Mukhopadhyay A, Basu N, Ghatak N, Gujral P. Anti-inflammatory and irritant activities of curcumin analogues in rats. Agents Actions 1982; 12: 508–515
25. Ghatak N, Basu N. Sodium curcuminate as an effective anti-inflammatory agent. Ind J Exp Biol 1972; 10: 235–236
26. Patacchini R, Maggi CA, Meli A. Capsaicin-like activity of some natural pungent substances on peripheral ending of visceral primary afferents. Arch Pharmacol 1990; 342: 72–77
27. Srivastava R, Srimal RC. Modification of certain inflammation-induced biochemical changes by curcumin. Indian J Med Res 1985; 81: 215–223
28. Srivastava R. Inhibition of neutrophil response by curcumin. Agents Actions 1989; 28: 298–303
29. Flynn DL, Rafferty MF. Inhibition of 5-hydroxy-eicosatetraenoic acid (5-HETE) formation in intact human neutrophils by naturally-occurring diarylheptanoids. Inhibitory activities of curcuminoids and yakuchinones. Prost Leukotri Med 1986; 22: 357–360
30. Rao DS, Sekhara NC, Satyanarayana MN, Srinivasan M. Effect of curcumin on serum and liver cholesterol levels in the rat. J Nutri 1970; 100: 1307–1316
31. Srinivasan K, Samaiah K. The effect of spices on cholesterol 7 alpha-hydroxylase activity and on serum and hepatic cholesterol levels in the rat. Int J Vitam Nutr Res 1991; 61: 364–369
32. Srivastava R, Dikshit M, Srimal RC, Dhawan BN. Anti-thrombotic effect of curcumin. Throm Res 1985; 40: 413–417
33. Srivastava R, Puri V, Srimal RC, Dhawan BN. Effect of curcumin on platelet aggregation and vascular prostacyclin synthesis. Arzneim Forsch 1986; 36: 715–717
34. Ramprasad C, Sirsi M. *Curcuma longa* and bile secretion. Quantitative changes in the bile constituents induced by sodium curcuminate. J Sci Indust Res 1957; 16C: 108–110
35. Kiso Y, Suzuki Y, Watanabe N et al. Antihepatotoxic principles of *Curcuma longa* rhizomes. Planta Med 1983; 49: 185–187
36. Lin SC, Lin CC, Lin YH et al. Protective effects of *Curcuma xanthorrihza* on hepatotoxin-induced liver damage. Am J Chi Med 1995; 23: 243–254
37. Rafatullah S, Tariq M, Al-yahya MA et al. Evaluation of turmeric (*Curcuma longa*) for gastric and duodenal antiulcer activity in rats. J Ethnopharmacol 1990; 29: 25–34
38. Lutomski VJ, Kedzia B, Debska W. Effect of an alcohol extract and active ingredients from *Curcuma longa* on bacteria and fungi. Planta Med 1974; 26: 17–19
39. Huang MT, Smart RC, Wong CQ, Conney AH. Inhibitory effect of curcumin, chlorogenic acid, caffeic acid, and ferulic acid tumor promotion in mouse skin by 12-O-tetradecanoylphorbol-13-acetate. Cancer Res 1988; 48: 5941–5946
40. Mukundan MA, Chacko MC et al. Effect of turmeric and curcumin on BP-DNA adducts. Carcinogenesis 1993; 14: 493–496
41. Kuttan R, Sudheeran PC, Josph CD. Turmeric and curcumin as topical agents in cancer therapy. Tumori 1987; 73: 29–31
42. Deodhar SD, Sethi R, Srimal RC. Preliminary studies on antirheumatic activity of curcumin (diferuloyl methane). Ind J Med Res 1980; 71: 632–634
43. Satoskar RR, Shah SJ, Shenoy SG. Evaluation of anti-inflammatory property of curcumin (diferuloyl methane) in patients with postoperative inflammation. Int J Clin Pharmacol Ther Toxicol 1986; 24: 651–654
44. Shankar TNB, Shantha NV, Ramesh HP et al. Toxicity studies on turmeric (*Curcuma longa*). Acute toxicity studies in rats, guinea pigs & monkeys. Indian J Exp Biol 1980; 18: 73–75
45. Wahlstrom B, Blennow G. A study on the fate of curcumin in the rat. Acta Pharmacol Toxicol 1978; 43: 86–92
46. Ravindranath V, Chandrasekhara N. Absorption and tissue distribution of curcumin in rats. Toxicology 1980; 16: 259–265

CHAPTER CONTENTS

81

Dehydroepiandrosterone

*Alan R. Gaby, MD**

INTRODUCTION

Dehydroepiandrosterone (DHEA) is a steroid hormone secreted by the adrenal glands and to a lesser extent by the testes and ovaries. First identified in 1934, DHEA was subsequently shown to be produced in greater quantity than any other adrenal steroid. However, although circulating levels of DHEA and its ester DHEA-sulfate (DHEA-S) are 20 times higher than those of any other adrenal steroid, the function of DHEA in the body was, until recently, unknown. Since DHEA can be converted into other hormones, including estrogen and testosterone, scientists assumed that DHEA is merely a "buffer hormone", a reservoir upon which the body can draw to produce the other hormones. However, the recent identification of DHEA receptors in the liver, kidney and testis of rats strongly suggests that DHEA has specific physiologic actions of its own.[1]

During the past several years, there has been a great deal of interest in DHEA as a possible anti-aging hormone and as a potential treatment for a wide array of medical conditions. This interest has been sparked by two different lines of evidence. First, circulating levels of DHEA decline progressively with age – the levels in 70-year-old individuals are only about 20% as high as those in young adults. This age-related decline does not occur with any of the other adrenal steroids. Furthermore, epidemiologic evidence suggests that higher DHEA levels are associated with increased longevity and prevention of heart disease and cancer. It has therefore been suggested that some of the manifestations of aging may be caused by DHEA deficiency.

Second, numerous animal studies have shown that administration of DHEA prevents obesity, diabetes, cancer, and heart disease; enhances the functioning of the immune system; and prolongs life.[2] Since most of these studies were carried out on rodents, which have little circulating DHEA, it is not clear whether the results

*Reprinted with permission from *Alternative Medicine Review* 1996; 1(2): 60–69

have relevance to human health. However, a growing body of human research, combined with the intriguing observations of innovative clinicians, suggests that DHEA may indeed have value in the treatment of various medical conditions. If this hormone can be convincingly shown to retard the aging process and to fight certain diseases, then DHEA therapy will be recognized as a major breakthrough in clinical medicine.

CLINICAL APPLICATIONS

Aging

Preliminary results in mice suggest that DHEA may retard the aging process. Animals treated with this hormone look younger and have glossier coats and less gray hair than control animals.[3]

In a recent study, 30 individuals between the ages of 40 and 70 years received 50 mg/day of DHEA or a placebo, each for 3 months, in double-blind cross-over fashion. During DHEA treatment, a remarkable increase in physical and psychological well-being was reported by 67% of the men and 84% of the women. There was no change in libido and no side-effects were seen.[4]

In this author's experience, elderly individuals who suffer from weakness, muscle wasting, tremulousness, fatigue, depression, declining memory and other signs of aging frequently have serum DHEA-S levels near or below the lower limit of normal. Treatment with DHEA (usually 5–10 mg/day for women and 10–20 mg/day for men) often results in improved mood, energy, memory, appetite, and skin color, sometimes after as little as 2 weeks. With continued treatment, the benefits may become even more pronounced and muscle wasting may be partially reversed.

Cancer prevention

Administration of DHEA inhibited tumor formation in a strain of mice that develops spontaneous breast cancer.[5] DHEA has also been shown to prevent chemically induced colon[6] and liver[7] cancer, as well as skin papillomas in mice.[8]

Premenopausal women with breast cancer had significantly lower plasma levels of DHEA than age-matched controls without breast cancer, whereas postmenopausal women had significantly higher DHEA levels than age-matched controls.[9] In another study, women with DHEA levels in the highest tertile were 60% less likely to develop breast cancer than were women in the lowest tertile.[10] In a prospective case–control study, serum DHEA and DHEA-S levels were significantly lower in individuals who subsequently developed bladder cancer than in those who did not.[11]

These findings suggest that DHEA has anti-cancer activity and that low DHEA levels may be a risk factor for cancer. However, further research is required before guidelines can be developed regarding DHEA therapy and cancer. The observation that some postmenopausal women with breast cancer have elevated DHEA levels, and the fact that DHEA is converted in part to estrogen and testosterone should be cause for concern. It is not known whether the anti-cancer effects of DHEA are stronger than the prostate cancer-promoting effects of additional testosterone or the breast cancer-promoting effects of additional estrogen. Until those questions can be answered, DHEA therapy should be approached with caution in patients who are at risk for developing hormone-dependent cancers.

Effects on immune function

DHEA exerts a number of different effects on the immune system. Some of these effects appear to result from the anti-glucocorticoid actions of DHEA. For example, DHEA antagonized the suppressive effects of dexamethasone on lymphocyte proliferation in mice[12] and prevented glucocorticoid-induced thymic involution.[13] Administration of DHEA has also been shown to preserve immune competence in burned mice,[14] an effect that extends beyond its anti-glucocorticoid action.[15] Administration of DHEA also protected against acute lethal infections with Coxsackie virus B4 and herpes simplex type 2 encephalitis in mice. DHEA appeared to act by preventing the suppression of immune competence caused by the viral infections.[16]

DHEA has also been shown to influence immune function in humans. In a double-blind study, administration of 50 mg/day of DHEA to postmenopausal women (mean age, 56.1 years) produced a twofold increase in natural killer cell activity and a 6% decrease in the proportion of helper T-cells.[17] While the increase in natural killer cell activity might be expected to enhance immune surveillance against cancer and viral infections, the decline in helper T-cells could have adverse consequences. On the other hand, since DHEA is known to mediate T-cell responses,[18] the decline in helper T-cells could merely be a reflection of enhanced T-cell function. Although the implications of these changes in immune function are not entirely clear, it should be noted that 50 mg/day of DHEA has been shown to produce supraphysiologic serum levels in postmenopausal women.[19] Lower doses may therefore be more appropriate and might result in more clear-cut improvements in immune function.

Autoimmune diseases

The potential value of DHEA as a treatment for autoimmune disease was suggested by the observation that DHEA reduced the severity of renal damage in the NZB × NZW mouse, an animal model of spontaneous lupus.

A clinical trial was therefore performed with 10 women suffering from mild or moderate systemic lupus erythematosus (SLE).[20] Each patient received 200 mg/day of DHEA for 3–6 months. Eight of the 10 patients reported improvements in overall well-being, fatigue, energy, and/or other symptoms. For the group as a whole, there was a significant improvement in the physician's overall assessment of disease activity. After 3 months, the average prednisone requirement had decreased from 14.5 to 9.4 mg/day. Of three patients with significant proteinuria, two showed marked reductions and one a modest reduction in protein excretion. There was no significant correlation between changes in serum DHEA or DHEA-S levels and clinical response. In addition, pre-treatment levels of these hormones did not predict clinical response. Side-effects were limited to mild or moderate acneiform dermatitis and mild hirsutism.

Administration of relatively large doses of DHEA has also been reported to increase stamina and improve the sense of well-being in patients with multiple sclerosis.[21]

During the past 5 years, a number of practitioners have been prescribing DHEA for patients with autoimmune disease. Pre-treatment plasma levels of DHEA or DHEA-S are usually below normal in patients receiving prednisone or related drugs, because these medications cause adrenal suppression. However, in my experience, DHEA-S levels are also frequently low in patients with autoimmune disease who are not receiving corticosteroids.

I have seen a 76-year-old woman with rheumatoid arthritis who was maintained on 5 mg/day of prednisone. After taking 10 mg/day of DHEA for several weeks, her joint symptoms improved and she was able to wean off the prednisone. Another woman with poorly controlled dermatomyositis had marked clinical improvement and was able to reduce her prednisone by 50% after receiving 10 mg of DHEA twice a day. A woman with a 3 year history of persistent bleeding due to inflammatory bowel disease reported no further bleeding after taking 15 mg/day of DHEA. Two other women with SLE had clinical improvements with DHEA. However, low doses were not effective in these cases; results became apparent only after the dose was increased to around 100 mg/day or more.

Dr Davis Lamson (personal communication) has given DHEA to six patients with ulcerative colitis who had failed to respond to a combination of conventional therapy and nutritional treatments. In all six cases, the bleeding, diarrhea, and overall condition improved.

Some patients with chronic fatigue syndrome (CFS) have also improved clinically with DHEA therapy. However, since cortisol deficiency appears to be the primary problem in some patients with CFS, and since DHEA can antagonize the effects of cortisol, DHEA therapy may actually make some patients with CFS worse. It is important, therefore, to measure both DHEA and cortisol levels before treating patients with CFS.

Acquired immunodeficiency syndrome

Preliminary evidence suggests that DHEA may play a role in acquired immunodeficiency syndrome (AIDS). In one study, DHEA inhibited the replication of HIV, the virus believed to cause AIDS.[22] In addition, DHEA has been shown to enhance the immune response to viral infections. Furthermore, DHEA levels are low in people infected with HIV and these levels decline even more as the disease progresses to full-blown AIDS.[23] In a study of 108 HIV-infected men with marginally low helper T-cell counts (between 200 and 499), those with serum DHEA levels below normal were 2.34 times more likely to progress to AIDS than were men with normal DHEA levels.[24] These studies suggest that DHEA deficiency may be one of the factors contributing to immune system failure in HIV-infected patients.

To date, only one clinical trial has tested the effect of giving DHEA to HIV-infected patients. Although DHEA did not improve CD4 counts or serum p24 antigen levels, the dosage used (750–2,250 mg/day) seems excessively large, possibly beyond the "therapeutic window" in which DHEA exerts its beneficial effects.[25] The concept of a therapeutic window has been clearly demonstrated for cortisol. For example, cortisol is known to enhance immune function at physiologic levels. However, both a deficiency and an excess of cortisol result in impaired immune function. Future trials of DHEA in HIV-infected patients should therefore use lower doses, perhaps 50–200 mg/day.

Allergic disorders

Eight patients with severe attacks of hereditary angioedema were treated with 37 or 74 mg/day of DHEA-S (equivalent to 25 or 50 mg, respectively, of DHEA) every 1–3 days, for 3–29 months. DHEA-S treatment resulted in a dramatic clinical improvement in all eight patients.[26]

Practitioners who use DHEA have observed that treatment sometimes reduces the severity of food or chemical allergies. I have seen several patients with multiple chemical sensitivities who responded to physiologic doses of DHEA (5–15 mg/day for women, 10–30 mg/day for men). However, it is difficult to predict which patients will improve.

Subnormal serum levels of DHEA-S are common in asthmatics. DHEA deficiency may result in part from corticosteroid-induced adrenal suppression. However, low levels of DHEA-S were also found in 21% of asthmatics who were not taking steroids.[27] DHEA deficiency may also result from long-term administration of inhaled corticosteroids. In a study of 36 postmenopausal asthmatic women, those who were receiving at least 1 mg/day of beclomethasone dipropionate had nearly a 50% reduction in serum DHEA levels, compared with women who were not receiving the drug. Apparently, inhaled corticosteroids are absorbed in amounts sufficient to cause some degree of adrenal suppression.[28]

I have seen two female patients with long-standing asthma who had clinical improvement after receiving 10 mg/day of DHEA. In one of these patients, chronic nasal polyps also disappeared, much to the surprise of her otolaryngologist.

Obesity

Administration of DHEA prevented the development of obesity in genetically obese mice.[29] However, studies in humans have so far failed to demonstrate a role for DHEA in the treatment of obesity.

Cardiovascular disease

Administration of DHEA reduced the severity of atherosclerosis in cholesterol-fed rabbits.[30] DHEA-S has also been shown to have digitalis-like activity, accounting for 62–100% of the total plasma digitalis-like factors in 11 healthy adults.[31]

Mean plasma DHEA-S levels were significantly lower in men with a history of heart disease than in men without such a history. In men with no history of heart disease at baseline, a low plasma DHEA-S level (less than 140 mcg/dl) was associated with a more than threefold increase in the age-adjusted risk of death from cardiovascular disease.[32] Similar findings were reported by others,[33] although another epidemiologic investigation found only a modest protective effect of DHEA.[34]

In women, no inverse association was found between DHEA-S levels and cardiovascular disease. In fact, cardiovascular death rates were highest in women in the highest tertile of DHEA-S levels and lowest in women in the middle tertile (a U-shaped distribution).[35]

Osteoporosis

At the time of menopause, the amount of DHEA manufactured by the ovaries declines. And, even though the ovaries are not the major source of DHEA, serum DHEA levels decline by more than 60% after menopause.[36]

The possible relationship between DHEA deficiency and osteoporosis was suggested by a study of women with Addison's disease. In these patients, the onset of menopause was followed by an unusually rapid rate of bone loss. This accelerated bone loss was associated with marked reductions in plasma concentrations of DHEA and testosterone (94 and 63% lower, respectively, than those of healthy postmenopausal women).[37] These findings suggest that DHEA and/or testosterone is essential for the maintenance of bone mass in postmenopausal women.

In another study, bone mineral density was measured at the lumbar spine, hip, and radius in 105 women aged 45–69 years. Fifty women had normal measurements, whereas 55 had low bone density. The average serum DHEA-S level was 60% lower in the women with low bone density than in those with normal bones. Women with low DHEA values were 40 times more likely to have osteoporosis than were women with normal DHEA levels. In contrast, there was no relationship between estrogen levels and bone density.[38] In a group of 29 postmenopausal women, there was a significant positive correlation between bone mineral content of the distal radius and ulna and age-adjusted serum DHEA levels.[39]

There are several mechanisms by which DHEA might prevent osteoporosis. First, one of the breakdown products of DHEA, 5-androstene-3β, 17β-diol, is known to bind strongly to estrogen receptors.[40] Therefore, DHEA, like estrogen, might exert an inhibitory effect on bone resorption. Second, there is evidence that androgens (a class of hormones that includes DHEA and testosterone) stimulate bone formation and calcium absorption.[41] Third, the partial conversion of DHEA to estrogen and testosterone would be expected to provide additional protection against bone loss.

I often recommend low doses of DHEA (usually 5–10 mg/day) for postmenopausal women whose serum DHEA-S levels are near or below the lower limit of normal. In some cases, DHEA relieves symptoms such as hot flashes that are usually attributed to estrogen deficiency. A combination of DHEA and identical-to-natural progesterone (usually given as a topical cream) may be more effective against hot flashes than either treatment alone.

Dementia

In one study, intracerebroventricular administration of DHEA or DHEA-S improved the results of certain memory tests in mice.[42] Some investigators have found low levels of DHEA in patients with Alzheimer's disease.[43] However, others have failed to confirm those observations.[44] In a small, uncontrolled trial, administration of DHEA appeared to produce modest improvements in cognition and behavior in a group of male patients with Alzheimer's disease.[45]

Diabetes

Administration of 0.4% DHEA in the diet reversed hyperglycemia, preserved beta-cell function, and increased insulin sensitivity in genetically diabetic mice.[46] Although DHEA has been reported to ameliorate insulin resistance in one patient with diabetes,[47] very large doses of DHEA (1,600 mg/day for 28 days) caused mild abnormalities of glucose metabolism.[48] The role of DHEA in the overall management of diabetes is therefore still unclear.

TOXICITY

For a steroid hormone, DHEA also appears to be relatively safe. Administration of 1,600 mg/day for 28 days to healthy volunteers resulted in some degree of insulin resistance, but no other significant side-effects occurred. In the SLE studies, 200 mg/day given for a number of months was well tolerated, with the exception of mild to moderate acne and occasional mild hirsutism.

Addition of 0.6% DHEA to the diet of rats reduced body weight and enhanced the development of chemically induced pre-neoplastic pancreatic lesions.[49] Although that dose of DHEA is extremely large (the equivalent human dose would be approximately 2,000 mg/day), this report indicates that DHEA is by no means innocuous and should therefore be treated with respect.

DOSAGE

As this review suggests, DHEA shows promise for preventing age-related decline and as a treatment for certain diseases. Innovative practitioners have therefore begun prescribing DHEA for their patients and the public is becoming increasingly interested in this purported "anti-aging pill".

Although DHEA appears to be safe, its long-term effects are unknown. It is possible that adverse consequences will become evident with chronic use. It is therefore important that we treat this hormone with respect and err on the side of caution. Although some practitioners are routinely prescribing 50 mg/day for healthy women and 100 mg/day for healthy men, those doses may be supraphysiologic and I am concerned about their long-term safety.

Unlike hydrocortisone (cortisol), for which the physiologic replacement dose is known, it is not clear what the physiologic dose of DHEA is. However, it may be lower than many doctors believe. I have treated one patient with severe adrenal insufficiency who had a clear response to 15 mg/day of DHEA. She experienced marked clinical improvement at that dose and her serum level of DHEA-S increased from barely detectable to well above the lower limit of normal. Another woman with a history of bilateral adrenalectomy reported marked symptom relief with DHEA doses as low as 5–10 mg/day.

In my practice, I usually prescribe 5–15 mg/day for women and 10–30 mg/day for men. Many patients have obvious improvements with these doses. Some patients who did not improve have tried larger doses, but in most cases, the larger doses were not helpful either. The one exception has been patients with lupus or other autoimmune diseases, who sometimes needed as much as 100 mg/day or more to obtain benefit. I have typically prescribed DHEA in capsule form, in a base of hydroxymethylcellulose, which is said to produce sustained release of the hormone and supposedly better results. With large doses, I recommend twice-a-day dosing, usually morning and evening.

Although serum measurements of DHEA and DHEA-S are available through most laboratories, it is not clear how closely one should rely on these measurements; nor is it clear whether DHEA or DHEA-S is the more reliable test. The normal range for DHEA-S as listed by my local laboratory is 350–4,300 ng/ml for women and 800–5,600 ng/ml for men. Many older individuals have values near or below the lower limit of normal. However, I prefer not to use an age-adjusted reference range (as published by some laboratories), since it seems that the age-related decline in serum DHEA-S is undesirable.

When DHEA therapy appears to be clinically indicated, I will consider treating women whose DHEA-S levels are below 600 ng/ml and men whose levels are below 1,200 ng/ml. There are as yet no data on what constitutes an optimum serum level. Consequently, I continue to err on the side of caution by using low doses of DHEA.

There are also no data available concerning long-term administration of DHEA. While lifetime replacement therapy seems appropriate for patients with age-related DHEA deficiency, other patients should be assessed on a case-by-case basis.

I have found that about 10% of patients who are taking thyroid hormone develop symptoms of thyrotoxicosis after starting DHEA therapy. That observation is consistent with a report that DHEA potentiates the action of thyroid hormones.[50] Symptoms of thyroid overtreatment responded to a reduction in the thyroid-hormone dosage, and patients reported that they felt better on DHEA plus lower-dose thyroid hormone than they did on thyroid hormone alone.

SUMMARY

In conclusion, DHEA appears to be one of the major therapeutic advances of the past 20 years. However, we must treat this powerful hormone with caution and respect, in order to maximize its benefits and minimize its risks.

REFERENCES

1. Kalimi M, Regelson W. Physicochemical characterization of [3H]DHEA binding in rat liver. Biochem Biophys Res Commun 1988; 156: 22–29
2. Nestler JE. DHEA: a coming of age. Ann NY Acad Sci 1995; 774: ix–xi
3. Anonymous. Antiobesity drug may counter aging. Science News 1981; 19: 39
4. Yen SSC, Morales AJ, Khorram O. Replacement of DHEA in aging men and women. Potential remedial effects. Ann NY Acad Sci 1995; 774: 128–142
5. Schwartz AG. Inhibition of spontaneous breast cancer formation in female C3H (A vy/a) mice by long-term treatment with dehydroepiandrosterone. Cancer Res 1979; 39: 1129–1132
6. Nyce JW, Magee, Hard GC, Schwartz O. Inhibition on 1,2-dimethylhydrazine-induced colon tumorigenesis in Balb/c mice by dehydroepiandrosterone. Carcinogenesis 1984; 5: 57–62
7. Mayer D, Weber E, Moore MA et al. Modulation of liver carcinogenesis by dehydroepiandrosterone. In: Kalimi M, Regelson W, eds. The biological role of dehydroepiandrosterone. New York: de Gruyter. 1990: p 361–385
8. Pashko LL, Rovito RJ, Williams JR et al. Dehydroepiandrosterone (DHEA) and 3-beta-methylandrost-5-en-17-one. Inhibitors of 7,12–dimethylbenz[a]anthracene (DMBA)-initiated and 12-O-tetradecanoylphorbol-13–acetate (TPA)-promoted skin papilloma formation in mice. Carcinogenesis 1984; 5: 463–466
9. Zumoff B, Levin J, Rosenfeld RS et al. Abnormal 24-hr mean plasma concentrations of dehydroisoandrosterone and dehydroisoandrosterone sulfate in women with primary operable breast cancer. Cancer Res 1981; 41: 3360–3363
10. Helzlsouer KJ, Gordon GB, Alberg AJ et al. Relationship of prediagnostic serum levels of dehydroepiandrosterone and dehydroepiandrosterone sulfate to the risk of developing premenopausal breast cancer. Cancer Res 1992; 52: 1–4
11. Gordon GB, Helzlsouer KJ, Comstock GW. Serum levels of dehydroepiandrosterone and its sulfate and the risk of developing bladder cancer. Cancer Res 1991; 51: 1366–1369
12. Blauer KL, Poth M, Rogers WN, Bernton EW. Dehydroepiandrosterone antagonizes the suppressive effects of dexamethasone on lymphocyte proliferation. Endocrinology 1991; 129: 3174–3179
13. May M, Holmes E, Rogers W, Poth M. Protection from glucocorticoid induced thymic involution by dehydroepiandrosterone. Life Sci 1990; 46: 1627–1631
14. Araneo BA, Shelby J, Li GZ et al. Administration of dehydroepiandrosterone to burned mice preserves normal immunologic competence. Arch Surg 1993; 128: 318–325
15. Araneo BA, Daynes R. Dehydroepiandrosterone functions as more than an antiglucocorticoid in preserving immunocompetence after thermal injury. Endocrinology 1995; 136: 393–401
16. Loria RM, Inge TH, Cook SS et al. Protection against acute lethal viral infections with the native steroid dehydroepiandrosterone (DHEA). J Med Virol 1988; 26: 301–314
17. Casson PR, Anserson RN, Herrod HG et al. Oral dehydroepiandrosterone in physiologic doses modulates immune function in postmenopausal women. Am J Obstet Gynecol 1993; 169: 1536–1539
18. Regelson W, Loria R, Kalimi M. Dehydroepiandrosterone (DHEA) – the "mother steroid". I. Immunologic action. Ann NY Acad Sci 1994; 719: 553–563
19. Casson PR, Faquin LC, Stenz FB et al. Replacement of dehydroepiandrosterone enhances T-lymphocyte insulin binding in postmenopausal women. Fertil Steril 1995; 63: 1027–1031
20. Van Vollenhoven RF, Engleman EG, McGuire JL. An open study of dehydroepiandrosterone in systemic lupus erythematosus. Arthritis Rheum 1994; 37: 1305–1310
21. Calabrese VP. Dehydroepiandrosterone in multiple sclerosis. Positive effects on the fatigue syndrome in a non-randomized study. In: Kalimi M, Regelson W, eds. The biological role of dehydroepiandrosterone. New York: de Gruyter. 1990: p 95–100
22. Henderson E, Yng JY, Schwartz A. Dehydroepiandrosterone (DHEA) and synthetic DHEA analogs are modest inhibitors of HIV-1 IIIB replication. AIDS Res Human Retrovir 1992; 8: 625–631
23. Merril CR, Harrington MG, Sunderland T. Reduced plasma dehydroepiandrosterone concentrations in HIV infection and Alzheimer's disease. In: Kalimi M, Regelson W, eds. The biological role of dehydroepiandrosterone. New York: de Gruyter. 1990: p 101–105
24. Jacobson MA, Fusaro RE, Galmarini M, Lang W. Decreased serum dehydroepiandrosterone is associated with an increased progression of human immunodeficiency virus infection in men with CD4 cell counts of 200–499. J Infect Dis 1991; 164: 864–868
25. Dyner TS, Lang W, Geaga J et al. An open-label dose-escalation trial of oral dehydroepiandrosterone tolerance and pharmacokinetics in patients with HIV disease. J Acq Immune Def Syndr 1993; 6: 459–465
26. Koo E, Feher KG, Geher T, Fust G. Effect of dehydroepiandrosterone on hereditary angioedema. Klin Wochenschr 1983; 61: 715–717
27. Dunn PJ, Mahood CB, Speed JF, Jury DR. Dehydroepiandrosterone sulphate concentrations in asthmatic patients. Pilot study. NZ Med J 1984; 97: 805–808
28. Smith BJ, Buxton JR, Dickeson J, Heller RF. Does beclomethasone dipropionate suppress dehydroepiandrosterone sulphate in postmenopausal women? Aust NZ J Med 1994; 24: 396–401
29. Cleary MP, Shepard A, Kenks B. Effect of dehydroepiandrosterone on growth in lean and obese Zucker rats. J Nutr 1984; 114: 1242–1251
30. Gordon GB, Bush DE, Weisman HF. Reduction of atherosclerosis by administration of dehydroepiandrosterone. J Clin Invest 1988; 82: 712–720
31. Vasdev S, Longerich L, Johnson E et al. Dehydroepiandrosterone sulfate as a digitalis like factor in plasma of healthy human adults. Res Commun Chem Pathol Pharmacol 1985; 49: 387–399
32. Barrett-Connor E, Khaw KT, Yen SS. A prospective study of dehydroepiandrosterone sulfate, mortality, and cardiovascular disease. N Engl J Med 1986; 315: 1519–1524
33. Mitchell LE, Sprecher DL, Borecki IB et al. Evidence for an association between dehydroepiandrosterone sulfate and nonfatal, premature myocardial infarction in males. Circulation 1994; 89: 89–93
34. Newcomer LM, Manosn JE, Barbieri RL et al. Dehydroepiandrosterone sulfate and the risk of myocardial infarction in US male physicians: a prospective study. Am J Epidemiol 1994; 140: 870–875
35. Barrett-Connor E, Khaw KT. Absence of an inverse relation of dehydroepiandrosterone sulfate with cardiovascular mortality in postmenopausal women. N Engl J Med 1987; 317: 711
36. Monroe SE, Menon KMJ. Changes in reproductive hormone secretion during the climacteric and postmenopausal periods. Clin Obstet Gynecol 1977; 20: 113–122
37. Devogelaer JP, Crabbe J, Nagant de Deuxchaisnes C. Bone mineral density in Addison's disease: evidence for an effect of adrenal androgens on bone mass. Br Med J 1987; 294: 798–800
38. Szathmari M, Szucs J, Feher T, Hollo I. Dehydroepiandrosterone sulphate and bone mineral density. Osteoporosis Int 1994; 4: 84–88
39. Brody S, Carlstorm K, Lagrelius A et al. Adrenal steroids in post-menopausal women: relation to obesity and to bone mineral content. Maturitas 1987; 9: 25–32
40. Taelman P, Kaufman JM, Janssns X, Vermeulen A. Persistence of increased bone resorption and possible role of dehydroepiandrosterone as a bone metabolism determinant in osteoporotic women in late post-menopause. Maturitas 1989; 11: 65–73
41. Taelman P, Kaufman JM, Janssns X, Vermeulen A. Persistence of increased bone resorption and possible role of dehydroepiandrosterone as a bone metabolism determinant in osteoporotic women in late post-menopause. Maturitas 1989; 11: 65–73
42. Flood JF, Morley JE, Roberts E. Memory-enhancing effects in male mice of pregnenolone and steroids metabolically derived from it. Proc Natl Acad Sci 1992; 89: 1567–1571

43. Sunderland T, Merril CR, Harrington MG et al. Reduced plasma dehydroepiandrosterone concentrations in Alzheimer's disease. Lancet 1989; 2: 570
44. Leblhuber F. Dehydroepiandrosterone sulphate in Alzheimer's disease. Lancet 1990; 336: 449
45. Schneider LS, Hinsey M, Lyness S. Plasma dehydroepiandrosterone sulfate in Alzheimer's disease. Biol Psychiatry 1992; 31: 205–208
46. Coleman DL, Leiter EH, Schwizer RW. Therapeutic effects of dehydroepiandrosterone (DHEA) in diabetic mice. Diabetes 1982; 31: 830–833
47. Buffington CK, Pourmotabbed G, Kitabchi AE. Case report. Amelioration of insulin resistance in diabetes with dehydroepiandrosterone. Am J Med Sci 1993; 306: 320–324
48. Mortola JF, Yen SSC. The effects of oral dehydroepiandrosterone on endocrine-metabolic parameters in postmenopausal women. J Clin Endocrinol Metab 1990; 71: 696–704
49. Tagliaferro AR, Roebuck BD, Ronan AM, Meeker LD. Enhancement of pancreatic carcinogenesis by dehydroepiandrosterone. Adv Exp Med Biol 1992; 322: 119–129
50. McIntosh MK, Berdanier CD. Influence of dehydroepiandrosterone (DHEA) on the thyroid hormone status of BHE/cdb rats. J Nutr Biochem 1992; 3: 194–199

CHAPTER CONTENTS

82

Echinacea species (narrow-leafed purple coneflower)

Michael T. Murray, ND

Joseph E. Pizzorno Jr, ND

Echinacea sp. (family: Asteraceae)

Echinacea angustifolia
Common names: narrow-leafed purple coneflower, black sampson, snakeroot

Echinacea purpurea
Common name: purple coneflower

Echinacea pallida
Common name: pale purple coneflower

GENERAL DESCRIPTION

Echinacea sp. are perennial herbs native to midwestern North America, from Saskatchewan to Texas. The genus derives its name from the Greek *echinos* (meaning sea urchin). This refers to the prickly scales of the dried seed head portion of the flower. There are nine species of *Echinacea* which have been taxonomically classified by McGregor based on comparative anatomy and morphology (see Table 82.1).[1]

Of the nine species, *E. angustifolia, E. purpurea,* and *E. pallida* are the most commonly used clinically. *E. angustifolia,* with a typical height of up to 2 feet, is shorter than *E. purpurea* (1.5–5 feet) and *E. pallida* (1–3 feet). Another

Table 82.1 Taxonomic formation of the genus *Echinacea*[3]

Species	Synonyms
Echinacea angustifolia	*Brauneria angustifolia*
Echinacea atrorubens	*Rudbeckia atrorubens*
Echinacea laevigata	*Brauneria laevigata*
Echinacea pallida	*Rudbeckia pallida*
Brauneria pallida	
Echinacea paradoxa	*Brauneria paradoxa*
Echinacea purpurea	*Rudbeckia purpurea*
Rudbeckia hispida	
Rudbeckia serotina	
Echinacea speciosa	
Echinacea intermedia	
Echinacea simulata	*Echinacea speciosa*
Echinacea sanguinea	
Echinacea tennesseensis	*Brauneria tennesseensis*

key to species identification is that *E. angustifolia* and *E. purpurea* have yellow pollen, while *E. pallida* is noticeably paler and has white pollen. The portions of the plant used for medicinal purposes includes the aerial portion, the whole plant including the root, and the root itself. The tap root *of E. angustifolia* can reach a length of 3–4 feet.[2,3]

E. angustifolia has thick, hairy, 1–3 inches long leaves found at the base of a purple seed head shaped like a cone. The only exception to the family of "purple" coneflower is *E. paradoxa* which has a yellow flower.

CHEMICAL COMPOSITION

Analysis of *Echinacea* sp. has yielded a wide assortment of chemical constituents with pharmacological activities. The broad chemical composition of this medicinal plant suggests possible synergistic effects among its constituents. For example, in some experimental models, while the water-soluble polysaccharides have shown greater stimulatory effects on the cellular immune system, the lipophilic components have demonstrated more potent effects on enhancing macrophage phagocytosis.[3,4]

The important constituents, from a pharmacological perspective, of *Echinacea* sp. can be divided into seven categories:

- polysaccharides
- flavonoids
- caffeic acid derivatives
- essential oils
- polyacetylenes
- alkylamides
- miscellaneous chemicals.

Polysaccharides

A number of immunostimulatory and mild anti-inflammatory polysaccharides have been isolated from *Echinacea* sp.[2,3,5–9] Most notable are inulin, which is found in a high concentration (5.9%) in *E. angustifolia* root, and the high molecular weight (25,000–50,000) polysaccharides found in the aerial part of *E. purpurea,* as these components possess significant immune-enhancing properties. Typically the most potent immune-enhancing polysaccharides are the water-soluble, acidic, branched-chain heteroglycans composed of many types of sugars rather than the polyfructose content of inulin.

Flavonoids

The leaves and stems of *E. angustifolia* and *E. purpurea* have been shown to contain numerous flavonoids, with rutoside being the most abundant.[3,9] The total flavonoid content (calculated as quercetin) for *E. angustifolia* and *E. purpurea* was 0.48 and 0.38% respectively.[2,3,9,10]

Caffeic acid derivatives

Caffeic acid serves as the backbone for a number of important medicinal plant compounds in other plants as well as *Echinacea* sp. (see Fig. 82.1). The first compound believed to be unique to *Echinacea* was echinacoside, a compound eventually shown to be composed of caffeic acid, a caffeic acid derivative (similar to catechol), glucose, and rhamnose, all attached to a central glucose molecule (see Figs 82.2 and 82.3).[11] Echinacoside accumulates in the roots, but is also found in smaller concentrations in the flowers. The roots *of E. angustifolia* contain 0.3–1.3%, while the roots of *E. pallida* contain a similar concentration of 0.4–1.7%.[12] It is assumed *that E. purpurea* has similar echinacoside levels as well.

Other caffeic acid derivatives important in the pharmacology of *Echinacea* include cichoric acid, chlorogenic

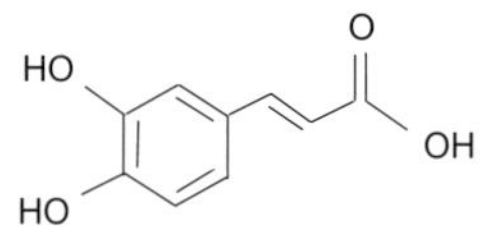

Figure 82.1 Caffeic acid.

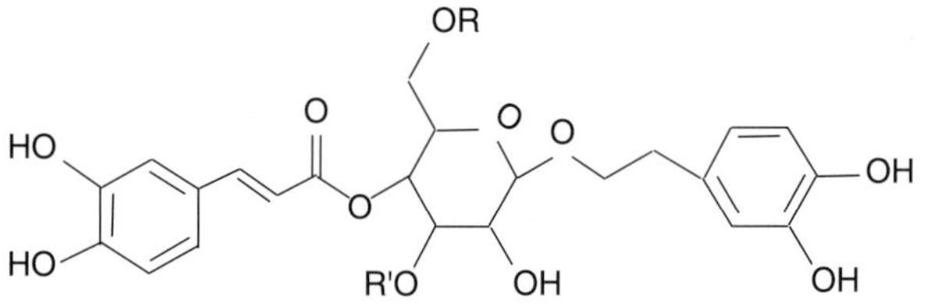

Compound	R	R′
Echinacoside	Glucose (1,6-)	Rhamnose (1,3-)
6-O-Caffeoyl-echinacoside	6-O-Caffeoyl-glucose	Rhamnose (1,3-)
Verbascoside	H	Rhamnose (1,3-)
Desrhamnosyl-verbascoside	H	H

Figure 82.2 Echinacoside and similar compounds.

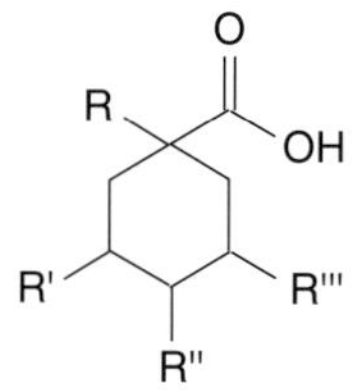

Compound	R	R′	R″	R‴
3-O-Caffeoly-quinic acid (cholorgenic acid)	OH	Caffeic acid	OH	OH
Isochlorogenic acids	OH	Caffeic acid	Caffeic acid	OH
	OH	Caffeic acid	OH	Caffeic acid
	OH	Caffeic acid	Caffeic acid	Caffeic acid
Cynarine	Caffeic acid	Caffeic acid	OH	Caffeic acid

Figure 82.3 Other caffeic acid derivatives.

acid, and cynarin.[3] Cichoric acid was originally isolated from *E. purpurea* and is found in much higher concentrations in this species compared with *E. angustifolia* and *E. pallida*.[2,3,9] However, *E. angustifolia* and *E. pallida* have higher amounts of other types of caffeic acid derivatives.[2,3,13] These differences are not thought to have much clinical significance; rather they may prove to be valuable in quick chemical differentiation of species.

Essential oils

The essential oil content varies among the three common species:[14]

- *E. angustifolia* root and leaves contain less than 0.1%
- *E. purpurea* root 0.2% and flowers and leaves contain 0.6%
- *E. pallida* root contains up to 2% and the leaves contain less than 1%.

Interestingly, in one study the essential oil content of *E. pallida* root was found to rise to 3.5–4% in April and May, but fall to 1–1.5% for the rest of the year.[15] The major essential oil components are sesquiterpene derivatives, borneol, alpha-pinine, and related aromatic compounds.[2,3]

Polyacetylenes

A number of polyacetylenes have been identified from the roots of all three commercial species.[16] The difference in the type of polyacetylene and susceptibility to breakdown may help to differentiate which species is best for commercial use. Since the polyacetylenes of *E. pallida* are quite susceptible to auto-oxidation, *E. angustifolia* may be better for commercial products.[17] Research has shown that long-term storage greatly decreases the content of polyacetylenes to only trace levels at best. However, the polyacetylene derivatives of auto-oxidation of *E. pallida* are quite characteristic and useful in differentiating *E. pallida* from *E. angustifolia*.

Alkylamides

Alkylamides typically exert a tingling sensation on the tongue. This is representative of their mild anesthetic effect. These compounds are found in highest concentrations in the roots. The roots of *E. angustifolia* contain higher concentrations (0.004–0.039%) than *E. purpurea* (0.009–0.151%) and *E. pallida* (.001%).[9,18]

Miscellaneous

There are undoubtedly other constituents which contribute to the pharmacology of *Echinacea*. The occurrence of a "colorless alkaloid" was first reported by the great John Uri Lloyd in 1897 and substantiated recently by the isolation of the alkaloids tussilagine and isotussilagine.[19] Other compounds isolated from *Echinacea* sp. include:[2,3]

- resins
- glycoproteins
- sterols
- minerals
- fatty acids.

HISTORY AND FOLK USE

Echinacea was used extensively by the native Americans living in areas where it grew. In fact, *Echinacea* was used by the American Indians against more illnesses than any other plant. The root was used externally for the healing of wounds, burns, abscesses, and insect bites; internally for infections, toothache and joint pains; and as an antidote for snake (rattlesnake) bites.[20]

A commercial product containing *Echinacea* was introduced to Americans around 1870 by H. C. F. Meyer, a German lay healer, who recommended it as a wonder cure called "Meyer's blood purifier".[2,3] Meyer recommended it for almost every conceivable malady and there were numerous case reports of successful treatments for snake bites, typhus, diphtheria, and other infections.

Echinacea angustifolia became a favorite with Eclectic physicians as it was thought to be greater in activity than other species. Eclectics used it externally as a local antiseptic, stimulant, deodorant, and anesthetic; and internally for "bad blood", i.e. to correct "fluid depravation with tendency to sepsis and malignancy".[21]

Although many physicians began to investigate and use *Echinacea* as a serious medicine, in 1909 the Council on Pharmacy and Chemistry of the American Medical Association refused to recognize *Echinacea* as an active drug stating: "In view of the lack of any scientific scrutiny of the claims made for it, *Echinacea* is deemed unworthy of further consideration until more reliable evidence is presented in its favor." Despite this opposition, *Echinacea* was included in the National Formulary of the US and remained there until 1950.[2,3]

With the demise of the Eclectic movement, the popularity of *Echinacea* in the US waned except amongst naturopathic physicians until around 1980 when *Echinacea* was rediscovered due to the increased consumer interest in immune system disorders such as candidiasis, chronic fatigue syndrome, AIDS, and cancer.[22] Although interest in *Echinacea* decreased in America between the 1930s and 1980s, European physicians continued research. Much of this research was initiated by a 1932 study by Gerhard Madaus. Madaus demonstrated immune-enhancing effects of a preparation from the fresh juice of the aerial portion of *E. purpurea*. This was followed by development of a commercial product and a great deal of scientific study. Thus, *E. purpurea* began to be as respected as *E. angustifolia* among herbal practitioners in Europe.[2,3]

PHARMACOLOGY

The chemistry, pharmacology and clinical applications of *Echinacea* have been the subject of over 200 scientific studies.[2,3] The overwhelming majority of the clinical studies have utilized an injectable form of a commercial product, Echinacin, containing an extract of the juice of the aerial portion *E. purpurea* along with 22% ethanol (for preservation). Other studies have utilized an oral Echinacin and another commercial product, Esberitox, which contains not only *E. purpurea* root extract, but also extracts of *E. pallida, Thuja occidentalis,* and *Baptisia tinctoria.* A recent review of published studies on the immunomodulating effects of *Echinacea* identified 26 controlled clinical studies, 16 of which featured Esberitox.[23]

This section summarizes some of the pharmacological information on *Echinacea* with attention to the species used, part of the plant used, solvent used for extraction, and other relevant features. When no species delineation is made, the activity described is similar in all species.

Tissue regeneration and anti-inflammatory properties

Echinacin, as well as polysaccharide components of *Echinacea*, have been shown to promote tissue regeneration and reduce inflammation in experimental studies.[8,24–27] This is apparently largely due to inhibition of the enzyme hyaluronidase via formation of a polysaccharide complex with hyaluronic acid, thereby maintaining the structure and integrity of the collagen matrix in connective tissue and ground substance. In addition to increased hyaluronic acid stabilization, *Echinacea* also stimulates fibroblast growth and manufacture of glycosaminoglycans, a critical goal in wound healing.[27]

Echinacea both exerts a mild direct cortisone-like effect and enhances the secretion of adrenal cortex hormones.[2,3,25] The polysaccharide portion appears to be responsible for the direct anti-inflammatory effects, although the alkylamide fraction has also demonstrated some activity.[28]

Immunostimulatory properties

Echinacea possesses a broad spectrum of effects on the immune system as a result of its content of a diverse range of active components affecting different aspects of immune function.[2,3] For example, inulin, the major component in the root of *E. angustifolia*, activates the alternative complement pathway and thus promotes chemotaxis of neutrophils, monocytes, and eosinophils; solubilization of immune complexes; neutralization of viruses; and bacteriolysis. *Echinacea* also increases the levels of properdin, the normal serum globulin that stimulates the alternative complement pathway.[2,3,29] Another non-specific immune enhancement is *Echinacea*'s enhancement of serum leukocyte and granulocyte counts.[2,3,30–33]

The high-molecular-weight heteroglycan polysaccharide components of *Echinacea* have profound immunostimulatory effects.[2,3,5–7] The majority of these effects appear to be mediated by the binding of active *Echinacea* polysaccharides to carbohydrate receptors on the cell surface of macrophages and T-lymphocytes. It should be noted, however, that some of the T-cell activation in early studies is now thought to be due to a contaminant protein. Later studies using a purer polysaccharide fraction have not shown significant results.[3]

Echinacea promotes non-specific T-cell activation, i.e. transformation, production of interferon, and secretion of lymphokines. The resultant effect is enhanced T-cell mitogenesis, macrophage phagocytosis, antibody binding, natural killer cell activity; and increased numbers of circulating PMNs.[2,3,5]

Echinacea polysaccharides have also been shown to enhance macrophage phagocytosis and stimulate macrophages to produce increased amounts of tumor necrosis factor (TNF), interferon, interleukin 1, to destroy tumor cells in tissue culture, and to inhibit *Candida albicans* infection in rats infected intravenously with a lethal dose (3×10^5 cells) of *C. albicans*.[2,3,6,7,34] The interactions with macrophages are most likely responsible for much of the immune system enhancement of *Echinacea* polysaccharides.

In addition to the polysaccharides, lipophilic alkylamides and caffeic acid derivatives like cichoric acid are thought to contribute to the immunostimulatory aspects of *Echinacea*, especially alcoholic extracts.[3,4,35] While most research has been devoted to the water-soluble components such as polysaccharides, the lipophilic fraction yields the most potent enhancement of macrophage phagocytosis.[3,4]

The carbon clearance test is often used to measure systemic macrophage activation. The method involves measuring the rate of disappearance of carbon granules from the blood at varying intervals following administration of the test substance. Root extracts of *Echinacea* administered orally tend to yield greater effects on phagocytic activity than the aerial portion with *E. purpurea* > *E. angustifolia* > *E. pallida*.[3,4]

Although many of the studies have utilized injectable preparations, oral preparations are generally thought to yield similar or even better results, although direct comparisons are apparently not available. For example, intramuscular Echinacin administered to healthy males on four successive days was shown to increase granulocytic phagocytosis by nearly 50%, while the oral administration of an *E. purpurea* root extract at a dose of 30 drops three times daily to healthy males for five consecutive days resulted in an increase of 120%.[29] This difference may, however, be due to the differing constituents of the forms used. The expressed juice of the aerial portion *E. pupurea*, as found in Echinacin, has lower concentrations of several of the phagocytosis-stimulating compounds characteristic to *Echinacea*, including polysaccharides, alkylamides and caffeic acid derivatives like cichoric acid compared with alcoholic extract.[3]

In general, *Echinacea* appears to offer benefit for all infectious conditions. An exception to this statement may be acquired immunodeficiency syndrome (AIDS). It is unclear at this time if *Echinacea* should be recommended for AIDS. Although this condition is associated with widespread depression of the immune system, presumably due to the human immunodeficiency virus (HIV), stimulation of T-cell replication may also stimulate replication of the virus as well. In addition, Echinacin has been shown to lower T-helper cells and decrease T-helper:suppressor cell ratios.[2,3] While there are some anecdotal reports of *Echinacea*'s efficacy in HIV-infected individuals, more research is necessary to determine *Echinacea's* effects in HIV.

Antiviral properties

The juice of the aerial portion of *E. purpurea* along with alcoholic and aqueous extracts of the roots have been shown to possess antiviral activity. Some of the viruses inhibited in cell cultures include influenza, herpes and vesicular stomatitis viruses.[3,36]

Although certain *Echinacea* components (e.g. echinacoside, other caffeic acid derivatives, polysaccharides, etc.) may block virus receptors on the cell surface, the antiviral effects may also be due to inhibition of hyaluronidases. The viral-inhibiting action of *Echinacea* is significantly diminished when hyaluronidase is added to the cell cultures.[3,24,37] Many organisms secrete hyaluronidase, which increases connective tissue permeability and allows the organism to become more invasive.[38]

Clinically, the inhibition of hyaluronidase coupled with general immunostimulation of *Echinacea* are probably more important than direct antiviral activity. The nonspecific antiviral action of *Echinacea* enhances cytotoxic killing of virus-infected cells and the release of interferon. Interferons bind to cell surfaces, where they stimulate synthesis of intracellular proteins that block the transcription of viral RNA.

Antibacterial properties

The direct antibacterial activity of *Echinacea* is quite mild. This is somewhat surprising as *Echinacea* has a long history of effective use in both internal and external bacterial infections. It is possible that it possesses some anti-infective properties which prevent bacterial adherence, though this has yet to be determined. Clearly its clinical efficacy is due to its strong immune-potentiating actions.

Echinacea does possess some mild antibacterial action due largely to echinacoside, the complex caffeic acid derivative, found in highest concentrations in the root of *E. angustifolia*. Echinacoside and caffeic acid have been shown to have antibacterial action against *Staphylococcus aureus, Corynebacterium diphtheria,* and *Proteus vulgaris.* Approximately 6.3 mg. of echinacoside is equivalent to 10 Oxford units of penicillin.[2,3,11]

Anti-neoplastic activity

Obviously, *Echinacea* possesses indirect anti-neoplastic activity via its general immuno-enhancing effects. Specifically important is its stimulation of macrophages to greater cytotoxic activity against tumor cells. (Z)-1,8-pentadecadiene, a lipid-soluble component found in the root of *E. angustifolia* and *E. pallida*, has been shown, in vivo, to possess significant direct anti-neoplastic activity.[39]

CLINICAL APPLICATIONS

Echinacea has long been used clinically for conditions where its pharmacological actions have proven efficacy, especially in infections. Clinical studies have demonstrated effectiveness in a number of infectious conditions using all three routes of administration: injectable, oral, and topical. Again, the majority of clinical studies have utilized Echinacin, containing an extract of the juice of the aerial portion *E. purpurea* along with 22% ethanol (for preservation) and Esberitox. A recent review of published studies on the immunomodulating effects of *Echinacea* identified 26 controlled clinical studies, 16 of which featured Esberitox.[23]

Infections

Numerous clinical studies have confirmed *Echinacea*'s immune-enhancing actions. Various *Echinacea* extracts or products have shown results in:

- general infectious conditions
- influenza
- colds
- upper respiratory tract infections
- urogenital infections
- other infectious conditions.

The common cold

One of the most popular uses of *Echinacea* is in the treatment of the common cold. Two recent studies offer considerable support for this clinical application. In one study, 180 patients with influenza were given either an extract of *E. purpurea* root at a daily dose of 450 mg or 900 mg, or a placebo. The 450 mg dose was found to be no more effective than a placebo; however the group taking the 900 mg dose showed significant reduction of cold symptoms.[40]

In the other study, 108 patients with colds received either an extract of the fresh-pressed juice of *E. purpurea* (4 ml twice daily) or placebo for 8 weeks.[41] The number of patients remaining healthy was as follows: *Echinacea*, 35.2%; placebo, 25.9%. The length of time between infections was: *Echinacea*, 40 days; placebo, 25 days. When infections did occur in patients receiving *Echinacea*, they were less severe and resolved quicker. Patients showing evidence of a weakened immune system (CD4/CD8 ratio <1.5) benefited the most from *Echinacea*.

Candidiasis

The effect of *Echinacea* against *C. albicans* noted in animal studies has been confirmed in several clinical studies.[2,3] A study featured in Table 82.2 demonstrated that Echinacin greatly accentuates the efficacy of a topical antimycotic agent (econazol nitrate), decreasing reoccurrence from 60.5% to 5–16.7%. The researchers used standardized skin tests to show that this enhancement was due to *Echinacea's* boosting of cell-mediated immunity.[42] Also of interest is the similarity in the efficacies of the oral and injectable forms.

Other applications

Snake bites

Echinacea has quite a reputation among naturopathic physicians and native American healers for the treatment of snake bites. No studies of this use were carried out, but *Echinacea*'s inhibition of hyaluronidase might account for much of its reputed efficacy since most snake venoms permeate the system as a result of hyaluronidase in the venom breaking down connective tissue of the ground substance.[24]

Wound healing

Several uncontrolled clinical studies have been reported to substantiate *Echinacea's* wound healing activities.[3,43–45] The largest (4,598 patients) demonstrated that a salve of the juice of the aerial portion of *E. purpurea* had an 85% overall success rate in the treatment of inflammatory skin conditions such as abscesses, folliculitis, wounds of all kinds, eczema, burns, herpes, and varicose ulcers of the leg.[3]

Table 82.2 Treatment of recurrent candidiasis with echinacin – rate of reoccurrence at 6 months[42]

Therapeutic scheme	No. of patients	Reoccurrence rate
Topical antimycotic alone	43	60.5%
Topical antimycotic + subcutaneous Echinacin	20	15.0
Topical antimycotic + intramuscular Echinacin	60	5.0
Topical antimycotic + intravenous Echinacin	20	15.0
Topical antimycotic + oral Echinacin	60	16.7

Arthritis

Echinacea's anti-inflammatory activity has been shown in uncontrolled studies to be useful in rheumatoid arthritis.[46] In one study, 15 drops of Echinacin three times daily resulted in a 21.8% decrease in inflammation. Although this improvement was less than cortisone (42%) and prednisone (49.2%), no side-effects were noted with Echinacin while the drugs have well known side-effects.

Cancer

Echinacea extracts have been shown to inhibit the growth of Walker carcinosarcoma and lymphocytic leukemia in experimental studies.[39]

Several studies have noted a stimulatory effect of *Echinacea* on leukocyte counts in patients receiving radiation for cancer therapy.[32,33] A study using Esberitox demonstrated that 85% of 55 patients showed a stabilization of leukocyte counts compared with the control group, which showed a steady decline in levels (starting at 6,000 and decreasing to 2,500 after 45 days).[32] This strongly supports the recommendation of *Echinacea* to patients undergoing orthodox cancer treatments.

COMMERCIAL PREPARATIONS

As evident from the above information, determining which *Echinacea* preparation is best is difficult to determine. It is not only difficult to determine which species is most effective – the portion of the plant used and how it is prepared are also serious issues. Dosage recommendations for all currently available forms are given below along with a few observations regarding the "preparations controversy".

Another problem needing to be addressed is quality control. Since as early as 1904, many commercial sources of *Echinacea* have contained adulterants and no *Echinacea*. For example, it has been estimated that due to supplier errors in collection, greater than 50% (and possibly as high as 90% at times) of the *Echinacea* sold in the US from 1908 to 1991 has actually been *Parthenium integrifolium*, Missouri snakeroot.[2,47] Some suggest that this adulteration is due to confusion of the common names. Others point out that while the *Parthenium integrifolium* plant looks quite different "... once the root is cut and sifted it has an uncanny resemblance to *E. angustifolia* or *E. Pallida* roots, though it possesses its own characteristic flavor and fragrance".[47] From a practical as well as a clinical viewpoint, physicians should require from suppliers adequate documentation that they are in fact supplying *Echinacea* as well as its species.

Species

Although studies have shown various *Echinacea* species, or components found in higher concentrations in one species, to be more effective than others, each commercial species has its advantages and disadvantages. No "best" species can at this time be recommended, as differing experimental models have at times yielded inconsistent results. Rather, the clinician must recognize the unique value of each species. Although *E. angustifolia* has long been considered the best species and to possess the greatest activity, some studies dispute this. For example, in one study *E. purpurea* demonstrated greater enhancement of phagocytosis.[4] In fact, in a recent study, an aqueous extract of *E. angustifolia* did not demonstrate any impact on phagocytic function in rats, whether it was administered orally, intraperitoneally, or intravenously.[48] As *E. purpurea* is the easiest to grow commercially, it may become the most utilized in the US, as it is Europe.

Part of the plant to use

Most laboratory studies report that the root possesses the greatest immune-enhancing properties. However, most of the actual clinical data are based on using Echinacin, a product containing the juice of the aerial portion, or Esberitox, a product that also contains baptisia and thuja. Therefore, this question can not be answered until more clinical research is done with mono-preparations obtained from the root.

Preparations

Echinacea products are available in many different forms:

- crude plant in either ground or powdered form
- freeze-dried
- alcohol-based tinctures and liquid extracts
- aqueous tinctures and liquid extracts
- dry powdered alcoholic or aqueous.

It is thought by some that dried powdered extracts offer the greatest shelf life and are therefore considered to be the "best". In addition, dry powdered extracts offer the greatest concentration of active compounds and a greater degree of product standardization. Others prefer using the fresh freeze-dried root, in the belief that it will provide the full range of active compounds in a active yet stable form.

In Europe, it is popular to standardize hydro/alcoholic extracts for echinacoside (for *E. angustifolia*) or cichoric acid (for *E. purpurea*). While these extracts are thought by their proponents to be the most potent, it must be noted that even 4–10× homeopathic preparations have been shown to produce activity, while the majority of clinical studies have utilized Echinacin and Esberitox.[31]

While Esberitox (containing *E. purpurea* root) has the highest quality of clinical research, it is hard to evaluate the role of *Echinacea* in this product as it also contains standardized extracts of *Thuja occidentalis* and *Baptisia tinctoria,* both of which exert significant effects on immune system cells.

Solvents

Again, this is extremely difficult to answer as both hydrophilic and lipophilic components have been shown to possess immune-enhancing activities. Even a small amount of ethanol results in precipitation or breakdown of the immuno-active polysaccharides, suggesting that aqueous extracts may be best. However, an aqueous extract would leave behind valuable lipophilic immune-enhancing alkylamides and caffeic acid derivatives. To optimize an extract's immune-enhancing effects, many manufacturers use low ethanol (10–20%) hydro/alcoholic mixtures. These extracts typically contain both polar and lipophilic compounds.

DOSAGE

As a general immune stimulant during infection, dosages are (three times/day):

- dried root (or as tea): 0.5–1 g
- freeze-dried plant: 325–650 mg
- juice of aerial portion of *E. purpurea* stabilized in 22% ethanol: 2–3 ml (0.5–0.75 tsp)
- tincture (1:5): 2–4 ml (1–2 tsp)
- fluid extract (1:1): 2–4 ml (1–2 tsp)
- solid (dry powdered) extract (6.5:1 or 3.5% echinacoside): 150–300 mg.

The question of whether *Echinacea* should be used on a long-term or continual basis really depends on the need. In a healthy individual with no apparent depression of the immune system, continual administration is certainly not indicated. However, as recent studies have shown, patients with impaired immune function experience long-term benefit.[40] The usual recommendation with long-term use is 8 weeks on followed by 1 week off.

TOXICOLOGY

When used at the recommended doses, there is no danger of toxicity, as no studies have reported acute or chronic toxicity reactions due to *Echinacea* extracts. Echinacin, given intravenously, has resulted in the production of fever (0.5–1°C elevation in body temperature) on occasion. This is presumably a result of secretion of interferon-alpha and interleukin 1 by activated macrophages.[2,3]

The LD_{50} of intravenous Echinacin has been determined to be 50 ml/kg body weight in mice and rats.

The polysaccharides in *E. purpurea* (aerial portion) were shown to have an LD_{50} of 1,000–2,500 mg/kg when given peritoneally to mice. Chronic administration of Echinacin to rats at doses many times the human therapeutic doses gave no evidence of any toxic effects.[49] Mutagenic tests with Echinacin demonstrated no mutagenic activity.[2,3]

A recent review of the safety and efficacy of *Echinacea* sp. found no toxicity in both adults and children in cases of both acute and long-term administration.[50] Extremely high dosages (1,000 times greater than those typically used) were found to be immunosuppressive.

SUMMARY

Echinacea is one of the most widely used botanical medicines. Its primary clinical applications have been in cases of infection or when immune system enhancement is desired. Clinical and experimental investigations have confirmed these applications. Although some of the clinical data are based on injectable formulations, oral administration is thought to yield similar results over time. In fact, there are some evidence indicating that oral administration may have a more profound effect on macrophage activity.

REFERENCES

1. McGregor RL. The taxonomy of the genus *Echinacea* (Compositae). Univ Kansas Sci Bull 1968; 48: 113–142
2. Hobbs C. The Echinacea handbook. Portland, OR: Eclectic Medical Publications. 1989
3. Bauer R, Wagner H. *Echinacea* species as potential immunostimulatory drugs. Econ Med Plant Res 1991; 5: 253–321
4. Bauer R, Jurcic K, Puhlmann J, Wagner H. Immunological in vivo and *in vitro* examinations of *Echinacea* extracts. Arzneim Forsch 1988; 38: 276–281
5. Wagner V, Proksch A, Riess-Maurer I et al. Immunostimulating polysaccharides (heteroglycans) of higher plants. Arzneim Forsch 1985; 35: 1069–1075
6. Stimpel M. Proksch A, Wagner H, Lohmann-Matthes ML. Macrophage activation and induction of macrophage cytotoxicity by purified polysaccharide fractions from the plant *Echinacea purpurea*. Infection Immunity 1984; 46: 845–849
7. Luettig B, Steinmuller C, Gifford GE et al. Macrophage activation by the polysaccharide arabinogalactan isolated from plant cell cultures of *Echinacea purpurea*. J Nat Cancer Inst 1989; 81: 669–675
8. Tubaro A, Tragni E, Del Negro P et al. Anti-inflammatory activity of a polysaccharide fraction of *Echinacea angustifolia* root. J Pharm Pharmacol 1987; 39: 567–569
9. Bauer R, Remiger P, Wagner H. Alkylamides from the roots of *Echinacea angustifolia*. Dtsch Apoth Ztg 1988; 128: 174–180
10. Christ B, Muller KH. Zur serienmabigen bestimmung dess gehhaltes an flavonol-derivaten in drogen. Arch Pharm 1960; 293/65: 1033–1042
11. Stoll A, Renz J, Brack A. Antibacterial substances II. Isolation and constitution of echinacoside, a glycoside from the roots of *Echinacea angustifolia*. Helv Chim Acta 1950; 33: 1877–1893
12. Bauer R, Remiger P. Der Einsatz der HPLC bei der standardisierung von echinacea-drogen Arch Pharm 1989; 322: 324
13. Bauer R, Reminger P, Alstat E. Alkamides and caffeic acid derivatives from the roots of *Echinacea tennesseensis*. Planta Medica 1990; 56: 533–534
14. Neugebuaer H. The constituents of *Echinacea*. Pharmazie 1949; 4: 137–140
15. Heinzer F, Meusy JP, Chavanne M. *Echinacea pallida* and *Echinacea purpurea*. Follow-up of weight development and chemical composition for the first two culture years. 36th Annual Congress of the Society of Medicinal Plant Research, Freiburg, Germany, September 12–16. 1988
16. Schulte KE, Ruecker G, Perlick J. The presence of polyacetylene compounds in *Echinacea purpurea* and *Echinacea angustifolia*. Arzneim Forsch 1967; 17: 825–829
17. Bauer R, Khan IA, Wagner H. TLC and HPLC analysis of *Echinacea pallida* and *E. angustifolia* roots. Planta Medica 1988; 54: 426–430
18. Bauer R, Remiger P. TLC and HPLC analysis of *Echinacea pallida* and *E. angustifolia* roots. Planta Medica 1989; 55: 367–371
19. Roder E, Wiedenfeld H, Hille T, Britz-Kistgen R. Pyrrolizidine in Echinaea angustifolia DC, und Echinacea purpurea MOENCH-Isolierung und Analytik, Dtsch. Apoth Atg 1984; 124: 2316–2318
20. Vogel VJ. *American Indian Medicine*. Norman, OK: University of Oklahoma Press. 1970: p 356–357
21. Felter H. The Eclectic Materia Medica, Pharmacology and Therapeutics. Portland, Or: Eclectic Medical Publications. 1983: p 347–351.
22. Kuts-Cheraux AW. Naturae Medicina and Naturopathic Dispensatory. Yellow Springs, OH: Antioch Press. 1953
23. Mechart D et al. Immunomodulation with Echinacea. a systematic review of controlled clinical trials. Phytomed 1994; 1: 245–254
24. Busing K. Hyaluronidasehemmung durch echinacin. Arzneim Forsch 1952; 2: 467–469
25. Bonadeo I, Lavazza M. Echinacin B. polisaccaride attivo dell' Echinacea. Riv Ital Essenze Profumi 1971; 53: 281–295
26. Tragni E, Tubaro A, Melis S, Galli CL. Evidence from two classic irritation tests for an anti-inflammatory action of a natural extract, *Echinacina* B. Food Chem Toxicol 1985; 23: 317–319
27. Koch FE, Uebel H. Experimentelle untersuchungen uber den einflur von *Echinacina purpurea* auf das hypophysennebennierenrinden-system. Arzneim Forsch 1953; 133–137
28. Wagner H, Breau W, Willer F et al. In vitro inhibition of arachidonate metabolism by some alkamides and phenylated phenols. Planta Medica 1989; 55: 566–567
29. Mose J. Effect of echinacin on phagocytosis and natural killer cells. Med Welt 1983; 34: 1463–1467
30. Djonlagic H, Feiereis H. Leukopoese und alkalische leukozytenphosphatase im echinacin-test bei colities ulcerosa. Z Gastroenterol 1975; 1: 19–22
31. Mose J. Effect of echinacin on phagocytosis and natural killer cells. Med Welt 1983; 34: 1463–1467
32. Pohl P. Therapy of radiation-induced leukopenia by Esberitox. Med Klin 1969; 64: 1546–1547
33. Chone B, Manidakis G. Echinacin-test zur leukozytenprovokation bei efict strahlentherapie. Deutsch Med Wschr 1969; 27: 1406
34. Roesler J, Steinmuller C, Kiderlen A et al. Application of purified polysaccharides from cell cultures of the plant *Echinacea purpurea* to mice mediates protection against systemic infections with *Listeria monocytogenes* and *Candida albicans*. Int J Immunopharmac 1991; 13: 27–37
35. Vomel V. Influence of a non-specific immune stimulant on phagocytosis of erythrocytes and ink by the reticuloendothelial system of isolated perfused rat livers of different ages. Arzneim Forsch 1984; 34: 691–695
36. Wacker A, Hilbig W. Virus-inhibition by *Echinacea purpurea*. Planta Medica 1978; 33: 89–102
37. Koch F, Haase H. Eine Modifikation des spreading-testes im tierversuch, gleichzeitig ein beitrag zum wirkungsmechanismus von echinacin. Arzneim Forsch 1952; 2: 464–467
38. Hopp E, Burn H. Ground substance in the nose in health and infection. Annals Oto Rhino Laryngol 1956; 65: 480–489
39. Voaden D, Jacobson M. Tumor inhibitors. 3. Identification and synthesis of an oncolytic hydrocarbon from American coneflower roots. J Med Chem 1972; 15: 619–623

40. Braunig B et al. *Echinacea purpurea* radix for strengthening the immune response in flu-like infections. J Z Phytother 1992; 13: 7–13
41. Schoneberger D. The influence of immune-stimulating effects of pressed juice from *Echinacea purpurea* on the course and severity of colds. Results of a double-blind study. Forum Immunologie 1992; 8: 2–12
42. Coeugniet EG, Kuhnast R. Recurrent candidiasis. adjuvant immunotherapy with different formulations of Echinacin. Therapiewoche 1986; 36: 3352–3358
43. Voaden D, Jacobson M. Tumor inhibitors. Identification and synthesis of an oncolytic hydrocarbon from American coneflower roots. J Med Chem 1972; 15: 619–623
44. Pohl P. Therapy of radiation-induced leukopenia by Esberitox. Med Klin 1969; 64: 1546–1547
45. Kinkel HJ, Plate M, Tullner HU. Effect of Echinacin ointment in healing of skin leasons. Med Klin 1984; 79: 580–583
46. Seidel K, Knobloch H. Nachweis und vergleich der antiphlogistischen wirkung antirheumatischer medikamente. Z fur Rheum 1957; 16: 231–238
47. Foster S. Echinacea. Nature's immune enhancer. Rochester, VT: Healing Arts Press. 1991
48. Schumacher A, Friedberg KD. Analysis of the effect of *Echinacea angustifolia* on unspecified immunity of the mouse. Arzniem Forsch 1991; 41: 141–147
49. Mengs U, Clare CB, Poiley JA. Toxicity of *Echinacea purpurea*. Arzneim Forsch 1991; 41: 1076–1081
50. Panrham MJ. Benefit-risk assessment of squeezed sap of the purple coneflower (*Echinaea purpurea*) for long-term oral immunostimulation. Phytomed 1996; 3: 95–102

CHAPTER CONTENTS

83

Eleutherococcus senticosus (Siberian ginseng)

Michael T. Murray, ND

Joseph E. Pizzorno Jr, ND

Eleutherococcus or *Acanthopanax senticosus* (family: Araliaceae)
Common names: Siberian ginseng, touch-me-not, devil's shrub, eleuthero ginseng

GENERAL DESCRIPTION

Eleutherococcus senticosus, or Siberian ginseng, is a shrub that stands 5–8.5 feet high. Its erect, spiny shoots, 1.5–2.5 inches in diameter, are covered with a light grey or brownish bark. The leaves are long-petioled in a compound, palmate configuration. The leaflets (five) are elliptic, and finely serrated at the margins on both sides, with scattered, minute spinules along the veins.[1,2]

Eleuthero grows abundantly in parts of the Soviet Far East, Korea, China, and Japan, north of latitude 38. Its distribution is much greater than that of *Panax ginseng* (see Ch. 100).[1]

The root is the most widely used component, with the highest concentration of biologically active substances occurring in the fall, just before defoliation. The leaves are also used medicinally, with their highest concentration of biologically active substances occurring in July, just before flowering.

CHEMICAL COMPOSITION

The initial phytochemical report on eleuthero was published in 1965 by members of the Institute of Biologically Active Substances, in Vladivostok, Russia.[1] Seven compounds, termed eleutherosides A–G, were isolated from a physiologically active fraction of the methanol extract of eleuthero. The total eleutheroside content of the root is in the range 0.6–0.9%, and of the stems is in the range 0.6–1.5%. The ratio of the eleutherosides A–G obtained is approximately 8:30:10:12:4:2:1 respectively. Their structure is shown in Fig. 83.1. Table 83.1, modified from Farnsworth et al's[1] excellent review of eleuthero, summarizes what is currently known about the components of *Eleutherococcus senticosus*. It is important to recognize

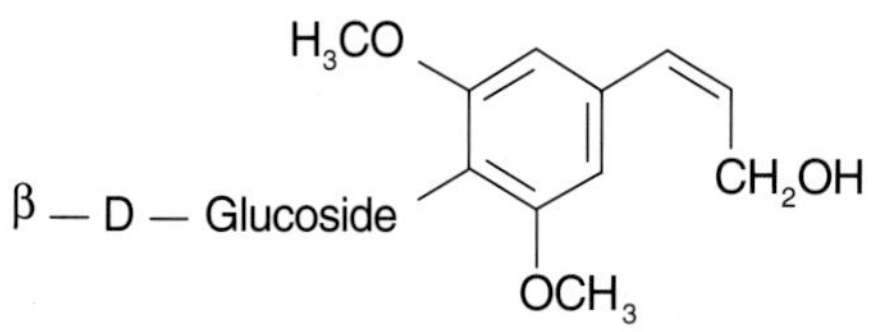

H_3CO — β — D — Glucoside — CH_2OH — OCH_3

Figure 83.1 Eleutheroside B.

that thin-layer chromatographic analysis has shown that the ginsenosides characteristic of *Panax* sp. (American, Chinese, Korean, Japanese ginsengs) are not present in the roots of *Eleutherococcus senticosus*.

HISTORY

The ginseng plants, i.e. members of the family Araliaceae, including *Eleutherococcus senticosus*, are among the most ancient and esteemed of all medicinal herbs. Their use in Chinese herbal medicine dates back more than 4,000 years.[1–3] References in ancient documents to members of the Araliacea family were imprecise, giving rise to some confusion in modern interpretation. However, the value of eleuthero as a medicinal agent was certainly known to the Chinese, as evidenced by the following ode [*Ode to Wujia* (*Eleutherococcus senticosus*) by Ye Zhishen (Qing Dynasty)]:[3]

From earth and heavens the quintessence originates,
Five folioles clustering your leaves,
And pretty little thorns wrapped whole your shoots;
Oh what a jackal's gaunt leg looks much alike.
How wonderful is Winzhang-grass, the Eleutheroginseng
Dispensing in liquor for drinking,
And decocting with burnet for daily using, It will keep your virgin face younger
And prolong your life for ever and ever;
Even if a cartload of gold and jewels,
That cannot estimate your price of nature.

The Chinese have long believed that the regular use of eleuthero would increase longevity, improve general health and appetite, and restore memory.

The Russians have a separate history of eleuthero and even go as far as saying, despite a long history of use by Chinese herbalists (references date back to 2,000 BC), that "Eleutherococcus was not known in Oriental folk medicine".[1] The Russian history of eleuthero begins in 1855 when a pair of Russian scientists, C. I. Maximovich and L. I. Shrenk, traveled from St Petersburg to the Ussuri region of Russia on the Amur river. It was in this area that Maximovich observed a vast thicket of unusual

Table 83.1 Compounds found in *Eleutherococcus senticosus*[1]

Compound	Type	Location
Eleutheroside A (daucosterol)	Sterol	Roots, stems
Eleutheroside B(syringin)	Phenylpropanoid	Roots, stems
Eleutheroside B_1 (isofraxidin-7-0-alpha-L-glucoside; also known as beta-calycanthoside)	Coumarin	Roots
Eleutheroside B_2	Unknown	Roots
Eleutheroside B_3	Unknown	Roots
Eleutheroside B_4 ((-)-sesamin)	Lignan	Roots
Eleutheroside C (methyl-alpha-D-galactoside)	Sugar	Roots, stems
Eleutheroside D ((-)-Syringarsinol di-0-beta-D-glucoside)	Lignan	Roots, stems
Eleutheroside E (different crystalline form of D; also known as acanthoside D)	Lignan	Roots, stems
Eleutheroside F	Unknown	Roots
Eleutheroside G	Unknown	Roots
Eleutheroside I (= mussenin B)	Triterpene	Leaves
Eleutheroside K	Triterpene	Leaves
Eleutheroside L	Triterpene	Leaves
Eleutheroside M (= hederasaponin B)	Triterpene	Leaves
Senticosides A–D (may be identical to eleutherosides I, K, L and M)	Triterpene	Leaves
Vitamin E	Benzofuran	Roots
Beta-carotene	Carotenoid	Roots
Isofraxidin	Coumarin	Roots
Coumarin X	Coumarin	Roots
Complex mixture	Essential oil	Roots
Copper	Mineral	Roots
(-)-Syringaresinol	Lignan	Roots
Caffeic acid	Phenylpropanoid	Roots
Caffeic acid ethyl ester	Phenylpropanoid	Roots
Coniferyl aldehyde	Phenylpropanoid	Roots
Synapyl alcohol	Phenylpropanoid	Roots
Beta-sitosterol	Sterol	Roots
Polysaccharides	Sugar	Roots, fruit
Galactose	Sugar	Roots
Glucose (alpha and beta)	Sugar	Roots
Maltose (alpha and beta)	Sugar	Roots
Sucrose	Sugar	Roots
Oleanolic acid	Triterpene	Roots

plants, with leaves resembling horse chestnut and young shoots resembling ginseng. Unable to identify the plant, the two scientists brought back samples to St Petersburg for classification. The plant was given the genus name of *Eleuthero*, or "free-berried shrub", and the species name of *senticosus*, which means "thorny" in Latin.

However, it wasn't until the middle of the 20th century that eleuthero was again "discovered", when Russian scientists began investigating substances which produce a "state of non-specific resistance" in the body. Substances with this effect were termed adaptogens. As defined by Brekhman in 1958, an adaptogen is a substance that:[1,4]

- must be innocuous and cause minimal disorders in the physiological functions of an organism
- must have a non-specific action (i.e. it should increase the resistance to adverse influences by a wide range of physical, chemical, and biochemical factors)
- usually has a normalizing action irrespective of the direction of the pathologic state (alterative action).

Brekhman's research with adaptogens began with *Panax ginseng*, since this was the best known natural adaptogen. After confirming the adaptogenic action of panax in human studies, Brekhman began searching for an alternative to this plant because of the difficulty and expense in obtaining panax. Initially, all six species of Araliaceae native to Russia were investigated, and eleuthero was found to be the most promising. Numerous studies (in vivo, in vitro, and human studies) have been conducted since the late 1950s, nearly all in the Soviet Union. These are not referenced here as they are not translated and not widely available. Instead, review articles and original articles in English are cited.[1–8]

PHARMACOLOGY

As mentioned above, a number of experimental and clinical studies have demonstrated that eleuthero does possess adaptogenic properties, i.e. the ability to increase non-specific body resistance to stress, fatigue, and disease. Additional experimental and clinical research supports other therapeutic applications of *Eleutherococcus senticosus*.

Experimental studies

Adaptogenic activity

An important characteristic of an adaptogen is its ability to "normalize", irrespective of the direction of pathology. *Eleutherococcus senticosus* has been found in experimental models to:

- impede the adrenal hypertrophy induced by ACTH and the adrenal atrophy induced by cortisone
- impede the thyroid hypertrophy induced by thyroidin and thyroid gland atrophy induced by 6-methylthiouracil
- reduce blood glucose levels in alimentary and adrenal hyperglycemia, and increase glucose levels in insulin-induced hypoglycemia
- reduce leukocytosis induced by the parenteral administration of milk, as well as leukopenia induced by endotoxins
- reduce erythrocytosis induced by cobaltous nitrate and erythropenia induced by phenylhydrazine.

These are summarized in Table 83.2. Similar results have been obtained with *Panax ginseng* (see Ch. 100).

Stress control

Another important action of adaptogens is the inhibition of the alarm phase of the stress reaction. Eleuthero has shown similar action to *Panax ginseng* in experiments designed to demonstrate an anti-alarm action. Specifically, eleuthero has been shown to increase the swimming time of rats, reduce activation of the adrenal cortex in response to stress (alarm phase reaction), and prevent stress-induced thymic and lymphatic involution.[1–7]

Radiation protection

In addition to its confirmed adaptogenic activity, eleuthero has also demonstrated both protective and therapeutic

Table 83.2 Abnormalities normalized by *Eleutherococcus senticosus*

Function	Normalization action of *Eleutherococcus*
Adrenal	Impedes hypertrophy induced by ACTH Impedes atrophy induced by cortisone
Thyroid	Impedes hypertrophy induced by thyroidin Impedes atrophy induced by 6-methylthiouracil
Kidney	Increases renal capacity in pyelonephritis
Blood pressure	Decreases high blood pressure through improvement of atherosclerosis Increases pressure in hypotension
Blood glucose	Reduces alimentary and adrenal hyperglycemia Increases blood sugar in insulin-induced hypoglycemia
Leukocyte	Reduces leukocytosis induced by the administration of milk Reduces leukopenia induced by endotoxins
Erythrocyte	Reduces erythrocytosis induced by cobaltous nitrate Reduces erythropenia induced by phenylhydrazine
Stress	Reduces activation of the adrenal cortex in response to stress Prevents stress-induced thymic and lymphatic involution
Radiation	Protects against radiation exposure
Cancer	Inhibits carcinogenesis from urethane, 6-methylthiouracil, indole
Cholesterol	Reduces hepatic biosynthesis
DNA	Stimulates synthesis

actions in animals exposed to both single and prolonged X-ray radiation. In one study, both *Eleutherococcus senticosus* and *Panax ginseng* were found to double the life span of rats exposed to prolonged radiation (total doses of 1620–7,000 rads). When eleuthero was combined with antibiotics, the lifetime of irradiated rats (total dose of 3,000 rads over 60 days) increased threefold.[8]

These results suggest that eleuthero may be of benefit in protecting against harmful radiation and as an adjunctive aid in radiation therapy in oncology. The latter suggestion is further supported by studies of eleuthero that have demonstrated an inhibition of carcinogenesis.

Carcinogenesis inhibition

Eleutherococcus preparations have been shown in experimental studies in animals to inhibit:[1,4]

- urethane-induced lung adenomas
- 6-methylthiouracil-induced tumors of the thyroid
- myeloid leukemia induced by indole
- the formation of spontaneous mammary gland tumors and leukemia
- transplantation of a variety of tumors.

As is evident from the discussion of eleuthero's adaptogenic activities, eleuthero shares many features with *Panax ginseng*. In addition to adaptogenic activities, eleuthero, like panax, has been shown to:[1]

- increase resistance to infection in animals
- reduce hepatic cholesterol biosynthesis
- increase reproductive capacity and sperm counts in bulls
- possess significant antioxidant activity
- stimulate DNA synthesis and cellular repair enzymes.

Part of eleuthero's anticancer effects may be due to its immuno-stimulating effects. In vitro, it increases phagocytosis of *Candida albicans* by granulocytes and monocytes from healthy donors by 30–45%.[9,10]

CLINICAL STUDIES

Adaptogenic activity in healthy individuals

Farnsworth et al[1] reviewed the results of clinical trials designed to evaluate the "adaptogenic" effects of eleuthero. In these studies, the fluid extract of *Eleuthero senticosus* root was administered to more than 2,100 healthy human subjects. The data indicated that eleuthero:

- increased the ability of humans to withstand many adverse physical conditions (i.e. heat, noise, motion, work load increase, exercise, and decompression)
- increased mental alertness and work output
- improved the quality of work under stressful conditions and athletic performance.

The male and female subjects ranged in age from 19 to 72 years. Dosages of the fluid extract (33% ethanol) ranged from 2.0 to 16.0 ml, one to three times a day, for periods of up to 60 consecutive days.

Adaptogenic activity in disease states

Farnsworth et al[1] also reviewed the results of clinical trials which evaluated the adaptogenic effects of eleuthero in patients with various diseases. A fluid extract (33% ethanol) of *Eleuthero senticosus* root was administered to more than 2,200 human subjects with a variety of illnesses, including angina, hypertension, hypotension, acute pyelonephritis, various types of neuroses, acute craniocerebral trauma, rheumatic heart disease, chronic bronchitis, and cancer.

Eleuthero appears to be effective in atherosclerotic conditions, as evidenced by its ability to lower elevated serum cholesterol and prothrombin levels, reduce blood pressure, and eliminate anginal symptoms in human subjects. Its action on blood pressure is truly adaptogenic, as eleuthero has also been shown to increase blood pressure in subjects with hypotension.[1]

Its effect in regulating blood pressure may be indicative of improved renal function; it has been demonstrated that patients with acute pyelonephritis given eleuthero extract demonstrate increased renal capacity, as measured by an increased secretion of phenol red.[1]

Eleuthero appears to have some psychotropic action, as it has been proven effective in the treatment of a variety of psychological disturbances. Eleuthero has consistently demonstrated an ability to increase the sense of well-being, regardless of the psychological complaint (insomnia, hypochondriasis, various neuroses, etc.). A possible explanation of this effect is improved balance of the biogenic amines (serotonin, dopamine, norepinephrine, epinephrine, etc.), as eleuthero extract administered to rats has been shown to increase biogenic amine content in the brain, adrenals, and urine.[1]

There is not yet sufficient data to fully evaluate eleuthero's action in other disease states. However, it must be kept in mind that an adaptogen is non-specific in its action and possesses a normalizing action irrespective of the direction of the changes from physiological norms.

TOXICOLOGY

Toxicity studies in animals have demonstrated that eleuthero extracts are virtually non-toxic. The LD_{50} of the 33% ethanol extract of eleuthero is 14.5 ml/kg in mice and greater than 20.0 ml/kg in rats. No long-term toxicity was observed when a daily dose of 5.0 ml/kg of the fluid extract was administered to rats. Teratogenicity has been studied in three species (rats, rabbits, and minks), with no adverse effects observed.[1]

In human clinical studies, it was demonstrated that eleuthero extracts (33% ethanol) in the recommended dosage range are well tolerated and side-effects are infrequent. A few studies found mild side-effects at higher dosages (4.5–6.0 ml three times daily) when used for long periods (60 days). The symptoms included insomnia, irritability, melancholy, and anxiety. In individuals with rheumatic heart disease, pericardial pain, headaches, palpitations, and elevations in blood pressure have been reported.[1] These symptoms are probably due to the mild stimulating effects of eleuthero and, while not serious, would indicate the need to decrease the dosage and/or allow a washout period.

DOSAGE

The standard dosage of the fluid extract (33% ethanol) of *Eleutherococcus senticosus* roots used in the majority of studies ranged from 2.0 to 4.0 ml (up to 16.0 ml), one to three times a day, for periods of up to 60 consecutive days. In multiple dosing regimens, there is usually a 2–3 week interval between courses.[1,4]

Dosages are as follows:

- dried root: 2–4 g
- tincture (1:5): 10–20 ml
- fluid extract (1:1): 2.0–4.0 ml
- solid (dry powdered) extract (20:1): 100–200 mg.

SUMMARY

Eleutherococcus senticosus, or Siberian ginseng, possesses significant adaptogenic action. Currently, it can be recommended as a general tonic and in the clinical situations mentioned above (angina, hypertension, hypotension, acute pyelonephritis, various types of neuroses, acute craniocerebral trauma, rheumatic heart disease, chronic bronchitis, and cancer), although it must be pointed out that its clinical application may turn out to be much broader, given its non-specific mechanisms of action.

REFERENCES

1. Farnsworth NR, Kinghorn AD, Soejarto D, Waller DP. Siberian ginseng (*Eleutherococcus senticosus*). Current status as an adaptogen. Econ Med Plant Res 1985; 1: 156–215
2. Leung AY. Encyclopedia of common natural ingredients used in food, drugs and cosmetics. New York, NY: John Wiley. 1980: p 186–189
3. Duke JA. Handbook of medicinal herbs. Boca Raton, FL: CRC Press. 1985: p 337–338
4. Baranov AI. Medicinal uses of ginseng and related plants in the Soviet Union. Recent trends in the Soviet literature. J Ethnopharmacol 1982; 6: 339–353
5. Brekhman II, Dardymov IV. New substances of plant origin which increase nonspecific resistance. Ann Rev Pharmacol 1969; 9: 419–430
6. Brekhman II, Dardymov IV. Pharmacological investigation of glycosides from ginseng and Eleutherococcus. Lloydia 1969; 32: 46–51
7. Brekhman II, Kirillov OI. Effect of Eleutherococcus on alarm-phase of stress. 1969; 8: 113–121
8. Ben-Hur E, Fulder S. Effect of P. ginseng saponins and *Eleutherococcus s.* on survival of cultured mammalian cells after ionizing radiation. Am J Chin Med 1981; 9: 48–56
9. Windfeuer A; Mayerhofer D. The effects of plant preparations on cellular functions in body defense. Arzneimittelforschung Mar 1994; 44: 361–366
10. Wagner H, Proksch A, Riess-Maurer I et al. Immunostimulating action of polysaccahrides (heteroglycans) from higher plants. Arzneimittelforschung 1985; 35: 1069–1075

CHAPTER CONTENTS

84

Ephedra species

Michael T. Murray, ND

Joseph E. Pizzorno Jr, ND

Ephedra sinica (family: Ephedraceae)
Common names: Chinese ephedra, Ma Huang, Chinese joint fir

Related species:
E. distacha (European ephedra)
E. trifurca or *E. viridis* (desert tea)
E. nevadensis (Mormon tea, cay note, canutillo, whorehouse tea, tapopote, teamster's tea)
E. americana (American ephedra)
E. gerardiana (Pakistani ephedra)

GENERAL DESCRIPTION

Ephedra spp. are erect, branching shrubs found in desert or arid regions throughout the world. The 1.5–4 foot shrubs typically grow on dry, rocky, or sandy slopes. The many slender, yellow-green branches of ephedra have two very small leaf scales at each node. The mature, double-seeded cones are visible in the fall.

CHEMICAL COMPOSITION

The chemical analysis of the stems and branches of *Ephedra* sp. has focused on their alkaloid content. In *Ephedra sinica*, the total alkaloid content can be up to 3.3%, with 40–90% of this being ephedrine. The remaining alkaloids are primarily pseudoephedrine and nor-pseudoephedrine.[1,2] In *Ephedra gerardiana*, the alkaloid content usually varies from 0.8 to 1.4%, about half ephedrine and half other alkaloids (pseudoephedrine, *N*-methylephedrine, norephedrine, etc.).[2] Mormon tea or *Ephedra nevadensis* is reported to contain little or no ephedrine.[2]

HISTORY AND FOLK USE

Ephedra sinica's medicinal use in China dates from approximately 2800 BC. Ma Huang (the stem and branch) was used primarily in the treatment of the common cold, asthma, hay fever, bronchitis, edema, arthritis, fever, hypotension, and urticaria.[1]

The Chinese believed the effect of the root and rhizome (Ma Huanggen) to be the opposite of the stem and branches, and limited its use to the treatment of profuse night sweating.[1] Two hypotensive principles (ephedradine A and B) have since been isolated from ephedra root, along with a hypertensive compound (1-tyrosine betaine or maokine).[1]

Western medicine's interest in ephedra began in 1923 with the demonstration that the isolated alkaloid ephedrine possessed a number of pharmacological effects. Ephedrine was synthesized in 1927 and has since been used extensively for clinical conditions in which sympathomimetic effects are desired.[3]

PHARMACOLOGY

The pharmacology of ephedra centers around its ephedrine content. Ephedrine and pseudoephedrine have been extensively investigated and are widely used in both prescription and over-the-counter medications for asthma, hay fever, and rhinitis. In 1973, over 20 million prescriptions contained one of these alkaloids.

Ephedrine

Ephedrine's basic pharmacological action is that of a sympathomimetic. Ephedrine stimulates both alpha- and beta-adrenergic receptors as well as the release of norepinephrine. Ephedrine shares many pharmacological actions with epinephrine, although ephedrine is much less active. Ephedrine also differs from epinephrine in its ability to be absorbed orally, its longer duration of action, and its more pronounced effect upon the central nervous system. The CNS effects of ephedrine are similar to those of amphetamine but, again, much less potent.[1–4] Its chemical structure is shown in Figure 84.1.

The cardiovascular effects of ephedrine are also similar to those of epinephrine. It increases both diastolic and systolic blood pressure, cardiac output, and heart rate, but for a longer (about 10 times) period. Like epinephrine, ephedrine will also increase coronary, cerebral, and muscle blood flow at the expense of renal and splanchnic blood flow.[1–5]

The bronchial muscle relaxation induced by ephedrine is much less than epinephrine, but, again, the duration of action is much longer. Other smooth muscles, with the exception of the human uterus, are generally affected by ephedrine in the same manner (mild relaxation) as epinephrine. Ephedrine relaxes the human uterus where the effects of epinephrine are more complex.[1–4]

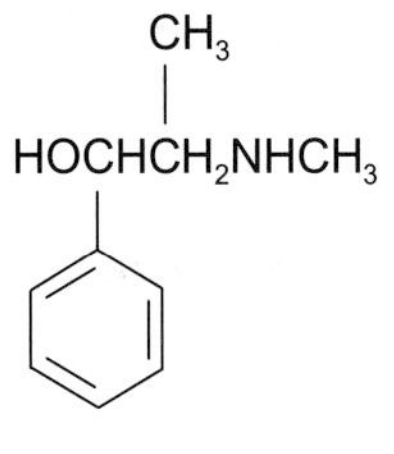

Extracts of ephedra have been shown to inhibit complement in vitro, and a Chinese herbal medicinal prescription, Makyo-kanseki-to, was found to inhibit cyclic AMP activity.[6,7]

The principle adverse effects of ephedrine are CNS stimulation, nausea, tremors, tachycardia, and urinary retention.[1–4]

The major route of elimination of ephedrine is as the unchanged drug in the urine. The average half-life is 6 hours, although acidifying the urine will decrease the half-life considerably. Alkalinization will increase the half-life.[8,9]

CH_3
|
$HOCHCH_2NHCH_3$
(attached to a phenyl ring)

Figure 84.1 Ephedrine.

Pseudoephedrine

Pseudoephedrine exhibits bronchodilating activity similar to ephedrine, but has weaker pressor, cardiac, and central nervous system effects. Pseudoephedrine is often recommended over ephedrine in the treatment of chronic asthma as it has fewer side-effects.[3,4]

Pseudoephedrine has also demonstrated significant anti-inflammatory effects in various experimental models.[8–10] Other ephedra alkaloids, including ephedrine, also exhibited anti-inflammatory activity, but at much lower potency. As the anti-inflammatory effect of pseudoephedrine is essentially identical in normal and adrenalectomized mice, the anti-inflammatory activity is not exerted via the adrenal glands. Instead, it appears that the anti-inflammatory activity of pseudoephedrine and other ephedra alkaloids is due to inhibition of prostaglandin E_2 synthesis.

CLINICAL APPLICATIONS

Asthma and hay fever

Ephedra and its alkaloids have proven effective as bronchodilators for the treatment of mild to moderate asthma and hay fever.[3,4] The peak bronchodilation effect occurs in 1 hour and lasts about 5 hours after administration.

The therapeutic effect of ephedra will diminish if used over a long period of time due to the weakening of the adrenal gland caused by ephedrine. Therefore it is often necessary to use ephedra in combination with herbs, such as *Glycyrrhiza glabra* and *Panax ginseng*; and nutrients, such as vitamin C, magnesium, zinc, vitamin B_6, and pantothenic acid, which all support the adrenal glands.

The folklore herbal treatment of asthma involved the use of ephedra in combination with herbal expectorants. (Expectorants are herbs that modify the quality and quantity of secretions of the respiratory tract, resulting in the expulsion of the secretions and an improvement in respiratory tract function.) Commonly used expectorants include:

- *Glycyrrhiza glabra* (licorice)
- *Grindelia camporum* (grindelia)
- *Euphorbia hirta* (euphorbia)
- *Drosera rotundifolia* (sundew)
- *Polygala senega* (senega).

Common cold

Ephedrine and pseudoephedrine are components of many OTC products for the self-treatment of the common cold.[4] In China, ephedra, in combination with various other herbs, has been found to be clinically effective in the treatment of cold symptoms as well as those of influenza, pneumonia, whooping cough, and bronchitis.[1]

Weight loss aid

In both human and animal studies, ephedrine has been shown to promote weight loss.[11–18] Although ephedrine has demonstrated an anorectic effect,[11] its main mechanism for promoting weight loss appears to be increasing the metabolic rate of adipose tissue.[11–16] Therefore, ephedra's weight-reducing effects are most significant in those individuals with a low basal metabolic rate.[13] These effects can be greatly enhanced when used in combination with methylxanthines caffeine and theophylline, as well as aspirin,[13–18] which potentiates the action of ephedrine and other ephedra compounds.

In one animal study, when ephedrine was used alone, it resulted in a 14% decrease in body weight and a 42% decrease in body fat. However, when used in combination with caffeine or theophylline, the decreases were 25 and 75%, respectively.[14] However, when either caffeine or theophylline were used alone, there was no significant loss in body weight. The reason for the greater decrease in body weight is the increased metabolic rate and fat cell breakdown promoted by ephedrine and enhanced by caffeine and theophylline.

It is recommended that, for methylxanthines, *Camellia sinensis* (green tea) or extracts of *Cola* sp. be used rather than coffee or black tea.

DOSAGE

The optimum dosage of ephedra depends on the alkaloid content in the form used. The average total alkaloid content of *Ephedra sinica* is 1–3%. When used in the treatment of asthma or as a weight loss aid, the ephedra dose should have an ephedrine content of 12.5–25.0 mg and be taken two to three times daily. For the crude herb, an equal dose would be approximately 500–1,000 mg three times per day. Standardized preparations are often preferred as they have more dependable therapeutic activity.

TOXICOLOGY

Ephedra can produce the same side-effects as ephedrine, i.e. increased blood pressure and heart rate, insomnia, and anxiety. A highly potent CNS stimulant, epehedrine may even induce toxic psychosis at high dosages.[19] But, according to the American Pharmaceutical Association: "There is far more discussion of ephedrine tachyphylaxis or tolerance than is evidenced as a significant problem in the scientific literature." A 1977 study of ephedrine therapy in asthmatic children concluded: "Ephedrine is a potent bronchodilator that, in appropriate doses, can be administered safely along with therapeutic doses of theophylline without the fear of progressive tolerance or toxicity."

The FDA advisory review panel on non-prescription drugs recommended that ephedrine not be taken by patients with heart disease, high blood pressure, thyroid disease, diabetes, or difficulty in urination due to enlargement of the prostate gland. Nor should ephedrine be used in patients on antihypertensive or antidepressant drugs.

Pregnant women should also avoid the use of ephedra and ephedrine. Ephedrine administered to chick embryos has resulted in cardiovascular teratogenicity and embryotoxicity at doses as low as 1 µmol/egg.[20] The teratogenic effect of ephedrine is potentiated by caffeine.[21] Presumably, this activity of ephedrine is the result of the production of nitrosamines.[22] Simultaneous vitamin C administration might reduce the formation of nitrosamines from ephedra alkaloids.[23,24]

REFERENCES

1. Chang HM, But PP. Pharmacology and applications of Chinese Materia Medica, vol 2. Teaneck, NJ: World Scientific Publishing. 1987. p 1119–1124
2. Duke JA. Handbook of medicinal herbs. Boca Raton, FL: CRC Press. 1985
3. Gilman AG, Goodman AS, Gilman A. The pharmacologic basis of therapeutics. New York, NY: MacMillan Publishing. 1980
4. American Pharmaceutical Association. Handbook of nonprescription drugs. 8th edn. Washington, DC: American Pharmaceutical Association. 1986
5. White LM, Gardner SF, Gurley BJ, Marx MA, Wang PL, Estes M. Pharmacokinetics and cardiovascular effects of ma-huang (*Ephedra sinica*) in normotensive adults. J Clin Pharmacol 1997; 37: 116–122
6. Ling M, Piddlesden SJ, Morgan BP. A component of the medicinal herb ephedra blocks activation in the classical and alternative pathways of complement. Clin Exp Immunol 1995; 102: 582–588
7. Nikaido T, Iizuka S, Okada N, Kuge T, Ohmoto T. The study of Chinese herbal medicinal prescription with enzyme inhibitory activity. VI. The study of makyo-kanseki-to with adenosine 3′,

5'-cyclic monophosphate phosphodiesterase. Yakugaka Zasshe 1992; 112: 124–128
8. Wilkinson GR, Beckett AH. Absorption, metabolism and excretion of the ephedrines in man. I. The influence of urinary pH and urine volume output. J Pharmacol Exp Ther 1968; 162: 139–147
9. Pickup ME, May CS, Sendagire R, Paterson JW. The pharmacokinetics of ephedrine after oral dosage in asthmatics receiving acute and chronic treatment. Br J Clin Pharmacol 1976; 3: 123–134
10. Hikino H, Konno C, Takata H, Tamada M. Anti-inflammatory principle of ephedra herbs. Chem Pharm Bull 1980; 28: 2900–294
11. Kasahara Y, Hikino H, Tsuru S, Watanabe M, Ohuchi K. Anti-inflammatory actions of ephedrines in acute inflammations. Planta Medica 1985; 54: 325–331
12. Zarrindast MR, Hosseini-Nia, Farnoodi F. Anorectic effect of ephedrine. Gen Pharmacol 1987; 18: 559–561
13. Astrup A, Madsen J, Holst JJ, Christensen NJ. The effect of chronic ephedrine treatment on substrate utilization, the sympathoadrenal activity, and expenditure during glucose-induced thermogenesis in man. Metabolism 1986; 35: 260–265
14. Bailey CJ, Thornburn CC, Flatt PR. Effects of ephedrine and atenol on the development of obesity and diabetes in ob/ob mice. Gen Pharmac 1986; 17: 243–246
15. Dulloo AG, Miller DS. The thermogenic properties of ephedrine/methylxanthine mixtures. animal studies. Am J Clin Nutr 1986; 43: 388–394
16. Pasquali R, Cesari MP, Melchionda N et al. Does ephedrine promote weight loss in low-energy-adapted obese women? Int J Obesity 1985; 11: 163–168
17. Miller DS. A controlled trial using ephedrine in the treatment of obesity. Int J Obesity 1986; 10: 159–160
18. Dulloo AG, Miller DS. Aspirin as a promoter of ephedrine-induced thermogenesis. potential use in the treatment of obesity. Am J Clin Nutr 1987; 45: 564–569
19. Daly PA, Krieger DR, Dulloo AG et al. Ephedrine, caffeine and aspirin. Safety and efficacy for the treatment of human obesity. International Journal of Obesity 1993; 17: S73–78
20. Kalix P. The pharmacology of psychoactive alkaloids from ephedra and catha. J Ethnopharmacol 1991; 32: 201–208
21. Nishikawa T, Bruyere HJ, Takagi Y et al. Cardiovascular teratogenicity of ephedrine in chick embryos. Toxicol Lett 1985; 29: 59–63
22. Nishikawa T, Bruyere HJ, Gilbert EF, Takagi Y. Potentiating the effects of caffeine on the cardiovascular teratogenicity of ephedrine in chick embryos. Toxicology Letters 1985; 29: 65–68
23. Alwan SM, Al-Hindawi MK, Abdul-Rahman SK, Al-Sarraj S. Production of nitrosamines from ephedrine, pseudoephedrine and extracts of ephedra foliata under physiological conditions. Cancer Lett 1986; 31: 221–226
24. Sever PS, Dring LG, Williams RT. The metabolism of (-)-Ephedrine in man. Europ J Clin Pharmacol 1975; 9: 193–198

CHAPTER CONTENTS

85

Fatty acid metabolism

Richard S. Lord, PhD

J. Alexander Bralley, PhD

INTRODUCTION

Fatty acids are common denominators for all life forms. The same oleic acid that is found in the cell membranes of olive trees is also critical for the cellular structure and functions of bacteria, fungi, and humans. Thin layers of fatty acids provide the separation of the inside from the outside of living cells. Plants fill their seeds with fatty acids because they are the most efficient storage form of energy.

Although a growing body of research is now documenting the critical importance of fatty acids for maintaining health, common food choices in modern society do not lead to appropriate levels or balances of these nutrients. Years of negative associations of dietary fat with calories, cholesterol and cancer have resulted in a general public attitude that foods containing fats are simply to be avoided. Many food manufacturers have taken advantage of this attitude by modifying fat content and labeling, wherever possible, to tout "low fat" foods. Advertisements for such foods further instill the notion that dietary fat is bad. Amid the clamor over the largely mistaken problems associated with dietary fats, many very real problems have been created by the large-scale use of modified fats by food suppliers. Individuals do not feel the effects of abusing dietary fats on the short term because of the presence of many protective mechanisms that make health threats from fat abuse a very insidious process.

Modern diets of fast foods and packaged dinners tend to be rich in saturated fats and hydrogenated oils and are frequently lacking in essential fatty acids. We now know that not only the amount, but also the type of dietary fat plays a major role in maintaining health. Some saturated fatty acids stimulate cholesterol formation but most do not.

The old concept of three essential fatty acids has been replaced by recognition of critical roles for multiple polyunsaturated fatty acids. Dietary fats simultaneously provide the major cellular energy source, control the passage of compounds into and out of cells, determine the integrity of nerve tissue, and serve to form powerful hormones.

The essential hormone function is mediated by some special fatty acids that affect energy flow, cell division, immune responses and many other body controls. These critical fatty acids are used to make powerful tissue-specific compounds called eicosanoids. The various roles of fatty acids are illustrated in Figure 85.1. More about these functions will be discussed after some basic fatty acid relationships are explained.

FATTY ACID STRUCTURE AND METABOLISM

There are about 30 structural isomers and homologs of fatty acids that occur in human tissues. They are named in various ways, including those with Latin prefixes (*penta-*, *hexa-*, ...) for the number of carbon atoms. These are the chemical names approved by the International Union of Pure and Applied Chemists (IUPAC). Many also have common names and, because the common name is in widest use among clinicians, they are used here. A lexicon of fatty acid terms is provided in Table 85.1.

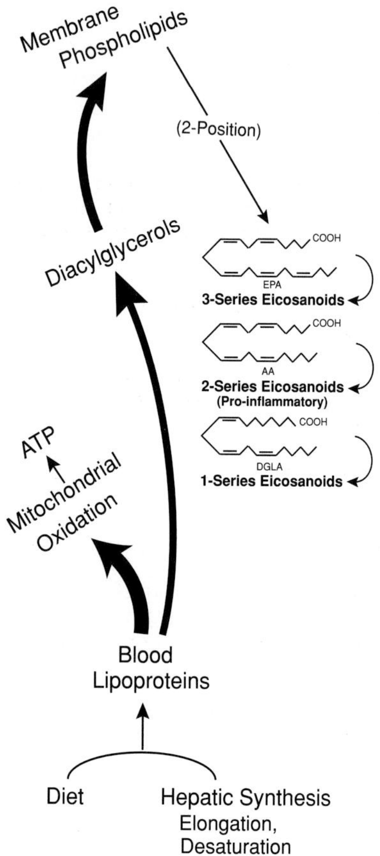

Figure 85.1 Metabolic roles of fatty acids.

Saturated fatty acids

Fatty acids containing the maximum number of carbon–hydrogen bonds are called saturated. They have higher energy or caloric yield than corresponding unsaturated fatty acids. They are present as major components of most foods and are very high in manufactured foods such as candy bars. The most abundant members in human tissues are those that are 12 (myristic), 14 (palmitic), or 18 (stearic) carbons long. The elongation process can be repeated to yield members that are 20, 22, and 24 carbons long. Although such very long-chain fatty acids are minor components of the lipid membranes of the body, they undoubtedly perform valuable functions, apparently helping to stabilize membranes, especially those in peripheral nerve cells.

Unsaturated fatty acids

Three major families of unsaturated fatty acids (UFA) are found in human tissues: the ω9, the ω6, and the ω3 UFAs (or n-9, n-6 and n-3). The ω6 and ω3 polyunsaturated fatty acids (PUFAs) are defined by the position of the double bond closest to the terminal methyl group of the fatty acid molecule. In the ω6 family, the first double bond occurs between the sixth and seventh carbons from the methyl group end of the molecule, whereas in the ω3 family the first double bond occurs between the third and fourth carbons.

The older delta (Δ) naming scheme gives the positions of all double bonds, counting from the carboxyl or number 1 carbon. The omega (ω) scheme takes advantage of the fact that the double bonds are always separated by three carbons and simply gives the total length and number of double bonds separated by a colon. The number following the ω symbol gives the position of the first double bond counting from the omega carbon (see Fig. 85.2 for naming conventions).

Fatty acids can be synthesized from acetyl-CoA derived from carbohydrate, protein, and other non-lipid sources. This pathway produces saturated fatty acids, predominantly palmitic acid (16:0). Palmitic acid can be desaturated, forming the ω7 class of unsaturated fatty acids. Palmitic acid can also be lengthened to stearic acid (18:0) and desaturated to from oleic of the ω9 class. Under ordinary metabolic conditions, these two classes are not further lengthened or desaturated to any appreciable extent. The ω6 and ω3 classes of unsaturated fatty acids are derived from dietary polyunsaturated fats. These classes can be further lengthened and desaturated. None of the four ω classes of unsaturated fatty acids, however, is interconvertible. These reactions can be repeated in various combinations, giving an array of saturated and unsaturated fatty acids for use in the essential functions of tissue maintenance.

Table 85.1 Lexicon of fatty acid terms

Term or abbreviation	Definition or explanation
AA	See arachidonic acid
ALA	See alpha linolenic acid
Alpha linolenic acid	Δ9,12,15 octadecatrienoic acid; 18:3 ω3
Arachidonic acid	Δ5,8,11,14 eicosatetraenoic acid; 20:4 ω6
Carnitine	The molecule to which fatty acids are attached in the process of their enzyme-mediated entry into the mitochondrial matrix. This enzyme is inhibited by malonyl-CoA formed during fatty acid synthesis from carbohydrate
Cerebronic acid	The 2-hydroxy derivative of lignoceric acid (24:0); found in glycosphingolipids in brain
Cervonic acid	Another name for DHA
cis	Geometrical isomer in which two substituents are on the same side of a double bond
Clupanodonic acid	Another name for Δ7,10,13,16,19-docosapentaenoic acid (DPA3), an ω3 series very long-chain, highly unsaturated fatty acid; found in fish oils and the phospholipids in brain
delta (Δ)	Used to describe the position of double bonds relative to the carboxyl end of a fatty acid
Desaturase	Tightly bound to the endoplasmic reticulum membrane, this enzyme, in association with cytochrome b5 and cytochrome b5 reductase utilizes NADH and O_2 to introduce double bonds into fatty acids. There are at least four separate desaturases, named according to the position in the fatty acid that they desaturate Delta-9-desaturase, delta-6-desaturase, and delta-5(4) desaturase act on fatty acyl-CoA thioesters, always inserting double bonds between the thioester bond (carboxylate group) and the double bond closest to it, leaving a three-carbon gap. Activities of these enzymes fluctuate according to dietary fat intake to maintain optimal fluidity state of the membrane lipids. Their concentrations decrease in starvation and increase greatly on re-feeding carbohydrate. They are suppressed when dietary unsaturated fatty acid intake (including *trans* isomers) is high
DGLA	See dihomogammalinolenic acid
Dihomogammalinolenic acid	Δ8,11, 4 eicosatrienoic acid; 20:3 ω6
DHA	Δ4,7,10,13,16,19 Docosahexaenoic acid; 22:6 ω3; an ω3 series very long-chain, highly unsaturated fatty acid; found in fish oils and the phospholipids in the brain (also known as cervonic acid)
Dienoic	Containing two double bonds
EFA	Essential fatty acid
Eicosanoid	A product of the specific, enzyme-directed oxidation of polyunsaturated fatty acids containing 20 (eicosa) carbons. This term encompasses the prostaglandins, thromboxanes, and leukotrienes
Eicosapentaenoic acid	Δ5,8,11,14,17 eicosapentaenoic acid; 20:5 ω3; one of the most abundant fatty acids in fish oils
Elongase	An enzyme that adds 2-carbon units (acetate) to the carboxyl end of an existing saturated or unsaturated fatty acid. Mitochondrial form utilizes acetyl-CoA while endoplasmic form has malonyl-CoA as substrate
EPA	See eicosapentaenoic acid
Gamma linolenic acid	Δ6,9,12 octadecatrienoic acid; 18:3 ω6
GLA	See gamma linolenic acid
HUFA	Highly unsaturated fatty acid; generally having five or six double bonds
LA	See linoleic acid
Lauric acid	Tetradecanoic acid; C12:O; first isolated and identified from the laurel plant
LCP	Long-chain polyunsaturated fatty acid
Linoleic acid	Δ9,12 octadecadienoic acid; 18:2 ω6
Meads acid	Δ5,8,11 eicosatrienoic acid; 20:3ω9. This compound is not normally produced in appreciable amounts due to the saturation of the desaturase enzymes with the more strongly binding essential fatty acids and their metabolic products. It accumulates, however, in essential fatty acid deficiency, making it a marker for this condition
Monoenoic	Containing one double bond
MUFA	Monounsaturated fatty acid
Omega (ω)	Used to describe the position of double bonds relative to the methyl end of a fatty acid
P+M/S ratio	Polyunsaturated + monounsaturated to saturated fatty acid ratio
P/S ratio	Polyunsaturated to saturated fatty acid ratio
Phospholipase A_2	An enzyme that catalyzes the hydrolysis of the fatty acid ester from position 2 of phosphoglycerides. Dependent on calcium, this enzyme is responsive to intracellular calcium, calmodulin, etc. It releases primarily polyenoic fatty acids (arachidonic acid, etc.) within membranes for eicosanoid synthesis
PUFA	Polyunsaturated fatty acid
Phosphatide	Diacylglycerol phosphate to which various groups may be attached through phosphoester linkage; the principal components of cell membranes
Polyenoic	Containing more than two double bonds
Saturated fatty acid	A fatty acid in which all of the carbon atoms except for the carboxyl carbon are fully hydrogenated as $-CH_2-$ (and $-CH_3$)
Beta (β)-oxidation	The mitochondrial metabolic pathway whereby fatty acids are converted into acetyl-CoA which enters the citric acid cycle to ultimately yield ATP. The carbon atoms of the fatty acid are oxidized to CO_2
Stearidonic acid	Δ6,9,12,15 octadecatetrienoic acid; 18:3ω3; a product of elongation of ALA and a precursor to EPA. A good source is black currant seed oil
Timnodonic acid	Another name for eicosapentaenoic acid (EPA) or 20:4ω6
trans	Geometrical isomer in which two substituents are on opposite sides of a double bond
Unsaturated fatty acid	A fatty acid in which two or more adjacent pairs of carbon atoms are lacking hydrogen atoms, having instead an additional carbon–carbon bond or double bond
Δ	The Greek letter, delta (see delta above)
ω	The Greek letter, omega (see omega above)

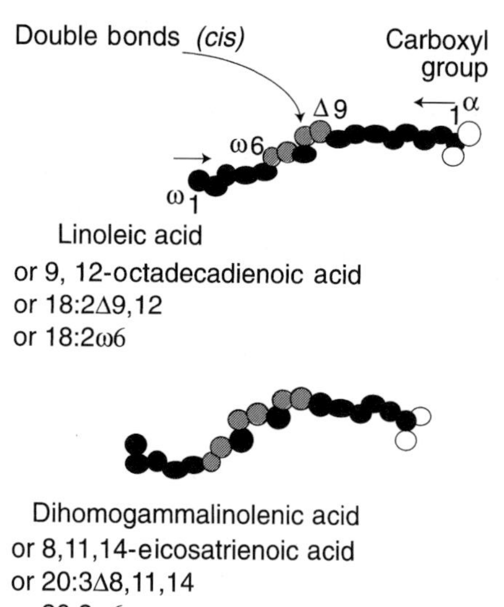

Figure 85.2 Naming conventions for unsaturated fatty acids.

The desaturase enzymes function to place double bonds at positions up to nine carbons from the carboxyl end of the molecules. When you count from the other end, the position varies, depending on the length of the fatty acid. Thus, for stearic acid with 18 carbons, a desaturase can form a double bond nine carbons from the carboxyl end which is also nine carbons from the methyl end (18 – 9 = 9). These differences become important because the type of eicosanoid hormones that can be formed later depend on the position of the first double bond from the methyl end.

The geometry of the desaturase will not allow insertion farther than nine carbons (Δ9) from the carboxyl group. This is the reason that linoleic acid (Δ9, 12) cannot be synthesized in humans. Fatty acids of various chain lengths can act as substrates as well as those that already posses double bonds at other positions. Figure 85.3 shows the products of the Δ9 desaturase acting on three saturated fatty acids.

The activity of the desaturase enzymes is critical for maintaining the ratio of saturated and unsaturated components in cell membranes. Tumor tissue and virus-transformed cells have a higher content of unsaturated fatty acids, especially oleic acid which increases relative to the amount of stearic acid. Such shifts increase the metabolic rates of many lipid-dependent enzymes and are associated with a higher capacity for cell division.[1] Individuals with recurrent tumors may already have too much oleic acid relative to stearic acid, and encouraging a diet high in olive oil or other highly unsaturated fatty acids is contraindicated.

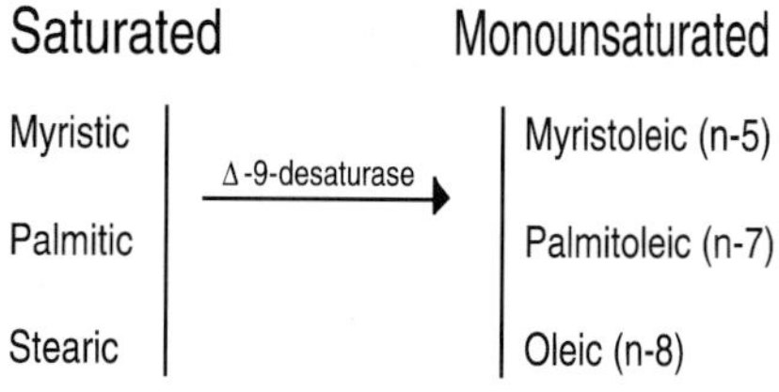

Figure 85.3 Formation of monounsaturated fatty acids.

Trans fatty acids

In the tissues of plants and higher animals, the insertion of double bonds always results in the *cis* geometry. The message "partially hydrogenated vegetable oil" on food labels indicates that a natural oil has been chemically modified in a process that converts some of the *cis* unsaturated fatty acids to the *trans* form. Oleic acid is transformed into its *trans* isomer, elaidic acid, which is the most abundant *trans* fatty acid in most hydrogenated oils. In human tissues, *trans* unsaturated fat behaves as if it were saturated, meaning more risk of heart disease, etc. Adverse impact on HDL or LDL cholesterol of *trans* fatty acids is well documented in the medical research literature.[2–4] Interference with eicosanoid production is also suspected and research in the area of health risks of *trans* fatty acids is accelerating. *Trans* fatty acid levels in cell membranes are determined by dietary intake of hydrogenated oils.[5] A person eating a doughnut for breakfast (3.19 g of *trans* fatty acids), a small order of French fries with lunch (3.43 g), two teaspoons of margarine on bread with dinner (1.24 g), and two cookies for a snack (1.72 g) would ingest a total of 9.58 g of *trans* fatty acids, enough to negate the serum cholesterol-lowering effects of a decrease in saturated fat of 10% of total energy intake.[6]

Elaidic acid is generally the most abundant of the *trans* fatty acids because it is produced by the hydrogenation of the most common oils used in the food industry, including corn, soybean, and safflower. These oils contain relatively high amounts of oleic and linoleic acids, both of which may convert to elaidic acid during the hydrogenation process. Hard margarine may contain as much as 60% of the total unsaturated fatty acids as elaidic acid. Palmitelaidic acid is a *trans* fat that can be formed from hydrogenation of natural fatty acids containing palmitoleic acid, or partial saturation of PUFAs with isomerization. The plasma level reflects body burden of *trans* fatty acids and is useful in monitoring intake of hydrogenated oils.

Polyunsaturated fatty acids (PUFAs)

Dietary PUFAs are largely composed of two classes of fatty acids, the ω6 family (e.g. LA), which is abundant in vegetable seed oils, and the ω3 family (e.g. ALA), which is high in vegetable leaves and modest in soybean oil.[7] When the diet supplies adequate linoleic and alpha linolenic acids, they may be used to form the eicosanoid precursors as shown in Table 85.2.

Table 85.2 Polyunsaturated fatty acid families

Family	Configuration	Name
ω6	18:2	Linoleic (LA)
	18:3	Gamma linolenic (GLA)
	20:3	Dihomogammalinolenic (DGLA)
	20:4	Arachidonic (AA)
ω3	18:3	Alpha linolenic (ALA)
	20:5	Eicosapentaenoic (EPA)
	22:5	Docosapentaenoic (DPA-3)
	22:6	Docosahexaenoic (DHA)

The Δ6 desaturase enzyme acts as a gateway for the flow of fatty acids through the desaturation and elongation pathway. Although it can act on any long-chain fatty acid, the substrate binding affinity increases greatly with the number of double bonds already present (Fig. 85.4). Thus 18:3 binds stronger than 18:2, which binds stronger than 18:1. The result is that ALA is quickly converted to EPA while oleic acid is slowly converted into 20:3ω9 in the presence of appreciable amounts of either LA or ALA. When the two essential fatty acids are absent, however, 20:3ω9 accumulates because the desaturase is free to act on oleic acid. Elevated 20:3ω9 (eicosatrienoic acid) is a marker of essential fatty acid deficiency that could be used in addition to the actual concentrations of the essential fatty acids in plasma and erythrocyte membranes.

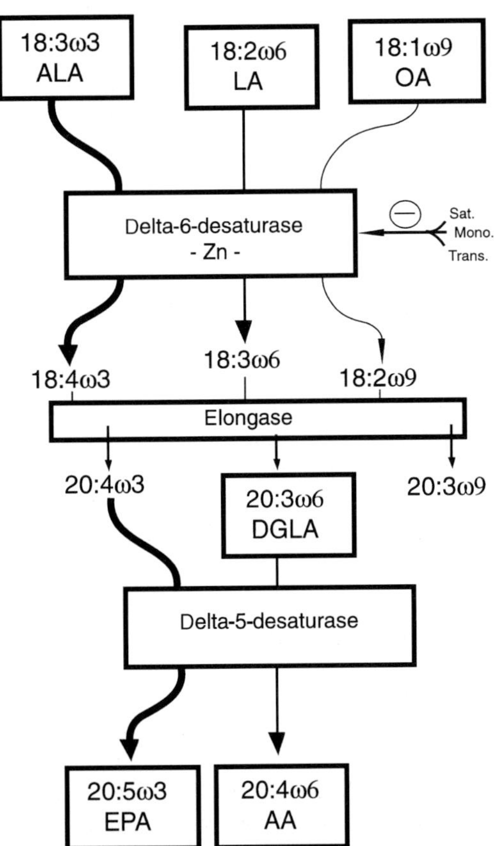

Figure 85.4 Formation of longer and more saturated fatty acids.

The Δ6 desaturase enzyme requires the zinc ion for activity. For this reason, supplementing a patient with sources of LA and ALA will do little good if zinc deficiency is present. The changes in body growth, organ weights and lipid concentrations of plasma and liver produced by zinc deficiency are reversed by the addition of primrose oil, but not safflower oil, showing the role of zinc in the Δ6 desaturase enzyme.[8] The enzyme is also inhibited by high concentrations of saturated fatty acids, monounsaturated and *trans* fatty acids, all of which compete for the enzyme binding site and yield products that are of less significance to the cell.

The primary function of the pathway described above is to supply the parent compounds for the 1-, 2-, and 3-series prostanoid and leukotriene pathways (see below). The PUFAs have great impact on health due to their conversion to these compounds collectively called eicosanoids. They possess extremely potent biological activities, and their homeostatic functions in regulating blood vessel leaking, lipid accumulation, inflammation and immune cell behavior are relevant to the initiation and progress of heart and blood vessel disease.[9] These compounds in turn are used to amplify and balance signals to the organs, the blood clotting system, and the immune system.

Production of eicosanoid hormones is shown in Figure 85.5. The parent compounds are the polyunsaturated fatty acids, DGLA, AA, and EPA, and the pathway utilizes the same enzyme for all three series of products. The concentrations of the three fatty acids present in the phospholipid of the cell membranes where the hormones are produced determine which product will predominate. There is direct substrate competition for the active site on the enzyme as depicted in Figure 85.5. In a similar manner, the lipoxygenase enzyme initiates the sequence of reactions leading to leukotriene formation. The 2-series that is derived from AA is by far the most pro-inflammatory. The effects of GLA and DGLA on rheumatoid arthritis and many other inflammatory diseases are mediated via this mechanism. Since dietary intake is a

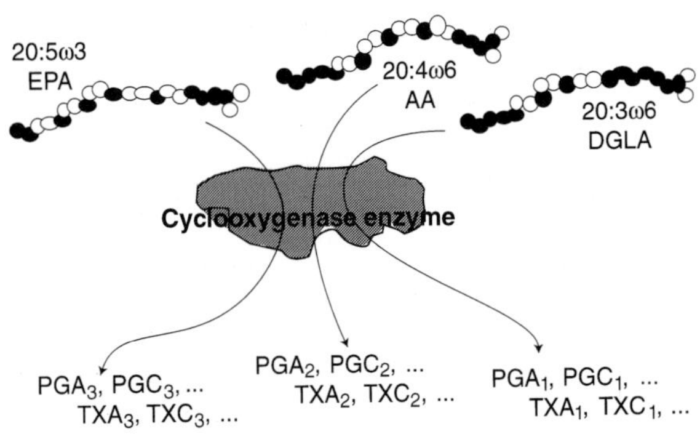

Figure 85.5 Fatty acid relationships to eicosanoid formation.

primary determinant of the fatty acids that go into this pathway, there is a direct link between the balance of specific fats in the diet and inflammatory responses and other local control processes. Long-term health maintenance is highly dependent on proper balance of dietary fatty acids.

Many people do not eat the fresh nuts, seeds, whole grain breads and seafood products that are the rich sources of essential fatty acids. The same individuals are likely to have high intakes of saturated and *trans* fatty acids. The recognition of vast health effects has led to the recent surge of interest in fatty acids. It is no longer adequate (or even correct) simply to recommend the replacement of fats high in saturated fatty acids with those that are high in unsaturated fatty acids. Balanced intake of the unsaturated fatty acids, not just a high PUFA/saturated ratio, is required for optimal control of almost every tissue in the body.[10]

While the actions needed to correct fatty acid abnormalities are quite straightforward, the subject of clinical applications of fatty acid profiling is complex. Those who seek to understand the underlying biochemical and physiological concepts are generally in need of good reference sources. Some that we have found helpful are listed in the "Further reading" section.

CONTROL OF FATTY ACID SUPPLY AND DISTRIBUTION

Fatty acids are present in the diet in the form of triglycerides in solid fats or liquid oils and as phosphatides in cell membranes of whole foods (Table 85.3). They are rarely present in nature as free fatty acids.

Digestion and assimilation

Fats are first digested by the action of bile acids and then pass into intestinal epithelial cells along with cholesterol where they are associated with proteins, becoming particles called chylomicrons. These are passed into the lymphatic system to flow directly through the heart into systemic circulation. Enzymes in capillary cell walls cause the transfer of fatty acids from the chylomicrons, which become greatly reduced in size and return for uptake by the liver as chylomicron remnants. By this process, the fatty acids in foods become directly incorporated into the membranes of all tissues.

Table 85.3 Dietary sources of even-numbered medium- and long-chain saturated fatty acids

Cs	Name	Source
10	Capric acid (C10:O)	Most plants and butter in small amounts
12	Lauric (C12:O)	Palm kernel, coconut, laurels
14	Myristic (C14:O)	Nutmeg, palm kernel, coconut, myrtle
16	Palmitic (C16:O)	Common in all animal and plant fats
18	Stearic (C18:O)	Common in all animal and plant fats
20	Arachidic (C20:O)	Peanut (arachis) oil
22	Behenic (C22:O)	Seeds
24	Lignoceric (C24:O)	Cerebrosides, peanut oil

Synthesis and distribution

Because of the critical life-supporting functions in forming cell membranes and supplying energy sources and hormone controls, there are several mechanisms for assuring that the supply of fatty acids will be continuous, even during short intervals between meals (see Fig. 85.6). In the fasting state, fatty acids are either produced from carbohydrate or protein or mobilized from adipose stores. The liver handles the role of supply depot by forming another class of lipid-protein particles called very low density lipoproteins (VLDL). These particles deliver fatty acids and cholesterol to the tissues by mechanisms similar to that for chylomicrons, except that the remnant LDL particles are taken up in total by binding to receptor sites on cell surfaces. By ensuring a constant supply of fatty acids, the body controls one of the most critical materials for carrying out the various life-sustaining functions of growth and repair.

Effect of low-fat diets

An individual on a low-fat, high-carbohydrate diet utilizes the fatty acid synthetic pathway extensively. As shown in Figure 85.7, this pathway requires citrate to leave the mitochondria to generate malonyl-CoA. The resultant high concentrations of malonyl-CoA inhibits the activity of the enzyme that is the gateway to fatty acid

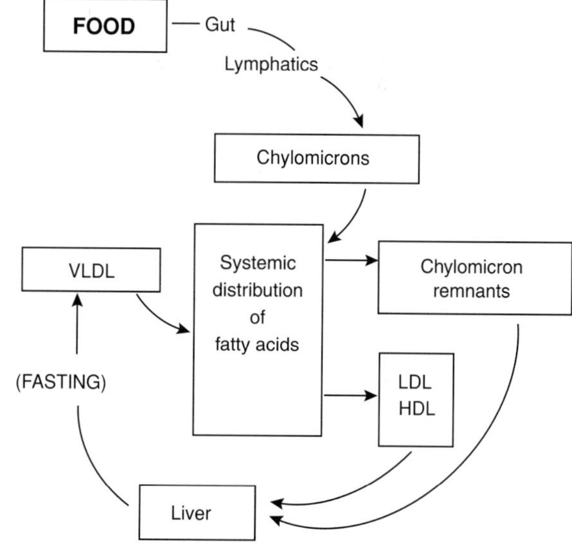

Figure 85.6 Mechanisms for continuous supply of fatty acids to all tissues.

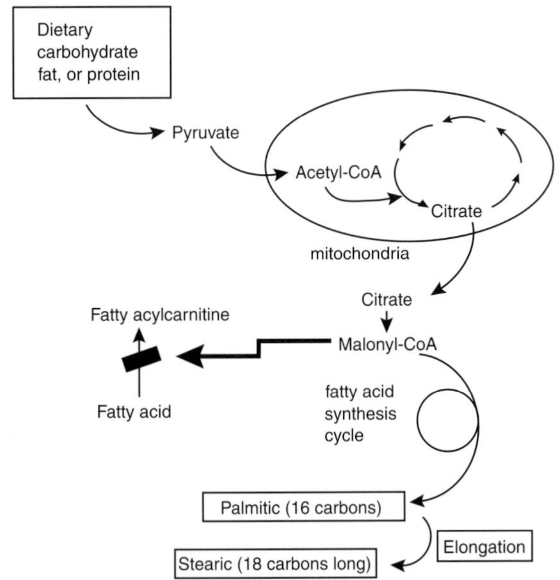

Figure 85.7 Carbohydrate conversion to fat; inhibition of fatty acid oxidation.

oxidation. It is for this reason that very low fat diets do not result in weight loss nearly as fast as one might expect. The burning of excess fat is actually inhibited by the high carbohydrate intake. In individuals with low body fat and good lean mass, high carbohydrate intake spares the use of fatty acids, and the medium-chain fatty acids that are otherwise so quickly used for energy may accumulate above normal in membranes.

Dramatically increased fatty acid oxidation occurs in starvation and diabetes mellitus with production of large amounts of ketone bodies that accumulate to give the ketoacidotic condition. Carnitine deficiency results in impairment of fatty acid oxidation and failure of gluconeogenesis, leading to hypoglycemia.

FATTY ACIDS AND HUMAN DISEASES

Quantification of the approximately 30 fatty acids that are present in human tissues is now routinely available. Both deficiencies and excesses of individual fatty acids lead to metabolic problems. Some specific clinical associations are discussed below (see Ch. 13 for additional discussion of specific fatty acid imbalances.) Table 85.4 lists typical signs and symptoms of fatty acid abnormalities while Table 85.5 lists the better documented clinical applications of supplemental fatty acids.

Developmental disorders

Children with attention-deficit hyperactivity disorder have lower concentrations of key fatty acids in plasma and in red blood cells.[11] Pre-term infants deprived of essential fatty acids during late pregnancy are likely to have failures of normal development, especially the visual system, unless ω3 fatty acids are supplemented.[12]

Table 85.4 Signs and symptoms associated with fatty acid abnormalities

Signs and symptoms	Fatty acid association	Action
Emaciation, weakness, disorientation	Caloric deprivation	Add balanced of fat, protein, and CHO
Reduced growth, renal dysplasia, reproductive deficiency, scaly skin	Classic essential fatty acid deficiency	Add good quality fats and oils
Eczema-like skin eruptions, loss of hair, liver degeneration, behavioral disturbances, kidney degeneration, increased thirst, frequent infections, poor wound healing, sterility (m) or miscarriage (f), arthralgia, cardiovascular disease, growth retardation	Linoleic acid insufficiency	Add corn or safflower oils
Growth retardation, weakness, impairment of vision, learning disability, poor coordination, tingling in arms/legs, behavioral changes, mental disturbances, low metabolic rate, high blood pressure, immune dysfunction	Alpha or gamma linolenic acid insufficiency	Add flax, primrose, borage, or black currant oils
Depression, anxiety, learning behavioral and visual development	Long-chain PUFA-dependent neuromembrane function	Add fish oils Avoid hydrogenated oils
Cardiovascular disease risk	Prostanoid balance	Add ω3 PUFAs
Cancer	Low stearic to oleic ratio Prostanoid imbalance	Use ω6 PUFAs with caution
Rheumatoid arthritis	Low GLA and DGLA	Add primrose oil
Deficiency of vitamin B_{12} and/or carnitine	Increased odd numbered FAs	Add B_{12} and/or carnitine
Myelinated nerve degeneration	Increased very long-chain FAs	Add high-erucate rape or mustard oils
Fatty liver	Saturated and ω9 accumulation in liver	Restrict alcohol Add lecithin Increase Methionine
Accelerated aging	High PUFA intake without increased antioxidants	Add vitamins E and C, Se, Mn, and Zn

Table 85.5 Clinical utilization of GLA and ALA (x, moderate; xx, strong clinical response)

Application	GLA	ALA
Lower blood pressure, lower blood cholesterol, and lower risk of stroke and heart attack	x	xx
Normalize fat metabolism in diabetes and decrease the amount of insulin required by diabetics	x	x
Prevent liver damage due to alcoholism and decrease withdrawal symptoms after discontinuing the habitual use of alcohol	x	x
Provide adjunctive treatment for schizophrenics	x	xx
Cause weight loss by increasing metabolic rate and fat burn-off	x	xx
Relieve premenstrual breast pain (mastalgia) and premenstrual syndrome of bloating, irritability, depression and aggressive behavior	xx	x
Prevent drying and atrophy of tear and salivary glands (Sjögren's syndrome)	x	
Prevent arthritis in animals	x	x
Improve the condition of hair, nails, and skin	x	xx
Improve certain kinds of eczema	x	x
Slow down or stop deterioration in multiple sclerosis	x	x
Help treat diabetic neuropathy in type II diabetes	x	x
Kill cancer cells in tissue culture without harming normal cells	x	xx

Heart disease

Higher palmitic and lower ω3 fatty acids in serum are correlated with higher incidence of coronary heart disease in middle-aged men at high risk for cardiovascular disease.[13] Improvements in plasma fatty acids and vitamins E and C were the only factors found to be related to improvements in life expectancy and 70% lowering of heart disease in a study population.[14]

Cancer

Tumor tissue and virus-transformed cells have a higher content of unsaturated fatty acids, especially oleic acid which increases relative to the amount of stearic acid. Such shifts increase the metabolic rates of many lipid-dependent enzymes and are associated with a higher capacity for cell division.[15] Changes in dietary fatty acid intake cause alterations in immune response, including antitumor activity.[16]

Neurological disorders

Adrenal leukodystrophy and related conditions are associated with the accumulation in nerve sheath membranes of fatty acids more than 20 carbons long. This situation may be made worse by the lack of sufficient long-chain polyunsaturated fatty acids. The indicator for this situation is the sum of the 22–26 carbon length even-numbered fatty acids.

SUMMARY

Many health problems are related to inappropriate fat intake and suboptimal fatty acid composition of the body. The therapeutic value of oils rich in specific fatty acids is being reported in the research literature with increasing frequency for a wide range of diseases. The availability of laboratory methodologies for accurate evaluation of fatty acid status now allows for sophisticated clinical manipulation of these important nutrients.

REFERENCES

1. Wood CB, Habib NA, Apostolov K et al. Reduction in the stearic to oleic acid ratio in human malignant liver neoplasms. Europ J Surg Onc 1995; 11: 347–348
2. Mensink RP, Zock PL, Katan MB, Hornstra G. Effect of dietary cis and trans fatty acids on serum lipoproteins levels in humans. J Lipid Res 1992; 33: 1493–1501
3. Longnecker M. Do trans fatty acids in margarine and other foods increase the risk of coronary heart disease? Epidemiology 1993; 4: 492–494
4. (Review). Trans fatty acids, blood lipids, and cardiovascular risk. Where do we stand? Nutr Rev 1993; 51: 340–343
5. Pettersen J, Opstvedt J. Fatty acid composition of lipids of the brain and other organs in suckling piglets. Lipids 1992; 27: 761–769
6. Litin L, Sacks F. Trans fatty acid content of common foods. New Engl J Med 1993; 329: 1969–1970
7. Kinsella JE. Requirements and sources of n-3 polyunsaturated fatty acids in the human diet. In. Karel M, Lees R, eds. Proceedings of the MIT conference on fish oils. New York: Marcel Dekker. 1989
8. Huang YS, Cunnane SC, Horrobin DF, Davignon J. Most biological effects of zinc deficiency corrected by g-linolenic acid, (18: 3 w6) but not by linoleic acid (18: 2w6). Atherosclerosis 1982; 41: 193–207
9. Stamler J. Nutrition related risk factors for the atherosclerotic diseases: present status. Prog Biochem Pharmacol 1983; 19: 245–252
10. Horrobin DF (Ed). Clinical uses of essential fatty acids. Montreal: Eden Press. 1981
11. Stevens LJ, Zentall SS, Deck JL et al. Essential fatty acid metabolism in boys with attention-deficit hyperactivity disorder. Am J Clin Nutr 1995; 62: 761–768
12. Innis S. n-3 Fatty acid requirements of the newborn. Lipids 1992; 27: 879–887
13. Simon JA, Fong J, Bernert JT, Browner WS. Serum fatty acids and the risk of stroke. Stroke 1995; 26: 778–782
14. Renaud S, deLorgeril M, Delaye J et al. Cretan Mediterranean diet for prevention of coronary heart disease. Am J Clin Nutr 1995; 61: 1360S–1376S
15. Wood CB, Habib NA, Apostolov K et al. Reduction in the stearic to oleic acid ratio in human malignant liver neoplasms. Europ J Surg Onc 1995; 11: 347–348
16. Erikson KL, Hubbard NE, Chakrabarti R. Modulation of signal transduction in macrophages by dietary fatty acids. J Nutr 1995; 125: 1683S–1686S

FURTHER READING

Murray RK, Granner DK, Mayes PA, Rodwell VW. Harpers review of biochemistry 20th edn. Stamford, CN: Appleton and Lange. 1985

Erasmus U. Fats that heal fats that kill. Burnaby, Canada: Alive Books. 1986

Spiller GA. Handbook of lipids in human nutrition. Boca Raton, FL: CRC Press. 1996

CHAPTER CONTENTS

86

Fish oils

Alexander G. Schauss, PhD

INTRODUCTION

A significant body of evidence now shows that consumption of fish oil may be beneficial to health.[1–5] Numerous studies have reported an inverse association between fish oil consumption, risk of cardiovascular disease, and various forms of cancer. Fish oil supplements have also been reported to ameliorate the signs and symptoms of other diseases, such as psoriasis and rheumatoid arthritis, and to play a role in the management of diabetes.

The unique health benefits of fish oil were first investigated in Greenland Eskimos who paradoxically consumed a very rich diet that was high in saturated animal fat from seals, whales, and fish, yet had very low rates of coronary heart disease. Later studies discovered that the Greenland Eskimos' diet contained large quantities of omega-3 fatty acids.

DESCRIPTION

Marine life is generally rich in the omega-3 fatty acids (also referred to as n-3 fatty acids) eicosapentaenoic acid (EPA) and docosahexanoic acid (DHA). These very long-chained and highly polyunsaturated fatty acids (PUFA) contain, respectively, 20 and 22 carbons and 5 and 6 double bonds, and are also referred to as 20:5n-3 PUFA and 22:6n-3 PUFA. The 20:5n-3 PUFAs and 22:6n-3 PUFAs are abundant in shellfish, sea mammals, and fish. EPA and DHA are very low or absent in domesticated land animals.

The source of EPA and DHA found in most marine foodstuffs are phytoplankton. The phytoplankton, naturally rich in EPA and DHA, serve as food for a variety of sea creatures. Fish oil from herring, cod liver, salmon, mackerel, and sardines is rich in omega-3 fatty acids, while containing varying levels of EPA and DHA. Table 86.1 lists the relative concentration of fatty acids in some common fish species.

The habitat in which fish grow has a major impact on their fatty acid composition.[7] In the wild, fish consume

Table 86.1 Relative concentration of fatty acids in fish oils[6]

		Unsaturated		n-3 PUFAs		
Oil	Cholesterol (mg/100 g)	Mono- (%)	Poly- (%)	18:3 (%)	20:5 (%)	22:6 (%)
Cod liver	570	18	51	0.7	9.0	9.5
Herring	760	19	60	0.6	7.1	4.3
Menhaden	600	34	32	1.0	12.7	8.0
Salmon	485	24	40	1.0	8.0	11.0
Pilchard	–	25	29	Trace	17.0	9.0
Mackerel	–	21	43	Trace	11.0	11.0
Anchovy	–	28	29	Trace	17.0	9.0
Sardine	–	24	34	Trace	15.0	10.0

food sources which contain higher levels of alpha-linolenic acid (18:3n-3). This is an important point given the increasing harvesting of fish reared in fish pens. In the natural ocean environment, phytoplankton, which are high in EPA and DHA, form the basis of the food chain. In contrast, commercial fish foods contain less DHA and EPA and hence result in lower concentrations of omega-3 fatty acids. Studies have shown that wild fish (hunted fish) have higher concentrations of omega-3 fatty acids than pond-reared/cultured fish fed commercial feedstuffs devoid in EPA/DHA.[8]

Another dietary omega 3 fatty acid is alpha-linolenic acid (LNA), an 18-carbon-chain fatty acid with three double bonds (18:3n-3 PUFA). Foods such as tofu, canola oil, black currant oil, flaxseed oil (the best non-fish source), nuts, and soybeans are important sources of LNA for those not eating seafood. However, soy-derived oils and foods and most nuts also contain large amounts of omega-6 fatty acids which will neutralize many of the therapeutic benefits of the omega-3 fatty acids.

Dietary requirement

The first suspected case of omega-3 fatty acid deficiency in humans was reported in 1988.[9] The patient was a 7-year-old girl with retarded growth who had been fed solely by gastric tube since 3 years of age. She began to experience normal growth after taking cod liver oil and linseed oil supplements.

Omega-3 fatty acid requirements in humans remain controversial. Some investigators contend that as little as one meal of fish a week is sufficient, while others suggest that a much higher intake level is necessary for individuals to fully profit from its multitudinous benefits.

Since the concentration of EPA and DHA in fish can vary depending on its growth environment, fish oil supplements offer a viable and reliable source of fish oil.

Fish oil supplements can supply high concentrations of eicosapentaenoic acid and docosahexanoic acid. The most popular combination of EPA- and DHA-rich fish oil is the brand "MaxEPA". MaxEPA (18% EPA and 12% DHA) and other fish oil supplements (e.g. blue-fin tuna oil which contains 7% EPA and 25% DHA) are derived from cold-water ocean fish. However, this does not imply that the beneficial fish are always pelagic (i.e. from deep ocean waters) since some freshwater fish contain higher levels of EPA and DHA than some salt-water species.

Most fish oil capsules contain between 300 and 500 mg of omega-3 fish oil per 1 g capsule. Patients using fish oil at the therapeutic levels discussed in this chapter may require between 15 and 30 capsules to derive the described benefits. At 9 calories/g of oil, this can represent a significant increase in caloric intake.

EPA/DHA-rich fish oil capsules should be kept in capsules (such as soft gelatin) capable of providing an oxygen barrier, otherwise toxic lipid peroxides (e.g. malondialdehyde) may form. Encapsulated liquid sources generally do not have this protection unless they contain antioxidants. Emulsified fish oils are preferred as they are better absorbed in humans.

Encapsulated products typically contain fish oil, not fish liver oil. This distinction is important since fish liver oil contains the fat-soluble vitamins A and D, which if taken in excessive amounts have the potential to cause toxicity. The lowest consistently reported daily intakes associated with chronic toxicity in adults are 50,000 IU for vitamin A and 10,000 IU for vitamin D (see Ch. 108). However, there is mounting evidence that vitamin D from sunlight and fish oil may reduce the incidence of certain cancers, such as breast cancer. Hence, some vitamin D residuals in the fish oil may actually increase its protective value against cancer as well as CHD.

Explaining inconsistent results of fish oil supplementation trials

There are many papers in the fish oil literature whose results are equivocal or contradictory. Much of these differences in outcomes can be explained by the use of olive oil as a placebo or the lack of control for saturated or omega-6 PUFA dietary intake.

Olive oil cannot be considered an inert placebo in trials that investigate effects on platelet function or CHD risk. Several studies have shown that olive oil supplementation has similar inhibitory effects on various aspects of platelet function, including decreased platelet aggregation and thromboxane TXA_2 release, increased platelet membrane oleic acid content, and decreased platelet membrane arachidonic acid content.[11,12] Further, an excess of oleic acid impairs incorporation of arachidonic acid into platelet phospholipids.

Another possible complicating factor is the squalene found in olive oil and some deep-water fishes, but not in other vegetable oils.[13] Other problems include the differing ratios of fatty acids, the position of the fatty acids on the glycerol backbone, and the susceptibility to peroxidation of the various fish oil preparations.[14]

PHARMACOLOGY

In general, the effects of supplemental and dietary unsaturated fatty acids appear to be mediated through changes in serum lipids, altered ratios of prostaglandins, decreased platelet aggregation, and modification of cell membrane activity.[14]

Fish oils appear to reduce undesirable circulating fats and decrease the production of the prothrombotic substance thromboxane (TXA_2) by occupying TXA_2 receptors and enhancing the production of the platelet anti-aggregatory substance prostacyclin. These actions play an important role in inflammation, atherogenesis, thrombosis, and CHD.

Through the vasodilatory effects of prostacyclin PGI_3, fish oils may improve peripheral circulation, thereby facilitating VLDL cholesterol removal. This may be accomplished by altering membrane fluidity in a specific manner, thus affecting the activity of membrane-bound enzymes and resulting in changes in receptor activity, specificity, and signal transduction.

Evidence also suggests that fish oils decrease hepatic synthesis of fatty acids and triglycerides, and reduce secretion of VLDL cholesterol, while displacing arachidonic acid from tissue phospholipids. This results in omega-3 EFA levels that inhibit thromboxane synthesis.

Researchers have noted that fish oil effects are selective. EPA and DHA not only displace arachidonic acid from phospholipid pools and inhibit cyclooxygenase, but EPA also becomes a preferred substrate for cyclooxygenase when peroxide tone is high. This results in decreased production of the vasoactive and aggregatory prostacyclin PGI_2 and increased production of PGI_3 which has more potent anti-aggregatory effects. According to some researchers, increased bleeding time is due to either less thromboxane (TXA_2) or higher prostacyclin I_3 levels,[15] although there are those who contend that EPA conversion to PGI_3 is the primary cause.[16] Many researchers believe this change is one of the primary factors that decrease the risk of atherosclerosis and thrombosis.[17–23] These findings may explain some of the epidemiological evidence of decreased coronary artery disease and prolonged bleeding time seen in some Eskimos and in those Japanese found eating a diet rich in fish.[24]

Fish oils rich in EPA and DHA have also been found to suppress production of inflammatory mediators found in patients with rheumatoid arthritis and psoriasis. The anti-inflammatory effect of the omega-3 fatty acids is probably due to reduced production of leukotrienes, interleukin-2, and tumor necrosis factor, all principal mediators of inflammation.

In relation to CAD, ingestion of fish oil and its effect on platelets, erythrocytes, neutrophils, monocytes, and liver cells are considered to be important in explaining its benefits. The increased concentrations of EPA and DHA from the ingestion of fish oil has been shown to:

- decrease production of prostaglandin E_2 (PGE_2) metabolites
- decrease production of thromboxane A_2 (an active vasoconstrictor and platelet aggregator)
- increase prostacyclin PGI_3 (an active vasodilator and inhibitor of platelet aggregation)
- increase production of leukotriene B_5 (a weak inducer of inflammation; weak chemotactic agent)
- decrease production of leukotriene B_4 (a weak inducer of inflammation; inducer of leukocyte adherence and chemotaxis.

CLINICAL APPLICATIONS

Cardiovascular disease

The EPA and DHA in fish oil inhibit the development of atherosclerosis which can increase the risk of primary cardiac arrest.[25] Evidence from large animal studies indicates that fish oil prevents atherosclerosis by mechanisms other than simply lowering cholesterol, including:

- stimulation of endothelial production of nitric acid
- decrease of cytokine and interleukin 1 production
- inhibition of monocyte migration into the plague.

These three events can, when uncontrolled, contribute to the characteristic yellowish plaques (atheromas) that contain the combination of cholesterol, lipophages, and lipoid material seen in the intima and inner media of large and medium-sized arteries found in atherosclerosis. Hence, the demonstrated ability of fish oil to control all three, combined with its ability to lower VLDL and elevated triacylglycerols, can be a useful approach in the prevention of ventricular fibrillation and sudden death.

That fish oil can perform this favorable reduction in risk of sudden death, not shown to be possible by the consumption of linolenic acid or linoleic acid from vegetable oils, has been shown in several double-blind, placebo-controlled, randomized trials conducted in human subjects, especially when compared with vegetable oils.[22]

In addition, diets rich in omega-3 fatty acids from fish oil lower triglyceride levels, especially in those with severe hypertriglyceridemia, for whom attempts to correct the cause through exercise, the drug gemfibrozil or other dietary modifications have proven inadequate. This benefit is not seen with plant source oils containing land-based alpha-linolenic fatty acid-rich polyunsaturated fat sources or the reduction of saturated animal fatty acids.[23]

The therapeutic use of fish oil supplements is also essential in patients with type V hyperlipidemia. At a 1994 scientific meeting on the role of fish oil in cardiovascular health, the following favorable mechanisms of action of omega-3 fatty acids in humans were reported:[21]

- inhibition of very-low-density lipoprotein (VLDL) triglyceride synthesis
- decreased apoprotein B synthesis
- enhancement of VLDL turnover with an increased fractional catabolic rate of VLDL
- depression of LDL synthesis
- reduction of postprandial lipidemia.

The incidence of diabetes is also low in Greenland Eskimos. Studies have shown that the type of fat consumed by humans may have a profound effect on insulin action in tissues. Patients with insulin-dependent diabetes mellitus (IDDM) are prone to disorders of lipoprotein and lipid metabolism, especially hyperlipidemias. The combination of low-density lipoprotein (LDL) cholesterol and elevated plasma cholesterol (hypertriacylglyceridemia) is associated with an increased risk of coronary heart disease. This combination is a major contributor to the morbidity and mortality associated with non-insulin-dependent diabetic (NIDDM) patients.[26] In individuals with NIDDM, fish oil ingestion has been demonstrated to favorably alter arterial wall compliance without adversely affecting cholesterol levels, blood pressure, or fasting blood sugar levels, thereby contributing to a reduced risk of vascular complications seen in IDDM and NIDDM patients.[27]

All of the above benefits of fish oil may not be conferred by only eating fish. Favorable therapeutic and preventive effects may require between 5 and 20 g/day of LNA and fish oil, which is unlikely in contemporary diets in industrialized societies – hence, the use of fish oil supplements.

The prevention of thrombosis by fish oil consumption is suggested by a number of studies, particularly in patients receiving coronary bypass surgery. In a randomized controlled trial of bypass patients who received warfarin or aspirin as anticoagulants, those subjects who also received fish oil had significantly less vein graft occlusions.[28]

Despite all of these findings as they relate to coronary heart disease (CHD), a 1997 American Heart Association (AHA) science advisory report on fish oil consumption states: "There is no convincing role for fish oil supplements in the prevention of CHD."[29] The AHA report does accept mounting evidence that sudden cardiac deaths may be prevented, although "further studies are needed to explore the potential of fish oil in the prevention of sudden cardiac death". Apparently, the American Heart Association's scientists require "compelling evidence" before they would recommend general usage of fish oil supplements to reduce CHD or sudden death. This, despite the conclusion of one of the studies they cite which finds that fish oils reduce myriad potential atherogenic processes associated with atherosclerosis, CHD, and sudden cardiac-related deaths.[30]

Researchers have focused more on fish oil supplements than on fish consumption as dietary surveys have found that less than half of the Australian, American, and Canadian populations regularly eat fish. In addition, some popular species of fish that are consumed by humans contain low levels of the omega-3 essential fatty acids.

Elevated serum lipids

The most consistent effect of fish oils on serum lipids is a reduction in total triglycerides and VLDL cholesterol, especially in patients with severe hypertriglyceridemia. In general, dietary fish oils appear to both reduce undesirable serum circulating fats and decrease the production of the prothrombotic thromboxanes. In most studies, fish oil supplementation causes a significant reduction of VLDL cholesterol, plasma triglycerides, plasma cholesterol, and LDL cholesterol. In hypertriglyceridemic patients, fish oil supplementation typically results in a significant decline in VLDL cholesterol levels, because large decreases in triglyceride levels lead to a decrease in VLDLs.[5,22,31–33]

There are some studies that do not find decreases of total cholesterol or LDL cholesterol following fish oil supplementation.[34–37] However, these equivocal studies used olive oil as a placebo, which, as discussed above, is not appropriate.

For patients with elevated serum cholesterol (7.75 mmol/L) or triglycerides (5.64 mmol/L), there is sufficient evidence to consider fish oil supplementation in the range of 5–10 g/day.[38] In one study of 365 patients, supplementation with 10 ml/day (9.2 g) of MaxEPA resulted in significant reductions in triglyceride levels which were maintained over a period of 4 years.[39] Continuing reductions were observed in persons remaining in the study more than 4 years. The authors concluded: "For triglycerides to remain depressed it seemed necessary to maintain a daily intake of 9.2 g MaxEPA."

In a Canadian study, triglyceride levels decreased 31% in 9 days following fish oil supplementation.[40] However, total and HDL cholesterol levels did not change. Nine days after supplementation ceased, triglyceride levels showed a trend of returning to baseline.

As total cholesterol and LDL cholesterol levels are predictors of death from cardiovascular and coronary heart disease, their control is crucial. Almost all epidemiologic studies show that populations eating fish have a reduced death rate from CHD.

By 1990, 22 primary and secondary prevention trials demonstrated that lowering serum total cholesterol and LDL cholesterol through either diet or drugs reduced the incidence of coronary heart disease among survivors of myocardial infarction. A 10 year prospective study of male mortality rates due to cardiovascular disease found that LDL cholesterol, HDL cholesterol, and total cholesterol levels are the most predictive indices of subsequent mortality from cardiovascular disease among men with and without pre-existing cardiovascular disease.[41]

Support for fish oil intake in the reduction of CHD comes primarily from epidemiological studies[1–3] and clinical and experimental studies in animals and humans.[5,22,42–48] A 20 year prospective study conducted in the Netherlands found that consuming as little as 35 g/day of fish (0.5 pounds/week) might be of benefit in preventing, and reducing mortality from, coronary heart disease.[49] In contrast, two epidemiological studies found no relationship between fish consumption and cardiovascular mortality.[50,51]

The effect of fish oil consumption on lowering serum lipids may account for the lower mortality rate due to cardiovascular disease found in coastal Alaskan natives, who, compared with mainland Americans, eat a diet rich in fish and other sea creatures. Autopsies on 339 Alaskan natives found that only 10.3% died of cardiovascular causes, compared with 50% of all deaths among those subjects who lived on the American mainland.[52]

The possibility of fewer fatal arrhythmias due to high fish consumption has also been proposed to explain the lower death rate of native Alaskans.[53] Two studies involving rats have shown that ingestion of either as much as 30% or as low as 0.4% of energy in the form of omega-3 fatty acids from fish decreased the incidence of ventricular fibrillation.[54,55] The anti-arrhythmic aspects of PUFAs are supported by a number of clinical and experimental studies in animals and humans.[42–46] Some investigators conclude that fish oil is more effective at reducing ventricular arrhythmias than pharmacologic agents in the prevention and management of cardiovascular disease.[47]

Recent evidence also suggests fish oil may prevent cardiovascular in Rhesus monkeys and hyperlipidemic pigs despite lack of improvement in serum cholesterol levels.[56,57] This retardation in the initiation and progression of atherogenesis may be due to fish oil's depression of inflammatory eicosanoid metabolism in platelets, macrophages, and monocytes.

The therapeutic dosage of fish oil for the treatment of cardiovascular disease should be 5 g/day or more.[23] One researcher has suggested that for both prophylactic and therapeutic applications, the most efficacious use of fish oil would be to concomitantly lower total fat intake to no more than 30% of calories and saturated fatty acids to no more than 30% of total fat, while limiting omega-6 fatty acids (vegetable oils) to a maximum of 10% of total fat intake.[23]

Hypertension

There is some evidence from placebo-controlled studies that fish oil reduces blood pressure in a dose–response fashion, especially in patients with hypercholesterolemia and hypertension, but not in subjects with normal blood pressure.[58]

Fish oil seems to have hypotensive effects, ranging from limited (at dosages of 5 g/day or less) to substantial (at larger dosages),[48,59–67] although there is some conflicting evidence.[68] It has been proposed that fish oil depresses vascular response to the hormones involved in hypertension.[38] Another suggestion is that fish oil acts by increasing vasodilatory prostaglandins PGI_1 and PGI_3, and that this increase accounts for observed reductions in blood pressure.[38]

To test this hypothesis, one study examined the effect of fish oil on blood pressure in men with mild, essential hypertension.[69] One group received 10 ml of fish oil (3 g of omega-3 fatty acids), a second group received 50 ml (9 g of EPA and 6 g of DHA), a third group received 50 ml of safflower oil (39 g of omega-6 fatty acids), and a fourth group received 50 ml of a mixture of coconut, olive, and safflower oils. The latter group represented the approximate amount and ratio of fatty acids consumed in the average American diet (39% saturated fat, 46% monounsaturated fat, and 15% polyunsaturated fat). The group receiving the highest dose of fish oil (50 ml) had an average reduction of 6.5 mmHg in systolic pressure and 4.4 mmHg in diastolic pressure. None of the other groups, including the low fish oil-supplemented group, demonstrated blood pressure reductions in the aggregate. The study did not find the expected association between increased production of PGI_1 and PGI_3 and sustained reduction in blood pressure. This suggests that vasodilatory prostaglandins are probably not the primary mediators of blood pressure reduction by fish oil consumption, although they may play a role.

Another proposed mechanism is that fish oils may facilitate excretion of sodium and fluid by the kidneys. This is supported by a reported but not published double-blind cross-over study in which researchers placed healthy, non-hypertensive men and women on a diet supplemented with approximately 1 g/day of PUFAs for 28 days.[70] Each participant received capsules with either fish oil or safflower oil. The fish oil dose was similar to the amount consumed in a single daily serving of tuna, lake trout, or salmon. After 2 weeks, the subjects crossed over to the other supplement. The study found an average 2–3 mmHg drop in both diastolic and systolic blood pressure in those who received fish oil supplements. The researchers also found that fish oil increased urine output by approximately 10%, performing much like a low-sodium diet. This resulted in a reduction in fluid volume. Unlike diuretics, the fish oil supplementation did not increase potassium excretion.

Angina pectoris

Significant rheological improvements in patients with

stable angina pectoris may occur following daily fish oil supplementation with 2.8 g of EPA and 1.8 g of DHA (15 capsules of MaxEPA).[71] In a double-blind, placebo-controlled study, fish oil supplementation resulted in increased red cell deformability, reduced whole blood viscosity, and prolonged bleeding time compared with olive oil supplementation. The frequency of angina attacks decreased in both groups. However, neither type of oil affected exercise capacity or hemodynamic response to exercise.

Myocardial infarction

Several studies of rodents have shown that dietary fats modulate the electrical stability of the myocardium. The appropriate fatty acids can reduce the vulnerability to arrhythmia during myocardial ischemia.[54,55,72] Raising the omega-3 fatty acids to higher levels in the myocardium may also prevent post-infarction ventricular fibrillation.[45,73,74]

One study evaluated the effect of dietary intervention in 2,033 men recovering from myocardial infarction.[75] Patients were randomly allocated to receive one of four types of dietary advice:

- lowered intake of dietary fat
- consumption of at least two portions of fatty fish (200–400 g) a day
- supplementation with three capsules (1.5 g) of MaxEPA a day
- increased dietary fiber intake.

At the end of 2 years, the group given fish were found to have increased their EPA intake to four times that of other subjects. This group also experienced significantly lower mortality. The fat advice and fiber advice produced no differences in mortality. Although the rate of recurrence of heart attack was similar in all groups, the fish and fish oil group had a 29% reduction in risk of death compared with the other groups. These findings are in direct conflict with an earlier study showing no such benefits.[76] However, it may be significant that the earlier study was conducted over the short period of 6 weeks.

Even in patients with no apparent clinical evidence of arterial disease, fish consumption has been shown to improve arterial wall function. One study found that, in both healthy and NIDDM patients, those who ate fish showed significantly better compliance of their left subclavian artery and femoral arteries.[77]

Immune function

Research in both animals and humans has not yet determined whether fish oil supplementation suppresses or enhances immune function. For example, recent laboratory animal experiments show that supplementation with GLA or fish oil results in marked changes in the structure and function of leukocyte membranes consistent with improved immune response.[78] In addition, animal studies have shown enhancement of the metabolic processes associated with resistance to infection and such diseases as cancer.[79] However, long-term supplementation with EPA results in pronounced inhibition of the oxidative processes necessary for the immune response.

In humans, an omega-3 enriched, low-fat, low-cholesterol diet suppresses immune function, possibly increasing susceptibility to infection. For example, increasing the typical American diet content of omega-3 fatty acid intake from 1 to 2.5% over a 6 week period results in decreased PGE_2 levels, helper cell activity, and other indices of immune function.[78] More research is needed to clarify the differences in animal and human responses to fish oils.

Pregnancy and lactation

During pregnancy, growth of new tissue raises the requirement for EFAs, as mobilization moves polyunsaturated fatty acids from maternal tissue stores to the fetus. A study of 19 normal pregnant women found an increased requirement for omega-3 EFA intake during pregnancy, lactation, and infancy.[80] The authors stated that because omega-3 EFA decreases in the maternal circulation during pregnancy and remains low for at least 6 weeks after pregnancy, "it may be reasonable to increase the omega-3 PUFA in the diet before, during, and after pregnancy". The authors further suggest that "dietary supplementation may be indicated", since maternal levels of eicosapentaenoic acid were 42% of normal value. The study concludes:

> It seems reasonable to suggest that 18:3 omega-3 intake be increased during pregnancy, lactation, and infancy, when requirements for omega-3 PUFA are highest, during the development of the nervous system, which is rich in lipids containing high proportions of omega-3 PUFA. The mental apparatus of the coming generation is developed in utero, and the time to begin supplementation is before conception. A normal brain cannot be made without an adequate supply of omega-3 PUFA, and there may be no later opportunity to repair the effects of an omega-3 fatty acid deficiency once the nervous system is formed.

Supplementation with either ALA or EPA would restore EFA levels in such individuals.

Nephrotic syndrome

Both hypertriglyceridemia and hypercholesterolemia are common in patients with nephrotic syndrome. This association results in an increased risk of coronary heart disease. Fish oils have been found to lower serum triglycerides in patients with nephrotic syndrome and may therefore be of clinical benefit.[40]

Autoimmune diseases

Fish oils may play a role in the treatment of autoimmune disease (e.g. lupus erythematosis, dermatomyositis, autoimmune nephritis, and multiple sclerosis)[81–83] and inflammatory disorders (e.g. rheumatoid arthritis,[84], psoriasis,[85] and atopic dermatitis[1]). At this time, no controlled studies have been completed using fish oil in the treatment of autoimmune diseases in humans. The evidence of fish oil's possible benefits is derived from animal studies using inbred mice strains.[38] Anecdotal reports by lupus patients suggest some benefit.

Rheumatoid arthritis

Rheumatoid arthritis is uncommon among Eskimos. There is mounting evidence that omega-3 fatty acids found in fish oil may beneficially influence the course of treatment in patients with rheumatoid arthritis due to their inhibition of inflammation upon incorporation into cell membanes.[86]

A population-based, case-controlled study in women found a decreased risk of rheumatoid arthritis in those who consumed the most fish.[84] A double-blind, placebo-controlled, study of rheumatoid arthritis patients given 1.8 g/day of fish oil showed less morning stiffness and tender joints. This particular study led to media coverage of the possible benefits of fish oil for this condition. However, analysis of the study showed that the possible benefits of the fish oil could have been due to the unusually rapid deterioration of the control group (placebo) rather than from any improvement by the fish oil group.[53]

Another double-blind, placebo-controlled, study of patients with rheumatoid arthritis found significant improvements in several clinical indices during the 12 weeks of fish oil supplementation.[87] Another study of patients with either rheumatoid arthritis or psoriasis also demonstrated improvement.[25] Patients taking 18 g of fish oil (containing 153 mg EPA and 103 mg DHA) for 6 weeks reported significant improvement in symptoms. Samples of peripheral blood mononuclear cells from these patients showed suppressed synthesis of two principal mediators of inflammation, interleukin-1, and tumor necrosis factor, as compared with patients receiving placebo. Of particular interest was the finding that the anti-inflammatory effect of the fish oils continued for up to 4 weeks after cessation of supplementation.

In another randomized double-blind placebo-controlled study conducted over a 24 week period, 49 patients with rheumatoid arthritis experienced significant clinical benefit, particularly in tender joints, from supplementation of either a low dose of 27 mg/kg EPA and 18 mg/kg DHA, or a high dose of 54 mg/kg EPA and 36 mg/kg DHA. Interleukin-1 levels decreased 54.7% in the high-dose group and 40.6% in the low-dose group.[66]

Psoriasis

Patients with psoriasis (vulgaris) have been successfully treated with a low-fat diet supplemented with fish oil.[88] An impressive 77% (23% did not respond) of the patients reported either excellent, moderate, or mild improvement. It was interesting to note that a number of patients did not show improvement until at least 4 months of supplementation. This may indicate the importance of allowing adequate time for clinical improvement after initiating fish oil therapy.

Fish oils presumably improve the condition by decreasing the levels of inflammatory leukotriene compounds, especially leukotriene B_4, a lipoxygenation product of arachidonic acid. The EPA in fish oil replaces the arachidonic acid in phospholipids, leading to the formation of leukotriene B_5 rather than B_4, resulting in a much weaker (at least 30 times less) inflammatory response.[89] This effect has been demonstrated in neutrophils isolated from the peripheral blood of patients given fish oil to treat their psoriasis.[88] Patients who showed evidence of clinical response to fish oil therapy for their psoriasis were shown to have higher levels of leukotriene B_5 than those failing to improve.

Cancer

Numerous animal studies have demonstrated anticancer activity by fish oil.[90] Experimental studies in rats have demonstrated that while corn oil-fed rats show an increased risk for colon cancer, fish oil-fed rats show both decreased risk and slowed progression of this cancer.[91] Fish oil appears to exert this anticancer effect by altering carcinogen metabolism and modifying prostaglandin synthesis.

In Japan, which enjoys the lowest breast cancer rate of the industrialized countries, fish consumption is highest. Conversely, in those countries where the risk of breast cancer is highest, the proportion of calories in the diet from fish is relatively low. A large epidemiological study of 23 dietary factors in countries with high and low risks of cancer found a strong association between the percentage of calories from fat and the risk of breast cancer.[92] Fish consumption was found to have the next most significant association, a negative correlation.

However, it remains premature to recommend fish oil as an anticancer substance until studies of its therapeutic efficacy are completed, especially in humans. Further, there is some conflicting evidence on the role of fish oil in oncogenic processes.[7]

Migraine headache

There are anecdotal reports that patients suffering from migraine headaches given 1 g/day of MaxEPA, particularly males, have significantly less frequent and/or less intense episodes. These results might be due to changes in prostaglandin synthesis and/or reduction in platelet serotonin release, with resultant reduction in cerebral vasospasm.

Malaria

Malaria afflicts more than 500 million people worldwide, with about 5% of victims dying each year. Unpublished studies at the US Department of Agricultural Research Service center in Beltsville, Maryland, have found evidence that the omega-3 fatty acids in fish oil may be beneficial in the treatment of malaria.[93] In their research, mice were fed dietary fish oils for 4 weeks and then inoculated with parasites, either *Plasmodium yoelii* or *Plasmodium berghei*. As the mice continued to eat the high-fish-oil diet, the parasites multiplied as usual. However, after 3–4 weeks, the mice were free of the parasites. The researchers suspected that the cause of the parasite's death was rupture of the parasites' cell membranes or red blood cell hosts. The researchers theorized that infected cells are more susceptible to rupture because the parasites foster a number of destructive oxidative reactions to which a diet high in fish oils makes them more vulnerable.

This finding is particularly promising since *P. berghei* is a chloroquine-resistant strain of malaria. Studies are underway by the World Health Organization to examine the benefits of treating malaria with dietary fish oil and qinghaosu, a Chinese botanical.

TOXICITY

A review of fish oil supplementation and CHD found that 10 MaxEPA capsules or 25 ml/day of cod liver oil (providing 1.8 g of EPA) is "safe over a long term".[94] Long-term studies of potentially adverse effects of fish oil supplementation in humans have not been published. However, this is also true of all other oils, such as vegetable oils and most currently prescribed hypolipidemic drugs.[38]

Care must also be taken to use fish oil, not fish liver oil, as the later can be excessively high in vitamins A and D, and cause toxicity.

Finally, large dosages of fish oil supplements may result in a significant increase in the total caloric intake.

Bleeding time

There have been concerns expressed about prolonged bleeding time in populations having a relatively high intake of fish. Several studies have shown that this effect appears to be dose-dependent, although collagen-induced platelet aggregation was not shown to be inhibited.[95] Many studies have shown that fish oil supplements prolong bleeding time, inhibit platelet aggregation, and decrease thromboxane A_2 production.[17,59,96–109]

Recent research suggests that, while the effect of fish oil supplementation on bleeding time is largely determined by the dosage, duration, and composition of the supplement, the typical treatment regimes are safe. In one double-blind placebo-controlled trial, daily supplementation with 30 ml of a Scandinavian fish oil formulation (ESKIMO-3: 35% n-3 fatty acids, 18% EPA, and 12% DHA) given for both short (4 weeks) and long (6 months) durations resulted in no changes in bleeding time.[20] Another controlled study used 1.5, 3, or 6 g of fish oils (SuperEPA) as a supplement for 3 months and found no effect on bleeding time in 45 healthy male volunteers with normal triglycerides.[110]

Caution should be taken when recommending fish oil supplementation to pregnant women (studies to date on bleeding time have all been carried out on males), individuals known or suspected of any bleeding disorder, or those prescribed therapeutic levels of aspirin or warfarin, who should consult with their physician.

There is conflicting evidence as to the degree to which fish oil may affect fibrinolysis. Plasma PAI-1 is an inhibitor of fibrinolysis. Increased PAI-1 activity has been linked to the development of myocardial infarction and thrombosis by several investigators. In at least one double-blind, randomized study conducted on an untreated essential hypertensive population, a modest increase in fibrinogen levels was observed after fish oil and corn oil intake was increased by 4 g of omega-3 PUFAs.[111] However, no change in PAI-1 activity or tissue plasminogen activator (tPA) activity was found.

Toxin contamination

While increased bleeding may not be a problem, there may be other risks from increased consumption of fish.[112] For example, some fish may be contaminated from industrial effluents and toxins. Many of these toxicants, such as PCB, are known to increase the risk of cancer. In animal experiments it has been demonstrated that eating such contaminated fish as infrequently as once a week may increase the risk of developing cancer and create a significant risk to pregnant women and infants.[113,114] With the growth of aqua-businesses, or fish farms, it remains unknown whether such exposure is being reduced. Some new fish varieties grow so quickly that the opportunity for toxic build-up in organs and fat is significantly decreased. However, as noted earlier, the EPA and DHA concentration and fatty acid balance of these fish oils may be adversely affected by the commercial feed they receive.

Oxidation

There is a possibility that a diet rich in fish oil taken for many months may induce a deficiency of vitamin E, which could contribute to cardiac necrosis.[115,116] For this reason, concurrent vitamin E supplementation appears warranted. However, there is no evidence that the incidence of cardiac necrosis is higher in Eskimos.

The omega-3 fatty acids found in fish oil are susceptible to oxidative breakdown. For this reason they must be protected from oxidation by proper extraction and storage, encapsulation or stabilization with an antioxidant, such as vitamin E. Inappropriately stored fish oils (i.e. exposure to oxygen) may result in the formation of toxic lipid peroxides.

DOSAGE

The dosages reported to be most effective range between 5 and 15 g/day of fish oil. Clinical results may require 4–6 months to manifest.

CONCLUSION

A substantial body of evidence now documents the beneficial effects of fish and fish oil consumption. The omega-3 fatty acids eicosapentaenoic acid and docosahexaenoic acid are the components of fish oil responsible for its preventive and therapeutic effects. These include:

- lowering of blood pressure
- improved plasma lipid profiles
- antithrombotic activity
- decreased risk of ventricular arrhythmias and atherosclerosis.

However, determining which source of fish oil, i.e. eating fish or supplementing with fish oil, and which fish species are most desirable is difficult, as the various species and sources have different levels and ratios of eicosanoid metabolites.

In an effort to resolve this question, one study compared the effects of fish oil (4.5 g EPA/DHA) from fish with fish oil supplements in 25 mildly hyperlipidemic men over a 5 week period. Both fish and fish oil supplements lowered serum triglycerides and raised HDL cholesterol. There was no difference between the two treatments in their effects on total cholesterol, apolipoprotein B, LDL cholesterol, or blood pressure. However, dietary fish did lower fibrinogen (15.6%) and thromboxane (10.5%) and increase bleeding time (10.8%), as compared with both controls and those receiving fish oil supplements.[117] These findings suggest that while both fish consumption and fish oil supplementation produce desirable effects on lipids and lipoproteins, fish consumption is more effective in improving several of the hemostatic factors involved in cardiovascular disease.

Which fish or fish oil products produce the most desirable combination of therapeutic effects remains unknown. Further research is needed. In the interim, it seems evident that humans could benefit from a diet containing fresh or fresh/frozen fish consumed at least three or four times a week, with additional fish oil supplementation when warranted. To ensure that fish is safe for consumption, either continued vigilance by regulatory agencies or effectively enforced industry standards are required to prevent contaminated fish containing toxicants from reaching the market place. Fish oil supplement manufacturers must provide sufficient information about the source of the fish oil. Information on the fish oil's source, EPA and DHA concentration and ratio, toxic residual levels (if any), and risk of oxidative activity should be provided.

REFERENCES

1. Kromann N, Green A. Epidemiological studies in the Upernavik district, Greenland. Acta Med Scand 1980; 208: 401–406
2. Yamori Y, Nara Y, Iritarri N et al. Comparison of serum phospholipids fatty acids among fishing and farming Japanese populations and American inlanders. J Nutr Sci Vitaminol 1985; 31: 417–422
3. Bulliyya G, Reddy KK, Reddy GPR et al. Lipid profiles among fish-consuming coastal and non-fish-consuming inland populations. Eur J Clin Nutr 1990; 44: 481–485
4. Kang, JX, Leaf, A. Antiarrhythmic effects of polyunsaturated fatty acids. Circulation 1996; 94: 1774–1780
5. Connor, WE. Do the n-3 fatty acids from fish prevent deaths from cardiovascular disease? Am J Clin Nutr 1997; 66: 188–189
6. Kinella JE, Lokesh B, Stone RA. Dietary n-3 polyunsaturated fatty acids and amelioration of cardiovascular disease: possible mechanisms. Am J Clin Nutr 1990; 52: 1–28
7. Erasmus U. Fats and Oils. Vancouver, BC: Alive. 1986: p 248–249
8. van Vliet T, Ketan MB. Lower ratio of n-3 to n-6 fatty acids in cultured than in wild fish. Am J Clin Nutr 1990; 51: 1–2
9. Bjerve KS, Thoresen L, Bursting S. Linseed and cod liver oil induce rapid growth in a 7-year old girl with omega-3 fatty acid deficiency. J Parenter Enteral Nutr 1988; 12: 521–525
11. Barradas MA. The effect of olive oil supplementation on human platelet function, serum cholesterol-related variables and plasma fibrinogen concentrations. Nutr Res 1990; 10: 403–411
12. Tichelaar HY. Eicosapentaenoic acid composition of different fish oil concentrates. Lancet 1990; ii: 1450
13. Budiarso IT. Fish oil versus olive oil. Lancet 1990; ii: 1313–1314
14. Allard JP, Kurian R, Aghdassi E et al. Lipid peroxidation during n-3 fatty acid and vitamin E supplementation in humans. Lipids 1997; 32: 535–541
15. Needleman P, Raz A, Minkes MS et al. Triene prostaglandin, prostacyclin and thromboxane synthesis and unique properties. Proc Natl Acad Sci (USA) 1979; 76: 944–949
16. Dyerberg J. Linolenate-derived polyunsaturated fatty acids and prevention of atherosclerosis. Nutr Rev 1986; 44: 125–134
17. Thorngren M, Gustafson A. Effects of 11–week increase in dietary eicosapentaenoic acid on bleeding time, lipid, and platelet aggregation. Lancet 1981; ii: 1190–1194
18. Sinclair HM. The importance of fish in the prevention of chronic degenerative diseases. Nahr Meer (International Symposium) 1980: p 201–210
19. Sinclair HM. Advantages and disadvantages of an Eskimo diet. In: Fumagalli R, Kritchevsky D, Paoletti R, eds. Drugs affecting lipid metabolism. Amsterdam: Elsevier. 1980: p 363–370

20. Haglund O. Effects of a new fluid fish oil concentrate, ESKIMO-3, on triglycerides, cholesterol, fibrinogen and blood pressure. J Int Med 1990; 227: 347–353
21. Conner WE. The impact of dietary omega-3 fatty acids on the synthesis and clearance of apo b lipoporteins and chylomicrons. Proceedings of Scientific Conference on Omega-3 Fatty Acids in Nutrition, Vascular Biology, and Medicine, Houston, TX, April 19 1994: p 19–32
22. Hwang, DH, Chanmugam, PS, Ryan, DH et al. Does vegetable oil attenuate the beneficial effects of fish oil in reducing risk factors for carviovascualr disease? Am J Clin Nutr 1997; 66: 89–96
23. Kestin, M, Clifton P, Belling GB, Nestel PJ. n-3 fatty acids of marine origin lower systolic blood pressure and triglycerides but raise LDL cholesterol compared with n-3 and n-6 fatty acids from plants. Am J Clin Nutr 1990; 51: 1028–1034
24. Weisburger, JH. Dietary fat and risk of chronic disease: mechanistic insights from experimental studies. J Am Diet Assoc 1997; 97(Suppl): S16–S23
25. Siscovick DS, Raghunathan TE, King I et al. Dietary intake and cell membrane levels of long-chain n-3 polyunsaturated fatty acids and the risk of primary cardiac arrest. JAMA 1995; 274: 1363–1367
26. Goh, YK, Jumpsen, JA, Ryan, EA et al. Effect of omega-3 fatty acid on plasma lipids, cholesterol and lipoprotein fatty acid content in NIDDM patients. Diabetologia 1997; 40: 45–52
27. Veigm GE, Brennan, GM, Cohn et al. Fish oil improves arterial compliance in non-insulin-dependent diabetes mellitus. Arterioscler Thromb 1994; 14: 1425–1429
28. Eritsland, J, Arnesen, H., Gronseth, K et al. Effect of dietary supplementation with n-3 fatty acids on coronary artery bypass graft patency. Am J Cardiol 1996; 77: 31–36
29. Stone NJ. Fish consumption, fish oil, lipids, and coronary heart disease. 1997; 65: 1083–1086
30. Harris, WS. Dietary fish oil and blood lipids. Curr Opin Lipidol 1996; 7: 3–7
31. Phillipson BE, Rothroch DW, Conner WE et al. Reduction of plasma lipids, lipoproteins and apoproteins by dietary fish oil in patients with hypertriglyceridemia. New Engl J Med 1985; 312: 1210–1216
32. Nestel PJ, Connor WE, Reardon MF et al. Suppression by diets rich in fish oil of very low density lipoprotein production in man. J Clin Invest 1984; 74: 75–89
33. Simons LA, Hickie JB, Balasubramaniam S. On the effects of dietary n-3 fatty acids (MaxEPA) on plasma lipids and lipoproteins in patients with hyperlipidemia. Atherosclerosis 1985; 54: 75–88
34. Dart AM, Riemersma RA, Oliver MF. Effects of MaxEPA on serum lipids in hypercholesterolemic subjects. Atherosclerosis, 1989; 80: 119–124
35. Riemersma RA, Sargent CA, Abraham RA et al. Fish and the heart. Lancet 1989; ii: 1450
36. Demke DM, Peters GR, Linet OI et al. Effects of a fish oil concentrate in patients with hypercholesterolemia. Atherosclerosis 1988; 70: 70–73
37. Bilo HJG, Gans ROB, Donker AJM. Fish oil for preventing coronary restenosis. Lancet 1989; ii: 693
38. Yetiv JZ. Clinical applications of fish oils. JAMA 1988; 260: 665–670
39. Saynor R, Gillott T. Fish oil. [Letter to editor] Lancet 1989; ii: 810–812
40. Bakker D, Haberstroh B, Philbrick D et al. Triglyceride lowering in nephrotic syndrome patients consuming a fish oil concentrate. Nutr Res 1989; 9: 27–34
41. Pekkanen J, Linn S, Heiss G et al. Ten-year mortality from cardiovascular disease in relation to cholesterol level among men with and without preexisting cardiovascular disease. New Engl J Med 1990; 322: 1700–1707
42. McLennan, PL, Bridle, TM, Abeywardena, MY et al. Dietary lipid modulation of ventricular fibrillation threshold in the marmoset monkey. Am Heart J 1992; 123: 1555–1561
43. McLennan, PL. Relative effects of dietary saturated, monounsaturated, and polyunsaturated fatty acids on cardiac arrhythmias in rats. Am J Clin Nutr 1993; 57: 207–212
44. Kang, JX, Leaf, A. Effects of long-chain polyunsaturated fatty acids on the contraction of neonatal rat cardiac myocytes. Proc Natl Acad Sci 1994; 91: 9886–9890
45. de Lorgeril, M, Renaud, S, Mamelle, N et al. Mediterranean alpha-linolenic acid-rich diet in secondary prevention of coronary heart disease. Lancet 1994; 343: 1454–1459
46. Kang, JX, Leaf, A. Prevention and termination of the beta-adrenergic agonist-induced arrhythmias by free polyunsaturated fatty acids in neonatal rat cardiac myocytes. Biochem Biophys Res Commun 1995; 208: 629–636
47. Simopoulos, AP. Omega-3 fatty acids in the prevention-management of cardiovascular disease. Can J Physiol Pharmacol 1997; 75: 234–239
48. Mori, TA, Beilin, LJ, Burke, V et al. Interactions between dietary fat, fish, and fish oils and their effects on platelet function in men at risk of cardiovascular disease. Arterioscler Throm Vasc Biol 1997; 17: 279–286
49. Kromhout D, Bosschieter EB, Coulander CL. The inverse relation between fish consumption and 20-year mortality from heart disease. New Engl J Med 1985; 312: 1205–1209
50. Vollset SE, Heuch I, Bjelke E. Fish consumption and mortality from coronary heart disease. New Engl J Med 1985; 313: 820–821
51. Curb JD, Reed DM. Fish consumption and mortality from coronary heart disease. New Engl J Med 1985; 313: 821
52. Arthaud JB. Cause of death in 339 Alaskan natives as determined by autopsy. Arch Pathol Lab Med 1970; 90: 433–438
53. Kremer JM, Bigauoetter JM Michalek AV et al. Effects of manipulation of dietary fatty acids on clinical manifestations of rheumatoid arthritis. Lancet 1985; i: 184–187
54. McLennan PJ, Abeywarden MY, Charnock JS. Dietary fish oil prevents coronary artery occlusion and reperfusion. Am Heart J 1988; 116: 709–717
55. Riemersma RA, Sargent CA. Dietary fish oil and ischaemic arrhythmias. J Intern Med 1989; 225(suppl 1): 111–116
56. Weiner BH, Ockene IS, Levine PH et al. Inhibition of atherosclerosis by cod-liver oil in a hyperlipidemic swine model. New Engl J Med 1986; 315: 841–846
57. Davis HR, Bridenstine RT, Vesselinovitch D et al. Fish oil inhibits development of atherosclerosis in rhesus monkeys. Atherosclerosis 1987; 7: 441–449
58. Morris, MC, Sacks, F, Rosner, B. Does fish oil lower blood pressure? A meta-analysis of controlled trials. Circulation 1993; 88: 523–533
59. Lorenz R, Spengler U, Fisher S et al. Platelet function, thromboxane formation and blood pressure control during supplementation of the Western diet with cod liver oil. Circulation 1983; 67: 504–511
60. Singer P, Wirth M, Volgt S et al. Clinical studies on lipid and blood pressure lowering effect of eicosapentaenoic acid-rich diet. Biomed Biochim Acta 1984; 43: S421–425
61. Rylance PB, Gordge MP, Saynor R et al. Fish oil modifies lipids and reduces platelet aggregability in hemodialysis patients. Nephron 1986; 43: 196–202
62. Lorenz R, Spengler U, Seiss W, Weber PC. Membrane fatty acids, platelet aggregation and thromboxane formation on dietary cod liver oil supplementation. In: Prostaglandins, Vth International Conference. Florence: Fondazione Giovanni Lorenzini. 1982: p 695–699
63. Singer R, Jaeger W, Wirth M, Voigt S. Lipid and blood pressure lowering effect of mackerel diet on man. Atherosclerosis 1983; 49: 99–108
64. Houwelingen ACV, Hornstra G. Effect of a moderate fish intake on blood pressure, platelet function and safety aspects. Agents Actions 1987; 22: 3–4
65. Krestin M, Clifton P, Belling GB, Nestel PJ. n-3 fatty acids of marine origin lower systolic blood pressure and triglycerides but raise LDL cholesterol compared with n-3 and n-6 fatty acids from plants. Am J Clin Nutr 1990; 51: 1028–1034
66. Kremer JM, Lawrence DA, Jubiz W et al. Dietary fish oil and olive oil supplementation in patients with rheumatoid arthritis. Arth Rheum 1990; 33: 810–820
67. Margolin G, Huster G, Glueck C et al. Blood pressure lowering

in elderly subjects: a double-blind crossover study of ω-3 and ω-6 fatty acids. Am J Clin Nutr 1991; 53: 562–572
68. Yetiv JZ. Clinical applications of fish oils. JAMA 1988; 260: 665–670
69. Knapp H, Fitzergerald G. The antihypertensive effects of fish oils. A controlled study of polyunsaturated fatty acid supplements in essential hypertension. New Engl J Med 1989; 320: 1037–1043
70. Raloff J. Fish oil lowers even normal blood pressure. Science News 1989; 135: 181
71. Solomon SA. A placebo-controlled, double-blind study of eicosapentaenoic acid-rich fish oil in patients with stable angina pectoris. Curr Med Res Opinion 1990; 12: 1–10
72. Lepran I, Nemecz G, Koltai M, Szekeres L. Effect of a linoleic acid-rich diet on the acute phase of coronary artery occlusion in conscious rats. influence of indomethacin and aspirin. J Cardiovascul Pharmacol 1981; 3: 747–753
73. Myerburg RJ. Epidemiology of ventricular tachycardia/ventricular fibrillation and sudden cardiac death. Pacing Clin Electrophysiol 1986; 9: 1334–1338
74. Buxton AE. Sudden cardiac death. Ann Intern Med 1986; 104: 716–718
75. Burr ML, Fehily AM, Gilbert JF et al. Effects of changes in fat, fish, and fibre intakes on death and myocardial reinfarction. Diet and reinfarction trial (DART). Lancet 1989; ii: 757–761
76. Hardarson T, Kristinsson A, Skuladottir G et al. Cod liver oil does not reduce ventricular extrasystoles after myocardial infarction. J Int Med 1989; 226: 33–37
77. Wahlvist ML, Lo CS, Myers KA. Fish intake and arterial wall characteristics in healthy people and diabetic patients. Lancet 1989; ii: 944–946
78. Fletcher M, Ziboh V. Effects of dietary supplementation with eicosapentaenoic acid or gamma-linolenic acid on neutrophil phospholipid fatty acid composition and activation responses. Inflammation 1990; 14: 585–597
79. Meydani S, Lichtenstein A, Cornwall S et al. Effects of low-fat, low-cholesterol diet enriched in N-3 fatty acids on the immune response of humans. FASEBJ 1991; 5: 1449A
80. Holman RT, Johnson SB, Ogburn PL. Deficiency of essential fatty acids and membrane fluidity during pregnancy and lactation. Proc Natl Acad Sci 1991; 88: 4835–4839
81. Rudin D. The dominant disease of modernized societies as omega-3 essential fatty acid deficiency syndrome. substrate beriberi. Med Hypothesis 1982; 8: 17–47
82. Vorhees JJ. Leukotrienes and other lypoxygenase products in the pathogenesis and therapy of psoriasis and other dermatoses. Arch Dermatol 1983; 119: 541–547
83. Rickett JD, Robinson DR, Steinberg AD. Effects of dietary enrichment with eicosapentaenoic acid upon autoimmune nephritis in female NZBXNZW/F1 mice. Arthritis Rheumatism 1983; 26: 133–139
84. Shapiro, JA, Koepsel, TD, Voigt, LF et al. Diet and rheumatoid arthritis in women. A possible protective effect of fish consumption. Epidemiol 1996; 7: 256–263
85. Isseroff RR. Fish again for dinner! The role of fish and other dietary oils in the therapy of skin disease. J Am Acad Dermatol 1988; 19: 1073–1080
86. Sperling RI. Dietary omega-3 fatty acids. Effects on lipid mediators of inflammation and rheumatoid arthritis. Rheum Dis Clin North Am 1991; 17: 373–389
87. van der Temple H, Tulleken JE, Limburg PC et al. Effects of fish oil supplementation in rheumatoid arthritis. Ann Rheum Dis 1990; 49: 76–80
88. Kragballe K, Fogh K. A low-fat diet supplemented with dietary fish oil (Max-EPA) results in improvement of psoriasis and in formation of leukotriene B5. Acta Derm Venereol 1989; 69: 23–28
89. Shils ME, Young VR. Modern nutrition in health and disease. 7th edn. Philadelphia, PA: Lea & Febiger. 1988: p 1473–1474
90. Karmali RA. Fatty acids. inhibition. Am J Clin Nutr 1987; 45: 225–229
91. Reddy B, Burill C, Rigotty J. Effects of diets high in omega-3 and omega-6 fatty acids on initiation and postinitiation stages of colon carcinogenesis. Cancer Res 1991; 51: 487–491
92. Kaizer L, Boyd N, Kriukov V et al. Fish consumption and breast cancer; an ecological study. Nutr Cancer 1989; 12: 61–68
93. Anonymous. Fish oil. New hope in fighting malaria. Science News 1989; 134: 237
94. Neutze JM, Starling MB. Fish oils and coronary heart disease. New Zealand Med J 1986; 99: 583–585
95. Ahmed AA, Holub BJ. Alteration and recovery of bleeding times, platelet aggregation and fatty acid composition of individual phospholipids in platelets of human subjects receiving a supplement of cod-liver oil. Lipids 1984; 19: 617–624
96. Goodnight SH, Harris WS, Connor WE. The effects of dietary ω3 fatty acids on platelet composition and function in man: a prospective, controlled trial. Blood 1981; 58: 880–885
97. Sanders TAB, Roshanai F. The influence of different types of omega-3 polyunsaturated fatty acids on blood lipids and platelet function in healthy volunteers. Clin Sci 1983; 64: 91–99
98. Ahmed AA, Holub BJ. Alteration and recovery of bleeding times, platelet aggregation and fatty acid composition of individual phospholipids in platelets of human subjects receiving a supplement of cod-liver oil. Lipids 1984; 19: 617–624
99. Knapp HR, Reilly I, Alessandrini P et al. In vivo indexes of platelet and vascular function during fish oil administration in patients with atherosclerosis. New Engl J Med 1986; 314: 937–942
100. Siess W, Roth P, Scherer B et al. Platelet-membrane fatty acids, platelet aggregation, and thrombosane formation during a mackerel diet. Lancet 1980; i: 441–444
101. Brox JH, Killie JE, Funnes S et al. The effect of cod-liver oil and corn oil on platelets and vessel wall in man. Thromb Haemost 1981; 46: 604–611
102. Hirai A, Terano T, Hamazaki T et al. The effects of the oral administration of fish oil concentrate on the release and the metabolism of 14C-arachidonic acid and 14C-eicosapentaenoic acid by human platelet. Thromb Res 1982; 28: 285–298
103. Bradlow BA, Chetty N, van der Westhuyzen J et al. The effects of a mixed fish diet on platelet function, fatty acids and serum lipids. Thromb Res 1983; 29: 561–568
104. Schimke E, Hildebrandt R, Beitz J et al. Influence of a cod liver oil diet in diabetics type I on fatty acid patterns and platelet aggregation. Biomed Biochim Acta 1984; 43: S351–353
105. Lands WEM, Culp BR, Hirai A et al. Relationship of thromboxane generation to the aggregation of platelets from humans: effects of eicosapentaenoic acid. Prostaglandins 1985; 30: 819–825
106. Von Schacky C, Fischer S, Weber PC. Long-term effects of dietary marine ω3 acids upon plasma and cellular lipids, platelet function, and eicosanoid formation in humans. J Clin Invest 1985; 76: 1626–1631
107. Srivastava KC. Docosahexaenoic acid (C22: 6ω3) and linoleic acid are anti-aggregatory and alter arachidonic acid metabolism in human platelets. Prostaglandins Leukotrienes Med 1985; 17: 319–327
108. Sanders TAB, Hochland MCA. Comparison of the influence on plasma lipids and platelet function of supplements of ω3 and ω6 polyunsaturated fatty acids. Br J Nutr 1983; 50: 521–529
109. Croft KD, Beilin LJ, Vandongen R. The effect of dietary fish oil on platelet metabolism of 14C-arachidonic acid. Thromb Res 1986; 42: 99–194
110. Blonk MC, Bilo HJG, Nauta JJP et al. Dose-response effects of fish-oil supplementation in healthy volunteers. Am J Clin Nutr 1990; 52: 120–127
111. Toft, I, Bonna, KH, Ingebretsen, OC et al. Fibrinolytic function after dietary supplementation with omega-3 polyunsaturated fatty acids. Arterioscler Throm Vasc Biol 1997; 17: 814–819
112. Foran JA, Glenn BS, Silverman W. Increased fish consumption may be risky. JAMA 1989; 262: 28
113. Foran JA, Cox M, Croxton D. Sport fish consumption advisories and projected cancer risks in the Great Lakes basin. Clinical Pediatrics 1989; 28: 322–325
114. Foran JA, VanderPloeg D. Consumption advisories for sport fish in the Great Lakes basin. Am J Public Health 1989; 79: 1435

115. Ruiter A, Jongbloed AW, van Gent CM et al. The influence of dietary mackerel oil on the condition of organs and on the blood lipid composition in the young growing pig. Am J Clin Nutr 1978; 31: 2159–2166
116. Gudbjarnason J, Hallgrimmson J. The role of myocardial membrane lipids in the development of cardiac necrosis. Acta Med Scand Suppl. 1976; 587: 17–27
117. Cobias L, Clifton PS, Abbey M et al. Lipid, lipoprotein, and hemostatic effects of fish vs fishoil ω-3 fatty acids in mildly hyperlipidemic males. Am J Clin Nutr 1991; 53: 1210–1216

CHAPTER CONTENTS

87

Flavonoids – quercetin, citrus flavonoids, and HERs (hydroxyethylrutosides)

Michael T. Murray, ND

Joseph E. Pizzorno Jr, ND

INTRODUCTION

The flavonoids are a group of plant pigments that are largely responsible for the colors of many fruits and flowers. Recent research suggests that flavonoids may be useful in the treatment and prevention of many health conditions. In fact, many of the medicinal actions of foods, juices, herbs, and bee pollen are now known to be directly related to their flavonoid content. Over 4,000 flavonoid compounds have been characterized and classified according to chemical structure. A few representatives of this class of useful clinical agents (quercetin, citrus bioflavonoids, and hydroxyethylrutosides) are discussed in this chapter.

One of the most beneficial group of plant flavonoids are the proanthocyanidins (also referred to as procyanidins). The most potent proanthocyanidins are those bound to other proanthocyanidins. Collectively, mixtures of proanthocyanidin dimers, trimers, tetramers, and larger molecules are referred to as procyanidolic oligomers or PCOs for short. The PCOs are discussed in Ch. 106.

HISTORICAL PERSPECTIVE

Flavonoids, as well as vitamin C, were discovered by Albert Szent-Gyorgyi (1893–1986), one of the most respected and honored biochemists of the 20th century. Szent-Gyorgyi received the Nobel Prize in 1937 for his discovery of some of the properties of these molecules.

It was during the process of isolating vitamin C that Szent-Gyorgyi discovered the flavonoids. A friend with bleeding gums had stopped the bleeding by taking a crude vitamin C preparation isolated from lemon. When the problem reappeared later on, Szent-Gyorgyi gave his friend a purer form of vitamin C. He expected to observe an even more impressive result, but the purer form of vitamin C did not work. Szent-Gyorgyi then isolated the flavonoid fraction from the original crude vitamin C preparation, gave it to his friend and observed complete healing.

Szent-Gyorgyi termed his discovery "vitamin P" due to its ability reduce vascular permeability, one of the hallmark features of scurvy. He went on to show that the clinical symptoms of scurvy are the result of a combined deficiency of vitamin C and flavonoids. However, because flavonoids could not fulfill all the requirements of a vitamin, the designation as vitamin P was abandoned. Although flavonoids are often referred to as "semi-essential" nutrients, their importance in human nutrition appears to be as important to good health as the essential vitamins and minerals.

Good dietary sources of flavonoids include citrus fruits, berries, onions, parsley, legumes, green tea, and red wine. The average daily intake in the United States for flavonoids is estimated to be between 150 and 200 mg.

CHEMICAL DESCRIPTIONS

Quercetin (Fig. 87.1)

Quercetin is a flavonoid that serves as the aglycone for many other flavonoids, including the citrus flavonoids rutin, quercitrin, and hesperidin. These derivatives differ from quercetin in that they have sugar molecules attached to the quercetin backbone. Quercetin is consistently the most active of the flavonoids in experimental studies and many medicinal plants owe much of their activity to their high quercetin content.

Citrus bioflavonoids

Citrus bioflavonoid preparations can include rutin, hesperidin, quercitrin, and naringin. Most of the clinical research on rutin and crude bioflavonoid complexes occurred before 1970. Since then, most of the clinical research has utilized a standardized mixture of rutinosides known as hydroxyethylrutosides (HERs). Impressive clinical results have been obtained in the treatment of capillary permeability, excessive bruisability, hemorrhoids, and varicose veins with HERs (discussed below). Citrus bioflavonoids can be viewed as providing similar effects to, but probably not as potent as, HERs or quercetin.

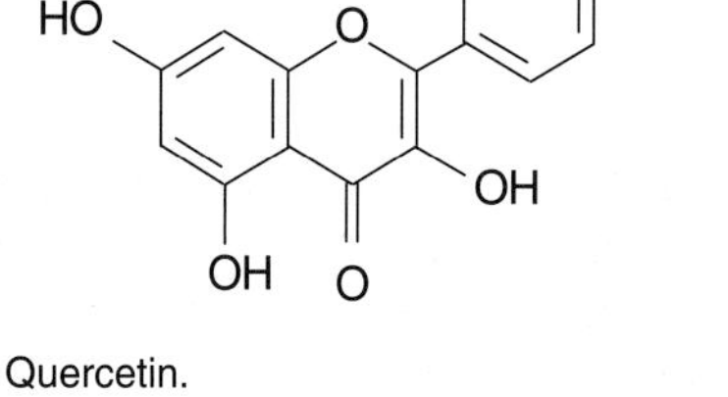

Figure 87.1 Quercetin.

PHARMACOLOGY

As a class of compounds, flavonoids have been referred to as "nature's biological response modifiers" because of their ability to modify the body's reaction to other compounds such as allergens, viruses, and carcinogens, as evidenced by their anti-inflammatory, anti-allergic, antiviral, and anticarcinogenic properties. In addition, flavonoids act as powerful antioxidants, providing remarkable protection against oxidative and free radical damage. The practical aspect of this antioxidant activity is highlighted by the results of a study in 805 men designed to determine the effect of dietary flavonoids on protecting against heart disease. The study demonstrated an inverse correlation between flavonoid intake and death from a heart attack.[1] This effect is probably a result of the potent antioxidant effects of the flavonoids preventing, similar to vitamins C and E, the formation of oxidized cholesterol. However, the antioxidant activity of flavonoids is generally more potent and effective against a broader range of oxidants than traditional antioxidant nutrients like vitamins C and E, selenium, and zinc.[2,3]

Because different flavonoids tend to provide different benefits, additional and more specific beneficial effects are discussed under the three selected categories. There is significant overlap among these flavonoids, however.

Quercetin

Quercetin consistently demonstrates the greatest activity among the flavonoids studied in experimental models, particularly in vitro studies. The primary actions that will be briefly reviewed here are its anti-inflammatory effects, inhibition of aldose reductase, antiviral activity, and anti-cancer properties.

Anti-inflammatory effects

Quercetin has demonstrated significant anti-inflammatory activity due to direct inhibition of several of the initial processes of inflammation via interaction with calcium channels and/or calmodulin (the intracellular calcium-binding protein) as well as through other mechanisms such as by inhibiting mast cell and basophil degranulation, neutrophil and monocyte lysosomal secretion, prostaglandin (most notably, leukotriene) formation, lipid peroxidation, and the resultant cascade of effects that are often a result of these processes. For example, it inhibits both the manufacture and release of histamine and other allergic/inflammatory mediators. In addition it exerts potent antioxidant activity and vitamin C-sparing action.[2–10]

Effect on histamine release

The release of histamine and other inflammatory mediators from mast cells and basophils is involved in the pathogenesis of acute allergic and inflammatory responses. Mast cells are widely distributed throughout the human body, but are found in higher concentrations in the blood vessels of the subepithelial connective tissue of the respiratory tract, conjunctiva, gastrointestinal tract, and skin. Mast cell and basophil degranulation is an active process that requires calcium influx. Quercetin and many other flavonoids have been shown to be potent inhibitors of mast cell, neutrophil and basophil degranulation.[6–9] A generally accepted hypothesis for this action is that quercetin inhibits receptor-mediated calcium influx, thereby inhibiting the primary signal for degranulation. However, quercetin is also active under conditions in which the calcium channel mechanism is not operative, indicating that other mechanisms are responsible as well.

Membrane stabilization, antioxidant activity, and hyaluronidase inhibition

Quercetin has been shown to inhibit many of the inflammatory processes attributed to activated neutrophils.[9] This is probably due to its membrane stabilizing action, potent antioxidant effect (which prevents the production of free radicals and inflammatory leukotrienes), and inhibition of the enzyme hyaluronidase (thus preventing the breakdown of the collagen matrix of connective tissue and ground substance). Quercetin's membrane stabilizing effect could also account for its action in preventing mast cell and basophil degranulation. This effect also inhibits inflammation by decreasing neutrophil lysosomal enzyme secretion.[9] Neutrophils and monocytes contain lysosomes that, upon secretion of their contents, contribute greatly to the inflammatory process.

Effects on eicosanoid metabolism

Excessive leukotriene formation has been linked to asthma, psoriasis, atopic dermatitis, gout, ulcerative colitis, and possibly cancer.[11,12] Quercetin has been shown to inhibit many steps in eicosanoid metabolism. Probably of most significance is its inhibition of phospholipase A2 and lipoxygenase enzymes (see Ch. 132 for diagram).[2,3,10] The net result is a significant reduction in the formation of leukotrienes. The leukotrienes C4, D4, and E4 (composing the slow-reacting substances of anaphylaxis (SRS-A)) are derived from arachidonic acid and are 1,000 times as potent as histamine in promoting inflammation. Leukotrienes promote inflammation by causing vasoconstriction (thereby increasing vascular permeability) and bronchoconstriction (thus inducing asthma), and by promoting WBC chemotaxis and aggregation. The reduction of leukotriene formation has significant anti-inflammatory effects.

Inhibition of aldose reductase

Quercetin is a strong inhibitor of aldose reductase, the enzyme responsible for the conversion of blood glucose to sorbitol This compound is strongly implicated in the development of diabetic complications, i.e. diabetic cataracts, neuropathy, and retinopathy.[13] The mechanism by which sorbitol is involved in the development of diabetic complications is best understood by considering its involvement in cataract formation. Although the lens does not have any blood vessels, it is an actively metabolizing tissue that continuously grows throughout life. Elevated blood sugar levels result in shunting of glucose to the sorbitol pathway. Since the lens membranes are virtually impermeable to sorbitol and lack the enzyme required to break down sorbitol (polyol dehydrogenase), sorbitol accumulates to high concentrations. These high concentrations persist even if glucose levels return to normal. This accumulation creates an osmotic gradient that results in water being drawn into the cells to maintain osmotic balance. As the water is pulled in, the cell must release small molecules like amino acids, inositol, glutathione, niacin, vitamin C, magnesium and potassium in order to maintain osmotic balance. Since these latter compounds function to protect the lens from damage, their loss results in an increased susceptibility to damage. As a result, the delicate protein fibers within the lens become opaque and a cataract forms.

Quercetrin, which is hydrolyzed by gut bacteria to yield quercetin and a sugar moiety, was shown to significantly decrease the accumulation of sorbitol in the lens of diabetic animals, effectively delaying the onset of cataracts.[14] In addition to its effect on aldose reductase, quercetin is also of value in diabetes for its ability to enhance insulin secretion and protect the pancreatic beta-cells from the damaging effects of free radicals, and for its inhibition of platelet aggregation.[2,3]

Antiviral activity

Flavonoids as a group possess significant antiviral activity, with quercetin having the greatest antiviral activity against herpes virus type I, para-influenzae 3, polio virus type I, and respiratory syncytial virus.[15–17] Quercetin has been shown, in vitro, to inhibit both viral replication and infectivity. In vivo studies in animals have also shown quercetin to inhibit viral infection.[17,18] This would suggest that quercetin may be of some benefit in viral infections, including the common cold.

Anti-cancer properties

Many flavonoids have also been shown to inhibit tumor formation, but again quercetin has consistently been shown to be the most effective. In experimental models, quercetin has demonstrated significant antitumor activity against a wide range of cancers, including squamous cell carcinoma, leukemia, and cancers of the breast, ovaries, colon, rectum, and brain. Unfortunately, there are no human studies to support the impressive results noted in animal and in vitro studies.[19–22]

Citrus flavonoids

In addition to possessing antioxidant activity and an ability to increase intracellular levels of vitamin C, rutin, hesperidin, and HER exert many beneficial effects on capillary permeability and blood flow, primarily via strengthening endothelial cells and supporting collagen structures. Collagen, the most abundant protein of the body, is responsible for maintaining the integrity of "ground substance" as well as the integrity of tendons, ligaments, and cartilage. Collagen is also the support structure of the skin and blood vessels. Citrus flavonoids affect collagen metabolism in several ways. They reinforce the natural cross-linking of collagen that forms the so-called collagen matrix of connective tissue and protect against free radical damage with their potent antioxidant and free radical scavenging action and inhibit enzymatic cleavage of collagen by enzymes secreted by leukocytes during inflammation, and microbes during infection. Like quercetin, citrus flavonoids also prevent the release and synthesis of compounds that promote inflammation and allergies, such as histamine, serine proteases, prostaglandins, and leukotrienes.[4]

CLINICAL APPLICATIONS

Their is much overlap between the clinical uses of flavonoid preparations. Most of the clinical research has focused on HER products.

Allergic and inflammatory conditions

Based largely on in vitro studies, quercetin appears to be indicated in virtually all inflammatory and allergic conditions, including asthma, hayfever, rheumatoid arthritis, and lupus, as well as in diabetes, and cancer. However, the main shortcoming is the limited number of clinical studies and poor absorption. Earlier pharmacokinetic studies in animals and humans indicated that very little quercetin is absorbed intact, with the majority of the oral dose (53%) being excreted in the feces.[23,24] One of the main problems in studying the absorption of quercetin and other flavonoids is their degradation by microorganisms in the colon. To side-step this issue, a recent study examined the absorption of quercetin in healthy ileostomy patients with complete small intestines.[25]

The study examined the absorption of quercetin from fried onions (a rich source of quercetin glycosides), rutin, or 100 mg of pure quercetin. Absorption was defined as oral intake minus ileostomy excretion and corrected for degradation within the ileostomy bag. Absorption results were as follows: 52% from onions, 17% from quercetin rutinoside, and 24% for pure quercetin. These results indicate that humans do absorb appreciable amounts of quercetin and that absorption (but not necessarily pharmacological activity) may be enhanced when quercetin is bound to glucose. In other words, citrus bioflavonoid preparations and/or HERs may prove to be more effective clinically.

Capillary fragility, excessive bruisabilty and hemorrhoids

Early studies demonstrated rutin to be effective in reducing capillary fragility, easy bruising, swelling and bruising after sports injuries, and nose bleeds.[26–29] More recent and much more extensive studies have been performed with HERs. Positive double-blind clinical studies exist in the treatment of venous insufficiency including varicose veins, hemorrhoids, diabetic vascular disease, and diabetic retinopathy.[30]

In double-blind studies in patients with chronic venous insufficiency, HER improves microvascular blood flow and clinical symptoms (pain, tired legs, night cramps, and restless legs) in 73–100% of patients.[31–36] Several of the studies were performed in pregnant women where HER was shown to be of great benefit in improving venous function as well as in helping to relieve hemorrhoidal signs and symptoms. In one study, 90% of the women given HER (1,000 mg daily for 4 weeks) had improved symptoms compared with only 12% in the placebo group.[37] Similar results in hemorrhoids not associated with pregnancy have been reported.[30,38]

Diabetes

Flavonoids appear to be quite important in the long-term care of diabetes. One of the hallmark features of diabetes is a significant disturbance of blood flow through small blood vessels. HERs appear to improve blood flow in diabetics significantly and can be useful in the treatment of diabetic microvascular disease and retinopathy. However, PCO or bilberry extracts may be better than quercetin, citrus flavonoids and HER in diabetics.[38–40]

COMMERCIALLY AVAILABLE FORMS

Quercetin

Quercetin is available alone in powder and capsule form. However, if the quercetin is being used for its anti-inflammatory properties, products which provide a combination of the pineapple enzyme bromelain may provide additional benefit. Bromelain exerts anti-allergy and anti-inflammatory activity on its own and it may also enhance the absorption of quercitin. Combination preparations of protein-digesting enzymes, like bromelain, and flavonoids have been shown to potentiate each other's anti-inflammatory activity.[41]

Citrus bioflavonoids

Mixed preparations of citrus bioflavonoids are the most widely used and least expensive flavonoid sources. However, mixed citrus flavonoids are the least active and generally the least quantified source of flavonoids, as most commercially available sources of mixed citrus flavonoids only contain 50% flavonoids. Preparations containing pure rutin and hesperidin or those which clearly state the levels of rutin and hesperidin are better than products which do not quantify the amount of the individual flavonoid components. HERs are probably the better choice when opting for the benefits in this class of flavonoids.

DOSAGES

The recommended dosage range for quercetin is 200–400 mg 20 minutes before meals (three times per day). If the quercetin is being used for its anti-inflammatory properties and bromelain is also indicated, administration with bromelain may enhance absorption. Combination preparations of proteolytic enzymes and flavonoids have been shown to have significant anti-inflammatory activity in experimental studies.[41] If used with bromelain, the amount of bromelain (1,800 mcu activity) should be equal to the amount of quercetin.

The dosage used for HERs in the double-blind clinical studies in the treatment of venous insufficiency and hemorrhoids has ranged from 1,000 to 3,000 mg daily. This translates to a dosage of citrus bioflavonoids, rutin, and hesperidin of 3,000–6,000 mg daily.

TOXICITY

Quercetin appears to be well tolerated in humans. Carcinogenic and teratogenic studies in rats and rabbits have shown that quercetin is without apparent side-effect, even when consumed in very large quantities (2,000 mg/kg body weight and 5–10% of total diet) for long periods of time (up to 2 years).[41–46] In addition, quercetin administration (up to 2,000 mg/kg body weight) to pregnant rats had no teratogenic effects.[47] As is true of any other compound, allergic reactions may occur. Although uncommon, if they occur, discontinue use.

Citrus bioflavonoids, rutin, hesperidin, and HER appear to be extremely safe and without side-effect even during pregnancy.[30]

INTERACTIONS

Quercetin, rutin, hesperidin, HER, and green tea polyphenols do not appear to interact with any drug. Citrus bioflavonoid preparations, if they contain naringin, may interact with drugs. This flavonoid is found in grapefruit juice, but not in orange juice. Studies in humans have shown grapefruit juice (i.e. naringin) to increase the oral bioavailability of drugs like nifedipine, felodipine, verapramil, and terfenadine, as well as inhibiting the breakdown of various drugs, particularly caffeine, coumarin, and estrogens.[48] Avoidance of grapefruit juice and flavonoid preparations containing naringin is recommended when taking any of these drugs.

REFERENCES

1. Hertog MG, Feskens EJ, Hollman PC et al. Dietary antioxidant flavonoids and risk of coronary heart disease. the Zutphen Elderly Study. Lancet 1993; 342: 1007–1011
2. Rice-Evans CA, Miller NJ, Paganga G. Structure-antioxidant relationships of flavonoids and phenolic acids. Free Radical Biol Med 1996; 20: 933–956
3. Havsteen B. Flavonoids, a class of natural products of high pharmacological potency. Biochem Pharmacol 1983; 32: 1141–1148
4. Ferrandiz ML, Alcaraz MJ. Anti-inflammatory activity and inhibition of arachidonic acid metabolism by flavonoids. Agents Action 1991; 32: 283–287
5. Middleton E, Drzewieki G. Flavonoid inhibition of human basophil histamine release stimulated by various agents. Biochem Pharmacol 1984; 33: 3333–3338
6. Middleton E, Drzewieki G. Naturally occurring flavonoids and human basophil histamine release. Int Arch Allergy Appl Immunol 1985; 77: 155–157
7. Amella M, Bronner C, Briancon F et al. Inhibition of mast cell histamine release by flavonoids and bioflavonoids. Planta Medica 1985; 51: 16–20
8. Pearce F, Befus AD, Bienenstock J. Mucosal mast cells. III. Effect of quercetin and other flavonoids on antigen-induced histamine secretion from rat intestinal mast cells. J Allergy Clin Immunol 1984; 73: 819–823
9. Busse WW, Kopp DE, Middleton E. Flavonoid modulation of human neutrophil function. J Allergy Clin Immunol 1984; 73: 801–809
10. Yoshimoto T, Furukawa M, Yamamoto S et al. Flavonoids. Potent inhibitors of arachidonate 5-lipoxygenase. Biochem Biophys Res Common 1983; 116: 612–618
11. Ford-Hutchinson AW. Leukotrienes. Their formation and role as inflammatory mediators. Fed Proc 1985; 44: 25–29
12. Ford-Hutchinson AW. Leukotriene involvement in pathological processes. J Allergy Clin Immunol 1984; 74: 437–440
13. Chaundry PS, Cambera J, Juliana HR, Varma SD et al. Inhibition of human lens aldose reductase by flavonoids, sulindac and indomethacin. Biochem Pharmacol 1983; 32: 1995–1998
14. Varma SD, Mizuno A, Kinoshita JH. Diabetic cataracts and flavonoids. Science 1977; 195: 87–89
15. Mucsi I, Pragai BM. Inhibition of virus multiplication and alteration of cyclic AMP level in cell cultures by flavonoids. Experentia 1985; 41: 930–931
16. Kaul T, Middleton E, Ogra P. Antiviral effects of flavonoids on human viruses. J Med VIrol 1985; 15: 71–79
17. Beladi I, Mucsi I, Pusztai R et al. In vitro and in vivo antiviral effects of flavonoids. In: Farkas L, Gabor M, Kallay F, Wagner H,

eds. Flavonoids and bioflavonoids. New York, NY: Elsevier. 1982: p 443–450
18. Guttner J, Veckenstedt A, Heinecke H, Pusztai R. Effect of quercetin on the course of mengo virus infection in immunodeficient and normal mice. A histological study. Arch Virol 1982; 26: 148–155
19. Elangovan V, Sekar N, Govindasamy S. Studies on the chemopreventive potential of some naturally-occurring bioflavonoids in 7,12-dimethylbenz(a)anthracene-induced carcinogens in mouse skin. J Clin Biochem Nutr 1994; 17: 153–160
20. Verma AK, Johnson JA, Gould MN et al. Inhibition of 7,12-dimethylbenz(a)anthracene and N-nitrosomethyl urea induced rat mammary cancer by dietary flavonol quercetin. Cancer Res 1988; 48: 5754–5758
21. Stavric B. Quercetin in our diet. From potent mutagen to probable anticarcinogen. Clin Biochem 1994; 27: 245–248
22. Larocca LM, Giustacchini M, Maggiano N et al. Growth-inhibitory effect of quercetin and presence of type II estrogen binding sites in primary human transitional cell carcinomas. J Urol 1994; 152: 1029–1033
23. Petrakis PL, Kallianos AG, Wender SH et al. Metabolic studies of quercetin labeled with C14. Arch Biochem Biophys 1959; 85: 264–271
24. Gugler R, Leshik M, Dengler HJ. Disposition of quercetin in man after single oral and intravenous doses. Europ J Clin Pharmacol 1975; 9: 229–234
25. Hollman PC, de Vries JH, van Leeuwen SD et al. Absorption of dietary quercetin glycosides and quercetin in health ileostomy volunteers. Am J Clin Nutr 1995; 62: 1276–1282
26. Lagrue E, Behar A, Maurel. Edematous syndromes caused by capillary hyperpermeability. J Mal Vasc 1989; 14: 231–235
27. Horoschak A. Nocturnal leg cramps, easy bruisability and epistaxis in menopausal patients. Treated with hesperidin and ascorbic acid. Del State Med J 1959; Jan: 19–22
28. Cragin RB. The use of bioflavonoids in the prevention and treatment of athletic injuries. Med Times 1962; 90: 529–530
29. Beretz A, Cazenave. The effect of flavonoids on blood vessel wall interactions. In: Cody V, Middleton E, Harborne JB, Beretz A, eds. Plant flavonoids in biology and medicine II: biochemical, cellular, and medicinal properties. New York, NY: Alan R Liss. 1988: p 187–200
30. Wadworth AN, Faulds D. Hydroxyethylrutosides. A review of its pharmacology, and therapeutic efficacy in venous insufficiency and related disorders. Drugs 1992; 44: 1013–1032
31. Poynard T, Valterio C. Meta-analysis of hydroxyethylrutosides in the treatment of chronic venous insufficiency. Vasa 1994; 23: 244–250
32. Boisseau MR, Taccoen A, Garreau C et al. Fibrinolysis and hemorheology in chronic venous insufficiency. A double blind study of troxerutin efficiency. J Cardiovasc Surg 1995; 36: 369–374
33. Neumann HA, van den Broek MJ. A comparative clinical trial of graduated compression stockings and O-(beta-hydroxyethyl)-rutosides (HR) in the treatment of patients with chronic venous insufficiency. Z Lymphol 1995; 19: 8–11
34. Renton S, Leon M, Belcaro G et al. The effect of hydroxyethylrutosides on capillary filtration in moderate venous hypertension. A double blind study. Int Angiol 1994; 13: 259–262
35. MacLennan WJ, Wilson J, Rattenhuber V et al. Hydroxyethylrutosides in elderly patients with chronic venous insufficiency. Its efficacy and tolerability. Gerontology 1994; 40: 45–52
36. Bergstein NAM. Clinical study on the efficacy of O-(beta-hydroxyethyl)-rutoside (HR) in varicosis of pregnancy. J Int Med Res 1975; 3: 189–193
37. Annoni F, Boccasanta P, Chiurazzi D et al. Treatment of acute symptoms of haemorrhoidal disease with high dose O-(beta-hydroxyethyl)-rutoside. Minerva Medica 1986; 77: 1663–1668
38. Wijayanegara H, Mose JC, Achmad L et al. A clinical trial of hydroxyethylrutosides in the treatment of haemorrhoids of pregnancy. J Int Med Res 1992; 20: 54–60
39. Belcaro G, Candiani C. Chronic effects of O-(beta-hydroxyethyl)-rutosides on microcirculation and capillary filtration in diabetic microangiopathy. Curr Ther Res 1991; 49: 131–139
40. Agolini G, Cavallini GM. Treatment of long-term retinal vasculopathies with high oral dosage of O-(beta-hydroxyethyl)-rutosides. Clini Therapeutica 1987; 120: 101–110
41. Tarayre JP, Lauressergues H. Advantages of a combination of proteolytic enzymes, flavonoids and ascorbic acid in comparison with non-steroid anti-inflammatory agents. Arzneim-Forsch 1977; 27: 1144–1149
42. Stoewsand GS, Anderson JL, Boyd JN et al. Quercetin. A mutagen, not a carcinogen, in Fischer rats. J Toxicol Env Health 1984; 14: 105–114
43. Hirono I, Ueno H, Hosaka S et al. Carcinogenicity examination of quercetin and rutin in ACI rats. Cancer Letters 1981; 13: 15–21
44. Kato K, Mori H, Fujii M et al. Lack of promotive effect of quercetin on methlazoxy acetate carcinogenesis in rats. J Toxicol Sci 1984; 9: 319–325
45. Kato K, Mori H, Tanaka T et al. Absence of initiating activity by quercetin in the rat liver. Ecotoxicol Environ Safety 1985; 10: 63–69
46. Hosaka S, Hirono I. Carcinogenicity test of quercetin by pulmonary-adenoma bioassay in Starin A mice. Gann 1981; 72: 327–328
47. Hirose M, Fukushima S, Sakata T et al. Effect of quercetin on two-stage carcinogenesis of the rat urinary bladder. Cancer Lett 1983; 21: 23–27
48. Willhite CC. Teratogenic potential of quercetin in the rat. Food Chem Toxicol 1982; 20: 75–79
49. Fuhr U, Kummert AL. The fate of naringin in humans. A key to grapefruit juice-drug interactions? Clin Pharmacol Ther 1995; 58: 365–373

CHAPTER CONTENTS

88

Ginkgo biloba (ginkgo tree)

Michael T. Murray, ND

Joseph E. Pizzorno Jr, ND

Ginkgo biloba (family: Ginkgoaceae)
Common names: ginkgo tree, maidenhair tree

GENERAL DESCRIPTION

Ginkgo biloba is a deciduous tree which, living as long as 1,000 years, may grow to a height of 100–122 feet and a diameter of 3–4 feet. The ginkgo has short horizontal branches with short shoots bearing fan-shaped leaves that measure 2–4 inches across. Because the leaf resembles a maidenhair fern, the ginkgo has been called "maidenhair tree". Ginkgo bears an inedible foul-smelling fruit and an edible ivory-colored inner seed that is sold in marketplaces in the Orient. Extracts from the leaves of the ginkgo tree are used medicinally.

CHEMICAL COMPOSITION

The active components of ginkgo leaves are the ginkgo-flavone glycosides or ginkgo heterosides (flavonoid molecules with sugars attached which are unique to the ginkgo), several terpene molecules unique to ginkgo (ginkgolides and bilobalide), and organic acids.[1]

The *Ginkgo biloba* extract (GBE), marketed in Europe under the trade names Tanakan, Rokan, Ginkgobil, Kaveri, and Tebonin, is a very well-defined and complex product prepared from the green leaves. Extracts identical to these preparations are available in the United States as food supplements. The culturing, harvesting, and extracting techniques have been thoroughly standardized and require careful control.

GBE is standardized to contain 24% flavonoid glycosides, as these molecules represent a convenient analytical reference group. Although they play a major role in the pharmacological activity of GBE, other components are also important. The three major backbone flavonoids of the *Ginkgo biloba* flavonols are quercetin, kaempferol, and isorhamnetine (see Fig. 88.1). The sugar (glucoside) components are glucose and rhamnose, which are present

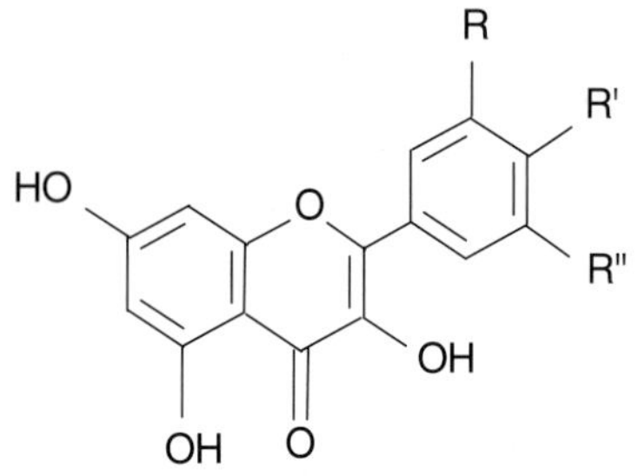

Compound	R	R′	R″
Kaempferol	H	OH	H
Quercetin	OH	OH	H
Isorhamnetine	OCH_3	OH	H

Figure 88.1 The major backbone flavonoids of GBE.

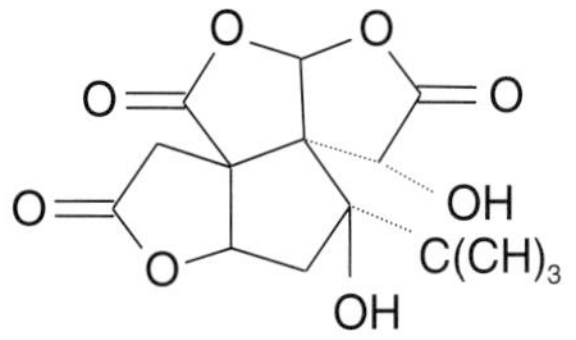

Figure 88.2 Bilobalide.

as single sugars or disaccharides (two sugar molecules attached to each other).

Other significant flavonoid components of the extract include proanthocyanidins, largely composed of dimers and oligomers of delphinidine and cyanidine. The major terpene molecules of GBE, which account for 6% of the extract, are the ginkgolides and bilobalide (see Fig. 88.2). These substances are unique to ginkgo and are not found in any other plants. Other constituents of GBE include a number of organic acids. These compounds contribute valuable properties to the extract by making the usually water-insoluble flavonoid and terpene molecules of ginkgo water-soluble.

HISTORY AND FOLK USE

Ginkgo biloba is the world's oldest living tree species. The sole surviving species of the family Ginkgoaceae, ginkgo tree can be traced back more than 200 million years to the fossils of the Permian period, and for this reason it is often referred to as "the living fossil".

Once common in North America and Europe, the ginkgo was almost destroyed during the Ice Age in all regions of the world except China, where it is has long been cultivated as a sacred tree.

In the late 17th century, Engelbert Kaempfer, a German physician and botanist, became the first European to discover and catalog the ginkgo tree. The flavonoid kaempferol is named after Kaempfer. In 1771, Linnaeus named the tree *Ginkgo biloba*.

The ginkgo tree was brought to America in 1784 to the garden of William Hamilton near Philadelphia. The ginkgo is now planted throughout much of the US as an ornamental tree. The ginkgo, which is the tree most resistant to insects, disease, and pollution, is frequently planted along streets in cities.[1]

Ginkgo biloba's medicinal use can be traced back to the oldest Chinese materia medica (2800 BC). The ginkgo leaves have been used in Traditional Chinese Medicine for their ability to "benefit the brain", relieve the symptoms of asthma and coughs, and help the body eliminate filaria.

Ginkgo leaf extracts are now among the leading prescription medicines in both Germany and France, where they account for 1 and 1.5%, respectively, of total prescription sales. In 1989 alone, over 100,000 physicians worldwide wrote over 10,000,000 prescriptions for GBE. The popularity of GBE has increased since.

PHARMACOLOGY

The standardized concentrated extract of the leaves of *Ginkgo biloba* (24% ginkgo heteroside content) has demonstrated remarkable pharmacological effects. Interestingly, the total extract is more active than single isolated components.[1,2] This suggests synergism between the various components of GBE, an explanation which is well supported in more than 400 clinical and experimental studies utilizing the extract.[1–4]

Tissue effects

GBE exerts profound, widespread tissue effects, including membrane-stabilizing, antioxidant, and free radical-scavenging effects. GBE also enhances the utilization of oxygen and glucose.[1–3]

Cellular membranes provide the first line of defense in maintaining the integrity of the cell. Largely composed of fatty acids (phospholipids), cellular membranes also serve as fluid barriers, exchange sites, and electrical capacitors. These membranes are fragile and vulnerable to damage, especially the lipid peroxidation induced by oxygenated free radicals. GBE is an extremely effective inhibitor of lipid peroxidation of cellular membranes.[1,2]

Red blood cells provide excellent models for evaluating the effects of substances on membrane functions. Red blood cell studies utilizing GBE have demonstrated that, in addition to directly stabilizing membrane structures and scavenging free radicals, GBE also enhances membrane transport of potassium into the cell and sodium out by activating the sodium pump. In essence, GBE leads to better membrane polarization. This effect is particularly important in excitable tissues, such as nerve cells.[1,2]

Nerve cell effects

GBE's membrane-stabilizing and free radical-scavenging effects are perhaps most evident in the brain and nerve cells. Brain cells contain the highest percentage of unsaturated fatty acids in their membranes of any cells in the body, making them highly susceptible to free radical damage.

The brain cell is also highly susceptible to hypoxia. Unlike most other tissues, the brain has very little energy reserves. Its functions require large amounts of energy which must be supplied by a constant supply of glucose and oxygen. Diminished circulation to the brain sets off a chain of reactions which disrupt membrane function and energy production and ultimately lead to cellular death.

GBE is remarkable in its ability to prevent metabolic and neuronal disturbances in experimental models of cerebral ischemia.[1,2,5–8] It accomplishes this by enhancing oxygen utilization and increasing cellular uptake of glucose, thus restoring energy production.

All of the above-mentioned metabolic effects are in addition to GBE's ability to re-establish effective tissue perfusion. Particularly interesting is GBE's ability to normalize the circulation in the areas most affected by microembolization, namely the hippocampus and striatum.[1,2]

Discussion of additional nervous tissues actions of GBE are incorporated into the clinical indications section below. Briefly, GBE promotes increased nerve transmission rate, improves synthesis and turnover of brain neurotransmitters, and normalizes acetylcholine receptors in the hippocampus (the area of the brain most affected by Alzheimer's disease).[1,2]

Vascular effects

The mechanisms of GBE's vascular effects have been investigated utilizing a number of in vivo and in vitro techniques (Table 88.1).[1,2] Isolated vessel techniques allow for separation of GBE's effects on different parts of the vascular system – e.g. arterial, arteriolar, microcirculatory, venular, and venous components – while in vivo studies provide information on the total circulatory phenomena, i.e. GBE's ability to increase the perfusion rate to various regions.

In general, GBE exerts its vascular effects primarily through its effects on the lining of the blood vessels (vascular endothelium) and the system which regulates blood vessel tone. Its vasodilating action is explained by direct stimulation of the release of endothelium-derived relaxing factor (EDRF) and prostacyclin (a beneficial prostaglandin). In addition, GBE inhibits an enzyme which results in relaxation of the blood vessel.[1,2]

On the venous system, GBE stimulates greater tone, thus aiding the dynamic clearing of toxic metabolites which accumulate during ischemia (times of insufficient oxygen supply)[1,2] (see Fig. 88.3).

GBE normalizes circulation by producing tonic effects. These effects are much more apparent in an ischemic vascular area than on a normally perfused area.[9]

Table 88.1 The cellular and membrane mechanisms of the vasoregulatory effects of *Ginkgo bioloba* extract

Site of action	Upstream flow (arteriole)			Exchange area (capillary)			Downstream flow (venous)	
Tissue pathological condition	Arterial spasm	Arterial thrombosis	Vascular atony	Hypoxic vasoparalysis	Capillary hyperpermeability and plasma	Debilitated capillary walls	Venous relaxation and vasoparalysis extravasation	Venular spasms
Effects found with Ginkgo biloba extract	Vasorelaxation	Diminished platelet hyperaggregability	Restitution of arterial tone	Diminished accumulation of toxic wastes: K^+, CO_2, and lactate	Amelioration of capillary hyperpermeability	Increased capillary resistance	Venous tonic effect	Antagonism of experimental venous spasms
Cellular and membrane mechanisms explaining *Gingko biloba's* effects	Release of EDRF from endothelium	Release of PGI_2	Direct effect	Consequence of venous tonic effect	Direct membrane effect	Direct membrane effect	Direct effect	Inhibition of PDE (?)
	Inhibition of PDE	Direct membrane effect	Potentiation of α-adrenergic effects*	Mitochondrial metabolic restart			Indirect effect via α-adrenergic effects	Release of dilating prostaglandins
	Potentiation of α-adrenergic effects*							

*Partly through COMT inhibition.

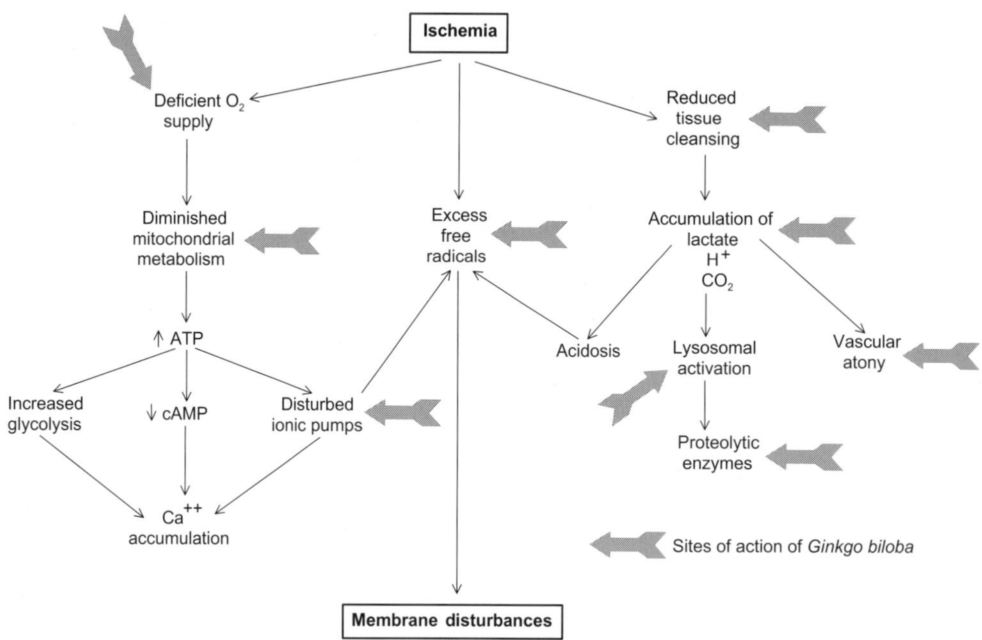

Figure 88.3 GBE's impact on ischemia.

However, despite intense investigation, many of GBE's tonic effects on vascular components are still largely unexplained. It is truly remarkable that a substance can simultaneously combat the phenomena resulting from vascular spasm and, with the same efficiency, restore circulation to areas subject to vasomotor paralysis.

The importance of this dual action is becoming more apparent in cerebral insufficiency, as single direction drugs, i.e. vasodilators, can often aggravate the condition by preferentially dilating the healthy areas, thereby deflecting blood and oxygen away from the ischemic area.

Platelet effects

GBE and isolated ginkgolides have profound effects on platelet function, including inhibition of platelet aggregation, adhesion, and degranulation.[3] These effects appear to be due to direct membrane and antioxidant effects, increased synthesis of prostacyclin and an antagonism of a substance known as platelet activating factor (PAF).

BE and the ginkgolides have been shown to be potent inhibitors of PAF.[3,10–12] PAF is a potent stimulator of platelet degranulation and is involved in many inflammatory and allergic processes, including neutrophil activation, increasing vascular permeability, smooth muscle contraction including bronchoconstriction, and reduction in coronary blood flow. GBE and ginkgolides compete with PAF for binding sites and inhibit the various events induced by PAF.[1,2,13,14] These actions may be responsible for many of the clinical effects of GBE. Interestingly, despite these effects on PAF, GBE exerts no inhibition of platelet aggregation in humans.

Absorption and distribution of GBE

The pharmacokinetics (absorption, distribution, and elimination) of GBE have been studied in rats using radiolabeled extracts.[1–3] Following oral administration, at least 60% of the radiolabeled extract was absorbed. Since blood levels peaked after 1.5 hours, upper gastrointestinal tract absorption was suspected.

The flavonoids appear to have an affinity for organs rich in connective tissues, such as the aorta, eyes, skin, and lungs. Levels of radioactivity in these tissues are two to three times higher than those in blood and decrease little over the course of time. Retained specific activity in the heart is twice that found in the skeletal muscles. Of the glands, the adrenals retained the greatest level of radioactivity.

At 72 hours, the hippocampus and the striated bodies show radioactivity five times greater than that of the blood. This deposition pattern, which parallels the circulation improvement observed after ischemia due to blood clot in rats, is alleviated by GBE extracts. Other areas of the brain such as the cerebral cortex, brain stem, and cerebellum do not show such high levels of radioactivity.

CLINICAL APPLICATIONS

Ginkgo biloba extract's primary clinical application has been in the treatment of vascular insufficiency. In over 50 double-blind clinical trials, both patients with chronic cerebral (brain) arterial insufficiency and peripheral arterial insufficiency have responded favorably to GBE. As described above, GBE exerts an extraordinary array of pharmacological activities which imply a broad spectrum of possible clinical applications, an implication borne out by the new applications of GBE which are constantly being discovered.

Cerebral vascular insufficiency and impaired mental performance

Cerebral vascular insufficiency is an extremely common condition in the elderly of developed countries, due to the high prevalence of atherosclerosis (hardening of the arteries). In well-designed studies, GBE has displayed a statistically significant regression of the major symptoms of cerebral vascular insufficiency and impaired mental performance. These symptoms included: [1–4,11–18]

- short-term memory loss
- vertigo
- headache
- ringing in the ears
- lack of vigilance
- depression.

The significant regression of these symptoms by GBE suggests that vascular insufficiency may be the major causative factor accounting for these so-called "age-related cerebral disorders" versus a true degenerative process.

In a comprehensive review, an analysis was made on the quality of research on over 40 clinical studies with GBE in the treatment of cerebral insufficiency. The results of the analysis indicate that GBE is effective in reducing all symptoms of cerebral insufficiency, including impaired mental function (senility), and the quality of research was comparable to Hydergine (dihydroergotamine), an FDA-approved drug used in the treatment of cerebral vascular insufficiency and Alzheimer's disease. Eight studies stood out as being extremely well-designed and are summarized in Table 88.2.[11–18]

It appears that by increasing cerebral blood flow, and therefore oxygen and glucose utilization, *Ginkgo biloba* extract offers relief of these presumed "side-effects" of aging and may offer significant protection against their development. Furthermore, *Ginkgo biloba*'s anti-aggregatory effect on platelets offers additional protection against a stroke. This has been supported in a clinical study of post-stroke patients which demonstrated that GBE improved blood flow and blood viscosity.[19]

As well as improving blood supply to the brain, experimental and clinical studies show that GBE increases the rate at which information is transmitted at the nerve cell level.[20–22] The memory-enhancing effects of GBE are not limited to the elderly. In one double-blind study, the reaction time in healthy young women performing a memory test was improved significantly after the administration of GBE.[22]

Alzheimer's disease

GBE is showing great benefit in many cases of senility

Table 88.2 Studies demonstrating the significant regression of the major symptoms of cerebral vascular insufficiency through the use of GBE

Principle author	Year	Diagnosis	No. of patients	Age	Duration (weeks)	Dosage (mg)	Type	Compared with:	Efficacy
Agnoli	1984	CCI	30	60	4	120	DB, CS	Placebo (*n* = 30)	76%
Arrigo	1984	CCI	80	40–80	7	120	DB, CS	Placebo (*n* = 40)	65%
Augustin	1976	Misc	99	77	24	120	DB	Placebo (*n* = 90)	44%
Bono	1975	CCI	14	65	5	120	DB	Placebo (*n* = 14)	65%
		CCI	40	67	5	120	Open	ED (*n* = 19)	90%
Boudouresques	1975	CCI,CVA	47	35–80	3	120	Open		80%
Choussat	1977	CCI	48	65–95	8	360	Open		60%
Dieli	1981	CCI	20	62	5	160	DB	Placebo (*n* = 20)	80%
Eckmann	1982	CVA	25	60	4	120	DB	Placebo (*n* = 20)	92%
Gessner	1983	Senescence	19	57–88	12	120	DB	Placebo (*n* = 19) Nicergoline (*n* = 19)	69%
Hofferberth	1989	COS	36	53–69	8	120	DB, CS	Placebo (*n* = 18)	83%
Israel	1977	D	48	72	8	240	Open		NS
Leroy	1978	CVA	27	78	8	120	DB	Raubasine + ED (*n* = 24)	74%
Moreau	1975	CCI	30	84	12	120	DB	Placebo (*n* = 30) ED (*n* = 30)	79%
Pidoux	1983	CCI	12	87	12	160	DB	Placebo	85%
Safi	1977	CCI	20	47–86	2	35 (IV)	Open		76%
Tea	1979	CVA	19	67	8	160	Open		
Terasse	1976	Misc	20	59–84	1–3	17.5 (IV)	Open		55%
Vorberg	1985	CCI	112	55–94	52	120	Open, M		68%
Wackenheim	1977	CCI	50	50	27	160	Open		76%
		CCT	50	50	27	160	Open		72%

CCI, chronic cerebral insufficiency; COS, cerebral organic syndrome; CVA, cerebral vascular accidents; D, dementia; CS, cross-over; DB, double-blind; ED, ergot derivatives; M, multicenter; NS, not specified.

including Alzheimer's disease.[1–4,20,23] In addition to GBE's ability to increase the functional capacity of the brain via the mechanisms described above, it also has been shown to normalize the acetylcholine receptor in the hippocampus of aged animals, increase cholinergic transmission, and to address many of the other major elements of Alzheimer's disease.[1,2]

Although preliminary studies in established Alzheimer's patients are quite promising, at this time it appears that GBE only helps to reverse or merely delay mental deterioration in the early stages of Alzheimer's disease. This may help to enable the patient to maintain a normal life for a while and stay away from being put in a nursing home.

The benefits of GBE in early-stage Alzheimer's is quite evident when looking at the results from a recent double-blind study.[23] In the study, 40 patients with a preliminary diagnosis of senile dementia of the Alzheimer's type received either 80 mg of *Ginkgo biloba* extract or placebo three times daily for 3 months. Patients were assessed by standard tests including the SKT, Sandoz Clinical Assessment Geriatric Scale, and EEG at baseline and at 1, 2, and 3 months. Results indicated that *Ginkgo biloba* extract improved all parameters, usually in the first month, compared with the placebo. Consistent with other studies involving *Ginkgo biloba* extract, the longer *Ginkgo biloba* extract is used, the more obvious the benefits become. *Ginkgo biloba* extract was well tolerated and no side-effects were noted in the trial.

In addition, to offering benefit in early-stage Alzheimer's disease, if the mental deficit is due to vascular insufficiency or depression and not Alzheimer's disease, GBE will usually be effective in reversing the deficit.[1–4]

Tinnitus

Permanent severe tinnitus is an extremely difficult condition to treat. Previous studies have shown contradictory results of GBE in the treatment of tinnitus. For example, in Meyer's study, GBE improved the condition in all patients regardless of prognostic factor.[24] However, in Coles' study, 21 patients with tinnitus took GBE for 12 weeks: 11 reported no change, four reported slight to very slight improvement, and five reported that their tinnitus was worse.[25] The explanation for these different results is that in Meyer's study the patients had recent onset tinnitus, while in Coles' study 18 patients had the tinnitus for at least 3 years.

The most recent study of GBE in tinnitus utilized a two part design: the first part was an open part, without a placebo control; the second part was a double-blind placebo-controlled cross-over study.[26] The 80 patients in the open study had been referred to the department of audiology, Sahlgren's Hospital, Goteborg, Sweden, due to permanent severe tinnitus. Twenty patients reporting a positive effect to *Ginkgo biloba* extract (14.6 mg twice daily) after 2 weeks were recruited for the double-blind study. Patients were given either the GBE or placebo for 2 weeks and were then crossed over into the other group. Evaluation indicated that six patients preferred GBE, seven preferred placebo, and seven had no preference.

On the surface, this study would seem to indicate that GBE is not effective for permanent severe tinnitus. However, the study was really designed for the GBE to fail. First of all the dosage used (14.6 mg twice daily or 29.2 mg daily) is far less the standard dosage of 40 mg three times daily (or roughly four times the daily dosage used in the study). Secondly, in studies in patients with cerebral vascular insufficiency it is well-established that GBE often takes at least 2 weeks before benefit becomes apparent. The longer that GBE is used, the more obvious the benefit. In a condition like permanent severe tinnitus, 2–4 weeks is simply not enough time. However, given the small insufficient dosage, it probably would not have mattered if the subjects had been studied for a longer period of time.

The degree to which GBE is of benefit in permanent severe tinnitus remains to be determined, but given GBE's excellent safety profile it is certainly worth a try.

Cochlear deafness

Ischemia is usually the underlying factor in acute cochlear deafness. GBE has been shown to improve recovery in cases of acute cochlear deafness due to unknown factors or due to sound trauma or pressure (barotrauma).[27]

Senile macular degeneration and diabetic retinopathy

GBE appears to address the multifactorial pathophysiology of senile macular degeneration, the most common cause of blindness in adults, quite effectively. In double-blind studies, GBE demonstrated a statistically significant improvement in long-distance visual acuity in both macular degeneration and diabetic retinopathy.[1,2,28]

GBE has demonstrated impressive protective effects against free radical damage to the retina in experimental studies. Furthermore, GBE has been shown to prevent diabetic retinopathy in diabetic rats, suggesting it may have a protective effect in human diabetics as well.[1,2]

Peripheral arterial insufficiency

Peripheral arterial disease has as its primary lesion the same cholesterol-containing plaque which is responsible for other conditions associated with atherosclerosis, e.g. coronary artery disease and cerebral vascular insufficiency.

The arterial obstruction or narrowing causes a reduction in blood flow during exercise or at rest. Clinical symptoms are caused by the consequent ischemia. The most common symptom of peripheral arterial disease is a pain upon exertion – intermittent claudication. The pain usually occurs in the calf and is described as a cramp or tightness or severe fatigue. The pain is usually bilateral. The cause of the pain is not only reduced oxygen delivery, but also an increase in the production of toxic metabolites and cellular free radicals. These free radicals accumulate and react with the lipid constituents of the cell membrane.

Pain at rest indicates serious reduction in resting blood flow. It is obviously a sign of severe disease. The pain may be localized to one or more toes, or it may have a stocking-type distribution. The character of the pain is usually described as burning or gnawing and is generally worse at night. Cyanosis or pallor of the extremity is usually apparent. In moderate to severe narrowing of the artery, there are trophic changes, including a dry, scaly, and shiny epidermis. The hair may disappear, and the toenails may become brittle, ridged, and deformed.

The standard medical approach to peripheral vascular disease and intermittent claudication includes avoidance of tobacco (which causes vasoconstriction), a regular exercise program consisting of walking, and/or a prescription for pentoxifylline (Trental). Surgery is also an option, though most patients with intermittent claudication need not take this risk.[29]

Trental has emerged as the "drug of choice" in the standard medical treatment of intermittent claudication.[30] A total of 17 placebo-controlled trials have shown that Trental will prolong the total and pain-free walking distance in patients with intermittent claudication. However, the level of improvement (approximately 65% for pain-free walking distance) is less than that achieved with exercise or with *Ginkgo biloba* extract.

In nine double-blind randomized clinical trials of GBE versus placebo in two matched groups of patients with peripheral arterial insufficiency of the leg, GBE was shown to be quite active and superior to placebo (eight studies) and equal to pentoxifylline (one study).[1–3,31–36] Not only were measurements of pain-free walking distance (75–110%) and maximum walking distance (52.6–119%) dramatically increased, but plethysmographic and Doppler ultrasound measurements also demonstrated increased blood flow through the affected limb, and blood lactate levels also dropped.[6–15]

The demonstration that *Ginkgo biloba* extract improves limb blood flow as well as improved walking tolerance (in studies following strict methodology and with sufficient patients for reliable evaluation) indicates that GBE is far superior to pentoxifylline and standard medical therapy in peripheral arterial insufficiency. This includes other peripheral vascular disorders such as diabetic peripheral vascular disease, Raynaud's syndrome, acrocyanosis, and post-phlebitis syndrome.

The longer the period over which GBE is used, the greater is the benefit. Table 88.3 below summarizes a 2 year trial of GBE (160 mg/day) in the treatment of peripheral arterial disease (Fontaine's stage IIb). Pain-free walking distance increased by 300%.[1]

Table 88.3 Effect of GBE on cardiovascular performance measures

Parameter	Time of measurement	
	Week 0	Week 104
Pain-free walking distance (m)	62.9	172.4
Total walking distance (m)	113.8	384.0
Rest flow (ml/100ml per min)	1.6	2.7
Peak flow (ml/100ml per min)	3.7	6.9
Doppler measurement after strain (mmHg)	46.5	72.6

The usual daily dosage of GBE is 120 mg (40 mg three times a day); however, some of the studies employed a dosage of 160 mg/day, including the study summarized in Table 88.3.

Impotence

Most cases of impotence (erectile dysfunction) are due to impaired blood flow to erectile tissue. Recent evidence indicates that *Ginkgo biloba* extract may be extremely beneficial in the treatment of erectile dysfunction due to lack of blood flow.[37] Sixty patients with proven erectile dysfunction who had not reacted to papaverine injections up to 50 mg were treated with *Ginkgo biloba* extract in a dose of 60 mg/day for 12–18 months. The penile blood flow was re-evaluated by duplex sonography every 4 weeks.

The first signs of improved blood supply were seen after 6–8 weeks. After 6 months' therapy, 50% of the patients had regained potency and in 20% a new trial of papaverine injection was then successful; 25% of the patients showed an improved blood flow, but papaverine was still not successful. The remaining 5% were unchanged.

According to the results in this preliminary study, *Ginkgo biloba* extract appears to be very effective in the treatment of erectile dysfunction due to lack of blood flow. The improvement of the arterial inflow to erectile tissue is assumed to be due to the known effect of *Ginkgo biloba* extract on enhancing blood flow through both arteries and veins without any change in systemic blood pressure.

It should be noted that ginkgo's effects are more apparent with long-term therapy and better results may have been obtained with a 120 mg/day dose in order to take full advantage of ginkgo's effect on improving blood flow.

Premenstrual syndrome and idiopathic cyclic edema

Premenstrual syndrome (PMS) is often characterized by fluid retention, vascular congestion, increased capillary permeability, and breast tenderness. A recent double-blind placebo controlled study sought to determine the effectiveness of GBE on these symptoms.[38] The population studied was a group of 165 women between the ages of 18 and 45 years who had suffered from these congestive symptoms for at least three cycles. The patients were then assigned to receive either the ginkgo extract (80 mg twice daily) or placebo from the 16th day of the period to day 5 of the next. Based on extensive symptom evaluation by the patients and physicians, it was concluded that the ginkgo extract was effective against the congestive symptoms of PMS, particularly breast pain or tenderness. Patients taking the ginkgo extract also noted improvements in neuropsychological assessments. These results indicate that *Ginkgo biloba* extract may hold some promise in the treatment of PMS.

Antidepressant effects

The ability of GBE to improve general mood in patients suffering from cerebral vascular insufficiency in double-blind studies has led researchers to begin investigating the antidepressive effects of GBE. In a recent double-blind study, 40 elderly patients (age range, 51–78 years) with depression who had not benefitted fully from standard antidepressant drugs were given either 80 mg of GBE three times daily or a placebo.[39] By the end of the eighth week study, the total score of the Hamilton Rating Scale for Depression in the *Ginkgo biloba* extract group had dropped from 14 to 4.5. In comparison, the placebo group dropped from 14 to only 13. This study indicated two things:

- *Ginkgo biloba* extract can be used with standard antidepressants
- it may enhance their effectiveness, particularly in patients over 50 years of age.

In addition, it is important to point out that the dosage used in the study (80 mg three times daily) is higher than the standard dosage of 40 mg three times daily.

Allergies

Mixtures of ginkgolides as well as the *Ginkgo biloba* extract standardized to contain 24% ginkgoflavonglycosides have shown clinical effects in allergic conditions due to their inhibition of platelet activating factor (PAF) – a key chemical mediator in asthma, inflammation, and allergies.[13,14]

In one double-blind placebo study, the ability of a mixture of ginkolides to block the effects of PAF when PAF was injected into the skin was investigated.[13] Normally, when PAF is injected it causes an immediate formation of a hive (classic wheal and flare reaction). However, if the ginkgolide mixture (120 mg) was given prior to PAF injection, it effectively counteracted the wheal and flare reaction. Specifically, the ginkgolide reduced the flare (reddened) area by a mean of 62.4% and the wheal (hive) volume by a mean of 60%.

Mixtures of ginkgolides, as well as purified ginkgolides, are under investigation in several European countries. The hope is that they will be shown to be clinically effective in asthma, eczema, and other allergies, as well as in many other conditions in which PAF plays a central role.[13,14]

Future applications of GBE

Experimental studies as well as some preliminary clinical evidence indicate that GBE may be of benefit in cases of angina, congestive heart failure, and acute respiratory distress syndrome. Its action on PAF may also make it useful for a great number of other applications in addition to allergies including various types of shock, thrombosis, graft protection during organ transplantation, multiple sclerosis, and burns.[1,2]

DOSAGE

Most of the clinical research on *Ginkgo biloba* has utilized a standardized extract, containing 24% ginkgo heterosides (flavoglycosides), at a dose of 40 mg three times a day. However, some studies have used the higher dosage of 80 mg two to three times daily.

It is difficult to devise a dosage schedule using other forms of ginkgo due to extreme variation in the content of active compounds in dried leaf and crude extracts. Whatever form of ginkgo is used, it appears to be essential that it is standardized for content and activity. For example, a standard 1:5 tincture obtained from the highest possible flavonoid content crude ginkgo leaf would require 1 ounce of the tincture/day to provide the equivalent dosage level of the standardized extract.

Clinical research clearly shows that GBE should be taken consistently for at least 12 weeks in order to determine effectiveness. Although most people report benefits within 2–3 weeks, some may take longer to respond.

TOXICITY

GBE is extremely safe and side-effects are uncommon. In 44 double-blind studies involving 9,772 patients taking GBE, the number of side-effects reported was extremely small. The most common side-effect, gastrointestinal discomfort occurred in only 21 cases, followed by headache (seven cases) and dizziness (six cases).[2–4]

In contrast to the tolerance of the leaf extract, contact with or ingestion of the fruit pulp has produced severe allergic reactions.[40] Contact with the fruit pulp causes erythema and edema, with the rapid formation of vesicles accompanied by severe itching. This is similar to an allergic reaction to the poison ivy-oak-sumac group, suggesting cross-reactivity between *Ginkgo biloba* fruit and this family. Ingestion of as little as two pieces of fruit pulp has been reported to cause severe gastrointestinal irritation from the mouth to the anus.

REFERENCES

1. DeFeudis FV, ed. *Ginkgo biloba* Extract (EGb 761). Pharmacological activities and clinical applications. Elsevier: Paris. 1991
2. EW Funfgeld, ed. Rokan (*Ginkgo biloba*). Recent results in pharmacology and clinic. New York: Springer-Verlag, 1988
3. Kleijnen J, Knipschild P. *Ginkgo biloba*. Lancet 1992; 340: 1136–1139
4. Kleijnen J, Knipschild P. *Ginkgo biloba* for cerebral insufficiency. Br J Clinical Pharmacol @ 34: 352–8, 1992
5. Schaffler VK, Reeh PW. Double-blind study of the hypoxia-protective effect of a standardized *Ginkgo bilobae* preparation after repeated administration in healthy volunteers. Arzneim-Forsch 1985; 35: 1283–1286
6. Chatterjee SS, Gabard B. Studies on the mechanism of action of an extract of *Ginkgo biloba*, a drug for the treatment of ischemic vascular diseases. Naunyn-Schmiedeberg's Arch Pharmacol 1982; 320: R52
7. Le Poncin, Lafitte M, Rapin J et al. Effect of *Ginkgo biloba* on changes induced by quantitative cerebral microembolization in rats. Archs Int Pharmacodyn Ther 1980; 243: 236–244
8. Karcher L, Zagerman P, Krieglstein J. Effect of an extract of *Ginkgo biloba* on rat brain energy metabolism in hypoxia. Naunyn-Schmiedeberg's Arch Pharmacol 1984; 327: 31–35
9. Schmidt U, Rabinovici K, Lande S. Einfluss eines *Ginkgo biloba* specialextraktes auf doe befomdlickeit bei zerebraler onsufficizienz. Munch Med Wockenschr 1991; 133: S15–18
10. Bruchert E, Heinrich SE, Ruf-Kohler P. Wirksamkeit von LI 1370 bei alteren patienten mit himleistungsschwache. Multizentrische doppelblindstudie des fachverbandes Deutscher Allegemeinaezte. Munch Med Wockenschr 1991; 133: S9–14
11. Meyer B. Etude multicentrique randomisee a double insu face au placebo due traitment des acouphenes par l'extrait de Gingko biloba. Presse Med 1986; 15: 1562–1564
12. Taillandier J et al. Traitment des troubles du vidillissement cerebral pal l'extrait *Ginkgo biloba*. Presse Med 1986; 15: 1583–1587
13. Koltai M, Hosford D, Guinot P et al. Platelet activating factor (PAF). A review of its effects, antagonists and possible future clinical implications (Part I). Drugs 1991; 42: 9–29
14. Koltai M et al. PAF. A review of its effects, antagonists and possible future clinical implications (Part II). Drugs 1991; 42: 174–204
15. Haguenauer JP, Canteno F, Koskas H et al. Traitment des troubles de l'equilibre par l'extrai *Ginkgo biloba*. Press Med 1986; 15: 1569–1572
16. Vorberg G, Schmidt U, Schenk N. Wirksamkeit eines neuen *Ginkgo biloba* extraktes bei 100 patienten mit zerebraler insuffizienz. Herg + Gefasse 1989; 9: 936–941
17. Eckmann F. Himleistungsstorungen – behandlung mit *Ginkgo biloba* extrakt. Fortsch Med 1990; 108: 557–560
18. Wesnes K et al. A double-blind placebo-controlled trial of Tanakan in the treatment of idiopathic cognitive impairment in the elderly. Hum Psychopharmacol 1987; 2: 159–169
19. Anadere I, Chmiel H, Witte S. Hemorrheological findings in patients with completed stroke and the influence of *Ginkgo biloba* extract. Clin Hemorheo 1985; 4: 411–420
20. Gessner B, Voelp A, Klasser M. Study of the long-term action of a *Ginkgo biloba* extract on vigilance and mental performance as determined by means of quantitative pharmaco-EEG and psychometric measurements. Arzneim Forsch 1985; 35: 1459–1465
21. Hofferberth B. Effect of *Ginkgo biloba* extract on neurophysiological and psychometric measurement in patients with cerebro-organic syndrome – A double-blind study versus placebo. Arzneim Forsch 1989; 39: 918–922
22. Hindmarch I, Subhan Z. The psychopharmacological effects of *Ginkgo biloba* extract in normal healthy volunteers. Int J Clin Pharmacol Res 1984; 4: 89–93
23. Hofferberth B. The efficacy of Egb761 in patients with senile dementia of the Alzheimer type. A double-blind, placebo-controlled study on different levels of investigation. Human Psychopharmacol 1994; 9: 215–222
24. Meyer B. A multicenter randomized double-blind study of *Ginkgo biloba* extract versus placebo in the treatment of tinnitus. In: Funfgeld EW, ed. Rokan (*Ginkgo biloba*) – recent results in pharmacology and clinic. New York, NY: Springer-Verlag. 1988: p 245–250
25. Coles RRA. Trial of an extract of *Ginkgo biloba* (EGB) for tinnitus and hearing loss. Clin Otolaryngol 1988; 13: 501–504
26. Holgers KM, Axelsson A, Pringle I. *Ginkgo biloba* extract for the treatment of tinnitus. Audiology 1994; 33: 85–92
27. Bascher V, Steinert W. Differential diagnosis of sudden deafness and therapy with high dose infusions of *Ginkgo biloba* extract. In: Clausen CF, Kirtane MV, Schlitter K, eds. Vertigo, nausea, tinnitus, and hypoacusia in metabolic disorders. Amsterdam: Elsevier. 1988: p 575–582
28. Lanthony P, Cosson JP. Evolution de la vision des couleurs dans la retinopathie diabetique debutante traitee par extait de *Ginkgo biloba*. J Fr Ophtalmol 1988; 11: 671–674
29. De Felice M, Gallo P, Masotti G. Current therapy of peripheral obstructive arterial disease. The non-surgical approach. Angiology 1990; 41: 1–11
30. Ernst E. Pentoxifylline for intermittent claudication. A critical review. Angiology 1994; 45: 339–345
31. Schneider B. *Ginkgo biloba* extract in peripheral arterial diseases. Meta-analysis of controlled clinical studies. Arzneim Forsch 1992; 42: 428–436
32. Thomson GJ, Vohra RK, Carr MH et al. A clinical trial of Gingko biloba extract in patients with intermittent claudication. Int Angiol 1990; 9: 75–78
33. Saudreau F, Serise JM, Pillet J et al. Efficacy of *Ginkgo biloba* extract in the treatment of lower limb obliterative artery disease at stage III of the Fontaine classification. J Mal Vasc 1989; 14: 177–182
34. Rudofsky VG. The effect of *Ginkgo biloba* extract in cases of arterial occlusive disease. A randomized placebo controlled double-blind cross-over study. Fortschr Med 1987; 105: 397–400
35. Bauer U. *Ginkgo biloba* extract in the treatment of arteriopathy of the lower limbs. Sixty-five week study. Presse Médicale 1986; 15: 1546–1549
36. Bauer U. 6-month double-blind randomized clinical trial of *Ginkgo biloba* extract versus placebo in two parallel groups in patients suffering from peripheral arterial insufficiency. Arzneim Forsch 1984; 34: 716–721
37. Sikora R, Sohn M, Deutz FJ et al. *Ginkgo biloba* extract in the therapy of erectile dysfunction. Journal of Urology 1989; 141: 188A
38. Tamborini A, Taurelle R. Value of standardized *Ginkgo biloba* extract (Egb 761) in the management of congestive symptoms of premenstrual syndrome. Rev Fr Gynecol Obstet 1993; 88: 447–457
39. Schubert H, Halama P. Depressive episode primarily unresponsive to therapy in elderly patients. Efficacy of *Ginkgo biloba* (Egb 761) in combination with antidepressants. Geriatr Forsch 1993; 3: 45–53
40. Becker LE, Skipworth GB. Ginkgo-tree dermatitis, stomatitis, and proctitis. JAMA 1975; 231: 1162–1163

89

Glucosamine

Michael T. Murray, ND

Joseph E. Pizzorno Jr, ND

CHAPTER CONTENTS

INTRODUCTION

Glucosamine is a simple molecule, manufactured in the body from glucose and an amine. One of the primary physiological roles of glucosamine is in the joints where it stimulates the manufacture of glycosaminoglycans, key structural components of cartilage. Glucosamine also promotes the incorporation of sulfur into cartilage. Because of this effect, glucosamine sulfate is thought to be the best source of glucosamine.

As some people age, they apparently lose the ability to manufacture sufficient levels of glucosamine. The result is that synthesis of glycosaminoglycans does not keep up with degradation. The inability to manufacture glucosamine at an adequate rate has been suggested to be the major factor leading to osteoarthritis.

Food sources

There are no food sources of glucosamine. Commercially available sources of glucosamine are derived from chitin – the exoskeleton of shrimp, lobsters, and crabs.

Deficiency signs and symptoms

As stated above, it is thought that a deficiency of glucosamine is a major factor in the development of osteoarthritis. The weight-bearing joints, like the knees and hips, and joints of the hands are the tissues most often affected with osteoarthritis. In affected joints, there is substantial cartilage destruction followed by hardening and the formation of large bone spurs in the joint margins. Pain, deformity, and limited joint motion result. The

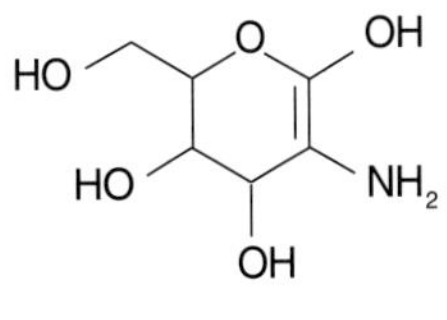

HO, O, OH, HO, NH_2, OH

Figure 89.1 Glucosamine.

onset of osteoarthritis can be very subtle; morning joint stiffness is often the first symptom. As the disease progresses, there is pain on motion of the involved joint that is made worse by prolonged activity and relieved by rest.

Available forms

Glucosamine is commercially available as glucosamine sulfate, glucosamine hydrochloride, and *N*-acetyl-glucosamine. Glucosamine sulfate, the only form of glucosamine that has been the subject of over 300 scientific investigations and over 20 double-blind studies, is the preferred form. Glucosamine sulfate has also been used by millions of people worldwide and is registered as an aid in osteoarthritis in over 70 countries.

When authors or manufacturers discuss glucosamine hydrochloride or *N*-acetyl-glucosamine (NAG), if references are provided all clinical studies have used glucosamine sulfate and no other form. Only glucosamine sulfate provides proven clinical effectiveness.

Glucosamine sulfate vs. NAG

NAG differs from glucosamine sulfate in that instead of a sulfur molecule, NAG has a portion of an acetic acid molecule attached to it. Glucosamine sulfate and NAG are entirely different molecules and appear to be handled by the body differently. Companies marketing *N*-acetylglucosamine (NAG) claim that this form is better absorbed, more stable, and is better utilized than glucosamine sulfate. These contentions are without support in the scientific literature. Detailed human studies on the absorption, distribution, and elimination of orally administered glucosamine sulfate have shown an absorption rate of as high as 98% and that once absorbed it is then distributed primarily to joint tissues where it is incorporated into the connective tissue matrix of cartilage, ligaments, and tendons.[1,2] In addition, there are impressive clinical studies on thousands of patients. In contrast, there has never been a double-blind study using NAG for any application. Nor have there ever been any detailed absorption studies on NAG in humans.

Further evidence of the superiority of glucosamine sulfate to NAG is offered by studies in laboratory animals. Several studies have demonstrated that glucosamine absorption and utilization is at least twice that of NAG.[3–14] The researchers have concluded that:[5]

> glucosamine is a more efficient precursor of macromolecular hexosamine [glycosaminoglycans] than N-acetylglucosamine. It is possible that N-acetylglucosamine does not penetrate the cell membranes and, as a result, is not available for incorporation into glycoproteins and mucopolysaccharides.

The body preferentially utilizes glucosamine sulfate rather than NAG. This preference appears largely due to the active processes which enhance absorption of glucosamine sulfate in the intestines.[15]

The absorption of NAG by humans is poor for several reasons:

- NAG is quickly digested by intestinal bacteria
- NAG binds with dietary lectins in the gut, resulting in a lectin-NAG complex which is excreted in the feces
- a large percentage of NAG is metabolized by intestinal cells.

In addition to the question of absorption, several studies have shown that the articular tissue is not able to utilize NAG as well as it does glucosamine.[4,5] These absorption and utilization problems suggest NAG is highly unlikely to possess the same kind of anti-arthritic and anti-inflammatory properties that glucosamine sulfate has been shown to possess.

Glucosamine sulfate vs. glucosamine HCl

Research has shown that sulfur is an extremely important component in the therapeutic effect of glucosamine sulfate, its substitution is likely to decrease the efficacy of supplemental glucosamine.[16] Sulfur is an essential nutrient for joint tissue where it functions in the stabilization of the connective tissue matrix of cartilage, tendons, and ligaments. Even healthy humans have low serum sulfate (0.3–0.4 mM) and synovial sulfur levels, but in osteoarthritis these concentrations are even lower. As far back as the 1930s, researchers demonstrated that individuals with arthritis are commonly deficient in this essential nutrient.[17,18] Restoring sulfur levels brought about significant benefit to these patients.[18] In addition to sulfur playing a critical role in the manufacture of glycosaminoglycans (GAGs) like chondroitin sulfate and keratan sulfate, sulfur has been shown to inhibit the various enzymes which lead to cartilage destruction in osteoarthritis (e.g. collagenase, elastases, and hyaluronidase).[16,19]

Because one of the primary effects of glucosamine sulfate is to promote the manufacture of GAGs, a lack of the sulfur moiety may mean less GAG synthesis when glucosamine HCl is used. Therefore, it is unlikely that glucosamine HCl will show the same excellent clinical results achieved with glucosamine sulfate, because it lacks this critical element.

In fact, preliminary results indicate that glucosamine hydrochloride may be no more effective than a placebo in relieving osteoarthritis. The results of the first clinical trial featuring glucosamine hydrochloride were announced at the 12th Panamerican Conference of Rheumatology by Joseph Houpt, Chief of Rheumatology, Mount Sinai Hospital in Toronto, Ontario, July 1998. The double-blind, placebo-controlled 10-week study examined the effects of glucosamine hydrochloride in patients with osteoarthritis of the knee. Patients received either 500 mg of glucosamine hydrochloride or a placebo three times daily. Forty-five patients received glucosamine hydrochloride, while 53 received the placebo. The results indicated that 49% of patients receiving glucosamine hydrochloride felt they had improved compared to 45% of the placebo group who said they felt improved. However, the difference between the two groups was not statistically significant. What these results call into question is the viability of glucosamine hydrochloride as an effective form of glucosamine.

The more than 20 published clinical trials with glucosamine sulfate have demonstrated a success rate of 72% to 95% in various forms of osteoarthritis. In osteoarthritis of the knee the success rate is over 80%. Clearly, the success rate noted by glucosamine hydrochloride in this preliminary study is much less than the rate reported with glucosamine sulfate.

CLINICAL APPLICATIONS

The primary use for glucosamine sulfate is in the treatment of osteoarthritis. Glucosamine is a safe and effective natural alternative to aspirin and other non-steroidal anti-inflammatory drugs (NSAIDs) in the treatment of osteoarthritis. Clinical and experimental research is indicating that current drugs being used in osteoarthritis may be producing short-term benefit, but actually accelerating the progression of the joint destruction. NSAIDs tend to inhibit cartilage repair by inhibiting glycosaminoglycan synthesis and the incorporation of sulfur into cartilage.[20,21] Since osteoarthritis is caused by a degeneration of cartilage, it appears that while NSAIDs are fairly effective in suppressing the symptoms, they possibly worsen the condition by inhibiting cartilage formation and accelerating cartilage destruction (see Ch. 176 for further discussion).[22–25]

Osteoarthritis

Numerous double-blind studies have shown glucosamine sulfate to produce much better results compared with NSAIDs and placebos in relieving the pain and inflammation of osteoarthritis. In one of the more recent studies comparing glucosamine sulfate with a placebo, 252 patients with osteoarthritis of the knee were given either a placebo or 500 mg of glucosamine sulfate three times daily for 4 weeks.[26] Results indicated that glucosamine sulfate was significantly more effective than the placebo in improving pain and movement after 4 weeks. Previous studies have shown that the longer glucosamine sulfate is used, the greater the therapeutic benefit. The rate and severity of side-effects with glucosamine did not differ from the placebo. These results are consistent with other double-blind studies versus a placebo.[27–30]

Head-to-head double-blind studies have shown glucosamine sulfate to produce much better results compared with NSAIDs in relieving the pain and inflammation of osteoarthritis, despite the fact that glucosamine sulfate exhibits very little direct anti-inflammatory effect and no direct analgesic or pain relieving effects.[31–34] While NSAIDs offer purely symptomatic relief and may actually promote the disease process, glucosamine sulfate appears to address the cause of osteoarthritis. By promoting cartilage synthesis, thus treating the root of the problem, glucosamine sulfate not only relieves the symptoms, but also helps the body to repair damaged joints. The clinical effect is impressive, especially when glucosamine's safety and lack of side-effects are considered.

In one of the earlier comparative studies in which glucosamine sulfate (1,500 mg/day) was compared with ibuprofen (1,200 mg/day), pain scores decreased faster in the first 2 weeks in the ibuprofen group. However, by week 4 the group receiving the glucosamine sulfate experienced a significantly better improvement than the ibuprofen group.[31] Physicians rated the overall response as good in 44% of the glucosamine sulfate-treated patients as compared with only 15% of the ibuprofen group.

Three more recent studies designed to further evaluate the comparative effectiveness of glucosamine sulfate to NSAIDs provide even better evidence. The first study consisted of 200 subjects with osteoarthritis of the knee given either glucosamine sulfate (500 three times daily) or ibuprofen (400 mg three times daily) for four weeks.[32] Consistent with previous studies, the ibuprofen group experienced quicker pain relief. However, by the end of the second week the group taking glucosamine sulfate experienced as good results as the ibuprofen group with one major exception – while the rate of side-effects with glucosamine were mild and only affected 6% of the group, ibuprofen produced more significant side-effects much more frequently, with 35% of the group experiencing them.

In the second study, 329 patients were given 1,500 mg glucosamine sulfate, 20 mg piroxicam, both compounds,

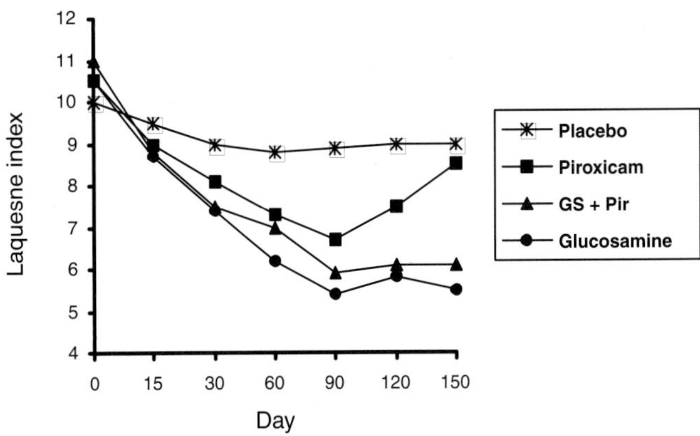

Figure 89.2 Symptom relief (Lequesne index) from glucosamine compared with piroxicam and placebo.

Table 89.1 Side-effects and drop-outs from glucosamine compared with piroxicam and placebo

	Placebo	GS	Piroxicam	GS + piroxicam
Incidence of side-effects	24.4%	14.8%	40.9%	5.9%
Drop-outs	3	0	20	3

GS, glucosamine sulfate.

or a placebo for 90 days.[33] The main efficacy variable was represented by the Lequesne index, a standard method of assessing disease activity. As can be seen in Figure 89.1, the results of the study were strikingly in favor of glucosamine sulfate alone.

These impressive results with glucosamine sulfate were achieved without side-effects. In fact, patients on glucosamine sulfate had fewer side-effects than the placebo and no drop-outs (the side-effect and drop-out values among the four groups are shown in Table 89.1).

In the third study, 178 patients suffering from osteoarthritis of the knee were randomized into two groups.[34] One group received 1,500 mg of glucosamine sulfate per day, the other received 1,200 mg of ibuprofen. Treatment lasted for 4 weeks. Outcome measurements included knee pain at rest, at movement, and at pressure; knee swelling; overall improvement rated by the investigators, and adverse effects.

Knee pain (average score)

Time	Glucosamine sulfate	Ibuprofen
Before treatment	8.42	8.46
Week 2	5.54	5.63
Week 4	3.60	4.18
2 weeks after treatment	3.26	3.84

Knee swelling (average score)

Time	Glucosamine sulfate	Ibuprofen
Before treatment	1.43	1.48
Week 2	0.77	0.89
Week 4	0.47	0.48
2 weeks after treatment	0.36	0.54

Clinical improvement

Effectiveness	Glucosamine sulfate		Ibuprofen	
	After 4 weeks	After 6 weeks	After 4 weeks	After 6 weeks
Symptom-free	45%	55%	32%	36%
Improved	39%	32%	45%	41%
Unchanged	11%	7%	15%	14%
Worsened	5%	6%	8%	9%

Side-effects

	Glucosamine sulfate	Ibuprofen
Side-effects	6%	16%
Drop-outs	0%	10%

Clearly these results confirm previous studies showing glucosamine sulfate is more effective and safer than conventional therapy for osteoarthritis.

In addition to showing benefit in double-blind studies, oral glucosamine sulfate was shown to offer significant benefit in an open trial involving 252 doctors and 1,506 patients in Portugal.[35] This large study provides valuable clinical information on the appropriate use of glucosamine sulfate. The patients received 500 mg of glucosamine sulfate three times daily over a mean period of 50 days. Symptoms of pain at rest, on standing, and on exercise and limited active and passive movements all improved steadily throughout the treatment period. Objective therapeutic efficacy was rated by doctors as "good" in 59% of patients, and "sufficient" in a further 36%. Although not a controlled study, a 95% response rate is very impressive. The results with glucosamine sulfate were rated by both doctors and patients as being significantly better than those obtained with previous treatment, including NSAIDs, vitamin therapy, and cartilage extracts. Glucosamine sulfate produced good benefit in a significant portion of patients who had not responded to any other medical treatment.

In the study, obesity was associated with a significant shift from good to fair. This finding may indicate that higher dosages may be required for obese individuals or that oral glucosamine is not enough to counteract the added stress of obesity on the joints. Patients with peptic ulcers and individuals taking diuretics were also associated with a shift from good to sufficient in efficacy, as well as tolerance. Individuals with current peptic ulcers should try and take glucosamine sulfate with foods. Individuals taking diuretics may need to increase the dosage to compensate for the reduced effectiveness. The improvement with glucosamine lasted for 6–12 weeks after the end of treatment.

DOSAGE

The standard dosage for glucosamine sulfate is 500 mg three times per day. Obese individuals may need higher dosages based on body weight (e.g. 20 mg/kg body weight daily). Also, individuals taking diuretics may also need to take higher dosages.

TOXICITY

Glucosamine sulfate has an excellent safety record in animal and human studies. Based on these studies, many experts have recommended that glucosamine sulfate "be considered as a drug of choice for prolonged oral treatment of rheumatic disorders". Side-effects, when they do appear, are generally limited to light to moderate gastrointestinal symptoms, including stomach upset, heartburn, diarrhea, nausea, and indigestion. If these symptoms occur, the glucosamine sulfate should be taken with meals.

In regards to people who are "sulfur-sensitive", an important distinction needs to be made. When patients report they are allergic to sulfur, what they usually mean is that they are allergic to the so-called sulfa drugs or sulfite-containing food additives. It is impossible to be allergic to sulfur as sulfur is an essential mineral. The sulfate form of sulfur is present in human blood. In short, glucosamine sulfate is extremely well-tolerated and no allergic reactions have been reported.

REFERENCES

1. Setnikar I, Palumbo R, Canali S et al. Pharmacokinetics of glucosamine in man. Arzneim Forsch 43 1993; 10: 1109–1113
2. Setnikar I, Palumbo R, Canali S et al. Pharmacokinetics of glucosamine in the dog and man. Arzneim Forsch 1986; 36: 729–735
3. Setnikar I. Antireactive properties of "chondroprotective" drugs. Int J Tissue React 1992; 14: 253–261
4. Karzel K, Domenjoz R. Effect of hexosamine derivatives and uronic acid derivatives on glycosaminoglycan metabolism of fibroblast cultures. Pharmacology 1971; 5: 337–345
5. Vidal y Plana RR, Bizzarri D, Rovati AL. Articular cartilage pharmacology. I. In vitro studies on glucosamine and non steroidal anti-inflammatory drugs. Pharmacol Res Comm 1978; 10: 557–569
6. Capps JC, Shertlar MR, Bradford RH. Hexosamine metabolism. II. Effect of insulin and phlorizin on the absorption and metabolism, in vivo, of D-glucosamine and N-acetyl-glucosamine in the rat. Biochim Biophys Acta 1966; 127: 205–212
7. Capps JC et al. Hexosamine metabolism. I. The absorption and metabolism, in vivo of orally administered D-glucosamine and N-aecetyl-D-glucosamine in the rat. Biochim Biophys Acta 1966; 127: 194–204
8. Shetlar MR, Capps JC, Hern DL. Incorporation of radioactive glucosamine into the serum proteins of intact rats and rabbits. Biochim Biophysica Acta 1964; 83: 93–101
9. Richmond JE. Studies on the metabolism of plasma glycoproteins. Biochemistry 1963; 2: 676–683
10. Capps JC, Shetlar MR. In vivo incorporation of D-glucosamine-1-C14 into acid mucopolysachharides of rabbit liver. Proc Soc Exptl Biol Med 1963; 114: 118–120
11. Shetlar MD, Hern DL, Bradford RH et al. Fate of radioactive glucosamine administered parenterally to the rat. Proc Soc Exptl Biol Med 1962; 109: 335–337
12. Kohn P, Winzler RJ, Hoffman R. Metabolism of D-glucosamine and N-acetyl-D-glucosamine in the intact rat. J Biol Chem 1962; 237: 304–308
13. McGarrahan JF, Maley F. Hexosamine metabolism. J Biol Chem 1962; 237: 2458–2465
14. Shetlar MD, Hern DL, Bradford RH et al. Incorporation of [1-14C]glucosamine into serum proteins. Biochim Biophys Acta 1961; 53: 615–616
15. Tesoriere G, Dones F, Magistro et al. Intestinal absorption of glucosamine and N-acetylglucosamine. Experientia 1972; 28: 770–771
16. Annefeld M. Personal communication. February 28, 1997, Chicago, IL
17. Sullivan MX, Hess WC. Cystine content of finger nails in arthritis. J Bone Joint Surg 1935; 16: 185–188
18. Senturia BD. Results of treatment of chronic arthritis and rheumatoid conditions with colloidal sulphur. J Bone Joint Surg 1934; 16: 119–125
19. Vignon E, Richard M, Annefeld M. An in vitro study of glucosamine sulfate on human osteoarthritic cartilage metabolism. Manuscript in preparation.
20. Brandt KD. Effects of nonsteroidal anti-inflammatory drugs on chondrocyte metabolism in vitro and in vivo. Am J Med 1987; 83: 29–34
21. Shield MJ. Anti-inflammatory drugs and their effects on cartilage synthesis and renal function. Eur J Rheumatol Inflam 1993; 13: 7–16
22. Brooks PM, Potter SR, Buchanan WW. NSAID and osteoarthritis – help or hindrance. J Rheumatol 1982; 9: 3–5
23. Newman, N.M., Ling, R.S.M. Acetabular bone destruction related to non-steroidal anti-inflammatory drugs. Lancet 1985; ii; 11–13
24. Solomon L. Drug induced arthropathy and necrosis of the femoral head. J Bone Joint Surg 1973; 55B: 246–251
25. Ronningen H, Langeland N. Indomethacin treatment in osteo-arthritis of the hip joint. Acta Orthop Scand 1979; 50: 169–174
26. Noack W, Fischer M, Forster KK et al. Glucosamine sulfate in osteoarthritis of the knee. Osteoarthritis Cartilage 1994; 2: 51–59
27. Crolle G, D'este E. Glucosamine sulfate for the management of arthrosis. a controlled clinical investigation. Curr Med Res Opin 1980; 7: 104–109
28. Pujalte JM, Llavore EP, Ylescupidez FR. Double-blind clinical evaluation of oral glucosamine sulphate in the basic treatment of osteoarthrosis. Curr Med Res Opin 1980; 7: 110–114
29. Drovanti A, Bignamini AA, Rovati AL. Therapeutic activity of oral glucosamine sulfate in osteoarthrosis. a placebo-controlled double-blind investigation. Clin Ther 1980; 3: 260–272
30. D'Ambrosia E, Casa B, Bompani R et al. Glucosamine sulphate. a controlled clinical investigation in arthrosis. Pharmatherapeutica 1982; 2: 504–508
31. Vaz AL. Double-blind clinical evaluation of the relative efficacy of ibuprofen and glucosamine sulfate in the management of osteoarthrosis of the knee in out-patients. Curr Med Res Opin 1982; 8: 145–149
32. Muller-Fassbender H, Bach GL, Haase W et al. Glucosamine sulfate compared to ibuprofen in osteoarthritis of the knee. Osteoarthritis Cartilage 1994; 2: 61–69
33. Rovati LC, Giacovelli G, Annefeld M et al. A large, randomized, placebo controlled, double-blind study of glucosamine sulfate vs piroxicam and vs their association, on the kinetics of the symptomatic effect in knee osteoarthritis. Osteoarthritis Cartilage 1994; 2: 56
34. Qiu GX, Gao SN, Giacovelli G et al. Efficacy and safety of glucosamine sulfate versus ibuprofen in patients with knee osteoarthritis. Arzneim Forsch 1998; 48: 469–474
35. Tapadinhas MJ, Rivera IC, Bignamini AA. Oral glucosamine sulfate in the management of arthrosis. report on a multi-centre open investigation in Portugal. Pharmatherapeutica 1982; 3: 157–168

CHAPTER CONTENTS

90

Glycyrrhiza glabra (licorice)

Michael T. Murray, ND

Joseph E. Pizzorno Jr, ND

Glycyrrhiza glabra (family: Leguminoseae)
Common names: licorice, glycyrrhiza

GENERAL DESCRIPTION

Glycyrrhiza is a perennial, temperate zone herb or subshrub, 3–7 feet high, with a long, cylindrical, branched, flexible, and burrowing rootstock with runners. The parts used are the dried runners and roots, which are collected in the fall.

CHEMICAL COMPOSITION

The major active component of licorice root is the triterpenoid saponin glycyrrhizin (also known as glycyrrhizic acid or glycyrrhizinic acid) (Fig. 90.1), which is usually found in concentrations ranging from 6 to 10%. The intestinal flora is believed to hydrolyze glycyrrhizin, yielding the aglycone molecule (glycyrrhetinic acid) and a sugar moeity, resulting in absorption of both.[1]

A processed licorice extract, deglycyrrhizinated licorice (DGL), which is used in the treatment of peptic and apthous ulcers, is made by removing the glycyrrhizin molecule. The active components of DGL are flavonoids. These compounds have demonstrated impressive protection against chemically induced ulcer formation in animal studies.[2]

Other active constituents of licorice include isoflavonoids (isoflavonol, kumatakenin, licoricone, glabrol,

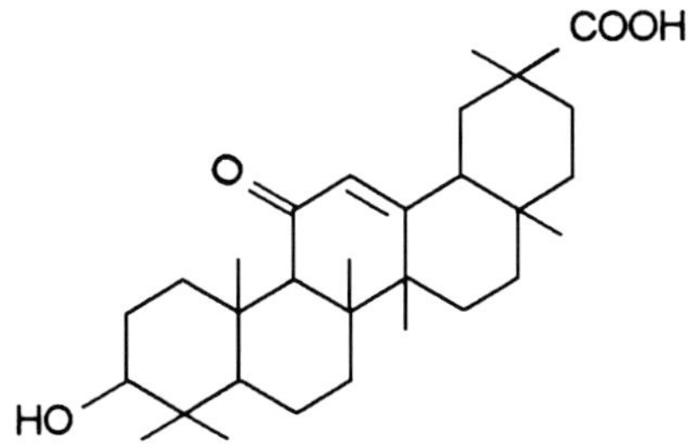

COOH
O
HO

Figure 90.1 Glycyrrhizinic acid.

etc.), chalcones, coumarins (umbelliferone, herniarin, etc.), triterpenoids and sterols, lignins, amino acids, amines, gums and volatile oils.[3]

HISTORY AND FOLK USE

The medicinal use of licorice in both Western and Eastern cultures dates back several thousand years. It was used primarily as a demulcent, expectorant, antitussive, and mild laxative. Licorice is one of the most popular components of Chinese medicines. Its traditional uses include treating peptic ulcers, asthma, pharyngitis, malaria, abdominal pain, insomnia, and infections.[3]

PHARMACOLOGY

Licorice is known to exhibit many pharmacological actions, including the following:[3]

- estrogenic
- aldosterone-like action
- anti-inflammatory (cortisol-like action)
- anti-allergic
- antibacterial, antiviral, and antitrichomonas
- antihepatotoxic
- anticonvulsive
- choleretic
- anti-cancer
- expectorant
- antitussive activities.

The majority of these actions are discussed individually below.

Although much of the pharmacology focuses on glycyrrhizin and glycyrrhetinic acid, it should be kept in mind that licorice has many other components, such as flavonoids, that may have significant pharmacological effects.

Estrogenic activity

Glycyrrhizin exhibits alterative action upon estrogen metabolism – i.e. when estrogen levels are too high, it will inhibit estrogen action, and when estrogens are too low, it will potentiate estrogen action when used in greater amounts.[4] Glycyrrhetinic acid has been shown to antagonize many of the effects of estrogens, particularly exogenous estrogens.[5] The estrogenic action of glycyrrhiza is due to its isoflavone content, as many isoflavone structures (e.g. daidzein and genistein from soy) are known to possess estrogenic effect. This effect has been demonstrated in experimental animal studies using the crude extract, suggesting that the estrogenic activity of the isoflavones are more significant than the estrogen antagonism of glycyrrhetinic acid.

Pseudoaldosterone activity

The chronic ingestion of glycyrrhiza in large doses leads to a well-documented pseudoaldosteronism syndrome, i.e. hypertension, hypokalemia, sodium and water retention, low plasma renin activity, and suppressed urine and serum aldosterone levels.[6–11] In normal subjects, the amount of glycyrrhizin needed to produce these side-effects is between 0.7 and 1.4 g, which corresponds to approximately 10–14 g of the crude herb.[7] Although glycyrrhiza possesses mineralocorticoid activity (about four orders of magnitude lower than aldosterone) and binds to aldosterone receptors, it is largely without effect in adrenalectomized animals or in patients with severe adrenocorticoid insufficiency. Therefore, it can be concluded that its primary effects are largely as a result of glycyrrhetinic acid inhibiting the breakdown of aldosterone in the liver.[12] Glycyrrhizin and glycyrrhetinic acid have been shown to suppress 5-beta-reductase, the main enzyme in humans responsible for inactivating cortisol, aldosterone, and progesterone. These effects can be put to good use in the treatment of Addison's disease, a severe disease of adrenal insufficiency.[11]

Anti-inflammatory and anti-allergic activity

Glycyrrhiza has significant anti-inflammatory and anti-allergic activity.[13,14] Although both glycyrrhizin and glycyrrhetinic acid bind to glucocorticoid receptors, and much of glycyrrhiza's anti-inflammatory activity has been explained by its "cortisol-like effects", many of the effects of glycyrrhiza actually antagonize or counteract cortisol.[15] Included are antagonism to such actions of cortisol as activation of tryptophan oxygenase, accumulation of hepatic glycogen, stimulation of hepatic cholesterol synthesis, inhibition of thymus atrophy, and inhibition of ACTH synthesis and secretion. Glycyrrhizin does, however, reinforce cortisol's inhibition of antibody formation, stress reaction, and inflammation. Like its mineralocorticoid effect, glycyrrhiza's major influence on glucocorticoid metabolism is probably related to its suppression of 5-beta-reductase activity, thus increasing the half-life of cortisol.

Glycyrrhiza's major cortisol-like effect relates to its ability to inhibit phospholipase-A2.[16] This enzyme is responsible for cleaving lipids from biomembranes for eicosanoid metabolism. In addition to this effect, glycyrrhizin has also been shown to inhibit cAMP-phosphodiesterase, thereby raising cAMP levels and prostaglandin formation by activated peritoneal macrophages from rats.[17,18] Glycyrrhizin has been shown to inhibit experimentally induced allergenic reactions, such as the Arthus' phenomenon, the Schwartzman's phenomenon, and Forssman's anaphylaxis, and to be an antidote against many toxins, including diphtheria, tetanus, and tetrodotoxin.[18,19]

Immunostimulatory and antiviral effects

Glycyrrhizin and glycyrrhetinic acid have been shown to induce interferon.[20] The induction of interferon leads to significant antiviral activity, as interferons bind to cell surfaces where they stimulate synthesis of intracellular proteins that block the transcription of viral DNA. The induction of interferon is also followed by activation of macrophages and augmentation of natural killer cell activity.

Glycyrrhizin has been shown to directly inhibit the growth of several DNA and RNA viruses in cell cultures (vaccinia, herpes simplex, Newcastle disease, and vesicular stomatitis viruses) and to inactivate herpes simplex 1 virus irreversibly.[21] Glycyrrhizin, as stated above, also inhibits the thymolytic and immunosuppressive action of cortisone.

Antibacterial activity

Alcohol extracts of glycyrrhiza have displayed antimicrobial activity in vitro against *Staphylococcus aureus, Streptococcus mutans, Mycobacterium smegmatis,* and *Candida albicans*.[22] The majority of the antimicrobial effects are due to isoflavonoid components, with the saponins having a lesser antibacterial effect.

Antihepatotoxic activity

Glycyrrhetinic acid inhibits carbon tetrachloride and galactosamine-induced liver damage. The mechanism of action is prevention of non-enzymatic lipid peroxidation and inhibition of the production of free radicals by the enzymatic action of NADPH-cytochrome P450 reductase on CCl4.[23]

CLINICAL APPLICATIONS

The clinical applications of licorice can be divided into three main categories:

- use of oral licorice preparations containing glycyrrhetinic acid
- use of deglycyrrhizinated licorice (DGL)
- use of topical prepations containing glycyrrhetinic acid.

Key uses of oral licorice include:

- viral infections (e.g. the common cold, HIV and AIDS, viral hepatitis)
- premenstrual syndrome (PMS)
- acute intermittent porphyria
- Addison's disease, inflammation
- as a sweetening agent.

The key use of DGL is in ulcerative conditions of the gastrointestinal tract (e.g. peptic ulcers, canker sores, and inflammatory bowel disease). Topical preparations containing glycyrrhetinic acid can be used in eczema, psoriasis, and herpes.

Preparations containing glycyrrhetinic acid

The common cold

Licorice has long been used in treating the symptoms of the common cold. This historical use is justified by its immune-enhancing and antiviral effects.

HIV and AIDS

Glycyrrhizin-containing preparations are showing promise in the treatment of human immunodeficiency virus (HIV) related diseases including AIDS. Although much of the research has featured intravenous administration, this route of administration may not be necessary, as glycyrrhizin and glycyrrhetinic acid are easily absorbed orally and are well-tolerated. This is most evident in a recent double-blind study on the clinical effectiveness of glycyrrhizin by long-term oral administration to 16 hemophiliac patients with evidence of HIV infection.[24] Patients received daily doses of 150–225 mg of glycyrrhizin for 3–7 years. Helper and total T-lymphocyte numbers, other immune system parameters, and glycyrrhizin and glycyrrhetinic acid levels in the blood were monitored. The results indicated that orally administered glycyrrhizin was converted into glycyrrhetinic acid which was detected in sera, without manifesting any side-effect. None of the patients given the glycyrrhizin had progression of immunologic abnormalities or development to AIDS. In contrast, the group not receiving glycyrrhetinic acid showed decreases in helper and total T-cell counts and antibody levels. Two of the 16 patients in the control group developed AIDS.

In another study, 10 HIV positive patients without AIDS took 150–225 mg glycyrrhizin daily.[25] After 1–2 years, none developed symptoms associated with AIDS or AIDS-related complex (ARC), while one of 10 patients of a matched control group developed ARC and two progressed to AIDS and subsequently died.

The result of glycyrrhizin in HIV-positive and AIDS patients is almost immediate improvement in immune function. In one study, nine symptom-free HIV-positive patients received 200–800 mg glycyrrhizin in vitro daily. After 8 weeks., the groups had increased helper T-cells, improved helper/suppressor ratios and improved liver function.[26]

In another study, six AIDS patients received 400–1,600 mg glycyrrhizin in vitro daily.[27] After 30 days, five of the six showed a reduction or disappearance of the P24 antigen which indicates active disease.

The results of these studies and others in HIV-positive and AIDS patients are encouraging.

Hepatitis

Some of the studies in HIV patients used an intravenous glycyrrhizin-containing product, Stronger Neominophagen C (SNMC), consisting of 0.2% glycyrrhizin, 0.1% cysteine and 2.0% glycine in physiological saline solution. This product is used in Japan primarily for the treatment of hepatitis. The other components, glycine and cysteine, appear to modulate glycyrrhizin's actions. Glycine has been shown to prevent the aldosterone effects of glycyrrhizin, while cysteine aids in the liver in detoxification reactions.

In addition to AIDS, SNMC has demonstrated impressive results in treating chronic hepatitis B, one of the most difficult infections for the body to clear.[19,28,29] SNMC has been shown to improve liver function and lower levels of liver enzymes. Approximately 40% of patients will have complete resolution.

Premenstrual syndrome

The symptoms of the premenstrual syndrome (depression, craving for sweets, weight gain due to water retention, breast tenderness, etc.) have been largely attributed to an increase in the estrogen to progesterone ratio. As licorice is considered to have alterative action on estrogen metabolism, and both glycyrrhizin and glycyrrhetinic acid possess anti-estrogenic effect and suppress the breakdown of progesterone, administration of licorice 2 weeks prior to the onset of menstruation (the mid-luteal phase) may help to reduce PMS symptomatology.

Acute intermittent porphyria (AIP)

This disorder of heme biosynthesis is characterized by recurrent attacks of neurological and psychiatric dysfunction. The symptoms include:

- abdominal complaints of nausea, vomiting and colicky pain, occasionally severe enough to present as an acute abdomen without fever or leukocytosis
- variable neurological signs and symptoms, e.g. paresthesia, hypesthesia, neuritic pain, wrist or foot drop, loss of deep tendon reflexes, etc.
- variable mental and emotional disturbances, typically restlessness, disorientation, and visual hallucinations (which are seen in one-third of the patients).

As estrogens are known to exacerbate or induce AIP, it is quite possible that some of the so-called PMS symptoms are exacerbations of AIP due to the midcycle estrogen surge.

A partial (50%) deficiency of uroporphyrinogen I synthase results in increased inducibilty of aminolevulinic acid (ALA) synthase by drugs and foreign chemicals and by 5-beta-reductase steroid metabolites (very potent inducers of ALA synthase). AIP is also associated with a marked deficiency in the activity of 5-alpha-reductase, resulting in increased 5-beta-reductase activity.[30] Glycyrrhetinic acid and glycyrrhizin have been shown to significantly reduce 5-beta-reductase while increasing 5-alpha-reductase.[31] (Note that lead also increases 5-beta-reductase activity, resulting in a presenting picture similar to AIP.[31] Chronic or acute lead toxicity must be ruled out in these patients.)

Addison's disease

As described above, licorice exerts an "aldosterone-like effect" useful in treating Addison's disease.

Inflammation

Virtually any inflammatory or allergic condition may be reduced by licorice by the mechanisms discussed above in the "Pharmacology" section (p. 768). Historically, licorice has been successfully used for treating asthma and other atopic conditions.[3,13]

Licorice has been shown to enhance the action of corticosteroids like prednisone and prednisolone, as well as the levels of the body's own corticosteroids.[32,33] In one study, six subjects received an i.v. dose of prednisolone with or without 200 mg glycyrrhizin. Glycyrrhizin was found to increase significantly the concentration of total and free prednisolone by inhibiting its breakdown. Furthermore, the effects of prednisolone appeared to be potentiated by glycyrrhizin.[33]

Sweetening agent

As glycyrrhizin is 50–100 times sweeter than sucrose, licorice can be used as a sweetening or flavoring agent to mask the bitter taste of other medications.[3]

Preparations without glycyrrhetinic acid

Peptic ulcer

By far, the most popular medicinal use of licorice in the United States is in the treatment of peptic ulcers. Original research focused on glycyrrhetinic acid. In fact, glycyrrhetinic acid was the first drug proven to promote healing of gastric and duodenal ulcers.[34] Most researchers and most physicians using licorice in the treatment of peptic ulcers now use deglycyrrhizinated licorice (DGL). DGL was actually shown to be more effective than glycyrrhetinic acid, without side-effects.[35]

DGL's mode of action is different than the current drugs, such as antacids and H_2-receptor antagonists, which focus on reducing gastric acidity. Though effective, these treatments can be expensive, carry some risk of toxicity, disrupt normal digestive processes, and alter the structure and function of the cells that line the digestive tract. The latter factor is just one of the reasons why peptic ulcers will develop again if antacids, cimetidine, ranitidine, and similar drugs are used.

Rather than inhibit the release of acid, DGL stimulates the normal defense mechanisms that prevent ulcer formation and stimulate healing of the damaged mucous membranes. Specifically, DGL:[36,37]

- increases the blood supply to the damaged mucosa
- increases the number of cells producing the mucous that protects the mucous membranes
- increases the amount of mucous the cells produce, and increases the life span of the intestinal cell.

Numerous clinical studies over the years have found DGL to be an effective anti-ulcer compound. DGL has been shown to be extremely effective in the treatment of gastric ulcers.[38–42] In one study, 33 gastric ulcer patients were treated with either DGL (760 mg, three times a day) or a placebo for 1 month.[41] There was a significantly greater reduction in ulcer size in the DGL group (78%), than in the placebo group (34%). Complete healing occurred in 44% of those receiving DGL, but only in 6% of the placebo group.

Comparison to conventional anti-ulcer drugs

In several head to head comparison studies, DGL has been shown to be more effective than cimetidine (Tagemet), ranitidine (Zantac), or antacids in both short-term treatment and maintenance therapy of peptic ulcers.[38,39,43] However, while these drugs are associated with significant side-effects (see above), DGL is extremely safe and is only a fraction of the cost.

Subsequent studies have shown DGL to be as effective as Tagemet and Zantac for both short-term treatment and maintenance therapy of gastric ulcer.[38–40] For example, in a head to head comparison with Tagamet, 100 patients received either DGL (760 mg, three times a day between meals) or Tagamet (200 mg, three times a day and 400 mg at bedtime).[39] The percentage of ulcers healed after 6 and 12 weeks were similar in both groups. Yet, while Tagamet is associated with some toxicity, DGL is extremely safe to use.

Gastric ulcers are often a result of the use of alcohol, aspirin or other non-steroidal anti-inflammatory drugs, caffeine, and other factors that decrease the integrity of the gastric lining. As DGL has been shown in human studies to reduce the gastric bleeding caused by aspirin, DGL is strongly indicated for the prevention of gastric ulcers in patients requiring long-term treatment with ulcerogenic drugs, such as aspirin, non-steroidal anti-inflammatory agents, and corticosteroids.[42]

Duodenal ulcers

DGL is also effective in duodenal ulcers. This is perhaps best illustrated by one study in patients with severe duodenal ulcers. In the study, 40 patients with chronic duodenal ulcers of 4–12 years' duration and more than six relapses during the previous year were treated with DGL.[44] All of the patients had been referred for surgery because of relentless pain, sometimes with frequent vomiting, despite treatment with bed rest, antacids, and anticholinergic drugs. Half of the patients received 3 g of DGL daily for 8 weeks; the other half received 4.5 g/day for 16 weeks. All 40 patients showed substantial improvement, usually within 5–7 days, and none required surgery during the 1 year follow-up. Although both dosages were effective, the higher dose was significantly more effective than the lower dose.

In another more recent study, the therapeutic effect of DGL was compared with that of antacids or cimetidine in 874 patients with confirmed chronic duodenal ulcers.[43] Ninety-one percent of all ulcers healed within 12 weeks; there was no significant difference in healing rate in the groups. However, there were fewer relapses in the DGL group (8.2%) than in those receiving cimetidine (12.9%), or antacids (16.4%). These results, coupled with DGL protective effects, suggest that DGL is a superior treatment of duodenal ulcers.

Apthous ulcers

Recurrent apthous stomatitis (canker sores) is a common problem. DGL may be effective in promoting healing. In one study, 20 patients were instructed to use a solution of DGL as a mouthwash (200 mg powdered DGL dissolved in 200 ml warm water) four times daily.[45] Fifteen of the 20 (75%) experienced 50–75% improvement within 1 day, followed by complete healing of the ulcers by the third day. DGL in tablet form may produce even better results.

Topical application

Eczema and psoriasis

Glycyrrhetinic acid exerts an effect similar to that of topical hydrocortisone in the treatment of eczema, contact and allergic dermatitis, and psoriasis. In fact, in several studies, glycyrrhetinic acid was shown to be superior to topical cortisone, especially in chronic cases. For example, in one study in patients with eczema, 93% of the patients applying glycyrrhetinic acid demonstrated improvement compared with 83% using cortisone.[46]

Glycyrrhetinic acid can also be used to potentiate the effects of topically applied hydrocortisone by inhibiting the 11-beta-hydroxysteroid dehydrogenase which catalyses the conversion of hydrocortisone to an inactive form.[47]

Herpes simplex

Topical glycyrrhetinic acid and derivatives have been shown, in clinical studies, to be quite helpful in reducing the healing time and pain associated with cold sores and genital herpes.[48,49] As mentioned earlier, glycyrrhizin inactivates herpes simplex 1 virus irreversibly and stimulates the synthesis and release of interferon.[21]

DOSAGE

The dosage of licorice for most clinical applications is based upon the content of glycyrrhetinic acid. The exception is in the treatment of peptic ulcer. In this application, deglycyrrhizinated licorice (DGL) is preferred as it produces equally effective results compared with glycyrrhetinic acid, but is free from any side-effects.

For most purposes, the goal is to achieve a high level of glycyrrhetinic acid in the blood without producing side-effects (discussed below). In general, the following three times a day dosages are safe and effective in raising glycyrrhetinic acid levels:

- powdered root: 1–2 g
- fluid extract (1:1): 2–4 ml
- solid (dry powdered) extract (4:1): 250–500 mg.

In the treatment of AIDS, pure glycyrrhetinic acid products or extracts standardized for glycyrrhetinic acid are recommended. Toxicity can become a problem for patients taking licorice for any period longer than 1 month (see below).

Dosage instructions for DGL

In order to be effective in healing peptic ulcers, it appears that DGL must mix with saliva. DGL may promote the release of salivary compounds which stimulate the growth and regeneration of stomach and intestinal cells. DGL in capsule form has not been shown to be effective.[50,51]

The standard dosage for DGL is two to four 380 mg chewable tablets between or 20 minutes before meals. Taking DGL after meals is associated with poor results.[52] DGL should be continued for 8–16 weeks, depending on the response.

TOXICITY

The main hazards of licorice administration are due to the aldosterone-like effects of glycyrrhetinic acid. If ingested regularly, licorice root (greater than 3 g/day for more than 6 weeks) or glycyrrhizin (>100 mg/day) may cause sodium and water retention, hypertension, hypokalemia, and suppression of the renin–aldosterone system. Monitoring of blood pressure and electrolytes and increasing dietary potassium intake is suggested.[6,7]

There is a great individual variation in the susceptibility to the symptom-producing effects of glycyrrhizin. Adverse effects are rarely observed at levels below 100 mg/day, while they are quite common at levels above 400 mg/day.[7]

Prevention of the side-effects of glycyrrhizin may be possible by following a high-potassium, low-sodium diet. Although no formal trial has been performed, patients who normally consume high-potassium foods and restrict sodium intake, even those with high blood pressure and angina, have been reported to be free from the aldosterone-like side effects of glycyrrhizin.[53]

Licorice should probably not be used in patients with a history of hypertension or renal failure, or those who are currently using of digitalis preparations.

REFERENCES

1. Hattori M, Sakamoto T, Kobashi K, Namba T. Metabolism of glycyrrhizin by human intestinal flora. Planta Med 1983; 48: 38–42
2. Yamamoto K et al. Gastric cytoprotective anti-ulcerogenic actions of hydroxychalcone in rats. Planta Med 1992; 58: 389–393
3. Chandler RF. Licorice, more than just a flavour. Can Pharmacy J 1985; Sept: 421–424
4. Kumagai A, Nishino K, Shimomura A et al. Effect of glycyrrhizin on estrogen action. Endocrinol Japon 1967; 14: 34–38
5. Kraus S. The anti-estrogenic action of beta-glycyrrhetinic acid. Exp Med Surg 1969; 27: 411–420
6. Farese RV et al. Licorice-induced hypermineralocorticoidism. N Engl J Med 1991; 325: 1223–1227
7. Stormer FC, Reistad R, Alexander J. Glycyrrhizic acid in liqourice – Evaluation of health hazard. Fd Chem Toxicol 1993; 31: 303–312
8. Takeda R, Morimoto S, Uchida K et al. Prolonged pseudoaldosteronism induced by glycyrrhizin. Endocrinol Japon 1979; 26: 541–547
9. Baron J. Side-effects of carbonoxolone. Acta Gastro-Enterol Belgica 1983; 46: 469–484
10. Epstein M, Espiner E, Donald R et al. Effect of eating liquorice on the renin-angiotensin aldosterone axis in normal subjects. Br Med J 1977; 1: 488–490
11. Armanini D, Karbowiak I, Funder J. Affinity of liquorice derivatives for mineralocorticoid and glucocorticoid receptors. Clin Endocrinol 1983; 19: 609–612
12. Tamura Y, Nishikawa T, Yamada K. Effects of glycyrrhetinic acid and its derivatives on delta4-5-alpha-and 5-beta-reductase in rat liver. Arzneim Forsch 1979; 29: 647–649
13. Kuroyanagi T, Sato M. Effect of prednisolone and glycyrrhizin on passive transfer of experimental allergic encephalomyelitis. Allergy 1966; 15: 67–75
14. Cyong J. A pharmacological study of the anti-inflammatory activity of chinese herbs. A review. Acupunct Electro-Ther 1982; 7: 173–202
15. Kumagai A, Nanaboshi M, Asanuma Y et al. Effects of glycyrrhizin on thymolytic and immunosuppressive action of cortisone. Endocrinol Japon 1967; 14: 39–42
16. Okimasa E, Moromizato Y, Watanabe S et al. Inhibition of phospholipase A2 by glycyrrhizin, an anti-inflammatory drug. Acta Med Okayama 1983; 37: 385–391
17. Amer S, Mckinney G, Akcasu A. Effect of glycyrrhetinic acid on the cyclic nucleotide system of the rat stomach. Biochem Pharmacol 1974; 23: 3085–3092

18. Ohuchi K, Kamada Y, Levine L et al. Glycyrrhizin inhibits prostaglandin E2 formation by activated peritoneal macrophages from rats. Prostagland Med 1981; 7: 457–463
19. Suzuki H, Ohta Y, Takino T et al. Effects of glycyrrhizin on biochemical tests in patients with chronic hepatitis – double blind trial. Asian Med J 1984; 26: 423–438
20. Abe N, Ebina T, Ishida N. Interferon induction by glycyrrhizin and glycyrrhetinic acid in mice. Microbial Immunol 1982; 26: 535–539
21. Pompei R, Pani A, Flore O et al. Antiviral activity of glycyrrhizic acid. Experientia 1980; 36: 304–305
22. Mitscher L, Park Y, Clark D. Antimicrobial agents from higher plants. Antimicrobial isoflavonoids from *Glycyrrhiza glabra* L. var. typica. J Nat Products 1980; 43: 259–269
23. Kiso Y, Tohkin M, Hikino H et al. Mechanism of antihepatotoxic activity of glycyrrhizin, I. effect on free radical generation and lipid peroxidation. Planta Medica 1984; 50: 298–302
24. Ikegami N, Akatani K, Yamazaki S et al. Prophylactic effect of long-term oral administration of glycyrrhizin on AIDS development of asymptomatic patients. Int Conf AIDS 1993; 9: 234[abstract no. PO-A25–0596]
25. Ikegami N, Akatani K, Yamazaki S et al. Clinical evaluation of glycyrrhizin on HIV-infected asymptomatic Hemophiliac patients in Japan. Fifth International Conference on AIDS. Abstract W.B.P. 298, June 1989. Cited in AIDS Treatment News 1990; 103: May 18
26. Mori K, Sakai H, Suzuki S et al. The present status in prophylaxis and treatment of HIV infected patients with hemophilia in Japan. Rinsho Byhori 1989; 37: 1200–1208
27. Hattori T, Ikematsu S, Koito A et al. Preliminary evidence for inhibitory effect of glycyrrhizin on HIV replication in patients with AIDS. Antiviral Res 1989; 11: 255–261
28. Eisenburg J. Treatment of chronic hepatitis B. Part 2. Effect of glycyrrhizinic acid on the course of illness. Fortschr Med 1992; 110: 395–398
29. Ahcarya SK, Dasarathy S, Tandon A et al. A preliminary open trial on interferon stimulator (SNMC) derived from *Glycyrrhiza glabra* in the treatment of subacute hepatic failure. Ind J Med Res 1993; 98: 75–78
30. Anderson K, Bradlow H, Sassa S, Kappas A. Studies in porphyria VII. Relationship of the 5-alpha-reductase metabolism of steroid hormones to clinical expression of the genetic defect in acute intermittent porphyria. Am J Med 1979; 66: 644–650
31. Tomita T, Sato T, Kazuo S, Takakuwa E. Effects of lead and arsenic on the formation of 5-beta-H steroids. Toxicol Lett 1979; 3: 291–297
32. MacKenzie MA, Jansen RW, Hoefnagels WH et al. The influence of glycyrrhetinic acid on plasma cortisol and cortisone in healthy young volunteers. J Clin Endocrinol Metab 1990; 70: 1637–1643
33. Chen MF, Shimada F, Kato H et al. Effect of glycyrrhizin on the pharmacokinetics of prednisolone following low dosage of prednisolone hemisuccinate. Endocrinol Japan 1990; 37: 331–341
34. Doll R, Hill I, Hutton C et al. Clinical trial of a triterpenoid liquorice compound in gastric and duodenal ulcer. Lancet 1962; ii: 793–796
35. Wilson JA. A comparison of carbenoxolone sodium and deglycyrrhizinated liquorice in the treatment of gastric ulcer in the ambulant patient. Br J Clin Pract 1972; 26: 563–566
36. van Marle J, Aarsen PN, Lind A et al. Deglycyrrhizinised liquorice (DGL) and the renewal of rat stomach epithelium. Eur J Pharmacol 1981; 72: 219–225
37. Goso Y, Ogata Y Ishihara K, Hotta K. Effects of traditional herbal medicine on gastric mucin against ethanol-induced gastric injury in rats. Comp Biochem Physiol 1996; 113C: 17–21
38. Morgan AG, Pacsoo C, McAdam WA. Maintenance therapy. A two year comparison between Caved-S and cimetidine treatment in the prevention of symptomatic gastric ulcer. Gut 1985; 26: 599–602
39. Morgan AG et al. Comparison between cimetidine and Caved-S in the treatment of gastric ulceration, and subsequent maintenance therapy. Gut 1982; 23: 545–551
40. Glick L. Deglycrrhizinated liquorice in peptic ulcer. Lancet 1982; ii: 817
41. Turpie AG, Runcie J, Thomson TJ. Clinical trial of deglycyrrhizinate liquorice in gastric ulcer. Gut 1969; 10: 299–303
42. Rees WD, Rhodes J, Wright JE et al. Effect of deglycyrrhizinated liquorice on gastric mucosal damage by aspirin. Scand J Gastroent 1979; 14: 605–607
43. Kassir ZA. Endoscopic controlled trial of four drug regimens in the treatment of chronic duodenal ulceration. Irish Med J 1985; 78: 153–156
44. Tewari SN, Wilson AK. Deglycyrrhizinated liquorice in duodenal ulcer. Practitioner 1972; 210: 820–825
45. Das SK, Gulati AK, Singh VP. Deglycyrrhizinated liquorice in aphthous ulcers. J Assoc Physicians India 1989; 37: 647
46. Evans FQ. The rational use of glycyrrhetinic acid in dermatology. Br J Clin Pract 1958; 12: 269–279
47. Teelucksingh S, Mackie AD, Burt D et al. Potentiation of hydrocortisone activity in skin by glycyrrhetinic acid. Lancet 1990; 335: 1060–1063
48. Partridge M, Poswillo D. Topical carbonoxolone sodium in the management of herpes simplex infection. Br J Oral Maxillofac Surg 1984; 22: 138–145
49. Csonka G, Tyrrell D. Treatment of herpes genitalis with carbonoxolone and cicloxolone creams. A double blind placebo controlled trial. Br J Ven Dis 1984; 60: 178–181
50. Bardhan KD, Cumberland DC, Dixon RA et al. Clinical trial of deglycyrrhizinised liquorice in gastric ulcer. Gut 1978; 19: 779–782
51. Multicentre Trial. Treatment of duodenal ulcers with glycyrrhinizin acid-reduced liquorice. Br Med J 1973; 3: 501–503
52. Feldman H, Gilat T. A trial of deglycyrrhizinated liquorice in the treatment of duodenal ulcer. Gut 1971; 12: 499–451
53. Baron J, Nabarro J, Slater J et al. Metabolic studies, aldosterone secretion rate and plasma renin after carbonoxolone sodium as biogastrone. Br Med J 1969; 2: 793–795

CHAPTER CONTENTS

91

Hydrastis canadensis (goldenseal) and other berberine-containing botanicals

Michael T. Murray, ND

Joseph E. Pizzorno Jr, ND

Hydrastis canadensis (family: Ranunculaceae)
Common names: goldenseal, yellow root, Indian turmeric, eye root, jaundice root

Berberis vulgaris (family: Berberidaceae)
Common name: barberry

Berberis aquifolium (family: Berberidaceae)
Common names: Oregon grape, trailing mahona

Coptis chinensis
Common name: goldthread

INTRODUCTION

The plants goldenseal (*Hydrastis canadensis*), barberry (*Berberis vulgaris*), Oregon grape (*Berberis aquifolium*), and goldthread (*Coptis chinensis*) share similar indications and effects due to their high content of berberis alkaloids. The chief berberis alkaloid, berberine, has been extensively studied in both experimental and clinical settings. Its pharmacological effects are reviewed below. The general description, history and folk use, chemical composition, and specific clinical indications for each plant are presented here. The pharmacology of these plants is primarily discussed in terms of the activity of berberine.

GENERAL DESCRIPTION

Hydrastis canadensis

Goldenseal is native to eastern North America and is cultivated in Oregon and Washington. It is a perennial herb with a knotty yellow rhizome from which arises a single leaf and an erect hairy stem. In early spring, it bears two five- to nine-lobed rounded leaves near the top, which are terminated by a single greenish-white flower. The parts used are the dried rhizome and roots.[1,2]

Berberis vulgaris

The common barberry is a deciduous spiny shrub that

may reach 16 feet in height. Native to Europe, it has been naturalized in eastern North America. Parts used are the barks of the stem and root.[1,2]

Berberis aquifolium

The Oregon grape is an evergreen spineless ornamental shrub, 3–7 feet in height, native to the Rocky Mountains from British Columbia to California. Parts used are the rhizome and roots.[1,2]

Coptis chinensis

Goldthread is a perennial herb native to China. The parts used are the rhizomes and root.[3]

CHEMICAL COMPOSITION

Hydrastis canadensis

Alkaloids isolated from hydrastis include:

- hydrastine (1.5–4.0%)
- berberine (0.5–6.0%)
- berberastine (2.0–3.0%)
- canadine
- candaline
- hydrastinine
- other related alkaloids.

Other constituents include meconin, chlorogenic acid, phytosterins, and resins.[1,2]

Berberis vulgaris

Barberry contains several alkaloids in its roots:

- jatrorrhizine
- berberine
- berberubine
- berbamine
- bervulcine
- palmatine
- columbamine
- oxyacanthine.

It also contains chelidonic, citric, malic, and tartaric acids.[1,2]

Berberis aquifolium

Oregon grape contains the alkaloids berbamine, berberine, canadine, corypalmine, hydrastine, isocorydine, mahonine, and oxyacanthine. Resins and tannins have also been reported.[1,2]

Coptis chinensis

Goldthread root contains berberine (5–8%) and other alkaloids similar to those found in goldenseal.[3]

HISTORY AND FOLK USE

Hydrastis canadensis

Native to North America, hydrastis was used extensively by the American Indian as an herbal medication and clothing dye. Its medicinal use centered around its ability to soothe the mucous membranes of the respiratory, digestive, and genitourinary tracts in inflammatory conditions induced by allergy or infection. The Cherokee and other Indian tribes used hydrastis in disorders of the eye and skin.[1,2]

Berberis vulgaris

This plant is native to most of Europe, and very similar species are found in North Africa and Asia. Barberry's historical use is as an antidiarrheal agent, bitter tonic, antipyretic, and antihemorrhagic.[1,2]

Berberis aquifolium

Oregon grape's historical and folk use is similar to that of hydrastis. In addition, Oregon grape was used in the treatment of chronic skin conditions such as acne, psoriasis, and eczema.[1,2]

Coptis chinensis

In China, goldthread was used in the traditional medicine system to "drain fire". It was used primarily in infectious conditions similar to the historical use of goldenseal. Some specific uses included fever, dysentery, gastrointestinal infection, furuncles, boils, and eye infections.[3]

PHARMACOLOGY

The medicinal value of hydrastis, barberry, Oregon grape root, and goldthread is thought to be due to their high content of isoquinoline alkaloids, of which berberine has been the most widely studied. Berberine has demonstrated antibiotic, immunostimulatory, anticonvulsant, sedative, hypotensive, uterotonic, cholerectic, and carminative activity. Berberine's pharmacological activities support the historical use of the berberine-containing herbs.

Antibiotic activity

Perhaps the most celebrated of berberine's effects has been its antibiotic activity. Although not as potent as many prescription antibiotics, berberine exhibits a broad spectrum of antibiotic activity. Berberine has shown antimicrobial activity against bacteria, protozoa, and fungi, including:[1–10]

- *Staphylococcus* sp.
- *Streptococcus* sp.

- *Chlamydia* sp.
- *Corynebacterium diphtheria*
- *E. coli*
- *Salmonella typhi*
- *Vibrio cholerae*
- *Diplococcus pneumonia*
- *Pseudomonas* sp.
- *Shigella dysenteriae*
- *Entamoeba histolytica*
- *Trichomonas vaginalis*
- *Neisseria gonorrhoeae*
- *N. meningitidiss*
- *Treponema pallidum*
- *Giardia lamblia*
- *Leishmania donovani*
- *Candida albicans*.

Its action against some of these pathogens is actually stronger than that of prescription antibiotics commonly used for these pathogens. Berberine's action in inhibiting *Candida*, as well as other pathogenic bacteria, prevents the overgrowth of yeast that is a common side-effect of antibiotic use. Table 91.1 lists the in vitro sensitivity of various organisms to berberine sulphate.

The antimicrobial activity of berberine increases with pH in all organisms studied.[5] At pH of 8.0, its antimicrobial activity in vitro is typically two to four times greater than it is at pH 7.0, which in turn is one to four times greater than at pH 6.0. This suggests that alkalinization will improve its clinical efficacy, particularly in the treatment of urinary tract infections.

Table 91.1 In vitro sensitivity of microorganisms to berberine sulphate[5,6,9]

Organism	Inhibitory concentration (μg/ml)*
Bacteria	
Bacillus cereus	25.0
B. cereus	50.0
B. subtilis	25.0
Corynebacterium diphtheria	6.2
Enterobacter aerogenes	2500.05
Escherichia coli	600.05
Klebsiella sp.	>100.0
K. pneumoniae	25.0
Proteus sp.	>100.0
Pseudomonas mangiferae	>100.0
P. pyocyanea	>100.0
Salmonella paratyphi	>100.0
S. typhimurium	>100.0
Shigella boydii	12.5
Staphylococcus aureus	6.2–50.0
Streptococcus pyogenes	12.5
Vibrio cholerae	25.0
Fungi	
Candida utilis	12.5
C. albicans	12.5
Cryptococcus neoformans	150.0 –
Microsporum gypseum	50.0 –
Saccharomyces cerevisiae	100.0 –
Sporothrix schenkii	6.2
Trichophyton mentagrophytes	100.0 –
Other	
Entamoeba histolytica	200.0
Erwinia carotovora	100.0
Leishmania donovani	5.08
Mycobacterium tuberculosis	200.0 –
Xanthomonas citri	3.1

*Minimum concentration that totally inhibits growth in a liquid medium at pH 8.0. Maximum concentration tested was 100 μg/ml, unless otherwise noted.
~Tested in a solid medium, which typically requires a four to 10 times greater concentration for the same level of inhibition.

Anti-infective activity

Researchers investigated berberine's ability to inhibit the adherence of group A streptococci to host cells based on the fact that the therapeutic effect of berberine appeared to be greater than its direct antibiotic effects.[11] Recent studies have shown that certain antimicrobial agents can block the adherence of microorganisms to host cells at doses much lower than those needed to kill cells or to inhibit cell growth.

Berberine's ability to inhibit the adhesion of streptococci to host cells has several modes of action. First, berberine causes streptococci to lose lipoteichoic acid (LTA). LTA is the major substance responsible for the adhesion of the bacteria to host tissues. Another important action of berberine is preventing the adhesion of fibronectin to the streptococci as well as eluting already bound fibronectin.

The significance of the results of this study are quite profound. It raises many questions and forces researchers as well as practitioners to look at the treatment of bacterial infections in a new light. Is it better to utilize a substance with bactericidal or bacteriostatic actions over a substance which prevents the adherence of bacteria to host cells? Is the true value of botanicals with "anti-infective" actions a multifactorial effect on all aspects of infections from immune stimulation to antimicrobial and anti-adherence actions?

The results of the study indicate that berberine interferes with infections due to group A streptococci not only by inhibiting streptococcal growth, but also by blocking these organisms to host cells. The study implies berberine-containing plants may be ideal in the treatment of "strep throat", a condition historically treated with goldenseal by American naturopathic physicians. Berberine's action in inhibiting *Candida albicans* prevents the overgrowth of yeast that is a common side-effect of antibiotic use.

Immunostimulatory activity

Berberine has been shown to increase the blood supply to the spleen.[12] This improved blood supply may promote optimal activity of the spleen by increasing the release of compounds, such as tuftsin, that potentiate immune function. Berberine has also been shown to activate macrophages, via both enhanced priming and triggering.[13]

Anti-cancer effects

Berberine exhibits potent anti-cancer activity both directly by killing tumor cells and indirectly by stimulating white blood cells.[13–15] The most impressive effect was noted in a study demonstrating antitumor activity against human and rat malignant brain tumors.[15] Several experimental approaches were used in the study. In vitro studies were performed on a series of six human malignant brain tumor cell lines and rat 9L brain tumor cells. Berberine used alone at a dose of 150 mcg/ml showed an average cancer cell kill of 91%. This kill rate was over twice that of 1,3-*bis*(2-chloro-ethyl)-1-nitrosourea (BCNU), the standard chemotherapeutic agent for brain tumors, which had a cell kill rate of 43%. Studies in rats harboring solid 9L brain tumors also showed that berberine has antitumor effects. Rats treated with berberine, 10 mg/kg, had a 81% cell kill. However, the combination treatment, berberine and BCNU, exihibited additive effects on killing cancer cells. These results indicate that berberine may prove to be more effective than BCNU or, at the very least, a valuable therapeutic addition in the treatment of difficult brain cancers.

Antipyretic activity

Historically, berberine-containing plants have been used as febrifuges. Berberine produces an antipyretic effect three times as potent as aspirin in a pyretic model in rats.[16] However, while aspirin suppresses fever through its action on prostaglandins, berberine appears to lower fever by increasing the immune system's handling of fever-producing compounds from microorganisms.

CLINICAL APPLICATIONS

The broad antimicrobial effects of berberine combined with its anti-infective and immune-stimulating actions supports the historical use of berberine-containing plants in infections of the mucous membranes. Berberine-containing plants may also be useful as an adjunct to standard cancer therapy.

Infectious diarrhea

Berberine has shown significant success in the treatment of acute diarrhea in several clinical studies. It has been found effective against diarrheas caused by *E. coli* (traveler's diarrhea), *Shigella dysenteriae* (shigellosis), *Salmonella paratyphi* (food poisoning), *Klebsiella* sp., *Giardia lamblia* (giardiasis), and *Vibrio cholerae* (cholera).[17–27] Studies in hamsters and rats have shown that berberine also has significant activity against *Entamoeba histolytica*, the causative organism of amebiasis.[7,8]

It appears that berberine is effective in treating the majority of common gastrointestinal infections. The clinical studies have produced results with berberine comparable to standard antibiotics in most cases. In fact, in several studies results were better.

For example, in a study of 65 children below 5 years of age with acute diarrhea caused by *E. coli, Shigella, Salmonella, Klebsiella* or *Faecalis aerogenes*, those given berberine tannate (25 mg/every 6 hours) responded better than those treated with standard antibiotic therapy.[22]

In another study, 40 children aged 1–10 years infected with the parasite giardia received either berberine (5 mg/kg body weight each day), the drug metronidazole (10 mg/kg body weight each day), or a placebo of vitamin B syrup in three divided doses.[23] After 6 days, 48% of patients treated with berberine were symptom-free and, on stool analysis, 68% were *Giardia*-free. In the metronidazole (Flagyl) group, 33% of patients were without symptoms and, on stool analysis, all were *Giardia*-free. In comparison, 15% of patients on placebo were asymptomatic and, on stool analysis, 25% were *Giardia*-free. These results indicate that berberine was actually more effective than metronidazole in relieving symptoms at half the dose, but was less effective than the drug in clearing the organism from the intestines.

And finally, in a study of 200 adult patients with acute diarrhea, the subjects were given standard antibiotic treatment with or without berberine hydrochloride (150 mg/day). The patients receiving berberine recovered more quickly.[24] An additional 30 cases of acute diarrhea were treated with berberine alone. Berberine arrested diarrhea in all of these cases with no mortality or toxicity.

Despite these results, due to the serious consequences of an ineffectively treated infectious diarrhea due to highly pathogenic organisms, the best approach may be to use berberine-containing plants as an adjunct to standard antibiotic therapy.

Much of berberine's effectiveness is undoubtedly due to a combination of its direct antimicrobial activity, inhibition of microbial attachment to mucous membranes and blocking of the action of toxins produced by several pathogenic bacteria.[28–30] The toxin-blocking effect is most evident in diarrheas caused by enterotoxins (e.g., *Vibrio cholerae* and *E. coli*), cholera and traveler's diarrhea respectively.[25–28]

While cholera is a serious disorder that needs standard antibiotic therapy, traveler's diarrhea is usually self-limiting. Good results with berberine in the treatment of traveler's diarrhea have been obtained. In one study, patients with traveler's diarrhea randomly received berberine sulfate 400 mg in a single dose or served as controls.[27] In treated patients, the mean stool volumes were significantly less than those of controls during three consecutive 8 hour periods after treatment. At 24 hours after treatment, significantly more treated patients stopped having diarrhea as compared with controls (42% vs. 20%).

For those patients planning to travel to an underdeveloped country or an area of poor water quality or sanitation, the prophylactic use of berberine-containing herbs during, and 1 week prior to and after visiting may be useful.

Trachoma

Water extracts of berberine-containing plants have been employed in a variety of eye complaints, including infectious processes, by cultures throughout the world. Recently, berberine has shown remarkable effect in the treatment of trachoma.[31,32] Trachoma, an infectious eye disease due to the organism *Chlamydia trachomatis*, is a major cause of blindness and impaired vision in underdeveloped countries. It affects approximately 500 million people worldwide, and results in blindness in 2 million.

The drug sulphacetamide is currently the most widely used anti-trachoma drug. In clinical trials comparing berberine (0.2%) and sulphacetamide (20.0% solution), sulphacetamide showed the best improvement (decrease in conjunctival discharge, edema, and papillary reactions), but the conjunctival scrapings of all patients receiving sulphacetamide were still positive for *Chlamydia trachomatis*. These patients had a high rate of recurrence of the symptoms. In contrast, patients treated with the berberine solution showed very mild ocular symptoms, which disappeared more gradually, but their conjunctival scrapings were always negative for *Chlamydia trachomatis*. These patients did not suffer relapse even 1 year after treatment, which suggests that berberine is probably curative for trachoma.[31,32]

Berberine's efficacy is believed to be due to stimulation of some host defense mechanism, rather than simply a direct action on the organism. As the berberine concentration used in these studies was 100 times less than the concentration of sulphacetamide, and berberine is much cheaper, it may be more cost-effective than other treatments for trachoma. Berberine (0.2% solution) is an appropriate therapy for many types of conjunctivitis.

Cholecystitis and cirrhosis of the liver

Berberine has been shown in several clinical studies to stimulate the secretion of bile (cholerectic effect) and bilirubin.[33–35] In one study of 225 patients with chronic cholecystitis, oral berberine doses of 5–20 mg three times a day before meals caused, over a period of 24–48 hours, disappearance of clinical symptoms, decrease in bilirubin level, and an increase in the bile volume of the gall bladder.

Berberine has been shown to correct the hypertyraminemia of patients with liver cirrhosis. It prevents the elevation of serum tyramine following oral tyrosine load by inhibiting the enzyme tyrosine decarboxylase found in bacteria in the large intestine.[35] Berberine inhibits tyrosine decarboxylase and tryptophanase activities of *Streptococcus faecalis* and *E. coli*, but not those of animal enzymes. Tyramine is believed to be responsible for some of the cardiovascular and neurological complications of liver disease, such as hepatic encephalopathy. The accumulation of tyramine and its derivatives may cause lowering of peripheral resistance, with resultant high cardiac output, reduction in renal function, and cerebral dysfunction. Berberine, by lowering plasma tyramine levels, helps prevent the complications of cirrhosis. This tyramine-lowering effect of berberine may have significance in other conditions as well.

Cancer

Berberine and another alkaloid found in berberine-containing plants, berbamine, have been shown to exert beneficial effects as adjuncts in cancer therapy. In fact, berbamine has been used in China since 1972 in the treatment of depressed white blood cell (WBC) counts due to chemotherapy and/or radiation.

In one study, 405 patients with WBC counts < 4,000 were given 150 mg of berbamine daily (50 mg orally three times daily) for 1–4 weeks. Berbamine was viewed as "significantly effective" if WBC increased to > 4,000 after 1 week or increased to > 1,000 after 2 weeks; "effective" if WBC increased to > 4,000 after 2 weeks or increased > 1,000 after 4 weeks; and "ineffective" if there was no change in WBC after 4 weeks of treatment. The overall results for the 405 patients are as follows:

- significantly effective in 163 cases (40.2%)
- effective in 125 cases (38.8%)
- ineffective in 117 cases (29%).

The total effective rate was 71%. However, WBC before therapy was related to overall effectiveness. The effective rate was only 54.8% in 31 cases where WBC was < 1,000 and 82.7% in cases where WBC count was between 3,100 and 3,800.[36]

DOSAGES

As no detailed clinical studies have differentiated which berberine-containing herb to use for specific conditions, the following is offered only as a guideline based on experimental studies and historical use. However, the plants can be viewed as interchangeable.

Hydrastis canadensis. This is used in the treatment of:

- infective, congestive and inflammatory states of the mucous membranes
- digestive disorders
- gastritis
- peptic ulcers
- colitis
- anorexia
- painful menstruation.

Berberis vulgaris. This is used in the treatment of gall bladder disease, including gallstones, and as a less expensive form of berberine in the treatment of the conditions listed above for hydrastis.

Berberis aquifolium. This is used in the treatment of chronic skin diseases and in the conditions listed above for hydrastis.

Coptis chinensis. This is used in the treatment of infective, congestive and inflammatory states of the mucous membranes, fever, and infectious disorders of the skin.

The dosage should be based on berberine content. As there is a wide range of quality in goldenseal preparations, standardized extracts are recommended. Three times a day dosages as follows:

- dried root or as infusion (tea): 2–4 g
- tincture (1:5): 6–12 ml (1.5–3 tsp)
- fluid extract (1:1): 2–4 ml (0.5–1 tsp)
- solid (powdered dry) extract (4:1 or 8–12% alkaloid content): 250–500 mg.

TOXICITY

Berberine and berberine-containing plants are generally non-toxic at the recommended dosages. However, berberine-containing plants are not recommended for use during pregnancy and higher dosages may interfere with B vitamin metabolism.

The oral LD_{50} in rats for berberine is greater than 1,000 mg/kg body weight, indicating that the toxicity is extremely low.[37]

REFERENCES

1. Duke JA. Handbook of medicinal herbs. Boca Raton, Fl: CRC Press. 1985: p 78, 238–239, 287–288
2. Leung AY. Encyclopedia of common natural ingredients used in food, drugs, and cosmetics. New York, NY: John Wiley. 1980: p 52–53, 189–190
3. Chang HM, But PPH. Pharmacology and applications of Chinese materia medica, Vol. 2. Teaneck, NJ: World Scientific. 1987: p 1029–1040
4. Hahn FE, Ciak J. Berberine. Antibiotics 1976; 3: 577–588
5. Amin AH, Subbaiah TV, Abbasi KM. Berberine sulfate. Antimicrobial activity, bioassay, and mode of action. Can J Microbiol 1969; 15: 1067–1076
6. Johnson CC, Johnson G, Poe CF. Toxicity of alkaloids to certain bacteria. Acta Pharmacol Toxicol 1952; 8: 71–78
7. Kaneda Y et al. In vitro effects of berberine sulfate on the growth of *Entamoeba histolytica, Giardia lamblia* and *Tricomonas vaginalis.* Annals Trop Med Parasitol 1991; 85: 417–425
8. Subbaiah TV, Amin AH. Effect of berberine sulfate on *Entamoeba histolytica*. Nature 1967; 215: 527–528
9. Ghosh AK. Effect of berberine chloride on *Leishmania donovani.* Ind J Med Res 1983; 78: 407–416
10. Majahan VM, Sharma A, Rattan A. Antimycotic activity of berberine sulphate. An alkaloid from an Indian medicinal herb. Sabouraudia 1982; 20: 79–81
11. Sun D, Courtney HS, Beachey EH. Berberine sulfate blocks adherence of *Streptococcus pyogenes* to epithelial cells, fibronectin, and hexadecane. Antimicrobial Agents and Chemotherapy 1988; 32: 1370–1374
12. Sabir M, Bhide N. Study of some pharmacologic actions of berberine. Ind J Physiol Pharm 1971; 15: 111–132
13. Kumazawa Y, Itagaki A, Fukumoto M et al. Activation of peritoneal macrophages by berberine alkaloids in terms of induction of cytostatic activity. Int J Immunopharmacol 1984; 6: 587–592
14. Sabir M, Akhter MH, Bhide NK. Further studies on pharmacology of berberine. Ind J Physiol Pharmacol 1978; 22: 9–23
15. Rong-xun Z et al. Laboratory studies of berberine used alone and in combination with 1,3-bis(2-chloroethyl)-1-nitrosourea to treat malignant brain tumors. Chinese Med J 1990; 103: 658–665
16. Nishino H et al. Berberine sulfate inhibits tumor-promoting activity of teleocidin in two-stage carcinogenesis on mouse skin. Oncology 1986; 43: 131–134
17. Gupta S. Use of berberine in the treatment of giardiasis. Am J Dis Child 1975; 129: 866
18. Bhakat MP, Nandi N, Pal HK et al. Therapeutic trial of berberine sulphate in non-specific gastroenteritis. Ind Med J 1974; 68: 19–23
19. Kamat SA. Clinical trial with berberine hydrochloride for the control of diarrhoea in acute gastroenteritis. J Assoc Physicians India 1967; 15: 525–529
20. Desai AB, Shah KM, Shah DM. Berberine in the treatment of diarrhoea. Ind Pediatr 1971; 8: 462–465
21. Sharma R, Joshi CK, Goyal RK. Berberine tannate in acute diarrhea. Ind Pediatr 1970; 7: 496–501
22. Sack RB, Froehlich JL. Berberine inhibits intestinal secretory response of *Vibrio cholerae* toxins and *Escherichia coli* enterotoxins. Infect Immun 1982; 35: 471–475
23. Choudry VP, Sabir M, Bhide VN. Berberine in giardiasis. Ind Pediatr 1972; 9: 143–146
24. Kamat SA. Clinical trial with berberine hydrochloride for the control of diarrhoea in acute gastroenteritis. J Assoc Physicians India 1967; 15: 525–529
25. Khin-Maung-U, Myo-Khin, Nyunt-Wai et al. Clinical trial of berberine in acute watery diarrhoea. Br Med J 1985; 291: 1601–1605
26. Gupte S. Use of berberine in treatment of giardiasis. Am J Dis Child 1975; 129: 866
27. Rabbani GH et al. Randomized controlled trial of berberine sulfate therapy for diarrhea due to enterotoxigenic *Escherichia coli* and *Vibrio cholerae.* J Infect Dis 1987; 155: 979–984
28. Akhter MH, Sabir M, Bhide NK. Possible mechanism of antidiarrhoeal effect of berberine, Ind J Med Res 1979; 70: 233–241
29. Tai YH, Feser JF, Mernane WG, Desjeux JF. Antisecretory effects of berberine in rat ileum. Am J Physiol 1981; 241: G253–258
30. Swabb EA, Tai YH, Jordan L. Reversal of cholera toxin-induced secretion in rat ileum by luminal berberine. Am J Physiol 1981; 241: G248–252
31. Babbar OP, Chatwal VK, Ray IB et al. Effect of berberine chloride eye drops on clinically positive trachoma patients. Ind J Med Res 1982; 76: 83–88
32. Mohan M, Pant CR, Angra SK, Mahajan VM. Berberine in trachoma. Ind J Opthalmol 1982; 30: 69–75
33. Preininger V. The pharmacology and toxicology of the papaveraceae alkaloids. Alkaloids 1975; 15: 207–251

34. Chan MY. The effect of berberine on bilirubin excretion in the rat. Comp Med East West 1977; 5: 161–168
35. Watanabe A, Obata T, Nagashima H. Berberine therapy of hypertyraminemia in patients with liver cirrhosis. Acta Med Okayama 1982; 36: 277–281
36. Liu CX et al. Studies on plant resources, pharmacology and clinical treatment with berbamine. Phytother Res 1991; 5: 228–230
37. Hladon B. Toxicity of berberine sulfate. Acta Pol Pharm 1975; 32: 113–120

CHAPTER CONTENTS

92

5-Hydroxytryptophan

Michael T. Murray, ND

Joseph E. Pizzorno Jr, ND

INTRODUCTION

5-Hydroxytryptophan (5-HTP) is the intermediate between tryptophan and serotonin. Although 5-HTP may be relatively new to most clinicians, it has been available through pharmacies for several years and has been intensely researched for the past three decades. It has been used clinically since the 1970s.

TRYPTOPHAN AND 5-HTP METABOLISM

Once tryptophan is absorbed from the intestines, it is carried by the blood to the liver along with the other amino acids consumed during the meal. Ingested tryptophan can pass into the general circulation, it can be metabolized into blood proteins, or it can be converted to kynurenine (which then goes on to form nicotinic acid, picolinate and other important metabolites) in the liver. After conversion to kynurenine, it cannot be converted to serotonin. The same is likely true if the tryptophan is incorporated into blood proteins. Unchanged tryptophan can be converted to 5-HTP and then to serotonin. However, if this conversion occurs outside the brain, brain chemistry will not be influenced, and even under the best-case scenario only 3% of a dosage of L-tryptophan in supplemental or dietary form is likely to be converted to serotonin in the brain.[1]

The manufacture of serotonin from tryptophan within the brain is highly dependent upon the level of tryptophan or 5-HTP which crosses the blood–brain barrier. While 5-HTP easily crosses the blood–brain barrier, the delivery of tryptophan into the brain is dependent upon several factors. The first factor of importance is the level of free tryptophan in the blood. There are a number of situations where the liver's conversion of tryptophan to kynurenine takes place at an elevated rate, i.e. stress, elevated cortisol levels, low B-vitamin status, and high dosages of L-tryptophan (i.e. greater than 2,000 mg). All of these situations lead to increased activity of the enzymes (tryptophan oxidase and kynurenine formamidase) that convert tryptophan to kynurenine. Elevated levels of kynurenine block the entry of tryptophan into the brain and lower brain serotonin levels. Increasing tryptophan intake makes matters worse when tryptophan oxidase activity is increased.

Unlike 5-HTP, which easily enters the brain, the transport of tryptophan across the blood–brain barrier involves the binding of tryptophan to a transport molecule. As tryptophan shares this transport vehicle with several other amino acids, when the ratio of tryptophan to these other amino acids is low (i.e. when the level of tryptophan is low and the level of the other amino acids is high), very little tryptophan is transported into the brain. The protein in almost all foods contains relatively small amounts of tryptophan and larger proportions of other amino acids. This low ratio of tryptophan to the other amino acids generally leads to low serotonin levels with a high-protein intake. Just the opposite occurs with a high-carbohydrate meal.

PHARMACOLOGY

Several pharmacokinetic studies have shown that about 70% of a dosage of 5-HTP taken orally is delivered to the bloodstream.[2,3] The remaining 30% is metabolized by intestinal cells.

Once absorbed, there is ample evidence from these pharmacokinetic studies as well as the clinical studies that 5-HTP is delivered to the brain, resulting in increased formation of not only serotonin, but also other brain chemicals such as other monoamines like melatonin, endorphins, dopamine, and norepinephrine. By raising brain serotonin levels (as well as by other effects), 5-HTP has shown positive effects in the various conditions associated with low serotonin levels.

Besides raising serotonin and melatonin levels, 5-HTP has been shown to raise beta-endorphin levels. Much of the pain-relieving and mood-elevating benefits of 5-HTP may be related more to its ability to enhance endorphin levels than to its ability to increase serotonin levels. This endorphin-increasing action is useful for both migraine and tension headache, fibromyalgia, as well other painful situations. In addition, raising endorphin levels produces significant effects on mood and behavior.

By raising serotonin (and melatonin) and beta-endorphin levels, 5-HTP produces a significant impact on helping to regulate and improve brain chemistry. But it goes well beyond affecting these systems, as 5-HTP has been shown also to raise the levels of other important neurotransmitters such as dopamine and norepinephrine.[4] The ability of 5-HTP to increase both serotonin (and other indoleamines) and catecholamines is quite significant and unique to 5-HTP. It is an effect that 5-HTP does not share with L-tryptophan. The effective treatment of depression requires more than simply raising serotonin levels; catecholamine levels must also be increased. 5-HTP provides the brain with both sets of tools.

In a head-to-head comparison study of 5-HTP and L-tryptophan in the treatment of depression, 5-HTP proved superior.[5] The proposed reason is the fact that 5-HTP easily crosses the blood–brain barrier and is not affected by competing amino acids and 5-HTP affects brain chemistry in a broader and more positive fashion. L-Tryptophan is often effective in cases of low serotonin, especially insomnia, but 5-HTP is more broadly effective.

5-HTP vs. L-tryptophan

Nutrition-oriented physicians have long used precursor therapy for affecting brain chemistry. Unfortunately, L-tryptophan has produced inconsistent results. These inconsistent results are likely due to its inconsistent elevation of brain serotonin level.

There are many advantages of 5-HTP over L-tryptophan. Chief among them are that 5-HTP easily crosses the blood–brain barrier and is one step further on the path to serotonin synthesis. The conversion of tryptophan to 5-HTP by tryptophan hydrolase is the most important step in the manufacture of serotonin. This enzyme is inhibited by a number of factors, including:

- stress
- vitamin B_6 insufficiency
- low magnesium levels
- insensitivity to insulin
- various hormones
- genetic factors.

In addition, as noted above, these same factors and others are known to increase the activity of tryptophan oxygenase, increasing the conversion of L-tryptophan to kynurenine.

Perhaps the biggest advantage of 5-HTP over L-tryptophan is that it is safer. Although L-tryptophan is safe if properly prepared and free of the contaminants linked to eosinophilia myalgia syndrome (EMS), 5-HTP is inherently safer. The reasons are that taking L-tryptophan to produce positive effects in the treatment of depression, insomnia, and other low serotonin conditions requires a relatively high dosage (e.g. a minimum of 2,000 mg in insomnia and 6,000 mg in depression). At high dosages such as these, L-tryptophan is potentially problematic, as more L-tryptophan will be shunted towards the kynurenine pathway and L-tryptophan promotes oxidative damage. Excessive levels of dietary tryptophan or high dosages of L-tryptophan result in tryptophan actually acting as a free radical.[6] By contrast, 5-HTP is an antioxidant.[7] This antioxidant difference is due to the additional molecule of oxygen and hydrogen in 5-HTP. This simple change in molecular structure allows the phenolic ring structure to effectively accept or quench the unpaired electron of a free radical.

CLINICAL APPLICATIONS

There is a massive amount of evidence that suggests that low serotonin levels are a common consequence of modern living. The lifestyle and dietary practices of many people living in this stress-filled era result in lowered levels of serotonin within the brain. As a result, many people are overweight, crave sugar and other carbohydrates, experience bouts of depression, get frequent headaches, and have vague muscle aches and pain. All of these maladies are correctable by raising brain serotonin levels. The primary therapeutic applications for 5-HTP are low serotonin states, as listed in Table 92.1.

Depression

Some of the first clinical studies on 5-HTP for the treatment of depression began in the early 1970s in Japan. The first study involved 107 patients with either unipolar depression or manic bipolar depression.[8] These patients received 5-HTP at dosages ranging from 50 to 300 mg/day. The researchers observed a very quick response (within 2 weeks) in more than half of the patients. Seventy-four of the patients either experienced complete relief or were significantly improved, and none experienced significant side-effects. These promising results were repeated in several other Japanese studies. One of the interesting aspects in two of these studies was the fact that 5-HTP was shown to be effective in some patients (50% in one study, 35% in another) who had not responded positively to any other antidepressant agent.[9,10]

Table 92.1 Conditions associated with low serotonin levels

- Depression
- Anxiety
- Obsessive compulsive disorder
- Obesity
- Carbohydrate craving
- Bulimia
- Insomnia
- Narcolepsy
- Sleep apnea
- Migraine headaches
- Tension headaches
- Chronic daily headaches
- Premenstrual syndrome
- Fibromyalgia
- Epilepsy
- Myoclonus
- Chronic pain disorders

The most detailed of the Japanese studies was conducted in 1978.[11] The study enrolled 59 patients with depression: 30 were male and 29 were female. The groups were mixed, in that both unipolar and bipolar depressions were included along with a number of other subcategories of depression. The severity of the depression in most cases was moderate to severe. Patients received 5-HTP in dosages of 50 or 100 mg three times daily for at least 3 weeks.

The antidepressant activity and clinical effectiveness of 5-HTP was determined by using a rating scale developed by the Clinical Psychopharmacology Research Group in Japan. The improvements among the various patients are detailed in Table 92.2. These results indicate that 5-HTP was helpful in 14 out of 17 patients with unipolar depression and 12 out of 21 patients with bipolar depression. The degree of improvement in most cases ranged from excellent to very good.

The results achieved in this open study are quite good, given how rapidly they were achieved. Thirty-two of the 40 patients who responded to 5-HTP did so within the first 2 weeks of therapy. Typically, in most studies with antidepressant drugs the benefits are not apparent until after 2 weeks to 1 month of use. For this reason, the length of study when assessing antidepressant drugs should be at least 6 weeks, because it may take that long to significantly affect brain chemistry in a positive manner. In contrast, many of the studies with 5-HTP were shorter than 6 weeks because statistically significant results were achieved so soon (Table 92.3). However, the longer 5-HTP is used, the better are the results. Some people

Table 92.2 Improvement in various subtypes of depression

Subtype	Improvement[a]						
	1	2	3	4	5, 6, 7	8	1+2+3/total[b]
First-episode depression	1	1	0	1	0	0	2/3
Unipolar depression	3	8	3	1	2	0	14/17
Bipolar depression	6	4	2	3	3	3	12/21
Mixed depression	0	1	0	1	0	0	1/2
Presenile or senile depression	3	2	0	3	1	0	5/9
Neurotic depression	0	1	2	1	0	0	3/4
Reactive depression	0	1	1	0	0	0	2/2
Schizophrenic depression	0	1	0	0	0	0	1/1
Total	13	19	8	10	6	3	40/59
Percentage of total (%)	22.0	32.2	13.6	16.9	10.2	5.1	67.8%

[a]Improvement: 1, marked improvement; 2, moderately improved; 3, slightly improved; 4, unchanged; 5, 6, 7 felt worse; 8, dropped out.
[b]The number of subjects that improved (improvement scores 1, 2 or 3) compared with the total number of subjects in that subtype.

Table 92.3 Day when improvements were first noticed

Improvement group	Day 1	Day 2	Day 3	Days 4–7	Days 8–14	Day 15
Marked	1	3	2	5	2	0
Moderate	0	1	13	1	4	0
Slight	0	2	2	2	1	1
Total	1	6	17	8	7	1

may need to be on 5-HTP for at least 2 months before they experience the benefits.

The only major side-effect noted in this study was mild nausea. The occurrence of nausea due to 5-HTP is actually less frequent than that experienced with other antidepressant drugs (roughly 10% of subjects taking 5-HTP at a daily dosage equal to or less than 300 mg experience nausea compared with about 23% taking Prozac) and about the same as that which occurs with a placebo. In double-blind studies, about 10% or so of people taking the placebo typically complain of nausea. Nonetheless, very mild nausea may be a natural consequence of elevated serotonin levels with 5-HTP. About 30% of the 5-HTP taken orally is converted to serotonin in the intestinal tract. This can lead to a mild case of nausea. Fortunately, this effect wears off after a few of weeks of use.

A 5-HTP dosage of 300 mg is sufficient in most cases, but in some cases a higher dosage may be necessary. For example, in one study it was shown that 13 out of 18 subjects with depression given 5-HTP at a level of 150 or 300 mg/day experienced good to excellent results.[12] This percentage of responders is quite good, but if we look at the level of serotonin in the blood as a rough indicator of brain serotonin levels, some interesting conclusions can be made (see Table 92.4).

The measurements in Table 92.4 suggest that serotonin levels in depressed individuals are considerably lower than those found in normal subjects and that individuals who respond to 5-HTP show a rise in serotonin to levels consistent with normal subjects. The level of serotonin in those who do not respond to 5-HTP remained quite low. These results imply that non-responders may require higher dosages to raise serotonin levels or that additional support may be necessary. When prescribing higher dosages, it is important that the 5-HTP be taken in divided dosages not only to reduce the problem with nausea, but also because rate of brain cell uptake of 5-HTP is limited.

Table 92.4 Level of serotonin in blood (ng/ml): controls, responders, and non-responders

	Before	After 1 week (150 or 300 mg/day 5-HTP)
Normal subjects	150	
Responders	78	148
Non-responders	56	77

The first studies of 5-HTP in a double-blind format (the Japanese studies) were open trials.[13] The antidepressive effects of 5-HTP were also compared with L-tryptophan in the early 1970s.[5] In one study, 45 subjects with depression were given L-tryptophan (5 g/day), 5-HTP (200 mg/day), or a placebo. The patients were matched in clinical features (age, sex, etc.) and severity of depression. The main outcome measure was the Hamilton Rating Scale for Depression (HDS), the most widely used assessment tool in clinical research in depression.

The HDS score is determined by having the test subject complete a series of questions where they rate the severity of their symptoms on a numerical basis, as follows:

- 0 – not present
- 1 – present but mild
- 2 – moderate
- 3 – severe
- 4 – very severe.

Symptoms assessed by the HDS include depression, feelings of guilt, insomnia, gastrointestinal symptoms and other bodily symptoms of depression (e.g. headaches, muscle aches, heart palpitations, etc.), and anxiety. The HDS is popular in research because it provides a good assessment of the overall symptoms of depression. Table 92.5 shows the results of the study.

A review of head-to-head comparison studies showed that 5-HTP, at a dosage of 200 mg/day, produced therapeutic success on a par with tricyclic antidepressant drugs.[14] Research has also shown that combining 5-HTP with clomipramine and other types of antidepressant drugs produces better results than any of the compound given alone.[15–20] For example, in one study, 5-HTP combined with a monoamine oxidase (MAO) inhibitor demonstrated significant advantages compared with the MAO inhibitor alone (see Table 92.6).[19]

This line of research suggests that 5-HTP might also be used in conjunction with St John's wort extract or *Ginkgo biloba* extract, two herbal medicines with proven antidepressant activity.

Table 92.5 HDS from a comparative study of HTP, L-tryptophan and placebo

	5-HTP	L-Tryptophan	Placebo
Beginning of the study	26	25	23
End of the study (30 days)	9	15	19

Table 92.6 Change in Hamilton Rating Scale for depression[19]

	5-HTP + MAO	MAO + placebo
Initial measurement	28.67	26.33
After 8 days	16.67	19.23
After 15 days	11.77	6.03

Because 5-HTP was very expensive back in 1972, researchers developed a test to determine who was most likely to respond to it, so that it would not be wasted on people who were unlikely to respond.[13,21–23] The test involved the patients first having a spinal tap to measure the level of 5-HIAA (the breakdown product of serotonin) in the cerebrospinal fluid (CSF). The drug probenecid, which prevents the transport of 5-HIAA from the CSF to the bloodstream, was given for the next 3 days. As a result of this blocking action the amount of serotonin produced over a 4 day period could be calculated by a repeat spinal tap on day 4. Since the 5-HIAA could not leave the CSF, it accumulated and provided a measure of serotonin manufacture.

The researchers discovered that the average level of 5-HIAA after 3 days of probenecid was significantly lower in depressed individuals than in controls matched for age, sex, and weight. This low level of serotonin reflected a decreased rate of manufacture within the brain. 5-HTP was most effective in patients with a low 5-HIAA response to 3 days of probenecid.[21–23] In other words, 5-HTP is most effective as an antidepressant when the amount of serotonin manufactured in the brain is reduced.

As stated above, 5-HTP will often produce very good results in patients who are unresponsive to antidepressant drugs. One of the more impressive studies involved 99 patients described as suffering from "therapy-resistant" depression.[24] These patients had not responded to any previous therapy including all available antidepressant drugs and electroconvulsive therapy. These therapy-resistant patients received 5-HTP at dosages averaging 200 mg/day but ranging from 50 to 600 mg/day. Complete recovery was seen in 43 of the 99 patients and significant improvement was noted in eight more. Such significant improvement in patients suffering from long-standing, unresponsive depression is quite impressive, prompting the author of another study to state:[25]

> L-5-HTP merits a place in the front of the ranks of the antidepressants instead of being used as a last resort. I have never in 20 years used an agent which: (1) was effective so quickly; (2) restored the patients so completely to the persons they had been and their partners had known; [and] (3) was so entirely without side-effects.

A 1987 review article on 5-HTP in depression highlighted the need for well-designed double blind, head-to-head studies of 5-HTP versus standard antidepressant drugs.[26] Although 5-HTP was viewed as an antidepressant agent with few side-effects, the authors of this review felt that the big question to answer was how 5-HTP compared with the new breed of antidepressant drugs, the selective serotonin reuptake inhibitors like Prozac, Paxil, and Zoloft. In 1991, a double-blind study comparing 5-HTP with a selective serotonin reuptake inhibitor (SSRI) was conducted in Switzerland.[27] 5-HTP was compared in the study with the SSRI fluvoxamine (Luvox). Fluvoxamine is used primarily in the United States as a treatment for obsessive compulsive disorder (OCD), an anxiety disorder characterized by obsessions and compulsions affecting an estimated 5 million Americans. Fluvoxamine exerts antidepressant activity comparable to (if not better than) other SSRIs like Prozac, Zoloft, and Paxil.

In the study, subjects received either 5-HTP (100 mg) or fluvoxamine (50 mg) three times daily for 6 weeks. The assessment methods used to judge effectiveness included the Hamilton Rating Scale for Depression (HSD), self-assessment depression scale (SADS), and physician's assessment (Clinical Global Impression). As can be seen in Table 92.7, the percentage decrease in depression was slightly better in the 5-HTP group (60.7% vs. 56.1%). 5-HTP was quicker acting than the fluvoxamine and a

Table 92.7 5-HTP vs. fluvoxamine in percentage changes in the HDS

	Decrease in HDS	5-HTP (*n* = 34)	Fluvoxamine (*n* = 29)
After 2 weeks	Mean decrease (%)	23	18.9
	Less than 35% decrease	20	19
	35–50% decrease	10	8
	50–75% decrease	4	2
After 4 weeks	Mean decrease (%)	46.2	46.1
	Less than 35% decrease	2	8
	35–50% decrease	7	3
	50–75% decrease	12	13
	More than 75% decrease	3	5
After 6 weeks	Mean decrease (%)	60.7	56.1
	Less than 35% decrease	4	5
	35–50% decrease	8	3
	50–75% decrease	12	8
	More than 75% decrease	10	13

higher percentage of patients responded to 5-HTP than to fluvoxamine.

The advantages of 5-HTP over fluvoxamine are evident when looking at the subcategories of the HDS: depressed mood, anxiety, physical symptoms, and insomnia. For depressed mood, 5-HTP produced a 65.7% reduction in severity compared with 61.8% for fluvoxamine; for anxiety, 5-HTP produced a 58.2% reduction in severity compared with 48.3% for fluvoxamine; for physical symptoms, 5-HTP produced a 47.6% decrease in severity compared with 37.8% for fluvoxamine; and, for insomnia 5-HTP produced a 61.7% decrease in severity compared with a 55.9% decrease for fluvoxamine. However, perhaps more important than simply relieving insomnia is 5-HTP's ability to improve the quality of sleep. By contrast, antidepressant drugs greatly disrupt sleep processes. On the self-assessment depression scale (SADS), 5-HTP produced a 53.3% drop in SADS values compared with a drop of 47.6% for the fluvoxamine group. Anything over a 50% drop is an excellent result. In fact, a 50% drop is the best SSRIs generally produce.

5-HTP is equal to or better than standard antidepressant drugs and the side-effects are much less severe (see Table 92.8). In the study comparing 5-HTP with fluvoxamine, this is how the physicians described the differences among the two groups:

> Whereas the two treatment groups did not differ significantly in the number of patients sustaining adverse events, the interaction between the degree of severity and the type of medication was highly significant: fluvoxamine predominantly produced moderate to severe, oxitriptan [5-HTP] primarily mild forms of adverse effects.

Fourteen (38.9%) of the patients receiving 5-HTP reported side-effects compared with 18 patients (54.5%) in the fluvoxamine group. The most common side-effects with 5-HTP were nausea, heartburn, and gastrointestinal problems (flatulence, feelings of fullness, and rumbling sensations). These side-effects were rated as being very mild to mild. In contrast, most of the side-effects experienced in the fluvoxamine group were of moderate to severe intensity. The only subject to drop out of the 5-HTP group did so after 35 days (5 weeks), while four subjects in the fluvoxamine group dropped out after only 2 weeks. Based on the studies in weight loss, the longer that 5-HTP is used (e.g. after 4–6 weeks of use), the less of a problem there is with any mild nausea.

5-HTP has been shown to have "equipotency" with SSRIs and tricyclic antidepressants in terms of effectiveness, but offers several advantages in that it is better tolerated and is associated with fewer and much milder side-effects; and because many people prefer to use a naturally occurring, natural substance like 5-HTP over synthetic drugs.

Table 92.8 5-HTP vs. antidepressant drugs: comparison of side-effects

Side-effect	Percentage of patients experiencing side-effects		
	5-HTP	Tricyclics	SSRIs
Nausea	9	15	23
Headache	5	16	20
Nervousness	2.5	11	16
Insomnia	2.5	7	17
Anxiety	2.5	9	14
Drowsiness	7	23	11
Diarrhea	2.5	4	12
Tremor	0	18	11
Dry mouth	7	64.5	12
Sweating	2.5	15	9
Dizziness	5	25.5	7
Constipation	5	25	5.5
Vision changes	0	14.5	4

L-Tyrosine: an adjunct to 5-HTP

In the early 1970s, researchers discovered that, in about 20% of patients who responded well to 5-HTP, the results tended to decrease after 1 month of treatment. The antidepressant effects of 5-HTP in these subjects began to wear off gradually after the first month despite the fact that the level of 5-HTP in the blood, and presumably the level of serotonin in the brain, remained at the same level as when they were experiencing benefit.[6]

The researchers discovered that while serotonin levels appeared to stay at the same levels after 1 month of treatment, the levels of the other important monoamine neurotransmitters, dopamine and norepinephrine, declined.[28] As discussed above, when depressed patients are treated with 5-HTP they experience a rise not only in serotonin, but also in catecholamines like dopamine and norepinephrine. In about 20% of subjects, the catecholamine-enhancing effects of 5-HTP tended to wear off. Providing these patients with L-tyrosine, the amino acid precursor to the catecholamines, helped to re-establish the efficacy of 5-HTP.[6,28] The dosage was 200 mg/day for 5-HTP and 100 mg/kg body weight for L-tyrosine. This dosage for L-tyrosine is quite high and would require substantial clinical supervision.

Weight loss

A considerable body of scientific evidence documents the major role serotonin in the brain plays in influencing eating behavior. One of the key findings is that when animals and humans are fed tryptophan-free diets, appetite is significantly increased, resulting in binge eating – carbohydrates would be preferable, but in fact the animals will binge on whatever is available.[1,2] A diet low in tryptophan leads to low brain serotonin levels; as a result the brain senses it is starving and so stimulates the appetite control centers in a powerful way. This stimulation results in a preference for carbohydrates. Researchers discovered that when animals or humans are fed a carbohydrate meal, more tryptophan is delivered to the brain, resulting in more serotonin being manufactured. This scenario has led to the idea that low serotonin levels leads to "carbohydrate craving" and plays a major role in the development of obesity as well as bulimia.[29]

Cravings for carbohydrate can be mild or quite severe. They may range in severity from the desire to nibble one piece of bread or cookie to uncontrollable binging. At the upper end of the spectrum of carbohydrate addiction is bulimia, a potentially serious eating disorder characterized by binge eating and purging of the food through forced vomiting or the use of laxatives. The serotonin theory of bulimia is that low serotonin levels trigger the binge eating which leads to a rush of serotonin being produced and released in the brain.[30,31] This increased serotonin effect produces a brief reduction in feelings of stress and tension. This serotonin "fix" is short-lived and is followed by feelings of guilt and low self-esteem. The current medical treatment for bulimia is the use of drugs which enhance the effects of serotonin. Although there are no reports in the medical literature of 5-HTP being used in the treatment of bulimia, given its effects on serotonin levels it merits consideration.

5-HTP may help to prevent the decline in serotonin levels associated with a reduced calorie intake. Concentrations of tryptophan in the bloodstream and subsequent brain serotonin levels plummet with dieting.[32] In response to severe drops in serotonin levels, the brain puts out a strong message to eat. This situation sets up the scenario to explain why most diets do not work.

As far back as 1975, researchers demonstrated that giving 5-HTP to rats who were genetically bred to overeat and be obese resulted in significant reduction in food intake.[33] It turns out that these rats bred to be fat have decreased activity of the enzyme which converts tryptophan to 5-HTP and subsequently to serotonin.

There is circumstantial evidence that many humans are genetically predisposed to obesity. This predisposition may involve the same mechanism as rats genetically predisposed to obesity. By providing preformed 5-HTP, this genetic defect is bypassed and more serotonin is manufactured.

The early animal studies with 5-HTP as a weight loss aid have been followed by a series of three human clinical studies. The first study involved 19 significantly overweight female subjects with a body mass index ranging between 30 and 40.[34] Analysis of the pretreatment dietary intake concluded that these women tended to overeat carbohydrates. Food intake and eating behavior were assessed using a 3 day diet diary at the beginning and end of the two treatment periods. All food was carefully weighed before meals and re-weighed if there were any leftovers. Participants also filled out a self-evaluation of appetite and satiety twice weekly, and mood was evaluated using standard psychological tests.

Table 92.9 The effect of 5HTP on food intake

	Food intake (calories/day)	Protein intake (g/day)	Carbohydrate intake (g/day)
Pretreatment	2,903	101	274
Placebo	2,327	85	223
5-HTP	1,819	79	176

The daily dosage of 5-HTP used in the study was 8 mg/kg body weight. Patients were given either the 5-HTP or a placebo 20 minutes before meals for 5 weeks, and after a 1 week interval were switched to receive the other treatment. No dietary restrictions were prescribed because the researchers wanted to answer the question, "Does 5-HTP reduce appetite and promote weight loss without any conscious effort?" To make sure that the women actually took the 5-HTP, researchers measured the level of the serotonin breakdown product, 5-hydroxy-3-indole acetic acid (5-HIAA), in the urine. The results of the study are listed in Table 92.9.

These results with 5-HTP were achieved without the women making any conscious effort to reduce food consumption. The average amount of weight loss during the 5 week period of 5-HTP supplementation was a little more than 3 pounds, compared with less than 1 pound of total weight loss during the placebo period.

Interestingly, evaluation of the various self-tests indicated that appetite or degree of initial hunger did not differ between the two groups. What differed was satiety. In other words, the 5-HTP did not reduce the appetite before a meal, but after consuming an adequate amount of food the satiety centers in the brain were stimulated and the women did not feel hungry. As a result their caloric intake was dramatically reduced.

The level of 5-HIAA, the breakdown product of serotonin, in the group receiving the 5-HTP increased by over 50-fold over the control group. This increase provided two things: (1) it assured researchers that subjects actually took the 5-HTP, and (2) it clearly indicated that 5-HTP increased serotonin manufacture.

The next study sought to determine if 5-HTP helped overweight individuals to adhere to dietary recommendations.[35] Fourteen overweight female subjects with a body mass index ranging between 30 and 40 were enrolled in the double-blind study.[8] Again, analysis of the pretreatment dietary intake concluded that these women tended to overeat. The women were randomly assigned to receive either 5-HTP (300 mg) or placebo 30 minutes before meals. The 12 week study was divided into two 6 week periods. For the first 6 weeks there were no dietary recommendations, and for the second 6 weeks the women were placed on a 1,200 calorie diet.

The women were seen every 2 weeks to evaluate body weight, diet diaries, self-evaluations of appetite and

Table 92.10 Impact of 5-HTP on weight loss

	Placebo	5-HTP group
Weight (pounds)		
Baseline	207.68	229.46
After 6 weeks	206.58	225.94
After 12 weeks	205.4	219.12
Total weight loss (pounds)		
After 6 weeks	1.1	3.52
After 12 weeks	2.28	10.34

satiety. The women were also asked if they experienced the presence of meat aversion, taste or smell alterations, early satiety, and nausea and/or vomiting. To verify patient compliance, urinary measurement of 5-HIAA was again determined. As shown in Table 92.10, the women taking the placebo lost 2.28 pounds while the women taking the 5-HTP lost 10.34 pounds.

Like the previous study, 5-HTP appeared to promote weight loss by promoting satiety. While some of the women reported some aversion to meat or altered taste and smell, every women (100%) reported early satiety (see Table 92.11). Most of the women receiving 5-HTP also experienced very mild nausea during the first 6 weeks of the trial, but during the last 6 weeks none complained of nausea. The fact that weight loss is accelerated during the second 6 week period makes it highly unlikely that 5-HTP promotes weight loss as a result of producing nausea.

The latest study with 5-HTP enrolled overweight women with a body mass index ranging between 30 and 40 and an overactive appetite.[36] The 28 subjects of the study were given either 5-HTP (300 mg three times daily before meals) or a placebo. For the first 6 weeks there were no dietary restrictions, and for the second 6 weeks the women were placed on a diet of 1,200 calories/day. Carbohydrates contributed to 53% of the calories, fats comprised 29%, and proteins provided 18%. No carbohydrate-rich foods were permitted between meals. Subjects were examined every 2 weeks to evaluate food intake and body weight. Routine blood measurements were also performed at the beginning, at 6 weeks, and at the end of the study. To verify patient compliance, urinary measurement of 5-HIAA was determined.

The results from this study were even more impressive than the previous studies for several reasons. The group receiving the 5-HTP lost an average of 4.39 pounds after the first 6 weeks and an average of 11.63 pounds after 12 weeks. In comparison, the placebo group lost an average of only 0.62 pounds after the first 6 weeks and 1.87 pounds after 12 weeks. The lack of weight loss during the second 6 week period in the placebo group obviously reflects the fact that the women had difficulty adhering to the diet.

Table 92.11 Impact of 5-HTP on appetite and satiety

	5-HTP		Placebo	
	Weeks 1–6	Weeks 7–12	Weeks 1–6	Weeks 7–12
Taste alteration	2/7	1/7	0/7	0/7
Smell alteration	2/7	1/7	0/7	0/7
Meat aversion	3/7	1/7	0/7	0/7
Early satiety	7/7	6/7	2/7	2/7
Nausea	5/7	0/7	1/7	2/7

Early satiety was reported by 100% of the subjects during the first 6 week period. During the second 6 week period, even with severe caloric restriction, 90% of the women taking 5-HTP reported early satiety. Once again, many of the women receiving the 5-HTP reported mild nausea during the first 6 weeks of therapy. However, the symptom was never severe enough for any of the women to drop out of the study. No other side-effects were reported.

Based upon the urinary measurements of 5-HIAA, the women took their 300 mg of 5-HTP with meals and as a result were able to achieve weight loss. The amount of weight loss was amplified by a better capability to adhere to a 1,200 calorie diet. The structure of the dietary changes reflected primarily a reduction in pasta, bread, and other carbohydrate-rich foods (the study was conducted in Rome).

Insomnia

Several clinical studies have shown 5-HTP to produce good results in promoting and maintaining sleep in normal subjects as well as in those experiencing insomnia.[36–40,42,43] One of the key benefits with 5-HTP in the treatment of insomnia is its ability to increase sleep quality. This effect is evident by its ability to increase REM sleep (typically by about 25%) while simultaneously increasing deep sleep stages 3 and 4 without increasing total sleep time.[36,38] The sleep stages that are reduced by 5-HTP to compensate for the increases are non-REM stages 1 and 2, the least important stages of sleep. In one of the studies, the subjects receiving 200 mg of 5-HTP increased the amount of REM sleep by 15.5 minutes during the 5 night study.[36] Those subjects taking 600 mg of 5-HTP increased REM sleep time by an average of 20 minutes for the 5 night study. These results indicate that 5-HTP increases the amount of dream time by about 3–4 minutes a night.

Although there was a clear dose-related effect, the lower dosage is sufficient in most cases. In addition, taking too much 5-HTP may increase REM sleep to an abnormal level, lead to an increased risk for disturbing dreams (i.e. nightmares), and cause mild nausea.

Migraine and tension headache

The relationship of serotonin and headaches is fully described in Chapter 172. Because migraine sufferers have low levels of serotonin in their tissues, some researchers refer to migraine as a "low serotonin syndrome".[43] Although the primary benefits of 5-HTP in the prevention of both migraine and tension headache is related to its ability to normalize underlying imbalances in the serotonin system, it also influences the endorphin system in a positive way.

There have been several clinical studies with 5-HTP in headaches, both vascular and non-vascular, that have showed excellent results. In particular, the use of 5-HTP in the prevention of migraine headache offers considerable advantages over drug therapy. Although a number of drugs have been shown to be useful in the prevention of migraine headaches, all of them carry significant side-effects.

The problem with drug therapy in the prevention of migraine headaches is perhaps best exemplified by one of the most commonly used drugs, methysergide (Sansert). Methysergide therapy for the prevention of migraine attacks is effective in about 60–80% of cases. However, this effectiveness is not without a high price as side-effects are quite common and can be quite severe. Retroperitoneal fibrosis, pleuropulmonary fibrosis and fibrotic thickening of cardiac valves may occur in patients receiving long-term methysergide maleate therapy. Therefore, this preparation must be reserved for prophylaxis in patients whose vascular headaches are frequent and/or severe and uncontrollable and for those who are under close medical supervision.

There have been several studies which have compared 5-HTP with methysergide in the prevention of migraine headaches. In one of the largest double-blind studies, 124 patients received either 5-HTP (600 mg daily) or methysergide (3 mg daily) in identically looking pills for 6 months.[44] Treatment was determined to be successful if there was a reduction higher than 50% in the frequency of attacks or in the number of severe attacks. Although 75% (30 of the remaining 40 patients) taking methysergide demonstrated significant improvement compared with 71% (32 of the 45 patients), this difference was not viewed as being statistically significant (see Table 92.12). The advantage of 5-HTP over methysergide was demonstrated when researchers looked at side-effects. Side-effects were more frequent in the group receiving methysergide than in the 5-HTP group. In fact, five patients in the methysergide group had to withdraw during the trial because of side-effects.

Table 92.12 5-HTP vs. methysergide: clinical effects of treatment in 124 patients

	Methysergide	5-HTP
No attacks (100% reduction)	35%	25%
Improvement (>50% reduction)	40%	46%
No improvement	12.5%	29%
Withdrawal due to side-effects	12.5%	0

Two other studies comparing 5-HTP with drugs used in the prevention of migraine headaches (pizotifen and propranolol) demonstrated that 5-HTP compared quite favorably in terms of effectiveness.[45,46] While these drugs have significant side-effects, 5-HTP is extremely well tolerated even at dosages as high as 600 mg/day. One of the other key differences noted in these studies between 5-HTP and the drugs was 5-HTP's ability to improve mood and relieve feelings of depression.

Juvenile headache

One of the best uses of 5-HTP is in chronic headaches in children. These headaches are a big problem because of the tremendous risk for side-effects of the current drugs used to treat as well as prevent these headaches in children. Fortunately, there have been several studies of 5-HTP in the treatment of chronic headaches in children and adolescents that have shown excellent results.[47–49] Given the risks of current drugs used in chronic childhood headaches, a trial of 5-HTP for 2 months certainly seems reasonable. If the headaches are also accompanied by sleep disorders, 5-HTP appears to be especially well-suited.

In one study, 48 elementary and junior high students suffering from recurrent headaches (at least one headache every 2 weeks) and sleep disorders, including difficulty it getting to sleep, frequent awakenings, sleep walking, nightmares, and bedwetting, were divided into two groups.[47] Group A was given 5-HTP for 2 months followed by a placebo for 2 months, while group B received just the opposite. It was necessary to divide group A into a nine patient subgroup, Group C. These nine patients did so well on the 5-HTP they did not want to switch over to the other medication even though they had no idea whether they were in fact taking 5-HTP or were on a placebo. The dosage of 5-HTP was based on the child's weight: 4.5 mg/kg per day.

The headache index was reduced by about 70% when the kids were taking 5-HTP compared with an 11.5% drop when they were taking the placebo. In the nine patients in group C, there was an 81.8% decrease in the headache index after the second month. Interestingly, these same patients only exhibited an 18.2% reduction after the first month. These results indicate that evaluation of the benefits of 5-HTP in the treatment of headaches requires at least a 2 month trial. The failure to show benefit with 5-HTP in some studies in headaches may be due to the fact that they lasted less than 2 months. The 25 patients experienced a modest reduction in frequent awakenings, nightmares, sleep walking, and talking while asleep and no change in difficulty falling asleep or in bedwetting.

Overall this study demonstrated very good effects in

these children. Perhaps the most impressive aspect to consider, however, was the fact that these benefits were achieved without side-effect. Not a single child reported a side-effect while taking 5-HTP. Interestingly, for some reason children rarely experience even mild nausea from 5-HTP.

The possible benefits of 5-HTP in children with recurrent headache and/or sleep disorders is far-reaching. Evaluation of the 48 children in the trial demonstrated inadequate school progress compared with their classmates. The children were shown to be of normal intellectual capacity, but demonstrated inattentiveness similar to that observed in depression. Many of the children may have been suffering from depression. The unwillingness of the nine subjects in Group C to switch to the other unknown medication (which was in fact the placebo) is a strong indicator that these children and their parents noted some rather dramatic improvements beyond simply a reduction in headaches or improved sleep.

The manner in which 5-HTP may be of benefit in migraine headaches may not simply be the overcoming of some defect in serotonin synthesis. As noted previously, part of the clinical benefit of 5-HTP may be via an ability to increase the levels of beta-endorphin. A decrease in beta-endorphin level in migraine as well as tension headache sufferers has been demonstrated by several investigators.[50,51]

A clinical trial measured the effects of 5-HTP on serotonin and beta-endorphin levels in 20 juvenile patients suffering from migraine or tension-type headaches.[52] Patients were monitored and evaluated for frequency and intensity of headache attacks for 3 months prior to 5-HTP treatment and 3 months of therapy. The researchers reported a statistically significant reduction in the headache score with 5-HTP treatment in both migraine and tension-type sufferers. These improvements were likely due to increased beta-endorphin levels as noted in Table 92.13. However, the level of beta-endorphin achieved with 5-HTP, especially as measured in the white blood cell, was still far less than that observed in control patients not suffering from recurrent headache. These results imply that longer periods of 5-HTP supplementation may be required before there is a normalization of beta-endorphin levels in children prone to headaches.

These results may indicate that 5-HTP alone is not able to raise beta-endorphin levels sufficiently to reduce or eliminate headaches, suggesting that other therapies designed to increase beta-endorphin levels should be used along with 5-HTP. Examples of other therapies which have been shown to raise beta-endorphin levels are exercise, acupuncture, and biofeedback.

Fibromyalgia

The history of the development of 5-HTP as an effective treatment for fibromyalgia began with studies on the drug fenclonine.[53] This drug blocks the enzyme which inhibits the conversion of tryptophan to 5-HTP and, as a result, blocks serotonin production. During the late 1960s and early 1970s, it was thought that increased serotonin formation may promote migraine headaches (the opposite of what was later proved, i.e. increasing serotonin levels reduce migraine headache occurrence). The researchers discovered that providing headache sufferers with fenclonine resulted in very severe muscle pain. This effect was the exact opposite of what was expected, but led to some important advances in the understanding of fibromyalgia – a way to induce its severe symptoms of (as well as symptoms nearly identical to) EMS, the condition caused by contaminated L-tryptophan. The researchers also discovered that migraine sufferers had a greater reaction to the drug than non-headache sufferers. In fact, in most normal subjects fenclonine produced no fibromyalgia. These occurrences highlight just how sensitive migraine sufferers are to low serotonin levels.

Migraine headaches and fibromyalgia share a common feature: both are low serotonin syndromes.[54] After over 25 years of research, one of the lead researchers has stated: "In our experience, as well as in that of other pain specialists, 5-HTP can largely improve the painful picture of primary fibromyalgia."[55]

A double-blind study in 50 patients with fibromyalgia found that 100 mg of 5-HTP three times per day significantly improved their symptoms.[56] As shown in Table

Table 92.13 Serotonin and beta-endorphin levels in juvenile patients with headaches before and after administration of 5-HTP

	Serotonin (serum, mcg/L)	Beta-endorphin (plasma, pmol/L)	Beta-endorphin (white blood cells, pmol/106 GB/L)
Migraine (13 subjects)			
Before	104.6	16.2	110.5
After	115.7	19.4	120.3
Tension-type (7 subjects)			
Before	90.7	14.5	142.3
After	97.2	17.6	152.4
Total (20 subjects)			
Before	100.5	15.7	129.3
After	108.3	18.4	140.4
Controls (17 subjects)	96	21.3	359.3

Table 92.14 Patients' and physicians' opinion on the effectiveness of 5-HTP vs. placebo in fibromyalgia

Response	5-HTP	Placebo
Good	11	1
Fair	8	5
Poor	4	8
None	0	9

92.14, 5-HTP was rated substantially better than placebo by subjects and evaluating physicians. Improvements were noted in all symptom categories: number of painful areas, morning stiffness, sleep patterns, anxiety, and fatigue. In another study, 100 mg of 5-HTP taken three times daily demonstrated maximum results by day 30 of the 90 day trial.[57]

One of the primary benefits with 5-HTP in fibromyalgia may be its ability to improve sleep quality. A key finding in patients with fibromyalgia is a reduced REM sleep and an increase in non-REM sleep.[58] In addition, the deeper levels (stages III and IV) are not achieved for long enough periods. As a result, people with fibromyalgia wake up feeling fatigued and in pain. The severity of the pain of fibromyalgia correlates with the rating of sleep quality. For example, a study of 50 women with fibromyalgia syndrome recorded their sleep quality, pain intensity, and attention to pain for 30 days, using palm-top computers programmed as electronic interviewers.[59] They described their previous night's sleep quality within 30 minutes of awakening each day, and at randomly selected times in the morning, afternoon, and evening rated their present pain. The researchers found that a night of poor sleep was followed by a significantly more painful day, and a more painful day was followed by a night of even poorer sleep. 5-HTP may help to break the cycle by addressing the low serotonin level as well as by promoting a restful sleep.

Parkinson's disease

The use of 5-HTP in Parkinson's disease provides some benefit, but only if used in combination with the drug Sinemet (the combination of L-dopa with the decarboxylase inhibitor, carbidopa). Although brain levels of serotonin are decreased in Parkinson's disease, the reduction in dopamine receptors is more severe. Increasing serotonin levels with 5-HTP in patients not taking Sinemet are associated with worsening of symptoms, especially rigidity.[60]

One of the key benefits of taking 5-HTP in Parkinson's disease is that it can help to counteract the negative effects that the L-dopa in the Sinemet has on sleep and mood.[61–63] In addition, 5-HTP has also been shown to improve the physical symptoms of Parkinson's disease.

About nine out of 10 people with Parkinson's disease suffer from depression. The degree of depression in Parkinson's disease is a reflection of their serotonin levels. The lower the level of serotonin, the more severe is their depression. One study examined the effect of 5-HTP in seven Parkinson's disease patients, all of whom were on Sinemet.[61] The initial dosage of 5-HTP was 75 mg, which was increased by 25 mg every 3 days until the patients reported a relief of their depression, or up to a maximum of 500 mg/day for 4 months. The impressive results obtained in these patients are shown in Table 92.15.

Table 92.15 The effect of HTP on depression in Parkinson's disease

Patient no.	L-dopa (mg/day)	Carbidopa (mg/day)	5-HTP (mg/day)	HDS	
				Before	After
1	1,000	175	125	22	11
2	300	75	75	14	3
3	400	150	100	21	13
4	1,000	100	100	12	6
5	500	125	500	18	22
6	1,125	112.5	300	18	7
7	500	50	100	17	13

Six out of seven patients responded to 5-HTP. Note that the dosages of 5-HTP in these five out of the six patients who responded ranged from only 75 to 125 mg. The only patient who did not respond took 500 mg of 5-HTP.

Seizure disorders

Most of the recent research on 5-HTP has focused on its use in the treatment of several seizure disorders.[64–68] 5-HTP has shown good results in most (but not all) studies in patients suffering from diseases characterized by myoclonus, with the exception of epilepsy which is not helped by 5-HTP.

The best response to 5-HTP for myoclonus occurs in people who have intention myoclonus, which is most often produced as a result of ischemic damage to the brain.[32] Intention myoclonus can be a problem after a stroke or heart attack, overdosage of a drug like heroin, a severe asthma attack, or an adverse reaction to anesthesia or other chemical. Improvements in intention myoclonus with 5-HTP have been demonstrated in patients. 5-HTP has also produced good results in patients with progressive myoclonus epilepsy, essential myoclonus, palatal myoclonus, and Friedreich's ataxia.[69]

In a 1983 article, one researcher of 5-HTP stated: "Some helpless bedridden patients dramatically improved to the extent that they could walk again and resume independent living."[70] Because of the phenomenal results, 5-HTP was the first compound to be evaluated as an orphan drug by the Pharmaceutical Manufacturing Associations Commission on Drugs for Rare Diseases.

TOXICOLOGY

The major concern with 5-HTP is a possible link to L-tryptophan and the eosinophilia-myalgia syndrome (EMS). However, an important distinction must be made in the manufacturing process. While L-tryptophan is produced via bacterial fermentation and filtration, 5-HTP is commercially available through an extraction process from the seed of *Griffonia simplicifolia*, an African plant. 5-HTP extracted from this natural source avoids the contamination problem associated with past manufacturing of L-tryptophan.

Detailed analyses of all the evidence by the Centers for Disease Control (CDC) and other experts have led to the conclusion that the cause of the EMS epidemic could be traced to a single Japanese manufacturer, Showa Denko.[71,72] Of the six Japanese companies which supplied L-tryptophan to the United States, Showa Denko was the largest (50–60% of all the L-tryptophan). The L-tryptophan was used not only as a nutritional supplement, but also in infant formulas and nutrient mixtures for intravenous feeding.

There was a single case report linking 5-HTP to a condition similar to EMS in 1980.[73] However, this case involved the use of very high dosages of 5-HTP (1,400 mg) over a 20 month period. Further examination of the patient indicated a defect in tryptophan metabolism that resulted in elevations in kynurenine. Such defects in tryptophan metabolism are common in patients with scleroderma, which shares many common features with EMS. It appeared that either the 5-HTP may have contained a contaminant to which this man was sensitive, or taking such high dosages of 5-HTP over a prolonged period of time aggravated his abnormal handling of L-tryptophan.

There has also been a report of a 28-year-old woman, her husband, and her two sons, 33 and 13 months old, developing an EMS-like illness in response to contaminated 5-HTP.[74] The young boys had inherited the inability to convert tryptophan to 5-HTP. As a result, they required daily administration of 5-HTP (5–7 mg/kg). Both boys had been receiving the 5-HTP almost from birth.

The mother was not taking 5-HTP, but she was preparing it for the young boys by opening the capsules, mixing the powder in juice or water, and giving it to them orally with a syringe. She never took the 5-HTP, she only touched it with her hands as she emptied the capsules.

When the second boy was about 9 months old, the mother began experiencing symptoms of EMS. Upon consulting a physician in July of 1991 it was noted that her eosinophil count was well over 30%. She continued to worsen and was hospitalized in August of 1991 with a tentative diagnosis of EMS. At this time she was referred to the National Institutes of Health (NIH) for further evaluation.

Because of the possible link between the mother's symptoms and the 5-HTP, the boys and the father were also evaluated. The older boy had an eosinophil count of 9% (normal is 1–4%) and the younger boy had a count of 6%. The father had no abnormalities.

The 5-HTP that the boys were using was analyzed by HPLC and found to contain an impurity not found in the 5-HTP that the NIH was using in their studies for ataxia and myoclonus. Switching the boys to the contaminant-free 5-HTP brought about normalization of eosinophil counts. The mother's case is interesting because she was the most severely affected and she was only coming into contact with the contaminated 5-HTP through her skin.

Evidence that uncontaminated 5-HTP does not cause EMS is also provided by researchers who have been using 5-HTP for over 25 years. They state that: "EMS has never appeared in the patients of ours who received only uncontaminated L-tryptophan or 5-hydroxtryptophan (5-HTP)."[75] Furthermore, researchers at the NIH studying the effects of uncontaminated 5-HTP on various metabolic conditions have not observed a single case of EMS nor has a case of elevated eosinophils been attributed to 5-HTP in these studies.[74] In short, there has never been a report of uncontaminated 5-HTP causing EMS.

Although there has never been a single person developing EMS from 5-HTP products proven to be free from the contaminants, and it is extremely unlikely that anyone would, nonetheless, to be on the safe side we recommend that long-term continual use of 5-HTP be monitored by regular (every 6 months) eosinophil determination. For any person suffering from scleroderma due to the problem with tryptophan metabolism noted in these patients, we recommend an eosinophil determination after the first month of 5-HTP use, especially if dosages are greater than 500 mg/day.

DOSAGE

The dosage should be started at 50 mg three times per day. If the response is inadequate after 2 weeks, increase the dosage to 100 mg three times per day. This recommendation will greatly reduce the mild symptoms of nausea often experienced during the first few weeks of 5-HTP therapy. Because 5-HTP does not rely on the same transport vehicle as L-tryptophan, it can also be taken with food.

For insomnia, prescribe 100–300 mg 30–45 minutes before retiring. Start with the lower dose for at least 3 days before increasing dosage.

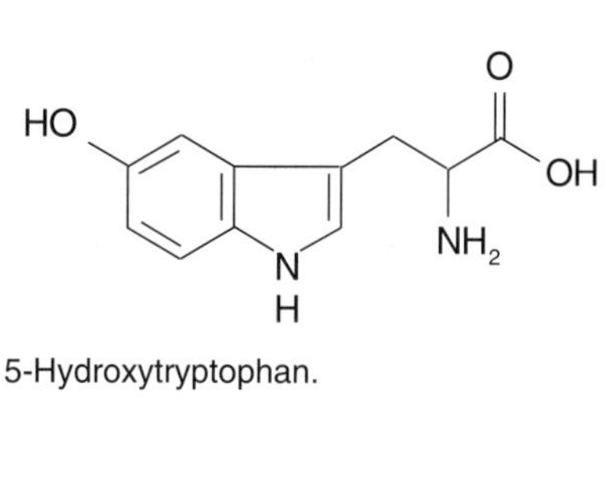

Figure 92.1 5-Hydroxytryptophan.

REFERENCES

1. Filippini GA, Costa CVL, Bertazzo A, eds. Recent advances in tryptophan research. tryptophan and serotonin pathways. Exp Biol Med 1996; 398: 1–762
2. Magnussen IE, Nielsen-Kudsk F. Bioavailability and related pharmacokinetics in man of orally administered L-5-hydroxy-tryptophan in a steady state. Acta Phamacol Toxicol 1980; 46: 257–262
3. Magnussen I, Jensen TS, Rand JH. Plasma accumulation and metabolism of orally administered single dose L-5-hydroxy-tryptophan in man. Acta Pharmacol Toxicol 1981; 49: 184–189
4. van Praag HM, Lemus C. Monoamine precursors in the treatment of psychiatric disorders. In: Wurtman RJ, Wurtman JJ, eds. Nutrition and the brain, vol. 7. New York, NY: Raven Press. 1986: p 89–139
5. van Praag HM. Studies on the mechanism of action with serotonin precursors in depression. Psychopharmacol Bull 1984; 20: 599–602
6. Aviram M, Cogan U, Mokady S. Excessive dietary tryptophan enhances plasma lipid peroxidation in rats. Atherosceloris 1991; 88: 29–43
7. Simic MG, al-Sheikhly M, Jovanovic SV. Inhibition of free radical processes by antioxidants – tryptophan and 5-hydroxytryptophan. Bibl Nutr Dieta 1989; 43: 288–289
8. Sano I. L-5-hydroxytryptophan therapy. Folia Psychiatr Neurol Japan 1972; 26: 7–17
9. Takahashi S, Kondo H, Kato N. Effect of L-5-hydroxytryptophan on brain monoamine metabolism and evaluation of its clinical effect in depressed patients. J Psychiatr Res 1975; 12: 177–187
10. Fujiwara J, Otsuki S. Subtype of affective psychosis classified by response on amine precursors and monoamine metabolism. Folia Psychiatr Neurol Japan 1974; 28: 94–100
11. Nakajima T, Kudo Y, Kaneko Z. Clinical evaluation of 5-hydroxy-L-tryptophan as an antidepressant drug. Folia Psychiatr Neurol Japan 1978; 32: 223–230
12. Kaneko M, Kumashiro H, Takahashi Y. L-5-HTP treatment and serum 5-HTP level after L-5-HTP loading on depressed patients. Neuropsychobioloby 1979; 5: 232–240
13. van Praag HM, Korf J, Dols LC. A pilot study of the predictive value of the probenecid test in application of 5-hydroxytryptophan as antidepressant. Psychopharmacologia 1972; 25: 14–21
14. van Praag HM. Management of depression with serotonin precursors. Biol Psychiatry 1981; 16: 291–310
15. Robie TR, Flora A. Anti-depressant chemotherapy, 1965. Rapid response to serotonin precursor potentiated by Ritalin. Psychosomatics 1965; 6: 351–354
16. Nardini M, De Stefano R, Iannuccelli M. Treatment of depression with L-5-hydroxytryptophan combined with chlorimipramine, a double-blind study. Int J Clin Pharmacol Res 1983; 3: 239–250
17. Rousseau JJ. Effects of a levo-5-hydroxytryptophan-dihydroergocristine combination on depression and neuropsychic performance. A double-blind placebo-controlled clinical trial in elderly patients. Clin Ther 1987; 9: 267–272
18. Mendlewicz J, Youdim MB. Antidepressant potentiation of 5-hydroxytryptophan by L-deprenil in affective illness. J Affect Disord 1980; 2: 137–146
19. Alino JJ, Gutierrez JL, Iglesias ML. 5-Hydroxytryptophan (5-HTP) and a MAOI (nialamide) in the treatment of depressions. A double-blind controlled study. Int Pharmacopsychiatry 1976; 11: 8–15
20. Angst J, Woggon B, Schoepf J. The treatment of depression with L-5-hydroxytryptophan versus imipramine. Results of two open and one double-blind study. Arch Psychiatr Nervenkr 1977; 224: 175–186
21. van Praag HM, Korf J. 5-Hydroxytrytophan as an antidepressant. The predictive value of the probenecid test. J Nerv Ment Dis 1974; 158: 331–337
22. Praag HM van, Korf J. Serotonin metabolism in depression. clinical application of the probenecid test. Int Pharmacopsychiatry 1974; 9: 35–51
23. van Praag HM. Central monoamine metabolism in depressions. I. Serotonin and related compounds. Compr Psychiatry 1980; 21: 30–43
24. van Hiele JJ. L-5-hydroxytryptophan in depression. The first substitution therapy in psychiatry? Neuropsychobiology 1980; 6: 230–240
25. Kielholz P. Treatment for therapy-resistant depression. Psychopathology 1986; 19: 194–200
26. Byerley WF, Judd LL, Reimherr FW. 5-Hydroxytryptophan. A review of its antidepressant efficacy and adverse effects. J Clin Psychopharmacol 1987; 7: 127–137
27. Poldinger W, Calanchini B, Schwarz W. A functional-dimensional approach to depression. Serotonin deficiency as a target syndrome in a comparison of 5-hydroxytryptophan and fluvoxamine. Psychopathology 1991; 24: 53–81
28. van Praag HM. In search of the mode of action of antidepressants. 5-HTP/tyrosine mixtures in depression. Adv Biochem Psychopharmacol 1984; 39: 301–314
29. Wurtman RJ, Wurtman JJ. Brain serotonin, carbohydrate-craving, obesity and depression. Adv Exp Med Biol 1996; 398: 35–41
30. Weltzin TE, Fernstrom MH, Kaye WH. Serotonin and bulimia nervosa. Nutr Rev 1994; 52: 399–408
31. Weltzin TE, Fernstrom MH, Fernstrom JD. Acute tryptophan depletion and increased food intake and irritability in bulimea nervosa. Am J Psychiatry 1995; 152: 1668–1671
32. Goodwin GM, Cowen PJ, Fairburn CG. Plasma concentrations of tryptophan and dieting. Br Med J 1990; 300: 1499–1500
33. Blundel JE, Leshem MB. The effect of 5-HTP on food intake and on the anorexic action of amphetamine and fenfluramine. J Pharm Pharmacol 1975; 27: 31–37
34. Ceci F, Cangiano C, Cairella M. The effects of oral 5-hydroxytryptophan administration on feeding behavior in obese adult female subjects. J Neural Transm 1989; 76: 109–117
35. Cangiano C, Ceci F, Cairella M. Effects of 5-hydroxytryptophan on eating behavior and adherence to dietary prescriptions in obese adult subjects. Adv Exp Med Biol 1991; 294: 591–593
36. Cangiano C, Ceci F, Cascino A. Eating behavior and adherence to dietary prescriptions in obese adult subjects treated with 5-hydroxytryptophan. Am J Clin Nutr 1992; 56: 863–867
37. Guilleminault C, Cathala HP, Castaigne P. Effects of 5-HTP on sleep of a patient with brain stem lesion. Electroencephalog Clin Neurophysiol 1973; 34: 177–184
38. Wyatt RJ, Zarcone J, Engelman K. Effects of 5-hydroxytryptophan on the sleep of normal human subjects. Electroencephalogr Clin Neurophysiol 1971; 30: 505–509
39. Autret A, Minz M, Bussel B. Human sleep and 5-HTP. Effects of repeated high doses and of association with benserazide. Electroencephalogr Clin Neurophysiol 1976; 41: 408–413
40. Zarcone VP, Jr, Hoddes E. Effects of 5-hydroxytryptophan on fragmentation of REM sleep in alcoholics. Am J Psychiatry 1975; 132: 74–76
42. Soulairac A, Lambinet H. Effect of 5-hydroxytryptophan, a serotonin precursor, on sleep disorders. Ann Med Psychol 1977; 1: 792–798
43. Sicuteri F. Migraine, a central biochemical dysnociception. Headache 1986; 16: 145–149
44. Titus F, Davalos A, Alom J. 5-Hydroxytryptophan versus methysergide in the prophylaxis of migraine. Randomized clinical trial. Eur Neurol 1986; 25: 327–329
45. Bono G, Criscuoli M, Martignoni E. Serotonin precursors in migraine prophylaxis. Adv Neurol 1982; 33: 357–363
46. Maissen CP, Ludin HP. Comparison of the effect of 5-hydroxytryptophan and propranolol in the interval treatment of migraine. Med Wochenschr 1991; 121: 1585–1590
47. De Giorgis G, Miletto R, Iannuccelli M. Headache in association with sleep disorders in children. a psychodiagnostic evaluation and controlled clinical study – L-5-HTP versus placebo. Drugs Exp Clin Res 1987; 13: 425–433
48. Santucci M, Cortelli P, Rossi PG. L-5-hydroxytryptophan versus placebo in childhood migraine prophylaxis. A double-blind crossover study. Cephalgia 1986; 6: 155–157

49. Longo G, Rudoi I, Iannuccelli M. Treatment of essential headache in developmental age with L-5-HTP (cross over double-blind study versus placebo). Pediatr Med Chir 1984; 6: 241–245
50. Fettes, Gawel M, Kuzniak S. Endorphin levels in headache syndromes. Headache 1984; 25: 37–39
51. Leone M, Sacerdote P, D'Amico D et al. Beta-endorphin levels are reduced in peripheral mononuclear cells of cluster headache patients. Cephalgia 1993; 13: 413–416
52. Battistella PA, Bordin A, Cernetti R. Beta-endorphin in plasma and monocytes in juvenile headache. Headache 1996; 36: 91–94
53. Sicuteri F. The ingestion of serotonin precursors (L-5-hydroxy-tryptophan and L-tryptophan) improves migraine. Headache 1973; 13: 19–22
54. Nicolodi M, Sicuteri F. Fibromyalgia and migraine, two faces of the same mechanism. Serotonin as the common clue for pathogenesis and therapy. Adv Exp Med Biol 1996; 398: 373–379
55. Nicolodi M, Sicuteri F. Eosinophilia myalgia syndrome. The role of contaminants, the role of serotonergic set up. Exp Biol Med 1996; 398: 351–357
56. Caruso I, Sarzi Puttini P, Cazzola M. Double-blind study of 5-hydroxytryptophan versus placebo in the treatment of primary fibromyalgia syndrome. J Int Med Res @ 18: 201–9, 1990
57. Puttini PS, Caruso I. Primary fibromyalgia syndrome and 5-hydroxy-L-tryptophan. A 90–day open study. J Int Med Res 1992; 20: 182–189
58. White KP, Harth M. An analytical review of 24 controlled clinical trials for fibromyalgia syndrome (FMS). Pain 1996; 64: 211–219
59. Affleck G, Urrows S, Tennen H. Sequential daily relations of sleep, pain intensity, and attention to pain among women with fibromyalgia. Pain 1996; 68: 363–368
60. Chase TN, Ng LK, Watanabe AM. Parkinson's disease. Modification by 5-hydroxytryptophan. Neurology 1972; 22: 479–484
61. Mayeux R, Stern Y, Sano M. The relationship of serotonin to depression in Parkinson's disease. Mov Disord 1988; 3: 237–244
62. Bastard J, Truelle JL, Emile J. Effectiveness of 5 hydroxy-tryptophan in Parkinson's disease. Nouv Presse Med 1976; 5: 1836–1837
63. Sano VI, Taniguchi K. L-5-hydroxytryptophan (L-5-HTP) therapy in Parkinson's disease. MMWR 1972; 114: 1717–1719
64. Pranzatelli MR, Tate E, Galvan I. A controlled trial of 5-hydroxy-L-tryptophan for ataxia in progressive myoclonus epilepsy. Clin Neurol Neurosurg 1996; 98: 161–164
65. Trouillas P, Serratrice G, Laplane D. Levorotatory form of 5-hydroxytryptophan in Friedreich's ataxia. Results of a double-blind drug-placebo cooperative study. Arch Neurol 1995; 52: 456–460
66. Wessel K, Hermsdorfer J, Deger K. Double-blind crossover study with levorotatory form of hydroxytryptophan in patients with degenerative cerebellar diseases. Arch Neurol 1995; 52: 451–455
67. Pranzatelli MR, Tate E, Huang Y. Neuropharmacology of progressive myoclonus epilepsy. Response to 5-hydroxy-L-tryptophan. Epilepsia 1995; 36: 783–791
68. Trouillas P, Brudon F, Adeleine P. Improvement of cerebellar ataxia with levorotatory form of 5-hydroxytryptophan. Arch Neurol 1988; 45: 1217–1222
69. Van Woert MH, Jutkowitz R, Rosenbaum D. Serotonin and myoclonus. Monogr Neural Sci 1976; 3: 71–80
70. Van Woert MH. Myoclonus and L-5-hydroxytryptophan (L-5HTP). Prog Clin Biol Res 1983; 127: 43–52
71. Kilbourne EM. Eosinophilia-myalgia syndrome. Coming to grips with a new illness. Epidemiologic Rev 1992; 14: 16–36
72. Kilbourne EM, Philen RM, Kamb ML. Tryptophan produced by Showa Denko and epidemic eosinophilia-myalgia syndrome. J Rheumatol Suppl 1996; 46: 81–88
73. Sternberg EM, Van Woert MH, Young SN. Development of a scleroderma-like illness during therapy with L-5-hyrdoxy-tryptophan and carbidopa. N Engl J Med 1980; 303: 782–787
74. Michelson D, Page SW, Casey R. An eosinophilia-myalgia syndrome related disorder associated with exposure to L-5-hydroxytryptophan. J Rheumatol 1994; 21: 2261–2265
75. Nicolodi M, Sicuteri F. Eosinophilia myalgia syndrome. The role of contaminants, the role of serotonergic set up. Exp Biol Med 1996; 398: 351–357

CHAPTER CONTENTS

93

Hypericum perforatum (St John's wort)

Michael T. Murray, ND

Joseph E. Pizzorno Jr, ND

Hypericum perforatum (family: Hypericaceae)
Common names: St John's wort, Klamath weed, hypericum

GENERAL DESCRIPTION

St John's wort (*Hypericum perforatum*) is a shrubby perennial plant with numerous bright yellow flowers. It is commonly found in dry, gravelly soils, fields, and sunny places. St John's wort is native to many parts of the world including Europe, Asia, and the United States. It grows especially well in northern California and southern Oregon.[1]

The plant is glabrous throughout, green or sometimes glaucescent; the stems are erect, branched at the top and 30–100 cm long; the leaves are oval or elliptic or oblong-ovate, or rather narrow, oblong-linear, subotuse, flat or more or less revolute-marginedated with numerous pellucid and a few black granular dots. The yellow flowers are numerous, forming a broadly paniculate, almost corymbose inflorenscence, 7–11 cm long and 5–11 cm broad. The lanceolate bracts are 0.5 cm long and acute. The calyx is deeply parted, 5 mm long and about two to three times shorter than corolla. The sepals are lanceolate or narrow lanceolate 4–5 mm long, 1 mm broad, as long as ovary, acute or acuminate, sparingly furnished with black oval dots, with a smooth or sparsely toothed margin. The petals are oblong to oblong-elliptic, 1.2–1.5 cm long and 0.5–0.6 cm broad, with or without numerous black granular dots and lines on the margin in the upper part, while the surface is full of yellow glandular dots, thin lines, and stripes. The three-bundled stames are numerous; the ovary is ovoid, 3–5 mm long. The seed is 1 mm long, cylindric, brown, and minutely pitted longitudinally.[1]

The whole plant is used medicinally. Harvesting time is generally July through August. The plant must be dried immediately to prevent degradation of active principles.[1]

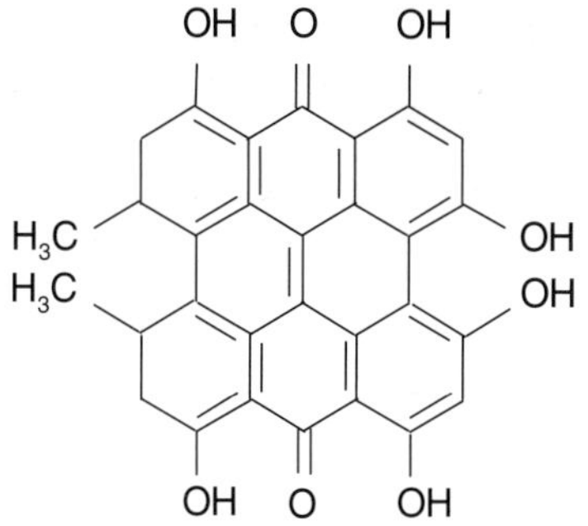

OH O OH

H_3C OH
H_3C OH

OH O OH

Figure 93.1 Hypericin.

CHEMICAL COMPOSITION

The major compounds of interest have been hypericin (see Fig. 93.1) and pseudohypericin. These compounds are typically found in very low concentrations, ranging from 0.0095 to 0.466% in the leaves and as much as 0.24% in the flowers.[1]

More recently, researchers have been interested in the other chemical constituents (especially the various flavonoid and xanthones). The interest in these other components stems largely from pharmacological studies with commercially available extracts demonstrating effects and benefits beyond hypericin and pseudohypericin. The other active components include:[1,2]

- flavonoids (flowers 16%, leaves 12%, and whole herb 9%)
- xanthones
- phenolic carboxylic acids (caffeic, chlorogenic, ferulic, and gentisic acids)
- essential oils (whole herb content 0.13%)
- carotenoids
- alkanes
- phloroglucinol derivatives
- phytosterols
- medium-chain fatty acid alcohols.

HISTORY AND FOLK USE

St John's wort has a long history of folk use. Dioscorides, the foremost physician of ancient Greece, as well as Pliny and Hippocrates, utilized St John's wort in the treatment of many illnesses. Its Latin name, *Hypericum perforatum,* is derived from Greek and means "over an apparition", a reference to the belief that the herb was so obnoxious to evil spirits that a whiff of it would cause them to depart.

The naming of St John's wort has its origins in folk traditions. One claims that red spots, symbolic of the blood of St John, appeared on the leaves of the plant on the anniversary of the saint's beheading. Another comes from a common medieval belief that if one slept with a piece of the plant under his pillow on St John's Eve, "the Saint would appear in a dream, give his blessing, and prevent one from dying during the following year".

Many people from the time of the ancient Greeks through the Middle Ages believed St John's wort to have magical powers. Recent research on St John's wort appears to offer some explanation of this "magical" power. Based on a long history of use as a mood-elevating substance and preliminary in vitro experiments and clinical studies, in 1984 the German Commission E permitted the medicinal use of St John's wort for depression, anxiety, or nervous excitement.

The Commission E evaluates efficacy of herbal medicines based on a doctrine of reasonable certainty versus the United States FDA's doctrine of absolute proof. Herbal products can be marketed with drug claims if they have been proven to be safe and effective. Whether the herbal product is available by prescription or OTC is based upon its application and safety of use. Herbal products sold in German pharmacies are reimbursed by insurance if they are prescribed by a physician.

Because the German system allowed companies to market their products according to the guidelines of the Commission E, many companies achieved success with their products allowing them to fund the necessary research to gain greater acceptance within mainstream conventional medicine. The case of St John's wort extract in the treatment of depression is a perfect case in point to illustrate how the Commission E monographs have fueled the science of botanical medicine. For example, originally it was thought that hypericin acted as an inhibitor of the enzyme monoamine oxidase (MAO) – thereby resulting in the increase of CNS monoamines such as serotonin and dopamine. However, newer information indicates that St John's wort possesses no in vivo inhibition of MAO (discussed below). It appears that the antidepressant activities are related more to modulating the relationship between the immune system and mood, as well as by inhibiting serotonin reuptake (discussed below). In addition, it appears that while hypericin is an important marker, there are other compounds such as flavonoids which are thought to play a major role in the pharmacology of St John's wort.

Over 25 double-blind randomized trials involving a total of 1,757 outpatients with mild to moderately severe depression have shown St John's wort extracts standardized for hypericin to yield excellent results in the treatment in depression with virtually no side-effects.[1,3] In 1994 a total of 66 million daily doses of St John's wort preparations were prescribed by German physicians.[4]

PHARMACOLOGY

St John's wort extracts (primarily of the flowering tops) have shown a wide variety of effects in experimental and clinical studies. Some of the activities demonstrated include:[1,2]

- antidepressant effects
- antiviral effects
- antibiotic effects
- increased healing of wounds and burns.

Antidepressant activity

Among the different biological hypotheses for depression, the biogenic amine hypothesis is the most widely accepted. This hypothesis suggests that depression is the result of a deficiency in function of the biogenic amines, e.g. serotonin, catecholamines, dopamine, etc. These neurotransmitters are stored in granules within neurons. After stimulation of the neurons, these neurotransmitters are released into the synaptic cleft via exocytosis. After binding to postsynaptic receptors, the neurotransmitters are either taken up again and re-stored in the vesicles or they are catabolized by the enzymes monoamine oxidase (MAO) or catechol-O-methyltransferase (COMT). Most antidepressant drugs increase the availability of these amines, particularly serotonin, by either inhibiting the re-uptake or blocking MAO.

As stated above, initial studies indicated that St John's wort extract's antidepressant action was based on the ability of crude hypericin preparations to inhibit both types A and B MAO.[5,6] As a result of this inhibition, there is an increase in the level of neurotransmitters within the brain that maintain normal mood and emotional stability including serotonin, catecholamines, and dopamine. These preliminary results identified hypericin as the supposed active constituent. However, later chemical analysis of these crude hypericin preparations identified a content of as much as 20% of other St John's wort constituents, with the flavonoids being the most important.[1] In other words, it is not known to what extent hypericin or the flavonoids individually contribute to any MAO inhibition.

To better understand the influence of hypericin, hypericum total extract, and hypericum fractions on the activity of MAO and COMT, a study was conducted.[7] An inhibition of MAO could be shown in the following concentrations:

- hypericin to 10^{-3} mol/L
- hypericum total extract to 10^{-4} mol/L
- one extract fraction up to 10^{-5} mol/L.

A COMT inhibition could not be shown for hypericin, with hypericum extract to 10^{-4} mol/L and with two extract fractions also up to 10^{-4} mol/L. The MAO inhibiting fraction contained hypericins as well as flavonols, the COMT-inhibition fraction being mainly flavonols and xanthones. The key result from this study, as well as in another in vitro/ex vivo study, is the demonstration that the concentrations of inhibition shown, particularly with regard to the inhibition of MAO activity, are likely not sufficient to explain the clinically proven antidepressive effect of St John's wort extract.[7,8] Therefore, additional mechanisms are likely responsible for these clinical benefits.

At least two other mechanisms have been proposed: modulation of interleukin-6 activity and inhibition of the re-uptake of serotonin. The modulating effect of St John's wort extract on interleukin-6 (IL-6) is the most interesting as it proposes a mechanism by which St John's wort interacts with the link between the immune system and mood. The immune system and the nervous system share many common biochemical features and regulatory interactions. In regards to IL-6, this cytokine is heavily involved in the communication between cells within and outside the immune system. With regard to the nervous system, IL-6 is known to modulate hypothalamic-pituitary-end organ axes, especially the hypothalamic-pituitary-adrenal (HPA) axis. The hypothesis is that an elevation in IL-6 results in activation of the HPA axis leading to elevations in CRH and other adrenal regulatory hormones – hallmark features in depression. St John's wort extract has shown an ability to reduce IL-6 levels, and hence this action may explain the clinical effectiveness of St John's wort extract.[9]

The study demonstrating reduction of IL-6 levels involved taking blood samples from five healthy volunteers and four depressive patients.[9] The release of interleukin-6 (IL-6), interleukin-1 beta (IL-1 beta) and tumor necrosis factor-alpha (TNF-alpha) was measured quantitatively after an incubation time of 24 hours on microtiter plates. A massive suppression of the interleukin-6 release was found for PHA-stimulated St John's wort extract. If these effects can be duplicated in vivo, it would provide a mechanism by which St John's wort extract modulates CRH release and, subsequently, mood.

St John's wort extract has also been shown to inhibit the re-uptake of serotonin similar in fashion to drugs like fluoxetine (Prozac), paroxetine (Paxil), and sertraline (Zoloft). The study demonstrating a 50% serotonin re-uptake inhibition utilized the 0.3% hypericin content standardized extract at a concentration of 6.2 mcg/ml and did not attempt to identify the active inhibitors.[10] The authors of the study concluded that "the antidepressant activity of Hypericum extract is due to inhibition of serotonin uptake by postsynaptic receptors". However, an important point must be made – until pharmacokinetic studies demonstrate that St John's wort components pass across the blood–brain barrier, a primary site of action outside the central nervous system cannot be ruled out.

Extracts of St John's wort have been tested in various animal models designed to study its antidepressant effects. In these studies, St John's wort extract was found to enhance the exploratory activity of mice in a foreign environment, extend the narcotic sleeping time in a dose-dependent fashion, antagonize the effects of reserpine, and decrease aggressive behavior in socially isolated male mice.[1,11] These activities are consistent with the expected effects of antidepressant compounds and appear to be the result of increased monoamine activity.

Anti-viral activity

In vitro studies have shown that hypericin and pseudohypericin exhibit strong antiviral activity against herpes simplex virus I and II as well as influenza types A and B, and vesicular stomatitis virus.[12] These compounds have also demonstrated remarkable antiviral activity against Epstein–Barr virus.[13]

A tremendous amount of excitement was generated when researchers from New York University Medical Center and the Weizmann Institute of Science in Israel demonstrated the anti-retroviral activity of hypericin and pseudohypericin.[14] This preliminary study examined the effect of these compounds on two animal retroviruses, Friend leukemia virus and radiation leukemia virus, both in vitro and in vivo (in mice). The researchers found the effective dose of hypericin in mice to be 1.5–2.0 mcg/ml. The researchers concluded:

> Hypericin and pseudohypericin display an extremely effective antiviral activity when administered to mice after retroviral infection. … The antiviral activity is remarkable both in its mechanism of action … and in the potency of one administration of a relatively small dose of the compounds. Availability … and the relatively convenient and inexpensive procedure for the extraction and purification of hypericin and pseudohypericin further enhance the potential of these compounds.

Later, two possible mechanisms were described to explain the antiviral activity of both hypericin and pseudohypericin.[15] First, inhibition of assembly or processing of intact virions from infected cells – released virions contain no detectable activity of reverse transcriptase. Second, these compounds also directly inactivate mature and properly assembled retroviruses.

The antiviral activity of hypericin against HIV appears to require the interaction with light to activate the hypericin.[16,17] Another requirement is sufficient concentrations, as entry of hypericin into infected cells is dependent upon the concentration of hypericin in the blood. At sufficient concentrations, hypericin incubated with HIV-infected whole blood decreases culturable HIV, indicating significant antiviral activity.[18]

Antibacterial activity

St John's wort extracts have broad-spectrum antimicrobial activity against both Gram-negative and Gram-positive bacteria.[19] The organisms they studied included *Staphylococcus aureus, Streptococcus mutans, Proteus vulgaris, Escherichia coli,* and *Pseudomonas aeruginosa.*

Pharmacokinetic studies

Recent pharmacokinetic studies have been published using the 0.3% hypericin content standardized extract.[1,20] The major drawbacks of these studies is the focus on hypericin and pseudohypericin. Nonetheless, these studies effectively demonstrated that hypericin and pseudohypericin are absorbed. In one of the studies, it was shown that after 4 days of taking the standard dosage of the extract (300 mg t.i.d.), a steady state is reached with mean maximal plasma levels during the steady-state period of 8.5 ng/ml for hypericin and 5.8 ng/ml for pseudohypericin.[20] Interestingly, even though pseudohypericin is found in higher concentrations in the extract than hypericin, higher blood levels are achieved with hypericin, indicating that hypericin is more bioavailable than pseudohypericin.

CLINICAL APPLICATIONS

The primary use of St John's wort is in the treatment of depression. It may also be of benefit in the treatment of chronic viral infections and, topically, in various skin products.

Depression

Extracts of St John's wort standardized for hypericin content (most studies used the 0.3% hypericin content extract) has significant support in the treatment of mild to moderate antidepressant.[1,3,21] The official German Commission E monograph for St John's wort lists psychovegetative disturbances, depressive states, fear, and nervous disturbances as clinical indications for St John's wort.

The clinical evaluation of St John's wort extract began with an initial clinical study of six depressed women, aged 55–65, which measured the change in urinary metabolites of noradrenaline and dopamine following administration of a standardized extract of St John's wort extract (0.14% hypericin content).[22] Researchers found a significant increase in the catecholamine metabolite 3-methoxy-4-hydroxyphenylglycol, a marker commonly used to evaluate the efficacy of antidepressant therapy. A follow-up study by the same researchers followed 15 women with depression taking the same standardized extract.[22] The results demonstrated a significant improvement in symptoms of anxiety, apathy, hypersomnia and insomnia, anorexia, psychomotor retardation, depression, and feelings of worthlessness. No side-effects were observed.

Since this initial study, a total of 1,592 patients have been studied in 25 double-blind controlled studies (15 compared with placebo, 10 compared with antidepressant drugs including five studies comparing St John's wort to tricyclics: two vs. imipramine; two vs. amitriptyline; and one vs. desipramine).[1,3,21,23]

In these studies, St John's wort extract was shown to produce improvements in many psychological symptoms, including:

- depression
- anxiety
- apathy
- sleep disturbances
- insomnia
- anorexia
- feelings of worthlessness.

Even more impressive is that St John's wort extract was able to achieve these benefits without producing significant side-effects.

The scientific investigation of St John's wort is not complete. From a clinical perspective, the major shortcomings of the existing clinical trials is their relatively short term (8 weeks) and the lack of studies in severely depressed patients.[23] Given the growing popularity of hypericum, studies which address these shortcoming are needed. The currently available information clearly supports the short-term use of St John's wort extract as an alternative to standard antidepressant drugs in cases of mild to moderate depression. Whether it will be shown to be suitable in the treatment of serious depressions (i.e. depressions associated with psychotic symptoms and/or depressions with serious risk of suicide) remains to answered.

As stated above, there have been over 25 double-blind studies with St John's wort extract in the treatment of depression. The methodological quality of this research, particularly the studies since 1989, has been judged as being acceptable by strict criteria.[3,21,23] The overall results have also been judged as providing good documentation of antidepressant activity.[3,21,23] The double-blind studies with the highest methodological quality rating are listed in Table 93.1. Several of the better studies are discussed below.

In the study with the highest methodological rating, 135 depressed patients were treated in 20 centers.[35] Patients were given either St John's wort extract (0.3% hypericin content, 300 mg t.i.d.) or imipramine (25 mg t.i.d.) for a period of 6 weeks. Inclusion diagnoses were typical depressions with single episode, several episodes, depressive neurosis, and adjustment disorder with depressed mood in accordance with DSM-III-R. Main assessment criteria were the Hamilton Depression Scale (HAMD), the Depression Scale according to von Zerssen (D-S) and the Clinical Global Impressions (CGI). In both treatment groups, there were significant decreases in the HAMD from 20.2 to 8.8 in the St John's wort group, and from 19.4 to 10.7 in the imipramine group. The D-S point value also dropped from 39.6 to 27.2 in the St John's wort group, and 39.0 to 29.2 in the imipramine group (see Table 93.2). The analysis of CGI revealed comparable results in both treatment groups. The main advantage, however, was not so much a difference in therapeutic outcome, but rather a significant advantage in terms of lack of side-effects and excellent patient tolerance in the St John's wort group.

Another high quality randomized, double-blind study examining the effectiveness and tolerance of the 0.3% hypericin content standardized St John's wort extract compared was maprotiline was performed in a group

Table 93.1 Summary of clinical trials with St John's wort extract in depression

Trial (ref no.)	No. of patients	Baseline HDS	Dose (mg/day)	Duration (weeks)	Responder rate (St John's wort)	Responder rate (placebo)
Trials comparing St John's wort with placebo						
Halama[24]	50	18.0	1.08	4	10/25	0/25
Hansgren et al[25]	72	20.4	2.7	4	27/34	9/38
Harrer & Sommer[26]	120	20.9	0.75	6	22/58	9/58
Hubner et al[27]	40	12.4	2.7	4	14/20	9/20
Quandt et al[28]	88	17.3	0.75	4	29/44	3/44
Reh et al[29]	50	20.0	1.0	8	20/25	11/25
Schmidt & Sommer[30]	65	16.4	1.08	6	20/32	6/33
Schmidt et al[31]	40	29.5	0.75	4	15/25	3/24
Sommer & Harrer[32]	105	15.8	2.7	4	28/50	13/55
Totals	630				185/313 (59%)	63/322 (20%)
Trials comparing St John's wort extract with an antidepressant drug						
Bergman et al[33]	80	15.4	0.75	6	32/40	28/40 (amitryptiline)
Harrer et al[34]	102	19.4	2.7	4	27/51	28/51 (maprotiline)
Vorbach et al[35]	135	9.4	2.7	4	42/67	37/68 (imipramine)
Totals	317				101/158 (64%)	93/159 (58%)

*Responder rate, a decrease in the HAMD of greater than 50% or achieving a value less than 10.

Table 93.2 Hypericum compared with imipramine

	St John's wort	Imipramine
Hamilton Depression Scale		
Initial measurement	20.2	19.4
Week 6	8.8	10.7
Depression Scale (von Zerssen)		
Initial measurement	39.6	39
Week 6	27.2	29.2

of 102 patients with depression.[34] Patients were given either St John's wort extract (300 mg t.i.d.) or maprotiline (25 mg t.i.d.) for a period of 4 weeks. Effectiveness was determined using the HAMD, D-S, and CGI scales. The total score of the HAMD scale dropped during the 4 weeks of therapy in both treatment groups by about 50%. The mean values of the D-S and the CGI scales showed similar results, and after 4 weeks of therapy, no significant differences in either treatment group were noticed. The onset of the effects occurred up to the second week of treatment, but were observed earlier with maprotiline than with the St John's wort extract. However, maprotiline treatment resulted in the typical side-effects with tricyclics, e.g. tiredness, mouth dryness, and heart complaints, while St John's wort caused no significant side-effects.

In a multicenter double-blind study, 72 depressive patients with a HAMD greater than 16 were given either St John's wort extract (0.3% hypericin content, 300 mg) or placebo three times daily for 4 weeks.[25] At the end of the trial period, there was a significant advantage for the St John's wort group as 27 out of 34 (81%) patients in this group responded based on a HAMD score less than 10, compared with nine out of 38 (26%) in the placebo group. Another way of looking at the results in this study is to examine the drop in the average HAMD in both groups. In the treatment group, the HAMD dropped from an average of 20.8 at the beginning of the trial to 9.2 after 4 weeks, while in the placebo group the drop was from 20.4 to 14.7. At the end of the 4 week trial, the placebo group and treatment group were subsequently treated for an additional 2 weeks with St John's wort extract in both groups, with the average HAMD in the treatment group dropping below 6 and the original placebo group dropping to below the responder rate of 10.

In another double-blind study, 105 patients with different types of mild to moderate depressions were given either 300 mg of the St John's wort extract standardized to contain 0.3% hypericin or an identically looking placebo three times daily for 4 weeks.[32] The effectiveness of treatment was judged after 2 and 4 weeks according to the HAMD scale, the standard measure to assess an antidepressant's effectiveness. The results are shown in Table 93.3.

Using the criteria of a decrease in the HAMD of greater than 50% or achieving a value less than 10 as identification of responders, 28 out of 42 patients (67%) in the St John's wort group responded, compared with 13 of 47 patients (27.7%) in the placebo group. The results of this study are consistent with other well-designed studies comparing St John's wort with placebo.

Table 93.3 Hypericum compared with palcebo

	St John's wort	Placebo
Baseline	15.81	15.83
Week 2	9.64	12.28
Week 4	7.17	11.30

Seasonal affective disorder

Seasonal affective disorder (SAD) represents a subgroup of major depression with a regular occurrence of symptoms in autumn/winter and full remission in spring/summer. Light therapy has become the standard treatment of this type of depression. Apart from this, pharmacotherapy with antidepressants also seems to provide an improvement of SAD symptoms. The aim of a controlled, single-blind study was to evaluate if St John's wort could be beneficial in treating SAD patients and whether the combination with light therapy would be additionally advantageous.[36] Patients who fulfilled DSM-III-R criteria for major depression with seasonal pattern were randomized in a 4 week treatment study with 900 mg of St John's wort extract/day (0.3% hypericin content) combined with either bright (3000 lux, $n = 10$) or dim light (<300 lux therapy). The significant reduction in the Hamilton Depression scale in both groups (72 and 60%, respectively) indicates that St John's wort extract may offer support to patients with SAD as a sole therapeutic agent as well as in combination with light therapy.

Insomnia

St John's wort has been shown to improve sleep quality and well-being in healthy elderly subjects.[37] With antidepressant drugs, particularly tricyclic antidepressants and MAO inhibitors, REM (rapid eye movement) sleep is reduced. St John's wort did not interfere with REM sleep like other antidepressants and was shown to increase the intensity of deep sleep during the total sleeping period as demonstrated by brain wave studies. While St John's wort improved sleep quality it did not act as a sedative (i.e. it did not reduce sleep onset) nor did it change total sleep duration.

Mental function

One of the most interesting comparative studies was a double-blind study where St John's wort extract (0.3%

hypericin content) was compared with maprotyline in 24 healthy volunteers by measuring resting brain wave (EEG) tracings and mental activity (visual and acoustic evoked potentials).[38] Interpretation of the differences in reactions indicated that, unlike maprotiline, which interferes with mental function, St John's wort actually improves memory and other mental activities.

AIDS and other viral infections

The research suggests that St John's wort may be a useful adjunctive treatment for herpes simplex, mononucleosis, and influenza, although further human studies are needed to establish the optimal dosage of the standardized extract. Combined with its antidepressant activity, St John's wort also appears to be a promising treatment for chronic fatigue syndrome.

The greatest promise of St John's wort, however, may be in the treatment of AIDS. In response to the in vitro and animal studies, many AIDS patients began self-administering St John's wort. Although most patients reported feeling better with a more positive outlook, more energy, and less fatigue, it was not known to what degree this was due to a placebo effect.[39,40] To better determine the benefits, a number of trials evaluated the efficacy of standardized extracts of St John's wort in the treatment of HIV-infected individuals.

In one study, St John's wort extracts providing approximately 1 mg of hypericin/day were studied in 31 patients.[41] Baseline and 4-monthly measurements, including physical exam, T-cell subsets, and other laboratory parameters, were performed. Concomitant use of AZT and other treatments was permitted. The results of the study were encouraging. In the subgroup of 10 patients who took no AZT either before or during the study ("AZT virgins"; none had AIDS), the mean helper T-cell count increased 13% from baseline after 1 month on St John's wort and maintained this increase for 4 months. Although these increases were not statistically significant, in contrast, helper T-cell counts of the 10 patients using AZT throughout the study fell significantly after an initial mild rise. Side-effects were limited to reversible liver enzyme elevations in five patients with all levels returned to baseline after 1 month without St John's wort extract.

In another open pilot study, 18 HIV patients (three with the CDC II, eight with CDC III, four with CDC IV B and three with CDC IV C1 classification) were treated solely with standardized St John's wort extract (weekly intravenous injection and daily oral intake), providing a daily intake of 2 mg of hypericin.[42] The 16/18 patients with good compliance showed stable or even increasing counts of absolute helper T-cells over the 40 months of observation. Also the helper to suppressor T-cell ratio showed an improvement in the majority of these patients. Clinically, it was noteworthy that only two of these 16 patients encountered an opportunistic infection during the 40 months of observation. The other 14/16 patients remained clinically stable and active in work and life. This steady-state situation of the HIV infection also correlated with stable values of hemoglobin, leukocytes and platelets. Furthermore, none of the otherwise known viral complications due to CMV, herpes or EBV was encountered in these 16 patients.

Despite these good preliminary results, the trials proved disappointing as significant blood levels of hypericin could not be achieved using the extract either orally or intravenously. Use of the standardized extract for the treatment of HIV infection has since been replaced by the use of intravenously administered synthetic hypericin. Preliminary studies are again producing some encouraging results with good safety, although photosensitivity may occur (see "Toxicity", p. 804) and long-term controlled evaluation is needed.[43,44] (for further discussion, see Ch. 141).

Topical application

St John's wort has a historical use as an aid in wound healing. Research has demonstrated antibacterial and wound healing activity.[2] St John's wort preparations have also been used in burns, as a sunscreen, and in the treatment of muscular pain.[2] Oil-based preparations are preferred for topical applications.

DOSAGE

The dosages of St John's wort preparations are based upon their hypericin content. The overwhelming majority of the studies in depression have used St John's wort extract standardized to contain 0.3% hypericin. This extract is produced via an extraction with 80% methanol (which is subsequently removed). Although hypericin is a key component, this extract is composed of a wide range of compounds constituting the remaining 99.7% of the extract. Manufacturers of these standardized extracts employ HPLC techniques to identify not only the hypericin and pseudohypericin, but also related compounds, flavonoid components, xanthones, cinnamic acid, and several other key components. The point is that although the dosage is based upon hypericin levels, assuring appropriate levels of these other constituents is also vitally important.

To achieve the benefits noted in the clinical trials, it is difficult to recommend any other forms beyond standardized extracts. Nonetheless, here are dosage recommendations for various forms of St John's wort:

- dried flowers: 2–4 g three times/day
- tincture (1:5): 3–6 ml three times/day
- fluid extract (1:1): 1–2 ml three times/day

- standardized fluid extract (0.14% hypericin–1.0 mg hypericin/3 cc): 0.5–0.9 ml three times/day
- standardized solid (dry-powdered) extract (0.14% hypericin): 600 mg three times/day
- standardized solid (dry-powdered) extract (0.3% hypericin): 300 mg three times/day.

TOXICITY

There is considerable evidence that St John's wort can cause severe photosensitivity in animals grazing extensively on the plant. The term "hypericism" has been used to describe a skin disease found in animals who graze on large quantities of St John's wort.[45] However, reports of photosensitivity in humans have been rare and have been limited to those taking excessive quantities for HIV infection. St John's wort is unlikely to be toxic to humans when used at recommended medicinal doses. However, individuals with AIDS taking large amounts of St John's wort extracts (or hypericin) have developed photosensitivity.[44]

Because of the possibility of photosensitivity, avoidance of exposure to strong sunlight and other sources of ultraviolet light when using St John's wort is often recommended to individuals, especially those with fair skin. However, while this recommendation may be appropriate, it must be pointed out that the therapeutic dosage of 2.7 mg/day of hypericin is about 30–50 times below the level required to produce phototoxicity.[46]

Historically, those taking St John's wort have been advised to avoid foods and medications that are known to negatively interact with MAO-inhibiting drugs such as tyramine-containing foods (cheeses, beer, wine, pickled herring, yeast, etc.) and drugs such as L-dopa and 5-hydroxytryptophan should be avoided. However, given the recent research demonstrating the lack of any in vivo MAO inhibition, this recommendation is no longer justified.

No significant side-effects have been reported in the numerous double-blind studies, but perhaps the best demonstration of the excellent safety record of St John's wort extract is a large-scale study involving 3,250 patients conducted in Germany.[47] Results were analyzed by means of a patient questionnaire. Pooled data indicated that symptoms of depression were reduced in frequency and intensity by approximately 50%. The frequency of undesired side-effects was reported in 79 patients (2.43%) and 48 (1.45%) discontinued therapy. The most frequently noted side-effects were gastrointestinal irritation (0.55%), allergic reactions (0.52%), fatigue (0.4%), and restlessness (0.26%).

The frequency and severity of side-effects with St John's wort extract are clinically insignificant, especially when compared with the well-known side-effects of tricyclics and other antidepressants. There have been no deaths due to St John's wort toxicity, a stark contrast to the 31 deaths per 1 million prescriptions produced by synthetic antidepressants.[48]

REFERENCES

1. Morazzoni P, Bombardellie E. *Hypericum perforatum*. Milan: Indena. 1994
2. Hobbs C. St John's wort , *Hypericum perforatum* L. HerbalGram 1989; 18/19: 24–33
3. Ernst E. St John's wort , an antidepressant? A systematic, criteria-based review. Phytomed 1995; 2: 67–71
4. De Smet PAG, Nolen W. St John's wort as an antidepressant. BMJ 1996; 313: 241–242
5. Suzuki O et al.: Inhibition of monoamine oxidase by hypericin. Planta Medica 1984; 50: 272–274
6. Holzl J, Demisch L, Gollnik B. Investigations about antidepressive and mood changing effects of *Hypericum perforatum*. Planta Med 1989; 55: 643
7. Thiede HM, Walper A. Inhibition of MAO and COMT by hypericum extracts and hypericin. J Geriatr Psychiatry Neurol 1994; 7: S54–56
8. Bladt S, Wagner H. Inhibition of MAO by fractions and constituents of hypericum extract. J Geriatr Psychiatry Neurol 1994; 7: S57–59
9. Thiele B; Brink I, Ploch M. Modulation of cytokine expression by hypericum extract. J Geriatr Psychiatry Neurol 1994; 7: S60–62
10. Perovic S, Muller WEG. Pharmacological profile of hypericum extract. Effect of serotonin uptake by postsynaptic receptors. Arzneim Forsch 1995; 45: 1145–1148
11. Okpanyi VSN, Weischer ML. Tierexperimentelle untersuchungen zur psychotropen wirksamkeit eines hypericum-extraktes. Arzneim Forsch 1987; 37: 10–13
12. Muldner VH, Zoller M. Antidepressive wirkung eines auf den wirkstoffkomplex hypericin standardisierten hypericum-extrakes. Arzneim Forsch 1984; 34: 918
13. Lavie D. Antiviral pharmaceutical compositions containing hypericin or pseudohypericin. European Patent Application, No. 87111467.4, filed 8/8/87, European Patent Office. Publ No. 0 256 A2. 175–177. 1987
14. Someya H. Effect of a constituent of *Hypericum erectum* on infection and multiplication of Epstein-Barr virus. J Tokyo Med Coll 1985; 43: 815–826
15. Meruelo D, Lavie G, Lavie D. Therapeutic agents with dramatic antiretroviral activity and little toxicity at effective doses. Aromatic polycyclic diones hypericin and pseudohypericin. Proc Natl Acad Sci 1988; 85: 5230–5234
16. Lavie G, Valentin F et al. Studies of the mechanism of action of the antiretroviral agents hypericin and pseudohypericin. Proc Natl Acad Sci 1989; 86: 5963–5967
17. Degar S, Prince A, Pascual D. Inactivation of the human immunodeficiency virus by hypericin. Evidence for photo-chemical alterations of p24 and a block in uncoating. AIDS Res Human Retrovir 1992; 8: 1929–1936
18. Valentine FT, Lavie G, Levin B et al. Synthetic hypericin enters blood lymphocytes and monocytes in vitro and decreases culturable HIV in blood obtained from infected individuals. Int Conf AIDS 1991; 7: 97 (abstract no. W.A.1022)
19. Barbagallo C, Chisari G. Antimicrobial activity of three Hypericum species. Filoterapia 1987; 58: 175–177
20. Staffeldt B et al. Pharmacokinetics of hypericin and pseudohypericin after oral intake of the *Hypericum perforatum* extract LI 160 in healthy volunteers. J Geriatr Psychiatry Neurol 1994; 7: S47–53
21. Muldner VH, Zoller M. Antidepressive wirkung eines auf den

wirkstoffkomplex hypericin standardisierten hypericum-extrakes. Arzneim Forsch 1984; 34: 918
22. Harrer G, Schulz V. Clinical investigation of the antidepressant effectiveness of Hypericum. J Geriatr Psychiatry Neurol 1994; 7: S6–8
23. Linde K et al. St John's wort for depression – an overview and meta-analysis of randomised clinical trials. BMJ 1996; 313: 253–258
24. Halama P. Efficacy of the Hypericum extract LI 160 in the treatment of 50 patients of a psychiatrist. Nervenheilkunde 1991; 10: 305–307
25. HansgrenD, Vesper J, Ploch M. Multicenter double-blind study examining the antidepressant effectiveness of the hypericum extract LI 160. J Geriatr Psychiatry Neurol 1994; 7: S15–18
26. Harrer G, Sommer H. Treatment of mild/moderate depressions with Hypericum. Phytomed 1994; 1: 3–8
27. Hubner WD, Lande S, Podzuweit H. Hypericum treatment of mild depressions with somatic symptoms. J Geriatr Psychiatry Neurol 1994; 7: S12–14
28. Quandt J, Scmidt U, Schenk N. Ambulante behandlung leichter und mittelschwerer depressiver verstiimmungen. Der Allgemeinarzt 1993; 2: 97–102
29. Reh C, Laux P, Schenk N. Hypericum-extrakt bei depressionen – eine wirksame alternative. Therapeiwoche 1992; 42: 1576–1581
30. Schmidt U, Sommer H. St John's wort extract in the ambulatory therapy of depression. Attention and reaction ability are preserved. Fortschr Med 1993; 111: 339–342
31. Schmidt U, Schenk N, Schwarz N et al. The therapy of depressive moods. Psycho 1989; 15: 665–671
32. Sommer H, Harrer G. Placebo-controlled double-blind study examining the effectiveness of an hypericum preparation in 105 mildly depressed patients. J Geriatr Psychiatry Neurol 1994; 7: S9–11
33. Bergman R, Nubner J, Demling J. Behandlung leichter gis mittelschwer depressionen. Therapiewoch Neurologie/Psychiatrie 1993; 7: 235–240
34. Harrer G, Hubner WD, Podzuweit H. Effectiveness and tolerance of the hypericum extract LI 160 compared to maprotiline. A multicenter double-blind study. J Geriatr Psychiatry Neurol 1994; 7: S24–28
35. Vorbach EU, Hubner WD, Arnoldt KH. Effectiveness and tolerance of the hypericum extract LI 160 in comparison with imipramine. Randomized double-blind study with 135 outpatients. J Geriatr Psychiatry Neurol 1994; 7: S19–23
36. Martinez B, Kasper S, Ruhrmann S et al. Hypericum in the treatment of seasonal affective disorders. J Geriatr Psychiatry Neurol 1994; 7: S29–33
37. Schulz H, Jobert M. Effects of hypericum extract on the sleep EEG in older volunteers. J Geriatr Psychiatry Neurol 1994; 7: S39–43
38. Johnson D, Ksciuk H, Woelk H et al. Effects of hypericum extract LI 160 compared with maprotiline on resting EEG and evoked potentials in 24 volunteers. J Geriatr Psychiatry Neurol 1994; 7: S44–46
39. James JS. AIDS Treatment News 1989; 74
40. James JS. AIDS Treatment News 1989; 91
41. Cooper WC, James J. An observational study of the safety and efficacy of hypericin in HIV+ subjects. Int Conf AIDS 1990; 6: 369 (abstract no. 2063)
42. Steinbeck-Klose A, Wernet P. Successful long term treatment over 40 months of HIV-patients with intravenous Hypericin. Int Conf AIDS 1993; 9: 470 (abstract no. PO-B26-2012)
43. Furner V, Bek M, Gold J. A Phase I/II unblinded dose ranging study of hypericin in HIV-positive subjects. Int Conf AIDS 1991; 7: 199 (abstract no. W.B.2071)
44. Gulick R, Lui H, Anderson R et al. Human hypericism. A photosensitivity reaction to hypericin (St John's wort). Int Conf AIDS 1992; 8: B90 (abstract no. PoB 3018)
45. Araya OS, Ford JH. An investigation of the type of photosensitization caused by the ingestion of St John's wort (*Hypericum perforatum*) by calves. J Comp Path 1981; 91: 135–141
46. Siegers CP, Biel S, Wilhelm KP. Zur frage der phototoxizitat von hypericum. 1993; 12: 320–322
47. Woelk H, Burkard G, Grunwald J. Benefits and risks of the hypericum extract LI 160. drug monitoring study with 3250 patients. J Geriatr Psychiatry Nerol 1994; 7: S34–38
48. Henry JA, Alexander CA, Sener EK. Relative mortality from overdose of antidepressants. Br Med J 1995; 310: 221–224

CHAPTER CONTENTS

94

Introduction to the clinical use of Chinese prepared medicines

M. Harrison Nolting, ND LAc

Qiang Cao, MD(China) ND LAc

INTRODUCTION

In traditional Chinese medicine, herbal medicines, which are considered synonymous with drugs, have been in use for more than 2,000 years.[1] Secret family (or company) recipes called "patent" medicines were first produced in the Song Dynasty (960–1234 AD) and were dispensed by government agencies such as the "Imperial Benevolence Pharmacy".[2] The long history and development of these prepared medicines, as well as their current widespread popularity, attest to the ancient adage that such preparations are convenient, effective, and economical.[3,4] In recent years, most of these "patent" medicine recipes have become part of the public domain, making it more appropriate to refer to this group as prepared medicines. But since the term "patent" has virtually become synonymous with all Asian produced medicines in pill, capsule, or liquid form, the term will certainly persist.[5]

History of use in the West

Yeung's Handbook of Chinese herbs and formulas[6] and Bensky & Gamble's Chinese herbal medicine[7] are major English works which provide basic Chinese herbal information. The introduction of Chinese prepared medicines and the books describing them have increased Western interest in Chinese herbs. The authors hope this growing interest in the prepared medicines will lead the serious student to closely study the history and development of the entire traditional Chinese materia medica. Mastering the art of herbal medicine practice requires lengthy study of the strategies as well as the formulas of Chinese herbal medicine.[6–10]

Although Chinese medicine and pharmacy began to spread outside of China's borders nearly 2,000 years ago, it is only in the last 20 years that interest has grown in North America. Much of this is due to former President Nixon's trip to the People's Republic of China in the early 1970s and subsequent reporters' visits and articles, especially those of James Reston of the *New York Times*.

The growth of acupuncture and oriental medical practices such as herbal medicine in the United States has been steady since that time.[11] In 1997, the number of practitioners of acupuncture and Oriental medicine, including those who utilize prepared medicines in their practice, had risen to over 20,000.

The traditional loose herb recipes used in Chinese herbal medicine are cooked and made into medicinal soups which are often quite bitter and difficult for the American palate. The Chinese solution to this dilemma is to increase the use of raw licorice in the formula and to offer sugar wafers to the patient to help offset the bitter taste, although most Chinese welcome a bitter taste as a normal part of Asian cuisine. The prepared medicines offer an alternative to the traditional preparations. A number of companies, particularly in Taiwan and California, have begun to popularize the manufacture and sale of powder and tincture formulas in single herb form to help "bridge" the traditional form and the prepared, more palatable, forms of medicine. This allows the practitioner to still utilize the traditional approach, that of mixing and adjusting the formulas tailored to the patient's individual diagnosis. Prepared formulas are fixed, of course, and do not allow any adjustments in the ingredients.

Prior to the mid-1970s, the FDA restricted the import and sale of traditional medicines by ethnic groups. New legislation and court rulings since then have lifted these restrictions, which, coupled with the explosion of acupuncture on the American health scene, has opened the door to the spread of prepared medicines.[12]

Now, due to this rapid growth in the sale and use of prepared medicines, problems with adulterants and false labeling are increasing, especially in California, where a multi-agency herbal medicine task force involving numerous California and federal government agencies was formed in response. In fact, it is stated in California Department of Health Services documents that "most imported Asian patent medicines do not fully comply with California laws".[13] While some of these violations are indeed potentially dangerous and may involve toxic ingredients and the inclusion of endangered species, many involve labeling issues and can often be sorted out by revising the labeling at the company of origin.

Market

The market for Chinese prepared medicines is huge. China will become the largest pharmaceutical market in the world within a few years. In herbal medicine, the Chinese sales alone were $2.3 billion in 1995. It is estimated that there are over 5,000 "licensed patent medicines" in China.[14] Outside of the enormous "inside China market", the growing interest and use of natural medicine worldwide are driving the consumption of prepared medicines rapidly upward. As mentioned already, this growth has sparked abuse and problems with product labeling and safety that the entire profession is working to counteract.

FORMULATIONS AND PREPARATIONS

Chinese patent medicines are prepared in a number of different forms. As far back as 200 BC, Chinese pharmaceuticals had developed a surprising level of sophistication. Pills were bound together using a wide variety of animal and human substances. Table 94.1 shows the 15 major dosage forms of Chinese prepared medicines.

In China, the prepared medicines are produced at factories located throughout the country. Reputation and awards are very important to these mainland Chinese operations. Factories such as the Chongqing Tong Jun Ge Medicine Works in Sichuan province, built in 1908, are quite proud of their products. This factory produces more than 200 medicines in 14 therapeutic categories.[16]

The most famous factory is at the Tong Ren Tang Pharmacy in Beijing. The Tong Ren Tang Pharmacy has been operated by the same family for 317 years. Prepared medicines produced in the factory hold the highest reputation in China, where the factory has supplied medicines to Chinese royalty over several centuries. The drug control acts implemented by the Chinese government in the 1970s and 1980s have helped to further guarantee quality control of prepared medicines in China.

Adulterants, endangered species

Many prepared medicines made outside mainland China lack the same quality controls as the factories within China. In 1975, an herbal-based preparation called Toukuwan was manufactured in Hong Kong by the Nan-Lien Pharmaceutical Company and widely promoted in the United States as a treatment for rheumatism and

Table 94.1 Major dosage forms of Chinese prepared medicines[15]

- Water paste pills
- Honey boluses
- Tablets
- Infusions (granules)
- Powders
- Capsules
- Medicated wines
- Injectables
- Plasters
- Semifluid extracts
- Oral liquids
- Suppositories
- Gelatins
- Syrups
- Tinctures (external, internal)

arthritis. The FDA banned the import of Toukuwan after it discovered four drugs including valium in the Chuifong preparation. Various prescription drugs have also been discovered in other prepared medicines. The *Journal of the American Medical Association* also reported four cases of agranulocytosis caused by prepared medicines in 1975 prior to the FDA ban.

The Chuifong product has continued to appear under various names such as "miracle herbs" since 1975.[17,18] Caution must be used when purchasing and prescribing prepared herbal medicines, and the authors recommend using only well-known and reputable manufacturers. If there is any doubt, utilize products produced at companies in America which are typically under far more quality control standards than those parts of Asia.

In May 1994, TRAFFIC USA and the World Wildlife Fund published *Prescription for Extinction: Endangered Species and Patented Oriental Medicines in Trade*.[19] This report gave insight into the vast number of endangered species being used in natural medicine. Bastyr University's Department of Acupuncture and Oriental Medicine has been conducting an in-depth study of the endangered species used in the practice of Chinese herbal medicine. The work at Bastyr has forged strong relationships with conservation groups, federal agencies, consumers, students, and others at institutions involved in the field of traditional Chinese medicine. The Bastyr project, called the Endangered Species Project (ESP), is creating a database listing all common Chinese herbal formulations, with their respective ingredients, sold in the United States. The database indicates which products and traditional formulas contain endangered or threatened species according to Appendices I, II, and III of the Convention on International Trade in Endangered Species Of Wild Fauna and Flora (CITES).[20]

DISPENSARY GUIDE

The 10 Chinese prepared medicines described in Table 94.2 represent a small sample of the most common and therapeutically effective formulations. Several common varieties of preparations such as pills, tablets, oral liquid, tincture and plaster are included. An attempt has been made to introduce preparations focusing on major human systems such as cardiovascular, respiratory, CNS, urinary, female, and dermatology. This systems approach is a common method of teaching prepared medicines.

Ingredients are listed with their Chinese (Pinyin) name, botanical name and percentage in formula. Actions are listed in terms of Traditional Chinese Medicine with Western activities when pertinent. Indications are given according to major Chinese sources. Administration and dosage information is provided with specific directions for adult as well as pediatric use. Packing information is also provided to help ensure proper recognition and dosage. A special notes section is included to highlight unique uses, cautions and contraindications of the preparations.

Due to the questionable standards of prepared medicines manufactured in Asia and generally outside of China, only mainland Chinese sources known to the authors are listed. The authors also urge practitioners to scrutinize the labels of products from unknown sources. With correct labeling, ingredients of prepared medicines should be obvious to anyone who can read Latin or Chinese herbal names.

In recent years, prepared medicine companies have become well established in the United States. Several high-quality manufacturers are now producing formulas in forms more suitable to Westerners. These tinctures, powders and capsules are usually based on the same classical formulas described in this chapter.

Table 94.2 Ten Chinese prepared medicines

Formula name	Ingredients	Actions	Indications	Dosage	Packaging	Notes
Yin Chiao Chieh Tu Pien (Lonicera and Forsythia dispel heat tablets)	Loniceral flower (Jin Yin Hua), 17.85% Forsythia fruit (Lian Qiao), 17.85% Arctium fruit (Niu Bang Zi), 10.72% Platycodon root (Jie Geng), 10.72% Mentha herb (Bo He), 10.72% Soja seed (Dan Dou Chi), 8.93% Licorice root (Gan Cao), 8.93% Lophaterum leaf (Zhu Ye), 7.14% Scizonepeta herb (Jing Jie), 7.14%	Antiphlogistic Disinfectant Carminative Refrigerant	Common cold and flu Fever and sensation of chill Pain and weariness of limbs Headache Cough Swelling sore throat Mumps Parotitis	Two to four tablets b.i.d. or t.i.d	0.6 g each tablet, eight tablets per tube, 12 tubes per box	This formula was made for wind heat invasion of the exterior in traditional Chinese medicine. It is a very popular and commonly used medicine throughout China for early stages of common cold and flu. The Chinese hold that it is the best medicine for common cold and flu. It is most effective when taken immediately or in the first day or two after onset of cold or flu. It may also produce a diaphoretic effect, so monitor use carefully Produced by Tien Jin Drug Manufactory, Tianjin, People's Republic of China
Pe Min Kan Wan (nasal allergy pills)	Xanthium fruit (Cang Er Zi) Magnolia flower (Xin Yi) Angelica root (Bai Zhi) Chrysanthemum (Ju Hua) Lonicera flower (Jin Yin Hua) Pogostemon herb (Huo Xiang) Ox gallstone (Niu Huang) Bear bile (Xiong Dan Zhi) Other herbal extracts This is a widely-known and used formula that is accepted as an herbal combination whose manufacturer maintains a patent on its exact formulation	Anti-inflammatory Anodyne Anti-asthmatic	Allergic rhinitis Sinusitis Chronic rhinitis Nasal obstruction Rhinorrhea Sneezing Cough Asthma Bronchitis	Two to three tablets each dose, b.i.d. or t.i.d. Taking this medicine consistently for 30 days is considered one course of treatment	Bottle of 50 tablets	Pe Min Kan Wan is an effective remedy for the treatment of acute or chronic sinusitis and rhinitis. It is particularly effective for hypersensitive sinusitis. In hypertrophic rhinitis, it will gradually reduce the size of the polyps in the nose. Marked amelioration of the symptoms can be seen after the patient has taken this medicine for 1 week in mild cases, and one or two courses of treatment are sufficient for recovery. In serious cases, several courses of treatment should be given Manufactured by the Fu Shan United Pharmaceutical Manufactory, Guang Dong, People's Republic of China
Renshenfengwangjiang (ginseng and Royal jelly oral liquid)	*Panax ginseng* (Ren Shen) Royal Jelly (Feng Wang Jiang) In a base of honey	Strengthen vital energy Tonify the digestive system Nourish the entire system	Fatigue Poor constitution Malnutrition Also used as supplementary treatment of coronary artery disease, chronic hepatitis, neurasthenia, arthritis, gastritis, stomach and duodenal ulcer, impotence, lower sexual drive	To be taken orally, one vial each time, in the morning and in the evening	Oral liquid, 10 ml each vial, 10 vials per box	This is a general tonic prepared medicine and is used to treat general weakness and to strengthen the immune system Produced by China National Medicine and Health Products Import and Export Corporation, Harbin Branch, Harbin, People's Republic of China.

continued overleaf

Table 94.2 (contd)

Formula name	Ingredients	Actions	Indications	Dosage	Packaging	Notes
Dan Shen Pian (*Salvia miltorrhiza* compound tablets)	*Salviae multiorrhiza* (Dan Shen) *Panax notoginseng* (San Qi) Borneolum (Bing Pian)	Promotes blood circulation Limits blood stasis Induces resuscitation by means of aromatics Regulates the blood flow of Qi to alleviate pain.	Coronary heart disease Angina pectoris Oppressed feeling in the chest	Three tablets t.i.d.	Bottle of 50 tablets	The most popular heart remedy in China. Laboratory and clinical research in China has shown that this remedy is able to improve heart muscle contractions, invigorate the blood, increase the blood supply to the coronary artery circulation, and regulate the heart function. This medicine may cause stomach irritation Produced by China National Chemicals Import & Export Company, Shanghai Branch, People's Republic of China
Wu Cha Seng tablet (*Eleutherococcus senticosus* tablets)	*Eleutherococcus senticosus* (Ci Wu Jia), 100%	Accelerates the function of the brain and kidney Improves the appetite Improves eyesight and hearing Sedative effect on the central nervous system	It has therapeutic effects for coronary heart symptoms such as dyspnea, dizziness, angina pectoris, etc. Satisfactory results for general debilitation, senility, sore limbs or arthritic pains This preparation also helps stimulate and restore the functions of the organs of the infirm or aged, and of those weakened after illness or childbirth According to the manufacturer, it is effective in curing leukopenia	Three to four tablets twice daily, to be taken in the morning and evening with warm boiled water. Desired effect is brought about in 2–3 weeks of administration. Prolonged administration will give better effects	Box of 60 tablets	Clinical research in China suggested that this herb is especially effective relieving fatigue and increasing the immune function. It can also reduce anxiety, mental depression and irritation. In China, anthropanax is preferred over ginseng in the treatment of cancer. Produced by Harbin Chinese Medicine Factory, Heilongjiang, People's Republic of China
Hsiao Yao Wan (Free and Easy pill)	*Bupleurum chinense* (Chai Hu), 14.3% *Angelica sinensis* (Dang Gui), 14.3% *Paeonia lactiflora* (Bai Shao), 14.3% *Atractylodes macrocephala* (Bai Zhu), 14.3% *Poria cocus* (Fu Ling), 14.3% *Glycyrrhiza uralensis* (Gan Cao), 11.5% *Zingiber* (Sheng Jiang), 14.3% *Herba mentha* (Bo He), 2.9%	Circulating the liver Qi and relieving depression of the liver Invigorating the spleen and regulating the nutrient system	Traditionally this remedy is used to treat depression of the liver Qi and deficiency of the liver blood which manifest as pain in the hypochondrial region, alternative fever and chills, headache, vertigo or dizziness, dry mouth and throat, fatigue, anorexia, irregular menstruation, distention of the breasts, wiry and weak pulse. Modern use includes treatment of anxiety, depression, irritability, dizziness, vertigo, PMS, and irregular menses	Eight to 10 pills, t.i.d. taken with warm water	Bottle of 200 pills	Produced by Lanzhou Fo Ci Pharmaceutical Factory, Lanzhou, People's Republic of China

continued overleaf

Table 94.2 (contd)

Formula name	Ingredients	Actions	Indications	Dosage	Packaging	Notes
Liu Wei Di Huang Wan (Rehmannia six formula)	*Rehmannia glutinosa* (Di Huang), 12% *Cornus officinalis* (Shan Zhu Yu), 16% *Dioscorea opposita* (Shan Yao), 16% *Alisma plantago* (Ze Xie), 12% *Poria cocus* (Fu Ling), 12% *Paeonia sufutricosa* (Mu Dan Pi), 12%	Nourishing yin Tonifying the kidney	Traditionally this remedy is used to treat deficiency of kidney yin, flaming up of deficient fire, with sore and weak back and knees, feverish and painful body, dizziness, tinnitus or deafness, spontaneous or night sweating, nocturnal emission with dream, thirst, dribbling of urine, dry tongue and soreness of throat, unstable teeth, and heel pain Modern use includes treatment of nephritis, diabetes, tuberculosis, hyperthyroidism, and hypertension	Eight to 10 pills t.i.d., taken with warm water	Bottle of 200 pills	Produced by Lanzhou Fo Ci Pharmaceutical Factory, Lanzhou, People's Republic of China
Fu Ke Ba Zhen Wan (women's precious pills)	*Angelica sinensis* (Dang Gui), 12.12% *Ligusticum wallichii* (Chuan Xiong), 9.10% White *Paaeonia lactiflora* (Bai Shao Yao), 12.12% *Rehmannia glutinosa* (Shou Di Huang), 18.18% *Codonopis pilosulae* (Dang Shen), 12.12% *Atractylodes macroephala* (Bai Zhu), 12.12% *Poria cocus* (Fu Ling), 12.12% *Glycyrrhiza uralensis* (Gan Cao), 6.06%	Replenishing both Qi and blood	Gynecological disorders with loss of blood, and deficiency of Qi and blood including pale face, fatigue, dizziness, vertigo, shortness of breath, irregular menstruation, hypermenorrhea, hypomenorrhea, dysmenorrhea, general deficiency during pregnancy, general deficiency in the postpartum period, chills and fever, restlessness and thirst	Eight to 10 pills t.i.d., taken with warm water	Bottle of 200 pills	Produced by Lanzhou Fo Ci Pharmaceutical Factory, Lanzhou, People's Republic of China
Tu Jin Liniment (complex hibisci tincture)	*Cortex hibisci* (Tu Jin Pi), 6 cc Benzoic acid, 1.8 g Salicylic acid, 0.9 g Alcohol, suitable amount Also contains safflower, dandelion, rhubarb extracts as inert ingredients as flavor and adjuvant in a base of myrrh gum mass	Eliminates damp and heat in the skin. Stops itching	Skin infections caused by fungus, tinea, or scabies Itch of toes and skin Athlete's foot, etc.	External application one to two times a day	In bottles of 15 cc; 12 bottles to a paper box	Rub on the skin (it is not necessary to cover the skin), and the liquid will dry quickly. Tighten the lid after use. Not to be taken orally or dropped into eyes Produced by The United Pharmaceutical Manufactory, Guangzhou, People's Republic of China.

continued overleaf

Table 94.2 (contd)

Formula name	Ingredients	Actions	Indications	Dosage	Packaging	Notes
Medicated herbal plaster	Menthol, 16% Methyl salicylate, 10%	Promotes the flow of Qi and blood circulation Dispels pathogenic factor Alleviates pain	Arthralgia Soreness of waist and pain of the back Sprain and local pain caused by rheumatism It also is used for acute bruises, sprains, fractures, and traumatic swelling	Remove attached film and apply to affected area. For adults and children 2 years of age and older. Apply to affected area not more than three or four times daily. It will remain effective for 24 hours; more effective if used after a bath. Remove patches while bathing. If needed, cut sheet into smaller patches to save plaster	3.9 × 11 inches, 10 pieces per box	Administer with care to pregnant women. Contraindicated for patients with local ulceration. If skin irritation occurs, move to adjoining area or discontinue use. In the case of an allergic reaction, immediately discontinue use Manufactured by the United Pharmaceutical Manufactory, Guang Zhong, People's Republic of China

REFERENCES

1. Fu W. Traditional Chinese medicine and pharmacology. Beijing, PRC: Foreign Languages Press. 1985
2. Gamble A. Chinese herbal formulations. Seattle, WA: Northwest Institute of Acupuncture and Oriental Medicine class notes. 1986
3. Zhu CH. Clinical handbook of Chinese prepared medicines. Brookline, MA: Paradigm Publications. 1989: p 2–34
4. Naeser MA. Outline guide to Chinese herbal patent medicines in pill form. Boston, MA: Boston Chinese Medicine. 1989: p 14–37
5. Asian patent medicines, questions and answers. California: California Department of Health Food & Drug Branch. 1991
6. Yeung, HC. Handbook of Chinese herbs and formulas, vols I & II. Los Angeles, CA: Institute of Chinese Medicine. 1983
7. Bensky D, Gamble A. Chinese herbal medicine. Seattle, WA: Eastland Press. 1986
8. Unschuld PU. Medicine in China – a history of pharmaceutics. Berkeley, CA: University of California Press. 1986
9. Fratkin J. Chinese herbal patent formulas. Portland, OR: Institute For Traditional Chinese Medicine. 1986
10. Bensky D, Barolet R. Chinese herbal formulations. Seattle, WA: Eastland Press. 1990
11. Wolpe PR. The maintenance of professional authority: acupuncture and the American Physician. Social Problems 1986; 32: 5
12. Dharmanada S. Update on herbs. J Inst Trad Med 1985; 2: 1–28
13. Important information for the sellers of Asian patent medicines. California: State of California, Department of Health Services. 1991
14. Traditional Chinese medicines: the Chinese market and international opportunities. London: Natural Medicine Marketing in Collaboration with Sino European Clinics Limited. 1996
15. Zhang E. Highly efficacious Chinese patent medicines. Shanghai, PRC: Publishing House of Shanghai College of Traditional Chinese Medicine. 1990
16. Chongqing Tong Jun Ge Medicine Works. Product Catalog, Chongqing, Sichuan, China. 1985
17. Rics CA, Sahud MA. Agranulocytosis caused by Chinese herbal medicines. JAMA 1975; 231: 252–255
18. McCaleb R, Blumenthal M. Black pearls lose luster. HerbalGram 1990; 22: 4–5, 38–39
19. Gaski A, Johnson K. Prescription for extinction: endangered species and patented oriental medicines in trade. Washington, DC: TRAFFIC USA. 1994
20. Convention on International Trade in Endangered Species of Wild Fauna and Flora (CITES), CITES Secretariat, Convention Documents, September 1997, Geneve, Switzerland

FURTHER READING

1. Fratkin J. Chinese herbal patent formulas. Portland, OR: Institute For Traditional Chinese Medicine. 1986
2. Hu X. Complete collection of TCM secret formulas, vol I, II, III [Chinese], Shanghai, PRC: Shanghai Weng Hui Bao Press. 1990
3. Leng F. China basic TCM patent medicine [Chinese]. Beijing, PRC: People's Health Press. 1988
4. Lu S. Complete collection of common TCM patent medicine [Chinese]. Harbin, China: Harbin Press. 1990
5. Naeser MA. Outline guide to Chinese herbal patent medicines in pill form. Boston, MA: Boston Chinese Medicine. 1989
6. Tu Guoshi. Pharmacopeia of the People's Republic of China (English edition), Bejing: American Overseas Book Co. 1993
7. Yeung HC. Handbook of Chinese herbs and formulas, vol. I, II. Los Angeles, CA: Institute of Chinese Medicine Institute of Chinese Medicine. 1983
8. Zhu CH. Clinical handbook of Chinese prepared medicine. Brookline, MA: Paradigm Publications. 1989

CHAPTER CONTENTS

95

Lobelia inflata (Indian tobacco)

Michael T. Murray, ND

Joseph E. Pizzorno Jr, ND

Lobelia inflata (family: Campanulaceae)
Common name: Indian tobacco

GENERAL DESCRIPTION

Lobelia is an indigenous North American annual or biennial plant with an erect, angular, hairy stem that contains a milky sap and grows from 6 inches to 3 feet in height. Numerous small, two-lipped, blue flowers grow in spike-like racemes from July to November.

CHEMICAL COMPOSITION

Lobelia contains about 0.48% pyridine (piperidine) alkaloids composed mainly of lobeline (see Fig. 95.1) with lesser amounts of lobelanine, lobelanidine, and other alkaloids. Other constituents include resin, gum, lipids, and chelidonic acid.[1–3]

HISTORY AND FOLK USE

Lobelia was used extensively by Thomsonians as an emetic, diaphoretic, expectorant, sedative, antispasmodic, and anti-asthmatic. Conditions for which it has been used include, among others:

- asthma
- whooping cough
- bruises
- sprains
- ringworm
- insect bites
- poison ivy symptoms.

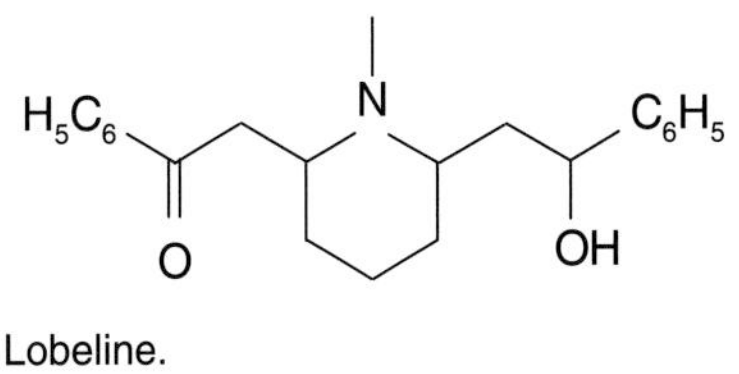

H_5C_6 N C_6H_5 O OH

Figure 95.1 Lobeline.

Thomson stated: "there is no vegetable which the earth produces more harmless in its effect on the human system, and none more powerful in removing disease and promoting health than lobelia".[4] Lobelia has also been used as an aid in stopping smoking.

PHARMACOLOGY

Lobeline has many of the same pharmacological actions as nicotine, but is generally regarded as being less potent.[5,6] These actions include stimulation of the autonomic ganglia (nicotinic receptors) followed by depression.

Gastrointestinal effects

The emetic action of lobeline is mediated by its stimulation of the emetic chemoreceptor trigger zone in the area postrema of the medulla oblongata (this area is outside the blood–brain barrier) and activation of the vagal and spinal afferent nerves that form the sensory input of the reflex pathways involved in vomiting.[7]

Respiratory effects

Indian tobacco is a very effective expectorant. Although it has a long history of use in asthma, it causes bronchoconstriction and is a respiratory stimulant in vitro,[8] suggesting a cholinergic effect in the respiratory system. However, it also binds to the nicotine acetylcholine receptors in ganglions, thus promoting the release of epinephrine and norepinephrine.[8] It is this action on adrenal hormone secretion that is responsible for lobelia's therapeutic effects in asthma.[9]

CLINICAL APPLICATIONS

Lobelia is primarily used as an expectorant in such conditions as pneumonia, asthma, and bronchitis. It appears that its major actions are mediated by the adrenal cortex.[8] Experimentally induced lung edema in rats is responsive to lobeline in many models that are unresponsive to any other medication.[8] Furthermore, although lobeline causes bronchoconstriction in dogs and rats, in guinea pigs and (presumably) humans the opposite – bronchodilation – occurs.[10] This is probably related to adrenal stimulation.

Although effective when used alone in the treatment of asthma, it has traditionally been used in combination with other botanical agents.[9] Typically it is combined with capsicum *frutescens* and *symphlocarpus factida*.

Lobelia is also used to lessen nicotine withdrawal, as it has a similar action to nicotine.[1,2]

DOSAGE

- Dried herb: 0.2–0.6 g three times/day
- Tincture: 15–30 drops three times/day
- Fluid extract: 8–10 drops three times/day.

TOXICOLOGY

Ingestion of toxic levels of lobelia usually results in vomiting, thereby lessening the likelihood of a fatal outcome.[4] Like nicotine poisoning, toxic symptoms include:

- nausea
- salivation
- diarrhea
- disturbed hearing and vision
- mental confusion
- marked weakness.

Faintness and prostration ensue; blood pressure falls; the pulse becomes weak, rapid, and irregular; breathing is difficult; and collapse occurs followed by convulsions. Death may result from respiratory failure.[5] The antidote in acute poisoning is 2 mg of atropine, which is given subcutaneously.[11]

REFERENCES

1. Leung A. Encyclopedia of common natural ingredients used in food, drugs, and cosmetics. New York, NY: John Wiley. 1980; p 220–223
2. Tyler V, Brady L, and Robbers J. Pharmacognosy. 8th edn. Philadelphia, PA: Lea & Febiger. 1981: p 68–70
3. Merck Index. 10th edn. Rahway, NJ: Merck. 1983: p 4374
4. Christopher J. School of natural healing. Provo, UT: BiWorld Publishers. 1976: p 358–367
5. Gilman A, Goodman L, Gilman A. The pharmacological basis of therapeutics. New York, NY: MacMillan. 1980: p 212–214
6. Mansuri S, Kelkar V, Jindal M. Some pharmacological characteristics of ganglionic activity of lobeline. Arzneim Forsch 1973; 23: 1271–1275
7. Laffan R, Borison H. Emetic action of nicotine and lobeline. J Pharmacol Exp Ther 1957; 121: 468–476
8. Halmagyi D, Kovacs A, Neumann P. Adrenocortical pathway of lobeline protection in some forms of experimental lung edema of the rat. Dis Chest 1958; 33: 285–296
9. Mitchell W. Naturopathic applications of the botanical remedies. Seattle, WA: Mitchell. 1983
10. Cambar P, Shore S, Aviado D. Bronchopulmonary and gastrointestinal effects of lobeline. Arch Int Pharmacodyn 1969; 177: 1–27
11. Dreisbach RH. Handbook of poisoning. Los Altos, CA: Lange Med Publ. 1983: p 553

CHAPTER CONTENTS

96

Melaleuca alternifolia (tea tree)

Michael T. Murray, ND

Joseph E. Pizzorno Jr, ND

Melaleuca alternifolia (family: Myrtaceae)
Common name: tea tree

GENERAL DESCRIPTION

Tea tree (*Melaleuca alternifolia*) is a small tree native to only one area of the world: the north-east coastal region of New South Wales, Australia. The leaves, the portion of the plant that is used medicinally, are the source of a valuable therapeutic oil. Although there are over 50 members of the Melaleuca family, the oil from the leaf of *Melaleuca alternifolia* has received the most research attention.

CHEMICAL COMPOSITION

Tea tree leaves contain about 1.8% of oil obtained via steam distillation.[1] This oil contains over 48 compounds, but is chiefly composed of:[2]

- 1-terpinen-4-ol
- 1,8-cineol
- gamma-terpinene (see Fig. 96.1)
- *p*-cymene
- other terpenes.

The Australian standard (AS 2782-1985) for "Oil of Melaleuca (Terpinen-4-ol type)" sets a minimum content of terpinen-4-ol at 30% and a maximum 1,8-cineol content of 15%.[1]

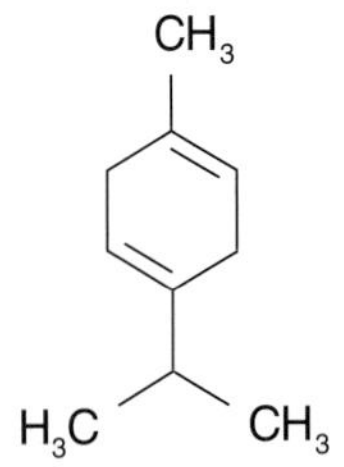

CH_3

H_3C CH_3

Figure 96.1 Gamma terpinene.

HISTORY AND FOLK USE

The medicinal properties of crushed tea tree leaves were known to the Bundjalung Aborigines of northern New South Wales, Australia. In fact, the waters of a lagoon where tea tree leaves had fallen and decayed for hundreds of years were viewed as having tremendous healing properties.[1]

The popular name of tea tree was first reported in 1777 Captain Cook's account of his second voyage entitled, A Voyage to the South Pole:[1]

> ... we at first made it [some beer] of a decoction of the spruce leaves; but finding that this alone made the beer too astringent, we afterwards mixed with it an equal quantity of the tea plant (a name it obtained in my former voyage from our using it as tea then, as we also did now), which partly destroyed the astringency of the other, and made the beer exceedingly palatable, and esteemed by everyone on board.

The leaves of *Melaleuca alternifolia* were also used by the early settlers of Australia to make tea, hence the further use of the popular name of "tea tree".[1]

The first report of tea tree's medicinal use appeared in the *Medical Journal of Australia* in 1930.[3] A surgeon in Sydney reported impressive results using a solution of tea tree oil to clean surgical wounds. According to the author:

> The results obtained in a variety of conditions when it (tea tree oil) was first tried were most encouraging, a striking feature being that it dissolved pus and left the surface of infected wounds clean so that its germicidal action became more effective without any apparent damage to the tissues. This was something new, as most efficient germicides destroy tissue as well as bacteria....

During World War II, tea tree oil was issued to soldiers to use as a disinfectant. The Australian Army went so far as to commandeer supplies of the oil and exempt leaf cutters from national service in order to maintain production. The production of tea tree oil during World War II was regarded as an "essential" industry.[1]

After World War II, the tea tree oil industry stagnated for more than 30 years. There were a number of reasons for this, including the general trend away from natural medicines toward synthetic medical drugs. However, during the late 1970s and early 1980s, the Australian tea tree oil industry was reborn as successful plantations growing *Melaleuca alternifolia* were established.[1]

Tea tree oil has been used in the treatment of:[1]

- acne
- aphthous stomatitis
- tinea pedis (athlete's foot)
- boils
- burns
- carbuncles
- corns
- gingivitis
- herpes
- impetigo
- infections of the nail bed
- insect bites
- lice
- mouth ulcers
- psoriasis
- root canal treatment
- ringworm
- sinus infections
- pharyngitis
- skin and vaginal infections
- thrush
- tonsillitis.

A variety of tea tree oil-based cosmetic products exist in the marketplace, including toothpastes, shampoos and conditioners, creams, hand and body lotions, soaps, gels, liniments, and nail polish removers.

PHARMACOLOGY

Tea tree oil possesses significant antiseptic properties and is regarded by many as the ideal skin disinfectant. This claim is supported by its efficacy against a wide range of organisms, its good penetration and lack of irritation to the skin.[1] The therapeutic uses of tea tree oil are based largely on its antiseptic and antifungal properties. Organisms inhibited by tea tree oil are listed in Table 96.1.

CLINICAL APPLICATIONS

The historical uses of tea tree oil demonstrate its wide range of applications as an antiseptic. Three of the more popular and documented uses are in the treatment of skin infections, vaginal infections, and common foot complaints.

Table 96.1 Organisms inhibited by *Melaleuca alternifolia oil*[1,4–6]

Organism	Mean inhibitory zone (mm)
Bacillus subtili	24.1
Bacteroides fragilis	26.1
Branhamell catarrhalis	56.4
Candida albicans	20.3
Clostridium perfingens	27.9
Escherichia coli	33.9
Enterococcus faecalis	16.9
Lactobacillus acidophilus	27.1
Mycobacterium smegmatsi	31.0
Propionibacterium acnes	
Pseudomonas aeruginosa	0
Serratia marcescens	24.8
Staphylococcus aureus	25.4
Streptococcus pyrogenes	
Trichomonas vaginalis	
Trichophyton mentagrophytes	

Skin infections

Tea tree oil is useful in a broad range of dermal infections, not only because of its broad-spectrum antiseptic properties, but also because of its capacity to mix with sebaceous secretions and penetrate the epidermis.

A clinical trial in patients with furuncles demonstrated that tea tree oil encouraged more rapid healing without scarring, compared with matched controls.[7] Presumably the positive clinical effects were due to the oil's germicidal activity against *Staphylococcus aureus*. The method of application included cleaning the site, followed by painting the surface of the furuncle freely with tea tree oil two or three times a day.

For most skin infections, the most effective treatment appears to be direct application of full-strength, undiluted oil at the site of infection. If irritation occurs, diluted preparations may be tried.

Acne

Topical application of tea tree oil is a suitable alternative to benzoyl peroxide preparations. In one study, 124 patients with mild to moderate acne randomly received either a 5% gel of tea tree oil or 5% benzoyl peroxide lotion to be applied topically daily. After 3 months, both treatments produced a significant improvement in the mean number of both non-inflamed and inflamed lesions, although with non-inflamed lesions benzoyl peroxide was found to be more effective. An important finding was that there were fewer reports of side-effects (dryness, pruritis, stinging, burning, and skin redness) with tea tree oil (44% vs. 79%).[8]

Common foot problems

Tea tree oil, in emollient form (8% tea tree oil) or in solution (40%), can be massaged into the feet daily for the treatment of tinea pedis, foot irritation, and bromhidrosis (severely foul-smelling feet).

One author concluded after 6 years of using different concentrations and preparations that tea tree oil eradicates or improves the symptoms of tinea pedis when used daily by the patient at home.[4] He also reported that even undiluted forms had little effect on onychomycosis (discussed further below). Diluted tea tree oil in solution was found to reduce foot irritation and promote wound healing with surgical incision in cases of corns, calluses, bunions, and hammer toes, and was extremely effective in diminishing bromhidrosis.

In tinea pedis, a double-blind study found that 10% tea tree oil cream compared quite favorably with the antifungal tolnaftate in relieving symptoms but was less effective in eliminating the fungi from cultures.[5] Specifically, both the tea tree group (24 out of 37) and the tolnaftate group (19 out of 33) showed significant improvement in the four clinical parameters of scaling, inflammation, itching, and burning, but only 30% of the subjects applying tea tree oil cream were culture negative, compared with 85% in the tolnaftate group.

Fungal nail infection

Fungal nail infections (onychomycosis) are the most frequent cause of nail disease, affecting approximately 2–13% of the population. Standard medical treatments include debridement, topical antifungals, and systemic antifungals. All current therapies have high recurrence rates. Oral therapy has the added disadvantages of high cost and potentially serious adverse effects. A recent study compared the efficacy and tolerability of topical application of 1% clotrimazole solution with that of 100% tea tree oil for the treatment of toenail onychomycosis.[9]

The 117 patients received twice daily applications of either 1% clotrimazole (CL) solution or 100% tea tree (TT) oil for 6 months. Debridement and clinical assessment were performed at 0, 1, 3, and 6 months. Cultures were obtained at 0 and 6 months. Each patient's subjective assessment was also obtained 3 months after the conclusion of therapy. After 6 months of therapy, the two treatment groups were comparable based on culture cure (CL = 11%, TT = 18%) and clinical assessment documenting partial or full resolution (CL = 61%, TT = 60%). Three months later, about one-half of each group reported continued improvement or resolution (CL = 55%, TT = 56%). These results indicate that topical therapy with tea tree oil, in conjunction with debridement, provides excellent improvement in nail appearance and symptomatology.

Vaginal infections

Tea tree oil demonstrates germicidal activity against a number of common vaginal pathogens and opportunistic organisms, including *Trichomonas vaginalis* and *Candida albicans*.[10,11]

A 40% solution of tea tree oil emulsified with isopropyl alcohol and water was found in a clinical study to be highly effective for the treatment of cervicitis, chronic endocervicitis, trichomonal vaginitis, and vaginal candidiasis.[11] Weekly in-office treatment (usually four to six were necessary) involved thorough washing of the perineum, labia, and vagina with a suitable scrub (the commercial product pHisoHex was used in the study). After drying, the affected areas were washed with a 1% tea tree oil solution. This was followed by insertion of a tampon (three 4 × 4 inch sponges) saturated with the 40% tea tree oil solution. Patients were instructed to remove the tampon after 24 hours.

For infectious processes, i.e. trichomonas and candidiasis, daily vaginal douches containing 1 quart of water with a 0.4% concentration of the oil were prescribed. No irritation, burning or other side-effects were reported or observed with either the office applications or the douches.

DOSAGE

A number of commercial products exist which contain tea tree oil. Tea tree oil can be used as a topical antiseptic for reducing microbial counts in wounds, surgical incisions, and skin and vaginal infections. In addition, tea tree leaves can be used to make teas which may be of benefit in cases of sore throat, tonsillitis, sinus infections, and colitis.

TOXICITY

Tea tree oil is extremely safe for use as a topical antiseptic. However, it may cause allergic contact dermatitis in some individuals. During a 3 year period, seven patients were seen in an outpatient dermatology clinic in Kona, Hawaii, for contact dermatitis due to the use of commercially available product containing 100% tea tree oil.[12] The patients were treating pre-existing skin conditions, which included foot fungus, dog scratches, insect bites, and rashes. All patients presented with an eczematous dermatitis. Patch tests indicated that all patients were sensitive to a 1% solution of tea tree oil. It is recommended that individuals apply the oil to a small area of skin before using tea tree oil for the first time to avoid the bother of developing contact dermatitis over a larger area.

The oral ingestion of tea tree oil cannot be recommended, as this could lead to a toxic reaction. However, folk use suggests that oral ingestion of tea from the leaves is reasonably safe.

REFERENCES

1. Altman PM. Australian tea tree oil. Australian J Pharmacy 1988; 69: 276–278
2. Swords G, Hunter GLK. Composition of Australian tea tree oil (*Melaleuca alternifolia*). J Agric Food Chem 1978; 26: 734–7
3. Humphery EM. A new Australian germicide. Med J Australia 1930; 1: 417–418
4. Walker M. Clinical investigation of Australian *Melaleuca alternifolia* oil for a variety of common foot problems. Current Podiatry 1972; 18: 30–35
5. Tong MM, Altman PM, Barnetson RS. Tea tree oil in the treatment of tinea pedis. Austral J Dermatol 1992; 33: 145–149
6. Carson CF, Riley TV. The antimicrobial activity of tea tree oil (letter to the editor). Med J Australia 1994; 160: 236
7. Feinblatt HM. Cajeput-type oil for the treatment of furunculosis. J Nat Med Assoc 1960; 52: 32–34
8. Bassett IB, Pannowitz DL, Barnetson RS et al. A comparative study of tea-tree oil versus benzoyl peroxide in the treatment of acne. Med J Aust 1990; 153: 455–458
9. Buck DS, Nidorf DM, Addino JG. Comparison of two topical preparations for the treatment of onychomycosis. *Melaleuca alternifolia* (tea tree) oil and clotrimazole. J Fam Pract 1994; 38: 601–605
10. Essential oils data search. *Melaleuca alternifolia*. Vancouver, WA. 1985
11. Pena EF. *Melaleuca alternifolia* oil. Ob Gynecol 1962; 19: 793–795
12. Knight TE, Hausen BM. Melaleuca oil (tea tree oil) dermatitis. J Am Acad Dermatol 1994; 30: 423–427

CHAPTER CONTENTS

97

Melatonin

Michael T. Murray, ND

Joseph E. Pizzorno Jr, ND

GENERAL DESCRIPTION

Melatonin (not to be confused with melanin, the compound responsible for skin pigment) is a hormone manufactured from serotonin and secreted by the pineal gland (see Fig. 97.1). The pineal gland, a small pea-sized gland at the base of the brain, has been a source of curiosity since antiquity. The ancient Greeks considered the pineal gland as the seat of the soul, a concept that was extended by the philosopher Descartes. In the 17th and 18th centuries, physicians associated "madness" with the pineal gland. Physicians in the early 1900s believed the pineal gland was somehow involved with the endocrine system. The identification of melatonin in 1958 provided the first solid scientific evidence of an essential role for the pineal gland. It is now thought that the sole function of the pineal gland is to manufacture and secrete melatonin.

The exact function of melatonin is still poorly understood, but it is critically involved in the synchronization of hormone secretion. The natural biorhythm of hormone secretion is referred to as the "circadian" rhythm. The human body is governed by an internal clock that signals the secretion of various hormones at different times to regulate body functions. Melatonin plays a key role as the biological time keeper of hormone secretion. Melatonin also helps to control sleep/wake cycles. Release of melatonin is stimulated by darkness and suppressed by light via a multisynaptic pathway which connects the pineal gland to the retina.

SYNTHESIS AND SECRETION

Melatonin secretion is largely related to the length of

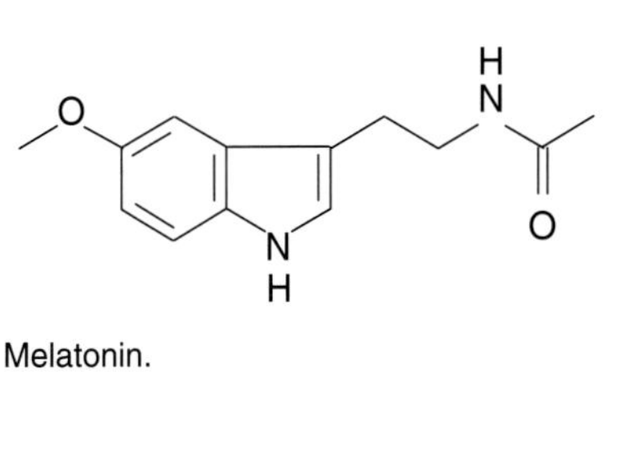

Figure 97.1 Melatonin.

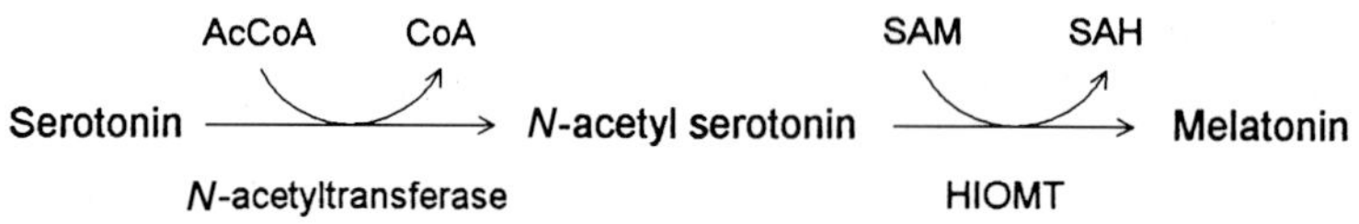

Figure 97.2 Melatonin synthesis.

the night, since most of the melatonin synthesis occurs during the dark phase as a result of increased activity of the enzyme serotonin-*N*-acetyltransferase.[1] Hence, there is a normal circadian pattern of melatonin synthesis and secretion (see Fig. 97.2). The longer the night, the longer the duration of synthesis and secretion. The most consistent observation in humans is that melatonin profiles show a phase change from winter to summer, with earlier secretion in summer than in winter. When humans are kept strictly in darkness for 14 hours/day for a period of 2 months, the melatonin secretion pattern expands to cover almost the entire dark period, and concomitantly, in extended periods of 14 hours of light, the rhythm contracts to less than 10 hours, with accompanying changes in body temperature and sleep.[2]

Light of sufficient intensity at night rapidly reduces melatonin production.[3] The most effective spectrum of light which produces melatonin-lowering effect is the green band (540 nm), corresponding to the rhodopsin absorption spectrum in the human eye.[4] This observation is of considerable importance, in understanding not only the physiological effects of melatonin, but also its importance in the control of circadian rhythms and the treatment of seasonal affective disorder (discussed further in Ch. 126).[5]

The antidepressant effect of light therapy in the treatment of seasonal affective disorder (SAD) is probably due to balancing of the altered circadian rhythm by restoring proper melatonin synthesis and secretion by the pineal gland. Disruption of pineal function is thought to be a major reason for seasonal affective disorder as well as jet-lag.[1,6]

Clinical evaluation of melatonin secretion

The circadian pattern of melatonin secretion and the response of body tissues to orally administered melatonin can be monitored by either salivary or serum levels, as saliva and serum melatonin concentrations correlate well.[7] However, salivary melatonin is preferable because it eliminates the need for multiple blood draws and allows the patient the luxury of collecting the sample at home. Typically, patients will be asked to collect saliva according to the laboratories own technique (either soaking a swab or simply expectorating saliva into a small container) at four different times (including nocturnal determination). Monitoring circadian secretion of melatonin is clinically indicated in the conditions in Table 97.1 and can assist the clinician in proper timing of melatonin dosage.

Table 97.1 Conditions where determining melatonin levels may be appropriate

- Insomnia related to disturbed circadian rhythm
- Seasonal affective disorder
- Delayed sleep phase syndrome
- Stress
- Cancer
- Multiple sclerosis
- Abnormal sexual development
- Administration and monitoring of melatonin therapy

PHARMACOLOGY

In addition to its role in synchronizing hormone secretion, melatonin has been shown to possess antioxidant effects.[8] This action may explain the studies in rats showing that melatonin supplementation led to longer lives (31 months vs. 25 months). However, the clinical significance of melatonin's antioxidant effects have not been fully determined. It is hard to imagine that its antioxidant effects would have greater significance than vitamin C, vitamin E, and a host of other antioxidants which can be delivered at much higher concentrations. Melatonin has also been shown to exert some sedative and anti-cancer effects (discussed below).

The pharmacokinetics of orally administered melatonin has recently been studied. Daytime serum melatonin levels in normal adults are in the range of 20 pg/ml rising to levels of about 150 pg/ml at night.[9] Oral dosages of 0.1–0.3 mg produce serum concentrations that are equivalent to normal physiologic night-time melatonin levels.[10] However, because melatonin demonstrates a large hepatic first-pass effect and a biphasic elimination pattern, therapeutic dosages are typically 1–3 mg.[2,11,12]

CLINICAL APPLICATIONS

The primary clinical uses of melatonin are in the treatment of jet-lag, insomnia, and as an adjunct in cancer therapy. In addition, the role of melatonin in depression is discussed. There are other possible indications for melatonin based on very preliminary studies. For example, low melatonin levels have been found in multiple sclerosis, coronary artery disease, epilepsy, and postmenopausal osteoporosis. The studies in multiple sclerosis and coronary artery disease are also briefly discussed below along with a discussion on the relationship to vitamin B_{12} and melatonin secretion.

Jet-lag

Several double-blind studies have shown melatonin to be very effective in relieving jet-lag.[13–16] Different dosage recommendations have been given. Some researchers have recommended that melatonin be taken at the beginning of the sleep period at the point of departure starting a few days before departure (especially when traveling eastward). Others have recommended taking melatonin just one time on the first evening upon arriving at the new destination. The later recommendation avoids the problem of extreme drowsiness sometimes produced by melatonin at an unwanted time.

A recent study was designed to answer the question of optimal timing of melatonin supplementation.[17] In the study, 52 members of an airline cabin crew flying an international route were randomly assigned to three groups:

- early melatonin – 5 mg started 3 days prior to arrival until 5 days after return home
- late melatonin – placebo for 3 days then 5 mg melatonin for 5 days at new destination)
- placebo.

Daily ratings in jet-lag, mood, and sleepiness measures demonstrated that the best recovery was in the late melatonin group. The early melatonin group actually demonstrated a worse recovery compared with the placebo group. This study suggests that the best way to use melatonin for jet-lag is 5 mg in the evening at the new destination for 5 days.

Insomnia

Melatonin plays an important role in the induction of sleep. Low melatonin secretion at night can be a cause of insomnia. Several double-blind trials have shown melatonin supplementation to be very effective in promoting sleep.[18–22] However, it appears that the sleep-promoting effects of melatonin are most apparent when melatonin levels are low.[23] In other words, melatonin is not like taking a sleeping pill. It will only produce its effects when melatonin levels are low. When melatonin is given just before going to bed in normal subjects or in patients with insomnia who have normal melatonin levels, it produces no sedative effect. This is because, normally, just prior to going to bed there is a rise in melatonin secretion. Melatonin supplementation is only effective as a sedative when the pineal gland's own production of melatonin is very low. However, low melatonin levels are thought to be an extremely common cause of insomnia in the elderly.[24]

In one of the most interesting studies, 26 elderly insomniacs with lower than normal melatonin levels were given 1–2 mg of melatonin 2 hours prior to the desired bedtime for 1 week. Rapid and slow release melatonin preparations were used. Both sleep latency and sleep quality were evaluated. While there was no discernible difference in sleep onset and sleep efficiency (percentage of time asleep of total time in bed) between the two forms, the timed-release form yielded better results on sleep maintenance.[25]

Cancer

Melatonin has been shown to inhibit several types of cancers, particularly hormone-related cancers like those of the breast and prostate.[26] It has been shown to inhibit both the initiation and promotion of cancer. It has been theorized that the increased cancer incidence reported in individuals living and/or working in an environment in which they are exposed to higher than normal artificial electromagnetic fields may be caused by suppression of melatonin synthesis.[27] The exposure of humans or animals to light (visible electromagnetic radiation) at night rapidly depresses pineal melatonin production and blood melatonin levels. Likewise, the exposure of animals to various pulsed static and extremely low-frequency magnetic fields also reduces melatonin levels. Reduction of melatonin by artificial electromagnetic field exposure may be a significant risk factor for cancer.

Melatonin has also been shown to exert anti-cancer effects in clinical trials in cancer patients. In these studies, melatonin has been given at moderate (e.g. 10 mg daily) to extremely high levels (i.e. greater than 40 mg daily). Melatonin has most often been used in combination with other anti-cancer agents, including interleukin 2 and interferon. The results are promising.

While interferon and interleukin 2 (IL-2) are often ineffective when used alone, in combination with melatonin very good results have been obtained. For example, in one study, 80 patients with advanced solid neoplasms were randomized to receive either IL-2 alone (3 million IU/day for 6 days a week for 4 weeks) or in combination with melatonin (40 mg/day orally at 8.00 p.m.).[28] A complete response was obtained in 3/41 patients treated with IL-2 plus melatonin compared with none of the patients receiving IL-2 alone. A partial response was achieved in 8/41 patients treated with IL-2 and melatonin compared with only one in the IL-2 only group. The survival rate after one year was 19/41 in the IL-2 and melatonin compared with only 6/30 in the IL-2 group. In another study of 100 patients with metastatic solid tumors, for whom no standard therapy was available, the percentage of survival at 1 year was significantly higher in patients treated with IL-2 and melatonin than in those receiving the supportive care alone (21/52 versus 5/48).[29]

Similar results have been shown with melatonin in combination with interferon, tumor necrosis factor, and tamoxifen, as well as when melatonin was used alone.[30–35] These preliminary results are quite encouraging, as improvements in survival time and quality of life assessments have been produced in approximately 30% of patients taking anywhere from 10–50 mg daily (at 8.00 p.m.). However, although melatonin has been shown to increase survival time in these studies, the results are good but not earth-shattering. For example, in one study of patients with solid tumors with brain metastasis 15/24 patients (63%) died within 1 year in the melatonin group compared with 21/26 (88%) in the group receiving supportive care only. These studies, although randomized, are not double-blind, indicating that a placebo response may be partially responsible for some of the improvements noted.

Depression

Initial studies performed in the 1980s demonstrated that melatonin levels are typically below normal in patients with clinical depression.[36–38] However, in all of these studies it turned out that antidepressant drugs or other factors were responsible for the depressed melatonin levels. More recent studies have not supported the association of low melatonin levels being common in patients with clinical depression.[39] These studies measured melatonin levels in drug-free, depressed patients and were careful to match these subjects with a comparable control group. In addition, it has been demonstrated that normal subjects secreting *no* melatonin do not frequently suffer from depression.[1]

Initially it was thought that melatonin may affect mood as a result of reducing cortisol levels by inhibiting the secretion by the pituitary hormone, ACTH, which then signals the adrenal glands to secrete cortisol. With melatonin deficiency, cortisol levels would be expected to be increased. This appears to be the case in many depressed patients, as both decreased melatonin and increased cortisol concentrations are frequently found.[39–41] However, it is unlikely that melatonin supplementation can significantly reduce cortisol levels as research has shown that melatonin supplementation does not suppress either ACTH or cortisol secretion.[42]

This research indicates that melatonin is unlikely to produce any significant positive effects in the treatment of depression in most patients. Clinical research seems to bear this out. In fact, one double-blind study conducted in 1973 demonstrated that melatonin supplementation actually dramatically worsened clinical depression in some cases.[43] Obviously worsening of depression is quite serious as it increases the risk for suicide. A possible explanation for the worsening is the fact that the melatonin was given two to four times during the day – a time when melatonin levels are typically low. Another study in non-depressed subjects demonstrated that when melatonin was given during the day it tended to cause fatigue, confusion, and sleepiness.[44]

Multiple sclerosis

Multiple sclerosis (MS) is the most common of the demyelinating diseases of the central nervous system. The clinical course and prognosis of the disease is extremely variable. The illness typically tends to progress in a series of relapses and remissions. The patient with MS seems, in most cases, to enter a phase of slow and steady deterioration of neurologic function. The pineal gland has been implicated recently in the pathogenesis and clinical course of MS. In a recent study, 32 MS patients randomly selected from consecutive hospital admissions to a neurology service due to exacerbation of symptoms had their nocturnal levels of melatonin monitored.[45] The study revealed that the progressive decline in melatonin may be relevant to the pathophysiology, and specifically to the course, of the disease. The specific role of melatonin in remission of MS is unknown, but what is known is that when melatonin levels decline it is associated with an exacerbation of symptoms. Patients with chronic progressive MS have been shown to have lower melatonin levels compared with those with a relapsing/remitting course. However, at this time it is not known whether melatonin therapy would have any benefit in MS.

Coronary artery disease

Melatonin levels are significantly lower in patients with coronary heart disease than in healthy controls. In a recent study, patients with coronary heart disease had nocturnal melatonin levels that were one-fifth that found in healthy controls. The absence of melatonin would cause increased night-time sympathetic activity which would increase the risk for coronary disease. Melatonin serves as a suppressor of sympathetic activity nocturnally. Lower levels of melatonin may lead to increased circulating epinephrine and norepinephrine, which has been implicated in damage to vessel walls. Atherogenic uptake of LDL cholesterol is accelerated by these amines at pathophysiological concentrations.[46] In another study melatonin was found to inhibit platelet aggregation.[47]

Interactions with vitamin B_{12}

Vitamin B_{12} has been shown to influence melatonin secretion.[48] The low levels of melatonin in the elderly may be a result of low vitamin B_{12} status. Vitamin B_{12} (1.5 mg/day of methylcobalamin) has been shown to produce good results in the treatment of sleep–wake rhythm disorders presumably as a result of improving melatonin secretion.[49]

DOSAGE

At this time, it appears that melatonin therapy is most appropriate for use when low melatonin levels are suspected, as occurs in some cases of insomnia and in jet-lag. Evaluation of salivary melatonin levels can provide valuable diagnostic insight as to the likely success or failure of melatonin in the treatment of insomnia. A dosage of 3 mg at bedtime is more than enough as dosages as low as 0.1 mg and 0.3 mg have been shown to produce a sedative effect when melatonin levels are low.[10] Higher dosages may be required to produce the anti-cancer benefits noted above.

TOXICOLOGY

Although there appear to be no serious side-effects at recommended dosages, conceivably melatonin supplementation could disrupt the normal circadian rhythm. In one study, a daily dosage of 8 mg/day for only 4 days resulted in significant alteration to the circadian rhythm.[42] It is not known what sort of effect would occur at commonly recommended dosages (i.e. 3 mg). In addition, as noted above, some depressed patients got much worse when they were given melatonin during the day.

REFERENCES

1. Yu HS, Reiter RJ, eds. Melatonin biosynthesis, physiological effects and clinical applications. Boca Raton: CRC Press. 1993.
2. Wehr TA. The durations of human melatonin secretion and sleep respond to changes in daylength (photoperiod). J Clin Endocrinol Metab 1991; 73: 1276–1280
3. Illnerova H. Entrainment of mammalian circadian rhythms in melatonin production by light. Pineal Res Rev 1988; 6: 173–217
4. Reiter RJ. Action spectra, dose response relationships and temporal aspects of light's effects on the pineal gland; the medical and biological effects of light. Ann NY Acad Sci 1985; 453: 215–230
5. Rosenthal NE, Sack DA, Gillin JC et al. Seasonal affective disorder. A description of the syndrome and preliminary findings with light therapy. Arch Gen Psychiatry 1984; 41: 72–79
6. Waldhauser F, Ehrhart B, Forster E. Clinical aspects of the melatonin action. Experentia 1993; 49: 671–681
7. Vakkuri O, Leppaluoto J, Kauppila A. Oral administration and distribution of melatonin in human serum, saliva and urine. Life Sci 1985; 37: 489–495
8. Reiter RJ et al. A review of the evidence supporting melatonin's role as an antioxidant. J Pineal Res 1995; 18: 1–11
9. Waldhauser F, Waldhauser M, Lieberman HR et al. Bioavailability of oral melatonin in humans. Neuroendocrinol 1984; 39: 307–313
10. Dollins AB, Zhdanova IV, Wurtman RJ et al. Effect of inducing nocturnal serum melatonin concentrations in daytime on sleep, mood, body temperature, and performance. Proc Natl Acad Sci USA 1994; 91: 1824–1828
11. Mallo C, Zaidan R, Galy G et al. Pharmacokinetics of melatonin in man after intravenous infusion and bolus injection. Eur J Clin Pharmacol 1990; 38: 297–301
12. Lane EA, Moss HB. Pharmacokinetics of melatonin in man. First pass hepatic metabolism. J Clin Endocrinology Metab 1985; 61: 1214–1216
13. Arendt J, Braodway J. Some effects of jet-lag and their alleviation by melatonin. Ergonomics 1987; 30: 1379–1393
14. Claustrat B, Brun J, David M et al. Melatonin and jet-lag. Confirmatory result using a simplified protocol. Biol Psyhiatry 1992; 32: 705–711
15. Petrie K, Conaglen JV, Thompson L et al. Effect of melatonin on jet-lag after long haul flights. Br Med J 1989; 298: 705–707
16. Lino A, Silvy S, Condorelli L et al. Melatonin and jet-lag. Treatment schedule. 1993; 34: 587
17. Petrie K, Dawson AG, Thompson L et al. A double-blind trial of melatonin as a treatment for jet-lag in international cabin crew. Biol Psychiatry 1993; 33: 526–530
18. Waldhauser F, Saletu B, Trinchard-Lugan I. Sleep laboratory investigations on hypnotic properties of melatonin. Psychopharmacology 1990; 100: 222–226
19. Zhdanova IV, Wurtman RJ, Lynch HJ et al. Sleep-inducing effects of low doses of melatonin ingested in the evening. Clin Pharmacol Ther 1995; 57: 552–558
20. Dahlitz M, Alvarez B, Vignau J et al. Delayed sleep phase syndrome response to melatonin. Lancet 1991; 337: 1121–1124
21. MacFarlane JG, Cleghorn JM, Brown GM et al. The effects of exogenous melatonin on the total sleep time and daytime alertness of chronic insomniacs. A preliminary study. Biol Psychiatry 1991; 30: 371–376
22. James SP, Sack DA, Rosenthal NE et al. Melatonin administration in insomnia. Neuropsychopharmacology 1990; 3: 19–23
23. Nave R, Peled R, Lavie P. Melatonin improves evening napping. Eur J Pharmacol 1995; 275: 213–216
24. Haimov I, Laudon M, Zisapel N et al. Sleep disorders and melatonin rhythms in elderly people. BMJ 1994; 309: 167
25. Haimov I, Lavie P, Laudon M et al. Melatonin replacement therapy therapy of elderly insomniacs. Sleep 1995; 18: 598–603
26. Molis TM, Spriggs LL, Jupiter Y et al. Melatonin modulation of estrogen-regulated proteins, growth factors, and proto-oncogenes in human breast cancer. J Pineal Res 1995; 18: 93–103
27. Reiter RJ. Melatonin suppression by static and extremely low frequency electromagnetic fields. relationship to the reported increased incidence of cancer. Rev Environ Health 1994; 10: 171–186
28. Lissoni P, Barni S, Tancini G et al. A randomized study with subcutaneous low-dose interleukin 2 alone vs interleukin 2 plus the pineal neurohormone melatonin in advanced solid neoplasms other than renal cancer and melanoma. Br J Cancer 1994; 69: 196–199
29. Lissoni P, Barni S, Fossati V et al. A randomized study of neuroimmunotherapy with low-dose subcutaneous interleukin-2 plus melatonin compared to supportive care alone in patients with untreatable metastatic solid tumour. Support Care Cancer 1995; 3: 194–197
30. Neri B, Fiorelli C, Moroni F et al. Modulation of human lymphoblastoid interferon activity by melatonin in metastatic renal cell carcinoma. A phase II study. Cancer 1994; 73: 3015–3019
31. Brackowski R, Zubelewicz B, Romanowski W et al. Preliminary study on modulation of the biological effects of tumor necrosis factor-alpha in advanced cancer patients by the pineal hormone melatonin. J Biol Regul Homeost Agents 1994; 8: 77–80
32. Lissoni P, Barni S, Meregalli S et al. Modulation of cancer endocrine therapy by melatonin. A phase II study of tamoxifen plus melatonin in metastatic breast cancer patients progressing under tamoxifen alone. Br J Cancer 1995; 71: 854–856
33. Lissoni P, Barni S, Ardizzoia A et al. Randomized study with the pineal hormone melatonin versus supportive care alone in advanced non-small cell lung cancer resistant to a first-line chemotherapy containing cisplatin. Oncology 1992; 49: 336–339
34. Lissoni P, Barni S, Cattaneo G et al. Clinical results with the

pineal hormone melatonin in advanced cancer resistant to standard antitumor therapies. Oncology 1991; 48: 448–450
35. Lissoni P, Barni S, Ardizzoia A et al. A randomized study with the pineal hormone melatonin versus supportive care alone in patients with brain metastases due to solid neoplasms. Cancer 1994; 73: 699–701
36. Maurizi C. Disorder of the pineal gland associated with depression, peptic ulcers, and sexual dysfunction. Southern Med J 1984; 77: 1516–1518
37. Wetterberg L. The relationship between the pineal gland and the pituitary-adrenal axis in health, endocrine and psychiatric conditions. Psychoneuroendocrinology 1983; 8: 75–80
38. Beck-Friis J, Kjellman BF, Aperia et al. Serum melatonin in relation to clinical variables in patients with major depressive mood and a hypothesis of low melatonin syndrome. Acta Psychiatr Scand 1985; 71: 319–30
39. Rubin RT, Heist EK, McGeoy SS et al. Neuroendocrine aspects of primary endogenous depression. XI. Serum melatonin measures in patients and matched control subjects. Arch Gen Psychiat 1992; 49: 558–567
40. Thompson C, Franey C, Arendt J et al. A comparison of melatonin secretion in depressed patients and normal subjects. Br J Psychiatry 1988; 152: 260–265
41. Waterman GS, Ryan ND, Perel JM et al. Nocturnal urinary excretion of 6-hydroxymelatonin sulfate in prepubertal major depressive disorder. Biol Psych 1992; 31: 582–590
42. Mallo C, Zaidan R, Faure A et al. Effects of a four-day nocturnal melatonin treatment on the 24 h plasma melatonin, cortisol and prolactin profiles in humans. Acta Endocrinologia 1988; 119: 474–480
43. Carman JS, Post RM, Buswell R et al. Negative effects of melatonin on depression. Am J Psychiatry 1976; 133: 1181–1186
44. Dollins AB, Lynch HJ, Wurtman RJ et al. Effect of pharmacological daytime doses of melatonin on human mood and performance. Psychopharmacology 1993; 112: 490–496
45. Sandyk R, Awerbuch GI. Relationship of nocturnal melatonin levels to duration and course of multiple sclerosis. Int J Neurosci 1994; 75: 229–237
46. Brugger P, Marktl W, Herold M. Impaired nocturnal secretion of melatonin in coronary heart disease. Lancet 1995; 345: 1408
47. Cardinali DP, Del Zar MM, Vacas MI. The effects of melatonin in human platelets. Acta Physiol Pharmacol Ther Latinoam 1993; 43: 1–13
48. Honma K, Kohsaka M, Fukuda N et al. Effects of vitamn B_{12} on plasma melatonin rhythm in humans. Increased light sensitivity phase-advances the circadian clock? Experentia 1992; 48: 716–20
49. Okawa M, Mishima K, Hishikawa Y et al. Vitamin B_{12} treatment for sleep-wake rhythm disorders. Sleep 1990; 13: 1–23

CHAPTER CONTENTS

98

Mentha piperita (peppermint)

Michael T. Murray, ND

Joseph E. Pizzorno Jr, ND

Mentha piperita (family: Labitae)
Common name: peppermint

GENERAL DESCRIPTION

Peppermint is a natural hybrid of garden spearmint (*M. spicata*) and water mint (*M. aquatica*). First described in England in 1696, peppermint now grows all over the world.[1] The two most popular varieties are white peppermint (*M. piperita* var. *officinalis*) and black peppermint (*M. Piperita* var. *vulgaris*). Both are typical members of the mint family, i.e. herbs with square stems, horizontal rhizomes, and lanceolated leaves with a serrated edge. Black peppermint has deep red stems with purplish-tinged dark green leaves, while the white has green stems with lighter green leaves. Both varieties produce purple flowers during the summer months. For medicinal effects, the aerial portion of the plant is the most widely used.

CHEMICAL COMPOSITION

The major medicinal component of peppermint is its volatile oil, which can be found in concentrations of up to 1.5% in the herb, but is usually present in the 0.3–0.4% range. The principal components of the oil are menthol (29–28%) (see Fig. 98.1), menthone (20–31%) and menthyl acetate (3–10%), although gas chromatographic analysis of peppermint oil will typically show more than 40 different peaks. Most of the volatile oil components are terpenoids.[1]

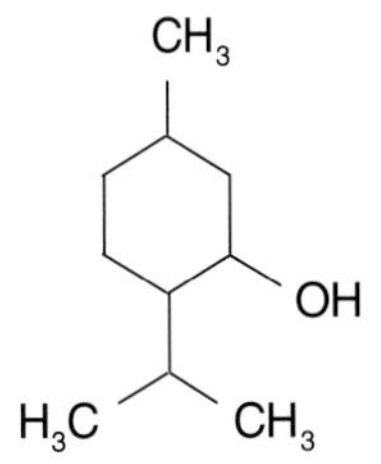

CH_3 — OH — H_3C — CH_3

Figure 98.1 Menthol.

The composition of menthol and other volatile oil components is sensitive to climate and latitude, as well as to the maturity of the plant. Pharmaceutical-grade peppermint oil is produced by distilling the fresh aerial parts of the plant harvested at the very beginning of the flowering cycle. The oil is standardized to contain not less than 44% free menthol and a minimum of 5% esters calculated as menthyl acetate. The ketone component (calculated as menthone) usually ranges from 15 to 30% with the remainder of the oil being composed of various terpenoids.[1] Menthol is also synthesized by hydrogenation of thymol.

Other components of peppermint herb which may contribute to its medicinal effects include polymerized polyphenols (19% of dry weight), flavonoids (12%), tocopherols, carotenes, betaine, and choline.[2]

HISTORY AND FOLK USE

Although peppermint was not officially recognized until the 17th century, mints have been used for their medicinal effects for thousands of years. Records from the ancient Egyptian, Greek, and Roman eras show that other members of the mint family, particularly spearmint (*Mentha spicata*), were used.[1]

The most popular uses of peppermint for medicinal purposes were in the treatment of indigestion and intestinal colic, colds, fever, and headache.

PHARMACOLOGY

The pharmacology of peppermint is attributed almost entirely to its menthol components. The major categories of actions for peppermint and menthol are:

- carminative
- antispasmodic
- choleretic
- external analgesic
- nasal decongestant.

Carminative effects

Carminatives promote the elimination of intestinal gas. Peppermint and peppermint oil are well-accepted carminatives. Although the exact mechanism of action has not been determined, one proposed mechanism is relaxation of the esophageal sphincter leading to the released gas pressure in the stomach.[3]

Antispasmodic effects

The mechanism behind peppermint oil's antispasmodic effects has been determined. Researchers have concluded that the ability of peppermint oil to inhibit contractions of isolated smooth muscles is via blockage of the influx of calcium into the muscle cells.[4,5] The researchers hypothesized that the clinical effectiveness of peppermint oil in the treatment of the irritable bowel syndrome is a result of inhibition of the hypercontractility of intestinal smooth muscle, thereby returning the muscle to its proper tone.

Choleretic effects

Choleretics stimulate the flow of bile. Menthol and related terpenes have been shown to exert a choleretic effect as well as improve the solubility of the bile.[6–10]

External analgesic effects

The external analgesic and counter-irritant effects of menthol are well accepted. When applied to the skin, peppermint oil or menthol stimulates the nerves which perceive cold, while simultaneously depressing those for pain. The initial cooling effect is followed by a period of warmth.

CLINICAL APPLICATIONS

Peppermint oil is the most extensively used of all the volatile oils. Pharmaceutical preparations often utilize peppermint oil or menthol for its therapeutic and flavoring properties. For example, it is used extensively in antacid products and irritant laxatives for both its flavor and its therapeutic effects. The same is true for its inclusion in mouthwash preparations and after-dinner mints.

The pharmacological effects of peppermint and peppermint oil are useful in a number of clinical situations. The most notable are:

- irritable bowel syndrome
- intestinal colic
- gallstones
- musculoskeletal pain
- the common cold.

Irritable bowel syndrome

Peppermint oil has been used in treating the irritable bowel syndrome (IBS) for many years. IBS can include a combination of any of the following symptoms:

- abdominal pain and dissension
- more frequent bowel movements with pain, or relief of pain with bowel movements
- constipation or diarrhea
- excessive production of mucus in the colon
- symptoms of indigestion such as flatulence, nausea, or anorexia
- varying degrees of anxiety or depression.

One of the central findings in IBS is a hypercontractility of intestinal smooth muscle. As described above, peppermint oil inhibits the hypercontractility of intestinal smooth muscle making it useful in cases of the irritable bowel syndrome as well as intestinal colic.

The preferred delivery of peppermint oil in the treatment of IBS is by enteric-coated preparations which prevent the oil from being released in the stomach. Without enteric coating, peppermint oil tends to produce heartburn. With the coating, the peppermint oil travels to the small and large intestine where it relaxes intestinal muscles. Several clinical studies have demonstrated that enteric-coated peppermint oil is quite effective in reducing the abdominal symptoms of the irritable bowel syndrome.[11–13]

Although effective on its own, enteric-coated peppermint oil is best used within a comprehensive treatment protocol for IBS (see Ch. 184).

Cholelithiasis

A formula containing menthol and related terpenes (menthone, pinene, borneol, cineol, and camphene) has demonstrated efficacy in several studies in dissolving gallstones.[6–10] This approach to gallstone removal offers an effective alternative to surgery and has been shown to be safe even when consumed for prolonged periods of time (up to 4 years). Terpenes, like menthol, help to dissolve gallstones by reducing bile cholesterol levels while increasing bile acid and lecithin levels in the gall bladder. As menthol was the major component of this formula, peppermint oil, especially if enteric-coated, may offer similar benefits.

External analgesic

Menthol and related substances can be used as counter-irritants in the treatment of arthritis, fibromyositis, tendonitis, and other inflammatory conditions involving the musculoskeletal system.

The common cold

Menthol and peppermint oils are often employed in the treatment of the common cold as components of topical nasal decongestants, cough and throat lozenges, ointments, salves, and inhalants. Whether the use of these products is of benefit has not been proven in clinical studies. However, their popularity appears to represent their ability to help make breathing easier during the common cold. The best method for using menthol or peppermint oil is by applying commercial preparations to the upper chest during periods of rest so that the vapors can be inhaled continuously.

Peppermint tea may also be of benefit during the common cold. Peppermint, as well as other members of the mint family, has demonstrated significant antiviral activity as well as a mild diaphoretic effect.[14] The most active antiviral components, the polyphenols, are concentrated in the tea.[2] Peppermint oil has shown antiviral activity against Newcastle disease, herpes simplex, and vaccina.

Headache

A recent study demonstrated another valuable use for peppermint oil – the relief of tension headaches. In a double-blind, placebo-controlled, randomized cross-over trial, topical application to the forehead and temples resulted in a statistically significant decrease in muscle tension as reported subjectively and measured objectively by EMG activity of the temporal muscle. In addition, the oil application resulted in decreased pain sensitivity.[15]

DOSAGE

Peppermint is most widely used as a tea (infusion), on its own or in combination with other botanicals. The infusion is usually prepared with 1 to 2 teaspoons of the dried leaves per 8 ounces of water.

The dosage of peppermint oil administered in an enteric-coated capsule for the treatment of the irritable bowel syndrome is one to two capsules (0.2 ml/capsule) three times daily between meals. This dosage is also appropriate for the treatment of gallstones.

The dosage of menthol as an external analgesic is 1.26–16% applied to the affected area no more than three or four times daily.

TOXICOLOGY

Peppermint herb is generally regarded as safe (GRAS) when used as a tea; however, hypersensitivity reactions have been reported. Adverse reactions to enteric-coated peppermint oil capsules are rare, but can include hypersensitivity reactions (skin rash), heartburn, bradycardia, and muscle tremor.

When applied topically, peppermint oil or menthol can induce contact dermatitis and hypersensitivity reactions. The likelihood of developing such a reaction is enhanced when heating pads are used in conjunction with topically applied preparations containing menthol.[16]

The LD_{50} of menthol in rats is 3,280 mg/kg. The fatal oral dose in humans is 1 g/kg. Repeated high dose feeding of rats for 28 days with peppermint oil produced signs of dose-related brain lesions, but the dosage (40 mg/kg) far exceeds those used in humans.[1,17,18]

REFERENCES

1. Briggs C. Peppermint. Medicinal herb and flavoring agent. Can Pharm J 1993; March: 89–92
2. Duband F, Carnat AP, Carnat A et al. The aromatic and polyphenolic composition of peppermint (*Mentha piperita*) tea. Ann Pharmaceutiques Franc 1992; 50: 146–155
3. Giachetti D, Taddei E, Taddei I. Pharmacological activity of essential oils on Oddi's sphincter. Planta Med 1988; 54: 389–392
4. Hills JM, Aaronson PI. The mechanism of action of peppermint oil in gastrointestinal smooth muscle. Gastroenterology 1991; 101: 55–65
5. Hawthorne M, Ferrante J, Luchowski E et al. The actions of peppermint oil and menthol on calcium channel dependent processes in intestinal, neuronal, and cardiac preparations. J Aliment Pharmacol Therap 1988; 2: 101–108
6. Hordinsky BZ. Terpenes in the treatment of gallstones. Minnesota Medicine 1971; 54: 649–651
7. Bell GD, Doran J. Gallstone dissolution in man using an essential oil preparation. Br Med J 1979; 278: 24
8. Doran J, Keighley RB, Bell GD. Rowachol – a possible treatment for cholesterol gallstones. Gut 1979; 20: 312–317
9. Ellis WR, Bell GD. Treatment of biliary duct stones with a terpene preparation. Br Med J 1981; 282: 611
10. Somerville KW, Ellis WR, Whitten BH et al. Stones in the common bile duct. experience with medical dissolution therapy. Postgrad Med J 1985; 61: 313–316
11. Somerville K, Richmond C, Bell G. Delayed release peppermint oil capsules (Colpermin) for the spastic colon syndrome. a pharmacokinetic study. Br J Clin Pharmacol 1984; 18: 638–640
12. Rees W, Evans B, Rhodes J. Treating irritable bowel syndrome with peppermint oil. Br Med J 1979; ii: 835–836
13. Lech U Olesen KM, Hey H et al. Treatment of irritable bowel syndrome with peppermint oil. A double-blind study with a placebo. Ugeskr Laeger 1988; 150: 2388–2389
14. Kerrman EC, Kucera L. Antiviral substances in plants of the mint family (III). Peppermint (*Mentha piperita*) and other mint plants. Proc Soc Exper Biol Med 1967; 124: 874–875
15. Gobel H, Schmidt G, Dworshak M et al. Essential plant oils and headache mechanisms. Phytomed 1995; 2: 93–102
16. Heng MC. Local necrosis and interstitial nephritis due to topical methyl salicylate and menthol. Cutis 1987; 39: 442–444
17. Olsen P, Thorup I. Neurotoxicity in rats dosed with peppermint oil and pulegone. Arch toxicol 1984; 7: 408–409
18. Thorup I, Wurtzen G, Carstensen J, Olsen P. Short-term toxicity study in rats dosed with peppermint oil. Toxicol Lett 1983; 19: 211–215

CHAPTER CONTENTS

99

Naturally occurring antioxidants

Robert A. Ronzio, PhD

INTRODUCTION

We depend on our oxygen-rich world for survival. Mitochondria use oxygen to maximize the energy yield in converting fuel molecules to carbon dioxide. Paradoxically, oxygen is such a powerful reactant that it can disrupt cellular function and impair homoeostatic mechanisms primarily through oxygen radicals. Recent research suggests that free radical attack and cumulative oxidative damage are associated with many degenerative conditions, including cancer,[1,2] atherosclerosis,[3,4] cataracts,[5] inflammation and autoimmune disease,[6,7] lung disease,[8] neurologic disorders,[9,10] aging,[11,12] and cell death.[13] Table 99.1 summarizes prominent examples of the more than 100 conditions that reflect oxidative damage. Free radicals may be a consequence of the disease process, or they may be a cause. The following discussion focuses on the formation and physiologic effects of free radicals and

Table 99.1 Conditions mediated by oxidative damage

- Alcohol-induced damage
- Atherosclerosis
- Autoimmune diseases (rheumatoid arthritis and others)
- Cancer
- Contact dermatitis
- Coronary artery bypass
- Diabetic cataracts
- Drug toxicity
- Emphysema
- Hypertensive cerebrovascular injury
- Immune deficiency of aging
- Inflammatory bowel disease
- Iron overload disease
- Liver cirrhosis
- Myocardial infarction
- Nephrotoxicity
- Nutrient deficiencies
- Obstructive lung disease
- Parkinson's disease
- Premature aging
- Premature retinopathy
- Senile dementia and neurologic degeneration
- Stroke
- Thermal injury
- Viral infections, including AIDS

oxygen-based reactants, and then addresses the body's antioxidant defenses.

FREE RADICALS AND REACTIVE OXYGEN SPECIES

Definitions

Free radicals

Free radicals are highly reactive molecules. Unlike most molecules, which contain pairs of electrons, free radicals possess at least one unpaired electron, an unstable condition. Consequently, free radicals will tear electrons from bystander molecules indiscriminately to make up for their own deficiency. Nitric oxide (NO•) and superoxide ($O_2•^-$), are examples of physiologically important radicals: NO• functions as a vasodilator and as a defensive chemical. It may also play a role in memory. Superoxide is a defensive compound. Furthermore, hydrogen peroxide and superoxide can influence growth, and the suggestion has been made that these species function as messengers. They may also regulate cellular redox state and cellular antioxidant levels (glutathione), thereby indirectly altering signal transduction and ultimately growth responses.[14] Hydroxyl radical (•OH) is one of the most reactive radicals occurring in the body. An initial event generates free radicals, and propagation steps repeated many times perpetuate their formation. Thus, free radical reactions tend to "snowball" unless held in check by antioxidant defenses.[15]

Reactive oxygen species

In addition to free radicals, the body generates an array of oxidizing agents, including hydrogen peroxide (H_2O_2), lipid peroxide (ROOH), and hypochlorite (OCl^-). Although $O_2•^-$ and H_2O_2 are not very reactive chemically, they can yield hydroxyl radical in the presence of transition metal ions. Reduced iron catalyzes the conversion of superoxide to singlet oxygen, an activated oxygen molecule with unstable electron configuration. Furthermore, nitric oxide and superoxide, in excess, form peroxynitrite ($ONOO^-$), an extremely powerful oxidizing agent and radical generator. It is useful to consider these metabolites collectively as "reactive oxygen species" (ROS) to include the various forms of more or less reactive oxidizing agents, whether or not they are free radicals.[14]

Likely targets of free radicals and ROS include polyunsaturated fatty acids in membrane lipids, serum lipoproteins, proteins and even DNA. (Fig. 99.1) The products may be lipid peroxides, protein carbonyls and altered purines such as 8-oxo-2-deoxyguanosine.[11,16] The consequences are often subtle: damage to membrane receptor proteins may alter cellular regulatory mechanisms such as signal transduction; inactivation of proteins required for ATP production, leading to an energy deficit; and inactivation of calcium ATPase, changing calcium homeostasis.[17] There is strong circumstantial evidence that ROS and free radicals also play a role in cancer initiation and promotion. While ROS often damage DNA and induce malignant transformation, the development of cancer depends on many factors, including the rates of damage and repair, the status of defenses, and alternative pathways for initiation and promotion. Apoptosis – programmed cell death – is regulated by a complex pathway involving activation of transcription factors. Oxidative stress induced by ROS is one of the triggers of apoptosis in several model systems.[18] Indeed, conditions ranging from diabetes mellitus and heart failure to HIV infection may entail apoptosis.[19]

The formation of free radicals and ROS

Although not plentiful, free radicals are surprisingly common in the body. Free radicals and ROS arise through a variety of mechanisms. Some sources are spontaneous chemical accidents: free radicals are generated by air pollutants such as ozone and nitric oxides, and by cosmic rays and radiation. On the other hand, oxygen may react with heme proteins such as myoglobin, hemoglobin and cytochrome C, as well as iron (Fe^{2+}) to generate superoxide, which yields H_2O_2. The extremely reactive hydroxyl radical can be formed from H_2O_2 in the presence of Fe^{2+}, or Cu^+. Therefore, the release of these ions from storage sites during inflammation and injury may promote the spontaneous production of free radicals.

In addition, normal metabolism yields free radicals and ROS:

- Approximately 1–3% of oxygen molecules passing through mitochondria end up as superoxide due to the leakage of electrons from the electron transport chain during damage, generating about 10 g/day of superoxide.[20] The aging process may be related to mitochondrial deterioration.
- Cells contain peroxisomes, organelles that oxidize fatty acids while producing H_2O_2. Drugs like clofibrate that cause peroxisome proliferation may act as promoters by stimulating the production of hydrogen peroxide.
- The oxidation of purines from DNA, RNA and ATP relies on the enzyme, xanthine oxidase, which produces superoxide. Various cytoplasmic oxidases generate ROS, including dopamine oxidase, beta hydroxylase, urate oxidase and others.
- The detoxication of metabolites and xenobiotics by microsomal mixed function oxidases (cytochrome P450) can generate ROS (1 mole of free radical is generated for each mole of toxin metabolized). Drugs such as penicillamine and phenylbutazone can be metabolized to free radicals. Also, several xenobiotics such as paraquat and alloxan catalyze the formation of superoxide through

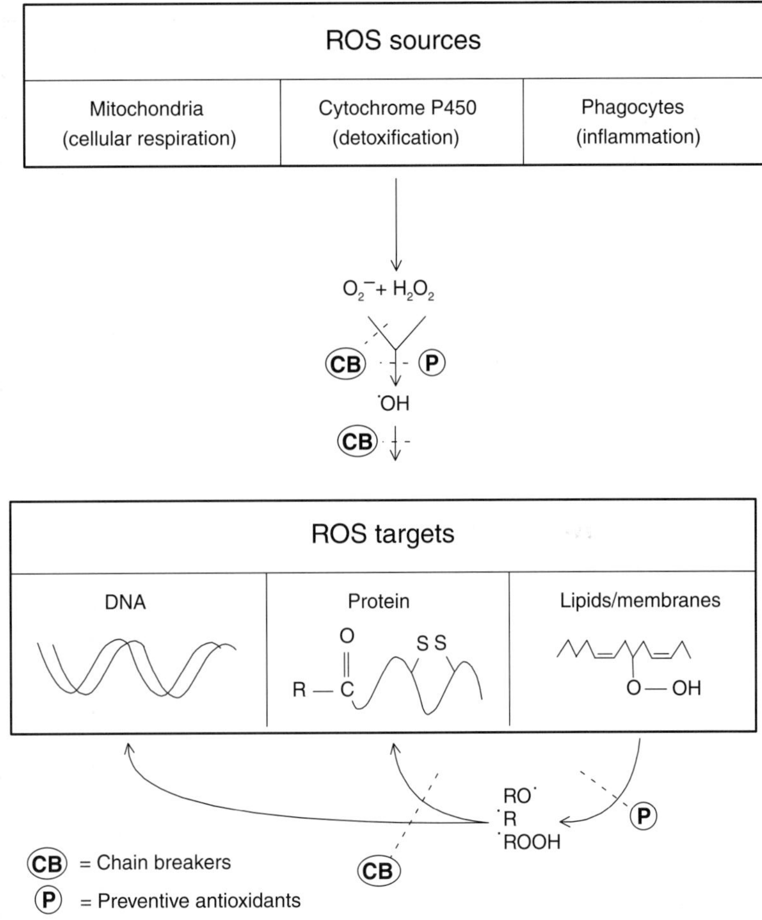

Figure 99.1 ROS sources, targets and sites of antioxidant neutralization.

cyclic reactions ("redox recycling"), promoting autooxidation. A number of pesticides and drugs are hepatotoxins for these reasons.[21]

In addition, ROS are made for useful purposes. Phagocytic cells, including macrophages, monocytes, neutrophils and eosinophils, create ROS as part of their defensive mechanism. The binding of immune complexes, bacterial endotoxins or other inflammatory agents to cell surface receptors triggers a "respiratory burst" in phagocytic cells. This localized production of highly reactive chemicals oxidizes viruses, bacteria and other foreign materials. Initially, plasma membrane NADPH oxidase releases superoxide, which dismutes to H_2O_2. Myeloperoxidase in lysosomes then transforms H_2O_2 and chloride ion to hypochlorite, the same powerful oxidizer found in commercial bleach. Hypochlorite spontaneously reacts with amines and ammonia to produce very reactive chloramines. In addition, nitric oxide is produced, which reacts with molecular oxygen to yield nitrogen oxides, NO_2 and N_2O_3 – potent oxidizing agents. Note that the respiratory burst can activate xenobiotics.[22]

Inflammation

Inflammation represents a major source of oxidants. Infection, toxic exposure, ischemia and trauma activate phagocytic cells.[6] Inappropriate activation of ROS production is potentially dangerous. Inflammation activates the arachidonic acid cascade, which converts polyunsaturated fatty acids to eicosanoids, lipid peroxides such as PGG_2 and PGH_2, leukotrienes and HETE via cyclooxygenase and lipoxygenase. Cyclooxygenase itself activates xenobiotics, creating an additional oxidant burden.[23] The autooxidation of polyunsaturated fatty acids with three or more double bonds in membranes yields pro-inflammatory PGG_2-like isomers called F_2 isoprostanes. The more or less continuous production of ROS by activated phagocytes during chronic, possibly low-level, inflammation may eventually deplete antioxidant defenses, thus allowing ROS to attack cells.[24] Ensuing tissue injury often impairs function in a downward spiral from health to disease. For example, free radicals and ROS are present at high levels in colons of patients with ulcerative colitis.[25]

Oxidative stress

The term "oxidative stress" refers to a shift in the ratio of prooxidant/antioxidant balance.[26] The imbalance can be due to excessive ROS production and/or to limited antioxidant defenses, which could be the result of inadequate dietary intake of antioxidant nutrients or chronic conditions such as malabsorption syndromes.

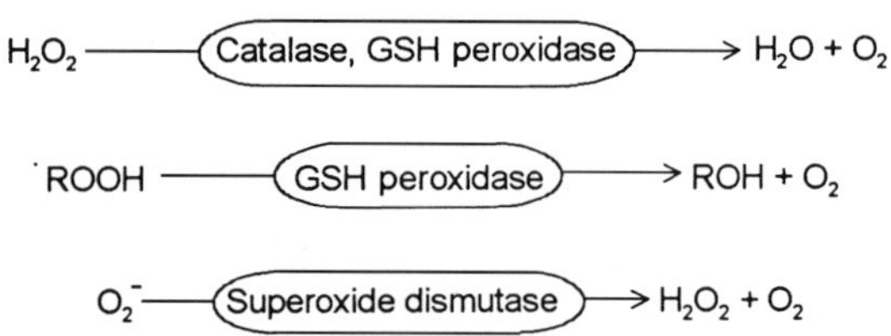

Figure 99.2 Preventive antioxidants.

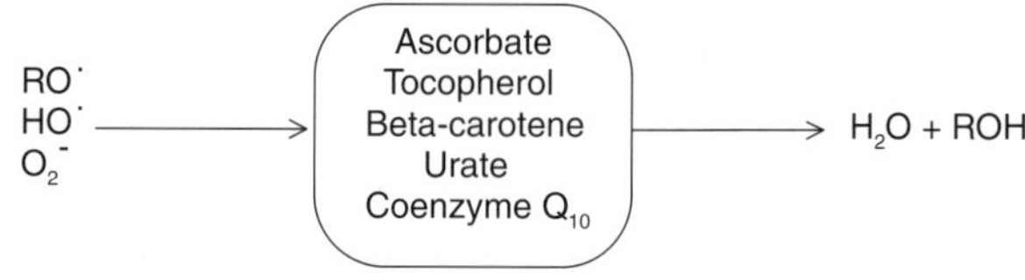

Figure 99.3 Chain-breaking antioxidants.

ANTIOXIDANTS

Antioxidants are substances that inhibit the oxidation of a target molecule, often by free radical attack.[15] Antioxidants are both lipid-soluble and water-soluble. In addition, there is a "pecking order" among antioxidants; some are more readily oxidized than others and will be consumed rapidly unless replenished or recycled.[27] Table 99.2 lists the primary and secondary antioxidant defenses that protect against free radicals and ROS, including enzymes, nutrients and metabolites. Certain antioxidants are "preventive inhibitors", which block the initiation of free radical attack (Fig. 99.2). Preventive inhibitors include defensive enzymes such as catalase, superoxide dismutase (SOD), peroxidases as well as the tripeptide glutathione. Beta-carotene, chelating agents such as organic acids, and plant polyphenols also represent preventive antioxidants when they quench singlet oxygen or sequester metal catalysts. Other antioxidants function as "chain breakers", which convert free radicals to stable products and thus block free radical chain reactions. Vitamin E and ascorbic acid are essential chain-breaking antioxidants (Fig. 99.3).

Table 99.2 Antioxidant defenses

Detoxication enzymes
• Superoxide dismutases (copper, zinc, manganese)
• Catalases (iron)
• Glutathione peroxidases (selenium)
• Glutathione transferase (glutathione)
Auxiliary proteins
• Glutathione reductase (niacin, glutathione)
• Glucose 6-phosphate dehydrogenase (niacin)
• Albumin
• Transferrin (iron)
• Ferritin (iron)
• Ceruloplasmin (copper)
• Metallothionein (cysteine)
Vitamin antioxidants
• Beta-carotene (provitamin A)
• Vitamin C
• Vitamin E (tocopherols)
Plant antioxidants (non-vitamins)
• Carotenoids and xanthophylls
• Phenolic acids and polyphenols
• Diketones
• Tocotrienols
Metabolites
• Coenzyme Q_{10}
• Uric acid
• Cysteine
• Glutathione
• Polyfunctional organic acids (citric acid, malic acid)
• Bilirubin, biliverdin
• Lipoic acid
• Histidine
• Melatonin
• Peptides (carnosine, anserine)

Enzyme antioxidants

Three types of enzymes detoxify ROS:

- superoxide dismutase (SOD)
- catalase
- glutathione peroxidase.

These enzymes occur throughout the body in cells, tissues and fluids. SOD very rapidly converts superoxide to H_2O_2. Because H_2O_2 may yield dangerous hydroxyl radicals, if allowed to accumulate, SOD cooperates with catalase to break down H_2O_2 to water, and with glutathione peroxidases to inactivate both H_2O_2 and lipid peroxides.

SOD

By "dismuting" superoxide to H_2O_2, SOD intervenes before ROS causes damage. The mitochondrial enzyme requires manganese, while the cytoplasmic form requires copper and zinc. These trace mineral nutrients are often classified as antioxidants, although it is their enzyme host that more accurately deserves this classification. Evidence for the role of SOD in preventing damage comes from a variety of sources. Aorta from copper-deficient rats contains less Cu-SOD activity and more lipid peroxidation than non-deficient animals[28]. Mn SOD is induced during acute inflammation.[29] Patients with a familial dominant form of amyotrophic lateral sclerosis possess a defective gene that decreases cytoplasmic SOD by 40%.[30] The level of SOD in the cerebral cortex of Alzheimer's disease patients is 25–35% lower than in the brains of healthy people.[31]

Liposomal SOD has been used therapeutically in patients with Crohn's disease.[32] Administering SOD bound to polyethylene glycol together with catalase reduced reperfusion injury in animals.[33] The SOD gene has been cloned, and chimeric enzymes with increased stability are being studied. Oral supplementation with coated plant or liver Cu/Zn SOD has anecdotally been noted to ameliorate symptoms in some patients with inflammatory conditions and sunburn. Others have reported no effect using ingested animal-derived, uncoated SOD.[34,35] Studies with supplemental SOD have been confounded by the observation that less than 20% of commercially available SOD met label claims for SOD, catalase or peroxidase activities.[36] Unlike mammalian enzymes, a coated, non-soy legume-derived SOD resists the action of pancreatic enzymes and a recent double-blind, placebo-controlled study suggested that oral ingestion of this material can increase the activity of erythrocyte SOD within 4 hours.[37]

Catalase

This iron-dependent enzyme occurs widely in cells and is a component of peroxisomes which generate H_2O_2 through oxidative metabolism. Catalase seems specifically designed to prevent a build-up of H_2O_2. Animal studies with catalase, usually in conjunction with SOD, suggest protection against ischemic injury to the retina,[38] intestinal ROS damage,[39] and radiation.[40] The transcytosis of catalase and SOD across capillaries has also been observed.[41]

Glutathione peroxidases

This family of enzymes work together with catalase. They require reduced glutathione to reduce peroxides cytoplasmic H_2O_2 as well as lipid peroxides. Unlike catalase and SOD, glutathione peroxidases use the trace mineral nutrient selenium in the form of selenocysteine. For this reason, selenium is sometimes referred to as an antioxidant nutrient. Glutathione peroxidases exist as several isoforms. A recently identified phospholipid hydroperoxide glutathione peroxidase can reduce membrane lipid peroxides to readily metabolized, non-toxic fatty acid alcohols.[42]

Selenium plays a role in the induction of glutathione-requiring enzymes, including the peroxidases. It should be noted that selenoprotein P, a plasma protein, seems to function in protecting endothelial cells of the liver and glomerular capillaries from oxidative damage, independent of peroxidases.[43] Defensive enzymes are often inducible. For example, in animal models, exhaustive exercise caused oxidative stress, leading to increased levels of SOD, glutathione peroxidase and glutathione transferase.[44] On the other hand, prior supplementation with vitamin E and selenium reduced ROS production and lesser amounts of detoxification enzymes were induced.[44]

Other defensive enzymes

Glutathione transferase adds glutathione to potentially toxic substances and is considered a component of phase II detoxification enzymes. Non-selenium-dependent glutathione peroxidase reduces aldehydes produced by radical-induced fragmentation of polyunsaturated fatty acids, epoxides produced during detoxification, in addition to peroxides. Like glutathione peroxidase, glutathione transferase requires a ready supply of reduced glutathione, produced by the action of glutathione reductase from oxidized glutathione. In turn, glutathione reductase requires NADPH, dependent on a robust glucose metabolism. NADPH and glutathione serve other reductases that help to regenerate tocopherol and ascorbate, demonstrating that overall metabolic balance is a prerequisite for adequate antioxidant defense.

Nutrient antioxidants

Vitamin E (tocopherols)

Vitamin E refers to eight fat-soluble compounds, of which alpha-tocopherol is the most active in the usual biological test systems (although some human models, such the RBC membrane stabilization test, suggest other forms may be more active). Vitamin E is acknowledged as the primary chain-breaking antioxidant of lipids, lipoproteins and membranes. Vitamin E contributes to membrane repair;[45] it blocks the formation of nitrosoamines,[46] helps protect LDL against oxidative damage,[47,48] reduces symptoms of tardive dyskinesia – perhaps by reducing nerve damage,[49] and decreases platelet aggregation and blood clot formation.[50]

According to the "oxidation hypothesis" of cardiovascular disease, the oxidation of LDL and other lipoproteins helps to initiate atherosclerosis, and an antioxidant role for vitamin E in preventing cardiovascular disease has been proposed.[51] Each molecule of LDL possesses on average seven molecules of alpha-tocopherol, while there is less than one molecule of beta-carotene per LDL molecule. One the other hand, vitamin E accounts for only 30% of total antioxidants present in LDL in some people. The oxidation of polyunsaturated fatty acids and cholesterol in LDL does not begin until tocopherol, beta-carotene and antioxidants have been consumed. Supplementation with 800 IU of alpha-tocopherol daily for 3 months increased the tocopherol level in isolated LDL and decreased the rate of LDL lipid peroxidation by 40%.[52] More recently, the Cambridge Heart Antioxidant Study demonstrated a large, significant reduction in nonfatal myocardial infarction among patients with atherosclerosis who had been supplemented with vitamin E (400 or 800 IU) compared with a placebo for a median of 1.4 years.[53] Alpha-tocopherol was administered at a daily level of 2,000 IU to patients with moderately severe Alzheimer's disease.[54] With vitamin E supplementation, there was a 230 day delay in the onset of severe dementia or death compared with controls, although there was no improvement in cognition with supplementation. These data lend support to the possible involvement of oxidative stress in neurodegenerative disease and a role of antioxidant supplementation in therapeutic programs. A protective role in cancer is less clear: the Nurses' Health Study failed to confirm a reduced risk of breast cancer in patients with high intakes of vitamins E and C.[55]

Whole foods provide mixtures of tocopherols, including alpha, beta and gamma isomers, and the typical US diet supplies twice as much gamma-tocopherol as the alpha form. Alpha-tocopherol predominates in the body, probably due to selection by tocopherol binding protein of the liver. Gamma-tocopherol, not the alpha form, selectively blocks peroxynitrite and acts as a radical sink. Gamma-tocopherol seems to complement the actions of alpha-tocopherol in blocking "electron-loving" mutagens and acting as an antioxidant.[56] Supplementing with alpha-tocopherol, a form common in supplements, may not be as effective as using natural mixed tocopherols.

Tocotrienols are a form of vitamin E having an unsaturated side chain. The antioxidant literature on these compounds is meager compared with vitamin E. They appear to complement tocopherols. Tissue distribution of tocotrienols, coenzyme Q_{10} and vitamin E differ, suggesting that selective mechanisms maintain the lipid antioxidants in various tissues.[57]

Tocopherol and other chain-breaker antioxidants become radicals as they deactivate potentially toxic substances. The tocopheryl radical (chromanoxyl radical) does not readily attack lipids and proteins and will decompose unless converted back to tocopherol by ascorbic acid, glutathione and coenzyme Q_{10}, illustrating the theme that antioxidant defenses complement each other.[58,59]

The current RDA (1997) for vitamin E of 15 IU (10 mg alpha-tocopherol equivalents, TE) for men and 12 IU (8 mg TE) for women was designed to prevent myopathy and neuropathy. However, the typical US diet provides less than the RDA of alpha-tocopherol. Healthy people consuming balanced diets supplying the RDA of vitamin E experienced decreased oxidative damage when supplemented with vitamin E at 10 times the RDA.[60] The daily vitamin E requirement varies dramatically according to factors that increase oxidative stress, including an increased consumption of polyunsaturated fatty acids, even with as little as 2.5 g of fish oil daily.[61] The best sources of vitamin E – such as unrefined vegetable oils, wheat germ, liver and eggs – represent high fat foods and it is difficult to provide high levels of vitamin E in the usual diet without supplementation. Synthetic alpha-tocopherol contains a mixture of D and L isomers; only the D form (actually RRR – alpha-tocopherol) is active in the body. Esterified alpha-tocopherol is considerably more stable than unesterified tocopherol, and supplemental forms incorporate acetate, succinate or palmitate, which are readily hydrolyzed and absorbed during digestion. Emulsified vitamin E is more readily assimilated than non-emulsified E. As with other fat-soluble vitamins, absorption of vitamin E depends on fat digestion and absorption. Therefore, conditions that impair fat digestion and assimilation will reduce tocopherol uptake.

Ascorbic acid (vitamin C)

This prominent, water-soluble antioxidant occurs in body fluids and the cytoplasm. Ascorbic acid is one of the most efficient chain-breaking antioxidants in human plasma,[59] and can react with a wide range of ROS and free radicals, including superoxide, singlet oxygen, hypochlorite, and sulfur radicals. Ascorbic acid protects lipids and membrane from oxidative damage by scavenging peroxyl and hydroxyl radicals. It is also reported to reduce the risk of cataracts and retinal damage,[62] increase immune function and detoxication,[63] and decrease heavy metal toxicity.[64] Ingested ascorbic acid reduces the gastrointestinal production of nitrosoamines and fecal mutagens.[65] These factors help to explain why increased ascorbic acid intake is linked to a reduced risk of cancer of the cervix, stomach, colon and lung.[66] Ascorbate supplementation can also reduce plasma LDL oxidation.[67]

Plasma ascorbic acid is a biomarker of oxidative stress. As an example, cigarette smoking depletes the ascorbic acid pool and decreases the body's reduction capacity to maintain plasma ascorbic acid in the reduced (bioactive) form.[68]

Ascorbic acid functions with glutathione and lipoic acid to regenerate alpha-tocopherol. Like the tocopheryl radical, the ascorbyl radical is relatively stable and has little tendency to attack cells. Dehydroascorbate can be reduced back to ascorbate by glutathione and NADPH by redox recycling. In animal models, high levels of ascorbate can compensate for low glutathione production, and vice versa. When exposed to catalytic levels of iron or copper ions, ascorbate promotes the formation of H_2O_2 and hydroxyl radicals.[11,68] In vivo, the effect requires high ascorbate and the depletion of tocopherol.[69] Possibly during inflammation, released iron or copper and ascorbate play a pro-oxidant role. Excessive dietary iron or iron accumulation could also promote ascorbate-induced oxidation.

The current (1997) RDA for vitamin C of 60 mg has long been challenged as inadequate. Convincing evidence that the RDA for (healthy young) men should be at least

200 mg is based upon careful tissue saturation studies.[70] Lifestyle choices such as cigarette smoking increase the need for vitamin C. Taking vitamin C with flavonoids can increase absorption and stabilize vitamin C.[71]

Carotenoids

Carotenoids represent over 500 different (red, orange, yellow) plant pigments and are conveniently divided into carotenes and xanthophylls (oxygenated carotenes). The most well-known carotenoid is beta-carotene. Although it is the most abundant in nature, beta-carotene does not stand alone: in green leafy vegetables xanthophylls make up 90% of the carotenoids. Beta-carotene represents only one-quarter to one-third of the carotenoids in plasma.

Carotenoids exhibit tissue specificity. Thus, beta-carotene is the major carotenoid in liver, adrenal gland, kidney, ovary and adipose tissue, while lycopene, a red carotene from tomatoes, is prevalent in testes and human plasma.[72] Lycopene effectively quenches free radicals, although it does not form vitamin A.[73]

Lutein and zeaxanthin are xanthophylls that accumulate in the body: they are the only carotenoids found in the retina and macula of primates. Lutein and lycopene are plentiful in blood. Levels of these carotenoids in blood are not affected by vitamin A status. Plasma alpha-carotene, beta-carotene and lutein are useful biomarkers of carotenoid-rich food consumption, while lutein may serve as an intake biomarker for the Cruciferae (cabbage) family.[74] There is a preferential uptake of lutein and zeaxanthin from the intestine into chylomicron, a general carrier of lipid nutrients.[75]

The beneficial effects of carotenoids in chemoprevention of cancer are thought to occur through protection against oxidative stress and immune enhancement.[76] In general, carotenoids are versatile antioxidants; lycopene, lutein, zeaxanthin, and others complement the antioxidant activity of beta-carotene. Beta-carotene absorbs energy from singlet oxygen and releases it as heat. It is especially effective at low oxygen tension, as found in tissues, where it can scavenge peroxyl radicals and alkoxyl radicals.[77] Carotenoids also enhance immune function, regardless of their provitamin activity. They quench ROS due to inflammation, help to maintain membrane receptors and they modulate the release of prostaglandins and leukotrienes.[78]

Increased carotenoid levels have been associated with decreased LDL oxidation,[79] and increased protection against coronary heart disease.[80] The increased consumption of carotenoids, especially lutein and zeaxanthin, correlates with a decreased risk of advanced, age-related macular degeneration.[81] Carotenoids and beta-carotene are linked to a decreased risk of some forms of cancer. Indeed, 29 of 31 lung cancer studies suggest that high dietary carotenoids offer significant protection.[82] Supplementation of healthy male non-smokers with 15 mg of beta-carotene daily for 26 days increased the function of isolated blood monocytes, suggesting that increased beta-carotene consumption could enhance cell-mediated immune function.[83] A study of Finnish men who had a decade long history of heavy cigarette smoking and alcohol use found an increased risk of lung cancer with beta-carotene supplementation, but not in those administered both vitamin E and beta-carotene.[84] Subjects who had the highest level of serum beta-carotene at the beginning of the study – indicative of a greater intake of fruits and vegetables – had the lowest risk of developing lung cancer. Beta-carotene could act as a pro-oxidant, unless protected by other antioxidants such as vitamin E, when there is excessive oxidative stress (smoking, alcohol consumption) and when diets are inadequate. The failure to find a reduced risk of lung cancer with beta-carotene supplements is also consistent with the generally accepted view of the chemopreventive properties of antioxidants; they can block cancer initiation and early promotion, but are less effective during very late stages of carcinogenesis.

It should be mentioned that another intervention trial also suggested that beta-carotene increased the risk of cancer in high risk groups (smokers or those exposed to asbestos).[85] In contrast, the Linxian China Study, which involved administering beta-carotene, vitamin E and selenium to marginally malnourished people, lowered the risk of cancer mortality.[86] The Physician's Health Study did not detect any effect on the incidence of cancer or heart disease after 12 years of supplementation with beta-carotene.

The synthetic form of beta-carotene represents the all *trans* isomer, while fruits, vegetables and algae provide varying amounts of the 9-*cis* isomer together with minor carotenoids. The 9-*cis* isomer appears to be a somewhat more efficient antioxidant.[87] Natural mixed carotenoids containing alpha and beta-carotenes, as well as xanthophylls, were better absorbed, and functioned as more effective antioxidants in vivo than synthetic (all trans) beta-carotene.[88] (For additional discussion of the broad impact of carotenoids on health, see Ch. 67.)

Vitamin A can act as a free radical trap and lipid peroxyl radical scavenger; it contributes to the antioxidant status of LDL, for example.[89] Vitamin A analogs, such as 13-*cis* retinoic acid and *trans* retinoic acid, can also reduce lipid peroxidation in vitro. However, the major role of vitamin A and its derivative in most tissues remains the regulation of transcription and translation in differentiation.

Antioxidants produced by the body

Glutathione

This sulfhydryl reducing agent is a tripeptide containing cysteine. Glutathione occurs in high (millimolar) concentrations in most cells and plays many roles. It serves as a detoxifying agent, assists amino acid transport, quenches free radicals, and helps regulate the internal redox environment of cells. As a substrate for glutathione peroxidases, glutathione plays a key role in antioxidant defenses. In addition, glutathione reacts directly with singlet oxygen, hydroxyl radicals and superoxide radicals to form oxidized glutathione (GSSG).[90] Glutathione reductases regenerate reduced glutathione (GSH) and the ratio of GSH/GSSG is normally >100:1.[90] Together with ascorbate, GSH participates in the regeneration of vitamin E, which emphasizes the cooperation of antioxidants. Oxidative stress decreases this ratio, activates transcription factors and increases production of interleukin 1 and tumor necrosis factor.[91] Depletion of intracellular glutathione is associated with immunodeficiency.

AIDS patients appear to have low levels of reduced glutathione, which could activate transcription factor NF-kappaB to increase transcription of the HIV genome.[92] A clinical study demonstrated that low GSH levels in CD4 T cells from HIV-infected subjects is associated with a decreased survival of 2–3 years.[93]

N-Acetylcysteine is an effective precursor for glutathione and can raise intracellular GSH.[94] Higher blood levels of glutathione correlate with higher degrees of health in elderly subjects.[95] Whether glutathione concentrations predict aging and whether low glutathione is a cause of aging remain to be determined.

There is evidence that dietary glutathione is absorbed and can increase plasma glutathione concentrations in animals and humans.[96,97] Oral supplementation of glutathione for maintenance and antioxidant protection ranges from 5 to 15 mg/kg body weight for antioxidant support. Detoxification protocols call for somewhat higher intakes, 15–25 mg/kg.[98]

Coenzyme Q_{10} (ubiquinone)

Ubiquinones are a family of fat-soluble antioxidants containing 1–12 isoprene units. The predominant form in humans is ubiquinone 10 or coenzyme Q_{10} (CoQ). Long recognized as a lipophilic electron carrier in mitochondrial ATP production, CoQ also functions as an important antioxidant, which can recycle tocopherol.[99] CoQ can enhance the immune system,[100] and has been used to improve status in patients with angina,[101] various cardiomyopathies and heart disease.[102] Ubiquinol, the reduced form of CoQ, protects LDL against lipid peroxidation.[103] Folkers noted that cancer patients are often low in CoQ.[104] CoQ deficiencies occur in the myocardium of older persons, especially those with heart disease.[105]

CoQ synthesis requires vitamins B_2, B_6, B_{12} and folate, and synthesis may not be optimal in people with a low intake of these important vitamins. The normal value for CoQ in plasma is approximately 0.4 µmol/L, mostly in the reduced form. Ubiquinol is readily oxidized, and dietary forms are ubiquinones, which are readily reduced after absorption. A decline in lipid peroxidation in plasma after supplementation with CoQ supports an antioxidative role for CoQ.[106] Because CoQ is not well absorbed, increasing plasma CoQ levels can be difficult. Oral supplementation with 30 mg of emulsified CoQ (CoQ-zyme) was as effective as 100 mg of powdered CoQ.[107]

Uric acid (urate)

Uric acid is a waste product of a purine metabolism, which occurs in high levels in plasma. Urate is a broad-spectrum antioxidant, capable of scavenging free radicals and of chelating transition metals.[108] Uric acid is responsible for 21–34% of the total plasma antioxidant activity, where it appears to protect alpha-tocopherol from peroxyl radicals.[109]

Polyfunctional organic acids

Citrate, fumarate, succinate, malate and tartrate can bind (chelate) transition metal ions and block ROS production, thus acting as preventive antioxidants. These acids require the presence of chain-breaking antioxidants for maximum effectiveness. Not all chelates confer antioxidant properties; for example, iron-ascorbate and iron EDTA complexes catalyze oxidation.[68]

Melatonin

In addition to helping to set the body biorhythms, this hormone quenches hydroxyl radicals very efficiently. The central nervous system consumes 20% of the oxygen used daily and thus is likely to generate ROS at a high rate. Melatonin production and sleep may play a pivotal part in preventing oxidative damage of nerves.[110] Though melatonin is sometimes sold as a food supplement, in reality it is a potent hormone.

Storage and transport proteins: ferritin, transferrin, ceruloplasmin

Free iron and copper ions catalyze the conversion of H_2O_2 to hydroxyl radicals; therefore proteins that bind these ions help to protect tissues against ROS. Under normal circumstances, it is questionable whether unbound iron is normally present in cells. However, with chronic inflammation, iron may be released from ferritin, and potentially this may pose a hazard. Iron storage disease is linked to oxidative damage. Transferrin (which has a high affinity for iron) and ceruloplasmin (which binds copper) can be considered part of the antioxidant defenses.[111] Iron stored in ferritin does not participate in free radical generation. Another intracellular sulfur-rich protein, metallothionein, binds many metals, including copper.

NON-NUTRITIVE ANTIOXIDANTS

Flavonoids

The typical diet provides a wide range of substances of plant origin that play important roles in maintaining health. Many act as antioxidants. One of the largest classes is the flavonoids, found mainly in fruits, leaves, stems and roots of vegetables, legumes and tea. Flavonoids potentiate the effects of vitamin C and protect other easily oxidizable substances. About 5,000 flavonoids have been reported; undoubtedly more remain to be discovered. Natural phenolics include: flavonoids (anthocyanidins, catechins, flavanones, flavones, flavonols and isoflavones); tannins (ellagic acid, gallic acid); phenyl isopropenoids (such as caffeic acid, coumaric acids, ferulic acid); lignans; and other substances, including catechol, resveratrol (grape skins), rosmarinic acid (rosemary) and others. Substantial amounts of ingested quercetin are absorbed by the GI tract in humans.[112] Quercetin and kaempferol are among the most abundant flavonoids in the diet.

Various flavonoids inhibit peroxidation in vitro by scavenging ROS, superoxide, hydroxyl radical and singlet oxygen. For example, rutin, myricetin and quercetin scavenge superoxide,[113] and block LDL oxidation.[114] Flavonoids from bilberries and grapes were able to protect collagen from superoxide-induced damage.[115] Flavonoids can also bind transition metals, limiting their ability to catalyze free radical formation.[116] The increased consumption of flavonoids correlated with the decreased risk of some forms of cancer and cardiovascular disease.[117] Quercetin inhibited melanoma cells, as a specific example.[118] Ascorbic acid enhances the inhibition of cancer cells by fisetin and quercetin in vitro, suggesting that ascorbate potentiates the action of flavonoids as chemoprotective agents.[119]

Previous estimates of daily consumption of total flavonoids ranged from 200 mg to 1,000 mg daily. However, accurate food consumption data and refined analytical methods based on high-performance liquid chromatography indicate that for northern European elderly men, the mean daily intake of the anti-cancer flavonoids was only about 23 mg daily, with quercetin being the predominant flavonoid.[120] Though quercetin consumption was low, this flavonoid level represents substantially more antioxidant activity than the typical daily consumption of vitamin E or beta-carotene. Furthermore, this level of flavonoid consumption correlated with a decreased risk of cardiovascular disease,[120] but not cancer[121](see Ch. 125 for further discussion).

Botanical extracts

Botanical extracts have been used for centuries by natural health care practitioners. Recent research has now demonstrated that much of their clinical efficacy is due to their flavonoid constituents, which are often organ-specific.

Silybum marianum *and other hepatoprotective botanicals*

Milk thistle extracts containing silymarin,[122] as well as extracts of Indian herbs such as *Picrorhiza kurroa,*[123] *Eclipta alba,*[124] and *Tinospora cordifolia,*[125] or combinations (Livotrit Plus™), concentrate flavonoids in the liver where they exert hepatoprotective effects. Since liver detoxication promotes autoxidation due to ROS produced by cytochrome P450,[126] the antioxidant properties of these botanical flavonoids largely explains the beneficial effects these plant extracts in normalizing liver function[127] (see Ch. 111 for a more in-depth discussion).

Proanthocyanidins

A variety of plant sources yield a family of flavonoids called proanthocyanidins. Often they are chained together (oligomers); hence the name oligomeric proanthocyanidins or OPCs. Pine bark and grape seeds are typical commercial sources. Animal experiments indicate that grape seed extracts can limit lipid peroxidation in the brain, suggesting that constituents or their colonic fermentation products, are absorbed and cross the blood brain barrier.[128] Preparations of European pine bark (Pycnogenol™) have been used as supplements for capillary dysfunction associated in patients with diabetes and for other venous abnormalities.[129] OPCs are also present in legume-derived polyphenols (Phytolens™), which inhibit peroxynitrite-induced apoptosis in human colonic cells, a model system for gut inflammation.[130]

Frenchmen consume a high fat diet, yet appear to have a lower mortality due to heart disease. Several explanations have been proposed for the so-called "French paradox". Of particular interest is the correlation of heart protection with wine consumption. The cholesterol-lowering effect of spirits is not unique to wine. However, red wine contains abundant tannins and other polyphenols, and drinking red wine increases the antioxidant capacity of serum.[131] Such experiments suggest the absorption of polyphenols. Red wine has a higher phenol antioxidant index measured against isolated LDL than white wine.[132] In addition, grape skins and red wine contain resveratrol, a phenolic compound, and phytoalexin, a compound produced by plants in response to environmental stressors. Resveratrol apparently inhibits platelet aggregation and eicosanoid syntheses and blocks cellular events linked to tumor initiation, promotion and progression.[133] These effects seem to be independent of its antioxidant properties (see Ch. 111 for further discussion).

Catechins

Tea is a rich source of polyphenols that are highly substituted with hydroxyl groups. Catechin and gallic acid derivatives – including epigallocatechin, epigallocatechin-3 gallate and epicatechin-3 gallate – which function as radical quenchers in vitro.[134,135] Tea consumption has been linked to a decreased risk of cancer, and antiproliferative effects seem to be a function of polyphenol content.[136] Urokinase, a proteolytic enzyme overexpressed in many cancers, can be inhibited by green tea flavonoids. Thus, green tea polyphenols probably have multiple effects in the body, including quenching radicals. Green tea extracts free of caffeine are now commercially available (see Chs 84 and 89).

Other botanicals

Extracts of *Ginkgo biloba* have long been known to support vascular function and cerebral insufficiency. It seems probable that active constituents, ginkgolides and related flavonoids reduce oxidative stress.[137,138] Turmeric has a long history of use in Eastern traditions. Curcuminoids are the bright yellow pigments isolated from this source. These lipids limit the metabolism of environmental mutagens. Consumption of extracts equivalent to 20 mg of curcuminoids for 45 days decreased serum lipid peroxides.[139] Animal studies suggest that consumption of curcumin can limit lipid peroxide induced cataracts and curcumin may suppress colon cancer.[140] Curcuminoids are diketones, not flavonoids, which emphasizes the point that many other plant ingredients besides polyphenols may function as antioxidants and as anticarcinogens (see Chs 97 and 105 for further discussion).

COMPARING ANTIOXIDANTS

There are several points to consider in comparing flavonoids. Studies of the quenching activity of antioxidants frequently employ single time points measured at a single concentration of antioxidant (end-point assay). This practice can lead to erroneous conclusions when comparing the effectiveness of antioxidants. A far more reliable approach evaluates the IC_{50}, the concentration of antioxidant yielding 50% inhibition of a given oxidant or radical. The smaller the IC_{50}, the more efficient the antioxidant. To illustrate, Table 99.3 compares IC_{50} values for several standardized botanical extracts and reference compounds using DPPH (diphenyl picrylhydrazyl radical), one of the test systems used for measuring free radical quenching.[141] Pine bark OPCs, grape seed OPCs, and polyphenols from non-soy legumes (Phytolens™) effectively quench organic free radicals.[130] It is important to compare antioxidant activity in several systems, such as superoxide, lipid peroxidation in LDL or microsomes, chemiluminence to detect the formation of reactive oxygen species, and so on. Table 99.3 presents additional data for quenching superoxide. Accordingly, the order of decreasing effectiveness of these superoxide quenchers is: legume-derived polyphenols (Phytolens™) > ascorbic acid > grape seed OPCs > pine bark OPCs > catechin.[127,130]

After demonstrating in vitro effectiveness, the question arises: "Does a given antioxidant improve cellular function?". Phytochemicals possess multiple effects, ranging from enzyme inhibition to enzyme induction via alteration of signal transduction. Flavonoids, in particular, often possess multiple effects, leading them to be considered as "biological response modifiers". There is also a growing awareness of the necessity of understanding the impact of flavonoids on the oxidative stress that contributes to mutagenesis and programmed cell death (apoptosis). Consumption of green tea and red wine flavonoids, and of oligomeric proanthocyanidins can decrease various indices of oxidative stress, such as plasma malondialdehyde or F_2-isoprostanes (from fatty acid peroxidation), tissue inflammation or urinary output of oxidized DNA bases.

Effectiveness of an antioxidant in vivo relies upon adequate absorption and assimilation. Water solubility of polyphenols would likely favor intestinal uptake; however, quercetin is readily absorbed, despite minimal water solubility.[112] The effects of bioactive ingredient or ingredients in botanical extracts are seldom completely

Table 99.3 Comparison of free radical quenching by plant antioxidants and reference compounds[127,130]

Test substance	DPPH* IC_{50} (ppm)	Superoxide# IC_{50} (ppm)
Pine bark oligomeric proanthocyanidins	4.4	17.8
Grape seed oligomeric proanthocyanidins	2.8–12.2	10.1–43.9
Phytolens™ legume polyphenols	4.9	5.6
Catechin	3.7	40.0
Ascorbic acid	14.5	7.0

*, 1,1-diphenyl-2-picrylhydrazl radical.
#, superoxide generated by phenazine methosulfate and NADH.
IC_{50} is the concentration of antioxidant able to reduce 50% of a given radical; therefore, the smaller the IC_{50}, the more effective the antioxidant.

understood. An additional complication is the fact that intestinal bacteria degrade complex polyphenols to simple phenolic acids. These may be more bioactive than the starting material.

THE ADEQUACY OF ANTIOXIDANT DEFENSES

Protection by free radical scavenging enzymes is limited and free radical damage is not completely prevented even in healthy people. All cells lack an enzyme defense against hydroxyl radicals, the most damaging species. Therefore, when free radical production exceeds the scavenging systems, hydroxyl radicals can be released, causing severe cellular damage. The body's ability to respond to oxidative stress is a function of age, inheritance, medical history, degree of exposure to pollutants and other environmental stressors, and diet.

Age

Because repair mechanisms decline with age, the body gradually loses functional resiliency, especially to oxidative stress. According to the free radical theory of aging, aging represents progressive oxidative damage.[142] Ames et al[11] have estimated that the average human cell sustains 10,000 DNA "hits" per day. Although most of these are repaired, unrepaired damage accumulates with age. Subtle structural alterations occur first, leading to decreased repair of damaged membranes and DNA, ultimately limiting the function of the nervous system, the endocrine system and the immune system.[11] A direct link between free radical scavenger enzymes and aging was suggested by the demonstration that transgenic fruit flies with extra copies of SOD and catalase genes produced elevated levels of these enzymes; they lived 30% longer than normal flies; and age-dependent oxidative damage also slowed down.[143]

Inheritance

Due to heredity, the levels of protective enzymes can vary among individuals. People who possess low levels of these enzymes face greater risks of free radical-induced disease. This distinction is blurred somewhat because these enzymes are often inducible, and increased enzyme synthesis occurs in many organs, such as liver and lung, as they adapt to increased oxidative burden (upregulation of antioxidant defense enzymes).[144]

Medical history and environmental exposure

Processes such as trauma, inflammation and infection generally increase ROS production. Oxidative stress sometimes accompanies drug treatment. Cigarette smoke, ozone, oxides of nitrogen, solvents and pesticides can cause toxicity when radicals are created during their detoxification. The gut epithelium does not appear to adapt to long-term oxidative stress and, because of low initial levels of defensive enzymes, may be especially susceptible to oxidative damage with even moderate inflammation.[145]

Strenuous physical exercise increases ROS production, and supplementing with antioxidant vitamins such as E, C and CoQ decreases associated oxidative damage, especially in older people,[146] and increases LDL antioxidant capacity in endurance athletes.[147] However, the paradox between exercise-induced oxidative stress and the obvious benefits of exercise has not been entirely resolved.

Nutritional status

Americans do not consume enough antioxidants, and the trend seems unlikely to change in the foreseeable future. Perhaps only 10–20% eat the minimum of five daily servings of fruits and vegetables recommended by federal agencies.[148,149] Median intakes of key antioxidants indicate that the consumption of vitamins C and E, beta-carotene, zinc, selenium, copper and manganese are low for specific segments of the population, and far below the RDAs for some. Furthermore, the RDAs do not address contributing factors concerning chronic diseases, lifestyle choices or medical history, nor do they address the issue of mutually supportive roles of antioxidants. The immune system, in particular, requires ample antioxidant nutrients.[150] They protect immune cells against oxidative damage and limit the production of non-inflammatory eicosanoids. As an example, supplementing apparently healthy, elderly people (who were consuming an otherwise typical diet), with 60–800 mg vitamin E improved several aspects of cell-mediated immunity within 4 months.[151,152] The research also suggested that consumption of 200 mg/day may be more effective than 800 mg/day. Overall studies indicate that the RDAs for this nutrient and other antioxidants are inadequate for optimal immune function (see Ch. 108 for an in-depth discussion of optimum nutrient levels).

GUIDELINES FOR USE OF ANTIOXIDANTS

Antioxidants represent powerful additions to the health-care practitioner's armamentarium. However, their application in treatment protocols requires an understanding of their strengths and limitations. No single supplement, nutrient or food can maintain the body's antioxidant defenses: there are simply too many oxidants to be neutralized, too many layers of antioxidant defenses to be sustained, and the range of reactivities of water- and lipid-soluble ROS is far too great. Multiple, complementary antioxidants are far more effective than large amounts of a single antioxidant. Often antioxidants work synergistically. An additional consideration: antioxidant requirements should be balanced against oxidant burden. Thus, exposure to pollutants such as cigarette smoke, nitric oxides and ozone as well as chronic inflammation increases oxidative stress. High intake of fish oil and polyunsaturated fatty acids increases the need for vitamin E. The goal is to support the body's defense system, rather than quenching all free radicals in the body, which would be counterproductive. Superoxide and nitric oxide play essential roles in maintaining the body's defenses and homoeostatic mechanisms, for example.

Precautions in using antioxidant supplementation

1. The uptake, assimilation and disposal or potential toxicity of polyphenols generally are not well studied.[153]
2. Flavonoids are metabolized and detoxified by liver enzymes, and pharmacologic doses may increase toxin burden. Some flavonoids can induce phase I detoxification enzymes, increasing the ability to transform toxins. The trade-off lies in the possible increased sensitivity to mutagens. In this context, quercetin at typical dietary levels appears to be a possible anticarcinogen.[154]
3. Vitamin E can exacerbate hypertension in susceptible people. High levels may antagonize other fat-soluble vitamins, thus decreasing bone mineralization. It may be contraindicated for patients receiving anticoagulants or for those with a vitamin K deficiency.[155]
4. Large amounts of vitamin C rarely increase oxalate production; the effects seems to be counterbalanced by increased vitamin B_6.[156]
5. Excessive iron and iron overload may cause hydroxyl radical production in vivo.[157]
6. Beta-carotene may increase the risk of lung cancer in high risk populations unless protected by antioxidants like vitamin E. In addition, beta-carotene may exacerbate liver abnormalities in patients with alcoholic liver disease. Fatal coronary heart disease increased in patients receiving 20 mg/day beta-carotene (with or without alpha-tocopherol).[158] Possibly high levels of beta-carotene are contraindicated for those with smokers with myocardial infarctions.
7. An antioxidant in one system is not necessarily an antioxidant in all systems. For example, vitamin C, vitamin E and beta-carotene exhibit pro-oxidant activity in vitro under certain conditions. Pro-oxidant effects of carotenoids are poorly understood and consumption of large amounts themselves could be hazardous in susceptible individuals. Depending on the concentration of supporting antioxidants, even flavonoids can become prooxidants.[159]
8. Vitamin A is a teratogen when the intake is 25,000 IU or more per day for several months. The general advice to women who are or who might become pregnant is to limit their daily intake of vitamin A from supplements to no more than 5,000 IU/day and to limit their consumption of liver and liver products.[160]

HOW TO CHOOSE ANTIOXIDANTS

The traditional definition of an essential (e.g. mineral or vitamin) nutrient is too restrictive from the perspective of life-long protection against chronic disease. The presence of vast numbers of non-vitamin antioxidants – in addition to established nutrients in vegetables, legumes, fruits and grains – poses the question of whether those antioxidants are in fact essential in the diet for optimal health and disease prevention. Consequently, antioxidant supplementation cannot substitute for a prudent diet, cessation of smoking and regular exercise. Supplementation may be most effective for those individuals who have the lowest baseline antioxidant levels, whether due to genetic or environmental causes. Foods supply a rich assortment of substances that can function as antioxidants. As an example, the total oxygen radical capacity of certain fruits has been determined.[161] Strawberry, plum, orange, red grapes, kiwi fruit and grape fruit possess high quenching activity. Blackberry, blueberry, raspberry, strawberry, plums, red wine and red grapes contain large amounts of anthocyanidins with strong antioxidant properties.[162] Further research will undoubtedly uncover many more phytochemical interactions.

Though the picture is far from complete, antioxidants apparently operate synergistically.[163] Thus, animal studies indicate that an increased diversity of antioxidants provides more antioxidant protection than single supplements.[164] Even members of the B complex, such as pantothenic acid, may indirectly stimulate antioxidant production.[165] It should be emphasized that many ingredients in foods play important physiologic roles in addition to their properties as antioxidants. Furthermore, their effects may be indirect; antioxidants and response elements help the cell to adapt to ROS exposure and to correct ROS-induced damage.[166] Exploration of the role of a major oxidant, peroxynitrite, and nitrogen oxides as NOS ("nitrogen reactive species") in chronic degenerative diseases is still in its infancy.[167] Consequently, the antioxidants that best defuse these reactive compounds have not yet been established.

Table 99.4 provides a summary of a recommended intake of antioxidants for maintenance as compiled by the European Federation of Health Product Manufacturers.[168] The levels often prescribed in treatment protocols may be considerably higher than those listed. Thus, the consumption of a broad spectrum of antioxidants in amounts geared to meet an individual's oxidant burden and nutritional status appears to be essential in order to promote optimal health and to minimize the effects of genetic predisposition that compromise defenses against aging, degenerative disease and toxic chemical exposure.

Table 99.4 Recommended safe upper limits of daily intake of antioxidants for maintenance[168]

Nutrient	Safe upper limit	Comments
Alpha-tocopherol	900 IU	No toxicity for alpha-tocopherol has been reported. Mild, reversible side-effects have been noted at intakes greater than 1000 mg/day
Beta-carotene	25 mg	Generally no adverse side-effects have been noted other than hypercarotenemia at levels of about 30 mg/day. One study noted an apparent slight increased risk of cancer at 20 mg/day with a high alcohol consumption[60]
Vitamin C	2,000 mg	There are generally no adverse effects with long-term consumption of up to several grams of vitamin C daily. High consumption may be contraindicated with renal insufficiency disease and iron overload
Vitamin A	9,000 RE	Toxicity with chronic consumption of 12,000–23,000 retinol equivalents/day can occur rarely
Copper	9 mg	Copper is interrelated with zinc. Contaminated water is often a source of toxic levels
Manganese	20 mg	Supplementation may raise blood pressure and chronic toxicity may cause neurologic disorders
Selenium	450 mcg	Excessive selenium can be toxic, though organic selenium seems safer. Selenite reportedly reacts with glutathione to produce ROS. Selenocysteine can enter amino acid pools directly, while selenomethionine may be funneled into protein with imbalanced dietary protein
Zinc	30 mg	Rigorous homoeostatic mechanisms regulate zinc balance Extremely high levels block copper assimilation and are immunosuppressive

REFERENCES

1. Menkes MS, Comstock GW, Vuilleumier JP et al. Serum beta-carotene, vitamins A and E, selenium, and the risk of lung cancer. N Eng J Med 1986; 315: 1250–1254
2. Weisburger JH. Nutritional approach to cancer prevention with emphasis on vitamins, antioxidants and carotenoids. Am J Clin Nutr 1991; 53: 226S–237S
3. Esterbauer H, Gebick J, Puhl H, Jurgens G. The role of lipid peroxidation and antioxidants in oxidative modification of LDL. Free Radic Biol Med 1992; 13: 341–390
4. Witztum JL. The oxidation hypothesis of atherosclerosis. Lancet 1994; 344: 793–795
5. Liles MR, Newsome DA, Oliver PD. Antioxidant enzymes in the aging human retinal pigment epithelium. Arch Opthalmal 1991; 109: 1285–1288
6. Grisham MB. Oxidants and free radicals in inflammatory bowel disease. Lancet 1994; 344: 859–861
7. Suryaprabha P, Das UN, Ramesh G et al. Reactive oxygen species, lipid peroxides and essential fatty acids in patients with rheumatoid arthritis and systemic lupus erythematosus. Prostaglandins Leukot Essent Fatty Acids 1991; 43: 251–255
8. Cross CE, van der Vliet A, O'Neill CA, Eiserich JP. Reactive oxygen species and the lung. Lancet 1994; 344: 930–933
9. Kogure, K, Arai H, Abe K, Nakano M. Free radical damage of the brain following ischemia. Prog Brain Res 1985; 63: 237–259
10. Jenner P. Oxidative damage in neurodegenerative disease. Lancet 1994; 344: 796–798
11. Ames BN, Shigenaga MK, Hagen TM. Oxidants, antioxidants, and the degenerative diseases of aging. Proc Natl Acad Sci USA 1993; 90: 7915–7922
12. Sohal RS, Sohal BH, Brunk UT. Relationship between antioxidant defenses and longevity in different mammalian species. Mech Ageing Dev 1990; 53: 217–227
13. Olanow CW, Arendash GW. Metals and free radicals in neurodegeneration. Curr Opin Neurol 1994; 7: 548–558
14. Burdon RH. Superoxide and hydrogen peroxide in relation to mammalian cell proliferation. Free Radic Biol Med 1995; 18: 775–794
15. Smith CV. Free radical mechanisms in tissue injury. In: Moslen MT, Smith CV, eds. Free radical mechanisms of tissue injury. Boca Raton, FL: CRC Press. 1992: p 2–22
16. Stadtman ER. Metal ion-catalyzed oxidation of proteins. biochemical mechanism and biological consequences. Free Radic Biol Med 1990; 9: 315–325
17. Orrenius S, Burkitt MJ, Kass GEN et al. Calcium ions and oxidative cell injury. Ann Neurol 1992; 32: S33–S42
18. Roberts RA, Soames AR, James NH et al. Dosing-induced stress causes hepaotcyte apoptosis in rats primed by the rodent nongenotoxid hepatocarcinogen cyproterone acetate. Toxicol Applied Pharmacol 1995; 135: 192–199
19. Narula J, Haider N, Virmani R et al. Apoptosis in myocytes in end stage heart failure. N Eng J Med 1996; 335: 1182–1189
20. Halliwell B. Free radicals, antioxidants, and human disease. curiosity, cause or consequence? Lancet 1994; 344: 721–724
21. Reed PJ. Mechanisms of chemically induced cell injury and cellular protection mechanisms. In: Hodgson E, Levi PE, eds. Introduction to biochemical toxicology. 2nd edn. Norwalk, CT: Appleton and Lange. 1994: p 267–295
22. Corbett MD, Corbett BR. Bioactivation of xenobiotics by the respiratory burst of human granulocytes. In: Moslen MT, Smith CV, eds. Free radical mechanisms of tissue injury. Boca Raton: CRC Press. 1992: p 144–151
23. Sivarajah K, Lasker JM, Eling TE, Abou-Donia MB. Metabolism of n-alkyl compounds during the biosynthesis of prostaglandins. n-dealkylation during prostaglandin biosynthesis. Mol Pharmacol 1982; 21: 133–141
24. Yamada T, Grisham MB. Role of neutrophil-derived oxidants in the pathogenesis of intestinal inflammation. Klin Wochenschr 1991; 69: 988–994
25. Keshavarzian A, Sedghi S, Kanotsky J et al. Excessive production of reactive oxygen metabolites by inflamed colon. Analysis by chemiluminescence probe. Gastroenterology 1992; 103: 177–185
26. Sies H. Oxidative stress. In: Sies H, ed. Introduction in oxidative stress: oxidants and antioxidants. San Diego: Academic Press. 1991: p. x–xxii
27. Buettner GR. The pecking order of free radicals and antioxidants. lipid peroxidation α-tocopherol and ascorbate. Arch Biochem Biophy 1993; 300: 535–543
28. Nelson SK, Huang CJ, Mathias MM, Allen KGD. Copper-marginal and copper-deficient diets decrease aortic prostacyclin production and copper-dependent superoxide dismutase activity and increase aortic lipid peroxidation in rats. J Nutr 1992; 122: 2101–2108
29. Visner GA, Dougall WC, Wilson JM et al. Regulation of manganese superoxide dismutase by lipopolysaccharide, interleukin-1, and tumor necrosis factor. J Biol Chem 1990; 265: 2856–2864
30. Deng H-X, Hentati A, Tainer JA et al. Amyotrophic lateral sclerosis and structural defects in Cu, Zn superoxide dismutase. Science 1993; 261: 1047–1051
31. Richardson SJ. Free radicals in the genesis of Alzheimer's disease. Ann NY Acad Sci 1993; 695: 73–76
32. Niwa Y, Sominya K, Michelson AM, Puget F. Effect of liposomal encapsulated superoxide dismutase on active oxygen-related human disorders. Free Radic Res Commun 1985; 1: 137–153
33. Rhee P, Waxman K, Clark L et al. Superoxide dismutase polyethylene glycol improves survival in hemorrhagic shock. Am Surg 1991; 57: 747–750

34. Giri SN, Misra HP. Fate of superoxide dismutase in mice following oral route of administration. Med Biol 1984; 62: 285–289
35. Zindenberg-Cherr S, Keen CL, Lonnerdal B, Hurely LS. Dietary superoxide dismutase does not affect tissue levels. Am J Clin Nutr 1983; 37: 5–7
36. Bucci LR, Klenda BA, Stiles JC. Nutritional supplements containing antioxidant enzymes: label claims and potencies. Paper Presented at the Third International Congress of Biomedical Gerontology, Acapulco, Mexico, 1989
37. Introna M, Moss J, Ronzio RA. The effect of oral supplementation with legume derived superoxide dismutase on human erythrocyte superoxide dismutase in healthy volunteers. J Applied Nutr 1997; 49: 12–17
38. Nayak MS, Kita M, Marmor MF. Protection of rabbit retina from ischemic injury by superoxide dismutase and catalase. Invest Ophthalmol Vis Sci 1993; 34: 2018–2022
39. Kohen R, Kakunda A, Rubinstein A. The role of cationized catalase and cationized glucose oxidase in mucosal oxidative damage induced in the rat jejunum. J Biol Chem 1992; 267: 21 349–21 354
40. Jones JB, Cramer HM, Inch WR, Lamps HB. Radioprotective effect of free radical scavenging enzymes. J Otolaryngol 1990; 19: 299–306
41. Chudej LL, Koke JR, Bittar N. Evidence for transcytosis of exogenous superoxide dismutase and catalase from coronary capillaries into dog myocytes. Cytobios 1990; 63: 41–53
42. Thomas JP, Geiger PC, Maiorino M et al. Enzymatic reduction of phospholipid and cholesterol hydroperoxides in artificial bilayers and lipoproteins. Biochem Biophys Acta 1990; 1043: 252–260
43. Burke RF, Hill KE. Selenoprotein P. A selenium-rich extracellular glycoprotein. J Nutr 1994; 124: 1891–1897
44. Veera-Reddy K, Kumar T, Prasad M, Reddanna P. Exercise-induced oxidant stress in the lung tissue. Role of dietary supplementation of vitamin E and selenium. Biochem Int 1992; 26: 863–871
45. Gonzalez-Flecha BS, Repetto M, Evalson P, Boveris A. Inhibition of microsomal lipid peroxidation by alpha tocopherol and alpha tocopherol acetate. Xenobiotica 1991; 21: 1013–1022
46. Mergens WJ, Kammi JJ, Newark HL. Alpha tocopherol. Uses in preventing nitrosoamine formation. In: Walker EA, Castegnaro M, Gricute L, Lyle RE, eds. Environmental aspects of n-nitroso compounds. Lyon: IARC Scientific Publications. 1978: p 190–212
47. Kagan VE, Serbinova EA, Forte T et al. Recycling of vitamin E in low density lipoproteins. J Lipid Res 1992; 33: 385–387
48. Wiklund O, Mattson L, Bjornheden T et al. Uptake and degradation of low density lipoproteins in atherosclerotic rabbit aorta. role of local LDL modifications. J Lipid Res 1991; 32: 55–62
49. Lohr JB, Caligiuri MP. A double blind, placebo-controlled study of vitamin E treatment of tardive dyskinesia. J Clin Psychiatry 1996; 57: 167–173
50. Seiner M. Influences of vitamin E on platelet function in humans. J Am Col Nutr 1991; 10: 466–473
51. Kritchevsky D. Antioxidant vitamins in the prevention of cardiovascular disease. Nutr Today 1992; 27: 1–4
52. Jialal I, Grundy SM. Effect of combined supplementation with alpha-tocopherol, ascorbate, and beta carotene on low-density lipoprotein oxidation. Circulation 1993; 88: 2780–2785
53. Stephens NG, Parsons A, Scholfield PM et al. Randomized controlled trial of vitamin E in patients with coronary disease. Cambridge Heart Antioxidant Study, Lancet 1996; 47: 781–786
54. Sano M, Ernesto C, Thomas K et al. A controlled trial of selegiline, alpha tocopherol or both as treatment for Alzheimer's disease. N Engl J Med 1997; 336: 1216–1222
55. Hunter DJ, Manson JE, Colditz GA et al. A prospective study of the intake of vitamins C, E and A and the risk of breast cancer. N Engl J Med 1993; 329: 234–240
56. Christen S, Woodall AA, Shigenaga MK et al. Gamma tocopherol traps mutagenic electrophiles such as Nox and complements alpha tocopherol. Physiologic implication. Proc Natl Acad Sci 1997; 94: 3217–3222
57. Podda M, Weber C, Taratve MG, Packer L. Simulateous determination of tissue tocopherols, tocotrienols, ubiquinols and ubiquiones. Lipid Res 1996; 37: 893–901
58. Chan AC. Partners in defense, vitamin E and vitamin C. Can J Physiol Pharmacol 1993; 71: 725–731
59. Frei B, England L, Ames BN. Ascorbate is an outstanding antioxidant in human blood plasma. Proc Natl Acad Sci 1989; 86: 6377–6381
60. Horwilt MK. Supplementation with vitamin E. Am J Clin Nutr 1988; 47: 1088–1089
61. Anti M, Armelao F, Marra G et al. Effects of different doses of fish oil on rectal cell proliferation in patients with sporadic colonic adenomas. Gastroenterology 1994; 107: 1709–1718
62. Chandra DB, Varma R, Ahmad S, Varma SD. Vitamin C in the aqueous human and cataracts. Int J Vit Nutr Res 1986; 56: 165–168
63. Jakob RA, Kelly DS, Piamalto FS et al. Immunocompetence and antioxidant defense during ascorbate depletion of healthy men. Am J Clin Nutr 1991; 54: 1302S–1309S
64. Calabrese EJ, Stoddard A, Leonard DA, Dinardi SR. The effect of vitamin C supplementation on blood and hair levels of cadmium, iron and mercury. Ann NY Acad Sci 1987; 498: 347–353
65. Tannenbaum SR, Wishnor JS. Inhibition of nitrosoamine formation by ascorbic acid. Ann NY Acad Sci 1987; 498: 354–363
66. Jialal I, Vega GL, Grundy SM. Physiological levels of ascorbate inhibit the oxidative modification of low-density lipoprotein. Atherosclerosis 1990; 82: 185–191
67. Bonorden WR, Pariza MW. Antioxidant nutrients and protection from free radicals. In: Kotsonis, FT, MacKey M, Hielle J, eds. Nutritional toxicology. New York: Raven Press. 1994: p 10–47
68. Chem LH. Interaction of vitamin E and ascorbic acid. In Vivo 1989; 3: 199–209
69. Levine M, Conry-Cantilena C, Wang Y et al. Vitamin C pharmokinetics in healthy volunteers. Evidence for a recommended dietary allowance. Proc Natl Acad Sci 199; 93: 3704–3709
70. Vinson JA, Bose P. Comparative bioavailability to humans of ascorbic acid alone or in a citrus extract. Am J Clin Nutr 1988; 48: 601–604
71. Parker RS. Analysis of carotenoids in human plasma and tissue. In: Packer L, ed. Carotenoids. Part B: metabolism, genetics and biosynthesis. Methods in Enzymology, vol. 124. San Diego: Academic Press. 1993: p 86–93
72. Stahl W, Schwarz W, Sundquist AR, Sies H. *Cis-trans* isomers of lycopene and beta-carotene in human serum and tissues. Arch Biochem Biophys 1992; 294: 173–177
73. Bendich A, Olson JA. Biological action of carotenoids. FASEB J 1989; 3: 1927–1932
74. Martin MC, Campbell DR, Gross MD et al. Plasma carotenoids as biomarkers of vegetable intake: the University of Minnesota Cancer Prevention Research Unit Feeding Studies. Cancer Epidemiol Biomarkers Prev 1995; 4: 491–496
75. Gartner C, Stahl W, Sies H. Preferential increase in chylomicron levels in xanthophylls lutein and zeaxanthan compared to beta carotene in the human. Internat J Vit Nutr Res 1996; 66: 119–125
76. Hughes DA, Wright JA, Fuglas PM et al. The effect of beta carotene supplementation on the immune function of blood monocytes from healthy male nonsmokers. J Lab Clin Med 1997; 129: 309–317
77. Vile GF, Winterbourn CC. Inhibition of adriamycin promoted microsomal lipid peroxidation by beta carotene, alpha-tocopherol and retinal at high and low oxygen partial pressure. FEBS Lett 1988; 238: 353–356
78. Bendich A. Carotenoids and the immune response. J Nutr 1989; 119: 112–115
79. Jialal I, Norju EP, Cristol L, Grundy SM. Beta carotene inhibits the oxidative modification of low-density lipoprotein. Biochem Biophys Acta 1991; 1086: 134–138
80. Morris DL, Kritchevsky SB, Davis CE. Serum carotenoids and coronary heart disease. JAMA 1994; 272: 1439–1441
81. Seddon JM, Ajani UA, Sperduto RD et al. Dietary carotenoids, vitamins A, C and E, and advanced age-related macular degeneration. JAMA 1994; 272: 1413–1420
82. Block G. The data support a role of antioxidants in reducing cancer risk. Nutri Rev 1992; 50: 207–213

83. Hughes DA, Wright JA, Finglas PM et al. The effect of beta carotene supplementation on the immune function of blood monocytes from healthy male nonsmokers. J Lab Clin Med 1997; 129: 309–317
84. The Alpha-Tocopherol, Beta Carotene Cancer Prevention Study Group. The effect of vitamin E and beta carotene on the incidence of lung cancer and other cancers in male smokers. N Engl J Med 1994; 330: 1029–1035
85. Omenn GS, Goodman GE, Thomquist MD et al. Effects of a combination of beta carotene and vitamin A in lung cancer and cardiovascular disease. N Eng J Med 1996; 334: 1150–1155
86. Blot WJ, Li J-Y, Taylor PR et al. Nutrition intervention trials in Linxian, China. Supplementation with specific vitamin/mineral combinations, cancer incidence and disease-specific mortality in a general population. J Natl Cancer Inst 1993; 85: 1483–1492
87. Levin G, Mokady S. Antioxidant activity of 9-cis compared to all trans β-carotene in vitro. Free Radic Bio Med 1994; 17: 77–82
88. Ben-Amotz A, Levy Y. Bioavailability of a natural isomer mixture compared with synthetic all trans beta carotene in human serum. Am J Clin Nutr 1996; 63: 729–734
89. Livrea MA, Tesoriere L, Bongiorno A et al. Contribution of vitamin A to the oxidation resistance of human low density lipoproteins. Free Radic Biol Med 1995; 18: 401–409
90. Akerboom TPM, Sies H. Assay of glutathione, glutathione disulfide and glutathione mixed disulfides in biological samples. In: Jakoby W, ed. Detoxication and drug metabolism: conjugation and related systems. Methods in enzymology, vol 77. New York: Academic Press. 1981: p 373–382
91. Peristeris P, Clark BD, Gatti S et al. N-acetylcysteine and glutathione as inhibitors of tumor necrosis factor production. Cell Immunol 1992; 140: 390–399
92. Greenspan HC. The role of reactive oxygen species, antioxidants and phytopharmaceuticals in human immunodeficiency virus activity. Med Hypothesis 1993; 40: 85–92
93. Herzenberg LA, DeRosa SC, Dubs JG et al. Glutathione deficiency is associated with impaired survival in HIV disease. Proc Natl Acad Sci 1997; 94: 1967–1972
94. Yim CY, Hibbs JR, Jr., McGregor JR et al. Use of N-acetyl cysteine to increase intracellular glutathione during induction of antitumor responses by IL-2: J Immunol 1994; 152: 5796–5805
95. Julius M, Lang CA, Gleiberman L et al. Glutathione and morbidity in a community-based sample of elderly. J Clin Epidmicol 1994; 47: 1021–1026
96. Hagen TM, Wierzbicka GT, Sillua AH et al. Bioavailability of dietary glutathione. Effect of plasma concentration. Am J Physiol 1990; 259: G524–529
97. Aw TY, Wierzbicka G, Jones DF. Oral glutathione increases tissue glutathione *in vivo*. Chem Cell Interact 1991; 80: 89–97
98. Pangborn J. Mechanisms of detoxication and procedures for detoxification. West Chicago, IL: Bionostics, Inc. 1994: p 115–118
99. Maguire JJ, Kagan V, Ackrell BA, Packer L. Succinate-ubiquinone reductase linked recycling of alpha-tocopherol in reconstituted systems and mitochondria. Requirement for reduced ubiquinone. Arch Biochem Biophys 1992; 292: 47–53
100. Sugimura K, Azuma I, Yamamura Y et al. Effect of ubiquinone and related compounds on immune response. In: Folkers K, Yamamura Y, eds. Biomedical and clinical aspects of coenzyme Q. Amsterdam: North-Holland Biomedical Press, Elsevier. 1977: p 151–163
101. Kamikawa T, Kobayashi A, Yamashita T et al. Effects of coenzyme Q_{10} on exercise tolerance in chronic stable angina pectoris. Am J Cardiol 1985; 56: 247–251
102. Mortensen SA, Vadhanavikit S, Muratsu K, Folkers K. Coenzyme Q_{10}: clinical benefits with biochemical correlates suggesting a scientific break-through on the management of chronic heart failure. Int J Tissue React 1990; 12: 155–162
103. Stocker R, Bowry VW, Frei B. Ubiquinol-10 protects human low density lipoproteins more efficiently against lipid peroxidation than does alpha tocopherol. Proc Natl Acad Sci USA 1991; 88: 1646–1650
104. Folkers K, Brown R, Judy WV, Morita M. Survival of cancer patients on therapy with coenzyme Q_{10}: Biochem Biophys Res Comm 1993; 192: 241–245
105. Folkers K, Vadhanaviki S, Mortensen SA. Biochemical rationale and myocardial tissue data on the effective therapy of cardiomyopathy with coenzyme Q_{10}. Proc Natl Acad Sci (USA) 1985; 82: 901–904
106. Weber C, Jakobsen TS, Mortensen SA et al. Antioxidative effect of dietary Coenzyme Q_{10} in human blood plasma. Internat J Vit Res 1994; 64: 311–315
107. Bucci LR, Klenda BA, Stiles JC, Sparks WS. Enhanced blood levels of coenzyme Q_{10} from an emulsified oral form. 3rd International Congress of Biomedical Gerontology Acapulco, Mexico. 1989
108. Ames BN, Cathcart R, Schwiers E, Hochstein P. Uric acid provides an antioxidant defense in humans against oxidant and radical caused aging and cancer: a hypothesis. Proc Natl Acad Sci 1981; 78: 6858–6862
109. Wayner DDM, Burton GW, Ingold KU, Locke S. Quantitative measurement of the total peroxyl radical-trapping antioxidant capability of human blood plasma by controlled peroxidation. FEBS Lett 1985; 187: 33–37
110. Reimund E. The free radical flux theory of sleep. Med Hypothesis 1994; 43: 231–233
111. Krsek-Staples JA, Webster RO. Ceruloplasmin inhibits carbonyl formation in endogenous cell proteins. Free Radic Biol Med 1993; 14: 115–125
112. Hollman PCH, Gaag MUD, Mengethers MJB et al. Absorption and disposition kinetics of the dietary antioxidant quercetin in man. Free Radic Bio Med 1996; 21: 703–707
113. Robak J, Gryglewski RJ. Flavonoids are scavengers of superoxide. Biochem Pharmacol 1988; 37: 837–841
114. DeWhalley CV, Rankin S, Hoult JRS et al. Flavonoids inhibit the oxidation modification of low density lipoproteins by macrophages. Biochem Pharmacol 1990; 39: 1743–1750
115. Monboissi JC, Braquet P, Pandoux A, Borel JB. Nonenzymatic degradation of acid soluble calf skin collagen by superoxide ion. protective effect of flavonoids. Biochem Pharmacol 1983; 32: 53–58
116. Afanasev JB, Dorozhko AI, Brodskii AV et al. Chelating and free radical scavenging mechanism of inhibition action of rutin and quercetin in lipid peroxidation. Biochem Pharmacol 1989; 38: 1763–1769
117. Stavric B, Matula TI. Flavonoids in foods. Their significance for nutrition and health. In: Ong ASH, Packer L, eds. Lipid-soluble antioxidants: biochemistry and chemical applications. Basel: Birkhauser Verlog. 1992: p 274–294
118. Piantelli M, Maggiano N, Ricci P et al. Tamoxifen and quercetin interact with type II estrogen binding sites and inhibit the growth of human melanoma cells. J Invest Dermatol 1995; 105: 248–253
119. Kandaswami C, Perkins E, Soloniuk DS et al. Ascorbic acid-enhanced antiproliferative effect of flavonoids on squamous cell carcinoma in vitro. Anti Cancer Drugs 1993; 4: 91–96
120. Hertog MGL, Feskens JM, Hollman RCH et al. Dietary antioxidant flavonoids and risk of coronary heart disease: the Zutphen elderly study. Lancet 1993; 342: 1007–1011
121. Hertog MGL, Feskens EJM, Hollman PCH et al. Dietary flavonoids and cancer risk in the Zutphen elderly study. Nutr Cancer 1994; 22: 175–184
122. Wagner H. Antihepatotoxic flavonoids. In: Cody V, Middleton E, Harbourne JB, eds. Plant flavonoids in biology and medicine: biochemical pharmacological and structure activity relationships. New York, Alan R Liss. 1986: p 545–558
123. Dwivedi Y, Rastogi R, Garg NK, Dhawan BN. Prevention of paracetamol-induced hepatic damage in rats by picroliv, the standardized active fraction from picrorhiza kurroa. Phytotherap Res 1991; 5: 115–119
124. Wagner H, Geyer B, Kiso Y et al. Coumestans as the main active principles of liver drugs Eclipta alba and Wedelia calendulacea. Plant Med 1986; 52: 370–374
125. Rege NN, Nazareth HM, Bapat RD, Dahanukar SA. Modulation of immuno suppression in obstructive jaundice. Indian J Med Res 1989; 90: 478–483
126. Kulkami AP, Byczkowski JZ. Hepatotoxicity. In: Hodgson E, Levi PE, eds. Biochemical toxicology. 2nd edn. Norwalk, CT: Appleton and Lange. 1994: p 460–490

127. Muanza DN, Ronzio RA. Comparison of antioxidant properties of Livotrit and Silymarin, herbal extracts that support liver function. Adjuvant Nutrition in Cancer Treatment Symposium, Tampa, September 1995
128. Bagchi D, Kortin RI, Garg A et al. Comparative *in vitro* and *in vivo* free radical scavenging abilities of grape seed proanthocyanidins and selected antioxidants. FASEB Proc Exp Biol 1997; New Orleans
129. Lagrue G, Olivier-Martin F, Grillot A. Etude des effects des oligomeres du procyamidol sur la resistance capillairie donas l'hypertension arteriella et certaines nephropathies. La Semaine de Hepitaux de Paris 1981; 57: 1399–1401
130. Sandoval M, Ronzio RA, Muanza DN et al. Protective action of plant antioxidants (Phytolenstm) against peroxynitrite-induced apoptosis in epithelial (T84) and macrophage (RAW264.7) cell lines. 3rd Annual Meeting, Oxygen Society, Miami. 1996
131. Whitehead TO, Robinson D, Allaway S et al. Effect of red wine ingestion on the antioxidant capacity of serum. Clin Chem 1995; 41: 32–36
132. Vinson JA and Hontz BA. Phenol antioxidant index. Comparative antioxidant effectiveness of red and white wines. J Agric Food Chem 1995; 43: 401–403
133. Jang M, Cai L, Udeani GO et al. Cancer chemopreventive activity of resveratrol, a natural product derived from grapes. Science 1997; 275: 218–220
134. Yen GC, Chen H-Y. Antioxidant activity of various tea extracts in relation to their antimutagenicity. J Agr Food Chem 1995; 43: 27–32
135. Lin Y-L, Juan I-M, Chen Y-L et al. Composition of polyphenols in fresh tea leaves and associations of their oxygen radical absorbing capacity with antiproliferative actions in fibroblast cells. J Agric Food Chem 1996; 44: 1387–1394
136. Hasegawa R, Chujo T, Sai-Kato K et al. Preventive effects of green tea against liver oxidative DNA damage and hepatotoxicity in rats treated with 2-nitropentane. Food Chem Toxic 1995; 33: 961–970
137. Rong Y, Geng Z, Lau, BHS. *Ginkgo biloba* attenuates oxidative stress in macrophages and endothelial cells. Free Radic Biol Med 1996; 20: 121–127
138. Otamiri T, Tagesson C. *Ginkgo biloba* extract prevents mucosal damage associated with small intestinal ischemia. Scand J Gastroenterol 1989; 24: 666–670
139. Ramirez-Bosca A et al. Antioxidant curcumin extracts decrease the blood lipid peroxide levels of human subjects. Age 1995; 18: 167–169
140. Swasthi S, Srivatava K, Piper JT et al. Curcumin protects against 4-hydroxy-2 trans nonenal-induced cataract formation in rat lenses. Am J Clin Nutr 1996; 64: 761–766
141. Halliwell B. How to characterize a biological antioxidant. Free Rad Res Commun 1990; 9: 1–32
142. Harman D. Aging. A theory based on free radical and radiation chemistry. J Gerontol 1956; 11: 288–300
143. Orr WE, Sohal RS. Extension of life span by over expression of superoxide dismutase and catalase in drosophila melanogaster. Science 1994; 263: 1128–1130
144. Visner GA, Dougall WC, Wilson JM et al. Regulation of manganese superoxide dismutase by lipopolysaccharide, interleukin-1 and tumor necrosis factor. J Biol Chem 1990; 265: 2856–2864
145. Grisham MB, MacDermott RP, Dietch EA. Oxidant defense mechanisms in the human colon. Inflammation 1990; 14: 669–680
146. Goldfarb AH. Antioxidants. Role of supplementation to prevent exercise induced oxidative stress. Med Sci Sports Exerc 1993; 25: 232–236
147. Vasankari TJ, Kujala UM, Vasankari TM et al. Increased serum and low density lipoprotein antioxidant potential after oxidant supplementation in endurance athletes. Am J Clin Nutr 1997; 65: 1052–1056
148. Block G. Antioxidant intake in the US. Toxicol Ind Health 1993; 9: 295–301
149. Patterson BH, Block G, Rosenberger WF et al. Fruit and vegetables in the American diet: data from the NHANES II Survey. Am J Public Health 1990; 80: 1443–1449
150. Meydani SN, Barklund MP, Liu S. Vitamin supplementation enhances cell-mediated immunity in healthy elderly subjects. Am J Clin Nutr 1990; 52: 557–563
151. Bogden JD, Bendich A, Kemp FW et al. Daily micronutrient supplements enhance delayed hypersensitivity skin test responses in older people. Am J Clin Nutr 1994; 60: 437–447
152. Meydani SN, Meydani M, Blumberg JB et al. Vitamin E supplementation and in vivo immune response in healthy elderly subjects. JAMA 1997; 277: 1380–1386
153. Canada AT, Watkins WDS, Nguyen TD. The toxicity of flavonoids to guinea pig enterocytes. Toxicol Applied Pharmacol 1989; 99: 357–361
154. Stavric B. Quercetin with our diet. From potent mutagen to probable anticarcinogen. Clinical Biochem 1994; 27: 245–248
155. Meydan SN. Vitamin E. Lancet 1995; 345: 170–177
156. Wright JV. High dose vitamin C and kidney stones. In: Dr. Wright's book of nutritional therapy. Emmanus, PA: Rodale Press. 1979: p 272–277
157. Tokokuni S. Iron-induced carcinogenesis. The role of redox regulation. Free Radic Bio Med 1996; 20: 553–566
158. Rapola JM, Virtamo J, Riatti S et al. Randomized trial of a-tocopherol and b-carotene supplements on incidence of major coronary events in men with previous myocardial infarction. Lancet 1997; 349: 1715–1720
159. Canada AT, Giannella E, Nguyen TD, Mason RP. The production of reactive oxygen species by dietary flavonoids. Free Radic Biol Med, 9: 441–9, 1990
160. Rothman KJ et al. Teratogenicty of high vitamin A intake. N Eng J Med 1995; 333: 1369–1373
161. Wang H, Cao G, Prior RL. Total antioxidant capacity of fruits. J Agr Food Chem 1996; 44: 701–705
162. Wang H, Cao G, Prior RL. Oxygen radical absorbing capacity of anthocyanidins. J Agr Food Chem 1997; 45: 304–309
163. May JM, Qu Z-C, Whitesell RR et al. Ascorbate recycling in human erythrocytes. Role glutathione in reducing dehydroascrobate. Free Radic Biol Med 1996; 20: 543–551
164. Chen H, Tappel AL. Protection by vitamin E, selenium, trolox c, ascorbic acid palmitate, acetylcysteine, coenzyme Q, beta-carotene, canthaxanthin, and (+,–) catechin against oxidative damage to liver slices measured by oxidized heme proteins. Free Radic Biol Med 1994; 16: 437–444
165. Slyshenkov VS, Moiseenok AG, Wojtczak L. Noxious effects of oxygen reactive species on energy-coupling processes in Ehrlich ascites tumor mitochondria and the protection by pantothenic acid. Free Radic Biol Med 1996; 20: 793–800
166. Ceruti P, Shah G, Peskin A, Amstad P. Oxidant carcinogenesis and antioxidant defense. Ann NY Acad Sci 1992; 663: 158–166
167. Yermilov V, Rubio J, Ohshima H. Formation of 8-nitroguanine in DNA treated with peroxynitrite in vitro and its rapid removal from DNA by depurination. FEBS Lett 1995; 376: 207–210
168. The Safety of Micronutrients. A review of the safety of vitamins and minerals provided in nutritional supplements for free sale in self-selection. European Federation of Health Product Manufacturers. 1994

CHAPTER CONTENTS

100

Panax ginseng (Korean ginseng)

Michael T. Murray, ND

Joseph E. Pizzorno Jr, ND

Panax ginseng C.A. Meyer (family: Araliaceae)
Synonym: *Panax schinseng* Nees
Common names: Korean ginseng, Chinese ginseng, Asiatic ginseng, Oriental ginseng

GENERAL DESCRIPTION

Korean or Chinese ginseng is a small perennial plant which originally grew wild in the damp woodlands of northern China, Manchuria, and Korea. Wild ginseng is now extremely rare. However, ginseng is a widely cultivated plant, especially in Korea, but also in Russia, China, and Japan. In addition to *Panax ginseng* C.A. Meyer, four other closely related species are often used:

- *Panax quinquefolium* (American ginseng)
- *Panax japonicum* C.A. Meyer (Japanese ginseng)
- *Panax pseudoginseng* (Himalayan ginseng)
- *Panax trifolium.*

Panax ginseng C.A. Meyer is the most widely used and most extensively studied species. Its pharmacology is the major focus of this chapter.[1,2]

Fully mature, Korean ginseng is a herbaceous plant with a tap-root, five-lobed palmate leaves, and greenish-white flowers in an umbel. In the first year, ginseng bears only a single leaf with three leaflets. In the second year, it bears a single leaf with five leaflets, and in its third year it bears two leaves with five leaflets. It usually starts flowering in its fourth year, while bearing three leaves. The roots of the cultivated plant are 3–4 mm in diameter and 10 cm long, while the roots of wild plants may attain 10 cm in diameter and a length of 50–60 cm.

Ginseng is often processed in two forms, white and red ginseng. White ginseng is the dried root whose peripheral skin is frequently peeled off. Red ginseng is the steamed root, which shows a caramel-like color.[2]

There are many types and grades of ginseng and ginseng extracts depending on the source, age, and parts of the root used, and the methods of preparation. Old, wild, well-formed roots are the most valued, while rootlets of cultivated plants are considered the lowest grade. For largely economic purposes, the majority of ginseng in the American marketplace is derived from the lowest grade root, diluted with excipients, blended with adulterants, or totally devoid of active constituents, i.e. ginsenosides.[3]

High quality preparations are available, however. These preparations are extracts of the main root of plants between 4 and 6 years of age and have been standardized for ginsenoside content and ratio to ensure optimum pharmacological effect.

CHEMICAL COMPOSITION

Ginseng contains at least 13 different triterpenoid saponins, collectively known as ginsenosides, which are believed to be the most important active constituents. The usual concentration of ginsenosides is between 2 and 3%. The ginsenosides have been designated R_0, R_{b1}, R_{b2}, R_{b3}, R_c, R_d, R_e, R_f, 20-gluco-R_f, R_{g1}, and R_{g2}. The ginsenosides originate from three fundamental aglycones:

- oleanolic acid (ginsenoside R_0)
- 20-S-protopanaxadiol (ginsenosides R_{b1} to R_d)
- 20-S-protopanaxatriol (ginsenosides R_e to R_{g2}).

As can be seen from Table 100.1, the ginsenosides differ primarily in their sugar groups.

Ginsenosides R_{b1}, R_{b2}, R_c, R_e, and R_{g1} are present in significant concentrations in Korean ginseng. In contrast, American ginseng (*Panax quinquefolius*) contains primarily ginsenosides R_{b1} and R_e, and does not contain ginsenosides R_{b2}, R_f, or, in some instances, R_{g1}. This allows for easy detection of species using HPLC (high-pressure liquid chromatography).[1,2,4]

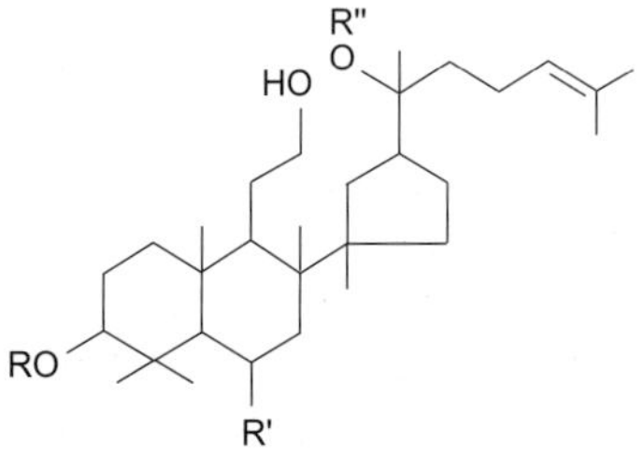

Ginsenoside	R	R′	R″
R_{a1}	Clc-^{2}Glc	H	Xyl-^{4}Ara(p)-^{6}Glc
R_{a2}	Clc-^{2}Glc	H	Xyl-^{4}Ara(f)-^{6}Glc
R_{b1}	Clc-^{2}Glc	H	Glc-^{6}Glc
R_{b2}	Clc-^{2}Glc	H	Ara(p)-^{6}Glc
R_{b3}	Clc-^{2}Glc	H	Xyl-^{6}Glc
R_c	Clc-^{2}Glc	H	Ara(f)-^{6}Glc
R_{d2}	Clc-^{2}Glc	H	Glc
R_e	H	Rha-^{2}Glc-O	Glc
R_f	H	Glc-^{2}Glc-O	H
R_{g1}	H	Glc-O	Glc
R_{g2}	H	Rha-^{2}Glc-O	H
20-Gluco-R_f	H	Glc-^{2}Glc-O	Glc
R_{h1}	H	Glc-O	H

Ara, arabinose; Glc, glucose; Rha, rhabinose; Xyl, xylose.

Figure 100.1 Ginsenosides of *Panax ginseng.*

Other components include:[1,2,4]

- panacene, a volatile oil
- free and glucoside-bound sterols (e.g. beta-sitosterol and its beta-glucoside)
- polyacetylene derivatives B-elemene and panaxinol
- 8–32% starch
- low molecular weight polysaccharides
- pectin
- vitamins (e.g. thiamin, riboflavin, B_{12}, nicotinic acid, pantothenic acid, and biotin)
- 0.1–0.2% choline
- minerals
- simple sugars (glucose, fructose, sucrose, maltose, trisaccharides, etc.)
- various flavonoids.

Although it had been reported that ginseng contains large amounts of germanium (i.e. 300 ppm), a follow-up study using highly sensitive (detection limit of 1 ppb), flameless atomic absorption spectrometry combined with solvent extraction demonstrated that the highest concentration of germanium measured in samples of ginseng purchased in the Osaka market was only 6 ppb.[5] More research is needed to accurately determine the germanium content of botanical medicines, as the reported concentrations vary widely. Such low levels suggest that a connection between the pharmacology of ginseng and its germanium content is unlikely.

HISTORY AND FOLK USE

Perhaps the most famous medicinal plant of China, ginseng has been generally used alone or in combination with other herbs to restore the "Yang" quality. It has also been used as a tonic for its revitalizing properties, especially after a long illness. Conditions for which ginseng is utilized in folk medicine are shown in Table 100.1 It has been used as an alterative, anodyne, aperitif, aphrodisiac, cardiotonic, carminative, emetic, estrogenic, expectorant, gonadotrophic, nervine, sedative, sialogogue, stimulant, stomachic, and tranquilizer.[1,6]

As can be seen from this list, ginseng has been used for most conditions, reflecting a broad range of nutritional and medicinal properties.

PHARMACOLOGY AND CLINICAL INDICATIONS

Since the 1950s, a great amount of research has been conducted worldwide to determine whether the therapeutic properties attributed to ginseng belong in the realm of legend or fact. Unfortunately, inconsistent results (due mostly to different procedures in the preparation of

Table 100.1 Conditions for which ginseng is utilized in folk medicine

• Amnesia	• Heart
• Anemia	• Hematoptysis
• Anorexia	• Hemorrhage
• Asthma	• Hyperglycemia
• Atherosclerosis	• Hypertension
• Boils	• Hypotension
• Bruises	• Impotence
• Cachexia	• Insomnia
• Cancer	• Intestinal complaints
• Convulsions	• Longevity promotion
• Cough	• Malaria
• Debility	• Menorrhagia
• Diabetes	• Nausea
• Diuretic	• Neurasthenia
• Divination	• Palpitations
• Dysentery	• Polyuria
• Dysmenorrhea	• Pregnancy
• Dyspepsia	• Puerperium
• Enterorrhagia	• Rectocele
• Epilepsy	• Rhinitis
• Epistaxis	• Rheumatism
• Fatigue	• Shortness of breath
• Fear	• Sores
• Fever	• Spermatorrhea
• Forgetfulness	• Splenitis
• Gastritis	• Swelling
• Hangover	• Vertigo
• Headache	

extracts, use of non-official parts of the plant, use of adulterants, and lack of quality control in the ginseng used) have made determination of ginseng's true properties difficult. Nonetheless, enough good research does exist to indicate that ginseng possesses pharmacological activity consistent with its near-legendary status, especially when high quality extracts, standardized for active constituents, are used.

Over the years, ginseng has been reported to have numerous pharmacological effects in humans and laboratory animals, including:[1,2,4,7]

- general stimulatory effects during stress
- decrease in sensitivity to stress
- increase in mental and physical capacity for work
- improved endocrine system function
- ameliorating radiation sickness, experimental neurosis, and cancer
- enhanced protein synthesis and cell reproduction
- improved glucose control in humans and alloxan-induced diabetes in rats
- modulation of various immune system parameters
- lowering of serum cholesterol
- protection of the liver from hepatotoxins.

Some of these actions are discussed in greater detail below.

Adaptogenic activity

Ginseng was originally investigated for its "adaptogen" qualities. An "adaptogen" was defined in 1957 by the Russian pharmacologist I. I. Brekhman as a substance that:[2]

- must be innocuous and cause minimal disorders in the physiological functions of an organism
- must have a non-specific action (i.e. it should increase resistance to adverse influences by a wide range of physical, chemical, and biochemical factors)
- usually has a normalizing action irrespective of the direction of the pathologic state.

According to tradition and scientific evidence, ginseng possesses this kind of equilibrating, tonic, anti-stress action, and so the term adaptogen is quite appropriate in describing its general effects.[2,7,8]

From a clinical perspective, ginseng can be used as a general tonic, especially in debilitated and feeble individuals. Use in this manner is consistent with its historic application.

Anti-fatigue (mental and physical) activity

Some of the first studies of ginseng's adaptogenic activities were performed during the late 1950s and early 1960s by Brekhman and Dardymov in the USSR, and by Petkov in Bulgaria.[7–11]

In one of Brekhman's experiments, Soviet soldiers given an extract of ginseng ran faster in a 3 km race than those given a placebo. In another, radio operators tested after administration of ginseng extract transmitted text significantly faster and with fewer mistakes than those given placebo. These and similar results found by European researchers, who demonstrated improvement in human physical and mental performance after the administration of ginseng extracts, prompted researchers to confirm the results in experimental models using mice.[2,7–9]

In perhaps the best known of these experiments, mice were subjected to swimming in cold water or running up an apparently endless rope to determine if ginseng could increase the time to exhaustion. The results indicated that ginseng possessed significant antifatigue activity, as a clear dose-dependent increase in time to exhaustion was noted in mice receiving ginseng.[2,8,12–15] In one study, the time to exhaustion was increased up to 183% in the mice given ginseng 30 minutes prior to exercising, compared with controls.[8]

Experimental animal studies indicated that much of the anti-fatigue action of ginseng was due to the stimulant effect of ginseng on the CNS. Stress coupled with ginseng ingestion induced alterations in energy metabolism during prolonged exercise.[10–15]

Ginseng has been shown to increase locomotor activity,[16] modify EEG tracings,[10] improve metabolic activity in the CNS,[17] and affect the hypothalamo-pituitary-adrenal axis (discussed below), all of which could be largely responsible for ginseng's anti-fatigue activity on mental and physical performance. The CNS activity of ginseng is essentially different from that of the usual stimulants. While stimulants are active under most situations, ginseng reveals its stimulatory action only under the challenge of stress.[17]

On the physical level, ginseng's anti-fatigue properties appear to be closely related to its ability to spare glycogen utilization in exercising muscle.[14] Exercise physiologists have clearly established that during prolonged exercise, the development of fatigue is closely related to the depletion of glycogen stores and the build-up of lactic acid, both in skeletal muscle and in the liver. If an adequate supply of oxygen is available to the working muscle, non-esterified fatty acids are the preferential energy substrate, thus sparing utilization of muscle glycogen, blood glucose, and, consequently, liver glycogen. The greater the ability to conserve body carbohydrate stores by mobilizing and oxidizing fatty acids, the greater the amount of time to exhaustion. Ginseng enhances fatty acid oxidation during prolonged exercise, thereby sparing muscle glycogen stores.[14]

Mental and physical anti-fatigue activity effects have been demonstrated in both animal studies and double-blind, clinical trials in humans. In addition to several Russian studies using soldiers and athletes as subjects, other studies have been published.[18,19]

In one double-blind, clinical study, nurses who had switched from day to night duty rated themselves for competence, mood, and general well-being, and were given an objective test of psychophysical performance, blood counts, and blood chemistry. The group administered ginseng demonstrated higher scores in competence, mood parameters, and objective psychophysical performance when compared with those receiving a placebo.[18]

In a double-blind, cross-over study on university students in Italy, ginseng extract was compared with placebo in various tests of psychomotor performance. A favourable effect of ginseng relative to baseline performance was observed in attention (cancellation test), mental arithmetic, logical deduction, integrated sensory-motor function (choice reaction time), and auditory reaction time. However, statistically significant superiority over the placebo group was noted only for mental arithmetic. It is interesting to note that in the course of the trial the students taking ginseng reported a greater sensation of well-being.[19]

From a clinical standpoint, ginseng's anti-fatigue properties may be useful whenever fatigue or lack of vigilance is apparent. Athletes, in particular, may derive some benefit from ginseng use.

Standardized extracts of *Panax ginseng* in combination with *Ginkgo biloba* (a formula called Gincosan) improved the retention of learned behavior in experiments on young (3 months) and old (26 months) rats. Results suggest *Panax* and *Gingko* extracts possess properties similar to those of nootropic drugs.[20]

Anti-stress activity

Ginseng has been shown to enhance the ability to cope with various stressors, both physical and mental. Presumably, as has been demonstrated in several animal studies, this is a result of delaying the alarm phase response in Selye's classic model of stress. These studies found that adrenal cholesterol levels are many times higher in animals given ginseng than in their matched controls, indicating increased tolerance to stress and delayed alarm phase response.[4,14,21,22]

Italian researchers have studied the effect of a standardized ginseng extract, whose ginsenosides composition was accurately determined, on the adrenal functions of rats exposed to cold.[4,21] The ginseng extract significantly counteracted body temperature decline without affecting blood glucose or cortisone levels. In a group of adrenalectomized rats, the ginseng extract had no significant effects. Administration of hydrocortisone to the adrenalectomized rats did, however, cause body temperature to be maintained when the rats were exposed to cold.

Histologically, it was noted that there was:

- evidence of hyperfunctioning in the supraoptic and paraventricular nuclei of the hypothalamus in rats fed the ginseng extract
- remarkable increase in corticotropic basophilic cells (ACTH-producing) in the pars distalis of the pituitary
- hyperplasia of the adrenal zona fasiculata, indicating that hyperfunctioning of the adrenal was promoted by the administration of the ginseng extract.

Other researchers have demonstrated that ginseng saponins significantly increase plasma ACTH and corticosteroids (in a parallel kinetic pattern).[23,24] Since this effect could be blocked by dexamethasone (which acts on the hypothalamus and pituitary to prevent ACTH release), it was concluded that ginsenosides act predominantly on the hypothalamus or pituitary to promote secretion of ACTH. This has been further confirmed by indirect studies. ACTH first stimulates an increase in cAMP in the adrenal and then promotes corticosteroid synthesis. Ginseng administration has been shown to increase adrenal cAMP in normal rats, but not in hypophysectomized rats.

These investigations make quite clear that ginseng's anti-stress action is mediated by the hypothalamo-pituitary-adrenal axis, as:

- the anti-stress action of ginseng is greatly reduced by adrenalectomy
- ginseng continues to exert its anti-stress action after hypophysectomy only if ACTH is administered
- histological and chemical evidence demonstrates a strong link between ginseng and the hypothalamo-pituitary-adrenal axis
- dexamethasone blocks the effects of ginseng.

This release of ACTH and associated pituitary substances (e.g. beta-lipoprotein, endorphins, enkephalins, etc.), coupled with their end-organ effects, is probably responsible for many of the anti-fatigue and anti-stress actions of ginseng, as ACTH and corticosteroids have been shown to bind directly to brain tissue to increase mental activities during stress. From a clinical perspective, it is apparent that ginseng has a balancing effect or alterative action on the hypothalamic-pituitary-adrenal axis by adjusting metabolic and functional systems governing hormonal control of homeostasis. This assists the body's response to the challenge of stress and therefore is indicated when disruption of this axis is apparent.

Ginseng may prove especially effective in restoration of normal adrenal function and prevention of adrenal atrophy associated with corticosteroid administration. In rats, ginseng has been found to inhibit cortisone-induced adrenal and thymic atrophy.[25] Ginseng could be combined with other botanicals with adrenal-enhancing activity (e.g. *Bupleuri falcatum*, *Glycyrrhiza glabra*, *Curcuma longa*, and *Eleutherococcus senticosus*) in the treatment of adrenal atrophy (a.k.a. exhaustion) (also see Chs 80 and 90).[26,27]

Diabetes

Ginseng, used either alone or in combination with other botanicals, has a long folk use in the treatment of diabetes. Ginseng has confirmed hypoglycemic activity. The constituents responsible for this effect include five types of substances:[28–32]

- five glycans (polysaccharides designated panaxans A to E)
- adenosine
- a carboxylic acid
- a peptide
- a fraction designated DPG-3-2.

The ginsenosides are devoid of hypoglycemic action. (This highlights the importance of using crude, standardized, extracts containing all active principles as opposed to using isolated ginsenosides or pure ginsenoside extracts.)

It is interesting to note that ginseng will increase serum cortisol levels in non-diabetic individuals, while in patients with diabetes, serum cortisol levels will be reduced.[33] As cortisol antagonizes insulin, this is presumably a beneficial effect. In addition, DPG-3-2 only exhibits hypoglycemic action or provokes insulin secretion in diabetic and glucose-loaded normal mice while having no effect on normal mice fed a standard diet.[28] This again demonstrates ginseng's non-specific balancing effect, baffling to researchers who are accustomed to investigating compounds with consistent pharmacological effects.

Ginseng is indicated as an adjunctive therapy in the treatment of diabetes, both for its hypoglycemic effect and for its ability to decrease the atherogenic index (see below).

Reproductive effects

Although it is claimed to be a "sexual rejuvenator", human studies supporting this belief are scanty. Ginseng has, however, been shown to:[34]

- promote the growth of the testes and increase spermatogenesis in rabbits
- accelerate the growth of the ovary and enhance ovulation in frogs
- stimulate egg-laying in hens
- facilitate lordotic response in female rats
- increase gonadal weight in both male and female rats
- increase testicular nucleic acid content in rats
- increase sexual activity and mating behavior in male rats.

These animal study results seem to support ginseng's use as a fertility and virility aid.

In other experimental animal studies, ginseng has been shown to increase testosterone levels while decreasing prostate weight.[35] This suggests that ginseng should have favorable effects in the treatment of benign prostatic hyperplasia; however, no clinical trials have yet been reported.

Ginsenosides have also been shown to bind to human myometrial receptor proteins, and they apparently exert estrogen-like action on the vaginal epithelium. These are significant enough to prevent the atrophic vaginal changes associated with postmenopause and other menopausal symptoms.[36]

Other clinical indications involving the reproductive system (based on historical use and experimental evidence) include decreased sperm counts, testicular atrophy or hypofunction, and other organic causes of male infertility, and ovarian atrophy or hypofunction, amenorrhea, and other organic causes of female infertility. It should be noted that several reports of mastalgia have been reported in women taking ginseng.[37,38]

Anti-cancer properties

Long-term oral administration of ginseng to newborn mice has been shown to reduce the incidence and also to inhibit the proliferation of tumors induced by various chemical carcinogens, including DMBA, urethane, and aflatoxin B1.[39]

Its anti-cancer effects in other experimental models can be summarized as follows:[39,40]

- it is observed only in slow-growing tumors, such as Ehrlich and sarcoma 180 ascites tumor
- it is not observed in rapidly growing tumors, such as L1210 and P388, and Walker carcinoma
- there is no dose–response relationship or cumulative effect.

The lack of a dose–response relationship suggests that ginseng's anti-cancer effects are indirect and subject to a threshold mechanism. Thus, ginseng once again appears to demonstrate non-specific effects.

Cell proliferating and anti-aging effects

Ginseng has a dual effect on cell growth: it stimulates cell division in an adequate nutritional environment, but it acts cytostatically under adverse conditions (as described above).[41] Furthermore, ginseng has yielded impressive results in lengthening the life span of cells in culture.[42]

This enhancement of cellular proliferation and function has been shown on a variety of cell types (epithelial, hepatic, lymphocyte, fibroblast, thymic, neural, etc.) and may be a result of potentiation of nerve growth factor (NGF) by ginsenosides.[3,43]

Clinically, these results indicate a potential use of ginseng in healing damage to virtually all tissue types. Again this demonstrates ginseng's non-specific action.

Immunostimulating effects

That ginseng possesses immunostimulating activity is evidenced by its ability to enhance:[44,45]

- antibody plaque forming cell response
- circulatory antibody titer against sheep erythrocytes
- cell-mediated immunity
- natural killer cell activity
- the production of interferon
- lymphocyte mitogenesis
- reticuloendothelial system proliferative and phagocytic functions.

Extracts of *Panax ginseng* were found to stimulate NK-function in normal individuals and patients with either chronic fatigue syndrome or acquired immunodeficiency syndrome.[46] Ginseng has been shown to prevent viral infections in experimental animals,[47] presumably a result of the combination of effects listed above.

Perhaps the most important immune system-enhancing effect of ginseng is its ability to produce a marked hyperplasia of the Kupffer cells of the liver and of the folliculi in the spleen and lymph nodes.[4,21] The hyperplastic folliculi show an increase in the number and volume of light centers, thus demonstrating morphological evidence of increased host defense capacity against a wide variety of external assaults.

It should be noted that large dosages of ginseng may be contraindicated in acute infections. This is due to its in vitro inhibition of lymphocyte transformation (similar to cortisone) at high (i.e. greater than 1 mg/ml), but not low, concentrations.[44,48,49] In fact, in vitro, ginseng at 1.6 mcg/ml has been shown to inhibit phytohaemagglutinin-induced transformation of peripheral blood lymphocytes to a greater degree than cortisone at 500 mcg/ml.[48] The greatest degree of inhibition, however, was observed when ginseng was used in combination with cortisone. These results suggest that ginseng at high doses may be effective against T-cell-mediated inflammatory diseases without producing glucocorticoid-like side-effects. It also suggests that a lower dose of cortisone could be used if ginseng is given simultaneously.

When using ginseng, it is important to remember that ginseng's in vitro effect on lymphocyte proliferation is biphasic, i.e. a strong inhibition at high concentrations and a moderate stimulation at low concentrations, and that while ginseng has demonstrated significant inhibition of lymphocyte proliferation in vitro, this has not been the observed effect in vivo, where lymphocyte proliferation has been enhanced.[44] These effects may be related to ginseng-induced elevation of interferon (which inhibits lymphocyte proliferation) which is dose-dependent.

From a clinical perspective, the chronic ingestion of ginseng by individuals with mild immunodeficiency may reduce the risk of viral infection. Use in this manner is consistent with the historical use of ginseng by debilitated individuals.

Cardiovascular effects

Ginseng has paradoxical effects on blood pressure. It appears that at low doses it possesses a hypertensive effect, but when administered at larger doses a hypotensive effect is noted.[50] Accordingly it has been reported useful in the treatment of essential hypertension in humans, but it has also been shown to have hypertensive effects as well.[51] This pressor effect must be kept in mind when administering ginseng to both normotensive and hypertensive individuals.

Ginseng administered to human subjects with hyperlipidemia has been shown to reduce total serum cholesterol, triglyceride, and non-esterified fatty acid levels, while raising serum HDL cholesterol levels. Platelet adhesiveness was also decreased.[52]

These results in humans confirmed earlier studies on rats fed high-cholesterol diets.[53,54] The mechanism of action appears to be through accelerated degradation, conversion, and excretion of cholesterol and triglyceride, despite increased lipogenesis and cholesterogenesis.

Ginseng has also been shown to be effective in inhibiting experimental disseminated intravascular coagulation in rats. It also inhibited platelet aggregation by various aggregating agents and the conversion of fibrinogen to fibrin. Its mechanism of action appears to be via promotion of urokinase's fibrinolytic activity.[55]

From a clinical perspective, it appears that ginseng may offer some protection against atherosclerotic disease, further supporting its use as a general tonic. It may also possess a blood pressure-regulating effect.

Hepatic effects

Obviously, any adaptogenic substance must impact the liver, due to the liver's central role in metabolic and detoxification reactions. Ginseng affects the liver in several ways. As was previously mentioned, ginseng promotes hyperplasia of Kupffer cells (hepatic macrophages).[4,21] As these cells are responsible for filtering out much of the toxins and debris from the portal circulation, increasing their number and activity could have profound effect.

Ginseng has also been shown to increase nuclear RNA biosynthesis, indicating increased protein synthesis.[3,56] In fact, ginseng has been shown to increase not only nuclear RNA synthesis, but also ribosomal and messenger RNA, the amount of rough endoplasmic reticulum, and the activity of RNA polymerase.[3,56–58] These results indicate that ginseng activates virtually every step in protein biosynthesis.

As protein synthesis is often reduced in the elderly, the significance of the above-described effects on enhancement of hepatic protein synthesis would be extremely high. However, these results have yet to be confirmed by clinical studies.

Ginseng has also been shown to reverse diet-induced fatty liver in animals and to possess significant antihepatotoxic action.[52,59]

The clinical indications of these hepatic actions of ginseng are quite broad and support its general tonic/adaptogen properties.

Radiation-protecting effects

Ginseng has been shown to offer some protection against harmful radiation, both in vivo and in vitro, and to hasten recovery from radiation sickness.[60,61] In wake of ever-increasing environmental radiation contamination, ginseng may be an appropriate prophylactic against radiation exposure.

TOXICOLOGY

The problem of quality control makes toxicology difficult to address. This is exemplified by a 1979 *JAMA* article entitled "Ginseng abuse syndrome".[62] In this article, a number of side-effects are reported, including:

- hypertension
- euphoria
- nervousness
- insomnia
- skin eruptions
- morning diarrhea.

Given the extreme variation in quality of ginseng in the American marketplace and the use of both non-official parts of the plant and adulterants, it is not surprising that side-effects were noted. None of the commercial preparations used in the trial had been subjected to controlled analysis. Furthermore, the species of ginseng used included *Panax ginseng*, *Panax quinquefolius*, *Eleutherococcus senticosus*, and *Rumex hymenosepalus* in a variety of different forms, i.e. roots, capsules, tablets, teas, extracts, cigarettes, chewing gum, and candies.

It is virtually impossible to derive any firm conclusions from the data presented in the *JAMA* article. The author's final words do, however, seem sensible and appropriate:

> An important caveat is that these GAS [ginseng abuse syndrome] effects are neither uniformly negative nor uniformly predictable. Nevertheless, long-term ingestion of large amounts of ginseng should be avoided, as even a panacea can cause problems if abused.

Studies have been performed on standardized extracts of ginseng which demonstrate the absence of side-effects and mutagenic or teratogenic effects.[4,13,63,64] These studies differ markedly from the trial reported in *JAMA* in that high quality extracts were used.

DOSAGE

The dosage is inversely proportional to the ginsenoside content, i.e. if an extract or ginseng preparation contains high concentrations of ginsenosides (and presumably other active components), a lower dose will suffice. The standard dose for ginseng is in the range of 4.5–6 g daily.

Currently, there is almost a total lack of quality control in ginseng products marketed in the United States. Independent research and published studies have clearly documented that there is a tremendous variation in the ginsenoside content of commercial preparations.[3,4] In fact, many products on the market contain only trace amounts of ginsenosides, and some formulations contain no ginseng at all. This has led to several problems, ranging from toxicity reactions[62] (discussed below) to lack of medicinal effect. The widespread disregard for quality control in the health food industry has done much to tarnish the reputation of ginseng as well as other important botanicals.

The authors recommend the use of standardized ginseng preparations to ensure sufficient ginsenoside content, consistent therapeutic results, and reduced risk of toxicity. Products should be standardized in their ginsenoside content. The typical dose (taken one to three times daily) for general tonic effects should contain a saponin content of at least 5 mg of ginsenosides with a ratio of R_{b1} to R_{g1} of 2:1. For example, for a high quality ginseng root powder containing 5% ginsenosides, the dose would be 100 mg.

As each individual's response to ginseng is unique, the patient should be monitored for signs of possible ginseng toxicity (see below). It is best to begin at lower doses and increase gradually. The Russian approach for long-term administration is to use ginseng cyclically for a period of 15–20 days followed by a 2 week interval without any ginseng.

REFERENCES

1. Leung AY. Encyclopedia of common natural ingredients used in food, drugs and cosmetics. New York, NY: John Wiley. 1980: p 186–189
2. Shibata S, Tanaka O, Shoji J, Saito H. Chemistry and pharmacology of Panax. Economic and Medicinal Plant Research 1985; 1: 217–284
3. Liberti LE, Marderosian AD. Evaluation of commercial ginseng products. J Pharm Sci 1978; 67: 1487–1489
4. Bombardelli E. Ginseng. Chemical, pharmacological, and clinical profile. Monograph from Indena S.p.A., Milan, Italy
5. Minmo Y, Ota N, Sakao S, Shimomura S. Determination of germanium in medicinal plants by atomic absorption spectrometry with electrothermal atomization. Chem Pharm Bull 1980; 28: 2687–2691
6. Duke JA. Handbook of medicinal herbs. Boca Raton, FL: CRC Press. 1985: p 337–338
7. Brekhman II, Dardymov IV. New substances of plant origin which increase nonspecific resistance. Ann Rev Pharmacol 1969; 9: 419–430
8. Brekhman II, Dardymov IV. Pharmacological investigation of glycosides from ginseng and Eleutherococcus. Lloydia 1969; 32: 46–51
9. Petkov W. Pharmacological studies of the drug P. ginseng C.A. Meyer. Arzniem Forsch 1959; 9: 305–311
10. Petkov W. The mechanism of action of P. ginseng. Arzniem Forsch 1961; 11: 288–95, 418–422
11. Petkov W. Effect of ginseng on the brain biogenic monoamines and 3′,5′-AMP system. Experiments in rats. Arzniem Forsch 1978; 28: 388–393
12. Saito H, Yoshida Y, Takagi K. Effect of *Panax ginseng* root on exhaustive exercise in mice. Jap J Pharmacol 1974; 24: 119–127
13. Kaku T, Miyata T, Uruno T et al. Chemicopharmacological studies on saponins of *Panax ginseng* C.A. Meyer. Arzniem Forsch 1975; 25: 539–547
14. Avakia EV, Evonuk E. Effects of *Panax ginseng* extract on tissue glycogen and adrenal cholesterol depletion during prolonged exercise. Planta Medica 1979; 36: 43–48
15. Sterner W, Kirchdorfer AM. Comparative work load tests on mice with standardized ginseng extract and a ginseng containing pharmaceutical preparation. Z Gerontol 1970; 3: 307–312
16. Hong SA, Park CW, Kim JH et al. The effects of ginseng saponin on animal behavior. Proceedings of the 1st International Ginseng Symposium. Seoul: Korean Ginseng Research Institute. 1975: p 33–44
17. Samira MMH, Attia MA, Allam M, Elwan O. Effect of the standardized ginseng extract G115 on the metabolism and electrical activity of the rabbit's brain. J Int Med Res 1985; 13: 342–348
18. Hallstrom C, Fulder S, Carruthers M. Effect of ginseng on the performance of nurses on night duty. Comp Med East & West 1982; 6: 277–282
19. D'Angelo L, Grimaldi R, Caravaggi M et al. A double-blind, placebo controlled clinical study on the effect of a standardized ginseng extract on psychomotor performance in healthy volunteers. J Ethnopharmacol 1986; 16: 15–22
20. Petkov VD, Kehayov R, Belcheva S, Konstantinova E, Petkov VV, Getova D, Markovska V. Memory effects of standardized extracts of *Panax ginseng* (G115), *Ginkgo biloba* (GK 501) and their combination Gincosan (PHL-00701). Planta Medica 1993; 59: 106–114
21. Bombardelli E, Cirstoni A, Lietti A. The effect of acute and chronic (Panax) ginseng saponins treatment on adrenal function; biochemical and pharmacological. Proceedings 3rd International Ginseng Symposium. Seoul: Korean Ginseng Research Institute. 1980: p 9–16
22. Fulder SJ. Ginseng and the hypothalamic-pituitary control of stress. Am J Chin Med 1981; 9: 112–118
23. Hiai S, Yokoyama H, Oura H. Features of ginseng saponin-induced corticosterone secretion. Endocrinol Japan 1979; 26: 737–740
24. Hiai S, Yokoyama H, Oura H, Kawashima Y. Evaluation of corticosterone secretion-inducing effects of ginsenosides and their prosapogenins and sapogenins. Chem Pharm Bull 1983; 31: 168–174
25. Tanizawa H, Numano H, Odani T et al. Study of the saponin of *P. ginseng* C.A. Meyer. I. Inhibitory effect on adrenal atrophy, thymus atrophy and the decrease of serum potassium ion concentration induced by cortisone acetate in unilaterally adrenalectomized rats. J Pharm Soc Jap 1981; 101: 169–173
26. Hiai S, Yokoyama H, Nagasawa T, Oura H. Stimulation of the pituitary-adrenocortical axis by saikosaponin of Bupleuri Radix. Chem Pharm Bull 1981; 29: 495–499
27. Farnsworth NR, Kinghorn AD, Soejarto DD, Waller DP. Siberian ginseng (*Eleutherococcus senticosus*). Current status as an adaptogen. Economic and Medicinal Plant Research 1985; 1: 156–215
28. Ng TB, Yeung HW. Hypoglycemic constituents of *Panax ginseng*. Gen Pharmacol 1985; 6: 549–552
29. Waki I, Kyo H, Yasuda M, Kimura M. Effects of a hypoglycemic component of ginseng radix on insulin biosynthesis in normal and diabetic animals. J Pharm Dyn 1982; 5: 547–554
30. Konno C, Sugiyama K, Kano M et al. Isolation and hypoglycaemic activity of panaxans A, B, C, D and E, glycans of *Panax ginseng* roots. Planta Medica 1984; 51: 434–436
31. Kimura M, Waki I, Tanaka O et al. Pharmacological sequential trials for the fractionation of components with hypoglycemic activity in alloxan diabetic mice from ginseng radix. J Pharm Dyn 1981; 4: 402–409
32. Kimura M, Waki I, Tanaka O et al. Effects of hypoglycemic components in ginseng radix on blood insulin level in alloxan diabetic mice and on insulin release from perfused rat pancreas. J Pharm Dyn 1981; 4: 410–417
33. Yamamoto M, Uemura T. Endocrinological and metabolic actions of *P. ginseng* principles. Proceeding 3rd International Ginseng Symposium. Seoul: Korean Ginseng Research Institute. 1980: p 115–119
34. Kim C, Choi H, Kim CC et al. Influence of ginseng on mating behavior of male rats. Am J Chinese Med 1976; 4: 163–168
35. Fahim WS, Harman JM, Clevenger TE et al. Effect of *Panax ginseng* on testosterone level and prostate in male rats. Arch Androl 1982; 8: 261–263
36. Punnonen R, Lukola A. Oestrogen-like effect of ginseng. Br Med J 1980; 281: 1110
37. Yonezawa M. Restoration of radiation injury by intraperitoneal injection of ginseng extract in mice. J Radiation Res 1976; 17: 111–113
38. Palmer BV, Montgomery ACV, Monteiro JCMP. Ginseng and mastalgia (letter). Br Med J 1978; i: 1284
39. Yun TK, Yun YS, Han IW. Anticarcinogenic effect of long-term oral administration of newborn mice exposed to various chemical carcinogens. Cancer Detect Prevent 1983; 6: 515–525
40. Lee KD, Huemer RP. Antitumoral activity of *Panax ginseng* extracts. Jap J Pharmacol 1971; 21: 299–302
41. Fulder SJ. The growth of cultured human fibroblasts treated with hydrocortisone and extracts of the medicinal plant *Panax ginseng*. Exp Gerontol 1977; 12: 125–131
42. Saito H. Ginsenoside-Rb1 and nerve growth factor (*P. ginseng*). Proceedings of the 3rd International Ginseng Symposium. Seoul: Korean Ginseng Research Institute. 1981: p 181–185
43. Yamamoto M, Masaka K, Yamada Y et al. Stimulatory effect of ginsenosides on DNA, protein and lipid synthesis in bone marrow. Arzneim Forsch 1978; 28: 2238–2241
44. Jie YH, Cammisuli S, Baggiolini M. Immunomodulatory effects of *Panax ginseng* C.A. Meyer in the mouse. Agents and actions 1984; 15: 386–391
45. Gupta S, Agarwal LB, Epstein G et al. Panax. A new mitogen and interferon producer. Clin Res 1980; 28: 504A
46. See DM, Broumand N, Sahl L, Tilles JG. In vitro effects of echinacea and ginseng on natural killer and antibody-dependent cell cytotoxicity in healthy subjects and chronic fatigue syndrome or acquired immunodeficiency syndrome patients. Immunopharmacology 1997; 35: 229–235

47. Singh VK, Agarwal SS, Gupta BM. Immunomodulatory activity of *Panax ginseng* extract. Planta Medica 1984; 51: 462–465
48. Chong SKF, Brown HA, Rimmer E et al. In vitro effect of *Panax ginseng* on phytohaemagglutinin-induced lymphocyte transformation. Int Arch Allergy Appl Immun 1984; 73: 216–220
49. Yeung HW, Cheung K, Leung KN. Immunopharmacology of Chinese medicine. I. Ginseng induced immunosuppression in virus infected mice. Am J Chin Med 1982; 10: 44–54
50. Oh JS, Lim JK, Park CW, Han MH. The effect of ginseng on experimental hypertension. Korean J Pharmacol 1968; 4: 27–31
51. Siegel RK. Ginseng and high blood pressure (letter). JAMA 1980; 243: 32
52. Yamamoto M, Uemura T, Nakama S et al. Serum HDL-cholesterol-increasing and fatty liver-improving action of *Panax ginseng* in high cholesterol diet-fed rats with clinical effect on hyperlipidemia in man. Am J Chin Med 1983; 11: 96–101
53. Yamamoto M, Kumagai. Plasma lipid lowering actions of ginseng saponins and mechanisms of the action. Am J Chin Med 1983; 11: 84–87
54. Joo CN. The preventative effect of Korean (*P. ginseng*) saponins on aortic atheroma formation in prolonged cholesterol-fed rabbits. Proceeding 3rd International Ginseng Symposium. Seoul: Korean Ginseng Research Institute. 1980: p 27–36
55. Matsuda H, Namba K, Fukuda S et al. Pharmacological study on *Panax ginseng* C.A. Meyer. III. Effects of red ginseng on experimental disseminated intravascular coagulation. (2). Effects of ginsenosides on blood coagulative and fibrinolytic systems. Chem Pharm Bull 1986; 34: 1153–1157
56. Oura H, Hiai S, Seno H. Synthesis and characterization of nuclear RNA induced by Radix ginseng extract in rat liver. Chem Pharm Bull 1971; 19: 1598–1605
57. Oura H, Hiai S, Nabatini S, Nakagawa H et al. Effect on ginseng on endoplasmic reticulum and ribosome. Planta Medica 1975; 28: 76–88
58. Oura H, Nakashima S, Tsukada K, Ohta Y. Effect of radix ginseng on serum protein synthesis. Chem Pharm Bull 1972; 20: 980–986
59. Hikino H, Kiso Y, Sanada S, Shoji J. Antihepatotoxic actions of ginsenosides from *Panax ginseng* roots. Planta Medica 1985; 52: 62–64
60. Kim TH, Lee YS, Cho CK et al. Protective effect of ginseng on radiation-induced DNA double strand breaks and repair in murine lympyhocytes. Radiopharm 1996; 11: 267–272
61. Ben-Hur E, Fulder S. Effect of *P. ginseng* saponins and *Eleutherococcus s.* on survival of cultured mammalian cells after ionizing radiation. Am J Chin Med 1981; 9: 48–56
62. Siegel RK. Ginseng abuse syndrome. JAMA 1979; 241: 1614–1615
63. Hess FG, Parent RA, Cox GE et al. Effects of subchronic feeding of ginsenoside extract G115 in beagle dogs. Food Chem Toxicol 1983; 21: 95–97
64. Hess FG, Parent RA, Cox GE et al. Reproduction study in rats of ginseng extract G115. Food Chem Toxicol 1982; 20: 189

CHAPTER CONTENTS

101

Pancreatic enzymes

Anthony J. Cichoke, MA DC

HISTORY

Pancreatic enzymes have a long history of clinical use. In the early 20th century, John Beard (a Scottish embryologist) successfully treated cancer using a pancreatic extract, which he described in his book, *The Enzyme Treatment of Cancer and its Scientific Basis*.

In 1934, Ernst Freund (a Viennese physician) found a substance which dissolved cancer cells in the blood of people free from cancer. Cancer patients did not have this material, which Freund called "normal substance".

It was Professor Doctor Max Wolf (considered by many to be the father of modern enzyme therapy) who identified "normal substance" as an enzyme which decomposes fatty materials and proteins. Wolf worked with Freund in Vienna in the early 1930s. This association and the work of John Beard sparked his interest in the possibilities of treating malignant diseases with enzymes. Dr Wolf founded the Biological Institute of New York City and, after studying various enzymes and enzyme combinations, developed what he considered an optimal preparation for the treatment of various acute and chronic conditions. His preparation was a combination of a fractionated hydrolysate of beef pancreas, calf thymus, *Pisum sativum* (common pea), *Lens esculenta* (edible lentil), mannitol, and papaya.

In the 1960s, Irving Innerfield conducted landmark research in the area of pancreatic enzymes, primarily relating to the clinical use of trypsin, chymotrypsin, and pancreatin, as well as streptokinase.

In 1971, Professor Heinrich Wrba, head of the Austrian Cancer Research Institute at the University of Vienna stated:

> Our present knowledge allows us to include this [enzyme] therapy into the small list of highly-effective causal anticancer compounds. It [enzyme therapy] will certainly play an important role in cancer treatment over the next few years.

However, it was Karl Ransberger who continued Wolf's research and refined it, bringing it to doctors, hospitals and patients throughout the world. Ransberger encouraged and funded research projects in numerous hospitals and universities in Europe, the Americas, and elsewhere. His research, and that of others, has validated enzyme therapy's effectiveness in treating numerous conditions, including arthritis, cancer, multiple sclerosis, cardiovascular disease, HIV / AIDS, and other diseases.

PANCREATIC ENZYMES

Pancreatic enzymes aid in a surprising variety of bodily functions, including:

- digestion
- detoxification
- bolstering the immune system
- slowing the aging process
- improving blood clot lysing
- enhancing tissue repair
- facilitating the inflammatory response
- fighting viruses.

Genetic weakness, illness, injury, exercise, aging and toxins (both endogenous and exogenous) may result in inadequate production or excessive need for pancreatic enzymes. In these and other situations, additional enzymes from an external source may be necessary.

Many variables influence the proper choice of pancreatic enzymes, including:

- therapeutic goals
- patient's health status
- product
  —type of enzyme(s)
  —activity levels
  —quality control (including pH and temperature ranges)
  —variables which affect therapeutic application (e.g. enteric coating).

Pancreatic enzymes play an integral role in the digestion of proteins, fats, and carbohydrates. Pancreatic juice contains numerous enzymes, including amylase, lipase, ribonuclease, and deoxyribonuclease;[1] and the proenzymes trypsinogen, chymotrypsinogen, and procarboxypeptidase, which are converted in the small intestine to their active forms, trypsin, chymotrypsin, and carboxypeptidase, respectively.

Protein leaves the stomach primarily in the form of proteases, peptones and large polypeptides.[2] Upon reaching the small intestine, these are further digested by the proteolytic enzymes, trypsin, chymotrypsin, and carboxypolypeptidase. Protein digestion mainly occurs in the duodenum and jejunum. Carbohydrates are digested by α-amylase in the pancreatic juice, which breaks down starches (converting them into maltose and other small glucose polymers), while pancreatic lipase digests fats.[2]

Pancreatic enzyme supplements

The pancreatic enzyme supplements most commonly used include chymotrypsin, trypsin, and pancreatin (which contains *proteolytic*, *amylolytic* and *lipolytic* properties), as well as pancrelipase (similar to pancreatin, but with a higher proportion of lipase). Primarily obtained from hog or ox pancreas, some of these enzymes (such as lipase) can also be obtained from microbial sources (e.g. *Aspergillus niger* and *Aspergillus oryzae*).

According to the *US Pharmacopoeia*, chymotrypsin and trypsin are crystallized from ox pancreas gland extract, and pancreatin from both hog and ox sources, while pancrelipase is derived from hog pancreas.[3] Porcine pancreas is especially rich in amylase and lipase and is similar to human pancreas.[1] Bovine pancreas contains considerable amounts of proteolytic enzymes but substantially lower amounts of lipase and amylase.[1]

Other countries (such as Germany, Japan, England, and India) utilize their own pharmacopoeia, and foreign companies may use other sources to formulate their enzyme products.

Age, sex and species of pork or ox can affect enzyme concentration and activity levels. For example, sow glands (from pork) are high in lipase, while butcher hogs (young male hogs, up to 90 kg and 6 months) are high in protease. Beef cows and bulls have different enzyme levels than steers or heifers. Beef, though providing all three basic enzyme types, does not exhibit the activity levels of pork (which has an activity level ⅓ to ½ higher). Further, hog physiology is more similar to humans than to that of any other animal.

Enzyme extraction processes

Because enzymes are particularly sensitive to environmental changes, it is especially important during extraction to control pH (usually with buffers), temperature (using pre-cooled solutions and apparatus), substrate, and proteolysis (controlled through the use of inhibitors) in order to render a product that is enzymatically active.[4] Several steps are typically involved in the production of pancreatic enzyme supplements:

- cell membrane rupture
- fractionation
- crystallization
- enzyme isolation.

Rupturing the cell membrane

Although a wide variety of methods are employed in enzyme extraction, most entail rupturing the cell membrane of the animal tissue. This can be achieved through mincing, homogenizing, shaking with fine glass beads (at high speed), grinding with sand, freezing (and subsequent thawing), oscillations (ultrasonic or sonic), autolysis (either alone or with toluene, ethyl acetate or sodium sulfide), treatment with solvents (e.g. acetone), or lysis with added enzymes.[5]

Extracting enzymes from animal tissues is easier than extracting from microorganisms, according to Dixon & Webb[5]. They state that, in many cases, simple extraction with water may be sufficient.

All extraction processes, however, must control pH and temperature to protect the enzymes from deactivation.

Fractionation

Once the enzyme is brought into a solution, it must be separated from the other substances in the solution. Gel filtration or dialysis can be used to remove the small molecules, leaving large molecules (primarily proteins, with some polysaccharides).[5] Various fractionation methods can be employed for purifying the enzymes, including changing the pH, heating, using organic solvents and/or salts, adsorption, column chromatography, and electrophoresis.[5] Inhibitor affinity chromatography and substrate affinity chromatography are also used.[6]

Crystallization

After an enzyme has been purified, it may be possible to crystallize it. Dixon & Webb[5] view this as a final stage method of fractionation. Crystallization can be achieved with ammonium sulfate solutions (the typical method), or at a constant salt concentration by gradually changing the temperature or the pH.[5]

Enzyme isolation

Chymotrypsin

One method (used in Germany) for extracting chymotrypsin (in the form of its inactive precursor chymotrypsinogen) is by fractionated extraction, ultrafiltration and subsequent chromatographic purification of pancreatic juice. The chymotrypsinogen is converted to the active chymotrypsin by treatment with trypsin in an acid environment.

Trypsin

Trypsinogen can be isolated from the animal pancreas by fractionated precipitation and then activation to trypsin in a slightly alkaline environment.

Pancreatin

Pancreatin can be obtained by an extraction procedure where, after elimination of the insoluble tissue, organic solvents dissolve and precipitate the enzymes.[1] However, because part of the lipase and other enzymes are inactivated during the manufacturing process, pancreatin, isolated in this way, is not very active.[1]

According to Ruyssen & Lauwers,[1] more effective pancreatin can be produced through lyophilization, i.e. by drying under reduced pressure or with acetone. At this low temperature, the enzymes are more stable and less likely to be denatured.[1]

After proper defatting, the pancreatin is stable, provided it contains not more than a small percentage of moisture.[1] However, it may contain undesirable microorganisms (such as *Salmonella*) and must, therefore, be decontaminated.[1] Under carefully controlled conditions, pancreatin can be decontaminated by a terminal heat treatment.[1]

According to the *US Pharmacopeia*,[3] each milligram of pancreatin should contain:

- not less than 25 USP units of amylase activity
- not less than 2.0 USP units of lipase activity
- not less than 25 USP units of protease activity.

The *US Pharmacopoeia* states that: "One USP unit [or 1×] of amylase activity is contained in the amount of pancreatin that decomposes starch at an initial rate such that one microequivalent of glucosidic linkage is hydrolyzed per minute" under the conditions listed in the USP to assay for amylase activity. "One USP unit [or 1×] of lipase activity is contained in the amount of pancreatin that liberates 1.0 μEq of acid per minute at a pH of 9.0 and 37°" under the conditions detailed in the USP to assay for lipase activity. "One USP unit [or 1×] of protease activity is contained in the amount of pancreatin that digests 1.0 mg of casein" under the conditions enumerated in the USP to assay for protease activity.[3] Therefore, a product labeled "4×" would be four times stronger than a product labeled "1×".

Pancrelipase

Pancrelipase is similar to pancreatin and according to the USP should contain:

- not less than 100 USP units of amylase activity
- not less than 24 USP units of lipase activity
- not less than 100 USP units of protease activity.

Pharmacology

Chymotrypsin and trypsin are proteolytic enzymes which break down proteins into peptides. Chymotrypsin liberates the amino acids, L-tyrosine, L-tryptophan, and L-phenylalanine, as well as other molecules including several synthetic esters and amides.[1] Trypsin hydrolyzes primarily lysyl and arginyl residues.[1]

Pancreatin contains amylase, lipase, and protease.

Amylase breaks down starch; lipase breaks down fats; and protease breaks down proteins.

Absorption

In the past, the efficacy of enzyme therapy has been discounted, since the intestinal epithelial mucosa had been thought to be impermeable to large protein molecules.[7–9] Research over the past two decades has shown that the intestinal epithelium can be crossed by macromolecules, including intact proteins such as proteolytic enzymes.[10]

These macromolecules normally penetrate the mucosal surface via the transcellular route as, in the healthy mucosa, the tight junctions (zonula occludens) between the enterocytes prohibit paracellular passage.[11–14] Binding to the luminal membrane of the interocyte is followed by phagocytosis.[15] Some of the vacuole membrane vesicles formed fuse with lysosomes, and within the resulting phagolysome, the peptides and proteins may be hydrolyzed by lysosomal enzymes.[13] Other macromolecules avoid intracellular digestion and are passed from the enterocytes through the basolateral membrane into the interstitial space.[16] In the interstitial space, the macromolecules become available to macrophages and lymphoid cells.[17] Those molecules not taken up by macrophages or lymphatic cells eventually pass from the interstitial space into the blood or lymph.[18]

The transport of macromolecular material from the lumen to the interstitium has been extensively studied in the epithelium covering the lymphatic structures, such as Peyer's patches or isolated follicles.[15] In these regions, specialized enterocytes, the follicle-associated epithelium cells (FAE cells)[12] or M-cells[19] (called M-cells because of their occurrence in the microfolds of the luminal surface), transport macromolecular material in both directions.[12] The gut-associated immune system is thus supplied with antigenic macromolecules from the intestinal lumen.[20–22] The immunoglobulins produced by the plasma cells in the lumina propria (mainly IgA) are transported transcellularly to the luminal surface.

The exact degree of the intestinal absorption of intact molecules or large breakdown products of dietary proteins is not yet totally clear.[23,24] Although it is generally assumed that, apart from a very small proportion, all protein is hydrolyzed into amino acids or small molecular weight peptides before absorption by the mucosa, some research supports the hypothesis that a considerable proportion of dietary protein is taken up in the form of macromolecules and is only then hydrolyzed intercellularly in the peripheral tissue into amino acids ("distributed digestion").[25–27]

Regardless of the nutritional significance, the transepithelial transfer of particulate matter is at least antigenically sufficient to elicit a response of the gut-associated immune system.[12] The production and secretion of the immunoglobulins promote binding and proteolysis of the antigen material on the mucosal brush-border, thereby reducing its absorption (immunological barrier).[28]

Absorption of enzymes

The intestinal transport of macromolecules is especially important for understanding the functions of enzymes.[29] Hydrolases such as trypsin or elastase can be transported functionally intact into the blood from the lumen of the gut. These circulating proteinases are bound to antiproteinases like alpha-2 macroglobulin or alpha-1 antiproteinase[20] and can be resorbed from the main stream by pancreatic cells (interopancreatic circulation as an enzyme conservation process).[29] Thus, the intestinal absorption of intact enzymes appears to be important for the balance between hydrolases and anti-proteinases in the intracellular space[30] and is an important factor for the establishment and maintenance of the internal stability in the body.

It should be kept in mind that, although there are a number of absorption mechanisms, the primary mechanism for enzymes and other macromolecular enteral absorption is pinocytotic transfer by the M-cells of the small intestinal epithelium. After connection to a receptor in the mucosa of the intestinal wall, the enzymes are then absorbed into the wall by pinocytosis, guided through the intestinal cells in vesicles, and finally released into the blood by exocytosis.[31]

To clarify rate of absorption, Steffen, et al,[32] investigated the absorption of an enzyme mixture "A" (EMA: pancreatin, 100 mg; papain, 60 mg; lipase, 10 mg; amylase, 10 mg; trypsin, 24 mg; chymotrypsin, 1 mg; bromelain, 45 mg; the bioflavonoid, rutin, 50 mg) in rabbits. Using electrophoresis, they found that entire enzyme molecules were absorbed. Although enzyme particles were also present, the ratio to the entire amount administered was not measured. EMA was found in both lungs and liver after 1–2 hours. After 1–4 hours, approximately twice as much EMA was found in the liver as in the lungs. The absorption maximum in all animals occurred approximately 1 hour after administration. After 24 hours, EMA was no longer found in either the lungs or liver.

The absorption rate of individual and combined enzymes can be seen in Table 101.1. The absorption rate of orally ingested EMA is about 20% within 6 hours.[21] (For additional discussion of the intestinal absorption of intact macromolecules, see Chs 21 and 66.)

Factors affecting enzyme activity

Factors affecting enzyme activity include:

- pH
- temperature

Table 101.1 Absorption rate of individual and combined enzymes (within 6 hours)[33,34]

Enzyme	Absorption rate
Amylase	45%
Chymotrypsin	14–16%
Pancreatin	18–19%
Papain	6%
Trypsin	26–28%
Enzyme combination (bromelain, chymotrypsin, pancreatin, papain, and trypsin, with the bioflavonoid rutin)	22%

- substrate and substrate concentration
- cofactors
- metal ions
- inhibitors and coating.

Optimal pH range

Each enzyme has an optimal pH range, depending upon such variables as temperature and substrate concentration, at which the enzymatic catalytic reaction occurs most rapidly.

Chymotrypsin is stable at a pH of 3 or 4, suffers reversible denaturation at a pH below 3.0, and becomes inactive at a pH of above 10.0.[1] Trypsin, stable at a pH of 3.0 (and at low temperature), is irreversibly denatured at a pH of 8.0 or higher.[1]

The effects of temperature

In general, an increase of 10°F (5.5°C) in the enzymatic environment will approximately double the rate of the chemical reaction.[35] However, since enzymes are proteins, excessively high temperatures denature enzymes, thus destroying their activity. Optimal temperature for an enzyme is the temperature at which the catalyzed enzymatic reaction progresses most rapidly without damage to the enzyme.

The enzymes in the human body develop high levels of activity at about body temperature, increasing to maximum at about the temperature of a severe fever, i.e. 104°F (40°C).

Substrate concentration

The rate of any reaction is accelerated by increasing the substrate concentration until the enzyme is saturated by substrate. At this level, the rate of reaction becomes independent of substrate concentration and is no longer accelerated by the addition of more substrate.

Cofactors

Although all enzymes consist of protein, some are complex proteins, i.e. they have a protein component and a "cofactor". If the cofactor is removed, the protein (no longer active enzymatically) is called the *apoenzyme*. A cofactor might be a metal (e.g. iron, magnesium, copper, or zinc), a prosthetic group (a moderately-sized organic molecule), or a coenzyme (small organic compounds). Prosthetic groups and metals can aid in the catalytic function of the enzyme, while coenzymes take part in the enzymatic reaction. Many vitamins, trace elements, and minerals essential to human bodily function are part of enzymatic cofactors.

Coenzymes are essential for the activity of many enzymes and serve as a type of substrate in certain reactions. In these reactions, the coenzyme is converted to a form no longer active in catalyzing the reaction. The reaction requires a mix which contains one molecule of cofactor for every molecule of substrate to be converted.

Metal ions

Specific metal ions are required for the activity of many enzymes. Certain metal ions increase activity while others decrease or inhibit activity. Calcium, cobalt, copper, iron, magnesium, manganese, molybdenum, potassium and zinc are the most frequent enzyme activators in humans.

Certain heavy metal ions inhibit enzyme reactions. These heavy metals include barium, lead and mercury, and they combine with the sulfhydryl reactive group (-SH) which is part of the active site of many enzymes.

Inhibitors

Ions, atoms, or molecules which terminate or retard enzyme activity are called inhibitors. These inhibitors are classified as non-competitive or competitive. Non-competitive inhibitors combine with the enzyme at a location other than the active site. The non-competitive inhibitor retards the conversion of the substrate by the enzyme, although it does not affect the bonding of the substrate of the enzyme.

An inhibitor is classified as *competitive* when it combines with the active site of the enzyme, preventing the substrate from having access to the active site.

Supplement coating

The normal human stomach has a pH of approximately 1.5–3.0.[36] This low pH inhibits bacterial growth and activates certain enzymes. This acidic nature, however, can destroy pH-sensitive supplemental enzymes. For this reason, many enzyme products are enterically coated. This coating allows the product to reach the small intestine before disintegrating.[1] Other products are encapsulated in "microspheres", which delays their disintegration.

In one study, cellulose acetate phthalate (CAP) and

maize starch were used as the coating materials for encapsulating pancreatic protease.[37] Results indicate that the coating materials were stable for at least 3 hours (time to pass through each part of the GI tract) in simulated gastric conditions (pH 3.97), but disintegrated rapidly under simulated intestinal conditions (pH of 6.82 and temperature of 39.5°C).

Measuring enzyme activity

When considering enzymes and enzyme applications, it is extremely important to understand the variables affecting their performance. When selecting an enzyme for therapeutic purposes, more than whether a given product contains amylase, protease, lipase, or other enzymes must be considered. The activity levels of the enzymes are of critical importance.

Unfortunately, the labels on most enzyme products sold in this country do not indicate the activity levels of the enzymes contained therein. In addition, when the activity is stated, the consumer has no way of knowing which enzyme assay the manufacturer used unless the label also indicates that the product conforms to the guidelines of the *USP*. This is particularly confusing because activity levels are greatly affected by the conditions under which the assay was performed (including temperature, pH and substrate).

Adding to the confusion, enzyme manufacturers utilize diverse assay methodologies. Therefore, directly comparing the enzymatic activity of competing products is difficult, if not impossible. The utilization of a single assay system (such as detailed in the USP) is probably necessary to directly compare competitive products. Several standardized assay systems are available for enzyme suppliers and are found in the *US Pharmacopoeia* (for a definitive assay), the *NFIA Laboratory Methods Compendium*, and the *Food Chemical Codex*.

Incomplete labeling and the inconsistent use of standardized assay methodologies make evaluation of competitive products extremely challenging. Price could be the first indication of inequities in assay procedures. For example, if company A is selling a product at 1,000 units/g for $30.00 a bottle, and company B is selling a product at 5,000 units/g for $10.00 a bottle, the units are most likely not the same.

For clinical reliability, utilize only appropriately labeled products or obtain the assay procedures from each of the manufacturers. If possible, compare competitor products by assays performed in an independent laboratory.

CLINICAL APPLICATIONS

Historically, enzyme therapy has been used in a wide variety of applications, ranging from the classic substitution of enzymes for intestinal deficiency to the centuries-old external application of enzymes to treat wound-healing disturbances (e.g. leg ulcers). Enzymes have been used individually or in complex enzyme mixtures. Clinical uses of individual enzymes can be seen in Tables 101.2–101.6.

Table 101.2 Clinical applications of chymotrypsin

- In debridement, treatment of abscesses and ulcerations, liquefaction of mucous secretions[38]
- In ophthalmic cataract surgeries and therapy of eyeball hematomas and ophthalmorrhagias[38,39]
- Before and after tooth extraction as well as in operative dentistry[40,41]
- After episiotomy surgeries[42]
- As an anthelmintic against enterozoic worms[43]
- In early recognition of tumor cells[44]
- In histologic gastroenteric diagnostics[45]
- In inflammatory conditions (local and systemic) to promote the dispersion of blood extravasates and effusions from fractures[39,46–53]
- Surgical trauma[42,51]
- Sporting injuries[46–50]
- Accidental soft tissue trauma[46–50,53]
- Intervertebral disc lesions[54]
- In uveitis vitreous hemorrhage, diabetic retinopathy and asthmatic symptoms[55]

Table 101.3 Clinical applications of trypsin

- In debridement of necrotizing wounds, ulcerations, abscesses, empyemas, hematomas, fistulas, and decubitus[56–59]
- To accelerate healing in injuries, inflammations, phlogistic edemas and traumatic changes[46–53]
- As an auxiliary agent in meningitis therapy[60]
- As an ointment or dressing (wet or dry)[1]
- As a liquid or an aerosol to liquefy sputum in bronchial disorders and in the preparation of sputum for cytological examination[1]
- As an anti-inflammatory agent, oily suspensions are injected intramuscularly[1]
- As an aid in the treatment of intraocular hemorrhage, thrombophlebitis, intestinal obstruction (due to cirrhosis or carcinoma)[61]

Table 101.4 Clinical applications of amylase (needs calcium ions for enzymatic activity)

- Acts on starch, glycogen and related poly- and oligosaccharides[5]
- In combination with other enzymes, as a digestant[38,62,63]
- As an anti-inflammatory[62]
- In treatment of deficiencies of exocrine pancreas, amylaceous dyspepsia and cystic fibrosis[1]

Table 101.5 Clinical applications of lipase

- In pancreatin-containing remedies to increase pancreatic/lipolytic activities (replacement therapy)[64–67]
- When given with pancreatin, it reduces fat level in stools[68–70]
- Synergistically intensifies the activity of lipoproteid-lipase in the blood[71] and migration of agranulocytes[72]
- As a digestive aid[70]

Table 101.6 Clinical applications of pancreatin

- In pancreatic insufficiency, inadequate secretion of exocrine pancreas, disturbed digestion and after gastrectomy[65,73–85]
- In chronic pancreatitis[86]
- Post-pancreatectomy[1,86]
- Ductal obstruction from neoplasm (e.g. of the pancreas or common bile duct)[86]
- To treat severe cases of steatorrhea (as found in cystic fibrosis patients)[87–91]

Inflammatory diseases

One of the basic concepts in systemic enzyme therapy is that all kinds of inflammatory processes (from sports injuries to arthritis to sinusitis to fibrocytis) respond to enzymes. The following is the postulated mechanism of action:

1. In the damaged area, various repair mechanisms are activated, resulting, among other effects, in fibrin surroundng the traumatized region.
2. After having been partly or completely sealed off by microthrombi, blood vessels become highly permeable, and the injured area is disconnected from the normal circulatory system. Stasis results, inhibiting the repair processes.
3. Supplemental enzymes, after absorption, are bound in complexes (e.g. alpha-2-macroglobulin-hydrolase) and circulate to the injured area from the bloodstream.
4. Hydrolytic enzymes directly attack the mircroclots breaking open the clogged vessels and re-establishing circulation.

By restoring normal blood flow, post-inflammatory pain and edema are reduced more rapidly and, equally important, the important physiological inflammatory repair process is not blocked or diminished (as with anti-inflammatory agents), but rather accelerated and reinforced.

Even inflammatory diseases, such as arthritis or herpes zoster, have been shown to respond to the systemic application of enzymes.[93–95] Despite the supportive research, the administration of enzymes in traumatology and injuries is not widely used. All types of injuries, e.g. sprains, strains, hematomas, dislocations, and even postoperative conditions can be effectively treated with enzymes.

Individual enzymes and enzyme combinations (particularly ones including trypsin, chymotrypsin, pancreatin, amylase, lipase, papain, and bromelain, with rutin) are effective in treating inflammation because they help limit the injury, aid its rectification, and promote new, healthy tissue formation. They are inflammation activators, not inflammation inhibitors. Enzymes can accelerate the inflammatory process which is a necessary component of wound healing. This acceleration means, on the one hand, that the work of damage control, damage repair, and new tissue construction is carried out more actively, and thus completed more swiftly. On the other hand, it also means that there can be a temporary increase in the visual and sensory effects produced by the inflammation (i.e. more redness, swelling, heat, and pain).

Since the inflammatory reaction is so universal, it appears that enzymes and enzyme mixtures can be effectively used to treat a wide variety of chronic disorders.

Autoimmune and immune complex-mediated diseases

In autoimmune disease, tissue-bound immune complexes activate the complement system. Activation of the enzyme cascade results in an intense protein-destroying inflammatory response, leading to significant local tissue destruction. For instance, when immune complexes collect in the kidneys, complement activation causes inflammation, resulting in glomerulonephritis.

Research shows that some enzymes can inhibit immune complex-mediated diseases, such as glomerulonephritis, by interrupting the complement cascade. Other disorders with similar mechanisms also respond to supplemental enzymes. Some are conditions, such as Crohn's disease, pulmonary fibrosis, chronic rheumatism, and ankylosing spondylitis, which have not responded well to conventional medical treatments.

Cardiovascular disorders

Cardiovascular disease, the number one killer in the US, kills nearly one in every two Americans. In 1988, heart and blood vessel diseases killed nearly 1 million Americans, almost as many as cancer, accidents, pneumonia, influenza, and all other causes of death combined. But cardiovascular disease is not limited to the elderly; nearly 175,000 Americans under the age of 65 die from this disease every year.[96]

In normal circulation, there is a constant dynamic balance between blood clotting and fibrinolysis.[97] If fibrinolysis is impaired, abnormal clot formation occurs. If fibrinolysis increases, a tendency toward excessive bleeding results. Therefore, maintenance of proper equilibrium is extremely important for the circulatory system.

One study examined the effects of various enzyme combinations on fibrinolysis and fibrin formation. The researchers induced fibrin deposition with calcium ions or staphylocoagulase in the plasma of centrifuged, acellular citrated blood from humans or rabbits and treated the clot with various concentrations of enzyme suspensions. The clots were degraded more rapidly the higher the enzyme content of the solution.[98,99]

Combination enzyme therapy

Because trypsin, chymotrypsin, lipase, and amylase are substrate-specific, combinations of enzymes are frequently employed for a broader spectrum of activity. In addition, when combined, some enzymes act synergistically with others – hence the use of pancreatin (from animal pancreas), as well as products which include both enzymes from different sources and activating substances. For example, one German product contains an enzyme extract consisting of proteinases, triacylglycerol lipase, and α-glycosidase (amylase), minor amounts of elastase, nuclease, and carboxypeptidase, and Ca^{2+} ions to increase activity.

Enzyme combinations should not be viewed as simply intensified forms of pancreatin. An enzyme combination has a number of therapeutic advantages as opposed to a preparation with only one or two components. Combining enzymes from diverse sources, i.e. animal, plant, and fungi, results in a wider range of optimal pH, synergism of the combined enzymes, increased percentage of absorption, increased level of effectiveness, and broader range of application.

Further, Streichhan states that enzyme combinations are better than single enzymes because:[92]

- isoenzymatic activity differences of single biocatalysts are more readily balanced by combining uniformly acting hydrolases of varying origins
- giant molecular substrates are more quickly and more intensively fragmented by a multihydrolytic preparation because the differently acting hydrolases are able to simultaneously disintegrate the giant molecular substrates at many different locations
- certain enzymatic mixtures have a broader range of action than pancreatin, bromelain, or any other standardized monohydrolytic preparation – this is because certain enzyme mixtures characteristically possess differences in optimal pH and also differences in reactive properties of the proteo-, lipo-, and/or glycolytic acting hydrolases.

Enzyme therapy (hydrolytic enzymes from plants, animals, and fungi) combined with rutin is a proven method for treating a number of conditions, as seen in Table 101.7.

Table 101.7 Clinical applications of enzyme combinations

- Soft-tissue injuries[100,101]
- Sprained ankle[101–103]
- Reabsorption of hematomas[100,104]
- Sports medicine[105–111]
- Meniscectomy (pre and post operative therapy)[112,113]
- Traumatology[114]
- Pancreatitis[115]
- Surgery[100,116]
- Lower extremity bypass surgery[117]
- Operative dentistry[118]
- Proctology[119]
- Sinusitis[120–123]
- Acute and chronic bronchitis[98,124,125]
- Cystitis and UTI (lower urinary tract infections)[120,126,127]
- Prostatitis[120,126,128]
- Pelvic inflammatory disease[129,130]
- Post-thrombotic syndrome[131–135]
- Pathologic venous processes[131,136–140]
- Occlusive arterial disease[141]
- Lymphedema[142–147]
- Soft tissue rheumatism (non-articular rheumatoid syndrome)[148,149]
- Rheumatoid arthritis (chronic polyarthritis)[95,99,120,124,133,144,150–163]
- Ankylosing spondylitis (Bekhterev's disease)[101,152,153,156]
- Degenerative rheumatic joint disease[108,120]
- Monoarticular, activated osteoarthrosis[108,125,164]
- Multiple sclerosis[98,165–169]
- HIV infections[170–174]
- Fibrocystic breast disease[146,175]
- Ulcerative colitis and Crohn's disease[120,124,176–177]

DOSAGE

Enzymes may be administered rectally, topically, orally, or by injection, depending on the condition being treated. Rectally, a retention implant or suppository is given. Topically, ointment is spread over the involved area. Orally, lozenges (dissolved in the mouth), oral tablets or enteric-coated tablets are used.

A wide range in daily dosage has historically been used because:

- there are individual differences in patient health
- the level of effective absorption in tablet strength can vary
- there are a wide variety of influencing ranges in pH
- enzyme activity levels vary between products.

For example, pancreatin dosage depends on the condition being treated, as well as the patient's diet and digestive requirements. Dosage can vary because of pancreatin's susceptibility to inactivation in the stomach and duodenum.[182]

Table 101.8 indicates the composition of three enzyme combinations ("A", "B", and "C"), while Table 101.9 lists several conditions effectively treated with these products, the dose required, and the treatment period.

Table 101.8 Composition of enzyme combinations (mg)[179]

Enzyme	"A"	"B"	"C"
Pancreatin	100	100	0
Papain	60	60	100
Bromelain	45	45	0
Lipase	10	10	0
Amylase	10	10	0
Trypsin	24	24	40
Chymotrypsin	1	1	40
Rutin	50	0	0
Thymus extract	0	0	40

Table 101.9 Dosage programs for specific conditions

Condition	Frequency × dosage	Treatment period	Combination
Post-thrombotic syndrome[180]	3 × 5	As needed	A
Oncology[181]	2 × 11	6 weeks or as needed	A
Lymphedema[143]	2 × 5	2 years	A
Fibrocystic breast disease[174]	2 × 10	6 weeks or as needed	A
Experimental hematoma[100]	3 × 10	24 hours	A
Prophylactic treatment of karate injuries[182]	3 × 5	During the season	A
Trauma and meniscus operation[112]	3 × 10	Average of 17.7 days	A
Soft tissue injuries and distortions of the ankle[101]	3 × 10 initially, then 3 × 1	As needed	A
Athletic soft tissue injuries[104]	2 × 5	Spring football season	A
Dental surgery[118]	4 × 5	Day before surgery to 7th postoperative day	A
Sports injuries[107]	3 × 10	As needed	A
Chronic polyarthritis[183]	4 × 8	6 months	A
Active arthoses[184]	4 × 7	6 weeks	A
Extra-articular rheumatism[148]	3 × 10	As needed	B
Adnexitis[129]	3 × 5	10–14 days	A
Prostatitis[120,126]	3 × 5	10 days	A
Mastopathy[185]	2 × 10		A
Multiple sclerosis[166–169,177]			
Initially	2 ampoules injection	Daily	C
As symptoms improve	2 ampoules injection	Every 2 to 3 days, then at longer intervals	C
On injection-free days	3 × 10		A
Later	3 × 5		A
Finally	3 × 3		A
Herpes zoster[94]			
Initially	2 ampoules injection	First 2 days	C
First two days	3–4 × 1	As indicated to 14 days	A
HIV[172,173]	3 × 10*	As indicated	A
HIV	25/day	12 months	A

*Ongoing studies insufficient to give effective dose levels.

TOXICOLOGY

Oral enzymes

In general, side-effects of orally administered enzymes are few and due primarily to excessive dosages or hypersensitivity reactions. According to Wolf & Ransberger, high dosages (70 tablets of 17.5 g each) of a proteolytic enzyme mixture have been given without long-term side effects.[187] Studies and literature searches commissioned by regulatory authorities such as the FDA have apparently confirmed that enzyme preparations obtained from suitable sources (e.g. non-toxic, non-pathogenic sources) are safe to consume.[188]

With normal use, stools can be pale or have a pungent odor. Transient intestinal upset, such as diarrhea and gas, may result from excessive dosage of pancreatin. Hyperuricosuria (excess uric acid in the urine) and hyperuricemia (excess uric acid in the blood) have been associated with extremely high doses of exogenous pancreatic enzymes.

If the pancreatin preparations are held in the mouth before swallowing, stomatitis can result, as well as ulcerations, and irritation of the mucosa, particularly in infants where pancreatin may also cause perianal soreness.[1,178]

It is not known whether pancreatin given to pregnant woman can harm the fetus since animal reproductive studies have not been conducted. Therefore, pancreatin should probably not be used during pregnancy.[178] Also, since it is not known if pancreatin is distributed into mother's milk, caution should be exercised with nursing women.[178]

Sneezing, lacrimation, rash and other hypersensitivity reactions have been reported in sensitive individuals. Pancrelipase (and any other enzyme derived from pork sources) is contraindicated in those who are hypersensitive or allergic to pork products.

Enzymes should not be used by hemophiliacs, nor immediately before or after operations with an increased risk of bleeding. Trypsin is especially contraindicated in those with blood-clotting mechanism disorders, in liver disease, and as an aerosol within a week of pulmonary hemorrhage.[1]

Enzyme enemas

Enzyme enemas can sometimes cause the rectum or anus to itch or burn. However, these are only minimal side-effects in relation to the positive benefits obtained.

Topical application

Enzymatic activity directed toward proteinaceous components of the epithelium can cause irritation. For example, prolonged skin contact with proteolytic enzymes may cause irritation of the skin, mucous membranes of the throat, nose, and eyes.[188]

Injectable enzymes

Injectable forms require more care. Chymotrypsin, when injected, can occasionally create anaphylactic reactions.[1] When injected, trypsin's toxicity is greatly increased, and rapid infusion is far more toxic than slower infusion.[1] In addition, trypsin must not be administered intravenously.[1] Further, intradermal or scratch testing is advised before parenteral administration.[1] Other contraindications to trypsin's use are pork allergy and pancreatitis.

It should be remembered that, at the beginning of therapy, an individual's symptoms may occasionally increase in severity. This is a sign that a therapeutic reaction is occurring and should be evaluated positively. The medication need not be discontinued, although a temporary reduction in dose might be advisable.

REFERENCES

1. Ruyssen R, Lauwers A, eds. Pharmaceutical enzymes: properties and assay methods. Ghent: Scientific Publishing. 1978: p 34–35, 45, 57–58, 70
2. Guyton AC. Textbook of medical physiology. 8th edn. Philadelphia, PA: WB Saunders. 1991: p 727–729
3. US Pharmacopoeia XXII. Rockville, MD: US Pharmacopoeia Convention. 1990
4. Eisenthal R, Danson MJ. Enzyme assays: a practical approach. Oxford: IRL Press. 1992: p 263–264
5. Dixon M, Webb EC. Enzymes. 3rd edn. New York: Academic Press. 1979: p 28–9, 40, 860–861
6. Beynon RJ, Bond JS. Proteolytic Enzymes, a Practical Approach. Oxford: IRL Press. 1989: p 20–21
7. Gardner MLG. Intestinal assimilation of intact peptides and proteins from the diet – a neglected field? Biol Rev 1984; 59: 289–331
8. Matthews DM. Memorial lecture. Protein absorption – then and now. Gastroenterol 1977; 73: 1267–1279
9. Volkheimer P. Persorption. Stuttgart: Thieme. 1972
10. Brambell FWR. The transmission of passive immunity from mother to young. Front Biol, vol. 18, Amsterdam: North-Holland. 1970
11. Bjarnason I, Peters TJ. Helping the mucosa make sense of macromolecules. Gut 1987; 28: 1057–1061
12. Bockman DE, Boydston WR, Beezhold DH. The role of epithelial cells in gut-associated immune reactivity. Ann NY Acad Sci 1983; 409: 129–143
13. Georgopoulou U, Dabrowski MF, Vernier JM. Absorption of intact proteins by the intestinal epithelium of trout, Salmo gairdneri. Cell Tissue Res 1988; 251: 145–152
14. Colony PC, Neutra MR. Macromolecular transport in the fetal rat intestine. Gastroenterol 1985; 89: 294–306
15. Adibi SA, Mercer DW. Protein digestion in human intestine as reflected in luminal, mucosal, and plasma amino acid concentrations after meals. J Clin Invest 1973; 52: 1586–1594
16. Borgstrom B, Dahlqvist A, Lundh G, Sjovall J. Studies of intestinal digestion and absorption in humans. J Clin Invest 1957; 36: 1521–1536
17. Seifert J, Sellschopp CH, Sass W. Werden makromolekule resorbiert und welchen einfluss hat dabei die immunitatslage? Z Hautkr 1987; 62: 55–59
18. Chung IL, Sleisenger MH. Protein digestion and absorption in human small intestine. Gastroenterol 1979; 76: 1415–1421
19. Pabst R. Anatomische grundlagen fur verdauung und immunfunktion im gastrointestinaltrakt. Z Hautkr 1987; 62: 39–44
20. LeFevre ME, Joel DD. Intestinal absorption of particulate matter. Life Sci 1977; 21: 1403–1408
21. Streichhan P. Resorption enteraler makromolekule. Verdauungskrankheiten 1989; 7: 28–38
22. Walker WA. Intestinal transport of macromolecules. In: Johnson LR, ed. Physiology of the gastrointestinal tract, vol 2. New York, NY: Raven; 1981: p 1271–1289
23. Hemmings C, Hemmings WA, Patey AL, Wood C. The ingestion of dietary protein as large molecular mass degradation products in adult rats. Proc R Soc Lond (Biol) 1977; 198: 439–453
24. Hemmings WA, Williams EW. Transport of large breakdown products of dietary protein through the gut wall. Gut 1978; 19: 715–713
25. Gruskay FL, Cooke RE. The gastrointestinal absorption of unaltered protein in normal infants and in infants recovering from diarrhea. Pediatrics 1955; 16: 763–769
26. Hemmings WA. Distributed digestion. Med Hypoth 1980; 6: 1209–1213
27. Kim YS, Erickson RH. Role of peptidases of the human small intestine in protein digestion. Gastroenterol 1985; 88: 1071–1073
28. Husby S, Foged N, Host A, Svehag SE. Passage of dietary antigen into the blood of children with coeliac disease. Quantification and size distribution of absorbed antigens. Gut 1987; 28: 1062–1072
29. Lake-Bakaar G, Smith-Laing G, Summerfield JA. Origin of circulating serum immunoreactive trypsin in man. Dig Dis Sci 1982; 27: 143–148
30. Seifert J, Ganser R, Brendel W. Die resorption eines proteolytischen enzyms pflanzlichen ursprungs aus dem magen-darm-trakt in das blut und die lymphe von erwachsenen ratten. Z Gastroenterol 1979; 17: 1–8
31. Gebert G. Physiologie. Stuttgart: Schattauer Publ. 1987
32. Steffen C, Menzel J, Smolen H. Untersuchungen uber intestinale resorption mit ^{3}H-markiertem enzymgemisch (Wobenzym). Acta Med Aus 1979; 6: 13–18
33. Seifert J, Siebrecht P, Lange JP. Quantitative untersuchungen zur resorption von trypsin, chymotrypsin, amylase, papain und pankreatin aus dem magen-darm-trakt nach oraler applikation. Allgemein Medizin Springer-Verlag, 1990; 19: 132–137
34. Papp M, Feher S, Folly G, Horvath EJ. Absorption of pancreatic lipase from the duodenum into lymphatics. Experienta 1977; 33: 1191
35. Hasselberger FX. Uses of Enzymes and Immobilized Enzymes. Chicago: Nelson-Hall. 1978
36. Burtis G, Davis J, Martin S. Applied Nutrition and Diet Therapy. Philadelphia: WB Saunders. 1988
37. Lin CW, Lee TG. A note on the micro-encapsulation of pancreatic protease for protection against gastric digestion. Anim Prod 1993; 56: 413–417
38. Reynolds JEP, ed. Martindale – the extra pharmacopoeia. London: The Pharmaceutical Press. 1982
39. Konotey-Ahulu FID. Enzyme treatment of vitreous haemorrhage. Lancet 1972; 2: 714–715
40. Sowray JH. An assessment of the value of lyophilized chymotrypsin in the reduction of post-operative swelling following the removal of impacted wisdom teeth. Br Dent J 1961; 110: 130–133
41. Frederick W, Messer E. Enzyme treatment of traumatic swelling in oral and maxillofacial surgery. Clin Med 1967; 74: 29–31
42. Bumgardner HD, Zatuchni GI. Prevention of episiotomy pain with oral chymotrypsin. Am J Obst Gyn 1965; 92: 514–517
43. Fiel RA. Tratamiento experimental de la trichuriasis masiva infantil con quimotripsina. Trop Dis Bull Bd 1968; 65: 917

44. Takahashi M, Hashimoto K, Osada H. Parenteral administration of chymotrypsin for the early detection of cancer cells in sputum. Acta Cytol Bd 1967; 11: 61–63
45. Brandborg LL, Tankersley CB, Uyeda F. "Low" versus "high" concentration chymotrypsin in gastric exfoliative cytology. Gastroenterol Bd 1969; 57: 500–505
46. Soule SE, Helman C, Wasserman RB. Oral proteolytic enzyme therapy (Chymoral) in episiotomy patients. Am J Obst Gyn 1966; 95: 820–833
47. Boyne PS, Medhurst H. Oral anti-inflammatory enzyme therapy in injuries in professional footballers. Practitioner 1967; 198: 543
48. Blonstein JL. Oral enzyme tablets in the treatment of boxing injuries. Practitioner 1967; 198: 547–548
49. Buck JE, Phillips N. Trial of chymoral in professional footballers. Br J Clin Pract Bd 1970; 24: 375–377
50. Rathgeber WF. The use of proteolytic enzymes (Chymoral) in sporting injuries. S African Med J 1971; 45: 181–183
51. De N'Yeurt A. The use of chymoral in vasectomy. J Coll Gen Pract 1972; 22: 633–637
52. Winsor T. Inhibition of the response to thermal injury by oral proteolytic enzymes. J Clin Pharmacol 1972; 12: 325–330
53. Rathgeber WF. The use of proteolytic enzymes in tenosynovitis. Clin Med 1973; 80: 39–41
54. Gibson T, Dilke TF, Grahame R. Chymoral in the treatment of lumbar disc prolapse. Rheumatol Rehabil 1975; 14: 186–190
55. Transcript from the Am Acad Ophthamology and Otolaryngology, Oct 11–16, 1959, Chicago, p16
56. Heinrich W. Trypsin und chymotrypsin – klinisches sachverstandigengutachten zur systemischen wirkung. Inst f angewante u exptl Onkologie d Univ Wien. Nov 1988
57. Stille G, Tuluwett K. Pharmakologisch-toxikologisches sachverstandigengutachten zut trypsin/chymotrypsin. Nov 1988
58. Gordon B. The use of topical proteolytic enzymes in the treatment of post-thrombotic leg ulcers. Br J Clin Pract Bd 1975; 29: 143–146
59. Sather MR, Weber Jr Ch E, George J. Pressure sores and the spinal cord injury patient. Drug Intell Clinic Pharm Bd 1977; 11: 154–169
60. Marquez OHD, Segur FG. The intrathecal use of proteolytic enzymes in tuberculous meningoencephalitis. Preliminary Communication; Abstr Wld Med 1968; 42: 800–801
61. Lichtman AL. Traumatic injury in athletes. In. Rec Med 1957; 170: 322–325
62. Windholz M, ed. The Merck Index – An Encyclopedia of Chemicals, Drugs, and Biologicals. Rahway, NJ: Merck. 1983
63. Auterhoff H, Knage J. Lehrouch der pharmazueutischen chemie. Verlagsgesellschaft (11 Auflk, Wissenschafel. Stuttgart). 1983
64. Graham DY. Enzyme replacement therapy of exocrine pancreatic insufficiency in man. New Engl J Med 1977 296: 1314–1317
65. Meyer JH. The ins and outs of oral pancreatic enzymes. New Engl J Med 1977; 296: 1347–1348
66. Yeh TL, Rubin ML. Potency of pancreatic enzyme preparations. New Engl J Med 1977; 297: 615–616
67. Kirshen R. Letter to the editor. New Engl J Med 1977; 297: 616
68. Mackie RD, Levine AS, Levitt MD. Malabsorption of starch in pancreatic insufficiency. Gastroenterol 1981; 80: 1220
69. Lankisch PG, Creutzfeldt W. Therapy of exocrine and endocrine pancreatic insufficiency. Clin Gastroenterol 1984; 13: 985–999
70. Schneider MU, Knoll-Ruzicka ML, Domschke S et al. Pancreatic enzyme replacement therapy. Comparative effects of conventional and enteric-coated micropheric pancreatin and acid-stable fungal enzyme preparations on steatorrhoea in chronic pancreatitis. Hepato Gastroenterol 1985; 32: 97–102
71. Hall DA, Zajac AR, Cox R, Spanswick J. The effect of enzyme therapy on plasma lipid levels in the elderly. Artheroscler 1982; 43: 209–215
72. Tylewska S, Tyski S, Hrynie-Wicz W. The effect of S. aureus lipase on granulocyte chemotaxis. Med Dos Microbio 1983; 35: 171–174
73. LeBauer E, Smith K, Greenberger NJ. Pancreatic influence and vitamin B_{12} malabsorption. Archs Intern Med 1968; 122: 423–426
74. Kataria MS, Bhaskarrao D. A clinical double-blind trial with a broad spectrum digestive enzyme product (Combinzym) in geriatric practice. Br J Clin Prac 1969; 23: 15–17
75. Karani S, Kataria MS, Barber AE. A double-blind clinical trial with a digestive enzyme product. Br J Pract 1971; 25: 375–377
76. Knill-Jones RP, Pearce H, Batten H, Williams R. Comparative trial of nutrizym in chronic pancreatic insufficiency. Br Med J 1970; 4: 21–24
77. DiMagno EP, Go VLW, Summerskill WHJ. Relations between pancreatic enzyme outputs and malabsorption in severe pancreatic insufficiency. New Engl J Med 1973; 288: 813–815
78. Saunders JHB, Wormsley KG. Progress report. Pancreatic extracts in the treatment of pancreatic exocrine insufficiency. Gut 1975; 16: 157–162
79. Bank S, Marks IN, Barbezat GO. Treatment of acute and chronic pancreatitis. Drugs 1977; 13: 373
80. DiMagno EP, Malagelada JR, Go VLW, and Moertel CG. Fate of orally ingested enzymes in pancreatic insufficiency; comparison of two dosage schedules. New Engl J Med 1977; 296: 1318–1322
81. Saunders JHB, Drummond S, Wormsley KG. Inhibition of gastric secretion in treatment of pancreatic insufficiency. Br Med J 1977; 1: 418–419
82. Anonymous. Pancreatic extracts. Lancet 1977; ii: 73–75
83. Regan PT, Malagelada JR, DiMagno EP et al. Comparative effects of antacids, cimetidine and enteric coating on the therapeutic response to oral enzymes in severe pancreatic insufficiency. New Engl J Med 1977; 297: 854–858
84. Regan PT, Malagelada JR, Dimagno EP, Go VL. Rationale for the use of cimetidine in pancreatic insufficiency. Mayo Clin Proc 1978; 53: 79–88
85. Austad WJ. Pancreatitis. The use of pancreatic supplements. Drugs 1979; 17: 480–7
86. Physicians' Desk Reference, vol. 47. Montvale, NJ: Medical Economics. 1993: p 1426
87. Anonymous. Pancreatic extracts. Br Med J, 1970; 2: 161–163
88. Anderson CM. Pancreatic enzyme replacement in the treatment of cystic fibrosis. Prescribers J 1972; 12: 45–49
89. Roy CC, Weber AM, Morin CL et al. Abnormal biliary lipid composition in cystic fibrosis. New Engl J Med 1977; 197: 1301–1305
90. Smalley AC, Brown GA, Parkes MET et al. Reduction of bile acid loss in cystic fibrosis by dietary means. Archs Dis Childh 1978; 53: 477–482
91. Goodschild MC, Sagaro E, Brown GA et al. Comparative trial of pancrex V. Forte and nutrizym in treatment of malabsorption in cystic fibrosis. Br Med J 1974; 3: 712–714
92. Streichhan P. Wobenzym®. An orally administered combination preparation consisting of hydrolytic enzymes and rutin acting in circulating body fluids. Inventory text Part A, Preclinical results. Geretsried: Mucos Pharma GmbH & Co.; 1993
93. Kleine MW, Pabst H. Enzymtherapie der lateralen sprunggelenksdistorsion. Dtsch Z Sportzmed 1990; 41: 126–134
94. Kleine MW. Therapie des herpes zoster mit proteolytischen. Enzymen Therapiewoche 1987; 37: 1108–1112
95. Miehlke K. Enzymtherapie bei rheumatoider arthritis. Natur-und Ganzheits-medizin 1988; 108–111
96. 1991 Heart and stroke facts. Dallas: American Heart Association. 1991
97. Haid-Fischer F, Haid H. Venenerkrankungen. Stuttgart: Thieme. 1985
98. Inderst R. Enzymtherapie – grundlagen und anwendungsmoglichkeiten. Naturund Ganzheitsmedizin 1991; 3
99. Inderst R. Enzymtherapie. Erfahrungsheilkunde, 1989; 38: 305
100. Kleine M-W, Pabst H. Die wirkung einer oralen enzymtherapie auf experimentell erzeugte hamatoma. Forum des Prakt und Allgemeinarztes 1988; 27: 42
101. Baumuller M. Der einsatz von hydrolytischen enzymen bei steumpfen weichteilverletzungen und sprunggelenksdistorsionen. Allgemeinmedizin 1990; 19: 178–182
102. Baumuller M. Enzyme zur widerherstellung nach sprunggelenkdistorsionen. Z Allg med 1992; 68: 61
103. Baumuller M. Therapy of ankle joint distortions with hydrolytic enzymes – results from a double blind clinical trial. In: Hermans GPH, Mosterd WL, eds. Sport, Med Health Excertpa Medica. New York: Amsterdam. 1990: p 1137

104. Cichoke AJ, Marty L. The use of proteolytic enzymes with soft tissue athletic injuries. Am Chiro 1981 Sept/Oct: 32–33
105. Helpap B. Leitfaden der Allgemeinen Entzundungslehre. Berlin: Springer. 1987
106. Kleine, M.-W. Systemische enzymtherapie in der sportmedizin. Dtsch Zeitschr f Sportmedizin 1990; 41: 126
107. Muller-Hepburn W. Anwendung von Enzymen in der Sportmedizin, Forum d. Prakt. Arztes 1970.; 18
108. Niethard FU, Pfeil J. Orthopadie. Stuttgart: Hippokrates Verlag. 1989
109. Hiss WF. Enzyme in der sport- und unfallmedizin. Continuing Education Seminars. 1979
110. Doenicke A, Hoernecke R. Wirksame behandlung von traumen mit schwellung und/oder hamatom im eishockeysport durch enzymtherapie. Dtsch Zeitschr f Sportmedizin 1993; 5: 214–219
111. Kleine M-W. Introduction to systemic enzyme therapy and results of experimental trials. In: Hermans GPH, Mostered WL, eds. Sports, medicine and health. Amsterdam: Excerpta Medica. 1990: 9 1131
112. Rahn H-D, Kilic M. Die Wirksamkeit hydrolytischer enzyme in der traumatologie. Ergebnise nach 2 prospektiven randomisierten doppelblindstudien. Allgemeinarzt 1990; 19: 183–187
113. Rahn H-D. Enzyme verkurzen rekonvaleszenz. Lecture given at 13th Systemische Enzymtherapie Symposium, Lindau. 1990
114. Carillo AR. Klinische untersuchung eines enzymatischen entzundungshemmers in der unfallchirurgie. Arztl Praxis 1972; 24: 2307
115. Chappa-Alvarez R. Pankreatitisbehandlung mit Wobenzym®. Working paper, 1992
116. Guggenbichler JP. Einfluss hydrolytischer enzyme auf thrombusbildung und thrombolyse. Die Medizinische Welt 1988; 39: 277
117. Rahn H-D. Wobenzym® nach gefassbypassoperationen am bein. Lecture given at 17th Systemische Enzymtherapie Symposium, Vienna, Austria, 1991
118. Vinzenz K. Odembehandlung bei zahnchirurgischen eingriffen mit hydrolytischen enzymen. Die Quintessenz 1991; 7: 1053
119. Werk W. Ein Polyenzympraparat zur Beschleunigung der Narbenbildung. Proktologie 1979; 3
120. Riede NU, Schaefer, HE, Wehner H. Allgemeine und Spezielle Pathologie. Stuttgart: Thieme. 1989
121. Rayn RE. A double-blind clinical evaluation of bromelain in the treatment of acute sinusitis. Headache 1967; 7: 13
122. Zollner N, Ed. Innere Medizin. Springer: Heidelberg, 1991
123. Wohlrab R. Enzymkombinationspraparat zur therapie der sinusitis acuta. Der Allgemeinarzt 1993; 15: 104–114
124. Zech R, Domagk G. Enzyme – Biochemie, Pathobiochemie, Klinik, Therapie. Weinheim: VCH Verlagsgesellschaft mbH. 1986
125. Grimminger A. Enzymtherapie bei thoraxerkrankungen. Erfahrungsheilkunde 1971; 1: 18
126. Barsom S, Sasse-Rollenhagen K, Bettermann A. Erfolgreiche prostatitisbehandlung mit hundrolytischen enzymen. Erfarungsheilkunde 1982; 31: 2
127. Barsom S, Sasse-Rollenhagen K, Bettermann A. Zur behandlung von zystitden und zystopyelitiden mit hydrolytischen enzymen. Acta Medica Empirica 1983; 32: 125
128. Rugendorff EW, Burghele A, Schneider H-J. Behandlung der chronischen abakteriellen prostatitis mit hydrolytischen enzymen. Der Kassenarzt 1986; 14: 43
129. Dittmar F-W, Weissenbacher ER. Therapie der adnexitis – unterstutzung der antibiotischen basisbehandlung durch hydrolytische enzyme. Int J Exper Clin Chemother 1992; 5: 73–82
130. Dittmar F-W. Enzymtherapie in der gynakologie. Allgemeinmedizin 1990; 19: 158
131. Rahn H-D. Wirksamkeit von enzymen bei gefasserkrankungen. Lecture given at 2nd Systemische Enzymtherapie Symposium, Dusseldorf, Germany, 1987
132. Ernst E, Matrei A. Orale therapie mit proteolytischen enzymen modifiziert die blutrheologie. Klin Wsch. 1987; 65: 994
133. Klein K. Proteolytisches Enzympraparat erfolgreich. Therapiewoche Osterreich 1989; 39: 448
134. Morl H. Behandlung des postthrombotischen syndroms mit einem enzymgemisch. Therapiewoche 1986; 36: 2443
135. Morl H. Therapie und prophylze des postthrombotischen syndroms mit Wobenzym®. Lecture given at 17th Systemische Enzymtherapie Symposium, Vienna, Austria, 1991
136. Valls-Serra J. Proteolytische enzyme in der behandlung von thrombophlebitis. Medicina Clinica 1967
137. Mahr H. Zur enzymtherapie entzundlicher venenerkrankungen der tiefen beinvenenthrombose und des postthrombotischen syndroms. Erfahrungsheilkunde 1983 117
138. Maehder K. Enzymtherapie venoser gefasserkrankungen. Die Arztpraxis 1972; 2
139. Kluken N. Venose krankheiten in klinik und praxis, systemische enzymtherapie, medizinische woche Baden-Baden, 1990. Natur-und Ganzheitsmedizin 1991; 2: 8
140. Vogler W. Enzymtherapie. Hessen. Hausarz, 1989; 4: 116
141. Rokitansky O, v. Ozontherapie und enzyme bei der chronisch-arteriellen verschlusskrankeit. Systemische Enzymtherapie am 31.10.90, Medizinische Woche, Baden-Baden, 1990, Natur-und Ganzheitsmedizin, Supplement, 14. 1991
142. Keim H et al. Methode zur linderung der lymphstauung am arm nach behandlung des mammakarzinoms. Rontgenberichte 1972; 1: 1
143. Scheef W, Pischnamazadeh M. Proteolytische enzyme als einfache und sichere methode zur verhutung des lymphodems nach ablatio mammae. Med Welt 1984; 35: 1032
144. Streichhan P, Inderst R. Konventionelle und enzymtherapeutische massnahmen bei der behandlung brustkrebsbedingter armlymphodeme. Der Prakt Arzt 1991; 13: 37–38
145. Ransberger K, Stauder G, Streichhan P. Wissenschaftliche monographie zur praklinik Wobenzym® N, Mulsal® N, Phlogenzym®. Forum Medizin. 1991
146. Konig W. Erfahrungen der Robert-Janker-Klinik, Bonn, mit systemischer enzymtherapie und emulgierten vitaminen. Acta Medica Emperica 1988; 37: 11
147. Konig W. Proteolytische enzyme verhindern lymphodem. In: Medizinische Enzym-Forschungesgesellschaft e.V., ed. Systemische Enzymtherapie, Symposium Munich, 1986; Medizin Aktuell (Enzyme Series,) Informed International Congress Report 53. 1986
148. Uffelmann K, Vogler W, Fruth C. Der eisatz hydrolytischer enzyme beim extraartikularen rheumatismus. Allgemeinmedizin 1990; 19: 151–153
149. Vogler W. Der stellenwert der enzymtherapie bei entzundlich-rheumatischen erkrankungen. Systemische Enzymtherapie, Medizinische Woche, Baden-Baden, 1990, Natur-und Ganzheitsmedizin 1991; 2: 23
150. Horger I, Moro V, van Schaik W. Zirkulierende immunkomplexe bei polyarthritis-patienten. Natur-und Ganzheitsmedizin 1988; 1: 117
151. Steffen C, Smolen J, Miehlke K, Horger J, Menzel J. Enzymtherapie im vergleich mit immunkiomplexbestimmungen bei chonischler polyarthritis. Zeitschr f Rheumatologie 1985; 44: 51
152. Reinbold H. Die biologische alternative in der therapie entzundlicher rheumatischer erkrankungen. Zeitschr Allgemeinmedizin 1981; 34
153. Reinbold H. Die therapie des morbus bechterew mit enzymen. Erfahrungsheilkunde 1980; 10
154. Ekerot L, Ohlsson K, Necking L. Elimination of protease-inhibitor complexes from the arthritic joint. In J Tissue Reac 1985; VII: 391
155. Ballachi G. Hydrolytische enzyme bei aktivierten polyarthrosen. Rheuma 1988; 8
156. Goebel KM. Enzymtherapie bei spondylitis ankylosans. Lecture given at 17th Systemische Enzymtherapie Symposium, Vienna, Austria, 1991
157. Horger I. Enzymtherapie bei einem rheumakollektiv. Therapiewoche 1983; 33: 3948
158. Panijel M. Entzundlich-rheumatische erkrankungen. Zeitschr f Allgemeinmedizin 1985; 61: 1305
159. Steffen C, Zeitlhofer J, Menzel J, Smolen J. Die antigen-induzierte experimentelle arthritis als prufverfahren fur entzundungshemmung durch oral appliqierte substanzen. Zeitschr Rheumatologie, 1979; 38: 264

160. Miehlke K. Enzymtherapie bei chronischer polyarthritis. Der Kassenarzt 1989; 46
161. Miehlke K. Rheumabahandlung mit enzymen ist mehr als nur antiphlogistische therapie. Lecture given at 17th Systemische Enzymtherapie Symposium, Vienna, Austria, 1991
162. Klein G, Schwann H, Kullich W. Enzymtherapie bei chronischer polyarthritis. Natur-und Ganzheitsmedizin 1988; 1: 112
163. Klein K. Behandlung der rheumatoiden arthritis mit Wobenzym® im vergleich zur basistherapie mit gold. Lecture given at 17th Systemische Enzymtherapie Symposium, Vienna, Austria, 1991
164. Singer F. Aktivierte arthrosen knorpelschonend behandeln. Lecture given at 10th Systemische Enzymtherapie Symposium, Frankfurt, Germany, 1990
165. Masuhr KF. Eurologie. Stuttgart: Hippokrates. 1989
166. Neuhofer CH, van Schaik W, Stauder G, Pollinger W. Pathogenetic immune complexes in MS: their elimination by hydrolytic enzymes. A therapeutic approach. International Multiple Sclerosis Conference, Rome. Bologna: Monduzzi Editore SPA. 1988
167. Ransberger K, van Schaik W. Enzymtherapie bei multipler sklerose. Der Kassenarz, 1986; 41: 42
168. Neuhofer CH. Enzymtherpie bei multipler sklerose. Hufeland J 1986; 47
169. Neuhofer CH. Systemische enzymtherapie bei encephalomyelitis disseminata. Der Prakt Arzt 1991; 702
170. Dirringer H. Unkonventionelle viruserkrankungen. Bundesgesundhbl 1990; 33: 188
171. Inderst R, Ransberger K, Brand G. Fortschritte in der therapie der erworbenen immunschwache durch naturheilkundliche methoden. Naturheilpraxis 1988; 41: 1050
172. Jager H, Popescu M, Samtleben W, Stauder G. Hydrolytic enzymes as biological response modifiers (BRM) in HIV-infection. In: San Marino Conferences – highlights in medical virology, immunology and oncology, vol. 1. Oxford: Pergamon Press. 1988
173. Jager H. Hydrolytische enzyme in der therapie der hiv-erkrankung. Zeitschr Allgemeinmedizin 1990; 19: 160
174. Ransberger K. Naturheilkundliche therapie von AIDS mit enzympraparaten. Forum des Prakt und Allgemeinarztes 1988; Heft 4. 27, Jahrgang, April 1988
175. Scheef W. Gutartige veranderungen der weiblichen brust. Therapiewoche 1985; 5090
176. Inderst R. Colitis ulcerosa und morbus crohn systemische enzymtherapie, medizinische woche Baden-Baden, 1990. Natur-und Ganzheitsmedizin 1991; 2: 28
177. Neuhofer CH. Autoimmunerkrankungen. Multiple sklerose, amyotrophe lateralsklerose, colitis ulcerosa. Erfahrungsheilkunde, 1988; 38: 451
178. McEvoy GK, ed. AHFS '94 Drug Information, American Hospital Formulary Service. Bethesda, MD: American Society of Hospital Pharmacists. 1994: p 20 814
179. Stauder G, Pollinger W, Fruth C. Systemische Enzymetherapie. Eine Ubersicht uber Neue Klinische Studient. Allgemein Medizin 1990; 19: 188–191
180. Inderst R. Enzymtherapie bei Gefasserkrankungen [Enzyme Therapy in Vascular Diseases]. Allgemein Medizin 1990; 19: 154–157
181. Wrba H. Kombinierte tumortherapie. Stuttgart: Hippokrates. 1992
182. Worschhauser S. Konservative Therapie der Sportverletzungen. Enzympraparate fur Therapie und Prophylaxe [Conservative Therapy for Sports Injuries. Enzyme Preparations for Therapy and Prophylaxis]. Allgemein Medizin 1990; 19: 173–177
183. Klein G, Pollmann G, Kullich W. Klinische Erfahrungen mit der Enzymtherapie bei Patienten mit Chronischer Polyarthritis im Vergleich Zur Oralen Goldtherapie [Clincal experience with enzyme therapy in patients with rheumatoid arthritis in comparison with oral gold]. Allgemein Medizin 1990; 19: 144–147
184. Gallacchi G. Der Einsatz Hydrolytischer Enzyme bei der Aktivierten Arthrose [The Use of Hydrolytic Enzymes in Activated Arthrosis]. Allgemein Medizin 1990; 19: 148–150
185. Dittmar F-W, Luh W, Phillipp E. Wobenzym® zur Behandlung der Mastopathie. Working paper. 1993
186. Sears A, Walsh G. Biotechnology in the feed industry: proceedings of alltech's ninth annual symposium. Nicholasville, KY: Alltech Technical Publ. 1993
187. Wolf M, Ransberger K. Enzyme therapy. Los Angeles: Regent House. 1972

FURTHER READING

Cichoke AJ. Enzymes and enzyme therapy: how to jump start your way to lifelong good health. New Canaan, CT: Keats. 1994

Cichoke AJ. Acute trauma and systemic enzyme therapy. Portland, OR: Seven C's Publ. 1993

Cichoke AJ. A new look at chronic disorders and enzyme therapy. Portland, OR: Seven C's Publ. 1993

Cichoke AJ. A new look at enzyme therapy. Portland, OR: Seven C's Publ. 1993

CHAPTER CONTENTS

102

Phage therapy: bacteriophages as natural, self-limiting antibiotics*

Elizabeth Kutter, PhD

INTRODUCTION

Phage therapy involves the use of specific viruses – viruses that can attack only bacteria – to kill pathogenic microorganisms. The art was first developed early in this century, but since the advent of chemical antibiotics in the 1940s, it has been little used in the West. Today, however, the growing incidence of bacteria which are resistant to most or all available antibiotics is leading to widespread renewed research interest in the possibilities of phage therapy.[1–4] Most of the recent articles appearing in the West reflect little knowledge of the extensive Eastern European research and clinical utilization of phage therapy. The good clinical results of Eastern European research provide a substantial basis for optimism and complement the limited recent animal work in the West. We need to draw as much as possible on the largely unknown body of knowledge that has accumulated in Poland and the former Soviet Union as we again explore phage therapy, and to give credit where it is due for the many years of hard, careful work in the field. This chapter has been written in order to put phage therapy into historical and ecological context and to explore some of the most interesting and extensive research in Eastern Europe.

*Special thanks to Drs Liana Gachechiladze, Zemphira Alavidze, Amiran Meipariani, Taras Gabisonia, Mzia Kutateladze, Rezo Adamia, Teimuraz and Nino Chanishvili and their colleagues at the Bacteriophage Institute, Tbilisi, for their hospitality and efforts to help me understand the extensive therapeutic work carried out there. Others who have been particularly helpful with information and communication include Dr Marina Shubladze, pediatrician in Tbilisi for 10 years, now residing in Seattle; Nino Mzavia, Nino Trapaidze, Timur and Natasha Zurabishvili, who have worked in my laboratory; Bill Summers (Yale), Hans-Wolfgang Ackermann (Laval University), Eduard Kellenberger (Basel) and Bruce Levin (Emory); Kathy d'Acci, clinical laboratory director, St Peter's Hospital, Olympia; physicians Jess Spielholz MD, and Robin Moore ND; and, especially, the many colleagues and students involved in our laboratory in Olympia, particularly Barbara Anderson, Pia Lippincot, Mark Mueller, Stacy Smith, Elizabeth and Chelsea Thomas and Jim Neitzel.

HISTORIC CONTEXT

Discovery

A century ago, Hankin[5] reported that the waters of the Ganges and Jumna rivers in India had a marked antibacterial action which could pass through a porcelain filter, an antibacterial activity destroyed by boiling. He particularly studied the water's effects on *Vibrio cholerae* and suggested that the substance responsible was what kept cholera epidemics from being spread by ingestion of the water of these rivers. However, he did not explore the phenomenon further. Edward Twort and Felix d'Herelle independently reported isolating filterable entities capable of lysing bacterial cultures and of producing small cleared areas on bacterial cultures, implying that discrete particles were involved.[6] They are jointly given credit for the discovery of bacteriophages.

Early research

It was d'Herelle, a Canadian working at the Pasteur Institute in Paris, who gave these newly discovered organisms the name *bacteriophages* – using the suffix *phage* "not in its strict sense of *to eat*, but in that of *developing at the expense of*".[7] He carefully characterized them as viruses which multiply in bacteria and worked out the details of infection of different bacterial hosts by various phages under a variety of environmental conditions. The 90th Annual Meeting of the British Medical Association in Glasgow featured a very interesting discussion among d'Herelle, Twort and several other eminent scientists of the day on the nature and properties of bacteriophages. The main question was whether the observed bacteriolytic principle was an enzyme produced by bacterial activity or a form of tiny virus. Gradually, it became clear that it is indeed viral in nature, able to reproduce and direct the synthesis of its own enzymes.

D'Herelle summarized the early phage work in a 300 page book, *The Bacteriophage*.[7] He wrote classic descriptions of plaque formation and composition, infective centers, the lysis process, host specificity of adsorption and multiplication, the dependence of phage production on the precise state of the host, isolation of phages from sources of infectious bacteria, and the factors controlling stability of the free phage. He quickly became fascinated with the apparent role of phages in the natural control of microbial infections. He noted, for example, the frequent specificities of the phages isolated from recuperating patients for disease organisms infecting them and the rather rapid variations over time of the phage populations. Throughout his life, he worked to develop the therapeutic potential of properly selected phages against the most devastating health problems of the day. However, he initially focused on simply understanding phage biology. Thus, the first known report of successful phage therapy came from Bruynoghe & Maisin,[8] who used phage to treat staphylococcal skin infections.

After much travel, including the study of epidemics in Latin America and a year at the Pasteur branch in Saigon, d'Herelle left the Pasteur Institute in 1922. He worked in Holland and then became employed as a health officer by the League of Nations, based in Alexandria, Egypt. Phage therapy and sanitation measures were the primary tools in his arsenal to deal with major outbreaks of infectious disease throughout the Middle East and India. In 1928, he was invited to Stanford to give the prestigious Lane lectures; his discussions were published as the monograph, *The Bacteriophage and its Clinical Applications*.[9] He gave many lectures for medical schools and societies as he crossed the country. He accepted a regular faculty position at Yale, where he was supported by George Smith who had translated his first two books into English. He continued to spend summers in Paris working with the phage company he had established there and returned permanently to France in 1933.

George Eliava, director of the Georgian Institute of Microbiology, saw bacteriocidal action of the water of the Koura river in Tbilisi (Tiflis) which he could not explain until d'Herelle's bacteriophage work was published. Eliava then spent 1920–21 at the Pasteur Institute and was a very early collaborator of d'Herelle's; several phage papers of his are cited in d'Herelle.[7] The two developed the dream of founding an Institute of Bacteriophage Research in Tbilisi – to be a world center of phage therapy for infectious disease, including scientific and industrial facilities and supplied with its own experimental clinics. The dream quickly became a reality due to the support of Sergo Orjonikidze, the People's Commissar of Heavy Industry, despite KGB opposition to this "foreign project". A large campus on the river Mtkvari was allotted for the project in 1926. D'Herelle sent supplies, equipment and library materials. In 1934 and 1935, he visited Tbilisi for a total of 6 months and wrote a book on *The Bacteriophage and the Phenomenon of Recovery*,[10] which was translated into Russian by Eliava. D'Herelle intended to move to Georgia; in fact, a cottage built for his use still stands on the institute's grounds. However, in 1937, Eliava was arrested as a "people's enemy" by Beria, then head of the KGB in Georgia and soon to direct the Soviet KGB as Stalin's much-feared henchman. Eliava was soon executed, sharing the tragic fate of many Georgian and Russian progressive intellectuals of the time, and d'Herelle, disillusioned, never returned to Georgia. However, their institute survived and is still functioning at its original site on the Mtkvari (which it now shares with the more modern Institutes of Molecular Biology & Biophysics and of Animal Physiology).

In 1938, the Bacteriophage Institute was merged with the Institute of Microbiology & Epidemiology, under the direction of the People's Commissary of Health of

Georgia. In 1951, it was formally transferred to the All-Union Ministry of Health set of Institutes of Vaccine and Sera, taking on the leadership role in providing bacteriophages for therapy and bacterial typing throughout the former Soviet Union. Under orders from the Ministry of Health, hundreds of thousands of samples of pathogenic bacteria were sent to the institute from throughout the Soviet Union to isolate more effective phage strains and to better characterize their usefulness. In 1988, an official Scientific Industrial Union "Bacteriophage" was formed, centered in Tbilisi with branches in Ufa, Habarovsk and Ghorki.

Initial attempts at commercialization

From the beginning, a major commercial use of phages has been for bacterial identification through a process called *phage typing* – the use of patterns of sensitivity to a specific battery of phages to precisely identify microbial strains. This technique takes advantage of the fine specificity of many phages for their hosts and is still in common use around the world. However, the sophisticated ability of phages to destroy their bacterial hosts can also have a very negative commercial impact; phage contaminants occasionally spread havoc and financial disaster for the various fermentation industries that depend on bacteria, such as cheese production and fermentative synthesis of chemicals.[11]

Phage therapy has been evaluated extensively, with many successes being reported for a variety of diseases, including dysentery, typhoid and paratyphoid fevers, pyogenic and urinary-tract infections and cholera. Phages have been given orally, through colon infusion, as aerosols, and poured directly in lesions. They have also been given as injections: intradermal, intravascular, intramuscular, intraduodenal, intraperitoneal, and even into the lung, carotid artery and pericardium. The early strong interest in phage therapy is reflected in some 800 papers published on the topic between 1917 and 1956. These have been reviewed in some detail by Ackermann & Dubow.[12] The reported results were quite variable. Many of the physicians and entrepreneurs who initially became excited by the potential clinical implications jumped into applications with very little understanding of phages, microbiology or basic scientific process. Thus, many of the studies were anecdotal and/or poorly controlled; many of the failures were predictable, and some of the reported successes did not make much scientific sense. Often, uncharacterized phages, at unknown concentrations, were given to patients without specific bacteriological diagnosis, and there is no mention of follow-up, controls or placebos.

Much of the understanding gained by d'Herelle was ignored in this early work, and inappropriate methods of preparation, "preservatives" and storage procedures were often used. On one occasion, d'Herelle reported testing 20 preparations from various companies and finding that not one of them contained active phages! On another occasion, a preparation was advertised as containing a number of different phages, but it turned out that the technician responsible had decided it was easier to grow them up in one large batch than in separate batches. Not surprisingly, checking the product showed that one phage had outcompeted all the others, and this was not, in fact, a polyvalent preparation. In general, there was no quality control except in a few research centers. Large clinical studies were rare, and the results of those that were carried out were largely inaccessible outside of Eastern Europe.

Specific problems of early phage therapy work

In the 1940s, the new "miracle" antibiotics such as penicillin became widely available, and phage therapy was largely abandoned in the Western world. Many believe (erroneously) that it was proven not to work; however, it simply was never adequately researched. It is thus important to carefully consider the reasons for the early problems and the question of efficacy. These included:

- paucity of understanding of the heterogeneity and ecology of either the phages or the bacteria involved
- failure to select phages of high virulence against the target bacteria before using them in patients
- use of single phages in infections which involved mixtures of different bacterial species and strains
- emergence of resistant bacterial strains – this can occur by selection of resistant mutants (a frequent occurrence if only one phage strain is used against a particular bacterium) or by lysogenization (if temperate phages are used, as discussed below)
- failure to appropriately characterize or titer phage preparations, some of which were totally inactive
- failure to neutralize gastric pH prior to oral phage administration
- inactivation of phages by both specific and non-specific factors in bodily fluids
- liberation of endotoxins as a consequence of widespread lysis of bacteria within the body (the Herxheimer reaction) – this can lead to toxic shock (which can also be caused by antibiotics)
- lack of availability or reliability of bacterial laboratories for carefully identifying the pathogens involved (necessitated by the relative specificity of phage therapy).

BACTERIOPHAGE PHYSIOLOGY

Viruses are like spaceships that are able to carry genetic material between susceptible cells and then reproduce

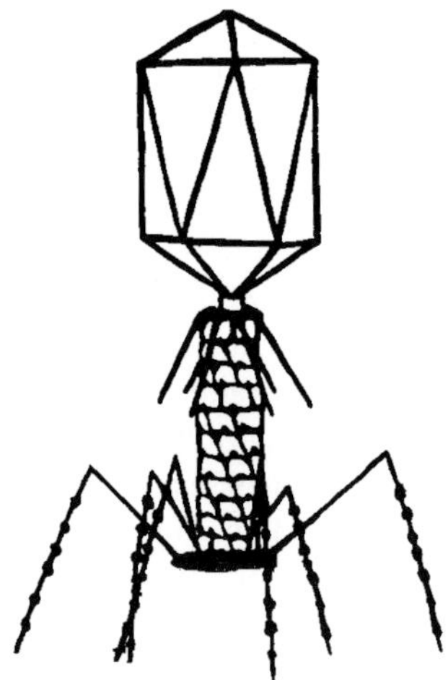

Figure 102.1 Phage diagram (bacteriophage T4).

in those cells, just as HIV specifically infects human T-lymphocytes which carry the CD-4 surface protein. In the case of bacteriophages, the targets are specific kinds of bacterial cells – they cannot infect the cells of more complex organisms. Each virus consists of a piece of genetic information, determining all of the properties of the virus, which is carried around packaged in a protein coat (Fig. 102.1). Most phages have tails, the tips of which have the ability to bind to specific molecules on the surface of their target bacteria (Fig. 102.2). The viral DNA is then ejected through the tail into the host cell, where it directs the production of progeny phages – often over 100 are produced in just half an hour. Each strain of bacteria has characteristic protein, carbohydrate and lipopolysaccharide molecules present in large quantities on its surface. These molecules are involved in forming pores, motility, and binding of the bacteria to particular surfaces. Each such molecule can act as a receptor for particular phages. Development of resistance to a particular phage generally reflects mutational loss of its specific receptor; this loss often has negative effects on the bacterium and does not protect it against the many other phages which use different receptors.

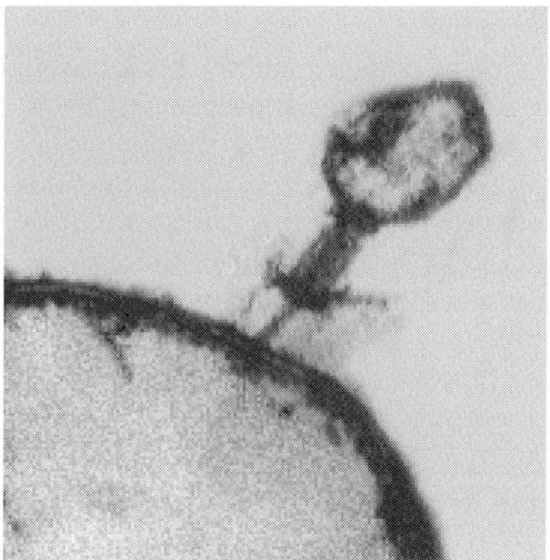

Figure 102.2 Electron micrograph of phage infecting a bacterium.

Each kind of bacterium has its own phages, which can be isolated wherever that bacterium grows: from sewage, feces, soil, even ocean depths and hot springs. The process of isolation is easy. The sample is placed in an appropriate salt solution; the supernate is separated, and then passed through a filter with a pore size small enough to remove the bacteria. The solution is then mixed (at several different dilutions) with a culture of the bacteria in question. A few drops are spread on a block of appropriate nutrient-agar medium. The next day, a dense lawn of bacteria is seen, dotted with round cleared areas called "plaques". Each plaque contains about a billion phages, all of them progeny of a single initial phage which multiplied at a high rate and destroyed the bacteria there in the process. An individual plaque is then transferred to a fresh culture of the bacteria in a liquid medium, allowing the culturing of a homogeneous stock of that particular phage, whose properties can then be studied.

Properties of phages

One major source of confusion in the early phage work was the perception that all phages were fundamentally similar, though subject to adaptive change depending on the recent conditions of growth. One consequence of this was that often new phages were isolated for each series of experiments, so there was little continuity or basis for comparison. Phages specific for virtually every known bacterial species have been isolated, but few have been well classified.

A second early source of confusion affecting therapeutic uses was the question of whether the lytic principle termed "bacteriophage" simply reflected an *inherent property* of the specific bacteria or required regular reinfection by an external agent. During the 1930s and 1940s, it became increasingly clear that in some senses both were true – that there were in fact two quite fundamentally different groups of bacteriophages. *Lytic* phages always have to infect from outside, reprogram the host cell and release a burst of phage through breaking open, or lysing, the cell after a relatively fixed interval. *Lysogenic* phages, on the other hand, have another option. They can actually integrate their DNA into the host DNA, much as HIV can integrate the DNA copy of its RNA.

Key technical developments that helped to clarify the general nature and properties of bacteriophages included:

- the concentration and purification of some large phages by means of very high-speed centrifugation and the demonstration that they contained equal amounts of DNA and protein[13]

- visualization of phages by means of the electron microscope (EM).[14,15]

Soon after, Ruska[12] reported the first attempts to use the EM for phage systematics.[16] This has since become a key tool of the field.[12] Each phage was found to have its own specific shape and size, from the "lunar lander"-style complexity of T4 and its relatives to the globular heads with long or short tails of lambda and T7, to the small filamentous phages that looked much like bacterial pili (see Fig. 102.3).

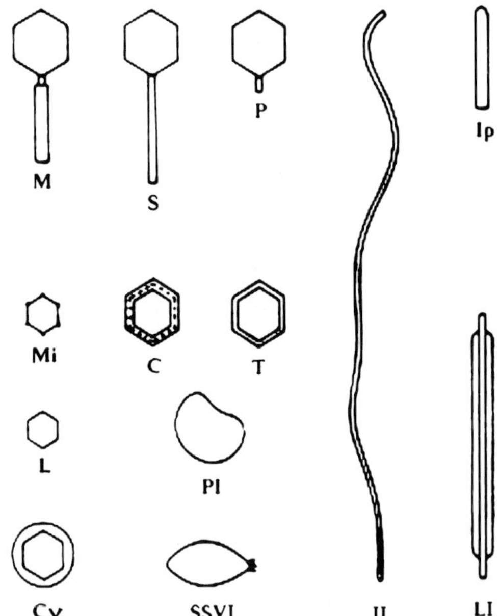

Figure 102.3 Various phages.

Lytic phages

A much better understanding of the interactions between lytic phages and bacteria began with one-step growth curve experiments.[17,18] These demonstrated an eclipse period during which the DNA began replicating, and there were no free phages in the cell; a period of accumulation of intracellular phages; and a lysis process which released the phage to go in search of new hosts. This phage infection cycle is outlined in Figure 102.4.

In 1943, an event happened which was to have a major impact on the orientation of phage research in the United States and much of western Europe, strongly shifting the emphasis from practical applications to basic science. Physicist-turned-phage biologist Max Delbrueck met with Alfred Hershey and Salvador Luria and formed the "Phage Group", which eventually expanded largely through the influence of the summer "Phage Course" at Cold Spring Harbor, Long Island, in 1945. Their influence on the origins of molecular biology has been well documented.[19,20] A major element of the successes of phages as model systems for working out fundamental biological principles was that Delbrueck convinced most phage biologists in the United States to focus on one bacterial host (*E. coli* B) and seven of its lytic phages. These were arbitrarily chosen and named T(type)1–T7. As it turned out, T2, T4 and T6 were quite similar to each

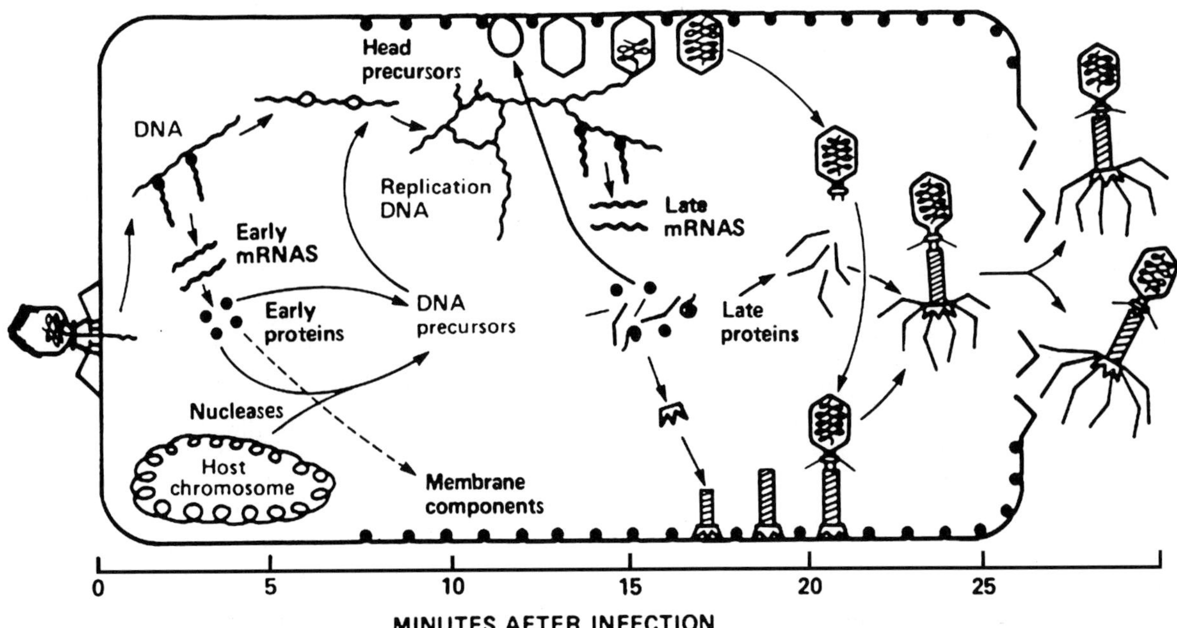

Figure 102.4 Bacteriophage intracellular growth cycle. Noteworthy features: nucleolytic action on host chromosome furnishes DNA precursors; replicating DNA is much longer than virion DNA; several phage-coded proteins become associated with the host membrane; maturation of phage head occurs at a membrane site.

other, defining a family now called the "T-even phages". These phages were key in demonstrating that DNA is the genetic material, that viruses can encode enzymes, that gene expression is mediated through special copies in the form of "messenger RNA", that the genetic code is triplet in nature, and many other fundamental concepts. The negative side of this strong focus on a few phages growing under rich laboratory conditions, however, was that there was very little study or awareness of the ranges, roles and properties of bacteriophages in the natural environment.

Lysogenic phages

The integration of lysogenic phage DNA into the host DNA leads to virtually permanent association as a *prophage* with a specific bacterium and all its progeny. The prophage directs the synthesis of a repressor, which blocks the reading of the rest of its own genes and also those of any closely related lysogenic phages – a major advantage for the bacterial cell, protecting it from infection by a significant class of phages and giving it a potential weapon against many competing bacteria. Occasionally, a prophage escapes from regulation by the repressor, cuts its DNA back out of the genome by a sort of site-specific recombination and goes ahead to make progeny phage and lyse open the cell. Sometimes the cutting-out process makes mistakes, and a few bacterial genes get carried along with the phage DNA to its new host; this process, called *transduction*, plays a significant role in bacterial genetic exchange. Such lysogenic phages are bad candidates for phage therapy, due both to their mode of inducing resistance and to the fact that they can potentially lead to transfer of genes involved in bacterial pathogenicity; this is discussed in more detail below. However, their specificity often makes them very useful for phage typing in distinguishing between bacterial strains.

CLINICAL APPLICATION

Current research

The growing understanding of phage biology has the potential to facilitate more rational thinking about the therapeutic process and the selection of therapeutic phages. However, there was generally little interaction between those who were so effectively using phages as tools to understand molecular biology and those working on phage ecology and therapeutic applications. Many in the latter group were spurred on by a concern about the increasing incidence of nosocomial infections and of bacteria resistant against most or all known antibiotics. This is particularly true in Poland, France and the former Soviet Union where use of therapeutic phages never fully died out and where there has been some ongoing research and clinical experience. In France, Dr Jean-François Vieu led the therapeutic phage efforts until his retirement some 10 years ago. He worked in the *Service des Entirobactiries* of the Pasteur Institute in Paris and, for example, prepared *Pseudomonas* phages on a case-by-case basis for patients. The experience there is discussed in Vieu[21] and Vieu et al.[22] Phage therapy was used extensively in many parts of eastern Europe as a regular part of clinical practice, and there is now a company in Moscow making phage for this purpose. However, most of the research and much of the phage preparation came under the direction of key centers in Tbilisi, Georgia, and Wroclaw, Poland. These two groups are discussed below.

Institute of Immunology and Experimental Medicine, Polish Academy of Sciences

The most detailed publications documenting phage therapy have come from Stefan Slopek's group at the Institute of Immunology and Experimental Medicine, Polish Academy of Sciences, Wroclaw. They published a series of extensive papers describing work carried out from 1981 to 1986 with 550 patients.[23–25] This set of studies involved 10 Polish medical centers, including the Wroclaw Medical Academy Institute of Surgery Cardiosurgery Clinic, Children's Surgery Clinic and Orthopedic Clinic, the Institute of Internal Diseases Nephrology Clinic, and Clinic of Pulmonary Diseases. The patients ranged in age from 1 week to 86 years. In 518 of the cases, phage use followed unsuccessful treatment with all available other antibiotics. The major categories of infections treated were:

- long-persisting suppurative fistulas
- septicemia
- abscesses
- respiratory tract suppurative infections and bronchopneumonia
- purulent peritonitis
- furunculosis.

In a final summary paper, the authors carefully analyzed the results with regard to such factors as nature and severity of the infection and monoinfection versus infection with multiple bacteria.[25] Rates of success ranged from 75 to 100% (92% overall), as measured by marked improvement, wound healing, and disappearance of titratable bacteria; 84% demonstrated full elimination of the suppurative process and healing of local wounds. Infants and children did particularly well. Not surprisingly, the poorest results came with the elderly and those in the final stages of extended serious illnesses, two groups with weakened immune systems and generally poor resistance.

The bacteriophages all came from the extensive collection of the Bacteriophage Laboratory of the Institute of

Immunology and Experimental Therapy, Polish Academy of Sciences, Wroclaw. In the later studies, some of the specific phages were named. All were virulent, capable of completely lysing the bacteria being treated. In the first study alone, 259 different phages were tested (116 for *Staphylococcus*, 42 for *Klebsiella*, 11 for *Proteus*, 39 for *Escherichia*, 30 for *Shigella*, 20 for *Pseudomonas*, and one for *Salmonella*); 40% of them were selected to be used directly for therapy. All of the treatment was in a research mode, with the phage prepared at the institute by standard methods and tested for sterility. Treatment generally involved 10 ml of sterile phage lysate orally half an hour before each meal, with gastric juices neutralized by taking (basic) Vichy water, baking soda or gelatum. In addition, phage-soaked compresses were generally applied three times a day where dictated by localized infection. Treatment ran for 1.5–14 weeks, with an average of 5.3. For intestinal problems, short treatment sufficed, while long-term use was necessary for such problems as pneumonia with pleural fistula and pyogenic arthritis. Bacterial levels and phage sensitivity were continually monitored, and the phage(s) were changed if the bacteria lost their sensitivity. Therapy was generally continued for 2 weeks beyond the last positive test for the bacteria.

Few side-effects were observed; those that were seen seemed to be directly associated with the therapeutic process. On about days 3–5, pain in the liver area was often reported, lasting several hours. The authors suggested that this might be related to the extensive liberation of endotoxins as the phage is destroying the bacteria most effectively. In severe cases with sepsis, patients often ran a fever for 24 hours on about days 7–8.[23]

Various methods of administration were successfully used, including oral, aerosols and infusion rectally or in surgical wounds. Intravenous administration was not recommended for fear of possible toxic shock from bacterial debris in the lysates.[23] However, it was clear that the phages readily entered the body from the digestive tract and multiplied internally wherever appropriate bacteria were present, as measured by their presence in blood and urine as well as by therapeutic effects.[26] This interesting and rather unexpected finding has been replicated in many studies and systems.[27–30]

Detailed notes were kept throughout on each patient. The final evaluating therapist also filled out a special inquiry form that was sent to the Polish Academy of Science research team along with the notes. The Computer Center at Wroclaw Technical University carried out extensive analyses of the data. They used the categories established in the WHO (1977) International Classification of Diseases in assessing results. They also looked at the effects of age, severity of initial condition, type(s) of bacteria involved, length of treatment and other concomitant treatments. The papers included many specific details on individual patients which helped to give some insight into the ways phage therapy was used, as well as an in-depth analysis of difficult cases.

Bacteriophage Institute, Tbilisi

The most extensive and least widely known work on phage therapy was carried out under the auspices of the Bacteriophage Institute at Tbilisi, in the former Soviet republic of Georgia. According to various physicians there, phage therapy is part of the general standard of care, used especially extensively in pediatric, burn and surgical hospital settings. Phage preparation was carried out on an industrial scale, employing 700 people just before the break-up of the Soviet Union, and many tons of a variety of products were shipped throughout the former Soviet Union. They were available both over the counter and through physicians. The largest use was in hospitals, to treat both primary and nosocomial infections, alone or in conjunction with other antibiotics and particularly when antibiotic-resistant organisms were found. The military is still one of the strongest supporters of phage therapy research and development because they have proven so useful for wound and burn infections as well as for preventing debilitating gastrointestinal epidemics among the troops.

From the institute's inception, the industrial part was run on a self-supporting basis, while its scientific branch was government-supported. The latter included the electron microscope facility, permanent strain collection, laboratories studying phages of the enterobacteria, staphylococci and pseudomonads and formulating new phage cocktails, and groups involved in immunology, vaccine production, *Lactobacillus* work and other therapeutic approaches. It also carried out the very extensive studies needed for approval by the Ministry of Health in Moscow of each new strain, therapeutic cocktail and means of delivery. This careful study of the host range, lytic spectrum and cross-resistance properties of the phages being used was a major factor in the reported successes of the phage therapy work carried out through the institute. All of the phages used for therapy are lytic, avoiding the problems engendered by lysogeny. The problems of bacterial resistance were largely solved by the use of well-chosen mixtures of phages with different receptor specificities against each type of bacterium as well as of phages against the various bacteria likely to be causing the problem in multiple infections. The situation was further improved whenever the clinicians typed the pathogenic bacteria and monitored their phage sensitivity. Where necessary, new cocktails were then prepared to which the given bacteria were sensitive. Not infrequently, using a phage in conjunction with other antibiotics was shown to give better results than either the phage or the antibiotic alone.

The depth and extent of the work involved are very

impressive. For example, in 1983–85 alone, the institute's Laboratory of Morphology and Biology of Bacteriophages carried out studies of growth, biochemical features and phage sensitivity on 2,038 strains of *Staphylococcus*, 1,128 of *Streptococcus*, 328 of *Proteus*, 373 of *P. aeruginosa*, and 622 of *Clostridium* received from clinics and hospitals in towns across the former Soviet Union. New broader-acting phage strains were isolated using these and other institute cultures and were included in a reformulation of their extensively used Piophage preparation; it now inhibited 71% of their *Staphylococcus* strains instead of 58%; 76% of *Pseudomonas* instead of 55%; 51% of *E. coli* instead of 11%; 30% of *Proteus* instead of 3%: 60% of *Streptococcus* instead of 38%; and 80% of *Enterococcus* instead of 3%.[31] In the years since, the formulation has continued to be improved based on further studies, and phages against *Klebsiella* and *Acinetobacter* have been isolated and developed into therapeutic preparations. One of the latest developments is their *IntestiPhage* preparation, which includes 23 different phages active against a range of enteric bacteria.

A good deal of work has gone into developing and providing the documentation for Ministry of Health approval of specialized new delivery systems, such as a spray for use in respiratory tract infections, in treating the incision area before surgery, and in sanitation of hospital problem areas such as operating rooms. An enteric-coated pill was also developed, using phage strains that could survive the drying process, and accounted for the bulk of the shipments to other parts of the former Soviet Union.

Much of the focus in the last 12 years has been on combating nosocomial infections, where multi-drug-resistant organisms have become a particularly lethal problem and where it is also easier to carry out proper long-term research. Clinical studies of the effectiveness of the phage treatment and appropriate protocols were carried out in collaboration with a number of hospitals, but little has been published in accessible form. Zemphira Alavidze and her colleagues, who are currently doing most of the actual therapeutic development and clinical application, have manuscripts in preparation which describe their work in institutions such as the Leningrad (St Petersburg) Intensive Burn Therapy Center, the Academy of Military Medicine in Leningrad, the Karan Trauma Center, and the Kemerovo Maternity Hospital. Some of the most intensive studies were carried out in Tbilisi at the Pediatric Hospital, the Burn Center, the Center for Sepsis and the Institute for Surgery. Special mixtures were developed for dealing with strains causing nosocomial infections in various hospitals, and they were very effectively used in sanitizing operating rooms and equipment, water taps and other sources of spread of the infections (most of them involving predominantly *Staphylococcus*). The number of sites testing positive for the problem bacteria decreased by orders of magnitude over the several months of the trial at each site.

Recent work in the West

Levin & Bull,[1] and Barrow & Soothill[4] have provided good reviews of much of the animal research carried out in Britain and the United States since interest in the possibilities of phage therapy began to resurface in the early 1980s. The results, in general, are in very good agreement with the clinical work described above in terms of efficacy, safety and importance of appropriate attention to the biology of the host–phage interactions, reinforcing trust in the reported extensive eastern European results.

In Britain, Smith & Huggins[27,28] carried out a series of excellent, well-controlled studies on the use of phages in systemic *E. coli* infections in mice and then in diarrhetic disease in young calves and pigs. For example, they found that injecting 10^6 colony-forming units of a particular pathogenic strain intramuscularly killed 10 out of 10 mice, but none died if they simultaneously injected 10^4 plaque-forming units of a phage selected against the K1 capsule antigen of that bacterial strain. This phage treatment was more effective than using such antibiotics as tetracycline, streptomycin, ampicillin or trimethoprim/sulfafurazole. Furthermore, the resistant bacteria that emerged had lost their capsule and were far less virulent. In calves, they found very high and specific levels of protection. They had to isolate different phages for each of their pathogenic bacterial strains, since they did not succeed in isolating phages specific for more general pathogenicity-related surface receptors such as the K88 or K99 adhesive fimbriae, which play key roles in attachment to the small intestine. Still, the phage was able to reduce the number of bacteria bound there by many orders of magnitude and to virtually stop the fluid loss. The results were particularly effective if the phage was present before or at the time of bacterial presentation, and if multiple phages with different attachment specificities were used. Furthermore, the phage could be transferred from animal to animal, supporting the possibility of prophylactic use in a herd. If the phage was given only after the development of diarrhea, the severity of the infection was still substantially reduced, and none of the animals died.[30]

Levin & Bull[1] carried out a detailed analysis of the population dynamics and tissue phage distribution of the 1982 Smith & Huggins[27] study, which can be helpful in assessing the parameters involved in successful phage therapy and its apparent superiority to antibiotics. They have gone on to do interesting animal studies of their own and conclude that phage therapy is at least well worth further study.[1]

Barrow & Soothill[4] carried out a series of studies preparatory to using phages for infections of burns patients.

Using guinea pigs, they showed that skin graft rejection could be prevented by prior treatment with phages against *Pseudomonas aeruginosa*. They also saw excellent protection of mice against systemic infections with both *Pseudomonas* and *Acinetobacter* when appropriate phages were used.[4] In the latter case, as few as 100 phages protected against infection with 10^8 bacteria – several times the LD_{50}!

Merrill et al[32] have carried out a series of experiments designed to better understand the interactions of phages with the human immune system, and have started a company called Exponential Therapeutics to explore the possibilities of phage therapy. Their published work has been with a lytic derivative of the lysogenic phage lambda – a poor choice for therapeutic use, as discussed above and below – but they have gathered some very interesting data about factors affecting interactions between phages and the immune system.

Bacterial pathogenicity

Most bacteria are not pathogenic; in fact, they play crucial roles in the ecological balance in the digestive system, mucous membranes and all body surfaces. They often actually help to protect against pathogens. This is one reason why broad-spectrum antibiotics have such a broad range of side-effects and why more narrowly targeted bacteriocidal agents would be highly advantageous. Interestingly, most of the serious pathogens are close relatives of non-pathogenic strains.

Studies clarifying the mechanisms of pathogenesis at the molecular level have progressed remarkably in recent years, crowned by the determination of the complete sequence of (non-pathogenic) *E. coli* K12 and several other bacterial species, and extensive cloning and sequencing of pathogenicity determinants. Generally, a number of genes are involved, and these are clustered in so-called "pathogenicity islands", or Pais, which may be 50,000–200,000 base pairs long. They generally have some unique properties indicating that the bacterium itself probably acquired them as a sort of "infectious disease" at some time in the past, and then kept them because they helped the bacterium to infect new ecological niches where there was less competition. Many of these Pais are carried on small extrachromosomal circles of DNA called *plasmids*, which can also be carriers of drug-resistance genes. Others reside in the chromosome where they are often found embedded in defective lysogenic prophages which have lost some key genes in the process and cannot be induced to form phage particles. However, they can sometimes recombine with related infecting phages. Therefore, it makes sense to avoid using lysogenic phages or their lytic derivatives for phage therapy to avoid any chance of picking up and moving such pathogenicity islands.

For bacteria in the human gut, pathogenicity involves two main factors:

- the production of toxin molecules, such as shiga toxin (from *Shigella* and some pathogenic *E. coli*) or cholera toxin; these toxins modify proteins in the target host cells and thereby cause the problem
- the acquisition of cell-surface adhesions which allow the bacterium to bind to specific receptor sites in the small intestine, rather than just moving on through to the colon.

They also all contain the components of so-called type III secretion machinery, related to those involved in the assembly of flagella (for motility) and of filamentous phages, and instrumental in many plant pathogens. For all of the pathogenic enteric bacteria, the infection process triggers changes in the neighboring intestinal cells. These include degeneration of the microvilli, formation of individual "pedestals" cupping each bacterium above the cell surface, and, in the case of *Salmonella* and *Shigella*, induction of cell-signalling molecules that trigger engulfment of the bacterium and its subsequent growth inside the cell.

Recently, *E. coli* O157 has been the subject of much concern, with contamination of such products as hamburgers and unpasteurized fruit juices leading to serious problems. Particularly in young children and the elderly, deaths have occurred from hemorrhagic colitis (bloody diarrhea) and from hemolytic-uremic syndrome, where the kidneys are affected. Antibiotic therapy has shown no benefit.[33] Our laboratory has found that the Jack-in-the-box version of O157, at least, is susceptible to several of our phages, and we plan to explore their potential use further, both as prophylactics and as therapeutic agents during outbreaks.[34]

T-even phages

A substantial fraction of the phages in the therapeutic mixes are relatives of bacteriophage T4, which has played such a key role in the development of molecular biology. This family is generally called the T-even phages, an historical accident reflecting the fact that T2, T4 and T6 from the original collection of Delbrueck's Phage Group all turned out to be related. Large sets of T-even phages have been isolated for study from all over the world: Long Island sewage treatment plants, animals in the Denver zoo, and dysentery patients in eastern Europe (the latter using *Shigella* as host). Members of the family are found infecting all of the enteric bacteria and their relatives.[35] Most of the T-even phages use 5-hydroxymethylcytosine instead of cytosine in their DNA, which protects them against most of the restriction enzymes that bacteria make to protect themselves against invaders and gives them a much more effective host range. T4's entire DNA sequence is known, and we know a great deal about its infection process in standard laboratory conditions and about the methods it uses to target bacteria so effectively.[36,37] We can potentially use this knowledge to develop more targeted approaches to phage therapy, particularly as more is learned about the similarities and differences in its extended family.[38,39] We know that different members of the T-even family use different outer membrane proteins and oligosaccharides as their receptors, and we understand the tail-fiber structures involved well enough to potentially predict which phages will work on given bacteria and to engineer phages with new specificities.[40,41]

The T-even bacteriophages share a unique ability which contributes significantly to their widespread occurrence in nature and to their competitive advantage. There have still been far too few studies of T4 ecology and its behavior under conditions more closely approaching the natural environment and the circumstances it will encounter in phage therapy – often anaerobic and/or with frequent periods of starvation. The limited available information in that regard was summarized by Kutter et al.[36,37] A variety of studies are shedding light on the ability of these highly virulent phages to coexist in balance with their hosts in nature. For example, they can reproduce in the absence of oxygen as long as their bacterial host has been growing anaerobically for several generations. They are also able to control the timing of lysis in response to the relative availability of bacterial hosts in their environment. When *E. coli* are singly infected with T4, they lyse after 25–30 minutes at body temperature in rich media, releasing about 100–200 phages/cell. However, when additional T-even phages attack the cell more than 4 minutes after the initial infection, the cell does not lyse at the normal time. Instead, it continues to make phages for as long as 6 hours.[42,43] We have found that they can also survive for a period of time in a hibernation-like state inside starved cells, allowing their host to readapt when nutrients are again supplied, and produce a few additional phages. This is particularly interesting and important since bacteria undergo many drastic changes to survive periods of starvation which increase their resistance to a variety of environmental insults.[44]

Thus, for many reasons, the T-even phages make excellent candidates for therapeutic use in enteric and other Gram-negative bacteria, and studies of their ecology and distribution are being carried out with these goals in mind both in Tbilisi and at Evergreen State College.

Advantages of phages

Phages have many potential advantages:

- They are self-replicating but also self-limiting because they will multiply only as long as sensitive bacteria are present.
- They can be targeted far more specifically than most antibiotics to the problem bacteria, causing much less damage to the normal microbial balance in the gut. The bacterial imbalance or "dysbiosis" caused by many antibiotic treatments can lead to serious secondary infections involving relatively resistant bacteria, often extending hospitalization time, expense and mortality (see Chs 7 and 9). Particular resultant problems include *Pseudomonads*, which are especially difficult to treat, and *Clostridium difficile*, the cause of serious diarrhea and membranous colitis.[45]
- Phages can often be targeted to receptors on the bacterial surface which are involved in pathogenesis, so any resistant mutants are attenuated in virulence.
- Few side-effects have been reported for phage therapy.
- Phage therapy would be particularly useful for people with allergies to antibiotics.
- Appropriately selected phages can easily be used prophylactically to help prevent bacterial disease at times of exposure or to sanitize hospitals and to help protect against hospital-acquired (nosocomial) infections.
- Especially for external applications, phages can be prepared fairly inexpensively and locally, facilitating their potential applications to underserved populations.
- Phages can be used either independently or in conjunction with other antibiotics to help reduce the development of bacterial resistance.

CONCLUSION

Clearly the time has come to look more carefully at the potential of phage therapy, both by strongly supporting new research and by looking carefully at the research already available.[46] As Barrow & Soothill[4] conclude:

> Phage therapy can be very effective in certain conditions and has some unique advantages over antibiotics. With the increasing incidence of antibiotic-resistant bacteria and a deficit in the development of new classes of antibiotics to counteract them, there is a need to investigate the use of phage in a range of infections.

Phages are quite specific as to the bacteria they attack, and the stipulations of Ackermann & DuBow[12] are important here. The specificity of phages means that:

> Phages have to be tested [against the bacteria] just as antibiotics, and the indications have to be right, but this holds everywhere in medicine. However, phage therapy requires the creation of phage banks and a close collaboration between the clinician and the laboratory. Phages have at least one advantage. ... While the concentration of antibiotics decreases from the moment of application, phage numbers should increase. Another advantage is that phages are able to spread and thus prevent disease. Nonetheless, much research remains to be done ... on the stability of therapeutic preparations; clearance of phages from blood and tissues; their multiplication in the human body; inactivation by antibodies, serum or pus; and the release of bacterial endotoxins by lysis. ... In addition, therapeutic phages should be characterized at least by electron microscopy.

While it seems premature to broadly introduce injectable phage preparations in the West without further extensive research, their carefully implemented use in gut and external applications and for a variety of agricultural purposes could potentially help to reduce the emergence of antibiotic-resistant strains. Furthermore, compassionate use of appropriate phages seems warranted in cases where bacteria resistant against all available antibiotics are causing life-threatening illness. They are especially useful in dealing with recalcitrant nosocomial infections, where large numbers of particularly vulnerable people are being exposed to the same strains of bacteria in a closed hospital setting. In this case, the environment as well as the patients can be effectively treated.

REFERENCES

1. Levin B, Bull JJ. Phage therapy revisited: the population biology of a bacterial infection and its treatment with bacteriophage and antibiotics. Am Nat 1996; 147: 881–898
2. Lederberg J. Smaller fleas ... *ad infinitum*: therapeutic bacteriophage. PNAS 1996; 93: 3167–3168
3. Radetsky P. Return of the good virus. Discover 1996; 17: 50–58
4. Barrow PA, Soothill JS. Bacteriophage therapy and prophylaxis: rediscovery and renewed assessment of the potential. Trends Microbiol 1997; 5: 268–271
5. Hankin EH. L'action bactericide des eaux de la Jumna et du Gange sur le vibrion du cholera. Ann de l'Inst Pasteur 1896; 10: 511
6. D'Herelle F, Twort FW, Bordet J, Gratia A. Discussion on the bacteriophage (bacteriolysin): from the Ninetieth Annual Meeting of the British Medical Association, Glasgow, July, 1922. Br Med J 1922; 2: 289–297; reproduced in Stent G. Papers on bacterial viruses. 2nd edn. Boston: Little, Brown. 1965
7. D'Herelle F. (trans. by G.H. Smith) The bacteriophage: its role in immunity. Baltimore: Williams and Wickens/Waverly Press. 1922
8. Bruynoghe R, Maisin J. Essais de therapeutique au moyen du bacteriophage du staphylocoque. C R Soc Biol 1921; 85: 1120–1121
9. D'Herelle F. The bacteriophage and its clinical applications. Springfield: CC Thomas. 1930
10. Eliava G. Bakteriofagi fenomenvyzdorovieniya. Tbilisi: Tbilis National University Publications. 1935
11. Saunders ME. Bacteriophages in industrial fermentationsin. In: Webster R, Granoff A, eds. Encyclopedia of virology. San Diego, CA: Academic Press. 1994: p 116–121
12. Ackermann HW, DuBow M. Viruses of prokaryotes I: general properties of bacteriophages, Ch. 7. Practical applications of bacteriophages. Florida: CRC Press, Boca Raton. 1987
13. Schlesinger M. Reindarstellung eines bakteriophagen in mit freiem auge sichtbaren mengen. Biochem. Z. 1933; 264: 6
14. Ruska H. Die sichtbarmachung der bakteriophagen lyse im ubermikroskop. Naturwissenschaften, 1940; 28: 45
15. Pfankuch E, Kausche G. Isolierung U. Uebermikroskopische abbildung eines bakteriophagen. Naturwissenschaften 1940; 28: 46
16. Ruska H. Ergeb. Hyg Bakteriol Immunforsch Exp Ther 1943; 25: 437
17. Ellis EL, Delbrueck M. The growth of bacteriophage. J Gen Physiol 1939; 22: 365–384
18. Doermann AD. The intracellular growth of bacteriophages. I. Liberation of intracellular bacteriophage T4 by premature lysis with another phage or with cyanide. J. Gen. Physiol. 1952; 35: 645–656
19. Cairns J, Stent G, Watson J. Phage and the origins of molecular biology. Long Island, NY: Cold Spring Harbor Laboratory Press. 1966
20. Fischer E, Lipson C. Thinking about science: Max Delbrueck and the origins of molecular biology. New York, NY: W.W. Norton. 1988
21. Vieu JF. Les bacteriophages. In: Fabre J., ed. Traite de therapeutique, Vol. Serums et vaccins. Paris: Flammarion. 1975: p 337–340b
22. Vieu JF, Guillermet F, Minck R, Nicolle P. Données actuelles sur les applications therapeutiques des bacteriophages. Bull Acad Natl Med 1979; 163: 61
23. Slopek S, Durlakova I, Weber-Dabrowska B et al. Results of bacteriophage treatment of suppurative bacterial infections I. General evaluation of the results. Arch Immunol Ther Exp 1983; 31: 267–291
24. Slopek S, Kucharewica-Krukowska A, Weber-Dabrowska B, Dabrowski M. Results of bacteriophage treatment of suppurative bacterial infections VI. Analysis of treatment of suppurative staphylococcal infections. Arch Immunol Ther Exp 1985; 33: 261–273
25. Slopek S, Weber-Dabrowska B, Dabrowski M, Kucharewica-Krukowska A. Results of bacteriophage treatment of suppurative bacterial infections in the years 1981–1986. Arch Immunol Ther Exp 1987; 35: 569–583
26. Weber-Dabrowska B, Dabrowski M, Slopek S. Studies on bacteriophage penetration in patients subjected to phage therapy. Archium Immunologiae et Therapiae Experimentalis 1987; 35: 363–368
27. Smith HW, Huggins RB. Successful treatment of experimental E. coli infections in mice using phage: its general superiority over antibiotics. J. Gen. Microbiology 1982; 128: 307–318
28. Smith HW, Huggins RB. Effectiveness of phages in treating experimental E. coli diarrhoea in calves, piglets and lambs. J. Gen. Microbiology 1983; 129: 2659–2675
29. Smith HW, Huggins RB. The control of experimental E. coli diarrhea in calves by means of bacteriophage. J Gen Microbiology 1987; 133: 1111–1126
30. Smith HW, Huggins RB, Shaw KM. Factors influencing the survival and multiplication of bacteriophages in calves and in their environment. J Gen Microbiology 1987; 133: 1127–1135
31. Alavidze Z. Personal communication.
32. Merrill C, Biswis B, Carlton R et al. Long-circulating bacteriophages as antibacterial agents. PNAS 1996; 93: 3188–3192
33. Greenwald D, Brandt L. Recognizing E. coli O157: H7 infection. Hospital Practice 1997; April 15: 123–140
34. Mueller M, Smith S, Kutter E. Unpublished data, 1997
35. Ackermann H, Krisch H. A catalogue of T4-type bacteriophages. Archiv Virol 1997; 142: 2329–2345
36. Kutter E, Kellenberger E, Carlson K et al. Effects of bacterial growth conditions and physiology on T4 infection. In: Karam JD, ed. Molecular biology of bacteriophage T4. Washington, DC: American Society for Microbiology. 1994: p 406–420
37. Kutter E, Stidham T, Guttman B et al. Genomic map of bacteriophage T4. In: Karam JD, ed. Molecular biology of bacteriophage T4. Washington, DC: American Society for Microbiology. 1994: p 491–519
38. Jacob F, Monod J. Genetic regulatory mechanisms in the synthesis of proteins. J Mol Biol 1961; 3: 318–356
39. Kutter E, Gachechiladze K, Poglazov A et al. Evolution of T4-related phages. Virus Genes 1996; 11: 285–297
40. Henning U, Hashemolhosseini S. Receptor recognition by T-even-type coliphages. In: Karam JD, ed. Molecular biology of bacteriophage T4. Washington, DC: American Society for Microbiology. 1994: p 291–298
41. Krisch H. Personal communication
42. Doermann AH. Lysis and lysis inhibition with *E. coli* bacteriophage. J Bacteriol 1948; 55: 257–275
43. Abedon S. Lysis and the interaction between free phages and infected cells. In: Karam JD, ed. Molecular biology of bacteriophage T4. Washington, DC: American Society for Microbiology. 1994: p 397–405
44. Kolter R. Life and death in stationary phase. ASM News 1992; 58: 75–79
45. Fekety R. Antibiotic-associated diarrhea and colitis. Cur Opin Infect Dis 1995; 8: 391–397
46. Alisky J, Iczkonski K, Rapoport A et al. Bacteriophage shows promise as antimicrobial agents. J Infection 1998; 36: 5–13

CHAPTER CONTENTS

103

Phosphatidylserine

Michael T. Murray, ND

Joseph E. Pizzorno Jr, ND

INTRODUCTION

Phosphatidylserine is the major phospholipid in the brain, where it plays a major role in determining the integrity and fluidity of cell membranes. Normally the brain can manufacture sufficient levels of phosphatidylserine, but if there is a deficiency of methyl donors like S-adenosylmethionine (SAM), folic acid, and vitamin B_{12}, or essential fatty acids, the brain may not be able to make sufficient phosphatidylserine. Low levels of phosphatidylserine in the brain are associated with impaired mental function and depression in the elderly.

PHYSIOLOGICAL FUNCTIONS

Phosphatidylserine is responsible for many functions essential to the structural matrix and function of cell membranes. With the help of phosphatidylserine and other phospholipid components, the cell membranes control:

- the cellular exchange of nutrients and waste products
- movement of electrolytes into and out of cells
- reception of molecular messages from outside the cell
- transformation of messages into enzymatic responses
- cell movement and shape
- cell-to-cell recognition and communication.

Although phosphatidylserine is found in every cell type in the body, it plays an especially vital role in nerve tissue. It is critical in membrane-to-membrane fusion – a key process in neurotransmitter release – as well as activating cell surface receptors and supporting the transmission of chemical signals.

PHARMACOLOGY

The pharmacology of phosphatidylserine appears to be a result of restoring proper levels of phosphatidylserine in cell membranes. As a result, cellular function improves. This improvement is most notable in brain tissue. Phosphatidylserine supplementation in animal studies has been shown to significantly improve acetylcholine release, memory, and age-related brain changes.[1–3] Presumably these effects are responsible for the positive effects noted in human clinical trials.

Absorption studies in animals indicate that phosphatidylserine is well absorbed orally. Absorption of phosphatidylserine is very similar to the absorption of phosphatidylcholine, the major component of soy lecithin. Like phosphatidylcholine, with absorption into the intestinal cell the lipid component at position 2 is cleaved from the glycerol backbone. This lysoform of phosphatidylserine is then re-esterified by the enterocyte and transported to various tissues where (presumably) it is reacylated with a specific fatty acid depending upon where it is being delivered. For example, in the brain most of the phosphatidylserine incorporates oleic acid (C18:1n9) or docosahexanoic acid (C22:6n3, DHA) while in the testes C:14:0 and arachidonic acid (C20:4n6) are the major forms.

Originally, phosphatidylserine was isolated from bovine brain, but with the concern for bovine spongiform encephalopathy (mad cow disease) an alternative preparation derived from soy was developed. Commercially available phosphatidylserine is now a semi-synthetic product manufactured from soy lecithin. In the United States phosphatidylserine is available in a complex containing the following:

- phosphatidylserine – 100 mg
- phosphatidylcholine – 45 mg
- phosphatidyethanolamine – 25 mg
- phosphatidylinositol – 5 mg.

The effectiveness of the soy-derived phosphatidylserine has yet to be proven as all of the published clinical studies to date have utilized bovine phosphatidylserine. The difference between the two is that the bovine source has predominantly DHA at the 2 position while the soy preparation has primarily linoleic acid (C18:2n6). Given DHA's critical role in brain metabolism, until soy phosphatidylserine is shown to produce results equal to that achieved with bovine phosphatidylserine, co-supplementation with DHA should be encouraged when using phosphatidylserine from soy sources.

CLINICAL APPLICATIONS

The primary use of phosphatidylserine is in the treatment of depression and/or impaired mental function in the elderly including Alzheimer's disease. To date there have been 11 double-blind studies completed with phosphatidylserine in the treatment of age-related cognitive decline, Alzheimer's disease or depression. Good results have been obtained with these studies.[4–9] In the largest study, a total of 494 elderly patients (aged between 65 and 93 years) with moderate to severe senility were given either phosphatidylserine (100 mg three times daily) or a placebo for 6 months.[4] The patients were assessed for mental performance, behavior, and mood at the beginning and the end of the study. Statistically significant ($P < 0.01$) improvements in mental function, mood, and behavior were noted in the phosphatidylserine-treated group.

Phosphatidylserine appears to positively affect mood in depressed elderly subjects.[10–14] This effect could also explain some of phosphatidylserine's positive effects on memory and cognition. The link between depression and impaired mental function is well-established in the geriatric population. In one small double-blind study of 10 depressed elderly patients, phosphatidylserine was shown to improve depressive symptoms, memory and behavior.[15] Unlike typical antidepressant drugs, phosphatidylserine promoted this improvement without influencing the levels of serotonin and other monoamine neurotransmitters, suggesting another mechanism of action. Improved brain cell membrane fluidity may be one explanation. Another is the fact that phosphatidylserine has been shown to reduce cortisol secretion in response to stress.[16–18] Typically, cortisol levels will be elevated in depressed patients.

DOSAGE

The standard dosage recommendation for phosphatidylserine is 100 mg three times daily.

TOXICOLOGY

No side-effects or adverse interactions have been reported. Animal studies have shown that phosphatidylserine from bovine sources given orally is extremely well tolerated. Dogs tolerated up to 70 g/day for 1 year without any apparent side-effect. In over 35 clinical studies involving more than 800 subjects, phosphatidylserine has been shown to be without side-effect at standard dosage (100 mg three times daily). Rarely, stomach upset has been reported and a large dose (e.g. 600 mg) taken prior to retiring may produce sleeplessness.

REFERENCES

1. Vannucchi MG, Casamenti F, Pepeu G. Decrease of acetylcholine release from cortical slices in aged rats. Investigations into its reversal by phosphatidylserine. J Neurochem 1990; 55: 819–825
2. Valzelli L, Kozak W, Zanotti A et al. Activity of phosphatidylserine on memory retrieval and on exploration in mice. Meth Find Exptl Clin Pharmacol 1987; 9: 657–660
3. Nunzi MG, Milan F, Guidolin D et al. Effects of phosphatidylserine administration on age-related structural changes in the rat hippocampus and septal complex. Pharmacopsychiat 1989; 22: 125–128
4. Cenacchi T, Betoldin R, Farina C et al. Cognitive decline in the elderly. A double-blind, placebo-controlled multicenter study on efficacy of phosphatidylserine administration. Aging 1993; 5: 123–133
5. Engel RR, Satzer W, Gunterh W et al. Double-blind cross-over study of phosphatidylserine vs. placebo in patients with early dementia of the Alzheimer type. Eur Neuropsychopharmacol 1992; 2: 149–155
6. Crook T, Petrie W, Ells C et al. Effects of phosphatidylserine in Alzheimer's disease. Psychopharmacol Bull 1992; 28: 61–66
7. Crook TH, Tinklenberg J, Yesavage J et al. Effects of phosphatidylserine in age-associated memory impairment. Neurology 1991; 41: 644–649
8. Funfgeld EW, Baggen M, Nedwidek P et al. Double-blind study with phosphatidylserine (PS) in parkinsonian patients with senile dementia of Alzheimer's type (SDAT). Prog Clin Biol Res 1989; 317: 1235–1246
9. Amaducci L. Phosphatidylserine in the treatment of Alzheimer's disease. Results of a multicenter study. Psychopharmacol Bull 1988; 24: 1030–1034
10. Nerozzi D, Aceti F, Meila E et al. Phosphatidylserine in age-related disturbance of memory. Clin Terapeutica 1987; 120: 399–404
11. Palmieri G. Double-blind controlled trial of phosphatidylserine in patients with senile mental deterioration. Clin Trials J 1987; 24: 73–83
12. Ransmayr G. Double-blind placebo-controlled trial of phosphatidylserine in elderly patients with arteriosclerotic encephalopathy. Clin Trials J 1987; 24: 67–72
13. Villardita C. Multicentre clinical trial of brain phosphatidylserine in elderly patients with intellectual deterioration. Clin Trials J 1987; 24: 84–93
14. Delwaide PJ, Gyselynck-Mambourg AM, Hurlet A et al: Double-blind, randomized controlled study of phosphatidylserine in senile demented patients. Effect of phosphatidylserine in senile demented patients. Acta Neurol Scand 1986; 73: 136–140
15. Maggioni M, Picotti GM, Bondiolotti GP et al. Effects of phosphatidylserine therapy in geriatric patients with depressive disorders. Acta Psychiatr Scand 1990; 81: 265–270
16. Monteleone P, Beinat L, Tanzillo C et al. Effects of phosphatidylserine on the neuroendocrine response to physical stress in humans. Neuroendocrinology 1990; 52: 243–248
17. Monteleone P, Maj M, Beinat L et al. Blunting chronic phosphatidylserine administration of the stress-induced activation of the hypothalamo-pituitary-adrenal axis in healthy men. Eur J Clin Pharamacol 1992; 41: 385–388
18. Nerozzi D, Aceti F, Melia E et al. Early cortisol escape phenomenon reversed by phosphatidylserine in elderly normal subjects. Clinical Trial J 1989; 26: 33–38

CHAPTER CONTENTS

104

Piper mythisticum (kava)

Michael T. Murray, ND

Joseph E. Pizzorno Jr, ND

Piper methysticum (family: Piperaceae)
Common name: kava

GENERAL DESCRIPTION

Kava is a hardy, slow-growing perennial that generally resembles other members of the pepper family. It is an attractive shrub and can attain heights of more than 9 feet. The plant does not have many leaves, but those it does have are thin, single, heart-shaped, alternate, petiolate, 4–10 inches long, and sometimes wider than they are long. Although *Piper methysticum* does flower, it is incapable of self-reproduction; its propagation is vegetative and now solely due to human effort.[1,2]

For medicinal purposes, it is the rootstock that is used. The rootstock is knotty, thick, and sometimes tuberous with holes or cracks created by partial destruction of the parenchyma. In other words, the rootstock is often somewhat pithy. From the main rootstock, there are extensions of lateral roots up to 9 feet long.[1,2]

CHEMICAL COMPOSITION

Analysis of the composition of the dried kava rootstock indicates that it contains approximately 43% starch, 12% water, 3.2% simple sugars, 3.6% proteins, 3.2% minerals (primarily potassium), and 15% kavalactones (see Table 104.1).[1,2]

Based on detailed analysis of the active ingredients of kava, a laborious process over the past 110 years, many experts now believe that the pharmacological activities of kava are due mostly, if not entirely, to the presence of compounds known as kavalactones (also referred to as kava alpha-pyrones). These compounds are found in the fat-soluble resin of the root. Although the kavalactones are the primary active components, other components appear to contribute to the sedative and anxiolytic activities of kava, as one study found the sedative activity of a crude preparation to be more effective than the

Table 104.1 Kavalactones

Compound	R	R′	R″	R‴	C5–6	C7–8
Kavain					–	=
7,8-Dihydrokavain					–	–
5,6-Dihydrokavain					–	=
Yangonin	OMe				=	=
5,6,7,8-Tetrahydroyangonin	OMe				–	–
Methysticin	O-CH_2-O				–	=
Dihydromethysticin	O-CH_2-O				–	–
5,6-Dehydromethysticin	O-CH_2-O				=	=
5,6-Dihydroyangonin	OMe				–	=
7,8-Dihydroyangonin	OMe				–	=
10-Methoxy-yangonin	OMe		OMe		=	=
11-Methoxy-yangonin	OMe	OMe			=	=
11-Hydroxy-yangonin	OMe	HO			=	=
Hydroxykavain				OH	–	=
11-Methoxy-12-hydroxy dehydrokavain	OH	OMe			=	=

Figure 104.1 Kavalactones.

isolated kavalactones (Fig. 104.1).[3] The kavalactone content of the root can vary between 3 and 20%.

HISTORY AND FOLK USE

Oceania, i.e. the Pacific island communities of Micronesia, Melanesia, and Polynesia, is one of the few geographic areas of the world that did not have alcoholic beverages before European contact in the 18th century. However, these islanders did possess a "magical" drink used in ceremonies and celebrations because of its calming effect and ability to promote sociability. The drink, also called kava, is still used today in this region of the world, where the people are often referred to as the happiest and friendliest in the world.

The origins of kava usage are not known as it predates written history in Oceania.[1,2] It was first described for the Western world by captain James Cook in the account of his voyage to the South Seas in 1768.

Many myths and legends surround the early use of kava. The plant itself probably originated in the New Guinea/Indonesia area and was spread from island to island by early Polynesian explorers in canoes, along with other plants. Each culture has its own story on the origins of kava. For example, in Samoa a story is told about the origins of kava and sugar cane. The story goes that a Samoan girl went to Fiji where she married a great chief. After some time, she returned to Samoa, but before doing so, she noticed two plants growing on a hill. She saw a rat chewing on one of the plants and noticed that the rat seemed to go to sleep. She concluded that the plant was a comforting food. She decided she would take this plant, sugar cane, back to Samoa, but then she noticed that the rat awoke and began to chew the root of another plant – kava. The animal which had been weak and shy became bold, strong, and more energetic. She decided that she would take both plants back with her to plant in Samoa. The plants grew very well in Samoa and soon a chief from a neighboring island exchanged two laying hens for roots of the two plants. Hence, the Samoans take credit for the spread of both the sugar cane and kava.

In Tonga, a legend is told about a great chief named Loau who lived on the island of Euaiki. He went to visit his servant Feva' anga, who wanted to give a feast in honor of the chief, but it was a time of great famine. In desperation, he and his wife killed and cooked their only daughter to be served to the chief. However, Loau recognized the human flesh in the food when it was served and would not eat it. He instructed Feva' anga to plant the food in the ground and to bring him the plant that would spring forth. On receiving the mature plant, Loau instructed that a drink be prepared from it and consumed with due ceremony.

The kava ceremony

Regardless of exactly how kava originated, it has been used in ceremonies by the Oceanic people for thousands of years. There are three basic kava ceremonies: the full ceremonial as enacted on every formal occasion; the one performed at the meeting of village elders, chiefs, and nobles and for visiting chiefs and dignitaries; and the less formal kava circle common on social occasions.[1,2]

The first step of any kava ceremony was the preparation of the beverage. A description of the classic process was written in 1777 by Georg Forster, a young naturalist on James Cook's second Pacific voyage:

[Kava] is made in the most disgustful manner that can be imagined, from the juice contained in the roots of a species of pepper-tree. This root is cut small, and the pieces chewed by several people, who spit the macerated mass into a bowl, where some water (milk) of coconuts is poured upon it. They then strain it through a quantity of fibres of coconuts, squeezing the chips, till all their juices mix with the coconut-milk; and the whole liquor is decanted into another bowl. They swallow this nauseous stuff as fast as possible; and some old topers value themselves on being able to empty a great number of bowls.

As this traditional method of preparation became frowned upon or made illegal by colonial governments and missionaries, more "sanitary" methods of preparation, involving grinding or grating, took its place in many parts of Oceania.

The full kava ceremony, reserved for very highly honored guests, involves leading all of the guests to a platform. The ceremony begins with the arrival of a group of young men dressed in ceremonial attire and carrying a bowl of the kava drink and necessary utensils. The bowl is placed between the kava preparers and the visitors. The kava is placed in a cup by a specially selected individual who then turns and faces the visitor and delivers the beverage to the chief guest. The guest is instructed to hold the cup with both hands and drink from it. If the whole cup is drained without stopping, everyone says "a maca" (pronounced "a matha," meaning "it is empty") and claps three times with cupped hands. The cup bearer then returns to the kava bowl and proceeds to serve the person next in rank or importance.

Important people who visit Fiji and other islands of Oceania still participate in the kava ceremonies. For example, during a 1992 presidential campaign visit to Hawaii, Hillary Clinton participated in a kava ceremony conducted by the Samoan community on O'ahu.

The effects of drinking kava

Kava drinkers relate a pleasant sense of tranquillity and sociability upon consumption. Subjective reports given by scientists who have sampled kava themselves are relatively abundant. One of the first scientific studies of kava was performed by the noted pharmacologist Louis Lewin in 1886. A later description written in 1927 is as follows:[1]

When the mixture is not too strong, the subject attains a state of happy unconcern, well-being and contentment, free of physical or psychological excitement. At the beginning, conversation comes in a gentle, easy flow and hearing and sight are honed, becoming able to perceive subtle shades of sound and vision. Kava soothes temperaments. The drinker never becomes angry, unpleasant, quarrelsome or noisy, as happens with alcohol. Both natives and whites consider kava as a means of easing moral discomfort. The drinker remains master of his consciousness and his reason. When consumption is excessive, however, the limbs become tired, the muscles seem no longer to respond to the orders and control of the mind, walking becomes slow and unsteady and the drinker looks partially inebriated. He feels the need to lie down.... He is overcome by somnolence and finally drifts off to sleep.

A more recent description is provided by researcher R. J. Gregory, who writes from his own experience:

Kava seizes one's mind. This is not a literal seizure, but something does change in the processes by which information enters, is retrieved, or leads to actions as a result. Thinking is certainly affected by the kava experience, but not in the same ways as are found from caffeine, nicotine, alcohol, or marijuana. I would personally characterize the changes I experienced as going from lineal processing of information to a greater sense of "being" and contentment with being. Memory seemed to be enhanced, whereas restriction of data inputs was strongly desired, especially with regard to disturbances of light, movements, noise and so on. Peace and quiet were very important to maintain the inner sense of serenity. My senses seemed to be unusually sharpened, so that even whispers seemed to be loud while loud noises were extremely unpleasant.

Drinking about half a coconut shell (100–150 mL) of certain varieties of kava is enough to put most people into a deep, dreamless sleep within 30 minutes. Unlike alcohol and other sedatives, kava does not produce any morning hangover. The kava drinker awakens having fully recovered normal physical and mental capacities.

PHARMACOLOGY

Many of the first comprehensive studies on the activities of kavalactones were conducted by a team of scientists from the Freiburg University Institute of Pharmacology in Germany, led by Hans J. Meyer, during the 1950s and 1960s.[3] This research determined that kavalactones exhibit sedative, analgesic, anticonvulsant, and muscle-relaxant effects in laboratory animals. These studies seemed to confirm earlier empirical and subjective observations. More recent studies have utilized better-defined kava extracts.

Isolated kavalactones compared with crude extracts

Some evidence suggests that the whole complex of kavalactones and other compounds naturally found in kava produce greater pharmacological activity. In addition, studies have shown that kavalactones are more rapidly absorbed when given orally as an extract of the root rather than as the isolated kavalactones. The bioavailability of lactones, as measured by peak plasma concentrations, is up to three to five times higher from the extract than when given as isolated substances.[3] Further evidence that kava root extracts are superior to isolated kavalactones is offered by an animal study showing that while isolated kavalactones are well absorbed by brain, crude kava preparations produce brain concentrations of lactones two to 20 times higher.[4] This evidence suggests that crude extracts standardized for kavalactone content may offer the greatest therapeutic benefit.

Several clinical trials have featured a kava extract standardized to contain 70% kavalactones. However, this high percentage of kavalactones may be sacrificing some of the other constituents that may contribute to the pharmacology of kava. More important than the actual percentage of kavalactones is the total dosage of the kavalactones and the assurance that the full range of kavalactones and other important constituents are present.

Standardized preparations of kava are now gaining greater popularity in Europe and the United States as mild sedatives and anxiolytics.

Sedative effects

Recent studies have confirmed and/or elaborated on the sedative effects of kava. Most notable are studies demonstrating that kavalactones exert many of their effects through non-traditional mechanisms. For example, most sedative drugs including the benzodiazepines (e.g. Valium, Halcion, Tranxene, etc.) work by binding to specific receptors (benzodiazepine or GABA receptors) in the brain which then leads to the neurochemical changes (potentiation of GABA effects) which promote sedation. Studies in animals have shown that the kavalactones do not bind to benzodiazepine or GABA receptors.[5] Instead, the kavalactones are thought to somehow modify receptor domains rather than interacting specifically with receptor binding sites. In addition, other studies have indicated that the kavalactones appear to act primarily on the limbic system, the ancient part of the brain which affects all other brain activities and is the principle seat of the emotions.[6] It is thought that kava may also promote sleep by altering the way in which the limbic system modulates emotional processes. It appears that many of the laboratory models of identifying how a substance works to promote a calming effect are simply not sophisticated enough to evaluate the physiological effects of kava.

Analgesic effects

In another example of the unusual pharmacological qualities of kava, a study designed to evaluate its pain-relieving effects could not demonstrate any binding to opiate receptors.[7] The significance of this finding is that the study used experimental models where non-opiate analgesics like aspirin and other non-steroidal anti-inflammatory drugs are ineffective. In addition, it was determined that the sedative or muscle-relaxing effects were not responsible for the pain-relieving effects. These findings indicate that kava reduces pain in a manner unlike morphine, aspirin, or any other pain reliever.

Anxiolytic effects

An interesting effect of kava compared with other anxiolytics is that unlike the drugs, kava does not lose effectiveness with time. Kavalactones, even when administered in large dosages, demonstrated no loss of effectiveness in animal studies.[8] Again, this is another example of the unusual qualities of kava.

Anti-ischemia effects

Another pharmacological activity of kava of importance is its ability to protect against brain damage due to ischemia.[9] This effect has been demonstrated in two animal models of focal cerebral ischemia. The effectiveness of the kavalactones was due to its ability to limit the infarct area as well as provide a mild anticonvulsant effect. Kava extract may prove useful in the recovery from a stroke.

CLINICAL APPLICATIONS

Several European countries have approved kava preparations in the treatment of nervous anxiety, insomnia, and restlessness on the basis of detailed pharmacological data and favorable clinical studies.

Anxiety

Early clinical trials used D,L-kavain, a purified kavalactone, at a dose of 400 mg/day. For example, in one double-blind placebo-controlled study of 84 patients with anxiety symptoms, kavain was shown to improve vigilance, memory, and reaction time.[10] In another double-blind study, kavain was compared to oxazepam (a drug similar to diazepam or Valium) in 38 patients.[11] Both substances caused progressive improvements in two different anxiety scores (Anxiety Status Inventory and the Self-rating Anxiety Scale) over a 4 week period. However, while oxazepam and similar drugs are addictive and cause side-effects, kavain appeared to be free of these complications.

In perhaps the most significant study, a 70% kavalactone extract was shown to exhibit significant therapeutic benefit in patients suffering from anxiety.[12] The study was double-blind; 29 patients were assigned to receive 100 mg of the kava extract three times daily, while another 29 patients received a placebo. Therapeutic effectiveness was assessed using several standard psychological assessments including the Hamilton Anxiety Scale. The result of this 4 week study indicated that individuals taking the kava extract had a statistically significant reduction in symptoms of anxiety including feelings of nervousness and somatic complaints such as heart palpitations, chest pains, headache, dizziness, and feelings of gastric irritation. No side-effects were reported with the kava extract.

In another double-blind study, two groups of 20 women with menopause-related symptoms were treated for a period of 8 weeks with the 70% kavalactone extract (100 mg three times daily) or placebo.[13] The measured variable was once again the Hamilton Anxiety Scale. The group receiving the kava extract demonstrated significant improvement at the end of the very first week of treatment. Scores continued to improve over the course of the 8 week study. In addition to improvement in symptoms of stress and anxiety, a number of other symptoms also improved. Most notably there was an overall improvement in subjective well-being, mood, and general symptoms of menopause, including hot flashes. Again, no side-effects were noted.

Two additional studies have shown that unlike benzodiazepines, alcohol, and other drugs, kava extract is not associated with depressed mental function or impairment in driving or the operation of heavy equipment.[14,15] In one of these studies, 12 healthy volunteers were tested in a double-blind cross-over manner to assess the effects of oxazepam (placebo on days 1–3, 15 mg on the day before testing, 75 mg on the morning of the experiment), the extract of kava standardized at 70% kavalactones (200 mg three times daily for 5 days), and a placebo on behavior and event-related potentials (ERPs) in electroencephalograph (EEG) readings on a recognition memory task. The subjects' task was to identify within a list of visually presented words those that were shown for the first time and those that were being repeated. Consistent with other benzodiazepines, oxazepam inhibited the recognition of both new and old words as noted by ERP. In contrast, kava showed a slightly increased recognition rate and a larger ERP difference between old and new words. The results of this study once again demonstrate the unusual effects of kava. In this case, it improves anxiety, but unlike standard anxiolytics, kava actually improves mental function and, at the recommended levels, does not promote sedation.

DOSAGE

In clinical studies using pure kavalactones or kava extracts standardized for kavalactones, the dosage is based on the level of kavalactones. As the kavalactone content of the root varies between 3 and 20%, preparations standardized for kavalactone content are preferred to crude preparations. A standard bowl of traditionally prepared kava drink contains approximately 250 mg of kavalactones, and in Oceania, several bowls may be consumed at one sitting. Dosages are as follows:

- anxiolytic dosage: 45–70 mg of kavalactones three times/day
- sedative dosage: 180–210 mg of kavalactones 1 hour before retiring.

TOXICOLOGY

Although no side-effects have been reported using standardized kava extracts at recommended levels in the clinical studies, several case reports have been presented indicating that kava may interfere with dopamine and worsen Parkinson's disease. Until this issue is resolved, kava extract should not be used in Parkinson's patients.[16]

Side-effects may also develop at high dosages. High daily dosages of kava consumed over a prolonged period (a few months to a year) are associated with "kava dermopathy" – a condition of the skin characterized by a peculiar generalized scaly eruption known as kani.[16] The skin becomes dry and covered with scales, especially the palms of the hands, soles of the feet, forearms, the back, and shins. It was thought at one time that kava dermopathy may be due to interference with niacin. However, in a double-blind, placebo-controlled study, niacinamide (100 mg/day) demonstrated no therapeutic effect.[17] It appears that the only effective treatment for kava dermopathy is reduction or cessation of kava consumption. No cases of kava dermopathy have been reported in those taking standardized kava extracts at recommended levels.

Other reported adverse effects of extremely high doses of kava (e.g. greater than 310 g/week) for prolonged periods include:[18]

- biochemical abnormalities (low levels of serum albumin, protein, urea, and bilirubin)
- presence of blood in the urine
- increased red blood cell volume
- decreased platelet and lymphocyte counts
- shortness of breath.

However, the validity of this report of adverse effects is questionable because the subjects were also heavy users of alcohol and cigarettes. Nonetheless, high doses of kava are unnecessary and should be avoided.

REFERENCES

1. Lebot V, Merlin M, Lindstrom L. Kava. The Pacific Drug. New Haven, CT: Yale University Press. 1992
2. Singh Y. Kava. An overview. J Ethnopharmacol 1992; 37: 13–45
3. Meyer HJ. Pharmacology of kava. In: Holmstedt B, Kline NS, eds. Ethnopharmacological search for psychoactive drugs. New York: Raven Press. 1979, p 133–140
4. Keledjian J, Duffield PH, Jamieson DD. Uptake into mouse brain of four compounds present in the psychoactive beverage kava. J Pharm Sci 1988; 77: 1003–1006
5. Davies LP, Drew CA, Duffield P. Kava pyrones and resin. Studies on GABAa, GABAb and benzodiazepine binding sites in rodent brain. Pharm Toxicol 1992; 71: 120–126
6. Holm E, Staedt U, Heep J. Studies on the profile of the neurophysiological effects of D,L-kavain. cerebral sites of action and sleep-wakefulness-rhythm in animals. Arzneim Forsch 1991; 41: 673–683
7. Jamieson DD, Duffield PH. The antinociceptive action of kava components in mice. Clin Exp Pharmacol Physiol 1990; 17: 495–508
8. Duffield PH, Jamieson D. Development of tolerance to kava in mice. Clin Exp Pharmacol Physiol 1991; 18: 571–578
9. Backhauss, Krieglstein J. Extract of kava (*Piper methysticum*) and its methysticum constituents protect brain tissue against ischemic damage in rodents. Eur J Pharmacol 1992; 215: 265–269
10. Scholing WE, Clausen HD. On the effect of d,l-kavain. experience with neuronika. Med Klin 1977; 72: 1301–1306
11. Lindenberg D, Pitule-Schodel H. D,L-kavain in comparison with oxazepam in anxiety disorders. A double-blind study of clinical effectiveness. Forschr Med 1990; 108: 49–50, 53–54
12. Kinzler E, Kromer J, Lehmann E. Clinical efficacy of a kava extract in patients with anxiety syndrome. Double-blind placebo controlled study over 4 weeks. Arzneim Forsch 1991; 41: 584–588
13. Warnecke G. Neurovegetative dystonia in the female climacteric. Studies on the clinical efficacy and tolerance of kava extract WS 1490. Forsch Med 1991; 109: 120–122
14. Herberg KW. The influence of kava-special extract WS 1490 on safety-relevant performance alone and in combination with ethylalcohol. Blutalkohol 1993; 30: 96–105
15. Munte TF, Heinze HJ, Matzke M. Effects of oxazepam and an extract of kava roots (Piper methysticum) on event-related potentials in a word recognition task. Neuropyschobiol 1993; 27: 46–53
16. Schelosky L, Raffauf C, Jendroska K. Kava and dopamine antagonism [letter]. J Neurol Neurosurg Psychiatry 1995; 58: 639–640
17. Norton SA, Ruze P. Kava dermopathy. J Am Acad Dermatol 1994; 31: 89–97
18. Ruze P. Kava-induced dermopathy. A niacin deficiency. Lancet 1990; 335: 1442–1445

CHAPTER CONTENTS

105

Probiotics

Michael T. Murray, ND

Joseph E. Pizzorno Jr, ND

INTRODUCTION

Probiotics, translated "for life", refer to bacteria in the intestine considered beneficial to health. At least 400 different species of microflora colonize the human gastrointestinal tract. The most important healthful bacteria are *Lactobacillus acidophilus* and *Bifidobacterium bifidum*. This chapter focuses on the principal uses of commercial probiotic supplements containing either or both *L. acidophilus* and *B. bifidum* as well as the fructo-oligosaccharides which facilitate their growth.

Foods fermented with lactobacilli have been, and still are, of great importance to the diets of most of the world's people. Most cultures use some form of fermented food in their diet such as yogurt, cheese, miso, and tempeh. The symbiotic relationship between humankind and lactobacilli has a long history of important nutritional and therapeutic benefits for humans.

DESCRIPTION

At the turn of the century, Metchnikoff[1] asserted that yogurt was the elixir of life. He theorized that putrefactive bacteria in the large intestine produce toxins which invite disease and shorten life. He believed that the eating of yogurt would cause the lactobacilli to become dominant in the colon and displace the putrefactive bacteria. For years, these claims of healthful effects from fermented foods were considered unscientific folklore. However, a substantial, and growing, body of scientific evidence has now demonstrated that lactobacilli and fermented foods play a significant role in human health.

Colonization of Gram-positive lactobacilli begins after birth, after which there is a dramatic increase in their concentration. *Bifidobacterium bifidum* is first introduced through breast-feeding to the sterile gut of the infant, and large numbers are soon observed in the feces. Later, other bacteria (including such beneficial strains as *L. casea*, *L. fermentum*, *L. salivores*, *L. brevis*, etc.) become

Table 105.1 Lactobacilli found in the human intestine

- *L. acidophilus*
- *L. bifidus (Bifidobacterium bifidum)*
- *L. brevis*
- *L. casei*
- *L. cellobiosus*
- *L. fermentum*
- *L. leichmannii*
- *L. plantarum*
- *L. salivaroes*

established in the gut through contact with the world (Table 105.1). Unfortunately, other, potentially toxic, bacteria also eventually cultivate the colon.[2]

Commercial forms

For clinical efficacy, products containing *L. acidophilus* and *B. bifidum* must provide live organisms in such a manner that they survive the commercial process (transportation, storage, etc.) and the hostile environment of the gastrointestinal tract. Several factors, such as species, strain, adherence, growth media, and diet, are involved in successful colonization.[3,4] Typically, a high-quality commercial preparation will produce greater colonization than simply eating yogurt. One of the key reasons that most currently available yogurts are not clinically very useful is that they are made with *L. bulgaricus* or *Streptococcus thermophilus*. While these two bacteria are friendly and possess some health benefits, they do not colonize the colon.

Proper manufacturing, packaging and storing of the product are necessary to ensure viability, the right amount of moisture, and freedom from contamination. Lactobacilli do not respond well to freeze-drying (lyophilization), spray drying, or conventional frozen storage. Excessive temperature during packaging or storage can dramatically reduce viability. Typically, unless the product has been shown to be stable, refrigeration is necessary. Some products do not have to be refrigerated until after the bottle has been opened.

While there are a number of excellent companies providing high-quality probiotic products, it is difficult to sort through all of manufacturer's claims of superiority, and some products have been shown to contain no active *L. acidophilus*. In fact, one study concluded: "Most of the lactobacilli-containing products currently available [1990] either do not contain the *Lactobacillus* species advertised and/or contain other bacteria of questionable benefit."[5] Another study evaluated 16 commercial lactobacillus products for actual microbial content. Four contained the *L. acidophilus* as stated on the label, while 11 were found to be contaminated with pathogens.[6] Clearly, the clinician needs documentation of product quality and content before prescribing for their patients.

CLINICAL APPLICATIONS

The intestinal flora plays a major role in the health of the host.[2–4] The intestinal flora is intimately involved in the host's nutritional status and affects immune system function, cholesterol metabolism, carcinogenesis, toxin load, and aging. Due to the importance of *L. acidophilus* and *B. bifidum* to human health, probiotic supplements can be used to promote overall good health. There are several specific uses for probiotics, however. The primary areas of use discussed here are:

- promotion of proper intestinal environment
- post-antibiotic therapy
- vaginal yeast infections
- urinary tract infections
- cancer prevention.

Promotion of proper intestinal environment

Lactobacilli have long been known to play an important role in the prevention of, and defense against, diseases, particularly those of the gastrointestinal tract and vagina. As part of the "normal flora", they inhibit the growth of other organisms through competition for nutrients, alteration of pH and oxygen tension to levels less favorable to pathogens (disease causing organisms), prevention of attachment of pathogens by physically covering attachment sites, and production of limiting factors such as antimicrobial factors.[2–4]

Lactobacilli produce a variety of factors which inhibit or antagonize other bacteria. These include metabolic end-products such as organic acids (lactic and acetic acid), hydrogen peroxide, and compounds known as bacteriocins.[7–18] Although some researchers have isolated substances from lactobacilli which they labeled antibiotics, these are probably more accurately described as bacteriocins. Bacteriocins are defined as proteins which are produced by bacteria which exert a lethal effect on closely related bacteria (Table 105.2). In general, bacteriocins have a narrower range of activity than antibiotics, but are often more lethal.

Some of the antimicrobial activity of *L. acidophilus* has been shown to be due to their production of hydrogen peroxide.[17,18] However, this reaction requires folic acid and riboflavin, which if in short supply will reduce H_2O_2 production. In addition to these direct effects, some researchers believe the antimicrobial activity is also due to immune system stimulation.[19–24]

The earliest reported therapeutic uses of *L. acidophilus* in the 1920s suggested that their proliferation in the gut was associated with a concomitant decrease in potentially harmful coliform bacteria. This effect has since been confirmed.[25–27] However, it is believed that many of the earlier commercial products were less reliable than those used in later published clinical trials because of

Table 105.2 Bacteria inhibited by *L. acidophilus*

- *Bacillus subtillis*
- *B. cerus*
- *B. stearothermophilus*
- *Candida albicans*
- *Clostridium perfringens*
- *E. coli*
- *Klebsiella pneumoniae*
- *L. bulgaricus*
- *L. fermentum*
- *L. helveticus*
- *L. lactis*
- *L. leichmannii*
- *L. plantarium*
- *Proteus vulgaris*
- *Pseudomonas aeruginosa*
- *P. flourescens*
- *Salmonella typhosa*
- *S. schottmuelleri*
- *Shigella dysenteriae*
- *S. paradysenteriae*
- *Sarcina lutea*
- *Serratia marcescens*
- *Staphylococcus aureus*
- *Streptococcus fecalis*
- *S. lactis*
- *Vibrio comma*

inappropriate strains and problems in production, storage, and distribution to consumers.[28]

Post-antibiotic therapy

Acidophilus supplementation is particularly important for preventing and treating antibiotic-induced diarrhea, *Candida* overgrowth, and urinary tract infections. *L. acidophilus* has been shown to correct the increase of Gram-negative bacteria observed following the administration of broad-spectrum antibiotics as occurs with any acute or chronic diarrhea.[2–4,29–31] Similarly, a mixture of *B. bifidum* and *L. acidophilus* inhibited the lowering of fecal flora induced by ampicillin and maintained the equilibrium of the intestinal ecosystem.[29]

Although it is commonly believed that acidophilus supplements are not effective if taken during antibiotic therapy, the research actually supports the use of *L. acidophilus* during antibiotic administration.[29,30] Reductions of friendly bacteria and/or superinfection with antibiotic-resistant flora may be prevented by administering *L. acidophilus* products during antibiotic therapy. A dosage of at least 15–20 billion organisms is required. Probiotic supplements should, however, be taken as far away from the antibiotic as possible.

Vaginal yeast infections

Lactobacillus acidophilus has been shown to retard the growth of *Candida albicans* – the major yeast involved in vaginal yeast infections.[32] Clinical studies have suggested that the introduction of yogurt or lactobacilli to the vagina can assist in clearing up and preventing recurrent vaginal yeast infections as well as bacterial vaginosis.[33]

Lactobacillus acidophilus is a normal constituent of the vaginal flora, where it contributes to the maintenance of the acid pH by fermenting vaginal glycogen to lactic acid.[34–37] It has been shown that suppression of *L. acidophilus* by broad-spectrum antibiotics leads to the overgrowth of yeast and other bacteria.[38]

Reestablishment of normal vaginal lactobacilli can be accomplished by having the woman douche twice a day with an acidophilus solution containing 10^8 live organisms/ml. However, the right strains must be used.

The appropriate lactobacilli produce hydrogen peroxide in the vaginal tract. It is present in 96% of normal vaginas but is absent in women suffering from chronic vaginosis. The production of hydrogen peroxide by lactobacilli is toxic to pathogens such as *Gardenerella vaginalis*.[39] Not all women's vaginas are colonized by the right strains of lactobacilli. One study evaluated the lactobacilli in 275 women in the second trimester of pregnancy by obtaining vaginal cultures to detect H_2O_2-production status as well as the presence of pathological organisms. Women colonized by H_2O_2-positive lactobacilli were less likely to have bacterial vaginosis, symptomatic candidiasis and vaginal colonization by *Gardnerella vaginalis, Bacteroides, Peptostreptococcus, Mycoplasma hominis, Ureaplasma urelurealyticum,* and *Viridans streptococci*.[40] The women who did not have any vaginal lactobacilli were also more likely to have *Chlamydia trachomatis*. The researchers also reported that most commercially available products contain lactobacilli that do not produce H_2O_2 or lactobacillus strains derived from dairy foods, which are unable to bind to vaginal epithelial cells.

While douching appears to be the preferred therapy for vaginal infections, even simple consumption of appropriate yogurt products appears beneficial. For example, one study of 33 patients with recurrent *Candida vaginitis*, found a threefold decrease in infections when they consumed 8 ounces/day of yogurt containing H_2O_2-producing *Lactobacillus acidophilus* for a period of 6 months. The mean number of infections per 6 months was 2.54 in the control group, and 0.38 in the yogurt-treated group. *Candida* colonization decreased from a mean of 3.23/6 months in the control group to 0.84/6 months in the yogurt group.[41] As might be expected, the researchers found an association between the presence of *Lactobacillus* sp. in the rectum and the vagina.

Urinary tract infection

One of the problems with antibiotic therapy for urinary tract infections is that the disturbance in the bacterial flora which protects against urinary tract infections leads to recurrent infections. The insertion of lactobaccilli suppositories into the vagina of women after they had been treated with antibiotics has been shown to significantly reduce the recurrence rate.[42] In one study, freeze-dried lactobacilli suppositories given intravaginally once weekly for 1 year to eight women with recurrent UTIs resulted in an impressive 78% reduction in the incidence of infection.[6]

Cancer

A series of population studies has suggested that the consumption of high levels of cultured milk products may reduce the risk of colon cancer.[43] *Lactobacillus bulgaricus,* the primary lactobacilli used for traditional yogurt, has demonstrated potent antitumor activity.[44] Feeding milk and colostrum fermented with *L. acidophilus* DDS1 has been reported to result in a 16–41% reduction in tumor proliferation in animal studies.[45] In human studies, ingestion of *L. acidophilus* resulted in reduced activity of the bacterial enzymes associated with the formation of cancer-causing compounds in the gut.[46] The beneficial effects of lactobacilli against cancer appear to extend well beyond the colon. In a double-blind trial conducted in 138 patients surgically treated for bladder cancer, patients were stratified into three groups: (A) with primary multiple tumors, (B) with recurrent single tumors, and (C) with recurrent multiple tumors.[47] In each group, patients were randomly allocated to receive the oral *Lactobacillus casei* preparation (LCP) or placebo. LCP showed a better effect than placebo in preventing cancer recurrences in subgroups A and B. However, no significant effect was noted in group C.

Lactobacillus acidophilus preparations are also of value in cancer patients receiving chemotherapy drugs or radiation therapy involving the gastrointestinal tract. In one study, 24 patients scheduled for internal and external irradiation of the pelvic area for gynecological cancers were selected for a controlled study to test the prevention of intestinal side-effects by administration of *L. acidophilus.*[48] The test group received 150 ml/day of a fermented milk product supplying them with live *L. acidophilus* bacteria in a 6.5% lactulose substrate, resulting in prevention of radiotherapy-associated diarrhea.

Traveler's diarrhea

Lactobacilli supplements are routinely recommended by nutritionally oriented doctors to their patients who travel to developing countries. However, one published report casts doubt on this practice. A randomized, double-blind, placebo-controlled trial was conducted on 282 British soldiers deployed to Belize. They received two capsules containing *L. fermentum, L. acidophilus* or a placebo daily for 3 weeks. There were 10^{11} colony-forming units of bacteria in each capsule of lactobacilli. No protection from traveler's diarrhea was provided by either species.[49] Unfortunately, the H_2O_2-producing status of the supplement was not reported.

Lactose intolerance

Lactose in yogurt with live bacteria is better tolerated in people who are lactose-intolerant than lactose in other dairy foods. This is primarily due to the activity of microbial B-galactosidase which breaks down lactose in vivo. Yogurt containing mixed strains of *Streptococcus salvarius* ssp. *thermophilus* and *L. delbrueckii* ssp. *bulgaricus,* and fermented milks containing *S. thermophilous, L. bulgaricus, L. acidophilus* or *B. bifidus* were evaluated. All the yogurt products dramatically improved lactose digestion regardless of their total or specific B-galactosidase activity. The fermented milks had marginal improvement with *B. bifidus* and almost complete lactose digestion with *L. bulgaricus.* These results suggest that B-galactosidase is not the only factor in promoting lactose digestion.[50]

Comparable results are found in children. One study of 14 lactose-malabsorbing children, with a mean age of 9.5 years, found that consumption of live yogurt containing *L. bulgaricus* and *S. thermophilous* resulted in significantly fewer symptoms than after consuming regular milk and pasteurized yogurt. Breath hydrogen correlated with the degree of symptoms.[51]

Crohn's disease

An interesting study found that four of five patients with disease went into remission for 22 months after having their bowel flora completely replaced with healthier bacteria. The researchers hypothesized that antigens or epitopes on host coliforms in Crohn's patients may cross-react with, or mimic, antigens or epitopes on epithelial cells of the colon or ileum. The five patients were initially treated with broad-spectrum oral and intravenous antibiotics to sterilize the bowel. They were then reinoculated by oral and rectal administration of two strains of non-pathogenic *E. coli* and lactobacilli. The clinical improvement lasted 3–4 months.[52]

DOSAGE

The dosage of a commercial probiotic supplement is based upon the number of live organisms. The ingestion of one to 10 billion viable *L. acidophilus* or *B. bifidum* cells daily is a sufficient dosage for most people. Amounts exceeding this may induce mild gastrointestinal disturbances, while smaller amounts may not be able to colonize the gastrointestinal tract.

PROMOTING GROWTH OF LACTOBACILLI

Fructo-oligosaccharides

Food components which may help to promote the growth of friendly bacteria include fructo-oligosaccharides (FOSs). These short-chain polysaccharides have only recently entered the US market. However, in Japan the number of consumer products containing purified FOSs reached 450 in 1991, and in 1990 the Japanese market for FOSs exceeded $46 million.[53]

FOS, which is not digested by humans, provides a preferred substrate for healthful bacteria. Human studies have shown FOS to increase bifidobacteria and lactobacilli while simultaneously reducing the colonies of detrimental bacteria. Other benefits noted with FOS supplementation include:[53,54]

- increased production of short-chain fatty acids like butyrate
- improved liver function
- reduction of serum cholesterol and blood pressure
- improved elimination of toxic compounds.

The dosage recommendation for pure FOS is 2,000–3,000 mg daily. Natural food sources of FOS include bananas, Jerusalem artichoke, onions, asparagus, and garlic. However, the estimated average daily ingestion of FOS from food sources is estimated to be only 800 mg. Thus, the supplementation of FOS may often be of clinical benefit.[54]

Spirulina

Another possible way to improve the conditions in the intestine is by the consumption of spirulina. While no human studies appear to have been published, intriguing veterinary research has shown that providing horses with spirulina stimulates the growth of *Lactobacillus* in the cecum. The researchers suggest that this may be due to the mucopolysaccharides in spirulina.[55]

TOXICITY

Probiotics are safe and are not associated with any side-effects other than a transient increase in gastrointestinal gas.

Interactions

Lactobacillus acidophilus and *B. bifidum* are negatively affected by alcohol and antibiotics.[56] Although there is no evidence that the organism interferes with the activity of most antibiotics, the metabolism of sulfasalazine, chloramphenicol palmitate, and phthalylsulfathiazole is affected by *L. acidophilus*.[57]

REFERENCES

1. Metchnikoff E. The prolongation of life. New York, NY: Arna Press. 1908 (1977 reprint)
2. Hentges DJ (ed). Human intestinal microflora. In: Health and disease. New York, NY: Academic Press. 1983
3. Shahani KM, Ayebo AD. Role of dietary lactobacilli in gastrointestinal microecology. Am J Clin Nutr 1980; 33: 2448–2457
4. Shahani KM, Friend BA. Nutritional and therapeutic aspects of lactobacilli. J Appl Nutr 1984; 36: 125–152
5. Hughes VL, Hillier SL. Microbiologic characteristics of *Lactobacillus* products used for colonization of the vagina. Obstet Gynecol 1990; 75: 244–248
6. Reid G, Bruce AW, Taylor M. Vaginal flora and urinary tract infections. Current Opinion in Infectious Disease 1991; 4: 37–41
7. Barefoot SF, Klaenhammer TR. Detection and activity of lacticin B, a bacteriocin produced by *Lactobacillus acidophilus*. Appl Environ Microbiol 1983; 45: 1808–1815
8. Klaenhammer TR. Microbiological considerations in the selection of preparations of lactobacillus strains for use in dietary adjuncts. J Dairy Sci 1982; 65: 1339–1349
9. Klaenhammer TR. Bacteriocins of lactic acid bacteria. Biochemie 1988; 70: 337–349
10. Upreti GC, Hinsdill RD. Isolation and characterization of a bacteriocin from a homofermentative *Lactobacillus*. Antimicrob Agents Chemotherapy 1973; 4: 487–494
11. Upreti GC, Hinsdill RD. Production and mode of action of lactocin 27. Bacteriocin from a homofermentative *Lactobacillus*. Antimicrob Agents Chemotherapy 1975; 7: 139–145
12. DeKlerk HC. Bacteriocinogency in *Lactobacillus fermenti*. Nature 1967; 214: 609
13. DeKlerk HC, Smit JA. Properties of a Lactobacillus fermenti bacteriocin. J Gen Microbiol 1967; 48: 309–316
14. Friend BA, Shahani KM. Nutritional and therapeutic aspects of lactobacilli. J Appl Nutr 1984; 36: 125–152
15. Shahani KM, Vakil JR, Kilara A. Natural antibiotic activity of *Lactobacillus acidophilus* and *bulgaricus*. II. Isolation of acidophilin from L. acidophilus. Cult Dairy Prod J 1977; 12: 8
16. Shahani KM, Vakil JR, Kilara A. Natural antibiotic activity of *Lactobacillus acidophilus* and *Lactobacillus bulgaricus*. Cult Dairy Prod J 1976; 11: 14–17
17. Dahiya RS, Speck ML. Hydrogen peroxide formation by lactobacilli and its effect on Staphylococcus aureus. J Dairy Sci 1968; 51: 1568
18. Price RJ, Lee JS. Inhibition of pseudomonas species by hydrogen peroxide producing lactobacilli. J Milk Food Technol 1970; 33: 13
19. Vesely R, Negri R, Bianchi-Salvadori B et al. Influence of a diet addition with yogurt on the mouse immune system. EOS J Immunol Immunopharmacol 1985; 5: 30–35
20. Vincent JG, Veonett RC, Riley RG. Antibacterial activities associated with *Lactobacillus acidophilus*. J Bacteriol 1959; 78: 477
21. Perdigon G, N de Macias ME, Alvarez S et al. Enhancement of immune response in mice fed with *Streptococcus thermophilus* and *Lactobacillus acidophilus*. J Diary Sci 1987; 70: 919–926
22. Weir D, Blackwell C. Interaction of bacteria with the immune system. J Clin Lab Immunol 1983; 10: 1–12
23. Perdigon G, N de Macias, Alvarez S et al. Systemic augmentation of the immune response in mice by feeding fermented milks with *Lactobacillus casei* and *Lactobacillus acidophilus*. Immunology 1988; 63: 17–23
24. Perdigon G, Alvarey S, Rachid M. Symposium. Probiotic bacteria for humans. Clinical systems for evaluation of effectiveness. Immune system stimulation by probiotics. J Dairy Sci 1995; 78: 1597–1606
25. Clements ML, Levine MM, Black RE et al. Lactobacillus prophylaxis for diarrhea due to enterotoxinogenic *Escherichia coli*.

Antimicrob Agents Chemotherap 1981; 20: 104–108
26. Dios Pozo-Olano JD, Warram JH, Gomez RG, Cavazos MG. Effect of a lactobacilli preparation on traveler's diarrhea. A randomized, double blind clinical trial. Gastroenterol 1978; 74: 829–830
27. Thompson GE. Control of intestinal flora in animals and humans: implications for toxicology and health. J Environ Path Toxicol 1977; 1: 113–123
28. Clements ML, Levine MM, Ristaino PA. Exogenous lactobacilli fed to man. Their fate and ability to prevent diarrheal disease. Prog Food Nutr Sci 1983; 7: 29–37
29. Zoppi G, Deganello A, Benoni G, Saccomani F. Oral bacteriotherapy in clinical practice. I. The use of different preparations in infants treated with antibiotics. Eur J Ped 1982; 139: 18–21
30. Gotz VP, Romankiewics JA, Moss J, Murray HW. Prophylaxis against ampicillin-induced diarrhea with a lactobacillus preparation. Am J Hosp Pharm 1979; 36: 754–757
31. Zoppi G, Balsamo V, Deganello A et al. Oral bacteriotherapy in clinical practice. I. The use of different preparations in the treatment of acute diarrhea. Eur J Ped 1982; 139: 22–24
32. Collins EB, Hardt P. Inhibition of Candida albicans by *Lactobacillus acidophilus*. J Dairy Sci 1980; 63: 830–832
33. Neri A, Sabah G, Samra Z. Bacterial vaginosis in pregnancy treated with yoghurt. Acta Obstet Gynecol 1993; 72: 17–19
34. Butler C, Beakley JW. Bacterial flora in the vagina. Am J Obstet Gynecol 1960; 79: 432
35. Lock FR, Yow MD, Griffith MI, Stout M. Bacteriology of the vagina in 75 normal young adults. Surg Gyn Obs 1948; 87: 410
36. Rogosa M, Sharp ME. Species differentiation of human vaginal lactobacilli. J Gen Microbiol 1960; 23: 197
37. Wylie JG, Henderson A. Identity of glycogen-fermenting ability of lactobacilli isolated from the vagina of pregnant women. J Med Microbiol 1969; 2: 363
38. Huppert M, Cazin J, Smith H. Pathogenesis of *C. albicans* infections following antibiotic therapy. J Bacterio 1955; 70: 440–447
39. Hydrogen peroxide-producing organisms toxic to vaginal bacteria. Infectious Disease News 1991; August 8: 5
40. Hillier SL, Krohn MA, Klebanoff SJ, Eschenbach DA. The relationship of hydrogen peroxide-producing lactobacilli to bacterial vaginosis in genital microflora in pregnant women. Obstet Gyn 1992; 79: 369–373
41. Hilton E, Isenberg HD, Alperstein P et al. Ingestion of yogurt containing *Lactobacillus acidophilus* as prophylaxis for candidal vaginitis. Ann Int Med 1992; 116: 353–357
42. Reid G, Bruce AW, Taylor M. Influence of three-day antimicrobial therapy and lactobacillus vaginal suppositories on recurrence of urinary tract infections. Clin Ther 1992; 14: 11–16
43. IARC Intestinal Microecology Group. Dietary fibre, transit time, fecal bacteria, steroids, and colon cancer in two Scandinavian populations. Lancet 1977; ii: 207–210
44. Bogdanov IG, Velichkov VT, Daley PG et al. Antitumor action of glycopeptides from cell wall of *Lactobacillus bulgaricus*. Bull Exp Biol 1977; 84: 1750
45. Bailey PJ, Shahani KM. Inhibitory effect of acidophilus cultured colostrum and milk upon the proliferation of ascites tumor. In: Proceedings of the 71st Annual Meeting of the American Dairy Science Association. 1979: p 41
46. Ayebo AD, Angelo IA, Shahani KM, Kies C. Effect of feeding *Lactobacillus acidophilus* milk upon fecal flora and enzyme activity in humans. J Dairy Sci 1979; 62 (suppl 1): 44
47. Aso Y, Akaya H, Katake T. Preventive effect of *Lactobacillus casei* preparation on the recurrence of superficial bladder cancer in a double-blind trial. Eur Urol 1995; 27: 104–109
48. Salminen E, Elomaa I, Minkiunen J. Preservation of intestinal integrity during radiotherapy using live *Lactobacillus acidophilus* cultures. Clin Radiology 1988; 39: 435–437
49. Katelaris PH, Salam I, Farthing MJ. Lactobacilli to prevent traveler's diarrhea? New Engl J Med 1995; 333: 1360–1361
50. Martini MC, Lerebours EC, Lin WJ et al. Strains and species of lactic acid bacteria and fermented milk products (yogurts): effect on in vivo lactose digestion. Am J Clin Nutr 1991; 54: 1041–1046
51. Shermak MA, Saavedra JM, Jackson TL et al. Effect of yogurt on symptoms and kinetics of hydrogen production in lactose-malabsorbing children. Am J Clin Nutr 1995; 62: 1003–1006
52. Substituting bowel flora eases Crohn's. Med Tribune 1992; June 11: 19
53. Tomomatsu H. Health effects of oligosaccharides. Food Tech 1994; October: 61–65
54. Gibson GR, Beatty ER, Wang X. Selective stimulation of bifidobacteria in the human colon by oligofructose and inulin. Gastroenterology 1995; 108: 975–982
55. Jones WE. Nutrition/spirulina and mucopolysaccharides. Equine Vet Data 1991; 12: 431–432
56. Daikos GK, Kontomichalou P, Bilalis D, Pimenidou L. Intestinal flora ecology after oral use of antibiotics. Chemotherapy 1968; 13: 146–160
57. Pradhan A, Majumdar MK. Metabolism of some drugs by intestinal lactobacilli and their toxicological considerations. Acta Pharmacol Toxicol 1986; 58: 11–15

CHAPTER CONTENTS

106

Procyanidolic oligomers

Michael T. Murray, ND

Joseph E. Pizzorno Jr, ND

GENERAL DESCRIPTION

The proanthocyanidins (also referred to as procyanidins) are one of the most beneficial groups of plant flavonoids. The most active proanthocyanidins are those bound to other proanthocyanidins. Collectively, mixtures of proanthocyanidin dimers, trimers, tetramers, and larger molecules are referred to procyanidolic oligomers or PCOs for short.[1,2]

Although PCOs exist in many plants, as well as red wine, commercially available sources of PCOs include extracts from grape seed skin (*Vitex vinifera*) and the bark of the maritime (Landes) pine.[1,2] This chapter reviews the benefits of PCOs from grape seeds and pine bark.

CHEMICAL COMPOSITION

Grape seed and pine bark PCO extracts are well defined chemically. Grape seed extracts are available which contain 92–95% PCOs while the pine bark extracts vary from 80 to 85%. Proanthocyanidin B_2 is shown in Figure 106.1.

HISTORY AND FOLK USE

In 1534, French explorer Jacques Cartier lead an expedition up the Saint Lawrence River. Trapped by ice,

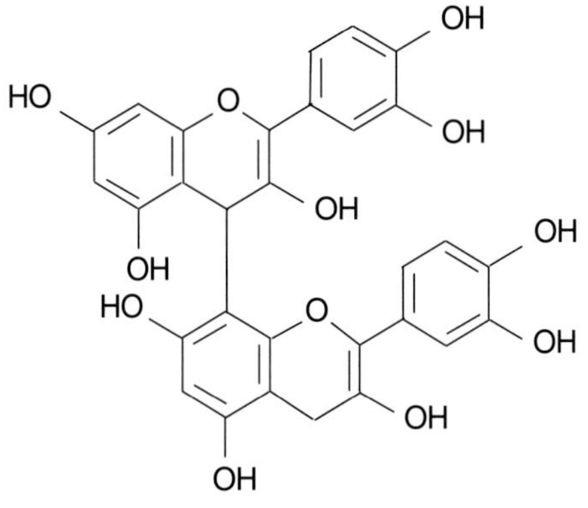

Figure 106.1 Proanthocyanidin B_2.

Cartier and his crew were forced to survive on a ration of salted meat and biscuits. Cartier's crew began to exhibit signs and symptoms of scurvy, the cause of which was unknown at that time. Fortunately for Cartier and the surviving members of his crew, they met a Native American who advised them to make a tea from the bark and needles of pine trees. As a result, Cartier and his men survived.

More than 400 years later, Professor Jacques Masquelier of the University of Bordeaux, France, read the book Cartier wrote detailing his expedition. Intrigued by Cartier's story, Masquelier and others concluded that pine bark must contain some vitamin C as well as bioflavonoids which can exert vitamin C-like effects.

Masquelier termed the active components of the pine bark "pycnogenols".[1,3] This term was used to describe an entire complex of proanthocyanidin complexes found in a variety of plants including pine bark, grape seeds, lemon tree bark, peanuts, cranberries, and citrus peels. The term "pycnogenols" has been replaced in the scientific community by the terms proanthocyanidins, oligomeric proanthocyanidin complexes (OPCs), and/or procyanidolic oligomers (PCO). In the United States, Pycnogenol® is a registered trademark of Horphag Ltd of Guernsey, UK, and refers to the procyanidolic oligomer (PCO) extracted from the bark of the French maritime pine.

Masquelier patented the method of extracting PCOs from pine bark in France in 1951, and from grape seeds in 1970. The PCO extract from grape seed emerged as the preferred source based on research between 1951 and 1971, as well as intensive research from 1972 to 1978.[1] The 1970s research was conducted with the goal of gaining approval for PCO as a medicinal agent by the French equivalent of the FDA. During this time, detailed analytical, toxicity, pharmacological, and clinical studies were performed on PCOs derived from grape seeds. PCOs from both grape seeds and pine bark have been marketed in France for decades where they have been promoted to improve retinopathies, venous insufficiency, and vascular fragility.

PHARMACOLOGY

Extracts of PCOs have demonstrated a wide range of activity as listed in Table 106.1.

Table 106.1 Pharmacological activity of proanthocyanidins[1,2]

- Increase intracellular vitamin C levels
- Decrease capillary permeability and fragility
- Scavenge oxidants and free radicals
- Inhibit destruction of collagen

Protection of collagen

Collagen, the most abundant protein of the body, is responsible for maintaining the integrity of ground substance as well as the integrity of tendons, ligaments, and cartilage. Collagen is also the support structure of the dermis and blood vessels. PCOs are remarkable in their effect in supporting collagen structures and preventing collagen destruction. They affect collagen metabolism in several ways. They have the unique ability to cross-link collagen fibers, resulting in reinforcement of the natural cross-linking of collagen that forms the so-called collagen matrix of connective tissue.[4,5] They also protect against free radical damage with their potent antioxidant and free radical scavenging action; and inhibit enzymatic cleavage of collagen by enzymes secreted by leukocytes during inflammation and microbes during infection.[6,7] PCOs also prevent the release and synthesis of compounds that promote inflammation and allergies such as histamine, serine proteases, prostaglandins, and leukotrienes.[1]

Antioxidant and free radical scavenging activity

Perhaps the most celebrated effects of PCOs in the United States are their potent antioxidant and free radical scavenging activity. Free radical damage has been linked to the aging process and virtually every chronic degenerative disease including heart disease, arthritis, and cancer. Fats and cholesterol are particularly susceptible to free radical damage. When damaged, fats and cholesterol form toxic derivatives known as lipid peroxides and cholesterol epoxides, respectively. The antioxidant and free radical scavenging effects of PCOs were discovered by Masquelier in 1986.[1]

A recent study evaluated the free radical scavenging activity of PCOs and determined their inhibitory effects on xanthine oxidase (a primary generator of oxygen-derived free radicals) and the lysosomal enzyme system (which governs the release of enzymes which can damage the connective tissue framework that acts as a protective sheath surrounding capillary walls).[7] This research, summarized in Table 106.2, provides a detailed explanation of the vascular protective action of PCOs and a strong rationale for their use in vascular disease.

In experimental models, the antioxidant activity of

Table 106.2 Antioxidant and free radical scavenging activities of PCOs

- Trap hydroxyl free radicals
- Trap lipid peroxides and free radicals
- Markedly delay the onset of lipid peroxidation
- Chelate free iron molecules, thereby preventing iron-induced lipid peroxidation
- Inhibit production of free radicals by non-competitively inhibiting xanthine oxidase
- Inhibit the damaging effects of the enzymes (e.g. hyaluronidase, elastase, collagenase, etc.) which can degrade connective tissue structures

PCOs is much greater (approximately 50 times) than that of vitamin C and vitamin E. From a cellular perspective, one of the most advantageous features of PCOs' free radical scavenging activity is that, because of their chemical structure, they are incorporated into cell membranes. This physical characteristic, along with their ability to protect against both water- and fat-soluble free radicals, provides significant cellular protection against free radical damage.

The researchers concluded their discussion with the following comment: "These findings, together [with] those of other investigators, provide a strong rationale for using these compounds in the therapeutic management of microvascular disorders."

CLINICAL APPLICATIONS

Venous and capillary disorders

The primary clinical applications of PCOs are in the treatment of:

- venous and capillary disorders including venous insufficiency
- varicose veins
- capillary fragility
- disorders of the retina, including diabetic retinopathy and macular degeneration.

Good clinical studies have shown positive results in the treatment of these conditions.[8–15]

Visual function

Increased intake of PCO is likely to benefit almost everyone. This suggestion is perhaps best illustrated by research evaluating the effects of grape seed PCOs extract on visual function in healthy subjects.[14,15] In the studies, 100 normal volunteers with no retinal disorder received 200 mg/day of PCOs or placebo for 5 or 6 weeks. The group receiving PCOs demonstrated significant improvement in visual performance in dark and after glare tests compared with the placebo group.

Atherosclerosis

There are now numerous studies demonstrating that an individual's level of antioxidants may be a more significant factor in determining the risk of developing heart disease than cholesterol levels. Antioxidants prevent the oxidation of cholesterol and its carrier proteins as well as preventing the initial damage to the artery which ultimately leads to the process of atherosclerosis. Large-scale studies with vitamin E, vitamin C, and beta-carotene have shown that these antioxidants are capable of significantly reducing the risk of dying of a heart attack or a stroke. For example, in one study of 87,245 nurses, it was discovered that nurses who took 100 IU of vitamin E daily for more than 2 years had a 41% lower risk of heart disease compared with non-users of vitamin E supplements.[16] Another study of 39,910 male health care professionals produced similar results: a 37% lower risk of heart disease with the intake of more than 30 IU of supplemental vitamin E daily.[17]

Since PCOs have a greater antioxidant effect than vitamins C and E, it is only natural to speculate they could offer greater protective effects. Support exists for this contention. For example, several studies have shown the protective effects of red wine against heart disease and stroke by protecting against LDL oxidation.[18] The active components in the wine are thought to be proanthocyanidins. Also, a recent study of 805 men beginning in 1985 demonstrated an inverse correlation between flavonoid intake and death due to heart attack.[19]

In addition to preventing damage to cholesterol and the lining of the artery, PCO extracts have been shown to lower blood cholesterol levels and shrink the size of the cholesterol deposit in the artery in animal studies.[1,20] Additional mechanisms of PCOs useful in preventing atherosclerosis include inhibition of platelet aggregation and inhibition of angiotensin-I-converting enzyme.[21,22] Presumably, PCO extracts may exert similar benefits in humans. PCO extracts, although in a supplement form, should be thought of as a necessary food in the prevention and treatment of atherosclerosis.

DOSAGE

As antioxidant support, a daily dose of 50 mg of either the grape seed or pine bark extract is suitable. For comparison, it is now estimated that the average daily intake of total flavonoids in the United States is about 25 mg. An intake greater than 30 mg offers significantly reduced risk for cardiovascular mortality.[19]

When being used for therapeutic purposes, the daily dosage should be increased to 150–300 mg.

TOXICITY

PCO extracts are without known side-effects.

REFERENCES

1. Schwitters B, Masquelier J. OPC in practice: biflavanols and their application. Rome: Alfa Omega. 1993
2. Masquelier J. Procyanidolic oligomers. J Parfums Cosm Arom 1990; 95: 89–97
3. Masquelier J. Pycnogenols. Recent advances in the therapeutical activity of procyanidins. Natural Prod Med Agents 1981; 1: 243–256

4. Masquelier J, Dumon MC, Dumas J. Stabilization of collagen by procyanidolic oligomers. Acta Therap 1981; 7: 101–105
5. Tixier JM, Godeau G, Robert AM. Evidence by *in vivo* and *in vitro* studies that binding of pycnogenols to elastin affects its rate of degradation by elastases. Biochem Pharmacol 1984; 33: 3933–3939
6. Meunier MT, Duroux E, Bastide P. Free-radical scavenger activity of procyanidolic oligomers and anthocyanosides with respect to superoxide anion and lipid peroxidation. Plant Med Phytother 1989; 4: 267–274
7. Facino RM, Carini M, Aldini G et al. Free radicals scavenging action and anti-enzyme activities of procyanidines from *Vitis vinifera*. A mechanism for their capillary protective action. Arzneim Forsch 1994; 44: 592–601
8. Henriet JP. Veno-lymphatic insufficiency. 4,729 patients undergoing hormonal and procyanidol oligomer therapy. Phlebologie 1993; 46: 313–325
9. Baruch J. Effect of Endotelon in postoperative edema. Results of a double-blind study versus placebo in 32 female patients. Ann Chir Plast Esthet 1984; 29: 393–395
10. Lagrue G, Oliver-Martin F, Grillot A. A study of the effects of procyanidol oligomers on capillary resistance in hypertension and in certain nephropathies. Sem Hosp Paris 1981; 57: 1399–1401
11. Gomez Trillo JT. Varicose veins of the lower extremities. Symptomatic treatment with a new vasculotrophic agent. Prensa Med Mex 1973; 38: 293–296
12. Soyeux A, Segiun JP, Le Devehat C. Endotelon. Diabetic retinopathy and hemorheology (preliminary study). Bull Soc Ophtalmol Fr 1987; 87: 1441–1444
13. Proto F et al. Electrophysical study of *Vitis vinifera* procyanoside oligomers effects on retinal function in myopic subjects. Ann Ott Clin Ocul 1988; 114: 85–93
14. Corbe C, Boisin JP, Siou A. Light vision and chorioretinal circulation. Study of the effect of procyanidolic oligomers (Endotelon). J Fr Ophtalmol 1988; 11: 453–460
15. Boissin JP, Corbe C, Siou A. Chorioretinal circulation and dazzling. use of procyanidol oligomers. Bull Soc Ophtalmol Fr 1988; 88: 173–174, 177–179
16. Stampfer MJ, Henneken SCH, Manson JE. Vitamin E consumption and the risk of coronary disease in women. New Engl J Med 1993; 328: 1444–1448
17. Rimm EB. Vitamin E consumption and the risk of coronary heart disease in men. New Engl J Med 1993; 328: 1450–1455
18. Frankel EN, Kanner J, German JB. Inhibition of oxidation of human low-density lipoprotein by phenolic substances in red wine. Lancet 1993; 341: 454–457
19. Hertog MG, Feskens EJ, Hollman PC. Dietary antioxidant flavonoids and risk of coronary heart disease. The Zutphen Elderly Study. Lancet 1993; 342: 1007–1011
20. Wegrowski J, Robert Am, Moczar M. The effect of procyanidolic oligomers on the composition of normal and hypercholesterolemic rabbit aortas. Biochem Pharmacol 1984; 33: 3491–3497
21. Chang WC, Hsu FL. Inhibition of platelet aggregation and arachidonate metabolism in platelets by procyanidins. Prostagland Leukotri Essential Fatty Acids 1989; 38: 181–188
22. Meunier MT, Villie F, Jonadet M. Inhibition of angiotensin I converting enzyme by flavanolic compounds. *In vitro* and *in vivo* studies. Planta Med 1987; 54: 12–15

CHAPTER CONTENTS

107

Pygeum africanum (bitter almond)

Michael T. Murray, ND

Joseph E. Pizzorno Jr, ND

Pygeum africanum (family: Rosaceae)
Synonym: *Prunus africanum*
Common names: bitter almond, red stinkwood

GENERAL DESCRIPTION

Pygeum africanum is an evergreen tree native to Africa that can grow to a height of 120–150 feet. It has pendulous branches with thick, oblong-shaped, leather-like, mat-colored leaves and creamy white flowers. The fruit (drupe) resembles a cherry when ripe. The dark brown to gray bark of the trunk is the part used for medicinal purposes.

CHEMICAL COMPOSITION

The major active components of the bark are:

- lipid-soluble pentacyclic triterpenes
- sterolic triterpenes
- fatty acids
- esters of ferulic acid (see Fig. 107.1).

The pentacyclic triterpenic components include ursolic acid (see Fig. 107.2), oleanolic acid, crataegolic acid, and their derivatives. The sterolic fraction is composed mainly of beta-sitosterol and beta-sitosterone (see Fig. 107.3). The fatty acids range from C12 to C24 and the important ferulic acid esters are those bound to *n*-tetracosanol and *n*-docosanol.[1–4]

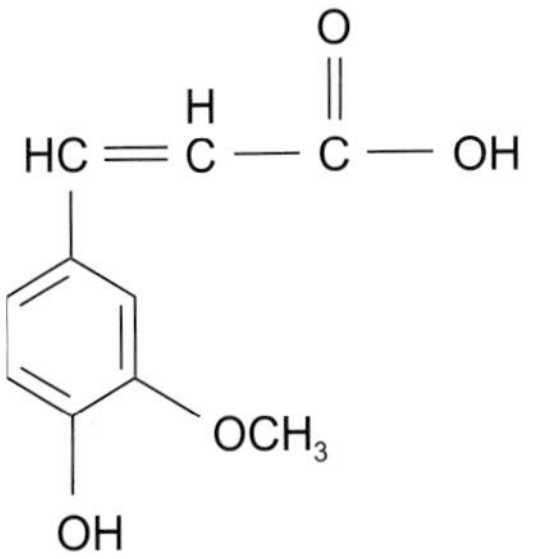

Figure 107.1 Ferulic acid.

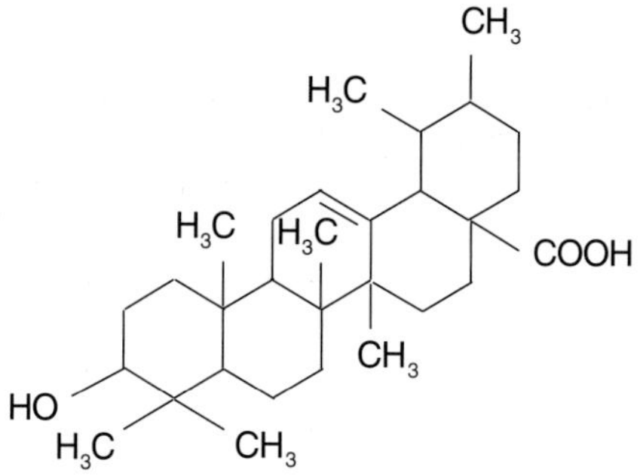

Figure 107.2 Ursolic acid.

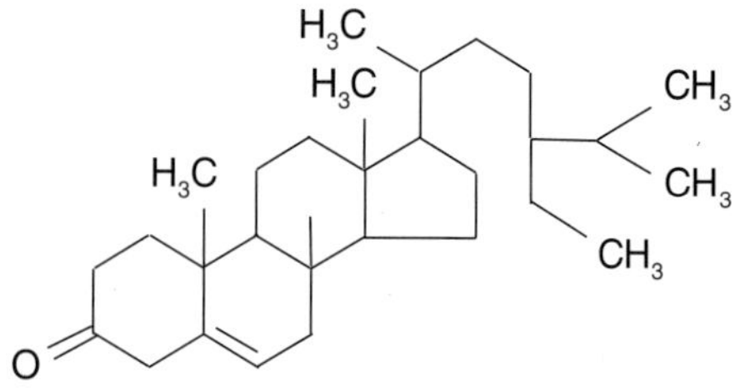

Figure 107.3 β-Sitosterone.

HISTORY AND FOLK USE

The powdered bark of *Pygeum africanum* was used by the natives of tropical Africa as a treatment for urinary disorders. It was often given with palm oil or milk.

PHARMACOLOGY

Pharmacological screening of various extracts prepared with solvents of differing degrees of polarity indicated that the highest activity was found in lipophilic extracts. This finding is interesting in light of pygeum's historical administration in lipophilic media (palm oil or milk). Virtually all of the pharmacological research has featured a pygeum extract standardized to contain 14% triterpenes including beta-sitosterol and 0.5% *n*-docosanol. This extract has been extensively studied in both experimental animal studies and clinical trials with humans.

The primary target organ for pygeum's effects in males is the prostate. The three major active components of pygeum appear to exert different, yet complementary, effects in benign prostatic hyperplasia (BPH). In addition, pygeum has been shown to enhance the secretions of the prostate and bulbourethral glands, in terms of both quantity and quality.

Ferulic acid esters

The esters of ferulic acid act primarily on the endocrine system. Studies in animals have shown docosanol to reduce levels of leutinizing hormone and testosterone while raising adrenal steroid secretion of both adrenal androgens and corticosteroids.[5,6] Docosanol also significantly reduces serum prolactin levels. This reduction of prolactin is quite significant as prolactin increases the uptake of testosterone and increases the synthesis of dihydrotestosterone within the prostate. The accumulation of testosterone within the prostate and its subsequent conversion to the more potent dihydrotestosterone is thought to be the major contributing factor to the hyperplasia of the prostatic cells observed in BPH.[7] Although traces of docosanol are present in pygeum, the esterification with ferulic acid results in greater bioavailability and activity.[2,4,8]

Ferulic acid esters, as well as the sterol fraction of pygeum, exert cholesterol-lowering action systematically, as well as reducing the intraprostatic cholesterol content.[8] Breakdown products of cholesterol have been shown to accumulate in the prostate tissue affected with either BPH or cancer.[7] These metabolites of cholesterol initiate degeneration of prostatic cells which can promote prostatic enlargement. Drugs which lower cholesterol levels have been shown to have a favorable influence on BPH, preventing the accumulation of cholesterol in the prostatic cells and limiting subsequent formation of damaging cholesterol metabolites. The lowering of intraprostatic cholesterol content is an important aspect of the pharmacology of pygeum.

The sterolic fraction is also endowed with competitive action against testosterone accumulation within the prostate. In addition, the sterols of pygeum have also been shown to reduce inflammation by preventing the intraprostatic formation of inflammatory prostaglandins.[8,9]

Other components

Other components of pygeum are also important. For example, the pentacyclic triterpenes exhibit anti-inflammatory effects within the prostatic epithelium and may be responsible for stimulation of the secretory cells of the prostate, seminal vesicles, and bulbourethral glands.[8–10] And finally, the fatty acids components are similar to those of *Serenoa repens* (see Ch. 110) and may exert similar effects as well as improve the oral bioavailability of other components of the lipophilic extract.

CLINICAL APPLICATIONS

Prostate disorders

The pharmacological actions of the standardized pygeum extract supports its use in prostate disorders, BPH in particular. Adding further support are the results from numerous clinical trials of over 600 patients.[11–33] Consistently, these studies have demonstrated pygeum to effectively reduce the symptoms and clinical signs of BPH, especially in early cases. However, it must be

Table 107.1 Results of the most significant open and double-blind studies of the last 20 years on outpatients with *Pygeum africanum* for 1–3 months

				Percentage of patients showing reduction (%)				
Author	mg/day	Days	No. of patients	Dysuria	Nocturia	Frequency	Residual urine	Prostate volume
Open trials								
Guillemin[11]	100	30	25	80	80	80	80	NC
Lange & Muret[12]	100	30	25	72	NC	72	NC	NC
Wemeau et al[13]	100	45	27	60	NC	71	NC	NC
Viollet[14]	75	60	20	64	NC	64	NC	NC
Lhez & Leguevague[15]	75	90	52	69	NC	NC	NC	NC
Thomas & Rouggilange[16]	75	50	33	60	57	57	NC	–
Huet[17]	50	30	55	85	85	85	NC	20
Rometti[18]	100	50	25	72	72	72	NC	25
Gallizia & Gallizia[19]	100	60	19	90	85	70	20	NC
Durval[20]	100	90	23	72	72	72	72	NC
Pansadoro & Benincasa[21]	75	90	35	94	94	94	94	–
Double-blind trials								
Maver[23]	100	60	60	77	70	57	23	–
Bongi[24]	75	60	50	88	88	88	88	88
Doremieuz et al[25]	100	60	77	85	NC	NC	NC	NC
Del Valio[26]	100	60	30	–	–	48	–	–
Colpi & Farina[27]	150	45	47	–	70	–	76	NC
Donkervoort et al[28]	150	90	20	80	80	80	NC	NC
Dufour & Choquenet[29]	100	45	120	–	78	45	65	NC
Legromandi et al[30]	100	45	104	89	89	89	NC	NC
Ranno et al[31]	200	60	39	75	75	75	NC	NC
Frasseto et al[32]	200	60	20	–	–	–	–	–
Bassi et al[33]	200	60	40	70	70	70	70	70

–, not measured; NC, no change.

pointed out that improvement is largely symptomatic, as the results on reducing the size of the prostate or the residual urine content of the bladder are modest. The results of the clinical trials on pygeum are given in Table 107.1. Below, there is a discussion of some of the most important aspects of these studies.

One of the major findings in evaluating the effectiveness of pygeum in BPH has been the high rate of responders to placebo. This is well-demonstrated in one of the larger double-blind studies.[29] Similar to the results in other double-blind studies, pygeum extract was shown to be statistically superior to a placebo in reducing the major symptoms of BPH (nocturnal frequency, difficulty in starting micturition, and incomplete emptying of the bladder). However, there was a high percentage of responders to the placebo (see Table 107.2 below). It seems that simply taking a capsule provides relief to many sufferers.

Another study highlights the importance of double-blind studies which feature both objective and subjective findings. In the study, both patients and physicians rated the placebo and pygeum extract to be effective in improving subjective symptoms of daytime frequency, nocturia, weak stream, after-dribbling, hesitation, and interruption of flow.[28] However, urodynamic variables (flow, frequency, and histogram) clearly demonstrated the superiority of pygeum over placebo.

Table 107.2 Patients responding to placebo and pygeum

Symptom	Placebo group	Pygeum group
Nocturia	26/52 = 50%	44/56 = 78%
Daytime frequency	16/50 = 33%	27/54 = 50%
Incomplete voiding	14/40 = 35%	21/32 = 66%
Dribbling	15/34 = 44%	13/33 = 39%
Urine flow rate	11/43 = 26%	21/38 = 55%

One of the shortcomings of some of the clinical research on pygeum is the lack, in many of the studies, of objective measures such as urine flow rate (ml/s), residual urine content, and prostate size. Studies that have used objective measurements have shown some good results. For example, in one open trial, 30 patients with BPH given 100 mg/day of the pygeum extract for 75 days demonstrated significant improvements in objective parameters: maximum flow rate increased from 5.43 to 8.20 ml/s and the residual urine volume dropped from 76 to 33 ml.[22]

Male infertility and impotence

Pygeum may be effective in improving fertility in cases where diminished prostatic secretion plays a significant role. Pygeum has been shown to increase prostatic secretions and improve the composition of the seminal fluid.[34–36] Specifically, pygeum administration to men with decreased prostatic secretion has led to increased levels of total seminal fluid plus increases in alkaline phosphatase and protein. Pygeum appears to be most effective in cases where the level of alkaline phosphatase activity is reduced (i.e. less than 400 IU / cm^3) and where there is no evidence of inflammation or infection (i.e. absence of white blood cells or IgA). The lack of IgA in the semen is a good predictor of clinical success. In one study, the patients with no IgA in the semen demonstrated an alkaline phosphatase increase from 265 to 485 IU / cm^3.[3,34] In contrast, those subjects with IgA showed only a modest increase from 213 to 281 IU / cm^3.

Pygeum extract has also shown an ability to improve the capacity to achieve an erection in patients with BPH or prostatitis as determined by nocturnal penile tumescence in a double-blind clinical trial.[37] BPH and prostatitis are often associated with erectile dysfunction and other sexual disturbances. Presumably by improving the underlying condition, pygeum can improve sexual function.

Pygeum vs. serenoa

The standardized liposterolic extract of *Serenoa repens* is another popular botanical treatment for BPH (see Ch. 110). In a double-blind study which compared the pygeum extract with the extract of serenoa, the serenoa extract produced a greater reduction of symptoms and was better tolerated.[38] In addition, the improvement of objective parameters, especially urine flow rate and residual urine content, is better in the clinical studies with serenoa. However, there may be circumstances where pygeum is more effective than serenoa. For example, serenoa has not been shown to produce the effects that pygeum has produced on prostate secretion. Although the two extracts have somewhat overlapping mechanisms of actions, they can be used in combination.

DOSAGE

The dosage of the lipophilic extract of *Pygeum africanum* standardized to contain 14% triterpenes including beta-sitosterol and 0.5% *n*-docosanol is 100–200 mg / day in divided doses. The crude herb is not used.

TOXICOLOGY

Acute and chronic toxicity tests in the rat and mouse have shown that the standardized extract of *Pygeum africanum* bark is non-toxic. Increasing doses from 1 to 6 g / kg in the mouse and from 1 to 8 g / kg in the rat caused no deaths within 48 hours. In chronic toxicity studies, dosing the animals with from 60 to 600 mg / kg for 11 months did not produce any negative effects.

In the human clinical trials, the pygeum extract also demonstrated no significant toxicity. The most common side-effect is gastrointestinal irritation, resulting in symptoms ranging from nausea to severe stomach pains; however, rarely does the presence of these side-effects result in discontinuation of therapy.

REFERENCES

1. Longo R, Tira S. Steroidal and other components of *Pygeum africanum* bark. Il Farmaco 1982; 38: 288–292
2. Martinelli EM, Seraglia R, Pifferi G. Characterization of *Pygeum africanum* bark extracts by HRGC with computer assistance. HRC & CC 1986; 9: 106–110
3. Pierini N. Identification and determination of n-docosanol in *Pygeum africanum* bark extract and in medicinal specialties containing them. Boll Chim Farm 1982; 121: 27–34
4. Uberti E. HPLC analysis of n-docosyl ferulate in *Pygeum africanum* extracts and pharmaceutical formulations. Fitotherapia 1990; 41: 342–347
5. Muntzing J, Eneroth P, Gustafsson JA, Liljekvist J. Direct and indirect effects of docosanol, the active principle in Tadenan, on the rat prostate. Invest Urol 1979; 17: 176–180
6. Thieblot L. Preventive and curative action of *Pygeum africanum* extracts on experimental prostatic adenoma in the rat. Therapie 1975; 26: 575–580
7. Hinman F. Benign Prostatic Hyperplasia. New York: Springer-Verlag. 1983
8. Bombardelli E. Methods, composition and compounds for the treatment of prostatic adenoma. EP Appl 8330491.3, June 10, 1985
9. Marcoli M. Anti-inflammatory and antiedemigenic activity of extract of *Pygeum afrcanum* in the rat. New Trends Androl Sci 1985; 1: 89
10. Latalski M. The ultrastructure of the epithelium of bulbourethral glands after administration of *Pygeum africanum* extract. Folia Morphol 1979; 1: 193–201
11. Guillemin P. Clinical trials of V1326, or Tadenan, in prostatic adenoma. Med Prat 1970; 386: 75–76
12. Lange J, Muret P. Clinical trial of V1326 in prostatic disease. Med 1970; 11: 2807–2811
13. Wemeau L, Delmay J, Blankaert J. Tadenan in prostatic adenoma. Vie Medicale 1970; Jan: 585–588
14. Viollet G. Clinical experimentation of a new drug from prostatic adenoma. Vie Medicale 1970; June: 3457–3458
15. Lhez A, Leguevague G. Clinical trials of a new lipid-sterolic complex of vegetal origin in the treatment of prostatic adenoma. Vie Medicale 1970; Dec: 5399–5404
16. Thomas JP, Rouffilange F. The action of Tadenan in prostatic adenoma. Rev Int Serv 1970; 43: 43–45
17. Huet JA. Prostatic disease in old age. Med Intern 1970; 5: 405–408
18. Rometti A. Medical treatment of prostatic adenoma. La Provence Medicale 1970; 38: 49–51
19. Gallizia F, Gallizia G. Medical treatment of benign prostatic hypertrophy with a new phytotherapeutic principle. Recent Med 1972; 9: 461–468
20. Durval A. The use of a new drug in the treatment of prostatic disorders. Minerva Urol 1970; 22: 106–111
21. Pansadoro V, Benincasa A. Prostatic hypertrophy. Results obtained with *Pygeum africanum* extract. Minerva Med 1972; 11: 119–144
22. Zurita IE, Pecorini M, Cuzzoni G. Treatment of prostatic hypertrophy with *Pygeum africanum* extract. Rev Bras Med 1984; 41: 364–366
23. Maver A. Medical therapy of the fibrous-adematose hypertrophy of the prostate with a new vegetal substance. Minerva Med 1972; 63: 2126–2136
24. Bongi G. Tadenan in the treatment of prostatic adenoma. Minerva Urol 1972; 24: 129–139

25. Doremieux J, Masson JC, Bollack C. Prostatic hypertrophy, clinical effects and histological changes produced by a lipid complex extracted from *Pygeum africanum*. J Med Strasbourg 1973; 4: 253–257
26. Del Valio B. The use of a new drug in the treatment of chronic prostatitis. Minerva Urol 1974; 26: 81–94
27. Colpi G, Farina U. Study of the activity of chloroformic extract of *Pygeum africanum* bark in the treatment of urethral obstructive syndrome caused by non-cancerous prostapathy. Urologia 1976; 43: 441–448
28. Donkervoort T, Sterling J, van Ness J, Donker PJ. A clinical and urodynamic study of Tadenan in the treatment of benign prostatic hypertrophy. Urol 1977; 8: 218–225
29. Dufour B, Choquenet C. Trial controlling the effects of *Pygeum africanum* extract on the functional symptoms of prostatic adenoma. Ann Urol 1984; 18: 193–195
30. Legramandi C, Ricci-Barbini V, Fonte A. The importance of *Pygeum africanum* in the treatment of chronic prostatitis void of bacteria. Gazz Medica Ital 1984; 143: 73–76
31. Ranno S, Minaldi G, Viscusi G et al. Efficacy and tolerability in the treatment of prostatic adenoma with Tadenan 50. Progresso Medico 1986; 42: 165–169
32. Frasseto G, Bertoglio S, Mancuso S et al. Study of the efficacy and tolerability of Tadenan 50 in patients with prostatic hypertrophy. Progresso Medico 1986; 42: 49–52
33. Bassi P, Artibani W, De Luca V et al. Standardized extract of *Pygeum africanum* in the treatment of benign prostatic hypertrophy. Minerva Urol 1987; 39: 45–50
34. Lucchetta G, Weill A, Becker N et al. Reactivation from the prostatic gland in cases of reduced fertility. Urol Int 1984; 39: 222–224
35. Menchini-Fabris GF, Giorgi P, Andreini F et al. New perspectives of treatment of prostato-vesicular pathologies with *Pygeum africanum*. Arch Int Urol 1988; 60: 313–322
36. Clavert A, Cranz C, Riffaud JP et al. Effects of an extract of the bark of *Pygeum africanum* on prostatic secretions in the rat and man. Ann Urol 1986; 20: 341–343
37. Carani C, Salvioli C, Scuteri A et al. Urological and sexual evaluation of treatment of benign prostatic disease using *Pygeum africanum* at high dose. Arch Ital Urol Nefrol Androl 1991; 63: 341–345
38. Duvia R, Radice GP, Galdini R. Advances in the phytotherapy of prostatic hypertrophy. Med Praxis 1983; 4: 143–148

CHAPTER CONTENTS

108

Recommended optimum nutrient intakes (RONIs)

Alexander G. Schauss, PhD

INTRODUCTION

In 1998, the Food and Nutrition Board of the US Institute of Medicine recommended that to reduce the likelihood of neural tube defects in children, "women should eat a varied diet *and take an extra 400 micrograms of folic acid* to be absolutely sure that they get enough of the nutrient".

That the public should use a dietary supplement, not just food, to reassure themselves that they are getting the necessary levels of a nutrient to prevent a disease or condition is nothing less than a paradigm shift in official public health policy.

In recent years a convincing link between the intake of folic acid and neural tube defects has been established. As a result, the National Institutes of Health and US Department of Health and Human Services have given special attention to the need for folic acid in the diet in the prevention of such neural tube defects as spina bifida.

Folic acid is but one of the B vitamins that in recent years has been the subject of research into the role that nutrients play in the prevention, mitigation or treatment of cancers, cardiovascular diseases, mental disorders, and other diseases or conditions. For example, researchers are continuing to unravel the association between levels of folate, pyridoxine (vitamin B_6) and inositol, and the reduction of excessive levels of blood homocysteine, a marker associated with the risk of cardiovascular disease.

This chapter will discuss the recommended optimal daily intake of nutrients necessary to maintain health and reduce the risk of disease. The conclusion reached by the author for each nutrient is based on a review of thousands of epidemiological, clinical, and experimental papers, offering evidence for optimal versus minimal intake levels.

The RDAs

The weaknesses of the RDAs

Since the mid-1940s, the US recommended daily allowances (RDAs) have served as a nutritional guideline.

These guidelines were developed from minimalist criteria aimed solely at the prevention of nutritionally related clinical deficiencies. More recently, in the mid-1990s, these guidelines were superseded by Food and Drug Administration (FDA) nutritional guidelines known as the recommended daily intake levels (RDIs). Curiously, the RDIs show no more promise than did the RDAs in providing the public with useful information on the intake of nutrients in the prevention, mitigation and treatment of a wide range of conditions and diseases for which diet does, or may, play a role. Hence, it is worthwhile to understand the limits of the RDAs and RDIs to fully appreciate the need for recommended optimal nutrition intake (RONIs). Since our understanding of the optimal level of each nutrient in the prevention, mitigation, and treatment of disease remains a somewhat primitive science, the discussion will be framed around the concept of recommended optimal nutrition intake (RONI). As our understanding of the role of each nutrient in disease processes becomes more sophisticated, the values for the RONIs are certain to change. Yet they certainly provide us with better guidelines to maintain health than the minimalist basis from which the RDAs were constructed.

The history of the RDAs

In May 1941, a committee of the National Academy of Sciences suggested for the first time that a "recommended daily dietary allowance" of essential nutrients be established. These guidelines were developed with the goal of reducing the incidence of nutritional deficiency diseases in the general population, such as scurvy (deficiency of vitamin C), pellagra (deficiency of niacin), and beri-beri (deficiency of vitamin B_1). Since then, nutritionists, dietitians, and physicians have relied on the RDAs, including nine revisions, as guidelines for advising public health officials and the public on recommended nutrient intake levels.

According to the committee that established the RDAs, they were intended:

- as guidelines for the prevention of nutritional deficiencies
- to be related to the nutrient status of population groups, not individuals.

In essence, the RDAs provide no information on the role of nutrients in the prevention, amelioration, or treatment of conditions or diseases.

A common mistake made by many public health practitioners is to use the RDAs to evaluate the adequacy of an individual's diet. Even worse is the assumption that maintaining a diet that provides an RDA level of nutrients will somehow ensure wellness over one's lifetime. Only recently has it become apparent that "healthy normal people" are an ideal. Among Americans aged 60 and over, more than 80% suffer from at least one or more chronic diseases, such as cancer, atherosclerosis, osteoporosis, macular degeneration, or diabetes.

Since at least 1951, critics of the RDAs have asserted that they lack the ability to recommend levels of nutrients sufficient to maintain health for a person seeking a healthy life span that is associated with a morbidity-free existence.

Studies used to determine the level of a nutrient that is sufficient to prevent a nutritional deficiency are typically conducted for only 6–9 months, about 1% of the average person's life span. This suggests that these minimalist dietary standards are based on data incapable of suggesting levels of nutrients essential to prevent many conditions and diseases associated with morbidity.

Even more germane to this issue is the attention focused in recent years on the role of substances not generally recognized as nutrients that appear to be directly involved in the prevention or mitigation of a diverse host of diseases from colon cancer to coronary heart disease, cataracts, birth defects, and stroke.

Early editions of the RDAs that where published in the 1940s clearly stated that the RDAs "vary greatly in disease". Yet in spite of this realization, the RDAs continue to focus only on the prevention of nutritional deficiencies in population groups. However, this began to change in 1989 with the release of the 10th edition of the RDAs by the National Academy of Sciences.

The 10th edition acknowledged for the first time that levels of a nutrient, specifically the nutrient vitamin C, may need to be higher than the RDA for groups at risk of developing chronic diseases, particularly, smokers. This welcome recommendation by the National Academy of Sciences has opened the door to an entirely new paradigm, namely, the determination of optimal nutrient intake levels needed to minimize the risk of developing conditions and diseases affecting various population groups (i.e. women at risk of birth defects).

Unfortunately, the RDAs' noble attempt remains inadequate because of its minimalist foundation. While a higher level of vitamin C intake for smokers is indeed suggested in the 10th edition, studies of the blood levels of vitamins and minerals in smokers have shown that low levels of other nutrients such as beta-carotene, zinc, vitamin B_6, and vitamin E may also be needed at significantly higher levels than that recommended for vitamin C or prescribed by the RDAs. Mounting evidence suggests that all of these nutrients, not just vitamin C, and probably many other nutrients and non-nutritive substances, may need to be taken by smokers to compensate for the nutrient loss such a habit produces.

The RDAs also fail to address excessive use of alcohol – yet another example of a common addiction that increases nutrient requirements. Individuals who chronically consume alcohol have been found to have lower levels of folate, vitamin B_1, vitamin B_6, vitamin A, beta-carotene, zinc, and vitamin C.

The lifestyles of individuals are also neglected in the RDAs. Dieters, for example, are a population who have frequently been found to have low nutrient status. Studies have shown that it is extremely difficult, if not impossible, to meet all of the RDAs for nutrients, let alone maintain health, when chronically consuming less than 1,200 calories/day. An analyses of 11 major reducing diets shows that none can provide 100% of the RDA for vitamins alone. What about individuals with eating disorders (i.e. bulimia nervosa)? Or those working under chronic conditions of stress? Individuals who smoke cigarettes? Or heavy alcohol consumers?

We have come to realize that individuals may have habits or lifestyles that require nutrient levels that are well in excess of those recommended by the RDAs.

It is important to understand the limits of the RDAs and to appreciate the potential benefits of higher nutrient intake levels. Table 108.1 outlines five limitations of the RDAs as dietary intake guidelines in the prevention of conditions and diseases that affect morbidity and mortality.

The need for a guideline to optimal intake levels of nutrients

A growing body of evidence indicates that intakes of certain vitamins and minerals at levels well above the RDAs may be necessary to protect against the development of certain conditions and diseases that affect our quality of life and/or life span. For example, antioxidants, such as vitamin C, beta-carotene, vitamin E, and selenium, may prevent free radical damage to vascular endothelial cells associated with the most common form of cardiovascular disease, atherosclerosis. These vitamins/minerals may be required in much higher amounts than the RDA to prevent atherosclerosis than those levels suggested by the RDAs to prevent deficiency symptoms, unless, of course, the development of atherosclerosis is a deficiency symptom of these vitamins. The same might be said of many cancers, heart disease, birth defects, eye diseases (e.g. macular degeneration and cataracts), hearing loss, diabetes, and other conditions and diseases.

Table 108.1 Limitations of the RDAs

- They are meant to serve as a guideline for the prevention of nutritional diseases, not the promotion of health
- The recommendations are based on the nutrient status of large population groups numbering in the millions, not as a guideline to determine individual dietary nutrient requirements
- The estimates of the RDAs are based only on short-term research that represents less than 1% of the average person's lifespan, so they cannot provide nutrient recommendations that may be of benefit over a lifetime in the prevention or amelioration of diseases associated with aging or certain lifestyles
- They do not make adjustments for variations in nutrient needs associated with conditions or diseases that affect nutrient requirements
- They provide no data on compensatory levels of nutrient intake needed to compensate for nutrient-demanding lifestyle factors such as: chronic stress, chronic intense exercise, cigarette smoking, alcoholism, restrictive dieting routines, polluted environments, exposure to chemical carcinogens, etc.

The development of recommended optimum nutrient intakes

As a result of numerous epidemiological, clinical and experimental studies, it is now possible to extrapolate a list of recommended optimum nutrient intakes, or RONIs, for all of the major vitamins and minerals essential to our health.

Nearly 20 years ago an attempt was made by Drs Cheraskin and Ringsdorf at the University of Alabama School of Medicine in Birmingham to establish RONIs. Their study of optimal intake levels of vitamins and minerals in humans spanned a period of 15 years. They examined the dietary intake and physiological levels of nutrients in over 13,500 male and female subjects living in six diverse regions of the United States. The results of their multimillion dollar study was compiled into over 49,000 pages found in 153 bound volumes.

A small but significant portion of their findings has been published, in a series of over 100 research papers, during a period of 20 years, ending in the early 1990s.

Cheraskin & Ringsdorf's research investigated the health status of its subjects through a relatively time-consuming evaluation of each person's health status. Each subject in the study completed the following test or procedure:

1. the 195 item Cornell Medical Index Health Questionnaire (CMI)
2. physical and anthropometric measurements
3. dental examination
4. eye examination
5. cardiac function tests, including an electroencephalogram (EKG)
6. a glucose tolerance test (GTT)
7. a panel of 50 blood chemistries
8. a comprehensive study of each subject's diet, including a study of food intake over a 7-day period.

Their study attempted to find evidence that there may exist an "ideal" diet consisting of micronutrients, carbohydrates, protein, and fat which could contribute to health and longevity. The hypothesis of the study concluded that relatively symptomless and disease-free individuals are healthier than those with clinical symptoms and signs and that this difference was due to the intake of nutrients from the diet and/or dietary supplementation.

Findings

Cheraskin & Ringsdorf's 15 year study of 13,500 subjects found that the healthiest individuals, meaning those with the least clinical symptoms and signs, were those who had consumed dietary supplements and eaten a diet nutritionally dense in nutrients relative to their caloric intake.

Nutritionally, density of the diet proved to be a key variable among the healthiest subjects. For example, Cheraskin & Ringsdorf discovered that the "healthiest" subjects had a mean vitamin C intake of 410 mg a day, a good portion of which was consumed from food. The finding of a vitamin C intake above 400 mg a day is particularly interesting in light of anthropological evidence of vitamin C intake in pre-agricultural diets. One study found that humans living prior to the dawn of agriculture (<10,000 BC) consumed approximately 392 mg of vitamin C a day, well above the 60 mg suggested by the RDAs.

This represents only a 4% difference in daily vitamin C intake between humans living many generations apart!

Equally intriguing is continuing evidence to suggest that the incidence of cancer and other chronic diseases of modern civilization is relatively rare in ancestral humans who lived prior to the advent of agriculture. Could the higher intake of vitamin C and other nutrients in primitive diets be related to the lower incidence of such chronic degenerative diseases? This is a question that may take years to be resolved, but it does warrant further inspection.

Epidemiologic evidence of a protective effect of vitamin C for non-hormone-dependent cancers is strong, according to a 1991 National Cancer Institute report. Of the 46 studies in which dietary vitamin C was calculated, 33 found statistically significant protection against cancer, with the highest vitamin C intake conferring the most protection. Of 29 additional studies that assessed fruit intake, 21 found significant protection. For cancers of the esophagus, larynx, oral cavity, and pancreas, evidence for a protective effect of vitamin C or some component in fruit (e.g. bioflavonoids and carotenoids) remains strong and consistent. For cancers of the stomach, rectum, breast, and cervix there is also strong evidence of a protective effect against cancer. Several recent lung cancer studies have found significant protective effects of vitamin C. Therefore, the concept of an "ideal" or suggested recommended optimum nutrient intake (RONI) of 410 mg/day of vitamin C or more may not be out of line, even though it is more than four times higher than the RDA.

The evidence in support of vitamin C at higher intake levels, along that with many similar findings for other nutrients, such as selenium, suggests that the RDAs may represent the nutritional equivalent of the minimum wage. Clearly, there is a profound need for a new paradigm to replace the minimalistic and outmoded RDAs.

RONIs present estimates of vitamin and mineral intake levels that may reduce the risk of conditions and diseases that impair our ability to function or increase our risk of illness.

RONIs survey questionnaire

The following questions can serve as a guideline to determine if higher nutrient requirements than the RDAs are warranted for an individual.

If the patient answers yes to any of the 16 items listed below, the RONIs that follow in the next section for each vitamin and mineral may be of benefit in determining a reasonable and safe daily intake of the respective nutrient. The asterisk (*) following any question indicates that there currently exists reasonable scientific evidence to support a nutrient intake of certain vitamins and minerals well above the RDAs:

1. Are you under chronic emotional stress?*
2. Do you have frequent colds and flus (more than three/year)?*
3. Do you wish to reduce your risk of developing cardiovascular disease?*
4. Do you wish to reduce your risk of developing cancer?*
5. Do you wish to reduce your risk of developing osteoporosis?*
6. Do you wish to reduce your risk of developing macular degeneration of the eye?*
7. Do you have skin problems?*
8. Do you smoke cigarettes?*
9. Are you regularly exposed to side-stream smoke at home or work?*
10. Do you frequently drink alcohol?*
11. Do you take birth control pills?*
12. Are you pregnant?*
13. Are you over the age of 50?*
14. Are you postmenopausal?*
15. Do you exercise more than three times a week for 1 hour at a time?
16. Is the air you breathe polluted?*

THE RONIs

The following sections discuss each nutrient for which a RONI could be determined based on existing scientific evidence. The format for each nutrient is identical, allowing you to contrast the RDA with the RONI for that nutrient. RONIs are divided by gender and age along the same parameters as the RDAs for easy comparison. The recommendations made are based on the median weight and height for each designated age group, as listed in Table 108.2. If the patient's height and weight are significantly higher or lower than the figures found for the age group, adjust accordingly.

Table 108.2 Median weight and height for US population of designated age

Category	Age (years)	Weight (lb)	Height (in)
Males	15–18	145	69
	19–24	160	70
	25–50	174	70
	51+	170	68
Females	11–14	101	62
	15–18	120	64
	19–24	128	65
	25–50	138	64
	51+	143	63

The nutrients discussed in the following sections are divided into three nutrient classifications in alphabetical order (Table 108.3). A comprehensive list of references for each nutrient is found in the reference section under the nutrient of interest.

Fat-soluble vitamins

Vitamin A (see Table 108.4)

Vitamin A is required for reproduction, embryonic development, the maintenance of epithelial tissue (i.e. skin, lung, vagina, uterus, gastrointestinal tract), cell differentiation, and vision. It may be important in cancer prevention and treatment of precancerous conditions. Illness, and particularly febrile conditions and lipid malabsorption, can markedly increase vitamin A requirements.

Table 108.3 Vitamin and mineral comparisons between RDAs and RONIs

Fat soluble vitamins
- Vitamin A/beta-carotene
- Vitamin D
- Vitamin E
- Vitamin K

Water-soluble vitamins
- Ascorbic acid (vitamin C)
- Cyanocobalamin (vitamin B_{12})
- Folic acid
- Niacin/niacinamide (vitamin B_3)
- Pyridoxine (vitamin B_6)
- Riboflavin (vitamin B_2)
- Thiamin (vitamin B_1)

Minerals
- Boron
- Calcium
- Chromium
- Copper
- Iodine
- Iron
- Magnesium
- Manganese
- Phosphorous
- Potassium
- Selenium
- Sodium
- Zinc

Table 108.4 Vitamin A (μg RE)

Category	Age	RDA	Optimal
Males	11–14	1,000	1,000
	15–18	1,000	1,000
	19–24	1,000	2,000
	25–50	1,000	2,000
	51+	1,000	2,000
Females	11–14	800	800
	15–18	800	800
	19–24	800	2,000
	25–50	800	2,000
	51+	800	2,000

Excessive intake of vitamin A, but not of the provitamin A carotenoids, can cause toxicity, the most serious of which are birth defects. Hence, women of child-bearing age should show prudence in taking excessive amounts of vitamin A without the advice of a health practitioner. Pregnant women should preferentially ingest foods rich in carotenoids or consume a mixed carotene supplement to ensure adequate vitamin A supplies, given the role of vitamin A in cell differentiation.

Vitamin A toxicity in adults is uncommon at doses below 100,000 IU/day. If toxicity does develop, symptoms disappear within a short period of time after reduction of intake.

Beta-carotene (see Table 108.5)

Beta-carotene is a source of vitamin A, since it is the most nutritionally active vitamin A precursor among carotenoids. Beta-carotene is also referred to as a "provitamin" since it converts to vitamin A in the body. Of the nearly 600 carotenoids which have been identified in natural sources, less than 50 are vitamin A precursors such as beta-carotene. Animal studies have shown that beta-carotene is not mutagenic, teratogenic, embryotoxic, or carcinogenic, nor does it cause hypervitaminosis A (vitamin A toxicity).

Table 108.5 Beta-carotene (mg)

Category	Age	RDA	Optimal
Males	11–14	n/a	50
	15–18	n/a	70
	19–24	n/a	100
	25–50	n/a	100
	51+	n/a	100
Females	11–14	n/a	50
	15–18	n/a	60
	19–24	n/a	80
	25–50	n/a	80
	51+	n/a	80

n/a, not available.
Retinol equivalents: 1 retinol equivalent = 1 μg retinol or 6 μg beta-carotene.

Beta-carotene and its related carotenoids protect against various cancers and can enhance cancer resistance directly as an antimutagen and anticarcinogen and indirectly as an antioxidant, reducing cell damage. In particular, increased beta-carotene levels seem to decrease the risk of developing lung cancer, important information for cigarette smokers or those regularly exposed to sidestream smoke. Individuals with low intakes of beta-carotene have a 30–220% higher risk of developing lung cancer than those with a high intake of this nutrient. A 12 year study of almost 3,000 men living in Switzerland found an association between low blood levels of vitamin A and beta-carotene and increased risk of lung cancer and death from all cancers. Men with low carotene levels had nearly twice the risk of developing lung cancer, as compared with men with normal levels, and nearly 3.5 times the risk of stomach cancer.

Beta-carotene also has non-vitamin A functions based on its ability to act as an antioxidant by scavenging free radicals. For example, carotenoids protect against the damage from excessive ultraviolet exposure that can lead to UV-related tissue damage and skin cancer.

Vitamin D (see Table 108.6)

Vitamin D is a prohormone classified as a vitamin. It is important for bone maintenance and the metabolism and absorption of phosphorous and calcium, while also contributing to the functioning of the reproductive system, the digestive system, and the immune system.

Vegetarians, the elderly, and individuals receiving limited exposure to sunlight ultraviolet, may be at risk of inadequate vitamin D levels. The elderly may be at particular risk of poor vitamin D status due to:

- decreased exposure to sunlight
- decreased intake of vitamin D fortified foods
- decreased absorption of the nutrient in the gastrointestinal tract
- decreased caloric intake.

The skin of elderly individuals also produces approximately half the vitamin D after exposure to the sun as produced by a young person.

Good vitamin D status may be associated with reduced risk of hypertension while also playing a role in regulating blood pressure. There is epidemiological evidence, including one very large study of US Navy personnel, that adequate vitamin D levels may decrease the chance of developing certain lethal skin melanomas (skin cancers) in adults with occupations and lifestyles that prevent regular exposure to sunlight for up to 15 minutes a day.

There is also increasing evidence that vitamin D combined with calcium might reduce the number of colorectal tumors. This is an important finding given the increasing incidence of colon cancer. Although those studying this phenomena conclude that optimal intake of calcium and vitamin D reduces colon cancer risk, they are unable as yet to explain the mechanism for this protective effect.

Vitamin D can be toxic at prolonged (several months) high intakes. No adverse effects, however, have been reported in healthy adults who have consumed up to 62 times the RDA of this nutrient. Since vitamin D has been shown to be teratogenic in animals, a pregnant, or potentially pregnant woman, should take vitamin D supplements with caution.

Sunlight ultraviolet exposure on the skin promotes vitamin D production. It is important to note that this process is self-limiting and will not cause vitamin D toxicity (hypervitaminosis D) in healthy people.

Vitamin E (tocopherols and tocotrienols) (see Table 108.7)

Vitamin E is essential to all mammals. The term vitamin E applies to a family of eight related compounds, the tocopherols and the tocotrienols. The four major forms of vitamin E are designated alpha, beta, delta, and gamma. The tocotrienols are less widely distributed in nature than the tocopherols. Tocotrienols are less biologically active than the tocopherols.

Table 108.6 Vitamin D*

Category	Age	RDA	Optimal
Males	11–14	10	10
	15–18	10	10
	19–24	10	12
	25–50	5	20
	51+	5	24
Females	11–14	10	10
	15–18	10	12
	19–24	10	12
	25–50	5	18
	51+	5	22

*As cholecalciferol.
10 μg cholecalciferol = 400 IU of vitamin D.

Table 108.7 Vitamin E (mg tocopherol)

Category	Age	RDA	Optimal
Males	11–14	10	70
	15–18	10	100
	19–24	10	400
	25–50	10	400
	51+	10	800
Females	11–14	8	70
	15–18	8	90
	19–24	8	400
	25–50	8	400
	51+	8	800

Alpha-tocopherol equivalents: 1 mg D-alpha tocopherol = 1 IU alpha-tocopherol.

One of the most important functions of vitamin E is to protect living cell membranes from damage by oxygen free radicals, a process known as "oxidative damage". By reacting with a free radical, the tocopherol molecule is converted into the tocopheroxyl radical, which can then be reduced back to harmless tocopherol by either vitamin C or glutathione. Any deficiency of this vitamin can affect the life span of red blood cells.

Vitamin E plays a role in preventing mutagenesis, in the repair of membranes and DNA, and in maintenance of immunocompetence, especially as it relates to normal T-lymphocyte function.

Many studies have found that the incidence of various cancers is higher in individuals with low levels of vitamin E. Evidence to date is strong that a low intake of vitamin E is a risk factor for cancer in many, but not all, organs. The expression of its protective effect may depend on the primary causes, which vary. This is particularly important for smokers or those exposed to cigarette smoke, since vitamin E is a respiratory tract antioxidant. There is evidence that vitamin E inhibits platelet aggregation, thereby reducing the risk of developing blood clots that can potentially lead to myocardial infarcts or stroke.

Immunity and infection resistance have been shown to be enhanced by vitamin E supplementation in elderly people. Adequate vitamin E levels may also protect against cataract development. In one study, vitamin E supplementation reduced the risk of cataracts by more than 50% compared with those not supplemented. The benefit of vitamin E supplementation is unclear for both recreational exercisers and high-intensity athletes. However, vitamin E may play an important role in preventing exercise-induced muscle injury.

Although vitamin E is required throughout an individual's life span, its levels decline with aging, probably due to lowered caloric intake or poor food choices.

In general, high intake of vitamin E seems very safe. Very few side-effects have been reported in any scientifically controlled studies, with intakes as high as 3,200 mg (3,200 IU). Vitamin E supplementation is not, however, recommended for individuals receiving anticoagulant therapy who may also be vitamin K-deficient. The suggested optimal levels are for natural vitamin E (D-alpha tocopherol, D-alpha tocopheryl acetate or D-alpha tocopheryl succinate). All forms of natural vitamin E become active antioxidants (free radical scavengers) inside the body. The synthetic forms of vitamin E have the DL-designations in front of the form provided.

Vitamin K (phylloquinone) (see Table 108.8)

Vitamin K is found in food and created by bacteria in normal intestines. Phylloquinone is the natural form of the vitamin and the primary dietary source of vitamin K.

Table 108.8 Vitamin K (mg)

Category	Age	RDA	Optimal
Males	11–14	45	45
	15–18	65	65
	19–24	70	70
	25–50	80	80
	51+	80	80
Females	11–14	45	45
	15–18	55	55
	19–24	60	60
	25–50	65	65
	51+	65	65

Vitamin K's primary function is in the production of blood clots and skeletal health. There is also growing evidence that vitamin K plays a role in bone development, especially loss of bone mass in postmenopausal osteoporosis.

A normal mixed diet contains 300–500 μg/day of vitamin K, well in excess of the RDA. The RDA recommends a daily intake of 1 μg/kg body weight of phylloquinone for adults and children. There is no known toxicity association with the administration of high doses of phylloquinone.

There is insufficient evidence to support supplemental intake of vitamin K beyond that found in most diets, except possibly in postmenopausal women and in women suffering from menorrhagia.

Water-soluble vitamins

Ascorbic acid (vitamin C) (see Table 108.9)

Adequate vitamin C (ascorbic acid) intake is necessary for immunity, maintenance of bones, formation of collagen, and a broad range of other biologic functions.

In a study which measured the vitamin C intake of

Table 108.9 Vitamin C (mg)

Category	Age	RDA	Optimal
Males	11–14	50	150
	15–18	60	200
	19–24	60	200
	25–50	60	400
	51+	60	800
Females	11–14	50	150
	15–18	60	200
	19–24	60	200
	25–50	60	400
	51+	60	1000

A new RDA for adults for vitamin C of 200 mg/day has been suggested, following US Department of Agriculture and National Cancer Institute recommendations for fruit and vegetable consumption that results in vitamin C intakes of greater than 210 mg/day.

1,038 doctors and their wives, those with the fewest signs and symptoms of illness or degenerative diseases consumed an average of 410 mg/day of vitamin C, about nine times the RDA. To achieve this level of intake usually requires supplementation. Cigarette smoking is associated with a significant decrease in vitamin C levels. For a typical smoker to attain the same vitamin C level as a non-smoker consumption of three to four times as much vitamin C is required. Alcoholics also have low vitamin C status, and may require considerably more vitamin C due to their condition. The elderly may especially benefit from vitamin C supplementation. Increased lipid (fat) peroxidation has been associated with accelerated aging and degeneration. One study demonstrated that supplementation over a 1 year period with vitamin C at levels much higher than the RDA significantly decreased lipid peroxide levels in elderly subjects.

Research suggests that vitamin C may decrease the risk of developing cataracts, cancers of the gastrointestinal tract, and cardiovascular disease. In a 12 year study of 3,000 men living in Switzerland, those with low blood levels of vitamin C had an increased risk of stomach and intestinal cancer. For people over 60, low vitamin C levels were associated with nearly a threefold increased risk of developing stomach cancer and twice the risk for intestinal cancer. The interest in vitamin C in the treatment of cancer is partially based on studies showing significantly reduced levels in patients with malignancies. Most evidence suggests that larger than RDA doses of vitamin C may be beneficial in reducing the risk of developing various cancers, rather than treating them. This may be due to the higher levels of vitamin C improving certain indices of immune competence and response that boost disease resistance.

High dietary intake of vitamin C has been reported to be associated with low death rates from cerebrovascular and cardiovascular diseases. A cohort study of 11,348 non-institutionalized US adults found that women and men with the highest vitamin C intake and regular vitamin C supplements had a 25 and 42% decrease in cardiovascular mortality, respectively. Vitamin C supplementation may reduce the risk of cardiovascular mortality by influencing cholesterol levels, platelets, and even blood pressure.

Since the levels of vitamin C decline with age after midlife, there is evidence that suboptimal levels of vitamin C may increase the risk of cataracts. Those individuals who consume the lowest levels of vitamin C seem to have the highest incidence of cataractous lenses. One study has shown that those subjects who supplemented with vitamin C significantly lowered their risk of developing cataracts.

Vitamin C markedly increases non-heme iron absorption. In some diets, only 3% of non-heme iron is absorbed compared with as much as 23% of the heme iron form. The addition of 50–100 mg of vitamin C with meals can double or triple non-heme iron absorption. Two grams (2,000 mg) of vitamin C taken throughout the day with meals increases the absorption of non-heme iron fivefold.

Bone density and vitamin C status decline after age 35. Vitamin C is an important nutrient in bone metabolism, especially in the synthesis of collagen which forms the structural framework of bones. A number of studies show that vitamin C supplementation results in improved maintenance of bone mineral density in postmenopausal women. Studies have also shown reductions in healing time of wounds with high-dose vitamin C supplementation.

Vitamin C taken at optimal ranges is virtually free of any known or observed side-effects. Doses of greater than 500 mg/day may increase urinary oxalate kidney stones in patients with a prior history of oxalate kidney stones, although this continues to be contested by conflicting evidence. Doses in excess of 1,000 mg at a time have been known to cause diarrhea (bowel tolerance), hyperuricosuria and hyperoxaluria in healthy individuals. There is also evidence that doses as high as 10,000 mg/day have no adverse side-effects.

Cyanocobalamin (vitamin B_{12}) (see Table 108.10)

Vitamin B_{12} is synthesized by bacteria and found in virtually all animals, but rarely in any plant foodstuffs. Vitamin B_{12} is essential for the functioning of the central nervous system and a number of enzymes involved in amino acid, nucleic acid, and fatty acid metabolism. It is also necessary in the metabolism of folic acid (folate), which is essential for thymidine, and thus DNA, synthesis.

Vitamin B_{12} deficiency is common among the elderly, due to lack of gastric intrinsic factor. This often results in neurological, cerebral, and psychiatric abnormalities. In such cases an injectable form of vitamin B_{12} has proven superior to oral vitamin B_{12} supplement. However, there is growing evidence that oral vitamin B_{12} (cyanocobalamin) is a completely safe alternative to vitamin B_{12} injections. One study has found that some individuals with gastric disease who poorly absorb vitamin B_{12} from food can absorb crystalline supplement form. Some experts have

Table 108.10 Vitamin B_{12} (Cyanocobalamin) (µg)

Category	Age	RDA	Optimal
Males	11–14	2.0	2.0
	15–18	2.0	2.0
	19–24	2.0	2.0
	25–50	2.0	2.0
	51+	2.0	3.0
Females	11–14	2.0	2.0
	15–18	2.0	2.0
	19–24	2.0	2.0
	25–50	2.0	2.0
	51+	2.0	3.0

argued that the only legitimate need for vitamin B_{12} supplementation is in patients with a congenital defect of vitamin B_{12} metabolism, such as vitamin B_{12}-responsive methylmalonic acidemia.

Vitamin B_{12} deficiency is more likely in very strict vegetarians, since the best sources of vitamin B_{12} are meat and meat products and, to a lesser extent, milk and milk products, some seafoods, and egg yolk.

There is increasing evidence that vitamin B_{12} may play a role in the prevention of some types of cancers. Smokers, for example, have been found to have significantly decreased levels of precancerous bronchial squamous metaplasia when given vitamin B_{12} (500 µg/day) and folic acid supplements as compared to those receiving placebo. Although there is increasing evidence that vitamin B_{12} may reduce one risk factor for arteriosclerosis, the accumulation of homocysteine (homocysteinemia), the actual risk reduction has not been definitively determined.

There is insufficient evidence to advocate an intake of vitamin B_{12} above the RDA in any population group, except in the elderly, or when there exists evidence of pernicious anemia. In the case of pernicious anemia, vitamin B_{12} injections (parenteral cobalamin) or weekly oral doses of 1,000 µg is suggested. However, during such treatment, care should be given to not take large amounts of folic acid, since this may mask the nerve damage associated with vitamin B_{12} deficiency.

Vitamin B_{12} is not carcinogenic, teratogenic, or mutagenic. It is considered safe even at 1,000 times the RDA.

Folic acid (pteroylglutamic acid) (see Table 108.11)

Recognition of the critical importance of folate for maintaining health is growing. It is essential not only in preventing the vitamin-related anemia, but in four dreaded conditions: heart disease, cancer, stroke, and neural tube defects.

Folic acid is required in the metabolism of some amino acids, for the synthesis of nucleic acids, and in a number of enzyme cofactors. Certain population groups are at particular risk of developing folate deficiency, especially pregnant women and adolescent females. Like newborn infants, which are also at risk, these groups experience considerable growth, confirming the importance of folic acid in protein synthesis and the DNA and RNA replication required in cell growth. Inadequate folic acid is also seen in the elderly, where it is less well absorbed.

Table 108.11 Folic acid (folate) (µg)

Category	Age	RDA	Optimal
Males	11–14	150	500
	15–18	200	750
	19–24	200	1,000
	25–50	200	2,000
	51+	200	2,000
Females	11–14	150	500
	15–18	180	750
	19–24	180	1,000
	25–50	180	1,000
	51+	180	2,000

Since folic acid deficiency is a well-documented cause of birth defects in animals, numerous studies have looked at its role in such human congenital malformations as neural tube defects, cleft palate, and cleft lip. Folic acid and multivitamin supplementation have been demonstrated in numerous studies to decrease or eliminate the recurrence of neural tube defects or cleft palate/cleft lip in human offspring.

Folic acid may also reduce a risk factor associated with atherosclerosis. Folic acid is required for the conversion of homocysteine to methionine. A deficiency of folic acid is associated with elevated homocysteine (homocystinemia), which is a risk factor for atherosclerosis. Normal subjects given 5 mg/day of folic acid for 2 weeks had significant decreases in homocysteine levels, especially in those whose initial homocysteine levels were high. There is also mounting evidence that smokers and heavy coffee drinkers require a higher intake of folic acid.

Folate is required for critical brain metabolic functions. Low folate levels have been implicated in poorer antidepressant response to selective serotonin reuptake inhibitors. Borderline to deficient serum or red blood cell folate levels have been detected in from 15 to 38% of adults diagnosed with depressive disorders.

Folic acid supplementation in healthy adults is safe even at high levels of intake, although such supplementation can mask clinical signs of pernicious anemia, which if left untreated can lead to permanent nerve damage. There is also some continuing controversy about whether folic acid supplementation of 400 µg or more reduces zinc absorption. To be on the safe side, until additional studies are completed, an optimal level of zinc intake is suggested.

Niacin (nicotinic acid) and (niacinamide) nicotinamide (see Table 108.12)

Niacin is the generic descriptor for nicotinic acid (pyridine-3-carboxylic acid) and derivatives exhibiting biological activity of nicotinamide (nicotinic acid amide). Niacin is critical in many biochemical processes, particularly those involving energy metabolism and lipid metabolism. Niacin is a vitamin whose requirements in humans is met in part by conversion of the essential amino acid tryptophan to niacin. Several studies have calculated that 39–86 mg of tryptophan produce the same levels of niacin metabolites as does 1 mg of niacin. For this reason the convention is to consider 1 mg of niacin as equivalent to 60 mg of tryptophan. Because most proteins contain at least 1–2% tyrptophan, it is possible to maintain adequate

Table 108.12 Niacin (mg)

Category	Age	RDA	Optimal
Males	11–14	17	25
	15–18	20	30
	19–24	19	30
	25–50	19	30
	51+	15	30
Females	11–14	15	25
	15–18	15	25
	19–24	15	25
	25–50	15	25
	51+	15	25

1 niacin equivalent = 1 mg niacin or 60 mg dietary tryptophan.

Table 108.13 Pyridoxine (mg)

Category	Age	RDA	Optimal
Males	11–14	1.7	2.0
	15–18	2.0	5.0
	19–24	2.0	10.0
	25–50	2.0	10.0
	51+	2.0	25.0
Females	11–14	1.4	2.0
	15–18	1.5	5.0
	19–24	1.6	10.0
	25–50	1.6	10.0
	51+	1.6	20.0

niacin status on a diet relatively devoid of niacin but containing at least 100 g/day of protein.

Its use as a drug-like agent that lowers low-density lipoprotein (LDL) and very low-density lipoprotein (VLDL) cholesterol and triglycerides, while increasing high-density lipoprotein (HDL) cholesterol has generated much interest. Nicotinic acid given in doses of 1.5–3.0 g/day has been shown to decrease total and LDL cholesterol and to increase HDL cholesterol concentrations. There is also interest in its notorious, but not harmful, vasodilatory or "flushing" effect in increasing blood flow to the extremities in certain circulatory disorders. This effect comes only from the nicotinic acid form, not from the amide. There is no evidence that levels above twice the RDA for niacin in healthy persons prevent disorders associated with high cholesterol (hypercholesterolemia) or other hyperlipidemias.

The only evidence for a significantly higher intake of niacin above the RDA in healthy asymptomatic individuals comes from the prospective study of Cheraskin & Ringsdorf discussed earlier in the introduction. In this study it was found that those individuals with the least number of signs and symptoms associated with physical illness or degeneration were consuming an average of 115 mg of niacin a day, or approximately six or seven times the RDA. A single study is inadequate, however, to suggest this amount is optimal; additional studies are needed.

Because nicotinic acid can increase blood sugar levels, nicotinic acid supplementation is contraindicated in diabetics. Also, large intakes of nicotinic acid (>1,000 mg) have been associated with stomach pain, diarrhea, cardiac arrhythmias, itching, and nausea. These side-effects have, however, have not been observed in humans supplementing with the esterified form of vitamin B_3 (inositol hexaniacinate).

Vitamin B_6 (pyridoxine, pyridoxal, pyridoxal 5′ phosphate, pyridoxamine, and corresponding phosphorylated forms) (see Table 108.13)

Vitamin B_6 is a group of nitrogen-containing compounds that occur naturally in three primary forms: pyridoxine, pyridoxal, and pyridoxamine.

Vitamin B_6 is required for growth and maintenance of almost every bodily function, amino acid metabolism, and production of neurotransmitters derived from amino acids. It also plays a role in glycogen breakdown, fatty acid metabolism, hormone metabolism, heme biosynthesis, and purine biosynthesis. Studies in humans indicate that the bioavailability of vitamin B_6 from natural sources is limited. In food, B vitamin levels vary. Vitamin B_6 levels in whole wheat bread and peanut butter are, respectively, 75 and 63% as available as that in tuna.

Supplementation of vitamin B_6 has been used in treating carpal tunnel syndrome, premenstrual syndrome (PMS), cardiovascular disorders, and diabetic neuropathy. Elderly people may have an increased requirement for vitamin B_6 to maintain health, particularly for their immune system. In one study, healthy elderly people were given either 50 mg/day of vitamin B_6 or placebo. Those supplemented had significant improvement in immunocompetence, especially lymphocytic activity.

There is preliminary evidence that inadequate vitamin B_6 status may contribute to the development of coronary heart disease by increasing plasma homocysteine. Homocysteine has been found to be highly atherogenic in animals and may contribute to atherosclerosis in humans. Added evidence that vitamin B_6 might be important in preventing cardiovascular diseases comes from experimental studies in animals. When these animals are given vitamin B_6-deficient diets, they develop atherosclerotic lesions similar to those found in human atherosclerosis.

While there is increasing evidence for a role in vitamin B_6 supplementation in preventing some kinds of cardiovascular diseases, and for enhancing immunity, optimal levels in healthy individuals need not exceed 12–15 times the RDA, even in the elderly. Supplementation of vitamin B_6 up to 250 mg/day is safe for most individuals.

Very high doses of vitamin B_6 have been associated with sensory and motor impairment. Daily intakes up to 500 mg/day, which is 250 times the RDA, for up to 6 months appear to be safe. Supplements of pyridoxal 5′ phosphate may be preferred over pyridoxine hydrochloric acid supplements in individuals wishing to avoid any reversible side-effects from vitamin B_6 supplementation.

Riboflavin (vitamin B_2) (see Table 108.14)

Riboflavin is a precursor of two coenzymes (riboflavin-5′-phosphate and flavin mononucleotide) needed for a wide variety of enzymes in intermediary metabolism. Riboflavin is also required as a precursor of several flavoenzymes that are needed by tissue proteins.

The need for riboflavin varies with energy requirements, explaining why riboflavin-deficient people tire easily and have a poor appetite. Riboflavin is especially important for tissue repair, vision, and blood.

There is growing evidence that riboflavin may be important in preventing the development of cataracts, commonly associated with aging. There is equivocal evidence that riboflavin supplementation may be required in those exercising regularly. This may be more of a consideration if the exerciser is on a calorie-restrictive diet.

Significantly higher than RONI or RDA levels of riboflavin have been employed in migraine prophylaxis with promising results. In one open pilot trial involving 25 patients with a history of migraine related to the syndrome of mitochondrial encephalomyopathy, lactic acidosis, or stroke-like episodes (MELAS), 400 mg/day of riboflavin was given as a prophylactic treatment for migraine. 68% of patients reported improvement on an index of severity. A second randomized, placebo-controlled trial involving 55 patients with similar migraines resulted in a reported 50% improvement among those receiving riboflavin versus a 15% response in the placebo group. It is theorized that riboflavin may in some migraine patients correct a mitochondrial dysfunction resulting from impaired oxygen metabolism. Therefore, the use of riboflavin at significantly higher than RONI levels may suggest that in this and other conditions, the RONI for riboflavin may be inadequate to meet metabolic needs essential in overcoming the pathogenic condition.

Evidence is building for a role for riboflavin as an antioxidant, due to its role as a precursor for glutathione reductase. A number of studies have demonstrated that certain vitamins, particularly riboflavin and retinol and their derivatives, have the ability to modify molecular reactivity and response to carcinogens. Dietary riboflavin has such an important role. The mechanism of action is through controlling the induction of repair enzymes (poly(ADP-ribose) polymerase, DNA polymerase beta and DNA ligase) responsive to carcinogens that cause damage to DNA. Studies have shown that DNA damage increases proportionate to a deficiency of riboflavin and that increased damage to DNA is reversed via riboflavin supplementation.

Riboflavin has no known toxicity, although its theoretical photosensitizing properties raise the possibility of potential risk. The basis for this concern is that riboflavin forms an adduct with tryptophan which increases its rate of photo-oxidation. There is insufficient evidence to support riboflavin supplementation in healthy adults above twice the RDA.

Thiamin (vitamin B_1) (see Table 108.15)

Thiamin consists of one pyrimidine and one thiazole ring linked by a methylene bridge. This is important to know because many processed foods are rich in sulfites which split the thiamine molecule into the pyrimidine and thiazole moieties, thus destroying its biological activity.

In a study of 1,009 dentists and their wives evaluated for daily thiamin intake, those subjects having the least number of signs or symptoms associated with illness or degenerative diseases consumed an average of 9 mg/day of thiamin, approximately eight times the RDA for this nutrient.

There is insufficient evidence to suggest intakes of thiamin above eight times the RDA in healthy persons. However, individuals regularly consuming high intakes of refined carbohydrates (i.e. refined sugar-sucrose, wheat flour products made with unfortified 70% extraction flour) may require supplemental intake of thiamin in the range of 5–15 mg/day until such time as the diet improves.

Manifestations of thiamin deficiency (beri-beri) can be induced by chronic alcoholism.

Table 108.14 Riboflavin (mg)

Category	Age	RDA	Optimal
Males	11–14	1.5	2.0
	15–18	1.8	2.2
	19–24	1.7	2.5
	25–50	1.7	2.5
	51+	1.4	2.5
Females	11–14	1.3	1.8
	15–18	1.3	1.8
	19–24	1.3	2.0
	25–50	1.3	2.0
	51+	1.2	2.0

Table 108.15 Thiamin (mg)

Category	Age	RDA	Optimal
Males	11–14	1.3	3.3
	15–18	1.5	3.5
	19–24	1.5	3.5
	25–50	1.5	7.5
	51+	1.2	9.2
Females	11–14	1.1	3.1
	15–18	1.1	3.1
	19–24	1.1	3.1
	25–50	1.1	7.1
	51+	1.0	9.0

To date, thiamin, when taken orally, has been reported as harmless in humans, although gastric upset can be experienced at high doses exceeding 100–200 times the RDA.

Minerals

This author has provided an extensive discussion of minerals and trace elements and their role in human health in *Minerals, Trace Elements and Human Health.* Readers interested in this topic are advised to consider this work as a source of information, especially as it relates to non-essential elements, such as aluminum, cadmium, lead, mercury and other potentially toxic elements.

Boron (see Table 108.16)

Boron has only recently been established to be of nutritional significance to humans. An insufficiency manifests only when the body is stressed in some way that enhances the need for boron. Boron is particularly important for optimal calcium, and thus bone metabolism. Most persons eating Westernized diets consume between 0.1 and 0.5 mg/day of boron. Human studies indicate that consuming less than 0.25 mg/day of boron, or less than one-half the estimated average minimum requirement for humans, may require supplementation. Thus an intake of between 1 and 4 mg/day may be appropriate to contribute to optimal health. There is no evidence to suggest that intakes above 10 mg are either beneficial or completely safe. Boron supplementation affects serum phosphorous and magnesium concentrations in young women and the effect is modified by exercise. Boron affects bone mineral density, along with calcium, phosphorous, and magnesium.

Supplementation of 3 mg/day of boron for postmenopausal women has resulted in improvement in both calcium and magnesium retention and elevation in circulating serum concentrations of testosterone and estrogen (17-beta-estradiol). This improvement is more marked in women who have been on low magnesium diets. Similar improvements might also be found if the women were vitamin D-deficient. There is preliminary evidence based on animal studies that boron has an effect in males on steroidogenesis (e.g. production of testosterone) and testicular function and development proportional to the boron concentration in the testes.

There is increasing interest in the role of boron on brain function. Results in animals and humans indicate that dietary boron influences brain electrical activity. Individuals in a low state of alertness consume less boron (<0.5 mg/day) than those found to be more alert (>3.0 mg/day).

Preliminary evidence in animals has demonstrated that boron may modulate immune function that might be of significance to humans. Adequate boron suppresses inflammatory processes.

There is some evidence that boron (as sodium tetraborate decahydrate) may prevent arthritis in sheep. In a randomized double-blind clinical trial of 20 patients with severe osteoarthritis given either 6 mg of boron or placebo, five improved and five did not, but only one of the 10 patients on the placebo improved. Boron deficiency in chicks results in a syndrome that resembles human arthritis.

There is evidence from other human studies that optimal intakes of boron can enhance memory and cognitive function. There is also preliminary evidence of an association between sufficient boron intake and resistance to dental caries (tooth decay).

In all human studies to date, patients reported no side-effects when consuming less than 10 mg/day of boron.

Calcium (see Table 108.17)

Calcium is primarily stored in bones (99%), where the ratio of calcium to phosphorous is nearly constant at slightly greater than 2:1. Calcium is involved in numerous vital functions throughout the body, including:

- protein and fat digestion
- energy production
- nerve transmission
- neuromuscular activity
- the absorption of other nutrients, such as vitamin B_{12}.

Table 108.16 Boron (mg)

Category	Age	RDA	Optimal
Males	11–14	n/a	1.5
	15–18	n/a	2.0
	19–24	n/a	2.5
	25–50	n/a	2.5
	51+	n/a	2.5
Females	11–14	n/a	1.5
	15–18	n/a	2.0
	19–24	n/a	2.5
	25–50	n/a	3.0
	51+	n/a	3.0

Table 108.17 Calcium (mg)

Category	Age	RDA	Optimal
Males	11–14	1,200	1,000
	15–18	1,200	1,000
	19–24	1,200	1,000
	25–50	800	700
	51+	800	700
Females	11–14	1,200	1,200
	15–18	1,200	1,200
	19–24	1,200	1,200
	25–50	800	800
	51+	800	800

Estimates of adult calcium requirements in humans vary from 300 to 400 mg/day to between 1200 and 1500 mg/day. The lowest requirements are usually seen in populations with low protein intakes. In general, persons with very low protein intakes require less calcium per day. High levels of protein, which are usually also high in phosphorous, require higher calcium intakes. An increase in protein intake affects urinary calcium and calcium retention. It is recommended that calcium intake be increased during adolescence, pregnancy and lactation.

In recent years, calcium has received considerable attention in the mass media because of age-related osteoporosis, which is occurring in epidemic proportions in many developed countries and has been linked in to calcium intake. Articles and advertisements suggest that high intakes of calcium via supplementation or enrichment of foods/beverages is essential to the development and maintenance of strong, healthy bones. The attention this nutrient has received is most important to women. Women are more prone to osteoporosis that men because of smaller skeletal mass at maturity and because the most rapid period of bone loss occurs after menopause. However, numerous studies do not show a relationship between levels of dietary calcium intake and the incidence of osteoporosis. In the largest prospective scientific study of bone in premenopausal women aged 20–40 years, no relationship could be found between calcium intake and bone mineral density. This is consistent with studies reported since 1985.

When developing or maintaining bone mineral density is a goal, optimal intake of all nutrients essential to bone formation and homeostasis is required. Diet, hormones, age, and gender are just some of the factors that influence calcium requirements and metabolism. Because of these variables and the interrelationships among calcium, protein, phosphorous, magnesium, zinc, vitamin D and boron, etc., it remains difficult to select a single calcium requirement for any age group or gender. Some new supplements incorporating the nutrients required for bone, including hydroxyapatite, have appeared in the marketplace, and may be superior to calcium supplementation alone to ensure adequate nutrient needs of bone.

New studies show that even moderate consumption of calcium in foods or as supplements can reduce both heme and non-heme iron absorption. These reductions could have important nutritional implications, especially for premenstrual and pregnant women who are already at risk for iron deficiency. Therefore, it is advisable that calcium supplements in excess of 250 mg not be consumed with meals.

Chromium (see Table 108.18)

Chromium is a trace element essential to the metabolism of lipids (e.g. cholesterol), glucose, and insulin regulation.

Table 108.18 Chromium (μg)

Category	Age	RDA*	Optimal
Males	11–14	50–200	200
	15–18	50–200	200
	19–24	50–200	300
	25–50	50–200	300
	51+	50–200	300
Females	11–14	50–200	200
	15–18	50–200	200
	19–24	50–200	300
	25–50	50–200	300
	51+	50–200	300

*Estimated safe and adequate daily dietary intake of mineral, National Research Council, 1989.

The long-term effects of a suboptimal intake of chromium has been related to:

- a decrease in tissue chromium associated with aging
- an increased incidence of diabetes and atherosclerosis, particularly in developed nations.

Illness, aging, stress (i.e. trauma, surgery, intense heat or cold), and strenuous exercise seem to increase chromium losses or needs.

Studies of humans with heart disease have demonstrated that chromium deficiency is associated with atherosclerosis, suggesting that optimal chromium levels may reduce the risk of heart disease. Tissues of humans who have died of heart disease have been found to have less chromium than tissues of humans who died of accidental causes. In those patients with atherosclerotic plaque who died of heart disease, no detectable chromium was found in these tissues. There is also evidence in humans that a diet sufficient in chromium along with selenium, copper, potassium, magnesium, and calcium reduces the risk of cardiovascular disease, by having a beneficial effect on serum cholesterol and triglyceride levels. Chromium taken with nicotinic acid (niacin) or the chromium supplement, chromium picolinate (200–400 μg/day), has been shown to lower cholesterol levels in individuals with elevated cholesterol.

Traces of chromium have been shown to be required for health as part of the glucose tolerance factor (GTF) involved in the regulation of blood glucose. The brain has high requirements for blood glucose as a fuel. The amount of chromium in foods decreases with processing. The widespread tendency toward increased consumption of highly processed foods, particularly refined sugar, which stimulates urinary losses of chromium, may result in a marginal intake of chromium and depletion of tissue chromium stores.

The safety of chromium supplementation is well established. Even in pharmacological doses (50–1,000 mg/day for 1–3 months), it has no toxicity in cats, rats or mice.

Copper (see Table 108.19)

Copper is an essential element in the human body. About 95% of copper is found in serum as part of ceruloplasmin. Copper is needed by all tissues, but is highest in the liver where it contributes to energy and detoxification mechanisms. The element is also required to absorb, utilize and synthesize hemoglobin, maintain the integrity of the outer covering of nerves (myelin), metabolize vitamin C, and oxidize fatty acids.

Both excess and deficiency of copper can result in problems such as:

- bone/joint and connective tissue disturbances
- cardiovascular degeneration
- abnormal electrocardiogram
- accelerated aging
- depigmentation and dermatitis
- anemia
- neurological impairments.

There is no evidence of a decline in copper status with age.

Proper balance of copper to zinc (and other trace elements) is necessary for good health. A low ratio of copper to zinc can result from dietary deficiency of copper or excessive zinc intake, and may result in hypercholesterolemia, myocardial and arterial damage, and increased mortality. High levels of serum copper found in humans living in areas with low selenium levels in their soil and high copper content in drinking water have been associated with a significantly elevated incidence of atherosclerosis. The zinc-to-copper ratio, should ideally be between 8:1 and 14:1.

Excess fructose consumption in the presence of inadequate copper intake has been shown in several mammalian species to lead to heart arrhythmias and even heart failure. The level of copper and amount of dietary fructose which results in such cardiovascular problems in humans remain unknown. However, it is known that dietary fructose exacerbates the signs associated with copper deficiency. These signs include anemia, hypercholesterolemia, impaired glucose tolerance, pancreatic atrophy, cardiomyopathy, and increased mortality. Fructose consumption during lactation also produces a significant reduction in copper concentrations in breast milk. Even the homeostasis of hormones is impaired by the consumption of fructose with a low-copper diet, which in animal studies has been shown to decrease levels of plasma thyroid hormones, insulin, epinephrine, norepinephrine, and an increase in the glucocorticoids.

Copper supplementation should be approached with caution since copper is amongst the most powerful producers of free radicals. However, in proper balance with zinc, the two elements act as antioxidants by removing damaging free radicals such as the superoxide radical. Excess copper supplementation suppresses immune function.

Table 108.19 Copper (mg)

Category	Age	RDA*	Optimal
Males	11–14	1.5–3.0	1.5–4
	15–18	1.5–3.0	1.5–4
	19–24	1.5–3.0	1.5–4
	25–50	1.5–3.0	1.5–4
	51+	1.5–3.0	1.5–4
Females	11–14	1.5–3.0	1.5–4
	15–18	1.5–3.0	1.5–4
	19–24	1.5–3.0	1.5–4
	25–50	1.5–3.0	1.5–4
	51+	1.5–3.0	1.5–4

*Estimated safe and adequate daily dietary intake of mineral, National Research Council, 1989

Iodine (see Table 108.20)

Iodine accumulates in thyroid tissue and is incorporated into thyroxine and triiodothyronine, the hormones of the thyroid gland. Iodine deficiency is the most common cause of endemic goiter and cretinism. Milk and dairy products, as well as bread and bakery products, are the main source of iodine in human food. Iodine is concentrated in milk and eggs, which are only second to seafood as the richest sources of iodine. Marine (sea) salt is a poor source of iodine. In conjunction with two enzymes (myeloperoxidase and hydrogen peroxide), iodine is known to be bactericidal. This bactericidal activity is accomplished by an abundant cellular halide, the chloride anion.

The RDA for iodine is 2 μg/kg body weight in adults and somewhat more in children. This amount seems optimal to ensure the biosynthesis of the thyroid hormones. An additional 25 and 50 μg may be required during pregnancy and lactation, respectively. The most common supplementation of iodine is via iodized salt, 1 g of which supplies approximately 75 μg of iodine. In the event of a nuclear reactor accident, a single dose of 300 mg of potassium iodide helps to block the uptake of radioactive iodine-131 by the thyroid.

Iodine in large amounts disturbs all thyroid functions.

Table 108.20 Iodine (mcg)

Category	Age	RDA	Optimal
Males	11–14	150	150
	15–18	150	150
	19–24	150	150
	25–50	150	150
	51+	150	150
Females	11–14	150	150
	15–18	150	150
	19–24	150	150
	25–50	150	150
	51+	150	150

Iron (see Table 108.21)

Most iron in the body is found in the hemoglobin of red blood cells. Some iron is also found in the myoglobin present in skeletal muscles and the heart. The remaining iron is found in enzymes essential to energy production.

Iron deficiency is one of the most common deficiency diseases in the world. Even in the US, repeated dietary surveys have found inadequate iron intake to meet even the RDA. The most common cause of this is nutritional, including inadequate absorption of iron due to poor iron intake, reduced bioavailability, etc. Iron loss, resulting from pregnancy, internal bleeding, parasitic infections (e.g. hook worm), low stomach acid (e.g. hypochlorhydria, achlorhydria), and malabsorption, is also an important factor contributing to iron deficiency. There are some data that suggest that iron deficiency anemia may be a secondary outcome of vitamin A deficiency which contributes to defective iron transport. The risk of iron deficiency is relatively high in menstruating women eating a diet inadequate in iron. This is one reason the RDA for iron is higher for women than for men. However, many women are on reduced calorie diets which are unable to provide enough iron and require supplementation.

Non-heme iron is the main source of iron in the diet, although it is much more poorly absorbed than heme iron, which is only found in animal sources. Meat, fish, and vitamin C enhance the absorption of non-heme iron, improving absorption. However, new studies are showing that even moderate consumption of calcium in foods or as supplements can reduce both heme and non-heme iron absorption. These reductions could have important nutritional implications, especially for those, such as premenstrual women and pregnant women, who may already be at high risk for iron deficiency. Symptoms of iron deficiency anemia include fatigue, irritability, paleness, intolerance to cold, and a general sense of lack of well-being. Brain function can also be impaired due to iron deficiency. Inadequate iron levels tend to affect the right hemisphere of the brain and have been linked to cognitive impairment, poor attention span, restlessness, and the inability of concentrate. Optimal levels of iron are also essential to immune function.

Table 108.21 Iron (mg)

Category	Age	RDA	Optimal
Males	11–14	12	15
	15–18	12	15
	19–24	10	20
	25–50	10	20
	51+	10	20
Females	11–14	15	20
	15–18	15	20
	19–24	15	22
	25–50	15	22
	51+	15	20

Table 108.22 Magnesium (mg)

Category	Age	RDA	Optimal
Males	11–14	270	300
	15–18	400	500
	19–24	350	500
	25–50	350	500
	51+	350	600
Females	11–14	280	300
	15–18	300	400
	19–24	280	450
	25–50	280	450
	51+	280	550

Iron supplementation is not safe for individuals with any iron storage disorder such as hemosiderosis, idiopathic hemochromatosis, or thalassemias.

Magnesium (see Table 108.22)

Magnesium, half of which is in the bone, is required for many metabolic functions. One of its most important is in maintaining the function of the nervous system and neuromuscular transmission and activity. Magnesium deficiency is associated with:

- tremors
- muscle spasms
- convulsions
- neuropsychiatric disturbances
- coronary artery disease
- angina pectoris
- cardiac arrhythmias
- hypertension.

Along with calcium, sodium and potassium, magnesium affects the muscle tone of blood vessels.

Blood levels of magnesium are low in patients with myocardial ischemia, coronary artery spasm, mitral valve prolapse, and cardiac tachyarrythmias. Low tissue and blood levels have also been observed in patients prior to, during and after myocardial infarction. Recent studies have also implicated lack of sufficient magnesium as a cause of pre-eclampsia and hypertension in pregnant women. Magnesium insufficiency directly and indirectly affects cardiac function through its effect on potassium, sodium and calcium concentrations in cells and surrounding fluids. Given that coronary and heart disease contribute profoundly to morbidity and mortality in developed countries, an intake above the RDA level is advocated by researchers who have studied this essential nutrient.

Manganese (see Table 108.23)

Manganese is involved in protein, fat and energy metabolism, and is required for bone growth and development,

Table 108.23 Manganese (mg)

Category	Age	RDA*	Optimal
Males	11–14	2–5	5
	15–18	2–5	5
	19–24	2–5	5
	25–50	2–5	5
	51+	2–5	10
Females	11–14	2–5	5
	15–18	2–5	5
	19–24	2–5	5
	25–50	2–5	5
	51+	2–5	10

* Estimated safe and adequate daily dietary intake of mineral, National Research Council, 1989.

and reproduction. Diets high in refined carbohydrates may provide inadequate intake of manganese. Addition of supplemental iron to the diet can depress manganese retention if iron nutriture is poor. Concentrations of manganese in tissues and organs remain relatively constant with age. Sources of dietary manganese are mainly plant foods since animal tissue contains very low amounts of this nutrient. One exceptionally rich dietary source for manganese is tea. However, tea can inhibit the uptake of iron.

Phosphorous (see Table 108.24)

About 85% of the phosphorous found in the body is in bone as calcium phosphate and hydroxyapatite. Deficiencies of this nutrient are extremely rare as foodstuffs seem to provide an ample supply. Both animal and plant food are rich in phosphates. However, a vitamin D deficiency may reduce absorption of phosphorous. Most adults consume between 1,000 and 1,500 mg of phosphorous each day of which 50–60% is usually absorbed.

A phosphorous intake greatly in excess of calcium, especially if the calcium intake is minimal (400 mg/day or less), can reduce calcium availability and contribute to calcium deficiency. In general, the calcium to phosphorous ratio should be about 1:1 and definitely above 1:2.

Potassium (see Table 108.25)

Potassium is an essential element in maintaining fluid balance in the cells, transmission of nerve impulses, skeletal muscle contractility, and normal blood pressure. However, it must exist in balance with sodium. During nerve transmission and muscle contraction, potassium and sodium exchange places. Together with high sodium intake, decreased potassium intake may be implicated in hypertension and heart disease. Potassium is also a catalyst in protein and carbohydrate metabolism. Diuretic drugs can deplete potassium and so can be dangerous. When sodium is lost with water from the body, the ultimate damage comes when potassium moves out of the cells with cell water.

There is no RDA for potassium. However, some believe that the minimum requirement should be between 1,600 and 2,000 mg/day. Since an intake of about 1,600 mg/day is required just to maintain normal body stores and a normal concentration in plasma and fluid, a higher level would ensure optimal levels. According to some researchers, a diet rich in fruits and vegetables and low in sodium should ensure the maintenance of optimal potassium levels. However, it has been calculated that due to the poor absorbability of potassium in fruit without chloride, only 40% of the potassium, e.g. in a banana, is retained. Unfortunately this finding is often not calculated into food value tables which estimate total potassium intake from foods. This is one reason why, when potassium supplementation is suggested by a physician, potassium chloride is recommended. A low-sodium diet enhances potassium conservation, whereas a high-sodium diet promotes potassium excretion.

In a study of vegetarians compared with non-vegetarians, significantly lower blood pressure was found in every decade of age and only 2% of the vegetarians had hypertension (higher than 160/95) as compared with 26% hypertensives in the non-vegetarians. This study further confirms the important role that potassium plays in the regulation of blood pressure. In a study of 10,000 subjects in the United States, it was found that those with the highest levels of calcium, potassium, vitamin A and

Table 108.24 Phosphorous (mg)

Category	Age	RDA	Optimal
Males	11–14	1,200	1,200
	15–18	1,200	1,200
	19–24	1,200	1,200
	25–50	800	800
	51+	800	800
Females	11–14	1,200	1,200
	15–18	1,200	1,200
	19–24	1,200	1,200
	25–50	800	800
	51+	800	800

Table 108.25 Potassium (g)

Category	Age	RDA	Optimal
Males	11–14	2	2
	15–18	2	2
	19–24	2	3
	25–50	2	3
	51+	2	3
Females	11–14	2	2
	15–18	2	2
	19–24	2	3
	25–50	2	3
	51+	2	3

vitamin C had the lowest incidence of hypertension, suggesting that potassium is not the only essential nutrient in maintaining normotensive status in humans.

Selenium (see Table 108.26)

Selenium is a trace element whose most important biologic function in maintaining health is as an antioxidant. Vitamin C intake of 600 mg/day has been shown to increase dietary selenium absorption by nearly 100%.

There is growing evidence that selenium may be protective against certain cancers (e.g. breast, colon, lung) and numerous tumors. Studies to date have given considerable credibility to the theory that decreased selenium status is associated with an increased risk of cancer. A landmark prospective study involving 1,312 subjects (75% of whom were male), reported in the December 1996 *Journal of the American Medical Association*, found that patients who took daily selenium supplementation at triple the RDA had 63% fewer cases of prostate cancer, 58% fewer colon or rectal cancers, and 47% fewer lung cancers than those who took the placebo. Overall in the selenium group there were 50% fewer cancer deaths than in the placebo group. It is believed that selenium may inhibit tumor growth and induce suicide in malignant cells.

There is evidence that in elderly people, several hundred micrograms of selenium and 400 mg of vitamin E improve their mental status, motivation, initiation, emotional stability, mental alertness, interest in the environment, and self-care, while decreasing anxiety, depression, poor appetite, and fatigue. This suggests that optimal selenium nutriture is increasingly important in the latter decades of life.

Adequate levels of selenium taken with chromium, copper, potassium, magnesium, and calcium have been found to reduce the risk of cardiovascular disease.

There are data suggesting that ingesting more than 750–1000 ug/day of selenium over an extended period of time may be harmful. Therefore optimal levels need to be below this level until there are assurances that higher intakes are safe.

Table 108.26 Selenium (mcg)

Category	Age	RDA	Optimal
Males	11–14	40	75
	15–18	50	150
	19–24	70	200
	25–50	70	200
	51+	70	250
Females	11–14	45	75
	15–18	50	100
	19–24	55	150
	25–50	55	175
	51+	55	200

Table 108.27 Sodium (mg)

Category	Age	RDA*	Optimal
Males	11–14	500	400
	15–18	500	400
	19–24	500	400
	25–50	500	400
	51+	500	400
Females	11–14	500	400
	15–18	500	400
	19–24	500	400
	25–50	500	400
	51+	500	400

* Estimated minimum requirement, National Research Council, 1989.

Sodium/sodium chloride (see Table 108.27)

Sodium chloride is the primary source of sodium (39% sodium by weight). The healthy adult can maintain sodium balance with an intake of approximately that required by an infant. Close regulation of the concentration and content of sodium within the body is crucial for health. Disorders of sodium regulation are a central feature of many human diseases. In general, the regulation of sodium in the body involves two processes: the control of sodium loss and the control of sodium intake. Sodium chloride occurs naturally in most foods. The problem is that sodium chloride is also added to most processed foods, often in amounts well in excess of that required physiologically or to maintain health. This added intake has been the subject of numerous studies. These studies have frequently found that the level of sodium chloride ingested by Americans is 10–20 times the level required to maintain health.

Many studies have found an association between excessive intake of salt and hypertension. The highest intakes (28 g/day) have been found in northern Japan where it is estimated that 38% of the population is hypertensive. In contrast, Alaska natives consume only 4 g/day and rarely develop hypertension. However, some studies do not show an association between salt and hypertension. These studies tend to be too small to discover the association and frequently fail to consider dietary potassium intake. Numerous studies have shown that potassium can limit some of the toxic effects of excessive sodium ingestion. For most individuals, the most prudent approach would be to limit salt intake by restricting salted processed foods. This alone should reduce daily salt intake by between 3 and 5 g, or about one-third the daily salt intake in the average American (10–14.5 g/day). Refraining from adding salt to food at the table would further reduce salt intake another one-third. This would leave only one-third remaining, or approximately that amount of salt per day found in populations with a very low incidence of hypertension. Potassium chloride may be an acceptable substitute to sodium chloride, especially when other agents, such as citric acid or other acids, have been added to mask its unpleasant bitter taste. However, it is important to recognize that some individuals with hypotension (low blood pressure) may benefit from added salt. Nevertheless, there remains no known benefit from large sodium or sodium chloride intake. Maintaining a low salt intake throughout life may decrease the risk of developing hypertension in the portion of the population at risk.

Zinc (see Table 108.28)

An adequate supply of zinc is essential for growth and physical development, and for the metabolism of proteins, fats and carbohydrates. Most aspects of reproduction in both males and females require zinc. This mineral is also vitally important to the immune system. Virtually every enzyme reaction in the brain involves zinc, and its essentiality in the development and function of the central nervous system and brain is uncontested. Zinc is antagonistic to such toxic elements as cadmium, mercury and lead. The highest concentrations of zinc are in the ear and eye. Disorders associated with impairment of either organ may benefit from continuous optimal intakes of zinc over a lifetime.

The typical intake of zinc in Western diets is around 10 mg, two-thirds of the RDA. The elderly often consume less than half the RDA for zinc. While some individuals seem to be poor absorbers, most cases of zinc deficiency, whether chronic or marginal, are self-inflicted. This may result from slimming diets, vegetarianism, or other lifestyle habits (e.g. alcoholism, excessive exercise). However, in some cases relative zinc deficiencies are induced by exposure to toxic metals, such as cadmium from cigarette smoke or excess copper from copper water pipes. There is increasing evidence that zinc levels decline following physical stress or injury. Zinc is one of the few minerals lost rapidly in the urine following acute or chronic psychological stress, which can lead to inadequate zinc status, despite RDA intake.

Impairments of taste, vision, smell, and appetite are often early signs of inadequate zinc status. There is a simple test for zinc status (Zinc Status, Ethical Nutrients, San Clemente, CA) which evaluates the ability to taste a pre-mixed solution of zinc. Individuals unable to taste this solution have been found to be zinc-deficient, in some cases despite being asymptomatic.

Insufficient zinc has multiple effects on the immune system, particularly T-lymphocytes, decreased number and activity of killer cells, and impaired antibody production.

There is insufficient evidence to suggest that zinc intake should be twice the RDA for zinc. However, since repeated studies of Westernized diets indicate that most populations consume less than the RDA of this essential mineral, it seems prudent that some supplementation of zinc, or increase in zinc-rich foods, be considered a part of maintaining an optimal level of this nutrient over a lifetime.

Zinc supplementation is generally safe if maintained at levels within two to eight times the RDA. Symptoms of zinc toxicity include gastrointestinal irritation, vomiting, adverse changes in HDL/LDL cholesterol ratios, and impaired immunity. The latter develops when levels above 180 mg/day are consumed for more than several weeks. Excess intake of zinc may either lower copper levels or aggravate an existing marginal copper deficiency.

Table 108.28 Zinc (mg)

Category	Age	RDA	Optimal
Males	11–14	15	15
	15–18	15	18
	19–24	15	20
	25–50	15	20
	51+	15	20
Females	11–14	12	12
	15–18	12	15
	19–24	12	17
	25–50	12	17
	51+	12	17

FURTHER READING

Introduction

1. National Research Council, Committee on Diet and Health. Diet and Health. Implications for reducing chronic disease risk. Washington, DC: National Academy Press. 1989
2. The Surgeon General's Report on Nutrition and Health, Department of Health and Human Services. DHHS publication [PHS] 50210. Washington, DC: Government Printing Office. 1988
3. Verschuren WM, Jacobs DR, Bloemberg BP et al. Serum total cholesterol and long-term coronary heart disease mortality in different cultures. Twenty-five year follow-up of the Seven Countries Study. JAMA 1995; 274: 131–136
4. Block G, Petterson B, Subar A et al. Fruit, vegetables, and cancer prevention. A review of the epidemiologic evidence. Nutr Cancer 1992; 18: 1–29
5. Giovannucci E, Rimm EB, Ascherio A et al. Alcohol, low-methionine-low-folate diets, and risk of colon cancer in men. J Natl Cancer Inst 1995; 87: 265–273
6. Chandra RK. Effect of vitamin and trace-element supplementation on immune responses and infection in elderly subjects. Lancet 1992; 2: 1124–1127
7. Rimm EB, Stampfer MJ, Ascherio A et al. Vitamin E consumption and the risk of coronary heart disease in men. New Engl J Med 1993; 328: 1450–1456
8. Food and Nutrition Board, National Research Council, National Academy of Science. Recommended dietary allowances. 10th edn. Washington, DC: National Academy Press. 1989
9. Kumpulainen JT, Salonen JT, eds. Natural antioxidants and food quality in atherosclerosis and cancer prevention. London: The Royal Society of Chemistry. 1996

Fat-soluble vitamins

Vitamin A/beta-carotene

1. Bendich A, Olson JA. Biological action of carotenoids. FASEB J 1989; 3: 1927–1932
2. Paganini-Hill A, Chao A, Ross RK et al. Vitamin A, beta carotene, and the risk of cancer. A prospective study. J Natl Cancer Inst 1987; 79: 443–448
3. Sommer A. New Imperatives for an old vitamin (A). J Nutr 1989; 119: 96–100
4. Bendich A. Symposium conclusions: biological actions of carotenoids. J Nutr 1989; 119: 112–5
5. Oson JA. Provitamin A function of carotenoids. The conversion of B-carotene to Vitamin A. J Nutr 1989; 119: 105–108
6. Pryor WA. The antioxidant nutrients and disease prevention – what do we know and what do we need to find out? Am J Clin Nutr 1991; 53: 391S–393S
7. Ziegler RG. Vegetables, fruits and carotenoids and the risk of cancer. Am J Clin Nutr 1991; 53: 251S–259S
8. DiMascio P, Murphy ME, Sies H. Antioxidant defense systems. the role of carotenoids, tocopherols and thiols. Am J Clin Nutr 1991; 53: 194S–200S
9. Stahelin HB, Gey KB, Eichholzer M et al. Beta-carotene and cancer prevention. The Basel Study. Am J Clin Nutr 1991; 53: 265S–269S
10. Connett JE, Kuller KH, Kjelsberg MO et al. Relationship between carotenoids and cancer. Cancer 1989; 64: 126–134
11. Colditz GA, Branch LJ, Lipnick RJ et al. Increased green and yellow vegetable intake and lowered cancer deaths in an elderly population. Am J Clin Nutr 1985; 41: 32–36
12. Gaby SK, Singh VN. Vitamin intake and health: a scientific review. New York: Marcel Dekker. 1991: p 29–57
13. Mobarhan S, Bowen P, Andersen B et al. Effects of beta-carotene repletion on beta-carotene absorption, lipid peroxidation, and neutrophil superoxide formation in young men. Nutr Cancer 1990; 14: 195–206
14. Burton GW, Ingold KU. Beta-carotene. an unusual type of lipid antioxidant. Science 1984; 224: 569–573
15. Bendich A, Olson, JA. Biological actions of carotenoids. FASEB J 1989; 3: 1927–1932
16. Palgi A. Association between dietary changes and morality rates: Israel 1949 to 1977; a trend-free regression model. Am J Clin Nutr 1981; 34: 1569–1583
17. Robertson J, Donner AP, Trevithick JR. Vitamin E: biochemistry and health implications, vol. 570. New York: Ann NY Acad Sci. 1989: p 372–382
18. Cheraskin E, Ringsdorf WM, Medford FH. The 'ideal' daily vitamin A intake. Int J Vit Nutr Res 1976; 46: 11–13
19. Goodman DS. Vitamin A and retinoids in heath and disease. N Eng J Med 1984; 310: 1023–1031
20. White WS, Kim CI, Kalkwarf HJ et al. Ultraviolet light-induced reduction in plasma carotenoid levels. Am J Clin Nutr 1988; 47: 879–883
21. Willette W. Nutritional epidemiology. New York: Oxford University Press. 1990: p 292–310
22. Salonen JT. Risk of cancer in relation to serum concentrations of selenium and vitamins A and E: matched case-control analysis of prospective data. Br Med J 1985; 290: 417–420
23. DiMascio P, Murphy M, Sies H. Antioxidant defense systems. The role of carotenoids, tocopherols, and thiols. Am J Clin Nutr 1991; 53: S19–S20
24. Weisburger J. Nutritional approach to cancer prevention with emphasis on vitamins, antioxidants, and carotenoids. Am J Clin Nutr 1991; 53: S226–237
25. Olson JA. Vitamin A. In: Present knowledge in nutrition. 7th edn. Washington DC: International Life Sciences Press. 1996: p 109–119
26. Sommer A., West, KP. The duration of the effect of vitamin A supplementation. [Letter] Am J Public Health 1997; 87: 467
27. Werler MA, Lammer EJ, Mitchell AA. Teratogenicity of high vitamin A intake. [Letter] N Eng J Med 1995; 334: 1195
28. Bates CJ. Vitamin A. Lancet 1995; 345: 31–35
29. Underwood BA. Was the 'anti-infective' vitamin misnamed? Nutr Rev 1994; 52: 140–143
30. Schauss AG. Beta-carotene and the incidence of lung cancer in Finnish male smokers. A critique. Q Rev Natural Med 1994; 191–195
31. Prince MR, Frisoli JK. Beta-carotene accumulation in serum and skin. Am J Clin Nutr 1993; 57: 175–181

Vitamin D

1. MacLaughlin J, Holick MF. Aging decreases the capacity of human skill to produce vitamin D3. J Clin Invest; 1985; 76: 1536–1538
2. Lips P, van Ginkel FC, Jongen MJ et al. Determinants of Vitamin D status in patients with hip fracture and in elderly control subject. Am J Clin Nutr 1987; 46: 1005–1010
3. Gaby SK, Singh VN. Vitamin intake and health: a scientific review. New York: Marcel Dekker. 1990: p 59–70
4. Chapuy MC, Chapuy P, Mennier PJ. Calcium and vitamin D supplements. effects on calcium metabolism in elderly people. Am J Clin Nutr 1987; 46: 324–328
5. Anonymous. Vitamin D supplementation in the elderly [editorial]. Lancet 1987; 1: 306–307
6. Webb AR, Holick MF. Influence of season and latitude on cutaneous synthesis of vitamin D3. Ann Rev Nutr 1988; 8: 375–399
7. Garland FC, Garland CF, Gorham ED et al. Geographic variation in breast cancer mortality in the United States. A hypothesis involving exposure to solar radiation. Arch Environ Health 1990; 45: 261–267
8. Sowers MR, Wallace RB, Lemke JH. The association of intakes of vitamin D and calcium with blood pressure among women. Am J Clin Nutr 1985; 42: 135–142
9. Garland C, Shekelle RB, Barrett-Connor E et al. Dietary vitamin D and calcium and risk of colorectal cancer. Lancet 1985; 1: 307–309
10. Garland CF, Comstock GW, Garland FC et al. Serum 25-hydroxy vitamin D and colon cancer. Lancet 1989; 2: 1176–1178
11. Sowers MF, Wallace RB, Hollis BW et al. Relationship between 1,25-dihydroxy vitamin D and blood pressure in our geographically defined population. Am J Clin Nutr 1988; 48: 1053–1056
12. Parfitt AM, Gallagher JC, Heaney RP et al. Vitamin D and bone health in the elderly. Am J Clin Nutr 1982; 36: 1014–1031
13. Omdahl JL, Garry PJ, Hunsaker LA et al. Nutritional status in a healthy elderly population: Vitamin D Nutritional status in a healthy elderly population: vitamin D. Am J Clin Nutr 1982; 36: 1225–1233
14. Wiedmann KH, Brattig NW, Diao GD et al. Serum inhibiting factors (SIF) are of prognostic value in acute viral hepatitis. Lancet 1985; i: 307–309
15. Garland CF, Garland FC. Do sunlight and vitamin D reduce the likelihood of colon cancer? Int J Epidemiol 1980; 9: 227–231
16. Garland CF, Gorham ED, Young JF. Geographic variation in breast cancer mortality in the United States: a hypothesis involving exposure to solar radiation. Prevent Med 1990; 19: 614–622
17. Crombie IK. Distribution of malignant melanoma on the body surface. Br J Cancer 1981; 43: 842–849
18. Vagero R, Ringback G, Kiveranta H. Vagero Melanoma and other tumors of the skin among office, other outdoor/indoor workers in Sweden. Br J Cancer 1986; 53: 507–512
19. Koh HK, Kligler BE, Lew RA. Sunlight and cutaneous malignant melanoma. Evidence for and against causation. Photochem Photobiol. 1990; 19: 614–622
20. Beaty M, Lee E, Glauart H. FASEB J 1991; 5: 926A
21. Norman AW. Vitamin D. In: Present knowledge in nutrition. 7th edn. Washington DC: International Life Sciences Press. 1996: p 120–129
22. Fraser DR. Vitamin D. Lancet 1995; 345: 104–107
23. Chapuy MC, Arlot ME, Duboeuf F et al. Vitamin D3 and calcium to prevent hip fractures in elderly women. N Engl J Med 1992; 327: 1637–1642

Vitamin E

1. Burton GW, Ingold KU. Vitamin E as an in vitro and in vivo antioxidant. In: Diplock AT, Machoin LJ, Parker L, Pryor WA, eds. Vitamin E: biochemistry and health implications. Ann NY Acad Sci 1989; 570: 7–22
2. Wald NJ, Boreham J, Hayward JL et al. Plasma retinol beta-carotene and vitamin E levels in relation to future risk of breast cancer. Br J Cancer 1984; 49: 321–324

3. Salonen JT, Salonen R, Lappetelainen R et al. Risk of cancer in relation to serum concentration of selenium and vitamins A and E. matched case control analysis. Br Med J 1985; 290: 417–420
4. Haenszel W, Correa P, Lopez A et al. Serum micronutrient levels in relation to gastric pathology. Int J Cancer 1985; 36: 43–48
5. Menkes MS, Comstock GW, Vuilleumier JP et al. Serum beta-carotene vitamins A and E, selenium, and the risk of lung cancer. N Eng J Med 1986; 315: 1250–1254
6. Miyamoto H, Araya Y, Ito M et al. Serum selenium and vitamin E. concentrations in families of lung cancer patients. Cancer 1987; 60: 1159–1162
7. Kok FJ, de Bruijn AM, Vermeeren R et al. Serum selenium, vitamin antioxidants, and cardiovascular mortality. N Eng J Med 1987; 316: 1416
8. Knekt P, Aromaa A, Maatela J et al. Serum vitamin E level and risk of cancer among Finnish men during a 10-year follow-up. Am J Epidemiol 1988; 127: 28–41
9. Gaby WK, Machlin LJ. Vitamin intake and health: a scientific review. New York: Marcel Dekker. 1991: p 71–101
10. Pacht ER, Kaseki H, Mohammed JR et al. Deficiency of vitamin E in the alveolar fluid of cigarette smokers. J Clin Invest 1986; 77: 789–798
11. Steiner M. Effect of alpha-tocopherol administration on platelet function in man. Thromb Haemostas 1983; 49: 73–77
12. Fong JSC. Alpha-tocopherol. Its inhibition on human platelet aggregation. Experientia 1976; 32: 639–641
13. Meydanin SN et al. FASEB J 1989; 3: A1057
14. Prasad JS. Effect of vitamin E supplementation on leukocyte function. Am J Clin Nutr 1980; 33: 606–608
15. Jacques PF. Chylack antioxidant status in persons with and without senile cataract. Arch Ophthalmol 1988; 106: 337–340
16. Taylor A. Associations between nutrition and cataract. Nutr Rev 1989; 47: 225–234
17. Robertson JM, Donner AP, Trevithick JR. Vitamin E intake and risk of cataracts in humans. Ann NY Acad Sci 1989; 570: 372–378
18. Pryor WA. Can vitamin E protect humans against the pathological effects of ozone in smog? Am J Clin Nutr 1991; 53: 702–722
19. Chavance M. Nutrition, immunity, and illness in the elderly. New York: Pergamon Press. 1985: p 137–142
20. Knekt P, Aromaa A, Maatela J et al. Vitamin E and cancer prevention. Am J Clin Nutr 1991; 53: 283S–286S
21. Van Den Berg JJ, Roelofsen B, OpdenKamp JAF et al. Vitamin E: biochemistry and health implications, vol. 570. New York: Ann NY Acad Sci. 1989: p 527–529
22. Riemersma RA, Wood DA, MacIntyre CCA et al. Low plasma vitamins E and C increased risk of angina in Scottish men. In: Diplock AT, Machlin LJ, Packer L et al, eds. Vitamin E: biochemistry and health implications, vol. 570. New York: Ann NY Acad Sci. 1989: p 291–295
23. Robertson J, Donner AP, Trevithick JR. Vitamin E: biochemistry and health implications, vol. 570. New York: Ann NY Acad Sci. 1989: p 372–382
24. Diplock AT, Machlin LJ, Packer L et al, eds. Daily vitamin E consumption and reported cardiovascular findings. New York: Ann NY Acad Sci. 1989: p 1–535
25. Cheraskin E, Ringsdorf WM, Jr. Nutr Rep Int 1970; 2: 107–117
26. Horwitt MK. Supplementation with vitamin E. Am J Clin Nutr 1988; 47: 1088–1089
27. Bendich A, Machlin LJ. Safety of oral intake of vitamin E. Am J Clin Nutr 1988; 48: 612–619
28. Dimitrov NV, Meyer C, Gilliland D et al. Plasma tocopherol concentrations in response to supplements vitamin E. Am J Clin Nutr 1991; 53: 723–729
29. Pascoe GA, Fariss MW, Olafsdottir K et al. A role of vitamin E in protection against cell injury. Maintenance of intracellular glutathione precursors and biosynthesis. Eur J Biochem 1987; 166: 241–247
30. Tolonen M, Markku H, Sarna S. Vitamin E and selenium supplementation in geriatric patients. A double-blind preliminary clinical trial. Biol Trace Elem Res 1985; 7: 161–168
31. Salonen JT, Salonen R, Lappetelainen R et al. Risk of cancer in relation to serum concentrations of selenium and vitamins A and E. matched case-control analysis of prospective data. Br Med J 1985; 290: 417–420
32. Giani E, Masi I, Galli C. Heated fat; vitamin E and vascular eicosanoids. Lipids 1985; 20: 439–448
33. Kneckt P. Serum vitamin E level and risk of female cancers. Int J Epidem 1988; 17: 281–286
34. Sword J, Pope A, Hoekstra W. Endotoxin and lipid peroxidation in vitro in selenium and vitamin E deficient and adequate rat tissue. J Nutr 1991; 121: 258–264
35. Sword J, Pope A, Hoekstra W. Endotoxin and lipid peroxidation in vitro in selenium and vitamin E deficient and adequate rat tissue. J Nutr 1991; 121: 251–257
36. Esterbauer H, Dieber-Rotheneder M, Striegl G et al. Role of vitamin E in preventing the oxidation of low-density lipoprotein. Am J Clin Nutr 1991; 53: 314S–321S
37. Niki E, Yamamoto Y, Komuro E et al. Membrane damage due to lipid oxidation. Am J Clin Nutr 1991; 53: S201–205
38. DiMascio P, Murphy M, Sies H. Antioxidant and defense systems. the role of carotenoids, tocopherols and thiols. Am J Clin Nutr 1991; 53: S194–200
39. Weisburger J. Nutritional approach to cancer prevention with emphasis on vitamins, antioxidants and carotenoids. Am J Clin Nutr 1991; 53: S226–237
40. Sokol RJ. Vitamin E. In: Ziegler EE, Filer LJ Jr, eds. Present knowledge in nutrition. 7th edn. Washington DC: International Life Sciences Press. 1996: p 130–136
41. Meydani M et al. Muscle uptake of vitamin E and its association with muscle fiber type. Nutr Biochem 1997; 8: 74–78
42. Losonczy, KG, Harris, TB, Havlik, RJ. Vitamin E and vitamin C supplement use and risk of all-cause and coronary heart disease mortality in older persons. The established populations for epidemiologic studies of the elderly. Am J Clin Nutr 1996; 64: 190–196
43. Veris Research Summary. The role of antioxidants in prevention of coronary heart disease. November, 1996: p 1–16

Vitamin K

1. Frick PG, Riedler G, Brogli H. Dose response and minimal daily requirement for vitamin K in man. J Appl Physiol 1967; 23: 387–389
2. Olson RE. The function and metabolism of vitamin K. Ann Rev Nutr 1984; 4: 281–327
3. Price PA. Role of vitamin K-dependent proteins in bone metabolism. Ann Rev Nutri 1988; 8: 565–583
4. Knapen MHJ, Hamuly'ak K, Vermeer C. The effect of vitamin K supplementation on circulating osteocalcin (bone Gla protein) and urinary calcium excretion. Ann Int Med 1989; 111: 1001–1005
5. Kuksis A. Fat absorption, vol. 2. Boca Raton, FL: CRC Press. 1987: p 65–86
6. Sadowski JA, Hood SJ, Dallal GE, Garry PJ. Phylloquinone in plasma from elderly and young adults. factors influencing its concentration. Am J Clin Nutr 1989; 50: 100–108
7. Jones DY, Koonsvitsky BP, Ebert ML et al. Vitamin K status of free-living subjects consuming olestra. Am J Clin Nutr 1991; 53: 943–946
8. Suttie, JW. Vitamin K. In: Present knowledge in nutrition. 7th edn. Washington DC: International Life Sciences Press. 1996: p 137–45
9. Binkley, NC, Suttie, W. Vitamin K nutrition and osteoporosis. J Nutr 1995; 125: 1812–1821
10. Ferland, G., Sadowski, JA., O'Brien, ME. Dietary induced subclinical vitamin K deficiency in normal human subjects. J Clin Invest 1993; 91: 1761–1768

Water-soluble vitamins

Vitamin C

1. Wartamowicz M, Panczenko-Kresowka B, Ziemlaski S et al. The effect of alpha-tocopherol and ascorbic acid on the serum lipid peroxide level in elderly people. Ann Nutr Metabol 1984; 28: 186–191
2. Calabrese EJ. Does exposure to environmental pollutants increase the need for vitamin C? J Environ Pathol Toxicol Oncol 1985; 5: 81–90

3. Tannenbaum SR, Wishnok JS, Leaf CD. Inhibition of nitrosamine formation by ascorbic acid. Am J Clin Nutr 1991; 53: 247S–250
4. Block G. Vitamin C and cancer prevention. The epidemiologic evidence. Am J Clin Nutr 1991; 53: 270S–282S
5. Gey KF. Scientific evidence for dietary targets in europe bibliotheca nutr deta, vol. 37. Basil: Karger. 1986
6. Ramirez J, Flowers NC. Leukocyte ascorbic acid and its relationship to coronary artery disease in man. Am J Clin Nutr 1980; 33: 2079–2087
7. Greco AM, Gentile M, DiFilippo O et al. Study of blood vitamin C in lung and bladder cancer patients before and after treatment with ascorbic acid. A preliminary report. Acta Vitaminol Enzymol 1982; 4: 155–162
8. Ghosh J, Das S. Evaluation of vitamin A and C status in normal and malignant conditions and their possible role in cancer prevention. Jpn J Cancer Res 1985; 76: 1174–1178
9. Romney SL, Duttagupta C, Basu J et al. Plasma vitamin C and uterine cervical dysplasia. Am J Obstet Gynecol 1985; 151: 976–980
10. Sergeev AV. Korrekksiia biokhimich eskilch i immunologicheskikh pokazatelei pri rake tolstoi kishki optimal nymi dozami retinilatseta i askorbinovoi kisloty. B Exp Biol Med 1984; 96: 90–92
11. Cameron E, Pauling L. Supplemental ascorbate in the supportive treatment of cancer. Reevaluation of prolongation of survival times in terminal human cancer. Proc Natl Acad Sci 1978; 75: 4538–4542
12. Bjelke E. Epidemiologic studies of cancer of the stomach, colon and rectum; with special emphasis on diet. Scand J Gastroenterol 1974; 9: 1–235S
13. Wassertheil-Smoller S, Romney SC, Wylie-Rosett J et al. Dietary vitamin C and uterine cervical dysplasia. Am J Epidemiol 1981; 114: 714–724
14. Marshall J, Graham S, Mettlin C et al. Diet in the epidemiology of oral cancer. Nutr Cancer 1982; 3: 145–149
15. Kune S, Kune GA, Watson LF. Case-control study of dietary etiological factors. The Melbourne Colorectal cancer study. Nutr Cancer 1987; 9: 21–42
16. Fontham ET, Pickle LW, Haenszel W et al. Dietary vitamins A and C and lung cancer risk in Louisiana. Cancer 1988; 62: 2267–2273
17. Lu SH, Otishima H, Fu HM, Tian Y, Li FM, Blettner M, Wahrendorf J, Bortsch H. Urinary excretion of N-nitrosamino acids and nitrate by inhabitants of high and low-risk areas of esophageal cancer in Northern China. Endogenous formation of nitrosoproline and its inhibition by vitamin C. Cancer Res 1986; 46: 1485–1491
18. O'Connor HJ, Habibzedah N, Schorah CJ et al. Effect of increased intake of vitamin C on the mutagenic activity of gastric juice and intrgastric concentrations of ascorbic acid. Carcinogenesis. 1985; 6: 1675–1676
19. Gaby SK, Singh VN. Vitamin intake and health: a scientific review. New York: Marcel Dekker. 1991: p 103–161
20. Sutor DJ, Johnston CS. FASEB J 1988; 2: A851
21. Shilotri PG, Bhat KS. Effect of mega doses of vitamin C on bactericidal activity of leukocytes. Am J Clin Nutr 1977; 30: 1007–1081
22. Anderson R, Oosthuizen R, Maritz R et al. Effects of increasing weekly doses of ascorbate on certain cellular and humoral immune functions in normal volunteers. Am J Clin Nutr 1980; 33: 71–76
23. Kennes B, Dumont I, Brohee D et al. Effect of vitamin C supplements in cell-mediated immunity in old people. Gerontology 1983; 29: 310
24. Ringsdorf WM Jr, Cheraskin E. Vitamin C and human wound healing. Oral Surg 1982; 53: 231–236
25. Schwartz PL. Ascorbic acid in wound healing: a review. J Am Diet Assoc 1970; 56: 497–503
26. Erden F, Gulenc S, Torun M et al. Ascorbic acid effect on some lipid fractions in human beings. Acta Vitaminol Enzymol 1985; 7: 131–138
27. Ziemlanski S, Wartanowicz M, Potrzebnicka K et al. Ascorbic acid and tocopherol levels in the organs and serum of guinea pigs with experimentally induced atherosclerosis. Acta Physiol Pol 1989; 40: 552–557
28. Ginter E, Cerna O, Budlovsky J et al. Effect of ascorbic acid on plasma cholesterol in humans in a long-term experiment. Int J Vit Nutri Res 1977; 47: 123–134
29. Lohmann W. Ascorbic acid and cataract. Ann NY Acad Sci 1987; 498: 307–311
30. Chandra DB, Varma R, Ahmad S et al. Vitamin C in the human aqueous humor and cataracts. Int J Vit Nutr Res 1986; 56: 165–168
31. Hallberg L, Rossander L. Absorption of iron from Western-type lunch and dinner meals. Am J Clin Nutr 1982; 35: 502–509
32. Cook JD, Watson SS, Simpson KM et al. The effect of high ascorbic acid supplementation on body iron stores. Blood 1984; 64: 721–726
33. Freudenheim JL, Johnson NE, Smith EL. Relationships between usual nutrient intake and bone-mineral content of women 35–65 years of age. longitudinal and cross-sectional analysis. Am J Clin Nutr 1986; 44: 863–876
34. Sowers MR, Wallace RB and Lemke JH. Correlates of mid-radius bone density among postmenopausal women. A community study. Am J Clin Nutr 1985; 41: 1045–1053
35. Cheraskin E, Ringsdorf WM Jr, Sisley EL. The vitamin C connection. New York: Harper & Row. 1983: p 1–279
36. Eaton SB, Shostak M, Konner M. The paleolithic prescription. New York: Harper & Row. 1988: p 82, 130–131
37. Riemersma RA, Wood DA, Macintyre CAC et al. Vitamin E. Biochemistry and health implications, vol. 570. New York: Ann NY Acad Sci. 1989: p 291–295
38. Robertson J, Donner AP, Trevithick JR. Vitamin E. Biochemistry and health implications, vol. 570. New York: Ann NY Acad Sci. 1989: p 372–82
39. Krumdieck C, Butterworth CE Jr. Ascorbate–cholesterollecithin interactions. Factors of potential importance in pathogenesis of atherosclerosis. Am J Clin Nutr 1974; 27: 866–876
40. Cheraskin E, Ringsdorf WM Jr. Vitamin C and chronologic versus bone age. J Tenn Dent Assoc 1974; 57: 177–178
41. Cheraskin E, Ringsdorf WM Jr, Medford FH. The 'ideal' daily vitamin C intake. J Med Assoc State Alabama 1977; 46: 39–40
42. Cheraskin E, Ringsdorf WM Jr. Vitamin C. Nutr Perspect 1978; 1: 34–36
43. Cheraskin E, Ringsdorf WM Jr. Vitamin C. J Can CA 1978; 22: 97–98
44. Cheraskin E. Vitamin C. J Orthomol Med 1986; 1: 241
45. Cheraskin E. Vitamin C. Nutr Report 1988; 6: 1–8
46. Cheraskin E, Ringsdorf WM Jr, Michael DW et al. Daily vitamin C consumption and reported respiratory findings. Int J Vit Nutr Res 1973; 43: 42–55
47. Yoshioka M, Matsushita T, Chuman Y. Inverse association of serum ascorbic acid level and blood pressure or rate of hypertension in male adults aged 30–39 years. Int J Vit Nutr Res 1984; 54: 343–347
48. Stamler J. Nutrition, lipids and coronary heart disease. New York: Raven Press. 1979: p 25
49. Weisburger J. Nutritional approach to cancer prevention with emphasis on vitamins, antioxidants, and carotenoids. Am J Clin Nutr 1991; 53: S226–237
50. Emstrom JE, Kanim LE, Klein MA. Vitamin C intake and mortality among a sample of the United States population. Epidem 1992; 3: 194–202
51. Levine M, Rumsey S, Wang Y, Park J et al. Vitamin C. In: Present knowledge in nutrition. 7th edn. Washington DC: International Life Sciences Press. 1996: p 146–159
52. Bendich A, Langseth L. The health effects of vitamin C supplementation. A review. J Am Col Nutr 1995; 14: 124–136
53. Weisburger JH. Vitamin C and disease prevention. J Am Col Nutr 1995; 14: 109–111
54. Hemilä H., Herman ZS. Vitamin C and the common cold. A retrospective analysis of Chalmers' review. J Am Col Nutr 1995; 14: 116–123
55. Johnston CS, Luo B. Comparison of the absorption and excretion of three commercially available sources of vitamin C. J Am Dietetic Assoc 1994; 94: 779–781
56. Hemilä H. Vitamin C and plasma cholesterol. Crit Rev Food Sci Nutr 1992; 32: 33–57
57. Moran JP, Cohen L, Greene JM et al. Plasma ascorbic acid concentrations relate inversely to blood pressure in human subjects. Am J Clin Nutr 1993; 57: 213–217

Vitamin B_{12}

1. Doscherholmen A, Swaim WR. Impaired assimilation of egg ^{57}Co vitamin B_{12} in patients with hypochlorhydria and achlorhydria and after gastric resection. Gastroenterol 1973; 64: 913–919
2. Carethers M. Diagnosing vitamin B_{12} deficiency, a common geriatric disorder. Geriatrics 1988; 43: 89–112
3. Nilsson-Ehle H, Landahl S, Lindstealt G et al. Low serum cobalamin levels in population study of 70- and 75-year-old subjects. Dig Dis Sci 1989; 34: 716–723
4. Brinton LA, Gridley G, Hrubec A et al. Cancer risk following pernicious anemia. Br J Cancer 1989; 59: 810–813
5. Heimburger DC, Alexander CB, Birch R, Bailey WC, Krumdieck CL. Improvement in bronchial squamous metaplasia in smokers treated with folate and vitamin B_{12}. J Am Med Assoc 1988; 259: 1525–1530
6. Chu RC, Hall CA. The total serum homocysteine as an indicator of vitamin B_{12} and folate status. Am J Clin Pathol 1988; 90: 446–449
7. Swift ME, Schultz TD. Vitamin B_{12}. Nutr Rep Int 1986; 34: 1–14
8. Olszewski AJ, Szostak WB, McCully KS. Plasma glucosamine and galactosamine in ischemic heart disease. Atherosclerosis 1989; 75: 1–6
9. Gaby SK, Bendich A. Vitamin intake and health: a scientific review. New York: Marcel Dekker. 1991: p 193–197
10. Richardson LR, Brock R. Studies of reproduction in rats using large doses of vitamin B_{12} and highly purified soybean proteins. J Nutr 1956; 58: 135–145
11. Omaye ST. Nutritional and toxicological aspects of food safety. New York: Plenum Press. 1984: p 169–203
12. Shils ME, Young VR. Modern Nutrition in Health and Disease. 7th edn. Lea and Febiger. 1988: p 401–404
13. Bendich A, Cohen M. Nutrition and Immunology. New York: Alan R. Liss. 1988: p 101–123
14. Lederle FA. Oral cobalamin for pernicious anemia. Medicine's best kept secret? JAMA 1991; 265: 94–95
15. Hathcock JN, Troendle GJ. Oral cobalamine for treatment of pernicious anemia? [editorial; comment] JAMA 1991; 265: 96–97
16. Inada M, Toyoshima M, Kameyama M. Brain content of cobalamin and its binders in elderly subjects. J Nutr Sci Vitaminol 1982; 28: 351–357
17. Herbert, V. Vitamin $B\text{-}_{12}$. In: Present knowledge in nutrition. 7th edn. Washington DC: International Life Sciences Press. 1996: p 191–205
18. Allen, LH, Casterline J. Vitamin B_{12} deficiency in elderly individuals. diagnosis and requirements. Am J Clin Nutr 1994; 60: 12–14

Folic acid

1. Anderson SA, Talbot JM. FDA technical report FDA/RF 82/13. Washington DC: FDA. 1981
2. Huber AM, Wallins LL, DeRusso P. Folate nutriture in pregnancy. J Am Diet Assoc 1988; 88: 791–814
3. Bailey LB, Wagner PA, Davis CG, Dinning JS. Food frequency related to folacin status in adolescents. J Am Diet Assoc 1984; 84: 801–804
4. Clark AJ, Mossholder S, Gates R. Folacin status in adolescent females. Am J Clin Nutr 1987; 46: 302–306
5. Bates CJ, Fleming M, Paul AA et al. Folate status and its relation to vitamin C in healthy elderly men and women. Age Aging 1980; 9: 241–248
6. Baker H, Jaslow SP, Frank O. Severe impairment of dietary folate utilization in the elderly. J Am Geriatr Soc 1978; 26: 218–221
7. Gaby SK, Bendich A. Vitamin intake and health: a scientific review. New York: Marcel Dekker. 1991: p 175–188
8. Smithells RW, Nevin NC, Seller MJ et al. Further experience of vitamin supplementation for prevention of neural tube defect recurrences. Lancet 1983; 1: 1027–1031
9. Laurence KM, James N, Miller MH et al. Double-blind randomized controlled trial of folate treatment before conception to prevent recurrence of neural-tube defects. Br Med J 1981; 282: 1509–1511
10. Milunsky A, Jick H, Jick SS, Bruell CL, MacLaughlin DS, Rothman KJ, Willette W. Multivitamin/folic acid supplementation in early pregnancy reduces the prevalence of neural tube defects. J Am Med Assoc 1989; 262: 2847–2852
11. Briggs RM. Vitamin supplementation as a possible factor in the incidence of cleft lip/palate deformities in humans. Clin Plast Surg 1976; 3: 647–652
12. Kang SS, Wong PWK, Norusis M. Homocysteinemia due to folate deficiency. Metabolism 1987; 36: 458–462
13. Brattstrom LE, Hultberg BL, Hardebo JE. Folic acid responsive postmenopausal homocysteinemia. Metabolism 1987; 34: 1073–1077
14. Brattstrom LE, Israelsson B, Jeppsson JO, Hultberg BL. Folic acid – an innocuous means to reduce plasma homocysteine. Scand J Clin Lab Invest 1988; 48: 215–221
15. Preuss HG. CRC Handbook series in nutrition and food. Section E: Nutritional disorders, vol. 1. Boca Raton, FL: CRC Press. 1978: p 61–62
16. Butterworth CE, Tamura T. Folic acid safety and toxicity. A brief review. Am J Clin Nutr 1989; 50: 353–358
17. Bendich A, Cohen M. Nutrition and immunology. New York: Alan R. Liss. 1988: p 101–123
18. Weisburger JH. Nutritional approach to cancer prevention with emphasis on vitamins, antioxidants, and carotenoids. Am J Clin Nutr 1991; 53: S226–S237
19. Selhub, J, Rosenberg, IH. Folic acid. In: Present knowledge in nutrition. 7th edn. Washington DC: International Life Sciences Press. 1996: p 206–219
20. Alpert JE, Fava, M. Nutrition and depression. The role of folate. Nutr Rev 1997; 55: 145–149
21. Nygard O, Refsum H, Ueland PM et al. Coffee consumption and plasma total homocysteine. The Hordaland homocysteine study. Am J Clin Nutr 1997; 65: 136–143
22. Center for Disease Control. Knowledge about folic acid and use of multivitamins containing folic acid among reproductive-aged women. Morbidity Mortality Weekly Report 1996; 45: 793–795
23. Murray, MT. Evaluating the many benefits of folic acid. Am J Natural Med 1996; 3: 8–11
24. Center for Disease Control. Recommendations for the use of folic acid to reduce the number of cases of spina bifida and other neural tube defects. Morbidity Mortality Weekly Report 1996; 41: RR–14

Niacin and niacinamide

1. Goldsmith GA, Miller ON, Unglaub WG. Efficiency of tryptophan as a niacin precursor in man. J Nutr 1961; 73: 172–176
2. Patterson JI, Brown RR, Lindswiler H et al. Exertion of tryptophan-niacin metabolites by young men. Effects of tryptophan, leucine, and vitamin B6 intakes. Am J Clin Nutr 1980; 33: 2157–2167
3. Alhadeff L, Gualtieri GT, Lipton M. Toxic effects of water-soluble vitamins. Nutr Rev 1984; 42: 33–40
4. Einstein N, Baker A, Galper J et al. Jaundice due to nicotinic acid therapy. Am J Digest Dis 1975; 20: 282–286
5. Cheraskin E, Ringsdorf WM Jr, Medford FH. The 'ideal' daily niacin intake. Int J Vit Nutr Res 1976; 46: 58–60
6. Gaby SK. Vitamin intake and health: a scientific review. New York: Marcel Dekker. 1991: p 189–192
7. Bendich A, Cohen M. Nutrition and immunology. New York: Alan R. Liss. 1988: p 114–115
8. Figge HL, Figge J, Souney PF et al. Nicotinic acid. A review of its clinical use in the treatment of lipid disorders. Pharmacotherapy 1988; 8: 287–294
9. Grundy SM. Drug therapy in dyslipidemia. Scand J Clin Lab Invest 1990; 50: 63–72
10. O'Hara J, Jolly PN, Nicol CG. The therapeutic efficacy of inositol nicotinate (Hexopal) in intermittent claudication of a controlled trial. Br J Clin Practice 1988; 42: 377–383
11. Jacob, RA, Swendseid, ME. Niacin. In: Present knowledge in nutrition. 7th edn. Washington DC: International Life Sciences Press. 1996: p 184–190.

Pyridoxine (vitamin B_6)

1. Ribaya-Mercado JD, Russell RM, Morrow FD et al. [Abstract.] FASEB J 1988; 2: A847

2. Driskell JA, Wesley RL, Hess IE. Effectiveness of pyridoxine hydrochloride treatment on carpal tunnel syndrome patients. Nutr Rep Int 1986; 34: 103–1040
3. Talbott MC, Miller LT, Kerkvliet NI. Pyridoxine supplementation. effect on lymphocyte responses in elderly persons. Am J Clin Nutr 1987; 46: 659–664
4. Gaby SK. Vitamin intake and health: a scientific review. New York: Marcel Dekker. 1991: p 163–74
5. Schaumburg H, Kaplan J, Windebank A et al. Sensory neuropathy from pyridoxine abuse. A new megavitamin syndrome. N Eng J Med 1983; 309: 445–448
6. Swift ME, Shultz TD. Relationship of vitamins B_6 and B_{12} to homocysteine levels: risk for coronary heart disease. Nutr Rep Int 1986; 34: 1–14
7. McCully KS. Vascular pathology of homocysteinemia: implications for the pathogenesis of arteriosclerosis. Am J Pathol 1969; 56: 111–128
8. Serofontein WJ, Ubbink JB, De Villers LS, Becker PJ. Depressed plasma pyridoxal-5′-phosphate levels in tobacco-smoking men. Atherosclerosis 1986; 59: 341–346
9. Rinehart JF, Greenburg LD. Vitamin B_6 deficiency in the Rhesus monkey. Am J Clin Nutr 1956; 4: 318–325
10. Parry GJ, Bredesen DE. Sensory neuropathy with low dose pyridoxine. Neurology 1985; 35: 1466–1468
11. Dalton K, Dalton MJT. Characteristics of pyridoxine overdose neuropathy syndrome. Acta Neurol Scand 1987; 76: 8–11
12. Cohen M, Bendich A. Safety of pyridoxine – a review of human and animal studies. Toxicol Letters 1986; 34: 129–139
13. Shultz TD, Santamaria AG, Gridley DS et al. Effect of pyridoxine and pyridoxal on the in vitro growth of human malignant melanoma. Nutr Res 1988; 8: 201–207
14. Gvozdova LG, Paramonova EG, Goriachenkova EV et al. The content of pyridoxal coenzymes in the blood plasma of patients with coronary atherosclerosis on a background of therapeutic diet and after supplemental intake of vitamin B_6. Vop Pitan 1966; 25: 40–44
15. Verrmaak WJ, Barnard HC, Potgieter GM et al. Plasma pyridoxal-5′-phosphate levels in myocardial infarction. S Afr Med J 1986; 70: 195–196
16. Bendich A, Cohen M. Nutrition and immunology. New York: Alan R. Liss. 1988: p 104–107
17. Gaby AR. The safe use of vitamin B_6. J Nutr Med 1990; 1: 153–157
18. Bassler KH. Megavitamin therapy with pyridoxine. Int J Vit Nutr Res 1988; 58: 105–118
19. Kabir H, Leklem JE, Miller LT. J Nutr 1983; 113: 2412–2420
20. Weisburger J. Nutritional approach to cancer prevention with emphasis on vitamins, antioxidant, and carotenoids. Am J Clin Nutr 1991; 53: S226–S237
21. Leklem, JE. Vitamin B-6. In: Present knowledge in nutrition. 7th edn. Washington DC: International Life Sciences Press. 1996: p 174–83

Riboflavin (vitamin B_2)

1. Joint, FAO/WHO Expert Group. Riboflavin. WHO Technical Report Series No. 362. 1967: p 86
2. Mats SGF. Vitamins in medicine, vol. I. 4th edn. 1980: p 398–438
3. Skalka HW, Prchal JT. Cataracts and riboflavin deficiency. Am J Clin Nutr 1981; 34: 861–863
4. Prchal JT, Conrad ME, Skalka HW. Association of presenile cataracts with heterozygosity for glactosaemic states and riboflavin deficiency. Lancet 1978; i: 12–143
5. Belko AZ, Meredith MP, Kalkwarf HJ et al. Effects of exercise on riboflavin requirements. Biological validation in weight reducing women. Am J Clin Nutr 1985; 41: 270–277
6. Belko AZ, Obarzanek E, Kalkwarf HJ et al. Effects of exercise on riboflavin requirements of young women. Am J Clin Nutr 1983; 37: 509–517
7. Belko AZ, Obazanek E, Roach R et al. Effects of aerobic exercise and weight loss on riboflavin requirements of moderately obese, marginally deficient young women. Am J Clin Nutr 1984; 40: 553–561
8. Beutler E. Glutathione reductase. Stimulation in normal subjects by riboflavin supplementation. Science 1969; 165: 614–615
9. Bendich A, Cohen M. Nutrition and Immunology. New York: Alan R. Liss. 1988: p 114
10. Goodwin JS, Garry PJ. Relationship between megadose vitamin supplementation and immunological function in a healthy elderly population. Clin Exp Immunol 1983; 51: 647–653
11. Tremblay A, Boilard F, Breton M-F et al. Nutr Res 1984; 4: 201–208
12. Weisburger J. Nutritional approach to cancer prevention with emphasis on vitamins, antioxidants, and cartenoids. Am J Clin Nutr 1991; 53: S226–227
13. Rivlin RS. Riboflavin. In: Ziegler EE, Filer LJ Jr, eds. Present knowledge in nutrition. 7th edn. Washington DC: International Life Sciences Press. 1996: p 167–173
14. Webster RP, Gawde MD, Bhattacharya RK. Modulation of carcinogen-induced DNA damage and repair enzyme activity by dietary riboflavin. Cancer Lett 1996; 98: 129–135
15. Salim-Hanna M, Edwards AM, Silva E. A photo-induced adduct between a vitamin and an essential amino acid: binding of riboflavin to tryptophan. Int J Vit Nutr Res 1987; 57: 155–159
16. Schoenen J, Jacquay J, Lenaerts M. Effectiveness of high-dose riboflavin in migraine prophylaxis: a randomized controlled trial. Neurology 1998; 50: 466–470
17. Schoenen J, Lenaerts M, Bastings E. High-dose riboflavin as a prophylactic treatment of migraine: results of an open pilot study. Cephalalgia 1994; 14: 328–329

Thiamin (vitamin B_1)

1. Lonsdale DA. Nutritionist's guide to the clinical use of vitamin B1. Tacoma, WA: Life Sciences Press. 1987: p 1–209
2. Cheraskin E, Ringsdorf WM Jr, Setyaadmadja AT et al. Thiamin consumption and cardiovascular complaints. J Am Geriatrics Soc 1967; 15: 1074–1079
3. Cheraskin E, Ringsdorf WM Jr, Setyaadmadja AT et al. Carbohydrate consumption and cardiovascular complaints. Angiology 1967; 18: 224–230
4. Cheraskin E, Ringsdorf WM Jr, Medford FH et al. The 'ideal' daily vitamin B_1 intake. J Oral Med 1978; 33: 77–79
5. Cheraskin E, Ringsdorf WM Jr. How much refined carbohydrate should we eat? Am Lab 1974; 6: 31–35
6. Lonsdale D. Red cell transketolase studies in a private practice specializing in nutritional correction. J Am Coll Nutr 1988; 7: 61–68
7. Iber FL, Blass JP, Brin M et al. Thiamin in the elderly–relation to alcoholism and to neurological degenerative disease. Am J Clin Nutr 1982; 6: 1067–1082
8. Shils ME, Young VR. Modern nutrition in health and disease. 7th edn. Philadelphia: Lea and Febiger. 1988: p 358
9. Cummings F, Briggs M, Briggs, M. Vitamins in human biology and medicine. Boca Raton, FL: CRC Press. 1981
10. Bendich A, Cohen M. Nutrition and Immunology. New York: Alan R. Liss. 1988: p 101–123
11. Rindi, G. Thiamin. In: Present knowledge in nutrition. 7th edn. Washington DC: International Life Sciences Press. 1996: p 160–166

Minerals

1. Schauss A. Minerals, treace elements and human health. 3rd edn. Tacoma, WA: AIBR Life Sciences. 1997

Boron

1. Nielsen FH. New essential trace elements for life sciences. Biol Trace Elem Res 1990; 26/7: 599–611
2. Newnham RE. Trace element in man and animals –5. Abstracts. Aberdeen, Scotland. 1984: p 26
3. Lovatt CJ, Dugger WM. Biochemistry of the essential ultratrace elements. New York: Plenum. 1984: p 389–421
4. Losee F, Bibby BG. Caries inhibition by trace elements other than fluorine. New York Dent J 1970; 36: 15–19
5. Nielsen FH. Ultratrace minerals: mythical elixirs or nutrients or concern. Contemp Nutr 1990; 15: 1–2
6. Nielsen FH, Shuler TR, Zimmerman TJ, Uthus EO. Magnesium and methionine deprivation affect the response of rats to boron deprivation. Biol Trace Elem Res 1988; 17: 91–99
7. Nielsen FH, Shuler TR, Zimmerman TJ, Uthus EO. Dietary

magnesium, manganese and boron affect the response of rats to high dietary aluminum. Magnesium 1988; 7: 133
8. Hunt CD, Nielsen FH. Interactions among dietary boron, magnesium, and cholecalciferol in the chick. Proc Natl Acad Sci 1987; 41: 50
9. Schuler TR, Nielsen FH. Effect of boron, calcium and magnesium and their interactions on the mineral content of kidney and liver from marginally methionine deficient rats. Proc Natl Acad Sci 1987; 41: 49
10. Nielsen FH, Hunt CD, Mullen LM, Hunt JR. Effect of dietary boron on mineral, estrogen, and testosterone metabolism in postmenopausal women. FASEB J 1987; 1: 394–397
11. Nielsen FH. [Abstract]. FASEB J 1989; 3: A760
12. Hunt CD. Dietary boron modified the effects of magnesium and molybdenum on mineral metabolism in the cholecalciferol-deficient chick. Biol Trace Elem Res 1989; 22: 201–220
13. Hegsted M, Keenan MJ, Siver F. Effect of boron on vitamin D deficient rats. Biol Trace Elem Res 1991; 28: 243–255
14. Nielsen FH. Ultratrace elements in nutrition. Ann Rev Nutr 1984; 4: 21–41
15. Nenham RE. Trace element metabolism in man and animals. Canberra: Australian Acad Sci. 1981: p 597–600, 400–402
16. Weir RJ, Fisher RS. Toxicol Appl Pharmacol 1972; 23: 351–364
17. Schroeder HA, Mitchell M. Life-term studies in rates. effects of aluminum, boriaum, beryllium, and tungsten. J Nutr 1975; 105: 421–424
18. Curzon MEJ. Trace elements and dental disease. Boston: John Wright/PSG. 1983: p 339–356
19. Elsair J, Merad M, Demine R. Boron as an antidote against fluoride intoxication in rabbits. Fluoride 1980; 13: 30–38
20. Chandra RK, Puri S. Trace elements in nutrition of children. New York: Raven Press. 1985: p 98
21. Tipton IH, Stewart PL and Martin PG. Trace elements in diet and excreta. Health Phys 1966; 12: 1683–1689
22. Curzon MEJ, Crocker DC. Relationships of trace elements in human tooth enamel and dental caries. Arch Oral Biol 1978; 23: 647–653
23. Varo P, Koivistinen P. Mineral element composition of Finnish foods. XII. General discussion and nutritional evaluation. Acta Agricult Scand 1980; 22: 165–171
24. Hamilton EI, Minski MJ. The concentration and distribution of some stable elements in healthy human tissues from the United Kingdom. Sci Total Environ 1972/73; 1: 375–394
25. Nielsen FH. Trace substances in environmental health – 18. Columbia: Univ Missouri Press 1984: p 47–52
26. Elsair J, Merad M, Demine R. Action of boron upon fluorosis and calcium-phosphorous metabolism: an experimental study. Fluoride 1982; 15: 75–78
27. Pinto J, Huang YP, McConnell RJ et al. Increased urinary riboflavin excretion resulting from boric acid ingestion. J Lab Clin Med 1978; 92: 126–134
28. Gilbert FA. Mineral nutrition of plants and animals. Norman: Univ OK Press. 1984: p 80–84
29. Travers RL, Rennie GC, Newnham RE. Boron and arthritis: the results of a double-blind pilot study. J Nutr Med 1990; 1: 127–132
30. Nielsen FH. Studies on the relationship between boron and magnesium which possibly affects the formation and maintenance of bones. Magnesium 1990; 9: 61–69
31. Meacham SL, Taper LJ, Volpe SL et al. Effect of boron supplementation on blood and urinary calcium, magnesium, and phosphorous, and urinary boron in athletic and sedentary women. Am J Clin Nutr 1995; 61: 341–345
32. Hunt CD, Herbel JL, Nielsen FH et al. Metabolic responses of postmenopausal women to supplemental dietary boron and aluminum during usual and low magnesium intake. Boron calcium, and magnesium absorption and retention and blood mineral concentrations. Am J Clin Nutr 1997; 65: 803–813
33. Effects of dietary boron and magnesium on brain function of mature male and female Long–Evans rats. J Trace Elem Exp Med 1993; 6: 53–64
34. Schauss, AG Boron. Essentiality, toxicity, and role in human health. Tacoma: Life Sciences Press. 1996
35. Usuda K, Kono K, Yoshida Y et al. Serum boron concentration from inhabitants of an urban area in Japan. Reference value and interval for the health screening of boron exposure. Biol Trace Elem Res 1997; 56: 167–178
36. Naghii, MR, Samman, S. The effect of boron supplementation on the distribution of boron in selected tissues and on testosterone synthesis in rats. Nutr Biochem 1996; 7: 507–512

Calcium

1. Arnaud, DC, Sanchez, SD. Calcium and phosphorous. Present knowledge in nutrition. 6th edn. Washington DC: Nutrition Foundation. 1990: p 212–221, 371–373
2. Linkswiler HM, Joyce CL, Anand CR. Calcium retention of young adult males as affected by level of protein & of calcium intake. Trans NY Acad Sci 1974; 36: 333–340
3. Chu JY, Margen S, Costa FM. Studies in calcium metabolism. Am J Clin Nutr 1975; 28: 1028–1035
4. Spencer H, Karmer L et al. Effect of a high protein (meat) intake on calcium metabolism in man. Am J Clin Nutr 1978; 31: 2167–2180
5. Adams P, Davies GT, Sweetnam P. Osteoporosis and the effects of aging on bone mass in elderly men and women. J Med New Series 1970; 39: 601–615
6. Heaney RP, Recker RR, Saville PD. Calcium balance and calcium requirements in middle-aged women. J Lab Clin Med 1978; 92: 964–70, 953–963
7. Jowsey J. Osteoporosis. dealing with a crippling bone disease of the elderly. Geriatrics 1977; 32: 41–50
8. Mazess RB, Barden HS. Bone density in premenopausal women. effects of age, dietary intake, physical activity, smoking, and birth-control pills. Am J Clin Nutr 1991; 53: 132–142
9. Dawson-Hughes B, Jacques P, Shipp C. Dietary calcium intake and bone loss from the spine in healthy postmenopausal women. Am J Clin Nutr 1987; 46: 685–687
10. Sowers MR, Wallace RB, Lemke JH. Correlates of mid-radius bone density among postmenopausal women. A community study. Am J Clin Nutr 1985; 41: 1045–1053
11. Sowers MR, Wallace RB, Lemke JH. Correlates of forearm bone mass among women during maximal bone mineralization. Prev Med 1985; 14: 585–596
12. Elders PJ, Netelenbos JC, Lips P et al. Perimenopausal bone mass and risk factors. Bone Miner 1989; 7: 289–299
13. Kanders B, Dempster DW, Lindsay R. Interaction of calcium nutrition and physical activity on bone mass in young women. J Bone Miner Res 1988; 3: 145–149
14. Nordin BE, Polley KJ. Metabolic consequences of the menopause. A cross-sectional, longitudinal, and intervention study on 557 normal postmenopausal women. Calcif Tissue Int 1987; 41: 1–59
15. Angus RM, Sambrook PN, Pocock NA, Eisman JA. Dietary intake and bone mineral density. Bone Miner 1988; 4: 265–277
16. Desai S, Baran D, Grimes J et al. Relationship of diet, axial, and appendicular bone mass in normal premenopausal women. Am J Med Sci 1987; 293: 218–220
17. Freudenheim JL, Johnson NE, Smith EL. Relationships between usual nutrient intake and bone-mineral content of women 35-65 years of age. Longitudinal and cross-sectional analysis. Am J Clin Nutr 1986; 44: 863–876
18. Garn SM, Rohmann CG, Wagner B. Continuing bone growth through life. A general phenomenon. Fed Proc 1967; 26: 1729–1736
19. Laval-Jeanet AM, Paul G, Bergot C et al. Correlation between vertebral bone density measurement and nutritional status. In: Proceedings – osteoporosis. Glostrup: Glostrup Hospital. 1984: p 953–963
20. Tylavsky FA, Anderson JJ. Dietary factors in bone health of elderly lactoovovetetarian and omnivorous women. B. Am J Clin Nutr 1988; 48: 842–849
21. Riggs BL, Wahner HW, Melton LJ 3rd et al. Dietary calcium intake and rates of bone loss in women. J Clin Invest 1987; 80: 979–982
22. Stevenson JC, Whitehead MI, Padwick M et al. Dietary intake of calcium and postmenopausal bone loss. Br Med J 1988; 297: 15–17
23. Nilas L, Christiansen C, Rodbro P. Calcium supplementation and postmenopausal bone loss. Br Med J 1984; 289: 1103–1106
24. Riis B, Thomsen K, Christiansen C. Does calcium supplementation

prevent post menopausal bone loss? A double-blind, controlled clinical study. New Eng J Med 1987; 316: 173–177
25. van Beresteijn EC, van't Hof MA, de Waard H. Relation of axial bone mass to habitual calcium intake and to cortical bone loss in healthy early postmenopausal women. Bone 1990; 11: 7–13
26. Kanis JA, Passmore R. Calcium supplementation of the diet – I. Br Med J 1989; 298: 137–140
27. Kanis JA, Passmore R. Calcium supplementation of the diet – II. Br Med J 1989; 298: 205–208
28. Arnaud CD, Sanchez SD. The role of calcium in osteoporosis. Ann Rev Nutr 1990; 10: 397–414
29. Fletcher MP et al. Nutrition and immunology. New York: Alan R. Liss. 1988: p 215–239
30. Hallberg L, Brune M, Erlandsson M et al. Calcium. Effect of different amounts on nonheme- and heme-iron absorption in humans. Am J Clin Nutr 1991; 53: 112–119
31. Cook J, Dassenko S, Whittaker P. Calcium supplementation. Effect on iron absorption. Am J Clin Nutr 1991; 53: 106–111

Chromium

1. Anderson RA, Polansky MM, Bryden NA et al. Urinary chromium excretion of human subjects. Effects of chromium supplementation and glucose loading. Am J Clin Nutr 1982; 36: 1184–1193
2. Stoecker, BJ Present knowledge in nutrition. 6th edn. Chromium. Washington DC: Nutrition Foundation. 1990: p 287–291
3. Offenbacher EG, Pi-Sunyer FX. Chromium in human nutrition. Ann Rev Nutr 1988; 8: 543–563
4. Wang M, Fox E, Stoecker B. Serum cholesterol of adults supplemented with brewer's yeast or chromium chloride. Nutr Res 1989; 9: 989–998
5. Urberg M, Parent M, Mill D et al. Evidence for synergism between chromium and nicotinic acid in normalizing glucose tolerance. Diabetes 1986; 35: 37a.
6. Anderson RA, Polansky MM, Bryden NA. Acute effects on chromium, copper, zinc and selected clinical variables in urine and serum of male runners. Biol Trace Elem Res 1984; 6: 327–336
7. Gibson RS, Scythes CA. Chromium, selelnium and other trace element intakes of a selected sample of Canadian premenopausal women. Biol Trace Eleme Res 1984; 6: 105–116
8. Kozlovsky AS, Moser PB, Reiser S, Anderson RA. Effects of diets high in simple sugars on urinary chromium losses. Metabolism 1986; 35: 515–518
9. Pekarek RS, Hayer EC, Rayfield EJ et al. Relationship between serum chromium concentrations and glucose utilization in normal and infected subjects. Diabetes 1975; 24: 350–353
10. Wedrychowski A, Ward WA, Schmidt WN, Hnilica LS. Chromium-induced cross-linking of nuclear proteins and DNA. J Biol Chem 1985; 260: 7150–7155
11. Borel JS, Anderson RA. Biochemistry of the essential ultratrace elements. New York: Plenum. 1984: p 175–199
12. Schroeder HA. The role of chromium in mammalian nutrition. Am J Clin Nutr 1968; 21: 230–244
13. Wolf W, Mertz W, Masironi R. Determination of chromium in refined and unrefined sugars. J Agr Food Chem 1974; 22: 1037–1042
14. Seaborn CD, Stoecker BJ. Effects of antacid or ascorbic acid on tissue accumulation and urinary excretion of 51chromium. Nutr Res 1990; 10: 1401–1407
15. Offenbacher EG, Rinko CJ, Pi-Sunyer FX. The effects of inorganic chromium and brewer's yeast on glucose tolerance, plasma lipids, and plasma chromium in elderly subjects. Am J Clin Nutr 1985; 42: 454–456
16. Anderson RA, Kozlovsky AS. Chromium intake, absorption and excretion of subjects consuming self-selected diets. Am J Clin Nutr 1985; 42: 1177–1183
17. Gordon JB. An easy and inexpensive way to lower cholesterol? [letter; comment] West J Med 1991; 154: 3
18. Reaven GM. Banting lecture 1988. Role of insulin resistance in human disease. Diabetes 1988; 37: 1595–1607
19. Press RI, Geller J, Evans GW. The effect of chromium picolinate on serum cholesterol and apolipoprotein fractions in human subjects. West J Med 1990; 152: 41–45
20. Evans GW. The effect of chromium picolinate on insulin controlled parameters in humans. Int J Biosocial Med Res 1989; 11: 163–180
21. Anderson RA. Chromium metabolism and its role in disease processes in man. Clin Physiol Biochem 1986; 4: 31–41
22. Uusitupa MI, Kumpulainen JT, Voutilainen E, Hersio K, Sarlund H, Pyorala KP, Koivistoinen PE, Lehto JT. Effect of inorganic chromium supplementation on glucose non-insulin-dependent diabetics. Am J Clin Nutr 1983; 38: 404–410
23. Simonoff M, Llabador Y, Hamon C et al. Low plasma chromium in patients with coronary artery and heart disease. Biol Trace Elem Res 1984; 6: 431–439
24. Bunker VW, Lawson MS, Delves HT, Clayton BE. The intake and excretion of chromium by the elderly. Am J Clin Nutr 1984; 39: 799–802
25. Evans GW, Ropginksi EE, Mertz W. Interaction of the glucose tolerance factor (GFW) with insulin. Biochem Biophys Res Commun 1973; 50: 718–722
26. Anderson RA, Polansky MM, Bryden NA, Patterson KY, Veillon C, Glinsmann. Effects of chromium supplementation on urinary Cr excretion with selected clinical parameters. J Nutr 1983; 113: 276–281
27. Offenbacher EG, Pi-Sunyer FX. Beneficial effect of chromium-rich yeast on glucose tolerance and blood lipids in elderly subjects. Diabetes 1980; 29: 919
28. Donaldson DL, Rennert OM. Metabolism of trace elements in man, vol. 2: genetic implications. Boca Raton, FL: CRC Press. 1984: p 113–132
29. Menendez CE, Stoecker BJ. Nutrition and diabetes. New York: Alan R. Liss. 1985: p 15–36
30. Anderson JW. Nutrition and diabetes. New York: Alan R. Liss. 1985: p 133–59
31. Singh RB et al. Trace Element Med 1991; 8: 29–33
32. Anderson RA. Chromium and its role in lean body mass and weight reduction. Nutrition Report 1991; 11: 41, 46
33. Stoecker BJ. Chromium. In: Present knowledge in nutrition. 7th edn. Washington, DC: Nutrition Foundation. 1996: p 344–352

Copper

1. O'Dell BL. Copper. In: Present knowledge in nutrition. 6th edn. Washington DC: Nutrition Foundation. 1990: p 261–265
2. Dowdy RP. Copper metabolism. Am J Clin Nutr 1969; 22: 887
3. Evans GW. Copper homeostasis in the mammalian system. Physiol Rev 1973; 53: 535
4. Zelkowitz M, Verghese JP, Antel J. Zinc and copper in medicine. Springfield IL: Charles C. Thomas. 1980: p 418–463
5. Stemmer KL, Petering HG, Murthy L et al. Copper deficiency effects on cardiovascular systems and lipid metabolism in the rat; the role of dietary proteins and excessive zinc. Ann Nutr Metabol 1985; 29: 332–347
6. Klevay LM. Metabolism of trace metals in man, vol. 1. Boca Raton, FL: CRC Press. 1984: p 129–157
7. Mertz LM. Nutrition and aging. New York: Alan R Liss. 1990: p 229–240
8. Fields M, Ferretti RJ, Smith JC Jr, Reiser S. The interaction of type of dietary carbohydrates with copper deficiency. Am J Clin Nutr 1984; 39: 289–295
9. Schroeder HA, Nason AP, Tipton IH. Essential trace metals in man. J Chron Dis 1966; 19: 1007–1034
10. Shamberger RJ. Nutrition and cancer. New York: Plenum. 1984: p 237–238
11. Fletcher MP, Gershwin ME, Keen CL et al. Trace element deficiences and immune responsiveness in human and animal models. In: Chandra RK, ed. Nutrition and immunology. New York: Alan R. Liss. 1988: p 215–239
12. Pocino M, Baute L, Malav'e I. Influence of oral administration of excess copper on the immune response. Fund Appl Therap 1991; 16: 249–256
13. Linder M.C. Copper. In: Present knowledge in nutrition. 7th edn. Washington, DC: Nutrition Foundation. 1996: p 307–319
14. Anonymous. Copper affects atherosclerosis. Med Tribune 1991; 32: 6
15. Percival S.S. Neutropenia caused by copper deficiency. Possible mechanisms of action. Nutr Rev 1995; 53: 59–66

16. Kelley DS, Dauda PA, Taylor PC et al. Effects of low-copper diets on human immune response. Am J Clin Nutr 1995; 62: 412–416
17. Reunanen A, Knekt P, Marniemi J et al. Serum calcium, magnesium, copper and zinc and risk of cardiovascular death. Eur J Clin Nutr 50: 431–437

Iodine

1. Hetzel, SC. Present knowledge in nutrition. 6th edn. Iodine deficiency. An international public health problem. Washington DC: Nutrition Foundation. 1990: p 308–312
2. Matovinovic J, Trowbridge FL. Endemic goiter and endemic cretinism. New York: John Wiley. 1980: p 37–67
3. Hunnikin C, Wood FO. Endemic goiter and endemic cretinism. New York: John Wiley. 1980: p 497–512
4. Wang YY, Yang SH. Improvement in hearing among otherwise normal schoolchildren in iodine-deficient areas of Guizhou, China, following use of iodized salt. Lancet 1985; 2: 518–520
5. Matovinovic J. Endemic goiter and cretinism at the dawn of the third millenium. Ann Rev Nutr 1983; 3: 341–412
6. Stanbury, JB. Iodine deficiency and the iodine deficiency disorders. In: Present knowledge in nutrition. 7th edn. Iodine. Washington, DC: Nutrition Foundation. 1996: p 378–383
7. Kearny, CH, Orient, JM. [Letter] Thyroid protection. Science 1996; 274: 1596–1597
8. Hetzel, B.S. Iodine deficiency and fetal brain damage. N Eng J Med 1994; 331: 1770–1771
9. Xue-Yi C, Xin-Min J, Zhi-Hong D et al. Timin of vulnerability of the brain to iodine deficiency in endemic cretinism. N Eng J Med 1994 331: 1739–1744

Iron

1. Dallman, PR. Iron. In: Present knowledge in nutrition. 6th edn. Washington DC: Nutrition Foundation. 1990: p 241–250
2. Green R, Charlton R et al. Body iron excretion in man; a collaborative study. Am J Med 1968; 45: 336–353
3. Hallberg L, Nilsson L. Constancy of individual menstrual blood loss. Acta Obstet Gynecol Scand 1964; 43: 352–359
4. Hallber L. Bioavailability of dietary iron in man. Ann Rev Nutr 1981; 1: 123–147
5. Magnusson B, Bjorn-Rasmussen E, Hallberg L et al. Iron absorption in relation to iron status. Model proposed to express results of food iron absorption measurements. Scand J Haematol 1981; 27: 201–208
6. Hallberg L, Rossander L, Persson H. Deleterious effects of prolonged warming of meals on ascorbic acid content and iron absorption. Am J Clin Nutr 1982; 36: 846–850
7. Dallman PR, Beutler E, Finch CA. Effects of Iron deficiency exclusive of anaemia Br J Haematol 1978; 40: 179–184
8. Prasad MK, Pratt CA. The effects of exercise and two levels of dietary iron on iron status. Nutr Res 1990; 10: 1273–1283
9. Kent S, Weinberg E. Hypoferremia. Adaptation to disease? New Eng J Med 1989; 320: 672
10. Kies C, Bylund DM. Nutr Rep Intl 1989; 40: 43–51
11. Zittoun J, Blot I, Hill C et al. Iron supplements versus placebo in pregnancy. Its effects on iron and folate status on mothers and newborns. Ann Nutr Metabol 1983; 27: 320–327
12. Ballott DE, MacPhail AP, Bothwell TH et al. Fortification of curry powder with NaFe(111) EDTA in an iron-deficient population. initial survey of iron status. Am J Clin Nutr 1989; 49: 156–161
13. Scrimshaw NS. Functional consequences of iron deficiency in human populations. J Nutr Sci Vitaminol 1984; 30: 47–63
14. Oski FA, Honig AS, Helu B, Howanitz P. Effect of iron therapy on behavior performance in nonanemic, iron-deficient infants. Pediatrics 1983; 71: 877–880
15. Oski FA, Honig AS. The effects of therapy on the developmental scores of iron deficient infants. J Pediatr 1978; 92: 21–25
16. Anonymous. Vitamin A deficiency and anemia. Nutr Rev 1979; 37: 38–40
17. Anonymous. Vitamin A deficiency and iron nutriture. Nutr Rev 1984; 42: 167–168
18. Edgerton VR, Ohira Y et al. Toleration of hemoglobin and work tolerance in iron deficient subjects. J Nutr Sci Vitaminol 1981; 27: 77–86
19. Ohira Y, Edgerton VR, Gardner GW et al. Work capacity after iron treatment as a function of hemoglobin and iron deficiency. J Nutr Sci Vitaminol 1981; 27: 87–96
20. Webb TE, Oski FA. Iron deficiency anemia and scholastic achievement in young adolescents. J Pediatr 1973; 82: 827–830
21. Beutler E, Larsh SE, Gurney CW. Iron therapy in chronically-fatigued, nonanemic women; a double-blind study. Ann Intern Med 1960; 52: 378–394
22. Pollitt E, Leibel RL. Iron deficiency and behavior. J Pediatr 1976; 88: 372–381
23. Webb TE, Oski FA. Behavioral status of young adolescents with iron deficiency anemia. J Spec Educ 1974; 8: 153–156
24. Voorhees ML, Stuart MJ et al. Iron deficiency anemia and increased urinary norepinephrine. J Pediatr 1974; 86: 542–547
25. Tucker DM, Sandstead HH, Penland JG et al. Iron status and brain function: serum ferritin levels associated with asymmetries of cortical electrophysiology and cognitive performance. Am J Clin Nutr 1984; 39: 105–113
26. Pollitt E, Leibel RL, Greenfield DB. Iron deficiency and cognitive test performance in preschool children. Nutr Behavior 1983; 1: 137–146
27. Pollitt E, Soemantri AG, Yunis F, Scrimshaw NS. Cognitive effects of iron-deficiency anaemia. Lancet 1985; 1: 158
28. Kies C, ed. Nutritional bioavailability of iron. Washington, DC: American Chemical Society. 1982
29. Hallberg L, Brune M, Erlandsson M et al. Calcium. Effect of different amounts on nonheme- and heme-iron absorption in humans. Am J Clin Nutr 1991; 53: 112–119
30. Cook J, Dassenko S, Whittaker P. Calcium supplementation. Effect on iron absorption. Am J Clin Nutr 1991; 53: 106–111
31. Yip, R, Dallman, PR. Iron. In: Present knowledge in nutrition. 7th edn. Washington, DC: Nutrition Foundation. 1996: p 277–292
32. Allen, LH. Pregnancy and iron deficiency. Unresolved issues. Nutr Rev 1997; 55: 91–100
33. Lynch, SR. Interaction of iron with other nutrients. Nutr Rev 1997; 55: 102–110
34. Walter T, Olivares M, Pizarro F et al. Iron, anemia, and infection. Nutr Rev 1997; 55: 111–124
35. Chua ACG, Morgan EH. Effects of iron deficiency and iron overload on manganese uptake and deposition in the brain and other organs of the rat. Biol Trace Elem Res 1996; 55: 39–54
36. Dalton MA et al. Calcium and phosphorous supplementation of iron-fortified infant formula. No effect on iron status of healthy full-term infants. Am J Clin Nutr 1997; 65: 921–926
37. Fairweather Tait SJ, Minihane AM, Eagles J et al. Rare earth elements as nonabsorable fecal markers in studies of iron absorption. Am J Clin Nutr 1997; 65: 970–976
38. Beard, JL, Dawson H, Pinero, DJ. Iron metabolism. A comprehensive review. Nutr Rev 1996; 54: 295–317
39. Sempos, CT, Looker, AC, Gillum, RF. Iron and heart disease. The epidemiologic data. Nutr Rev 1996; 54: 73–88
40. McCord, JM. Effects of positive iron status at a cellular level. Nutr Rev 1996; 54: 85–88
41. Gleerup A, Rossander-Hulthen L, Gramatkovski E et al. Iron absorption from the whole diet: comparison of the effect of two different distributions of daily calcium intake. Am J Clin Nutr 1995; 61: 97–104
42. Sheard, NF. Iron deficiency and infant development. Nutr Rev 1994; 52: 137–140
43. Hunt, JR, Gallagher, SK, Johnson, LK. Effect of ascorbic acid on apparent iron absorption by women with low iron stores. Am J Clin Nutr 1994; 59: 1381–1385
44. Kies, C, Bylund, DM. Iron status of adolescent boys and girls as influenced by variations in dietary ascorbic acid and iron intakes. Nutr Rep Intl 1989; 40: 43–51

Magnesium

1. Seelig MS. The requirement of magnesium by the normal adult. Am J Clin Nutr 1964; 14: 342–390
2. Jones JE, Manalo R, Flink EB et al. Magnesium requirements in adults. Am J Clin Nutr 1967; 20: 632
3. Wacker WEC, Parisi AF. Magnesium metabolism. N Eng J Med 1968; 278: 658–663, 712–717, 772–786

4. Sjogren A, Edvinsson L, Fallgren B. Magnesium deficiency in coronary artery diseases and cardiac arrhythmias. J Int Med 1989; 226: 213–222
5. Tucker MM, Turco SJ. Human nutrition. Philadelphia: Lea & Febiger. 1983: p 25–28
6. Shils ME. Magnesium. In: Present knowledge in nutrition. 6th edn. Washington, DC: Nutrition Foundation. 1990: p 224–232
7. Seelig MS, Heggtveit H. Magnesium interrelationships in ischemic heart disease. Am J Clin Nutr 1974; 27: 59–79
8. Dunn MJ, Waber M. Magnesium depletion in normal man. Metabolism 1966; 15: 884–895
9. Shils ME. Experimental human magnesium depletion. I. Clinical observations and blood chemistry alterations. Am J Clin Nutr 1964; 15: 133–143
10. Hodgkinson A, Marshall DH, Nordin BEC. Vitamin D and magnesium absorption in man. Clin Sci 1979; 57: 121–123
11. Watson WS, Lyon TDB, Hilditch TE. Red cell magnesium as a function of cell age. Metabol Clin Exp 1980; 29: 397–399
12. Shine KI. Myocardial effects of magnesium. Am J Physiol 1979; 237: H413–H423
13. Abraham AS, Eylath U et al. Serum magnesium levels in patients with acute myocardial infarction. New Eng J Med 1977; 296: 862–863
14. DeLuca HF. The Vitamin D system in the regulation of calcium and phosphorus metabolism. Nutr Rev 1979; 37: 161–193
15. Shils ME. Experimental human magnesium depletion. Medicine 1969; 48: 61–85
16. Fletcher MP, Gershwin ME, Keen CL et al. Trace element deficiences and immune responsiveness in humans and animal models. In: Chandra RJ, ed. Nutrition and immunology. New York: Alan R. Liss. 1988: p 215–239
17. Gaby AR. Magnesium. New Canaan, CT: Keats Publications. 1994
18. Howard JMH. Magnesium deficiency in peripheral vascular disease. J Nutr Med 1990; 1: 39–49
19. Singh RB, Cameron EA. Relation of myocardial magnesium deficiency to sudden death in ischemic heart disease (letter). Am Heart J 1982; 103: 399–450
20. Laban E, Chardon GA. Magnesium and cardiac arrhythmias. nutrient or drug? J Am Coll Nutr 1986; 5: 521–532
21. Sheehan JP, Seelig MS. Interactions of magnesium and potassium in the pathogenesis of cardiovascular disease. Magnesium 1984; 3: 301–314
22. Brenton DP, Gordon TE. Fluid and electrolyte disorders. Magnesium. Br J Hospital Med 1984; 1: 60–69
23. Resnick LM, Gupta RK, Laragh JH. Intracellular free magnesium to erythrocytes of essential hypertension. Relation to blood pressure and serum divalent cations. Proc Nat Aca Sci 1984; 81: 6511–6515
24. Shils, ME. Magnesium. In: Present knowledge in nutrition. 7th edn. Washington, DC: Nutrition Foundation. 1996: p 256–264
25. Lemke, MR. Plasma magnesium decrease and altered calcium/magnesium ratior in severe dementia of the Alzheimer type. Biol Psychiatry 1995; 37: 341–343
26. Dahle LO, Berg G, Hammar M et al. The effect of oral magnesium substitution on pregnancy-induced leg cramps. Am J Obstet Gynecol 1995; 173: 175–180
27. Seelig MS. Magnesium in oncogenesis and in anti-cancer treatment interaction with minerals and vitamins. In: Quillian, P, Williams, RM, eds. Adjucant nutrition in cancer treatment. Publ Cancer Treatment Res Foundation, 1993; 15: 238–318
28. Dreosti, IE. Magnesium status and health. Nutr Rev 1995; 53: S23–S27

Manganese

1. Beisel WR. Single nutrients and immunity. Am J Clin Nutr 1982; 35: 456
2. Keen, CL, Zidenberg-Cherr, S. Present knowledge in nutrition. 6th edn. Washington, DC: Nutrition Foundation. 1990: p 279–286
3. Gruden N. Suppression of transduodenal manganese transport by milk diet supplemented with iron. Nutr Metabol 1977; 21: 305–309
4. Greger JL, Baligar P, Abernathy RP et al. Calcium, magnesium, phosphorus, copper, and manganese balance in adolescent females. Am J Clin Nutr 1978; 31: 117–121
5. Spencer H, Asmussen CR, Holtzman RB et al. Metabolic balances of cadmium, copper, manganese, and zinc in man. Am J Clin Nutr 1979; 32: 1867–1875
6. Guthrie BE, Robinson MF. Daily intakes of manganese, copper, zinc and cadmium by New Zealand women. Br J Nutr 1977; 38: 55–63
7. Wenlock RW, Buss DH, Dixon EJ. Manganese in British food. Br J Nutr 1979; 41: 253–261
8. Schlage C, Wortberg B. Manganese in the diet of healthy preschool and school children. Acta Paediatr Scand 1972; 61: 648–652
9. McLeod BE, Robinson MF. Metabolic balance of manganese in young women. Br J Nutr 1972; 27: 221–227
10. Engel RW, Price NO, Miller RF. Copper, manganese, cobalt, and molybdenum balance in pre-adolescent girls. J Nutr 1967; 92: 197–204
11. Bertinchamps AJ, Miller ST, Cotzias GC. Interdependence of routes excreting manganese. Am J Physiol 1966; 211: 217–224
12. Britton AA, Cotzias GC. Dependence of manganese turnover on intake. Am J Physiol 1966; 221: 203–206
13. Kies C, ed. Nutritional bioavailability of manganese. Washington, DC: American Chemical Society. 1982
14. Baly DL, Curry DL, Keen CL, Hurley LS. Effect of manganese deficiency on insulin secretion and homeostasis in rats. J Nutr 1984; 114: 1438–1446
15. Davidsson L, Almgren A, Juillerat MA et al. Manganese absorption in humans. The effect of phytic acid and ascorbic acid in soy formula. Am J Clin Nutr 1995; 62: 984–987
16. Keen, CL, Zidenberg-Cherr, S. Manganese. In: Present knowledge in nutrition. 7th edn. Washington, DC: Nutrition Foundation. 1996: p 334–343

Phosphorous

1. Knochel JP. The pathophysiology and clinical characteristics of severe hypophosphatemia. Arch Intern Med 1977; 137: 203–220
2. Walling MW. Intestinal inorganic phosphate transport. Adv Exp Med Biol 1977; 103: 131–147
3. Harrison HE, Harrison HC. Sodium, potassium and intestinal transport of glucose, l-tyrosine, phosphate and calcium. Am J Physiol 1963; 205: 107–111
4. Arnaud CD, Sanchez SD. The role of calcium in osteoporosis. Ann Rev Nutr 1990; 10: 397–414
5. Veis A, Subsay B. Bone and mineral research, vol. 5. New York: Elsevier. 1987: p 1–63
6. Marel GM, McKenna MJ, Frame B. Bone and mineral research, vol. 4. New York: Elsevier. 1986: p 335–412
7. Heaney RP. Bone and mineral research, vol. 4. New York: Elsevier. 1986: p 255–301
8. Portale AA, Halloran BP, Murphy MM, Morris RC Jr. Oral intake of phosphorus can determine the serum concentration of 1,25-dihydroxyvitamin D by determining its production rate in humans. J Clin Invest 1986; 77: 7–12
9. Portale AA, Booth BE, Halloran BP, Morris RC, Jr. Effect of dietary phosphorus on circulating concentrations of 1,25-dihydroxyvitamin D and immunoreactive parathyroid hormone in children with moderate renal insufficiency. J Clin Invest 1984; 73: 1580–1589
10. Lutwak L. Metabolic and biochemical considerations of bone. Ann Lab Clin Sci 1975; 5: 185–194
11. Bell RR, Draper HH, Tzeng DY et al. Physiological responses of human adults to foods containing phosphate activities. J Nutr 1977; 107: 42–50
12. Spencer H, Kramer L, Norris C et al. Effect of small doses of aluminum-containing antacids on calcium and phosphorus metabolism. Am J Clin Nutr 1982; 36: 32–40
13. Arnaud, CD, Sanchez, SD. Calcium and phosphorous. In: Present knowledge in nutrition. 7th edn. Washington, DC: Nutrition Foundation. 1996: p 245–255

Potassium

1. Sebastian A, McSherry E, Morris RC, Jr. Renal potassium wasting in renal tubular acidosis (RTA): its occurrence in types 1 and 2 RTA despite sustained correction of systemic acidosis. J Clin Invest 1971; 50: 667–678

2. Pennington JA, Wilson DB, Newell RF et al. Selected minerals in food surveys, 1974–1981/82. J Am Diet Assoc 1984; 84: 771–780
3. Massry SG, Friedler RM, Coburn JW. Excretion of phosphate and calcium. Arch Intern Med 1973; 131: 828
4. Tuckerman MM, Turco SJ. Human Nutrition. Philadelphia: Lea & Febiger. 1983: p 20–24
5. Ophir O, Peer G, Gilad J, Blum M, Aviramt. Low blood pressure in vegetarians. the possible role of potassium. Am J Clin Nutr 1983; 37: 755–762
6. Prior IA, Evans JG, Harvey HP et al. Sodium intake and blood pressure levels in two Polynesian populations. N Eng J Med 1968; 279: 515–520
7. Sacks FM, Rosner B, Kass EH. Blood Pressure in vegetarians. Am J Epidemiol 1974; 100: 390–398
8. Armstrong B, Van Merwyk AJ, Coates H. Blood pressure in Seventh-day Adventist vegetarians. Am J Epidemiol 1977; 105: 444–449
9. Armstrong B, Phil D, Clarke H. Urinary sodium and blood pressure in vegetarians. Am J Clin Nutr 1979; 32: 2472–2476
10. McCarron DA, Morris CD, Henry HJ, Stanton JL. Blood pressure and nutrient intake in the United States. Science 1984; 224: 1392–1398
11. Tannen RL. Effects of Potassium on blood pressure control. Ann Intern Med 1983; 98: 773
12. Kuriyama H, Ito Y, Suzuki H et al. Factors modifying contraction-relaxation cycle in vascular smooth muscles. Am J Physiol 1982 243: H641
13. Webb RC, Bohr DF. Mechanism of membrane stabilization by calcium in vascular smooth muscle. Am J Physiol 1978; 235: C227
14. Meneely GR, Batarbee HD. High sodium-low potassium environment and hypertension. Am J Cardiol 1976; 38: 768–785
15. Grim CE, Luft FC, Miller JZ et al. Racial differences in blood pressure in Evans county, Georgia. Relationship to sodium and potassium intake. J Chronic Dis 1980; 33: 87–94
16. Sullivan JM, Ratts TE, Taylor JC et al. Hemo dynamic effects of dietary sodium in man. A preliminary report. Hypertension 1980; 2: 506–514
17. Kassirer JP, Berkman PM et al. The critical role of chloride in the correction of hypokalemic alkalosis in man. Am J Med 1965; 38: 172–189
18. Kopyt N, Dalal F, Narins RG. Renal retention of potassium in fruit. New Eng J Med 1985; 313: 582–583
19. Anonymous. Potassium. the kitchen revisited (letter). Lancet 1983; 1: 362–363
20. Grimm RH Jr, Neaton JD, Elmer PJ et al. The influence of oral potassium chloride on blood pressure in hypertensive men on a low-sodium diet. N Eng J Med 1990; 322: 569–574
21. Luft, FC. Potassium and its regulation. In: Present knowledge in nutrition. 7th edn. Washington, DC: Nutrition Foundation. 1996: p 272–276

Selenium

1. Levander OA. Trace substances in environmental health – 23. Springfield: University of Missouri. 1990: p 11–19
2. Jackson ML. Selenium. Present status and perspectives in biology and medicine. Clifton, NJ: Humana Press. 1988: p 13–21
3. Levander OA. A global review of human selenium nutrition. Ann Rev Nutr 1987; 7: 227–250
4. Olson OE. Selenium toxicity in animals with emphasis on man. J Am Coll Toxicol 1986; 5: 45–70
5. Shamberger RJ, Frost DV. Possible protective effect of selenium against human cancer. Can Med Assoc J 1969; 100: 682
6. Overad K, Thorling EB, Bjerring P, Ebbesen P. Selenium inhibits UV-light-induced skin carcinogenesis in hairless mice. Cancer Lett 1985; 27: 163–170
7. Chen X, Xiaoshu, Chen X et al. Selenium in biology and medicine. New York: AVI/Van Nostrand Reinhold. 1987: p 589–607
8. Longnecker GF. Nutrition and cancer prevention: investigating the role of micronutrients. New York: Marcel Dekker. 1989: p 389–420
9. Winnefeld K, Dawczynski H, Schirrmeister W et al. Selenium in serum and whole blood in patients with surgical interventions. Biological Trace Element Res 1995; 50: 149–155
10. Sunde RA. Molecular biology of selenoproteins. Ann Rev Nutr 1990; 10: 451–474
11. Yang GQ, Wang SZ, Ahou RH, Sun SZ. Endemic selenium intoxication of humans in China. Am J Clin Nutr 1983; 37: 872–881
12. Shamberger RJ. Biochemistry of selenium. New York: Plenum. 1983
13. Glover JR. Proceedings of the symposium on selenium-tellurium environments. Pittsburgh: Industrial Health Foundation. 1976: p 279–292
14. Fletcher MP, Gershwin ME, Keen CL et al. Trace element deficiences and immune responsiveness in humans and animal models. In: Chandra RK, ed. Nutrition and immunology. New York: Alan R. Liss. 1988: p 215–239
15. Clark LC. The epidemiology of selenium and cancer. Fed Proc 1985; 44: 2584–2589
16. Salonen JT, Alfthan G, Huttunen JK, Puska P. Association between serum selenium and the risk of cancer. Am J Epidem 1984; 120: 342–349
17. Sword J, Pope A, Hoekstra W. Endotoxin and lipid peroxidation in vitro in selenium- and vitamin E-deficient and -adequate rat tissues. J Nutr 1991; 121: 258–264
18. Sword J, Pope A, Hoekstra W. Endotoxin and lipid peroxidation in vivo in selenium- and vitamin E-deficient and -adequate rats. J Nutr 1991; 121: 251–257
19. Levander, OA, Burk, RF. Selenium. In. Present knowledge in nutrition. 7th edn. Washington, DC: Nutrition Foundation. 1996: p 320–328
20. Winnefeld K, Dawczynski H, Schirrmeister W et al. Selenium in serum and whole blood in patients with surgical interventions. Biol Trace Elem Res 1995; 50: 149–155
21. Benton D, Cook R. The impact of selenium supplementation on mood. Biol Psychiatry 1991; 29: 1092–1098
22. Vanderpas JB, Contempre B, Duale NL et al. Iodine and selenium deficiency associated with cretinism in northern Zaire. Am J Clin Nutr 1990; 52: 1087–1094
23. L'Abbe M, Fischer W, Trick K et al. Dietary Se and tumor glutathione peroxidase and superoxide dismutase activities. J Nutr Biochem 1991; 2: 430–436
24. Clark L, Combs GF Jr, Turnbull BW et al. Effects of selenium supplementation for cancer prevention in patients with carcinoma of the skin. JAMA 1996;

Sodium

1. Dahl LK. Salt and hypertension. Am J Clin Nutr 1972; 25: 231–244
2. Meneely GR, Ball COT. High sodium-low potassium environment and hypertension. Am J Med 1958; 25: 713–725
3. Grollman A. The role of salt in health and disease. Am J Cardiol 1961; 8: 593–602
4. Dahl LK. Salt in processed baby foods. Am J Clin Nutr 1968; 21: 787–792
5. Meneely GR, Battarbee HD. Sodium. Am J Cardiol 1976; 38: 768–785
6. Battarbee HD, Meneely GR. CRC Crit Rev Toxicol 1977/78; 5: 355–576
7. Luft, FC. Sodium. Present knowledge in nutrition. 6th edn. Washington, DC: Nutrition Foundation. 1990: p 233–240
8. Gros G, Weller JM, Hoohler SW. Relationship of sodium and potassium intake to blood pressure. Am J Clin Nutr 1971; 24: 605–608
9. Marsh AC, Koons PC. The sodium and potassium content of selected vegetables. J Am Diet Assoc 1983; 83: 24–27
10. Sanchez-Castillo CP, Branch WJ, James WP. A test of the validity of the lithium-marker technique for monitoring dietary sources of salt in man. Clin Sci 1987; 72: 87–94
11. Sanchez-Castillo CP, Warrender S, Whitehead TP, James WP. An assessment of the sources of dietary salt in a British population. Clin Sci 1987; 72: 95–102
12. Luft, FC. Salt, water, and extracellular volume regulation. In: Present knowledge in nutrition. 7th edn. Washington, DC: Nutrition Foundation. 1996: p 265–271
13. Trials of Hypertension Prevention Collaborative Research Group. The effects of nonpharmacologic interventions on blood pressure of persons with high normal levels. Results of the trials of hypertension prevention, phase I. JAMA 1992; 267: 1213–1220

14. Cutler JA, Follmann D, Elliott P et al. An overview of randomized trials of sodium reduction and blood pressure. Hypertension 1991; 17: I-27–I-33

Zinc

1. Underwood EJ. Trace elements in human and animal nutrition. 4th edn. New York: Academic Press. 1977
2. Simmer K, Thompson RP. Maternal zinc and intrauterine growth retardation. Clin Sci 1985; 68: 395–399
3. Meadows NJ, Ruse W, Smith MF et al. Zinc and small babies. Lancet 1981; 2: 1135–1137
4. Masters DG, Keen CL, Lonnerdal B, Hurley LS. Zinc deficiency teratogenicity. The protective role of maternal tissue catabolism. J Nutr 1983; 113: 905–912
5. Wagner PA, Bailey LB, Christakis GJ, Dinning JS. Serum zinc concentrations in adolescents as related to sexual maturation. Human Nutr. Clin Nutr 1985; 39C: 459
6. Takihara H, Cosentino MJ, Cockett AT. Effect of low-dose androgen and zinc sulfate on sperm motility and seminal zinc levels in infertile men. Urology 1983; 22: 160
7. Soltan MH, Jenkins DM. Maternal and fetal plasma zinc concentration and fetal abnormality. Br J Obstet Gynaecol 1982; 89: 56
8. Sandstead HH. WO Atwater memorial lecture. Zinc. essentially for brain development and function. Nutr Rev 1985; 43: 129–137
9. Aamodt RL, Rumble WF, Johnston GS et al. Absorption of orally administrated ^{65}Zn by normal human subjects. Am J Clin Nutr 1981; 34: 2648–2652
10. Prasad ASP. Clinical biochemical and nutritional spectrum of zinc deficiency in human subjects: an update. Nutr Rev 1983; 41: 197–208
11. Taper LJ, Oliva JT, Ritchey SJ. Zinc and copper retention during pregnancy. The adequacy of prenatal diets with and without dietary supplementation. Am J Clin Nutr 1985; 41: 1184–1192
12. Schauss AG, Bryce-Smith D. Nutrients and brain function. Basil: Karger. 1987: p 151–162
13. Gibson RS, Anderson BM, Scythes CA. Regional differences in hair zinc concentrations. A possible effect of water hardness. Am J Clin Nutr 1983; 37: 37–42
14. Sandstead HH. Trace element interactions. J Lab Clin Med 1981; 98: 457–462
15. Haring BSA, Van Delft W. Changes in the mineral composition of food as a result of cooking in 'hard' and 'soft' waters. Arch Environ Health 1981; 36: 33–35
16. Moser-Veillon PB, Reynolds RD. A longitudinal study of pyridoxine and zinc supplementation of lactating women. Am J Clin Nutr 1990; 52: 135–141
17. Bales CW, Freeland-Graves JH, Askey S et al. Zinc, magnesium, copper, and protein concentrations in human saliva. Age- and sex-related differences. Am J Clin Nutr 1990; 51: 462–469
18. Fosmire GJ. Zinc toxicity. Am J Clin Nutr 1990; 51: 225–227
19. Shambaugh GE Jr. Zinc. The neglected nutrient. Am J Otol 1989; 10: 156–160
20. Shambaugh GE Jr. Zinc for tinnitus, imbalance, and hearing loss in the elderly. Am J Otol 1986; 7: 476–477
21. Shambaugh GE Jr. Zinc and presbycusis. Am J Otol 1985; 6: 116–117
22. Cunnigham-Rundles S, Cunningham-Rundles WF. Nutrition and immunology. New York: Alan R. Liss. 1988: p 197–214
23. Cousins RJ, Hempe JM. Zinc. In: Present knowledge in nutrition. 6th edn. Washington, DC: Nutrition Foundation. 1990: p 251–260
24. Shambaugh GE. Zinc, an essential nutrient for hearing and balance. Int J Biosocial Med Res 1991; 13: 192–199
25. Cousins RJ. Zinc. In: Present knowledge in nutrition. 7th edn. Washington, DC: Nutrition Foundation. 1996: p 293–306
26. Thomas EA, Bailey LB, Kauwell GA et al. Erythrocyte metallothionein response to dietary zinc in humans. J Nutr 1992; 122: 2408–2414
27. King JC, Hambidge KM, Westcott JL et al. Daily variation in plasma zinc concentrations in women fed meals at six-hour intervals. J Nutr 1994; 124: 508–516
28. Taylor CM, Bacon JR, Aggett PJ et al. Homeostatic regulation of zinc absorption and endogenous losses in zinc-deprived men. Am J Clin Nutr 1991; 53: 755–763
29. Nishi Y. Anemia and zinc deficiency in the athlete. J Am Col Nutr 1996; 15: 323–324
30. Nishi Y. Zinc and growth. J Am Col Nutr 1996; 15: 340–344
31. Reunanen A, Knekt P, Marniemi J et al. Serum calcium, magnesium, copper and zinc and risk of cardiovascular death. Eur J Clin Nutr 50: 431–437
32. Hambidge KM. Zinc deficiency in young children. Am J Clin Nutr 1997; 65: 160–161
33. Mossad SB, Macknin ML, Medendorp SV et al. Zinc gluconate lozenges for treating the common cold. A randomized, placebo-controlled study. Ann Intern Med 1996; 125: 81–88
34. King JC. Does poor zinc nutriture retard skeletal growth and mineralization in adolescents? Am J Clin Nutr 1996; 64: 375–376
35. Mahajan S, Prasad A, Brewer G et al. Effect of changes in dietary zinc intake on taste acuity and dark adaptation in normal human subjects. J Trace Elem Exp Med 1992; 5: 33–45
36. Kondo T, Toda Y, Matsui H. Effects of exercise and sleep deprivation on serum zinc. J Trace Elem Exp Med 1990; 3: 324–354
37. Zlotkin SH, Casselman CW. Urinary zinc excretion in normal subjects. J Trace Elem Exp Med, 1990; 3: 13–21
38. Berg JM, Shi Y. The galvanization of biology. A growing appreciation for the roles of zinc. Science 1996; 271: 1081–1085
39. Tuormaa TE. Adverse effects of zinc deficiency. A review from the literature. J Orthomol Med 1995; 10: 149–164
40. Krebs NF, Reidinger CJ, Hartley S et al. Zinc supplementation during lactation. Effects on maternal status and milk zinc concentrations. Am J Clin Nutr 1995; 61: 1030–1036
41. Sturniolo GC, Montino MC, Rossetto L et al. Inhibition of gastric acid secretion reduces zinc absorption in man. J Am Col Nutr 1991; 4: 372–375
42. Koyama H, Hosokai H, Tamura S et al. Positive association between serum zinc and apolipoprotein A-II concentrations in middle-aged males who regularly consume alcohol. Am J Clin Nutr 1993; 57: 657–661

CHAPTER CONTENTS

109

Sarsaparilla species

Michael T. Murray, ND

Joseph E. Pizzorno Jr, ND

Smilax aristolochiifolia (family: Liliaceae)
Synonym: *Smilax medica*
Common name: Mexican sarsaparilla

Smilax officinalis (family: Liliaceae)
Synonym: *Smilax regelii*
Common name: Honduras sarsaparilla

GENERAL DESCRIPTION

Sarsaparilla is a tropical American perennial plant. Its long slender root and short thick rhizomes produce a vine which trails on the ground and climbs by means of tendrils growing in pairs from the petioles of the alternate, obicular to ovate, evergreen leaves. The root is the part of the plant utilized for medicinal purposes.

CHEMICAL COMPOSITION

Sarsaparilla contains 1.8–2.4% steroid saponins, including:

- sarsaponin
- smilasaponin
- sarsaparilloside and its aglycones sarsapogenin (see Fig. 109.1), smilagenin, pollinastanol.

Other constituents include starch, resins, and a trace of volatile oil.[1]

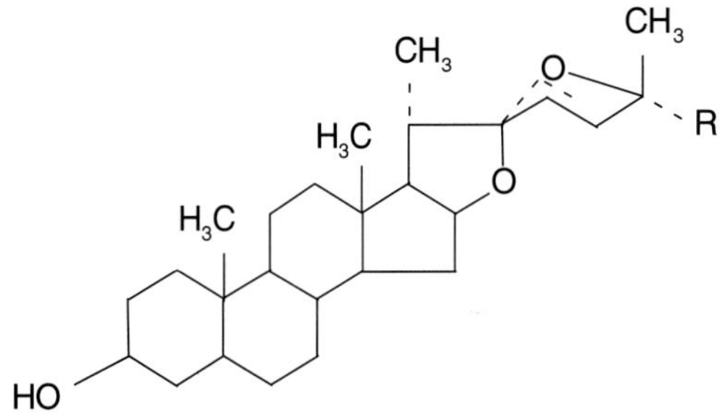

Figure 109.1 Sarsasapogenin.

HISTORY AND FOLK USE

Sarsaparilla's medicinal use has been as a tonic and blood purifier. Tonics are defined as agents:[2]

> ... which permanently exalt the energies of the body at large, without vitally affecting any one organ in particular. ... In short, tonics tone the whole system.

A blood purifier or depurative refers to an agent which cleanses and purifies the system.[2] Sarsaparilla's reputation in this regard probably stems from its importation from the Caribbean and South America to Europe in the 16th century for the treatment of syphilis.[3]

Historical use in the treatment of syphilis

A French physician, Nicholas Monardes, published a comprehensive account of sarsaparilla and several other "new" drugs in the treatment of syphilis in 1574. Many Europeans at the time believed that syphilis had come to Europe from the West Indies with Columbus' sailors, and since there was a general belief that whatever disease was native to a country might be cured by the medicinal herbs growing in that region, it was only natural for sarsaparilla to become a popular remedy. Furthermore, the standard treatment for syphilis, mercury, often resulted in greater morbidity and mortality than the disease itself.

Sarsaparilla was a welcome alternative, but despite initial excitement, Monardes' sarsaparilla cure sank in favor. This was probably due to other aspects of the cure, which included confinement to a warm room for 30 days, followed by 40 days of abstinence from both wine and sexual intercourse.[3]

However, sarsaparilla continued to be used in the treatment of syphilis. During military operations in Portugal in 1812, a British Inspector General of Hospitals noted that the Portuguese soldiers suffering from syphilis who used sarsaparilla recovered much faster and more completely than their British counterparts who were treated with mercury.[3]

Sarsaparilla was also used by the Chinese in the treatment of syphilis. Clinical observations in China demonstrated that sarsaparilla is effective, according to blood tests, in about 90% of acute cases and 50% of chronic cases.[1,4]

Although sarsaparilla was clearly more beneficial in the treatment of syphilis, it was mercury that established itself as the standard treatment for over four and a half centuries. It has been stated that "the use of mercury in the treatment of syphilis may have been the most colossal hoax ever perpetrated" in the history of medicine. Mercury represented a new kind of medicine, one formulated and prepared in a laboratory using the new techniques of chemistry. It helped to prepare the way for the future use of drugs rather than herbal medicines.[3]

An interesting note is that sarsaparilla species have been used all over the world in many different cultures for the same conditions, namely gout, arthritis, fevers, digestive disorders, skin disease, and cancer.[1]

PHARMACOLOGY

The mechanism of action of sarsaparilla is largely unknown, although the plant does contain several saponins and has been shown to be clinically effective in the treatment of psoriasis.[1,5,6] This evidence points to a possible effect on binding of cholesterol and bacterial toxins in the intestines.

Endotoxin binding

Evidence seems to support sarsaparilla as an endotoxin binder. Endotoxins are cell wall constituents of bacteria that are absorbed from the gut. Normally, the liver plays a vital role by filtering these, and other, gut-derived compounds before they reach the general circulation. If the amount of endotoxin absorbed is excessive or if the liver is not functioning adequately, the liver can become overwhelmed, and endotoxins will spill into the blood.

If endotoxins are allowed to circulate, activation of the alternate complement system occurs. This system plays a critical role in aggravating inflammatory processes, and activation of complement is responsible for much of the inflammation and cell damage that occurs in many diseases, including gout, arthritis, and psoriasis. Historically, these conditions have been treated with sarsaparilla.

In further support of sarsaparilla's effect as a binder of endotoxin is its historical use in the treatment of fever, as absorbed endotoxins produce fever. Sarsaparilla also exhibits some antibiotic activity, but this is probably secondary to its endotoxin-binding action.[1]

CLINICAL APPLICATION

Sarsaparilla's medicinal action appears to be a result of its binding of bacterial endotoxins in the gut, which makes them unabsorbable. This greatly reduces the stress on the liver and other organs and is probably responsible for sarsaparilla's historical use as a tonic and blood purifier. This ability to bind endotoxins is also the probable reason why sarsaparilla is effective in many cases of psoriasis, gout, and arthritis.

Psoriasis

Individuals with psoriasis have been shown to have high levels of circulating endotoxins. Binding of endotoxin in the gut is associated with clinical improvement in these individuals. In a controlled study of 92 patients, an endotoxin-binding saponin (sarsaponin) from sarsaparilla greatly improved the psoriasis in 62% of the patients and resulted in complete clearance in 18%.[6]

DOSAGE

- Dried root: 1–4 g or by decoction three times/day
- Liquid extract (1:1): 8–15 ml three times/day
- Solid extract (4:1): 250 mg three times/day.

TOXICOLOGY

Although no adverse effects have been reported, it is possible that problems could arise if large doses are used over a long period of time.

REFERENCES

1. Leung AY. Encyclopedia of common natural ingredients used in food, drugs and cosmetics. New York, NY: John Wiley. 1980
2. Felter HW. The eclectic materia medica, pharmacology and therapeutics. Portland, OR: Eclectic Medical Publications. 1983
3. Griggs B. Green pharmacy, a history of herbal medicine. London: Jill Norman & Hobhouse. 1981
4. Bensky D, Gamble A. Chinese herbal medicine materia medica. Seattle, WA: Eastland Press. 1986
5. Duke JA. Handbook of medicinal herbs. Boca Raton, FL: CRC Press. 1985
6. Thurman FM. The treatment of psoriasis with sarsaparilla compound. New Engl J Med 1942; 227: 128–133

CHAPTER CONTENTS

110

Serenoa repens (saw palmetto)

Michael T. Murray, ND

Joseph E. Pizzorno Jr, ND

Serenoa repens (family: Arecaceae)
Common names: saw palmetto, palmetto scrub, sabal serrulata

GENERAL DESCRIPTION

Serenoa repens is a small palm tree native to the West Indies and the Atlantic coast of North America from South Carolina to Florida. The plant grows from 6–10 feet high, with a crown of large, 2–4 feet high spiny-toothed leaves which form a circular, fan-shaped outline. The berries of the plant are the components used for medicinal purposes. The deep red-brown to black berries are wrinkled, oblong, and 0.5–1 inch long with a diameter of 0.5 inch.[1]

CHEMICAL COMPOSITION

The saw palmetto berries contain about 1.5% of a fruity-smelling oil containing saturated and unsaturated fatty acids and sterols.[1] About 63% of this oil is composed of free fatty acids including capric, caprylic, caproic, lauric, palmitic, and oleic acids. The remaining portion is composed of ethyl esters of these fatty acids and sterols, including beta-sitosterol and its glucoside. The lipid-soluble compounds are thought to be the major pharmacological components. Other components of the berries include carotenes, lipase, tannins, and sugars.

The purified fat-soluble extract is used medicinally and contains between 85 and 95% of fatty acids and sterols. It is made up predominantly of a complex mixture of saturated and unsaturated free fatty acids, their methyl- and ethyl-esters (approximately 7%), long chain alcohols in free and esterified form, and various free and esterified sterol derivatives.

The free fatty acids in this extract are identified by gas chromatography and mass spectrometry as:

- caproic acid (C6)
- capric acid (C8)

- caprylic acid (C10)
- lauric acid (C12)
- myristic acid (C14)
- isomyristic acid (C14)
- palmitic acid (C16)
- oleic acid (C18:1)
- stearic acid (C18).

Lauric and myristic acid are the major fatty acids, accounting for approximately 30% of the fatty acid content.

The identified alcohols include those with *n*-C22, *n*-C23, *n*-C24, *n*-C26, *n*-C28, and *n*-C30 chains, phytol, farnesol, and geranylgeraniol, in addition to high molecular weight unsaturated polyphenols.

The sterolic fraction is composed of beta-sitosterol, stigmasterol, cycloartenol, lupeol, lupenone, and 24-methylcycloartenol. Many of these sterols are esterified with the fatty acids of the extract.

HISTORY AND FOLK USE

The American Indians, and later Eclectic and Naturopathic physicians, used saw palmetto berries in the treatment of genitourinary tract disturbances and as a tonic to support the body nutritionally.[2,3] It was used in men to increase the function of the testicles and relieve irritation in mucous membranes, particularly those of the genitourinary tract and prostate. It has been used in women with disorders of the mammary glands; long-term use was reputed to cause the breasts to enlarge slowly.[2] Many herbalists have considered it to be an aphrodisiac.[1]

PHARMACOLOGY

A standardized liposterolic (fat-soluble) saw palmetto berry extract has demonstrated numerous pharmacological effects relating to its primary clinical application in the treatment of the common disorder of the prostate gland, benign prostatic hyperplasia (BPH). BPH is thought to be caused by an accumulation of testosterone in the prostate. Once within the prostate, testosterone is converted to the more potent hormone dihydrotestosterone (DHT). This compound stimulates the cells to multiply excessively, eventually causing the prostate to enlarge.

The primary therapeutic action of saw palmetto extract in the treatment of BPH has been thought to be a result of inhibition in the intraprostatic conversion of testosterone to dihydrotestosterone (DHT and inhibition of its intracellular binding and transport.[4,5] However, more recent research has suggested additional mechanisms of action, including anti-estrogenic and receptor site-binding effects.[6]

Estrogen contributes to BPH because it inhibits the hydroxylation and subsequent elimination of DHT. Serenoa appears to inhibit the activity of estrogen in the prostate. For example, in a double-blind study of 35 men with BPH, 18 were given the saw palmetto extract at 160 mg twice daily and 17 were given placebo.[4] At the end of the 90 day study, androgen, estrogen, and progesterone receptors from prostate tissue samples were evaluated by two different techniques. The men receiving the saw palmetto extract had significantly lower cytosol and receptor values for estrogen and progesterone compared with the placebo group. Since the progesterone receptor content is linked to estrogenic activity, the results of the evaluation imply that at least part of the efficacy of the saw palmetto extract is through its anti-estrogenic effect.

The results from the androgen receptor analysis were quite interesting: there was no change in the number of cytosol androgen receptors, but the number of nuclear androgen receptors was significantly lower in the saw palmetto group (60% of the placebo group were positive for the nuclear receptor compared with 10% in the saw palmetto group). These results indicate that the saw palmetto extract probably competitively blocks the translocation of the cytosol androgen receptor to the nucleus.

The overall results of the study indicate that the standardized extract of saw palmetto exerts both anti-androgenic and anti-estrogenic activities. Preliminary analysis of the extract indicate that separate fractions are responsible for these effects. Researchers in this study concluded:

> It cannot be excluded, however, that the primary effect is antiestrogenic and that the inactivation of androgen receptors and progesterone receptors and of the 5-alpha-reductase activity is secondary to the estrogen receptor blockade.

The standardized extract has also demonstrated anti-edematous effects and the polysaccharide components have demonstrated immunostimulatory effects.[7,8]

CLINICAL APPLICATION

Currently, the primary clinical application of saw palmetto berries (specifically the fat-soluble extract) is in the treatment of benign prostatic hyperplasia (BPH). Based on its pharmacology, this extract may also be of benefit in conditions of androgen excess in women, such as hirsutism and polycystic ovarian disease.

Benign prostatic hyperplasia

In the United States, between 50 to 60% of men between the ages of 40 and 59 years have BPH. This disorder is characterized by increased urinary frequency, night-time awakening to empty the bladder, and reduced force and caliber of urination (see Ch. 138). These major symptoms have been shown to be significantly improved in over

Table 110.1 Clinical studies demonstrating the efficacy of *Serenoa repens* extract (85–95% fatty acids and sterols at a dosage of 320 mg/day)

Authors	Type of study	No. of patients	Length of study	Results
Boccafoschi & Annoscia[9]	Double-blind, placebo	22	60 days	Significant difference for volume voided, maximum flow, mean flow, dysuria, nocturia
Cirillo-Marucco et al[10]	Open	47	4 months	Significant difference for dysuria, nocturia, urine flow
Tripodi et al[11]	Open	40	30–90 days	Significant difference for dysuria, nocturia, volume of prostate, voiding rate, residual urine
Emili et al[12]	Double-blind, placebo	30	30 days	Significant difference for number of voided, strangury, maximum and mean urine flow, residual urine
Greca & Volpi[13]	Open	14	1–2 months	Significant difference for dysuria, perineal heaviness, nocturia, volume of urine per voiding, interval between two diurnal voidings, sensation of incomplete voiding
Duvia et al[14]	Controlled trial vs. *Pygeum africanum*	30	30 days	Significant difference for voiding rate
Tasca et al[15]	Double-blind, placebo	30	31–90 days	Significant difference for frequency, urine flow measurement
Cukier et al[16]	Double-blind, placebo	168	60–90 days	Significant difference for dysuria, frequency, residual urine
Champault et al[17]	Double-blind, placebo	168	60–90 days	Significant difference for objective and subjective parameters
Crimi & Russo[18]	Open	32	4 weeks	Significant difference for dysuria, nocturia, volume of prostate, voiding rate
Champault et al[19]	Double-blind, placebo	110	28 days	Significant difference for: dysuria, nocturia, flow measurement, residual urine
Mattei et al[20]	Double-blind	40	3 months	Significant difference for dysuria, nocturia, residual urine
Braeckman[21]	Open	305	3 months	Significant difference for maximum urine flow, prostate volume, and international prostate score

a dozen double-blind, placebo-controlled clinical trials (summarized in Table 110.1).[9–20]

In one of the larger studies involving 110 patients with BPH, impressive clinical results were reported: nocturia decreased by over 45%, flow rate (ml/s) increased by over 50%, and post-micturition residue (ml) decreased by 42% in the group receiving the serenoa extract.[18] In contrast, those on placebo showed no significant improvement in nocturia or flow rate, and post-micturition residue actually worsened.

Significant improvements were also noted in self-rating by the patients and global rating by the physicians. Of the 50 treated subjects completing the 30 day study, physicians rated 14 greatly improved, 31 improved, and only five unchanged or worsened. In contrast, no subjects in the placebo group had greatly improved, 16 showed some improvement, and 28 remained unchanged or worsened.

Although the saw palmetto extract has shown excellent results in numerous double-blind, placebo-controlled clinical trials, results from a recent open, multicenter study are perhaps the most revealing.[21] The results corroborate those from numerous double-blind, controlled studies showing that the liposterolic extract of saw palmetto (*Serenoa repens*) standardized to contain 85–95% fatty acids and sterols is an effective treatment for benign prostatic hyperplasia (BPH). While drugs like finesteride (Proscar) typically take up to a year to produce significant benefit, the saw palmetto extract produces better results in a much shorter period of time. Most patients achieve some relief of symptoms within the first 30 days of treatment with the saw palmetto extract. In this study, 305 men were given a dosage of 160 mg twice daily. The subjective evaluations of treatment made by patients after 45 and 90 days of treatment were quite favorable. After 45 days, 83% of patients estimated that the drug was effective. After 90 days, the percentage increased to 88%. Similarly, global evaluations made by physicians after 45 and 90 days demonstrated 81 and 88% effectiveness, respectively. The objective evaluations demonstrated remarkable improvements in all measurements. Maximum urinary flow increased from 9.8 to 12.2 ml/s, mean urinary flow rate increased from 5.8 to 7.4 ml/s, prostatic volume decreased from 40,348 to 36,246 mm^3; and the international prostate symptom score decreased from 19.0 to 12.4. No serious adverse reactions were reported.

While these results are impressive, perhaps the most impressive changes occurred in the quality of life scores as shown in Table 110.2. These improvements in quality of life scores demonstrate just how powerful an effect improving bothersome symptoms such as nocturia can have on an individual's mental outlook. Another important finding was that the saw palmetto extract had no demonstrable effect on serum prostatic specific antigen levels.

A recently reported study has now evaluated the long-term efficacy of saw palmetto. This 3 year, multicenter,

Table 110.2 Quality of life scores

Evaluation	Day 0	Day 90
Delighted	0.6%	5.4%
Happy	2.3%	24.0%
Satisfied	9.7%	36.8%
Mitigated	22.7%	20.9%
Unsatisfied	43.8%	9.5%
Unhappy	18.5%	2.4%
Hopeless	2.3%	1.0%

open-label study evaluated 160 mg of a standardized extract (Strogen®) in 435 men (aged 41–89 years) with stage I or II BPH. By the end of the study, 120 patients had withdrawn – 12 due to lack of efficacy, 41 due to the need for surgery, 41 lost to follow-up and eight due to adverse reactions. In the remaining 315, the following were reported:

- nocturia normalized or improved in 73%
- daytime frequency improved in 54%
- feeling of incomplete emptying improved in 75%
- rectal examination revealed improvement in prostate congestion in 55%
- average residual volume decreased from 64 to 38 ml
- peak urine flow increased by an average of 6.1 ml/s.

A total of 14.7% of the men experienced a continued deterioration of their prostate function. The primary adverse events were mild gastrointestinal disturbance.

DOSAGE

The dosage for the liposterolic extract of saw palmetto berries (containing 85–95% fatty acids and sterols) is 160 mg twice daily. A similar dose using fluid extracts and tinctures would require extremely large quantities of alcohol and therefore cannot be recommended. Dosages are as follows:

- crude berries: 10 g twice daily
- liposterolic extract (standardized at 85–95% fatty acids and sterols): 160 mg twice daily.

TOXICOLOGY

No significant side-effects have been reported in the clinical trials of the saw palmetto berry extract or with saw palmetto berry ingestion.

REFERENCES

1. Duke JA. Handbook of medicinal herbs. Boca Raton, FL: CRC Press. 1985: p 118
2. Felter HW, Lloyd JU. King's American dispensatory (1898). Portland OR: Eclectic Med Publ (reprint). 1983: p II: 1750–1752
3. Kuts-Cheraux AW. Naturae medicina and naturopathic dispensatory. Yellow Springs, OH: Antioch Press. 1953: p 249
4. Carilla E, Briley M, Fauran F et al. Binding of Permixon, a new treatment for prostatic benign hyperplasia, to the cytosolic androgen receptor in the rat prostate. J Steroid Biochem 1984; 20: 521–523
5. Sultan C, Terraza A, Devillier C et al. Inhibition of androgen metabolism and binding by a liposterolic extract of *Serenoa repens* B in human foreskin fibroblasts. J Steroid Biochem 1984; 20: 515–519
6. Di Silverio F, D'Eramo G, Lubrano C. Evidence that *Serenoa repens* extract displays antiestrogenic activity in prostatic tissue of benign prostatic hypertrophy. Eur Urol 1992; 21: 309–314
7. Tarayre JP, Delhon A, Lauressergues H et al. Anti-edematous action of a hexane extract of the stone fruit of *Serenoa repens* Bartr. Ann Pharm Franc 1983; 41: 559–570
8. Wagner H, Proksch A. Immunostimulatory drugs of fungi and higher plants. Econ Med Plant Res 1985; 1: 113–153
9. Boccafoschi, Annoscia S. Comparison of *Serenoa repens* extract with placebo by controlled clinical trial in patients with prostatic adenomatosis. Urologia 1983; 50: 1257–1268
10. Cirillo-Marucco E, Pagliarulo A, Tritto G et al. Extract of *Serenoa repens* (Permixon^R) in the early treatment of prostatic hypertrophy. Urologia 1983; 5: 1269–1277
11. Tripodi V, Giancaspro M, Pascarella M et al. Treatment of prostatic hypertrophy with *Serenoa repens* extract. Med Praxis 1983; 4: 41–46
12. Emili E, Lo Cigno M, Petrone U. Clinical trial of a new drug for treating hypertrophy of the prostate (Permixon). Urologia 1983; 50: 1042–1048
13. Greca P, Volpi R. Experience with a new drug in the medical treatment of prostatic adenoma. Urologia 1985; 52: 532–535
14. Duvia R, Radice GP, Galdini R. Advances in the phytotherapy of prostatic hypertrophy. Med Praxis 1983; 4: 143–148
15. Tasca A, Barulli M, Cavazzana A et al. Treatment of obstructive symptomatology caused by prostatic adenoma with an extract of *Serenoa repens*. Double-blind clinical study vs. placebo. Minerva Urol Nefrol 1985; 37: 87–91
16. Cukier (Paris), Ducassou (Marseille), Le Guillou (Bordeaux) et al. Permixon versus placebo. C R Ther Pharmacol Clin 1985; 4/25: 15–21
17. Champlault G, Patel JC, Bonnard AM. A double-blind trial of an extract of the plant *Serenoa repens* in benign prostatic hyperplasia. Br J Clin Pharmacol 1984; 18: 461–462
18. Crimi A, Russo A. Extract of *Serenoa repens* for the treatment of the functional disturbances of prostate hypertrophy. Med Praxis 1983; 4: 47–51
19. Champault G, Bonnard AM, Cauquil J, Patel JC. Medical treatment of prostatic adenoma. Controlled trial. PA 109 vs placebo in 110 patients. Ann Urol 1984; 18: 407–410
20. Mattei FM, Capone M, Acconcia A. *Serenoa repens* extract in the medical treatment of benign prostatic hypertrophy. Urologia 1988; 55: 547–552
21. Braeckman J. The extract of *Serenoa repens* in the treatment of benign prostatic hyperplasia. A multicenter open study. Curr Ther Res 1994; 55: 776–785
22. Bach D, Ebeling L. Long-term drug treatment of benign prostatic hyperplasia – results of a prospective 3-year multicenter study using Sabal extract IDS89. Phytomed 1996; 3: 105–111

CHAPTER CONTENTS

111

Silybum marianum (milk thistle)

Michael T. Murray, ND

Joseph E. Pizzorno Jr, ND

Silybum marianum (family: Compositae)
Synonym: *Carduus marianum*
Common names: milk thistle, marian thistle, St Mary's thistle

GENERAL DESCRIPTION

Silybum marianum is a stout, annual or biennial plant, found in dry rocky soils in southern and western Europe and some parts of the United States. The branched stem grows 1–3 feet high and bears alternate, dark green, shiny leaves with spiny, scalloped edges that are markedly streaked with white along the veins. The solitary flower heads are reddish-purple with bracts ending in sharp spines. Flowering season is from June to August. The seeds, fruit, and leaves are used for medicinal purposes.

CHEMICAL COMPOSITION

Silybum marianum contains silymarin, a mixture of flavanolignans, consisting chiefly of silibin, silydianin, and silychristine.[1–3] The concentration of silymarin is highest in the fruit, but it is also found in the seeds and leaves. Other flavanolignans are contained in silybum, including silandrin, silyhermin, silymonin, and neosilyhermin.[1] Silibin is the silymarin component which yields the greatest degree of biological activity (see Fig. 111.1).

HISTORY AND FOLK USE

Perhaps the most widespread folk use of this plant has

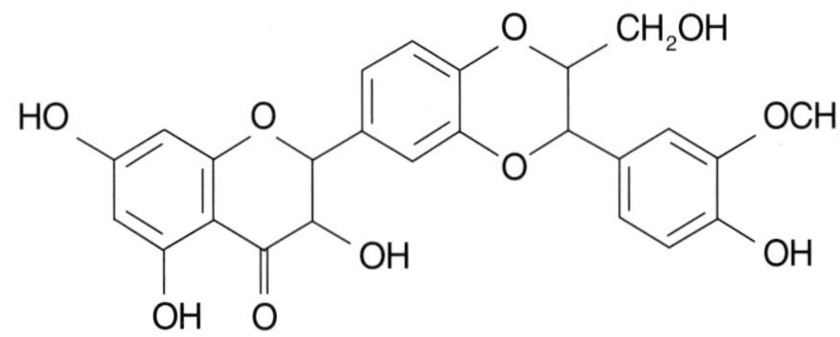

Figure 111.1 Silibin.

been in assisting the nursing mother in the production of milk. It was also used in Germany for curing jaundice and biliary derangements. It is interesting to note that the discovery of the liver-protecting flavanolignans in *Silybum marianum* was not the result of systemic pharmacological screening, but rather of investigation of silybum's empirical effects in liver disorders.[1]

PHARMACOLOGY

Silybum marianum extracts (usually standardized to contain 70% silymarin) are currently widely used in European pharmaceutical preparations for hepatic disorders. Silymarin is one of the most potent liver-protecting substances known.[1–7,9]

Hepatoprotection effects

Free radical scaveging

Silybum's ability to prevent liver destruction and enhance liver function is due largely to silymarin's inhibition of the factors that are responsible for hepatic damage, i.e. free radicals and leukotrienes, coupled with its ability to stimulate liver protein synthesis.

Silybum components prevent free radical damage by acting as antioxidants.[1–4] Silymarin is many times more potent in antioxidant activity than vitamin E.

Effects on hepatic glutathione

Silymarin prevents the depletion of glutathione (GSH) induced by alcohol and other liver toxins. Even in normals, it increases the basal GSH level of the liver by 35% over controls.

Protection from liver-damaging chemicals and drugs

The protective effect of silybum against liver damage has been demonstrated in a number of experimental and clinical studies. Experimental liver damage in animals can be produced by such diverse toxic chemicals as carbon tetrachloride, galactosamine, ethanol, and praseodymium nitrate. Silymarin has been shown to protect the liver from all of these toxins.[1–4,7]

Perhaps the most impressive of silymarin's protective effects is against the severe poisoning of *Amanita phalloides* (the deathcap or toadstool mushroom), an effect which has long been recognized in folk medicine.[5–7] Ingestion of *Amanita phalloides* or its toxins causes severe poisoning and, in approximately 30% of victims, death.

Among the experimental models for measuring protection against liver damage, those based on amanitin or phalloidin toxicity are the most important, because these two peptides from *Amanita phalloides* are the most powerful liver-damaging substances known. Silymarin has demonstrated impressive results in these experimental models. When silymarin was administered before amanita toxin poisoning, it was 100% effective in preventing toxicity.[5,7] Even if given 10 minutes after the amanita toxin, it completely counteracted the toxic effects.

Two cases reported in the literature found that silymarin still prevents death and greatly reduces the amount of liver damage as long as 24 hours after ingestion.[6] This study reported on a husband and wife who ate toxic mushrooms and developed gastrointestinal symptoms 18 hours later. Despite initial conventional treatment with gastric emptying, intravenous fluids, activated charcoal and a duodenal tube, both patient's laboratory work showed deteriorating liver and renal function. One patient developed mild hepatic encephalopathy. Treatment with intravenous silibinin at a dose of 20 mg/kg of body weight, penicillin and glucose for 3 days resulted in reversal of both the organ failures and encephalopathy.

Silymarin may also be of great value as an adjunct for patients receiving long-term drug therapy. A very interesting study found that providing psychiatric patients receiving phenothiazines or butyrophenones with the unusually high dose of 800 mg/day of silymarin resulted in significant protection of the liver as measured by malondialdehyde serum liver enzyme levels.[10] The silymarin did not interfere with the efficacy of the antidepressants.

Stimulation of hepatic protein synthesis

Perhaps the most interesting effect of silybum components on the liver is their ability to stimulate protein synthesis.[4,11,12] This results in an increase in the production of new liver cells to replace the damaged old ones. It has been suggested that:[12]

> silibinin imitates in some way a physiological regulator in animal cells, so that the structure fits into a specific binding site on the polymerase and in such a way causes the observed effects on rRNA synthesis making the drug from *Silybum marianum* indeed interesting for liver therapy.

Interestingly enough, silybinin does not have a stimulatory effect on malignant hepatic tissue.[11]

Anti-inflammatory effects

Leukotrienes, key chemical mediators of inflammation, produced by the transfer of oxygen to polyunsaturated fatty acids (a reaction catalyzed by the enzyme lipoxygenase) can also damage the liver. Silymarin has been shown to be a potent inhibitor of this enzyme, thereby inhibiting the formation of damaging leukotrienes.[13]

Silymarin has also been shown to inhibit prostaglandin synthesis during inflammation.[14] Free radical damage to membrane structures due to organic disease or intoxication results in increased release, by lipolysis, of fatty acids. This leads, among other things, to increased prostaglandin and leukotriene synthesis. Silymarin counteracts this deleterious process by suppressing the pathological decomposition of membrane lipids and inhibiting prostaglandin formation.[14] As leukotrienes and inflammatory prostaglandins are also involved in the damage of the liver by toxins, their neutralization by silybin is another mechanism for its protection of the liver.

Other pharmacological actions

Silymarin has demonstrated several other physiologic effects. It is a strong inhibitor of cyclic AMP phosphodiesterase: 13–50 times more active than theophylline and one to three times more active than papaverine.[15] Silymarin has also been shown to prevent the toxic effects of a variety of compounds, e.g. hemolysis induced by phenylhydrazine, X-radiation-induced damage, and brain edema induced by triethyltinsulfate (TZS).[16–18] Presumably, these effects are related to silymarin's significant membrane-stabilizing and antioxidant actions. Its action in increasing the osmotic resistance of RBCs is also quite significant.[19]

CLINICAL APPLICATIONS

Silymarin's primary use is as an aid to the liver, although additional clinical applications are regularly being discovered. It can be used to support detoxification reactions or in the treatment of more severe liver disease. In numerous clinical studies, silymarin has been shown to have positive effects in treating several types of liver disease, including:[20–38]

- cirrhosis
- chronic hepatitis
- fatty infiltration of the liver (chemical- and alcohol-induced fatty liver)
- subclinical cholestasis of pregnancy
- cholangitis and pericholangitis.

The therapeutic effect of silymarin in these disorders has been confirmed by histological, clinical, and laboratory data. Silymarin may also be useful in improving the solubility of the bile in the treatment of gallstones and in psoriasis.

Chemical-induced liver damage

In one of the first extensive double-blind clinical trials investigating silymarin's therapeutic effect in liver disorders, silymarin demonstrated impressive results for 129 patients with toxic metabolic liver damage, fatty degeneration of the liver of various origin, or chronic hepatitis, as compared with a control group comprised of 56 patients. The results might have been even more impressive if the study had lasted longer than 35 days.[20]

A follow-up study of patients with liver damage due to alcohol, diabetes viruses, or toxic exposure demonstrated even more striking results. Patients were followed for a long period of time (e.g. 7 weeks). Not only were clinical findings markedly improved in the silymarin-treated groups, but laboratory and liver biopsy data improved as well. Highly significant results were obtained in bromsulphalein retention, SGPT, iron, and cholesterol levels. There were remarkable tissue restorative effects as evidenced by biopsy. Upon completion of silymarin therapy, the liver showed restitution of normal cell structure even in severely damaged livers. These effects on the tissue level correlated well with improvements in blood chemistry.[21]

Another study highlighted the benefit of silymarin in individuals exposed to toxic chemicals. In this study, abnormal results of liver function tests (elevated levels of AST, ALT activity) and/or abnormal hematological values (low platelet counts, increased white blood cell counts, and a relative increase of lymphocytes compared with other white blood cells) were observed in 49 of 200 workers exposed to toxic toluene and/or xylene vapors for 5–20 years.[33] Thirty of the affected workers were treated with silymarin, and the remaining 19 were left without treatment. Under the influence of silymarin, the liver function tests and the platelet counts significantly improved. The white blood counts also showed a tendency towards improvement.

Cirrhosis

As described above, silymarin is quite effective in treating alcohol-related liver disease. There is a tremendous range in severity of alcohol-related liver disease from relatively mild to serious damage, such as cirrhosis. Even in this severe state, silymarin has shown benefit. Perhaps the most significant benefit is extending the life span of these patients.

In one study, 87 cirrhotics (46 with alcoholic cirrhosis) received silymarin, while 83 cirrhotics (45 with alcoholic cirrhosis) received a placebo.[34] The mean observation period was 41 months. In the treatment group, there were 24 deaths with 18 related to liver disease while, in the controls, there were 37 deaths with 31 related to liver disease. The 4-year survival rate was 58% in the treatment group compared with 39% in the controls.

Silymarin can also improve immune function in patients with cirrhosis.[35] Whether this effect is involved in the hepatoprotective action or a result of improved liver function has yet to be determined.

Viral hepatitis

Silymarin is useful in helping reverse viral-induced liver damage. It is effective in both acute and chronic viral hepatitis. In one study of acute viral hepatitis, 29 patients treated with silymarin showed a definite therapeutic influence on the characteristic increased serum levels of bilirubin and liver enzymes compared with a placebo group.[36] The laboratory parameters in the silymarin group had regressed more than in the placebo group by the fifth day of treatment. The number of patients attaining normal liver values after 3 weeks of treatment was significantly higher in the silymarin group than in the placebo group.

In a study in chronic viral hepatitis, silymarin was shown to result in dramatic improvement. Used at a high dose (420 mg of silymarin) for periods of 3–12 months, silymarin resulted in a reversal of liver cell damage (as noted by biopsy), an increase in protein level in the blood, and a lowering of liver enzymes. Common symptoms of hepatitis (e.g. abdominal discomfort, decreased appetite, and fatigue) were all improved.[37]

Gallstones

Silymarin may help to prevent or treat gallstones via its ability to increase the solubility of the bile. In one study, the composition of the bile was assayed in 19 patients with a history of gallstones (four) or removal of the gall bladder due to gallstones (15) before and after silymarin (420 mg/day for 30 days) or placebo. Silymarin treatment led to significant reduction in the biliary cholesterol concentration and bile saturation index.[38]

Psoriasis

Correction of abnormal liver function is indicated in the treatment of psoriasis. Silymarin has been reported to be of value in the treatment of psoriasis, and this may be due to its ability to inhibit the synthesis of leukotrienes, and improve liver function.[39]

The connection between the liver and psoriasis relates to one of the liver's basic tasks – filtering the blood. Psoriasis has been shown to be linked to high levels of circulating endotoxins, such as those found in the cell walls of gut bacteria. If the liver is overwhelmed by an increased number of endotoxins or chemical toxins, or if the liver's functional ability to filter and detoxify is decreased, the psoriasis is aggrevated.

Another factor in psoriasis is excessive production of leukotrienes. Silymarin has been shown to reduce leukotriene formation by inhibiting lipoxygenase.[13] Therefore, silymarin would inhibit one of the causes of the excessive cellular replication.

Silymarin has other effects of value in patients with psoriasis. Most of these effects revolve around correcting the abnormal cAMP to cGMP ratio observed in the skin of patients with psoriasis. The ratio of these two cellular control agents controls cellular replication. In psoriasis, cGMP levels are high relative to cAMP levels. Silymarin works to lower cGMP levels while raising cAMP levels.[15]

Protection against chemical-induced renal damage

Recent research has indicated that the anti-toxin, free radical scavenging effects of silymarin may be of value in protecting the kidneys.[40] In a very provocative study, female rats were given the anti-cancer drug cisplatin either with or without silibinin (300 mg/kg). Compared to the drug-only group, the silibinin-treated group lost significantly less weight, experienced no loss in creatinine clearance, no changes in urea level or magnesium excretion, and only slight degenerative changes in the glomerulus and tubules. Considering the significant problem of serious nephrotoxicity from cisplatin and other chemotherapeutic agents, silibinin may be of great value as an adjunct in the treatment of cancer.

Silibin bound to phosphatidylcholine

In the past decade, a new form of silymarin has emerged that may provide the greatest benefit. The new form binds silybin to phosphatidylcholine. Preliminary research indicates that phosphatidylcholine-bound silybin is better absorbed and produces better clinical results.

Absorption studies

Several human and animal studies have shown phosphatidylcholine-bound silybin is better absorbed. In one study, the excretion of silybin, the major component of silymarin, in the bile was evaulated in patients undergoing gall bladder removal (cholecystectomy). A drainage tube, the T-tube, was used to sample the bile. Patients were given either a single oral dose of the silybin–phosphatidylcholine complex or silymarin. The amount of silybin recovered in the bile in free and conjugated form within 48 hours was 11% for the silybin–phosphatidylcholine group compared with 3% for unmodified silybin.[41]

One of the significant features of this study is the fact that silymarin has been shown to improve the solubility of the bile. Since more silybin is being delivered to the liver and gall bladder when the phosphatidylcholine-bound silybin is used, this form is the ideal form for individuals with gallstones or fatty infiltration of the liver, two conditions characterized by decreased bile solubility.

In another study, plasma silybin levels were determined after administration of single oral doses of silybin–phosphatidylcholine complex and a similar amount of silymarin to nine healthy volunteers. Although absorption was rapid with both preparations, the bioavailability of the silybin–phosphatidylcholine complex was much greater than that of silymarin, as indicated by higher plasma silybin levels at all sampling times after intake of the complex. The authors concluded that complexation with phosphatidylcholine greatly increases the oral bioavailability of silybin, probably by facilitating its passage across the gastrointestinal mucosa.[42]

Clinical studies

Several clinical studies have shown phosphatidylcholine-bound silybin to be more effective. In one study, eight patients with chronic viral hepatitis (three with hepatitis B, three with both hepatitis B and hepatitis C, and two with hepatitis C) were given one capsule of phosphatidylcholine-bound silybin (equivalent to 140 mg silymarin) between meals for 2 months.[43] After treatment, serum malondialdehyde levels (an indicator of lipid peroxidation) decreased by 36% and the quantitative liver function evaluation, as measured by galactose elimination capacity, increased by 15%. A statistically significant reduction of liver enzymes was also seen: AST decreased 17% and ALT decreased 16%.

In another study designed primarily to evaluate the dose–response relationship of phosphatidylcholine-bound silybin, positive effects were again displayed.[44] In this study, patients with chronic hepatitis due to either a virus or alcohol were given different doses: 20 patients received 80 mg twice daily, 20 patients received 120 mg twice daily, and 20 patients received 120 mg three times daily for 2 weeks. At all tested doses, phosphatidylcholine-bound silybin produced a remarkable and statistically significant decrease of mean serum and total bilirubin levels. When used at the dose of 240 or 360 mg/day, it also resulted in a remarkable and statistically significant decrease in ALT and GGTP liver enzymes. These results indicate that even short-term treatment of viral or alcohol-induced hepatitis with relative low doses of phosphatidylcholine-bound silybin can be effective, but for the best results higher doses are indicated.

DOSAGE

The standard dose of milk thistle is based on its silymarin content (70–210 mg three times daily). For this reason, standardized extracts are preferred. The best results are achieved at higher dosages, i.e. 140–210 mg of silymarin three times daily.

The dosage for silybin bound to phosphatidylcholine is 120–240 mg twice daily.

Alcohol-based extracts are virtually always contraindicated in liver disease, as a relatively large amount of alcohol is administered in order to obtain an adequate dose of silymarin.

TOXICITY

Silymarin preparations are widely used medications in Europe, where a considerable body of evidence points to very low toxicity.[1] When used at high doses for short periods of time, silymarin given by various routes to mice, rats, rabbits, and dogs has shown no toxic effects. Studies in rats receiving silymarin for protracted periods have also demonstrated a complete lack of toxicity.[1]

As silymarin possesses choleretic activity, it may produce a looser stool as a result of increased bile flow and secretion. If higher doses are used, it may be appropriate to use bile-sequestering fiber compounds (e.g. guar gum, pectin, psyllium, oat bran, etc.) to prevent mucosal irritation and loose stools. Because of silymarin's lack of toxicity, long-term use is feasible when necessary.

REFERENCES

1. Wagner H. Antihepatotoxic flavonoids. In: Cody V, Middleton E, Harbourne JB, eds. Plant flavonoids in biology and medicine: biochemical, pharmacological, and structure-activity relationships. New York, NY: Alan R Liss. 1986: p 545–558
2. Adzet T. Polyphenolic compounds with biological and pharmacological activity. Herbs Spices Medicinal Plants 1986; 1: 167–184
3. Hikino H, Kiso Y, Wagner H, Fiebig. Antihepatotoxic actions of flavanolignans from Silybum marianum fruits. Planta Medica 1984; 50: 248–250
4. Wagner H. Plant constituents with antihepatotoxic activity. In: Beal JL, Reinhard E, eds. Natural products as medicinal agents. Stuttgart: Hippokrates-Verlag. 1981
5. Vogel G, Tuchweber B, Trost W, Mengs U. Protection against Amanita phalloides intoxication in beagles. Toxicol Appl Pharm 1984; 73: 355–362
6. Serne EH, Toorians AWF, Gietema JA et al. *Amanita phalloides*, a potentially lethal mushroom. Its clinical presentation and therapeutic options. Netherlands J Med 1996; 49: 19–23
7. Vogel G, Trost W, Braatz R et al. Studies on pharmacodynamics, site and mechanism of action of silymarin, the antihepatotoxic principle from *Silybum marianum* (L.) Gaert. Arzneim-Forsch 1975; 25: 179–185
9. Sarre H. Experience in the treatment of chronic hepatopathies with silymarin. Arzneim-Forsch 1971; 21: 1209–1212
10. Palasciano G, Protinacasa P et al. The effect of silymarin on plasma livels of malondialdehydyde in patients receiving long-term treatment with psychotropic drugs. Curr Ther Res 1994; 55: 537–545
11. Sonnenbichler J, Goldberg M, Hane L et al. Stimulatory effect of silibinin on the DNA synthesis in partially hepatectomized rat livers. non-response in hepatoma and other malignant cell lines. Biochem Pharm 1986; 35: 538–541
12. Sonnenbichler J, Zetl I. Biochemical effects of the flavanolignane silibinin on RNA, Protein and DNA synthesis in rat livers. In: Cody V, Middleton E, Harbourne JB, eds. Plant flavonoids in biology and medicine: biochemical, pharmacological, and structure-activity relationships. New York, NY: Alan R Liss. 1986: p 319–331
13. Fiebrich F, Koch H. Silymarin, an inhibitor of lipoxygenase. Experentia 1979; 35: 148–150
14. Fiebrich F, Koch H. Silymarin, an inhibitor of prostaglandin synthetase. Experentia 1979; 35: 150–152

15. Kock HP, Bachner J, Loffler E. Silymarin. Potent inhibitor of cyclic AMP phosphodiesterase. Meth Find Exptl Clin Pharm 1985; 7: 409–413
16. Valenzuela A, Barria T, Guerra, Garrido A. Inhibitory effect of the flavonoid silymarin on the erythrocyte hemolysis induced by phenylhydrazine. Biochem Biophys Res Comm 1985; 126: 712–718
17. Flemming K. Effect of silymarin on X-radiated mice. Arzneim-Forsch 1971; 21: 1373–1375
18. Zoltan OT, Gyori I. Studies on the brain edema of the rat induced by triethyltinsulfate. Part 7: The therapeutic effect of silymarin, theophylline, and mannitol in the conditioned reflex test. Arzneim-Forsch 1970; 20: 1248–1249
19. Seeger R. The effect of silymarin on osmotic resistance of erythrocytes. Arzneim-Forsch 1971; 21: 1599–1605
20. Schopen RD, Lange OK, Panne C, Kirnberger EJ. Searching for a new therapeutic principle. Experience with hepatic therapeutic agent legalon. Med Welt 1969; 20: 888–893
21. Schopen RD, Lange OK. Therapy of hepatoses. Therapeutic use of silymarin. Med Welt 1970; 21: 691–698
22. Sarre H. Experience in the treatment of chronic hepatopathies with silymarin. Arzneim-Forsch 1971; 21: 1209–1212
23. Canini F, Bartolucci, Cristallini E et al. Use of silymarin in the treatment of alcoholic hepatic steatosis. Clin Ter 1985; 114: 307–314
24. Salmi HA, Sarna S. Effect of silymarin on chemical, functional, and morphological alteration of the liver. A double-blind controlled study. Scand J Gastroenterol 1982; 17: 417–1421
25. Scheiber V, Wohlzogen FX. Analysis of a certain type of 2 × 3 tables, exemplified by biopsy findings in a controlled clinical trial. Int J Clin Pharm 1978; 16: 533–535
26. Boari C, Montanari M, Galleti GP et al. Occupational toxic liver diseases. Therapeutic effects of silymarin. Min Med 1981; 72: 2679–2688
27. Grossi F, Viola F. Protettori di membrana e silimarina nella terapia epatologica. Cl Terap 1981; 96: 11–23
28. Maneschi M, Tiberio C, Cittadini E. Impegno metabolico dell'epatocita in gravidanza. profilassi e terapia con un farmaco stabilizzante di membrana. Cl Terap 1981; 97: 625–630
29. Bulfoni A, Gobbato F. Evaluation of the therapeutic activity of silymarine in alcoholic hepatology. Gazz Med Ital 1979; 138: 597–608
30. Cavalieri S. A controlled clinical trial of Legalon in 40 patients. Gazz Med Ital 1974; 133: 628–635
31. Saba P, Galeone GF, Salvadorini F et al. Therapeutic effects of silymarin in chronic liver diseases due to psychodrugs. Gazz Med Ital 1976; 135: 236–251
32. De Martis M, Fontana M, Sebastiani F et al. La silymaina, farmaco membranotropo. Ossevazioni cliniche e sperimentali. Cl Terap 1977; 81: 333–362
33. Szilard S, Szentgyorgyi D, Demeter I. Protective effect of Legalon in workers exposed to organic solvents. Acta Med Hung 1988; 45: 249–256
34. Ferenci P, Dragosic SB, Dittrich H. Randomized controlled trial of Silymarin treatment in patients with cirrhosis of the liver. J Hepatology 1989; 9: 105–113
35. Deak G, Muzes G, Lang I. Immunomodulator effect of silymarin therapy in chronic alcoholic liver diseases. Orv Hetil 1990; 131: 1291–2, 1295–1296
36. Magliulo E, Gagliardi B, Fiori GP. Results of a double blind study on the effect of silymarin in the treatment of acute viral hepatitis, carried out at two medical centres. Med Klin 1978; 73: 1060–1065
37. Berenguer J, Carrasco D. Double-blind trial of silymarin versus placebo in the treatment of chronic hepatitis. Munch Med Wochenschr 1977; 119: 240–260
38. Nassauto G et al. Effect of silibinin on biliary lipid composition. Experimental and clinical study. J Hepatol 1991; 12: 290–295
39. Weber G, Galle K. The liver, a therapeutic target in dermatoses. Med Welt 1983; 34: 108–111
40. Gaedeke J, Fels LM, Bokemeyer C et al. Cisplatin nephrotoxicity and protection by silibinin. Nephrol Dial Transplant 1996; 11: 56–62
41. Schandalik R, Gatti G, Perucca E. Pharmacokinetics of silybin in bile following administration of silipide and silymarin in cholecystectomy patients. Arzneim Forsch 1992; 42: 964–968
42. Barzaghi N, Crema F, Gitti G. Pharmacokinetic studies on IdB 1016, a silybin-phosphatidylcholine complex, in healthy human subjects. Eur J Drug Metab Pharmacokinet 1990; 15: 333–338
43. Mascarella S, Giusti A, Marra F et al. Therapeutic and antilipoperoxidant effects of silybin-phosphatidylcholine complex in chronic liver disease. Preliminary results. Curr Ther Res 1993; 53: 98–102
44. Vailati A, Aristia L, Sozze E et al. Randomized open study of the dose-effect relationship of a short course of IdB 1016 in patients with viral or alcoholic hepatitis. Fitoterapia 1993; 44: 219–228

CHAPTER CONTENTS

112

Soy isoflavones and other constituents*

Kathi Head, ND

INTRODUCTION

In the past several years, soy and its constituents have received considerable attention, from both researchers and health practitioners. Epidemiological data which indicated that people from Asian cultures have lower rates of certain cancers, including cancer of the breast, prostate and colon, sparked an interest in soy as a contributing factor. While soy constituents, including saponins, lignans, phytosterols, protease inhibitors, and phytates, have come under investigation, the constituents which seem to hold the most promise from a therapeutic standpoint are the two isoflavones, genistein and daidzein. Numerous epidemiological, human, animal, and in vitro studies have demonstrated that soy isoflavones are effective chemopreventive agents for certain types of cancer. Mechanisms involved include:

- antiangiogenesis
- estrogen receptor binding
- modulation of sex hormone binding globulin (SHBG)
- anti-inflammatory and antioxidant effects
- inhibition of the enzymes protein tyrosine kinase (PTK) and 5 alpha-reductase.

Interaction with many other enzymes has been suggested. Evidence also points to the beneficial effects of soy, particularly the isoflavones, in prevention of cardiovascular disease. Isoflavones appear to inhibit platelet-activating factor and thrombin formation. They also increase HDL cholesterol and decrease triglycerides, LDL, VLDL, and total cholesterol. Other potential health benefits of soy include prevention of osteoporosis, via the phytoestrogen effects of isoflavones, and prevention of neovascularization in ocular conditions, via inhibition of angiogenesis.

*Reprinted with permission from *Alternative Medicine Review* 1997; 2: 433–450

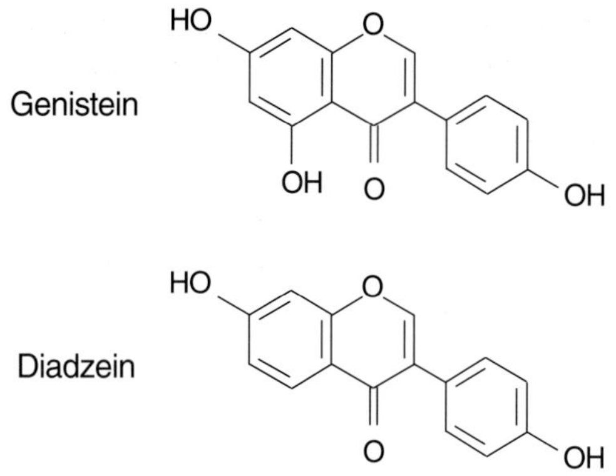

Figure 112.1 Structure of genistein and diadzein.

CHEMICAL COMPOSITION

Recent interest in the constituents of soybeans, particularly the isoflavones, has catapulted soy to the status of a promising nutraceutical with potentially significant health benefits. The principal isoflavones in soy are genistein (4′,5,7-trihydroxyisoflavone), daidzein (4′,7-dihydroxyisoflavone) (see Fig. 112.1), and their metabolites. In addition, soy products are a source of lignans, coumestans, saponins, plant sterols, phytates (inositol hexaphosphate), and protease inhibitors, all of which are also receiving attention for their health-promoting benefits.[1]

Isoflavones

Classification

Flavonoids are a subgroup of the larger group of plant constituents, the polypenols. Flavonoids are further differentiated into isoflavonoids, with isoflavones a subcategory of isoflavonoids (see Fig. 112.2). Isoflavonoids differ from other classes of flavonoids by their greater structural variability, their frequent presence in plants in their free form, rather than as a glycoside, and by the greater frequency of isoprenoid substitution. They are not as ubiquitous in nature as some of the other flavonoids, such as flavones and flavonols, being found primarily in one subfamily of Leguminosae, the Papilionoideae.[2] Approximately 600 isoflavonoids have been identified. They are divided into subclasses depending on the oxidation level of the central pyran ring. Isoflavones are the most abundant of the subclasses of isoflavonoids. Genistein and daidzein are two important isoflavones in soy. As can be seen in Figure 112.1, genistein has a hydroxy group in the 5 position, giving it three hydroxy groups, while

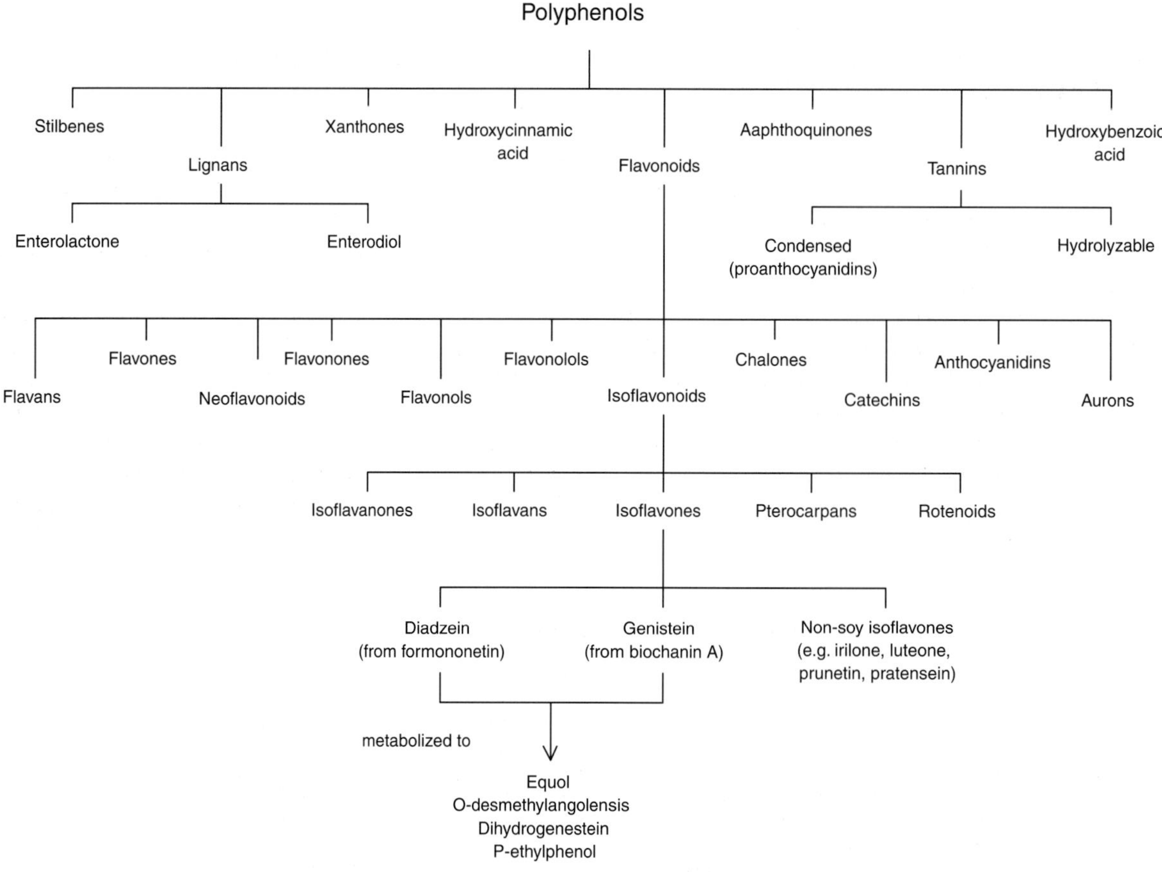

Figure 112.2 Polyphenol classification.

daidzein has just two. Due to the fact that the 5 hydroxy group on the genistein binds to the 4 ketonic oxygen, genistein is a more hydrophobic molecule than daidzein. This affords genistein some of its unique therapeutic effects.

Absorption, metabolism and excretion

Isoflavones undergo extensive metabolism in the intestinal tract prior to absorption. Genistein is formed from biochanin A, and daidzein from formononetin.[1] Genistein and daidzein also occur in soy products in the form of their glycosides, genistin and daidzin. In the case of the glycosides, intestinal bacterial glucosidases cleave the sugar moieties, releasing the biologically active isoflavones, genistein and daidzein. In adults, these are further transformed by bacteria to specific metabolites: equol, O-desmethylangolensis, dihydrogenistein, and p-ethylphenol. Due to soy intake by livestock, isoflavone metabolites are also consumed indirectly in a diet high in dairy products and meat.[3]

In at least one study, genistein was found to be well-absorbed in the small intestines by human subjects fed a soy beverage.[4] After absorption, the isoflavones are transported to the liver where they are removed from the portal blood. However, a percentage of the isoflavones in the portal blood can escape uptake by the liver and enter the peripheral circulation. The effectiveness of this hepatic first-pass clearance influences the amount which reaches peripheral tissues.[4] The isoflavones are then eliminated, primarily via the kidneys, similar to endogenous estrogens.[5]

After examining plasma, fecal and urinary concentrations of isoflavones in healthy volunteers, Xu et al[6] concluded that the bioavailability of soy isoflavones is influenced by an intact, healthy gut, with microflora capable of converting these isoflavones to their active forms. Wheat fiber appears to decrease the bioavailability of genistein. A small cross-over study of seven healthy women found that a more fiber-rich diet resulted in 55% less plasma genistein 24 hours after soy intake and a 20% reduction in total urinary genistein. The researchers postulated that fairly insoluble wheat fiber reduced the absorption of genistein by its bulking effect and hydrophobic binding.[7] Karr et al[8] found urinary excretion of isoflavones to be reflective of the type and amount of soy ingested. A study conducted on healthy male subjects between the ages of 20 and 40 found that urinary excretion of genistein and daidzein was greater after consumption of 112 g of tempeh, a fermented soy product, than after 125 g of unfermented soy pieces.[9] This finding seems to indicate that fermentation of soy products increases bioavailability of the isoflavones. Plasma levels of soy isoflavones are also increased after consumption of soy and certain other leguminous plants, such as clover.[10]

Levels in soy products

Fukutake et al[11] analyzed soy products for genistein and genistin (the glycoside of genistein) content. The results are outlined in Table 112.1. In general, they found that fermented soy products contain more genistein than soybeans, soy milk and tofu. Alcohol extraction, a process used in the production of many soy protein concentrates and isolates (used in soy protein powders), results in the removal of up to 90% of the isoflavones.[12] The isoflavone content of soybeans varies considerably depending on the variety of soybean (there are over 10,000 varieties of soybeans), the year harvested, geographic location, and the plant part in question.[13] Non-soy legumes, such as lentils and other beans, do not contain appreciable amounts of isoflavones.[14]

Other soy constituents

Protease inhibitors

Researchers have looked with interest at protease inhibitors (PI) and their potential anti-cancer and anti-inflammatory effects. Two prominent protease inhibitors from soybeans are Bowman–Birk inhibitor (BBI) and Kunitz–Trypsin inhibitor (KTI). BBI is a 71-residue inhibitor which has two independent inhibitory sites involving binding with the proteases, trypsin and chymotrypsin.[15] BBI has been found to inhibit expression of certain oncogenes in irradiated animal models[16] and to inhibit chemically induced carcinogenesis.[17,18] Both in vitro and in vivo animal models have demonstrated that BBI appears to exert its effects directly on the target organ rather than by a non-specific effect on metabolism.[19,20]

Table 112.1 Levels of genistein and its glycoside, genistin, in soy foods[11]

	Genistein	Genistin
Soybeans, soy nuts, soy powder	4.6–18.2 mcg/g*	200.6–968.1 mcg/g*
Soy milk, tofu	1.9–13.9 mcg/g	94.8–137.7 mcg/g
Fermented soy miso and natto†	38.5–229.1 mcg/g	71.7–492.8 mcg/g
Calculated daily Japanese dietary intake	1.5–4.1 mg/day	6.3–8.3 mg/day

*mcg/g raw food.
†Soy sauce contains both genistein and genistin, but at lower levels than other fermented soy products.

Some researchers have hypothesized that the dietary intake of exogenous PIs indirectly increases endogenous PI formation.[21] Other researchers have questioned the concept that PIs contribute significantly to the anti-cancer effects of soy. This is due, in part, to the fact that both raw and cooked soy products are equally effective in reducing cancer incidence, even though heating virtually destroys all protease activity.[22] Another reason for skepticism is that ingested PIs (such as purified BBI) are very poorly absorbed from the digestive tract.[22] Some researchers have postulated that the formation of these protease:protease inhibitor complexes might interfere with protein absorption, offering some cancer protection (epidemiological studies indicate that high-fat and high-protein diets increase cancer risk).[23]

Protease inhibitors in soy products have been implicated in pancreatic hypertrophy and hyperplasia in animal models.[24] Whether it is the protease inhibitors and whether this hyperplasia contributes to increased rates of pancreatic cancer in these animals are still subjects of debate.

Lignans

Lignans are capable of exerting a phytoestrogenic effect in humans. In addition, they exhibit antitumor and antiviral activity.[2] The most prevalent lignans in mammals are enterolactone and enterodiol, formed by gut bacteria, from the plant precursor lignans, matairesinol and secoisolariciresinol, respectively.[3] Oil seeds, such as flaxseed, contain about 100 times the lignan content of other plants. Other sources of lignans in descending order of importance are dried seaweed, whole legumes (including soy), cereal bran, legume hulls, whole grain cereals, vegetables, and fruit.[1] Gender differences in urinary lignan excretion have been observed, with men excreting more enterolactone and less enterodiol than women. The researchers felt this implied a difference in colonic bacterial metabolism of lignans between the genders.[25] Administration of antibiotics nearly completely eliminates the formation of these mammalian lignans from their precursors.[3]

Phytosterols

Phytosterols, such as β-sitosterol, are found in high concentrations in soy products. Although poorly absorbed, they bind cholesterol in the gut.[22] Dietary content of phytosterols differs widely among populations. The typical Western diet contains about 80 mg/day, while the traditional Japanese diet contains approximately 400 mg/day.[26,27]

Coumestans

The phytoestrogen, coumesterol, and other coumestan isoflavonoids have been found by some researchers in significant quantities in soy foods of all types, including:[28]

- soybeans
- soy flour
- soy flakes
- isolated soy protein
- tofu
- soy drinks
- soy sprouts.

On the other hand, Adlercreutz & Mazur[3] reports its presence only in soy sprouts. The most abundant source is mung bean sprouts. It is also found in significant quantities in other members of the Leguminosiae family, including *Trifolium* and *Medicago* spp.[2]

Saponins

Saponins are distributed widely in the plant kingdom, including in soybeans. They appear to have anti-cancer properties by virtue of their antioxidant and antimutagenic properties.[29] They also bind cholesterol and bile acids in the gut.[22] An in vitro study demonstrated that saponins isolated from soybeans exhibited potent antiviral effects on the HIV virus. Saponin B1 completely inhibited HIV-induced cytopathic changes and virus-specific antigen expression within 6 days of infection. Saponin B2 exhibited similar, although less potent, effects.[30]

Phytates

Although phytic acid (inositol hexaphosphate) has been implicated in blocking the absorption of minerals, the phytate content of plants, including soy, seems to be responsible for some of the anti-cancer properties of vegetable-based foods. Phytic acid is a highly charged antioxidant, capable of scavenging hydroxyl radicals and chelating metal ions such as the pro-oxidant, iron. Graf & Eaton[31] reported the iron-chelating ability of phytate to be more important than the fiber in dietary colon cancer prevention. Vucenik et al[32] reported antitumor effects of phytic acid both in vitro and in animal models. Phytates also appear to enhance natural killer cell activity.[33] Rao et al[34] found these potent antioxidant effects to protect against cardiac ischemia and reperfusion injury in animal models. For a summary of soy constituents and their functions, see Table 112.2.

PHARMACOLOGY

Soy constituents have been shown to have estrogenic, anti-estrogenic, antiviral,[35] anticarcinogenic,[36–38] bacteriocidal, and antifungal[39] effects. Isoflavones also have antimutagenic,[37] antioxidant,[40,41] mild anti-inflammatory,[42] antihypertensive,[42] and antiproliferative effects.[36,43] This

Table 112.2 Soy constituents and their functions

Constituent	Function
Protease inhibitors (Bowman–Birk inhibitor, Kunitz–Trypsin inhibitor)	Inhibit oncogene expression Inhibit chemically induced carcinogenesis Implicated in pancreatic hypertrophy (animal studies)
Lignans (enterolactone, enterdiol)	Phytoestrogen effects (agonistic/antagonistic) Antitumor Antiviral
Phytosterols (β-sitosterol)	Binds cholesterol in the gut
Coumestans (coumesterol)	Phytoestrogen effects (agonistic/antagonistic)
Saponins	Antioxidant Bind cholesterol and bile acids in the gut Antiviral (HIV)
Phytates	Antioxidant Chelate metal ions (e.g. iron) Enhance natural killer cell activity
Isoflavones (genestein, daidzein and their metabolites)	Phytoestrogen effects (agonistic/antagonistic) Anti-mutagenic Antioxidant Anti-inflammatory Antiproliferative Antihypertensive Angiogenesis inhibition

chapter focuses primarily on isoflavones as these are the constituents found in greatest quantity in soy products. Brief reference will be made to other beneficial constituents.

Hormonal effects

Infants

Recent advances in understanding the phytoestrogen content of soy foods have led researchers to examine the isoflavone content in commonly consumed infant formulas. A recent study examined the isoflavone content of 25 randomly selected samples from five major brands of soy-based infant formulas. There were significant levels of isoflavones, particularly in the form of the glycosides of genistein and daidzein, in all samples tested. The plasma concentrations of genistein and daidzein were compared in 4-month-old infants fed exclusively soy formula, cow's milk formula, and breast milk. A 4-month-old infant consuming soy milk was estimated to be ingesting between 4.5 and 8.0 mg/kg body weight per day of total isoflavones. This is a proportionately greater concentration per body weight than that found in adults consuming soy foods.

Additionally, the researchers estimated the daily exposure of infants to soy isoflavones was 6–11 times higher, with body weight factored into the equation, than the typical dose necessary to exert hormone-like effects in adults. They found negligible concentrations of isoflavones in breast milk and cow's milk.[5] There was some evidence of the daidzein metabolite, equol, in the infants who were fed cow's milk, confirming previous observations that cow's milk also contains some isoflavones. In this study, the plasma concentration of isoflavones in breast-fed babies was 1/200 the level in soy-formula fed babies. Franke & Custer,[44] on the other hand, reported in 1996 that human breast milk from mothers consuming soy foods provided significant levels of isoflavones. Some researchers have concluded that the isoflavone content of human breast milk appears to be a reflection of the mother's diet.

These findings have raised some interesting questions and stimulated lively debate. Adverse effects of phytoestrogens on development and reproductive capacity of livestock, wildlife and experimental animals have been reported.[45] There has been very little clinical experience with human infants and phytoestrogens, however. In animal models, phytoestrogens have had effects similar to other estrogens, included interfering with normal reproductive system development.[46] On the other hand, phytoestrogenic isoflavones have been found to possess some important anti-cancer properties. Genistein, given in only three doses to newborn mice, decreased breast cancer incidence and tumor numbers significantly.[44] Although millions of Asians have consumed large quantities of soy foods for hundreds of years without any apparent health risk and seemingly with health benefits, long-term studies are needed to clarify the safety of using soy-based infant formulas and to assess the potential beneficial or adverse effects of consuming phytoestrogens in the form of soy isoflavones early in life.

Adults

Plant lignan and isoflavonoid glycosides are converted by gut bacteria in the intestines to compounds with molecular weights and structures similar to steroid hormones (see Fig. 112.3). The pattern of isoflavonoid and lignan excretion in the urine is similar to endogenous estrogens.[47] Studies of the effects of phytoestrogens on hormone levels are conflicting.

Lu et al[48] found that the consumption of soy products by premenopausal women resulted in decreased circulating ovarian steroids and adrenal androgens, as well as increased length of the menstrual cycle. Six healthy females, aged 22–29, were given 12 ounces of soy milk three times daily with meals for 1 month. Daily isoflavone intake was approximately 100 mg each of daidzein and genistein (in the form of their glycosides, daidzin and genistin). The estradiol levels decreased by 31% on days 5–7 of the cycle, 81% on days 12–14, and 49% on days 20–22. Luteal phase progesterone levels decreased by 35%, and DHEA sulfate levels decreased progressively during the month by 14–30%. The length of the menstrual cycle increased during the soy feeding month from 28.3 ± 1.9 to 31.8 ± 5.1 days.

In another study, also on premenopausal women, Lu et al found that 60 g of soy protein, with 45 mg of isoflavones daily, resulted in the suppression of midcycle surges of FSH and LH. Plasma concentrations of estradiol increased during the follicular phase in the soy group, while cholesterol decreased by 9.6%. The researchers noted that a similar effect occurs in women given tamoxifen. There were no significant differences in estradiol levels between the soy and control groups at midcycle or during the luteal phase.[49] At least one study found soy protein isolate to have a stimulatory effect on breast tissue in premenopausal women, characterized by increased breast secretions, epithelial cell hyperplasia, and elevated levels of serum estradiol.[50]

Wang et al[51] found that genistein competed with estradiol binding to estrogen receptors, with 50% inhibition occurring at 5×10^{-7} M. A study of soy-supplemented postmenopausal women found a small estrogenic effect on vaginal cytology. However, no difference between soy-supplemented subjects and controls, with regard to serum FSH, LH, sex hormone binding globulin, endogenous estradiol or body weight, was observed.[52]

Many studies on phytoestrogens focus on the use of coumestrol, as it has more potent phytoestrogenic effects than lignans, genistein and daidzein. In vitro studies have found that both genistein and coumestrol inhibit the conversion of estrone to 17-beta estradiol. Coumestrol exhibited the strongest inhibition.[53] An in vitro study monitoring the expression of the estrogen-responsive protein pS2 in breast cancer cell MCF-7 tissue culture, to assess the estrogenic response of various plant substances, found that the following substances elicited estrogen-like activity:

- daidzein
- equol
- nordihydroguaiaretic acid
- enterolactone
- kaempferol.

The substances tested that did not appear to have estrogen-like activity were quercetin and enterodiol.[54]

The effects of phytoestrogens vary greatly depending on the species of animal, the particular phytoestrogen compound being tested, the age of the animal, the length

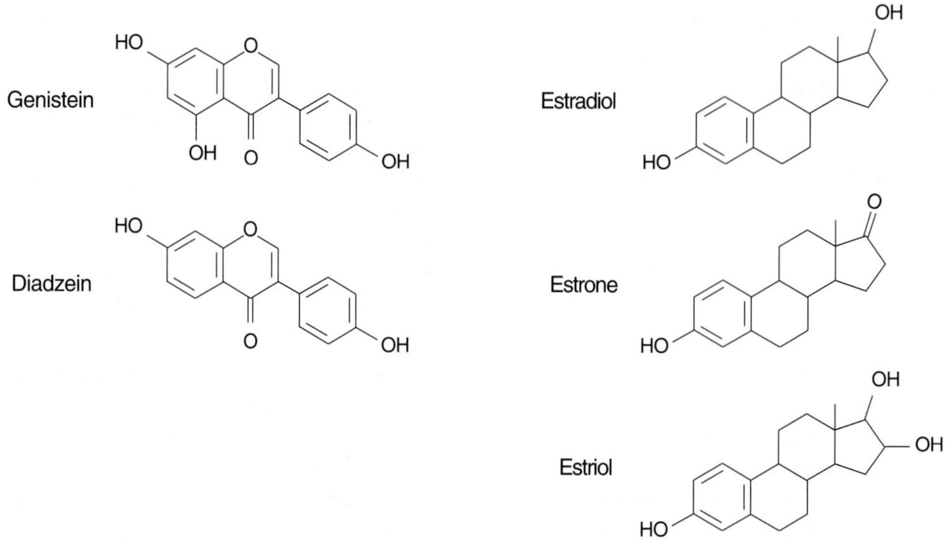

Figure 112.3 Structure of soy isoflavones compared with estrogens.

of time of ingestion, the presence or absence of exogenous estrogen, the target tissue in question, and the dosage used. The phytoestrogen, coumestrol, was found to have an estrogenic effect, as demonstrated by changes in uterine and brain tissue, when given to prepubescent rats; however, when given to adult female rats, ovarian cycling was inhibited. When given for 10 days to neonatal rats, there was no effect on estrous cycling, but when given for 21 days, it interfered with normal cycling once the rats reached adulthood. The females exhibited persistent estrous and lack of an LH surge, while the males demonstrated a decrease in sexual behavior.[55]

Historically, the consumption of soy products in Asian cultures, from a very young age, has not resulted in any apparent negative effects related to hormone imbalances. It is unlikely that animal studies are effective at predicting the effects of phytoestrogens in the human model.[56]

The mechanisms for the anti-estrogenic effect of phytoestrogens are largely unknown, but some experts believe it is unlikely to be a direct receptor-mediated effect.[3] One mechanism of action of lignans and isoflavonoids is to stimulate sex hormone-binding glubulin (SHBG) (also known as sex steroid-binding protein (SBP)) synthesis in the liver. SHBG binds to cell surface receptors, resulting in regulation of bioavailability and activity of hormones.[3] In vitro, in MCF-7 human breast cancer cells, SHBG has been found to downregulate estradiol.[57]

It appears that phytoestrogens exert mild agonistic and antagonistic effects on estrogen, depending on the level of endogenous estrogen present and on the tissue being tested. In vitro studies demonstrate an estrogenic effect in the absence of endogenous estrogen, and an anti-estrogenic effect in the presence of estrogen.[3] Much research in this area remains to be done.

Much of the effect of phytoestrogens might be due to enzyme inhibitions. It appears that phytoestrogens have an inhibitory effect on many enzymes involved in the biosynthesis and metabolism of steroid hormones. The effect on enzymes is further discussed below.

Mechanism of action of soy isoflavones

Soy's inhibition of cancer cell growth does not seem to be entirely estrogen-dependent.[58] There are many proposed mechanisms for the therapeutic effects of isoflavones. The mechanisms include:

- inhibition of protein tyrosine kinase (PTK)
- binding of estrogen receptors (although soy's inhibition of cancer cell growth does not seem to be entirely estrogen-dependent)[58]
- inhibition of production of reactive oxygen species[59]
- induction of DNA strand breakage resulting in apoptosis or cell death[58]
- inhibition of angiogenesis[60]
- modulation of sex steroid-binding protein[61]
- inhibition of 5-alpha-reductase[62]
- inhibition of P-form phenolsulfotransferase (PST)-mediated sulfation[63]
- inhibition of thrombin formation and platelet activation[64]
- increased LDL receptor activity.[65]

The therapeutic implications of each of these mechanisms is elaborated below.

CLINICAL APPLICATIONS

Cancer

The first clues that soy diets might provide protection from cancer came from epidemiological studies, in which people from Asian cultures eating a diet high in soy foods, such as tofu, demonstrated lower rates of several types of cancers, including types not typically considered to be hormone- or diet-related. Messina et al[66] reviewed 21 epidemiological studies which evaluated the effect of soy diets on 26 different cancer sites. An evaluation of the effect of non-fermented soy products in these studies found that 10 showed decreased risks for rectal, stomach, breast, prostate, colon, and lung cancers, while 15 showed no significant effect. Only one, in which fried bean curd was evaluated, showed an increased risk for esophageal cancer. On the other hand, the effects of fermented soy products – miso soup and soybean paste – were much less consistent. In 21 studies evaluating fermented soy products, involving 25 cancer sites, an increased cancer risk was found in four, mixed results were obtained in four, no significant effects were found in 14, and a decreased risk was found in three. The increased risks of cancer from consumption of fermented soy products appear to involve primarily the gastrointestinal tract – esophageal, stomach, colorectal, and pancreatic cancers.[66] These studies are summarized in Table 112.3.

To put the epidemiological studies into some perspective, Adlercruetz et al[67] found high urinary excretion of the soy isoflavones, equol, daidzein, and O-desmethylangolensin, in both men and women living in rural Japan. Most soy foods contain about 1–2 mg/g of genistein. In Asian cultures people tend to consume 20–80 mg/day. The usual dietary intake of genistein in Western cultures is 2–3 mg/day. Messina et al[66] examined 26 animal studies and reported that 17 (65%) of them demonstrated a protective effect of soy from experimental carcinogensis.

There are many proposed mechanisms for the anticancer benefits of soy-based foods. Inhibition of PTK activity has been proposed as a major mechanism in the prevention of carcinogenesis. While synthetic PTK inhibitors have been proposed for the treatment of cancer, expected toxicity has restricted their development. In

Table 112.3 Summary of epidemiological studies of soy and cancer (From Messina et al[66])

Cancer location	Fermented miso/soybean paste	Unfermented tofu/bean curd	Other soy products
Breast (five studies)	1. Risk 2. Risk, premenopausal No effect, postmenopausal 3. Risk 4. No significant effect*	5. Risk	
Prostate (three studies)	1. No significant effect 2. No significant effect 3. No significant effect	3. No significant effect	
Colorectal (six studies)	1. No significant association* 2. Risk (colon) 3. Risk (rectal) 5. No significant association	3. No significant association 4. Risk (not significant) 6. Risk (rectal, colon, not significant)	3. No significant association 5. Risk (rectal, not colon)
Lung (four studies)	1. No significant association	1. No significant association 2. Risk 3. Risk	4. Risk (soy in general)
Stomach (16 studies)	1. Risk (miso) 1. No effect (bean paste) 2. Risk (not significant) 3. No significant association 4. Risk (soybean paste) 5. Risk (miso) 6. Risk 7. Risk 8. No significant association 9. No significant association 10. Risk	1. Risk 2. Risk 3. Risk (not significant) 12. Risk 14. No significant association	1. No effect (soybean, fried curd) 11. Risk (soybean) 13. Risk (soy milk) 15. No significant association (non-miso soy products) 16. Risk (soy milk, other soy products)
Esophageal (two studies)	1. Risk (males, no effect females)	1. No significant association	2. Risk (fried bean curd)
Gall bladder/bile duct (two studies)	1. No significant effect (all soy products) 2. Risk (bile duct, not significant) No effect (gall bladder)		
Liver (one study)	1. No significant association		
Pancreatic (one study)	1. Risk		

*Type of soy not reported.

1987, genistein was discovered to be a natural PTK inhibitor.[58] Tyrosine kinase inhibition results in the inhibition of leukotriene production, (products of inflammation which have been implicated in the stimulation of tumor growth). In vitro studies found that pretreatment of cancer cell lines with genistein completely inhibited leukotriene production.[68]

Influence on a number of other enzymes has been suggested as a possible mechanism for the anti-cancer properties of isoflavones. Some of these enzymes include DNA topoisomerases,[69,70] ribosomal S6 kinase activity,[71] phospholipase C-gamma,[72] phosphatidylinositol kinases,[73] and mitogen-activated protein kinase.[74] In addition, genistein demonstrated in vitro inhibition of phenolsulfotransferase, an enzyme involved in sulfation-induced carcinogensis.[63]

In vitro studies have found genistein to be a very potent inhibitor of neovascularization or angiogenesis, one of the proposed mechanisms for cancer growth inhibition.[60] Isoflavone effects on hormone regulation, expression and metabolism have been elaborated above and are discussed further below in the sections on breast and prostate cancer.

At issue in the study of soy isoflavones in the treatment of cancer is whether the concentration achieved by dietary consumption of soy products is enough to influence tumor growth. Studies on human volunteers consuming soy beverages, which provided 42 mg genistein and 27 mg daidzein daily, resulted in peripheral blood concentrations of 0.5–1.0 μM,[4] a concentration much lower than that necessary to inhibit growth of cultured cancer cells.[75] However, these same researchers found non-transformed mammary epithelial cell cultures to be much more sensitive to genistein, with inhibition of growth stimulation occurring in the range of 1–2 μM. This suggests a role of isoflavones as chemopreventive rather than chemotherapeutic agents.

Breast cancer

Case-controlled, epidemiological, in vitro, and animal studies point to effectiveness of soy isoflavones in the prevention of breast cancer. A recent case-controlled study, examined the effect of phytoestrogens on breast cancer risk. One hundred and forty-four women with early diagnosed breast cancer were paired with age- and area-of-residency-matched controls. Prior to treatment, a questionnaire, and 72 hour urine and blood tests were administered. Urine was assayed for the isoflavones daidzein, genistein, and equol, and the lignans enterodiol, enterolactone, and matairesinol. Adjustments were made for age at menarche, parity, and alcohol and total fat intake. Increased excretion of daidzein, equol, and enterolactone was associated with a reduction in the risk for development of breast cancer. The most significant correlation was between the levels of the soy isoflavone, equol, and the risk of breast cancer, with those in the highest quartile of equol excretion exhibiting only one-quarter the risk of those in the lowest quartile – a fourfold reduction in risk. The lignan, enterolactone, and the isoflavone, daidzein, were associated with a threefold reduction in risk. The daidzein results were insignificant, after correcting for confounding variables. Similar trends were noted for both pre- and postmenopausal groups. Unfortunately, no reliable data for genistein were available due to instability of the derivative of genistein being tested and interference by an unknown compound.[76] Two case-controlled studies, one in Singapore[77] and one in Japan,[78] found significant protection from soy intake for pre- but not postmenopausal women.

Epidemiological studies demonstrate an inverse relationship between soy intake and incidence of breast cancer (see Table 112.3). Americans have two to three times the breast cancer rate of Asians eating a traditional diet.[79] An epidemiological study of Asian-American women found tofu intake to correlate inversely with breast cancer incidence, after adjustment for other dietary, menstrual and reproductive factors.[80] This effect was observed in both pre- and postmenopausal women. In summary, all four of the human studies examined seemed to indicate a protective effect of soy against breast cancer in premenopausal women. The effect on postmenopausal women was significant in two of the four studies.

In vitro experiments with human breast cancer cells confirm genistein to be a potent inhibitor of cell growth, regardless of estrogen receptor status. Other isoflavones, daidzein and biochanin A, demonstrated weaker growth inhibition.[81–83] Pagliacci et al[84] reported that the in vitro inhibition of MCF-7 human breast cancer cells occurred through blocks at critical points in cell cycle control as well as via induction of apoptosis. Wang et al[51] found that genistein produced a concentration-dependent effect on breast cancer cell cultures. At lower concentrations (10^{-8}–10^{-6} M), genistein stimulated growth, while higher concentrations ($>10^{-5}$) inhibited growth. They concluded that the effect of genistein at the lower concentrations appeared to be estrogen receptor-mediated, while effects at higher concentrations were independent of estrogen receptors.

Genistein, when administered to neonatal[85] or prepubescent rats,[86] suppressed the development of chemically induced mammary tumors without causing toxicity to the development of the endocrine or reproductive systems. Barnes et al[87] found that soy in the form of raw soybeans as well as soy protein isolate inhibited mammary tumors in experimental models.

Prostate cancer

Epidemiological evidence points to the benefits of soy constituents in the prevention of prostate cancer. Japanese men who consume a low-fat, high-soy diet have low mortality rates from prostate cancer. Isoflavones in the plasma of Japanese men were between seven and 110 times higher than in Finnish men, with genistein present in the highest concentrations.[88] Mechanisms suggested include genistein-induced prostate cancer cell adhesion, direct growth inhibition, and induction of apoptosis. Growth inhibition appears to be independent of genistein's estrogenic effects.[89] An in vitro study indicated that the isoflavones genistein, biochanin A, and equol were potent inhibitors of 5-alpha-reductase,[62] the enzyme necessary for the conversion of testosterone to dihydrotestosterone (implicated in prostate cancer).

Studies have found that animals fed soy isolates high in the isoflavones, genistein and daidzein, demonstrated a lower incidence of prostate cancer and a 27% longer disease-free period after exposure to chemical carcinogens than animals fed a soy isolate low in isoflavones.[90] This not only points to the potential chemoprotective effects of soy, but seems to point to the importance of the isoflavones over other soy constituents. Peterson & Barnes[91] found that the isoflavones, genistein and biochanin A, but not daidzein, inhibited several human prostate cancer cell lines.

NIH recommendations

The committee of the National Institutes of Health (NIH) studying chemoprevention from soy products made the following recommendations:

- Future dietary studies involving soybeans should be carried out using soy products rather than isolated compounds, since soybeans appear to contain several potential anticarcinogens.
- Standardized and improved analytical methods are needed so that the contents of all soy-based materials employed in soybean research, whether soybean fractions or soy products, can be accurately described.
- Basic research in the absorption, metabolism, and physiology of potential anticarcinogens in humans should be conducted.

Cardiovascular disease

Lipid effects

A large meta-analysis of 38 controlled studies of the effects of soy diets, with animal protein diets serving as the controls, found a statistically significant decrease in serum lipids in the soy group. The changes were most significant in hypocholesterolemic subjects[92] (see Table 112.4). The intake of energy, fat, saturated fat, and cholesterol was similar between the two groups. Gooderham et al[93] reported no effect on platelet aggregation or serum lipid levels in healthy, normocholesterolemic men fed soy protein compared with casein.

One of the proposed mechanisms for the hypolipidemic effect involves an increase in LDL receptor activity in both humans and animals.[65] Other metabolic changes which have been noted in animals and humans on soy diets include increased cholesterol and bile acid synthesis, increased apolipoprotein B and E receptor activity, and decreased hepatic secretion of lipoproteins (associated with increased clearance of cholesterol from the bloodstream).[94] Proposals for the specific constituents involved include the amino acid profile, saponins, phytic acid, fiber, as well as the effects of isoflavones discussed below.[94]

In one study, monkeys were fed soy isolates high in isoflavones and compared in a cross-over trial with a soy isolate in which the isoflavones had been removed via alcohol extraction. LDL, VLDL, and total cholesterol:HDL ratios were significantly lowered, while HDL was significantly elevated in the group on the isoflavone-rich diet.[12] No lipid-lowering effect occurred in the group on the casein diet.

Table 112.4 Results of a meta-analysis of the effects on serum lipids of soy diet compared with meat protein diet[92]

Total cholesterol	23.2 md/dl decrease	9.3% decrease
LDL cholesterol	21.7 mg/dl decrease	12.9% decrease
Triglycerides	13.3 mg/dl decrease	10.5% decrease
HDL cholesterol	1.2 mg/dl increase (NS)	2.4% increase

Effects on the atherosclerotic process

Arterial thrombus formation is generally initiated by an injury to the endothelial cells lining the blood vessels. One of the first events after an injury is thrombin formation. This leads to a cascade of events including platelet activation, resulting in thrombus formation. Genistein has been found to inhibit thrombin formation and platelet activation.[64] The pathogenesis of atherosclerotic plaque formation also involves, in addition to lipid accumulation, the infiltration of monocytes and T-lymphocytes into the artery wall, contributing to the thickening of the wall and occlusion of the vessel. Monocytes and lymphocytes are able to adhere to the endothelial cell surfaces via the expression of certain "adhesion molecules". The infiltration and proliferation appear to be controlled by peptide growth factors. Increased levels of isoflavones, genistein in particular, appear to alter the growth factor activity, and inhibit cell adhesion and proliferation, all activities necessary for lesion formation in the intima of the blood vessels (see Fig. 112.4).[95]

Cardioprotective effects

Animal studies with monkeys have confirmed the cardioprotective effects of soy. Soy protein diets, when compared with casein diets, resulted in significant improvements in lipid profiles, insulin sensitivity, and a decrease in arterial lipid peroxidation.[96] Furthermore, animal studies also indicate the isoflavone content of the soy is an important factor.

Other potential therapeutic benefits

While research on the health benefits of soy constituents has focused primarily on the chemopreventive effects for cancer and cardiovascular disease, there are a few other conditions which might benefit from the addition of soy isoflavones to the diet.

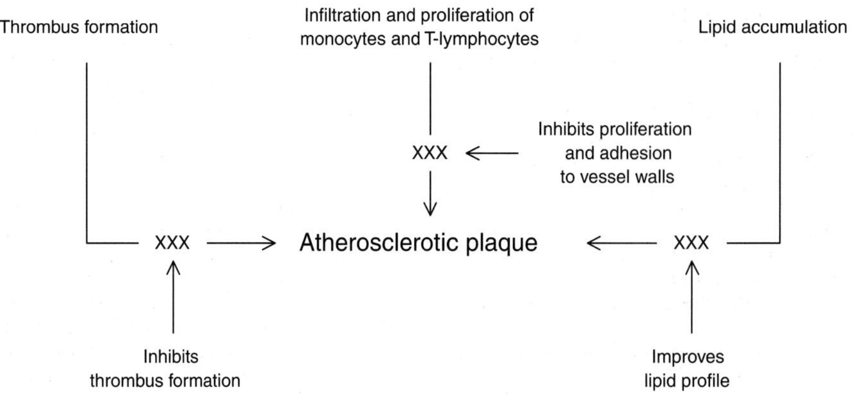

Figure 112.4 Impact of soy on atherosclerotic plaque formation.

Osteoporosis

Animal studies indicate that soy isolates enhance bone density. Ovariectomized rats fed a high-soy diet demonstrated enhanced bone density of the vertebral bodies and femoral bone compared with the group fed a casein diet. While there was considerable bone turnover in the soy-fed group, bone densities suggest that formation exceeded resorption.[97] Further studies on the use of soy isoflavones for the prevention and treatment of osteoporosis are warranted.

Eye disorders

Neovascularization complicates many eye disorders, such as proliferative diabetic retinopathy, and is responsible for corneal transplant rejection. Substances which exhibit the capacity to inhibit angiogenesis could play an important role in preventing this vascularization. An animal study demonstrated that genistein, when injected subconjunctivally, inhibited corneal neovascularization.[98] While this was not a human study with the use of oral doses, this study has opens the door for future investigation.

CONCLUSION

Research indicates that soy and its individual constituents have several potential health benefits. The primary isoflavones, genistein and daidzein, as well as their metabolites, exert a wide array of effects which appear to offer protection against cancer, cardiovascular disease, osteoporosis, and ocular neovascularization. Many of the studies to date have been epidemiological, animal, or in vitro. Further controlled human trials are needed to confirm the preliminary findings reported in these studies. Soy constituents, particularly the isoflavones, have come under scrutiny, due to their phytoestrogen effects. Because in some cases they act as estrogen agonists, and at other times as antagonists, the use of these isoflavones in cancer patients and in infant formulas is controversial. Further study to determine whether their use in these situations is harmful or beneficial is indicated.

REFERENCES

1. Knight DC, Eden JA. A review of the clinical effects of phytoestrogens. Obstet Gynecol 1996; 87: 897–904
2. Harbone JB, Baxter H, eds. Phytochemical dictionary. Basingstoke, England: Burgess Science Press. 1995
3. Adlercreutz H, Mazur W. Phyto-oestrogens and Western diseases. Ann Med 1997; 29: 95–120
4. Barnes S, Sfakianos J, Coward L, Kirk M. Soy isoflavonoids and cancer prevention. Underlying biochemical and pharmacological issues. Adv Exp Med Biol 1996; 401: 87–100
5. Setchell KD, Zimmer-Nechemias L, Cai J, Heubi JE. Exposure of infants to phyto-oestrogens from soy-based infant formula. Lancet 1997; 350: 23–27
6. Xu X, Harris KS, Wang HJ et al. Bioavailability of soybean isoflavones depends upon gut microflora in women. J Nutr 1995; 125: 2307–2315
7. Tew BY, Xu X, Wang HJ et al. A diet high in wheat fiber decreases the bioavailability of soybean isoflavones in a single meal fed to women. J Nutr 1996; 126: 871–877
8. Karr SC, Lampe JW, Hutchins AM, Slavin JL. Urinary isoflavonoid excretion is dose dependent at low to moderate levels of soy-protein consumption. Am J Clin Nutr 1997; 66: 46–51
9. Hutchins AM, Slavin JL, Lampe JW. Urinary isoflavonoid phytoestrogen and lignan excretion after consumption of fermented and unfermented soy products. J Am Diet Assoc 1995; 95: 545–551
10. Morton MS, Wilcox G, Wahlqvist ML, Griffiths K. Determination of lignans and isoflavonoids in human female plasma following dietary supplementation. J Endocrinol 1994; 142: 251–259
11. Fukutake M, Takahashi M, Ishida K et al. Quantification of genistein and genistin in soybeans and soybean products. Food Chem Toxicol 1996; 34: 457–461
12. Anthony MS, Clarkson TB, Hughes CL et al. Soybean isoflavones improve cardiovascular risk factors without affecting the reproductive system of peripubertal rhesus monkeys. J Nutr 1996; 126: 43–50
13. Messina M, Barnes S. The role of soy products in reducing risk of cancer. J Natl Cancer Inst 1991; 83: 541–546
14. Franke A. Isoflavone content of breast milk and soy formula: benefits and risks [letter]. Clin Chem 1997; 43: 850–851
15. Hatano K, Kojima M, Tanokura M,, Takahashi K. Solution structure of bromelain inhibitor IV from pineapple stem. Structural similarity with Bowman-Birk trypsin/chymotrypsin inhibitor from soybean. Biochemistry 1996; 30: 5379–5384
16. St Clair WH, St Clair DK. Effect of the Bowman-Birk protease inhibitor on the expression of oncogenes in the irradiated rat colon. Cancer Res 1991; 51: 4539–4543
17. St Clair WH, Billings PC, Carew JA et al. Suppression of dimethylhydrazine-induced carcinogenesis in mice by dietary addition of the Bowman-Birk protease inhibitor. Cancer Res 1990; 50: 580–586
18. Messadi DV, Billings P, Shklar G, Kennedy AR. Inhibition of oral carcinogenesis by a protease inhibitor. J Natl Cancer Inst 1986; 76: 447–452
19. Oreffo VI, Billings PC, Kennedy AR, Witschi H. Acute effects of the Bowman-Birk protease inhibitor in mice. Toxicology 1991; 69: 165–176
20. Billings PC, St Clair W, Owen AJ, Kennedy AR. Potential intracellular target proteins of the anticarcinogenic Bowman-Birk protease inhibitor identified by affinity chromatography. Cancer Res 1988; 48: 1798–1802
21. Schelp FP, Pongpaew P. Protection against cancer through nutritionally-induced increase of endogenous proteinase inhibitors – a hypothesis. Int J Epidemiol 1988; 17: 287–292
22. Clawson GA. Protease inhibitors and carcinogenesis. A review. Cancer Invest 1996; 14: 597–608
23. Yavelow J, Finlay TH, Kennedy AR, Troll W. Bowman-Birk soybean protease inhibitor as an anticarcinogen. Cancer Res 1983; 43: 2454S–2459S
24. Kennedy AR. The evidence for soybean products as cancer preventive agents. J Nutr 1995; 125: 733S–743S
25. Kirkman LM, Lampe JW, Campbell DR et al. Urinary lignan and isoflavonoid excretion in men and women consuming vegetable and soy diets. Nutr Cancer 1995; 24: 1–12
26. Nair PP, Turjman N, Kessie G et al. Diet, nutrition intake, and metabolism in populations at high and low risk for colon cancer. Dietary cholesterol, beta-sitosterol, and stigmasterol. Am J Clin Nutr 1984; 40: 927–930
27. Hirai K, Shimazu C, Takezoe R, Ozeki Y. Cholesterol, phytosterol

and polyunsaturated fatty acid levels in 1982 and 1957 Japanese diets. J Nutr Sci Vitaminol 1986; 32: 363–372
28. Reinli K, Block G. Phytoestrogen content of foods – a compendium of literature values. Nutr Cancer 1996; 26: 123–148
29. Elias R, De Meo M, Vidal-Ollivier E et al. Antimutagenic activity of some saponins isolated from *Calendula officinalis* L., *C. arvensis* L. and *Hedera helix* L. Mutagenesis 1990; 5: 327–331
30. Nakashima H, Okubo K, Honda Y et al. Inhibitory effect of glycosides like saponin from soybean on the infectivity of HIV in vitro. AIDS 1989; 3: 655–658
31. Graf E, Eaton JW. Dietary suppression of colonic cancer. Fiber or phytate? Cancer 1985; 56: 717–718
32. Vucenik I, Tomazic VJ, Fabian D, Shamsuddin AM. Antitumor actitivity of phytic acid (inositol hexaphosphate) in murine transplanted and metastatic fibrosarcoma, a pilot study. Cancer Lett 1992; 659–613
33. Baten A, Ullah A, Tomazic VJ, Shamsuddin AM. Inosito-phosphate-induced enhancement of natural killer cell activity correlates with tumor suppression. Carcinogenesis 1989; 10: 1595–1598
34. Rao PS, Liu XK, Das DK et al. Protection of ischemic heart from reperfusion injury by myo-inositol hexaphosphate, a natural antioxidant. Ann Thorac Surg 1991; 52: 908–912
35. MacRae WD, Hudson JB, Towers GH. The antiviral action of lignans. Planta Med 1989; 55: 531–535
36. Hirano T, Fukuoka K, Oka K et al. Antiproliferative activity of mammalian lignan derivatives against the human breast carcinoma cell line, ZR-75–1. Cancer Invest 1990; 8: 595–602
37. Hartman PE, Shankel DM. Antimutagens and anticarcinogens: a survey of putative interceptor molecules. Environ Mol Mutagen 1990; 15: 145–182
38. Hirano T, Gotoh M, Oka K. Natural flavonoids and lignans are potent cyto-static agents against human leukemic HL-60 cells. Life Sci 1994; 55: 1061–1069
39. Naim M, Gestetner B, Zilkah S et al. Soybean isoflavones. Characterization, determination, and antifungal activity. J Agric Food Chem 1974; 22: 806–810
40. Jha HC, von Recklinghausen G, Zilliken F. Inhibition of in vitro microsomal lipid peroxidation by isoflavonoids. Biochem Pharmacol 1985; 34: 1367–1369
41. Wei H, Wei L, Frenkel K et al. Inhibition of tumor promoter-induced hydrogen peroxide formation in vitro and in vivo by genistein. Nutr Cancer 1993; 20: 1–12
42. Wu ES, Loch JT 3rd, Toder BH et al. Flavones. 3. Synthesis, biological activities, and conformational analysis of isoflavone derivatives and related compounds. J Med Chem 1992; 18: 3519–3525
43. Hirano T, Oka K, Akiba M. Antiproliferative effects of synthetic and naturally occurring flavonoids on tumor cells of the human breast carcinoma cell line, ZR-75–1. Res Commun Chem Pathol Pharmacol 1989; 64: 69–78
44. Franke AA, Custer LJ. Daidzein and genistein concentrations in human milk after soy consumption. Clin Chem 1996; 42: 955–964
45. Sheehan DM. Isoflavone content of breast milk and soy formulas. benefits and risks [letter]. Clin Chem 1997; 43: 850
46. Medlock KL, Branham WS, Sheehan DM. The effects of phytoestrogens on neonatal rat uterine growth and development. Proc Soc Exp Biol Med 1995; 208: 307–313
47. Adlercreutz H, van der Wildt J, Kinzel J et al. Lignan and isoflavonoid conjugates in human urine. J Steroid Biochem Mol Biol 1995; 52: 97–103
48. Lu LJ, Anderson KE, Grady JJ et al. Effects of soya consumption for one month on steroid hormones in premenopausal women. Implications for breast cancer risk reduction. Cancer Epidemiol Biomarkers Prev 1996; 5: 63–70
49. Cassidy AR, Bingham S, Setchell KD. Biological effects of a diet of soy protein rich in isoflavones on the menstrual cycle of premenopausal women. Am J Clin Nutr 1994; 60: 333–340
50. Petrakis NL, Barnes S, King EB et al. Stimulatory influence of soy protein isolate on breast secretion in pre- and postmenopausal women. Cancer Epidemiol Biomarkers Prev 1996; 5: 785–794
51. Wang TT, Sathyamoorthy N, Phang JM. Molecular effects of genistein on estrogen receptor mediated pathways. Carcinogenesis 1996; 17: 271–275
52. Baird DD, Umbach DM, Lansdell L et al. Dietary intervention study to assess estrogenicity of dietary soy among postmenopausal women. J Clin Endocrinol Metab 1995; 80: 1685–1690
53. Makela S, Poutanen M, Lehtimaki J et al. Estrogen-specific 17 beta-hydroxysteroid oxidoreductase type 1 (E.C. 1.1.1.62) as a possible target for the action of phytoestrogens. Proc Soc Exp Biol Med 1995; 208: 51–59
54. Sathyamoorthy N, Wang TT, Phang JM. Stimulation of pS2 expression by diet-derived compounds. Cancer Res 1994; 54: 957–961
55. Whitten PL, Lewis C, Russel E, Naftolin F. Potential adverse effects of phytoestrogens. J Nutr 1995; 125: 771S–776S
56. Price KR, Fenwick GR. Naturally occurring oestrogens in foods – a review. Food Addit Contam 1985; 2: 73–106
57. Fortunati N, Fissore F, Fassari A et al. Sex steroid binding protein exerts a negative control on estradiol action in MCF-7 cells (human breast cancer) through cyclic adenosine 3′5′-monophosphate and protein kinase A. Endocrinology 1996; 137: 686–692
58. Barnes S, Peterson TG, Coward L. Rationale for the use of genistein-containing soy matrices in chemoprevention trials for breast and prostate cancer. J Cell Biochem Suppl 1995; 22: 181–187
59. Wei H, Bowen R, Cai Q et al. Antioxidant and antipromotional effects of the soybean isoflavone genistein. Proc Soc Exp Biol Med 1995; 208: 124–130
60. Fotsis T, Pepper M, Adlercreutz H et al. Genistein, a dietary-derived inhibitor of in vitro angiogenesis. Proc Natl Acad Sci USA 1993; 90: 2690–2694
61. Martin ME, Haourigui M, Pelissero C et al. Interactions between phytoestrogens and human sex steroid binding protein. Life Sci 1996; 58: 429–436
62. Evans BA, Griffiths K, Morton MS. Inhibition of 5 alpha-reductase in genital skin fibroblasts and prostate tissue by dietary lignans and isoflavonoids. J Endocrinol 1995; 147: 295–302
63. Eaton EA, Walle UK, Lewis AJ et al. Flavonoids, potent inhibitors of the human P-form phenolsulfotransferase. Potential role in drug metabolism and chemoprevention. Drug Metab Dispos 1996; 24: 232–237
64. Wilcox JN, Blumenthal BF. Thrombotic mechanisms in atherosclerosis. Potential impact of soy proteins. J Nutr 1995; 125: 631S–638S
65. Potter SM. Soy protein and serum lipids. Curr Opin Lipidol 1996; 7: 260–264
66. Messina MJ, Persky V, Setchell KD, Barnes S. Soy intake and cancer risk: a review of the in vitro and in vivo data. Nutr Cancer 1994; 21: 113–131
67. Adlercreutz H, Honjo H, Higashi A et al. Urinary excretion of lignans and isoflavonoid phytoestrogens in Japanese men and women consuming a traditional Japanese diet. Am J Clin Nutr 1991; 54: 1093–1100
68. Hagmann W. Cell proliferation status, cytokine action and protein tyrosine phosphorylation modulate leukotriene biosynthesis in a basophil leukaemia and a mastocytoma cell line. Biochem J 1994; 299: 467–472
69. Okura A, Arakawa H, Oka H et al. Effect of genistein on topoisomerase activity and on the growth of [Val 12]Ha-ras-transformed NIH 3T3 cells. Biochem Biophys Res Commun 1988; 157: 183–189
70. Markovits J, Linassier C, Fosse P et al. Inhibitory effects of the tyrosine kinase inhibitor genistein on mammalian DNA topoisomerase II. Cancer Res 1989; 49: 5111–5117
71. Linassier C, Pierre M, Le Pecq JB, Pierre J. Mechanisms of action in NIH-3T3 cells of genistein, an inhibitor of EGF receptor tyrosine kinase activity. Biochem Pharmacol 1990; 39: 187–193
72. Nishibe S, Wahl MI, Rhee SG, Carpenter G. Tyrosine phosphorylation of phospholipase C-II in vitro by the epidermal growth factor receptor. J Biol Chem 1989; 264: 10 335–10 338
73. Cochet C, Filhol O, Payrastre B et al. Interaction between the epidermal growth factor receptor and phosphoinositide kinases. J Biol Chem 1991; 266: 637–644
74. Nishida E, Hoshi M, Miyata Y et al. Tyrosine phosphorylation by

the epidermal growth factor receptor kinase induces functional alteration in microtubule-associated protein 2. J Biol Chem 1987; 262: 16 200–16 204
75. Barnes S, Peterson TG. Biochemical targets of the isoflavone genistein in tumor cell lines. Proc Soc Exp Biol Med 1995; 208: 103–108
76. Ingram D, Sanders K, Kolybaba M, Lopez D. Case-control study of phyto-oestrogens and breast cancer. Lancet 1997; 350: 990–994
77. Lee HP, Gourley L, Duffy SW et al. Dietary effects on breast-cancer risk in Singapore. Lancet 1991; 337: 1197–1200
78. Hirose K, Tajima K, Hamajima N et al. A large-scale, hospital-based case-control study of risk factors of breast cancer according to menopausal status. Jpn J Cancer Res 1995; 86: 146–154
79. Barnes S, Peterson TG, Grubbs C, Setchell K. Potential role of dietary isoflavones in the prevention of cancer. Adv Exp Med Biol 1994; 354: 135–147
80. Wu AH, Ziegler RG, Horn-Ross PL. Tofu and risk of breast cancer in Asian-Americans. Cancer Epidemiol Biomarkers Prev 1996; 5: 901–906
81. Peterson G, Barnes S. Genistein inhibition of the growth of human breast cancer cells. independence from estrogen receptors and the multi-drug resistance gene. Biochem Biophys Res Commun 1991; 179: 661–667
82. Peterson G, Barnes S. Genistein inhibits both estrogen and growth factor-stimulated proliferation of human breast cancer cells. Cell Growth Differ 1996; 7: 1345–1351
83. Peterson TG, Coward L, Kirk M et al. The role of metabolism in mammary epithelial cell growth inhibition by the isoflavones genistein and biochanin A. Carcinogenesis 1996; 17: 1861–1869
84. Pagliacci MC, Smacchia M, Migliorati G et al. Growth-inhibitory effects of the natural phyto-oestrogen genistein in MCF-7 human breast cancer cells. Eur J Cancer 1994; 30A: 1675–1682
85. Lamartiniere CA, Moore J, Holland M, Barnes S. Neonatal genistein chemoprevents mammary cancer. Proc Soc Exp Biol Med 1995; 208: 120–123
86. Murrill WB, Brown NM, Zhang JX et al. Prepubertal genistein exposure suppresses mammary cancer and enhances gland differentiation in rats. Carcinogenesis 1996; 17: 1451–1457
87. Barnes S, Grubbs C, Setchell K, Carlson J. Soybeans inhibit mammary tumors in models of breast cancer. Prog Clin Biol Res 1990; 347: 239–253
88. Adlercreutz H, Markkanen H, Watanabe S. Plasma concentrations of phyto-oestrogens in Japanese men. Lancet 1993; 342: 1209–1210
89. Kyle E, Neckers L, Takimoto C et al. Genistein-induced apoptosis of prostate cancer cells is preceded by a specific decrease in focal adhesion kinase activity. Mol Pharmacol 1997; 51: 193–200
90. Pollard M, Luckert PH. Influence of isoflavones in soy protein isolates on development of induced prostate-related cancers in L-W rats. Nutr Cancer 1997; 28: 41–45
91. Peterson G, Barnes S. Genistein and biochanin A inhibit the growth of human prostate cancer cells but not epidermal growth factor receptor tyrosine autophosphorylation. Prostate 1993; 22: 335–345
92. Anderson JW, Johnstone BM, Cook-Newell ME. Meta-analysis of the effects of soy protein intake on serum lipids. N Engl J Med 1995; 333: 276–282
93. Gooderham MH, Adlercreutz H, Ojala ST et al. A soy protein isolate rich in genistein and daidzein and its effects on plasma isoflavone concentrations, platelet aggregation, blood lipids and fatty acid composition of plasma phospholipid in normal men. J Nutr 1996; 126: 2000–2006
94. Potter SM. Overview of proposed mechanisms for the hypocholesterolemic effect of soy. J Nutr 1995; 125: 606S–611S
95. Raines EW, Ross R. Biology of atherosclerotic plaque formation. Possible role of growth factors in lesion development and the potential impact of soy. J Nutr 1995; 125: 624S–630S
96. Wagner JD, Cefalu WT, Anthony MS et al. Dietary soy protein and estrogen replacement therapy improve cardiovascular risk factors and decrease aortic cholesteryl ester content in ovariectomized cynomolgus monkeys. Metabolism 1997; 46: 698–705
97. Arjmandi BH, Alekel L, Hollis BW et al. Dietary soybean protein prevents bone loss in an ovariectomized rat model of osteoporosis. J Nutr 1996; 126: 161–167
98. Kruse FE, Joussen AM, Fotsis T et al. Inhibition of neovascularization of the eye by dietary factors exemplified by isoflavonoids. Ophthalmologe 1997; 94: 152–156 (in German)

CHAPTER CONTENTS

113

Tabebuia avellanedae (LaPacho, Pau D'Arco, Ipe Roxo)

Terry Willard, PhD

Tabebuia avellanedae (family: Bignoniaceae)
Tabebuia ipe
Tabebuia cassinoides
Tecoma ochracea
Common names: LaPacho, Pau D'Arco, Ipe Roxo

INTRODUCTION

The taxanomical division of plants with medicinal uses in the Bignoniaceae family is confused. The literature often interchanges the genera of *Tecoma* and Tabebuia. At least four species have been called LaPacho:

- *Tecoma ochracea*
- *Tecoma ipe*
- *Tabebuia cassinoides*
- *Tabebuia avellanedae.*

This chapter considers the *Tabebuia* genus.

GENERAL DESCRIPTION

The tree from which LaPacho is obtained is a member of the Bignoniaceae family known as *Tabebuia avellanedae* or *Tabebuia ipe*. This tropical tree, native to Brazil, can grow up to 125 feet tall and has rose to violet-colored flowers which bloom in profusion just before the new leaves appear.

There are about 100 species of these evergreen trees or shrubs, native to tropical America. The leaves are opposite, long-petiolate, digitately five- or seven-foliate. The leaflets are entire or toothed; the flowers large in terminal cymes or panicles; the calyx tubular or campanulate, closed in bud, variously cleft or toothed in anthesis; the corolla tubes ampliate, the limb somewhat bilate; the stamens four; the capsule slender-cylindric, suterete; and the seeds broadly winged.

The trees of this genus are very showy when in flower as they usually blossom when leafless. Because the taxonomy of these plants is so difficult, it is quite possible that there is confusion among even trained gatherers.

One specific way to distinguish the species is at the seedling stage. The four-leaf clover-like cotyledons are distinctively deeply cleft.[1]

CHEMICAL COMPOSITION

Many of the studies and chemical analyses on *Tabebuia* spp. have been performed on the heart wood, while the bark is the product available in the market place and the part utilized in folklore. The major components of *Tabebuia avellanedae* are 16 quinones (mostly with C_{15} skeleton) containing both naphthoquinones (seven, C_{10}–C_5) and anthraquinones (nine, C_{14}–C_1). Both of these groups of quinones rarely occur in the same plant. The lapachol content is usually 2–7%. The quinones are listed in Table 113.1.

Other compounds found in the heart wood include lapachenole, quercetin, and *o*- and *p*-hydroxybenzoic acids.[2]

Lapachol content can be estimated by study of the yellowish flaky powder found on the surface of the fractured wood chips or bark. If the lapachol content is over 1–2%, mixing with dilute (5%) NaOH generates, due to a litmus-type reaction, a red-brown solution. There is no color if the content is below 0.5%. Exact concentration can be determined by titrating the NaOH reaction or by chromatography.[3]

A recent analysis of 10 products found in the market place showed that only one contained lapachol (and only in trace amounts) and the other nine had none. This suggests that many of the products now present on the market are not truly *Tabebuia* spp., that the wrong part of the plant is being marketed, or that processing and transportation have damaged the product. This might explain the variation in results practitioners have experienced. Standardization of LaPacho products for lapachol or naphthoquinone content is needed to solve this problem.

Table 113.1 Quinones in *Tabebuia avellanedae*

Naphthoquinones
- Lapachol
- Menaquinone-l
- Deoxylapachol
- Beta-lapachone
- Alpha-lapachone
- Dehydro-alpha-lapachone

Anthraquinones
- 2-Methylanthraquinone
- 2-Hydroxymethylanthraquinone
- 2-Acetoxymethylanthraquinone
- Anthraquinone-2-aldehyde
- 1-Hydroxyanthraquinone
- 1-Methoxyanthraquinone
- 2-Hydroxy-3-methylquinone
- Tabebuin (a newly discovered compound)

HISTORY AND FOLK USE

The native Indians of Brazil also refer this tree as Pau D'Arco or Ipe Roxo. The inner bark has been used for medicinal purposes for centuries as a folk remedy for a wide variety of afflictions, including:[4,5–7]

- boils
- chlorosis
- colitis
- diarrhea
- dysentery
- enuresis
- fever
- pharyngitis
- snakebite
- syphilis
- wounds
- ulcers
- respiratory problems
- arthritis
- cystitis
- constipation
- prostatitis
- poor circulation
- constipation
- cancer of the esophagus, head, intestine, lung, prostate and tongue.

It is reported to be alexiteric, analgesic, anodyne, antidotal, antimicrobial, diuretic, and fungicidal.[4]

PHARMACOLOGY

During the past century, LaPacho has been subjected to scientific scrutiny. The first active constituent to be studied, lapachol, was isolated by Paterno in 1882 (see Fig. 113.1). Its structure was determined by Hooker in 1896. In 1927, Fieser synthesized lapachol. It has since been studied by numerous researchers.

It is interesting to note that many of the scientific studies have found LaPacho and lapachol to be more effective in treating malaria and cancerous tumors through oral ingestion rather than intravenous or intramuscular injection.[8]

An herbalist's interpretation would be that the body's recuperative powers are more effectively stimulated

Figure 113.1 Lapachol.

by the more natural route of nutrient plant material absorption through the digestive tract. Although most of the studies are on individual chemicals, some show significantly better results with the whole extract and diminishing effectiveness as the extracts are refined or individual chemicals are tested.[8]

Antimicrobial activity

Antibacterial activity

In 1956, a research team at the Universidade do Recife in Brazil reported that lapachol isolated from the *Tabebuia avellanedae* tree exhibited antimicrobial activity against Gram-positive and acid-fast bacteria, and *Brucella* sp.[9]

It is important to note that the research team found that progressive purification reduced the antimicrobial activity of the extract. This led to the conclusion that there was more than one active substance present in the original extract.

Later that year the researchers published a paper proclaiming a new antibiotic substance from *Tabebuia avellanedae* which demonstrated "strong anti-*Brucella* activity and fungistatic behavior".[10] They eventually found that, along with lapachol, the extract of the Tabebuia tree contained alpha-lapachone, beta-zlapachone, and a newly discovered quinone which they named xyloidone.

In 1967, another group of researchers discovered seven naphthoquinones, nine anthraquinones, lapachenole, quercetin and *o*- and *p*-hydroxybenzoic acids in the heartwood of the tree.[11] Several of these exhibit strong microbicidal and fungicidal activities (see Table 113.2). Naphthoquinones are highly effective against *Candida albicans* and *Tricophyton mentagrophytes*.[12]

Lapachol has been shown to have both antimicrobial and antiviral activity.[13–15] Beta-lapachone shows diversified antiparasitic activity as well as antiviral action.[16,17] Alpha-lapachone is also active against certain parasites, and xyloidone is active against numerous bacteria and fungi.[18,19] Another LaPacho component, the flavonoid quercetin, is cytotoxic for certain parasites.[20]

Xyloidone is effective against a wide array of organism, such as *Staphylococcus aureus* and the *Brucella* species. The causative agents of tuberculosis, dysentery, and anthrax are also inhibited by xyloidone. In addition to its activity against a variety of bacteria, this quinone inhibits several species of fungus (including *Candida albicans*, *C. kruzei*, and *C. neoformans*).

Mechanism of action

Lapachol, like many naphthoquinones, acts as a respiratory poison by interfering with electron transport in microbes.[21] Research showed in 1946 that drug suppression of malarial parasites could usually be correlated with the inhibition of their oxygen uptake.[22] In 1947, lapachol was found, at concentrations of 100 mg/L, to inhibit O_2 uptake by *Plasmodium knowles* by 74% and succinate oxidase systems by 26%.[23] In the following year, lapachol was found to exhibit antimalarial activity against *Plasmodium lophurae*,[24] suggesting respiratory poisoning as a likely mechanism.

Mitochondrial respiration is inhibited by 50% at a lapachol concentration of less than 110 μmol/L.[25] Increasing doses of lapachol produced progressive respiratory inhibition in tumor cells isolated from animals. Oxygen consumption and oxygen metabolite production

Table 113.2 Antimicrobial activity of *Tabebuia avellanedae**

Microorganism	Lapachol	Chorohidro-lapachol	Alpha-lapachone	Beta-lapachone	Xiloidona
B. sutilus	60.0–80.0	8.0–10.0	40.0–50.0	1.0–2.0	4.0–6.0
B. mycoides	40.0–60.0	10.0–15.0	40.0–50.0	5.0–8.0	20.0–30.0
B. anthracis	40.0–60.0	20.0–30.0	40.0–50.0	4.0–6.0	20.0–30.0
S. aureus	60.0–80.0	30.0–40.0	30.0–40.0	2.0–4.0	15.0–20.0
Sar. lutea	40.0–60.0	15.0–20.0	30.0–40.0	4.0–6.0	20.0–30.0
S. hemolyticus	>100.0	60.0–80.0	60.0–80.0	10.0–15.0	>50.0
M. tuberculosis	80.0–100.0	40.0–60.0	30.0–50.0	10.0–15.0	10.0–15.0
M. smegmatis	80.0–100.0	60.0–80.0	30.0–50.0	15.0–20.0	15.0–20.0
M. phisi	60.0–80.0	40.0–60.0	20.0–30.0	10.0–15.0	8.0–10.0
N. asteroides	>100	40.0–60.0	60.0–80.0	10.0–15.0	20.0–30.0
N. catarrhalis	40.0–60.0	30.0–50.0	80.0–100.0	10.0–15.0	<20.0
E. coli	>100.0	>100.0	>100.0	>100.0	>100.0
K. pneumonia	>100.0	>100.0	>100.0	>100.0	>100.0
S. typhosa	>100.0	>100.0	>100.0	>100.0	>100.0
Br. suis	15.0–20.0	2.0–4.0	20.0–30.0	0.6–1.0	0.8–1.0
Br. abortus	15.0–20.0	2.0–4.0	30.0–40.0	1.0–2.0	1.5–2.0
Br. melitensis	10.0–15.0	2.0–4.0	30.0–40.0	1.0–2.0	1.5–2.0
C. albicans	>100.0	40.0–60.0	80.0–100.0	80.0–100.0	30.0–50.0
C. kruzei	>100.0	40.0–60.0	80.0–100.0	80.0–100.0	50.0–60.0
C. neoformans	>100.0	40.0–60.0	50.0–80.0	30.0–50.0	40.0–60.0

*Minimum concentration of inhibition (mcg/ml).

are inhibited in neutrophils upon administration of lapachol.[26]

The exact site at which lapachol acts has been the subject of some controversy. Some researchers have concluded that 2-hydroxy-3-alkyl-1,4 naphthoquinones, such as lapachol, act just after cytochrome c in the respiratory chain,[27] while others suggest that lapachol exhibited an oligomycin-like action in mitochondria, acting just after cytochrome b.[21] It has been hypothesized that naphthoquinones either prevent an interaction between cytochromes b and c, or act directly on an unknown enzyme between the two.[28] The inhibitory action can be reversed by the addition of 2,4-dinitrophenol, suggesting that lapachol may act on energy conservation reactions.[18]

Lapachol has now been shown to act as an uncoupler of oxidative phosphorylation. Lapachol prevents ATP synthesis by stimulating respiration in the absence of a phosphate acceptor. This effect is most pronounced at a high pH level where lipid solubility is the lowest.[29]

Hadler & Moreau[25] studied lapachol in combination with showdomycin and demonstrated that lapachol exposes a mitochondrial thiol group which occupies a pivotal position between the cycle that meshes with the respiratory chain and the cycle that meshes with ATP. They believe the side chain acts as a swinging arm while the remainder of the lapachol molecule is embedded in a lipid matrix.[30]

In addition to inhibiting cellular respiration and uncoupling oxidative phosphorylation, lapachol inhibits certain enzymes. In particular, it is a competitive inhibitor of glycolase I in erythrocytes. The side chain is again thought to be significant in this action. Lapachol also demonstrates non-competitive inhibition of alpha-ketoaldehyde dehydrogenase, leading to the accumulation of toxic alpha-ketoaldehydes.[30] Lapachol demonstrated 64% inhibition of 3-alpha-hydroxysteroid mediated transhydrogenase at a concentration of 10^{-5} M (well within dosage range).[31]

Antiviral activity

Lapachol has proven to be active against certain viral strains, including herpes virus hominis types I and II.[31] Hydroxynaphthoquinone has been shown to effectively inhibit four influenza viruses. Lapachol also significantly inhibits poliovirus and vesicular stomatitis virus.[14]

Studies of beta-lapachone's antiviral activity have offered insights into the mechanism of this powerful quinone. In experiments with viruses, beta-lapachone demonstrated its ability to inhibit certain enzymes, such as DNA and RNA polymerases.[32] Beta-lapachone was tested against avian myeloblastosis virus and Rauscho murine leukemia virus and found to inhibit retrovirus reverse transcriptase.[33] In the presence of dithioreitol, beta-lapachone inhibits eukaryotic DNA polymerase-alpha activity. Although the mechanism of action for enzyme inhibition is complex, it may be related to superoxide production.[32] This in turn may aid in explaining the structural changes in the DNA of the epimastigotes. The site of action appears to be the enzyme protein. This has great significance for possible treatment of both HIV and HLBV (the implicated viruses in AIDS and Epstein–Barr syndrome).

Beta-lapachone also inhibits Friend virus and was the only substance among a number tested which prolonged survival time of chickens infected intraperitoneally with Rous sarcoma virus.[34]

Antiparasitic activity

The trematode *Schistosoma mansoni* is the causative agent of the common tropical disease schistosomiasis. The cercariae of this blood fluke live in water and enter the host by penetrating the skin. This debilitating disease, a serious problem in many tropical areas, causes weakening of the host and increases susceptibility to a variety of other pathogens, some of which may be fatal.

Lapachol has been tested as a topical barrier to the cercariae and has been found to be highly effective at preventing its penetration.[32,35] Oral lapachol was also tested and found to significantly reduce penetration. After being consumed, the lapachol was secreted onto the skin, apparently by the sebaceous glands, where it again acted as a topical barrier. The cercariae seek to penetrate the host through or near the sebaceous glands, which suggests that dietary administration of lapachol would be an efficient means of protecting against infection. Although the mechanism for this anti-schistosomal activity is relatively unknown, Pinto thought that the side chain was involved, and noted that effective barriers are liposoluble.

Alpha-lapachone and beta-lapachone, also components of LaPacho, both exhibited activity against *S. mansoni*.[13] The activity of beta-lapachone against viruses and parasites has been studied in an attempt to understand the mechanism by which this quinone works. Beta-lapachone is notably effective against *Trypanosoma cruzi*, a zoomastigote responsible for trypanosomiasis, or Chaga's disease. This disease occurs in both acute and chronic forms and has no known cure.

Beta-lapachone causes complete inhibition of *T. cruzi* at concentrations of 0.8–5.0 μg/mL and progressively inhibits motility with increasing concentrations. When *T. cruzi* epimastigotes were incubated with the quinone, they were subject to nuclear, mitochondrial, endoplasmic reticular, and cytoplasmic membrane damage, and underwent alterations in the chromatin distribution. Respiration rates were lowered, the mitochondria became swollen, and glucose and pyruvate oxidation was inhibited. Lipid peroxidation was stimulated, which resulted in decreased cell viability.

In addition, in vitro testing resulted in the rapid decay of DNA, RNA, and protein, and DNA breakage in *T. cruzi*. This was accompanied by inhibition of DNA, RNA, and protein synthesis and instigation of "unscheduled" DNA synthesis.[36]

It is thought that this toxic action against parasites is at least partly due to superoxide production.[37] Both O_2^- and H_2O_2 are intermediates of oxygen reduction and both are toxic to living organisms. When beta-lapachone is introduced to *T. cruzi*, it rapidly enters the epimastigote and is reduced to its semiquinone form in the mitochondria and microsomes of the pathogen.[38] Superoxide is produced by the reduction of molecular oxygen, which is facilitated by auto-oxidation of the semiquinone free radical. Superoxide is then converted to hydrogen peroxide via SOD (superoxide dismutase). Stimulation of lipid peroxidation follows and the cell degenerates.

Anti-neoplastic effects

Due to the folklore information surrounding the tumor-reducing qualities of the herb LaPacho, it underwent extensive study by the National Cancer Institute (NCI). After initial positive results, it was felt that lapachol was the most active anti-neoplastic agent. Lapachol entered phase I clinical trials at NCI in 1968, based on its activity against Walker 256 tumors (with over a 90% confidence rate). During these trials it was difficult to obtain therapeutic blood levels of lapachol without some mild toxic side-effects such as nausea, vomiting, and anti-vitamin K activity. This is quite hard to understand, as latter studies found the toxicity to be very low, with an LD_{50} of 487 mg, about the same as caffeine.[4] The IND (investigative new drug status) for the drug was closed in 1970.[39]

It has been shown, however, that some of the anthraquinones in LaPacho have vitamin K activity, and therefore use of the whole herb would compensate for lapachol's effect on vitamin K.[40]

An analog, dichloroallyl lawsone, which had a better in vivo activity in the Walker 256 system, was selected to replace lapachol with IND approval in 1975. It was found, as was lapachol, to be an inhibitor of oxidative phosphorylation. In Rhesus monkeys it was observed to have some cardiac toxicity. It was decided subsequently that there was little point to any further analog development and the case was closed.[41]

The approach described above indicates a flaw in the underlying philosophy of the pharmaceutical sciences and the NCI program. Since the initial studies came from a whole plant, the detailed studies should have been undertaken on the whole plant: some of the other quinones have also been shown to have anti-neoplastic activities. Was it too complex to consider the chemical reactions of the over 20 components found in the LaPacho? Or was the standard economic/political incentive for patenting an analog an impediment to the investigation of a plant species?

Lapachol is rapidly absorbed through the gastro-intestinal tract after oral administration to rats bearing W-256 tumors. It is taken up by all tissues except the brain and blood cells. A significant amount appears in the tumor after 6 hours, with most of the drug disappearing from the other body tissue. The half-life of i.v. lapachol in mice is 33 minutes (75 minutes in dogs). Lapachol is extensively metabolized and excreted mostly in the feces.[1] Most other analogs had little effect on cancer.[42]

The theories on how lapachol works as an anti-neoplastic agent vary considerably. One of the most prominent involves redox cycle capabilities. The redox function of lapachol was known as early as 1936.[43] In 1947, Ball et al[44] studied the respiratory poison mechanism of naphthoquinones in the i.v. killing of malarial parasites. In 1966, lapachol was shown to stimulate mitochondrial ATPase activity (in the general fashion of uncouplers), while being without effect on ATPase stimulation by dinitrophenol. Its maximum activity is at a high pH where lipid solubility might be expected to be lowest.[10] Lapachol was found to be an in vivo inhibitor of respiration at chemotherapeutic doses.[7] Later, lapachol was shown to augment the flow of electrons from reduced NADP to form oxygen-related free radicals. These seem to be site-specific free radicals that bind to the cancerous DNA or RNA producing either superoxides or free hydroxyl radicals.[45,46]

There seems to be a redox potential which is important for the inhibition of electron transfer in coenzyme Q_{10}.[47] It is argued by Bennett et al[48] that this respiration poisoning is not the mechanism of antitumor activity. Lapachol was shown to significantly reduce the pool of uridine triphosphate (UTP), the largest pool of the pyrimidine nucleotides (exposure time was very short, 2–4 hours).

Lapachol is theorized to be like dichloroallyl lawsone (DCL) in that it blocks pyrimidine biosynthesis through inhibition of dihydroorotate dehydrogenase.[21] It is also believed that the anti-neoplastic activities of lapachol might stem from its interaction with nucleic acids[49] and it is proposed that interaction of the naphthoquinone moiety between base pairs of the DNA helix occurs with subsequent inhibition of DNA replication and/or RNA synthesis. Free amino groups in the sugar moiety are necessary for DNA binding.[49]

Beta-lapachone was shown to decrease the viability of sarcoma cells by stimulating lipid peroxidation. This was accomplished through:[37]

- reduction of lapachone at the mitochondrial and microsomal membranes with generation of the semiquinone form

- autooxidation to produce O_2
- production of H_2O_2 via SOD.

Anti-inflammatory activity

Extracts of the bark from *Tabebuia avellanedae* demonstrate clear anti-inflammatory activity with low toxicity.[50] Tampons soaked in an alcoholic extract of LaPacho have been shown to be very successful against a wide range of inflammations, such as cervicitis and cervicovaginitis.[2,33]

Quercetin

Quercetin is a highly active flavonoid which inhibits a wide range of enzymes and suppresses the synthesis of DNA, RNA, and proteins.[51] Quercetin's cytotoxicity may be due to the fact that it inhibits mitochondrial electron transport.[52] Hodnick et al have noted that quercetin produced a substrate-independent, KCN-insensitive, respiratory burst in mitochondria. Other flavonoids which demonstrated this activity produced O_2^- and H_2O_2, suggesting that quercetin may also generate these cytotoxic chemicals.

Among the enzymes inhibited by quercetin are:[36,37,53]

- NADH oxidase
- phosphodiesterase
- cAMP-independent protein kinases
- Ca^{2+} phospholipid-dependent protein kinase
- tyrosine protein kinases.

Shapiro et al suggested that the cytotoxicity of quercetin may be due to its chelating abilities.[20] It is trypanocidal to *Trypanosoma brucei*, a livestock parasite belonging to the same genus as *Trypanosoma cruzi*. Soon after the parasite enters the host, the host's unsaturated iron-building proteins remove iron from the hemoflagellate. Since the parasite is unable to synthesize heme, it encounters a shortage of iron. By chelating the host's iron, quercetin blocks utilization by the parasite, yet does not adversely affect the host. This flavonoid is also cytotoxic against *Crithidia fasiculata*. The fact that it is small and lithophilic seems to be significant to its activity.

Like lapachol, quercetin inhibited O_2 consumption and H_2O_2 production in neutrophils.[28]

Many flavonoids exhibit antiviral activity. When mice that had been intracerebrally infected with attenuated viruses, including rabies, were given quercetin in their diet, a prophylactic effect was observed.[54] Quercetin inactivates the following viruses:

- herpes simplex type 1
- respiratory syncytial virus
- pseudorabies/Aujesky's virus
- poliovirus type 1
- parainfluenza type 3
- Sindbis virus
- potato virus X.

(Inactivation is defined as reducing viral infectivity tenfold.)

CLINICAL APPLICATION

The spectrum of clinical applications of *Tabebuia avellanedae* is quite broad. Current use has focused on LaPacho's anti-neoplastic and antimicrobial activity. Its use is extremely popular in the treatment of intestinal candidiasis and vaginal candidiasis (topically and internally). There are also many anecdotal reports of remission of different forms of cancer from use of this botanical.[28]

Unfortunately, due to lack of quality control and confusion about the portion of the plant to use (any of the studies and chemical analyses have been done on the heart wood, while the bark is the product available in the market place and discussed in the folklore), it is highly likely that most practitioners are not using effective materials. This could explain varying clinical results.

DOSAGE

The usual form of administration of LaPacho is as a decoction, with the standard dose being 1 cup of decocted bark two to eight times/day. The decoction is made by boiling 1 tsp of LaPacho for each cup of water for 5–15 minutes.

A more precise dosage based on a lapachol content of 2–4% would be 15–20 g of bark boiled in 500 ml or 1 pint of water for 5–15 minutes three to four times daily.

Dosages of other forms (aqueous extract, fluid extract, solid extract) should be based on lapachol content, providing a daily lapachol intake of 1.5–2.0 g/day.

A tampon which has been soaked in the decoction or fluid extract is used in the treatment of vaginitis and cervicitis. The tampon is inserted vaginally and changed every 24 hours until resolution.

TOXICOLOGY

Although anti-vitamin K activity has been reported for lapachol, the presence of several vitamin K-like substances in the whole plant suggests this is not a problem. Lapachol has been reported to have an oral LD_{50} of 1.2–2.4 g/kg in albino rats and 487–621 mg/kg in mice.[55] In comparison, the oral LD_{50} of caffeine is 192 mg/kg in rats and 620 mg/kg in mice.[5]

Chronic administration of lapachol at a dose of 0.0625–0.25 g/kg per day to monkeys produces moderate to severe anemia. The anemia was most pronounced during the first 2 weeks of treatment. Death occurred in monkeys after six doses of lapachol at 0.5 g/kg per day and after five doses of 1.0 g/kg per day.[8]

There have been no reports in the literature of human toxicity when the whole bark as a decoction is used.

REFERENCES

1. Duke JA. Interview. Saturday, February 24, 1984
2. Burnett AR, Thomson RH. Naturally occurring quinones. part x. the quinonoid constituents of *Tabebuia avellanedae* (Bignoniaceae). J Chem Soc (C) 1967: 2100–2104
3. Pfizer C. Antitumor composition from lapachol and its salts, CA70: 9075B. 156
4. Canadian Health Protection Branch. Herbs and botanical preparations. Information Letter 726, Aug 13 1987
5. Duke JA. CRC Handbook of medicinal herbs. Boca Raton, FL: CRC Press. 1985: p 470–473
6. Bernarde A. A Pocket book of Brazilian herbs (folklore – history – uses). Rio de Janeiro: Shogun Editora. 1984: p 22–23
7. Hartwell JL. Plants used against cancer. A survey. Lawrence, MA: Quarterman Publications. 1982
8. Morrison RK, Brown DE, Oleson JJ, Cooney DA. Oral toxicology studies with lapachol. Toxicol Appl Pharmacol 1970; 17: 1–11
9. de Lima OG, d'Albuquerque IL, Machado MP et al. Primeiras Observacoes sobre a acao antimicrobiana do lapachol. Anais da Sociedade de biologica de pernambuco 1956; XIV: 129–135
10. de Lima OG, d'Albuquerque IL, Machado MP et al. Uma Nova substancia Antibiotica isolada do "Pau D'Arco", Tabebuia sp. Anais da Sociedade de biologica de pernambuco 1956; XIV: 136–140
11. Burnett AR, Thomson RH. Naturally occurring quinones. Part X. The Quinonoid Constituents of Tabebuia avellanedae (Bignoniaceae). J Chem Soc (C) 1967; 2100–2104
12. Gershon H, Shanks L. Fungitoxicity of 1,4-naphthoquinones to Candida albicans and Trichophyton mentagrophytes. Can J Microbiol 1975; 21: 1317–1321
13. de Lima OG, d'Albuquerque IL, Machado MP et al. Primeiras Observacoes sobre a acao antimicrobiana do lapachol. Anais da Sociedade de biologica de pernambuco 1956; XIV: 129–135
14. Lagrota M et al. Antiviral activity of lapachol, Rev Microbiol 1983; 14: 21–26
15. Guiraud P, Steinman R, Campos-Takaki GM. Comparison of antibacterial and antifungal activities of lapachol and b-lapachone. Planta Med 1994; 60: 373–374
16. Lopes JN, Cruz FS, Docampo R et al. *In vitro* and *in vivo* evaluation of the toxicity of 1,4-naphthoquinone and 1,2-naphthoquinone derivatives against *Trypanosoma cruzi*. Ann Trop Med Parasit 1978; 72: 523–531
17. Schuerch AR, Wehrli W. β-Lapachone, an inhibitor of oncornavirus reverse transcriptase and eukaryotic DNA polymerase-a. Inhibitory effect, thiol dependency and specificity. Eur J Biochem 1978; 84: 197–205
18. Pinto AV, Pinto MDR, Gilbert B. Schistosomiasis mansoni. blockage of cercarial skin penetration by chemical agents. I. naphthoquinones and derivatives. Trans Royal Soc Trop Med Hyg 1977; 71: 133–135
19. de Lima OG, d'Albuquerqul IL, de Lima CG, Dalia Maia MH. Comunicacao XX. Antividade antimicrobiana de alguns derivados do lapachol em comparacao com a xiloidona, Nova ortonaftoquinona natural isolada de extractos do cerne do "Pau d'Arco" roxo, Tabebuia avellanedae Lor. ex. Griseb. Substancias antimicrobianas de plantas superiores. Revista do Instituto de Antibioticos Recife 1962; 4
20. Shapiro A, Nathan HC, Hunter SH et al. In vivo and in vitro activity by diverse chelators against Trypanosoma brucei. J Protozool 1982; 29: 85–90
21. Howland JL. Uncoupling and inhibition of oxidative phosphorylation by 2-hydroxy-3-alkyl-1,4-naphthoquinones. Biochim Biophys Acta 1963; 77: 659–662
22. Wendel WB. The influence of naphthoquinones upon the respiratory and carbohydrate metabolism of malarial parasites. Fed Proc 1946; 5: 406–407
23. Ball EG, Anfinsen CB, Cooper O. The inhibitory action of naphthoquinones on respiratory processes. J Biol Chem 1947; 168: 257–270
24. Fieser LF, Richardson AP. Naphthoquinone antimalarials. II. Correlation of structure and activity against Plasmodium lophurae in ducks. J Am Chem Soc 1948; 70: 3156–3165
25. Gosalvez M, Garcia-Canero R, Blanco M, Guru charri-Lloyd C. Effects and specificity of anticancer agents on the respiration and energy metabolism of tumor cells. Canc Treat Rep 1976; 60: 1–8
26. Crawford DR, Schneider DL. Identification of ubiquinone-50 in human neutrophils and its role in microbicidal events. J Biol Chem 1982; 257: 6662–6668
27. Wendel WB. The influence of naphthoquinones upon the respiratory and carbohydrate metabolism of malarial parasites. Fed Proc 1946; 5: 406–407
28. Weed B. Second Opinion, Lapacho fight against cancer. Vancouver: Rostrum Communication. 1984
29. Howland JL. Influence of alkylhydroxynaphthoquinones on the mitochondrial oxidation of tetramethyl-p-phenylenediamine. Biochim Biophys Acta 1967; 131: 247–254
30. Hadler HI, Moreau TL. The induction of ATP energized mitochondrial volume changes by the combination of the two antitumour agents showdomycin and lapachol, J Antibiot 1969; 513–520
31. Koide SS. Inhibition of 3a-hydroxysteroid-mediated transhydrogenase of rat liver by various quinones and flavonoids. Biochim Biophys Acta 1962; 59: 708–710
32. Austin FG. Schistosoma mansoni chemoprophylaxis with dietary lapachol. Am J Trop Med Hygiene 1974; 23: 412–419
33. Wanick MC et al. Acao antiinflamatoria e cicatrizante do extrato hidroalcoolico do liber do pau d'arco roxo (*Tabebuia avellanedae*), em pacientes portadoras de cervicites e cervico-vaginites. Separata da Revista do Instituto de Antibioticos 1970; 10: 41–46
34. Schaffner-Sabba K, Schmidt-Ruppin KH, Wehrli W. β-Lapachone. Synthesis of derivatives and activities in tumour models. J Medicinal Chem 1984; 27: 990–994
35. Gilbert B, de Souza JP, Fascio M et al. Schistosomiasis. Protection against infection by terpenoids. An Acad Brasil Cienc 1970; 42: 397–400
36. Goijman SG, Stoppani AOM. Oxygen radicals and macromolecule turnover in Trypanosoma cruzi. Life Chem Rep 1984; 2: 216–221
37. Docampo R, Cruz FS, Boveris A et al. β-Lapachone enhancement of lipid peroxidation and superoxide anion and hydrogen peroxide formation by sarcoma 180 ascites tumor cells. Biochem Pharmacol 1979; 28: 723–728
38. Boveris A, Stoppani AOM, Docampo R, Cruz FS. Superoxide anion production and trypanocidal action of naphthoquinones on Trypanosoma cruzi. Comp Biochem Phys 1978: 327–329
39. Block JB, Serpick AA, Miller W, Wiernik PH. Early clinical studies with lapachol (NSC-11905). Cancer Chemo Rep 1974; 4: 27–28
40. Preusch PC, Suttie J W. Lapachol inhibition of vitamin K epoxide reductase and vitamin K quinone reductase. Arch Biochem Biophys 1984; 234: 405–412
41. McKelvey EM, Lomedica M, Lu K et al. Dichloroallyl lawsone. Clin Pharmacol Ther 1979; 586–590
42. Rao KV. Quinone natural products. Streptonigrin (NSC-45383) and lapachol (NSC-11905) structure-activity relationships. Cancer Chemo Rep 1974; 4: 11–17
43. Ball EG. Studies on oxidation-reduction. XXII. Lapachol, lomatiol, and related compounds. J Biol Chem 1936; 114: 649–655
44. Ball EG, Anfinsen CB, Cooper O. The inhibitory action of naphthoquinones on respiratory processes. J Biol Chem 1947; 168: 257–270
45. Bachur NR, Gordon SL, Gee MV, Kon H. NADPH cytochrome P-450 reductase activation of quinone anticancer agents to free radicals. Proc Natl Acad Sci USA 1979; 76: 954–957
46. Bachur NR, Gordon SL, Gee MV. A general mechanism for microsomal activation of quinone anticancer agents to free radicals. Cancer Res 1978; 38: 1745–1750
47. Iwamoto Y, Hansen IL, Porter TH, Folkers K. Inhibition of coenzyme Q_{10}-enzymes, succinoxidase and NADH-oxidase, by adriamycin and other quinones having antitumor activity. Biochem Biophys Res Comm 1974; 58: 633–638
48. Bennett LL, Smithers D, Rose LM et al. Inhibition of synthesis of pyrimidine nucleotides by 2-hydroxy-3-(3,3-dichloroallyl)-1,4-naphthoquinone. Cancer Res 1979; 39: 4868–4874

49. Lee S-H, Sutherland TO, Deves R, Brodie AF. Restoration of active transport of solutes and oxidative phosphorylation by naphthoquinones in irradiatiated membrane vesicle from Mycobacterium phlei. Proc Natl Acad Sci USA 1980; 77: 102–106
50. Oga S, Sekino T. Toxicidade e Atividade Anti-inflamatoria de Tabebuia avellanedae Lorentz e Griesbach ("Ipe Roxo"). Rev Fac Farm Bioquim S Paulo 1969; 7: 47–53
51. Graziani Y, The effect of quercetin of pp60$^{v\text{-}src}$ kinase activities. Plant flavonoids in biology and medicine: biochemical, pharmacological, and structure–activity relationships. New York: Alan R Liss. 1986: p 301–313
52. Hodnick WF, Roettger WJ, Kung FS. Inhibition of mitochondrial respiration and production of superoxide and hydrogen peroxide by flavonoids. A structure activity study. Plant Flavonoids in Biology and Medicine. Biochemical, Pharmacological, and Structure-Activity Relationships. New York: Alan R Liss. 1986: p 249–252
53. Srivastava AK, Chiasson JL. Effect of quercetin on serine/threonine and tyrosine protein kinases. Plant flavonoids in biology and medicine: biochemical, pharmacological, and structure–activity relationships. New York: Alan R Liss. 1986: p 315–318
54. Selway JWT. Antiviral activity of flavones and flavins. Plant flavonoids in biology and medicine: biochemical, pharmacological, and structure–activity relationships. New York: Alan R Liss. 1986: p 521–536
55. Ball EG. Studies on oxidation-reduction. XXII. Lapachol, Lomatiol, and related compounds. J Biol Chem 1936; 114: 649–655

CHAPTER CONTENTS

114

Tanacetum parthenium (feverfew)

Michael T. Murray, ND

Joseph E. Pizzorno Jr, ND

Tanacetum parthenium (family: Compositae)
Synonym: *Chrysanthemum parthenium*
Common names: feverfew, featherfew

GENERAL DESCRIPTION

Feverfew (*Tanacetum parthenium*) is a composite plant that is cultivated in flower gardens throughout Europe and the United States. The round, leafy, branching stems bear alternate, bipinnate leaves with ovate, hoary-green leaflets. The flowers are small and daisy-like, with yellow disks and from 10 to 20 white, toothed rays. The name feverfew is a corruption of the word febrifuge used to signify its tonic and fever-dispelling properties.

CHEMICAL COMPOSITION

The major active chemicals in the plant are sesquiterpene lactones, principally parthenolide. The flowering herb also contains 0.02–0.07% essential oils (L-camphor, L-borneol, terpenes, and miscellaneous esters).[1,2]

HISTORY AND FOLK USE

Feverfew has been used for centuries as a febrifuge and for the treatment of migraines and arthritis. Other historical uses of feverfew have been in the treatment of anemia, earache, dysmenorrhea, dyspepsia, trauma, and intestinal parasites.[1] It has also been used as an abortifacient, and in gardens to control noxious pests (its pyrethrin component is an effective insecticide and herbicide).

PHARMACOLOGY

Feverfew has demonstrated some remarkable pharmacological effects in experimental studies. Its long folk history of use in the treatment of inflammatory conditions such as fever, arthritis, and migraine suggests that it acts in a fashion similar to that of the more common non-steroidal anti-inflammatory agents (NSAIDs), such as aspirin. Extracts of feverfew have been shown to inhibit the synthesis of compounds which promote inflammation, including inflammatory prostaglandins, leukotrienes, and thromboxanes. Unlike aspirin and other NSAIDs, inhibition by feverfew at the initial stage of synthesis is more like that of cortisone than NSAIDs.[3]

Feverfew also has a favorable effect on the behavior of blood platelets.[3,4] The favorable effects include inhibition of platelet aggregation and the secretion of inflammatory and allergic mediators like histamine and serotonin. Parthenolide components also exert a tonic effect on vascular smooth muscle.[5]

The combined effect on smooth muscle and platelets is probably the factor responsible for feverfew's effect in preventing and treating migraine headaches.

CLINICAL APPLICATIONS

Feverfew has been used for centuries to relieve fever, migraines and arthritis. The only condition with confirmed scientific documentation at the present time is in the prevention and treatment of migraine headache.

Migraine headache

Physician John Hill, in his book *The family herbal* (1772) noted: "In the worst headache this herb exceeds whatever else is known." Recently, there has been tremendous increase in the interest in feverfew for migraine headache. This renewed interest began in 1970s in Britain. Increased public awareness of the herb led to scientific investigation. A 1983 survey found that 70% of 270 migraine sufferers who had eaten feverfew daily for prolonged periods claimed that the herb decreased the frequency and/or intensity of their attacks.[6] Many of these patients had been unresponsive to orthodox medicines. This prompted two clinical investigations of the therapeutic and preventive effects of feverfew in the treatment of migraine.

The first double-blind study was done at the London Migraine Clinic, using patients who reported being helped by feverfew.[6] Those patients who received the placebo (and as a result stopped using feverfew) had a significant increase in the frequency and severity of headache, nausea, and vomiting during the 6 months of the study, while patients taking feverfew showed no change in the frequency or severity of their symptoms. Two patients in the placebo group who had been in complete remission during self-treatment with feverfew leaves developed recurrence of incapacitating migraine and had to withdraw from the study. The resumption of self-treatment led to renewed remission of symptoms in both patients.

The second double-blind study was performed at the University of Nottingham.[7] The results of the study clearly demonstrated that feverfew was effective in reducing the number and severity of migraine attacks. In the study, 72 patients were randomly allocated to receive either one capsule of dried feverfew leaves (82 mg) daily or placebo. After 4 months, patients were transferred to the other treatment for another 4 months. Treatment with feverfew was associated with a reduction in the mean number and severity of attacks and in the degree of vomiting; duration of single attacks was unaltered. The efficacy of feverfew in the prevention of migraine headaches has now been demonstrated in several controlled studies.[8]

Rheumatoid arthritis

Inflammatory compounds released by white blood cells and platelets contribute greatly to the inflammation and cellular damage found in rheumatoid arthritis. The inhibition of the release of inflammatory particles by feverfew is much greater than that achieved by NSAIDs like aspirin.[4] This, coupled with many of feverfew's other effects, indicates that feverfew could greatly reduce inflammation in rheumatoid arthritis.

Although a double-blind, placebo-controlled study demonstrated no apparent benefit from oral feverfew in rheumatoid arthritis, the dosage used was small (76 mg dried, powdered feverfew leaf corresponding to two medium-sized leaves), the level of parthenolide was not determined in the product, and patients continued to take NSAIDs, a practice that has been suggested to reduce the efficacy of feverfew.[9] Therefore, the benefit of feverfew in rheumatoid arthritis has not yet been determined.

DOSAGE

The effectiveness of feverfew is dependent upon adequate levels of parthenolide, the active principle. Unfortunately, recent analyses of the parthenolide content of over 35 different commercial preparations indicate a wide variation in the amount of parthenolide.[10] The majority of products contained no parthenolide or only traces.

The preparations used in successful clinical trials had a parthenolide content of 0.4–0.66%. In order to achieve the benefits noted in the migraine studies, the dosage of parthenolide must be similar. The dosage of feverfew used in the London Migraine Clinic study was one capsule containing 25 mg of the freeze-dried pulverized leaves twice daily. In the Nottingham study it was one capsule containing 82 mg of dried powdered leaves once daily. Therefore, the daily dosage of parthenolide which may be effective in the prevention of a migraine headache is roughly 0.25–0.5 mg.

While these low dosages may be effective in preventing an attack, a higher dose (1–2 g) is necessary during an acute attack:

- dried pulverized leaves: 25–50 mg two times/day.

TOXICITY

There were no reports of toxic reactions in patients taking feverfew in the 6 month migraine study. Feverfew has been used by large numbers of people for many years without reports of toxicity. Chewing the leaves, however, may result in aphthous ulcerations, and some sensitive persons will develop an exudative dermatitis from external contact.[11]

REFERENCES

1. Duke JA. Handbook of medicinal herbs. Boca Raton, Fl: CRC Press. 1985: p 118
2. Bohlmann F, Zdero C. Sesquiterpene lactones and other constituents from *Tanacetum parthenium*. Phytochemistry 1982; 21: 2543–2549
3. Makheja AM, Bailey JM. A platelet phospholipase inhibitor from the medicinal herb feverfew (*Tanacetum parthenium*). Prostagland Leukotri Med 1982; 8: 653–660
4. Heptinstall S, White A, Williamson L, Mitchell JRA. Extracts of feverfew inhibit granule secretion in blood platelets and polymorphonuclear leukocytes. Lancet 1985; i: 1071–1074
5. Barsby RWJ, Salan U, Knight BW, Hoult JRS. Feverfew and vascular smooth muscle. Extracts from fresh and dried plants show opposing pharmacological profiles, dependent upon sesquiterpene lactone content. Planta Medica 1993; 59: 20–25
6. Johnson ES et al. Efficacy of feverfew as prophylactic treatment of migraine. Br Med J 1985; 291: 569–573
7. Murphy JJ, Heptinstall S, Mitchell JRA. Randomized double-blind placebo-controlled trial of feverfew in migraine prevention. Lancet 1988; ii: 189–192
8. Gawel MJ. The use of feverfew in the prophylaxis of migraine attacks. Today's Ther Trends 1995; 13: 79–86
9. Pattrick M et al. Feverfew in rheumatoid arthritis. A double blind, placebo controlled study. Ann Rheum Dis 1989; 48: 547–549
10. Heptinstall S et al. Parthenolide content and bioactivity of feverfew (*Tanacetum parthenium* (L.) Schultz-Bip.). Estimation of commercial and authenticated feverfew products. J Pharm Pharmacol 1992; 44: 391–395
11. Awang DVC. Feverfew. Can Pharm J 1989; 122: 266–270

CHAPTER CONTENTS

115

Taraxacum officinale (dandelion)

Michael T. Murray, ND

Joseph E. Pizzorno Jr, ND

Taraxacum officinale (family: Compositae)
Common names:

- English: dandelion, wet-a-bed, Lion's tooth
- French: dent-de-lion, pissenlit
- German: lowenzahn, pfaffenrohrlein
- Spanish: diente de leon
- Italian: tarassaco
- Chinese: p'u kung ying, Ching p'o po, chiang-nou-ts'ao, huang-hua-tii-ting

GENERAL DESCRIPTION

Dandelion (*Taraxacum officinale*) is a member of the Compositae family and is closely related to chicory.[1] Several origins have been attributed to the name *Taraxacum,* among them the most likely being from the Greek *taraxo* (disorder, disturbance) and *akos* (remedy), *akeomai* (I heal) and from *tharakhcharkon,* possibly a derivative of a Persian-Arabic word for "edible" and the name by which the plant is referred to in a 13th-century Arabian botanical work.

Taraxacum is known around the world by a variety of names. In English speaking countries, dandelion (from the French *dent-de-lion,* referring to the plant's lion's tooth leaves) is its most common name. It is also known as wet-a-bed (after its diuretic action), Lion's tooth, fairy clock, priest's crown, swine's snout, blowball, milk gowan, wild endive, white endive,[4] cankerwort,[5] puffball, and Irish daisy.[1]

Dandelion is a variable perennial, growing to a height of 12 inches. Its spatula-like leaves are deeply toothed, shiny, and hairless, and are arranged in a ground level rosette. The yellow flowers bloom for most of the year, are sensitive to light and weather – opening at daybreak and closing at night fall, and opening in dry weather and closing in wet (a closed dandelion flower signals rain). When the flower matures, it closes up, the petals wither, and it forms into a puffball containing seeds which are dispersed by the breeze.

The rosette formation of grooved leaves channels rainwater into its center and down to a taproot which is thick, dark brown and almost black on the outside. The root is cylindrical, tapering, and somewhat branched. It has a slight odor and a sweetish taste. The inside of dried dandelion root is yellowish, very porous and without pith.

It is believed that the plant originated in Central Asia and spread throughout most of the world, preferring the cooler climates.[1] Although *Taraxacum* is very adaptable, it prefers moist nitrogen-rich soils at altitudes less than 6,000 feet. Most species occur in the temperate zones of the northern hemisphere, with the greatest concentration in north-west Europe.

The portion of the plant that is most commonly used is the root; however, the leaves and whole plant can also be used. In addition to its medicinal use, dandelion is also used as a nutritious food and beverage. Tender leaves are used raw in salads and sandwiches, or lightly cooked as a vegetable. Tea is made from the leaves, coffee substitute from the roots, and wine and schnapps from the flowers.

CHEMICAL COMPOSITION

The primary therapeutic actions of dandelion are believed to be due to the bitter principle taraxacin, various terpenoids, inulin, and its high concentration of nutrients. Other constituents of dandelion which may contribute to its pharmacology include resins, pectin, taraxanthin (a carotenoid pigment in the flowers), fatty acids, and flavonoids.

Many studies show that dandelion is a rich source of vitamins and minerals.[1] The leaves have the highest vitamin A content (14,000 IU/100 g raw) of all greens, as well as ample amounts of vitamins D, B complex, C and minerals such as iron silicon, magnesium, sodium, potassium, zinc, manganese, copper and phosphorus.[1,2] Dandelion also contains relatively high amounts of choline, an important nutrient for the liver.[3]

Taraxacum officinale roots contain the triterpenes β-amyrin, taraxasterol, taraxerol and the sterols sitosterin, stigmasterin and phytosterin (Figs 115.1 and 115.2).[4]

More recent research is now eliciting several compounds which are likely to be clinically significant. Three

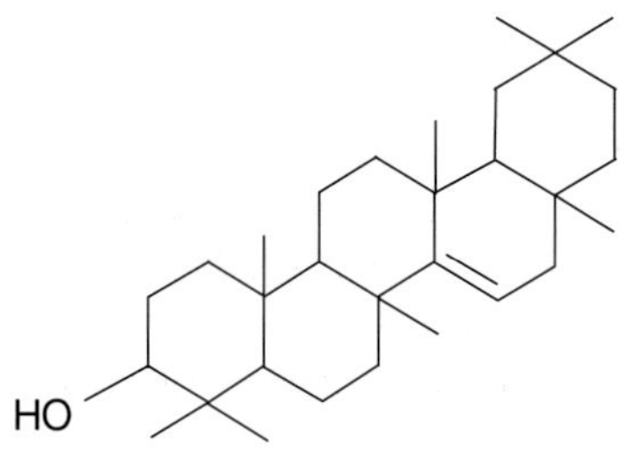

HO

Figure 115.1 Taraxerol.

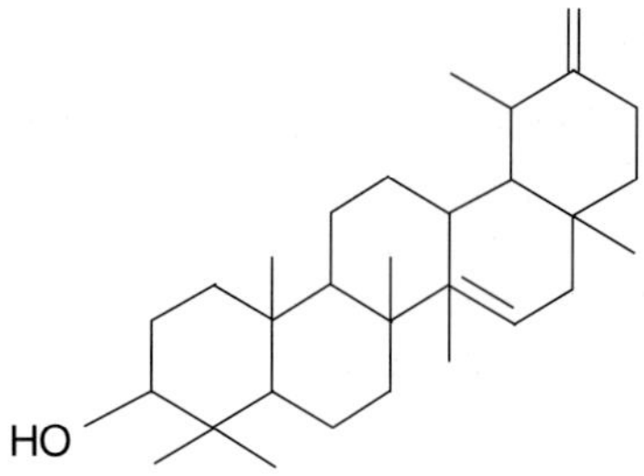

HO

Figure 115.2 Taraxasterol.

flavonoid glycosides – luteolin 7-glucoside and two luteolin 7-diglucosides – have been isolated from dandelion flowers and leaves together with free luteolin and chrysoeriol in the flower tissue. Three hydroxycinnamic acids – chicoric acid, monocaffeyltartaric acid and chlorogenic acid – have been found throughout the plant, and the coumarins, cichoriin and aesculin, have been identified in leaf extracts. Chicoric acid and the related monocaffeyltartaric acid were found to be the major phenolic constituents in flowers, roots, leaves and involucral bracts and also in the medicinal preparations tested.[5]

HISTORY AND FOLK USE

While many individuals may consider the common dandelion an unwanted weed, herbalists all over the world have revered this valuable herb. Generally regarded as a liver remedy, dandelion has a long history of folk use throughout the word. In Europe, dandelion was used in the treatment of:

- fevers
- boils
- eye problems
- diarrhea
- fluid retention
- liver congestion
- heartburn
- various skin problems.

In China, dandelion has been used to treat:

- breast problems (cancer, inflammation, lack of milk flow, etc.)
- liver diseases
- appendicitis
- digestive ailments.

Dandelion's use in India, Russia, and most other parts of the world revolved primarily around its action on the liver.

PHARMACOLOGY

The primary pharmacological activities relate to digestion, liver function, and diuresis.

Digestive effects

Bitter herbs like dandelion are used to aid digestion based on the belief that bitter principles stimulate the initial phase of digestion including the secretion of salivary and gastric juices. Dandelion goes beyond this initial stimulation by stimulating the release of bile by the liver and gall bladder.

Liver effects

Studies in humans and laboratory animals have shown that dandelion root enhances the flow of bile, improving such conditions as liver congestion, bile duct inflammation, hepatitis, gallstones, and jaundice.[6–8] Dandelion's action on increasing bile flow is twofold: it has a direct effect on the liver, causing an increase in bile production and flow to the gall bladder (choleretic effect), and a direct effect on the gall bladder, causing contraction and release of stored bile (cholagogue effect). The high choline content of the root may be a major factor in dandelion's ability to act as a "tonic" to the liver. Historically, dandelion's positive effect on such a wide variety of conditions is probably closely related to its ability to improve the functional ability of the liver.

Diuretic and weight-loss effects

The leaves of dandelion have confirmed diuretic activity. In one study in mice, dandelion exerted a diuretic activity comparable to furosemide (Lasix).[9] Because dandelion replaces potassium lost through diuresis, it does not have the potential side-effects of furosemide such as hepatic coma and circulatory collapse. The dose given was 8 ml/kg body weight of the aqueous fluid extract of the leaves. This dose produced a 30% loss of body weight in mice and rats in a 30 day period. Much of the weight loss was attributed to the significant diuretic effects.

Hypoglycemic effects

Dandelion and inulin have demonstrated experimental hypoglycemic activity in animals.[10] Since inulin is composed of fructose chains, it may act to buffer blood glucose levels, thus preventing sudden and severe fluctuations.

CLINICAL APPLICATIONS

Although dandelion's specific action is on the liver, as an alterative or tonic it benefits the body as a whole. It is often used as:

- a diuretic
- a laxative
- a cholagogue
- a general stimulant for the urinary system
- a choleretic
- a depurative (purifier)
- a hypoglycemic
- an antitumor agent.

Liver conditions

Two human studies have demonstrated the liver-healing properties of dandelion. In a 1938 study in Italy, 12 patients with severe liver imbalances, many exhibiting classical symptoms of loss of appetite, low energy and jaundice, were treated with dandelion extract (one 5 ml injection per day for 20 days).[1] Eleven of the 12 patients showed a considerable drop in blood cholesterol. In the other study, dandelion extract was shown to successfully treat hepatitis, swelling of the liver, jaundice and dyspepsia with deficient bile secretion.[6]

Dandelion's effects on the liver, particularly its lipotropic effects, may be put to good use in the treatment of premenstrual syndrome. Decreased clearance of estrogen and other hormones by the liver is believed to be responsible for these symptoms in some women. If dandelion can improve the liver's ability to detoxify these hormones, symptoms may be likewise improved.

Cancer

A Japanese study in 1979 found that dandelion alcoholic extract administered to mice for 10 days markedly inhibited the growth of inoculated Ehrlich ascites cancer cells within a week of treatment.[11] A freeze-dried warm-water extract of the root for use as an antitumor agent was patented by the Japanese in 1979, and TOf-CFr, a glucose polymer isolated by Japanese researchers in 1981, was found to have antitumor properties in laboratory mice.[1] These findings lend support to the Chinese use of dandelion for breast cancers.

Kidney stones

One study, using female Wistar rats, evaluated seven botanicals historically used to prevent and treat stone kidney formation:

- *Verbena officinalis*
- *Lithospermum officinale*
- *Taraxacum officinale*
- *Equisetum arvense*
- *Arctostaphylos uva-ursi*
- *Arctium lappa*
- *Silene saxifraga.*

Variations of the main urolithiasis risk factors – citraturia, calciuria, phosphaturia, pH and diuresis – were measured. The researchers concluded that the beneficial effects caused by these herbal infusions on urolithiasis can be attributed to some disinfectant action, and, tentatively, to the presence of saponins.[12]

DOSAGE

As a general tonic and mild liver remedy, the root can be used at the following dosages three times/day:

- dried root: 2–8 g by infusion or decoction
- fluid extract (1:1): 4–8 ml (1–2 tsp)
- tincture: alcohol-based tinctures of dandelion are not recommended because of the extremely high dosage required
- juice of fresh root: 4–8 ml (1–2 tsp)
- powdered solid extract (4:1): 250–500 mg.

Preparations of the leaves can be used as a mild diuretic and weight-loss agent at the following dosages three times/day:

- dried leaf: 4–10 g by infusion
- fluid extract (1:1): 4–10 ml.

TOXICITY

No toxic or adverse effects have been reported, for either external or internal use. It is considered safe to use, even in large amounts.[1]

REFERENCES

1. Hobbs C. *Taraxacum officinale*: a monograph and literature review. In: Alstadt E, ed. Eclectic dispensatory. Portland, OR: Eclectic Medical. 1989
2. Leung AY. Encyclopedia of common natural ingredients used in food, drugs and cosmetics. New York, NY: John Wiley. 1980
3. Broda B, Andrzejewska E. Choline content in some medicinal plants. Farm Polska 1966; 22: 181–184
4. Devys M. Triterpene alcohols from dandelion (T. dens-leonis) pollen. CR Acad Sci Ser D. 1969; 269: 798–801
5. Williams CA, Goldstone F, Greenham J. Flavonoids, cinnamic acids and coumarins from the different tissues and medicinal preparations of *Taraxacum officinale*. Phytochemistry 1996; 42: 121–127
6. Faber K. The dandelion *Taraxacum officinale*. Pharmazie 1958; 13: 423–436
7. Susnik F. Present state of knowledge of the medicinal plant *Taraxacum officinale* Weber. Med Razgledi 1982; 21: 323–328
8. Bohm K. Choleretic action of some medicinal plants. Arzneimittel-Forsch 1959; 9: 376–378
9. Racz-Kotilla E, Racz G, Solomon A. The action of *Taraxacum officinale* extracts on the body weight and diuresis of laboratory animals. Planta Medica 1974; 26: 212–217
10. Yamashita K, Kawai K, Itakura M. Effects of fructo-oligosaccharides on blood glucose and serum lipids in diabetic subjects. Nutr Research 1984; 4: 491–496
11. Kotobuki Seiyaku KK. *Taraxacum* extracts as antitumour agents. Chem Abst 1979; 94: 14 530
12. Grases F, Melero G, Costa-Bauza A et al. Urolithiasis and phytotherapy. Int Urol Nephrol 1994; 26: 507–511

CHAPTER CONTENTS

116

Taxus brevifolia (Pacific yew)

Cathy Flanagan, ND

Taxus brevifolia (family: Taxaceae)
Common names: Pacific yew, taxol, paclitaxel

GENERAL DESCRIPTION

Paclitaxel (also known as taxol) and taxotene (docetaxel) are a complex diterpenoid taxanes extracted from *Taxus brevifolia*, the Pacific yew. They have been cited as some of the most promising plant compounds tested for anti-cancer properties to date.[1] First collected in 1962 by a USDA team in Washington state as part of the large natural products screening program of the US National Cancer Institute, confirmed activity against the KB cell line in tissue culture was reported in 1964. Isolation studies began in 1965 and by 1971 Wall and co-workers at the Research Triangle Institute (Durham, NC) identified taxol as the active constituent.[2] Taxol became big news in 1989, when investigators at the Johns Hopkins Oncology Center in Baltimore reported a 30% response rate in cases of refractory ovarian cancer, a remarkable rate for this type of cancer.[3] Taxanes used in conjunction with chemotherapy and radiation have demonstrated improved results to either therapy alone along with improved tolerance to the therapies.

Yews are evergreen trees or shrubs which produce a seed surrounded by an edible red fleshy aril. The yew is difficult to class taxonomically as its appearance is similar to conifers, but because of the absence of cones and resin ducts, it is placed in a separate order.

Although the yew appears to be tenacious, it is slow to reproduce. The species is dioecious, with female trees producing relatively scarce fruits. Seedlings are rare. Most often, new yew trees come from offshoots of a "mother tree", which is why they are usually found in clusters. They grow best on deep, moist, rich rocky or gravelly soils. The largest known living Pacific yew is in Lewis County, Washington, near Mount Rainier. It stands 21.3 m tall, has a girth of 4.5 m, and is estimated to be 1,000 years old.[2]

Although taxol is found in species other than the

Pacific yew, its concentration is too low to warrant the extensive extraction processing required. Initially, it was thought that the most consistently stable and highly active constituent came from bark isolates, followed by root isolates. Currently, taxol and another compound, baccatin III (from the English yew, *T. baccata*), are being extracted from needles and twigs of 3- to 5-year-old cuttings being grown for this purpose. Taxol, a complex molecule, can be synthesized from baccatin III, but to date eludes efforts at total synthesis.[4,5]

Harvesting of a sufficient natural source is unrealistic for long-term use, as the Pacific yew, an inhabitant of old-growth stands, is in limited supply. The demand for taxol is estimated at 50–200 kg/patient, which would require 500,000–635,000 kg of bark yearly. One 200-year-old tree, with a 25 cm diameter yields only 2.7 kg of bark.[2] The National Cancer Institute had requested 340,200 kg of dried bark in 1991 for 25 kg to be used in clinical trials alone. Environmentalists are concerned about the decimation of the little old-growth habitat which has survived logging efforts. Ironically, the Pacific yew had been previously regarded as a trash tree, left behind or burnt after logging operations. Now it is sought for its bark, and accessible stands are being harvested for maximum yield.

The future of taxol as a viable anti-cancer agent depends either on it, or a molecule similar enough to retain the therapeutic properties, being synthetically produced or on improved harvesting and extraction techniques that will maximize yield while perpetuating the natural source. Researchers at Stanford University have overcome many hurdles in the synthesis, but have not yet been totally successful. Extraction from needles looks promising, as it takes only 27.2 kg of foliage (produced from one tree) versus 4.1 kg of bark (consuming three trees) to obtain 2 g of taxol, the necessary dose for one patient. Harvesting trees in a manner that allows for sprouting of new trees is another way to sustain a supply and the survival of the species.

A collaborative research and development agreement between the National Cancer Institute and the Bristol-Myers Squibb Company has made it possible for taxol to be the first drug available through the treatment referral center to designated comprehensive cancer centers for eligible patients before being commercially available.[3] The National Cancer Institute announced (newsletter, September 1992) that taxol had been reclassified as a group C drug, making it available with Medicare reimbursement to women with refractory ovarian cancer.

CHEMICAL COMPOSITION

Yew is poisonous because of at least 11 alkaloids, known collectively as taxines. The structure of only two of the alkaloid constituents is known: taxine A, which accounts

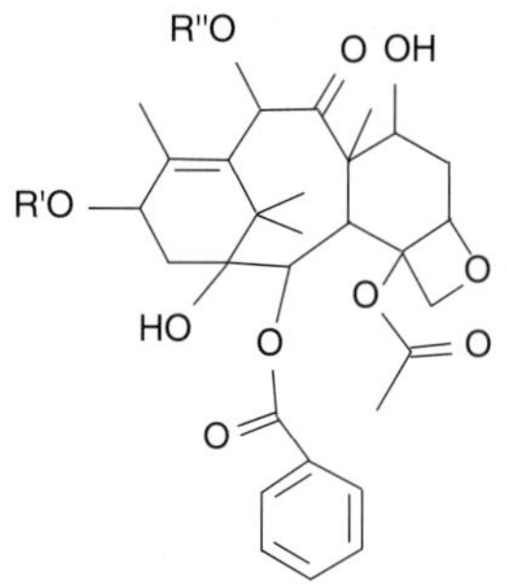

	R′	R″
10-Deacetylbaccatin III	H	H
Taxol	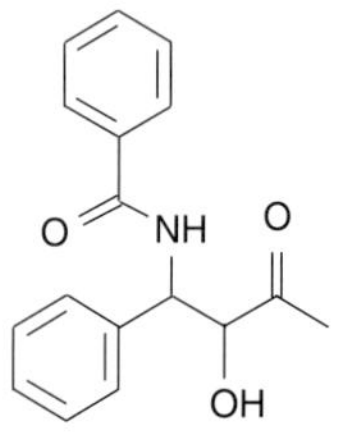	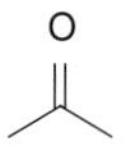

Figure 116.1 Paclitaxel.

for 30%, and taxine B, which accounts for 2%. Paclitaxel (Fig. 116.1) is a pseudoalkaloid, but not a constituent of taxine since its nitrogen is acylated with benzoic acid and has no basic principle. The concentration of paclitaxel in yew bark is low, only 0.01%.

Taxenes have now been found in species other than the Pacific yew, but at lower concentrations. The harvesting of 500,000–635,000 kg/year of the bark is required to provide the estimated placitaxel needed. Therefore, development of analogs synthesized from natural turpenes are important for long-term use.

In the search for precursors for paclitaxel synthesis, the much more prevalent yew needles have been analyzed for paclitaxel analogs. Several have been identified (e.g. 10-deacetyltaxol III, cephalmannine, 10-deacetyltaxol, 10-deacetylcephalomannine, and baccatin-III). As all yew species contain these highly oxygenated diterpenoids based on the unique taxane skeleton, most of the over 100 yew varieties are being screened, as are other members of the *Taxus* species. Other analogs, like docefaxel, are made by altering compounds extracted from the yew tree needles.

Paclitaxel is synthesized from cyclization of the universal diterpenoid precursor, geranylgeranyl diphosphate to taxa-4(5),11(12)-diene. This olefin is hydroxylated via cytochrome P450 catalysts to taxa-4(20), 11(12)-dien-5 alpha-ol. Then this alcohol is converted via an acetylCoA-dependent process to the corresponding acetate ester. Further genetic identification and isolations are targeted to improve the yield of taxol from the *Taxus* species.[6]

HISTORY AND FOLK USE

Historically, the yew has been highly valued for its dense, resilient, decay-resistant, tight-grained wood, and its medicinal properties. The Greeks named the yew *toxus* in reference to its use for making strong bows (toxon), and its poisonous nature (toxikon).[2] It was used as an animal and fish poison by primitive cultures, as well as for murder and suicide. In the 1st century AD, Claudius suggested its use as an antidote for viper bites. Europeans used it as an abortifacient, and for heart ailments and hydrophobia.[2] Native Americans used the yew for many ailments such as:

- rheumatism
- lung ailments
- colds
- fever
- pain
- scurvy
- numbness
- paralysis
- stomach ache
- bowel ailments
- dysmenorrhea
- clots
- gonorrhea.

Women ate yew berries to prevent conception. Youths rubbed smooth sticks of yew on their developing bodies to gain its strength. Both the bark and the leaves have been brewed for tea, and powders made from the bark alone. The fleshy red aril (berry) that surrounds the seed is not poisonous, although the seed itself is.[7]

There is a lot of folklore about the yew's supernatural powers. As it is a slow-growing, long-lived tree, it was associated with immortality. It was used in spells to raise the dead.[8] Because it was regarded as among the most potent of trees for protection against evil, it was considered unlucky to cut down or damage a yew tree. Many were planted in churchyards/graveyards and alongside homes for protection. Specimens survive today in spite of main trunks being hollowed out from decay following hundreds of years of existence.

PHARMACOLOGY

Paclitaxel's anti-cancer action is unique in that it inhibits cell division by promoting the formation of microtubules, the rod-like structures that function as a cell skeleton, making cells more stable and resistant to depolymerization. In contrast, other anti-cancer phytoagents (i.e. colchicine and vinca alkaloids) induce polymerization of microtubules. In addition, under the influence of paclitaxel, the microtubules polymerize independently of the microtubule-organizing center (MTOC), which is in a perinuclear area, and instead localize predominantly in the cell periphery.[9] This interferes with the mitotic spindle and selectively blocks cells in the G_2 and M phases of the cell cycle, the most radiosensitive phases. Additionally, paclitaxel induces the formation of abnormal spindle asters that do not require centrioles for enucleation and are reversible following treatment.[10,11] Discovery of this unique mechanism of action by Horowitz and co-workers in 1979 kindled interest in paclitaxel, despite the inherent problems in the utilization of a scarce natural product.[12,13]

In addition, paclitaxel has demonstrated, in vivo, an ability to activate a local release of an apoptosis-inducing cytokine.[14] Studies on cancer cell lines induced with *gml*, a novel gene, demonstrated a marked increase in sensitivity to paclitaxel via apoptosis. An assay for *gml* expression could serve as a clinically useful predictor of chemotherapeutic sensitivity.[15]

Docetaxel (taxotene) manifests its maximum inhibitory effect against cells that are in S phase.[46] Other analogs (particularly IDN5109) are showing anti-proliferative activity 20- to 30-fold higher than paclitaxel in multi-drug-resistance-positive cancer cells.[16]

CLINICAL APPLICATION

Paclitaxel has demonstrated a broad spectrum of anti-tumor activity. Phase I trials, which began in 1983, demonstrated paclitaxel's anti-neoplastic activity against several tumor types, such as:[17–24]

- melanoma
- adenocarcinoma of unknown origin
- refractory ovarian carcinoma
- small-cell and non-small-cell lung carcinoma
- gastric, colon, prostate, breast, head and neck carcinomas
- lymphoblastic and myeloblastic leukemias.

Trials are also being conducted with impressive results, using paclitaxel in combination with other anti-neoplastic agents, such as cisplatin.[25] The Gynecology Oncology Group (GOG) reports a 33% response rate in patients who were previously resistant to cisplatin, when they are treated with the combination of cisplatin and paclitaxel.[26] Trials are being conducted on small-cell and non-small-cell lung, renal, gastric, breast, advanced ovarian, colon, and cervical carcinomas; head and neck cancers; small cell lung and prostate carcinomas and low-grade non-Hodgkin's lymphoma.[27] Table 116.1 lists the short-term partial or complete response rates of various types of cancer to paclitaxel alone or in combination with other chemotherapeutic drugs.

Table 116.1 Results of clinical trials of paclitaxel or paclitaxel combinations[28]

Cancer type	Response range (%)
Ovarian cancer	20–50
Breast cancer	56–62
Lung cancer	21–46
Melanoma	28
Renal carcinoma	0 (small numbers)
Prostate	50 (small numbers)

TOXICITY

Human poisoning from the deliberate consumption of yew leaves or seeds is now rare. Recently published cases, from psychiatric patients and prisoners, describe the first symptoms of intoxication as appearing 1 hour after ingestion. The manifestations include mydriasis, nausea, vomiting, abdominal cramping and arrhythmia. Death occurs from cardiac arrest 3–24 hours after ingestion.[28] The lethal dose in humans is approximately four or five handfuls of leaves, corresponding to 150 needles. No specific antidote is known.

Paclitaxel binds 95–98% with plasma proteins, yet is readily eliminated through hepatic metabolism, biliary excretion, and/or extensive tissue binding. Total urinary excretion has been insignificant, indicating that renal clearance contributes minimally to systemic clearance.[24,29–31] Hepatic metabolism via cytochrome p450 (CYP) is involved for both paclitaxel and docetaxel. However, the former is hydroxylated by CYP2C8 while the latter is hydroxylated by CYP3A4.[32]

Toxicity in clinical trials manifests as:

- bone marrow suppression
- hypersensitivity
- cardiovascular abnormalities
- neurotoxicity
- arthralgias and myalgias
- alopecia
- gastrointestinal upset.

Junctional tachycardia via conduction block rather than direct primary toxicity on myocytes has been suggested.[33] Hypersensitivity, skin reactions and accumulated fluid retention syndrome are minimized with a 3–5 day corticosteroid regime prior to paclitaxel infusions.[34]

Leukemia patients treated with high doses of paclitaxel exhibited mucositis, which also appeared in response to lower, cumulative dosing. An accumulation of epidermal cells with paclitaxel-induced asters has been evident in ulcerated mucosa, indicating that the cell cycle was arrested in mitosis.[35]

Paclitaxel has been known to inhibit neurite growth and induce prominent morphological effects, such as microtubule bundles in neurons, in satellite cells and in Schwann cells in organotypic dorsal root ganglion cultures.[36–41] Clinically, the most common symptoms have been glove-and-stocking paresthesia and perioral numbness. Distal sensory loss to large- (proprioception, vibration) and small-fiber (pin-prick, temperature) modalities and lost or decreased distal deep tendon reflexes have been noted, although motor nerves seem to be spared. In general, the clinical incidence and severity of peripheral neurotoxicity have been dose-related. Patients with a history of substantial alcohol use have appeared to be more predisposed to the development of neurosensory toxic effects of cisplain and paclitaxel.[17–20,42–44]

The development of a suitable clinical formulation has been hampered by paclitaxel's poor aqueous solubility. Cremophor is being used as the vehicle for administration and has been implicated in side-effects such as type 1 hypersensitivity reactions.[45] Neutropenia is the principle dose-limiting toxic effect of paclitaxel and resolves rapidly (15–21 days) after treatment is stopped.[42] The major clinical risk factor for neutropenia seems to be the extent of prior myelotoxic chemotherapy and/or irradiation.

Bradyarrhythmias, which have been noted as transient and asymptomatic, have been reported during paclitaxel infusions in at least 29% of ovarian cancer patients, as reported by Mcguire et al.[42] This appears to be more related to paclitaxel, as other agents formulated with Cremophor have not been associated with similar arrhythmias. Atypical chest pains during paclitaxel infusion have been observed, but they are believed to be a manifestation of a hypersensitivity reaction.[29,43]

Other paclitaxel or Cremophor-related side-effects include sudden and complete alopecia – often occurring in a single day – local venous toxic effects such as erythema, tenderness and cellulitis in areas of dermal extravasation, fatigue, headaches, taste perversions, significant elevations in serum triglyceride levels, and minor elevations in hepatic and renal functions.[24]

Lipid-coated microbubbles may be an effective way of providing selective affinity for tumor cells, thus reducing systemic effects while maintaining antitumor actions.[46] Additional precautions may be necessary with

Table 116.2 Medications which interact with paclitaxel[47]

- Amphotericin B by injection (e.g. Fungizone)
- Antithyroid agents
- Azathioprine (e.g. Imuran)
- Chloramphenicol (e.g. Chloromycetin)
- Colchicine
- Flucytosine (e.g. Ancobon)
- Ganciclovir (e.g. Cytovene)
- Interferon (e.g. Intron A, Roferon A)
- Plicamycin (e.g. Mithracin)
- Zidovudine (e.g. AZT, Retrovir)

the concurrent use of the medications listed in Table 116.2. Medical problems which may affect the use of paclitaxel are listed in Table 116.3. Studies in rats and rabbits have shown that taxol causes miscarriages and fetal deaths. Breast-feeding is contraindicated while receiving paclitaxel.[47]

Table 116.3 Medical problems which may affect the use of paclitaxel

- Chickenpox
- Herpes zoster
- Cardiac arrythmias
- Infection

REFERENCES

1. Bolsinger C, Jaramillo AE. *Taxus brevifolia* Nutt. Pacific Yew, 1990 In: Silvis of forest trees of North America (rev.). Portland: Pacific Northwest Research Station 1990: 17
2. Hartzell H, Jr. The yew tree: a thousand whispers. Eugene, OR: Hulogosi. 1991: p 31, 80, 154–156, 176, 230
3. Rowinsky EK, Donehower RC. Taxol: twenty years later, the story unfolds. J Natl Cancer Inst 1991; 83: 1055–1056, 1780
4. Denis JN, Greene AE. A highly efficient approach to natural taxol. J Am Chem Soc 1988; 110: 5917–5919
5. Blume E. Investigators seek to increase taxol supply (News). J Natl Cancer Inst 1989; 81: 1122–1123
6. Hezari M, Croteau R. Taxol biosynthesis: an update. Planta Med 1997; 63: 291–295
7. Duke J. Handbook of northeastern Indian medicinal plants. Lincoln, MA: Quarterman. 1986: p 156
8. Cunningham S. Encyclopedia of magical herbs. St. Paul, MO: Llewelyn Publications. 1985: p 228
9. Wehland J, Henkart M, Klausner R, Sandoval IV: role of microtubules in the distribution of the Golgi apparatus. taxol and microinjected anti-alpha-tubulin antibodies. Proc Nat Acad Sci USA 1983; 80: 4286–4290
10. Rowinsky EK, Donehower RC, Jones RJ et al Microtubule changes and cytotoxicity in leukemic cell lines created with taxol. Cancer Res 1988; 48: 4093–4100
11. Debrabander M, Geuens G, Nuuydens R et al. Taxol induces the assembly of free microtubules in living cells and blocks the organizing capacity of the centrosome and kinetochores. Proc Nat Acad Sci USA 1981; 78: 5608–5612
12. Brasch RC, Rockoff SD, Kuhn C et al. Contrast media as histamine liberators. II. Histamine release into venous plasma during intravenous urography in man. Invest Radiol 1970; 5: 510–513
13. Shedadi WH. Adverse reactions to intravenous administration of contrast media: a comparative study based on a prospective study. Am J Roentgenol 1975; 124: 145–151
14. Lanni JS, Lowe SW, Licitra EJ et al. p53-independent apoptosis induced by paclitaxel through an indirect mechanism. Proc Natl Acad Sci USA 1997; 94: 9679–9683
15. Kimura Y, Furuhata T, Shiratsuchi T et al. GML sensitizes cancer cells to taxol by induction of apoptosis. Oncogene 1997; 15: 1369–1374
16. Distefano M, Scambia G, Ferlini C et al. Anti-proliferative activity of a new class of taxanes (14-beta-hydroxy-10–deacetylbaccatin III derivatives) on multidrug-resistance-positive human cancer cells. Int J Cancer 1997; 72: 844–850
17. Koeller J, Brown T, Havlin K et al. A phase I/pharmacokinetic study of taxol given by prolonged infusion without premedication Proc ASCO 1989; 8: 82
18. Donehower RC, Rowinsky EK, Grochow LB et al. Phase I trial of taxol in patients with advanced cancer. Cancer Treat Rep 1987; 71: 1171–1177
19. Wiernik PH, Schwartz EL, Strauman JJ et al. Phase I clinical and pharmacokinetic study of taxol. Cancer Res 1987; 47: 2486–2493
20. Wiernik PH, Schwartz EL, Einzig A et al. Phase I trial of taxol given as a 24-hour infusion every 21 days: responses observed in metastatic melanoma. J Clin Oncol 1987; 5: 1232–1239
21. Legha SS, Tenney DM, Krakoff IR. Phase I study of taxol using a 5-day intermittent schedule. J Clin Oncol 1986; 4: 762–766
22. Grem JL, Tutsch KD, Simon KJ et al. Phase I study of taxol administered as a short i.v. infusion daily for 5 days. Cancer Treat Rep 1987; 71: 1179–1184
23. Ohnuma T, Zimet AS, Coffey VA et al. Phase I study of taxol in a 24-hour infusion schedule. Proc Am Assoc Cancer Res 1985; 26: 662
24. Kris MG, O'Connell JP, Gralla RJ et al. Phase I trial of taxol given as a 3-hour infusion every 21 days. Cancer Treat Rep 1986; 70: 605–607
25. Rowinsky EK, Gilbert M, McGuire WP et al. Sequences of taxol and cisplatin: a phase I/pharmacological study. Proc ASCO 1990; 9: 290
26. Thigpen T, Blessing J, Ball H et al. Phase II trial of taxol as second-line therapy for ovarian carcinoma: a gynecologic oncology group study. Proc ASCO 1990; 9: 604
27. Dustin P. Microtubules. Sci Am 1980; 243: 66–76
28. Appendino G. Taxol. Historic and ecological aspects. Fitoterapia 1993; 64(suppl 1): 5–25
29. Jacrot M, Riondel J, Picot F et al. Action of taxol on human tumors transplanted in athymic mice. R Seances Acad Sci III 1983; 297: 597–600
30. Riondel J, Jacrot M, Nissou MF et al. Antineoplastic activity of two taxol derivatives on an ovarian tumor xenografted into nude mice. Anticancer Res 1988; 8: 387–390
31. Sternberg CN, Sordillo PP, Cheng E et al. Evaluation of new anticancer agents against human pancreatic carcinomas in nude mice. Am J Clin Oncol 1987; 10: 219–221
32. Dorr RT. Pharmacology of the taxanes. Pharmacotherapy 1997; 17(5 Pt 2): 96S–104S
33. Faivre S, Goldwasser F, Soulie P, Misset JL. Paclitaxel (Taxol)-associated junctional tachycardia. Anticancer Drugs 1997; 8: 714–716
34. Von Hoff DD. The taxoids. same roots, different drugs. Semin Oncol 1997; 24(4 Suppl 13): 3–10
35. Hruban RH, Yardley JH, Donehower RC et al. Taxol toxicity. Epithelial necrosis in the gastrointestinal tract associated with polymerized microtubule accumulation and mitotic arrest. Cancer 1989; 63: 1944–1950
36. Masurovsky EB, Peterson ER, Crain SM et al. Microtubule arrays in taxol-treated mouse dorsal root ganglion-spinal cord cultures. Brain Res 1981; 217: 392–398
37. Masurovsky EB, Peterson ER, Crain SM et al. Morphological alterations in satellite and Schwann after exposure of fetal mouse dorsal root ganglia-spinal cord culture to taxol. IRCS Med Sci Libr Compend 1981; 9: 968–969
38. Masurovsky EB, Peterson ER, Crain SM et al. Morphological alterations in dorsal root ganglion neurons and supporting cells of organotypic mouse spinal cord-ganglion cultures exposed to taxol. Neuroscience 1983; 10: 491–509
39. Letourneau PC, Ressler AH. Inhibition of neurite initiation and growth by taxol. J Cell Biol 1984; 98: 1355–1362
40. Letourneau PC, Shattuck TA, Ressler AH. Branching of sensory and sympathetic neuritis in vitro is inhibited by treatment with taxol. J Neuroscience 1983; 10: 491–509
41. Roytta M, Horwitz SB, Raine CS. Taxol-induced neuropathy: short-term effects of local injection. J Neurocytol 1984; 13: 685: 701
42. Mcguire WP, Rowinsky EK, Rosenshein NB et al. Taxol: a unique antineoplastic agent with significant activity in advanced ovarian epithelial neoplasms. Ann Intern Med 1989; 111: 373–379
43. Rowinsky EK, Burke PJ, Karp JE et al. Phase I and pharmacodynamic study of taxol in refractory acute leukemias. Cancer Res 1989; 49: 4640–4647
44. Burgoyne RD, Cumming R. Taxol stabilizes synaptosomal

microtubules without inhibiting acetylcholine release. Brain Res 1983; 280: 190–193
45. Laussus M, Scott D, Leyland-Jones B. Allergic reactions (ar) associated cremophor (c) containing antineoplastic (anp). Proc ASCO 1985; 4: 1042
46. Ho SY, Barbarese E, D'Arrigo JS et al. Evaluation of lipid-coated microbubbles as a delivery vehicle for Taxol in brain tumor therapy. Neurosurgery 1997; 40: 1260–1266
47. US Pharmacopeia, Rockville, MD. Drug interactions, vol. II. 1997: p 1237–1238

CHAPTER CONTENTS

117

Uva ursi (bearberry)

Michael T. Murray, ND

Joseph E. Pizzorno Jr, ND

Arctostaphylos uva ursi (family: Ericaceae)
Common names: bearberry, upland cranberry

GENERAL DESCRIPTION

Uva ursi is a small evergreen shrub found in the northern US and in Europe. A single long, fibrous main root sends out several prostate or buried stems 4–6 inches high. The bark is dark brown, the leaves are obovate to spatulate 0.5–1 inch long, the flowers are pink or white growing in sparse terminal clusters, and the fruit is a bright red or pink.

CHEMICAL COMPOSITION

Uva ursi's most active ingredient is arbutin, which typically composes 7–9% of the leaves. Other constituents include:

- tannins (6–7%)
- flavonoids (quercetin)
- allantoin
- gallic and ellagic acids
- volatile oils
- a resin (urvone).[1,2]

HISTORY AND FOLK USE

This plant has a long history of use for its diuretic and astringent properties. Conditions for which it was used include chronic cystitis, nephritis, kidney stones, and bronchitis.[1]

PHARMACOLOGY

Antimicrobial

Although pharmacological research has primarily focused on arbutin, the pharmacology of the whole plant is different from that of just arbutin alone. The crude plant extracts are much more effective medicinally than the isolated constituent arbutin. This appears to be related to the activity of gallic acid, which prevents the splitting of arbutin by such enzymes as beta-glucosidase.[2] Arbutin undergoes hydrolysis to produce its aglycone, hydroquinone, which has urinary antiseptic properties.[3] This hydrolysis of arbutin is responsible for much of the therapeutic effect of *uva ursi*.[1,3] By preventing the splitting of arbutin, the flavonoid components allow more arbutin to be hydrolyzed than when arbutin is administered as an isolated component.

Arbutin alone has been reported to be an effective urinary antibiotic, but only if taken in large doses and if the urine is alkaline (once again documenting the value of whole plant medicines).[1] It is reported to be active against *Candida albicans* and *S. aureus*, and especially active against *E. coli*.[4] *Uva ursi* also has diuretic properties.[1]

Anti-inflammatory effects

Some early animal research is now showing that arbutin, and possibly other constituents of *uva ursi*, potentiate the activity of commonly prescribed anti-inflammatory drugs. One study found that an aqueous extract increased the inhibitory activity of dexamthasone in allergic and inflammatory models without increasing any of the side-effects.[5] Similar results have been demonstrated with isolated arbutin when combined with indomethacin.[6]

Inhibition of melanin synthesis

Another recently discovered property of *uva ursi* is the inhibition of tyrosinase by a 50% alcoholic extract.[7] This effect impairs melanin synthesis, which leads the authors to suggest it could be used as a whitening agent for the skin. However, no clinical trials have been reported.

CLINICAL APPLICATIONS

Crude extracts are widely used in Europe as components in certain diuretic and laxative products, but the major use of *uva ursi* is as a urinary disinfectant in cases of urinary tract infection.[1]

Uva ursi is reported to be especially active against *E. coli*.[3] It can be used in both the acute treatment and the prevention of recurrent cystitis. In one double-blind study, the prophylactic effect of a standardized *uva ursi* extract compared to a placebo on recurrent cystitis was evaluated in 57 women.[8] At the end of one year, 5/27 women in the placebo group had a recurrence while 0/30 women receiving *uva ursi* extract had a recurrence. No side-effects were reported in either group. These impressive results indicate that regular use of *uva ursi* is a safe and effective measure to prevent recurrent cystitis.

DOSAGES

- Dried leaves or as an infusion: 1.5 to 4.0 g (1 to 2 tsp)
- Freeze-dried leaves: 500 to 1,000 mg
- Tincture (1:5): 4 to 6 ml (1 to 1.5 tsp)
- Fluid extract (1:1): 1 to 2 ml (¼ to ½ tsp)
- Powdered solid extract (10% arbutin): 250 to 500 mg

TOXICOLOGY

The toxicology of *uva ursi* is proportional to the conversion of arbutin to hydroquinone. Hydroquinone has been shown to be toxic at 1 g (equivalent to approximately 0.5 ounce of the fresh leaves), with signs and symptoms of:[2]

- tinnitus
- nausea
- vomiting
- sense of suffocation
- shortness of breath
- cyanosis
- convulsions
- delirium
- collapse.

REFERENCES

1. Leung A. Encyclopedia of common natural ingredients used in food, drugs, and cosmetics. New York, NY: John Wiley. 1980: p 316–317
2. Merck Index, 10th edn. Rahway, NJ: Merck. 1983: p 112–113, 699
3. Frohne V. Untersuchungen zur frage der harndesifizierenden wirkungen von barentraubenblatt-extracten. Planta Medica 1970; 18: 1–25
4. Mitchell W. Naturopathic applications of the botanical remedies. Seattle, WA. 1983: p 8
5. Matsuda H, Nakamura S, Tanaka T, Kubo M. Pharmacological studies on leaf of *Arctostaphylos uva-ursi* (L.) Spreng. V. Effect of water extract from *Arctostaphylos uva-ursi* (bearberry) on the antiallergic and antiinflammatory activities on dexamethasone ointment. Yakugaku Zasshi 1994; 112: 673–677
6. Matsuda H, Tanaka T, Kubo M. Pharmacological studies on leaf of *Arctostaphylos uva-ursi* (L.) Spreng. III. Combined effect of arbutin and indomethacin on immuno-inflammation. Yakugaku Zasshi 1991; 111: 256–258
7. Matsuda H, Higashino M, Nakai Y et al. Studies of cutical drugs from natural sources. IV. Inhibitory efffects of *Arctostaphylos* plants on melanin biosynthesis. Biol Pharm Bull 1996; 19: 153–156
8. Larsson B, Jonasson A, Fianu S. Prophylactic effect of UVA-E in women with recurrent cystitis: A preliminary report. Curr Ther Res 1993; 53: 441–443

CHAPTER CONTENTS

118

Vaccinium myrtillus (bilberry)

Michael T. Murray, ND

Joseph E. Pizzorno Jr, ND

Vaccinium myrtillus (family: Ericaceae)
Common names: bilberry, huckleberry, European blueberry, whortleberry, blueberry

GENERAL DESCRIPTION

The genus *Vaccinium* in the family Ericaceae comprises nearly 200 species, most of which are found in the Northern Hemisphere. This chapter focuses on *Vaccinium myrtillus* and the medicinal use of extracts of its fruit.

Vaccinium myrtillus, or bilberry, is a shrubby perennial plant that grows in the sandy areas of the northern US and in the woods and forest meadows of Europe. The angular, green, branched stem grows from a creeping rootstock to a height of 1–1.5 feet. The 0.5–1.0 inch long leaves are oval, slightly dentate, and bright green, while the flowers are reddish- or greenish-pink and bell-shaped. The flowering season is April–June. The fruit is a blue-black berry.[1]

CHEMICAL COMPOSITION

The pharmacologically active constituents of bilberries are its flavonoid components, specifically its anthocyanosides. Anthocyanosides are composed of an aglycone (e.g. anthocyanidin) bound to one of three glycosides (arabinoside, glucoside, or galactoside). Over 15 different anthocyanosides originate from the five aglycones found in *Vaccinium myrtillus* (see Fig. 118.1).[2] Other members of the genus *Vaccinium*, as well as *Ribes nigrum* (blackcurrant) and *Vitis vinifera* (grape), contain similar anthocyanosides.[3] Extracts of these fruits are also used for medicinal purposes in Europe.

The concentration of anthocyanosides in the fresh fruit is approximately 0.1–0.25%, while concentrated extracts of *Vaccinium myrtillus* are produced which yield an anthocyanidin content of 25%.[2] An extract with an anthocyanidin content of 25% actually contains about 37% anthocyanosides due to the conjugation of the anthocyanidin with a glycoside. (For analytical purposes, the

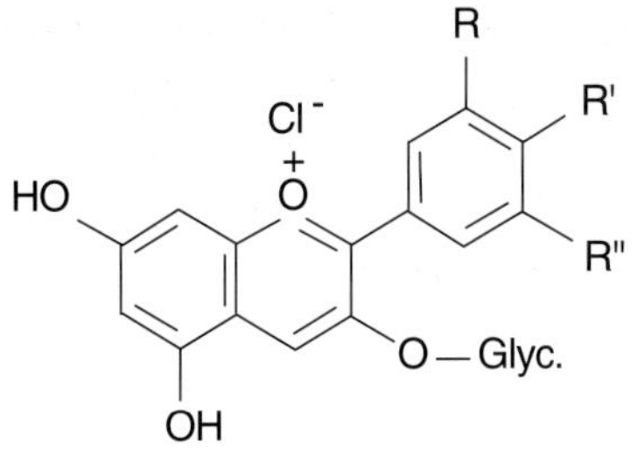

Anthocyanin	R	R′	R″
Delphinidin 3-O-glycoside	OH	OH	OH
Cyanidin 3-O-glycoside	OH	OH	H
Petunidin 3-O-glycoside	OH	OH	OCH_3
Peonidin 3-O-glycoside	OCH_3	OH	H
Malvidin 3-O-glycoside	OCH_3	OH	OCH_3

Figure 118.1 Structures of *V. myrtillus* anthocyanins[2]
Glyc. = arabinoside, glucoside or galactoside

anthocyanosides content should always be expressed in terms of anthocyanidin.) Only very small amounts of free anthocyanidins exist in nature and in *V. myrtillus* extracts.

HISTORY AND FOLK USE

Bilberries have, of course, been used as food and for their high nutritive value. Medicinally, they have been utilized in the treatment of scurvy and urinary complaints (including infection and stones).[1] The dried berries have been used primarily for their astringent qualities in the treatment of diarrhea and dysentery. Decoctions of the leaves have been used in the treatment of diabetes.[1]

PHARMACOLOGY

The pharmacology of *Vaccinium myrtillus* is discussed almost entirely in relationship to its anthocyanoside content, as research has focused primarily on the anthocyanosides.

Collagen-stabilizing action

Anthocyanosides possess significant collagen-stabilizing action.[4–10] Collagen, the most abundant protein of the body, is responsible for maintaining the integrity of "ground substance" as well as tendons, ligaments, and cartilage. Collagen is destroyed during the inflammatory processes that occur in rheumatoid arthritis, periodontal disease, and other inflammatory conditions involving bones, joints, cartilage, and other connective tissue.

Anthocyanidins, proanthocyanidins and other flavonoids are remarkable in their ability to prevent collagen destruction. The anthocyanidins in *Vaccinium myrtillus* extracts have been shown to affect collagen metabolism in several ways:

- Anthocyanosides cross-link collagen fibers, resulting in strengthening of the natural cross-linking of collagen that forms the collagen matrix of connective tissue (ground substance, cartilage, tendon, etc.).[4–7,8]
- Anthocyanosides prevent free radical damage with their potent antioxidant and free radical scavenging action.[4–7,9]
- Anthocyanosides inhibit enzymatic cleavage of collagen by enzymes secreted by leukocytes during inflammation.[4–6,8–10]
- Anthocyanosides and other flavonoid components of *V. myrtillus* prevent the release and synthesis of compounds that promote inflammation, such as histamine, serine proteases, prostaglandins, and leukotrienes.[4–6,11,12]
- Anthocyanosides promote mucopolysaccharide and collagen biosynthesis and stimulate reticulation of collagen fibrils.[13–15]

Normalization of capillary permeability

Anthocyanosides have strong "vitamin P" activity.[4] Included in their effects are an ability to increase intracellular vitamin C levels and to decrease capillary permeability and fragility.[4–6] Their effect in reducing capillary fragility and permeability is roughly twice that of rutin, in both intensity and duration of action.[16]

Vaccinium myrtillus extracts have been widely used in Europe in the treatment of various arterial, venous, and capillary disorders. Clinical studies have demonstrated a positive effect in the treatment of:[17–22]

- capillary fragility
- blood purpuras
- various encephalic circulation disturbances (similar to *Ginkgo biloba*)
- venous insufficiency
- varicose veins
- microscopic hematuria caused by diffused and kidney capillary fragility.

V. myrtillus's efficacy in the treatment of a variety of venous disorders relates to the ability of anthocyanosides to protect altered veins (postphlebotic veins as well as varicose veins) via two mechanisms:[15]

- increasing the endothelium barrier-effect through stabilization of the membrane phospholipids
- increasing the biosynthesis of the acid mucopolysaccharides of the connective ground substance, thus restoring the altered mucopolysaccharide pericapillary sheath.

This latter effect leads to a marked increase in newly formed capillaries and collagen fibrils.

One interesting effect of the normalization of collagen structures and capillaries is the demonstration that anthocyanosides from *Vaccinium myrtillus* decrease the permeability of the blood–brain barrier.[8,23] Increased blood–brain permeability has been linked to autoimmune diseases of the central nervous system, schizophrenia, "cerebral allergies", and a variety of other CNS disorders. Presumably, the anthocyanosides inhibit both enzymatic and non-enzymatic degradation of the basement membrane collagen of brain capillaries, thus helping to maintain or restore the brain's protection from drugs, pollutants, naturally occurring degradation products, and other cerebral toxins.[7–10, 23]

Another recent study further demonstrates the remarkable efficacy of bilberry in protecting and strengthening the capillaries and microcirculation. In this study, the effects of anthocyanidins on hamster cheek microcirculation were investigated after ischemia and reperfusion. The treated group had decreased adherence of leukocytes to the venules after reperfusion, resulting in prevention of the markedly increased capillary permeability seen in the placebo group.[24]

Anti-aggregation effect on platelets

Anthocyanosides, like many other flavonoids, have been shown to possess significant anti-aggregation effects on platelets.[25–27] Their action in vivo appears to be direct anti-aggregation effects on the platelets and an indirect effect via prostacyclin-like action.[25–27] Prostacyclin (PGI_2) is a potent stimulator of adenyl cyclase, the enzyme which catalyzes the production of cAMP from ATP. cAMP prevents platelets from aggregating and adhering to the endothelial surface.

Smooth muscle relaxing activity

Anthocyanoside extracts have demonstrated significant vascular smooth muscle-relaxing effects in a variety of experimental models.[28–30] The clinical application of this research may be in the treatment of dysmenorrhea, for which a preliminary study has demonstrated positive effects.[31]

CLINICAL APPLICATIONS

The primary clinical application of bilberry extracts has been in the prevention and treatment of a diverse group of disorders of the eye and vision. However, the same mechanisms of action which benefit the eye are of value to other health problems, especially those involving capillary dysfunction or inflammation.

Ophthalmological applications

Night vision

Perhaps the most significant clinical applications for *Vaccinium myrtillus* extracts are in the field of ophthalmology. Interest in *V. myrtillus* anthocyanosides was first aroused when it was observed that the administration of bilberry extracts to healthy subjects resulted in improved night-time visual acuity, quicker adjustment to darkness, and faster restoration of visual acuity after exposure to glare.[32,33]

Further studies confirmed these results.[34–37] Results were most impressive in individuals with pigmentary retinitis and hemeralopia. (Hemeralopia refers to "day blindness" or an inability to see as distinctly in bright light as in dim light.)

It appears that, in addition to their effect on capillaries, *V. myrtillus* anthocyanosides have an affinity for the pigmented epithelium of the retina, which composes the optical or functional part of the retina.[38] This is consistent with several of the clinical effects observed.

Anthocyanoside extracts of *V. myrtillus* appear to be of great value in both poor night vision and poor day vision.

Glaucoma

Vaccinium myrtillus may play a significant role in the prevention and treatment of glaucoma via its effect on collagen structures in the eye. In the eye, collagen provides tensile strength and integrity to the tissues, i.e. cornea, sclera, lamina cribosa, trabecular meshwork, vitreous, etc.

Morphological changes in the collagen of the eye precede clinically detectable abnormalities. These changes may result in elevated intraocular pressure (IOP) readings or, perhaps more significantly, the progression of peripheral vision loss. Changes in collagen structure would explain why there is:

- similar peripheral vision loss in patients with normal and elevated IOP
- cupping of the optic disc even at low IOP levels
- no apparent anatomical reason for decreased aqueous outflow (see Ch. 153 for complete discussion and references).

Therefore, primary prevention of glaucoma involves maintaining ground substance and collagen framework integrity. It appears the prevention of collagen matrix breakdown is important here, as it is in other conditions involving collagen abnormalities, i.e. atherosclerosis, rheumatoid arthritis, and periodontal disease.

Vaccinium myrtillus consumption may offer significant protection against the development of glaucoma, due to its collagen-enhancing actions. In addition, anthocyanosides may be of benefit in the treatment of chronic glaucoma, as rutin has been demonstrated to lower IOP when used as an adjunct in patients unresponsive to miotics alone.[39] *V. myrtillus* anthocyanosides are, in general, much more biologically active than rutin.[16]

Cataracts and retinal degeneration

Vaccinium myrtillus anthocyanosides may offer significant protection against the development of retinal (macular) degeneration and cataracts, particularly diabetic retinopathy and cataracts. Both the rate of retinal degeneration and the occurrence of cataracts in rats can be retarded by changing their diet from a commercial laboratory chow to a "well-defined diet".[40,41] Preliminary research suggests that flavonoid components in the well-defined diets may be responsible for the protective effects against cataracts and retinal degeneration.[42] Limited research has shown that, when combined with vitamin E, bilberry significantly slowed the progression of senile cataracts in humans.[43]

Vaccinium myrtillus anthocyanoside extracts are widely used in Europe in the prevention of diabetic retinopathy.[43–45] The positive effects noted in clinical trials may be due to improved capillary integrity as well as inhibition of sorbitol production (see Ch. 147). Flavonoids have been shown to be potent in vitro and in vivo inhiitors of sorbitol accumulation. In laboratory experiments they have been shown capable of inhibiting the development of diabetic cataracts.[46–48]

Other clinical applications

Diabetes mellitus

A decoction of blueberry leaves has a long history of folk use in the treatment of diabetes. This use is supported by research, which has shown that oral administration reduces hyperglycemia in normal and depancreatized dogs, even when glucose is concurrently injected intravenously.[45,49]

The anthocyanoside myrtillin (3-glucoside of delphinidin) is apparently the most active hypoglycemic component of *V. myrtillus*. Upon injection, it is somewhat weaker than insulin, but it is also less toxic, even at 50 times the 1 g/day therapeutic dose. It is of interest to note that a single dose can produce beneficial effects lasting for several weeks.[45]

The most important benefits from use of anthocyanosides in the treatment of diabetes, however, relate to their ability to improve collagen integrity and capillary permeability. Benefit also possibly derives from their ability to inhibit sorbitol accumulation, thus providing protection from the serious vascular and neurological sequelae of diabetes.

Vaccinium myrtillus anthocyanosides have also been shown to have a protective effect on capillary fragility in diabetics and to reduce serum cholesterol and triglyceride levels in primary dyslipidemia.[50]

Although studies in rabbits have not confirmed a cholesterol-lowering effect, the anthocyanosides significantly decrease the proliferation of the intima, extracellular matrix production, and calcium and lipid deposition found in the aorta of untreated atherosclerotic rabbits. Presumably, this is a result of increasing collagen cross-linking, thus diminishing the permeability in small, as well as in large, blood vessels.[51]

Inflammatory joint disease

The effects of anthocyanosides on collagen structures and their potent antioxidant activity make *V. myrtillus* anthocyanoside extracts very useful in the treatment of a wide variety of inflammatory conditions, most notably rheumatoid arthritis. Bioflavonoids have been found to increase collagen synthesis and inhibit collagen catabolism in rats with adjuvant-induced arthritis (a chronic progressive polyarthritis with some similarities to rheumatoid arthritis).[13]

Blueberries, like cherries, are particularly indicated in the treatment of gout, as their flavonoid components are able to reduce both uric acid levels and tissue destruction (see Ch. 154).[52]

Microscopic hematuria

The effect of *V. myrtillus* in the reduction of microscopic hematuria may be reflective of its tissue distribution. Pharmacokinetic studies in rats have demonstrated an affinity for the skin and kidneys.[53] Anthocyanosides' affinity for these tissues reflects the high concentration of collagen and mucopolysaccharides in the skin and kidneys and the fact that they are excreted via the kidneys.

DOSAGE

The standard dose for *V. myrtillus* is based on its anthocyanoside content, as calculated by its anthocyanidin percentage. Widely used pharmaceutical preparations in Europe are typically standardized for a 25% anthocyanidin content. Dosages are as follows:

- anthocyanosides (calculated as anthocyanidin): 20–40 mg three times/day
- *Vaccinium myrtillus* (25% extract): 80–160 mg three times/day
- fresh berries: 55–115 g three times/day.

TOXICOLOGY

Extensive toxicological investigation has demonstrated that *V. myrtillus* anthocyanoside extracts are devoid of toxic effects. Administration to rats of dosages as high as 400 mg/kg produces no apparent side-effects, and excess levels are quickly excreted through the urine and bile.[16,24]

SUMMARY

Vaccinium myrtillus anthocyanosides exhibit significant pharmacological activity, particularly on collagen structures. Research has demonstrated a positive effect in the treatment of:

- capillary fragility
- blood purpuras
- various encephalic circulation disturbances
- venous insufficiency
- varicose veins
- microscopic hematuria caused by diffused and kidney capillary fragility
- poor night vision
- hemeralopia
- diabetic retinopathy.

Experimental studies indicate that anthocyanoside should also be useful in most inflammatory or degenerative conditions involving connective tissues (e.g. osteoarthritis, gout, rheumatoid arthritis, periodontal disease, etc.), glaucoma, diabetes, cataracts, retinal degeneration, and schizophrenia.

REFERENCES

1. Grieve M. A modern herbal, vol. 1. New York, NY: Dover Publications. 1971: p 385–386
2. Baj A, Bombardelli E, Gabetta B, Martinelli EM. Qualitative and quantitative evaluation of *Vaccinium myrtillus* anthocyanins by high-resolution gas chromatography and high-performance liquid chromatography. J Chromatogr 1983; 279: 365–372
3. Andersen OM. Anthocyanins in fruits of *Vaccinium uliginosum* L. (bog whortleberry). J Food Sci 1987; 52: 665–666, 680
4. Kuhnau J. The flavonoids. A class of semi-essential food components. Their role in human nutrition. Wld Rev Nutr Diet 1976; 24: 117–191
5. Gabor M. Pharmacologic effects of flavonoids on blood vessels. Angiologica 1972; 9: 355–374
6. Havsteen B. Flavonoids, a class of natural products of high pharmacological potency. Biochem Pharmacol 1983; 32: 1141–1148
7. Monboisse JC, Braquet P, Randoux A, Borel JP. Non-enzymatic degradation of acid-soluble calf skin collagen by superoxide ion. Protective effect of flavonoids. Biochem Pharmacol 1983; 32: 53–58
8. Detre A, Jellinek H, Miskulin M, Robert AM. Studies on vascular permeability in hypertension. Action of anthocyanosides. Clin Physiol Biochem 1986; 4: 143–149
9. Monboisse JC, Braquet P, Borel JP. Oxygen-free radicals as mediators of collagen breakage. Agents Actions 1984; 15: 49–50
10. Jonadet M, Meunier MT, Bastide J, Bastide P. Anthocyanosides extracted from Vitis vinifera, *Vaccinium myrtillus* and *Pinus maritimus*. I. Elastase-inhibiting activities in vitro. II. Compared angioprotective activities in vivo. J Pharm Belg 1983; 38: 41–46
11. Middleton E. The flavonoids. Trends in Phramaceutical Science 1984; 5: 335–338
12. Amella M, Bronner C, Briancon F et al. Inhibition of mast cell histamine release by flavonoids and biflavonoids. Planta Medica 1985; 51: 16–20
13. Rao CN, Rao VH, Steinman B. Influence of bioflavonoids on the collagen metabolism in rats with adjuvant induced arthritis. Ital J Biochem 1981; 30: 54–62
14. Ronziere MC, Herbage D, Garrone R, Frey J. Influence of some flavonoids on reticulation of collagen fibrils in vitro. Biochem Pharmacol 1981; 30: 1771–1776
15. Mian E, Curri SB, Lieti A, Bombardelli E. Anthocyanosides and the walls of the microvessels. Further aspects of the mechanism of action of their protective effect in syndromes due to abnormal capillary fragility. Minerva Med 1977; 68: 3565–3581
16. Lietti A, Forni G. Studies on *Vaccinium myrtillus* anthocyanosides. I. Vasoprotective and anti-inflammatory activity. Arzneim Forsch 1976; 26: 829–832
17. Ghiringhelli C, Gregoratti F, Marastoni F. Capillarotropic activity of anthocyanosides in high doses in phlebopathic stasis. Min Cardioangiol 1978; 26: 255–276
18. Treviso A. Therapeutic value of the association of anthocyanin glucosides with glutamine and phosphorylserine in the treatment of learning disturbances at different ages. Gazz Med Ital 1979; 138: 217–232
19. Grismond GL. Treatment of pregnancy-induced phlebopathies. Minerva Ginecol 1981; 33: 221–230
20. Piovella F, Almasio P, Ricetti MM, Trpin L, Cavanna L. Results with anthocyanidins in the treatment of haemorrhagic diathesis due to defective primary haemastasis. Gazz Med Ital 1981; 140: 445–449
21. Pennarola R, Roco P, Matarazzo G et al. The therapeutic action of the anthocyanosides in microcirculatory changes due to adhesive-induced polyneuritis. Gazz Med Ital 1980; 139: 485–491
22. Amouretti M. Therapeutic value of *Vaccinium myrtillus* anthocyanosides in an internal medicine department. Therapeutique 1972; 48: 579–581
23. Robert AM, Godeau G, Moati F, Miskulin M. Action of the anthocyanosides of *Vaccinium myrtillus* on the permeability of the blood brain barrier. J Med 1977; 8: 321–332
24. Bertuglia S, Malandrino S, Colantuoni A. Effect of *Vaccinium myrtillus* anthocyanoside on ischemia reperfusion injury in hamster cheek pouch microcirulcation. Pharmacol Res 1995; 31: 183–187
25. Zaragoza F, Iglesias I, Benedi J. Comparison of thrombocyte antiaggregant effects of anthocyanosides with those of other agents. Arch Pharmacol Toxicol 1985; 11: 183–188
26. Morazzoni P, Magistretti MJ. Effects of *Vaccinium myrtillus* anthocyanosides on prostacyclin like activity in rat arterial tissue. Fitoterapia 1986; 57: 11–14
27. Bottecchia D, Bettini V, Martino R, Camerra G. Preliminary report on the inhibitory effect of *Vaccinium myrtillus* anthocyanosides on platelet aggregation and clot retraction. Fitoterapia 1987; 48: 3–8
28. Bettini V, Mavellaro F, Ton P, Zanella P. Effects of *Vaccinium myrtillus* anthocyanosides on vascular smooth muscle. Fitoterapia 1984; 55: 265–272
29. Bettini V, Mavellaro F, Patron E et al. Inhibition by *Vaccinium myrtillus* anthocyanosides of barium-induced contractions in segments of internal thoracic vein. Fitoterapia 1984; 55: 323–327
30. Bettini V, Mayellaro F, Pilla I et al. Mechanical responses of isolated coronary arteries to barium in the presence of *Vaccinium myrtillus* anthocyanosides. Fitoterapia 1985; 56: 3–10
31. Colombo D, Vescovini R. Controlled clinical trial of anthocyanosides from *Vaccinium myrtillus* in primary dysmenorrhea. G Ital Obstet Ginecol 1985; 7: 1033–1038
32. Jayle GE, Aubert L. Action des glucosides d'anthocyanes sur la vision scotopique et mesopique du sujet normal. Therapie 1964; 19: 171–185
33. Terrasse J, Moinade S. Premiers resultats obtenus avec un nouveau facteur vitamininique P 'les anthocyanosides' extraits du *Vaccinium myrtillus*. Presse Med 1964; 72: 397–400
34. Sala D, Rolando M, Rossi PL, Pissarello L. Effect of anthocyanosides on visual performances at low illumination. Minerva Oftalmol 1979; 21: 283–285
35. Gloria E, Peria A. Effect of anthocyanosides on the absolute visual threshold. Ann Ottalmol Clin Ocul 1066; 92: 595–607
36. Junemann G. On the effect of anthocyanosides on hemeralopia following quinine poisoning. Klin Monatsbl Augenheilkd 1967; 151: 891–896

37. Caselli L. Clinical and electroretinographic study on activity of anthocyanosides. Arch Med Int 1985; 37: 29–35
38. Wegmann R, Maeda K, Tronche P, Bastide P. Effects of anthocyanosides on photoreceptors. Cytoenzymatic aspects. Ann Histochim 1969; 14: 237–256
39. Stocker F. New ways of influencing the intraocular pressure. NY St J Med 1949; 49: 58–63
40. Pautler EL, Ennis SR. The effect of diet on inherited retinal dystrophy in the rat. Curr Eye Res 1984; 3: 1221–1224
41. Hess H, Knapka JJ, Newsome DA et al. Dietary prevention of cataracts in the pink-eyed RCS rat. Lag Anim Sci 1985; 35: 47–53
42. Pautler EL, Maga JA, Tengerdy C. A pharmacologically potent natural product in the bovine retina. Exp Eye Res 1986; 42: 285–288
43. Bravetti G. Preventive medical treatment of senile cataracts with vitamin E and anthocyanosides. Clinical evaluation. Ann Ottalmol Clin Ocul 1989; 115: 109
44. Scharrer A, Ober M. Anthocyanosides in the treatment of retinopathies. Klin Monatsbl Augenheilkd 1981; 178: 386–389
45. Bever B, Zahnd G. Plants with oral hypoglycemic action. Quart J Crude Drug Res 1979; 17: 139–196
46. Chaundry PS, Cambera J, Juliana HR, Varma SD. Inhibition of human lens aldose reductase by flavonoids, sulindac and indomethacin. Biochem Pharmacol 1983; 32: 1995–1998
47. Varma SD, Mizuno A, Kinoshita JH. Diabetic cataracts and flavonoids. Science 1977; 195: 87–89
48. Varma SD, El-aguizy HK, Richards RD. Refractive change in alloxan diabetic rabbits control by flavonoids I. Acta Ophthalmol 1980; 58: 748–759
49. Allen FM. Blueberry leaf extract. Physiologic and clinical properties in relation to carbohydrate metabolism. JAMA 1927; 89: 1577–1581
50. Passariello N, Bisesti V, Sgambato S. Influence of anthocyanosides on the microcirculation and lipid picture in diabetic and dyslipidic subjects. Gazz Med Ital 1979; 138: 563–566
51. Kadar A, Robert L, Miskulin M et al. Influence of anthocyanoside treatment on the cholesterol-induced atherosclerosis in the rabbit. Paroi Arterielle 1979; 5: 187–206
52. Blau LW. Cherry diet control for gout and arthritis. Tex Rep Biol Med 1950; 8: 309–311
53. Lietti A, Forni G. Studies on *Vaccinium myrtillus* anthocyanosides. II. Aspects of anthocyanins pharmacokinetics in the rat. Arzneim Forsch 1976; 26: 832–835

CHAPTER CONTENTS

119

Valeriana officinalis (valerian)

Michael T. Murray, ND

Joseph E. Pizzorno Jr, ND

Valeriana officinalis (family: Valerianaceae)
Common names: valerian, all heal

GENERAL DESCRIPTION

Valerian is a perennial plant native to North America and Europe. The yellow-brown tuberous rootstock produces a flowering stem 2–4 feet high. The stem is round, but grooved and hollow, with leaves arranged in pairs. The small rose-colored flowers are in bloom from June to September. The rootstock is the portion used medicinally.

CHEMICAL COMPOSITION

The important active compounds of valerian are the valepotriates (iridoid molecules; see Fig. 119.1) and valerenic acid. These compounds are found exclusively in valerian. Originally it was thought that just the valepotriates were responsible for valerian's sedative effects, but recently an aqueous extract of valerian has also been shown to have a sedative effect. Since the valepotriates are not soluble in water, it was concluded that valerenic acid also possesses sedative action and is the chemical factor responsible for the sedative effect noted in human clinical trials with aqueous extracts of valerian root (see below).

R'O
O
CH_2OR''
RO
O

Compound	R	R′	R″
Valtrate	Isovaleroyl	Isovaleroyl	Acetyl
Isovaltrate	Isovaleroyl	Acetyl	Isovaleroyl
Homovaltrate	Isovaleroyl	Methyl-valeroyl	Acetyl
Acevaltrate	Isovaleroyl	O-acetyl-valeroyl	Acetyl

Figure 119.1 Valepotriates in *Valeriana officinalis.*

Moreover, because the safety of valepotriates was questioned after studies demonstrated mutagenicity, most commercial extracts feature water-soluble extracts standardized for valerenic acids.[1–3]

Other components of valerian include a volatile oil (0.5–2%), choline (3%), flavonoids, sterols, and several alkaloids (actinidine, valerianine, valerine, and chatinine).[1]

HISTORY AND FOLK USE

Valerian's primary traditional use has been as a sedative for the relief of insomnia, anxiety, and conditions associated with pain. Specific conditions for which it was used include migraine, insomnia, hysteria, fatigue, intestinal cramps, and other nervous conditions.

PHARMACOLOGY

Valerian has demonstrated a number of pharmacological effects including:[4–7]

- normalizing of the central nervous system (it acts as a sedative in states of agitation and a stimulant in cases of extreme fatigue)
- lowering of blood pressure
- enhancement of the flow of bile (choleretic effect)
- relaxing intestinal muscles
- antitumor and antibiotic activity.

Its prime pharmacological effect, however, is consistent with its historical use as a sedative.

A recent pharmacological study indicated that both valepotriates and valerenic acid are capable of binding to GABA receptors in a similar fashion to benzodiazepines.[8] However, valerian does not appear to act in a similar fashion, in that side-effects such as impaired mental function, morning hangover, and dependency have not been reported with valerian. In addition, valerian compounds which do not bind to GABA receptors have also been shown to produce sedative effects.

CLINICAL APPLICATIONS

The primary clinical application for valerian is as a sedative in the treatment of insomnia. It can also be used in the treatment of stress and anxiety.

Insomnia

Several recent clinical studies have substantiated valerian's ability to improve sleep quality and relieve insomnia.[9–13]

The first studies were performed on subjects who did not have insomnia. In the first double-blind study involving 128 subjects, an extract of valerian root improved subjective ratings for sleep quality and sleep latency (the time required to go to sleep) but left no "hangover" the next morning.[9]

In another study, the effects of valerian on sleep were studied in two groups of healthy young subjects.[10] One group slept at home, the other in a sleep laboratory. Sleep was evaluated on the basis of questionnaires, self-rating scales and night-time motor activity. Under home conditions, both doses of an aqueous valerian extract (450 and 900 mg) reduced perceived sleep latency and wake time after sleep onset. Night-time motor activity was enhanced in the middle third of the night and reduced in the last third. The data suggest a dose-dependent effect. In the sleep laboratory, where only the higher dose of valerian was tested, no significant differences from placebo were obtained. However, the direction of the changes in the subjective and objective measures of sleep latency and wake time after sleep onset, as well as in night-time motor activity, corresponded to that observed under home conditions. There was no evidence for a change in sleep stages and EEG spectra. The results indicate that the aqueous valerian extract exerts a mild sedative effect.

While these two studies demonstrated that valerian could improve sleep quality in normal subjects, they failed to answer the question whether valerian could improve sleep patterns in people suffering from insomnia. In a follow-up to these two preliminary studies, valerian extract was shown to significantly reduce sleep latency, improve sleep quality, and reduce night-time awakenings in sufferers of insomnia.[11] This study, performed under strict laboratory conditions, demonstrated that valerian is as effective in reducing sleep latency as small doses of barbiturates or benzodiazepines. However, while these latter compounds also increase morning sleepiness, valerian usually reduces morning sleepiness.

In another study of insomniacs, subjects received either a valerian preparation placebo.[12] Compared with the placebo, valerian showed a significant effect, with 44% reporting perfect sleep and 89% reporting improved sleep.

And finally, in another double-blind study of insomniacs, 20 subjects received a combination of valerian root (160 mg) and *Melissa officinalis* (80 mg), a benzodiazepine (triazolam 0.125), or placebo.[13] In the insomniac group, the valerian preparation showed an effect comparable to that of the benzodiazopine, as well as an increase in deep sleep stages 3 and 4. The valerian preparation did not, however, cause daytime sedation and there was no evidence of diminished concentration based on the Concentration Performance Test or impairment of physical performance.

DOSAGE

As a mild sedative, valerian may be taken at the following dosages 30–45 minutes before retiring:

- dried root (or as tea): 1–2 g
- tincture (1:5): 4–6 ml (1–1.5 tsp)

- fluid extract (1:1): 1–2 ml (0.5–1 tsp)
- solid (dry powdered) extract (4:1): 250–500 mg
- valerian extract (1.0–1.5% valtrate or 0.5% valerenic acid): 150–300 mg.

For the rare patient with increased morning sleepiness, reducing the dosage will eliminate the problem. For best results, eliminate dietary factors such as caffeine and alcohol which disrupt sleep (see Ch. 164).

TOXICITY

Valerian is generally regarded as safe and is approved for food use by the United States Food and Drug Administration.[14] A major concern for any sedative or anti-anxiety medication is its potential to affect a person's ability to drive or operate potentially dangerous machinery. A randomized, placebo-controlled, double-blind study evaluated the impact of a valerian/lemon balm preparation on psychomotor and mental performance tests.[15] No impact was found on reaction time, concentration or attentiveness.

One case of valerian overdose has been reported in the literature.[16] The patient presented with mild symptoms, all of which disappeared within 24 hours after taking an overdose of approximately 20 times the recommended therapeutic dose.

Since the safety of the valepotriates have been questioned, until there is better information, the best choice is to use water-soluble extracts standardized for valerenic acid content.

REFERENCES

1. Houghton PJ. The biological activity of Valerian and related plants. J Ethnopharmacol 1988; 22: 121–142
2. von der Hude W, Scheutwinkel-Reich M, Braun R. Bacterial mutagenicity of the tranquilizing constituents of Valerianaceae roots. Mut Research 1986; 169: 23–27
3. von der Hude W, Scheutwinkel-Reich M, Braun R. In vitro mutagenicity of valepotriates. Arch Toxicol 1985; 56: 267–271
4. Takeda S, Endo T, Aburada M. Pharmacological studies on iridoid compounds. III. The choleretic mechanism of iridoid compounds. J Pharm Dyn 1981; 4: 612–623
5. Hendriks H, Bos R, Allersma DP et al. Pharmacological screening of valerenal and some other components of essential oil of *Valeriana officinalis*. Planta Medica 1981; 42: 62–68
6. Hazelhoff B, Malingre TM, Meijer DK. Antispasmodic effects of valeriana compounds. An in vivo and in vitro study on the guinea pig ileum. Arch Int Pharmacodyn 1982; 257: 274–287
7. Bounthanh C, Bergmann C, Beck JP et al. Valepotriates, a new class of cytotoxic and antitumor agents. Planta Medica 1981; 41: 21–28
8. Mennini T, Bernasconi P, Bombardelli E et al. In vitro study on the interaction of extracts and pure compounds from *Valeriana officinalis* roots with GABA, benzodiazepine and barbiturate receptors in rat brain. Fitoterapia 1993; 54: 291–300
9. Leathwood P, Chauffard F, Heck E et al. Aqueous extract of valerian root (*Valeriana officinalis* L.) improves sleep quality in man. Pharmacol Biochem Behavior 1982; 17: 65–71
10. Balderer G, Borbely AA. Effect of valerian on human sleep. Psychopharmacol 1985; 87: 406–409
11. Leathwood PD, Chauffard F. Aqueous extract of valerian reduces latency to fall asleep in man. Planta Medica 1985; 54: 144–148
12. Lindahl O, Lindwall L. Double blind study of a valerian preparation. Pharmacol Biochem Behav 1989; 32: 1065–1066
13. Dressing H, Riemann D, Low H. Insomnia. Are Valerian/Melissa combinations of equal value to benzodiazepine? Therapiewoche 1992; 42: 726–736
14. Leung A. Encyclopedia of common natural ingredients used in food, drugs, and cosmetics. New York, NY: John Wiley. 1980
15. Albrecht M, Berger W et al. Psychopharmaceuticals and safety in traffic. Zeits Allegmeinmed 1995; 71: 1215–1221
16. Wiley LB, Mady SP, Cobaugh DJ, Wax PM. Valerian overdose. A case report. Vet Hum Toxicol 1995; 37: 364–365

CHAPTER CONTENTS

120

Viscum album (European mistletoe)

Michael T. Murray, ND

Joseph E. Pizzorno Jr, ND

Viscum album L. (family: Loranthaceae)
Common names: European mistletoe, all-heal, birdlime, devil's fuge

GENERAL DESCRIPTION

Viscum album or European mistletoe is an evergreen, semi-parasitic plant found on the branches of deciduous trees in Europe and northern Asia. The roots of the plant penetrate through the bark into the wood of the host tree. The green branches are 1–2 feet long and form pendent bushes with leaves that are opposite, leathery, yellow-green and narrowly obovate. Inconspicuous pale yellow or green flowers appear from March to May, the female developing into sticky white berries which ripen from September to November.[1,2]

Viscum is most commonly seen on old apple, ash, and hawthorn trees. Traditionally, mistletoe from oak has been the most widely used, although it does not grow as well on oak as the previously mentioned trees.[1,2]

CHEMICAL COMPOSITION

Viscum album contains a variety of pharmacologically active substances including alkaloids, polysaccharides, phenylpropanes, lignins, lectins, and viscotoxins.[3–10] Specific compounds found in viscum include:[2,5,6,10]

- a wide range of carbohydrates, including simple sugars as well as polysaccharides
- phenolic compounds such as flavonoids, caffeic acid, syringin, and eleutherosides
- sterols, including beta-sitosterol, stigmasterol, and triterpenes
- various amino acids as well as vasoactive amines, including tyramine, phenylethylamine, and histamine
- fatty acids such as linoleic, palmitic, and oleic acids.

The alkaloids isolated from viscum appear to be related to those found in the host plant.[3,4] For example, mistletoes growing on solanaceae shrubs contain nicotine alkaloids like hyoscine, anabasine, and isopelletierine; cardiac glycosides have been found in mistletoe growing on *Nerium oleander*; strychnine has been found in mistletoe growing on *Strychnos* sp.; and caffeine in mistletoe growing on coffee plants.

Since pharmacologically active compounds appear to be concentrated within the mistletoe, different host trees, providing diverse chemical constituents, could be used for different therapeutic action.

Also of importance is the fact that the proteins/lectins are present only in aqueous extracts, indicating that therapeutic activity would differ from the alcoholic/aqueous extracts. The alcoholic/aqueous extracts also demonstrate considerably less toxicity.

HISTORY AND FOLK USE

Mistletoe was held in great reverence by the Druids who, dressed in white robes, would search for the sacred plant. When some was discovered, a great ceremony would ensue, culminating in the mistletoe's separation from the oak with a golden knife. The Druids believed that mistletoe protected them from all evil, and that the oaks on which it was seen growing were to be respected because of the wonderful cures which the priests were able to produce with it.[1]

Mistletoe's use has been recorded in the Middle East, Africa, India, and Japan, and it was mentioned as an anti-cancer drug by Pliny, Dioscorides, and Galen.[3]

In 1720, an English physician, Sir John Colbatch, extolled the virtues of viscum in a pamphlet entitled *The treatment of epilepsy by mistletoe*. For many years, mistletoe was used in the treatment of a variety of nervous system disorders, including convulsions, delirium, hysteria, neuralgia, and nervous debility.[1,3] It has been used in naturopathic medicine in the treatment of hypertension and vascular disorders of the uterus, bladder, and intestines.

Probably due to its potential toxicity, viscum use appeared to fall into some disrepute shortly after Colbatch's work. For many years it was used only in external preparations for the treatment of dermatitis. Then in 1906 a study demonstrating viscum's hypotensive effect in animals and humans was published. This appears to have restored viscum's medical prestige, initially in France and eventually throughout Europe.[3]

PHARMACOLOGY

Viscum album exhibits diverse pharmacological actions. The herb and various extracts have demonstrated the following activities:

- hypotensive
- vasodilating
- cardiac depressant
- sedative
- antispasmodic
- immunostimulatory
- anti-neoplastic.

It is interesting to note that purified mistletoe lectins are, in general, not as active in experimental studies as crude preparations.[21,22] Presumably, there are a number of compounds in viscum which act synergistically. It has also been proposed that alkaloidal components are responsible for the maintenance of lectin structure and activity.[5] During isolation and purification procedures, alkaloidal linkages are cleaved from the lectins, resulting in a loss of specificity for target molecules. Unfermented viscum preparations typically demonstrate a greater direct cytotoxicity to tumor cells due to higher concentrations of the viscotoxin ML I.[14,23,24]

Cardiovascular effects

Viscum has exhibited a variety of effects on components of the cardiovascular system.[3,11] In particular, viscum has repeatedly demonstrated hypotensive action in animal studies. The mechanism of action for its hypotensive effect is still not entirely clear, and no recent investigations have been published. Viscum has been shown to inhibit the excitability of the vasomotor center in the medulla oblongata and to possess cholinomimetic activity.[11]

The hypotensive activity may be dependent on the form in which the mistletoe is administered and the host tree from which it was collected. Studies indicate that aqueous extracts are more effective; the highest hypotensive activity was demonstrated by a macerate of leaves of mistletoe parasitizing on willow and gathered in January.[11]

Viscum's non-protein components, e.g. flavonoids, phenol carboxylic acids, phenylpropanes, and lignins, have been shown to possess hypotensive action. Alcoholic solutions (tinctures and fluid extracts) contain these compounds, but not viscotoxins or lectins. However, as stated above, aqueous extracts appear to be more effective.

Currently, in Europe, several viscum preparations for hypertension exist. In fact, in Britain alone over 150 different mistletoe preparations can be found in the marketplace.[3] These preparations typically have small amounts of viscum in combination with other botanicals with hypotensive action, e.g. garlic, *Crataegus oxyacantha*, and *Tilia platyphyllos*.

Anti-neoplastic and immunostimulatory effects

Viscum preparations have been used clinically in Europe for the treatment of cancer since 1926 when Iscador, a fermented product made from the crude pressed juice, was introduced as an immunotherapeutic agent for cancer. This work was carried out under the direction of Rudolph Steiner. Since that time, numerous studies have shown that Iscador, and other viscum preparations and components, are effective anti-neoplastic and immunostimulatory agents.[12–31]

Iscador and other fermented viscum preparations differ from non-fermented extracts in their greater effectiveness and their decreased toxicity.[12] Specifically, the major viscotoxin, ML I, is not found in Iscador.[13] It is thought, that fermentation transforms ML I to its A and B chains, which have important immunological properties.[14] The A chain has mitogenic effects and the B chain stimulates macrophages and the release of lymphokines. In addition, there is a rapid decrease of lectin concentration during fermentation.

The pharmacological activity of Iscador has been shown to be due to its viscum components, rather than to other constituents such as lactobacilli, which possess adjuvant activity. The lectins have been clearly demonstrated to be the viscum components largely responsible for Iscador's adjuvant activity. Although in vitro unfermented plant juice has demonstrated a 10-fold greater cytotoxicity to tumor cells than Iscador, fermented Iscador contains a great number of substances which may act synergistically. In vivo studies in mice have demonstrated Iscador to be of greater adjuvant activity than purified mistletoe lectin, and without secondary toxic effects.[15,16]

Viscum's adjuvant activity is demonstrable in both delayed-type hypersensitivity and antibody responses of mice to sheep red blood cells.[15,16] Similar to other adjuvants (BCG, levamisole, muramyl dipeptide, bacterial and yeast components, etc.), Iscador is most effective when administered near the tumor, although systemic administration has also yielded positive results. Upon local administration, an inflammatory process ensues which promotes WBC infiltration and an encapsulation of the tumor.

The non-specific host defense factors stimulated by *Viscum album* include:

- enhanced macrophage phagocytic and cytotoxic activity[12,16]
- increased neutrophil production[12]
- increased thymic weight and enhanced cortical thymocyte activity and proliferation[17,19]
- enhanced natural killer cell activity[12,18,20]
- increased antibody-dependent, cell-mediated cytotoxicity.[12,18]

Iscador's effects on these immunological parameters have been confirmed in patients with cancer.[12,18]

Iscador's effect on stimulating the thymus gland has been demonstrated in several studies.[17,19] Its ability to induce hyperplasia of the thymic cortex and to accelerate the regeneration of hematopoietic cells following X-irradiation is much greater than any other agent reported to date.[17] In addition, thymic lymphocytes became 29 times more responsive to concanavalin A as a result of Iscador administration.

In summary, *Viscum album* exhibits numerous cytotoxic, adjuvant, and immunostimulatory effects which indicate a therapeutic effect in human cancer. These effects have been confirmed in vivo against murine tumors, Lewis lung carcinoma, colon adenocarcinoma 38, and C3H mammary adenocarcinoma 16/C.[4]

CLINICAL APPLICATIONS

Cancer

The only clinical application with any significant scientific documentation is the use of viscum preparations as adjuncts in cancer therapy. It must be pointed out that the route of the administration of viscum preparations used in published studies as adjuncts in cancer treatments is subcutaneous or intravenous. It is not known to what degree (if any) the effects noted for Iscador, as well as other preparations and viscum compounds, can be achieved with oral administration.

Early clinical investigations of viscum preparations, i.e. Iscador, were not very well documented. Due to the shortage of acceptable controlled clinical trials, the use of Iscador and other viscum preparations as a cancer treatment in Europe has remained controversial, even though positive effects with Iscador in the postoperative treatment of lung, breast, colon, and cervical carcinomas has been shown in several controlled studies.[25] The problem is that the methodological criteria in these studies are quite poor. Until their benefits are better documented, at this time, mistletoe preparations appear most useful as adjuncts to standard therapy.

A new generation of mistletoe preparations standardized on mistletoe lectin I (e.g. Eurixor) is emerging. This greater standardization offers significant advantages. Mistletoe lectin I is a potent inducer of cytokines like interleukin 1, interleukin 6, and tumor necrosis factor. Its cytotoxic effects are also related to its ability to induce apoptosis (programmed cell death).[26]

In one study, the effect of Eurixor was examined in 40 patients with advanced carcinoma of the breast. Along with standard chemotherapy (VEC regimen), 21 patients were assigned to receive mistletoe (treatment group) while 19 patients were given a placebo (control group).[27] After the fourth cycle of chemotherapy, the treatment group had statistically significantly higher leukocyte levels ($P < 0.001$) compared with the control group. The treatment group had an average white blood cell count of 3,000, while the control group had an average count of 1,000. Furthermore, the parameters of the quality of life and anxiety strain revealed significantly better values in the treatment group than in the control group. These results show that the adjuvant treatment with mistletoe extracts, in this case Eurixor, is a valuable addition to standard chemotherapy for advanced breast cancer patients. These results are quite important as advanced breast cancer carries with it a very poor prognosis. Similar results have been shown in advanced pancreatic cancer.[28] These results in better designed studies are quite encouraging.

Clearly, additional investigations into the pharmacology of *Viscum album* are needed. Specifically, it must be determined whether the effects noted both in vitro and in vivo in animals, as well as in patients receiving injectable viscum preparations, can be attained by oral administration.

In addition, greater clarification is needed to determine optimal viscum preparations. What host tree should be selected for which condition? What is the optimal harvesting time? In what form should the viscum be administered – crude herb, aqueous or alcoholic extract, fermented or non-fermented?

Viscum is undoubtedly one of the most complex botanicals, yet, after examining currently available data, it can be said with much confidence that the future medicinal use of *Viscum album* is quite promising.

DOSAGE

The standard dose of *Viscum album*, based on the *British herbal pharmacopoeia*, is as follows:[32]

- dried leaves: 2–6 g (or by infusion) three times/day
- tincture 1:5 (45% alcohol): 1–3 ml three times/day
- fluid extract 1:1 (25% alcohol): 0.5 ml three times/day
- dried aqueous extract 4:1: 100–250 mg three times/day.

TOXICITY

Viscum album possesses significant toxicity. Historically, the berries have been regarded as being considerably more toxic than the leaves and stems despite the fact they both contain similar toxic compounds. The reason the toxicity of the berries is considered to be greater probably stems from fatal poisonings of children resulting from ingestion of the berries.

Lethal doses of viscum lectins administered by various routes to mice produce two types of toxicity:

- a typical type characterized by death after 3–4 days with marasmus-like symptoms
- an atypical type characterized by immediate death from respiratory paralysis.[19]

In mice, the LD_{50} of the plant juice administered intraperitoneally is 32 mg (dry weight)/kg body weight.[29]

The LD_{50} values of orally administered *Viscum album* or extracts of *Viscum album* have not yet been determined. As stated earlier, alcohol-based extracts contain virtually no viscum proteins. This would imply significantly less toxicity with these preparations. However, this would also imply loss of activity, as much of the pharmacology of viscum relates to its protein content, especially immuno-enhancing activity.

It is interesting to note that the toxicity of Korean mistletoe, *Viscum album coloratum*, appears to be lower than that of European mistletoe.[30,31] This species has also demonstrated anti-cancer effects, but the effects appear to be due to highly cytotoxic alkaloids rather than to lectins.[5,30] Studies comparing Korean viscum extracts with European extracts, as well as their alkaloid components, have demonstrated that the Korean mistletoe has greater activity in inhibiting cancer cells. In addition, fresh Korean mistletoe extracts exhibited greater activity compared with fermented extracts.[5,30] In the future Korean mistletoe may prove to be superior to European mistletoe.

REFERENCES

1. Grieve M. A modern herbal. New York, NY: Dover Publications. 1971: p 547–548
2. Becker H. Botany of European mistletoe (*Viscum album* L.). Oncology 1986; 43: 2–7
3. Anderson LA, Phillippson JD. Mistletoe – the magic herb. From the Department of Pharmacognocy, School of Pharmacy, University of London, 1982
4. Khwaja TA, Dias CB, Pentecost S. Recent studies on the anticancer activities of mistletoe (*Viscum album*) and its alkaloids. Oncology 1986; 43: 42–50
5. Jordan E, Wagner H. Structure and properties of polysaccharides from *Viscum album* (L.). Oncology 1986; 43: 8–15
6. Wagner H, Jordan E, Feil B. Studies on the standardization of mistletoe preparations. Oncology 1986; 43: 16–22
7. Franz H, Ziska P, Kindt A. Isolation and properties of three lectins from mistletoe (*Viscum album* L.). Biochem J 1981; 195: 481–484
8. Olsnes S, Stirpe F, Sandvig K, Phil A. Isolation and characterization of viscumin, a toxic lectin from *Viscum album* L. (mistletoe). J Biol Chem 1982; 257: 13,263–13,270
9. Petricic J, Kalogjera Z. Isolation of glucosides from mistletoe leaves (*Viscum album* L.). Acta Pharm Jugosl 1980; 30: 163
10. Wagner H, Feil B, Kalogjera Z, Petricic J. Phenylpropanes and lignins of *Viscum album*. Planta Medica 1986; 2: 102
11. Petkov V. Plants with hypotensive, antiatheromatous and coronarodilatating action. Am J Chin Med 1979; 7: 197–236
12. Hajto T. Immunomodulating effects of Iscador. A *Viscum album* preparation. Oncology 1986; 43: 51–65
13. Jordan E, Wagner H. Detection and quantitative determination of lectins and viscotoxins in mistletoe preparations. Arzneim Forsch 1986; 36: 428–433
14. Ribereau-Gayon G, Jung ML, Di Scala D, Beck JP. Comparison of

the effects of fermented and unfermented mistletoe preparations on cultured tumor cells. Oncology 1986; 43: 35–41
15. Bloksma N, Dijk HV, Korst P, Willers JM. Cellular and humoral adjuvant activity of a mistletoe extract. Immunobiol 1979; 156: 309–319
16. Bloksma N, Schmiermann P, Reuver MD, Dijk HD, Willers J. Stimulation of humoral and cellular immunity by viscum preparations. Planta Medica 1982; 46: 221–227
17. Rentea R, Lyon E, Hunter R. Biological properties of Iscador. A *Viscum album* preparation. Lab Invest 1981; 44: 43–48
18. Hajto T, Lanzrein. Natural killer and antibody-dependent cell-mediated cytotoxicity activities and large granular lymphocyte frequencies in *Viscum album*-treated breast cancer patients. Oncology 1986; 43: 93–97
19. Nienhaus J, Stoll M, Vester F. Thymus stimulation and cancer prophylaxis by Viscum proteins. Experentia 1970; 26: 523–525
20. Hamprecht K, Handretinger R, Voetsch W, Anderer FA. Mediation of human NK-activity by components in extracts of *Viscum album*. Int J Immunopharm 1987; 9: 199–209
21. Evans MR, Preece AW. *Viscum album* – a possible treatment for cancer? Bristol Med Chir J 1973; 88: 17–20
22. Klamerth O, Vester F, Kellner G. Inhibitory effects of a protein complex from Viscum album on fibroblasts and HeLa cells. Z Physiol Chem 1968; 349: 863–864
23. Hulsen H, Doser C, Mechelke F. Differences in the in vitro effectiveness of preparations produced from mistletoes of various host trees. Arzneim Forsch 1986; 36: 433–436
24. Hulsen H, Mechelke F. The influence of a mistletoe preparation on suspension cell cultures of human leukemia and human myeloma cells. Arzneim Forsch 1982; 32: 1126–1127
25. Kleijnen J, Knipschild P. Mistletoe treatment for cancer. Review of controlled trials in humans. Phytomedicine 1994; 1: 255–260
26. Janssen O, Scheffler A, Kabelitz D. In vitro effects of mistletoe extracts and mistletoe lectins. Arzneim Forsch 1993; 43: 1221–1225
27. Heiny BM. Adjuvant treatment with standardized mistletoe extract reduces leukopenia and improves the quality of life of patients with advanced carcinoma of the breast gettin palliative chemotherapy (VEC regimen). Krebsmedizin 1991; 12: 3–14
28. Friess H et al. Treatment of advanced pancreatic cancer with mistletoe. Results of a pilot trial. Anticancer Res 1996; 16: 915–920
29. Duke JA. *Handbook of medicinal herbs.* Boca Raton, FL: CRC Press. 1986: p 512–513
30. Khwaja TA, Varven JC, Pentecost S, Pande H. Isolation of biologically active alkaloids from Korean mistletoe *Viscum album,* coloratum. Experentia 1980; 36: 599–600
31. Manjikian S, Pentecost S, Khwaja TA. Isolation of cytotoxic proteins form Viscum album, coloratum. Proc Am Ass Cancer Res 1986; 27: 266
32. British Herbal Medicine Association, Scientific Committee. British Herbal Pharmacopoeia. Cowling: British Herbal Medicine Association. 1983: p 235–236

CHAPTER CONTENTS

121

Vitamin A

Michael T. Murray, ND

Joseph E. Pizzorno Jr, ND

INTRODUCTION

Vitamin A was the first fat-soluble vitamin to be recognized. Although identified as a necessary growth factor in 1913, it was not chemically characterized until 1930. The initial discovery of vitamin A was made almost simultaneously by two groups of research workers, McCollum & Davis at the University of Wisconsin, and Osborne & Mendel at Yale University. They found that young animals fed a diet deficient in natural fats became very unhealthy, as evidenced by their inability to grow and poor immune function. These researchers also noted that the animals' eyes would become severely inflamed and infected on the restricted diet and that this could be quickly relieved by the addition to the diet of either butterfat or cod liver oil. Once known as the "anti-infective vitamin", vitamin A has recently regained recognition as a major determinant of immune status.

NOMENCLATURE

When isolated in its pure form, vitamin A is a pure, lipid-soluble, yellow crystal with a condensed formula of $C_{20}H_{29}OH$. Vitamin A is termed retinol, signifying that it is an alcohol that is intricately involved in the function of the retina of the eye. All-*trans* retinol is found in nature primarily as long-chain retinyl esters. The aldehyde form of all-*trans* retinol is commonly designated retinaldehyde or retinal, while the acidic form is termed retinoic acid. It has been suggested that retinol serves only as a precursor to these two active forms of vitamin A – retinal being primarily involved with vision and reproduction, while retinoic acid is important in other somatic functions, such as growth and differentiation.

Synthetic derivatives of retinoic acid have been developed to treat many dermatological conditions and, more recently, certain forms of cancer. Isotretinoin (13-*cis* retinoic acid) is used in treating severe cystic acne and disorders of keratinization, such as Darier's disease and lamellar ichthyosis. Etretinate, an aromatic derivative of retinoic acid, has no appreciable activity against acne, but is claimed to be more potent than isotretinoin in the treatment of psoriasiform diseases. These compounds, however, are not without side-effects.[1,2]

RECOMMENDED DIETARY ALLOWANCE (RDA)

Vitamin A was originally measured in international units, with 1 IU being defined as 0.3 mcg of crystalline all-*trans* retinol or 0.6 mcg beta-carotene. In 1967, an FAO/WHO Expert Committee recommended that vitamin A activity be referred to in terms of retinol equivalents rather than in IU, with 1 mcg of retinol being equivalent to 1 retinol equivalent (RE). The amount of beta-carotene required for 1 RE is 6 mcg, while the amount required for other provitamin A carotenoids is 12 mcg. In 1980, The Food and Nutrition Board of the NRC/NAS adopted this recommendation, and the 1980 RDA for vitamin A is stated in mcg and RE. For the adult male the RDA is set at 1000 RE (750 as retinol and 250 as beta-carotene, 5000 IU), while the RDA for women is lower at 800 RE (4000 IU). Children need 400–1000 RE (2000–5000 IU), increasing from infancy to 14 years.[1–3] The RDAs for different age groups are shown in Table 121.1.

DIETARY SOURCES

The most concentrated sources of preformed vitamin A are liver, kidney, butter, whole milk, and fortified skim milk, while the leading sources of provitamin A are dark green leafy vegetables (collards and spinach), and yellow-orange vegetables (carrots, sweet potatoes, yams, and squash) (see Table 121.2). Ingestion of excessive amounts of liver, i.e. 2.7–11 kg/week, has been reported to cause hypervitaminosis A.[4]

DEFICIENCY

Vitamin A deficiency may be due to inadequate dietary intake (primary deficiency) or some secondary factor that interferes with the absorption, storage, or transportation of vitamin A. Some factors known to induce a vitamin A deficiency include:

- malabsorption due to bile acid or pancreatic insufficiency
- protein-energy malnutrition
- liver disease
- zinc deficiency
- abetalipoproteinemia.

Table 121.1 Recommended dietary allowances

Group	Retinol equivalents	International Units
Infants		
0–1 year	375	1,875
Children		
1–3 years	400	2,000
4–6 years	500	2,500
7–10 years	700	3,500
Young adults and adults		
Males 11+ years	1,000	5,000
Females 11+ years	800	4,000
Pregnancy	800	4,000

Table 121.2 Food sources of Vitamin A[4]

Food	Portion size	IU/portion
Meats		
Beef liver, fried	100 g	50,375
Calf liver, cooked	100 g	26,872
Chicken liver, cooked	2 livers	25,760
Vegetables		
Sweet potatoes, baked	1 medium	14,600
Carrots, raw	1 large	11,000
Spinach, raw	100 g	8,100
Carrots, cooked	½ cup	8,000
Pumpkin, cooked	½ cup	8,000
Spinach, cooked	½ cup	7,300
Collard greens	½ cup	5,400
Broccoli, cooked	½ cup	1,900
Fruits		
Watermelon	1/16 melon	5,310
Cantaloupe	¼ melon	3,400
Apricots, dried	4 halves	2,275
Apricots, raw	2–3 medium	2,700
Nectarines, raw	1 medium	1,650

Immune system effects

Immune system abnormalities associated with a vitamin A deficiency include impaired ability to mount an effective antibody response, decreased levels of helper T-cells, and alterations in the mucosal linings of the respiratory and gastrointestinal tract. Vitamin A-deficient individuals are more susceptible to infectious diseases and have higher mortality rates. It appears that while a vitamin A deficiency may predispose an individual to an infection, during the course of an infection vitamin A stores are severely depleted. Thus, a vicious cycle ensues. Infectious conditions associated with vitamin A deficiency include the measles, chicken pox, respiratory synctial virus (RSV), AIDS, and pneumonia.

Other effects

Prolonged vitamin A deficiency results in the characteristic signs of follicular hyperkeratosis (build-up of cellular debris in the hair follicles giving the skin a goose bump appearance, which occurs most often at the back of the upper arm), night blindness, and increased rate of infection. As the condition worsens, the mucous membranes of the respiratory tract, gastrointestinal tract, and genitourinary tract also become affected, and the classic eye disease known as xerophthalmia due to vitamin A deficiency ensues. Even a mild vitamin A deficiency is associated with a significant increase in mortality. This is extremely significant, as vitamin A deficiency is particularly widespread in developing countries, especially in Asia where as many as 10 million children develop xerophthalmia every year.[1,2,5]

Xerophthalmia

The term xerophthalmia is generally used to cover all the ocular manifestations of vitamin A deficiency. Blindness is one of the most serious consequences of vitamin A deficiency. Although it rarely occurs in the United States, it is the major preventable cause of blindness in Asia. The xerophthalmia of vitamin A deficiency is staged, as shown in Table 121.3.

In an effort to prevent vitamin A deficiency in underdeveloped countries, large prophylactic doses (200,000 IU) are given by the World Health Organization to children every 6 months.

Determination of deficiency

The rapid dark adaptation test (see Ch. 26) is perhaps the most sensitive of the currently available tests designed to determine vitamin A deficiency. Measurement of serum retinol levels is usually not useful, since they may not become lowered until marked deficiency occurs. Deficiency in the United States and other developed countries is usually secondary to malabsorption, liver disease, or proteinuria.[1,2]

METABOLISM

Absorption

A variety of factors are known to influence the absorption efficacy of vitamin A and carotenoids. Although retinol does not require bile acids to facilitate absorption, carotenoids do. Other factors that affect vitamin A and carotenoid absorption include:

- the presence of fat, protein, and antioxidants in the food
- the presence of bile and a normal complement of pancreatic enzymes in the intestinal lumen
- the integrity of the mucosal cells.

The absorption efficiency of dietary vitamin A is usually quite high (80–90%), with only a slight reduction in efficiency at high doses. In contrast, beta-carotene's absorption efficiency is much lower (40–60%), and it decreases rapidly with increasing dosage.[1,2] Carotene supplements are better absorbed than the carotenes from foods.[6]

Table 121.3 The staging of the xerophthalmia

Stage	Diagnosis	Signs and symptoms
XO	Night blindness	Poor dark adaptation
X1A	Xerosis of conjuctiva	Dryness with "lackluster" appearance, thickening, wrinkling, and diffuse pigmentation of conjunctiva
X1B	Bitot's spots	Usually triangular-shaped collections of desquamated keratinized epithelial cells and mucus
X2	Xerosis of cornea	Dryness of cornea leading to keratinization and a hazy milky appearance
X3	Keratomalacia	Ulceration, distortion, and softening of the cornea with eventual perforation and iris prolapse and infection

Transformation in the intestinal mucosa

The majority of absorbed retinol is esterified with palmitic acid or another free fatty acid within the intestinal mucosal cells. It is then incorporated, along with triglycerides, phospholipids, and cholesterol esters, into chylomicra. The chylomicron is transported through the lymphatic channels into the general circulation and eventually is removed from the circulation by the liver.

Transport, storage and excretion

Upon reaching the liver, vitamin A is stored primarily in special perisinusoidal lipocytes (Ito cells), while the hepatocytes contain only a minor fraction of the total vitamin A stored in the liver. Although small amounts of vitamin A are found in most tissues (see Table 121.4), more than 90% of the total body vitamin A content is stored in the liver. It is stored as a lipoglycoprotein complex consisting of 96% retinyl esters and 4% unesterified retinol. The retinyl esters are hydrolyzed by a tightly bound retinyl ester hydrolase which transfers the released all-*trans* retinol to intracellular retinol binding protein (RBP). The bound retinol is then processed through the Golgi apparatus and secreted into the plasma where it forms a reversible 1:1 molar complex with prealbumin.[1,2]

Table 121.4 Distribution of vitamin A in some human tissues (mcg/kg)

Tissue	Vitamin A
Adrenal	10.4 ± 7.1
Liver	149 ± 132
Testis	1.14 ± 1.23
Fat	1.46 ± 1.55
Pancreas	0.52 ± 0.28
Spleen	0.89 ± 0.88
Lung	0.91 ± 1.89
Thyroid	0.43 ± 0.33

Adequate dietary protein and zinc are necessary for proper retinal mobilization. The half-lives of RBP and prealbumin are less than 12 hours, making them particularly likely to be deficient during protein-calorie malnutrition or other situations in which protein metabolism is abnormal. A zinc or vitamin E deficiency will also severely impair vitamin A metabolism, as these two nutrients function synergistically in many physiological processes of vitamin A metabolism (absorption, transport, and mobilization in particular).[2]

Retinol is transferred into the cell after RBP binds to a cell surface receptor. The retinol is then quickly bound by cellular retinol binding protein (CRBP) in the cell cytosol.

Retinoic acid is metabolized differently from retinol. It is absorbed through the portal system and transported in the plasma bound to albumin. It does not accumulate in the liver or other tissues in any appreciable amounts. It is metabolized quite rapidly to more polar oxygenated compounds. Intracellularly, it is bound to the cellular retinoic acid binding protein (CRABP).[7]

Vitamin A metabolites are excreted mainly through the feces (via the bile) and the urine. During periods of deficiency there appears to be an adaptation in utilization, as evidenced by a reduction in the rate of vitamin A catabolism.[1,2]

PHYSIOLOGICAL ROLES OF VITAMIN A

Vision

The best understood physiological role of vitamin A is its effects on the visual system. The human retina has four kinds of vitamin A-containing photopigments:

- rhodopsin, present in the rods (maximum absorption at 498 nm)
- three iodopsins, present in the cones
  —blue cones (maximum absorption 420 nm)
  —green cones (maximum absorption 534 nm)
  —red cones (maximum absorption 563 nm).

The vitamin A form found in these pigments is the 11-*cis* isomer of vitamin A aldehyde (retinal). When a photon of light strikes the dark-adapted retina, the 11-*cis* configuration is converted to the all-*trans* form of the retinaldehyde and split from the rhodopsin molecule to yield opsin and all-*trans* retinol. This leads to a change in membrane potential and subsequent visual excitation. During light adaptation, as the visual processes are largely dependent on the cone cells, the released all-*trans* retinal or retinol from the rod cells is transported to pigment epithelial cells and stored as retinyl palmitate. During dark adaptation these processes are reversed, and, in addition, the retinal is isomerized to the 11-*cis* form. As the rod cells are particularly sensitive to vitamin A deficiency, night blindness or poor dark adaptation is an early consequence of vitamin A deficiency (see Ch. 26).[1,2]

Growth and development

Vitamin A is believed to affect growth and development by its necessary role in the synthesis of many glycoproteins (e.g. mucus), some of which may control cellular differentiation, and by its function as CRBP in controlling gene expression.[1,2]

The adhesion between cells is apparently related to glycoprotein synthesis, which is markedly depressed in vitamin A deficiency. Consequently, during deficiency there is a loss of normal stimuli for cellular growth and differentiation. CRBP is transferred directly into the nucleus and may function in a fashion similar to some of the steroid hormones. The effects of a vitamin A deficiency most readily seen at the cellular level are in those differentiating tissues that have a rapid turnover rate, i.e. epithelial cells of the oral cavity, respiratory tract, urinary tract, and ducts of secretory glands.[1,2]

Epithelial tissue development and maintenance

The role of vitamin A and carotenoids in the development and maintenance of epithelial tissue cannot be overstated. Vitamin A status determines whether mucin or keratin is synthesized in epidermal cells – the presence of adequate vitamin A results in mucin production, while a lack results in hyperkeratinization of the skin, cornea, upper respiratory tract, and genitourinary tract. Mucopolysaccharide synthesis also appears to be dependent on adequate vitamin A status.[1,2,8]

Reproduction

The requirement of vitamin A for reproductive functions in higher animals has been known since 1922.[2] Beta-carotene has also been reported to have a specific effect in fertility distinct from its role as a precursor to vitamin A.[9–11] In bovine nutritional studies, cows fed beta-carotene-deficient diets exhibited delayed ovulation and an increase in the number of follicular and luteal cysts.[9,10] The corpus luteum has the highest concentration of beta-carotene of any organ measured.[11] The carotene cleavage activity changes with the ovulation cycle, with the highest activity occurring during the midovulation stage. It has been speculated that a proper ratio of carotene to retinol must be maintained to ensure proper corpus luteum function.

As the corpus luteum produces progesterone, inadequate corpus luteum function could have significant deleterious effects. Inadequate corpus luteum secretory function is one of the characteristic features of infertile and/or irregular menstrual cycles.[12] Furthermore, an increased estrogen to progesterone ratio has been implicated in a variety of clinical conditions, including ovarian cysts, premenstrual tension syndrome, fibrocystic breast disease, and breast cancer.[13] Since supplemental beta-carotene given to cows significantly reduced the incidence of ovarian cysts (42% in control group vs. 3% in the beta-carotene group), it may have a similar effect in humans.[10,11] Another bovine condition that benefited from increased dietary beta-carotene levels is cystic mastitis.[12] It appears that farmers have a greater appreciation of beta-carotene than do many nutritionists. Of course, there are significant financial reasons, as the annual monetary loss from bovine mastitis in the United States has been estimated to be at least $1.5–2.0 billion and ovarian cysts represent the major cause of infertility in cattle.

Immune system

Vitamin A is absolutely essential to proper immune function. The first way in which vitamin A affects the immune system is that it plays an essential role in maintaining the epithelial and mucosal surfaces and their secretions. These systems constitute a primary non-specific host defense mechanism. Furthermore, vitamin A has been shown to stimulate and/or enhance numerous immune processes, including induction of antitumor activity, enhancement of white blood cell function, and increased antibody response.[14] These effects are not due simply to a reversal of vitamin A deficiency, since many of these effects are further enhanced by (supposedly) excessive amounts of vitamin A. Retinol has also demonstrated significant antiviral activity and has prevented the immunosuppression induced by glucocorticoids, severe burns, and surgery. Some of these effects are probably related to vitamin A's ability to prevent stress-induced thymic involution and to promote thymus growth. As carotenes are better antioxidants, they may turn out to be even better in protecting the thymus gland than vitamin A, since the thymus gland is particularly susceptible to free radical and oxidative damage. The clinical uses of vitamin A and beta-carotene in infectious diseases are discussed below.

CLINICAL APPLICATIONS

Adequate tissue vitamin A levels are vital for optimum health. In addition, this nutrient can be used beyond its "physiological" role in the treatment of various conditions. Supplemental vitamin A is used primarily to enhance the immune system in viral illnesses and in the treatment of numerous skin disorders.

Natural vitamin A is available either as retinol or retinyl-palmitate. Absorption may be improved via either micellization or emulsification. Micellization is the process of making the fat-soluble vitamin A into very small droplets (micelles) so that the material is dispersed in water. Emulsification is the process of emulsifying the vitamin A with another chemical (such as lecithin) so that it can mix with water. Despite manufacturers' claims, it is important to remember that regular vitamin A is absorbed at a rate of 80–90%.

Viral illnesses

As discussed above, vitamin A is absolutely critical to a healthy functioning immune system. Vitamin A-deficient individuals are more susceptible to infectious diseases in general, but especially viral infections. While vitamin A deficiency may predispose an individual to an infection, during the course of an infection vitamin A stores are severely depleted.

Measles

Vitamin A deficiency is a major problem in many developing countries as 5–10 million children in these countries exhibit severe vitamin A deficiency. Recently, a number of well-designed studies have confirmed an effect first noted in 1932 – vitamin A supplementation can significantly reduce infant mortality among measles patients by at least 50%. Typically the dosage of vitamin A in double-blind studies has been 200,000–400,000 IU administered only once or twice to replenish body stores.[15,16]

The benefits of vitamin A supplementation in the treatment of measles is not limited to developing countries. A study of "well nourished" children in Long Beach, California, suffering from measles indicated that 50% were deficient in vitamin A.[17] This finding supports the use of vitamin A supplementation even in the US.

Infants with RSV infections

Wide-scale immunization programs have reduced the risk of measles in children. However, vitamin A therapy appears appropriate for other childhood viral illnesses. One of the more common viruses is the respiratory syncytial virus (RSV), a common cause of severe respiratory disease in young children. Studies have shown that children with RSV have low serum vitamin A levels. Furthermore, the lower the vitamin A level, the greater the severity of the disease, similar to the relationship shown in measles. Because vitamin A supplementation diminishes the morbidity and death caused by measles, a group of researchers decided to determine vitamin A's safety and absorption pattern in RSV as a first step in determining the therapeutic effectiveness.[18]

Twenty-one children with a mean age of 2.3 months

(range, 1–6 months) with mild RSV infection were treated with 12,500–25,000 IU of oral micellized vitamin A. Baseline vitamin A levels were shown to be low, but within 6 hours of receiving 25,000 IU, but not 12,500 IU, of vitamin A normal levels were re-established. Despite the young age, none of the children experienced any obvious signs or symptoms of vitamin A toxicity. Although the study was not designed as a therapeutic trial, the subjects receiving vitamin A had hospital stays that were shorter than those of children with a similar severity of illness who were not enrolled in the study.

Although vitamin A supplementation is an attractive treatment of RSV infections, due to its low cost, wide availability, and ease of administration, recent placebo-controlled trials are suggesting it may be of value only in the most severe cases. A placebo-controlled study of 180 children in Chile with RSV provided 50–200,000 IU of retinyl palmitate (according to age) within 2 days of admission.[19] Supplementation resulted in no significant benefit, except for those children suffering from hypoxemia. These children experienced substantial benefit – a more rapid resolution of tachypnea and shortening of their hospital stay from 9.3 to 5.5 days.

AIDS

Another viral illness that may benefit from vitamin A supplementation is AIDS. It was recently shown that a vitamin A deficiency is quite common during HIV infection and that vitamin A deficiency is clearly associated with a decreased level of circulating helper T-cells, one of the hallmark features of AIDS.[20]

Analysis of vitamin A levels, helper T-cells, and other blood parameters in HIV individuals indicated that more than 15% had low serum vitamin A levels. When vitamin A levels were low, helper T-cell levels were much lower than the levels in HIV-infected individuals who had normal levels of vitamin A. Vitamin A deficiency was also shown to be associated with a higher rate of mortality due to HIV.

Increasing beta-carotene may be the preferred form of vitamin A for supplementation in HIV patients as there is concern that retinoic acid, the active form of vitamin A, may actually increase HIV replication in humans. Low beta-carotene levels are common in AIDS, presumably as a result of fat malabsorption. Low beta-carotene levels are associated with greater impairment of immune function.[21]

Skin disorders

The use of high-dose vitamin A therapy for acne and other skin disorders was introduced in dermatology in the late 1930s. It is still used by a few dermatologists, although, since the advent of the synthetic retinoids, this type of therapy is not as popular as it once was. Vitamin A therapy has been shown to be quite effective in treating skin conditions associated with excessive formation of keratin (hyperkeratosis), a skin protein which can clog the pores of the skin to produce a "goose bump" effect. Examples of some skin conditions associated with hyperkeratosis include acne, psoriasis, ichthyosis, lichen planus, Darier's disease, palmoplantar keratoderma, and pityriasis rubra pilaris. The dosages of vitamin A used to treat these conditions have typically been quite high (300,000–500,000 IU/day for 5–6 months in the treatment of acne, and 1–3.5 million IU/day for 1–2 weeks for the other conditions).[22–25] The use of these high dosages usually results in the development of significant toxicity (see below). Although there is some evidence that carotenes may be more useful, and less toxic, in some of these conditions, the pharmacological activity responsible for the effects of vitamin A in hyperkeratosis are believed to result when serum retinol levels exceed serum retinol binding protein capacity, causing destabilization of membranes and destruction of the keratin-producing cells.[21]

In monitoring for vitamin A toxicity, laboratory tests appear unreliable until obvious toxicity symptoms are apparent. The first significant toxic symptom is usually headache followed by fatigue, emotional instability, and muscle and joint pain. Chapped lips (cheilitis) and dry skin (xerosis) will generally occur in the majority of patients, particularly in dry weather. Because high doses of vitamin A during pregnancy can cause birth defects, women of child-bearing age should use effective birth control during vitamin A treatment and for at least 1 month after discontinuation.

High doses of vitamin A may not be necessary if other nutritional factors like zinc and vitamin E are included. These nutrients work with vitamin A in promoting healthy skin. A safe and effective recommendation for vitamin A in the treatment of acne is less than 25,000 IU/day.

Dry eyes

Dry-eye disorders are a complex group of diseases characterized by a localized water deficiency in the tear ducts; a mucin deficiency; or a combination of the two. Despite the diversity of underlying causes, the changes in the conjunctiva of the eye are similar in all cases, i.e. loss of goblet cells (mucin-producing cells), abnormal enlargement of non-goblet epithelial cells, and an increase of cellular layers and keratin deposition, stratification and keratinization.

Apart from topical vitamin A therapy, all other non-surgical therapies of dry eye, i.e. the frequent application of artificial tears, lubricants, or slow-releasing polymers, and the therapeutic use of soft contact lenses, are not directed toward reversing the underlying process, but rather toward alleviating the symptoms.

The hypothesis that a localized vitamin A deficiency in the lining of the outer eye may be responsible for dry eye, considering vitamin A's vital role in epithelial tissue, seems obvious. Clinical studies featuring commercial vitamin A eye drops (Viva-Drops from Vision Pharmaceuticals) have yielded impressive clinical results in the treatment of dry eyes.[26,27]

DOSAGE

Dosage ranges for vitamin A reflect the intent of use. For general health purposes, a dosage of 5,000 IU for men and 2,500 IU for women appears reasonable. During an acute viral infection, a single oral dosage of 50,000 IU for 1 or 2 days appears to be safe even in infants (note, however, that women who might be pregnant must not use vitamin A supplements; beta-carotene is fine). For the treatment of acne and hyperkeratotic skin disorders, high-dose therapy may be useful but should be monitored closely by a physician.

TOXICITY

Vitamin A supplementation must be avoided during pregnancy. Vitamin A in large doses has been shown to be teratogenic. Unfortunately, the safe dosages for pregnant women have not yet been determined. According to recent studies, dosages greater than 10,000 IU during pregnancy (specifically during the first 7 weeks after conception) have probably been responsible for one out of every 57 cases of birth defects in the United States. Women who are at risk of becoming pregnant should keep their supplemental vitamin A levels below 5,000 IU or, better yet, look to carotenes.[28]

Acute toxicity with vitamin A is most often seen in children as a result of the accidental ingestion of a single large dose of vitamin A (100,000–300,000 IU) and manifests as:[1]

- raised intracranial pressure with vomiting
- headache
- joint pain
- stupor
- occasionally papilledema.

Symptoms rapidly subside upon withdrawal of the vitamin, and complete recovery always results.[1]

Vitamin A toxicity may occur in adults when taking an excess of 50,000 IU/day for several years. Smaller daily doses may produce toxicity symptoms if there are defects in storage and transport of vitamin A such as occurs in cirrhosis of the liver, hepatitis, or protein calorie malnutrition, and in children and adolescents.[29,30] Signs of vitamin A toxicity generally include:

- dry, fissured skin
- brittle nails
- alopecia
- gingivitis
- cheilosis
- anorexia
- irritability
- fatigue
- nausea.

Serum levels of vitamin A of 250–6,600 IU/dl are typical of toxicity. Prolonged, severe hypervitaminosis A will result in bone fragility and thickening of the long bone.

Toxicity is typically encountered during high-dose vitamin A therapy for various skin conditions. Although dosages below 300,000 IU/day for a few months rarely cause toxicity symptoms, early recognition is still very important. Cheilitis (chapped lips) and xerosis (dry skin) will generally appear in the majority of patients, particularly in dry weather. The first significant toxicity symptom is usually headache, followed by fatigue, emotional lability, and muscle and joint pain. Laboratory tests are of little value in monitoring toxicity, as serum vitamin A levels correlate poorly with toxicity, and SGOT and SGPT are elevated only in symptomatic patients.[21]

Interactions

Vitamin E and zinc are particularly important to the proper function of vitamin A. A deficiency of zinc, vitamin C, protein, or thyroid hormone will impair the conversion of provitamin A carotenes to vitamin A.

Studies have demonstrated a link between exposure to toxic chemicals and vitamin A nutrition. Administration of compounds such as polybrominated biphenyls, dioxin, and other toxic chemicals to rats results in a decrease in the hepatic content of vitamin A. Administration of vitamin A concurrently with the xenobiotics partially prevents the symptoms of toxicity. Exposure to these compounds results in an increased vitamin A requirement due to the enhanced degradation of vitamin A in the liver.[31,32]

REFERENCES

1. Olson R, ed. Nutrition reviews. Present knowledge in nutrition. 6th edn. Washington, DC: Nutrition Foundation. 1989: p 96–107
2. Underwood B. Vitamin A in animal and human nutrition. In: Sporn M, Roberts A, Goodman S, eds. The retinoids, vol 1. Orlando, Fl: Academic Press. 1984: p 282–392

3. Krause MV, Mahan LK. Food, nutrition and diet therapy. 5th edn. Philadelphia, PA: WB Saunders. 1984: p 103–107, 224
4. Selhorst JB, Waybright EA, Jennings S et al. Liver lover's headache. Pseudotumor cerebri and vitamin A intoxication. JAMA 1984; 252: 3365
5. Sommer A, Tarwato I, Hussaini G et al. Increased mortality in children with mild vitamin A deficiency. Lancet 1983; ii: 584–588
6. Brown ED, Micozzi MS, Craft NE. Plasma carotenoids in normal men after a single ingestion of vegetables or purified beta-carotene. Am J Clin Nutr 1989; 49: 1258–1265
7. Goodman DS. Overview of current knowledge of metabolism of vitamin A and carotenoids. JNCI 1984; 73: 1375–1379
8. Zile MH, Cullum ME. The function of vitamin A. Current concepts. Proc Soc Exp Biol Med 1983; 172: 139–152
9. Folman Y, Rosenberg M, Ascarelli M et al. The effect of dietary and climatic factors on fertility, and on plasma progesterone and oestradiol-17B levels in dairy cows. J Steroid Biochem 1983; 19: 863–868
10. Editor. Metabolism of beta-carotene by the bovine corpus luteum. Nutr Rev 1983; 41: 357–358
11. Lotthammer KH. Importance of beta-carotene for the fertility of dairy cattle. Feedstuffs 1979; 51: 16–19
12. O'Fallon JV, Chew BP. The subcellular distribution of B-carotene in bovine corpus luteum. Proc Soc Exp Biol Med 1984; 177: 406–411
13. Sherman BM, Korenman SG. Inadequate corpus luteum function: a pathophysiological interpretation of human breast cancer epidemiology. Cancer 1974; 33: 1306–1312
14. Semba RD. Vitamin A, immunity, and infection. Clin Inf Dis 1994; 19: 489–499
15. Fawzi WW et al. Vitamin A supplementation and child mortality. JAMA 1993; 269: 898–903
16. Hussey GD, Klein M. A randomized, controlled trial of vitamin A in children with severe measles. N Engl J Med 1990; 323: 160–164
17. Arrieta AC, Zaleska M, Stutman HR. Vitamin A levels in children with measles in Long Beach, California. J Pediatr 1992; 121: 75–78
18. Neuzil KM, Gruber SC, Chytil F. Safety and pharmacokinetics of vitamin A therapy for infants with respiratory syncytial infections. Antimicrob Agents Chemother 1995; 39: 1191–1193
19. Dowell SF, Papic Z, Bressee JS et al. Treatment of respiratory syncytial virus infection with vitamin A. A randomized, placebo-controlled trial in Santiago, Chile. Ped Inf Dis J 1996; 15: 782–786
20. Semba RD et al. Increased mortality associated with vitamin A deficiency during human immunodeficiency virus type 1 infection. Arch Intern Med 1993; 153: 2149–2154
21. Ullrich R et al. Serum carotene deficiency in HIV-infected patients. AIDS 1994; 8: 661–665
22. Kligman AM, Mills OH, Leyden JJ et al. Oral vitamin A in acne vulgaris. Int J Derm 1981; 20: 278–285
23. Thomas JR, Cooke J, Winkelmann RK. High-dose vitamin A in Darier's disease. Arch Dermatol 1982; 118: 891–894
24. Randle HW, Diaz-Perez J and Winkelmann RK. Toxic doses of vitamin A for pityriasis rubra pilaris. Arch Dermatol 1980; 116: 888–892
25. Winkelmann RK, Thomas JR, Randle HW. Further experience with toxic vitamin A therapy in pityriasis rubra pilaris. Cutis 1983; 31: 621–629
26. Rengstorff RH. Topical treatment of external eye disorders with preparations containing vitamin A. Practical Optometry 1993; 4: 163–165
27. Westerhout D. Treatment of dry eyes with aqueous antioxidant eye drops. Contact Lens J 1989; 19: 165–173
28. Rothman KJ, Moore LL, Singer MR. Teratogenecity of high vitamin A intake. N Engl J Med 1995; 333: 1369–1373
29. Hatoff DE, Gertler SL, Miyai K et al. Hypervitaminosis A unmasked by acute viral hepatitis. Gastroenterol 1982; 82: 124–128
30. Harris WA, Erdman JW. Protracted hypervitaminosis. A following long-term, low level intake. JAMA 1982; 247: 1317–1318
31. Cullum ME, Zile MH. Acute polybrominated biphenyl toxicosis alters vitamin A homeostasis and enhances degradation of vitamin A. Toxicol Appl Pharmacol 1985; 81: 177–181
32. Thunberg T, Ahlborg Ug, Wahlstrom B. Comparison of the effects of 2,3,7,8–tetrachlorodibenzo-p-dioxin and six other compounds on vitamin A storage, the UDP–gluconosyltransferase and aryl hydrocarbon hydroxylase activity in the rat liver. Arch Toxicol 1984; 55: 16–19

CHAPTER CONTENTS

122

Vitamin toxicities and therapeutic monitoring

Michael T. Murray, ND

Joseph E. Pizzorno Jr, ND

INTRODUCTION

When nutrients such as vitamins are being used at high doses for pharmacological effects, the physician must be vigilant for possible toxicity or side-effects. In general, vitamin therapy is virtually "non-toxic" and the small risk of developing any toxicity can be further reduced by careful monitoring of the patient. The physician should also be aware of toxicity resulting from self-administered vitamins. The primary signs and symptoms of vitamin toxicity are listed in Tables 122.1 and 122.2, which are complemented by a more detailed discussion of toxicity and guidelines for monitoring selected vitamins.

VITAMIN TOXICITY

Lipid-soluble vitamins

Vitamin A

The majority of the cases of hypervitaminosis A involve acute ingestion by young children.[1,2] Adverse reactions to acute ingestion are usually transient. Chronic ingestion in children, usually a result of administration by a parent, may result in long-lasting changes in bone formation.

When large doses of vitamin A are being given, careful monitoring is necessary. Rather than using sudden large doses, a gradual stepwise increase in dosage is indicated, with a symptom evaluation made before increasing the dose. Usually, the first recognized symptom of hypervitaminosis is frontal headache. If signs or symptoms appear, supplementation should be discontinued until they disappear. Therapy may be carefully resumed at a lesser dose. Periodic liver enzyme levels should be determined to check for hepatic damage. Typically, SGOT levels are the first to be affected.[1–4]

As vitamin A has been shown to have teratogenic effects in animals (e.g. resorption of fetus, cleft palate, spina bifida, anencephaly, etc.), supplementation above the RDA is not warranted in pregnant, or potentially pregnant, women. According to recent studies (see

Table 122.1 Toxic doses and side-effects of lipid-soluble vitamins

Vitamin	Toxic dose	Toxic signs and symptoms
Carotene	Chronic: none	No apparent toxicity, even at large doses (250 mg/day); synthetic form may be a problem for heavy smokers not taking other antioxidants
Vitamin A	Acute	
	—infants: 75–300,000 IU	Anorexia, bulging fontanelles, hyperirritability, vomiting
	—adults: 2–5 million IU	Headache, drowsiness, nausea, vomiting
	Chronic	
	—infants: 18–60,000 IU/day	Premature epiphyseal bone closing, long bone growth retardation
	—adults: 100,000 IU/day	Anorexia, headache, blurred vision, loss of hair, bleeding lips, cracking and peeling skin, muscular stiffness and pain, severe hepatic damage and enlargement, anemia, teratogenesis
Vitamin D	Acute: 1–3,000 IU/kg	Anorexia, nausea, vomiting, diarrhea, headache, polyuria, polydipsia
	Chronic: 10–50,000 IU/day	Weight loss, pallor, constipation, fever, hypercalcemia, calcium deposits in soft tissues
Vitamin E	Chronic: >800 IU/day	Severe weakness, fatigue, exacerbation of hypertension, potentiation of anticoagulants
Vitamin K	Chronic: none	Phylloquinone (K_1), unlike menadione (K_3), is not associated with side-effects when given orally

Table 122.2 Toxic doses and side-effects of water-soluble vitamins

	Toxic dose	Toxic signs and symptoms
Ascorbic acid	Acute: usually >10 g	Nausea, diarrhea, flatulence
	Chronic: >3 g/day	Increased urinary oxalate and uric acid levels in extremely rare cases, impaired carotene utilization, chelation and resultant loss of minerals may occur
Biotin	Chronic: >10 mg/day	No side-effects from oral administration at therapeutic doses have been reported
Folic acid	Chronic: 15 mg/day	Abdominal distension, anorexia, nausea, sleep disturbances (see discussion)
Niacin	Acute: >100 mg	Transient flushing, headache, cramps, nausea, vomiting
	Chronic: 3–7 g/day	Anorexia, abnormal glucose tolerance, increased plasma uric acid levels, gastric ulceration, elevated liver enzymes
Niacinamide	Chronic: >1,000 mg/day	Same as for niacin
Pantothenic acid	Chronic	Occasional diarrhea
Pyridoxine	Acute	No acute effects are noted at therapeutic doses
	Chronic: 300 mg/day	Sensory and motor neuropathy
Riboflavin	Chronic	No toxic effects have been noted
Thiamin	Chronic	No toxic effects noted for humans after oral administration
Vitamin B_{12}	Chronic	No side-effects from oral administration have been reported

Ch. 121), dosages greater than 10,000 IU during pregnancy (specifically during the first 7 weeks after conception) have probably been responsible for one out of every 57 cases of birth defects in the United States.

Carotenoids

Carotenoids appear to be without toxic effects at the therapeutic doses usually used and are therefore more appropriate than vitamin A for most conditions. The only effect of large dosages is an apparently benign yellowing of the skin.

Three large, recent, widely publicized therapeutic trials with synthetic beta-carotene have found that it appears to increase the risk of cancer for heavy smokers. However, several factors complicate the interpretation of these results. The significance of the these trials is fully discussed in Ch. 121.

Vitamin D

Large doses of vitamin D are rarely used clinically; self-administration is the usual cause of toxicity. Vitamin D has great potential to cause toxicity. Dosages greater than 1,000 IU/day are certainly not recommended. Toxicity is characterized by hypercalcemia, deposition of calcium into internal organs, and kidney stones. It has also been suggested that long-term overconsumption of vitamin D_2 in fortified foods contributes to atherosclerosis and heart disease, possibly as a result of decreasing magnesium absorption.[5]

Vitamin E

Although vitamin E is a fat-soluble vitamin it has an excellent safety record. Recent clinical trials of vitamin E supplementation at doses as high as 3,200 IU/day in a wide variety of subjects for periods of up to 2 years have not shown any unfavorable side-effects. Detailed safety assessments have been carried out in several studies. For example, in one double-blind trial in 32 elderly (>60 years old) people, the effect of daily supplementation of 800 IU of D,L-alpha-tocopheryl acetate for 30 days was assessed by measuring general health, nutrient status, liver and kidney function, metabolism, blood cell status, blood nutrient and antioxidant status, thyroid hormones, and urinary function.[6] The only significant effect noted was an increase in serum vitamin

E levels. Vitamin E at this dose was extremely well-tolerated and no side-effects were reported. The results of this study are not surprising and are consistent with a large body of knowledge demonstrating that vitamin E supplementation is extremely safe.

Vitamin K

Large doses of the synthetic, water-soluble vitamin K_3 (menadione), when administered to infants, may cause hemolytic anemia, hyperbilirubinemia, hepatomegaly, and possibly death. Adults with G6PD deficiency may show hemolytic reactions.[7] The natural vitamin K_1 (phytadione or phylloquinone) does not appear to have any toxicity when given orally, until huge doses (200 mg) are given.[8]

Water-soluble vitamins

Ascorbic acid

Vitamin C has been reported to have perhaps the lowest toxicity of all vitamins. Diarrhea and intestinal distension or gas are the most common complaints at higher dosages. High doses have been shown to:

- increase the urinary excretion of calcium, iron and manganese
- increase the absorption of iron
- increase urinary oxalate or uric acid levels, but only in an extremely small subgroup of the population
- alter many routine laboratory tests, i.e. serum B_{12}, aminotransferases, bilirubin, glucose, stool occult blood.

It is necessary to take these effects into consideration when supplementing with mega-doses of vitamin C.

The primary concern with high dosages of vitamin C often cited in the medical literature is the development of calcium oxalate kidney stones. However, numerous studies have now demonstrated that in persons not on hemodialysis or suffering from recurrent kidney stones, severe kidney disease, or gout, high dosage vitamin C therapy will not cause kidney stones. Vitamin C administration of up to 10 g/day has not shown any effect on urinary oxalate levels.[9,10]

There have been reports that abrupt cessation of high dosage vitamin C intake leads to "rebound scurvy", or in pregnant women to the presence of rebound scurvy after birth in their babies. However, other studies do not support the existence of rebound scurvy with sudden cessation or after pregnancy with high doses of vitamin C. While the existence of rebound scurvy is controversial (some experts question its existence), it is better to err on the side of caution. At this time a safe recommendation to pregnant women would be a daily dosage of 500 mg.

Folic acid

It has been reported that eight out of 14 healthy human subjects who consumed 15 mg/day of folic acid for 1 month developed abdominal distension, flatulence, nausea, anorexia, sleep disturbances with vivid dreams, malaise, and irritability.[11] This, however, has not been confirmed in a double-blind clinical study[12] and other investigations.[13–15] Folic acid supplementation appears to be without side-effects, even at high doses (e.g. 15 mg/day).

Niacin

The acute side-effects of niacin are well known. The most common and bothersome is the skin flushing that typically occurs 20–30 minutes after the niacin is taken. Long-term consequences of niacin therapy include gastric irritation, nausea, and liver damage. In an attempt to combat the acute reaction of skin flushing, several manufacturers began marketing "sustained-release", "timed-release" or "slow-release" niacin products. These formulations allow the niacin to be absorbed gradually, thereby reducing the flushing reaction. However, while these forms of niacin reduce skin flushing, they have actually proven to be more toxic to the liver. In a recent study, it was strongly recommended that the use of sustained-release niacin be restricted because of the high percentage (78%) of patient withdrawal due to side-effects – 52% of the patients taking the sustained-release niacin developed liver damage, compared with none of the patients taking immediate-release niacin.[16]

Because niacin can impair glucose tolerance, it should probably not be used in diabetics unless they are under close observation. Niacin should also not be used in patients with pre-existing liver disease or elevation in liver enzymes, gout, or peptic ulcers.

Side-effects can occur with any form of niacin, including niacinamide. Although niacinamide does not cause the acute flushing of the skin, it can cause liver damage. Inositol hexaniacin is the safest form of niacin currently available. Both short- and long-term studies have shown it to be virtually free of side-effects other than an occasional mild gastric upset or mild flushing of the skin.

Regardless of the form of niacin being used, periodic checking (at least every 3 months) of liver function tests are indicated when high-dose (i.e. 2–6 g/day) niacin, inostitol hexaniacinate, or niacinamide therapy is being used.

Pyridoxine

Vitamin B_6 is one of the few water-soluble vitamins that is associated with some toxicity when taken in large doses or moderate dosages for long periods of time.

Large doses of vitamin B_6 are currently being used for a wide variety of conditions.

Doses greater than 2,000 mg/day can produce symptoms of nerve toxicity (tingling sensations in the feet, loss of muscle coordination, and degeneration of nerve tissue) in some individuals. Chronic intake of dosages greater than 500 mg/day can be toxic if taken daily for several months.[17] There are also a few rare reports of toxicity occurring at chronic long-term dosages as low as 150 mg/day.[18–20] The toxicity is thought to be a result of supplemental pyridoxine overwhelming the liver's ability to add a phosphate group to produce the active form of vitamin B_6 (pyridoxal-5-phosphate). As a result, it is speculated either that pyridoxine is toxic to the nerve cells or that it actually acts as an anti-metabolite by binding to pyridoxal-5-phosphate receptors thereby creating a relative deficiency of vitamin B_6. It appears to make sense to limit dosages to 50 mg. If more than 50 mg are desired, then the dosages should be spread throughout the day.

LABORATORY TESTS FOR VITAMIN TOXICITY

Only a limited number of routine laboratory tests are available for detecting vitamin toxicity. These are presented in Table 122.3.

Table 122.3 Laboratory tests for vitamin toxicity

Vitamin	Laboratory test
Vitamin A	SGOT, serum vitamin A
Vitamin D	Serum calcium
Niacin	SGOT, SGPT
Vitamin C	Urinary oxalate and uric acid

REFERENCES

1. Miloslav R. CRC handbook series in nutrition and food, section E: nutritional disorders, vol. 1. Cleveland, OH: CRC Press. 1978
2. Omaye S. Safety of megavitamin therapy. Adv Exp Med Biol 1984; 177: 169–203
3. DiPalma J and Ritchie D. Vitamin toxicity. Ann Rev Pharmacol Toxicol 1977; 17: 133–148
4. Buist R. Vitamin toxicities, side effects and contraindications. Int Clin Nutr Rev 1984; 4: 159–171
5. Seelig MS. Magnesium deficiency with phosphate and vitamin D excess: role in pediatric cardiovascular nutrition. Cardio Med 1978; 3: 637–650
6. Meydani SN et al. Assessment of the safety of high-dose, short-term supplementation with vitamin E in healthy older adults. Am J Clin Nutr 1994; 60: 704–709
7. Krupp MA, Chatton MJ. Current medical diagnosis and treatment. Los Altos, CA: Lange Medical. 1984: p 803–808
8. Bicknell F, Prescott F. The vitamins in medicine. 3rd edn. Milwaukee, WI: Lee Foundation. 1953: p 694
9. Rivers JM. Safety of high level vitamin C ingestion. Int J Vitamin Nutr Res 1989; 30: 95–102
10. Wanzilak TR et al. Effect of high dose vitamin C on urinary oxalate levels. J Urol 1994; 151: 834–837
11. Hunter R, Barnes J. Toxicity of folic acid given in pharmacological doses to healthy volunteers. Lancet 1970 i: 61–63
12. Hellstrom L. Lack of toxicity of folic acid given in pharmacological doses to healthy volunteers. Lancet 1971; i: 59–61
13. Sheehy T. Folic acid. Lack of toxicity. Lancet 1973; i: 37
14. Richens A. Toxicity of folic acid. Lancet 1971; i: 912
15. Boss G, Ragsdale R, Zettner A and Seegmiller J. Failure of folic acid (pteroglutamic acid) to affect hyperuricemia. J Lab Clin Med 1980; 96: 783–789
16. McKenney JM et al. A comparison of the efficacy and toxic effects of sustained- vs immediate-release niacin in hypercholesterolemic patients. JAMA 1994; 271: 672–677
17. Cohen M, Bendich A. Safety of pyridoxine – A review of human and animal studies. Toxicol Lett 1986; 34: 129–139
18. Parry GJ, Bredesen DE. Sensory neuropathy with low-dose pyridoxine. Neurol 1985; 35: 1466–1468
19. Waterston JA, Gilligan BS. Pyridoxine neuropathy. Med J Aust 1987; 146: 640–642
20. Dalton K, Dalton MJT. Characteristics of pyridoxine overdose neuropathy syndrome. Acta Neurol Scand 1987; 76: 8

CHAPTER CONTENTS

123

Vitex agnus castus (chaste tree)

Donald J. Brown, ND

Vitex agnus castus (family: Verbenaceae)
Common name: chaste tree

GENERAL DESCRIPTION

Vitex agnus castus, also known as chaste tree, is a shrub with finger-shaped leaves and slender violet flowers. *Vitex agnus castus* grows in creek beds and on river banks in valleys and lower foothills in the Mediterranean and central Asia. The plant blooms in high summer and, after pollination, develops dark-brown to black fruit the size of a peppercorn. The fruit possess a pepper-like aroma and flavor. The ripe, dried fruit of *Vitex agnus castus* is the part of the plant used in medicinal preparations today.[1]

CHEMICAL COMPOSITION

The fruit of Vitex contains essential oils, iridoid glycosides, and flavonoids.[2] The essential oils include limonene, 1,8 cineole, and sabinene.[3] The primary flavonoids include castican, orientin, and isoVitexin. The two isolated iridoidglycosides are agnuside and aucubin (see Figs 123.1 and 123.2).[4] Agnuside serves as a reference material for quality control in the manufacture of Vitex extracts.

One study found delta-3-ketosteriods in the flowers and leaves of Vitex. The authors reported (albeit in a somewhat vague manner) that this fraction of the leaves and flowers "probably" contained progesterone and 17-hydroxyprogesterone. Testosterone and epitestosterone were also presumed to be present.[5] Additional research is needed.

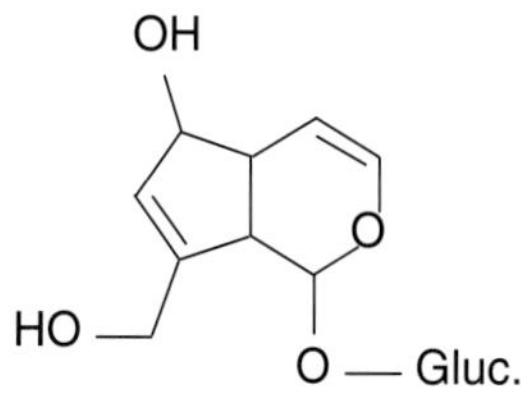

Figure 123.1 Aucubin.

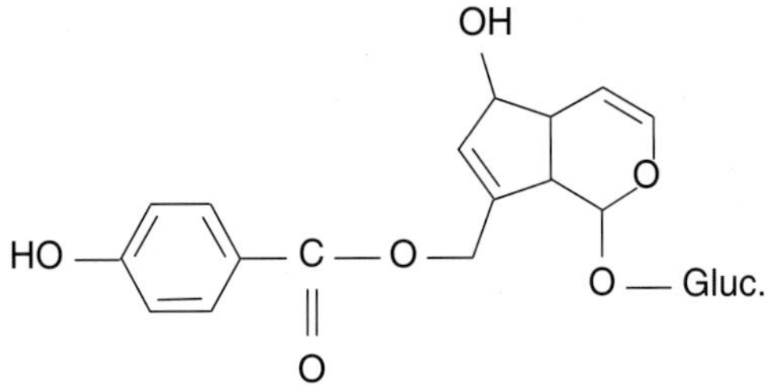

Figure 123.2 Agnuside.

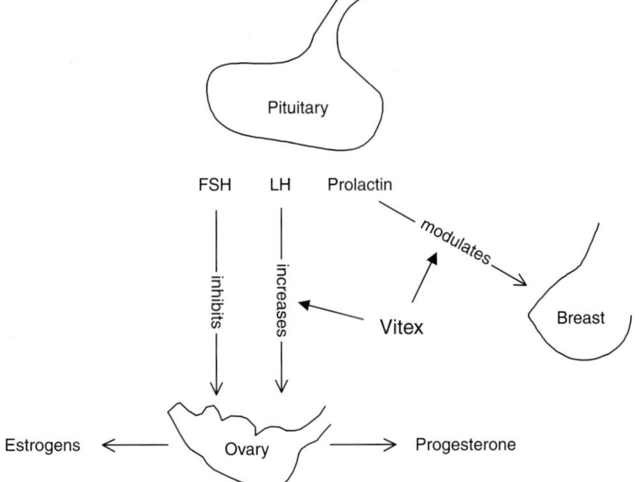

Figure 123.3 Impact of Vitex on pituitary hormone secretion.

HISTORY AND FOLK USE

The genus name *Vitex* is derived from the "vitilium" which means plaiting. The flexible, but tough and hard, branches were used for construction of wattle fences. Plinius, 1st century AD, has the earliest reference to the plant as Vitex. The species name *agnus castus* originates from the Latin "castitas" (chastity) and the equating of the Greek "agnos" with the Latin "agnus" (lamb).

Vitex agnus castus belonged to the official medicinal plants of antiquity and is mentioned in the works of Hippocrates, Dioscorides, and Theophrast. The first specific medicinal indications can be found in the writings of Hippocrates, 4th century BC. He recommends the plant for injuries, inflammation, and swelling of the spleen, and the leaves in wine for hemorrhages and the "passing of afterbirth". In the *Corpus Hippocratum* he states:

> If blood flows from the womb, let the woman drink dark red wine in which the leaves of the chaste tree have been steeped. A draft of chaste leaves in wine also serves to expel a chorion held fast in the womb.

Dioscorides attributed to the fruit a hot and astringent activity and recommended it for wild animal bites, swelling of the spleen, and dropsy. Decoctions of the fruit and plant were used as sitz baths for diseases of the uterus.

The English name for *Vitex agnus castus*, "chaste tree", is derived form the belief that the plant would suppress libido in women taking it. In Greek cities, festivals in the honor of Demeter included a vow of chastity by the local women. The Catholic church in Europe developed a variation on this theme by placing the blossoms of the plant in the clothing of novice monks to supposedly suppress libido. It is interesting to note that another common name for *Vitex agnus castus*, "monk's pepper", derived from the fact that monks in southern Europe commonly used the fruit as a spice in their cooking.

PHARMACOLOGY

According to Dr Rudolf Fritz Weiss, Vitex acts on the diencephalohypophyseal system. Vitex increases LH production (see Fig. 123.3). The result is a shift in the ratio of estrogen to progesterone, in favor of progesterone. This is, in fact, a corpus luteum-like hormone effect.[6] The ability of Vitex to increase or modulate progesterone levels in the body is therefore an indirect effect and not a direct hormonal action.[7] This is in contrast to other phytomedicines, like Black cohosh, frequently used in gynecology, which directly bind to estrogen receptors through their content of phytoestrogens.[8]

Vitex also modulates the secretion of prolactin from the pituitary gland. Early animal studies indicated an increase in lactation and enlargement of the mammary gland following administration of Vitex.[7]

Current research with Vitex indicates usefulness in hyperprolactinemia. In studies with rats, Vitex was shown to inhibit prolactin release by the pituitary gland – particularly under stress. The mechanism of action appears to involve the ability of Vitex to directly bind dopamine receptors and subsequently inhibit prolactin release in the pituitary.[9,10] Slight hyperprolactinemia is commonly associated with corpus luteum insufficiency.[11]

CLINICAL APPLICATIONS

The causes of menstrual disorders are multifaceted and can vary greatly in their manifestation. Frequently, therapeutic interventions must be used on a trial and error basis over the duration of a number of menstrual cycles to determine their efficacy. Nutritional interventions like vitamin B_6, magnesium, and vitamin E, as well as phytomedicines such as dong quai and evening primrose oil, have all shown greater efficacy when used over time periods of several months. This reflects the gradual balancing effect that many of these interventions have on the female hormonal system. Vitex certainly fits this mould.

The majority of clinical studies completed with Vitex have been non-controlled studies with large populations of female patients in European gynecology practices. Vitex, which has a Commission E Monograph in Germany, is frequently used in these practices as an initial intervention in a number of menstrual disorders, including:

- premenstrual syndrome
- hypermenorrhea
- polymenorrhea
- anovulatory cycles
- secondary amenorrhea
- infertility
- hyperprolactinemia.

Many of these cases can be linked to corpus luteum insufficiency. Vitex is also used in cases of poor lactation, uterine fibroids, and climacteric.

Corpus luteum insufficiency

Corpus luteum insufficiency (also referred to as luteal phase defect) is a manifestation of suboptimal ovarian function. In laboratory terms, corpus luteum insufficiency is usually defined as an abnormally low progesterone level 3 weeks after the onset of menstruation (serum progesterone below 10–12 ng/ml). This state is normal during puberty and at menopause. However, it is usually considered abnormal when occurring in women between the ages of 20 and 40 years.[12]

Corpus luteum insufficiency points to abnormal formation of ovarian follicles, an abnormality that may be so pronounced that no secondary or tertiary follicles are produced, with a resulting lack of ovulation (anovulation). Corpus luteum insufficiency also leads to a relative deficiency of progesterone. Insufficient levels of progesterone may also result in the formation of ovarian cysts.

Corpus luteum insufficiency may result in a myriad different menstrual abnormalities. Table 123.1 lists the most common clinical conditions in 1,592 women diagnosed with corpus luteum insufficiency. Foremost are hypermenorrhea (heavy periods), polymenorrhea (abnormally frequent periods), and persistent anovulatory bleeding. It is interesting to note that secondary amenorrhea (lack of a period) may sometimes be observed in women with corpus luteum insufficiency.

Disturbances of other hormones may also be associated with corpus luteum insufficiency. One study found hyperprolactinemia in 70% of cases.[13] Also noted is an exaggerated response to the thyroid-releasing hormone (TRH) test which is associated with manifest or latent hypothyroidism.

Premenstrual syndrome

Premenstrual syndrome (PMS) is one of the most frequent complaints found in gynecology practices. According to some estimates, 30–40% of menstruating women are affected by PMS.[14] Table 123.2 lists the different categories for PMS and the symptoms associated with them.

Two monitoring surveys of gynecology practices in Germany examined the effect of Vitex on 1,542 women with a diagnosis of PMS.[15] The mean age of the patients was 34.7 with a range of 13–62 years. Additional diagnoses noted with these patients included corpus luteum insufficiency (n = 1016) and uterine fibroids (n = 170). Patients were placed on a proprietary Vitex liquid extract known as "Agnolyt®" and were instructed to take 40 drops daily. The average duration of treatment was 166 days. The efficacy of treatment was assessed by both patients and their physicians. These assessments are listed in Table 123.3. In over 90% of the cases, symptoms were completely relieved, with a report of side-effects in only 2% of the patients (listed in Table 123.3). Only 17 of the 1,542 women studied had to stop treatment due to side-effects. Improvement in symptoms began after an average treatment duration of 25.3 days. After completion on the monitoring period, 562 patients continued taking Agnolyt.

Another study with 36 patients with a diagnosis of

Table 123.1 The most common clinical conditions in 1,592 women diagnosed with corpus luteum insufficiency

Diagnosis	No. of patients	Percentage of total
Hypermenorrhea	418	26.3
Polymenorrhea	369	23.2
Persistent anovulatory bleeding	216	13.6
Secondary amenorrhea	202	12.7
Dysmenorrhea	186	11.7
Anovulatory cycles	175	11.0
Involuntary sterility	145	9.1
Oligomenorrhea	69	4.3
Menorrhagia/metrorrhagia	66	4.1
Irregular menstrual cycles	32	2.0
Primary amenorrhea	1	0.1

Table 123.2 PMS subgroups

Subgroup	Symptoms	Prevalence
PMS-A	Anxiety Nervous tension	75–80%
PMS-H	Irritability Fluid retention Weight gain Swollen extremities Abdominal bloating Breast tenderness	60–70%
PMS-C	Increased appetite Sweet craving Headache Fatigue Fainting spells	35–40%
PMS-D	Depression Insomnia Forgetfulness	30–35%

Table 123.3 Efficacy of Vitex

Outcome	Percentage of patients
Patient assessment	
Improved	57%
Relieved	33%
No change	4%
No data	5%
Physician assessment	
Very good/good	71%
Satisfactory	21%
Unsatisfactory	4%
No data	3%

PMS used 40 drops of Vitex liquid extract (Agnolyt®) daily over 3 cycles. A reduction was noted in physical symptoms (headaches, pressure and tenderness in the breasts, bloating and fatigue) and psychological changes (increased appetite, craving for sweets, nervousness/restlessness, anxiety, irritability, lack of concentration, depression, mood swings, and aggressiveness). Additionally, the interval of the luteal phase was normalized from an average of 5.4 days to one of 11.4 days and a diphasic cycle was established.[16]

A recent study compared the efficacy of Vitex (3.5–4.2 mg/day of dried fruit extract – Agnolyt®) with vitamin B_6 (200 mg/day) in 175 women with premenstrual tension symdrome.[17] While both were effective (symptom scale decreased from 15.2 to 5.1 in the Vitex group and from 11.9 to 5.1 in the B_6 group), 24.5% reported excellent results, compared with only 12.1% with B_6. However, over twice as many women (12) reported side-effects from Vitex than from B_6 (5).

Abnormal menstrual cycles

The first major clinical study on Vitex was published in 1954. Fifty-seven women suffering from a variety of menstrual disorders were given Vitex on a daily basis. Fifty patients developed a cycle in phase with menses while seven women did not respond. Of the 50 women, six with secondary amenorrhea demonstrated one or more cyclic menstruations. Of nine with oligomenorrhea (scant or infrequent menstrual flow), six experienced a shortening of the menstrual interval and an increase in bleeding.

Most striking was a dramatic improvement in menstrual regularity among 40 patients with cystic hyperplasia of the endometrium. This condition is associated with a relative deficiency of progesterone and is characterized by dysfunctional uterine bleeding. No side-effects were observed with Vitex treatment.[18]

An observational study of 126 women with menstrual disorders utilized 15 drops of Vitex liquid extract three times daily over several cycles. In 33 women suffering from polymenorrhea, the duration between periods lengthened, on average, from 20.1 days to 26.3 days. In 58 patients with menorrhagia, a statistically significant shortening of menses was achieved. Fourteen patients became pregnant during the study; among them were three women with primary infertility over 2, 3, and 8 years, as well as two patients with secondary infertility over 4 and 15 years.[19]

Twenty patients with secondary amenorrhea were admitted to a 6 month study using Vitex liquid extract at 40 drops daily. Laboratory monitoring of progesterone, FSH, LH, and pap smears were performed at pre-study, 3 months, and 6 months. At the end of the 6 month study, data were available in 15 patients. The onset of cycles with menstruation was observed with Vitex treatment in 10 out of 15 patients. The hormone values showed increased values for progesterone and LH, while FSH values either did not change or decreased slightly.[20]

Two non-blind uncontrolled trials studied the effect of Vitex on corpus luteum function in 48 infertile women between 23 and 39 years of age. The inclusion criteria were normal prolactin levels (below 20 ng/ml), normal results in the prolactin and thyroid-stimulating hormone (TSH) stimulation tests and an abnormally low serum progesterone (below 12.0 ng/ml on the 20th day of the cycle). Treatment consisted of Vitex liquid extract, 40 drops daily, without any other medication for 3 months. Forty-five women completed the studies (three were excluded because of concurrent hormone use). The outcome of therapy was assessed by the normalization of the midluteal progesterone level and by correction (lengthening) of any pre-existing shortening of the phases of the cycle. Treatment was deemed successful in 39 of the 45 patients. Seven women became pregnant, serum progesterone was restored to normal (>12 ng/ml) in 25 patients and there was a trend toward normalization of progesterone levels in seven cases.[21]

Hyperprolactinemia

A mentioned previously, Vitex has shown a modulating effect on prolactin. A double-blind, placebo-controlled study examined the effect of a proprietary Vitex preparation ("Strotan®") on 52 women with luteal phase defects due to latent hyperprolactinemia. The daily dose of the Vitex extract was 20 mg and the study lasted for 3 months. Hormonal analysis was performed at days 5–8 and day 20 of the menstrual cycle before and after 3 months of therapy. After 3 months of therapy, 37 cases were available for analysis (20 placebo and 17 Vitex). Prolactin release was significantly reduced in the Vitex group. Shortened luteal phases were normalized and deficits in progesterone production were normalized. No side-effects were noted and two women in the Vitex group became pregnant.[22]

Potential indications

Anecdotal clinical reports have indicated a potential use for Vitex in the management of climacteric (hot flashes) in the early stages of menopause.[24] Uterine fibroids which are embedded into the muscle or are subserous may have their growth arrested by use of Vitex. Submucosal fibroids, however, are not likely to respond. Mild cases of endometriosis for which progesterone therapy are indicated also may respond to Vitex.

DOSAGE

The majority of clinical studies with *Vitex agnus castus* (Vitex) have been performed with a tincture of the fruit. Most medicinal texts, as well as monographs in Europe, list the entire preparation as "medicinally active".[1] This is an indication that the medical activity of the fruit is examined as a whole and that specific "active constituents" have not been individually isolated.

Since the early 1950s, the standard Vitex extract used for clinical research and treatment in Europe has been an alcohol-based tincture of the fruits of the plant known as Agnolyt®. A 100 ml amount of the solution is standardized to contain 9 g of the fruit. The recommended dosage is 40 drops with some liquid in the morning over several months without interruption. It is recommended that treatment with this extract be continued over several weeks after relief of symptoms is determined. The recent development of a solid extract equivalent of the tincture has allowed used by alcohol-sensitive women. The capsules, which contain 4.2 mg of the dried extract, have a one-a-day recommendation also.

It is important to note that Vitex is not a fast-acting medication. In cases of anovulatory cycles and infertility, treatment duration may be as long as 5–7 months before inception occurs. For secondary amenorrhea of more than 2 years' duration, Vitex should be administered for at least 1.5 years. In other conditions mentioned, however, first indications of efficacy with Vitex are usually seen within one or two cycles. Extensive or complete freedom of symptoms usually occurs after 4–6 months of treatment.

TOXICOLOGY

Human and animal studies have determined Vitex to be safe for most women of menstruating age. Vitex should not be used during pregnancy, but it is safe for use during lactation. Safety has not been determined in children. Vitex is not recommended in women taking hormone replacement therapy.

Side-effects noted in one large population study are listed in Table 123.4. Side-effects noted in other clinical observations have included itching and an occasional rash. Again, these side-effects are rare and have been noted in only 1–2% of the patients monitored on Vitex. Some women also report that menstrual flow increases during Vitex treatment. This is often an indication of therapeutic efficacy.

Table 123.4 Side-effects from Vitex in 1,542 women

Side effect	No. of patients reporting
No information	7
Nausea	5
Gastric complaints	3
Acne	3
Changes in menses rhythm	2
Diarrhea	2
Erythema	2
Allergy	1
Weight gain	1
Giddiness	1
Heartburn	1
Hypermenorrhea	1
Pruritis	1
Alopecia	1
Cardiac palpitations	1

REFERENCES

1. Monograph *Agni casti* fructus (Chaste tree fruits). Bundesanzeiger No. 90, May 15, 1985
2. *Agni cast* fructus (chaste tree fruits). Commission E Monograph, December 2, 1992
3. Kustrak KJ, Balzevic N. The composition of the essential oil of *Vitex agnus castus*. Planta Medica 1992; 58: A 681
4. Gomaa CS. Flavonoids and iridoids from *Vitex agnus castus*. Planta Medica 1978; 33: 277
5. Saden-Krehula M, Kustrak D, Blazevic N. Delta-3-ketosteroids in flowers and leaves of *Vitex agnus castus*. Planta Medica 1990; 56: 547
6. Weiss RF. Herbal medicine. Sweden: Ab Arcanum. 1988
7. Amann W. Removing an ostipation using Agnolyt. Ther Gegenew 1965; 104: 1263–1265
8. Reichert RG. Phyto-estrogens. Quart Rev Nat Med Spring 1994, pp. 27–33
9. Sliutz G, Speiser P et al. Agnus castus extracts inhibit prolactin secretion of rat pituitary cells. *Horm Metab Res* 1993; 25: 253–255
10. Jarry H, Leonhardt S, Wuttke W. *Agnus castus* as dopaminergous effective principle in mastodynon N. Zeitschrift Phytother 1991; 12: 77–82
11. Schneider HPG, Goeser R, Cirkel U. Prolactin and the inadequate corpus luteum. In: Lisuride and other dopamine agonists. New York: Raven Press. 1983: p 113–120
12. Propping D, Katzorke T, Beliken L. Diagnosis and therapy of corpus luteum deficiency in general practice. Therapiewoche 1988; 38: 2992–3001
13. Muhlenstedt D, Wutke W, Schneider HPG. Short luteal phase and prolactin. Fertil Steril 1977; 373–374
14. Lurie SR. The premenstrual syndrome. *Obstet Gynecol* 1990; 45: 220–228
15. Dittmar FW, Bohnert KJ et al. Premenstrual syndrome: treatment with a phytopharmaceutical. TW Gynakol 1992; 5: 60–68
16. Coeugniet E, Elek E, Kuhnast R. Premenstrual syndrome (PMS)

and its treatment. Arztezeitchr Naturheilverf 1986; 27: 619–622
17. Lauritzen CH, Reuter HD, Repges R et al. Treatment of premenstrual tension syndrome with *Vitex agnus castus*: controlled, double-blind study versus pyridoxine. Phytomed 1997; 4: 183–189
18. Probst V, Roth OA. On a plant extract with a hormone-like effect. Dtsch Med Wschr 1954; 79: 1271–1274
19. Bleier W. Phytotherapy in irregular menstrual cycles or bleeding periods and other gynecological disorders of endocrine origin. Zentralblatt Gynakol 1959; 81: 701–709
20. Losh EG, Kayser E. Diagnosis and treatment of dyshormonal menstrual periods in the general practice. Gynakol Praxis 1990; 14: 489–495
21. Propping D, Katzorke T. Treatment of corpus luteum insufficiency. Zeits Allgemeinmedizin 1987; 63: 932–933
22. Milewicz A, Gejdel E et al. *Vitex agnus castus* extract in the treatment of luteal phase defects due to hyperprolactinemia: results of a randomized placebo-controlled double-blind study. Arzneim-Forsch Drug Res 1993; 43: 752–756
23. Mohr H. Clinical investigations of means to increase lactation. Dtsch Med Wschr 1954; 79: 1513–1516
24. Du Mee C. *Vitex agnus castus*. Aust J Med Herbalism 1993; 5: 63–65

CHAPTER CONTENTS

124

Zingiber officinale (ginger)

Michael T. Murray, ND

Joseph E. Pizzorno Jr, ND

Zingiber officinale (family: Zingiberaceae)
Common name: ginger

GENERAL DESCRIPTION

Ginger is an erect perennial herb with thick tuberous rhizomes (underground stems) from which the aerial stem grows to a height of 2–4 feet. Grass-like alternate leaves, 6–12 inches long and 0.75 inch wide, shoot off from the aerial stem. Wild ginger will produce a beautiful flower, but cultivated ginger rarely flowers.

Although ginger is native to southern Asia, it is now extensively cultivated throughout the tropics (e.g. India, China, Jamaica, Haiti, and Nigeria). Jamaica is the major producer, with exports to all parts of the world amounting to more than 2,000,000 lb annually.

The knotted and branched rhizome, commonly called the "root", is the portion of ginger used for culinary and medicinal purposes. Extracts and the oleoresin are produced from dried unpeeled ginger, as peeled ginger loses much of its essential oil content.[1,2] Ginger oil is produced from the fresh ginger via steam distillation.

CHEMICAL COMPOSITION

The following compounds have been isolated from ginger:[1,2]

- starch (up to 50%)
- protein (~ 9%)
- lipids (6–8%) composed of triglycerides, phosphatidic acid, lecithins, and free fatty acids
- a protease (2%)
- volatile oils (1–3%), the principal components of which are sesquiterpenes (bisabolene, zingiberene and zingiberol) and various "pungent" principles, aromatic ketones, known collectively as gingerols vitamins (especially niacin and vitamin A)
- resins.

The pungent principles are thought to be the most

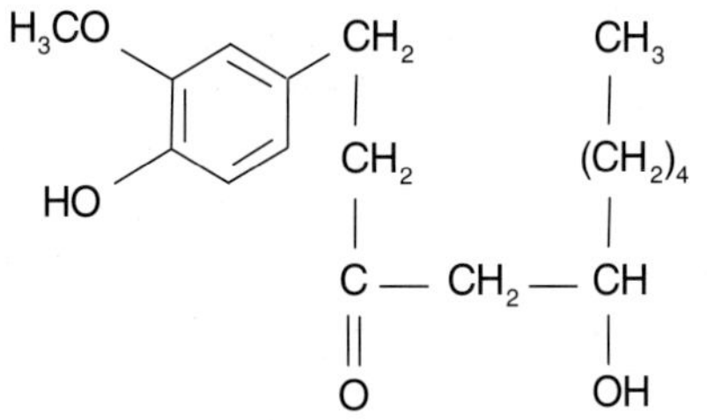

Figure 124.1 Gingerol.

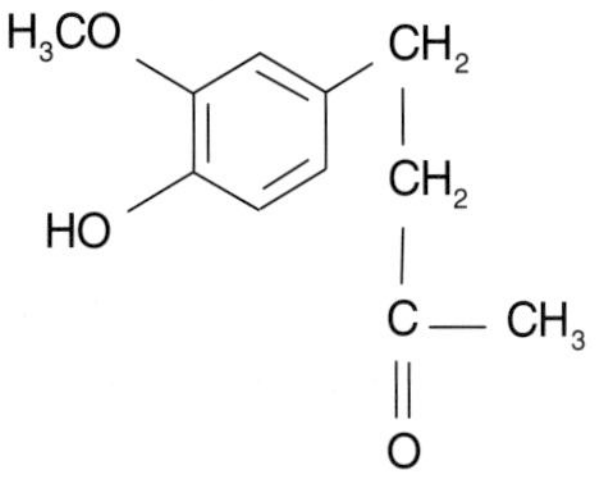

Figure 124.2 Zingerone.

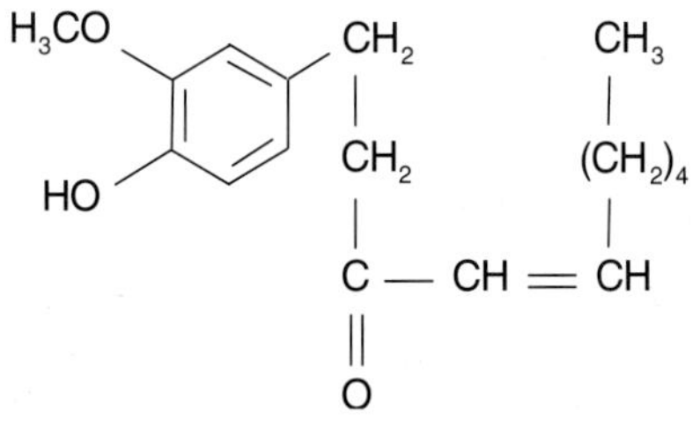

Figure 124.3 Shogaol.

pharmacologically active components of ginger. Gingerol and its derivatives can be found in concentrations as high as 33% in ginger oleoresin (see Fig. 124.1). The fresh oleoresin will have a higher percentage of the more pungent gingerol, as gingerol can be dehydrated during storage to form shogaol or have its fatty acid moiety cleaved to form zingerone (see Figs 124.2 and 124.3). The oleoresin is made by extracting the oily and resinous materials with the aid of a solvent (alcohol, hexane, or acetone).

HISTORY AND FOLK USE

Ginger has been used for thousands of years in China for medicinal purposes. Chinese records dating from the 4th century BC indicate that it was used to treat numerous conditions:[1]

- stomach ache
- diarrhea
- nausea
- cholera
- hemorrhage
- rheumatism
- toothache.

It was used by Eclectic physicians in the US in the late 1800s as a carminative, diaphoretic, appetite stimulant, and local counter-irritant.[3]

Ginger is widely used as a spice, especially in Asian and Indian dishes. It is also used in many baked goods, beverages (ginger ale), candy, liqueurs, and cosmetic products (perfumes, soaps, creams, etc.).

PHARMACOLOGY

Ginger possesses numerous pharmacological properties, the most relevant are:

- its antioxidant effects
- inhibition of prostaglandin, thromboxane, and leukotriene synthesis
- inhibition of platelet aggregation
- cholesterol-lowering actions
- choleretic effects
- cardiotonic effects
- gastrointestinal actions
- thermogenic properties
- antibiotic activities.

Antioxidant effects

Ginger's strong antioxidant properties have led to its being investigated for preventing the development of rancidity in meat products.[4] Ginger has been shown to prolong the shelf life of fresh, frozen, and pre-cooked pork patties. Since the use of many synthetic antioxidants is prohibited by law, ginger may one day be used commercially to extend the shelf life of meats and other foods.

Presumably the antioxidant components of ginger are absorbed in vivo where they undoubtedly contribute greatly to the pharmacology of ginger. In comparison, curcumin is about 30 times more potent in preventing lipid peroxidation than zingerone.[5]

Effects on prostaglandin and leukotriene metabolism

Numerous constituents in ginger have been shown to be potent inhibitors of prostaglandin and leukotriene synthesis.[6–8] The most potent components appear to be the pungent principles, although the aqueous extract has also demonstrated inhibition. Inhibition of prostaglandin and leukotriene formation could explain some of ginger's historical use as an anti-inflammatory agent. However, ginger and its extracts also have strong antioxidant activities, and fresh ginger contains a protease that may have similar action to other plant proteases (e.g. bromelain, ficin, papain, etc.) on inflammation.[1]

Effects on platelets

Ginger, like garlic and onions, is an inhibitor of platelet aggregation. However, ginger's effects may be far more powerful. In a comparison, an aqueous extract of ginger was shown to exert greater inhibitory effects on platelet aggregation than aqueous garlic and onion extracts.[9] Ginger was shown to produce a greater inhibition on thromboxane formation and pro-aggregatory prostaglandins. Ginger, but not onion or garlic, also significantly reduced platelet lipid peroxide formation.

The superiority of ginger over onions was also demonstrated in a controlled study.[10] Female volunteers given either 70 g raw onions or 5 g raw ginger demonstrated that ginger has a pronounced effect in lowering platelet thromboxane production while onion actually produced a mild elevation (pooled results).

Cholesterol-lowering and hepatic effects

Ginger has been shown to significantly reduce serum and hepatic cholesterol levels in cholesterol-fed rats by impairing cholesterol absorption as well as stimulating cholesterol-7-alpha-hydroxylase, the rate-limiting enzyme of bile acid synthesis.[11–13] In addition, ginger has also been shown to increase bile secretion.[14] Therefore, ginger works to lower cholesterol by promoting excretion and impairing absorption.

Cardiotonic and hypotensive properties

Gingerol has shown potent cardiotonic activity (positive ionotropic and chronotropic effects) on isolated guinea pig left atria.[15,16] These effects are a result of acceleration of calcium uptake by the sarcoplasmic reticulum. Gingerol was the first substance shown to produce these effects.

Individuals with heart problems or high blood pressure are probably better off using fresh ginger rather than the dried preparation. This recommendation is based not only on the fact that gingerol is the more potent cardiotonic, but also because shogaol has been shown to produce a blood pressure-elevating effect in animals.[17] Gingerol is found predominantly in fresh ginger while shogaol is rarely found in fresh ginger.

Analgesic effects

Ginger has demonstrated analgesic effects in experimental studies in animals.[18] This effect is thought to be a result of shogaol inhibiting the release of substance P in a similar fashion to capsaicin, the pungent principle of red pepper (*Capsicum frutescens*).

Gastrointestinal smooth muscle effects

One interesting aspect of ginger is its ability to simultaneously improve gastric motility while exerting antispasmodic effects. This is consistent with its use as a gastrointestinal tonic. A lipophilic ginger extract was shown in one study to enhance gastric motility, as evidenced by increased intestinal transport of a charcoal meal fed to rats,[19] and various fat-soluble components of ginger, such as galanolactone, demonstrated antagonism of serotonin receptor sites.[20] This latter mechanism may be responsible for ginger's antispasmodic effects on visceral and vascular smooth muscle. Ginger has been shown to inhibit serotonin-induced diarrhea.[21]

Anti-ulcer effects

Ginger has demonstrated significant anti-ulcer effects in a variety of animal models.[22–24] Ginger prevents ulcer formation due to ethanol, indomethacin, aspirin, and other common ulcerogenic compounds. The pungent principles appear to be responsible for this effect. Interestingly, in one study, roasted ginger demonstrated inhibition of ulcer formation in three gastric ulcer models while dry ginger had no such effect.[25]

Thermogenic properties

Ginger is noted for its apparent ability to subjectively warm the body and has historically been used as a diaphoretic. In animal studies, ginger has been shown to help maintain body temperature and to inhibit serotonin-induced hypothermia.[21,26]

Crude extracts and the pungent components of ginger have been shown to increase oxygen consumption, perfusion pressure, and lactate production in the perfused rat hind limb.[27] These effects signify increased thermogenesis. Gingerol is the most potent thermogenic component of ginger. A human study demonstrated that consuming a ginger sauce (containing unspecified amounts of ginger principles) with a meal produced no significant effect on metabolic rate.[28] However, there were two problems with this study: (1) the concentration of gingerol in the preparation used was probably low or zero; and (2) the effective concentration range of gingerol for its thermogenic effects is quite narrow.

Given ginger's historical use as a "warming" substance, these scientific investigations appear to support its use as a diaphoretic and thermogenic aid, although confirmation in humans is still lacking.

Antibiotic activity

Ginger, shogaol, and zingerone have been shown to be strongly inhibitory against *Salmonella typhi*, *Vibrio cholerae*, and *Tricophyton violaceum*, while aqueous extracts at 2.5, 5, and 25% concentration have been shown to be effective against *Trichomonas vaginalis*.[29]

CLINICAL APPLICATIONS

Ginger is widely used as a condiment for its unique flavors, but from the above-described pharmacology it obviously has important medicinal effects as well. In general, like many other culinary herbs and spices such as garlic and onions, ginger provides many health-promoting effects. Specifically, ginger provides benefit to many body systems including the digestive, hepatobiliary, and cardiovascular systems.

Historically, the majority of complaints for which ginger was used concerned the gastrointestinal system. A clue to ginger's efficacy in alleviating gastrointestinal distress is offered in several recent double-blind studies in motion sickness, hyperemesis gravidum, and post-operative nausea and vomiting. Human studies have also shown a positive effect in arthritis and migraine headaches.

Motion sickness

Ginger was first shown to be effective in treating motion sickness by Mowrey & Clayson in 1982.[30] In their study, ginger (940 mg) was shown to be far superior to Dramamine (100 mg) in relieving symptoms of nausea and vomiting. Since this initial study, several better designed follow-up studies have evaluated the effectiveness of ginger as a motion sickness medication.

The appearance of motion sickness trials using ginger prompted an interest in ginger by NASA, which subsequently funded a study at Louisiana State University. This study compared ginger, both fresh and dried powdered, with scopolamine by measuring the number of head movements experimental subjects could make in a rotating chair until they reached an end-point of motion sickness short of vomiting. Ginger was not shown to produce any protection against motion sickness in this model or in two additional protocols (vestibular stimulation only and combined vestibular-visual stimulation).[31] However, in perhaps a more "real life" test, ginger (1 g) given to naval cadets, unaccustomed to sailing in heavy seas, was shown to reduce the tendency to vomiting and cold sweating compared with a placebo in a double-blind trial.[32]

Mowrey & Clayson proposed that the anti-motion sickness effects of ginger were due to local gastrointestinal tract effects rather than to central nervous system effects. Although ginger's mechanism of action in alleviating gastrointestinal distress has yet to be fully elucidated, there is evidence to support this hypothesis. Ginger has been shown to partially inhibit the excessive gastric motility characteristic of motion sickness.[31] To further support a gastric versus a CNS mechanism of action, one study clearly demonstrated that neither the vestibular nor the oculomotor system, both of which are of critical importance in the occurrence of motion sickness, was influenced by ginger (1 g).[33] However, in a double-blind cross-over placebo-controlled study, ginger (1 g) was shown to produce significant reductions in induced vertigo, but not nystagmus.[34] These results suggest that ginger may dampen the vestibular impulses to the autonomic centers of the brain.

The overall effectiveness of ginger in motion sickness has yet to be determined. Issues that the studies have raised include the variability in the quality of commercial ginger preparations and the time required for ginger to produce its effects. Commercial preparations vary widely in chemical composition and often contain adulterants, and in the ginger study conducted at sea, ginger only reduced symptoms of cold sweating and vomiting at the end of 4 hours. In other words, it appears that ginger may prove to be more effective when well-defined preparations are given at least 4 hours prior to experiencing motion.

Nausea and vomiting

Ginger's anti-emetic actions has been studied in hyperemesis gravidum, the most severe form of pregnancy-related nausea and vomiting. This condition usually requires hospitalization. In a double-blind randomized cross-over trial, ginger root powder at a dose of 250 mg four times a day brought about a significant reduction in both the severity of the nausea and the number of attacks of vomiting in 19 of 27 cases of early pregnancy (less than 20 weeks).[35] These clinical results, along with the safety and the relatively small dose of ginger required and the problems (e.g. teratogenicity) with anti-emetic drugs in pregnancy, support the use of ginger in nausea and vomiting in pregnancy. This is becoming a well-accepted prescription even in orthodox obstetrical practices – ginger (as well as vitamin B_6) was recommended as an effective treatment of early nausea and vomiting of pregnancy in a 1992 review of current drug therapy during pregnancy published in the medical journal *Current Opinion in Obstetrics and Gynecology*.

The anti-emetic action of ginger was also observed in women who had undergone major gynecological surgery. In a double-blind study, 500 mg of dry powdered ginger root was shown to significantly reduce the incidence of nausea compared with placebo in a manner similar to the drug metoclopramide.[36]

Inflammatory conditions

Ginger's ability to inhibit the formation of inflammatory prostaglandins, thromboxanes, and leukotrienes, along with its strong antioxidant activities and protease component, suggests a possible benefit in inflammatory conditions. To test this hypothesis, a preliminary clinical study was conducted on seven patients with rheumatoid arthritis, in whom conventional drugs had provided only temporary or partial relief.[37] One patient took 50 g/day of lightly cooked ginger while the remaining six took either 5 g of fresh or 0.1–1 g of powdered ginger daily. All patients reported substantial improvement, including pain relief, increased joint mobility, and decreased swelling and morning stiffness.

In the follow-up to this study, 28 patients with rheumatoid arthritis, 18 with osteoarthritis, and 10 with muscular discomfort who had been taking powdered ginger for periods ranging from 3 months to 2.5 years were evaluated.[38] Based on clinical observations, Srivastava & Mustafa reported that 75% of the arthritis patients and 100% of the patients with muscular discomfort experienced relief in pain or swelling. The recommended dosage was 500–1,000 mg/day, but many patients took three to four times this amount. Patients taking the higher dosages also reported quicker and better relief.

Srivastava & Mustafa[39] have also reported ginger to be beneficial in migraine headache. Given ginger's effects on platelets, eicosanoids, and serotonin inhibition, this recommendation makes sense.

DOSAGE

There remain many questions concerning the best form of ginger and the proper dosage. Most research studies have utilized 1 g of dry powdered ginger root. Practically speaking, this is a small dose of ginger. For example, ginger is commonly consumed in India at a daily dose of 8–10 g. Furthermore, although most studies have used powdered ginger root, fresh (or possibly freeze-dried) ginger root or extracts concentrated for gingerol at an equivalent dosage may yield even better results because they may deliver higher levels of gingerol as well as the active protease.

In the treatment of nausea and vomiting due to motion sickness, pregnancy, or postoperatively, a dosage of 1–2 g of dry powdered ginger may be effective. This would be equivalent to approximately 10 g or one-third of an ounce of fresh ginger root, roughly a quarter-inch slice. For inflammatory conditions like rheumatoid arthritis, the dosage should be double this amount.

For ginger extracts standardized to contain 20% gingerol and shogaol, an equivalent dosage in treating motion sickness or nausea and vomiting would be 100–200 mg. For inflammatory conditions like rheumatoid arthritis, the dosage is 100–200 mg three times daily.

TOXICOLOGY

Ginger does not appear to produce any toxicity problems when used at normal dosages. Although ginger extracts and several components in ginger have been shown to possess potent mutagenic activity, ginger also contains several equally potent anti-mutagenic substances.[40,41] The significance of this mutagenicity (the study was conducted in *E. coli* not the Ames test) has not been entirely determined, but the long historic use and lack of carcinogenic or toxic effect in animals suggest that it is not a problem.

In acute toxicity tests in mice, ginger extract administered as a lavage was tolerated up to 2.5 g/kg with no mortality or side-effects during a 7 day trial period.[42] Increasing the dosage to 3.0–3.5 g/kg resulted in a 10–30% mortality. In comparison, 0.6 g/kg of aspirin produced mortality in 25%, stomach ulcers in 40%, and hypothermia in 60% of subjects.

Some individuals consuming high doses, i.e. greater than the equivalent of 6 g of dried powdered ginger alone on an empty stomach, may experience some gastrointestinal discomfort. Administration of 6 g of dried powdered ginger has been shown to increase the exfoliation of gastric surface epithelial cells in human subjects.[43] This may cause some gastric distress and ultimately could lead to ulcer formation. Therefore, it is recommended that dosages on an empty stomach be less than 6 g.

REFERENCES

1. Leung A. Encyclopedia of common natural ingredients used in food, drugs, and cosmetics. New York, NY: John Wiley. 1980: p 184–186
2. Tyler V, Brady L, Robbers J. Pharmacognosy. 8th edn. Philadelphia, PA: Lea & Febiger. 1981: p 156–157
3. Felter H. The eclectic materia medica, pharmacology and therapeutics. Portland, OR: Eclectic Medical Publications. 1983: p 702
4. Lee YB, Kim YS, Ashmore CR. Antioxidant property in ginger rhizome and its application to meat products. J Food Sci 1986; 51: 20–23
5. Reddy AC, Lokesh BR. Studies on spice principles as antioxidants in the inhibition of lipid peroxidation of rat liver microsomes. Mol Cell Biochem 1992; 111: 117–124
6. Kiuchi F, Iwakami S, Shibuya et al. Inhibition of prostaglandin and leukotriene biosynthesis by gingerols and diarylheptanoids. Chem Pharm Bull 1992; 40: 387–391
7. Kiuchi F, Shibuyu M, Sankawa U. Inhibitors of prostaglandin biosynthesis from ginger. Chem Pharm Bull 1982; 30: 754–757
8. Srivastava KC. Isolation and effects of some ginger components on platelet aggregation and eicosanoid biosynthesis. Prostaglandins Leurotri Med 1986; 25: 187–198
9. Srivastava K. Effects of aqueous extracts of onion, garlic and ginger on the platelet aggregation and metabolism of arachidonic acid in the blood vascular system. In vitro study. Prost Leukotri Med 1984; 13: 227–235
10. Srivastawa KC. Effect of onion and ginger consumption on platelet thromboxane production in humans. Prost Leukotri Ess Fatty Acids 1989; 35: 183–185
11. Gujral S, Bhumra H, Swaroop M. Effect of ginger (*Zingebar officinale* Roscoe) oleoresin on serum and hepatic cholesterol levels in cholesterol fed rats. Nutr Rep Intl 1978; 17: 183–189

12. Giri J, Sakthi Devi TK, Meerarani S. Effect of ginger on serum cholesterol levels. Ind J Nutr Diet 1984; 21: 433–436
13. Srinivasan K, Sambaiah K. The effect of spices on cholesterol 7 alpha-hydroxylase activity and the serum and hepatic cholesterol levels in the rat. Int J Vitam Nutr Res 1991; 61: 364–369
14. Yamahara J, Miki K, Chisaka T et al. Cholagogic effect of ginger and its active constituents. J Ethnopharmacol 1985; 13: 217–225
15. Shoji N, Iwasa A, Takemoto T et al. Cardiotonic principles of ginger (*Zingiber officinale* Roscoe). J Pharm Sci 1982; 10: 1174–1175
16. Kobayashi M, Ishida Y, Shoji N, Ohizumi Y. Cardiotonic action of [8]-gingerol, an activator of the Ca^{++}-pumping adenosine triphosphatase of sarcoplasmic reticulum, in guinea pig arterial muscle. J Pharmacol Exp Ther 1988; 246: 667–673
17. Suekawa M, Aburada M, Hosoya E. Pharmacological studies on ginger. II. Pressor action of (6)-shogoal in anesthetized rats, or hindquarters, tail and mesenteric vascular beds of rats. III. Effect of spinal destruction on (6)-shagoal-induced pressor response in rats. J Pharmacobio Dyn 1986; 9: 842–860
18. Onogi T, Minami M, Kuraishi Y, Staoh M. Capsaicin-like effect of (6)-shagoal on substance P-containing primary afferents of rats. A possible mechanism of its analgesic action. Neuropharmacol 1992; 31: 1165–1169
19. Yamahara J, Huang QR, Li YH et al. Gastrointestinal motility enhancing effect of ginger and its active constituents. Chem Pharm Bull 1990; 38: 430–431
20. Huang QR, Iwamoto M, Aoki S et al. Anti-5-hydroxytryptamine effect of galanolactone, diterpinod isolated from ginger. Chem Pharm Bull 1991; 39: 397–399
21. Huang Q, Matsuda H, Sakai K et al. The effect of ginger on serotonin induced hypothermia and diarrhea. Yakugaku Zasshi 1990; 110: 936–942
22. Al Yahya MA, Rafatullah S, Mossa JS et al. Gastroprotective actitivity of ginger, Zingiber officinale Rosc., in albino rats. Am J Chin Med 1989; 17: 51–56
23. Yamahara J, Mochizuki M, Rong HQ et al. The anti-ulcer effect in rats of ginger constituents. J Ethnopharmacol 1988; 23: 299–304
24. Yamahara J, Hatakeyama S, Taniguschi K et al. Stomachic principles in ginger. II. Pungent and anti-ulcer effects of low polar constituents isolated from ginger, the dried rhizome of *Zingiber officinale* Roscoe cultivated in Taiwan. The absolute stereostructure of a new diarylheptanoid. J Pharm Soc Japan 1992; 112: 645–655
25. Wu H, Ye D, Bai Y, Zhao Y. Effect of dry ginger and roasted ginger on experimental gastric ulcers in rats. China J Chinese Materia Medica 1990; 15: 278–280, 317–318
26. Kano Y, Zong QN, Komatsu K. Pharmacological properties of galenical preparation. XIV. Body temperature retaining effect of the Chinese traditional medicine, "goshuyu-to" and component crude drugs. Chem Pharm Bull 1991; 39: 690–692
27. Elderhsaw TPD, Colquhoun EQ, Dora KA et al. Pungent principles of ginger (*Zingiber officinale*) are thermogenic in the perfused rat hind limb. Int J Obesity 1992; 16: 755–763
28. Henry CJK, Piggott SM. Effect of ginger on metabolic rate. Human Nutr Clin Nutr 1987; 41C: 89–92
29. Chang HM, But PPH. Pharmacology and applications of Chinese materia medica, vol. 1. Philadelphia, PA: World Scientific. 1986: p 366–369
30. Mowrey D, Clayson D. Motion sickness, ginger, and psychophysics. Lancet 1982; i: 655–657
31. Stewart JJ, Wood MJ, Wood CD, Mims ME. Effects of ginger on motion sickness susceptibility and gastric function. Pharmacology 1991; 42: 111–120
32. Grontved A, Brask T, Kamskard J, Hentzer E. Ginger root against seasickness – a controlled trial on the open sea. Acta Otolaryngol 1988; 105: 45–49
33. Holtman S, Clarke AH, Scherer H, Hohn M. The anti-motion sickness mechanism of ginger. Acta Otolaryngol 1989; 108: 168–174
34. Grontved A, Hentzer E. Vertigo-reducing effect of ginger root. ORL 1986; 48: 282–286
35. Fischer-Rasmussen W, Kjaer SK, Dahl C, Asping U. Ginger treatment of hyperemesis gravidarum. Eur J Obstet Gynecol Reprod Biol 1990; 38: 19–24
36. Bone ME, Wilkinson DJ, Young JR et al. Ginger root – a new antiemetic. The effect of ginger root on postoperative nausea and vomiting after major gynecological surgery. Anaesthesia 1990; 45: 669–671
37. Srivastava KC, Mustafa T. Ginger (*Zingiber officinale*) and rheumatic disorders. Med Hypothesis 1989; 29: 25–28
38. Srivastava KC, Mustafa T. Ginger (*Zingiber officinale*) in rheumatism and musculoskeletal disorders. Med Hypothesis 1992; 39: 342–348
39. Mustafa T, Srivastava KC. Ginger (*Zingiber officinale*) in migraine headaches. J Ethnopharmacol 1990; 29: 267–273
40. Nakamura H, Yamamoto T. Mutagen and antimutagen in ginger, *Zingiber officinale*. Mutation Res 1982; 103: 119–126
41. Nagabhushan M, Amonkar AJ, Bhide SV. Mutagenicity of gingerol and shogaol and antimutagenicity of zingerone in salmonella/microsome assay. Cancer Lett 1987; 36: 221–233
42. Macolo N, Jain R, Jain SC, Capasso F. Ethnopharmacologic investigation of ginger (*Zingiber officinale*). J Ethnopharmacol 1989; 27: 129–140
43. Desai HG, Kalro RH, Choksi AP. Effect of ginger and garlic on DNA content of gastric aspirate. Ind J Med Res 1990; 92: 139–141

Index

A

E

F

H

P

Q

R

S

T

U

V